From
Miss Dall. H. Garside
27.11.61.

pe 6/.

T.W. GREENWOOD
WILSON HOUSE.
(St. Mary's Hospital)
SUSSEX GARDENS
Paddington W.2.

A Textbook of

PATHOLOGY

Structure and Function in Diseases

By

WILLIAM BOYD

M.D., Dipl. Psychiat., M.R.C.P. (Edin.), Hon. F.R.C.P. (Edin.), F.R.C.P. (Lond.),
F.R.C.S. (Can.), F.R.S. (Can.), LL.D. (Sask.), (Queen's), D.Sc. (Man.), M.D., (Hon.) (Oslo).

Professor Emeritus of Pathology, The University of Toronto; Visiting Professor of Pathology,
The University of Alabama; Formerly Professor of Pathology, The University
of Manitoba and the University of British Columbia.

Seventh Edition, Thoroughly Revised
792 Illustrations and 20 Plates in Colour

LONDON
HENRY KIMPTON
134 GREAT PORTLAND STREET, W.1
1961

Library of Congress Catalog Card Number: 61-9368
Printed in the United States of America

Preface

There is more than one way to revise a medical textbook. The author can collect all the new material he would like to insert. This is patching the old coat. At the same time he can delete material which he thinks is no longer of value. Dead wood must be pruned, as every gardener knows, leaving room for the new shoots. Or he can attempt something more drastic. I have tried to rewrite rather than merely to revise the book, with function as well as structure in mind. The difference between the new and the old is illustrated by a comparison of Chapter I, dealing with the Pathology of the Cell, with the corresponding Chapter 2 of the previous edition describing Degenerative Processes.

I have sought to emphasize the general principles governing disease processes, and have entitled the first part of the book Principles of Pathology rather than the more customary General Pathology, used in previous editions. General pathology may be regarded in a sense as representing the theory of disease, while special or regional pathology is the practical application of that theory to individual instances. The reader of Part I is a student of disordered biology. When he comes to Part II he becomes the future doctor of medicine. The student who has mastered such subjects as inflammation, thrombosis and neoplasia can apply his knowledge to disease problems like acute appendicitis, coronary thrombosis and bronchogenic carcinoma without much outside assistance. He will also learn to recognize that ignorance, however aptly veiled in an attractive phraseology, still remains ignorance.

Disease, whether of the heart, the kidney or the brain, is disturbed function, not merely disordered structure, for pathology in the modern sense is physiology gone wrong, and not just the morphological changes we call lesions. A world of disordered function lies revealed in any lesion, if only we have the eye to see it. It is the high function of the pathologist not merely to attach correct labels to the lesions which he sees, but to reconstruct the course of events from the earliest inception of the disease to the final moment when we fall out of "the splendid procession of life." Altered structure corresponds to the *lesions* studied by the pathologist, but it is disordered function that is responsible for the *symptoms* which bring the patient to the doctor. It is the functioning of the lung rather than its structure which determines whether or not a person is short of breath. It is for this reason that I have devoted what may seem at times an inordinate amount of space to physiological considerations.

This concept is of course in no sense new. In 1847 Rudolf Virchow, the father of modern pathology and then only twenty-six years of age, wrote these words: "Pathological physiology is the main fortress of medicine, while pathological anatomy and the clinic are outlying bastions." Unfortunately those who followed Virchow were apt to forget this great truth, and indeed prided themselves on being "morbid anatomists," an unpleasant term in itself. To be able to give a name to some pathological lesion, and to make it fit into some accepted scheme of classification, is a very limited concept of pathology. But morbid anatomy is not dead and never has been, except in the hands of those whose dull minds would take the breath of life from the most vital subject. The world of medicine did not think that there was anything dead about cellular pathology when Virchow poured the new wine of his vital spirit into the old bottles of tradition. And today the bottles are not yet full. It is *pathological processes* with their morphological basis with which we are concerned, both as biologists and physicians. Let us not forget that pathology is a discipline in its own right, not merely a diagnostic tool.

With this in view I have opened several chapters in Part I and almost every chapter in Part II with a section on General Considerations, a conveniently vague and non-commital term which allows a review of anatomical, physiological and biochemical facts that may have a bearing on the diseased states which are presently to be considered. In such a disease as diabetes it is physiology rather than morphology that concerns us. These sections afford a convenient place to consider the startlingly new details of fine structure which electron micrography has introduced, suggesting that we stand on the threshold of a new era in our concept of the cell, as indicated in the opening chapter. No better illustration of the importance of this new technique can be imagined than in studies of the changes in the glomeruli and tubules of the kidney in various forms of renal disease.

As we have already suggested, the day of morphological pathology is by no means past, a fact evidenced by the emphasis placed by the radiologist on gross morbid anatomy, more particularly in relation to disease of the lungs. Examples of new techniques opening doors for further exploration in microscopic morphology are afforded by the application of fluorescence antibody methods in the study of immunity, the demonstration of abnormalities of individual sex chromosomes and autosomes in cytogenetic studies, and the laying bare of too much or too little enzyme activity by new cytochemical and histochemical staining methods. In these days of multiple authorship, not only of books but also of articles, the solitary author takes on himself a heavy burden and responsibility for which he may well be criticized for undue presumption at at a time when explosive advances are shattering the boundaries and frontiers of knowledge.

Although clinical diagnosis is still dependent on the recognition of the presence of structural changes, from the point of view of the patient damaged structure and disturbed function are only of significance in relation to the symptoms from which he suffers. The sections on the Relation of Symptoms to Lesions which close the account of most diseases have been expanded in many instances and introduced for the first time in others, with emphasis on the concept that disease is a manifestation of disordered function rather than altered structure. To enumerate a list of symptoms and then a list of lesions is not enough. It is the relation of one to the other which counts, just as in a well ordered clinical pathological conference it is to the explanation of the clinical picture in all its aspects that the pathologist should bend his energies, rather than merely to lay bare the lesion which he thinks was responsible for death. Sometimes this is easy, sometimes difficult, and sometimes impossible at the present time. The value of a persistent endeavour to correlate symptoms with lesions lies not so much in the number of facts the student may succeed in memorizing, as in the development of an attitude of mind which may color the whole of his future career. In Osler's memorable words: "As is our pathology, so is our practice." For the student of medicine, then, pathology has a threefold interest, for it comprises a study of: (1) structural changes, (2) disturbance of function, and (3) the relation of the lesions to the symptoms which represent disease in the patient. This has been the aim of the present edition.

An Outline of Contents has been placed at the beginning of each chapter. I have found the compilation of this outline of great value to myself, because it has enforced on me a more orderly arrangement of material, as well as a due regard to classification. These considerations may also prove of value to the student, particularly in the revision of his work before having to face the examiners. It is perhaps in the chapters dealing with such complex subjects as immunity and hypersensitivity, carcinogenesis, ionizing radiation, and diseases of the kidneys, the lungs, the blood and the nervous system that a review of the outlines may be of value. Even the pathogenesis of atherosclerosis becomes slightly less confusing when the possibilities are listed. A glance at the Outline of Contents of Chapter 1 will show that the subject of pathological calcification has been omitted inadvertently. It is discussed in connection with diseases of bone in Chapter 43.

New chapters have been introduced on immunity and hypersensitivity, derangements of body fluids, pigments and pigmentation, ionizing radiation, and a fuller discussion of medical genetics, because of the dominant place which these play in the science of pathology today. The chapter on tumors now becomes two, the first on the principles of neoplasia, the second on specific tumors. The kidney, as a member of the cardio-vascular-renal system, is now considered in Chapter 23, a more fitting position for it, and the lower urinary tract in Chapter 31.

I have endeavoured, perhaps unsuccessfully, to curtail the second part of the book dealing with Regional Pathology, formerly called Special Pathology, partly by abbreviating the accounts of a number of diseases regarded as of lesser importance, partly by omitting many of the rarer conditions which the undergraduate, once he becomes a doctor, may not see once in a lifetime. In other cases I have merely mentioned the condition, giving a reference to some review article which may be consulted if desired for any special reason.

The references are intended for the student who has to prepare a paper or write a thesis on a particular subject. Knowledge is of two kinds: we may know a subject ourselves, or we may know how and where to find the necessary information. The value of what has been termed the "look-it-up technique" is becoming more generally recognized. It has been said that an educated man is one who knows how to use a library. The student should be provided with a living stream of knowledge, not a stagnant pool from which to drink. The references are indicated in the text by the name of the author rather than by a number, because it is felt that the reader should become familiar with the names of some of those who have advanced the science of pathology, even though he may never have time to consult the original paper. For the same reason I have sometimes quoted a sentence or two from a writer, because to do so makes the man more living. The list of references at the end of the chapter are now arranged alphabetically rather than grouped according to subjects.

Use of the library makes us aware of the fact that the picture of disease is changing before our very eyes. Old diseases are pass-ing away as the result of the assaults of modern therapy, but new ones are continually taking their place. The inn that shelters for the night is not the journey's end. Many of these new diseases are iatrogenic (*iatros*, a physician) in nature, that is to say, they are the result of the well-meant but injudicious use of therapeutic agents. In these days when tranquilisers take the place of baby-sitters, blood transfusions are given thoughtlessly, indiscriminately and often needlessly, exposure to diagnostic or therapeutic ionizing radiation has become so universal, antibiotics are regarded as the cure-all for the most minor infections, and steroid therapy is the refuge of the destitute, it is small wonder that the old maladies are replaced by new man-made ones, and that allergies to a multitude of antigens have become so commonplace that they are said to exceed pathogenic microorganisms in number. I must apologize for the too frequent use of the words "what is powerful for good can be potent for evil," but this is true of so many situations created by modern therapy that I have been unable to resist the temptation. If we continually interfere with nature, we must pay the penalty. The idea is of profound importance to the medical student who is to become the future doctor with the safety and welfare of his patient at heart.

It may not be out of place to remark here that the student, beguiled by the fascination of pathology, must not regard clinical medicine as merely the application of physics, chemistry and physiology to the sick person. Medicine can never be purely a science; it contains too many immeasurables. The patient with heart disease is not just an internal combustion engine with a leaking valve but a sensitive human being with a diseased heart. Disease in man is never exactly the same as disease in the experimental animal, for in man the emotions come into play. It may be the man or woman rather than the disease that needs to be treated. There is always the psyche to be considered as well as the soma.

The use of small print is always a contentious subject. Some textbooks of pathology do without it, while others use it liberally. The object of small print is two-fold, partly to save space, partly to indicate to the student what is of lesser importance and need not be read if time is limited. The difficulty is to decide what is unimportant. What is rare in one part of the world may be very common in another, and in these days when air travel between distant countries has become an everyday affair, the geographic demarcation of disease is no longer as sharp as it used to be. For better or worse, I have used small print to a much less extent than formerly. The book is designed for the medical student who is going to devote his life to the diagnosis and treatment of disease. In spite of that it has been difficult to resist the temptation to include a few conditions which the reader will almost certainly never encounter. Kuru is an example of such a disease which, because of its unusual and dramatic character, makes an irresistible appeal. At least I have put it in small type.

A number of the old pictures and one-half of the color plates have been discarded. Many new ones have been introduced, including a selection of electron micrographs. Some of these pictures have been taken from my book, *Pathology for the Physician*. I am much indebted to the W. B. Saunders Company for permission to use both color plates and black and white photographs from my *Pathology for the Surgeon*, as well as a number of extracts from that book, more particularly the account of shock.

One of the pleasant features of writing a preface is the opportunity it affords the author to express his appreciation to those who have made the final result possible.

Of my associates in the University of Toronto I wish in particular to thank Dr. John Hamilton for suggesting the desirability of including a chapter on immunity and hypersensitivity, to Dr. Henry Z. Movat for criticism and help with that chapter and for a number of electron micrographs, and to Dr. John Paterson and Dr. H. A. Hunter for invaluable suggestions regarding the chapters on the Respiratory System and the Teeth respectively. Much stimulus has come from the men I have worked with at the University of Alabama Medical Center. I must thank Dr. J. F. A. McManus for acting as my guide in the labyrinth of histochemistry, especially in relation to the kidney, Dr. Sidney P. Kent for much needed assistance with the chapter on Ionizing Radiation, and, in particular, Mr. Ralph F. Coleman, an undergraduate student who has helped to give me the point of view of the medical student, has read the entire manuscript, has provided most of the tables summarizing a subject, and has impressed on me the value of italics for emphasizing the salient features of a subject, an emphasis particularly useful when reviewing the work later.

Without a library an author would be helpless. In this respect I am deeply indebted to Miss Marian Patterson of the Academy of Medicine, Toronto, and to Mrs. Hilda Harris of the University of Alabama Medical Center. I am grateful to those who have sent me reprints of their papers, and I would very much appreciate others following their example.

For the laborious and exacting task of transcribing illegible writing to type script I must thank Miss Linda Cox of Toronto and Mrs. Carol Cross of Birmingham.

Finally I must thank my long-suffering publishers, Lea and Febiger, for having completely reset the type, which is in double column, and in particular Mr. John F. Spahr and Mr. V. J. Boland for the remarkable patience they have displayed with the endless demands of an author who insists in making last minute additions not only of manuscript, but also of illustrations, in an endeavour to bring the book more or less up-to-date at the moment of publication.

WILLIAM BOYD

Toronto, Canada

Contents

Part I. Principles of Pathology

CHAPTER   PAGE

1. Pathology of the Cell 9
2. Inflammation 34
3. Repair 65
4. The Intercellular Substance and its Reactions 79
5. Immunity and Hypersensitivity 97
6. Coagulation, Thrombosis and Embolism 126
7. Derangements of Body Fluids 149
8. Neoplasia I: General Principles 173
9. Neoplasia II: Specific Tumors 226
10. Growth and its Disorders 249
11. Bacterial Infections 255
12. Fungal Infections 316
13. Viral and Rickettsial Infections 330
14. Animal Parasites 354
15. Deficiency Diseases 377
16. Pigments and Pigmentation 393
17. Physical Irritants 407
18. Ionizing Radiation 412
19. Chemical Poisons 427
20. Medical Genetics 431

Part II: Regional Pathology

21. The Heart 445
22. The Blood Vessels 500
23. The Kidneys 545
24. The Respiratory System 622
25. The Mouth, Neck and Esophagus 702
26. The Stomach and Duodenum 721
27. The Intestine 744

CHAPTER   PAGE

28. The Liver and Gall Bladder 781
29. The Pancreas 831
30. The Peritoneum and Abdominal Wall 852
31. The Lower Urinary Tract 859
32. The Male Reproductive System 873
33. The Female Reproductive System 896
34. The Breast 941
35. The Pituitary 964
36. The Adrenals 980
37. The Thyroid 1000
38. The Parathyroids 1026
39. The Blood 1032
40. The Spleen 1092
41. The Lymphatic System 1103
42. The Nervous System 1122
43. The Bones 1221
44. The Joints 1268
45. The Muscles 1302
46. The Skin 1314
47. The Teeth 1344

Part I. Principles of Pathology

Chapter 1

Pathology of the Cell

Introduction
The Normal Cell
  CELL MEMBRANE
  NUCLEUS
  MITOCHONDRIA
  ENDOPLASMIC RETICULUM
  CYTOPLASMIC INCLUSIONS
The Sick Cell: Cellular Degenerations
  CLOUDY SWELLING
  HYDROPIC DEGENERATION
  FATTY DEGENERATION

FATTY INFILTRATION
  Lipoidal Degeneration
  Progressive Lipodystrophy
GLYCOGEN INFILTRATION
  Von Gierke's Disease
MUCOID DEGENERATION
HYALINE DEGENERATION
The Dying and Dead Cell: Necrosis
COAGULATION NECROSIS
LIQUEFACTION NECROSIS
CASEATION

AUTOLYSIS
FAT NECROSIS
Gangrene
  DRY GANGRENE
  MOIST GANGRENE
  Gas Gangrene
  Bed Sores
Postmortem Changes
  RIGOR MORTIS
  POSTMORTEM DECOMPOSITION
  WEIGHTS AND MEASUREMENTS

INTRODUCTION

IT is not necessary to impress on the medical student the importance of the cell. His study of histology and embryology has already made him fully conscious of that fact. Life on earth began with the appearance of the first cell, and to this day each of us begins life as a single cell, the fertilized ovum. The origin of modern pathology, on which present day medicine is based, dates from the publication of Rudolf Virchow's "Cellular Pathology" in 1858, over one hundred years ago.

Before commencing a study of the pathology of the cell, it might be well if we paused for a moment to enquire as to the meaning and connotation of the term pathology. Pathology is *the study of disease by the methods of the laboratory,* just as medicine and surgery are the study of disease by the methods of the bedside. The practice of medicine is, will always be, and always should be both an art and a science. The clinician studies illness, while the pathologist studies disease. It is with the *science* of medicine that pathology, is concerned, for, in the telling words of Sir Roy Cameron, its aim is a "welding together of structural and functional observations into a coherent story." When a clinician makes a diagnosis he is merely expressing an opinion as to the underlying pathology, so it is evident that he must become familiar with the fundamentals of that science.

Pathology is concerned with answering, or trying to answer, the questions What, How and Why in relation to disease. The answer to *What* consists in a description of the structural changes produced by the disease process. In the beginning, and indeed until recent years, such a description of the gross and microscopic changes, known as the *lesions,* constituted the bulk of the science, and the pathologist was known as a morbid anatomist (suggesting a diseased anatomist) or morbid histologist. But the student of pathology must not content himself with such a description. He must also try to answer the much more difficult questions, *How* and *Why.* As a matter of fact, when we read a complete autopsy report we may find ourselves asking how the patient continued to live, not why he died, so roughly has the sharp tooth of time dealt with his body. In the following pages the student must ask what is going on inside the cell. The present day pathologist, studying sections of the kidney with modern histochemical technique, is as much concerned with fundamental changes involving the enzyme systems of the cells of the convoluted tubules as in the structural changes he sees under the microscope. Disease may be defined as merely a summation of chemical reactions that have gone wrong.

In the course of his clinical studies the student will soon realize that in many cases it is not possible to demonstrate a gross or even a cellular organic basis for the patient's symptoms. Such cases have been classified in the past as examples of "functional disease." With advances in knowledge this vague group is undergoing a wholesome shrinkage. Much of the failure to demonstrate a structural change has been due to inability to lay bare submicroscopic changes in the cell or disturbance of its enzyme systems. These *biochemical lesions* are now being revealed by the demonstration of the fine structure of the cell by the electron microscope, by remarkable advances in cytochemistry, and by what is termed molecular pathology. For disease may be produced at a molecular level, the level of the constituent metabolic units. One of the best known examples of a molecular disease is sickle-cell anemia with its abnormal hemoglobin molecule which is genetically inherited. We shall encounter a biochemical lesion in the poisoning of the enzymatic activity of the mitochondria by arsenic. All hereditary diseases have as their basis a genetic abnormality which expresses itself as an altered metabolic pathway, another example of a biochemical lesion. There can be little doubt that such an apparently purely functional mental disease as schizophrenia, with its distressing delusions and hallucinations and split personality, has a biochemical lesion as its basis. These are some of the things which make pathology so exciting a study at the present time.

But the student in his new-found enthusiasm for pathology must not forget that it is the whole patient who comes to consult the doctor, not just a disordered liver, a cardiac lesion, a lump in the breast, or a painful knee. In the words of an Old French proverb: "There are no diseases, but only sick people."

With this brief review of the content of pathology and the changes which it has undergone since the publication of Virchow's "Cellular Pathology" one hundred years ago, we may now pass to a consideration of the cell in health and in disease. In this chapter we shall consider the normal cell, the sick cell, and the dying and dead cell. The sick cell is likely to show changes which are grouped under the rather old fashioned term, the *degenerations*, but we have already seen that sometimes the change is a biochemical lesion rather than a histological one, in which case the microscope will reveal no abnormality. As a matter of fact all lesions are primarily biochemical, but some also become visible. The changes associated with the death of a cell are known as necrosis. They demand time to develop. Every cell we see under the microscope is of course dead, killed by the fixative, but it is not necrotic. Before considering the sickness and death of cells it may be useful to recall one or two simple facts about normal cell structure and function. The student who wishes to delve deeper into the subject of the cell in health and disease could not do better than read Sir Ray Cameron's pleasantly small book "New Pathways in Cellular Pathology." If he wishes more detailed information he may consult "The Cell" by the same author, 840 pages long with 126 pages of references.

THE NORMAL CELL

The three principal constituents of the cell are: (1) cell membrane, (2) nucleus, and (3) cytoplasm. The nucleus contains (a) the chromosomes, which are the carriers of the genes, and (b) the nucleolus. The cytoplasm contains a variety of structural constituents known as *organelles* or little organs. Of these we shall consider the *mitochondria* and the *endoplasmic reticulum*. Two others may be mentioned: the *microsomes*, which are innumerable submicroscopic particles, and the *Golgi apparatus or complex*, an assembly depot of various kinds of secretions. As so little is known of their function and next to nothing of their reaction to injury, they will be passed by.

In recent years enormous advances have been made in our knowledge of the structure and function of the cell in health and to a lesser degree in disease. We owe these advances in the main to two new methods of technique. (1) When cells are disrupted by mechanical means, the contents are liberated, and when these are suspended in a suitable medium and the homogenate is spun in a centrifuge, the largest and heaviest particles come down first, followed later by the smaller and lighter particles. By this means first the nuclei, then the mitochondria, and finally the microsomes can be separated, and examined histologically and biochemically. (2) The electron microscope has given us a new insight into the structure of these units and brought the microsomes into view.

The cells are not the static structures that they appear when viewed in fixed tissues under the microscope. They are as alive and active as the animal or person from whom they are removed. Each cell, which is really a biochemical machine, contains chemical and physical mechanisms designed to obtain material from its environment to satisfy the nutritional and energy requirements of the organ concerned. When these mechanisms, which involve a relationship between structure and function, are impaired, the result is sickness and it may be death.

Metabolism (*metabole*, change) is the sum total of the chemical reactions which proceed in the cells. The tools of these reactions are the *enzymes* or metabolic catalysts which are present in vast numbers in every cell. Protoplasm consists largely of enzymes, each of which is extraordinarily specific, acting on its own particular substrate by combining with it. Part of the activity is *anabolic*, involving the synthesis of protein, whilst part is *catabolic*, being concerned with the breaking down of food substances and protoplasm. The energy yielded by catalysing reactions is used in part for the resynthesis of the enzymes concerned. The enzyme reactions are extremely sensitive to injurious influences such as poisons, loss of nutrition, *etc*. The breakdown of the enzyme systems results in sickness or death of the cell.

Chemical poisons such as carbon tetrachloride can pass through the surface membrane as through a sieve, finally reaching the mitochondria and disrupting the respiratory enzymes, so that the whole complex structure of the cell crumbles. For instance, the nitrophenols lead to an increased consumption of energy in the cell, but the enzymes are not able to use the energy so liberated, with the result that adenosine triphosphate, the great energy-carrier, is not synthesized, and the life of the cell suffers.

Bacterial toxins may also inhibit the enzyme systems, as we see in the case of Cl. welchii, tetanus, botulinus and diphtheria. Botulinus toxin causes severe muscular paralysis without any observable structural changes even in fatal cases. The same is true of tetanus toxin. These are examples of *biochemical lesions, in which the function of an enzyme but not the structure of the cell is disrupted*, with "jamming" of the metabolism as the result.

We have already enumerated the structural elements in the cell which interest the student of pathology. These are the cell membrane, the nucleus with its chromosomes, and the cytoplasm with its organelles, more particularly the mitochondria, and cell inclusions. In cell death the nucleus claims our attention as pathologists, whereas disorders of the cytoplasm are more likely to result in sickness of the cell. As Ham puts it in his chapter on The Cell, the nucleus is the heart of the cell, so that when it dies, the cell dies, whereas the cytoplasm performs the ordinary day-to-day work of the cell.

Amongst the dominant constituents of both nucleus and cytoplasm are the *nucleic acids*, complexes of bases, sugars and phosphoric acid. They are divided into two groups, namely ribose nucleic acid (RNA) and deoxyribose or desoxyribose nucleic acid (DNA), the two groups being distinguished by their sugar component. Both are basophilic, but they can be differentiated by means of the Feulgen reaction which is based on the difference in the sugars. Mild hydrolysis liberates aldehydes from DNA but not from RNA, and these aldehydes stain purple or magenta with the Schiff reagent. DNA is said to be Feulgen-positive, whilst RNA is Feulgen-negative. The two nucleic acids can also be distinguished by observing the action of the specific enzymes desoxyribonuclease and ribonuclease on the constituents of the cell. By the use of these methods it becomes evident that DNA is confined to the nucleus, and in particular the chromosomes, whereas RNA is present mainly in the mitochondria of the cytoplasm, but also in the nucleolus. It is the DNA of the fertilized ovum which determines the species of animal that will develop, as well as the individual characteristics of that animal. The nucleoproteins of cells can be changed by the incorporation of nucleoproteins of viruses, as well as by chemical and even physical agents such as radiation, a point to which we shall return when we consider the causation of cancer.

A working model of DNA (Watson-Crick model) has been devised to fit the fact that it seems to represent what has been called "the hereditary codescript" of the cell. The giant molecule is pictured as consisting of a pair of chains wound in a double helix. Each chain consists of alternate desoxyribose and phosphoric acid groups. The chains are cross-connected by two pairs of four nitrogenous bases, namely adenine with thymine and guanine with cytosine. If a molecule contained a large number of these nucleotide pairs, their arrangement could be varied almost endlessly, and such a structure could code an organism's characteristics for hereditary transmission. It seems sufficient to dictate the formation of every kind of protein to be formed from a choice of 20 amino acids, thus every possible enzyme, thus every sort of cellular organization and function. The genes consist of DNA, and the chromosomes are assemblies of genes, so that the part played by chromosomes in determining structure and function is evident.

Just as the body as a whole operates on the principle of the division of labor, so also does the secret of the complex activity of the individual cell lie in the isolation of its various activities. If the cell is a biochemical machine, its separate parts such as the nucleolus and the mitochondria are similarly distinct machines. This isolation is achieved by the presence of various membranes (Bourne). Thus the *nuclear membrane* isolates the activities of the nucleus from those of the cytoplasm. It is now known that this is only a partial isolation, for the electron microscope has shown the membrane to be perforated with pores, through which materials are transferred from the nucleus to the cytoplasm. RNA molecules labelled with radioactive atoms have been followed from the nucleolus through these pores to the endo-

plasmic reticulum. where they preside over protein synthesis, while DNA presides over the synthesis of RNA in accord with the genetic plan borne by the chromosomes. This migration can be best seen in the gigantic cells of the salivary glands of Drosophila, the fruit fly. The mitochondria and the Golgi complex also have their membranes, so that their activities are carried on in partial but not complete seclusion.

With this review of what is going on inside the cell we are in a better position to appreciate the meaning of its finer structure, and we shall now consider in more detail the cellular constituents which have already been mentioned.

Cell Membrane.—With the light microscope the cell membrane is only visible in red blood cells from which the hemoglobin has been removed, but the electron microscope reveals that every cell has its membrane. It is an all-important structure, for it regulates the internal environment of the cell, determining what goes in and what comes out. It is at this surface structure that many reactions take place. If the cells are very active they need a correspondingly large surface, so that they may be studded with microvilli in the intestine or show infoldings in the renal tubules, much as the cerebral cortex is thrown into convolutions to gain increased surface without expanding the skull unduly. Water and all food particles must pass through the membrane freely, whilst metabolites must pass out. The membrane consists largely of lipid molecules, polysaccharides, and a much smaller number of protein molecules. Cameron pictures the lipid molecules as behaving like swing doors hinged to the protein molecules. A chemical poison is not toxic for the cell unless it can penetrate the cell membrane. Unfortunately the lipids of the membrane can act as a solvent for many hydrocarbons, amongst which are some powerful carcinogenic (cancer-producing) agents.

It is to the surface structure that many substances such as chemical dyes become attached. Effective drugs probably react first with specific surface constituents. An enzyme seems to fit into the cell surface in which its substrate is embedded. Antigens react at the surface of the cell with the for-

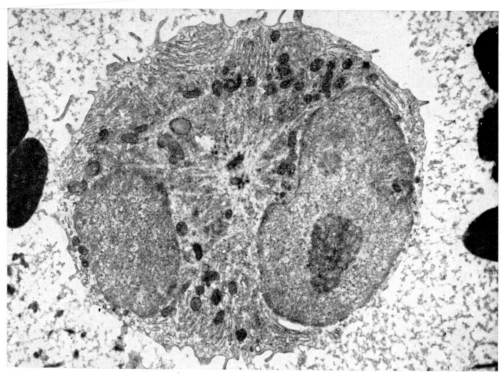

Fig. 1.—Electron photomicrograph of plasma cell. Note the wealth of fine detail barely suggested in the same cell seen with the light microscope. To the right is the eccentric nucleus containing a prominent nucleolus of dense reticular composition. To the left there is a second nucleus. The cytoplasm is filled with organelles, including a highly developed endoplastic reticulum and dense mitochondria. The structure in the center is the centrosome. The cell membrane shows slender projections and invaginations. × 22,000. (Kindness of Dr. Alice Smith, Wadley Research Institute, Dallas).

mation of antibodies which are then cast off to enter the blood stream. This is the basis of Ehrlich's side-chain theory which marked the beginning of our modern concepts of immunity, a subject to which we shall return in Chapter 5. Virus particles are adsorbed to the surface of the cell before penetrating to the interior. Poisons can alter the permeability of the cell membrane, so that some ions stream in and become attached to the mitochondria, whilst other ions stream out, with resulting sickness of the cell or it may be death. From these facts it becomes apparent that the cell membrane is a structure of paramount importance.

The Nucleus.—We have already seen that the nucleus may be regarded as the heart of the cell, although a cell from which the nucleus has been removed may live for three days. If such a cell is given another nucleus by modern microsurgery, it will continue to live. The nucleus houses the apparatus for maintaining the genetic constitution of the cell, namely the *chromosomal network* with its infinite tally of *genes*, the arbiters of hereditary characteristics. It is also concerned with cellular reproduction and multiplication, the development of separate chromosomal threads from the network being the first step in mitosis or cell division (*mitos*, a thread). We shall return to the subject of normal and abnormal cell division when we come to the subject of cancer or neoplasia in Chapter 8. Finally, the nucleus is believed to control the production of the cytoplasmic enzymes which are responsible for the chemical transformations associated with life. Reference has already been made to the nucleolus with its rich RNA content, and the fenestrated character of the nuclear membrane.

Mitochondria.—The principal organelles of

the cytoplasm with which we are concerned are the mitochondria and the endoplasmic reticulum (Fig. 1), although the Golgi complex and the centrosome deserve mention. The ground substance in which the organelles are suspended is known as the cytoplasmic matrix.

The mitochondria are not visible with hematoxylin and eosin staining, yet they are present in enormous numbers, with an average of 2500 in the normal rat liver cell. As seen with the electron microscope they are far from threadlike (*mitos*, thread; *chondros*, granule), but are rod-shaped or like a cucumber. They are surrounded by a double-layered membrane, and folds of the inner membrane project inward in the form of shelves termed *cristae*. They are in constant motion, change their size and shape very readily, and provide a sensitive indicator of cell injury. Mitochondria have been likened to the main power plants of the cell, because by virtue of the 25 or so different enzyme systems they contain, they utilize molecular oxygen and distribute energy-yielding components to other organelles; in other words, they are responsible for cell respiration.

In *cellular respiration* the enzymes catalyze the oxidation of pyruvic acid to CO_2 and H_2O by way of the citric-acid Krebs cycle. It must be borne in mind that oxidation no longer refers merely to the addition of oxygen to a substance, but now includes the removal of hydrogen atoms from a substance, and indeed any process in which electrons are lost. The enzymes of the Krebs cycle have been pictured as arranged in an orderly way on the inner surface of the mitochondrion and on the shelves of the cristae. The ultimate purpose of the mechanism is oxidative phosphorylation and the synthesis of adenosine triphosphate. When a fat-soluble poisonous compound such as carbon tetrachloride enters the liver cells, it attacks the mitochondria physically, so that they lose the power of retaining enzyme co-factors, and this disrupts the Krebs cycle. It may be noted in passing that cancer cells have fewer mitochondria than normal, because these cells unfortunately are more concerned with reproduction (mitotic division) than with functional activity.

Cell respiration seems to govern *water*

balance in the cell, because not only is water formed together with carbon dioxide by the reaction of oxygen with food, but some of the energy released is used for the active transport of water from the cells. As water is continually entering the cells it is obvious that this transport mechanism is of importance. As Cameron puts it, the cell is like a leaking ship kept steady by the pumps. If cell respiration decreases, the water content will increase and the cell will become waterlogged. This is the condition known as *hydropic degeneration*, which is discussed later in this chapter.

It must be realized that energy can be furnished in the absence of oxygen by means of *fermentation*. Oxidation suppresses fermentation, but this does not mean that fermentation and oxidation are two different mechanisms; they are rather two steps in normal cell respiration. Fermentation is glycolysis without the aid of oxygen. Glycolysis is the first step in cell respiration and is followed by oxidation. The enzymes concerned with the glycolysis of fermentation seem to be situated in other parts of the cytoplasm than the mitochondria. Cyanide is a deadly poison because it instantly arrests the oxygen transport system in the cells. It is of interest to note that cancer cells use anaerobic glycolysis more than do normal cells, and we have already seen that cancer cells have fewer mitochondria than normal cells.

Endoplasmic Reticulum.—This is a series of vesicles and intercommunicating canals, whose primary function is the manufacture of protein. It probably also provides a large amount of floor and wall space for the placement of the enzymes which constitute the machinery of the cell. The elements of the reticulum do not extend into the outer layer of cytoplasm known as the ectoplasm—hence the term endoplasmic. The membranous vesicles are usually flattened, so that with the electron microscope they are seen as double black lines, but sometimes they are in a distended form. Many of the vesicles are dotted on their outer surface with fine dark granules known as *Palade granules*. Such vesicles are called rough-surfaced vesicles, the smaller vesicles near the surface of the cell being smooth-surfaced. The granules consist of RNA, and are responsible for the basophilia of cytoplasm. They constitute a pattern or template for the manufacture of proteins. The amino acid building blocks are first arranged in proper order, and are then united by the enzymes in the wall of the endoplasmic reticulum to form the needed protein.

Cytoplasmic Inclusions.—Inclusions are not, like organelles, part of the living systems of the cell. They are of three main types: (1) stored foods, (2) secretion granules and globules, (3) pigments. It is the stored foods which are of interest in relation to sickness of the cell, but pigments will be discussed later in this chapter. Food stored in the cell can be drawn on during periods of starvation, allowing the body to survive as long as there is a sufficient supply of water. The food may be protein, carbohydrate or fat. *Protein* does not need to be in the form of inclusions, because cytoplasm is composed mainly of protein which can be consumed when the need arises.

Carbohydrates are absorbed from the bowel as glucose and stored in the liver cells as glycogen. As glycogen is highly soluble in water the cytoplasmic inclusions are dissolved out when the tissue has been fixed in an aqueous solution such as 10 per cent formalin, being represented merely by spaces with a ragged outline. When alcohol is used as a fixative the glycogen is preserved, and can be stained by the periodic acid-Schiff technique. We have already seen that the Feulgen reaction for demonstrating DNA depends on the staining of aldehyde liberated by mild hydrolysis, using the Schiff reagent. When it was demonstrated by McManus and independently in the same year by Hotchkiss that periodic acid, a strong oxidizing agent, can liberate aldehydes from polysaccharides, it was then possible to stain the aldehyde with the Schiff reagent. This is the best method of staining cytoplasmic inclusions of glycogen, but of course the tissue must be fixed in alcohol. It must be noted that in the ordinary hospital patient who has died of a wasting disease we see very little glycogen in the liver cells, so that the medical student may come to think that this is the normal appearance. It is only when a well nourished person dies suddenly that we see

the proper foamy appearance of the liver cells caused by the presence of glycogen.

Fat is stored in specialized fat cells and to a lesser degree in the liver, although in dietary deficiency cytoplasmic fat inclusions in the liver may dominate the picture. Just as glycogen is removed by aqueous fixatives, so fat is dissolved by the clearing agents used for paraffin sections It can be demonstrated in the cells in one of two ways: (1) by using frozen sections stained red with Scharlach R or some similar stain for fat; (2) by fixing the fat with osmic acid, which at the same time stains it black, after which paraffin sections can be cut. In ordinary routine sections we recognize fat in the cytoplasm as small spherical spaces with a smooth outline, which, when larger, may displace the nucleus to one side, in this respect differing from glycogen inclusions. The small droplets may fuse together, with rupture of the intervening walls and the formation of large spaces called by Hartroft *fatty cysts*, which are surrounded by the crescentic segments of the original cells that still persist (Fig. 2).

From this brief review of the structure and working of the normal cells of which the entire body is composed we can agree with Hamlet when he exclaims: "What a piece of work is a man!" Nor is it small wonder that this complex mechanism should sometimes go out of order.

THE SICK CELL: CELLULAR DEGENERATIONS

The infinitely complex and delicate structural and functional mechanism of the cell may be damaged by a variety of influences. If the damage is slight, the cell becomes sick with structural evidence of the sickness visible in the sections, although the very earliest lesions are purely biochemical in character, but the changes are reversible and recovery is possible. The fingerprints of disease can be seen in the tissue, but these prints can be erased. The changes in structure (and presumably in function) are described by the terms *degeneration* and *infiltration*. In the degenerations the primary change is presumed to be in the tissue elements, whilst in the infiltrations something unusual has been brought and added to the cell. As we shall

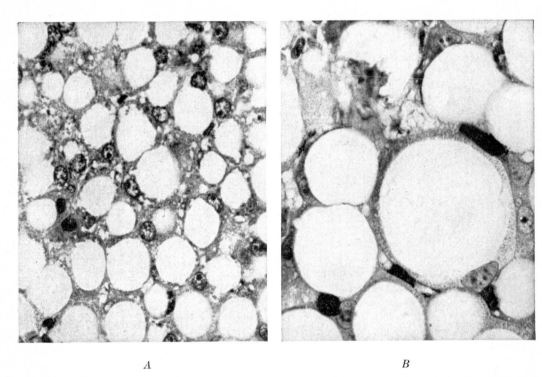

A   B

Fig. 2.—*A*, Photomicrograph of a section of liver from a rat which had experienced a choline deficiency for 12 days. McGregor stain, × 600. The liver cells that are distended with fat are almost twice as wide as normal cells.

B, A similar preparation from a rat that experienced the same kind of deficiency for 45 days. Observe that individual cells have liberated their fat into a cyst which is surrounded by several cells. The black structures seen are capillaries that have been injected with India ink. (Hartroft, courtesy of Anat. Rec.)

soon see, this distinction is not as simple and clear as the foregoing statement would suggest. When the damage is more severe the changes are irreversible and we have a dying or dead cell, the condition described below as *necrosis*. If lime salts are deposited in the dead tissue we speak of *pathological calcification*.

A few years ago the student was expected to be familiar with various abnormal appearances of cells under the microscope. These were empirically grouped together as degenerations, and the subject was generally ranked as perhaps the most dull in the entire study of pathology, because most of the changes seemed to have little if any connection with practical medicine. Advances in biochemistry and electron microscopy have begun to lift the curtain on their significance, and we are looking on the so-called "degenerations" with new interest, for they are

sign-posts of various disturbances of the countless enzymes governing cellular activity. Sometimes they baffle us by their nonspecificity, sometimes they are so specific that a glance down the microscope at a single cell will tell us that the patient was suffering from potassium deficiency (the clear-cell vacuolation of the renal tubules in potassium loss), or a disturbance of phenylalanine metabolism (pigmentation of cartilage in alcaptonuria).

Most of these cytological changes depend on the appearance in the nucleus or cytoplasm of the normal components of the cell, components which are not usually visible because they normally occur in intricate combinations with the other components. When one or more enzyme system is damaged or blocked these intimate combinations may be broken down, or raw materials coming to the cell may remain unprocessed and

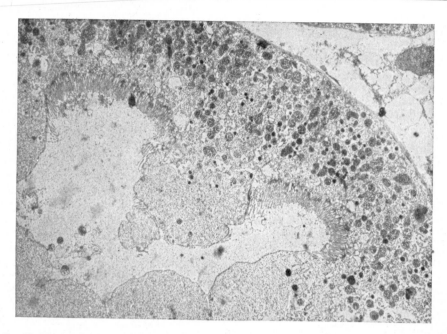

Fig. 3.—Cloudy swelling of kidney. Low power electron micrograph of proximal convoluted tubule. The affected areas are homogeneous and granular, bulging into the lumen and having lost their covering brush border. There are no organelles in the swollen parts. × 2900. (Kindness of Dr. Henry Z. Movat).

therefore accumulate in visible form. Thus the appearance of fatty vacuoles tells us that something is wrong with fat metabolism, of glycogen that carbohydrate metabolism is disturbed, and of excess water that the number and distribution of electrolytes is faulty. They are not really degenerations, therefore, but signs of dysfunction.

Cloudy Swelling.—The term cloudy swelling, a relic of the past, is about as vague and unsatisfactory as could be conceived. As a matter of fact, it was originally applied to the gross appearance of the organs involved, but it now connotes a microscopic change. It is closely related to hydropic or vacuolar degeneration, described below. Indeed the two appear to represent some sort of water and protein disturbance in cells as the result of many forms of mild injury. Cloudy swelling is so common a manifestation of minor sickness of the cell that it may be compared with the furring of the tongue which used to attract the attention of the doctor not so long ago. Being a manifestation of a disturbance of protein metabolism, it is also called *albuminous degeneration.* Cloudy swelling is the commonest of the cellular degenerations,

and it may be caused by bacterial toxins, chemical poisons, malnutrition, *etc.*

The principal organs showing cloudy swelling are the kidney, the liver, and the heart muscle. The organ affected is slightly enlarged, owing to swelling of the cells of which it is composed. It is pale, the blood vessels being compressed by the swollen cells. The cut surface has a rather cloudy appearance, slightly opaque, as if scalded in hot water.

The *microscopic appearance* can best be studied in the highly specialized cells of the convoluted tubule of the kidney. (Fig. 3). The cell presents two abnormal features: (1) it is unduly granular, and (2) it is swollen so that it projects unevenly into the lumen of the tubule. As the condition advances the cell may break down and the granular material is discharged into the lumen of the tubule. The granules are albuminous in character, and can be distinguished from fatty granules by the fact that they are soluble in acetic acid and insoluble in lipid solvents such as chloroform. The swelling of the cell is due to edema.

Hydropic Degeneration.—This condition is closely related to cloudy swelling. The per-

2

meability of the cell membrane is damaged and altered, so that unusually large amounts of water accumulate in the cytoplasm and may form vacuoles, either many small ones or one large clear space which must not be mistaken for a fat globule. At the same time potassium ions are lost and sodium ions enter the cell. The mitochondria appear to be specially involved in this hydropic change in the cytoplasm. They may be converted into bags of fluid or may actually disintegrate. There are two reasons for believing that the mitochondria are involved in hydropic degeneration and the closely related cloudy swelling. (1) When ultracentrifugation is applied to liver cells rendered hydropic by poisoning with carbon tetrachloride or chloroform, the mitochondira released are seen to be vacuolar (Judah *et al.*). (2) Cell respiration is a function of the mitochondria, and some of the energy released is used for active transportation of water out of the cells. If the mitochondrial power stations break down, the water content of the cell naturally increases. This relationship between respiration and water content can be demonstrated in surviving slices of rat liver. It has also been suggested that cloudy swelling may be a result of disturbance of the active transport of water from cells.

Fatty Infiltration and Degeneration.—The position of fat in relation to what we have been calling cell sickness is a peculiar dual one, which is not seen in the case of protein and carbohydrate. (1) Fat may accumulate in the cell or at least become visible because of a local breakdown of the mitochondrial metabolism of fat produced by disruption of the enzymes concerned. This is *fatty degeneration*. (2) The cell may be healthy, but it may be presented with an overload of fat as a result of some systemic metabolic derangement. As it cannot deal with this overload, fat accumulates within the cytoplasm, and in turn damages the cellular mechanism. This is *fatty infiltration*.

The fat in the food is not absorbed as such, but is broken down in the duodenum by the intestinal juice, the pancreatic secretion and the bile to simpler forms, mainly fatty acids and glycerol. After absorption these are recombined to form neutral fats, passing by the portal vein to the liver. In the liver the fat is phosphorylated, one of its fatty-acid groupings being replaced by phosphoric acid to form phospholipids, which are more readily metabolized. Phosphorylation is one of the basic functions of the liver cell, a function in which choline plays an integral part. After the fat has been dealt with by the liver it is carried throughout the body to be used. Some of it is stored in the fat depots known as adipose tissue, where the connective cells are so distended with fat that they constitute what we are accustomed to refer to as fat cells. In spite of the name, it must not be supposed that the fat in the depots is static, for experiments with isotope-labelled fat show that there is a constant turn over and flow of fat between the depots, the liver and the cells where it is used. Fat destined for the cells of the body is taken first to the liver to be conditioned by phosphorylation. It will be evident that part of the fat reaching the cells via the liver will come from the diet and part from the circulating pool represented by the depots.

Lipotropic factors are necessary for the removal from the liver of fat brought to it by the blood (Best). The most powerful of these agents is choline. An animal fed on a choline-deficient diet rapidly accumulates enormous amounts of fat in liver cells. Phospholipids are essential for the transport of fat and as choline promotes the formation of phospholipids, absence of this food factor from the diet leads to the rapid accumulation of liver fat. This is true also of choline precursors such as methionine. The effect of dietary protein on fat transport seems to be due to the transfer of methyl groups from methionine for the synthesis of choline. Pregnancy damages the liver because the lipotropic factors are sidetracked to the fetus. It is evident that a long-continued dietary deficiency in protein may damage the liver owing to an excessive accumulation of fat, damage which can be repaired if treated in time by the administration of choline or methionine. We shall return to this subject when discussing cirrhosis of the liver in Chapter 28. For further information on lipotropic factors the reader is referred to reviews by Best and by McHenry and Patterson.

Fatty Degeneration.—This is a true sickness of the cell caused by some injurious influence. It is seen best in the liver, kidney and myocardium. The fat metabolism of the cell is interfered with, and fat accumulates in the cell. In some cases there is merely an unmasking of fat already present.

The *causes* of fatty degeneration are: (1) poisons and (2) anoxia. The *poisons* may be *organic* in the form of any bacterial toxin which interferes with the cellular enzymes, or *inorganic*, of which the best examples are phosphorus, carbon tetrachloride and chloroform. *Anoxia* may occur in a number of diseases. Perhaps the most striking example is the fatty degeneration of the myocardium which used to develop in pernicious anemia before the days of liver therapy as the result of the long-continued anoxemia due to the lack of red blood cells.

Lesions.—The *gross appearance* of the organs principally involved, namely the liver, kidney and heart, could be described in the main by the student from his previous knowledge. As might be expected, the organs look and feel fatty. The liver and to a lesser degree the kidney are paler, yellow and softer than normal. The heart is soft and flabby, and the endocardial surface presents a speckled appearance which suggested to the more fanciful minds of our predecessors in pathology the expression "the thrush breast heart." This is most marked in the left ventricle and particularly the papillary muscles. This used to be a common finding in autopsies on cases of pernicious anemia before the days of liver therapy, but is now seldom seen—a good example of the changing picture of pathology.

The *microscopic picture* is equally simple and could be suggested by the student who had never seen an example of the condition. The cytoplasm of the *liver cells* contains innumerable fine vacuoles, for the most part grouped around the nucleus which is not misplaced. When in doubt these vacuoles can be shown to be fat with appropriate technique (Fig. 4). Owing to the action of the toxin the cytoplasm may also show some of the granularity which we have already recognized as characteristic of cloudy swelling. In the *kidney* the tubular cells show a similar appearance. In the *myocardium* the muscle cells contain numerous droplets of fat often arranged in longitudinal rows. In the

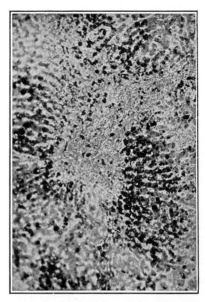

Fig. 4.—Fatty liver stained with osmic acid. The fat is at the periphery of the lobules. × 75.

profound toxemia of diphtheria fatty degeneration of the myocardium may reflect a change so severe that it is responsible for death.

Fatty Infiltration.—We have already seen that when an undue load of fat is presented to the liver or when the all-important lipotropic factors are lacking the cells become filled up with fat. In clinical practice the condition is most commonly seen in cases of chronic alcoholism, where alcohol takes the place of food, so that there is a long-continued dietary deficiency of protein, including choline and methionine. Dietary deficiency for other reasons will naturally lead to a similar result. The liver is the only organ the parenchymal cells of which present the picture of fatty infiltration. The gross appearance of the liver is much more striking than in fatty degeneration. The organ may be greatly enlarged, the softness and yellow color are more striking, and the texture may be friable.

The *microscopic appearance* is different from that of fatty degeneration of the liver. Large globules of fat occupy the cytoplasm and displace the nucleus to one side, so that the liver cell may assume the appearance of an adult fat cell. The distended liver cells may fuse together to form much larger

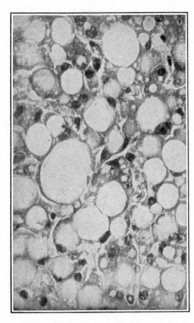

FIG. 5.—Fatty liver. Note Similarity to condition produced by choline deficiency in rat in Fig. 2. ×375

masses at the margin of which the original nuclei can still be discerned. These are known as "fatty cysts" (Fig. 5). Such a process may naturally result in the destruction of large areas of liver cells. This condition is discussed more fully in relation to cirrhosis of the liver in Chapter 28.

It might be thought from what has just been said that the distinction between fatty degeneration and fatty infiltration of the liver was clear-cut. In many cases this is not so, and the features of both conditions may be combined. The very presence of large quantities of infiltrating fats is apt to damage the enzymatic mechanism and lead to fatty degeneration. For this reason the noncommittal term *fatty metamorphosis* is used, or the simpler *fatty changes*, or the simplest of all, namely *fatty liver*.

Stromal fatty infiltration is seen in the heart, the pancreas, and the voluntary muscles in muscular dystrophy. Fat accumulates in the connective tissue cells and converts them into adult fat cells. This is usually an accompaniment of obesity, but not necessarily so. In the *heart* the fat collects under the epicardium, particularly that of the right ventricle, and extends between the muscle bundles until it reaches the endocardium. In extreme cases this accumulation of fat may interfere with the heart's action. In the *pancreas* the accumulation of fat may be so great that on gross inspection the parenchymatous tissue may seem to have disappeared. Under the microscope the pancreatic glands are seen to be widely dispersed by the fat.

Staining of Fat.—Reference has already been made to the methods by which the pathologist demonstrates the presence of fat in cells. The usual procedure is to cut frozen sections, thus avoiding use of the fat solvents inseparable from the paraffin section technique, and staining with Scharlach R or Oil red O (Plate I). Tissues embedded in carbowax, which is miscible with water, can be cut more easily. If more permanent paraffin sections are desired, the tissue can be fixed in osmic acid, which at the same time stains the fat an intense black (Fig. 4); paraffin sections can then be cut without danger of losing the fat. Special methods such as those of Marchi and Weigert designed to stain myelin will be described in connection with diseases of the nervous system in Chapter 42. The student will usually be satisfied with recognizing fat in his paraffin sections as clear spherical vacuoles of varying size in the cytoplasm. To distinguish these spaces from those due to glycogen or even water, the special techniques outlined above are required.

Lipoidal Degeneration.—In ordinary fatty degeneration and infiltration the fats concerned are neutral fats. There is in addition an important group of pathological changes involving the lipids, mainly cholesterol and cholesterol ester. These lipoidal changes may be both in the nature of degeneration and infiltration. Cholesterol, which is not a true fat but an alcohol, is a constituent of all the cells of the body, but in an invisible form. When the cell undergoes autolysis the cholesterol is not destroyed, so that it may become visible either as a needle-shaped crystal or as a flat plate with one corner bitten out. The nature of these crystals as well as that of the ester can be beautifully demonstrated by examining frozen sections under crossed Nicol's prisms; the brilliantly white anisotropic material stands out against the black background. Cholesterol crystals may be found in caseous tissue, infarcts, old hem-

PLATE I

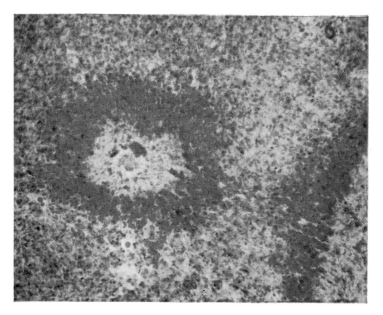

Fatty liver.   The fat has accumulated mainly around the central veins
Oil red O and hematoxylin. (Kindness of Dr. Henry Z. Movat.)

orrhages, atheroma, degenerating goiters, dermoid cysts, hydrocele fluid, *etc.* The yellow patches on the inner surface of the aorta in atheroma consist mainly of lipids, but neutral fats are also present. The characteristic spindle-shaped clefts in the tissue are often associated with giant cells, indicating a foreign body giant-cell reaction. This reaction is best seen in the tumor-like masses called xanthomas. The cholesteatomatous masses which occasionally occur in the ear and the cranial cavity consist largely of cholesterol. Two conditions which more closely resemble true fatty metamorphosis than those already mentioned are cholesterolosis of the gallbladder and those forms of Bright's disease which are associated with marked albuminuria and edema, *i. e.*, nephrosis and wet nephritis. In these conditions there is a remarkable collection of cholesterol in the epithelial cells of the gallbladder and kidney respectively, which will be considered in detail when these diseases are described. When cholesterol ester is set free as the result of lipoidal degeneration it is often taken up by phagocytic cells, giving the cytoplasm of these cells a vacuolated appearance. These *foam cells* are seen to best advantage around an area of brain softening, but they are found in degenerating goiter and many other situations.

Tissue reactions to lipids, a term which signifies a heterogeneous group that includes fats, oils, waxes, phospholipids and sterols, are varied. These reactions occur when the fats are not completely metabolized. The reaction about unhydrolyzed fat is similar to that against an inert oil-like petrolatum. With hydrolysis of the fat and liberation of fatty acids there may be acute necrosis or a non-specific reaction on the part of fibroblasts and macrophages. Insoluble soaps excite a foreign body giant-cell reaction. The various reactions have been fully discussed by Hirsch.

PROGRESSIVE LIPODYSTROPHY.—This strange disturbance of fat metabolism is characterized by a symmetrical and progressive loss of subcutaneous fat in the face, arms and upper part of the body, associated with undue deposition of fat in the buttocks and lower limbs, occurring in children, usually girls. In extreme cases the skin rides loosely over the muscles, giving the patient a cadaver-like expression. To the eyes of one observer the lower half of the body looked like a model of one of Rubens' paintings, while the upper half resembled one of the witches in Macbeth. The adipose tissue of the affected parts is unable to store fat, no matter how much the patient may eat. The cause is unknown.

GLYCOGEN INFILTRATION

Glycogen is the storage form of carbohydrates, and corresponds to the starch of plants. It occurs in the body in a labile and a stable form. The *labile form*, which represents by far the greatest amount, is present in abundance in the liver (38 per cent of the total amount in the body) and in the muscles (44 per cent). It is converted into glucose with great ease, and rapidly disappears from the tissues after death. As it is soluble in water, the tissue should be fixed in alcohol. The *stable form* occurs in minute quantity in many tissues, and under pathological conditions it may be greatly increased in amount. Glycogen is the only carbohydrate which can be demonstrated under the microscope, and is of particular interest on that account. It is colored reddish-brown with iodine, and is beautifully shown by Best's carmine stain which colors it crimson. Even better is the McManus PAS stain (periodic acid-leukofuchsin reaction of Schiff) with diastase digestion of duplicate slides as a control. This is a particularly sensitive method capable of demonstrating the minute amount of glycogen left in the cell after the use of watery fixatives.

Unlike the case of fat, glycogen is of interest to us only as an infiltration, not as a degeneration. It accumulates as the result of too much carbohydrate being presented to the cell, that is to say a condition of hyperglycemia, commonly diabetic in origin, not of inability on the part of the cell to deal with the carbohydrate. To this general truth there is one possible exception, namely von Gierke's disease, which is discussed below. The increased glycogen content of the liver and kidney does not appear to interfere with their function.

Lesions.—Glycogenic infiltration is seen in the liver and kidney. The situation is different in the two organs, because the liver cells normally contain an abundance of glycogen,

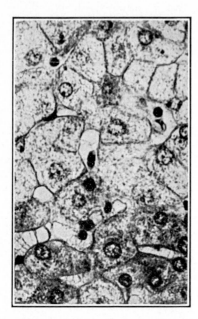

FIG. 6.—Glycogen in liver cells (pale and vacuolated) × 500.

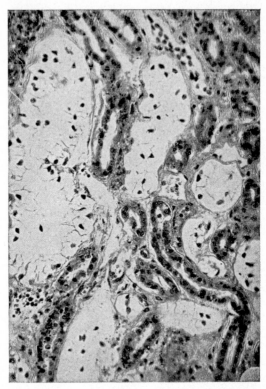

FIG. 7.—Armanni-Ebstein lesion.   Deposits of glycogen in the cells of the loop of Henle.   × 225. (Boyd, *Pathology for the Physician*)

whereas renal tubular cells do not . The liver cells of a person who has died of a sudden accident are seen to have a foamy vacuolated appearance which is apt to be mistaken by the ignorant for a pathological condition. It is in reality the normal picture of a healthy liver, and is identical with the appearance seen in a piece of liver removed surgically or for biopsy, especially if the patient happens to have received a preoperative injection of glucose (Fig. 6).   The liver seen in the ordinary hospital autopsy is one which is depleted of glycogen, as the patient is likely to have eaten little during the preceding twelve hours.

In glycogen infiltration of the *liver* the glycogen is contained principally in the nuclei of the hepatic cells.   The nuclei are distended, and are so clear that they may appear empty in sections of tissue fixed in a watery fixative such as formalin, the chromatin being displaced to the margin.   In very severe cases the cytoplasm is finely vacuolated.

In the *kidney* the degree of infiltration is related not only to the degree of hyperglycemia, but also to the duration and intensity of the glycosuria which forms an integral part of diabetes mellitus.   The glycogen deposited in the cells of the tubules represents the glucose reabsorbed from the sugar-loaded urine passing along the lumen of the tubules.   The cytoplasm becomes filled with glycogen, which is dissolved out by the water of aqueous fixatives, so that the interior of the cell appears absolutely clear, leaving the nucleus intact (Fig. 7). The principal change is in the terminal straight segment of the proximal convoluted tubules with extension into the contiguous portion of the thin limb of the loop of Henle.   Ritchie and Waugh have shown by microdissection of individual nephrons that marked glycogenic vacuolation is confined to the epithelium of the tubules in the outer layer of the medulla and the inner layer of the cortex, so that the lesions are astride the cortico-medullary junction.   This lesion which used to be known as the *Armanni-Ebstein lesion* from the men who described it many years ago, but is now referred to as *glycogen nephrosis*, was an invariable accompaniment of diabetes before the days of insulin. Now it has disappeared with the sugar in the urine of the well-controlled diabetic. Another disturbance of carbohydrate metabolism in the kidney has been reported in cases where solutions of glucose and more particularly sucrose have been given intravenously in large amount. In this so-called *sucrose nephrosis* the cytoplasm of the cells of the convoluted tubules contains large numbers of small vacuoles in place of the empty appearance of the cells in glycogen infiltration.

von Gierke's Disease.—This is a strange condition in children, characterized by an excessive storage of glycogen, especially in the liver and to a lesser degree in the kidney. The liver becomes enormous, and this great hepatomegaly in a child unaccompanied by splenomegaly, jaundice, or any marked constitutional disturbance is highly characteristic. There is hypoglycemia, but without the usual clinical symptoms. The injection of adrenalin fails to mobilize the glycogen in the liver as it should do in a normal person. Acetone and diacetic acid may be present in the urine but without glycosuria. The cause of this ketosis is fundamentally the same as that of diabetes, although brought about in a different way. In diabetes the sugar, although present in abundance in the blood, is unable to play its proper part in the combustion of fats. In this disease the fats are not properly burnt because the sugar is held in the liver in the form of glycogen. The liver cells are greatly distended, the cytoplasm clear or vacuolated and, in one case which I studied, the cell boundaries in many places appeared to be broken down (Fig. 8). In von Gierke's original case the kidneys were markedly enlarged owing to accumulation of glycogen in the epithelium of the convoluted tubules. The disease appears to depend on a defective transformation of glycogen into glucose owing to absence of the glycogenolytic enzyme, hexose-6-phosphatase, so that it accumulates in the glycogen depots. The condition is, therefore, analogous to the lipid storage disease (Gaucher's disease, Niemann-Pick's disease, Christian's syndrome) in which the cells of the reticuloendothelial system become loaded with lipid. Glycogen storage, like lipid storage, may show a familial tendency and may be regarded as a congenital anomaly of metabolism.

Another very rare manifestation of glycogen storage is known as *glycogen storage disease of the heart*, also called glycogenic tumor of the heart. This is one variety of idiopathic hypertrophy of the heart in infants. The heart of the child may

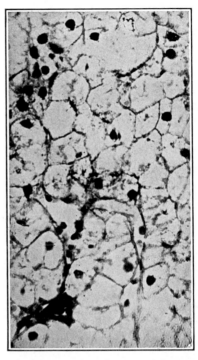

Fig. 8.—Von Gierke's disease. Liver cells distended with glycogen, which has been dissolved out. × 400.

be as much as seven times the normal weight. The muscle cells present a characteristic vacuolated or empty appearance. The cause of this congenital lesion is not known, the hexose-6-phosphatase being present in normal amount.

An analysis of the whole subject of glycogen storage disease will be found in the papers of von Creveld, who, it may be noted, reported two clinical cases one year before the publication of von Gierke's autopsy report.

Mucoid Degeneration.—Mucus, the viscid watery secretion of mucous glands, is a loose combination of protein with mucopolysaccharides of high molecular weight. Mucin, a glycoprotein, is its chief constituent. Mucous granules appear to be produced by the mitochondria, then moving to the Golgi area or apparatus, where they are changed into mature mucin granules. When this process is exaggerated with excessive secretion of mucus associated with degeneration of the cells, we speak of mucoid degeneration. Mucin is produced normally both by the epithelial cells of mucous membranes and mucous glands, and also by certain connective tissue cells, especially in the fetus. Mucoid degeneration may involve both of these types of mucin.

Epithelial Mucin.—In catarrhal inflammation of the mucous membrane of the respiratory tract, the gastrointestinal canal, and the uterus, there is an excessive secretion of mucin, the cells are distended with this substance, and their outlines may disappear. The cells of a cystadenoma of the ovary produce pseudomucin in enormous amount so that a huge cyst may be formed; many of these cells degenerate and are cast off into the cyst. Cancer of the stomach, the large bowel, and more rarely the breast may produce mucin to such an extent that the tumor is converted into a mass of mucoid material. Mucin is a slimy substance which is precipitated by acetic acid; it is basophilic, *i.e.*, stains with basic dyes, and gives a metachromatic reaction with toluidin blue, staining reddish-purple. Pseudomucin is not precipitated by acetic acid, and is stained by acid stains. Newer stains for acid mucopolysaccharides stain both mucin and pseudomucin.

Connective-tissue Mucin.—The only place where intercellular connective-tissue mucin normally occurs is in the umbilical cord. The cells are stellate with branching processes and are separated by an abundance of clear mucin. Mucinoid or myxomatous degeneration may occur in the stroma of various tumors, most notably in the myxoma. In conditions of malnutrition a similar change may affect the bone-marrow, adipose tissue, and cartilage. In myxedema, a disease due to deficiency of thyroid secretion, the connective tissue of the skin and elsewhere becomes swollen and gelatinous, and in the early stages contains mucin. Mucin may be formed in the intercellular substance of synovial membranes and tendon sheaths; the development of this process is beautifully illustrated in the early stages of a ganglion of the wrist.

Hyaline Degeneration.—Hyaline degeneration is the commonest of the degenerations and the most obscure. In one sense it is perhaps unfortunate that the expression was ever coined. Hyalinization is perhaps a better term. It seems to represent an end stage of many degenerative processes, both cellular and connective tissue. Unfortunately we know nothing of the origin or chemistry of hyaline. The term denotes a physical rather than a chemical constitution, and includes many substances which are translucent or hyaline and stain bright red with eosin or blue (or green) with a trichrome stain. It seems to correspond to a coagulation of protein, and is therefore found in a variety of conditions. With the electron microscope the cell organelle mainly involved seems to be the smooth-surfaced variety of endoplasmic reticulum (and therefore free of ribonucleoprotein particles), agglomerates of the tubules of the reticulum corresponding to the hyaline bodies seen in light microscopy (Bruni), although in the opinion of others these bodies represent swelling of mitochondria with uptake of protein.

Hyaline degeneration affects chiefly collagenous connective tissue and the fibrous tissue in the walls of blood vessels. This may be called connective-tissue hyaline. Other forms can be grouped together as cellular hyaline. The tissue dies before becoming changed into hyaline. *Connective-tissue hyaline* appears as a homogeneous swelling of collagen and in the walls of vessels in arteriosclerosis. It is seen in chronic malnutrition and in old age, but the exact factors responsible are not certain. The change is well seen in arteriosclerosis. The subendothelial layer of the arterioles shows marked hyaline thickening in vascular hypertension. In chronic nephritis the renal glomeruli become converted into hyaline masses. Scar tissue undergoes a similar change. The stroma of tumors may show hyaline degeneration, and the same may be seen in the reticulum of lymph nodes draining a focus chronic inflammation (Fig. 9). In all of these instances the fibrous tissue loses its structure, the fibers are swollen and homogeneous, and stain red with acid stains. The appearance may resemble that of amyloid, but the material does not give the amyloid staining reactions.

Cellular hyaline is a heterogeneous group with no special meaning. Small hyaline masses are often seen in the cells of the renal tubules, especially in amyloid disease. The cells of the islets of Langerhans in the

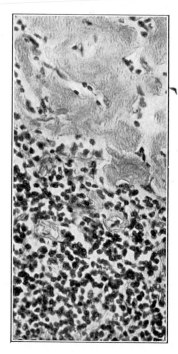

FIG. 9.—Hyaline degeneration of a lymph node. × 350.

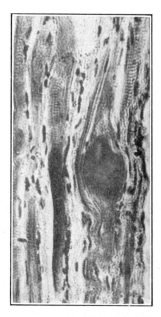

FIG. 10.—Zenker's degeneration of muscle in typhoid fever. The affected parts of the fibers have lost their transverse striations and are dark and swollen. × 400.

pancreas may become converted into a hyaline mass in diabetes. Hyaline thrombi in vessels are formed largely by fusion together of blood platelets which then undergo hyaline degeneration. *Corpora amylacea*, so-called because like starch they stain deeply with iodine (*amylon*, starch), are hyaline spherical masses made up of concentric laminæ. They are seen in the normal prostate, in old infarcts of the lung, in the brain and spinal cord in old age and in degenerative conditions, and occasionally in other situations. They represent masses of degenerative cells and sometimes merely the secretion of cells. In necrosis of voluntary muscle and sometimes of cardiac muscle the protoplasm may become coagulated, the striations are lost, and the fiber is converted into a swollen homogeneous hyaline mass (Fig. 10). This condition, known as *Zenker's degeneration*, is best seen in the rectus abdominis muscle and diaphragm in typhoid fever, but it is also seen in other muscles and other infections.

NECROSIS

We may turn now from the sick or degenerating cell to the dying and dead cell. By necrosis is meant, as the word implies, the local death of cells. Now although death may be regarded as the final degeneration, a cell which has been suddenly killed shows no sign of degeneration. It looks exactly like a normal cell. This after all is natural, for the fixed cells of microscopic sections have all been killed. Moreover the cells removed from the body at autopsy (or necropsy) are, of course, dead. The cellular changes characteristic of necrosis are changes which the cell undergoes *after* it has died while still remaining in the body. These changes are very similar to those undergone by living cells when they are removed from the body and allowed to die, being due to the same cause, namely, the action of enzymes. It is evident that necrotic changes may easily be confused with those of postmortem degeneration, and the distinction is sometimes hard to make.

The complex system of enzymes to which reference has already been made cease to take part in the metabolism of food stuffs brought to the cell and turn their energies on the framework of the cell itself, a process known as *autolysis*. It is the nucleoproteins of the chromatin of the nucleus which suffer most, so that it is in this "heart of the cell" that the changes about to be described are most evident. Secondary changes in the cytoplasm follow as a matter of course. The products of autolysis are readily diffusable, so that they pass into the surrounding fluid and eventually the cell disappears. It is evident that necrotic changes may easily be confused with those of postmortem degeneration, especially if the dead body has not been efficiently refrigerated. The subject of postmortem changes is discussed presently.

Causes.—1. *Loss of Blood Supply.*—When the supply of oxygen and food is cut off, the cells of the part rapidly undergo necrosis. This is well seen in an infarct caused by blockage of a vessel by a blood clot, which produces immediate ischemia or loss of blood supply with consequent anoxia. Even though the cutting-off of the blood is only transient, the cells may be killed. The time necessary varies with the tissue; the secreting cells of the kidney may be killed, while the connective tissue survives. Thrombosis of the vessels to a part is followed by necrosis unless a collateral circulation can be quickly established.

2. *Bacterial Toxins.*—The action of toxins is the commonest cause of necrosis. The student can supply examples for himself. As the toxins act on the vessels of the part and are apt to produce thrombosis, it is evident that ischemia and toxemia are often combined. Much depends on the concentration of the toxin; if the toxin is weak inflammation is produced; if strong the result is necrosis.

3. *Physical and Chemical Agents.*—The various physical and chemical irritants which may produce inflammtion may also lead to necrosis. Heat is much more injurious than cold. Heat above 45°C. will kill cells, whereas freezing may leave them unaffected. The death of tissue following frostbite is due to injury to the vessels and thrombosis rather than to any direct action on the cells. Electricity, roentgen-rays, and radium rapidly cause cell death if in sufficient concentra-

tion. The subject of radiation necrosis has assumed pressing importance in this atomic age. Profound necrosis may be produced by therapeutic radiation. Caustics and other poisons, trauma, and continued pressure may produce the same result.

Structural Changes.—Necrosis can be recognized by changes in the cell body and in the nucleus. The *cellular changes* are swelling of the cytoplasm which becomes homogeneous and loses its normal reticulated appearance. There is loss of the normal sharp contour and obliteration of the cell boundaries. Muscle fibers lose their striations and become swollen and homogeneous. *Zenker's degeneration*, which is best seen in the rectus abdominis and diaphragm in typhoid fever, is an example of necrosis with hyaline changes. The *nuclear changes* are even more striking, and should be looked for in determining the presence of necrosis. There are three possible changes (Figs. 11 to 13). (1) *Chromatolysis* or *karyolysis*, in which the nuclear chromatin appears to be dissolved and the nucleus gradually fades from sight. This is the commonest change. (2) *Karyorrhexis*, in which the nucleus is broken up into a number of small fragments, well seen at the edge of an infarct. (3) *Pyknosis*, in which the nuclear material is condensed into a small deeply-staining mass. This may be attributed to hydrolysis of the nucleoprotein, with liberation of nucleic acid which stains densely with basic dyes. The student must learn to recognize necrosis under the microscope, because he will encounter tissue death in most diseases and in every organ of the body.

The gross appearance also varies, there being two main types known as coagulation necrosis and liquefaction or colliquative necrosis.

Coagulation Necrosis.—Coagulation necrosis is the common form, and is characteristically seen in infarcts of the kidney or spleen. The part becomes dry, homogeneous, and opaque. There is coagulation of the cytoplasm by intracellular enzymes. Perhaps some of the surrounding lymph may be absorbed and coagulated in the same way. The process is similar to coagulation of the blood. Architectural outlines (glomeruli, tubules) may be preserved though all cellular

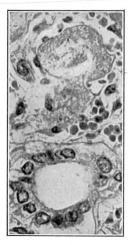
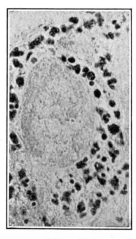
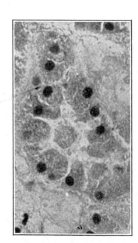

Fig. 11   Fig. 12   Fig. 13

Figs. 11 to 13.—Forms of nuclear degeneration in the tubules of the kidney.

Fig. 11.—Chromatolysis. The nuclei of the upper tubule have disappeared.
Fig. 12.—Karyorrhexis. The nuclei are broken up into small fragments.
Fig. 13.—Pyknosis. The nuclear material is collected into small compact masses. × 500.

detail is lost. The coagulated material may remain unchanged for long periods of time, but at the margin of the infarcted area there is a gradual process of absorption owing to the action of proteolytic enzymes in the leukocytes brought by the circulating blood. In the course of time calcification may occur.

Liquefaction Necrosis.—Liquefaction necrosis occurs in the central nervous system. The necrotic area becomes softened and liquefied, and the fluid material is absorbed leaving a cyst-like space. The change is probably in some way dependent on the high lipid content of the nervous tissue.

Caseation.—Caseation is a form of necrosis in which all details of structure are wiped out, with the production of a dry, cheesy, granular material, completely amorphous. In ordinary necrosis, on the other hand, though the cells are destroyed the stroma is spared, so that the architecture is preserved. Caseation is the characteristic necrotic change of tuberculosis and syphilis. Tuberculous caseous tissue is not chemotactic, so that it attracts no leukocytes; the material therefore remains unchanged owing to the absence of leukocytic ferments. If secondary infection occurs there is invasion of leukocytes and softening may rapidly follow.

Caseous material has a high fat content, and calcification is a frequent sequel.

Autolysis.—Autolysis plays an important part in producing the picture of necrosis. Take two pieces of fresh tissue, heat one for an hour at 55° C. or boil it for a few minutes, then insert both pieces in the abdominal cavity of an animal. The fate of the two pieces will be very different. The heated piece in which the enzymes have been destroyed will undergo little change, the nuclei staining well after a lapse of months. The unheated piece will pass through the usual changes characteristic of necrosis owing to the autolytic action of its enzymes. If the two pieces are placed in normal saline and incubated, the heated piece will show no change, but the cells of the unheated piece will undergo enormous swelling due to the enzymes breaking down the large molecules into a greater number of small molecules with increase of the osmotic pressure and imbibition of fluid. For this reason dead cells floating in a fluid medium become very swollen. Autolysis proceeds much more quickly outside the body than in necrotic areas such as infarcts, because the plasma contains substances which inhibit the action of the enzymes.

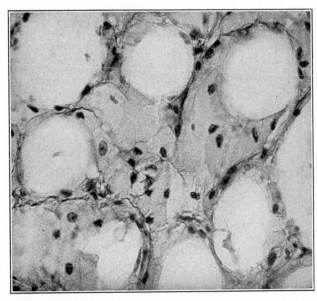

Fig. 14.—Fat necrosis. The necrotic fat cells have a cloudy appearance. × 400.

Fat Necrosis.—When the pancreatic secretion is liberated in the abdomen owing to inflammation (acute pancreatitis) or injury to the pancreas, the fat-splitting ferment, lipase, acts upon the fat on the surface of the pancreas and in the omentum with the production of small opaque white areas of fat necrosis. The fat is split into glycerin and a fatty acid. The former is absorbed, while the latter remains in the cells as acicular crystals. The necrotic fat cells are easily recognized, because the material which they contain is much less soluble than normal fat, and is therefore not dissolved away in paraffin sections, giving the cells a cloudy appearance (Fig. 14). The patches may be rapidly removed; in experimental fat necrosis they have disappeared in eleven days. Calcium may unite with the fatty acid to form a calcium soap, and lime salts may be deposited in the patches of necrosis rendering them permanent. Recent patches are surrounded by a zone of leukocytes. Owing to postmortem changes in the pancreas, lipase may be liberated after death and produce fat necrosis. These postmortem patches can be distinguished from those produced during life as the result of disease by the absence of the zone of leukocytes.

Traumatic fat necrosis is quite a different matter. As a result of injury the fat cells of subcutaneous tissue may be injured, and an area of induration partly necrotic, partly inflammatory in character, is produced. The fat cells resemble those in the opaque patches of pancreatic fat necrosis, containing insoluble material in paraffin sections. A well-marked inflammatory reaction is seen around and within the affected area; foreign body giant cells often form a striking feature so that the lesion may be mistaken for tuberculosis or syphilis. The breast is the most common site.

GANGRENE

Gangrene is death of a part with putrefaction superadded.

The essence of the process is putrefaction. In the student's mind and in that of the surgeon there is often confusion as to the difference between gangrene, necrosis and infarction. In gangrene the tissues become putrid and rotten owing to the action of saprophytic putrefying bacteria. Necrosis is a microscopic term indicating cellular death, whilst infarction is a gross term signifying death of a part owing to sudden ischemia. An infarct is of course necrotic, but bacteria play no part in the process.

Saprophytes grow only in dead tissue, so that gangrene can only occur in parts which are already dead and which are exposed to these bacteria. It is therefore found in skin surfaces, and in the mouth, bowel, lung, cervix, etc. It does not occur in the heart, liver or spleen. Gangrene may be moist (wet) or dry. In moist gangrene there is abundant fluid in the part due to venous obstruction, lack of evaporation, etc., a condition which favors the prolific growth of putrefying bacteria. It therefore occurs in internal organs (bowel, lung), or in an extremity when veins as well as arteries are occluded. Dry gangrene occurs where there is little fluid in the tissues owing to evaporation or good venous drainage. It is therefore confined to the extremities and is caused most characteristically by the gradual narrowing of the lumen of an artery by arteriosclerosis, so that the tissues have time to become dried out. Sudden obstruction of an artery by an embolus may lead to moist gangrene. A common belief is that bacterial infection plays no part in dry gangrene. This is a mistake. The classical color change of the part (see below) is due to the action of saprophytes on the blood, and these bacteria can be demonstrated if the part is incubated in a fluid medium.

Causes.—The two great factors are loss of blood supply and bacterial infection; often these two are combined. *Senile gangrene* occurs in old people with arteries narrowed by arteriosclerosis, but the thrombosis is often responsible for the final occlusion. The gangrene begins in the foot, commonly in the big toe, and is naturally of the dry variety. *Diabetic gangrene* is very similar in type, though occurring in younger persons. Here again the arteries are narrowed, but in addition the sugar in the tissues favors bacterial growth. *Thromboangiitis obliterans* is often complicated by dry gangrene, usually in the lower limb but occasionally in the upper limb. The spasmodic narrowing of the arterioles in *Raynaud's disease* and in chronic *ergot poisoning* may lead to dry gangrene of the extremities. Sudden occlusion of an artery by *embolism* or *thrombosis* may result in gangrene, but only if the collateral circulation is insufficient for the needs of the part. In a limb with healthy vessels there is no danger of gangrene, but embolism of the superior mesenteric artery is certain to be followed by moist gangrene. *Inflammation* may be com-

plicated by gangrene, especially when the vessels become thrombosed. Gangrene of an inflamed appendix is a good example. *Frostbite* may cause gangrene of such extremities as the fingers, toes, nose and ears. Necrosis is first produced by thrombosis in the vessels, and infection is superadded. *Escharotics* (strong acids and alkalis) kill the tissues by direct action. Acids produce dry gangrene as they coagulate the fluids in the tissues; alkalis produce moist gangrene as they cause liquefaction of the tissue. *Carbolic acid* applications to a finger may be followed by death and gangrene in the course of a few hours.

Dry Gangrene.—Dry gangrene is seen in typical form when the arteries to the foot are closed off in old age as the result of arteriosclerosis. The part is cold and pulseless, there is no collateral circulation, and with or without a slight injury gangrene begins in one of the toes, as these are farthest from the blood supply. The part contains so little blood that invading bacteria grow with difficulty in the dead tissue, and the spread of the gangrene is slow. The part becomes dry, shrivelled and dark like the foot of a mummy. Hemolysis of the red blood cells liberates the hemoglobin, which is acted on by the hydrogen disulphide produced by the bacteria with the formation of black sulphide of iron so that the tissues are stained black. The gangrene extends slowly upward until it reaches a point where the circulation is sufficient to keep the part alive. At this level a line of separation is formed between the living and dead tissue. The line consists of inflammatory granulation tissue, which erodes the dead tissue and finally brings about complete separation. The microscopic picture is one of complete necrosis, but in addition there is usually a blurring and smudging of outline, a disintegration and breaking-up of tissue beyond what is seen in simple necrosis.

Moist Gangrene.—Moist gangrene is the same process in a part containing fluid, but the effect on the patient is very different. Gangrene of internal organs (lung, bowel, etc.) is always of the moist variety. It rapidly develops when the venous as well as the arterial flow is blocked and the part becomes filled with blood. This is seen in the limbs (injury to a main artery and vein) as well as in the viscera (strangulated hernia). It may also develop in naturally moist external regions (vulva). The tissue becomes rotten and putrid, in sharp contrast to the necrosis of such a lesion as an infarct. Owing to the abundant moisture there is rapid growth of putrefactive bacteria which break down the dead tissue with the formation of foul-smelling nitrogenous end-products such as indol and skatol. The organisms cause liquefaction of the tissues and sometimes gas formation, so that blebs of fluid form under the skin, and bubbles of gas give an emphysematous crackling when the part is palpated. Sulphide of iron is formed from the decomposed hemoglobin as in dry gangrene, and the parts are stained dark blue, green, and black. The local spread of the condition is very rapid and there is no attempt to form a line of demarcation. The most serious feature is the great absorption of toxic products which cause profound toxemia and finally death. In dry gangrene little or no absorption takes place.

Gas Gangrene.—This variety of moist gangrene merits separate consideration. It used to be one of the most important complications of war wounds, and is occasionally seen after wounds in civil life and following surgical operations. The tissue is killed by trauma or the action of pathogenic bacteria. The dead tissue is then decomposed by saprophytic anaërobic bacilli with the formation of foul-smelling gas and fluid. The chief of these anaërobes are: (1) Bacillus welchii (Bacillus aërogenes capsulatus), (2) Vibrion septique (probably identical with the bacillus of malignant edema), and (3) Bacillus oedematiens. The gangrene, which is of the moist variety, affects principally the muscles. Gas can be pressed up and down the fibers, and softening and liquefaction soon follow. Microscopically the sarcolemma is seen to be separated from the fiber by a space filled with toxic fluid, so that the fiber loses its blood supply and quickly dies. As this fluid passes up and down the entire length of the fibers, the spread of the condition is very rapid.

Bed Sores.—These troublesome lesions are a form of gangrene of particular importance to the future doctor, because he must prevent them rather than treat them, and for prevention a knowledge of causation is essential. The principal cause is pressure, the localized patches of gangrene developing over the sacrum, buttocks and heels. The best way to prevent pressure is to provide the patient with a good nurse. But pressure alone is not enough, for a healthy person may lie in bed for a year without developing a bed sore. The additional factors are a devitalized condition as the result of old age, long illness, malnutrition with protein deficiency, and, above all, stasis of the blood stream in the lower extremities with superadded thrombosis. When the dead tissue is cast off, a sore is left which may be of any depth and not infrequently exposes the underlying bone. Bacterial infection is invariable, and the resulting septic absorption is a serious feature of the condition.

POSTMORTEM CHANGES

The changes which the body undergoes after death are of great importance to the pathologist who performs the autopsy and subsequently examines sections of the tissues. They are not so important to the student who is concerned with the processes of disease. For this reason small print has been used for this account. Without a knowledge of postmortem changes it is possible to make grave errors in performing an autopsy by mistaking the results of these changes for the lesions of disease produced during life. They are also of great importance in medico-legal work in determining how long a body has been dead. The changes unfortunately depend on a number of variable factors, of which the most important are the temperature of the air, the temperature of the body at the time of death, and the presence of widespread bacterial infection. In spite of what one reads in detective stories it is seldom possible to fix the hour of death with any exactness. The two principal changes are rigor mortis and postmortem decomposition.

Rigor Mortis.—This is a unique example of function (contractility) being not only maintained but actually exaggerated for a period after death. Contraction of muscle so firm as to immobilize the joints generally appears in two to four hours after death, attaining its full intensity within forty-eight hours, and disappearing within another forty-eight hours. The time of development is shortened in a warm atmosphere and when death occurs at a time of marked muscular activity as during combat. Reduc-duction in adenosine triphosphate (A T P) is the chemical event which precipitates rigor mortis, a phenomenon which is also observed in the heart, gastrointestinal tract, bladder and arteries. The adsorption of a considerable quantity of A T P to the muscle proteins is necessary for the relaxation of the fibers. There is a rapid turnover of A T P in muscle immediately after death, but at first the breakdown is balanced by resynthesis in the glycogen cycle. There is a long delay in the onset of rigor in well-fed animals with a high glycogen content in the muscle. As the glycogen stores become ex-hausted, which occurs sooner in starved animals, resynthesis of the A T P cannot keep pace with the degradation, and rigor is the result. Finally there is complete exhaustion of the energy necessary to sus-tain chemical activity in the muscle fibers, and the rigor passes off. When A T P is added with the correct proportion of potas-sium and magnesium ions in the experimental animal, contractility is restored.

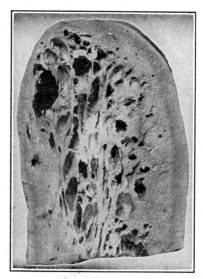

FIG. 15.—Foamy liver. Gross specimen showing the vacuolated appearance.

Postmortem Decomposition.—Decomposition of the body causes two main changes: (1) discolora-tion, and (2) softening. *Discoloration* is due to blood pigments and their derivatives. The red blood cells are hemolyzed after death, and the hemoglobin stains the vessel walls and the sur-rounding tissues. This is most marked in septicemia due to hemolytic bacteria, but in these cases some of the pink staining of the lining of the large vessels may have been antemortem. With the onset of putrefaction sulphuretted hydrogen is formed in the intestinal canal and combines with the iron of the breaking-down hemoglobin to form black sulphide of iron which stains the tissues green and black. The color is first seen in the skin of the abdominal wall and on the surface of the abdominal organs.

Postmortem softening is due to the action of ferments, partly autolytic ferments in the tissues, partly the proteolytic ferments of the saprophytic bacteria causing putrefaction. The process is similar to that which occurs in moist gangrene. As the result of this ferment action the tissues are first softened and finally liquefied. This *postmortem digestion* may thin the stomach wall and cause actual perforation, so that the stomach contents are found in the abdominal cavity. The hole in the stomach wall must not be mistaken for an antemortem lesion, traumatic or otherwise. The distinction is made by microscopic examina-tion of the edge of the opening; in the postmortem lesion there is no inflammatory reaction. Soften-ing of the pancreas may also occur, and the pancreatic juice may escape and produce areas of fat necrosis, but these also show no leukocytic reaction. The change proceeds very rapidly in hot weather, and when death has been due to some septicemic condition, invasion of the body by putrefactive bacteria may occur even before death. When bacteria are found in the tissues at autopsy it must be realized that this may be merely a terminal invasion with no causal rela-tion to the disease from which the patient died. Gas may be formed by the anaërobic saprophytes as in gas gangrene, and the liver may be full of bubbles like a sponge, a condition known as *foamy liver* (Fig. 15). When a body is kept in cold storage autolysis and bacterial growth are greatly delayed, and when it is injected with chemical poisons as in the process of embalming, both ferments and bacteria are destroyed, and the tissues are preserved for long periods. In the kidney of an embalmed body which had been buried for nine months I found that the red blood cells stained perfectly and showed no evidence of hemolysis. The fixation of tissues for microscopic examination depends on the same principle of destroying autolytic ferments and bacteria as quickly as possible.

The *technique of the autopsy* is a subject to which special monographs are devoted. The object of the autopsy is not only to deter-mine the cause of death, but to throw light if possible on the clinical manifestations of the disease from which the patient suffered and to trace the development of the lesions and morbid processes involved. From the point of view of the advancement of medical science the latter investigation may be of much greater importance than the former.

The student in his undergraduate course must attend a certain number of autopsies and observe how they are performed, in particular how the various organs are removed, opened and examined. To give detailed instructions as to how this should be done would be out of place in this book. Moreover each department of pathology has

its own concept of how the autopsy should be performed, and often issues written instructions on the subject to the class.

WEIGHTS AND MEASUREMENTS

In the course of his work, however, the student will continually encounter statements regarding the size and weight of diseased organs. He cannot form an opinion as to the meaning and significance of these figures unless he is familiar with the normal. I have therefore appended a list of normal figures modified from *The Autopsy*, published

WEIGHTS AND MEASUREMENTS OF NORMAL ADULT ORGANS

Organ	Weight	Measurements
Adrenal Gland	5.7 gm.	0.5 × 3 × 4.5 cm.
Brain	1250–1400 gm.	16.5 × 12.5 cm.
Duodenum (length)		30 cm.
Esophagus (length)		25 cm.
Heart	275– 325 gm.	L.V. 8–10 mm.; R.V. 2–3 mm.
Intestine (length)		
Large		150–170 cm.
Small		550–660 cm.
Kidney	140– 160 gm.	3.5 × 5.5 × 11.5 cm.
Liver	1500–1700 gm.	27 × 20 × 8 cm.
Lungs		
Right	375– 550 gm.	
Left	325– 450 gm.	
Nulliparous uterus	40– 60 gm.	
Ovary	8– 12 gm.	
Pancreas	90– 120 gm.	3.8 × 4.5 × 23 cm.
Parathyroid glands (4)	115– 130 mg.	
Parotid Gland	30 gm.	
Parous Uterus	75– 125 gm.	
Pineal Gland	140– 170 mg.	
Pituitary Gland	610 mg.	
Prostate	14– 16 gm.	2.7 × 3.6 × 1.9 cm.
Spinal Cord	27– 28 gm.	Length 45 cm.
Spleen	125– 175 gm.	3.5 × 8.5 × 13 cm.
Stomach (length)		25–30 cm.
Submaxillary Gland	17 gm.	
Testis and Epididymis	17– 27 gm.	2.5 × 3 × 4.5 cm.
Thymus	19– 23 gm.	
Thyroid Gland	40 gm.	

WEIGHTS OF NORMAL ORGANS OF THE NEWBORN AT TERM

Organ	Weight
Adrenals	9.3 gm.
Brain	429.6 gm.
Heart	21.7 gm.
Kidneys	26.6 gm.
Liver	151.5 gm.
Lungs	59.4 gm.
Pancreas	3.6 gm.
Spleen	11.1 gm.
Thymus	10.8 gm.
Thyroid	2.4 gm.

by the Armed Forces Institute of Pathology, Washington, D. C., together with a list of weights of normal organs in the newborn taken from Edith Potter's *Pathology of the Fetus and Newborn*.

REFERENCES

BEST, C. H. and HUNTSMAN, M. E.: J. Physiol., 1935, *83*, 255. (Lipotropic factors).

BRUNI, C.: Lab. Invest., 1960, *9*, 209. (Hyaline degeneration seen with the electron microscope).

CAMERON, G. R.: *New Pathways in Cellular Pathology*, London, 1952.

————.: *Pathology of the Cell*, London, 1952.

HAM, A. W.: *Histology*, Philadelphia, 4th ed., 1961.

HIRSCH, E. F.: Arch. Path., 1941, *31*, 516. (Tissue reaction to lipids).

McHENRY, E. W. and PATTERSON, J. M.: Physiol. Rev., 1944, *24*, 128. (Lipotropic factors).

POTTER, E. S.: *Pathology of the Fetus and the Newborn*, Chicago, 1952.

RITCHIE, S. and WAUGH, D.: Am. J. Path., 1957, *33*, 1035. (Glycogen infiltration of renal tubules).

The Autopsy, Armed Forces Institute of Pathology, Washington, D. C., 1951.

VAN CREVELD, S.: Arch. Dis. Child., 1952, *27*, 113. Medicine, 1939, *18*, 1. (Glycogen storage disease).

Chapter 2

Inflammation

Introduction
DEFINITION
CAUSES
The Vascular Phenomena
DILATATION OF VESSELS
EMIGRATION OF LEUKOCYTES
ESCAPE OF BLOOD PLASMA
MECHANISM OF THE VASCULAR
    CHANGES
    Chemotaxis
The Cells of the Inflammatory
Exudate
THE NEUTROPHIL LEUKOCYTE
THE EOSINOPHIL LEUKOCYTE
THE MAST CELL
THE LYMPHOCYTE
THE PLASMA CELL

THE MACROPHAGE
    Giant Cells
PHAGOCYTOSIS
INTERRELATIONSHIPS OF THE
    INFLAMMATORY CELLS
The Lymph of the Exudate
FIBRIN
The Localization of Infection
General Discussion of the
Inflammatory Process
The Tissue Changes in
Inflammation
DEGENERATIONS
INFLAMMATION OF SEROUS
    MEMBRANES
SUPPURATION
    Abscess

    Ulcer
    Cellulitis
Varieties of Acute Inflammation
    Serous
    Purulent
    Membranous
    Fibrinous
    Catarrhal
ALLERGIC INFLAMMATION
INFLUENCE OF CORTISONE ON
    THE CELLS OF INFLAMMATION
Chronic Inflammation
The Granulomata
INFECTIVE GRANULOMAS
FOREIGN BODY GRANULOMAS

INTRODUCTION

INFLAMMATION is the most common, the most carefully studied, and the most important of the changes which the body undergoes as the result of disease. Its history is the history of pathology, and the last chapter has by no means been written. Not until Rudolf Virchow in 1858 laid the solid foundation of modern pathology by his doctrine of Cellular Pathology was it possible to lift even the hem of the curtain which shrouded the mystery. "For the development of the sound pathologist," as Adami remarked, "a full knowledge of the factors concerned in the inflammatory process and a right appreciation of the doctrine of inflammation is as essential as to the orthodox theologian is a right attitude in respect to the doctrine of the Trinity." That was written at the beginning of this century, and our "appreciation of the doctrine" has changed appreciably since then.

The word inflammation takes us back a long way in the history of medicine. Literally it means a burning. The condition was studied clinically hundreds of years before any true insight was obtained as to the inner pathological meaning of the process. It was Celsus in the first century A.D. who named the famous "cardinal signs" of

inflammation as calor, rubor, tumor and dolor in words which have subsequently become celebrated: "Now the characteristics of inflammation are four—redness and swelling, with heat and pain." In the course of time it became evident that these cardinal signs were the outward expression of vascular changes. In the middle of the nineteenth century Cohnheim applied the experimental method to the study of inflammation and showed with a brilliance and conclusiveness which left no room for doubt the all-important part played by the vessels in the process.

But the vascular changes are not the essence of inflammation. It remained for Metchnikoff in 1882 to demonstrate in his great work on the Comparative Pathology of Inflammation that the central theme of inflammation was the reaction of the wandering mesodermal cells against the irritant. In the higher animals which possess a vascular system these cells are for the most part contained within the blood vessels. They are the leukocytes of the blood. The object and meaning of the vascular phenomena is to bring these mesodermal defense cells from the interior of the vessels to the outside where they can meet and cope with the irritant. The vascular changes are very striking; for the clinician they provide the cardinal signs of inflammation, but they are not essential. In a non-vascular tissue such as the cornea the wandering cells of the part gather around the irritant and cope with it just as surely as if they had come from inside the vessels.

It is worth while noting that, like Pasteur, Metchnikoff was not a physician. He was a Russian zoologist with no medical training. At the time of his great discovery he was in no way interested in problems of immunity, being engaged on a biological research into the intracellular digestion of mesodermal cells in lowly organized animals. One evening Metchnikoff introduced some rose thorns into the transparent body of a star-fish larva, and next morning, after a restless night, he had the joy of observing that the thorns were surrounded by the cells whose function he had been trying to determine. In that hour Metchnikoff was transformed from a zoologist into a pathologist.

Definition.—Inflammation may be defined as the reaction of living tissue to injury. As some degree of tissue injury occurs in almost every pathological condition, it is but natural that inflammation should be one of the commonest changes observed, although not necessarily in acute or severe form. In essence it is a defense reaction. The suggestion of flaming in the name is a heritage from the days when the only students of inflammation were clinicians. The injurious agent is referred to as an irritant. The student will realize that the reaction is a beneficial one, for without inflammation life would be impossible. It is evidently an evolutionary adaptive response having survival value for the species. Only those animals survived who were capable of this response.

The local inflammatory reaction presents two phases. The object, or perhaps we should say the effect, of the first is to destroy and remove the irritant; the object of the second is to repair the damage done to the tissues. The first is subserved by the wandering mesodermal cells whether of the blood or the tissues, the second by the fixed cells of the part. Repair is often considered together with inflammation, but for the sake of convenience we shall discuss it in a separate chapter.

Causes.—From our definition it is evident that any irritant may act as a cause of inflammation, so that a full list of causes would include every known irritant. These irritants may be divided into two great groups, the living and the non-living. Of the *living* irritants by far the most important are the *pathogenic* or disease-producing *microörganisms*. Of less importance are the *animal parasites*. Both of these act as irritants mainly by virtue of chemical poisons which they produce, and to a lesser degree by the mechanical irritation which they excite. The pathogenic bacteria usually excite an acute reaction, as a result of which both the cells and the fluid part of the blood pass from the vessels into the tissues. Some produce a more chronic form of reaction, characterized in the main by proliferation of the tissue cells; examples of such chronic irritants are the microörganisms of tuberculosis and syphilis. These chronic inflammations constitute the important group of the *granulomata*. The *non-living* irritants may be divided into physical and chemical. Among the *physical* irritants may be mentioned trauma, the presence of a foreign body, the action of undue heat and cold (burns and frostbite), of pressure, of light, of electricity, of roentgen rays, of the radiations from radium, etc. *Chemical* irritants include strong acids and alkalis, and poisons of every description.

In the discussion which follows it should be borne in mind that there is no hard and fast line between an irritant and a stimulant. If an irritant is sufficiently weakened it becomes a stimulant. It follows, therefore, that while at the center of the inflammatory stage we shall find every evidence of intense irritation, away at the wings the tissues may respond as to a stimulant.

In man and other vertebrates the mesodermal cells of defense may be divided into the wandering cells of the blood (the leukocytes) and the resting wandering cells of the tissue. It is the former which play the major part in the earliest stages of acute inflammation. They represent the police force which appears promptly on the scene when trouble develops. Moreover there is a *humoral factor* of defense as well as a *cellular factor*, and the constituents of the humoral factor are contained in the blood plasma. It thus becomes necessary for both the white blood cells and the blood plasma to escape from the interior of the vessels in order that they may reach the irritant. This escape is brought about by the vascular phenomena of inflammation. At the present day attention is being directed not so much to the changes seen down the microscope, important as they are, as to the more subtle chemical and physical mechanisms involved in these changes. We now translate the clinical and microscopic phenomena into chemical and physical terms. These matters are discussed on page 53.

Before proceeding to the details of the process, we may pause to take a look at the battle ground in which the conflict of opposing forces takes place. This battle ground is the ground substance of the connective tissue which separates the cells and fibers. It consists mainly of hyaluronic acid, a highly polymerized acid mucopolysaccharide. The degree of polymerization imparts to it a marked viscidity which constitutes a barrier to the spread of infection. The microorganisms of markedly invasive infections such as erysipelas or gas gangrene produce an enzyme, hyaluronidase, which depolymerizes and breaks down the barrier. The state of the barrier seems to be under the influence of the pituitary-adrenal system. Cortisone certainly decreases the resistance thus increasing the permeability of the barrier.

The pathology of inflammation may conveniently be described under three headings: (1) vascular phenomena, (2) inflammatory exudate, and (3) tissue changes.

THE VASCULAR PHENOMENA

We owe our present complete knowledge of the vascular changes in inflammation to the experimental researches of Cohnheim, whose Lectures on General Pathology, published in 1877 and now available in English translation, should be consulted by anyone interested in inflammation. It is remarkable how little has been added by subsequent workers to Cohnheim's original observations, although there is plenty of difference of opinion as to the mechanism by which the changes are produced.

Cohnheim's method was to draw out the intestine of a curarized frog through an opening in the abdominal wall and spread the mesentery on the stage of the microscope. Or he shaved off the papillary surface of the frog's tongue and observed the vessels in the base of the wound. Or the web of the foot may be used to which a mild irritant such as dilute acetic acid is applied. Whichever of these methods are employed, soon, as Cohnheim remarks, "a succession of appearances will be developed which are well calculated to fully engross your attention."

Dilatation of Vessels.—There may be a brief contraction of the vessels due to the stimulating effect on the vessel wall produced by the irritant when still weak in its action, but the first thing to attract attention is a dilatation of the exposed vessels, most marked in the arteries, then in the veins, and last of all in the capillaries. This paralytic dilatation is accompanied by a temporary acceleration of the blood stream, followed later by slowing. At this stage the vascular dilatation is very marked and innumerable capillaries come into view, because though previously empty they are now filled with blood, so that the active capillary bed is greatly increased and the vascularity of the part may actually be doubled. The increased vascularity is responsible for such cardinal signs as redness and heat. The slowing of the blood stream in the still dilated vessels becomes more and more marked, and if the action of the irritant is sufficiently intense there may be complete stasis or stoppage of the local circulation. This condition is known as *sludging* of the red blood corpuscles (Knisely). The red cells become sticky and adhere to one another in masses (sludging), at the same time sticking to the walls. The effect of sludging may be disastrous, for the capillary circulation is the key to tissue respiration, and the tissues cannot survive when their blood supply is cut off, and death of the part (necrosis or gangrene) is certain. In the slower blood stream it now becomes possible to distinguish the individual corpuscles. It is then seen that a rearrangement of the formed elements of the blood has taken place. Under normal conditions

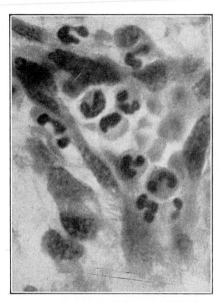

Fig. 16.—Swollen endothelial cells with leukocytes passing between them. × 1300.

the red and white cells flow intermingled in the central part of the vessel, forming an *axial stream* which is separated from the wall of the vessel by a clear *plasmatic zone* free from cells. In the veins of the inflamed part the leukocytes fall out of the axial stream and come to occupy the plasmatic zone. They tend to adhere to the vessel wall, and seem to drag themselves along with difficulty. In this way the inner wall of the vein becomes paved by an unbroken line of leukocytes without the admixture of a single red blood cell. This arrangement is spoken of as the *pavementing* of the leukocytes.

The vascular endothelium does not remain passive during this period of excessive activity. The lining cells become enlarged and proliferate, they assume a rounded form so as to project into the lumen of the vessel, and they exhibit amoeboid movement. In sections of inflamed tissue this swelling of the endothelium is a striking feature (Fig. 16), and if the observer is fortunate he may detect evidence of cell division (mitosis).

Emigration of Leukocytes.—The next step is the *emigration* or *diapedesis* of the leukocytes. The ground substance or cement of the swollen endothelial cells becomes loosened, the sharpness of outline of the individual elements of the vessel wall is lost, and its outer limit is nebulous. Through this protoplasmic sponge flows the cytoplasm of the polymorphonuclear leukocytes just as smoke floats through a keyhole (Fig. 17). Numbers of red blood cells may follow in the wake of the leukocytes, but these numbers vary widely, depending on the nature of the irritant. When particularly numerous the inflammation is said to be hemorrhagic. It will be seen that the essence of inflammation, the central point of the whole process, is the increased permeability of the walls of the small veins and capillaries.

It is worth recalling that the oxygen-carrying red blood cells and the defensive white blood cells have not always been fellow travellers. At the bottom of the animal scale we find phagocytic cells loose in the tissues. As we ascend the evolutionary ladder we encounter a vascular system in the earthworm which contains respiratory hemoglobin but no cells, whilst in the arthropods there are colorless macrocytes but no elements with a respiratory function. Finally in man and the higher animals the two bloods are combined in a single organ (Dible).

Escape of Blood Plasma.—The outward movement is not confined to the solid particles of the blood. The blood plasma also passes out into the tissues, the amount varying much with the nature of the irritant. In the tissues it may be responsible for much of the swelling, causing an *inflammatory edema*. The subject of the plasma in the tissues will be taken up when the inflammatory exudate is considered.

In inflammation there is not only an opening up of preëxisting capillaries, but also a formation of new vascular channels. This is accompanied by new formation of lymphatic capillaries (Pullinger and Florey). An astonishingly rich plexus of lymphatics is formed by the end of ten days. These vessels are only visible when injected owing to the colorless nature of their contents. They disappear as healing occurs.

It is evident that the more rapidly and completely a condition of hyperemia can be induced, the more satisfactory will be the inflammatory response, the less damage will be done, and the more complete will be the

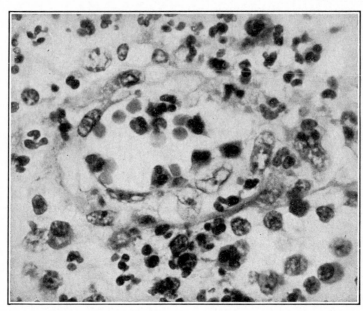

FIG. 17.—Separation of elements of vessel wall; emigration of leukocytes. × 800.

return to normal. This provides an explanation of the value of hot moist applications to an inflamed part. The fomentations act through the local vasodilator nerves, increasing the hyperemia, hastening the formation of an exudate, and limiting the spread of the infection. It is possible that there may be a liberation of acetylcholine at the nerve endings, and that this may produce a local action on the vessels.

Mechanism of the Vascular Changes.—The result of the vascular changes which have just been described is to bring both the solid and the fluid constituents of the blood from the interior to the exterior of the vessels, where they encounter the irritant responsible for the reaction. The varied changes of inflammation both in the vessel walls and in the blood and tissue cells are due to chemical stimuli produced at the site of irritation. The commonest of all irritants are bacteria, and these produce chemical substances which indirectly act upon the vessels. Even in aseptic inflammation caused by mechanical or thermal injuries there is destruction of tissue with the liberation of disintegration products which exert a similar action.

The vascular changes, both dilatation and exudation, are influenced by *nervous impulses*. If in one ear of a rabbit the vasoconstrictor nerve be cut and in the other ear the vasodilator nerve, and inflammation of both ears be then produced by means of hot water, a marked difference in reaction on the two sides can be observed. In the ear where the constrictor fibers are cut, hyperemia is marked and complete recovery ensues. In the ear where the dilator fibers are cut, the vessels remain constricted, stasis soon develops, and there will be a considerable amount of necrosis of tissue. When the nerve to a part is divided the normal constrictor impulses are cut off, and inflammation develops much more rapidly than usual. In such a part the capillaries permit a greater emigration of leukocytes and a greater transudation of lymph through their walls.

Sir Thomas Lewis showed that the vascular dilatation which follows firm stroking of the skin is due to the liberation of a histamine-like or "H"-substance. He suggested that in the tissue destruction of inflammation a similar substance is liberated and sets in motion the vascular mechanism. "The agent that alarms the garrison and mobilizes the first or vascular defenses is a chemical agent derived from the tissues. The perfection of this mechanism is such that the defense is organized immediately and at every threatened point; it is arranged and carried through locally, being independent of higher systems of control (nervous) and of distribution (cardiovascular)."

Chemotaxis.—The two striking phenomena for which an explanation must be sought are the dilatation of blood vessels and the emigration of leukocytes. In the early days of research on the inflammatory process the magic word *chemotaxis* made its appearance. For very many years this term sufficed to silence discussion. The leukocytes emigrated from the blood into the connective tissues because they were drawn out by chemotaxis. This was as satisfying as saying that inflammation is caused by an irritant or that cancer is caused by a carcinogen. All three statements are merely a play on words.

Bowing to custom and using this convenient if nebulous term, we recognize that there is a *negative* as well as a *positive chemotaxis.* Such substances as quinine, alcohol, and lactic acid repel rather than attract the leukocytes. The result depends to some extent on the concentration of the material. If the solution is made sufficiently dilute, the negative action is changed into a positive one. When bacteria are extremely virulent they cease to exercise any positive chemotactic power, and merely paralyze the leukocytes. If the two ears of a rabbit are inoculated with an attenuated and a virulent culture respectively, in the former there will be a great accumulation of leukocytes with very little fluid, while in the latter there will be an abundant effusion of fluid but hardly any leukocytes.

The various leukocytes show different degrees of response to chemotaxis. The polymorphonuclear leukocytes are the most readily affected. The lymphocytes are much less active probably because of the small amount of mobile cytoplasm which they contain. Of particular interest is the behavior of the white cells in an inflammatory focus in a patient with lymphatic leukemia. In this disease there may be 99 per cent of lymphocytes in the blood to 1 per cent of polymorphonuclears, and yet if an inflammatory blister of the skin is produced, the exudate consists of polymorphonuclear forms

with hardly a single lymphocyte. The products of animal parasites attract the *eosinophil leukocytes* more than any other variety, so that these increase in number both in the blood and in the tissue affected.

Of late years a large amount of experimental work has provided a number of more concrete suggestions regarding chemotaxis. Menkin, one of the principal workers in this field, has isolated from inflammatory exudates a polypeptide which he names leukotaxine because it induces both increased capillary permeability and diapedesis of leukocytes. Similar material has been obtained by the digestion of fibrin, and here it has been possible to dissociate the two properties, that producing vascular dilatation and that producing leukotaxis. Finally it has been shown that substances derived from damaged cells attract leukocytes into the area, in addition to causing hyperemia and edema (Moon and Tershakovec). It would appear that the injured cells may issue their own call for help and thus mobilize the forces of defense before the action of leukotaxine derived from the inflammatory exudate comes into play. It must be added that other workers, employing a somewhat different technique, do not agree that dead tissue fragments or autolyzing tissue exert chemotactic power for mammalian granulocytes (Harris).

Another line of work on altered capillary permeability in acute inflammation is that of Spector, who measured permeability in the rat by means of labelled serum albumin. The increased permeability coincides with the presence in the exudate of a soluble globulin factor which has a powerful effect on the vessel wall. This disappears later owing to suppression of its activity by a specific protein inhibitor. Two fractions exist in the globulins of the blood serum, one of which increases capillary permeability, whilst the other inhibits the process. The *permeability factor* exists in the serum as a precursor which has to be activated before it can achieve its effect, just as is the case with prothrombin. It is activated by blood clot, platelet extract, incubation with isolated mitochondria, and extract of minced tissue. It is suggested that after tissue injury the damaged cells release substances which lead first to the liberation of 5-hydroxy-tryptamine (serotonin) and histamine, and then to activation of the permeability globulin precursor. This seems to overwhelm the amount of globulin inhibitor available and to increase the state of permeability possibly initiated by histamine and 5-hydroxytryptamine. Later the activation is slowed down, and the relative concentration of the inhibitor becomes sufficient to restore capillary permeability to normal.

A third concept of the mechanism of inflammation focusses attention on the *mast cells* of the vessel wall (McGovern). In experimental inflammation in the rat's foot increased permeability of the vessels is associated with rapid and marked reduction in the granules of the mast cells or complete degranulation. The mast cells are thought to be a source of heparin, histamine, and a permeability factor, and that injury causes release of these substances. *Heparin*, which bears a negative charge, is believed to be held in solution normally in the endothelial cement, and thus repels the leukocytes which are also negatively charged. *Histamine*, released from the mast cells as the result of injury, increases the blood supply by vascular dilatation, the *permeability factor* alters the consistency of the cement film on the endothelial surface of the capillaries allowing fluid to pass through, whilst heparin is no longer held in the damaged cement, so that the negatively charged barrier is removed, and leukocytes collect on the capillary wall. When the mast cells of the perivascular tissues have exhausted their supply of heparin, these tissues again become positively charged, and attract the negatively charged leukocytes congregated on the damaged endothelium. Thus it would appear that changes in electrical potential may play a part in the mechanism of inflammation, a concept which has been called the *electrical potential theory*.

THE CELLS OF THE EXUDATE

The exudate which collects at the site of irritation is partly derived from the blood (hematogenous), partly from the tissues (histogenous). The various forms of leukocytes of the blood migrate through the vessel walls; the blood plasma also passes out and gives rise to the formation of fibrin; the wandering cells of the tissues accumulate at the site of irritation. These three components constitute the inflammatory exudate. Red blood cells may be present in varying degree, but have no functional part to play. Let us now examine these various elements in greater detail.

The Neutrophil Leukocyte.—These cells, commonly called the polymorphonuclears, although the eosinophil and basophil are also polymorphonuclear, are the active agents in acute inflammation, especially in its earlier stages. They are called forth in particular by the pyogenic group of bacteria, and form the chief constituent of pus. The ordinary *pus cell* is a polymorphonuclear leukocyte. The great increase in the number of leukocytes in the blood which occurs during inflammation is an increase of the neutrophils. In sections of inflamed tissue the vessels may be packed with these leukocytes. They are attracted not only by bacteria but also by their toxins, as can be shown by the experimental injection of a toxin freed from the microörganisms by which it is produced. The cells collect in great numbers around the dilated vessels (Fig. 18), and they pass through the tissue spaces by their amœboid movement. They are actively amœboid and actively phagocytic. Their power of movement is remarkable, but they cannot swim through fluid with any degree of effectiveness. They must have a framework on which to crawl. It is fibrin which provides the interlacing pathways that bridge across the fluid-distended spaces on which the leukocytes can move. The phagocytic power is shown towards bacteria rather than to dead and disintegrating cells. They form the first line of defense of the body against pyogenic bacteria. Having devoured the bacteria they digest them by means of an enzyme, which brings about solution of the bacterial bodies. Large numbers of the leukocytes are killed by the bacterial toxins, but even in their death they serve the body, for on disintegrating they liberate a proteolytic enzyme which dissolves the dead tissue, and thus hastens the process of ultimate recovery. This ferment has a similar action on fibrin, and also tends to prevent

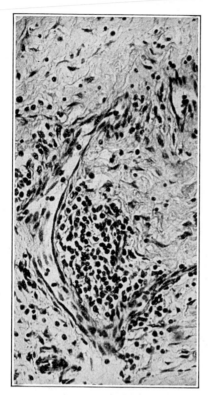

Fig. 18.—Leukocytes collected at point of bifurcation of a dilated vessel. × 200.

its formation. In a fresh exudate the cell outline is sharp and the nucleus distinct, but as degeneration proceeds the cytoplasm becomes granular, the outline indistinct, and the nucleus eventually disappears. Many of the cells which survive pass back into the lymphatics and blood vessels and reënter the general circulation.

The Eosinophil Leukocyte.—The eosinophils of the blood are few in number, constituting only from 2 to 4 per cent of the total white count. They appear early in the inflammatory exudate, and may disappear entirely from the blood. A marked increase in the number of eosinophils in the blood (eosinophilia) is characteristic of infection by many animal parasites. Large numbers of these cells are found in the tissue in which the parasite is lodged. In bronchial asthma the mucosa of the bronchi is often crowded with eosinophils. In both of these instances the eosinophilia may be a reaction against a foreign protein. A marked tissue eosino-

philia is sometimes seen in appendicitis in the subacute or chronic stage. Eosinophils are frequently present in the lesions in the lymph nodes in Hodgkin's disease. In these latter instances the cells may be derived from the tissues rather than from the blood. Eosinophilia, both in the tissue and the blood, is a constant accompaniment of the allergic reaction. These cells may serve as a factor in causing the allergic response. The antibodies rather than the antigen may be responsible for the eosinophilia, which in post-infection states rises with the rise of antibody titer. Eosinophils on breaking down release histamine, with resulting increase of capillary permeability and outpouring of more antibodies and neutralization of the antigen. Clinical manifestations of allergy may result. In support of the idea that there is a relationship between the eosinophils and histamine is the fact that the eosinophilia which follows injection of extracts of the worm Ascaris is completely prevented by the use of antihistamine drugs.

It is common knowledge that the administration of ACTH or cortisone produces a rapid and remarkable disappearance of the eosinophils of the blood, so much so that this reaction is used as an indication of the response of the body to these hormones.

The Mast Cell.—This is a cell with coarse basophilic granules in the cytoplasm, and an indented or even polymorphonuclear nucleus. Mast cells have no relation to the basophils of the blood which are derived from the bone marrow, whereas the tissue mast cells are born, live and die in the connective tissues. Although present in very great numbers in connective tissue they are easily overlooked, because of the great solubility of the specific granules in water, so that the tissue must be fixed in alcohol and stained with an aniline dye such as toluidine blue. It may interest the student to know that the cells were first discovered by Paul Ehrlich when as a medical student he was playing with basic aniline dyes. He called them mast cells from the German word, *mast*, meaning food, because they occurred in connective tissue where nutrition seemed to be enhanced as the result of lymph stasis, as in elephantiasis. Cells with basophil granules are encountered in the lowest forms of life, and they are particularly numerous in the soft flesh of the fish. In higher forms they are most abundant in perivascular tissue. It will be appreciated that in inflammatory lesions mast cells are of tissue and not of hematogenous origin.

The *function* of the mast cell in the normal individual is by no means clear, and what Ehrlich nearly one hundred years called "the riddle of the mast cell" has not yet been solved. It is known for certain that mast cells produce the acid mucopolysaccharide, *heparin*. Indeed the small mast-cell tumor in the skin of a dog can yield more heparin than the dog's entire liver, the organ from which heparin first received its name. The mast cells contain not only heparin but the bulk of the *histamine* in the body. The exaggerated "triple response" which can be provoked in the skin of a patient with *urticaria pigmentosa* is dependent on the very abundant mast cells which are present in the skin lesions of that disease. Finally, small quantities of a second amine, 5-hydroxytryptamine or *serotonin*, are present, although this occurs mainly in the enterochromaffin cells of the intestine. It cannot be said that all of this new chemical knowledge has provided us with a solution of the riddle. In some species the mast cell is concerned with the anaphylactic reaction, but not in others, such as the rat. Whether it plays a part in immunological processes in man is not known.

The great wheel of time has perhaps completed its full circle, and brought us back to the original idea of Ehrlich that the mast cell is concerned with the nutrition of connective tissue. Heparin is believed to represent the building blocks of hyaluronic acid, and the mast cell seems to play the part of a unicellular gland which elaborates the mucinous intercellular cement of the connective tissue.

Reference has already been made to the part which the liberation of histamine and heparin from mast cells bears to the mechanism of inflammation. It is in *acute* inflammation that the mast cells function most actively, and with this active function they rapidly lose their granules and become unrecognizable. Indeed it has been said that the primary response to injury is an immediate and sudden degranulation of the mast cells with resulting changes in the vascular endothelium.

In conclusion we may remark that in two rare pathological conditions the essential lesion is a great increase in the number of mast cells. These are *urticaria pigmentosa*, a skin disease of infants where copper-colored spots when traumatized become red and intensely itchy due to liberation of histamine from the great numbers of mast cells, and *mast-cell tumors* in the dog, which are extraordinarily rich in histamine, as well as heparin.

The Lymphocyte.—The lymphocyte is one of the problem cells of the body. It is present in enormous numbers in the tissues, being congregated particularly in such organs as the spleen and thymus, in lymph nodes, and in non-encapsulated nodules scattered all over the body. Next to the neutrophils the lymphocytes are the most numerous of the white cells of the blood. They are produced in vast quantities by the lymphoid tissues, it being estimated that they disappear at the approximate rate of 25 billion every day, the life of a lymphocyte being estimated at 24 hours. Yet the lymphocyte is unable to perpetuate itself, and it does not show mitotic division. This tremendous daily turnover must mean something. The administration of cortisone or ACTH controls the rate of dissolution of the lymphocytes, from one-third to one-half disappearing from the blood in the course of one hour. Various forms of stress also cause shrinkage of lymphoid tissue and loss of lymphocytes.

The lymphocyte is the predominant cell in chronic inflammation and in the late stages of acute inflammation. Together with its close relative, the plasma cell, it constitutes the so-called "small round cell infiltration" which dominates the picture. What part do these cells play in the process? Not so long ago Arnold Rich, in a notable discussion of the inflammatory process, pointed out that they do not phagocytose bacteria nor other particulate matter, and that, "congregated often in the more peripheral parts of the lesion, they have the appearance of phlegmatic spectators pas-

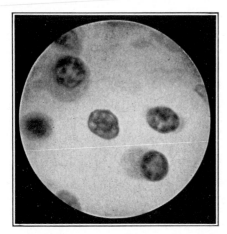

FIG. 19.—Two plasma cells showing polygonal shape and eccentricity of nucleus. The other two cells in the center are lymphocytes. × 1600.

sively watching the turbulent activities of the phagocytes."

The outstanding feature of the small lymphocyte is its very high nucleocytoplasmic ratio. The nucleus constitutes about 70 per cent of the cell, compared with about 10 per cent in the case of the liver cell. The lymphocyte, together with the plasma cell, is now believed to play the part of a trophocyte, that is to say a feeding or nutritive cell (Kelsall and Crabb), for it stores nucleoproteins manufactured either by itself or by the plasma cell, and acting as a humble carrier, it deposits a supply of trephones in packaged form in sites where its components are used by other cells. Lymphocytes are also believed to be carriers of antibody manufactured by reticuloendothelial cells and plasma cells. This would account for their great numbers in chronic inflammatory lesions. The lymph nodes, with their afferent and efferent lymphatics, represent nucleoprotein storage systems interposed between the tissue fluid and the blood vascular system. The relation of the lymphocyte to the plasma cell is discussed in the next section.

The Plasma Cell.—The plasma cell has a highly characteristic appearance. It is larger than the lymphocyte, with a more abundant cytoplasm and an eccentric nucleus so that the cell has a lop-sided appearance (Fig. 19). The chromatin is collected in small masses around the periphery of the nucleus like the figures on a clock-face, although this may possibly be an artefact due to fixation. The cytoplasm is intensely basophilic, and presents a clear space on the side of the nucleus which faces the center of the cell. This space corresponds to the Golgi apparatus. The abundant cytoplasm gives a characteristic bright red staining with pyroninmethyl green (pyroninophilia). Under the electron microscope the cytoplasm is seen to contain a well developed endoplasmic reticulum, known as rough-surfaced vesicles, which are coated with ribonucleic acid granules. The combination of intense basophilia by light microscopy and endoplasmic reticulum by electron microscopy is believed to indicate a cell with the ability to manufacture and secrete protein (Movat and Wilson).

The Origin of the Plasma Cell.—Unlike the lymphocyte it is non-mobile, and yet it may be present in great numbers in chronic inflammations, particularly those in which an immune mechanism is believed to operate. The general view has been that plasma cells develop from lymphocytes by synthesizing an increased amount of R N A and gamma globulin in their cytoplasm. There is now some evidence that plasma cells develop from primitive reticulum and mesenchymal cells.

The *function* of the plasma cell has also been a matter of debate. Modern advances in technology indicate that these cells are a very important source of globulin antibodies. The Coons technique, which will be discussed again in Chapter 5, is of particular value in this respect. It is known that the molecules of certain fluorescent dyes can be coupled with antibody molecules without impairing the ability of the latter to react specifically with the antigen. If frozen sections of the tissue of an immunized animal are exposed to the antigen which has been employed it becomes attached to cells containing antibody. When the sections are now flooded with the corresponding antibody labelled with a fluorescent dye, it in turn becomes attached to the antigen (*fluorescent antibody technique*). The fluorescence of the dye indicates with startling clarity the cells in which the immune reaction has occurred.

These cells prove to be plasma cells, indicating that it is they which are responsible for the production of antibody.

A consideration of the nucleic acids also points to the importance of the plasma cell in antibody formation. When an antigen is injected into a rabbit's foot the popliteal lymph nodes become enlarged, reaching a maximum size in from 5 to 6 days. By the end of this time the nodes contain 5 or 6 times as much antibody as the surrounding lymph plasma. Antibody formation seems to be related to the nucleic acids, which govern the synthesis of proteins, desoxyribonucleic acid (D N A) being associated with multiplication of chromosomes, whilst ribonucleic acid (R N A) is concerned with cytoplasmic protein. The pyronin-stained material in the cytoplasm of plasma cells is R N A, and the cells in the enlarged antibody-rich nodes are either adult plasma cells or less developed cells with pyronin-stained cytoplasm (Ehrich).

The plasma cell has been called *the key to the allergic process*. Hypersensitivity, both experimental and clinical, is associated with a marked increase in plasma cells. There is an invariable relationship between plasmacytosis and hyperglobulinemia, which is an important feature of many immunologic processes. Plasma cells in the tissues are increased in the lesions of long-continued infections with marked immunological response such as syphilis and rheumatoid arthritis, in hypersensitivity states, and in multiple myeloma, a bone marrow tumor, where they seem to be related to the presence of Bence-Jones protein in the urine.

The Macrophage.—Many names have been given to the large mononucleated cells which play so important a part in the later stages of acute inflammation and in some types of chronic inflammation. Some of these names reflect doubt as to their origin. It is probably twofold: from the blood and from the tissue.

There is reason to believe that many lymphocytes derived from the blood become converted into macrophages at the site of inflammation by increase in the cytoplasm and enlargement of the nucleus. Ebert and Florey, using Clark's transparent observation chamber in the rabbit's ear and moving picture technique, observed monocytes marked by vital dye and traced their passage through capillary walls into the tissues, where they became converted into macrophages.

It is probable that the bulk of the macrophages are histogenous in origin, particularly from the reticuloendothelial system. They are derived not only from cells lining blood sinuses, such as the Kupffer cells of the liver, but from the tissue cells of that system known as *histiocytes*. In addition to the fixed cells there are nomadic mesodermal cells which have no fixed abode, but wander through the tissues by virtue of their amœboid powers. The distinction between the fixed and the wandering cells can be most readily realized by studying tissue cultures, and can be demonstrated in a dramatic manner by projecting a moving picture of the culture on the screen, when the actively amœboid and actively phagocytic nature of these cells becomes vividly apparent.

MacCallum has given an unsurpassed description of such a picture. "The connective tissue cells grow out majestically and smoothly from the margin of the field, crossing and interlacing until a firm new structure is formed. Among these cells one may see others of quite different aspect worming their way with no thought of building. Arrived at the margin where they escape from the entanglement of these more serious fibroblasts, they show their true characters. Some are polymorphonuclear leucocytes, and they hop about within a limited area in a sort of ecstatic frenzy, evidently throwing out and retracting pseudopods at a great rate. Then there are lymphocytes which move humbly, like slugs crawling only a little way with head to the ground. But also there are macrophages which reach out great arms, perhaps in two or more directions, and at the end of these arms there is a flourish of clear protoplasm with outflung streamers that wave and search about for whatever can be seized, or else the whole advancing margin of the cell flows out and comes back like a wave, sucking in any particle that comes in its way." In the fixed and stained tissue of a microscopic preparation the cells lose all this vivid character, and appear as large pale rounded bodies with a vesicular nucleus and abundant cytoplasm. The marginal portion of the cytoplasm when viewed with dark-field illumination is seen to be an extremely delicate membrane, which undulates incessantly like a delicate silk veil when blown by the wind. It is from this membrane that the pseudopods are formed, and it appears to play the part of the spider's web which envelops foreign particles in its voluminous folds.

It is these cells which form the scavenger cells of ordinary inflammation, the epithelioid cells of tuberculosis and syphilis, the compound granular corpuscles which surround an area of brain softening, the heart failure cells which take up blood pigment in the lung when the heart is failing, the large phagocytes which form a zone around a chronic abscess, and finally, when the utmost in phagocytic action is needed, they fuse together to form giant cells. Their amoeboid and phagocytic character is better seen in smears made from inflammatory exudates and immediately fixed than in sections of inflamed tissue, in which the pseudopodia are retracted and the outline becomes rounded. A rather different picture of the part played by the macrophage in inflammation is given by the experimental work of Tompkins and Grillo, who injected suspensions of particulate matter (India ink, dead tubercle bacilli, etc.) into the subcutaneous tissue of the mouse and made smears from excised pieces of tissue. It was found that macrophages collected and showed marked phagocytic activity for two or three hours before the neutrophils put in an appearance. Even then the neutrophils were outdistanced by the macrophages as phagocytes except for bacteria. The first thing needed for phagocytosis is cohesion between the cells and the suspensoid, and this is brought about by muscular movements. This raises the question as to whether some degree of mobility may not be more desirable than complete immobility in the early hours of inflammation. Tompkins and Grillo say that in experimental inflammation in the mouse produced by particulate matter, the macrophages carry the burden of phagocytosis before the arrival of the polymorphonuclears, they share that burden later, and

for twelve hours, until the arrival of the monocytes of the blood, they alone must phagocytose those invading substances which can not be taken up by the polymorphonuclears.

Giant Cells.—When the individual macrophages are unable to deal with particles to be removed, they fuse together and form multinucleated giant cells. Excellent examples of giant cell formation can be seen around a foreign body such as a fragment of bone, a piece of ligature, a crystal of cholesterol, or even a splinter of wood (Fig. 20). For this reason the cells are called foreign body giant cells. They may contain enormous numbers of nuclei, which cannot all be seen in one section, since the cell is spherical.

It must not be supposed from this brief summary that the subject of giant-cell formation is as simple as it sounds. Haythorn's excellent review of the whole subject contains 391 references. Three great classes of giant cells must be distinguished: (1) tumor giant cells, (2) foreign body giant cells, (3) a miscellaneous group (Figs. 22 and 23).

Tumor giant cells are best seen in osteogenic sarcoma of bone, in glioblastoma multiforme (a malignant tumor of the neuroglia), in rhabdomyosarcoma (a malignant tumor of muscle), and in primary carcinoma of the liver. They are large cells, and have one or several nuclei, but these are never very numerous. The nuclei are often hyperchromatic so that they stain very darkly, and may vary considerably in size and shape, so that the cell has a more atypical neoplastic appearance than the Langhans' type of cell. The genesis is also different, for tumor giant cells are formed by the nucleus of the cell dividing, while the body of the cell fails to divide. These giant cells are not derived from the macrophages but from the cells of the tumor, whether connective tissue or epithelial in nature.

The *foreign body giant cell* is larger than an ordinary cell and may be of enormous size; it contains numerous nuclei, sometimes as many as 50 or 100. The nuclei are regular in size and seldom large. In the ordinary type of giant cell engaged in removal of a foreign body, the nuclei are scattered through the cytoplasm. In the giant cells so char-

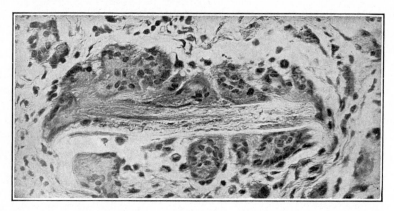

FIG. 20.—Sliver of wood surrounded by giant cells. × 300.

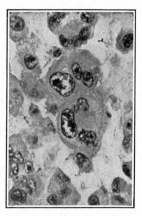

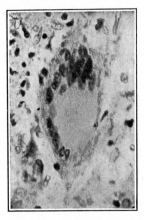

FIG. 21   FIG. 22

FIGS. 21 and 22.—Types of giant cells.

FIG. 21.—Tumor giant cell with several large nuclei. × 400.

FIG. 22.—Foreign body giant cell with a large number of smaller nuclei arranged around the periphery and at one pole. × 700.

acteristic of tuberculosis, also known as the *Langhans' type of giant cell*, the nuclei tend to be arranged around the periphery or are collected at one or both poles of the cell. Identical cells are seen in the granulomatous lesions of sarcoidosis.

Foreign body giant cells may be found in a great variety of conditions. Of these the commonest is tuberculosis, but it is a great mistake to jump to the conclusion that a lesion containing giant cells must be tuberculous. They are found in other chronic destructive inflammations such as syphilis, leprosy, actinomycosis, blastomycosis, and sarcoidosis. In leprosy the cells may be crowded with bacilli (lepra cells), and in tuberculosis they may contain a smaller number of tubercle bacilli. Any destructive lesion of bone may contain giant cells. They form the most striking feature of the giant-cell tumor of bone. Giant cells may be found at the site of old hemorrhages, but they are more often associated with attempted removal of cholesterol crystals. I have seen examples of this in atheroma of the aorta. The lesions of traumatic fat necrosis often show numerous giant cells, and are easily mistaken for the lesions of tuberculosis.

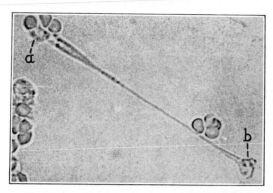

Fig. 23.—Photograph of living leukocyte showing stretching of cytoplasm: (*a*) portion of leukocyte containing 3 red cells attached to slide; (*b*) migrating portion. (Mudd and Mudd, Jour. Gen. Physiology.)

Asteroid inclusions or radial inclusions are observed in giant cells in tubercle-like formations in a variety of conditions. These are most characteristically seen in sarcoidosis, but are also found in subcutaneous tissues containing paraffin, in the wall of dermoid cysts, in old hemorrhages, etc. They have been observed in the liver, spleen and lymph nodes. Hirsch, from an exhaustive examination of human and experimental material, came to the conclusion that the star-like inclusions represent crystalline forms of fat separated from an oil system containing cholesterol. Chemical changes take place in the composition of the crystals in the tissues so that they become insoluble in fat solvents. Cunningham believes that they are organic protein structures present in many foreign body reactions. They are best stained with phosphotungstic acid hematoxylin.

In addition to the two great groups of tumor giant cells and foreign body giant cells, a *third miscellaneous group* may be recognized. In certain conditions of continued irritation the mesodermal cells become larger and may contain several nuclei. The large Aschoff cells of the rheumatic nodule offer one example. Another is the Reed-Sternberg cell of Hodgkin's disease.

Phagocytosis.—A unicellular organism such as an amoeba shows to a marked degree the power of taking foreign particles into its body. The cell of which the organism is composed swallows or devours the particle. Hence the process is known as phagocytosis (*phagein*, to eat). The mechanism is that of amoeboid motion, the same by which the leukocytes pass through the vessel walls.

The cytoplasm of the cell flows out in one or more processes or *pseudopodia*, which surround the particle and draw it within the body of the cell. Here it undergoes digestion, a vacuole being formed around it which contains a digestive enzyme. If the particle can be dissolved and digested it gradually disappears; if not, it is discharged from the cell.

Stuart Mudd and his associates have shown that phagocytosis involves the spreading of the leukocyte over the surface of the particle until the latter is completely enclosed; the capacity of spreading is the principal factor (Fig. 23). The deposition of serum protein on the surface of the particle greatly increases this power. When leukocytes are examined at the interface of an oil-water mixture, their remarkable deformability at once becomes evident. This appears to depend on the wetting properties of the leukocytes; they are hydrophilic. Red blood cells, on the other hand, are hydrophobic and exhibit no deformability.

In vertebrates the phagocytes are represented by the polymorphonuclear leukocytes of the blood and the large mononuclear phagocytes of the blood and of the tissues, those cells called by Metchnikoff the macrophages. The former engulf bacteria, both alive and dead. If a mixture of leukocytes and bacteria is incubated and a film is then spread and stained, numbers of the bacteria will be seen lying within the leukocytes (Fig. 24). The macrophages devour dead cells, blood pigment, inorganic particles, etc.

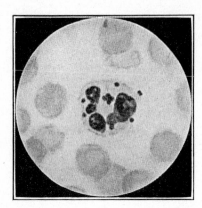

Fig. 24.—Polymorphonuclear leukocyte containing bacteria. × 1250.

They are true scavengers. They may also engulf protozoal parasites. In acute inflammation the polymorphonuclears play the chief part in the early stages, the macrophages taking their place in the later stages. The two sets of cells react differently to different bacteria. Thus the mononuclears will not take up streptococci or gonococci which the polymorphonuclears readily devour, but they will take up tubercle bacilli or leprosy bacilli.

We have already seen that when foreign particles which cannot be digested have to be removed, such for instance as pieces of bone or cholesterol crystals, the macrophages fuse together so as to form giant cells. Such a foreign body giant cell is a cytoplasmic syncytium containing a large number of nuclei. In this form it seems to have greater phagocytic power than when the cells act singly.

Metchnikoff naturally considered phagocytosis of transcendent importance. In his own words: "The *primum movens* of inflammation consists in a phagocytic reaction on the part of the animal organism. All the other phenomena are merely accessory to this process, and may be regarded as means to facilitate the access of phagocytes to the injured part." At the present time we would regard this as a distinct overstatement; nevertheless the theory became and remains today one of the most creative forces in the field of pathology. We may be astonished at the very strong opposition with which pathologists greeted his theory—perhaps

because it came from a zoologist. Pasteur suffered the same fate at the hands of the medical profession. Ziegler, one of the leading pathologists of his day, wrote as follows: "I look upon the phagocytosis which occurs in an inflammation as a purely accidental phenomenon which is often brought about for the simple reason that mobile cells happen to be present, together with a material capable of being ingested by them."

Barry Wood has shown beautifully and conclusively the importance of what he calls *surface phagocytosis*. In free fluid a phagocyte is unable to engulf encapsulated microorganisms such as pneumococci unless they are sensitized by serum; it merely pushes the organism ahead of it. When, however, it can crawl along some form of trellis and pin the coccus against a tissue surface, such as the wall of a pulmonary alveolus, or can force it against other leukocytes, or catch it against strands of fibrin, phagocytosis readily occurs (Figs. 25 and 26). In acute bacterial pneumonia phagocytosis operates even in the early stages when no immune bodies can be demonstrated either at the site of infection or in the serum. As might be expected, surface phagocytosis is relatively inefficient in potentially open serous cavities (pleura, peritoneum, etc.), and in the center of an abscess. An additional factor is the lack of oxygen at these sites, for in the absence of oxygen polymorphonuclears quickly become immobile and lose the power of phagocytosis.

The cellular side of inflammation is not the only side, as Metchnikoff in his enthusiasm was apt to imagine. There is a humoral immunity as well as a cellular immunity. If leukocytes are washed free from blood plasma and are then mixed with bacteria, no phagocytosis will occur. Evidently substances in the plasma known as *opsonins* (from the Greek word meaning to prepare food for) are necessary for the reaction between phagocyte and bacterium to occur. On the other hand antibodies by themselves do not possess bactericidal power; they merely sensitize the bacteria for phagocytosis or for attack by complement-like substances.

Interrelationships of the Inflammatory Cells.—Although we have discussed the vari-

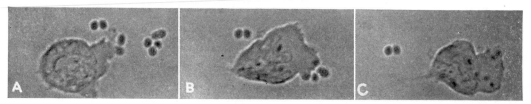

FIG. 25.—Phagocytosis of pneumococci in hanging drop containing type-specific opsonin. In photomicrograph *A*, seven pneumococci are readily seen, two of them apparently adhering to pseudopod of leukocyte. Two minutes later (*B*) the cell has ingested the first two organisms (in between lobes of nucleus) and has come into contact with the clump of four. The third picture in the series (*C*), taken at 4 minutes, shows the cell after it has phagocyted six of the seven pneumococci in the field. The only organism that has escaped phagocytosis is the one which the cell failed to touch ($\times$ 800). (Wood, Smith and Watson, courtesy of Journal of Experimental Medicine.)

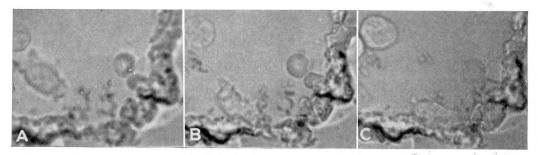

FIG. 26.—Series showing surface phagocytosis of unopsonized Friedländer's bacilli in section of normal rat lung. (*A*) Polymorphonuclear leukocyte is seen approaching bacilli near alveolar wall. (*B*) Having reached the alveolar wall, the leukocyte is about to trap the bacilli against the tissue surface. (*C*) Cell has trapped some of the bacilli against the wall and is in the process of phagocyting them. The photomicrographs in this series were taken at 12:30, 12:31, and 12:32 P.M., respectively ($\times$ 735). (Smith and Wood, courtesy of Journal of Experimental Medicine.)

ous cells of the inflammatory exudate separately, there is reason to believe that they influence one another. There is a regular sequence in the inflammatory cycle which is independent of the irritant responsible. An early accumulation of histogenous wandering cells is followed within an hour by an outpouring of neutrophils, which are succeeded in turn by macrophages. Observations on cases of neutropenia, both natural and induced, show the existence of a relationship between neutrophils and lymphocytes (Page and Good). In a patient with cyclic neutropenia every 21 days a small area of the skin was denuded of cornified epithelium, a drop of antigen applied, and a cover slip taped over the area but removed at frequent intervals. The absence of neutrophils inhibited the early stages of the acute inflammatory cycle, with delay or absence of the lymphocytes, and in consequence a deficit

of the hematogenous macrophages derived from lymphocytes (Figs. 27 and 28). The addition of viable neutrophils to the antigen was followed by the prompt appearance of lymphocytes. Similar results were obtained with experimentally induced neutropenia in the rabbit. It is suggested that the neutrophils may act on connective tissue elements to induce the production of substances which are chemotactic for lymphocytes. As the local edema of connective tissue which occurs in the normal inflammatory cycle fails to take place when neutrophils are absent from the circulation, it is possible that a similar mechanism may be responsible in part for increased capillary permeability.

One last point must be borne in mind regarding the cells of the exudate. Polymorphonuclear cells are unable to reproduce themselves, whereas the reproductive power of the macrophages is very great. It is true

4

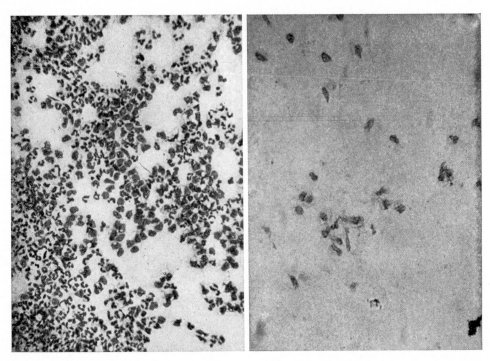

FIG. 27.—Sampling of the inflammatory exudate at 12 hours, obtained by Rebuck's cover slip technique, when the patient had normal numbers of circulating neutrophils, showing the abundant neutrophil and mononuclear cell exudation. Wright's and Giemsa stains. × 150. (Page and Good, courtesy of Am. J. Path.)

FIG. 28.—Sampling of the inflammatory exudate at 12 hours, obtained by Rebuck's cover slip technique, when neutrophils were absent from the patient's circulation, showing only a few mononuclear cells. Wright's and Giemsa stains. × 150. (Page and Good, courtesy of Am. J. Path.)

that the polymorphonuclears migrate at first in vast numbers compared with the macrophages, but in time the balance is readjusted. In tissue cultures of the buffy coat of the blood there is a great preponderance of polymorphonuclear cells during the first two days, but as these cannot multiply they soon disintegrate, and become replaced by the multiplying macrophages (Rich).

THE LYMPH OF THE EXUDATE

Under normal conditions a certain amount of blood plasma passes through the vessel walls into the tissue spaces where it constitutes the lymph. From these spaces it is absorbed into the lymphatics, and passes *via* the thoracic duct back into the blood stream. There is thus a continuous flow from the blood into the tissues, but the fluid is absorbed at an equal rate so that it does not accumulate in the tissue spaces.

The lymph which escapes from the vessels is not the same as the plasma which remains; it is thinner and contains much less protein, owing to the selective action of the vascular endothelium.

In inflammation the outward flow is enormously increased. By inserting a cannula into one of the chief lymphatics of the leg and then producing inflammation of the foot by immersing it in hot water, Cohnheim was able to show that the flow of lymph might be increased to eight times the normal. Field and his associates have amplified these observations. They found that the lymph flow in the inflamed part showed an extraordinary increase, and that the subcutaneous lymphatics were so greatly dilated that they could be injected with ease. It is evident

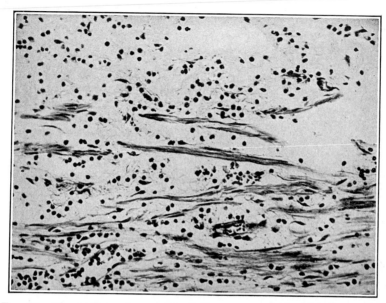

Fig. 29.—Muscle fibers of appendix widely separated by fluid exudate. × 200.

that the lymphatics do not collapse as the result of pressure of the fluid in the tissues, as is sometimes supposed. The normal lymph pressure in the leg of a dog is too low to be measured, but in sterile inflammation it rose to 120 cm. of lymph. The increased lymph flow lasted as long as twenty-four hours. The production of fluid is so great that it cannot be carried away by the lymphatics, and therefore accumulates in the tissue spaces. Here it gives rise to *inflammatory edema*, which is the chief cause of the swelling of the part in acute inflammation. The lymphatic channels tend to become blocked with the inflammatory products; this increases the accumulation in the tissues. Inflammation of the lymphatics (lymphangitis) will still further aggravate the condition.

The principal factors in the production of inflammatory edema are changes in the capillary wall and increased osmotic pressure in the tissues.

The dispute regarding the filtration and secretion theories of the production of lymph must be left to the physiologists. We may take refuge in that non-committal term, the *permeability of the capillaries*. This is greatly increased by the action of the products of irritation on the vascular endothelium, so that the plasma is no longer held back within the vessels. Not only is the amount of lymph which escapes greatly increased; its quality is also changed. Normal lymph usually contains less than 1 per cent of protein, whereas in inflammation the lymph may contain as much as 8 per cent.

Of much greater importance is the *increased osmotic pressure* of the tissue fluids at the site of inflammation, which is a far more powerful force than the pressure inside the vessels. Early in the inflammatory process as the result of tissue disintegration metabolic products are liberated, for the most part *acid in reaction*, and these so raise the osmotic pressure that fluid is drawn from the vessels to dilute them.

The *amount* of the fluid exudate varies greatly, depending on two main factors, the irritant and the site. (1) The bite of a mosquito and the sting of a nettle are examples of irritants which cause a marked outpouring of fluid. In a blister the exudate is almost entirely serous. Influenzal pneumonia is characterized by an extreme degree of inflammatory edema in the pulmonary alveoli. (2) The more open the tissue, the greater will be the exudate. It is most marked in serous sacs (pleurisy, peritonitis). In loose cellular tissues the fluid may be

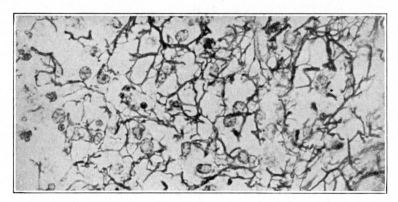

FIG. 30.—Exudate consisting mainly of fibrin.   × 600.

abundant. It may separate the muscle fibers of the appendix in acute appendicitis (Fig. 29). In such dense structures as bone the amount is negligible.

Fibrin.—Fibrin is intimately associated with the inflammatory lymph. The fibrinogen of the plasma passes out of the capillaries with the lymph, and this is acted on by the thrombin liberated by the disintegration of the polymorphonuclear leukocytes with the production of fibrin. This takes the form of a series of fine threads interlacing with one another (Fig. 30). The amount of fibrin varies with the irritant and the location, just as does the amount of lymph. Some bacteria such as the pneumococcus and the diphtheria bacillus excite an abundant formation of fibrin. Much fibrin is formed on serous surfaces such as the pleura and the peritoneum. Proteolytic ferments liberated by the leukocytes tend to prevent its formation, so that in an abscess crowded with pus cells no fibrin will be formed. The fibrin plays an important part in the process of healing, acting as a temporary scaffold on which the new tissue is built up. It may serve as a barrier against spread of the infection, so that in pneumonia the pneumococci do not readily pass from the lung into the pleural cavity. The formation of fibrinous thrombi in the efferent lymphatics may also play some part in localizing the infection. An offset to these advantages is the fact that adhesions take their origin in the fibrin. Such adhesions are of value at first, for they serve to localize the inflammation as in the case of an inflamed appendix. Later they may exact a penalty by undergoing contraction and thus gravely interfering with the function of the part affected. We have already seen that the network of fibrin provides an invaluable trellis over which the phagocytes can move, for they do not swim like goldfish in a free fluid.

THE LOCALIZATION OF INFECTION

The inflammatory reaction tends to prevent the dissemination of infection. Speaking generally, the more intense the reaction, the more likely is the infection to be localized. Staphylococci produce an acute inflammatory lesion in which the bacteria tend to remain confined to the lesion. Streptococci may have spread to a distance before a reaction manifests itself. In addition to the element of acuteness of reaction bacteria differ in their inherent tendency to become disseminated.

An important element in the spread of bacterial infection seems to be the ability of some of the most highly invasive organisms (hemolytic streptococci, *Cl. welchii*) to produce the spreading factor, *hyaluronidase*. This enzyme has the ability to depolymerize the long chains of the mucopolysaccharide, hyaluronic acid, which is an important constituent of the ground substance between the cells and fibers. It is a secret weapon in the hands of virulent bacteria. As the cement between the fibers melts away, the bacteria are free to move or be carried by edema fluid through the tissues.

Menkin has drawn attention in experimental inflammation to the part which mechanical obstruction may play in limiting the spread of infection. This obstruction is due partly to the formation of a network of fibrin, partly to occlusion of the lymphatic vessels. These factors tend to cause what may be called fixation of the infective agent in the early stages before phagocytes have time to accumulate. If iron salts are injected into the peritoneal cavity, they can soon be demonstrated in the regional lymph nodes; if an aseptic peritonitis is first produced, the iron does not reach the nodes, as the channels to the nodes are blocked. In the immunized animal, however, as Rich has shown experimentally, fixation is mainly due to the action of immune bodies, which cause the bacteria to be agglutinated and held in situ.

Related to the question of the success or failure of localization is that of *absorption of bacteria and toxins* from the tissues. It might be thought that bacteria introduced into a freshly made wound would readily enter the open ends of the divided vessels, but such is not the case. McMaster and Hudack examined such a wound under the microscope and observed that the blood vessels shut down within a few minutes, whilst the lymph vessels remained patent for over forty-eight hours. The experimental work of Barnes and Trueta has shown that bacteria and toxins of large molecular weight are absorbed from the tissues only by the lymphatics, and that such absorption will occur much less readily if the limb is immobilized. It is well known that no lymph will flow from an immobilized leg. Russell viper venom and tetanus toxin, with molecular weights over 20,000, are not absorbed from an immobilized limb, indicating absorption by lymphatics, whereas cobra venom (molecular weight under 5000) and strychnine are absorbed with equal rapidity from a normal limb and from one whose lymphatics are obstructed or from one that is immobilized, indicating absorption by blood vessels. In inflammatory or other forms of edema, the lymph flow, and therefore absorption, is greatly increased.

GENERAL DISCUSSION OF THE INFLAMMATORY PROCESS

From our account of the details of the process of inflammation it becomes evident that two main factors are involved, the one cellular, the other chemical. It is but natural that one or other of these has been emphasized, perhaps unduly, by different workers. When the inflammatory lesion is studied under the microscope it is the cellular factor which commands attention. Certain it is that without the phagocytes and other cells of the exudate the defense of the body would indeed be feeble in many instances. When we come to study diseases of the heart we shall see that in subacute bacterial endocarditis the causal streptococci are out of reach of phagocytes and are able to proliferate enormously on the surface of the valvular lesions, even though they are bathed with plasma rich in specific antibodies. Yet these same streptococci are unable to colonize and produce lesions in other tissues to which leukocytes have access, unless bacteria-laden vegetations are swept away and become lodged in a distant vessel, and even then the organisms become destroyed by phagocytic action (Rich).

With advances in knowledge and technique, however, the importance of chemical factors becomes more and more apparent. Although the value of the phagocyte is obvious and unquestioned, it is also true that many bacteria and protozoa and perhaps all viruses find the intracellular environment to their liking, as it protects them against noxious influences (including chemotherapeutic agents) and allows them to multiply. Under these conditions the phagocyte tends to spread rather than to limit the infection.

One of the many puzzling aspects of the problem is the fact that the antibacterial power of leukocytes is highly selective, some germs being readily destroyed, whilst others closely related flourish in the self-same cells. Thus coagulase-positive staphylococci multiply within polymorphonuclear leukocytes, whereas coagulase-negative strains die immediately. Obviously this is a chemical problem, but the explanation so far eludes us.

Apart from the function of phagocytosis it is known that the cells of the exudate may liberate soluble antibacterial substances either by secretion or as a result of necrosis and disintegration. This brings us to the subject of the metabolic characteristics of the environment of the inflammatory lesion, what has been termed the micro-environment by Dubos, whose masterly paper on the subject should be consulted. Phagocytosis is often accompanied by a marked increase in acidity, both intracellular and extracellular. The source of energy used in phagocytosis appears to be glycogen, which yields lactic acid through glycolytic fermentation. The increase of acidity within the phagocyte must contribute to destruction of the ingested bacteria. The extracellular environment also becomes markedly acidic owing to production of lactic acid, and the local reaction may fall as low as pH 5.3. Pathogenic bacteria and animal parasites are highly sensitive to acidity and this is true of many viruses. The glycolytic activity of inflammatory cells is impaired in uncontrolled diabetes, and this may partly account for the serious character of infections in this disease. The well-known enhancement of infection by over-doses of cortisone is due to the anti-inflammatory action of the hormone, and this may be due in turn to interference with cellular metabolism. It is evident that the response of the body to infection is under the control of factors which may be metabolic or originally even psychic in origin. In other words, the physiological state of the patient may determine the outcome of infection just as much as the intensity of the infectious agent.

It becomes apparent from the foregoing discussion that inflammation is not only the most important but one of the most fascinating of disease processes, indeed *the* most fascinating with the exception of neoplasia.

THE RELATION OF SYMPTOMS TO LESIONS

It now becomes a simple matter to picture the pathological basis of the cardinal signs of inflammation. The *heat* is due to the increased amount of blood flowing through the part. The *redness* is also caused by the local hyperemia. The *swelling* is to be attributed in part to the vascular dilatation, but much more to the accumulation of exudate in the tissues. The chief constituent of the exudate responsible for the swelling is the lymph, the accumulation of which leads to inflammatory edema. There may be marked enlargement of an inflamed appendix, even though the cellular exudate is slight.

Pain is one of the most common accompaniments of inflammation. Undoubtedly tension with pressure on nerve endings is a major factor. Inflammation in loose tissue may be painless, whereas inflammation in bone can be agonizing. Stretching of a serous membrane rich in nerves will also cause much pain. But other and more subtle factors may be involved. It is known that when 5-hydroxytryptamine (serotonin), a substance released in the inflammatory reaction, is applied to a raw surface, pain is experienced. A pain-producing substance resembling the polypeptide bradykinin has been found in human plasma, developing in plasma collected in glass or metal apparatus. It is present in inflammatory exudates, and seems to be formed within a few minutes when plasma escaping from capillaries comes in contact with damaged tissues.

Fever of varying degree is likely to be present if the inflammation is at all severe. We might think that the explanation of the fever was a simple matter, the culprit being bacterial exotoxins or endotoxins, but that is far from the case. In 1943 Menkin isolated from inflammatory exudates a pyrogenic globulin fraction which he named *pyrexin*. Like bacterial pyrogens it was heat-stable. It is now known that the principal source of endogenous pyrogens in the exudate is the polymorphonuclear leukocyte, which discharges its pyrogenic component into the surrounding medium while still motile and apparently otherwise functionally intact (Barry Wood). This leukocytic pyrogen passes by way of the thoracic duct to the circulating blood, and thus reaches and activates the thermo-regulatory centers of the brain.

Leukocytosis is another of the puzzling features of the inflammatory process. In addition to the accumulation of white cells in the inflamed tissue there is a striking increase in the total number of circulating leukocytes in the blood, which in severe infections may amount to 30,000 or 40,000 per cubic millimeter. This condition is known as leukocytosis. The mechanism by which this remarkable increase is produced is obscure. Menkin has extracted from the inflammatory exudate a polypeptide which he calls a leukocytosis promoting factor. When this substance is injected into the body it causes a marked increase in the circulating white cells. The factor, which is probably released from disintegrating cells of the exudate, particularly neutrophils, seems to stimulate the bone marrow to pour out great supplies of white cells, some of which are utilized at the site of inflammation. In a few infections, notably typhoid fever, the production of leukocytes is depressed, so that the number in the blood drops to a low level, a condition known as *leukopenia*. We have no explanation for this diminution in circulating leukocytes.

THE TISSUE CHANGES IN INFLAMMATION

The vascular phenomena and the formation of an exudate do not constitute the whole pathology of inflammation. There are also tissue changes. These may be of two types, (1) degenerative and (2) proliferative. If the irritant is intense, the effect is degeneration and destruction. If it is mild it acts as a stimulant, and the effect is proliferation. Growth will either be impaired or enhanced, the result depending on the intensity of the irritant. At the center of the inflammatory area the action of the irritant is severe, so that degeneration predominates; at the periphery the action is mild, so that the tissue may be stimulated to proliferate. This part of the inflammatory process is known as repair or healing.

Degenerations.—The bacterial toxins poison the tissues of the inflamed part, leading either to degeneration or death (*necrosis*). Both of these processes have been discussed in Chapter 1. The two most common degenerations are *albuminous degeneration* or *cloudy swelling* and *fatty degeneration*. If either of these is carried too far the affected tissue will die and become necrosed. Should

thrombosis of the vessels occur, necrosis will be hastened, as the tissues have lost their food supply. In addition to the bacterial toxins, the proteolytic ferments liberated by the broken-down leukocytes play an important part in the destructive processes, although they are unable to act on living cells. These ferments produce liquefaction of the dead tissues. The result is the formation of the fluid known as *pus*. It must not be supposed that every inflammation goes on to the formation of pus, and so becomes *purulent* in type. Some bacteria are pyogenic or pus-producing. Most of the pathogenic cocci are in this class and many bacilli. But some bacilli, such as the tubercle bacillus, lead to a proliferative reaction with little or no attempt at pus formation. Even the pyogenic cocci when few in number or of mild virulence may fail to produce a purulent inflammation. Large numbers of leukocytes are necessary for the formation of pus. If the exudate consists mainly of lymph or of fibrin, not sufficient leukocytes are present to produce the liquefaction which is necessary for pus formation. The serum contains an antibody which tends to inhibit the proteolytic enzyme of the leukocytes, so that in serous exudates there will be no autolysis. The leukocytes of some animals, such as the rabbit, contain but little enzyme; such animals usually fail to produce liquid pus. Living cells are not affected by digestive enzymes. Thus in lobar pneumonia the dead cells of the exudate undergo autolysis (resolution), but the living walls of the alveoli are left intact.

Inflammation of Serous Membranes.—Inflammation of the pericardium, pleura, peritoneum, etc., is usually serofibrinous in type, *i. e.*, the exudate in the cavity is serous, but fibrin produced by coagulation of the exudate is laid down on the smooth surface of the membrane, covering it with a sticky, shaggy exudate or in milder cases merely robbing it of its normal sheen and imparting to it a frosted or ground-glass appearance. Microscopically the exudate consists mainly of fibrin, with a varying number of polymorphonuclears and some serum. As a result of the relative absence of pus cells from which the proteolytic ferments of inflammation are derived, the fibrinous exu-

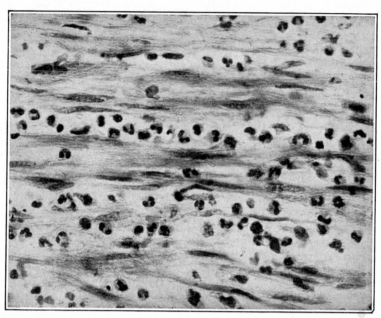

FIG. 31.—Muscle fibers of appendix separated by leukocytes but without suppuration. × 500.

date is not removed by autolysis. Instead, it undergoes the process known as *organization* which will be studied in connection with repair. New fibroblasts grow into the exudate and remove it in part or whole. If some of the exudate remains it is converted into dense fibrous tissue. If the two serous surfaces are stuck together by the exudate, as is often the case, the invasion of fibroblasts will sew the surfaces together at this point with permanent *adhesions*.

Suppuration.—If the dead tissue in an inflamed area undergoes softening and liquefaction the process is known as *suppuration* and the fluid formed is *pus*. This is the method by which the dead material is removed from the body. There are three requisites for suppuration: (1) *necrosis*; (2) the presence of sufficient leukocytes; (3) digestion of the dead material by proteolytic ferments. If any one of these is absent suppuration will not occur. Anything which will produce both positive chemotaxis and necrosis will produce suppuration. Not only pyogenic bacteria and their toxins, but aseptic irritants such as turpentine and croton oil will cause typical suppuration. *The presence of leukocytes does not constitute suppuration.* The tissues may be crowded

with polymorphonuclear leukocytes, but suppuration and pus formation need not be present (Fig. 31).

The digestive enzymes are produced mainly by the leukocytes, and to a lesser extent by the necrosed tissue cells and the infecting bacteria. The part played by the leukocytes is readily shown by testing the action of pus on fibrin or egg albumen. This is easily dissolved by pus or purulent sputum, whereas non-purulent sputum has no effect. The action of the protease of the leukocytes tends to be inhibited by the antienzymes of the serum. On this account, if the exudate be rich in serum and poor in leukocytes, no liquefaction and suppuration will occur. Drainage of the serum with removal of the antienzymes may lead to liquefaction and removal of the dead tissue. In some animals such as the rabbit the leukocytes are poor in protease and the serum is rich in antienzymes. In such an animal infection with the ordinary pyogenic cocci does not result in the formation of pus. The antienzymes appear to be of lipoid character, such as unsaturated fatty acids. Tuberculous caseous material is rich in unsaturated fatty acids and therefore resists liquefaction. The toxins of the tubercle bacillus appear also to destroy the autolytic ferments. Another reason why the ordinary tuberculous lesion does not suppurate is that it does not contain leukocytes. If secondary infection occurs, or even if leukocytes are attracted to the part by the injection of iodoform, liquefaction and suppuration will soon follow.

Pus is the fluid product of suppuration. It is alkaline in reaction and usually yellowish in color. It consists of pus cells and pus serum, but in addition it contains the débris of tissue destruction and bacteria living or dead. The *pus cells* are leukocytes, for the most part polymorphonuclear in type. If the exudate is fresh as in the discharge from a recent gonorrhea, the details are sharp and the cells are well preserved. If the exudate is old, all details may be lost.

The *pus serum* is inflammatory lymph to which are added the products of cell disintegration. It does not coagulate, because the fibrinogen of the blood plasma is destroyed by the enzymes of the leukocytes. It is for this reason that the exudate of a serous pleurisy when removed from the body will clot into a jelly-like mass, while the much thicker exudate of a purulent pleurisy (empyema) will remain uncoagulated.

Abscess.—An abscess is an example of localized suppuration. The inflammation is limited to one area, and as the irritant is a pyogenic one, pus is produced. When staphylococci lodge in the kidney, an acute inflammatory reaction results, the cells in the center of the focus are killed, and are liquefied by the proteolytic enzymes (Fig. 32). In this way a cavity is produced which contains fluid pus. The wall of the abscess cavity consists of damaged but still living tissues. It is here that the struggle goes on to limit the spread of the infection (Fig. 33). This limiting zone is crowded with polymorphonuclear leukocytes and with macrophages filled with débris. Pus cells are continually discharged from this zone into the abscess, so that it is called the *pyogenic membrane*. If the abscess is chronic, or if the infection is dying out, the macrophages will greatly outnumber the polymorphonuclears. Further out the tissue becomes more normal.

If the infection continues active, more and

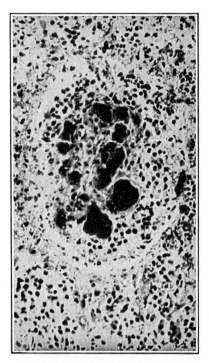

Fig. 32.—Abscess of kidney showing dark masses of bacteria and destruction of tissue. × 275.

more material is added to the abscess, so that the pressure within it rises. It therefore tends to extend or "point" in the direction of least resistance. In the kidney it may discharge into the renal pelvis or on to the surface of the kidney. If the abscess enters a muscle sheath such as that of the psoas it may track along it for a considerable distance.

A *boil* is an abscess of a hair follicle or a sebaceous gland, caused by the Staphylococcus aureus which has penetrated the opening of a duct, due perhaps to repeated friction, so that it is commonest on the buttocks or the back of the neck. There is marked fibroblastic proliferation, which, with intercellular formation of fibrin, causes the characteristic induration. The tension thus becomes high and is responsible for the pain. There may be very little liquefaction of the necrosed tissue, so that the center of the boil is composed of a solid "core" instead of pus. In a *carbuncle* the infection spreads to the subcutaneous tissue where it causes a more diffuse lesion which discharges

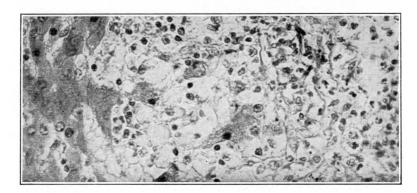

Fig. 33.—Wall of abscess in liver. At the left the liver cells are comparatively uninjured.
At the right there is an acute inflammatory exudate. × 300.

on the surface by a series of openings, and from which toxic absorption is more liable to occur. The pus serum is absorbed into the lymphatics, the pus becomes inspissated, and the dead tissue is converted into a mass of fatty débris in which lime salts may be deposited. This fatty change with calcification is seen much more commonly in tuberculous lesions than in acute inflammation.

The path formed by an abscess in its effort to discharge on a free surface is known as a *sinus*. Should the abscess discharge simultaneously on to both a skin and a mucous surface, the path which connects these surfaces is called a *fistula*. If the mucous surface is in the bowel, feces will be discharged on the skin, and the fistula is a *fecal fistula*. A good example is the abscess which may form when an inflamed appendix ruptures, and which may eventually discharge both into the bowel and on to the abdominal wall. When an abscess reaches a surface, either skin or mucous membrane, the overlying tissue becomes necrosed, forming a *slough*, and when the slough is discharged an open sore or *ulcer* is produced. This used to be the usual fate of an abscess before the days of modern chemotherapy. An ulcer, which is an open sore, an interruption of surface continuity of skin or mucous membrane with accompanying inflammation, is, of course, frequently produced by injurious agents acting directly on the surface.

Ulcer.—An acute inflammatory lesion which discharges on the surface generally heals quickly. Such a healing ulcer is called a *healthy ulcer*. Its floor is covered by pink granulations composed of the vascular connective tissue known as *granulation tissue*, any discharge which comes from it is slight and contains only a few pus cells, the edges are sloping and are bordered by a bluish-white line of ingrowing epithelium, and the surrounding parts are not inflamed. An ulcer may fail to heal and be *unhealthy* because of continued infection or defective circulation in the part. In such an ulcer the base is bathed with pus, the edges are ragged owing to continued tissue destruction, the epithelium shows no sign of covering the ulcer, the surrounding parts are inflamed and edematous or may be hard and sclerotic from fibroblastic proliferation (Fig. 34).

Cellulitis.—So far we have only considered suppuration limited to a circumscribed area. The suppuration may spread through the tissues, a condition known as cellulitis. Streptococci are more likely to cause a spreading inflammation, staphylococci a limited one. This difference depends in part on the intensity of the local inflammatory reaction; this is much more severe in staphylococcal than in streptococcal infections. Menkin claims that this is on account of blocking of the lymph channels by fibrin. Staphylococci produce a clotting principle or staphylocoagulase which favors fibrin formation, whereas streptococci produce a fibrinolytic principle which breaks down and prevents the formation of fibrin. For these reasons the constitutional reaction (due to widespread bacterial invasion) may be in

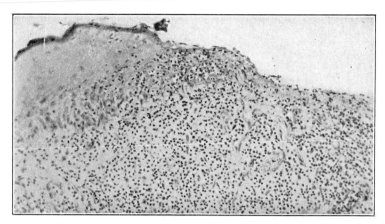

FIG. 34.—Non-healing ulcer. The epithelium on the left shows no sign of growing over the inflamed floor of the ulcer. × 125.

inverse proportion to the intensity of the local reaction.

Varieties of Acute Inflammation.—A multitude of descriptive names have been applied to the various forms of inflammation. The meaning of most of these is self-evident, so that they need only be mentioned. An understanding of the principles which underlie the variations is far more important than any string of names. *Serous* inflammation is characterized by an exudate composed chiefly of serum. Pleurisy with effusion is an example. In *fibrinous* inflammation the chief element is fibrin. It is seen in dry pleurisy, in diphtheria, and in pneumonia. *Purulent* inflammation is suppuration. *Catarrhal* inflammation is a mild inflammation of a mucous membrane; the mucous cells pour out mucus with which are mingled desquamated epithelial cells and a certain number of leukocytes, but the process stops short of suppuration. A cold in the head is an example. *Membranous* or *diphtheritic* inflammation is a condition where the cells of a mucous surface are killed, an exudate is laid down on the surface, and the whole necrotic layer is bound by fibrin to the underlying tissue to form a "false membrane."

Allergic Inflammation.—When an animal or person is sensitized to bacteria by previous inoculation (*i.e.*, is in a state of allergy), a subsequent injection of the same organisms will cause a violent local reaction with inflammatory changes which are much more extreme than in the normal animal. This condition may be called allergic inflammation. Its two main features are: (1) the large amount of exudate and the tendency to necrosis and destruction of tissue, owing to the union of antigen and antibody within the cells; (2) the increased phagocytic power of the leukocytes and macrophages, as a result of which the infection is more readily overcome. In the chapter on Immunity and Hypersensitivity we shall have occasion to observe that only the first of these features is a manifestation of allergy, the second being dependent on the acquired immunity which accompanies the allergic state. If the condition is of benefit to the animal it is on account of the second, not the first, of these features.

Influence of Cortisone on the Cells of Inflammation.—Far-reaching effects upon the dynamics of inflammation have been ascribed to secretions of the adrenal cortex (Dougherty and Schneebeli, Rebuck and his associates). These effects are produced both by cortisone and ACTH, and have been observed in the experimental animal and in man. The cortisone may be used topically as well as parenterally. In the human subject the technique of skin windows has been used effectively (Rebuck *et al.*). This consists of scraping the epidermis over a small area, the application of an antigen (egg white, diphtheria toxoid, old tuberculin, etc.) to the denuded surface, and overlaying the lesion with a small cover-slip. The exudative cells migrate to the undersurface of the cover-slip within thirty minutes. The cover-slip is removed, stained, and replaced by others as often as is desired.

The most striking changes concern the lymphocytes. There is marked depletion of these cells at the period when they should appear (eight to twelve hours), and later of the macrophages. These results seem to be brought about by injury to the lymphocytes in the lymphopoietic tissues, depletion of lymphocytes in the circulating blood and inhibition of lymphocytic migration. Phagocytic activity is diminished to a marked degree. This involves both the polymorphonuclears directly and the macrophages. Other well-known results of the administration of cortisone and ACTH are inhibition of the growth of granulation tissue and depletion of eosinophils in those cases in which these cells form part of the inflammatory exudate. The antispreading effect of cortisone due to inhibition of the spreading factor hyaluronidase, may also have to be considered.

The basic disturbances are damage to the organ sources of lymphocytes, inhibition of phagocytosis, decrease of the margination and migration of leukocytes in the vessels, possible interference with transport of the white blood cells, and local inhibition of the defense mechanism.

Most of the changes described above are likely to be deleterious in effect, especially if the exciting agent is virulent and capable of reproduction. Both the morbidity and mortality are increased in many experimental infections induced by bacteria (pneumococci, staphylococci, streptococci, tubercle bacilli) and by viruses (poliomyelitis, vaccinia, influenza). The incidence of spontaneous infections is increased and there is recrudescence of chronic and latent infections. If, on the other hand, the antigen is not virulent nor capable of reproduction, the toning down or inhibition of the normal inflammatory response can protect such delicate structures as arterioles, glomeruli and the eye. The remarkable effect of cortisone on the lesions of chronic arthritis are well known and a similar beneficial

result may be obtained with the vascular lesions of periarteritis nodosa (Baggenstoss). It is evident that cortisone and ACTH are two-edged tools, not to be used lightly, for though they are powerful for good they are also potent for evil.

CHRONIC INFLAMMATION

When an irritant of low-grade intensity acts upon the tissues the result is said to be chronic inflammation, because it does not run the rapid acute course characteristic of acute inflammation. The tissue reaction is quite different from that of the acute form. It is often said to be productive in character, but the cells which collect in response to the irritation either come from the blood stream (lymphocytes, etc.), or are derived from those wandering tissue cells which go by the alternative names of histiocytes, mononuclears and macrophages. The only cells which proliferate are the fibroblasts. The cells most characteristic of chronic inflammation and on which the microscopic diagnosis is based are lymphocytes, plasma cells and macrophages. In the center of the lesion there is often a varying number of polymorphonuclear leukocytes, whilst at the periphery there may be a fibroblastic reaction. The microscopic picture is much more variable than in acute inflammation.

In an organ such as the liver or kidney an intense irritant producing acute inflammation will destroy both the highly specialized parenchymatous cells and the more lowly developed connective tissue. An irritant of low intensity may kill the special cells, but only stimulate the fibrous tissue to proliferate (fibrosis), just as a degree of cold which will kill a race horse may merely stimulate a cart horse. John McCrae, the poet pathologist who wrote "In Flanders Fields," compares the parenchymatous cell to the professional man in a community, specially trained, not prone to be physically hard, nor overgiven to reproduction. The supporting cell is its laboring-class brother, physically strong, not readily injured, and ready in reproduction.

A chronic inflammatory lesion is cellular at first, but becomes more and more fibrous as the irritation subsides and collagen is laid down. It follows the usual course of healing. But it is obvious from the nature of the process that the resulting fibrosis is likely to be much more marked than in acute inflammation. Newly-formed fibrous tissue invariably contracts as it becomes older, so that the affected organ will be shrunken as well as hard. Examples of these changes are healed tuberculosis of the lung and cirrhosis of the liver.

One word regarding nomenclature. A healed inflammatory lesion is not an example of chronic inflammation. It is not an "itis," so that when the surgeon finds a firm and shrunken appendix it does not follow that the patient is suffering from chronic appendicitis. The appendix may be chronically inflamed, or it may be merely a fibrosed appendix; microscopic examination is necessary to settle the question. This subject is brought up because of a loose habit, all too common, of speaking of chronic appendicitis, chronic myocarditis, of chronic pleurisy when the speaker really means a fibrosed appendix, myocardium, or pleura.

THE GRANULOMATA

It is difficult if not impossible to give a short satisfying definition of a granuloma. It is a variety of chronic inflammation characterized by lesions which tend to be distinctly circumscribed and by cells rather of histiocytic than of hematogenous type. Granulomatous inflammation is a highly specific reaction of the reticuloendothelial system. The cells of this system have a great ability to change their form, to proliferate, and to move through the tissues. The result is a granuloma. As the reaction is defensive in character it is called inflammatory, but it must be realized that there is no true exudate, nor are the vascular changes of inflammation present. If, however, inflammation is considered as a process by means of which cells (and serum) accumulate around an injurious substance, it is obvious that granulomas must be regarded as a special example of inflammation. Obviously it will be a reaction to a wide variety of agents. The circumscribed lesions first

appear as tiny *granules*, which later fuse to form quite large lesions; hence the term granuloma.

The process is in the main productive rather than exudative: the cells come from the tissues rather than the blood. The histiocytes belong to the reticuloendothelial system, although to the wandering rather than the fixed members of that group. These large polyhedral cells, being designed for phagocytosis, have abundant cytoplasm. *Epithelioid cells* are merely histiocytes with abundant pale cytoplasm like that of epithelium. The lipid content may be high, accounting for the abundance and pallor of the cytoplasm. The epithelioid cells have a tendency to fuse, forming large multinucleated giant cells of the foreign body or Langhans type.

Other cells may enter into the formation of a granuloma. In syphilis plasma cells and lymphocytes may preponderate, while in actinomycosis there is an acute exudative element. But by and large the histiocyte is the characteristic cell. It is well seen in tuberculosis, but in its purest form in sarcoidosis. Necrosis and actual caseation of the central part of the lesion may occur, usually in tuberculosis, almost never in sarcoidosis. Collagen may be formed at the periphery, and eventually the entire lesion may be converted into dense scar tissue. This is seen in the most striking degree in silicosis.

The granulomas may be divided according to the causal agent into infective granulomas and foreign body granulomas. The infective granulomas in turn may be due to (1) bacteria, (2) fungi or (3) viruses. In addition there are a few examples of unknown etiology, of which the best examples are sarcoidosis and regional ileitis.

Infective Granulomas. — These granulomas are caused by living agents, which, as just mentioned, may be bacteria, fungi or yeasts, and viruses. Amongst the *bacterial granulomas* the most important are tuberculosis, syphilis and brucellosis. These diseases are described in Chapter 11. Sarcoidosis possibly belongs to this group, a matter which is discussed in the same chapter. The important *mycotic granulomas* are actinomycosis and blastomyces, but to these may be added sporotrichosis, coccidioidomycosis and histoplasmosis. The only *virus granuloma* which need be mentioned is lymphogranuloma venereum.

Different causal agents may stimulate tissue reactions which are identical histologically, and a given species of microorganism may produce a wide variety of histological patterns. This is apt to present a difficult problem to the pathologist who is asked to make a precise diagnosis from a fragment of a granulomatous lesion removed during life. In former days when the specific therapy of infections was limited, an exact bacteriological diagnosis was often largely academic. In these days of chemotherapy and antibiotics it has now become of pressing practical importance. In addition to the usual microscopic examination, the biopsy material may have to be examined bacteriologically by culture and by animal inoculation. This is particularly true of cases of suspected tuberculosis (MacDonald and Weed). If the histological picture alone is relied on, mistakes may occur in two ways: (1) tuberculous tissue may resemble granulomas produced by other agents; (2) other infectious agents, both bacterial and mycotic, may cause histological changes which may readily be mistaken for tuberculosis unless bacteriological techniques are employed.

Foreign Body Granulomas.—The foreign bodies which may excite a localized histiocytic reaction are numerous and varied. This group of granulomas is therefore a miscellaneous and heterogeneous one. The histological diagnosis depends on the demonstration of the foreign body in the tissue, usually clustered around by very large foreign body giant cells with numerous nuclei scattered throughout their cytoplasm but lacking the peripheral or polar arrangement seen in the Langhans type of giant cell characteristic of tuberculosis. The material may be solid or semi-fluid, organic or inorganic, dead or living. The following is a partial list: talc, lycopodium, sutures, silica, beryllium, oils and paraffin, wood ticks, insect venom, and necrotic material as in fat necrosis of the breast. These need not be considered separately and in detail, for the general principles are the same in all.

Dusting powder granuloma is caused by the material used by the surgeon as a lubricant for rubber gloves. Talcum powder containing crystals of magnesium silicate and lycopodium powder containing spores have gone out of fashion, but foreign body granulomas caused by these powders left in the tissue continue to be removed. Starch powder, which is now popular, is much less irritating, but in some persons it may excite a granulomatous reaction. In all of these instances the causal agent can be detected in the histiocytic cells.

Lint granuloma is caused by fragments of lint remaining in a surgical wound or even after a hypodermic injection, the needle having been presumably wiped with gauze before being used. *Beryllium granuloma* is a modern industrial hazard usually affecting the lungs, but sometimes causing skin lesions in janitors and children handling broken fluorescent bulbs. *Lipogranulomas* are seen when antibiotics in a fatty base are injected into the buttocks, or when paraffin is injected into the tissues in face-lifting, etc.

Some of the more important granulomatous infections and their key differential characteristics are outlined in the table opposite. These may be compared with the various foreign body granulomata. Many of the conditions mentioned are discussed in subsequent chapters.

PRINCIPAL GRANULOMATOUS INFLAMMATIONS

Common Diseases	Causative organism	Special characteristics
Tuberculosis	Mycobacterium tuberculosis	Tubercle: central caseation with loss of cellular detail.
Syphilis	Treponema pallidum	Gumma: central necrosis and caseation without complete loss of cellular detail.
Brucellosis (Undulant Fever)	Brucella	Non-specific g anuloma; positive tissue culture. (A systemic disease).
Leprosy (Clinically: nodular lesions and anesthetic patches)	Bacillus lepræ	Cellular granuloma; mainly large, pale, foamy, mononuclear cells (*lepra cells*) with a high lipid content.
Tularemia (Clinically: glandular and typhoidal forms)	Pasteurella tularensis	*Acute*: focal necrosis and suppuration. *Chronic*: Focal granuloma; central necrosis, epithelioid cells, giant cells.
Glanders	Bacillus mallei	Infective granuloma without caseation; rare giant cells.
Cat Scratch Disease	Virus	Lymphadenitis; reticuloendothelial hyperplasia followed by necrosis.
Actinomycosis	Streptothrix fungus: (1) A. bovis (2) rarely: Nocardia asteroides	Granuloma plus suppuration with "sulfur granules." Abscesses and multiple sinuses common.
Blastomycosis	Blastomyces dermatididis	(1) Cutaneous form: papules with suppuration, ulceration, and frequent epithelial hyperplasia simulating carcinoma.
Cryptococcosis (Torulosis; European blastomycosis)	Cryptococcus neoformans (Torula histolytica)	Less tissue destruction and cellular exudation than in blastomycosis. Sections show clear halo around organism due to capsule.
Coccidioidomycosis	Coccidioides immitis (thick-walled spherule filled with endospores	Granulomatous masses and abscesses; usually in lungs. Less cavitation than tuberculosis but bone lesions more extensive.
Sporotrichosis	Sporotrichum schenckii (fungus demonstrated by culture, not smears)	Usually nodules along lymphatics of forearm, later suppuration. No visible organisms in sections or smears
Granuloma Inguinale	Donovanii granulomatis (coccobacilli)	Usually in anal and genital area. Granulation tissue with ulcerated necrotic center and intracellular Donovan bodies

Other granulomatous reactions which should be mentioned are: Sarcoidosis, Histoplasmosis, Regional enteritis and Foreign body granulomas.

Less common diseases with granulomatous lesions are: Streptothricosis, Aspergillosis, Yaws, and other rare conditions.

REFERENCES

ADAMI, J. G.: *Inflammation*, London, 1909.

BAGGENSTOSS, A. H., SHICK, R. M. and POLLEY, H. F.: Am. J. Path., 1951, *27*, 537. (Cortisone and inflammation).

CLARK, E. L. and CLARK, E. R.: Am. J. Anat., 1935, *57*, 385. (Emigration of leukocytes).

COHNHEIM, J.: *Lectures on General Pathology*, (English translation), London, 1889.

CUNNINGHAM, J. A.: Am. J. Path., 1951, *27*, 761. (Stellate inclusions in giant cells).

DIBLE, J. H.: Ann. Roy. Coll. Surg. England, 1950, *6*, 120. (Inflammation and repair).

DOUGHERTY, T. F. and SCHNEEBELI, G. L.: Proc. Soc. Exper. Biol. and Med., 1950, *75*, 854. (Cortisone and inflammation).

DUBOS, R. J.: Lancet, 1958, *2*, 1. (The microenvironment of inflammation).

EBERT, R. H. and FLOREY, H. W.: Brit. J. Exper. Path., 1939, *20*, 342. (Development of the monocyte).

EHRICH, W. E., DRABKIN, D. L. and FORMAN, C.: J. Exper. Med., 1949, *90*, 157. (Plasma cells and antibody formation).

FIELD, M. E., DRINKER, C. K. and WHITE, J. C.: J. Exper. Med., 1932, *56*, 363. (Lymph flow in inflammation).

HARRIS, H.: J. Path. and Bact., 1953, *66*, 135. (Chemotaxis).

HAYTHORN, S. R.: Arch. Path., 1929, *7*, 651. (Giant cells).

KNISELY, M., BLOCK, E. H. and WARNER, L.: Science, 1947, *106*, 431. (Sludged blood in inflammation).

KELSALL, M. A. and CRABB, E. D.: Ann. New York Acad. Sci., 1958, *72*, 295. (Lymphocytes and plasma cells in nucleoprotein metabolism).

LEWIS, T.: *The Blood Vessels of the Human Skin and Their Responses*, London, 1927. (Observations on the mechanism of the vascular changes in inflammation).

MACCALLUM, W. G.: *Textbook of Pathology*, Philadelphia, 1940. (Macrophages in inflammation).

McDONALD, J. R. and WEED, L. A.: Am. J. Clin. Path., 1951, *21*, 223. (Bacteriological differentiation of the granulomas).

McGOVERN, V. J.: Path. and Bact., 1957, *73*, 99. (Mast cells and capillary permeability in inflammation).

MENKIN, V.: *Dynamics of Inflammation*, New York, 1940. *Newer Concepts of Inflammation*, Springfield, Ill., 1950.

METCHNIKOFF, E.: *The Comparative Pathology of Inflammation*. (English translation), London, 1893.

MOON, V. H. and TERSHAKOVEC, G. A.: Arch. Path., 1951, *52*, 369. (Dynamics of inflammation).

MOVAT, H. Z. and WILSON, D. R.: Can. Med. Ass. J., 1959, *81*, 154. (Fine structure of plasma cells in relation to their function).

MUDD, E. B. H. and MUDD, S.: J. Gen. Physiol., 1933, *16*, 625. (Phagocytosis).

PAGE, A. R. and GOOD, R. A.: Am. J. Path., 1958, *34*, 645. (Neutrophils in inflammation).

REBUCK, J. W. and MELLINGER, R. C.: Am. J. Path., 1953, *29*, 599. (Cortisone and inflammation).

RICH, A. R.: Arch. Path., 1936, *22*, 228. (A general discussion of the inflammatory process).

RILEY, J. F.: *The Mast Cells*, Edinburgh, 1959.

SPECTOR, W. G.: J. Path. and Bact., 1956, *72*, 367. 1957, *74*, 67. (Capillary permeability in inflammation).

TOMPKINS, E. H. and GRILLO, M. A.: Am. J. Path., 1953, *29*, 217. (The macrophages in inflammation).

WOOD, W. B., JR.: Lancet, 1958, *2*, 53; New England J. Med., 1958, *258*, 1023. (The genesis of fever in inflammation). The Harvey Lectures, 1951, *47*, 72. (Cellular immunity).

WOOD, W. B., JR., SMITH, M. R. and WATSON, B.: J. Exper. Med., 1946, *84*, 387. (Phagocytosis).

Chapter 3

Repair

Introduction
  STIMULI TO REPAIR
  INHIBITING FACTORS
    General
    Local

Healing of a Wound
  PRIMARY UNION
  SECONDARY UNION
    Granulation Tissue
Organization of a Surface Exudate

Organization of a Thrombus
Parenchymal Repair
  LABILE CELLS
  STABLE CELLS
  PERMANENT CELLS
Repair in Different Tissues

INTRODUCTION

THE repair of injured tissue is an even more fundamental process than inflammation. It is seen throughout the animal and vegetable kindgom. The lower in the scale the animal, the more complete is the regeneration. When the head of the earthworm is severed, a new one is formed, and this process can be repeated many times. Some of the most remarkable examples of repair are seen in the star-fish. In this and other animals in which repair is particularly complete, reproduction is of the asexual type; indeed repair may be regarded as a special example of asexual reproduction. The process of repair is so commonplace that we seldom pause to enquire what induces cells which have remained dormant for years suddenly to take on active growth. When looked at closely this is seen to be a remarkable phenomenon. Incise the most quiescent of fibrous tissue, and in twenty-four hours the connective-tissue cells have developed from mere nuclei into actively dividing fibroblasts. What is the cause of this sudden transformation? What is the *vis medicatrix naturæ*, the healing power of Nature? To which we may add an equally awkward question: why do repair processes stop when they have reached their goal and not go on indefinitely as we see in neoplasia?

Before proceeding farther we may pause to consider the connotation of the three words, repair, healing and regeneration. *Repair* is the most inclusive of these. It signifies the restitution of the part to a more or less complete replica of its former structure. *Healing* is an aspect of repair, but it suggests the closure of some gap, as in a wound or an ulcer. A wound of the skin may heal perfectly, but the new tissue is a scar, lacking sweat and sebaceous glands and other specialized structures. *Regeneration* implies a complete renewal of tissue, and is more applicable to a parenchymatous organ such as the liver, which is endowed with remarkable regenerative power.

It is difficult to draw a hard and fast line between repair and inflammation. Both represent the reaction of the tissues to an irritant. Repair usually follows inflammation, and is usually preceded by it, but not always so. An irritant of some intensity produces inflammation and death of the tissues. At a distance the action is weakened, and the irritant becomes a stimulant, so that the tissue response now is proliferation. In this way reparative processes may go on at the same time as inflammation. Mac-Callum compares inflammation to a fire in which, while the flames are still burning fiercely in one part of the building and the fire engines are pouring on floods of water, gangs of carpenters have already begun to arrive, and are busy with reconstructive work on the burnt-out portions. We shall see that this analogy is a particularly apt one.

In the past we have had to reconstruct the march of events in healing from the study of microscopic sections of dead fixed tissue. Now it is possible to witness the fascinating sight of living tissue undergoing repair, and if we cannot see this at first hand, we can at least see moving pictures which speed up the process. The observations of Clark and his associates are of particular interest. By

5

inserting a double-walled transparent chamber constructed of celluloid in a rabbit's ear they have been able to watch under the microscope the injured tissues recovering from the blow and setting themselves to reconstruct the part. By this means new vessels can be seen differentiating and beginning to contract and dilate. Using intravital injections of methylene blue they could demonstrate the development of non-medullated nerve fibers going to the arteries; only when the vessels were supplied with nerves were they capable of contraction. The ingrowth of capillaries is followed by a remodelling of the indifferent plexus of vessels into an adult pattern, and a change into definite arteries and veins. The same is true of lymphatics, which also grow by sprouting, and appear later than the blood vessels. Even the different stages of mitosis were seen and photographed. After injury associated with edema definite holes could be seen in the lymphatics which remained open for several days, allowing free passage of fluid and red blood cells into the injured lymphatics. This passage was not observed when the ear was splinted, thus demonstrating the importance of immobilization in the treatment of localized injuries and infections in order to prevent the entrance of bacteria into the lymphatics, although, as has been pointed out in the preceding chapter, this immobilization can be overdone.

Stimuli to Repair.—It is obvious that the cells which proliferate so abundantly and so quickly to effect regeneration and repair must do so on account of stimuli they receive, stimuli which are presumably chemical in nature. It has long been known that if in an aseptic wound all débris and blood clots are removed and the wound completely protected from outside irritation, no healing will occur (Carrel and Ebeling). Even at the end of three weeks no change may have occurred. But when the wound is covered with a slightly irritating dressing such as dry gauze or when a few staphylococci are introduced, healing commences very shortly.

The chemical stimulus appears to be liberated by degenerating cells in the injured tissue. The frustrating fact is that we are ignorant as to the character of this substance, although a number of high-sounding names have been suggested for it. One result of our ignorance is that we are unable to expedite the healing of a wound or the repair of destroyed tissue, much as we could wish to do so. It is said that moderate exposure to ultraviolet light increases the rate of wound healing in man and in the common laboratory animals.

Inhibiting Factors.—It is easier to say what may interfere with the healing process than what makes it work. Unfortunately quite a number of conditions may interfere with the process of repair. These may either be general or local.

GENERAL FACTORS.—Under conditions of ordinary health, repair proceeds at a uniform rate providing there is no local interference. The following general factors may be detrimental.

Age.—When we consider the very rapid growth of tissue in the child compared with the adult, it is small wonder that wounds in children heal quickly. With advancing years the rate of wound healing may be considerably impaired. One factor may be the less adequate blood supply in the aged.

Diet.—The supply of food to a part influences its reparative power. This is most easily observed in the experimental animal, but prolonged malnutrition in man, as occurs in malignant disease, has an adverse effect on healing. This is probably connected with *low serum protein* levels. It would appear that a food factor of special importance is the amino acid methionine (Perez-Tamayo and Ihnen). When animals with experimental wounds are kept on a protein-free diet for a short time, only a narrow zone of reaction develops, the new capillaries and fibroblasts are few in number, and there is a marked delay in the formation of fibers. The result is a weak scar with decreased tensile strength. When, however, methionine is added to the diet normal connective tissue of normal tensile strength is formed. As regards wound healing protein deficiency seems to mean methionine deficiency. This amino acid increases the rate of utilization of the protein available, and its sulphur radicle may also be used for the formation of chondroitin sulfate which imparts firmness to the ground substance.

Vitamin C deficiency is an important cause of poor and delayed wound healing in the experimental animal and to a lesser degree in man. In the early stage of wound healing acid mucopolysaccharides (hyaluronic acid) are produced. In the absence of vitamin C this substance is lacking, but it reappears on injection of the vitamin. *Scurvy*, which is due to lack of vitamin C, is characterized by atrophy of connective-tissue fibers, and under scorbutic conditions fibroblasts produce little collagen, and what is produced is of poor quality. It is evident, therefore, that an adequate supply of vitamin C is necessary for good healing. It has been shown clinically that when the vitamin supply is insufficient the healing of wounds is delayed and they tend to break open again (Crandon, Lund and Dill).

Endocrines.—Cortisone interferes with the process of repair in the experimental animal, as well as inhibiting the vascular and exudative changes of inflammation. There is an almost complete lack of fibroblastic and vascular proliferation, migration of histiocytes, foreign body giant cell formation, and development of adhesions. Some workers find that these effects are only observed after a lag of a day or two (Lattes *et al.*). It seems probable that the cortisone interferes with chemical changes in the mucopolysaccharides of the ground substance of connective tissue, changes which are initiated by release of agents as the result of injury and are indicated by metachromasia of the ground substance. Other steroid hormones also influence repair. Thus desoxycorticosterone stimulates the proliferation of fibroblasts and encourages the formation of collagen in the wall of a chemically-produced abscess, whilst testosterone and estradiol have the opposite effect (Taubenhaus and Amronin). The sex hormones may act by inhibiting the anterior pituitary. The experimental observations outlined above may not be of importance in human pathology. The dose of cortisone used on the animals is very much greater than the dose used in humans. Surgical evidence in man suggests that a wound in a person on cortisone therapy should heal well. On the other hand there seems to be a tendency for perforation of a gastric ulcer, and for inter-ference with reparative fibrosis in pulmonary tuberculosis.

One of the most interesting examples of the influence of general systemic factors on repair is the *healing of a fracture*. Here the osteoclasts are working at top speed, but they demand the most favorable conditions. Insufficiency of amino acids and protein, of vitamin C (as in scurvy) and vitamin D, interferes with their work. Vitamin C is concerned with the formation of collagen, and vitamin D with calcification. Parathyroid hormone is necessary for proper calcification and so to a lesser degree is thyroxin. The healing of a fracture is considered more fully in Chapter 43.

LOCAL FACTORS.—In the ordinary case of delayed healing the cause is more likely to be local than general.

*Ischemia.—*Repair or healing is a manifestation of an outburst of cellular activity. It is obvious that if the cells have an inadequate supply of nutriment, vitamins, etc. because of arterial narrowing or venous thrombosis, normal healing cannot be expected. Complete and prolonged immobilization of the part will impair the circulation because of lack of muscular contraction. Finally, the formation of dense scar tissue deep to a surface wound or ulcer will tend to interrupt the flow of blood to that lesion.

Local Irritants.—Bacterial infection of a wound sufficient to cause active inflammation will make healing impossible, just as the masons and carpenters cannot begin the work of reconstruction at a spot where the fire is burning fiercely, though it may be possible to start such work at a safe distance. Necrotic débris, collections of pus, etc. may interpose a barrier between two surfaces which cannot grow together until such material has been removed by the surgeon. Finally foreign bodies, including fragments of gauze or unabsorbed surgical sutures, will delay healing or make it impossible.

Repair after injury occurs in every part of the body, but not equally in every tissue. In this respect we shall consider separately repair of the connective and the parenchymatous tissues. Nearly every form of injury involves connective tissue, but it is convenient to consider the subject in relation to the healing of wounds, obviously a most important practical matter. A very thorough survey of normal repair and of the factors which may interfere with it will be found in a review by Edwards and Dunphy. The early literature is reviewed in a paper by Arey.

Systemic Effects of Trauma.—Before turning our attention to the healing of a wound, we may consider the systemic effects of serious trauma such as that of a major surgical procedure or a compound fracture of the femur. Soon after receipt of the injury a state of post-traumatic metabolism is established (Moore). This may be reflected presently all too clearly in the clinical state of the patient. The principal features of the metabolic change are as follows.

(1) Loss of nitrogen from the skeletal muscles due to catabolic breakdown in the muscle with resulting negative nitrogen balance. This loss of nitrogen may be far greater than that which occurs in starvation. It is mediated by adrenal hydroxycorticosteroids by way of the hypothalamic-pituitary-corticosteroid system. A patient who has no adrenals cannot tolerate trauma, passing into hypotensive, hypovolemic shock owing to lack of corticosteroid hormones. The amount of nitrogen lost depends on the severity of the injury.

(2) Diversion of protein substrates from the lean body mass to the wound, where an active build up takes place. The wound seems to have a high priority on bodily substances, and succeeds in maintaining a state of anabolism while the rest of the tissues are in one of catabolism.

(3) Mobilization of carbohydrate from the liver. This is mediated through the action of epinephrine and norepinephrine from the adrenal medulla, secretion of which is stimulated by apprehension and fright.

(4) Decreased sodium excretion, with a lowered sodium-potassium ratio in the urine. This is due to increased renal tubular resorption of sodium, caused in turn by an increased production of aldosterone.

(5) Marked water retention. It is common knowledge that even slight degrees of trauma will interfere with free water clearance by the kidneys. This is due to the antidiuretic hormones acting through the renal tubular system.

It becomes apparent that four hormonal mediators bring to the organs and tissues the message of bodily injury. These are the adrenal corticosteroids, aldosterone, the hormones of the adrenal medulla, and the antidiuretic hormones. It is also evident that the healing of a wound, and more especially a major surgical operative wound as in the resection of viscera, involves a good deal more than merely bringing together two cut surfaces, although that is the particular aspect which we shall now proceed to consider.

HEALING OF A WOUND

The process of healing is fundamentally the same in all wounds, but there are marked quantitative differences, depending on the amount of tissue destruction and to a certain extent on the presence of sepsis. It consists of two parts: (1) removal of inflammatory material and necrotic débris, which may be much or little; (2) replacement or reconstruction of the original tissue to as great a degree as possible. It involves the invasion and replacement of dying and dead tissue by immature mesenchyme called *granulation tissue*. "The essential function of granulation tissue is to replace useless material by living mesenchyme" (Hadfield). It derives its name from the fact that it is seen in abundance as tiny red granules on the surface of a clean open wound beginning to heal. The process of the conversion of inflammatory débris into granulation tissue and finally into fibrous tissue is known as *organization*. A similar process is involved in dealing with an inflammatory exudate on a serous surface, the healing of an abscess, the removal of tissue devitalized by arterial ischemia, and the replacement of extravasated blood and intravascular thrombi.

It is convenient to consider wound healing under two headings: (1) the healing of a clean incised wound, which used to be known by the old clinical name of "healing by first intention," but is now termed primary union; (2) healing of a wound with loss of substance formerly known as "healing by secondary intention," and now called secondary union or union by granulation tissue. In all varieties of healing we encounter a trilogy of factors, each one of which appears to be essential. These are: (1) the *ground substance* becomes more basophilic and rich in acid mucopolysaccharides, so that it resembles embryonic ground substance; (2) the *endothelium of capillaries* proliferates, so that new capillaries grow into the gap; (3) *fibroblasts* follow the capillaries, with a resulting formation first of fibrils and later of collagen. The complex of ground substance, new capillaries and new fibroblasts has been named the *blastema*. Reestablishment of the capillary circulation is the primary requisite of healing. Replacement of the parenchymatous cells of the part is secondary, desirable but not essential. We have already considered some factors which may delay the process. In our subsequent studies we shall encounter examples of impaired healing which are a great trial to the doctor as well as to the patient. Intestinal epithelium is continually being renewed. Ulcers of the bowel in typhoid fever heal readily, and yet peptic ulcer of the duodenum may refuse to heal in some patients, while it readily does so in others. We shall have to seek the answer to this and similar riddles in later chapters, although all too often our search will be without success.

Primary Union.—Here the cut surfaces are brought together by stitches, so that the process is direct, with no intermediary material playing a part. There is no appreciable loss of substance, bleeding is at a minimum, infection is absent, and if the edges are brought into apposition there is hardly any exudate between the surfaces. The knife acts as an irritant, so that the edges will show slight inflammatory changes in the shape of vascular dilatation and exudation, and a small quantity of plasma, fibrin, and leukocytes will be present in the thin gap. Although the wound is strictly *aseptic*, it is not bacteriologically *sterile*, and Staphylococcus albus may be present in small numbers. We have already seen that this tends to favor healing rather than to retard it.

Perhaps the earliest evidence of repair is the appearance of mitosis in the *vascular endothelial cells* and the formation of protoplasmic buds formed from the preexisting endothelium. These capillary buds always grow in the direction of the dead material

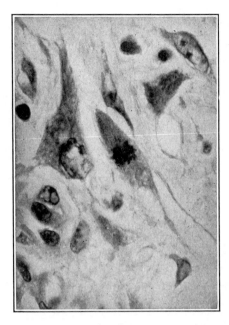

FIG. 35.—Proliferating fibroblasts, one of which shows a mitotic figure. × 800.

requiring replacement, as if directed by some compelling force. Healing tissue is therefore highly vascular to begin with, so that the surface of a wound which is still unclosed is bright red in color. These new capillaries appear to be unduly permeable, so that plasma proteins and enzymes pass through the walls more readily than normally, giving a plasma clot similar to that which is so suitable for the growth of cells in tissue culture. When the need for increased vascularization has passed, the capillaries become closed, devascularization proceeds, and the wound is now pale.

Almost at the same time the fibroblasts at the edges of the wound show mitotic activity (Fig. 35). The connective-tissue cell or fibrocyte of adult fibrous tissue is little more than a narrow nucleus surrounded by a thin layer of cytoplasm and wedged between dense bundles of collagen fibers, but it rapidly changes into a plump fusiform cell, the fibroblast, with a large nucleus and well-developed cytoplasm which may end in branching processes. The sudden change from complete quiescence to extreme activity denotes the action of a powerful stimulant.

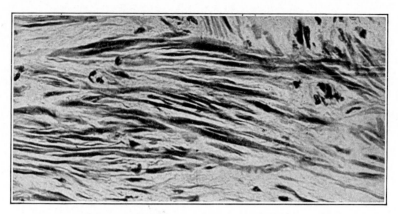

FIG. 36.—Fibroblasts separated by scanty collagen. × 275.

The mode of growth of the fibroblasts may best be studied by the method of *tissue culture*. The colonies of fibroblasts in culture medium tend to grow toward one another, as if the cells of one attracted the cells of the other. The coagulated plasma between the edges of the wound plays the part of a medium into which the fibroblasts grow and establish connection with those on the other side. The cells when photographed and projected on a screen can be seen to move through the medium in straight lines in the same fashion which we have already seen to characterize the growth of the capillary buds. The anterior process streams through the medium; then the nucleus and cytoplasmic body move forward. From such a picture it is easy to understand how the fibroblasts will rapidly unite the opposing surfaces. In culture the fibroblasts are seen always to keep in touch with their fellows, thus differing from the macrophages which wander about and live as independent units.

Collagen fibers are now laid down (Fig. 36). It used to be thought that the new and all-important fibrils were formed by a splitting off from the cytoplasm of the fibroblasts. That idea has been given up. It now appears that the fibrils develop from the metachromatic ground substance of the granulation tissue, which, after an initial period of shock of 12 to 24 hours duration, rapidly increases in amount about the fifth or sixth day. The formation of collagen appears to depend on two factors in the ground substance. (1) A soluble protein procollagenous substance secreted by the fibroblasts, which eventually becomes converted into collagen. (2) A carbohydrate component, a complex mucopolysaccharide which provides a medium in which the procollagen is converted into collagen. It has been suggested that mast cells are responsible for this material, but it seems more probable that fibroblasts are in control of the process (Taylor and Saunders). Ascorbic acid appears to be essential to this change. An acid solution of collagen can be made to precipitate into collagen fibers in the presence of an acid polysaccharide such as chondroitin sulfuric acid, fibers which can be demonstrated with the electron microscope.

In *summary* of the discussion so far we may say that two main phases of wound healing may be recognized: (1) A *productive or substrate phase* which begins shortly after wounding and lasts about 5 days, being characterized by the ingrowth of capillary buds and fibroblasts, together with the production of soluble precursors of collagen and of mucopolysaccharides; (2) a *collagen phase* in which normal collagen fibers are formed, beginning about the 5th day and lasting until healing is complete (Dunphy and Udupa) (Plate II).

In *ascorbic acid deficiency* the production phase is greatly extended and there is no collagen phase. The concentration of mucopolysaccharides rises greatly, and the building blocks of collagen are produced in

PLATE II

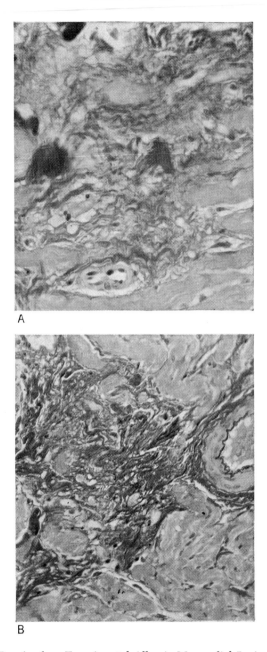

A

B

Repair of an Experimental Allergic Myocardial Lesion.

A, Substrate phase, early repair. The young repair tissue which replaces the site of previous necrosis, is composed mainly of blue-staining fibrillar ground substance, scattered through which are newly formed red collagen fibers. The orange-yellow fibers represent surviving myocardium.

B, Collagen phase, scar tissue. The ground substance with its blue-staining acid mucopolysaccharides has all been converted into collagen. Pentachrome II stain. (Kindness of Dr. Henry Z. Movat.)

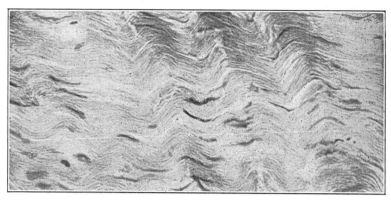

Fig. 37.—Scar tissue. Bundles of collagen fibers, between which are flattened fibroblasts. × 400.

abundance, but an all-important key to synthesis is lacking.

In *protein deficiency* the productive phase is again unduly prolonged, the collagen phase not beginning till the eighth day, and even then being slow in development. In this instance there is a deficiency of building blocks, so that collagen formation is delayed and inadequate. As we have already seen, both forms of deficiency interfere seriously with the healing of wounds.

In normal healing, which we can almost always expect in our patients, the collagen fibers form wavy bundles of *scar tissue* (Fig. 37). By this process of fibroblastic proliferation and immigration together with the formation of fibrils of increasing density the two surfaces of the wound are firmly sewn together. When the fibers are fully formed they shorten, and this contraction continues for some months, so that the scar which was at first raised becomes puckered.

Early in the healing process *macrophages* also crowd into the wound, and no doubt play an important part in the removal of dead material. It is of interest to note that these cells always maintain an intimate relationship with the developing capillary loops, which is not seen with any granulocytes or lymphocytes which may happen to be present.

We have already seen that the capillary buds and fibroblasts grow in remarkably straight lines in the direction of the dead material requiring replacement. We are ignorant of the cause of this movement, nor do we know what makes the endothelial cells and fibroblasts proliferate. We read of "wound hormones," but that sounds like a modern version in these less reverent days of Ambroise Paré's famous saying in the year 1537: "I dressed the wound; God healed it." It is true that a substance has been extracted from plants (string-bean pods) which causes renewed cell division. The chemical constitution is known, it has been synthesized, and has been christened traumatic acid. Unfortunately in mammals repair is much more complex, and there has been no purification of chemical stimulators, much as the surgeon would like to lay his hands on such a substance.

Hormonal control does seem to play some part in the healing process. Somatotrophin of the pituitary appears to facilitate capillary vascularization, thus creating an environment in which cells can multiply, whereas cortisone inhibits vascularization and the synthesis of mucopolysaccharides and collagen in the wound (Edwards and Dunphy).

Pullinger and Florey using the transparent chamber in the mouse's ear introduced by Smith, found by direct observation that lymphatic capillaries proliferate in the same manner as the blood vessels. A remarkably rich capillary network is established in ten to twelve days which can be demonstrated by injection. These new lymphatics no doubt play an important part in removal of the exudate. As healing proceeds they retrogress and finally disappear.

The epithelium from the sides grows over the narrow gap. In incised wounds the epithelinm does not merely bridge the gap but grows down to the deeper structures, where it proliferates irregularly, and, only after collagen fibers appear regresses to be arranged in a normal pattern (Hartwell). It might be thought that the new epithelial cells were produced by mitosis. This is not the case. The defect is made good by the migration or sliding of cells from the edge of the wound. Mitoses are found regularly at some distance from the edge. At first the epithelial layer is thin and bluish in color, a mere layer or two of cells, but soon it becomes thick and white. The specialized structures of the skin such as hair follicles and sweat glands are not replaced. The scar is pale, without hair and without sweat.

The time at which the various steps occur differs with differing conditions, but on an average it may be said that fibroblastic and endothelial proliferation occurs by the end of *twelve hours*, the epithelium has covered the surface and the edges are firmly sewn together by the *fourth day*, and at the end of *three weeks* there is fully formed non-vascular scar tissue. The active process of primary union takes about five days, and nothing but a thin line of connective tissue remains to indicate the site of the wound. If the wound is irritated there will be a more abundant exudate, more fibroblasts are formed, and the scar will be thicker. If the wound is badly infected suppuration will occur, and there will be no primary union.

Secondary Union.—This is healing of an open wound with loss of substance. The fibroblasts are unable to sew the surfaces together, and the gap is filled from below by a mass of granulation tissue. The principles of the healing process are the same as in primary union. The only difference is the loss of a mass of tissue, with in consequence an *open surface* and the likelihood of bacterial infection.

The gap is first filled with a mixture of coagulated blood, fibrin, and inflammatory exudate, and upon this scaffold the fibroblasts and vascular endothelium build the

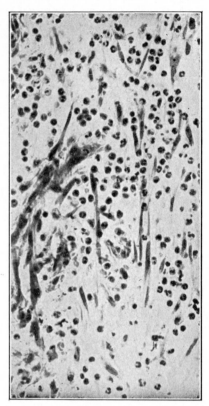

Fig. 38.—Granulation tissue. Young vascular connective tissue consisting of new capillaries and fibroblasts, together with many inflammatory cells. × 350.

granulation tissue. (Fig. 38). The process commences at the base and works to the surface, so that the youngest tissue is always at the surface. It is on the surface that the granulations are formed which give the name to the whole mass of young vascular connective tissue. When the surface of a clean open wound is examined at the end of the second day, it is seen to be covered with tiny red granules, so that it has the appearance of a pile of rough velvet. This red, finely granular surface is an indication of normal and healthy healing. Such a surface is highly vascular and bleeds very readily. If a dry gauze dressing sticks to the surface and is then torn off, the capillary loops are ruptured, and the process of healing is materially interfered with.

In addition to the fixed cells of the part (fibroblasts and vascular endothelium), wandering cells also form an important element of granulation tissue.

In the early stages these are mainly polymorphonuclear leukocytes, which migrate from the new capillaries in response to the irritation and appear on the surface in large numbers in the scanty exudate which our forefathers used to call "laudable pus." They doubtless serve to keep the surface free from infection. In the later stages and in the deeper layers the wandering cells are mainly macrophages and lymphocytes. The macrophages provide an even greater protection than the polymorphonuclears, for it can be shown experimentally that if an aseptic inflammation be produced and infection be added later, the substances which call forth macrophages in the aseptic inflammation give much better protection than those which call forth polymorphonuclears. Not until the leukocytes have overcome the infection does the epithelium begin to cover the surface, and true healing can be said to have commenced.

On account of its cellularity a granulating surface has a remarkable power of resisting bacterial infection. It presents so powerful a barrier that septicemia (blood invasion) cannot occur once an intact wall of granulation tissue has been formed. Billroth demonstrated this experimentally as long ago as 1865 by applying septic dressings soaked in putrid pus to the surface of a granulating wound. No infection resulted; but if the dressings were stitched in position, the stitch holes in the healthy skin at once became infected. When virulent streptococci are injected into the freshly epilated skin of a rabbit severe inflammation resulted, but if there is an interval of five days between the two procedures, no inflammation develops. Crystalline substances in solution are rapidly absorbed, probably on account of the great vascularity of the surface, so that death may follow the application of a poisonous substance like mercuric chloride, and it is said that opium will occasion sleep nearly as quickly as when given by mouth.

The granulation tissue grows in maturity from below upward. In the superficial layers the fibroblasts run at right angles to the surface and therefore parallel to the vessels, but in the deeper parts of the wound where the process is older they are arranged parallel with the surface, and eventually all the fibroblasts and the fibers which they produce run in this direction. The direction depends largely on the pull which is exerted on them. If this be altered experimentally, the direction of the fibroblasts will be correspondingly changed.

When the wound is aseptic the *epithelium* will grow in from the edge in two or three days, first as a delicate blue pellicle, gradually becoming thick and opaque. To say that the wound is aseptic does not mean of course that it is bacteriologically sterile. If there is sepsis and active inflammation the surface is bathed in pus, and the epithelium shows no sign of activity. In a chronic ulcer, where for some reason healing is long delayed, the epithelium sends long processes down into the deeper tissues. These may appear to be detached from the surface in a microscopic section, and may be very suggestive of carcinoma. In some cases a malignant growth may actually commence in such a chronic ulcer.

When the surface is covered by epithelium the process of *devascularization* begins. The new vessels being no longer needed gradually disappear, and the scar which is first red and angry-looking becomes white and bloodless.

Scar Hypertrophy and Keloids.—There may be too much as well as too little collagen formation. A *scar* may undergo hypertrophy which remains localized and after a time slowly regresses; if the condition spreads progressively it is known as a *keloid*. Whether these two conditions are basically the same or fundamentally different is still uncertain. Scar hypertrophy has been called "the plastic surgeon's nightmare." The keloid is a firm, smooth, pink, raised patch from which extend claw-like processes, and it may cover a considerable area (Fig. 39). It consists of very dense collagen, the bundles of which run parallel with the surface. It tends to recur when removed.

There seem to be two *etiological factors*, the one systemic, the other local. A *systemic* influence or individual sensitivity appears to be a prerequisite. This may be familial or racial. In one reported case over 400 keloids developed. Colored races are particularly liable to develop keloids. Indeed they capi-

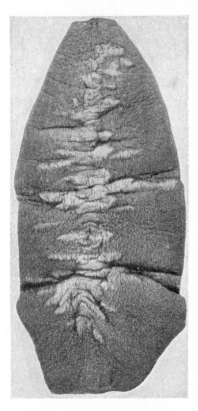

Fig. 39.—Keloid; excessive scar formation. (Boyd, *Pathology for the Surgeon*, courtesy of W. B. Saunders Company.)

talize on this trait in producing "ornamental keloids" by rubbing foreign material into skin incisions, by this means adding appreciably to their marriage value. Scar hypertrophy is commoner in women, and may occur as the result of pregnancy, suggesting the possible action of steroid hormones.

Local factors are more difficult to assess. The work of Glücksmann and his associates at Cambridge suggests that scar hypertrophy and scar keloids are due, at least in many instances, to a spreading proliferative inflammatory process elicited in sensitive persons by various particles acting as foreign bodies. In this view keloids should not be regarded as autonomous and neoplastic in nature, but rather as a peculiar type of foreign body granuloma. In 45 out of 50 cases of scar hypertrophy Glücksmann found a foreign body reaction associated with dislocated hairs, keratin débris, dust, cotton wool fibers,

etc. Keloids may follow burns, where there is dislocation of hair follicles, and tattooing with dyes containing sulfide of mercury. Similar reactions can be produced in rats by introducing grafts containing keratin into the dermis.

Healing of an Abscess.—All repair is fundamentally the same, whether in an open wound or in an abscess in the center of the kidney. If the infection is destroyed, attempts at repair begin. These are much more successful if the pus can discharge on to a surface, as into the pelvis of the kidney. If the cavity is small it becomes filled up first with granulation tissue, then with scar tissue. If the cavity is large it cannot be filled in, but a fibrous wall is built around it. Surgical drainage of the pus in the abscess is, of course, the first requisite for healing.

Organization of an Exudate on a Serous Membrane.—When a serous membrane such as the peritoneum is inflamed the endothelial covering is destroyed, and an exudate is formed on the surface consisting mainly of fibrin. This is invaded by fibroblasts and new capillaries, so that the exudate is replaced by granulation tissue, which in turn is fibrosed. The surface endothelium may again cover the fibrous patch, restoring the integrity of the membrane. Or two fibrinous surfaces, *e. g.*, two inflamed loops of bowel, may coalesce and become adherent. The *fibrinous adhesions* become *fibrous*, and although the sides of the adhesions are clothed with endothelium the integrity of the surface cannot be restored, and the adhesions are permanent. The fibrous bands contract, and may cause kinking and obstruction of the bowel.

Organization of a Thrombus.—A blood clot or thrombus in a vessel undergoes the same changes as an inflammatory exudate. It is invaded from the side of the vessel by fibroblasts and endothelial buds. New capillaries are formed, and a vascular connective tissue gradually takes the place of the clot. As cicatrization occurs the fibrous mass may shrink from the vessel wall, so that a space is formed which becomes lined by the endothelium of the vessel. In this way a certain flow of blood may be reëstablished through the vessel. Occasionally new channels are opened through the clot; these become lined with endothelium, and the clot is said to be *canalized*.

PARENCHYMAL REPAIR

The parenchymal structures differ enormously in their capacity for repair or regeneration. At one end of the line we have the liver, which can replace large portions of the organ when these are removed, whilst at the other end there are the nerve cells which are irreplaceable. In the latter case "the moving finger writes, and, having writ, moves on." It would almost seem as if this were the penalty of extreme differentiation. The nerve cell has one type of function to perform, motor, sensory, *etc.*, whereas the liver cell has such a bewildering variety of duties that it must be quickly replaced if destroyed. It has been found convenient to divide the parenchymatous cells into three main groups with differing powers of regeneration. To these three have been attached the rather unimaginative labels of labile, stable and permanent cells.

Labile Cells.—These cells line the various *epithelial and mucous surfaces* of the body, including the cells lining the ducts of glands. The cells may be squamous stratified, columnar or transitional in type. They are essentially expendable, being continually cast off and replaced by multiplication of the underlying cells. The situation is obviously ideal for complete repair (regeneration), provided that the underlying tissues have not been extensively damaged. No better example of this could be afforded than the desquamation and perfect replacement of the endometrium every month. Perhaps the erythrocytes should be included among the labile cells, because they are continually being destroyed and replaced in enormous numbers, and the same is true of the lymphocytes.

Stable Cells.—These epithelial cells constitute the various glands of the body. They retain the power of multiplication, but evidence of this power is rarely in evidence. In the case of the liver, an organ endowed with a remarkable capactiy for regeneration, it is said that if some 20,000 cells are examined, one may be found to show mitosis. These cells are not immortal, but replacement of

dying cells is so slow that it is not detected. Destruction of an area of the liver at once awakens the remaining cells to a high pitch of regenerative activity. If the hepatic cells alone are destroyed, as may happen in viral hepatitis, the architecture of the liver lobule is restored to perfection. Mitoses are seen in the epithelium of the smaller bile ducts, and buds of these cells grow outwards into the portal tracts, so that the liver cells of the lobule become linked up with their own excretory duct system. This is regeneration in perfection. When, however, the supporting stroma is also destroyed, although the hepatic cells are replaced the structure of the lobule is not restored, so that the cells are unable to establish connection with the bile ducts and fail to excrete bile. There is more or less formation of scar tissue, with resulting distortion of the architecture of the organ, a matter which will be discussed more in detail in connection with cirrhosis of the liver.

Permanent Cells.—These cells have lost the power of multiplication in postnatal life. When destroyed they cannot be replaced. Regeneration is therefore impossible. Repair of an injury is attempted by proliferation of the connective tissue of the part. This may serve to restore the structural integrity of the part, but the loss of function is permanent. The two important members of this group are the nerve cells and heart muscle cells.

Cells of the Central Nervous System when destroyed, as in poliomyelitis, are not replaced, nor can the loss of power be restored. In the case of the *peripheral nerves* a certain amount of regeneration is possible, provided the corresponding nerve cells remain intact. The distal part of the nerve degenerates, but the proximal portion of the axis cylinder may grow along the channel of the degenerated nerve, and once more resume function. The matter will be discussed more fully in relation to diseases of the nervous system.

Muscle Cells are in the same class as nerve cells and are unable to replace cells which may be killed, although this is more true of the cells of heart and plain muscle than of striated muscle. The muscle as a whole, however, has one great advantage over the nerve cells, for neighbouring cells hypertrophy to meet the need, and much of the lost power may be regained. The dead tissue

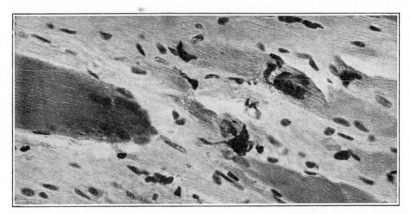

Fig. 40.—Regeneration of muscle showing syncytial masses of sarcolemma. × 300.

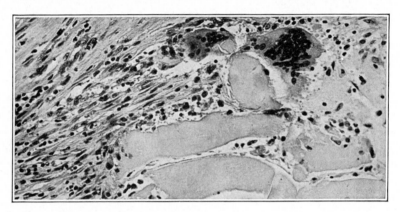

Fig. 41.—Necrotic muscle fibers being removed by giant cells and replaced by fibrous tissue. × 180.

is replaced by scar. The local destruction of myocardium is nearly always caused by ischemia due to coronary artery obstruction by thrombosis or arteriosclerosis. *Striated muscle* has greater reparative power. The extent of regeneration depends on the type of injury. In an incised wound with no loss of substance the nuclei of the sarcolemma proliferate and form multinucleated syncytial masses (Fig. 40), while the sarcous substance puts out bands which bridge the gap and eventually become striated. On the other hand when the muscle fibers have been destroyed the débris is removed by mononuclear phagocytes which may form foreign body giant cells, and the gap is closed by fibrous tissue (Fig. 41).

REPAIR IN DIFFERENT TISSUES

The healing of certain tissues and organs having been considered in some detail, we may glance briefly at the repair process in a number of other tissues. Greater detail will be found in the chapters devoted to the individual organs.

Epithelium as it occurs in the skin is repaired rapidly and completely. The more specialized epithelial skin structures such as hair follicles are not replaced. *Connective tissue* is completely replaced, as fibroblasts are the cells of connective tissue. *Elastic tissue* is replaced very slowly, but fairly completely. *Fat* destroyed in a wound is usually not reformed, but if the fat cells are only partially destroyed new cells smaller in size and containing fine droplets may be formed within them. *Cartilage* is so avascular that healing is very slow and imperfect. If the damage is at all extensive, the replacement is by scar tissue. New cartilage can be formed from the cells of the perichondrium, and small gaps may be filled in this way. *Bone* presents such an important example of healing that it is considered in connection with the repair of a fracture in Chapter 43. *Tendon* is very avascular so that healing is very slow, but it is remarkably complete, though it may take as long as two months. If the gap is small it is filled completely by tendon cells; if large, scar tissue has to be used. Sepsis is fatal to healing, because necrosis occurs so readily in the non-vascular tendon. Injury of a *serous membrane* is repaired by fibrous tissue which becomes covered by the endothelium of the membrane. A fibrinous exudate is formed on the surface at the site of injury, and the two surfaces tend to be united by adhesions which are at first fibrinous but soon become converted into fibrous tissue. A *mucous membrane* is repaired quickly and well. The surface epithelium is completely replaced, and simple tubular glands can be reformed from this epithelium, but complete restoration of such glands as those of the stomach only occurs when portions of the glands have escaped destruction. Healing in the *liver* has already been considered. In the *kidney* there is no regeneration of glomeruli although the tubular epithelium may be replaced; any extensive repair is confined to the formation of scar tissue.

A rather special form of repair is afforded by the case of *pneumococcal* (lobar) *pneumonia.* Here a lobe or an entire lung may be rendered completely solid by an acute inflammatory exudate which fills all the acini, yet it is the rule for the lung to be restored to normal in the course of a few weeks. There are two reasons for this remarkable and satisfactory outcome (1) the acute exudate of fibrin and polymorphonuclears is completely removed as the result of proteolytic digestion combined with coughing up of the material, this removal of the exudate being known as *resolution;* (2) the fact that the alveolar wall is not destroyed by the pneumococcal infection. Organization instead of resolution of the exudate may occasionally develop with disastrous results. This may be (1) the result of destruction of the alveolar walls in other types of bacterial pneumonia, or (2) it may follow pneumococcal pneumonia for no apparent reason.

When some organs, such as liver and pancreas, are injured by brief freezing, the necrotic tissue is removed quickly and completely and replaced by reparative tissue. With other tissues, such as testis and kidney, the process is very much slower (Cameron and Mehrotra). In the liver polymorphonuclear infiltration is marked in twelve hours, a wide layer of granulation tissue is formed in two days, and there is complete replacement by scar in five days. In the testis, on the other hand, although necrosis is complete in twelve hours, polymorphonuclears are few in number, there is little change during the next few days, and only a small amount of granulation tissue is formed by the end of five days. This variation in tissue response may be referred either to the injured cells or to the cell environment. If the necrotic piece of liver is inserted in the omentum or testis, replacement by fibrous tissue is not complete until the end of twenty-eight days, and when the piece of frozen testis is inserted in the liver the time of replacement is the same as in the testis itself. These experiments indicate that a change in environment prolongs the inflammatory and reparative reaction in the case of the one tissue but not of the other, so that the cells throughout the body should be thought of in terms of their immediate environment as well as their own characteristics. Cameron and Mehrotra suggest that for this dual and reciprocal relationship the term "field" is suitable. The result of cellular injury may vary with the environment, which is itself affected by the products of cell injury. This also suggests the question of the reaction to various kinds of injury in diseased tissues as opposed to the response in normal tissues, quite a different state of affairs. The relation of the cells of an epithelial tumor to the surrounding stroma is also another matter, yet related to the concept of field of influence.

A century and a half ago Virchow introduced us to the concept of cellular pathology, which marked the birth of modern pathology. Today we are beginning to realize that the ground substance with its mucopolysaccharides is the foster parent of the cellular parenchyma, determining the state of health or disease of the cells to a degree that no parent can ever attain.

REFERENCES

AREY, L. B.: Physiol. Rev., 1936, *16*, 327. (Wound healing).

CAMERON, G. R. and MEHROTRA, R. M. L.: J. Path. and Bact., 1953, *65*, 1. (Response to injury in different tissues.)

CARREL, A. and EBELING, A. H.: J. Exper. Med., 1926, *44*, 285 (Wound healing.)

CRANDON, J. H., LUND, C. C. and DILL, D. B.: New Eng. J. Med., 1940, *223*, 353. (Deficiency of vitamin C in healing.)

DUNPHY, J. E., Ann. Roy. Coll. Surg. Eng., 1960, *26*, 69.

DUNPHY, J. E. and UDUPA, K. N.: New Eng. J. Med., 1955, *253*, 847. (Wound healing.)

EDWARDS, L. C. and DUNPHY, J. E.: New Eng. J. Med., 1958, *259*, 224, 275. (Wound healing.)

GLÜCKSMANN, A.: Brit. J. Plastic Surg., 1951, *4*, 88. (Keloid formation.)

HADFIELD, G.: Ann. Roy. Coll. Surg. England, 1951, *9*, 397. (Granulation tissue.)

HARTWELL, S. W.: *The Mechanisms of Healing in Human Wounds*, Springfield, Ill, 1955.

LATTES, R., *et al.*: Am. J. Path., 1953, *29*, 1. (Effect of cortisone on healing.)

MOORE, F. D.: Can. Med. Ass. J., 1958, *78*, 85. (Systemic mediators of surgical injury.)

PEREZ-TAMAYO, R. and IHNEN, M.: Am. J. Path., 1953, *29*, 233. (Effect of protein deficiency in healing.)

PULLINGER, B. D. and FLOREY, H. W.: J. Path. and Bact., 1937, *45*, 157. (Formation of new lymphatics in granulation tissue.)

TAUBENHAUS, M. and AMRONIN, G. D.: Endocrinology, 1949, *44*, 359. (Cortisone and repair.)

TAYLOR, H. E. and SAUNDERS, A. M.: Am. J. Path., 1957, *33*, 525. (Formation of fibrous tissue from ground substance).

Chapter 4

Intercellular Substance Reactions

The Intercellular Substance
  Cells
  Fibers
  Ground Substance
    Hyaluronidase
    Ascorbic Acid
    Hormones
Infection

Localization of Infection
Spread of Infection
Recovery from Infection
The Diffuse Collagen Diseases
  Fibrinoid
Amyloidosis
  Staining Reactions
  Generalized Secondary
    Amyloidosis

Generalized Primary
  Amyloidosis
Localized Primary
  Amyloidosis
Pathogenesis
The Patient
Pseudoxanthoma Elasticum

In the opening chapter we have considered the cells of the body and some of the degenerative processes to which they are liable. We now turn to the intercellular substance, without which cell life would be impossible. This substance of course is not synonymous with connective tissue, which consists of cells (fibroblasts), fibers, and ground substance, the two latter comprising the intercellular substance.

The living body is composed of cells and fibers, just as a house is composed of bricks or stones and wood. But if a house consisted of nothing else, if it were lacking in cement and glue and nails it would be like a house of cards. The frail house in which we live depends for its welfare upon its cement and ground substance as well as on the bricks and stones, the cells and fibers, of which it is composed.

Cells.—While we are concerned in this place more particularly with ground substance and to some extent with fibers, it would be well to devote a moment to the cells of connective tissue, although many of these have been discussed in relation to the inflammatory reaction. Three of the principal cells are fibroblasts, histiocytes and plasma cells. The fibroblast is concerned with the formation of connective tissue, the histiocyte is a phagocyte, commonly called a macrophage, and the plasma cell is the producer of antibodies. The *fibroblasts* are the sites of the origin of collagen, the building blocks being manufactured in these cells, and then liberated to the extracellular compartment, where the molecules become oriented to form collagenous fibrils.

Macrophages have been discussed in connection with inflammation. *Plasma cells* will be considered in the next chapter which deals with the mechanism of immunity. *Mast cells* are characterized by their cytoplasmic granules containing acid mucopolysaccharides which take a metachromatic stain with aniline dyes such as toluidine blue. Taken together, the mast cells constitute a mass larger than the liver. They produce heparin, and they are rich in histamine and serotonin. The eosinophils and the mysterious lymphocytes have already been considered.

Fibers.—There are three main groups of cellular fibers: (1) dense bundles of collagen fibers, (2) a fine network of reticular fibers which require silver staining for their demonstration, and (3) elastic fibers. In the present discussion we shall confine ourselves to the first group. Collagen fibers consist of the protein collagen, and are characterized by their toughness. Tough meat has an overabundance of collagen, which can be softened by prolonged boiling, thus converting the collagen into gelatin by hydration. With the electron microscope it can be seen that collagen fibers are really composed of fine cross-striated fibrils bound together by cement substance, the fibers themselves being connected by this type of ground substance into bundles. In the group of conditions to be considered later in this chapter under the heading of the collagen diseases, we shall see that loosening and solution of this glue marks the beginning of the degrading and downfall of the fibers themselves.

Ground Substance.—The ground substance of connective tissue is an amorphous mucoid gel-like material which is not apparent with ordinary stains, but may show metachromasia with appropriate stains. It is a material of amazing chemical complexity and biological versatility. Ground substance is composed of *acid mucopolysaccharides* (hyaluronic acid and chondroitin sulfates in varying proportions) bound to *protein*. Proteins containing less than 4 per cent carbohydrate are known as *glycoproteins* and those containing more than 4 per cent as *mucoproteins*. The degree of polymerization naturally affects the consistency. The long-chained polymers ordinarily give it a gel-like consistency, but if depolymerization occurs the gel becomes more fluid. The principal mucopolysaccharides are (1) hyaluronic acid, so named because it was first obtained from the hyaloid or vitreous humor of the eye, and (2) chondroitin sulfuric acid, which derives its name from the fact that it is abundant in cartilage, to the cement of which it imparts a characteristic hardness. The sulfated form shows marked *metachromasia* with certain basic dyes such as toluidin blue. Metachromatic staining was indeed the first histochemical method for demonstrating the ground substance. Newer methods of staining acid mucopolysaccharides are alcian blue and colloidal iron.

This ubiquitous material is not a mere glue or filler-in. It may be non-living, but it is not inert. Through it has to pass the nutrient material from capillaries to parenchymatous cells, as well as metabolites passing in the reverse direction. When it is remembered that 7000 liters of fluid a day pass from the vascular bed to the extravascular space through this filtration barrier, its importance for the preservation of cell health becomes apparent. Interference with this transport leads to depression of cellular respiration, with, it may be, necrosis and ultimate sclerosis. It is in the ground substance that the inflammatory process takes place, it forms a medium or an obstacle to the passage of invading microorganisms and cancer cells, and it appears to be a principal site of antigen-antibody reaction. Indeed it is not too much to say that the concept of a cell is not complete without a consideration of the all-embracing ground substance.

The ground substance appears to be formed by fibroblasts, although Scandinavian workers favor an origin from mast cells. The fibroblasts are believed to secrete a procollagen into the ground substance, where the acid mucopolysaccharides provide a medium for the conversion of this soluble precursor into insoluble collagen fibers bound together into tough bundles by cement. Ascorbic acid or vitamin C is necessary for this reaction, assisting in the polymerization of the mucopolysaccharides. In the absence of ascorbic acid the ground substance and collagen are not properly formed, and this is the basis of the disease, scurvy.

Regeneration and repair of connective tissue is initiated by the formation of ground substance. There is first mucinous organization of an edema fluid. The early dominant role is played by hyaluronic acid, but after a few days the content of chondroitin sulfate increases. These mucopolysaccharides stimulate the deposition of fibrils, and this is followed by fibrous organization.

The health of the ground substance and collagen fibers depends on the regulating action of enzymes, vitamins and hormones.

Hyaluronidase.—This enzyme degrades hyaluronic acid and chondroitin sulfuric acid, depolymerizing the long-chain molecules. As it breaks down the ground substance barrier and reduces its viscosity it is known as the *spreading factor*. It was first isolated from the testis, then from the ciliary body of the eye. It is now known to be produced by bacteria with an ability to spread readily through the tissue, such as hemolytic streptococci and Cl. welchii. Certain types of cancer cells produce the enzyme, and this may facilitate their spread. There appears to be more than one variety of the enzyme. Thus chondroitin sulfuric acid is hydrolyzed by testicular hyaluronidase, but not by pneumococcal hyaluronidase, whilst collagenase, a hyaluronidase produced by Cl. welchii, dissolves the mucopolysaccharides of ground substance, basement membrane, and collagen fibers. *Antihyaluronidase* is an inhibitor of the enzyme. It may be present in specific or nonspecific form. The specific antihyaluronidases are antibodies which reside in gamma globulin, and are increased in rheumatic fever. The nonspecific anti-enzymes are raised in the acute stage of most of the collagen diseases. It is evident that the health of the ground substance will depend on the balance between the activity of the enzyme and the anti-enzyme.

Ascorbic Acid.—Reference has already been made to the part played by ascorbic acid or vitamin C in the formation of collagen. In the complete absence of this vitamin no collagen is laid down. The fibroblasts show fatty degeneration and reduction in phosphatase activity. There is failure in the production of acid mucopolysaccharides. The activity of this vitamin is closely related to the adrenal cortical hormones, stress and ACTH releasing ascorbic acid from the adrenals.

Hormones.—As might be expected, the ground substance is under the influence of various hormones. The lack of the *thyroid hormone* is responsible for the condition known as myxedema, in which there is marked softening and increase of the ground substance. *Testosterone* has the same effect, so also do the *estrogens*, as evidenced by changes in the sex skin of our cousin, the monkey. The *gonadotropins* have the opposite effect, depolymerizing the hyaluronic acid, and increasing the permeability of the ground substance.

It is evident that the ground substance is in a constant state of flux through removal and replacement by virtue of depolymerization and the reverse. *Ageing* produces a natural effect. Just as a house does not last forever, so the passing years bring a slow but inevitable change in the ground substance. From the abundant jelly-like condition of the fetus, there is a gradual building up of the fibrous elements, until the dessicated state of old age is reached.

An interesting example of the interrelationship between structure and ground substance is provided by the effect of *papain* on the elastic cartilage of the rabbit's ear (Thomas). When this enzyme is injected intravenously there is a rapid collapse of the animal's normally upright ears. This is associated with a liberation of the sulfated polysaccharide chondroitin sulfate from the cartilaginous matrix into the perichondrial spaces and lymph vessels (Spicer and Bryant).

6

One hundred years ago (1858) Virchow introduced us to the concept of cellular pathology, which marked the birth of modern pathology. Today we are beginning to realize that the ground substance with its mucopolysaccharides is the foster parent of the cellular parenchyma, determining the state of health or disease to a degree which no parent could ever approach.

INFECTION

It is evident from what has been said that the state of the ground substance, depending as it does on a delicate balance between enzyme and substrate, a balance influenced by many factors, will vary depending on age, hormonal stimulation or deprivation, and other factors. When depolymerization occurs the linkage of the polymers is broken, the viscidity reduced, and the permeability increased with loss of metachromasia. The permeability of the ground substance may be a deciding factor in the *spread of infection*. If bacteria of low virulence are unable to spread in the skin owing to an increase in the gel-like state at adolescence, they may multiply locally and give rise to the lesions of acne. Bacteria such as certain strains of hemolytic streptococci and Cl. welchii which produce much hyaluronidase might be expected to spread widely, as indeed they do.

Localization of Infection.—Once infection has occurred, its localization depends on a number of factors. When the organisms have entered the body, as through a wound in the skin, they may be held more or less *in situ* or they may drift through the ground substance with amazing rapidity. It is evident that the consequences to the patient will be entirely different in the two cases. Local fixation is seen in a striking form in an animal which has been actively immunized, and of course even more so in an animal which is naturally immune. When tubercle bacilli are injected into the skin of a normal animal they spread from the site of inoculation in the course of an hour, so that excision of the area after that time fails to save the animal, and when placed in the peritoneal cavity they are found in the regional lymph nodes in the course of five minutes. If the animal has previously been immunized, the bacilli remain, for a time at least, at the site of inoculation.

The use of small numbers of washed bacteria more closely resembles the primary lodgment of bacteria in natural infection. In a study of 9 different bacterial infections in the skin of the guinea pig the maximum death rate of injected bacteria occurred during the first two hours of infection, and after five hours most of the reactions determining the ultimate size of the lesions had occurred (Miles, Miles and Burke). During the first two hours of this "decisive period" macroscopic signs of inflammation were negligible; they did not become obvious until the third or fourth hour, and were not fully developed for several more hours. In these experiments it may be noted that there was no thrombosis in the blood vessels or lymphatics in the first five hours, although an increase of capillary permeability and endothelial stickiness was evident within half an hour. An infection with living bacteria will be limited and localized only if the bacteria are prevented from escaping and are killed on the spot. This is done by phagocytes and by destructive antibody which may be generated locally and possibly rapidly.

Menkin is of the opinion that the local fixation is due to the formation of a fibrinous network both in the lymphatics and the tissues, although many lymphatics still remain open so that the lymph flow from the part may be accelerated, as Drinker has demonstrated. The network of fibrin is abundant in staphylococcal infection, scanty or absent in streptococcal infection, thus perhaps accounting for the localized character of the former and the spreading character of the latter.

On the other hand Miles and Miles showed by means of micro-injection of the lymphatic plexus with dyes and opaque inks that, whilst thrombosis of blood and lymphatic vessels together with coagulation necrosis of the extravascular tissues undoubtedly hinder the spread of infection, this coagulation and necrosis commonly occur only in the center of an inflammatory focus, so that there is no blockade to the more peripheral lymphatic channels. In many cases the area of obstruction involves only 10 per cent of the total area of pronounced inflammation. Only

lymphatic channels traversing lesions undergoing coagulation necrosis were blocked. In mature staphylococcal abscesses of the skin living staphylococci were demonstrated well outside the central area of lymphatic occlusion. Finally, as we have already seen, no evidence of lymphatic occlusion was observed until after the end of five hours, that is to say the period during which the general spread of the infection is largely determined.

The beautiful experiments of Rich are of particular interest in connection with the localization of infection. Working with the pneumococcus, an organism which rapidly spreads through the tissues of the rabbit and kills it in from twenty-four to thirty-six hours, he compared the local lesions produced by inoculation of normal animals and of animals which had been rendered immune but not allergic to the pneumococcus. In the normal animal the organisms at once began to drift through the ground substance as each one divided into two and the pair separated, while in the immunized animal they rapidly clumped together and remained *in situ*, as if glued to the part. The process is one of agglutination, an increase of stickiness, as a result of which the bacteria adhere to one another and to the tissues with which they come in contact. Large clumps were formed in the course of thirty minutes, but at that time there was no inflammatory exudate, no fibrin formation.

So far we have discussed the mechanism by which bacteria which gain entrance to the tissues are held locally and prevented from setting up a general blood infection. Now we may turn to the converse of this question. When organisms are circulating in the blood their localization in the tissues depends largely on the permeability of the capillaries, which in turn is governed by such a factor as *trauma*, causing the liberation of histamine and resulting local capillary paralysis with increased permeability. When trypan blue is injected intraperitoneally in rats, and the animals are then struck on the head repeatedly, the dye is found to be localized in the brain. When the dye is injected intravenously and a hot-water bag is applied to the abdomen, the dye will stain not only the abdominal wall but also the subjacent coils of bowel. As the result of a similar mechan-

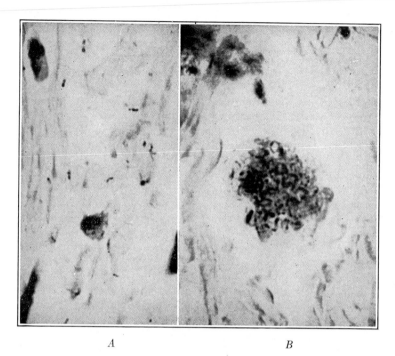

A   *B*

Fig. 42.—*A*, Site of infection in non-immune rabbit four hours after injection of pneumococci; cocci drifting through the tissue; *B*, the same in an immune rabbit four hours after injection; the proliferating cocci are clumped together. (Rich, Bull. Johns Hopkins Hospital.)

ism, bacteria circulating in the blood will tend to become localized at the site of injury. Should hemorrhage have occurred, the bacteria will leave the blood stream still more readily. A common clinical example is the relation of trauma to acute osteomyelitis, that is to say, inflammation of bone.

Bacterial invasion usually produces a local lesion at the site of entry, but there may be no indication of a lesion to the naked eye. Tubercle bacilli when placed in the eye may cause enlargement of the cervical lymph nodes with no disturbance in the eye. The same bacilli may pass through the wall of the bowel and infect the mesenteric lymph nodes. An unrecognizable lesion of the finger may give rise to fatal streptococcal blood poisoning. Even in these instances, however, microscopic examination will show some change in the tissue.

An even more rapid spread may occur along the lymphatics, and lymph nodes at a distance may be infected in a few hours. The microörganisms may be arrested and destroyed in the lymph nodes; they may

cause suppuration and breaking-down of the nodes, or they may pass through the nodes and enter the blood stream. The infection then becomes a general blood infection.

We have already seen that the invasiveness of bacterial infection depends partly on the permeability of the ground substance, partly on the spreading factor, hyaluronidase, which Duran-Reynals showed can be extracted from invasive strains of staphylococci as well as streptococci and other microörganisms. Non-invasive strains of the same species of staphylococci and streptococci do not contain the spreading factor, so that the long chains of hyaluronic acid are not depolymerized, and the barrier to the spread of infection remains intact.

The common result of infection is *local inflammation.* This may be acute, as in the case of the pyogenic bacteria, or the reaction may be chronic in type, as in tuberculosis and syphilis. The microörganisms may be killed by the inflammatory leukocytes, so that the infection ceases there and then. Sometimes the infection becomes quiescent but does not die out, and may at any time re-awaken into activity; a chronic abscess of bone or a quiescent tuberculous lesion in the lung is a sleeping volcano of this kind.

Spread of Infection.—Instead of remaining localized and giving rise to an abscess, the infection may spread. Streptococcal infections show a marked tendency to spread, and the most virulent strains may spread at an appalling speed. When the first natural barrier of defence, namely the hyaluronic acid of the ground substance, is broken down by hyaluronidase, the offensive weapon of the microörganisms, a spreading *cellulitis* is the result. An even more rapid spread may occur along the lymphatics, and lymph nodes at a distance may be infected in a few hours. The microörganisms may be arrested and destroyed in the lymph nodes; they may cause suppuration and breaking-down of the nodes, or they may pass through the nodes and enter the blood stream. The infection then becomes a general blood infection.

Septicemia is a commonly used term, but it is most difficult to define. When microörganisms circulate in the blood stream the patient has a *bacteremia*. This does not necessarily mean that he is ill. It is probable that bacteria continually gain access to the blood from the mouth and through the intestinal wall, but the life of these bacteria is short. When bacteria are injected into the subcutaneous tissue of an animal they can be found within a few minutes in the liver, heart, and lungs, but they soon disappear. It is probable that in all infections a bacteremia occurs at some stage. In typhoid fever the blood is flooded with bacilli at the beginning of the illness and the same is true of lobar pneumonia. To none of these conditions is the term septicemia applied. Septicemia is a clinical rather than a pathological conception. In addition to the presence of a bacteremia, the patient manifests symptoms which are known as septicemia, such as high fever, chills, and petechial hemorrhages in the skin. The prognosis at once becomes much more serious. Microörganisms are present in the blood in large numbers. They are readily demonstrated by blood culture, and when the infection is very heavy they can be seen in blood smears, as in some cases of streptococcal and meningococcal septice-

mia. Their great numbers may be due partly to multiplication in the blood, but mainly to a continual pouring of bacteria into the blood stream from some focus of infection. Good examples are the heavily infected vegetations on the heart valves in acute endocarditis, the thrombosed open blood sinuses of the septic puerperal uterus, and the bacteria-laden bone-marrow of acute osteomyelitis. When the focus is removed or even drained, the bacteria may rapidly disappear from the blood stream. The picture which has just been painted was of course very much more common and important before the days of modern chemotherapy and antibiotics.

Pyemia is one step further in the septicemic process. Clumps of bacteria lodge in the tissues and set up secondary abscesses in the kidney, liver, myocardium, skin, *etc.* (Fig. 43). The condition is usually caused by thrombi infected with pyogenic bacteria breaking up and being discharged into the circulation, only to be arrested when they reach the capillaries of the lungs, the renal glomeruli, and so on.

Toxemia connotes changes in the parenchymatous cells caused by toxins without the bacteria which produced these toxins entering the blood stream or necessarily being present at the site of damage. Diphtheria is an excellent example. Here the bacteria remain in the mucous membrane of the throat, but profound toxemic changes are found in the heart, liver, and kidneys. These changes are degenerative in character, ranging from cloudy swelling and fatty degeneration to necrosis and disintegration of the cells, processes which have been described in the opening chapter. In toxemias of long duration amyloid degeneration may develop.

Recovery From Infection.—Recovery from infection is so common that it is taken for granted and never excites wonder. It is none the less remarkable. When pathogenic bacteria enter the body they find ideal culture conditions both for food and incubation. They multiply exceedingly and may bring the patient to death's door, yet recovery is the rule. Apart from the action of phagocytes which has already been studied, the body responds to infection by producing

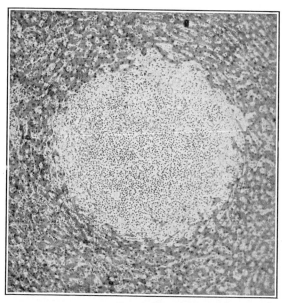

Fig. 43.—Pyemic abscess in liver. × 200.

protective substance antagonistic to the invader and known as antibodies. These will be considered in detail in the section on Immunity.

Antibodies are of many varieties, but those concerned in recovery from infection fall into two main groups: (1) Antitoxic antibodies or antitoxins which act against the bacterial toxins, and (2) antibacterial antibodies which act against the bacteria themselves, often bringing about their destruction (bacteriolysis). A few bacteria, e.g., the bacilli of diphtheria and tetanus, produce an extracellular toxin or exotoxin which circulates in the blood. Against such an exotoxin a specific antitoxin is produced, which will neutralize some or all of the toxin. With most bacteria, e.g., Bacillus typhosus, the toxin is intracellular, an endotoxin, which is only liberated when the bacterial bodies are broken down. In such a case the antibodies are mainly antibacterial in nature, leading to destruction of the microörganisms; no doubt some antitoxins are also produced, though difficult to demonstrate.

Some of the principal symptoms of infectious disease are due to toxins, both exotoxins and endotoxins. This toxemia is combatted by antitoxins. Recovery from infection, on the other hand, is due mainly to antibacterial antibodies. Thus in scarlet fever the general toxemia is due to action of toxins, which are neutralized by antitoxins, but the pyogenic effects are due to the presence of the streptococci, against which antibacterial antibodies are produced. Antitoxic immunity must be distinguished from antibacterial immunity. A person may have no diphtheria antitoxin in his blood, and yet may resist infection from diphtheria by virtue of the presence of antibacterial antibodies. Antitoxic immunity develops slowly, and the antitoxins may continue to be produced after the patient has made a complete recovery.

Many infectious diseases are self-limited in their course. Pneumonia usually lasts about eight days, and typhoid fever about three weeks. The mode of recovery in these two diseases differs markedly. In the classical case of untreated pneumonia the fever ends abruptly, signs of toxemia disappear, and the patient makes a sudden passage from a grave condition to one of comparative safety. This is recovery by crisis, and is not due to destruction of the pneumococci, for they disappear from the blood some days previously. There must be a sudden detoxication; the equilibrium of the toxin-antitoxin system is apparently governed by the laws of mass action, so that the end-result is abrupt, a crisis. In typhoid, on the other hand, the fever drops day by day, and it may be a week before the temperature reaches normal. This is recovery by *lysis*, and it is evident that the biochemical change involved must be of a different order. As to the nature of that difference we are completely in the dark.

The chronic infectious diseases are not self-limited. A balance is struck between the attack and the defense, and the defense slowly gains or slowly loses; there is no sudden change. The invader may live in a state of equilibrium or symbiosis with the host, causing little or no evidence of disease. This may occur in tuberculosis and syphilis, and probably in several of the virus diseases. Such a patient cannot be reinfected as long as the microörganisms remain alive. He enjoys what may be called a symbiotic immunity.

An acute bacterial infection usually terminates in one of two ways. The infection may triumph and the patient dies, or the patient may recover and the microörganisms are destroyed. There is a *third possibility*, for the patient may recover, but continue to harbor the organisms in his body. Such a person is called a *carrier*. He is a constant though usually unconscious source of danger. Examples of this condition are provided by typhoid, diphtheria, and meningococcal infections. A person may be a carrier, but may be unaware that he has ever suffered from the disease, for the original attack may have been too slight to be diagnosed. A diphtheria carrier may never have been truly infected; simple contact with a diphtheria patient may be sufficient. In epidemics of meningococcal meningitis and poliomyelitis a carrier epidemic accompanies the disease epidemic and greatly exceeds it in extent.

THE DIFFUSE COLLAGEN DISEASES

From the days of Morgagni we have been accustomed to think of disease in terms of organ pathology; we speak of tuberculosis of the lung or cancer of the breast. The cellular pathology of Virchow, as Duff points out in his admirable review, supplemented but did not supplant the concept of organ pathology. Rheumatic fever is a disease of the fibrous connective tissue or collagen, whether it occurs in the heart, arteries, joints, skin, serous membranes or internal organs. It was in 1941 that Klemperer and his associates pointed out that the common denominator of the multiform lesions of disseminated lupus erythematosus was degeneration of the collagenous connective tissue in many organs, and that the same common denominator was present in polyarteritis nodosa, rheumatic fever, rheumatoid arthritis, serum sickness, diffuse scleroderma and dermatomyositis. These constitute the group of what is now known as the diffuse collagen diseases, or, to use Rich's more accurate expression, the collagen-vascular diseases. The term diffuse signifies the wide distribution of the lesions, which themselves tend to be focal in character. The name can readily be criticized. If we spoke of necrosis as cellular disease it would hardly be satisfying. Nevertheless the name is convenient and is here to stay. Some writers have included other diseases in this group, but if it becomes a wastepaper basket for conditions that are little understood the concept will lose its value.

Fibrinoid.—The most characteristic lesion in the diffuse collagen diseases is so-called *fibrinoid degeneration and necrosis* of connective tissue. The usual concept of this condition is that there are two components of the lesion, the first an increase and *swelling of the ground substance*, the second a loosening and *separation of the collagen bundles* which later undergo *disintegration* into granular material that finally merges with the swollen ground substance. Fibroblasts and elastic fibers share in the general downfall. The necrotic material stains bright red with eosin and reacts with the special stains for fibrin, hence the name fibrinoid necrosis or degeneration.

There is much controversy as to the nature of fibrinoid material, whether it represents degenerated collagen, altered ground substance, or simply fibrin deposited in the area. The fundamental lesion may be an alteration in the physical character (depolymerization) of the acid mucopolysaccharides of the ground substance with secondary changes in the fibers (Altshuler and Angevine). It is the

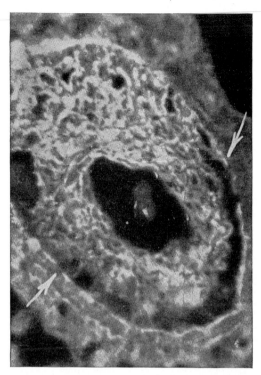

Fig. 44.—Fibrinoid in renal artery from poly-arteritis nodosa treated with fluorescent antibody method. (Gitlin, Craig and Janeway, courtesy of Am. Jour. Path.)

altered mucopolysaccharide which is responsible for the intensely positive reaction with the McManus periodic acid-Schiff (PAS) stain. On the other hand it is possible to show by the use of fluorescein-labelled rabbit anti-serum against human fibrin that the fibrinoid material found in the lesions associated with the collagen diseases is, at least in part, fibrin (Gitlin *et al.*). Even in sections which show no reaction with the conventional stains for fibrin, brilliant fluorescence is at once evident in these lesions, indicating an antigen-antibody reaction for fibrin (Fig. 44). The presence of fibrin shows that there has been a local conversion of fibrinogen into fibrin, and suggests a local increase in vascular permeability, together with an abnormal release of thromboplastic substances in the area as a result of local tissue deterioration or necrosis. For a detailed and well illustrated discussion on the origin and nature of fibrinoid the reader is referred to the paper by Movat and More

(1957), who consider on morphological and histochemical grounds that fibrinoid material represents the homogenization of a fibrinous exudate and is therefore of plasma protein origin, a view originally expressed by Marchand in 1896, and one with which I agree. Fibrin is not formed from acid mucopolysaccharides, because these are decreased in the early exudative lesions. They can only be demonstrated in advanced lesions with marked fibrinoid degeneration, because they are associated with repair, for they furnish the matrix for the formation of young connective tissue which is later converted into collagenous scar tissue. The formation of fibrinoid as a result of the inspissation of exudate plasma has been observed in the experimental animal in physical, chemical and irradiation injury (Movat *et al.*, 1960). The necrotic areas become invaded with fibroblasts which lay down dense collagen, and thus healing occurs. Even without necrosis there may be marked fibroblastic proliferation with eventual formation of scar tissue. There is a third component of the lesion, namely an inflammatory reaction to the primary connective tissue injury. In *polyarteritis nodosa* the *inflammatory reaction* is a striking feature, in *disseminated lupus erythematosus fibrinoid formation* is the dominant lesion, in *diffuse scleroderma*, as the name suggests, *collagenous sclerosis* overshadows the other components, whilst in *rheumatic fever all three* are well represented. "These differences, together with differences in the anatomical distribution of the lesions, permit the recognition of distinct disease entities on pathological as well as on clinical grounds. The same theme runs through all of them, but the variations on the theme are distinctive for each disease." (Duff).

The acute lesion is in the nature of an allergic inflammation with rapid and massive exudation of protein-rich fluid. This may go on to fibrinoid formation, or it may remain as a *mucoid edema*, which in turn may undergo *hyaline* transformation with eventual *sclerosis* or collagenization. This last phase is best seen in scleroderma, and to a lesser degree in the formation of *pannus* in rheumatoid arthritis.

Although the lesions described above justify the inclusion on morphological grounds of a number of different clinical entities in one common group, it does not follow that they have a common etiology. Identity of lesions is no proof of identity of etiology or pathogenesis. There is a tendency to regard the presence of fibrinoid necrosis as an indication of an antigen-antibody reaction allergic in nature in the tissue involved. This is too sweeping a generalization, for classical fibrinoid degeneration of the arterioles is seen in malignant hypertension, a condition in which allergy certainly plays no part. Collagen disease is not a disease entity "in spite of the impatience of clinical investigators and a peculiar worship of diagnostic terms which has led to an exaggerated popularity of the diagnosis collagen disease. There is a danger that it may become a catch-all term for maladies with puzzling clinical and anatomical features" (Klemperer). There is every reason to believe that the lesions of rheumatic fever and polyarteritis nodosa are manifestations of an antigen-antibody reaction in the target organs and therefore allergic in nature, but there is no *clinical* evidence to support the view that disseminated lupus erythematosus and scleroderma have an allergic basis, although the clinical and pathological manifestations of the former are similar to those of known hypersensitivity reactions. In the next chapter we shall discuss the pathogenesis of the collagen diseases and consider the much more convincing *experimental* evidence in support of the view that these conditions are in the nature of allergic reactions. In that place also we shall review some of the main features of the "big six," namely rheumatic fever and rheumatoid arthritis, polyarteritis nodosa and disseminated lupus erythematosus, scleroderma and dermatomyositis, a convenient grouping from the point of view of recall. A more detailed account of the lesions and the clinical features will be found in the chapters on the heart, arteries, joints, skin, *etc.*

AMYLOIDOSIS

The condition formerly known as amyloid degeneration and amyloid infiltration but better referred to as amyloidosis is one of the enigmas of pathology, and all the more fas-

cinating on that account. It was described by Rokitansky well over one hundred years, and first named by Virchow under the mistaken belief that the material involved was starch (Gr. *amylon*, starch), because, like starch, it stained brown with iodine. The reasons for including the condition in this chapter will become apparent presently. We have retained the name, but it has become completely noncommittal and it indicates nothing as to the chemical nature of the material involved, differing in this respect entirely from such terms as fatty degeneration and glycogen infiltration. The material appears to be a *glycoprotein*, consisting mainly of protein, probably globulin, combined with a sulfated polysaccharide, which is not chondroitin sulfuric acid as used to be thought.

Amyloid is a homogenous, translucent, acidophilic material, resembling and easily mistaken for hyaline degeneration of connective tissue in sections stained with hematoxylin and eosin. Unlike fat and glycogen, amyloid does not collect within the cells but *in the ground substance* between the cells and fibers. When present in large amount the affected part is swollen, waxy in appearance, and of increased consistence.

Staining Reactions.—Amyloid can be stained, but unfortunately the staining does not have the invariable character of staining for fat or glycogen. Three methods are employed: (1) iodine, (2) methyl or cresyl violet, (3) congo red. *Iodine solution* produces a dark, mahogany brown color when poured over the cut surface of an organ. *Methyl violet* and *cresyl violet* which belong to the rosanilin group of basic dyes, give a metachromatic reaction, the amyloid material staining rose red whilst the surrounding tissue is colored blue. This metachromasia is the most reliable reaction for amyloid. *Congo red* produces a brilliant or salmon pink color. This dye stains amyloid in the living body. When it is injected intravenously into an animal in which amyloidosis has been produced experimentally, all the amyloid is found to be stained bright red at autopsy. This reaction with congo red is the basis of a valuable clinical test which will be referred to later. The periodic acid-Schiff method sometimes gives an intense positive red re-

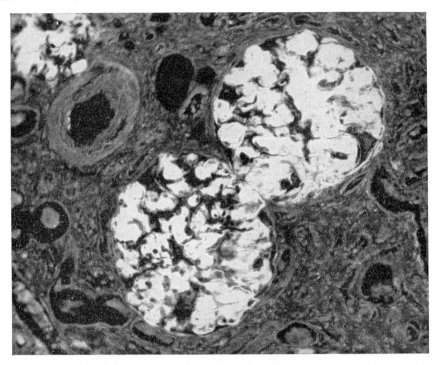

Fig. 45.—Amyloidosis of kidney. The amyloid glomeruli stained with thioflavine T fluoresce with ultraviolet light. (Kindness of Dr. Philip S. Vassar).

action, but often little or none. Van Gieson's stain, which colors amyloid a curious khaki shade, is especially useful when there is little or no metachromasia with the rosanilin dyes, and is of particular value for distinguishing amyloid from hyalinized collagenous tissue, for which it is easily mistaken. From this discussion it becomes apparent that no one staining method is entirely reliable. With ultraviolet light amyloid gives a specific bright yellow fluorescence, even when methyl violet and congo red staining are inconclusive (Vassar *et al.*) (Fig. 45). There are different groups of amyloidosis which react differently, and we have no assurance that the chemical composition of amyloid is identical in the various groups.

Classification.—There is no general agreement as to the best classification of the various manifestations of amyloidosis. The one suggested by Symmers in his excellent review of the subject will be followed here. Three main groups can be recognized: (1) generalized secondary amyloidosis; (2) generalized

primary amyloidosis; (3) localized amyloidosis. A fourth group, amyloidosis associated with myelomatosis or multiple myeloma, a plasma cell tumor of bone, is recognized as a separate group by many authors. It seems better to include these cases with our first group. In the first group there is a recognized predisposing disease to which the amyloidosis is regarded as secondary, whilst in the second group there is no recognized predisposing disease, so that the amyloidosis is referred to as primary or idiopathic. There is of course a cause, but we do not know what it is.

In the first group the *lesions* are generalized involving the parenchymatous organs, the order of involvement being spleen, kidneys, adrenals, liver, lymph nodes and pancreas. In the second group mesodermal structures of mesenchymatous origin, such as plain and skeletal muscle, the cardiovascular and alimentary systems and the skin, are mainly involved. The lesions of the so-called primary or idiopathic group are sometimes more localized than generalized, thus resembling the third group. The staining reactions for amyloid are much more variable and unreliable in the primary than in the secondary group. In the third or localized group the lesions tend to be confined to mesodermal structures. One cannot but agree with Symmers when he points out that the differences, both pathological and clinical, between the primary and secondary forms are not greater than the differences between individual cases in each category, from which we may conclude that all varieties are probably related to one fundamental disturbance, the nature of which is still unknown. In spite of these thoughts it will probably help the student if he considers the lesions of amyloidosis under the three main headings already indicated.

Generalized Secondary Amyloidosis.— This form is called secondary because it is associated with or follows some well developed disease. If we consider the subject of causation under the headings of etiology and pathogenesis we at once realize that we are unable to name any etiological agent, whilst as regards pathogenesis or method of production we are only now beginning to form a few vague concepts. A great change has come over the associated diseases in my own lifetime. When I was a student secondary amyloidosis was fairly common, being associated with long-continued sepsis, extensive tuberculosis, and ulcerating syphilitic lesions, all conditions characterized by marked loss of protein. This was even more true in the days of Rokitansky and Virchow. The triumphs of modern medicine and surgery have for the most part eliminated these conditions, so that the incidence of secondary amyloidosis has fallen sharply. Their place has been taken by a bewildering variety of conditions such as rheumatic and rheumatoid affections, ulcerative colitis, pyelonephritis, Hodgkin's disease, and multiple myeloma, in which there is a significant disturbance of protein metabolism or actual loss of protein. We shall return to the subject of pathogenesis a little later.

The *organs chiefly affected* are the liver, spleen, and kidney, the change usually beginning in the spleen. An additional group of three comprises the adrenals, the pancreas, and the intestinal mucous membrane. In addition to these almost every organ in the body may show some degree of change. It is the ground substance of the organs, particularly in the media of the arterioles, which is attacked. The affected tissues undergo a hyaline homogeneous swelling, so that the organ looks as if molten wax had been poured into the interstices and had hardened there. As a result of this swelling the parenchymatous cells become compressed and atrophic. The walls of the small vessels are thickened and their lumen may be greatly narrowed. The liver and spleen are enlarged, dense and elastic, resembling hard India rubber, the edges remaining hard and sharp in contrast to the rounded contours of the fatty liver. The cut surface is smooth, and has a translucent waxy appearance, so that the condition is sometimes known as waxy degeneration. In the kidney other degenerative changes complicate the picture, so that its gross appearance will be described separately.

The *liver* is enlarged, sometimes to a great degree. It seems to have been fixed in formalin, so firm is its consistence and so sharply marked its borders, but it is elastic rather than hard. The cut surface presents the usual translucent appearance. Microscopically, the change commences in the intermediate zone of the lobule. The amyloid appears between the sinus endothelium and the liver cells. This tissue becomes enormously swollen, so that on the one hand the liver cells are so compressed that they atrophy and may finally disappear, while on the other hand the sinusoids become narrowed. (Fig. 46).

The *spleen* is also enlarged, firm, elastic, and translucent. The amyloid may be distributed in two ways. In the common form it appears in the walls of the arteries in the Malpighian bodies (Fig. 47) and these lymphoid masses are gradually replaced by translucent masses of amyloid which are scattered over the surface like grains of boiled sago, so that this form is known as the *sago spleen*. (Fig. 48). In the rarer form, the *diffuse amyloid spleen*, the change affects the connective tissue of the venous sinuses and the reticulum of the pulp, so that the enlargement of the organ is much greater.

The *kidney* presents a special problem

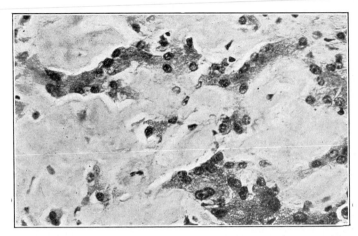

FIG. 46.—Amyloid degeneration of liver. The liver cells are greatly compressed by the abundant amyloid material. × 350.

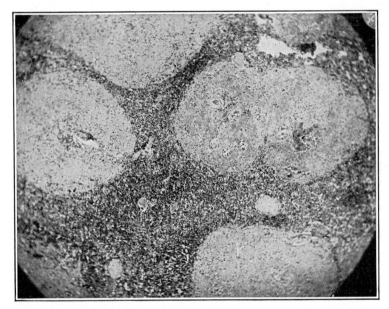

FIG. 47.—Sago spleen, showing large masses of amyloid. × 45.

because of secondary changes. It may be enlarged like the liver and spleen, or normal in size, or even contracted. Fatty degenerative changes in the tubules are common, and these interfere with the waxy look of the cortex, giving it a streaked or spotty appearance. Microscopically the change begins in the connective tissue of the vessels in the glomerular tufts, and also involves the walls of the arterioles and the connective tissue under the basement membrane of the collecting tubules. When a solution of iodine is poured over the cut surface the affected glomeruli stand out as little brown dots. The glomeruli become converted into masses of amyloid, as a result of which all circulation through the glomerulus may be stopped, but usually some patent vessels still remain. In cases in which there is a "nephrotic syndrome" with edema, albuminuria and hypercholesterolemia, there is a marked deposition of lipids from the blood stream, so that the

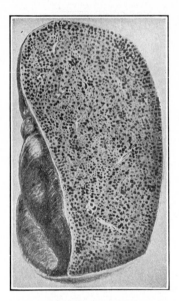

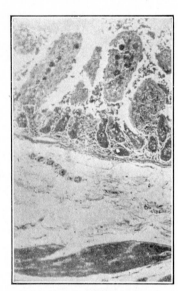

Fig. 48.—Amyloid spleen of the sago type. The numerous small areas of amyloid are stained darkly with iodine.

Fig. 49.—Amyloid degeneration of intestine. The villi are much enlarged by amyloid deposits. × 60.

condition has been called amyloid nephrosis. It is these tubular changes which are responsible for the gross appearance already described. The tubules may gradually atrophy and be replaced by fibrous tissues, which by shrinking produce a picture of a contracted kidney like that of chronic Bright's disease. In the earliest stages the patient may present the features of the condition which the clinician calls the nephrotic syndrome, whilst in the later stages the patient is likely to die of renal failure.

Many *other organs* may show the amyloid change. The adrenals may be converted into solid masses of amyloid so that they become considerably enlarged. In the intestine the change affects the connective tissue in the villi (Fig. 49), so that when treated with iodine the mucosa may have an appearance of brown velvet. The thyroid may be converted into an almost solid mass of amyloid. The heart may be the seat of extensive amyloid deposits between the muscle fibers. In addition to these principal sites, small deposits of amyloid may be found in almost any of the other organs. There may be widespread amyloidosis of the lymph nodes. In one obscure case of enlarged liver with palpable superficial lymph nodes I found

amyloid in an excised node, thereby enabling a correct diagnosis of amyloid degeneration of the liver to be made.

Generalized Primary Amyloidosis.—Here the amyloidosis is not preceded or accompanied by any predisposing disease, so that the condition is called idiopathic, which by derivation means "self-originated," but actually signifies without a known cause. As a rule the distribution is quite different from that of secondary amyloidosis in which the parenchymatous organs are involved. Here the lesions are in the mesodermal structures. The staining reactions are also usually anomalous. We have already seen, however, that there are exceptions to these generalizations, for in about 25 per cent of cases the distribution and staining character of the primary lesions are identical with those of the secondary group. It may be mentioned here that the amyloid lesions associated with multiple myeloma are of the primary type.

Heart.—The heart is most commonly involved, and death is usually due to cardiac failure. The myocardium presents translucent streaks or patches, nodules may be scattered throughout it, and sometimes the entire organ may be of an extraordinary waxen rigidity, as if it had been fixed in formalin. I have seen a case in which the heart weighed

775 gm., the wall of the left ventricle measured 30 mm., the valves were the seat of verrucose endocarditis, and pin-head translucent nodules were scattered under the endocardium and epicardium. In this case nearly every tissue and organ of the body were involved in amyloidosis. *Microscopically* the earliest lesions are minute deposits in the intercellular substance and on the cell membranes and reticulin fibers, leading to pressure atrophy and disappearance of the muscle cells.

Alimentary Tract.—The esophagus, stomach and intestine may be involved in the amyloid process. These lesions need not be described individually, as the student can provide these descriptions for himself, but it may be mentioned that gastric ulcers of the peptic ulcer type may develop. There are often widespread subserosal deposits with resulting adhesions. The *tongue* deserves special mention. *Macroglossia* (big tongue) may be a striking feature owing to deposits of amyloid between the muscle fibers, and in some cases the enlargement may be so great that the unhappy patient is not able to close his mouth. Macroglossia is sometimes seen in secondary amyloidosis.

Respiratory System.—Involvement of this system may dominate the entire clinical picture. The commonest lesions are in the *layrnx*, and these are also seen in the localized form of the disease. In other cases there are tumor-like masses in the *lungs*, readily seen in the X-ray picture, or there may be widespread involvement of the alvolar septa, with obstruction to the pulmonary circulation and right-sided heart failure.

Urinary System.—*Renal lesions* may resemble those of the secondary form, with amyloid casts in the tubules sometimes surrounded by multinucleated giant cells. The *ureters* may be converted into rigid tubes. In the *bladder* there may be tumor-like masses of amyloid.

Endocrine System.—As in the case of secondary amyloidosis there may be involvement of the adrenals, pituitary and thyroid.

Skeletal Muscles.—These may show widespread involvement, with great enlargement of the individual muscles.

Skin.—Amyloid masses in the skin may be the main feature in the clinical picture.

Nervous System.—The central nervous system provides a striking exception to the general involvement, probably because of the absence of mesodermal elements. The *peripheral nerves* are not infrequently involved, with accompanying neuritis symptoms (Chamers *et al.*).

Localized Primary Amyloidosis.—The rarest form of amyloidosis is that confined to a single organ or system. The sites for such localized lesions are (1) the upper respiratory tract, especially the larynx; (2) the lower respiratory tract; (3) the bladder; (4) the skin and mucous membranes of the orifices (mouth, vagina). The lesions are similar to those in generalized amyloidosis, but they must not be mistaken for hyalinized collagenous nodules, especially in the larynx. It is in this differentiation that the van Gieson stain is of greater value than the ordinary stains for amyloid. The lesions are usually tumor-like in character. In true localized amyloidosis no amyloid deposits are found in other organs.

Pathogenesis of Amyloidosis.—I have not used the term etiology in this discussion of causation, because we know nothing about an etiological agent in any of the three major forms. We can, however, hazard a guess as to the method of production of the lesions.

The early workers succeeded in producing amyloidosis in a variety of animals in a number of ways. This was done by injecting bacterial toxins over a number of months, by the subcutaneous injection of nutrose (sodium caseinate) into mice, even by feeding the animal on a diet rich in cheese. Horses injected with diphtheria toxin for the production of antitoxin often die from generalized amyloidosis.

These observations on the experimental animal do not throw much light on the disease in man, but they do serve to direct our thoughts towards the field of immunity with the formation of antibodies. At the present time this idea is receiving increasing support. "The view which is now most generally held is that amyloidosis is a manifestation of an immunological disturbance, with the deposition in prepared situations of amyloid, a substance of somewhat varied composition which may be the insoluble glycoprotein product of a local antigen-antibody reaction"

(Symmers). The polysaccharides and connective tissue of the ground substance as well as the serum globulins may play a part in this reaction, which serves to justify the inclusion of a discussion of amyloidosis in this chapter. The condition may be a manifestation of a hypersensitivity mechanism in which antibody is precipitated with polysaccharides of the ground substance. This would bring the formation of amyloid into line with that of fibrinoid. In fibrinoid degeneration the protein appears to come from the fibrinogen, as already suggested, whereas in amyloidosis it seems to be normal or abnormal globulin formed by normal, or more probably abnormal, plasma cells (Ehrich). As seen with the electron microscope amyloid seems to be fibrillar in structure, the fibrils appearing to originate in the cytoplasm of the cells. With the fluorescent antibody technique the amyloid deposits of secondary amyloidosis stain strongly for the corresponding gamma globulin but weakly for albumin, and the same is true of experimental casein amyloidosis in the rabbit. This may be contrasted with such a condition as acute appendicitis, where there is considerably more albumin than gamma globulin (Vazquez and Dixon). It is reasonable to suppose that in secondary amyloidosis associated with long-continued destruction of tissue there should be increased production of antibodies owing to the formation of autogenous antigens. In the primary form there may be a reaction between some component of the serum globulin and tissue elements in the mesoblastic structures, a reaction which may have a basis of autosensitization with the production of autoimmune bodies. Hyperglobulinemia is certainly a striking feature of some cases of generalized amyloidosis, being most marked in multiple myeloma, a tumor of plasma cells which are known to be a chief source of antibody formation. In other cases a transitory hyperglobulinemia may play a part, but be no longer present at the time the patient is examined. There is known to be an increase of serum globulin associated with the development of amyloidosis in horses used for the production of various antisera.

The Patient.—So far we have considered the disease process. The diagnosis of this process in the living patient is usually far from easy, because of the endless variety of symptoms, sometimes it is difficult and often impossible. It is obvious that the physician has a much better chance of arriving at a correct conclusion if the amyloidosis is of the secondary type. In the primary form the patient, usually a middle-aged man is likely to show the gradual onset of impaired function of the myocardium, kidneys or peripheral nerves. Three organs merit special mention, the kidney, the adrenals and the heart.

The *kidney* is very frequently involved in secondary amyloidosis. As already mentioned, the earlier stages are marked by the albuminuria and edema of the nephrotic syndrome, the passage of albumin from blood to urine being caused by the amyloid lesions of the glomerular filter, whilst the edema is due to the lower osmotic pressure of the plasma from the loss of protein. In the late stages destruction and atrophy of the kidney may give rise to hypertension and renal failure terminating in death. The *adrenals* are also frequently involved in the secondary form. In only occasional cases is the destruction sufficiently great to give the clinical picture of chronic adrenal insufficiency known as Addison's disease. The *heart* is the organ most often involved in primary generalized amyloidosis, particularly in men over fifty years of age. The condition should at least be considered in all cases of intractable congestive heart failure and obscure cardiomegaly without obvious cause and associated with nonspecific electrocardiographic changes.

Other clinical features which will be evident to the student from his consideration of the pathology are enlargement of the *tongue*, dyspnea (shortness of breath) and perhaps right-sided heart failure due to *pulmonary lesions*, diarrhea from involvement of the *intestine*, raised and indurated patches in the *skin*. The lymph nodes may be enlarged, and pain in the limbs due to involvement of the peripheral nerves (amyloid neuropathy) occurs in about 25 per cent of the primary cases. The presence of hyperglobulinemia may give a lead, and amyloid, generally of primary distribution, occurs in up to 30 per cent of cases of multiple mye-

AMYLOIDOSIS

A review of the principal sites of involvement in the different types of amyloidosis is given in the following table.

Major Groups	Principal Sites of Involvement
Generalized Secondary*	Parenchymatous organs (Spleen, kidneys, liver, adrenals, lymph nodes, pancreas)
Generalized Primary	Mesodermal structures of mesenchymatous origin (Heart, tongue, larynx, skeletal muscle, kidneys, intestine, skin)
Localized	Mesodermal structures (Larynx, bladder, lungs, skin, oral mucosa, vaginal mucosa).

*The amyloidosis associated with the various myelomatous disorders are included in this category.

loma. It has been said that amyloidosis, which used so often to be due to syphilis, has now supplanted syphilis as the great mimic of other diseases.

Biopsy may be of great value, especially in the primary form where diagnosis is often so difficult. The skin, tongue, gum or skeletal muscle may provide material of diagnostic value. All three types of staining already described must be used, because primary amyloid may be stained by one and not by the others. In the secondary form needle biopsy of the liver, spleen or kidney may be of value.

The *Congo red test* may prove of great assistance, but clinical suspicion of amyloidosis must of course be first aroused. A negative result is not significant because of the variability with which amyloid, particularly in the primary form, takes up the stain. The test depends on the affinity of amyloid deposits for the dye. A measured amount of Congo red solution proportioned to the patient's body weight is injected intravenously; one hour later a sample of blood is withdrawn and the serum tested for the presence of dye. The test is positive if almost all the dye has disappeared from the blood; in the absence of amyloid disease only 15 to 30 per cent disappears. The result will depend, of course, on the amount of amyloid. Large deposits such as occur in the liver will give a positive result, whereas the smaller deposits in the renal glomeruli are likely to prove negative.

Remissions apparently occur in some cases of secondary amyloidosis when the predisposing disease is cured or removed, the amyloid material being resorbed. They do not occur in the primary form, which kills the patient in around three years, although the time may be shorter or very much longer.

PSEUDOXANTHOMA ELASTICUM

An interesting but rare example of disturbance of intercellular tissue is pseudoxanthoma elasticum. This hereditary and familial condition is characterized, as it name suggests, by the presence of yellow papules and plaques in abnormally lax skin (neck, axilla, groin, antecubital and popliteal fossæ), and elastic tissue changes. As a matter of fact, there is difference of opinion as to whether the basic lesion is: (1) a degeneration of elastic tissue, or (2) a degeneration of connective tissue as a result of which it takes on the staining character of elastic tissue. It is a systemic condition, with special involvement of the skin and cardiovascular system, and associated with angioid streaks in the retina in about 50 per cent of cases (Robertson and Schroder). The *microscopic* condition has been described as *elastorrhexis*, the corium of the skin presenting great numbers of swollen, fragmented, curled fibers taking elastic tissue stains. The blood vessels, particularly those of the mesentery, share this degeneration of elastic-staining tissue, with secondary mucosal involvement of the gastrointestinal tract at any level. The chief *clinical* features are small yellow nodules in the skin giving a "plucked chicken" appearance, progressive amblyopia which may end in blindness, and gastrointestinal hemorrhage.

REFERENCES

ALTSHULER, C. H. and ANGEVINE, D. M.: Am. J. Path., 1949, *25*, 1061. (Pathogenesis of fibrinoid).

CHAMBERS, R. A., MEDD, W. E. and SPENCER, H.: Quart. J. Med., 1958, *27*, 207. (Amyloid neuropathy.)

DIXON, F. J.: Am. J. Clin. Path., 1955, *25*, 1182. (Sites of antigen-antibody reaction in hypersensitive states).

DUFF, G. L.: Can. Med. Ass. J., 1948, *58*, 317. (Diffuse collagen disease).

GITLIN, D., CRAIG, J. M. and JANEWAY, C. A.: Am. J. Path., 1957, *33*, 55. (Fibrinoid in collagen diseases.)

GODDARD, J. W.: Am. J. Path., 1947, *23*, 943. (Granuloma in focal anaphylactic inflammation).

KLEMPERER, P., POLLACK, A. D., and BAEHR, G.: Arch. Path., 1941, *32*, 569. J.A.M.A., 1942, *119*, 331. (Diffuse collagen disease).

MILES, A. A. and MILES, E. M.: J. Path. and Bact., 1958, *76*, 21. (Lymphatic obstruction in acute inflammation).

MOVAT, H. Z. and MORE, R. H.: Am. J. Clin. Path., 1957, *28*, 331. (Nature and origin of fibrinoid).

MOVAT, H. Z., MORE, R. H. and WOLOCHOW, D.: Brit. J. Exper. Path., 1960, *41*, 97. (Fibrinoid formation in various injuries of connective tissue.)

McMANUS, J. F. A.: *Connective Tissue in Health and Disease*, Ed. by Asboe-Hansen, Copenhagen, 1954.

ROBERTSON, M. G. and SCHRODER, J. S.: Am. J. Med., 1959, *27*, 433. (Pseudoxanthoma elasticum.)

SPICER, S. S. and BRYANT, J. H.: Am. J. Path., 1957, *33*, 1237: 1958, *34*, 61. (Effect of papain on chondroitin sulfate of cartilage.)

SYMMERS, W. ST. C.: J. Clin. Path., 1956, *9*, 187. (Primary amyloidosis).

THOMAS, L.: J. Exper. Med., 1956, *104*, 2 to 5. (Effect of papain on cartilage).

VASSAR, P. S. and CULLING, C. F. A.: Arch. Path., 1959, *68*, 487. (Fluorescent staining of amyloid).

Chapter 5

Immunity and Hypersensitivity

General Principles
ANTIGENS
ANTIBODIES
  Gamma Globulins
   Agammaglobulinemia
   Hypergammaglobulinemia
TISSUE IMMUNITY
Hypersensitivity
IMMEDIATE TYPE
  Anaphylactic Shock
  Serum Sickness
  Arthus Reaction
  Shwartzman Phenomenon

Atopy
DELAYED TYPE
CLINICAL FEATURES
HYPERSENSITIVITY LESIONS
Auto-Immunity
ACTIVELY ACQUIRED
  TOLERANCE
Auto-Immune Disease
BLOOD
  Acquired Hemolytic Anemia
  Idiopathic Hemorrhagic
   Purpura
ENDOCRINES

Hashimoto's Disease
Addison's Disease
CONNECTIVE TISSUE
  Systemic Lupus Erythematosus
  Rheumatoid Arthritis
OTHER DISEASES
  Ulcerative Colitis
  Chronic Hepatitis
  Multiple Sclerosis
MISCELLANEOUS LESIONS
Tissue Transplantation
CANCER

GENERAL PRINCIPLES

IT is not easy at the present time to give a concise definition of immunity. In its original legal sense it meant exemption from the need to pay certain taxes or perform certain duties. The early bacteriologists adopted it to signify resistance to infection. A person was immune because of a natural or acquired resistance. Very early in the course of evolution the struggle for survival became bitter and relentless, as it has continued to the present day. It was the universal law of eat or be eaten. Animals learned to protect themselves against external enemies by developing armor, spines or poison. But some discovered the gentle art of parasitism, by means of which they were saved the labor of seeking their own food from an outside world. Resistance to these invaders evolved as the result of the development of the mechanism of immunity.

Within recent years, our concept of immunity has widened its scope immeasurably. Considering immunity merely as a defense against infection, our thinking can be best summarized by two sentences from Burnet (1953). "In the broadest terms, the development of immunity is a process by which the body learns from experience of past infections to deal more efficiently with subsequent ones." "Antibody appears in the blood, but it is even more important that the antibody-producing cells are so modified that they can rapidly produce fresh supplies of antibody on renewed contact with the antigen."

Basically we may say that immunology depends on the recognition of differences in the chemical structure of substances. Moreover, the interaction of antibody with antigen, which constitutes the obvious feature of the defense mechanism, may occasionally result in a harmful or even fatal effect instead of a beneficial one, an illustration of the fact, of which we shall encounter all too many examples, that what is powerful for good can be potent for evil. The body may react in a certain way when exposed for the first time to foreign substances, but in a qualitatively different way when re-exposed. From the immunological point of view, the person has become a new man, although he does not know it. This change is expressed by the term *allergy*, which means altered energy (*allos*, other, and *ergon*, energy). It is also expressed, less accurately, by the word *hypersensitivity*, a term which has a quantitative connotation, whereas allergy indicates a qualitative change. The whole subject of immunology has been expanding in explosive fashion, and now includes such subjects as tissue and organ transplantation, the tagging of antigens and antibodies, thus tracing them to individual cells, and, above all, the concept of auto-immunity. This extraordinary expansion can be gathered from the volume of articles on the subject

7

in the current literature, and from the fact that the second edition of that mine of information, W. C. Boyd's *Fundamentals of Immunology*, published in 1947, contained 503 pages and no reference to auto-immunity, whereas the third edition in 1956 contains 776 pages and a chapter on auto-immunity with 111 references.

Reference has already been made to *natural* and *acquired immunity*. The difference between the two is more apparent than real. It is probable that natural immunity is in the main a result of minimal infections, not large enough to produce actual disease, but sufficient to stimulate the production of immune substances. In this way an immunity to diphtheria and other infections can gradually be built up, so that the immunity is really acquired. The infant has a certain degree of immunity transmitted from the mother *via* the placenta or the breast milk, but this is transient. When it passes away the child becomes highly susceptible to infection.

Species immunity is of a different nature. Some diseases such as gonorrhea and typhoid fever are peculiar to man, and have not been reproduced in animals. Other diseases, *e.g.*, chicken cholera, are limited to certain animals. It is a matter of chemical relationship between the tissues and the microorganisms. If there is no affinity between the infective agent and the cells of the body, the animal will possess perfect immunity against that particular infection. Tetanus toxin is extremely virulent for man; it unites firmly with his nerve cells. On the other hand, it is quite harmless to the hen, because it forms no union with these cells in the hen.

In *passive immunity* the tissues of the patient take no active part in the process. When an immune serum, *i.e.*, the serum of a highly immunized animal, is injected into the blood, the patient is immunized against that particular infection. The immunity is only temporary, passing off in a few weeks, for it is dependent only on the antibodies which have been injected, and the cells of the body have undergone no change. Its great value in practice depends on the fact that the immunity is immediate, whereas an active immunity takes time to be built up. The use of diphtheria antitoxin is the best example of the application of passive immunity to medicine, but passive immunity can be produced by antibacterial as well as antitoxic serum.

The *properdin system* appears to be an important element in natural immunity. Properdin is a serum macroglobulin, with a molecular weight eight times greater than that of gamma globulin. It acts only in conjunction with complement and magnesium, hence the term properdin system (Pillemer). It is intimately involved in the destruction of bacteria, the neutralization of viruses, and the lysis of red blood cells. The importance of the properdin system lies in its lack of specificity and therefore wide range of defense. Amongst laboratory animals the rat, which is remarkably resistant to infection, has the highest titer of properdin, whereas the guinea pig, notoriously susceptible to infection, has the lowest. Human serum is highly bactericidal to dysentery bacilli, but not if properdin is completely removed. Nor has properdin alone any bactericidal action; it must be combined with complement and magnesium.

The antibacterial properties of properdin are not due to specific antibodies. There is a marked depression of the properdin serum level in shock, viremia, bacteremia, surgical trauma, and total body radiation. The parenteral administration of zymosan, a polysaccharide isolated from yeast, which was at first used in isolating properdin from the serum, raises the serum level after an initial reduction, with a corresponding increase in resistance to pneumococci and other bacteria (Ross). Properdin can now be derived from serum by chemical methods not requiring the use of zymosan adsorption.

Antigens.—An antigen, as its name implies, is a substance, usually foreign in character and protein in structure, although sometimes a polysaccharide, which when introduced into the body excites the formation of neutralizing substances or antibodies. As Rich points out, the crucial test of whether a given effect on the tissues is actually the result of an antigen-antibody reaction depends upon the production of the effect by *passive transfer*, *i.e.* by introducing into a normal animal the antigen together with the corresponding antibody from a sensitized animal. The formation of anti-body occurs when the tissues recognize the material as foreign or "not-self," the reaction corresponding to a demonstration of nationalism or tribalism. We now recognize that the reaction is not confined to foreign material, but may under some circumstances be elicited by the cells of the body. This phenomenon, known as auto-immunity, has rapidly assumed outstanding importance, and is responsible for many of the so-called immunological diseases considered later in this chapter.

Antibodies.—The antibodies which provide the key to the complex problems of immunity are gamma globulins. The antibody molecule is synthesized from the amino-acid pool of the body by cells of the reticuloendothelial system. The saying that ignorance, however aptly veiled in an attractive terminology, remains ignorance, is particularly applicable to the science of immunology, but the following word picture drawn by Burnet has much to back it up. "The antibody-producing mechanism is initiated by the entry of the antigen into phagocytic cells of the reticuloendothelial system (macrophages). Antibody-producing units are transferred to reticulum cells or other relatively undifferentiated mesenchymal cells in the immediate vicinity of the macrophages. These cells multiply freely, and take on the staining qualities of plasma cells. They are responsible for the actual production of antibody during the peak phase of the response. The reticulum cells also give rise to lymphocytes which are probably responsible for the maintenance of low levels of antibody long after the antigenic stimulus." Antibody production runs parallel with the concentration of immature plasma cells in the tissue. The antibody gamma globulin is believed to be made by the endoplasmic reticulum of the plasma cells, which are therefore well named.

It is perhaps somewhat surprising that antibodies may persist in the blood and that the cell may retain its ability to produce antibody long after the infecting organism (antigen) has disappeared. So long as the antigen is also present in the cells, a fresh dose of antigen produces only a minor effect. But if the original antigen has disappeared, the persisting antibody may react violently with the new antigen, particularly if the antibodies in the blood have disappeared.

If the host has previously been exposed to the antigen, there is a specific response of eosinophils. It has been suggested that the antigen induces specific enzyme formation in the eosinophil cells, which are then subjected to phagocytosis by reticuloendothelial cells, and that these in turn utilize the specific enzymes from the ingested eosinophils to form antibodies (Speirs). While antibody is being formed by the ribonucleic acid of the cytoplasm of the reticuloendothelial cells, these cells become more and more readily stained with pyronin and are transformed into mature plasma cells.

Labelled antibody is a development which has provided the basis for the formulation of such concepts as those which have just been outlined. Dye molecules can be chemically linked with antibody globulin molecules without impairing the capacity of the latter to reaction with antigen, as was first clearly demonstrated by Marrack in 1934. The most useful method depends on the use of the *fluorescent-labelled antibody* technique of Coons and his associates. By this method the globulin fraction of a hyperimmune serum is conjugated with fluorescein isocyanate. The labelled antibody combines with the appropriate antigen, and the antigen-antibody reaction can be seen and photographed because of the fluorescence. The formation of antibody in plasma cells can be demonstrated by treating frozen sections with antigen, and then rendering the antigen-antibody so formed fluorescent by further treatment with fluorescent antibody. It is obvious that such a method is equally valuable for demonstrating the site of the antigen with which the labelled antibody reacts, and by this means we can photograph bacteria which are unrecognizable by ordinary methods of staining. With the use of labelled rabbit antibodies against rat kidney it is possible to see that the reaction is localized not merely in the glomeruli of the rat but with maximum concentration in the glomerular basement membrane (Mellors, *et al.*) (Fig. 50). Fluorescence labelling has also been used in the investigation of tumors,

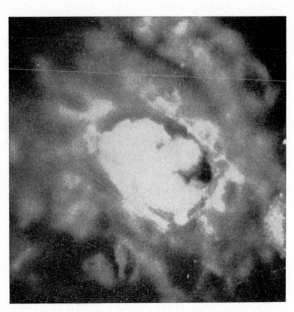

Fig. 50.—Kidney of rabbit which received injections of bovine gamma globulin and developed glomeru-lonephritis. The glomeruli in sections treated with the fluor (fluorescein-labeled chicken antisera to rabbit globulin) show intense fluorescence which is due to the glomerular localization of antibodies. (Flurorescence photomicrograph, × 200) (Mellors, Siegel and Pressman, courtesy of Laboratory Investigation.)

a subject which will be discussed in the chapter on Neoplasia.

Antigen can also be labelled, but by a very different technique. It is made radio-active by being linked with the radioisotope I^{131}, and the rate of loss of radioactivity of the plasma indicates the degree to which the antigen is being incorporated in the tissue.

Gamma Globulins.—The gamma globulins are so important a source of antibodies that a few words of general discussion may not be out of order in this place. Electro-phoresis separates the serum proteins into 4 major fractions, namely albumin and 3 distinct globulins. The gamma globulins migrate more slowly during electrophoresis, because they have a very low negative charge, and therefore stay close to the point of origin. The gamma globulins form a heterogeneous family as shown by immuno-electrophoretic analysis, hence the wide variety of specific antibodies which they represent (Gitlin *et al.*). Most of the anti-bacterial, antiviral, and antitoxic antibodies in the serum migrate slowly as gamma globu-lins, but others do not. Rats raised in a germ-free environment have serum gamma

globulin levels only one-third of that of controls. Patients with agammaglobulinemia, who cannot synthesize gamma globulins, do not synthesize antibodies. In multiple myeloma, however, gamma globulins may be in normal or usually in increased amount, but they do not produce antibodies. It looks, therefore, as if some antibodies may not be gamma globulins, and some gamma globulins may not be antibodies.

Antibodies alone may not be sufficient to resist infection, as the ultimate result may depend on the interaction of antibodies with other defense mechanisms, such as comple-ment, phagocytes and properdin, acting in conjunction with complement and magnes-ium ions. About 55 per cent of the gamma globulin present in the body is in the inter-stitial fluid, for about half of the gamma globulins present in the vascular system pass into the interstitial fluid every day.

The newborn infant synthesizes little gamma globulin or antibodies until between three or twelve weeks of age. The level is the same as that of the mother at birth, but it falls quickly. The lymphoid tissue of the newborn resembles that of the individual with agammaglobulinemia, with poor cortical development in the lymph nodes, absence of secondary germinal follicles, and absence of plasma cells.

Agammaglobulinemia is a deficiency of the gamma globulin fraction of the plasma proteins, which illustrates in a striking manner the important part which this fraction plays in resistance to infection. The condition may be congenital or acquired. The *congenital* and usual form is not only congenital, but also familial and sex-linked, occurring only in males. The symptoms occur early in life, and are probably due to a sex-linked recessive gene. The children have a very low resistance to infection, and are apt to die of infections which in normal people are of a trivial nature. The inability to synthesize gamma-globulin antibodies is reflected, as in the newborn, in atrophy of the lymphoid tissue, failure in the formation of secondary lymphoid follicles, and differentiation of plasma cells on antigenic stimulation. There is also absence of isoagglutinins for appropriate blood groups. The *acquired form* may occur in either sex, usually comes on in later life, and is not familial. There may or may not be an absence of isohemagglutinins.

Hypergammaglobulinemia, as its name implies, is a condition in which the gamma globulins are above the normal level. The most striking examples are seen in *multiple (plasma cell) myeloma*, sarcoidosis and the collagen or connective tissue diseases, in all of which plasma cells form an outstanding feature of the microscopic lesions. *Chronic granulomas*, such as those of tuberculosis, leprosy, lymphogranuloma venereum and kala-azar, show a marked rise in gamma globulins. In *chronic liver disease*, particularly cirrhosis, elevated gamma globulins are one of the commonest signs, directly correlated with the mesenchymal reaction in the liver and the increased number of plasma cells in the bone marrow. Indeed the so-called liver function tests are more the result of a disproportion among the serum protein fractions than a true index of disturbed liver function. Finally, in the *collagen diseases* an increase in the gamma globulins may be expected. This is particularly true of systemic lupus erythematosus

and scleroderma. It is the basis of the L.E. factor in systemic lupus and the rheumatoid factor in rheumatoid arthritis.

Tissue Immunity.—It is a common mistake to imagine that immunity is simply a matter of the blood plasma and the circulating leukocytes. The immunological tests of the laboratory show the presence of various antibodies in the blood, but it must be remembered that we know little of the part which test-tube phenomena actually play in the immunity of the living body. Agglutinins are abundant in the blood after typhoid inoculation, and yet the inoculated person may develop typhoid fever. On the other hand the antibodies may completely disappear from the blood when the patient has recovered from typhoid fever, and yet he is immune from a second attack. Practically all infections begin and end in the tissues. Our knowledge of resistance to infection is largely confined to antibodies and phagocytes, especially in the case of toxin-producing organisms. Humoral and cellular concepts dominate immunology, but we know little of what goes on in the tissues. One hears more about the hypersensitiveness of tissues than about their powers of defense. It is evident that the whole of the defense mechanism is not contained in the blood. The cells of the body form the background of immunity, and the antibodies of the blood are only a reflection of the more fundamental processes which have gone on in these cells, just as the fundamental changes in leukemia are to be looked for in the myeloid and lymphoid tissue rather than in the circulating blood. An interesting example of *cellular* as opposed to *humoral* immunity is provided by subacute bacterial endocarditis. In this disease the masses of bacteria on the surface of the vegetations attached to the heart valves are continually bathed with blood, but remain uninjured. When they are carried in the form of emboli to the kidney and lodge in the glomeruli they are soon killed, and the lesion heals with scarring.

The antibodies are produced by tissue cells, and there is little doubt that the main, perhaps the only, source are the cells comprising the *reticuloendothelial system*, for when these cells are "blockaded" by the intravenous injection of dyestuffs for which they have an affinity, there is a temporary rupture of immunity. The importance of the spleen, which is the greatest single collection of reticulo-endothelial cells, is strikingly shown by the experimental work on *Bartonella anemia of rats*. When albino rats are infected with Bartonella muris they remain apparently quite healthy, but the spleen becomes enlarged, an enlargement due to proliferation of its reticuloendothelial elements. If splenectomy is performed, this animal develops an acute fatal infectious anemia and small cocco-bacillary bodies are found in the red blood cells in blood smears. Adequate blockade of the entire reticuloendothelial system by the injection of India ink is followed by an anemia of the same type. It is evident that the spleen and the rest of the reticulo-endothelial system in some way prevent the development of the Bartonella organism.

The reticuloendothelial cells play a dual role, for in addition to manufacturing antibodies they are the most important agents concerned with the clearing of infectious agents from the blood stream. This can be shown in a striking manner by injecting a small quantity of India ink into the ear vein of a rabbit. If the animal is killed shortly afterward, all the ink particles are found collected in a few organs, particularly the spleen, the bone marrow, and the Kupffer cells of the liver. When bacteria are injected they are filtered out of the circulation in exactly the same manner. It is probable that the spleen prevents the development of Bartonella anemia in this way, holding the organism attached to its cells.

So far we have been thinking about antibodies produced against invading bacteria. But what about protection against virus infections? In many such infections antibodies can play little part in the early stage of defense, because viral antibodies appear very late in an infection in relation to the time at which recovery starts. Patients with hypogammaglobulinemia may recover in a normal manner from many virus infections without forming any detectable antibodies. The answer seems to be that cellular resistance to virus infection is mediated by the production of *interferon* by the infected cells (Isaacs and Hitchcock). This was first shown in the case of influenza, but it has also been demonstrated in a number of other virus infections, including vaccinia and poliomyelitis.

HYPERSENSITIVITY

We have seen that the body tends to protect itself against foreign protein invasion, including bacterial and viral infection, by certain processes which may be grouped under the common heading of immunity. But during the development of immunity there may appear a very different and indeed opposite type of reaction, namely hypersensitivity. This reaction is a hypersensitivity to bacterial protein and to any *foreign protein* (horse serum, egg albumin) which may be injected. The first injection may produce no evident effect (although in some cases it does so), but a second injection is followed by the development of striking and often dramatic phenomena, which may be local or general in their manifestations. *Immunity* is a manifestation of the *wisdom of the body*, to use Cannon's famous phrase, but *hypersensitivity* might well be called the *stupidity of the body*.

The conditions of life in modern "civilization" have vastly multiplied the chances of a person developing hypersensitivity. This is due partly to our industrial environment, but even more to the unbelievable number and variety of chemicals and drugs which it has become fashionable to swallow, to inhale, to apply to the skin, or to have injected. Manifestations of such hypersensitivity are said to be allergic in nature, and their number has increased to such an extent that a doctor can now make a comfortable living by diagnosing and treating them. Hypersensitivity is in essence an altered state of reactivity of the body.

To the student of hypersensitivity the question of nomenclature presents a problem. In the course of his reading he will encounter three terms: hypersensitivity, allergy and anaphylaxis. Payling Wright says that hypersensitivity and allergy are used almost interchangeably, adding that the brevity and euphony of allergy make it preferable, yet his chapter dealing with the subject is entitled Hypersensitivity Reactions.

The manifestations of hypersensitivity may be (1) *immediate* (*early*) or *anaphylactic*, or (2) *delayed* (*late*) or *tuberculin* in type. The term allergic is sometimes applied to the delayed type, in contrast to the anaphylactic or immediate type. This is unfortunate, for allergy is synonymous with hypersensitivity, of which anaphylaxis is a subdivision. Both are manifestations of hypersensitivity to different antigens, in different animals, and under different conditions. The main contrasting characteristics of the two types are shown in the accompanying table.

phenomenon or reaction, serum sickness, and some forms of experimental glomerulonephritis and polyarteritis.

Anaphylactic Shock.—The word anaphylaxis (*ana*, backward, and *phulaxis*, protection) means the opposite of protection. The response is immediate, evidence of inflammation developing in a matter of minutes. The combination of antigen with circulating antibody on sensitized cells apparently results in the release of histamine, which causes a spasmodic contraction of smooth muscle in the walls of the bronchioles, the pulmonary arteries and the gastrointestinal tract, and to increased capillary permeability with resulting edema, particularly in the

Anaphylactic Hypersensitivity	*Tuberculin Hypersensitivity*
Immediate reaction	Delayed reaction
Circulating antibody in serum	No circulating antibody
Passive transfer by serum possible	Transfer by cells
Not heritable	Heritable
Artificially induced	Naturally induced
Short duration of hypersensitivity	Long duration
Symptoms mainly due to smooth muscle spasm	Symptoms mainly due to edema
Desensitization easy	Desensitization difficult

Anaphylactic (Immediate) Hypersensitivity.—We have already seen that this form of hypersensitivity is marked by the presence of circulating antibodies in the peripheral blood which can be demonstrated by test-tube reactions. For this reason *passive transfer* of the hypersensitivity to a normal animal can readily be accomplished. Although antibodies are found in the blood, it is necessary that antigen be present in excess, and the type of hypersensitivity induced seems to be dependent on the amount of antigen. It is natural to suppose that anaphylactic shock requires the actual interaction of antigen and antibody in the tissues, but this does not appear to be the case, for shock may be induced by the use of preformed *antigen-antibody complexes* acting on susceptible cells (Germuth and McKinnon). The supernatent fluid from an antigen-antibody mixture is used. It is only effective if there is excess of antigen. If antibody is present in excess, shock does not result. In the anaphylactic group we may include anaphylactic shock, the Arthus

lungs, as a consequence of which the animal passes into a condition of anaphylactic shock which may end in death. All the major manifestations of anaphylactic shock can be reproduced by the intravenous injection of histamine. The condition has been studied for the most part in the sensitized experimental animal, but it also has its human counterpart. Human anaphylaxis is much less striking, because, fortunately, man is far less sensitive than the guinea pig. A person may, however, become sensitized against horse serum (diphtheria and other antitoxins), so that a second injection may be followed rapidly by symptoms of anaphylactic shock and even death.

Serum Sickness. — Experimental serum sickness is the best laboratory model for the study of a variety of human diseases of presumed hypersensitivity origin (Dixon *et al.*). When a foreign serum is injected into an animal such as a guinea pig, and a minute second dose is given after an interval of eight to twelve days, the animal may die in anaphylactic shock. In man the second injection is more likely to be followed by the development of an urticarial rash, fever, pains in the joints, and swelling of the lymph nodes. The histological picture may be identical with that of polyarteritis nodosa and other conditions believed to have an immunological basis. Sometimes the picture resembles that of anaphylactic shock, with death in rare cases. The symptoms are attributed to a reaction of the foreign antigen with sessile antibodies resulting from the first injection. Occasionally the clinical picture develops after a single injection. In such a case we must presume the presence of already existing antibodies.

As regards the *mechanism* of serum sickness, it is easy in the experimental animal to test for the pres nce of antigen, which can be labelled with I^{131}, and for antibody, which can be labelled with the fluorescent antibody technique of Coons, but it is difficult or impossible in human disease where the antigen is unknown. Dixon and his associates point out that there are three possibilities: (1) Antigen may be localized in the sites of the lesions, where antibody is then formed, resulting in an antigen-antibody reaction which causes tissue changes. (2) Antibody might become fixed in certain sites, and then react with circulating antigen to produce lesions. (3) There may be no fixation of either antigen or antibody, the antibody reaching the site of the lesions in the form of soluble antigen-antibody complexes. The third possibility appears to be the most probable, the development of the lesions and the concentration of complexes progressing simultaneously.

Arthus Reaction.—One year after Richet first described anaphylactic shock in 1902, Arthus showed in 1903 that when horse serum was injected into the skin of a rabbit which had been previously sensitized by injections of the same serum, a violent *local* reaction was produced, characterized first by constriction of the arterioles in the general anaphylactic reaction, followed by slowing of the blood stream in the veins, exudation of plasma, blocking of the vessels by plugs of leukocytes, and finally necrosis and sloughing of tissue. The condition, known also as the *Arthus phenomenon*, may be regarded as a local anaphylactic reaction in reverse. The essence of the reaction is that the tissues are locally damaged and killed by an amount of protein which is harmless to the normal body. The injections need not be given at the same place; the first may be given intraperitoneally and the second into the skin. It is evident that all the tissues become sensitized, and the reaction is an *antigen-antibody reaction in the cell itself.*

Shwartzman Phenomenon.—This puzzling condition does not depend, as do the others just described, on an antigen-antibody reaction. In 1928 Shwartzman showed that when a bacterial endotoxin, especially one of the Gram-negative group of bacteria, is injected into the skin, followed twenty-four hours later by an intravenous injection of the same *or some other* bacterial filtrate, a severe hemorrhagic and necrotizing inflammation develops at the site of the local injection. This obviously differs from the ordinary immunological reaction in its lack of specificity. Moreover, the provocative dose must be given intravenously. No adequate explanation of this peculiar phenomenon is as yet forthcoming, but it has been suggested that a similar mechanism may be involved in the hemorrhagic rashes in fulminating blood infections such as meningococcemia, the hemorrhagic adrenal lesions of the Waterhouse-Friderichsen syndrome in meningococcal infection, acute hemorrhagic pancreatitis, and the flare-up of a tuberculous lesion as the result of an intercurrent nontuberculous infection.

Atopy.—Certain persons have an idiosyncrasy, a *natural* rather than an acquired hypersensitivity, to pollens, to some kinds of foods, and to the emanations of animals. This idiosyncrasy is a quantitative rather than a qualitative difference from the normal. The greater the concentration of the substance, the more people are found to be hypersensitive. Idiosyncrasy has been described as *individuality run wild.* To this form of protein hypersensitivity the name of atopy (*atopia,* a strange disease) has been given. The most clear-cut examples are *asthma* and *hay fever.* In the former the bronchial mucosa, in the latter the nasal mucosa, is hypersensitive to pollens of various kinds, which differ with different people. The condition is an *inherited predispostion,* and this hereditary tendency forms one of its most striking characteristics. The tendency follows the laws of Mendelian inheritance. The atopy is not present at birth, and takes some years to develop. Cases are on record of identical twins who have been hypersensitive to the same protein, the atopy appearing at the same age. An increase in the eosinophils of the blood is characteristic of these persons.

Hypersensitivity to foods of various descriptions, especially shellfish (shrimps, oysters), may be included in this group, but the manifestations are different, nor does heredity play a part of importance. The symptoms which follow the ingestion of the food may be eczema, urticaria, angioneurotic edema, or gastrointestinal disturbances, but the patient does not suffer from asthma or hay fever.

Hypersensitivity to plant poisons is a rather common affliction. Such plants as poison ivy, poison oak, and the primula family may set up a severe inflammation of the skin (*dermatitis venenata*) when the sensitive person touches the leaves. Even the smoke of burning poison ivy will produce the same result. It often happens that florists only develop hypersensitivity after they have been handling primulas for many years.

Delayed Hypersensitivity.—This is also known as the *bacterial* or *tuberculin* type of hypersensitivity. The delayed reaction is seen in many diseases caused by bacteria, viruses, fungi, spirochetes, and parasites. It occurs most frequently in conjunction with living organisms. The *entire microbial cell* is necessary as the sensitizing agent, in contrast to the relatively simple antigens such as soluble products of microorganisms or soluble proteins alone which produce the immediate reaction. The maximum inflammatory response does not develop for twenty-four hours or more after the application of the test antigen. As we have seen previously, the reaction has no relation to circulating antibody. Indeed antibody, produced by plasma cells after specific stimulation and released as gamma globulin, plays no part either in this or in the Shwartzman type of reaction.

Bacterial allergy can be readily studied in the case of *tuberculosis*. When tuberculin is injected into the skin of a normal animal there is no reaction, but if the animal is already tuberculous a small dose will cause redness and swelling (the basis of the *von Pirquet tuberculin test* in man), while if the dose of antigen is larger there will be extensive necrosis and sloughing (the *Koch phenomenon*). In the natural disease as it occurs in man the same sequence of events takes place. The initial lesion, providing the infecting dose be sufficiently small, may be insignificant, but reinfection of the allergic tissues results in a lesion which may be destructive and progressive. This may occur in the lung, kidney, bone, and other organs. It is interesting to note, as well as of practical clinical importance, that in the last stages of tuberculosis, and also in general miliary tuberculosis in which there is an overwhelming infection, the allergic skin reaction is lost.

Syphilis, a disease which is discussed in Chapter 11, offers an interesting combination of immunity (resistance) and hypersensitivity. Three clinical stages are recognized. The *primary stage*, in which an infective lesion develops at the site of inoculation and swarms with treponemata (spirochetes), yet complete healing with some scarring occurs in a few weeks. The *secondary* skin and mucous membrane lesions which develop in the course of a couple of months appear relatively mild and heal without a trace, yet they are teeming with organisms. On the other hand, in the markedly destructive type of lesion of the *tertiary stage* it is rare to find a single treponema. It may be added that the more severe the tissue reactions in the primary and secondary stages, the less frequent and severe are the late manifestations, especially those in the central nervous system.

In a paper by Hamilton on the tissue lesions of hypersensitivity the phrase *cellular hypersensitivity* is used to denote this type of allergic reaction. As a result of the primary bacterial infection all the cells of the body become sensitized, and a subsequent reinfection with the antigen causes a hypersensitivity reaction on the surface of or possibly within the cell, with cellular degeneration and necrosis and an accompanying acute inflammatory response. The essential feature is the intracellular biochemical change in the enzyme systems which progresses to death of the cell. As there is no excess of circulating antibodies, passive transfer to a normal animal is only possible with the use of living or killed mesenchymal cells. That the reaction is essentially a cellular one independent of circulating antibody is shown by the observations of Rich and Lewis on cells isolated from an animal rendered sensitive to tuberculin and grown in tissue culture. When a minute amount of tuberculin was added to this culture, the same tissue destruction and necrosis occurred that is seen in the living animal. Hamilton suggests that the difference between the cellular and anaphylactic types of hypersensitivity may depend on the slow solubility of the antigen in the former variety. It may be that the essential difference between immunity and hypersensitivity is that in the former the union of antigen and antibody takes place in the serum, whilst in the latter it takes place on or in the cells.

Clinical Features of Hypersensitivity.— Many common diseases in man are manifestations of hypersensitivity to exogenous stimulating agents. A few of these are mentioned below. The subject of autoimmunity and the diseases associated with it is considered separately.

Hay fever is a reaction of hypersensitive tissue to the pollens of trees, grasses and weeds. *Bronchial asthma* with obstruction of the smaller bronchioles due to spasm of the bronchial muscles or swelling of the mucosal lining, is often allergic in origin. The allergens (antigens) may be inhaled or ingested. Among the inhalants are house dust, orris root in face powder, pollens, animal danders, glue in furniture, etc. Ingested irritants include foods, particularly in children, and drugs in adults. The result may occasionally be sudden death. In such cases the lungs are voluminous and emphysematous, and the smaller and medium-sized bronchi are occluded with thick, tough and tenaceous mucus (Walton *et al.*). A striking infiltration of the bronchial wall with eosinophils is in keeping with the allergic nature of the disease. *Loeffler's pneumonia*, a transitory pulmonary infiltration with eosinophilia, may be caused by a number of allergens, including animal parasites, fungi,

dusts and pollen. *Dermatitis* and *urticaria* (nettle rash) may be caused by many of the irritants already enumerated. *Drug allergy* may be due to a wide variety of medicinal substances, even aspirin, which may be a cause of bronchial asthma. *These are not in themselves antigenic, but by becoming linked with protein molecules they acquire antigenic properties. Sulfonamide allergy* deserves special mention. When these drugs become conjugated with serum proteins they may cause serious and sometimes fatal disturbances (More *et al.*). In addition to fever, chills and a skin eruption there may be failing renal function with anuria about a week after the administration of the sulfonamide, more especially sulfathiazole. The principal lesions are in the kidney, liver and heart, but almost any organ may be involved, and the lesions are often widespread in fatal cases. The lesions are often similar to or identical with those of polyarteritis nodosa. As Rich points out, modern civilization has greatly increased the chances of the development of hypersensitivity by reason of the multitude of synthetic sensitizing agents which are being continually introduced and avidly taken up by the public.

Hypersensitivity Lesions.— From what has already been said it is evident that the lesions encountered in various hypersensitivity states will not be uniform. In *acute anaphylactic shock* death is due to respiratory spasm and vascular collapse, so that little or nothing may be seen save commencing pulmonary edema.

In the localized lesion of the Arthus phenomenon, serum sickness, and the *allergic* forms of the collagen diseases the changes are striking and characteristic. They may be acute or more chronic in character, involving the vascular endothelium and basement membrane, collagen fibers, intercellular cement substance, and smooth muscle. The endothelial cells swell and occlude the lumen of the capillaries, the basement membrane becomes broadened and blurred and may eventually rupture, while in the arteries there is necrosis of the muscle. Some of the most important changes are in the intercellular substance, which intervenes not only between the cells and the collagen fibers, but between the fibrils of those fibers and the fibers of the smooth muscle. The mucopolysaccharides of the ground substance may well be the site of the antigen-antibody reaction which is the basis of allergy, and these are normally concentrated in the skin, synovial membranes, heart valves and perivascular stroma of the myocardium, which are the sites of the lesions in rheumatic fever and the other collagen diseases about to be described.

There are three principal *acute changes* in or connected with the *ground substance*. (1) *Mucoid swelling or edema*, which refers to actual increase of the basophilic mucopolysaccharides or a shifting of their distribution. (2) *Fibrinoid formation (? degeneration) in the intercellular substance*, which will be discussed more fully in connection with the collagen diseases. (3) *Degeneration and necrosis of the vascular endothelium and smooth muscle*, the elements of which are separated by ground substance. These lesions are characterized by an acute inflammatory exudate. In the *chronic reaction*, which is conditioned by the slow solubility of the necrotic material, there is a productive inflammation with proliferation of vascular endothelium, best seen in the glomerular capillaries in experimental nephritis.

It is probable that undue emphasis has been laid in the past on intercellular changes at the expense of the cellular response, both in the collagen diseases in man and in experimental hypersensitivity. The rather incongruous association of acute destructive lesions of connective tissue, often fibrinoid in character, with a granulomatous type of cellular response, mainly mononuclear in type, is highly suggestive, possibly pathognomonic, of the hypersensitive state in the laboratory animal and possibly a similar condition in human collagen disease. Fibrinoid evidently develops following the interaction between antigen and antibody, for it is seen best when the free antibody titer in the serum is on the decline, with the antibody becoming fixed to the tissues.

The *mast cell* appears to be a key factor in allergic reactions (Weiser). This cell is extremely susceptible to injury by numerous physical and chemical agents which are harmless to other types of cells. By injury

is meant either disintegration of the cells or merely loss of granules without disruption of the cellular membrane. Serotonin, histamine, heparin, and perhaps other components responsible for immunological lesions may be released by mast cells. The distribution of mast cells varies greatly in different species of animals. This together with the substances released may account for the confusingly different results observed in experimental work on laboratory animals. Thus histamine is thought to be the principal mediator of anaphylaxis in the guinea pig and dog, whilst serotonin may be chiefly responsible in rats and mice. Rats are extremely sensitive to serotonin but resistant to histamine. The extreme fragility of the mast cell may represent a defense mechanism, since histamine and serotonin are inflammatory agents.

Special forms of hypersensitivity reaction will be considered in connection with the individual organs in the Special Pathology section of this book. In this place brief reference may be made to one or two of these lesions. *Myocarditis* is seen in cases of drug sensitivity and in serum sickness. Allergic *pneumonitis* is marked by damage to alveolar capillaries with exudation of fluid and leukocytes, and the formation of hyaline alveolar membranes. *Glomerulonephritis* following scarlet fever and streptococcal tonsillitis is characterized, after a lapse of time needed for the production of a sufficient amount of sensitizing antibody, by a proliferation of glomerular capillary endothelium and later epithelium, changes in the basement membrane, and a varying amount of inflammatory exudate. Experimental glomerulonephritis can be produced by the introduction of small amounts of protein into the sensitized animal.

AUTO-IMMUNITY

When foreign organic material, usually bacteria, enters the body, processes are set in motion which have been evolved throughout the ages to rid the body of the foreign element, and to prevent future invasion by the same intruder. It has long been recognized that the immunity mechanism is a reaction against substances of foreign origin, and it used to be taken for granted that the body would never make the grave mistake of responding immunologically to its own antigens by the formation of antibodies. The very idea of such a thing happening was so abhorrent to Ehrlich that he coined the famous phrase, *horror autotoxicus.* Horse serum when injected into human beings acts as a powerful antigen, but it does not elicit antibody formation when injected into a horse. The same holds true for the injection of human serum into horses and into humans. A skin graft from a child to its mother is rejected because it is a *homograft,* not an *autograft,* on account of the presence of paternal antigens in the cells of the graft, but of course it is accepted by the child itself, for whom it is an autograft.

Burnet has formulated a challenging concept to account for the fact that antigens originating in the body itself are recognized and therefore ignored by the antibody-forming cells. This he calls the *self-marker hypothesis.* The *molecular pattern* of the body proteins seems to be marked "self," thus presenting a passport to the defense cells which is accepted. Organic material from outside is marked "not-self," its passport is not acceptable, and antibodies are formed against it. Those cells of the body which are of very short life such as the red blood cells and the lymphocytes, the so-called "expendable cells," seem to carry not a passport but a death warrant, which is recognized by the reticuloendothelial cells whose function it is not only to dispose of the expendable cells but to initiate the mechanism for the formation of antibodies. Another and perhaps more acceptable explanation, that of *immunological paralysis,* suggests that antigenic constituents of the body reach antibody-forming cells in such large amounts that these cells are kept saturated and are unable to respond.

Acquired Tolerance.—A very important fact brought out by Medawar and his associates is that the self-marker stamp is not placed on the cells until *late in embryonic life.* When an antigen is injected into an adult for the first time the result will be a reaction either of immunity or hypersensitivity. In 1951 Billingham showed that non-identical twin calves, whose circulations had mingled while in utero, would accept skin grafts from each other. This observation gave rise to the concept of *"actively acquired tolerance."* It was then found that in the mouse, before a certain point of embryonic development, the entry of foreign cells provokes a specific tolerance in later life. This may be related to the absence in the fetus of plasma cells which form antibody in the process of maturation, so that acquired tolerance may represent an inability of plasma cells to mature in response to stimulation by an antigen to which the animal is tolerant.

Acquired tolerance applies not only to cells, but also to bacteria, viruses and protozoa. As a result of being inoculated with an antigen during fetal life, an animal is unable to react normally to subsequent doses of the same antigen given in postnatal life; its capacity to make antibody to this antigen is weakened or suppressed. Thus the intrauterine infection of mice with the virus of lymphocytic choriomeningitis results in the birth of apparently healthy offspring whose tissues contain large amounts of the virus, but with no evidence of reaction. This example of symptomless congenital lymphocytic choriomeningitis in mice may serve to explain some cases of serum hepatitis in man, a point which will be discussed in the chapter on the liver. After a certain stage of development has been reached, a point of no return, the entry of foreign material gives rise to *specific intolerance,* that is to say, an immune reaction with formation of antibody. Homologous grafts of skin or other tissue from another individual of the same species are rejected. Medawar has shown, however, that *a skin graft of a strain B mouse is tolerated and accepted in an A strain animal if mouse A has been prepared by the fetal inoculation of B cells.* This tolerance is lost if a normal lymph node from an *untreated* A mouse is grafted into the B mouse, for in a few weeks the graft is destroyed. It has now become "not self." From the immunological point of view, the eye seems to be in a class by itself, probably by reason of the isolation of the lens and anterior chamber from the circulation. It is for this reason that cancer transplants can be made successfully into the anterior chamber of the eye of another species.

It is now recognized that under certain conditions not at present clearly understood antigenic substances *formed in the body* (*auto-antigens*) may excite the formation of antibodies, with a resulting antigen-antibody reaction. Using saline suspensions of human tissues as antigens, an auto-immune reaction for auto-antibodies with specific complement fixation may be obtained with human serum in a number of diseases, especially those associated with hyperglobulinemia (Gajdusek). In many instances the condition develops after an acute streptococcal or other infection, as in acute glomerulonephritis or in rheumatic fever. It would appear as if the bacterial products had altered the molecular pattern of the glomerular or synovial proteins, thus obliterating their self-recognition character and giving them an antigenic character, so that they come to be regarded by the defense system of cells as not-self and are treated accordingly. A foreign non-antigenic substance or *hapten* such as a drug may combine with an endogenous protein and modify it enough to make it antigenic, so that antibodies are formed to this complex. The initial stimulus can start a mechanism which is self-perpetuating, thus suggesting an explanation for the continuance of the lesions and clinical manifestations long after the original injury has passed away and been forgotten. This, of course, is entirely different from what occurs in syphilis or tuberculosis, where the long-continued sojourn of living microorganisms in the tissue ensures the presence of lesions for months or years. Some of the collagen diseases are just as protracted, but we cannot explain the marked chronicity by the presence of the original causal agent. In the case of the various collagen diseases the course of events will be determined by the nature of the original target organ or tissue.

The concept of auto-immunity, which might more appropriately be termed *auto-sensitivity*, is one of far-reaching importance, and at the present moment we only stand on its threshold. It is possible that a number of diseases which in the past have been labelled as idiopathic, that is to say of unknown etiology, may prove to be caused by an auto-immune mechanism. In the following brief account of diseases believed or suspected to be of auto-immune origin the student must forgive me for referring to conditions which may be unknown to him. Should he return to the subject at a later date the matter will appear a good deal simpler. To explain fully the various conditions about to be mentioned would give rise to needless repetition. These will be discussed in detail in later sections of the book.

AUTO-IMMUNITY DISEASE

The disease conditions referred to in the preceding paragraph may be grouped under a common heading, but it is difficult to find a perfect name for the group. They have been called the *immunological diseases*. The objection to that term is that the hypersensitivity reactions caused by *exogenous* antigens (allergens) which we have already studied might well claim admission to the group of immunological diseases. The most grammatical and euphonious expression is *auto-allergic disease*, but it has not won general favor, although used for one recent book on the subject.

Much more difficult than the question of nomenclature is the lack of correlation between the clinical and the laboratory evidence in support of the concept of auto-immune disease, of an immunological reaction directed, in defiance of Ehrlich's *horror auto-toxicus*, against one or more of the antigenic constituents of an individual's own tissues. This has been done in the experimental animal with brain, spinal cord and peripheral nerves, thyroid, adrenals, testes and kidney, often making use of the adjuvant effect of killed acid-fast bacilli or of fractions obtained from them. Inert oils are included to slow down absorption and produce persistent areas of productive inflammation. This factor, known as *Freund's adjuvant*, helps to overcome the usual resistance to the development of an auto-immune reaction, although by what means is not clear. It would appear that the adjuvant is helpful in causing some injury or chemical alteration of the cells which assists in the formation of antibodies.

In the experimental animal the reaction is regarded as one of delayed type hypersensitivity, with the same fundamental lesions as are seen in hypersensitivity reactions to exogenous antigens. Though the antigens may be very different, *e.g.* thyroglobulin, lens protein, proteo-lipid of myelin and carbohydrate of sperms, all have one major point of similarity, namely separation from the vascular bed and connective tissue by more or less impermeable cellular barriers such as the follicular thyroid epithelium and the pial-glial membrane, or by poor lymphatic drainage. This physiological remoteness, together, perhaps, with the special nature of their metabolism, prevents the antigens from reaching the blood stream in more than negligible concentrations, so that the immune apparatus treats them as strangers and interlopers. If delayed reactivity results from this, an auto-allergic disease process develops, in which a perivascular inflammatory reaction of mononuclear cells is the primary event, with a secondary parenchymal destruction. As the antigen persists, the disease tends to be prolonged or intermittent.

But what are we to say about the disease in man? The immunological evidence for the clinical parallels of most of the conditions to be discussed is far from conclusive, with the exception of Hashimoto's disease of the thyroid. The resemblance between the experimental lesions produced by immunological measures and those of autoimmune human disease may be more apparent than real. The instances in which the clinical evidence for an immunological mechanism is best are worst for the experimental reproduction in lower animals, and vice versa. Thus the best examples in man involve erythrocytes and blood platelets, but we are unable to reproduce auto-immune hemolytic anemia or thrombocytopenia in the laboratory animal, although the fact that acquired hemolytic anemia was due to hemolysis by auto-antibodies was recognized fifty years ago, although largely forgotten. The evidence for an immunological type of demyelination of the central nervous system is conclusive in the laboratory animal, but so far there is no evidence of an immune mechanism in human demyelinating disease such as multiple sclerosis. In rheumatoid arthritis and in systemic lupus erythema-

tosus serum factors are present which resemble antibodies against body antigens, *e.g.* denatured gamma globulin in rheumatoid arthritis and components of cell nuclei and cytoplasm in systemic lupus. Unfortunately there is a lack of correlation between the clinical state and the level of these antibodies. The most direct experimental proof of the action of auto-antibodies on tissue cells is obtained in Hashimoto's disease, where the injection of homologous thyroid extract together with adjuvants into rabbits results in a serum containing iso-antibodies to the thyroid.

The *criteria which should be satisfied* before acceptance of an auto-immune disease are as follows: (1) circulating antibodies should be demonstrated in the serum of the patient, or cell-bound antibodies by indirect means; (2) the antigen should be known; (3) specific antibodies should be produced against the same antigen in the experimental animal. These high standards can seldom be met in human supposedly auto-immune disease, some examples of which we shall now consider. In most of these there is often a history of a preceding infection, the condition is often familial, the symptoms are often relieved by ACTH and cortisone, and the serum often gives false-positive tests for syphilis.

Blood.—We are on safe ground in saying that circulating auto-antibodies to erythrocytes are present in forms of *acquired hemolytic anemia*, and that union of the antibodies with antigens in the red cells is responsible for the hemolysis and the anemia. The antibody may be of the "warm" or "cold" variety, depending on the temperature at which it operates. The first auto-immune disease to be clearly demonstrated as such was *paroxysmal cold hemoglobinuria*, in which the serum contains an autohemolysin that unites with red cells only at a low temperature. Union occurs when the body is chilled, but hemolysis does not take place until it gets warmed again. This is the only condition in which properdin, complement and the magnesium ion are required for full effectiveness of the hemolytic system. The most constant finding in the auto-immune blood diseases is a positive Coombs test for antiglobulins.

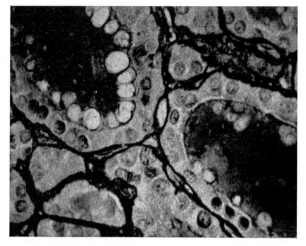

A

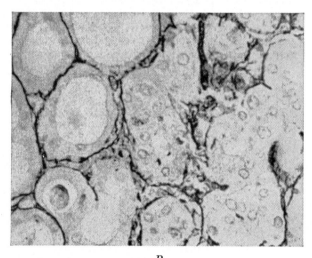

B

Fig. 51.—*A*, Photomicrograph of thyroid gland to show the normal relationship of the basement membrane to the capillary vessels. (Silver. × 650.)

B, Fragmentation of the basement membrane in thyroid tissue from a patient with thyrotoxicosis and a high antibody titer. (Silver. × 500.) (Stuart and Allen, courtesy of Lancet.)

Idiopathic thrombocytopenic purpura, as its name implies, is marked by purpuric hemorrhages associated with a marked drop in the number of circulating blood platelets. Here again anti-platelet antibodies can be demonstrated in the serum. It is of interest that the condition may develop after such viral infections as chicken pox and measles, or after vaccination against poliomyelitis or influenza.

Leukemia may be associated with auto-immunization, but we shall defer a consideration of this subject until we come to diseases of the blood in general.

Blood groups present one of the best examples of the principle of self and not-self. Red blood cells contain one (A) or another (B) antigen (agglutinogen) or both (A B) or neither (O), on the basis of which human beings can be classified into four groups. In the serum there are corresponding antibodies (agglutinins) to A and B. A person's serum does not contain the antibody for the antigen present in his own red cells, but it does carry antibodies against the antigens he does not possess (self and not-self). When red cells not carrying the correct passport are injected into the blood stream, there is danger of an antigen-antibody reaction with agglutination of red cells, hemolysis, serious shock, and even death. Group antigens are determined genetically, depending on the presence of 3 allelic genes, A, B and O. The question of the blood groups is considered in detail in Chapter 39.

Endocrine Glands.—The two endocrine diseases in which auto-immunity seems to play a part are Hashimoto's disease of the thyroid and Addison's disease of the adrenals. The evidence is much more convincing in the case of the former than of the latter.

Hashimoto's Disease.—This is a form of chronic inflammation of the thyroid gland marked by the presence of great numbers of lymphocytes and plasma cells in the gland. It is practically confined to the female in the child-bearing period of life. This form of thyroiditis remained an idiopathic enigma until Witebsky and his associates showed that auto-immunization to thyroglobulin may be the answer. When thyroglobulin is injected into the rabbit or guinea pig it acts as an antigen, stimulating the formation of antibodies which react with the thyroid to produce lesions similar to those of Hahimoto's disease (Roitt *et al.*). The presence of circulating antibodies can be demonstrated in the human disease, whilst antithyroglobulin antibodies can be shown in the gland of the patient by means of the Coons fluorescent antibody technique, and intradermal tests with extract of human thyroid as antigen give a strongly positive Arthus type of reaction (Buchanan *et al.*).

Thyroid auto-antibodies may sometimes be present in other thyroid disorders, and even in persons with no apparent thyroid disease. It is known that thyroid disease tends to run in families, and circulating thyroid antibodies are found in the relatives of patients with auto-immune thyroid disease. It would appear that there is a distinct genetic predisposition to thyroid auto-immunity, which is inherited as a dominant characteristic.

The still unanswered question is: How does the thyroglobulin escape from the follicles and act as an antigen? It may be due to changes in the basement membranes of the follicles, which are correlated with the circulating antibody titer (Stuart and Allan).

Thyroglobulin seems to be immunologically inert when contained within the follicles, but when it escapes into the interstitial tissue it is treated as a foreign protein (not-self). The basic question is: How does the thyroglobulin make its escape and act as an antigen? If the basement membrane maintains the immunological integrity of the follicle, a break in this membrane would provide an anatomical basis for thyroid antibody formation. That such a break does occur in Hashimoto's disease has now been demonstrated (Stuart and Allan) (Fig. 51).

Idiopathic Addison's Disease.—In the past Addison's disease was most often due to tuberculosis of the adrenals. Within recent years a so-called idiopathic variety has been replacing the tuberculous form. Its chief features are atrophy of the adrenals and replacement by great numbers of lymphoid cells (Fig. 52). By means of the complement fixation test antibodies to human adrenal cortex can be demonstrated in the blood of some cases of idiopathic Addison's disease (Anderson *et al.*). It may be that auto-immune anti-adrenal antibodies are responsible for the progressive destruction of the adrenal cortex.

In strong support of this concept is the production of lesions in the guinea pig adrenal by the injection of autologous and homologous pooled adrenal tissue with Freund's adjuvant, lesions similar to those of idiopathic Addison's disease in man (Steiner *et al.*). The lesions consist of a focal and later a diffuse proliferation of mesenchymal cell derivatives with secondary disintegration of the architecture of the deep cortex and medulla of the gland (Fig. 53). The adrenal reaction produced by a circulating adjuvant-bound antigen followed the same pattern as would obtain if the antigen had been liberated within the adrenal cortex.

Connective Tissue: Collagen.—The general subject of the group of conditions known as the *diffuse collagen diseases* has already

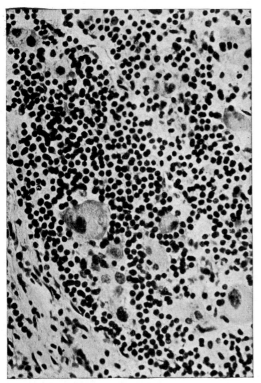

Fig. 52.—Round-cell infiltration of the adrenal in idiopathic Addison's disease. × 350. (Boyd, *Pathology for the Physician.*)

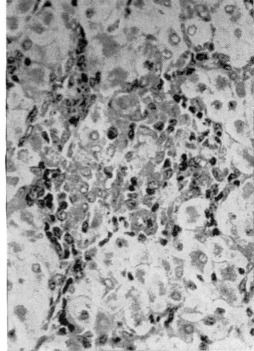

Fig. 53.—Experimentally produced auto-immune lesion of adrenal cortex. Parenchyma replaced by plasma cells and lymphocytes. × 284. (Steiner *et al.*, courtesy Jour. Exper. Med., 1960.)

been considered in the previous chapter on Intercellular Substance Reactions. This is a convenient blanket term to describe the pathological lesions in a variety of clinical conditions, in which the changes are not confined to an organ, or even to a system, but affect collagenous connective tissue in widely separated parts of the body. There is a certain danger, however, that the term may become a mere label, a refuge for the diagnostically destitute. The feature which the different members of the group have in common is the presence of *fibrinoid*. Marked differences of opinion still exist as to the origin of fibrinoid. The two most popular views are: (1) that it represents a change in the mucopolysaccharides in the ground substance so that they come to have the staining character and physical appearance of fibrin; (2) that, in part at least, it really is fibrin, being derived from the fibrinogen in the plasma. The arguments for and against these ideas will be found in the general

discussion on collagen disease in Chapter 4, page 86. The consensus of opinion at the present time seems to be that fibrinoid is the result of exudation, precipitation and inspissation of plasma proteins, somehow related to an immune mechanism, rather than an intrinsic alteration of connective tissue (Movat) (Figs. 54 and 55).

The *etiology* of the diffuse collagen diseases is also a matter of doubt. There is no reason to think that there is one single causal agent, any more than there is reason to look for a single cause of the various granulomata. Throughout the variations, however, there seems to run a fairly constant theme of hypersensitivity, an antigen-antibody reaction in the cells and ground substance of the connective tissue and vessel walls. The antigens will vary, some being possibly exogenous, others autogenous, but the reaction will be of the same type as the generalized Shwartzman phenomenon in the experimental animal, which also is characterized

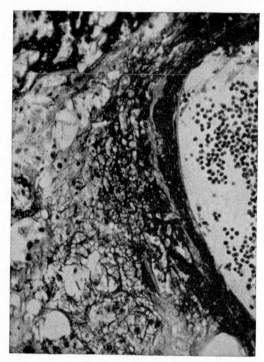

Fig. 54.—Formation of fibrinoid from condensation of fibrin following injection of trypsin into the rabbit's skin. The fibrin is seen to form a dense mesh work in the upper part of the photograph and a band along the wall of a vein. Phosphotungstic Acid Hematoxylin. (Kindness of Dr. H. Z. Movat.)

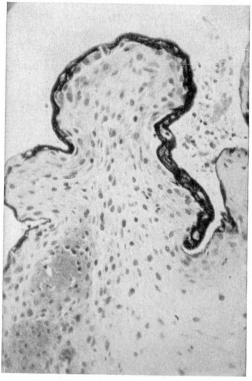

Fig. 55.—An irregular band of fibrinoid is deposited onto the surface of the knee joint of a rabbit which has received multiple injections of horse serum. (Kindness of Dr. H. Z. Movat.)

pathologically by the occurrence of widespread fibrinoid lesions involving the cardiovascular system. It has indeed been suggested that *systemic fibrinoid diseases* would be a more descriptive name than diffuse collagen diseases (Brunson and Davis). It may well prove to be that the most important element in the pathogenesis of the collagen diseases is an auto-immune reaction.

The *experimental evidence* points to the intimate and frequent association of fibrinoid necrosis with allergic reactions. The lesions of polyarteritis nodosa can readily be produced in animals in this way, and similar lesions are observed in human cases of serum sickness (Rich). More and Movat adduce morphological evidence for the pathogenesis of collagen disease on an allergic basis. Horse serum was injected as an antigen into a series of animals, and the ensuing histological changes analyzed with regard to time of appearance and the phase of the immunological reaction. The three

basic changes observed were: (1) *Proliferation of plasma cells*, first immature, later mature, best seen in the spleen; this morphological counterpart of antibody formation is seen in human as well as experimental material. (2) *Swelling of the interstitial tissue* of the myocardium with an increase of acid mucopolysaccharides, accompanied by proliferation of histocytes; these changes coincided with the appearance of circulating antibody. (3) *Fibrinoid "necrosis"* together with an acute inflammatory reaction; this was observed at the time the circulating antibody began to decrease. Similar lesions are found in the human collagen diseases. These facts are highly suggestive, but the pathologist knows from hard experience and the clinician should learn that similarity of histological appearance does not necessarily imply identity of etiology.

Even more striking confirmation of the allergic reaction concept is afforded by application of the fluorescent antibody technique already alluded to. As the antigens which may be responsible for the collagen diseases are almost always unknown, specific identification of the antigen or the corresponding antibody in the lesion is not possible. An antigen-antibody reaction should, however, result in a local increase of gamma globulin, since most antibodies are gamma globulins. Using fluorescent anti-human gamma globulin it is possible to demonstrate a significant concentration of fluorescent material in the lesions of rheumatic fever, disseminated lupus erythematosus, and to a lesser degree rheumatoid arthritis, as well as in the inclusions in L.E. cells (Vazquez and Dixon).

Biochemical changes are a feature of the various collagen diseases. The most characteristic change is increase in gamma globulins, probably due to proliferation of plasma cells, which are the cellular source of antibodies and other gamma globulins. Alpha globulin, C-reactive protein, and fibrinogen are all raised in the acute and subacute manifestations, although normal during remissions. The rise in alpha globulin seems to correspond with injury to the connective tissue. It is normal in scleroderma, but this is a very chronic disease. In contrast to the globulins, serum albumin is depressed in the collagen diseases, suggesting some form of liver injury. Some of these changes may be due to leakage through connective tissue membranes whose permeability is altered by depolymerization or destruction of their mucoproteins.

Cortisone and *hydrocortisone*, which are so valuable in several of the collagen diseases, seem to be effective through their action on the pathogenetic mechanism. In sufficient doses they can destroy plasma cells, with rapid degradation of antibodies. They also suppress the permeability of connective tissue membranes, thus interfering with the exchange of components between the blood and the tissues. As Ehrich puts it in his remarkably comprehensive review of the whole subject: "The common denominator of the various collagen diseases lies in their pathogenesis, or, more precisely, in the production in these diseases of abnormal gamma globulins apparently by plasma cells

causing injury of the general mesenchyme." If we wished to be fanciful we might speak of the collagen diseases as dysgammaglobulinemias.

In *conclusion* we may say that "the collagen diseases are etiologically heterogeneous but pathogenetically well-defined maladies, characterized morphologically by systemic alterations of the connective tissue, and chemically by changes in the composition of blood, reflecting both cause and effect of the injury" (Ehrich).

The principal examples of the diffuse collagen (fibrinoid) group are polyarteritis nodosa, systemic or disseminated lupus erythematosus, and Wegener's granulomatosis; rheumatic fever, and rheumatoid arthritis; scleroderma and dermatomyositis. It will be obvious from their names that some of these conditions are discussed more appropriately in relation to the system which is involved. Thus polyarteritis nodosa is considered in relation to the arteries, rheumatoid arthritis to the joints, scleroderma to the skin, and dermatomyositis to the muscles. The lesions of disseminated or systemic lupus erythematosus are so widespread, as again the name indicates, that it may be taken as a prototype of the diffuse collagen group and considered here.

Systemic Lupus Erythematosus.—Perhaps the most intriguing member of the collagen disease group is systemic or disseminated lupus. The name, which is from the Latin meaning a wolf, has a curious history. It was first given in 1305 to a destructive skin condition, in which the disease ate away the skin and "devoured it like a wolf." Several centuries later another skin lesion, distinguished by erythema rather than destruction, received the same name. Then two erythematous types were differentiated, one chronic, local and circular, often involving the bridge of the nose and the adjacent cheeks (*discoid lupus*), the other with acute widely scattered lesions, often with no involvement of the skin (*disseminated lupus*). Finally it was recognized that the disseminated form may have no skin lesions. In rare instances the local discoid eventually develops into the disseminated form.

Our present day concept of disseminated or systemic lupus has been built up over

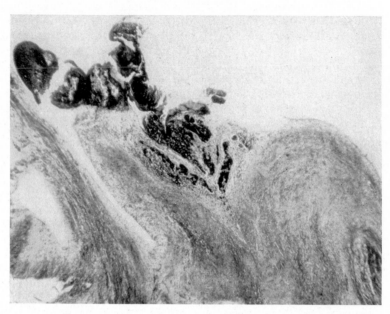

Fig. 56.—Libman-Sacks endocarditis in acute disseminated lupus erythematosus. The fibrinoid is seen in black. Some fibrinoid is adherent to the valve and some has become incorporated into the valve substance. × 35. (Kindness of Dr. H. Z. Movat.)

many years, piece by piece being added until now we have a complex and fascinating whole. The so-called "typical," fully fledged case, (which is in reality quite atypical), has more or less of the following *characteristics*. (1) A butterfly-like erythematous rash on the skin of the face, (2) the Libman-Sacks type of non-bacterial endocarditis (p. 117), (3) nephritis, and (4) enlargement of the spleen and lymph nodes. The *course* may be short and stormy (death in six to eight weeks), or chronic with acute exacerbations. It appears to represent a hyperimmune state to antigens, either external or even more probably autogenous, including nuclei of the patient's cells. From the clinical standpoint it has been described as "an overwhelming mass of organized confusion." It used to be said: "know syphilis and all other things clinical will be added unto you." Today we substitute systemic lupus for syphilis, the reason for the confusion being the widespread and variable character of the lesions. Evidence of renal involvement, even though quite mild at first, is the most serious prognostic sign, renal failure being the most frequent cause of death. Other manifestations

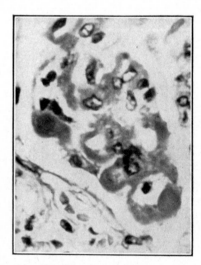

Fig. 57.—Wire loop lesions in systemic lupus.

of the disease are pericarditis, myocarditis, encephalitis, hemolytic anemia and thrombocytopenic purpura, the last two indicating an auto-immune mechanism.

Lesions.—The lesions are widespread in many organs, and are particularly marked in the vessels, in these respects resembling

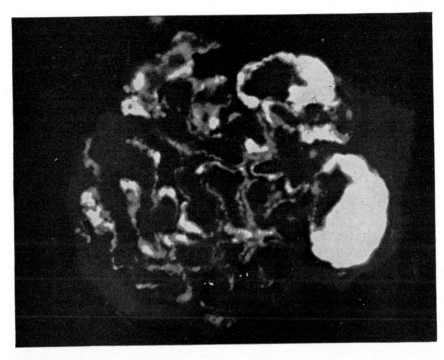

Fig. 58.—Specific fluorescence of glomeruli in lupus erythematosus. The white areas indicate the site of gamma globulin in the basement membranes and 2 wire loop lesions. Frozen section, stained with fluorescent antibody for human V-globulin. × 575. (Mellors, courtesy of J. Exper. Med.)

polyarteritis nodosa. Although a classical case of disseminated lupus differs greatly from a classical case of polyarteritis nodosa it is doubtful if the distinction is fundamental. I have encountered a number of instances where the features and lesions of the two diseases were combined. In general *the lesions of lupus tend to be more degenerative (necrotic) and those of polyarteritis more inflammatory* in type, but combinations occur. In polyarteritis the medium-sized vessels (coronary, mesenteric) are affected, in lupus the small arteries and arterioles and even the capillaries. Perhaps the most important difference is in sex, polyarteritis being predominantly a male disease, and lupus largely though not exclusively female. Sex may be a conditioning factor which determines the target organ and the character of the lesions. The basic lesion is a widespread *fibrinoid formation*, to which may be added a minor degree of reactive inflammation. One of the striking effects of the involvement of the capillaries is an increased permeability, which is seen particularly in the skin. As disseminated lupus is one of the collagen diseases, it is natural that arthritis may be a feature. Heavy deposits of fibrin are found on the synovial membrane of the affected joints.

For descriptive purposes the principal lesions are cardiac, renal, vascular, and cutaneous. In the *heart* (in less than half the cases) the striking gross lesion may be the flat warty vegetations described by Libman and Sacks in 1923 extending on to the mural endocardium, now known as *Libman-Sacks endocarditis* (Fig. 56). Microscopically the basic lesion is fibrinoid change of the connective tissue of the endocardium, myocardium and pericardium. In the *kidney* the characteristic microscopic lesions are in the glomerular tufts: (1) the so-called "wire loop capillaries," (2) focal necrosis of the tuft. The wire loop appearance is due to thickening of the basement membrane of the capillaries giving a resemblance to bent wire similar to that of early amyloidosis

(Fig. 57). With haematoxylin and eosin the wire loop appearance seems to be due to a thickening of the basement membrane of the capillaries giving a resemblance to bent wire. With finer differential staining, however, and also with phase microscopy, the wire loop material is seen to be deposited between the epithelial and the endothelial basement membranes (Churg and Grishman). An appearance suggesting hyaline thrombi in the capillaries is probably due to protrusion into the lumen of the fibrinoid material in the vessel wall; true thrombosis is rare. By means of the fluorescent specific antibody method of Coons it can be shown that the thickened basement membrane, the wire loop lesions, and even the "hyaline thrombi" represent deposition of serum gamma globulin (Mellors *et al.*) (Fig. 58). In the *spleen* the small arteries show a periarterial fibrosis, swollen bands of collagen giving a characteristic "onion-skin" type of lesion (Fig. 59). Teilum suggests that the periarterial hyalinization in the spleen and the hyaline wire-loop capillaries in the kidneys may be related to the hyperglobulinemia, representing indeed a *hyperglobulinosis*. This concept is supported by the results of the fluorescent antibody technique just mentioned. As a result of these changes there is a varying degree of splenomegaly. The *lymph nodes*, both superficial and deep, may be enlarged, and they may show the same onion-skin thickening of the arteries as the spleen. The *vascular* lesions are most common and severe in the kidneys, but they may be present in any organ in the body. In advanced cases there may be complete fibrinoid necrosis of all the coats of the arterioles. Marked thickening of the intima may cause great narrowing of the lumen. A fulminating necrosis may be accompanied or preceded by an inflammatory cellular reaction of lymphocytes, plasma cells, and a few polymorphonuclears. In the *skin* fibrinoid occurs in the upper layer of the corium involving both collagenous fibers and ground substance. The arterioles and capillaries show the usual changes. Klemperer has called attention to hematoxylin-stained bodies, first described by Libman and Sacks in 1924 and again by Gross in 1932. The *hematoxylin bodies* are believed to be pathognomonic of dissemin-

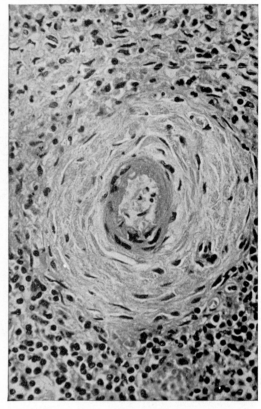

FIG. 59.—Onion-skin thickening of splenic arteriole in disseminated lupus erythematosus. (Kindness of Dr. S. Hanson, Edmonton, Alberta.)

ated lupus (Fig. 60). In *summary*, the *four most characteristic lesions* of the disease are: (1) the *Libman-Sacks endocarditis*, (2) the *wire-loop capillaries* in the renal glomeruli, (3) the *onion-skin arterioles* in the spleen, and (4) the *hematoxylin bodies*.

Pathogenesis.—In many respects disseminated lupus resembles polyarteritis nodosa, although the sex incidence is very different, but the clinical evidence of hypersensitivity, such as a history of asthma, urticaria and eosinophilia which is so characteristic of polyarteritis, is lacking in disseminated lupus. Strong evidence is accumulating, however, that an *auto-immune mechanism* is responsible for all of the varied manifestations of the disease. Auto-antibodies seem to develop against various antigens both in the blood cells and in the plasma (Dameshek). The Coombs test is positive, thus indicating the presence of an antibody globulin on the

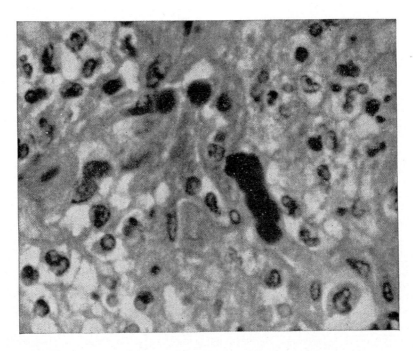

Fig. 60.—Hematoxylin bodies characteristic of disseminated lupus in section of the lung. × 1500.
(Ogryzlo and Smythe, courtesy of Pediatrics, 1957).

surface of the red blood cells, while leuko-penia, thrombocytopenic purpura, and other conditions believed to have a hypersensitivity basis may sometimes be present.

Strong evidence in support of a hyper-immune mechanism is afforded by the fluorescent antibody technique (conjugation of the globulin fraction to fluorescein isocyanate) by which the serum gamma globulin can be shown to possess a reactive affinity with intranuclear material, probably desoxyribonucleoprotein (Bardawil). Sensitization may be against either intrinsic or extrinsic nucleoprotein. Gamma globulin is incriminated in the L.E. cell phenomenon (*see* below), and it is probable that L.E. cell inclusions and hematoxylin bodies are interrelated phenomena. Similar results are obtained in scleroderma and dermatomyositis, which suggests that these diseases, and possibly rheumatoid arthritis which may occasionally show the L.E. phenomenon, may be manifestations of a common disease process initiated by sensitization against nucleoprotein which may be intrinsic or

extrinsic. Sensitization may begin as a response to heterologous proteins, continuing thereafter as an auto-immunity reaction against one or more native intranuclear substances. One possible pathway for development may be through intrauterine sensitization against fetal or placental tissues. Bacterial or viral nucleoproteins from invading microorganisms must be included in the list of possible heterologous antigens. Once established, a state of sensitivity may be maintained by the small amounts of nucleoprotein which are liberated when cells die normally or are destroyed by disease.

The *lupus erythematosus (L.E.) phenomenon* or reaction consists in the demonstration of (a) a characteristic inclusion-containing cell, the *L.E. cell*, or (b) *rosettes* or clumps of leukocytes around inclusion material. It is an *in vitro*, not an *in vivo*, phenomenon, being occasioned by a change in the serum, not the leukocytes, of the patient. In the test the L.E. factor in the blood can be allowed to react with the white blood cells of the patient, or the cells of human or

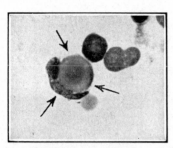

Fig. 61.—L. E. cell. (Kindness of
Dr. A. J. Blanchard.)

animal bone marrow, the cells of the buffy coat of myelogenous leukemia, and even the cells of joint effusions. As the reaction almost never takes place *in vivo*, it appears to be activated by the breakdown of platelets during coagulation when the blood is drawn. The reaction consists of two phases.

The first phase is *nucleolysis*, in which the L.E. factor in the gamma globulin depolymerizes the desoxyribonucleic acid of the chromosomes, converting the nucleus into a homogeneous structureless mass. The second phase is *phagocytosis* of the extruded nuclear material by polymorphonuclear and other leukocytes. The engulfed homogeneous material displaces the nucleus of the leukocyte to the rim of the cell, giving the highly characteristic appearance of the L.E. cell (Fig. 61). It gives a positive Feulgen reaction, indicating its nuclear origin. Some of the amorphous material may remain extracellular, where it can still be recognized. *Rosettes* represent an attempt at phagocytosis of free nuclear material by three or four leukocytes, which form a cluster of cells around the mass. The L.E. factor disappears in remissions and reappears during exacerbations, a feature of great diagnostic value, but it must be realized that the test is really a test for abnormal globulins in the blood. The reaction is seen in the acute form of the disease, being rarely if ever encountered in the chronic stage. The condition giving the next highest positive reaction is chronic rheumatoid arthritis, another member of the diffuse collagen group.

While the L.E. phenomenon occurs most characteristically in acute disseminated lupus erythematosus, it cannot always be demonstrated in this disease, and may occasionally be positive in other disorders. In a careful study of a large amount of material in Toronto, Ogryzlo found the reaction to be positive in 17 patients with rheumatoid arthritis, 3 patients with chronic hepatitis, and isolated cases in other diseases.

The importance of the L.E. phenomenon, apart from its diagnostic value, is the light which it throws on the nature of the disease. It is dependent on a serum factor which has many of the characters of an auto-antibody, being comparable in this respect to the "rheumatoid factor" causing sheep red cell agglutination in rheumatoid arthritis. The factor resides in the gamma globulin fraction of the serum, and this factor with its affinity for tissue nuclei seems to be responsible for the widespread cellular lesions (Holborow *et al.*). It would appear that the reaction is an immunological one in which the L.E. factor is the antibody and the nucleoprotein is the antigen. When the antibody is adsorbed to the nucleoprotein, the latter is phagocytozed by viable white cells to form an inclusion body, with a resulting L.E. cell.

The *hematoxylin bodies*, which have already been described, contain depolymerized desoxyribonucleic acid, so that they may represent a disturbance of nucleoprotein metabolism comparable to the L.E. reaction.

It is of interest to note, as we have already seen, that the Coombs test, an indicator of the presence of antibody-globulin on the surface of the red blood cell, is also positive. The Coombs test points to involvement of the erythrocytes, just as the L.E. factor points to the leukocytes. More than one or even several auto-immune antibodies may be concerned, some being responsible for the vascular and skin lesions, as well as the nephritis, endocarditis, and arthritis, whilst others are involved in such hematological phenomena as the L.E. reaction, positive Coombs test and hematoxylin bodies, as well as the occasional occurrence of such blood disturbances as thrombocytopenic purpura, leukopenia, and hemolytic anemia. Disseminated lupus, is therefore, a complex of immunological disturbances involving not only small blood vessels but also the red and white blood cells. Dameshek suggests that the development of antigens responsible for the formation of these auto-immune antibodies may take place in the menstruating endometrium, where at monthly intervals there is destruction of red and white blood cells, plasma constituents, and small blood vessels. In the occasional unfortunate male, other mechanisms must be responsible.

The *Sjögren syndrome* is characterized by keratoconjunctivitis sicca, arthritis, and a dry mouth, with or without enlargement of the salivary glands. It is first cousin or even more closely related to Mikulicz's disease, in which the main salivary as well as the lachrymal glands are enlarged. It is considered in this place because the autopsy findings are very similar to those of systemic lupus, the L.E. cell test is positive in perhaps one-third of the cases, and even hematoxylin bodies have been reported (Bain). Biopsy of the salivary glands shows the acinar tissue to be replaced by a dense lymphocytic infiltration known as the "benign lympho-epithelial lesion."

Rheumatoid Arthritis.—Here again is a member of the collagen disease group that is a disease of mystery, but in which accumulating evidence points to an element of hypersensitivity. In the beginning the reaction may be due to some external antigen, but the extremely chronic nature of the condition with recurring exacerbations suggests an element of auto-immunity. A specific agglutination test points to the presence of a *rheumatoid factor* in the blood. The test uses sheep's red cells treated with tannic acid and coated with human gamma globulin, or latex particles coated with gamma globulin. Rheumatoid arthritis is again a disease mainly of women in the child-bearing age, and the symptoms may be greatly relieved by the occurrence of pregnancy.

Other Diseases.—*Idiopathic Ulcerative Colitis.*—Marked anemia is a constant feature of ulcerative colitis, and in some cases an auto-immune mechanism seems to be responsible, as a positive Coombs reaction can be demonstrated. Indeed one wonders if the destructive lesions of the bowel in this very distressing and obscure form of colitis may themselves be a manifestation of a similar mechanism.

Multiple Sclerosis.—Nothing is known regarding the causation of multiple sclerosis. We shall see in Chapter 42, however, that this belongs to the group of demyelinating diseases, in which the axis cylinders gradually lose their myelin sheaths, and that in the experimental animal an acute disseminated encephalomyelitis with demyelination can be induced by the injection of emulsions of normal brain and cord with the production of anti-brain antibodies. Moreover in Japan anti-rabies inoculation, which involves the injection of an emulsion of spinal cord, has produced an acute form of demyelination in man in a number of cases. It is possible that various forms of *polyneuritis* are also the result of an auto-immune reaction. In multiple sclerosis there is a significant elevation of globulins in the cerebrospinal fluid, leading to characteristic changes in the colloidal gold curve, and antibrain-antibodies have been demonstrated in the blood (Raskin).

Chronic Hepatitis.—There is every reason to believe that the ordinary forms of *chronic hepatitis* are caused by viral infection. It is customary, however, for a virus to attack a cell explosively, with rapid subsidence of the evidence of infection. In many cases of hepatitis there appears to be a continuance or recurrence of cellular damage as indicated by the presence of a high level of circulating complement-fixing antibodies to human liver or a raised glutamic oxalo-acetic transaminase level in the plasma, the latter being reduced by cortisone therapy. In some cases the L.E. cell reaction has been present. It is believed that certain liver-cell components become antigenic; antibodies to these antigens are produced which react in a damaging manner with the liver cells, thus perpetuating the hepatitis (Mackay). Even cases of so-called primary biliary cirrhosis may present a high auto-antibody titer in the serum.

Miscellaneous Lesions.—It would be possible to discuss the possibility of an auto-immune mechanism in a number of other conditions. Some of these will merely be mentioned in this place. *Glomerulonephritis* is undoubtedly the immunological response of the sensitized kidney to streptococcal insult, but the continuance of the lesions over a period of months may well have an auto-immune basis. It has been known for fifty years that the intravenous injection of serum containing antibodies prepared against the animal's kidney tissue can produce lesions resembling those of glomerulonephritis. *Sympathetic ophthalmia* is the dreaded complication where a granulomatous lesion in the uveal tract of one eye develops after injury involving the uveal tract of the other. The most probable explanation is on an auto-immunity basis. *Interstitial myocarditis* is known in many cases to represent a hypersensitivity reaction on the part of the myocardium to drugs, especially the sulfonamide group, but those cases labelled as *idiopathic myocarditis* may perhaps be explained as an auto-immune reaction. *Sarcoidosis* is a granulomatous reaction, usually generalized, which resembles tuberculosis histologically, but for which no cause is known, although pine pollen has been suspected. Here again, an auto-immune reaction may be responsible for the picture.

In summarizing the various conditions which have as their pathogenetic basis, at least in part, auto-immune mechanisms, the student is referred to the table of contents at the beginning of this chapter. Still other examples of apparent auto-immunity will be found in a paper by McMaster and in Boyd's *Fundamentals of Immunology*.

Many diseases suspected of being due to auto-immune reactions follow infections or the development of drug allergy, conditions which appear to trigger the auto-immune mechanism. The agent seems to make certain constituents of a person's own tissues antigenic for him. This is well seen in the relationship of hemolytic streptococci to rheumatic fever and also in the case of the sulfonamides. Nearly all cases of paroxysmal nocturnal hemoglobinuria are syphilitic. Most members of the auto-immune group have the following features in common. (1) They often *follow an infectious disease*; (2) they are often *familial*, suggesting an inherited tendency to produce antibodies too readily; (3) they commonly show an *elevated gamma globulin* level; (4) they often give rise to *"false-positive" tests for syphilis*; (5) they are often *relieved by cortisone* and ACTH.

A word of warning must be sounded in concluding this discussion. It is dangerously, if not fatally, easy to be seduced by the concept of auto-immunity as an explanation for many so-called idiopathic diseases. When I was an undergraduate student everything that was obscure was blamed on "focal infection." Now these obscurities have become "psychosomatic." Auto-immune reactions are going to prove of great value in explaining a number of obscure conditions, but they will not provide a key to every mystery.

Moreover it must not be forgotten that we are still in the dark as to the mechanism responsible for the formation or liberation of auto-antigens. Even in Hashimoto's disease, one of the easiest examples to understand, we can say that small quantities of thyroglobulin escaping from the follicles encounter lymphoid tissue where antibodies are formed, and that these damage the surrounding tissues, thus releasing more thyroglobulin, so that a chain reaction is started. But when we are asked what is responsible for the original release of the thyroglobulin, we are embarrassed and have only a stumbling answer. Moreover, there is no relation between the amount of circulating antibody which we can demonstrate in the laboratory and the severity of the clinical disease. It is possible that the circulating antihuman tissue antibodies may be the result rather than the cause of the continuing tissue damage. It is true that the auto-immune process may possibly be initiated by some *subclinical* viral infection or drug sensitivity, but of this there is as yet no proof. Finally there is the possibility that the lesions may be the result of a cell-fixed antibody, as in tuberculin sensitivity, the circulating antibody being merely an epiphenomenon (Gajdusek).

These ideas are mentioned, not with the object of discouraging the student in his search into the unknown, but to stimulate him to distinguish between hypothesis and fact.

TISSUE TRANSPLANTATION

In the general subject of auto-immunity, of the recognition of self and not-self, one question of particular importance is that of tissue transplantation. This is a subject which will be of greater interest to the student when he encounters the problem of the transplantation (grafting) of tissues and even of organs in his surgical studies. Each of us is so different from anyone else that we can recognize, and reject, the tissues of another person when they are introduced into ourselves. We recognize them as foreign in nature, refuse integration, produce antibodies, and reject the intruder. This is even true of red corpuscles in a blood transfusion. If the antigens of the donor do not belong to the same blood group as those of the recipient, antibodies are produced and the red cells are destroyed. Self will not accept not-self.

The same holds true for tissue transplants. In the case of inbred strains of mice, where brothers have been mated with sisters for 100 generations or more, the transplanted tissue will take and grow. These transplants made within a pure inbred strain are known as *isologous* (*isos*, equal), and behave like *autogenous* grafts (*auto*, self) made from one part of an individual's own body to another part. Transplantation from one member of a species in which random breeding is practiced, as in man, to another is known as *homologous* (*homo*, same), whilst *heterologous* grafts (*heteros*, another) are transplants made between different species. Heterologous grafts are rejected for reasons we have just considered. The obstacle can be overcome by a number of devices. *Total body radiation* destroys the immunity mechanism to such a degree that death will come from infection. If, however, a less than lethal dose is administered, the capacity of antibody production is interfered with to such a degree that homologous and even heterologous transplants are accepted. *Cortisone*, and particularly hydrocortisone, has a similar effect, so that human tissue may be transplanted into and accepted by rats. In Chapter 8 we shall see that human cancers may be transplanted into and grow in rats whose power of antibody production has been impaired to such a degree that they fail to distinguish between self and not-self. The value and importance of this advance will become apparent when we come to study the subject of neoplasia.

The matter of the transplantation of tissues and organs is also vitally important to the surgeon. If both kidneys of a patient have been destroyed by disease, the obvious thing to do would be to transplant a kidney from a healthy donor or cadaver. This procedure will work in the case of identical twins (self and self), but not under other circumstances (self and not-self). As we have already seen, tissue can be transplanted with success into the fetus which has not yet learned how to produce antibodies, but this is of small comfort to the surgeon. It is possible, however, that in the near future, by virtue of some of the theoretical considerations outlined above, we may succeed in solving the problem. Indeed success has already attended kidney transplantation between *nonidentical* twins (Merrill *et al.*). A condition of at least partial acquired tolerance was induced by subtotal whole-body irradiation, sufficient to impair temporarily but not completely the ability of the lymphopoietic tissues to elaborate antibody and to reproduce themselves. The transplanted kidney was then accepted, and beginning rejection of the homograft eight months later was aborted by a second course of low-dose irradiation, together with adrenocorticoid therapy.

It must not be supposed from what has been said that tissue transplants in the past have been of no value. Autogenous transplants in man are of course most desirable, and these are used in skin grafts. Heterologous transplants, however, have also proved of great use, particularly in the case of bone, fascia, nerves, blood vessels, and the cornea. In these instances we are using the *intercellular substance* of the transplant, and even though antibodies may destroy the cells of the foreign transplant, the intercellular substance acts as a scaffold on which the cells of the host can build a new structure. This is particularly well exemplified in arterial transplants, which provide a temporary skeleton on which a new vessel can be constructed, the skeleton itself being later discarded.

Cancer.—Here we are on the most uncertain ground of all. There is reason to believe, however, that the body frequently or usually has a defense mechanism against cancer, and that the cases we see clinically develop in persons lacking this defense or in whom the defense has broken down. Cancer of the prostate in latent form is found in nearly 50 per cent of men over fifty years of age, and yet it usually does not develop so as to manifest itself clinically. So-called carcinoma-in-situ is a not infrequent finding in the cervix uteri, but it seems to be held in check and only occasionally becomes invassive. Cancer transplants inoculated into other laboratory animals of the same strain often die. The same is true of human cancer inoculated into healthy volunteers, yet these transplants grow in cancer patients lacking the necessary immunity. Finally, as we shall see when we come to the discussion of neoplasia, in rare cases human cancers may undergo spontaneous regression and disappear (Boyd). All of these facts suggest the existence of an immune mechanism present in most people. It is obvious that if we could learn more about the nature of this mechanism we might make a big step forward in our ability to control cancer, as we have already done in the control of infectious disease.

REFERENCES

ANDERSON, J. R., et al.: Lancet, 1957, 2, 1123. (Auto-antibodies in Addison's disease).

BAIN, G. O.: Can. Med. Ass. J., 1960, 82, 143. (Sjögren's syndrome)

BARDAWIL, W. A.: Am. J. Path., 1958, 34, 607. (Nucleo-protein sensitization in disseminated lupus).

BILLINGHAM, R. E., BRENT, L. and MEDAWAR, P. B.: Nature, 1953, 172, 603. (Immunological reactions).

BOYD, W. C.: Fundamentals of Immunology, 3rd ed., New York, 1957.

BOYD, W.: J. Canad. Ass. Radiol., 1957, 8, 45, 63. (Spontaneous regression of cancer).

BRUNSON, J. G. and DAVIS, R. L.: Arch. Path., 1955, 60, 593. (Systemic fibrinoid diseases).

BUCHANAN, W. W., et al.: Lancet, 1958, 2, 928. (Skin test in Hashimoto's disease).

BURNET, F. M.: Natural History of Infectious Disease, Cambridge, 1953.

————.: Enzyme, Antigen and Virus, Cambridge, 1956. Brit. Med. J., 1954, 2, 189. (Self-markers in immunological reactions).

COONS, A. H. and KAPLAN, M. H.: J. Exper. Med., 1950, 91, 1. (Fluorescent labelled antibody.)

————: Internal, Rev. of Cytology, 1956, 5, 1. (Histochemistry and technic of labelled antibody).

CHURG, J. and GRISHMAN, E.: Am. J. Path., 1953, 29, 190. (Renal lesion in disseminated lupus erythematosus).

DAMESHEK, W.: Blood, 1953, 8, 382. (Platelet-destroying factor in idiopathic thrombocytopenic purpura.)

————.: Ann. Int. Med., 1958, 48, 707. (Disseminated lupus erythematosus as an autoimmune disorder).

DIXON, F. J., et al.: Arch. Path., 1958, 65, 18. (Pathogenesis of serum sickness).

EHRICH, W. E.: Am. Heart J., 1952, 43, 121. (Hypersensitivity and the collagen diseases).

GAJDUSEK, D. C.: Arch. Int. Med., 1958, 101, 9. (Auto-immunity in disease production).

GERMUTH, F. G., JR. and McKINNON, G. E.: Bull. Johns Hopkins Hosp., 1957, 101, 13. (Soluble antigen-antibody complexes).

GITLIN, D., GROSS, P. A. M. and JANEWAY, C. A.: New Eng. J. Med., 1959, 260, 21, 72, 121, 170. (Gamma globulins).

HACKETT, E., BEECH, M. and FORRES, I. J.: Brit. Med. J., 1960, 2, 17. (Auto-immune complement-fixation reaction).

HAMILTON, J. D.: Can. Med. Ass. J., 1958, 78, 834. (Tissue lesions in hypersensitivity).

HOLBOROW, E. J., WEIR, D. M. and JOHNSON, G. D.: Brit. Med. J., 1957, 2, 655. (A serum factor in lupus erythematosus with affinity for tissue nuclei).

KING, E. S. J., et al.: Brit. J. Cancer, 1958, 12, 5. (Antigen-antibody fluorescence in cancer).

KLEMPERER, P., POLLACK, A. D. and BAEHR, G.: Arch. Path., 1941, 32, 569. J.A.M.A., 1942, 119, 331. (Diffuse collagen disease).

————.: Am. J. Path., 1950, 26, 505. (Diffuse collagen disease).

MACKAY, I. R.: New Eng. J. Med., 1958, 258, 185. (Auto-immune reaction in chronic hepatitis).

MARRACK, J.: Nature, 1934, 133, 292. (Labelled antibody).

McMASTER, P. R. B.: New York State J. Med., 1958, 58, 2980. (Auto-antibodies and autosensitivity).

MELLORS, R. C., SIEGEL, M. and PRESSMAN, D.: Lab. Invest., 1955, 4, 69. (Histochemical demonstration of antibody localization in tissues)

MERRILL, J. P., et al.: New Eng. J. Med., 1960, 262, 1251. (Homotransplantation of kidney between nonidentical twins).

MORE, R. H. and MOVAT, H. Z.: Arch. Path., 1959, 67, 679. (Cellular and intercellular changes in local hypersensitivity).

————.: J. Path. and Bact., 1958, 75, 127. (Plasma cells in acute polyarteritis nodosa.

MORE, R. H., McMILLAN, G. C. and DUFF, G. L.: Am. J. Path., 1946, 22, 703. (Sulphonamide allergy).

MOVAT, H. Z.: Can. Med. Ass. J., 1960, 83, 683, 747, 799. (Pathology and pathogenesis of the diffuse collagen diseases).

OGRYZLO, M. A.: Can. Med. Ass. J., 1956, 75, 980. (The L. E. cell reaction).

OGRYZLO, M. A. and SMYTHE, H. A.: Pediatrics, 1957, 19, 1109. (Systemic lupus erythematosus and related conditions.)

PILLEMER, L., *et al.*: Science, 1954, *120*, 279. (Properdin system immunity).

RAITT, I. M., *et al.*: Lancet, 1956, *2*, 820. (Autoimmunity in Hashimoto's disease).

RASKIN, N.: Arch. Neurol. and Psychiat., 1955, *73*, 6. (Antibrain-antibodies in multiple sclerosis).

RICH, A. R.: Can. Med. Ass. J., 1958, *78*, 163. (Studies on hypersensitivity).

RICH, A. R. and LEWIS, M. R.: Bull. Johns Hopkins Hosp., 1932, *50*, 115. (Hypersensitivity in tissue culture cells).

ROSS, O. A.: Am. J. Path., 1958, *34*, 471. (The properdin system in resistance to infection).

SPEIRS, R. S.: Nature, 1958, *181*, 681. (Site of antibody production).

STEINER, J. W., *et al.*: J. Exper. Med., 1960, *112*, 187. (Experimental immunological adrenal injury).

STUART, A. E. and ALLAN, W. S. A.: Lancet, 1958, *2*, 1204. (Basement membrane changes in Hashimoto's disease).

TEILUM, G.: Am. J. Path., 1948, *24*, 409. (Disseminated lupus erythematosus).

VAZQUEZ, J. J. and DIXON, F. J.: New York Acad. Sci., 1960, *86*, 1025. (Immunopathology of hypersensitivity).

————.: Lab. Invest., 1957, *6*, 205. (Immunohistological study of lesions of collagen diseases.

WEISER, R. S.: J. Allergy, 1957, *28*, 475. (The mast cell in immunological reactions).

WITEBSKY, E., *et al.*: J.A.M.A., 1957, *164*, 1439. (Autoimmunization in chronic thyroiditis).

Chapter 6

Coagulation, Thrombosis and Embolism

Blood Coagulation
  ANTICOAGULANTS
Thrombosis
  INTRODUCTION
  CAUSES
    Slowing of the Blood Stream
    Changes in the Vessel Wall
    Changes in the Blood
  SITES
    Veins
      Venous thrombosis

Septic thrombophlebitis
Simple thrombophlebitis
Phlegmasia caerulea dolens
Thrombophlebitis migrans
Axillary vein thrombosis
Arteries
Heart
FIBRINOLYSIS
CLINICAL EFFECTS
SUBSEQUENT FATE OF THE
  THROMBUS

Embolism
  PULMONARY EMBOLISM AND IN-
    FARCTION
  PARADOXICAL EMBOLISM
  FAT EMBOLISM
  AIR EMBOLISM
  AMNIOTIC FLUID EMBOLISM
  ATHEROMATOUS EMBOLISM
  BONE MARROW EMBOLISM

BLOOD COAGULATION

IT is convenient to consider coagulation and thrombosis separately, although the two are usually inextricably combined. *Coagulation* or *clotting* can occur in the test tube or in the vessels after the blood has ceased to flow, as well as in blood which is still in motion. Its primary constituent is *fibrin*, in the network of which are entangled the various formed elements of the blood. Chief amongst these are the red cells, so that the clot or coagulum is red and soft, and is referred to as a red clot, or sometimes (unfortunately) as a red thrombus A better term is a fibrin or coagulation clot. A *true thrombus*, as we shall see presently, consists primarily of *platelets*, but these are associated with fibrin and a limited number of blood cells. It is correctly described as a white or firm thrombus. If the end result, the clot and the thrombus, may resemble one another, the processes by which they are produced are entirely distinct.

The classical theory of clotting, which has been in vogue for the past fifty years, states that fibrin is formed by the action of thrombin on fibrinogen, and that the circulating blood contains two special proteins, prothrombin and fibrinogen. When the blood is shed and comes in contact with damaged tissue, a third substance, thromboplastin, is formed, which, in association with ionized calcium, leads to the formation of thrombin. There are thus four factors involved: (1)

prothrombin, (2) *thromboplastin*, (3) *calcium*, and (4) *fibrinogen*. The first three form *thrombin*, whilst the fourth is acted on by thrombin to form fibrin. This is brought about by polymerization of fibrinogen units. The fibrinogen molecule is a long, slender rod which rotates rapidly on its long axis. The rods join together end to end and side to side to form a sticky fibrin network.

The classical theory still remains true, but it has become enormously complicated by the introduction of many additional factors and the use of an obscure jargon. It is now recognized that the thrombin-fibrinogen reaction is the last and most important link in a long chain of reactions (MacFarlane). The justification for mentioning these factors here is that the absence of any one of them may be the basis of a defect in coagulation with a resulting "bleeding disease." Two of the main difficulties are the origin of the thromboplastin and the activation of prothrombin. We now recognize that two additional factors in the plasma in addition to the original four are required for the conversion of prothrombin into thrombin by thromboplastin. These are known as factors V and VII; fortunately an original factor VI has now been discarded. A depression of either of these factors or of prothrombin will cause marked lengthening of the "prothrombin time," with corresponding interference with blood clotting. So also will a deficiency in platelets, calcium, antihemophilic globulin (AHG), and Christmas factor. Deficiency of AHG is responsible for the bleeding of hemophilia, and of Christmas factor for the bleeding of Christmas disease, conditions which are discussed in Chapter 39.

In our concentration on the subject of coagulation we must not forget the most remarkable fact about the blood in this respect, namely that it remains fluid even in the finest capillaries under normal conditions, yet the moment it is shed it clots and plugs the hole in the vessel wall. The spontaneous transformation of fluid blood to solid clot has something in the nature of a conjuring trick. It is like a fire-sprinkler system, unnoticed as long as all goes well, but ready for any emergency at a moment's notice. The cause of the continuing fluidity in the vessels is the absence of contact with an activating surface and the presence of inhibitors.

As Biggs and Macfarlane point out in their classic monograph on *Blood Coagulation*, the hemostatic mechanism is so unobtrusively efficient that we are hardly aware of its existence. It is essentially concerned with bleeding from the small vessels, *i.e.* the capillaries, the venules and arterioles which are liable to be injured by such trivial everyday procedures as brushing the teeth, and more obviously by the scratches, knocks and cuts which everyone sustains. Such injuries stop bleeding of their own accord. Even in an operation after the surgeon has applied his ligatures to the wounds he has made, he forgets that nature has quietly sealed the countless small vessels he has also divided. Without that hemostatic mechanism the patient would die from hemorrhage. Failure of the mechanism means that a normal life becomes almost impossible, and that he may die at any time from some small injury. Examples of such failure are discussed in connection with diseases of the blood (Chapter 39).

We have already seen that *thromboplastin* is essential for the conversion of prothrombin into thrombin, and is therefore the key substance in the process of clotting. It is released as the result of injury, mainly to platelets, but also to tissue. It is this fact which links clotting with thrombosis. When a vessel is opened the platelets at once stick together in clumps and at the same time release thromboplastin. It is now believed that this matter also is no longer as simple

as was once thought and that, as in the case of the activation of prothrombin, other factors such as factors V and VII and the Christmas factor must also come to the assistance of the platelets. If these are lacking, clotting is interfered with. It used to be supposed that injured tissue could also release thromboplastin, but it would now appear that all the elements involved are in the blood itself.

Anticoagulants.—We cannot live without clotting of the blood, but often we cannot live with it, particularly when it is associated with thrombosis. Various agents which are known to interfere with clotting and to prevent the extension of the process are available, and have been used in cases of coagulation and thrombosis in the veins of the leg and the coronary arteries, and particularly in vascular surgery. The two most generally used are heparin and Dicumarol.

Heparin, so-called because it was first obtained from the liver, but now known to be secreted by the mast cells, helps to maintain the fluidity of the blood in the vascular bed. It prevents the agglutination of platelets to form platelet thrombi, and it neutralizes the action of thrombin, thus preventing the formation of a soft fibrin clot. It is therefore of great value in blood vessel surgery, permitting end-to-end anastomosis, suture of vessels, *etc.*, without subsequent thrombosis.

Dicumarol has a similar action to heparin, prolonging the coagulation time to a much greater degree. It has the advantage that it can be taken by mouth instead of being injected intravenously. Cattle suffer from a hemorrhagic disease caused by eating decayed sweet clover, and it was from this material that Dicumarol was first obtained, although now it is synthesized.

THROMBOSIS

Introduction.—Thrombosis is one of the most important conditions which the student has to study, and one of the most important with which the physician and surgeon have to deal. It has been said with truth that "throughout his entire existence man is almost constantly hemorrhaging and thrombosing" (Wright). As we have seen to be the case in the associated condition of coagulation, thrombosis can be both helpful and harmful. Without thrombosis life would be impossible, but thrombosis at the wrong time and the wrong place leads to death.

Thombosis is in essence platelet deposition, whereas clotting or coagulation is a reaction by which a sol, fibrinogen, is converted into a gel, fibrin, through the action of thromboplastin. As the platelets (thrombocytes) elaborate thromboplastin, it is evident that the two processes may be combined. If the blood flow is sufficient in volume and velocity to wash away the thromboplastin, clotting will not occur. Both thrombosis and clotting are necessary for the arrest of hemorrhage, but the platelet reaction is the more immediate. Indeed platelets begin to appear for the occlusion of an opened vessel within from ten to thirty seconds. Both, as we shall see, have the potentiality for evil, which merely illustrates the profound truth that pathology is merely physiology gone wrong. All the elements of the blood, platelets, fibrin, red cell and leukocytes, may enter into the formation of a thrombus. A thrombus is commonly spoken of as a clot, and, while this is not strictly accurate, it is convenient to bow to customary usage.

It is rather sobering for us to learn that in 1888 Eberth and Schimmelbusch watched the whole process of thrombus formation in the small veins of the translucent mesentery under the microscope, and published the most important single contribution to the literature on thrombosis. They showed that a mass of platelets was built up in the course of one hour of sufficient size to project into the lumen. When the stream was rapid, as in the arteries, clumps of platelets were torn away, but quickly replaced. If the flow was slow, as in the veins, the lumen became closed. Eberth and Schimmelbusch proved above all that a thrombus is not primarily an intravascular coagulum. When the lumen is closed and the flow stops, two stagnating columns of blood are formed, the one in front and the other behind the next collateral vessels. Thromboplastin is liberated from the mass of platelets, and then, and only then, does true coagulation occur. Since 1888 little of fundamental importance has been added to our knowledge of thrombosis.

In a stained blood smear the platelets

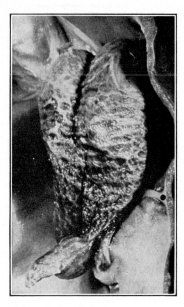

Fig. 62.—Thrombus showing lines of Zahn.

appear as small nuclear bodies arranged in clumps, but moving pictures of streaming blood show that the nucleus is a very small part of the platelet, and that it is surrounded for some distance by a thin veil-like cytoplasm which is actively ameboid and throws out pseudopodia that are arrested by any irregularity of surface. Above a critical velocity the platelets are evenly distributed, but below it they show a remarkable tendency to stick together and to adhere to the intima, more especially if the intimal surface is roughened. When the number of platelets is increased (thrombocytosis) the stickiness is increased, because of the many young forms present. Heparin causes the platelets to lose their stickiness. *Thrombocytosis* always follows tissue injury, particularly that of parturition, fractures, and surgical operations. The greater the injury, the more marked is the thrombocytosis and the tendency to thrombosis.

As the platelets fall out of the streaming blood they form a kind of snowdrift, which smoothes over any roughness of the surface. Then a series of ridges or laminæ of platelets grow across at right angles to the stream. These give to the thrombus the appearance of a piece of coral, and the edges of the lam-

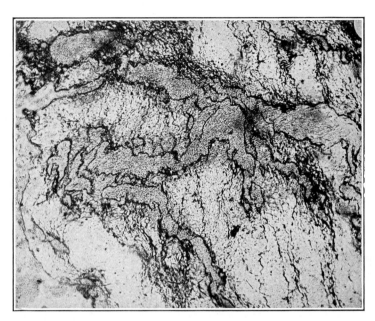

FIG. 63.—Antemortem thrombus, showing laminæ of platelets outlined by fibrin
and connected by fibrin threads. Fibrin stain. × 100.

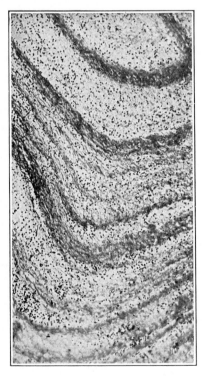

FIG. 64.—Antemortem thrombus. Numerous cells
between the strands of platelets × 75.

9

inæ are seen as ripples known as the *lines of Zahn* (Fig. 62). Leukocytes stick to the laminæ as flies to sticky fly-paper. The adherent platelets liberate thromboplastin, and this sets in motion the machinery of fibrin formation, so that festoons of fibrin threads hang between the ridges and entangle many red cells and more leukocytes (Fig. 63). As Hadfield points out, the object of thrombosis is the restoration of the integrity of the vascular bed, but it may be complicated by fibrin formation, which is both purposeless and progressive. The thrombus is now composed of platelets and fibrin, with an admixture of red cells and leukocytes (Fig. 64). In time the various elements are fused to form a hyaline mass.

When occlusion of the lumen occurs, true thrombosis ceases, because streaming blood is no longer available. Clotting, however, continues, and the clot is "propagated" to the next side branch if the vessel is an artery, the next tributary if it is a vein (Fig. 65). This propagated soft red clot lies floating free in the lumen, though still anchored to the thrombus. In the case of a leg vein the propagated clot may be from $1\frac{1}{2}$ to 2 feet in

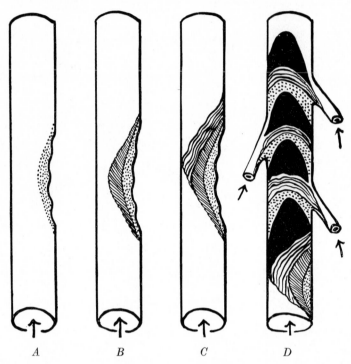

FIG. 65.—Stages in the formation of a thrombus. *A*, primary platelet thrombus. *B*, coralline thrombus. *C*, fibrin formation and occlusion. *D*, propagated clot. (Modified from G. Hadfield: Annals of the Royal College of Surgeons of England, 1950, *6*, 219, in Boyd's, *Pathology for the Surgeon*, W. B. Saunders Company.

length. Progagation occurs when the stream is slow and sluggish. If it is rapid, due to inflow from tributaries, a new platelet thrombus may be formed on the propagated fibrin clot so that there is segmental formation of alternate white and red thrombus (Fig. 65). It is the soft propagated clot, not the firm adherent platelet thrombus, that is likely to become detached and form an embolus.

The process of thrombosis can be observed microscopically through the transparent wall of a celloidin tube connecting the carotid artery and the jugular vein. In these observations one is struck by the speed with which a thrombus is formed, often only a matter of a few minutes.

Causes.—Thrombosis is the result of an upset in a delicate balance. More than a hundred years ago Rudolf Virchow, who gave us our first understanding of the process and introduced the all-important concept of embolism, stated that there were three factors (*Virchow's triad*) involved in its causation.

These were: (1) slowing of the blood stream, (2) changes in the vessel wall, and (3) changes in the blood itself. In the intervening years almost nothing of real importance has been added to our knowledge. Of the three the last is perhaps the most important and the one of which we know the least.

1. *Slowing of the Blood Stream.*—This is the important factor in veins, and it may be added that thrombosis is much commoner in veins than in arteries. When in a snowstorm the wind drops, the snowflakes pile up in masses; so it is with the blood platelets. The venous circulation is a low-pressure, low-velocity system which is dependent on the strength of the left ventricle, the depth of respiration, muscular contraction, and the adequacy of the valves in the veins. Venous thrombosis may be a post-operative complication, but it is practically confined to patients with an ageing heart muscle. It is even commoner in congestive heart failure, especially when combined with general muscular immobility owing to the patient being

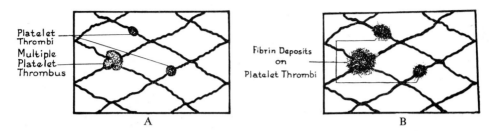

FIG. 66.—Diagrammatic representation of the development of platelet thrombi and fibrin on an injured endothelial surface. *A*, pure platelet thrombi. *B*, fibrin added to platelet thrombi. (Samuels and Webster, courtesy of Ann. Surg.,)

confined to bed. The calf muscles have been called "the peripheral heart" and it is only natural that venous thrombosis should be commonest in the veins of the leg, often starting in the valve pockets. Shallow breathing due to pulmonary disease, shock, or abdominal distension interferes with the venous flow and therefore predisposes to thrombosis. As Hadfield remarks, even in health there is only a narrow margin between movement and stasis in the outlying parts of the venous system, a margin which is dependent on general circulatory and respiratory efficiency. The vein walls are weak and thin, with little elastic tissue and therefore easily collapsed by pressure; they are superficial and easily injured; they are readily invaded by bacteria. In all these respects they differ from the deeply-placed arteries with their turbulent high-velocity flow, whilst in the intervals of flow the lumen remains empty, thanks to their thick elastic walls. In health the blood manifests a laminar type of flow, with the large leukocytes at the center, then the red cells, and farthest out the platelets, which are normally separated from the vessel wall by a clear zone of plasma. If the laminar flow and the clear plasmatic zone are disrupted by slowing of the stream or by turbulence and eddies such as may occur in the auricles, the platelets are brought in direct contact with the vascular bed.

2. *Changes in the Vessel Wall.*—This is not so important a factor as slowing of the blood stream, as is shown by the fact that disease is rare in the wall of a vein as compared with an artery, and yet we have seen that venous thrombosis is very much commoner than arterial. Injury to the intima may recur in

the arteries, the veins or the heart. In the arteries the smooth intima may be roughened by atheroma, which also narrows the lumen and slows the stream; it may become necrotic as the result of malignant hypertension, periarteritis nodosa, or disseminated lupus; or it may be injured by the surgeon's knife or ligature. In the arteries, with the exception of the aorta, there can, of course, be no propagated clot nor danger of embolism. The veins are liable to injury by trauma, by pressure, and by infection. In the heart the valves are injured by inflammation, so that thrombi are deposited on the surface.

The absence of any apparent change in the vein wall has always been a puzzle. Samuels and Webster have now shown that in the experimental animal there is a significant reaction of the vein wall to mechanical trauma, to chemical injury, and to stripping of the sheath. The intracellular substance of the endothelium becomes sticky, so that particles adhere to it. At first discrete platelet thrombi are formed, followed by the development of more vague masses of fibrin which spread along the intercellular lines (Fig. 66). These observations serve to support the idea that the continued pressure of a hard mattress on the calf of the leg may be a contributory factor to the development of venous thrombosis, as also may more obvious trauma.

Experimental injury to a vessel wall also stimulates the endothelium to produce a granular material which closely resembles the intercellular cement (McGovern). At the same time a metachromatic substance, thought to be heparin and probably produced by mast cells in the adventitia, diffuses through the endothelium, unites with the newly formed granular cement, and causes the granules to coalesce and form a protective film on the endothelial surface. If this mechanism is impaired either by severe trauma or by anoxia, thrombosis may result.

3. *Changes in the Blood.*—This is perhaps the most decisive but certainly the least known factor. Some persons with diseased arterial walls or slow stream in the veins develop thrombosis, while others do not. There is even an idiopathic group in which persons who appear to be in perfect health develop venous thrombosis. What does all this mean? It must point to a third factor, which probably lies in the character of the blood. Little is known about this matter, but it may involve the *stickiness of the platelets*, the *viscosity of the blood*, or the *heparin content*. It is well recognized that thrombocytosis follows any severe injury such as a surgical operation and child birth, conditions which are frequently associated with venous thrombosis. Moreover, the stickiness of the young platelets is much greater than that of ageing ones, so that they tend to stick together and to the wall of the vessel, just as do snow flakes when they become wet. The viscosity of the blood is increased as the result of the dehydration which may accompany severe injury or major surgery, especially on the stomach and intestines. Trauma in the experimental animal causes the intravascular agglutination of red cells known as *sludging;* normally the circulating red blood cells tend to repel each other. The plasma fibrinogen is raised as the result of trauma. Finally the possibility of a temporary decrease in the output of heparin has to be considered.

Spontaneous Venous Thrombosis deserves special mention, inasmuch as we are accustomed to take for granted the presence of predisposing factors responsible for the process. In a study of venous thrombosis in 90 apparently healthy individuals there was no preceding trauma, heart failure, cancer, surgical operation, or other precipitating episode (De Camp *et al.*). The incidence was 4.5 per cent in a large series of cases of acute venous thrombosis. The ages of the persons affected ranged from 13 to 88 years. The

frequency of pulmonary embolism was low, and the fatality rate was still lower. There is at present no reasonable explanation for these cases.

SITES.—Thrombosis may occur in the veins, the arteries and the heart. We have already seen that the method of causation is not the same in these three sites, and the clinical effects are even more different. In arteries the chief damage to be feared is from ischemia, whereas in the case of the veins and of the heart embolism is the great threat.

Veins.—The veins are the commonest site of thrombosis for reasons already given. The thrombosis may be divided into two groups: (1) venous thrombosis, and (2) thrombophlebitis.

Venous thrombosis is by far the more important. It is associated with such factors as general circulatory failure, interference with respiration, and trauma. This is the type likely to be followed by pulmonary embolism, which may cost the patient his life. We have already seen that it is the soft friable propagated clot which is the source of danger rather than the firm adherent thrombus. About 40 per cent of instances of fatal pulmonary embolism occur in surgical cases, whereas 60 per cent occur in medical cases, but even in the surgical cases the causal factors responsible for the thrombosis are mainly medical in character. An exception is the increased number and stickiness of the platelets due to production of a large number of young forms. This occurs during the first week following operations or delivery; thrombosis and pulmonary embolism are most frequent between the fourth and tenth day. The common initial site of venous thrombosis is the deep veins of the calf muscles, with a propagated clot occupying the femoral vein. In fatal pulmonary embolism the veins of one leg may be filled with thrombus, whilst those of the other leg are empty. In such a case it is probable that the fatal embolus came from the empty vein. One barrel of the gun has been discharged; the other remains loaded. When a person is confined to a hospital bed the veins of the leg tend to collapse, and the pressure of the calf on a hard mattress brings the walls of the vein together with possible injury to the intima and liberation of thromboplastic substances which induce coagulation in the thin stream of blood that percolates through the crack-like lumen (Frykholm). In support of this idea is the fact that during the bombing of London venous thrombosis of the leg veins with subsequent fatal pulmonary embolism occurred in elderly persons who spent long winter nights sitting in air-raid shelters on deck chairs which pressed on the back of the leg.

In 100 complete dissections of the veins of the pelvis and leg carried out by McLachlin and Paterson on middle-aged and elderly men, thrombi were found in 34 per cent of cases, in 56 per cent of which there was pulmonary embolism. Seventy-three per cent of the thrombi arose in the veins of the thigh and pelvis.

Septic Thrombophlebitis has lost the importance it used to possess before the days of antisepsis and antibiotic therapy. Here the thrombosis is secondary to infection and inflammation of the vein wall (phlebitis). It is still seen in such conditions as cavernous sinus thrombosis in infection of the face and thrombosis of the pelvic veins in puerperal sepsis. The thrombus is firmly attached to the inflamed vein wall, so that there is no danger of massive fatal pulmonary embolism. Infection, however, causes the thrombus to break up, in which case there may be multiple small infected infarcts in the lung.

It may be added that the condition which first directed the great Rudolph Virchow's attention to research was septic thrombophlebitis, because of its fearful prevalence in those far-off days of putrid hospital surgical infection. Times change and so does medicine. But out of that research came our concept of embolism.

In addition to venous thrombosis or phlebothrombosis and septic thrombophlebitis which have just been discussed, four other conditions involving thrombosis in the veins may be briefly considered, since the student will encounter them in his clinical studies.

Simple Thrombophlebitis is marked by an inflammatory reaction in the vein wall, mostly lymphocytic in type, without any demonstrable bacterial infection. The clinical evidence suggesting inflammation (fever, redness, swelling and tenderness) is more striking than the histological changes. The

thrombus is attached to the wall of the vein, so that pulmonary embolism is uncommon. There may be painful swelling of an entire limb, as in *phlegmasia alba dolens* or "milk leg" which may develop after delivery. This appears to be the result of a lymphedema, the venous block throwing more work on the lymphatic system than it can deal with. There is also a marked perivascular inflammatory reaction which involves the lymphatics.

Phlegmasia Caerulea Dolens (literally the hot, blue, painful condition) or blue phlebitis is in essence thrombophlebitis with gangrene, fortunately a very rare condition. The clinical picture resembles an acute arterial occlusion, and indeed appears to be due to arterial spasm complicating deep venous thrombosis. A more modern and less pretentious name is *massive venous occlusion*.

Thrombophlebitis Migrans or migrating venous thrombosis is a pathological puzzle but a useful clinical indicator. It is characterized by repeated attacks of thrombosis, now one, now another short segment of vein being involved in different parts of the body, often in recurring attacks extending over a period of months or even years. It may occur at any age. I have seen a case in the Vancouver General Hospital of a young man in whom the common iliac, inferior vena cava, splenic, mesenteric and cerebral veins were all involved, death being finally due to infarction of the brain. In this case a correct diagnosis was made by the neurologist. There is a curious relation between the condition and visceral malignancy, which may involve the body and tail of the pancreas (most frequent), the stomach, the lung, the prostate, and more rarely other organs. The great Trousseau observed and recorded the condition in himself when he was dying of carcinoma of the pancreas, so that the term *Trousseau's syndrome* has been fittingly applied to the association. Thrombophlebitis associated with malignancy is characteristically resistant to anticoagulant therapy, a feature which may put the clinician on his guard when the signs of malignancy have not yet become apparent. The cases can be divided into two groups: those which are primary or idiopathic and those secondary to other conditions, particularly malignant neoplasms. The secondary cases are the commoner. When the condition occurs for the first time in a patient of the cancer age group, it should be considered malignant unless proved otherwise. The primary group involves relatively young people, predominantly males, the superficial and deep veins of the legs being most commonly involved, followed by the arms and superficial veins of the abdomen. The majority of the primary cases recover, so that autopsy reports are very rare.

Axillary Vein Thrombosis is a rare but readily recognized condition. It is characterized by a history of recent trauma or exceptional effort, swelling of the affected arm from the fingers to the base of the axilla, slight cyanosis of the skin, dilatation of the superficial veins over the anterior and lateral aspects of the chest wall, and the presence of a firm tender cord which can be felt along the line of the axillary vein. The patient is usually young, robust, and engaged in heavy labor. The chief etiological factor appears to be overstretching and contusion of the axillary vein between the clavicle and the first rib, the costocoracoid ligament and the subclavius muscle. It is rather remarkable that pulmonary embolism is not a complication of primary axillary thrombosis, as might have been confidently expected.

Arteries.—Arterial thrombosis is due to *local causes*, in distinction to venous thrombosis where such general causes as failing circulation and embarrassed respiration are important factors. Roughening of the intima due to atheroma is the common causal agent. The most frequent site is in the *coronary arteries*, where the thrombus blocks the lumen, and may or may not lead to myocardial infarction, depending on the excellence of the collateral circulation. An atheromatous *cerebral artery* may become thrombosed, with softening of the brain. A thrombus may be deposited on an atheromatous patch in the *aorta*, and may be carried as an embolus into the arteries of the leg with disastrous results; this is the one example of embolism from an arterial thrombus. Inflammation or necrosis of the wall of an artery is likely to be followed by thrombosis; examples in the arteries of the leg are Buerger's disease, in the visceral arteries

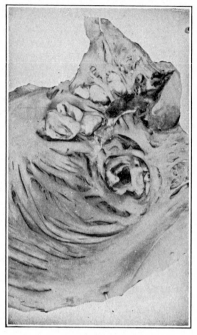

FIG. 67.—Pale thrombi adherent to auricle and auricular appendix.

polyarteritis nodosa, and in the arterioles malignant hypertension.

Heart.—True thrombi are found in three sites in the heart. When the *valves* are inflamed (endocarditis), platelets are deposited on the roughened surface to form masses known as vegetations. On the necrotic surface of a *myocardial infarct* of the left ventricle a large thrombus may be deposited. In both of these cases portions of the thrombus may become detached and form emboli in the systemic circulation. In the *left auricle* a thrombus may form in mitral stenosis, owing to the eddying and poor flow of blood in the auricle due to the extreme narrowing of the lumen of the valve (Fig. 67).

Postmortem Clots.—It is important to realize that postmortem clots are not true thrombi. If sufficient time is allowed to elapse following death, the blood elements will settle out into various layers and form a clot that is loosely, if at all, attached to the vessel wall. Thus, depending on the rapidity with which they are formed, they may be of the *"chicken-fat"* type (firm and yellow) or the *"current-jelly"* type (soft and red). Some of their more important characteristics are summarized in the following table.

Fibrinolysis.—Fibrinolysis is the process by which the organism dissolves and removes deposits of fibrin, a process which is now recognized to be of fundamental physiological importance and of corresponding pathological significance. The body is being continually exposed to minute injuries, so that the formation of fibrin deposits is a regular phenomenon in the healthy organism. These

The active agent, plasmin, appears to be adsorbed on to the fibrin threads. The transformation of plasminogen into plasmin can be effected by various activators, or it may involve the activation of pro-activators, by kinases in the blood, in the tissue, produced by hemolytic streptococci, *etc.* It is known that *fibrinolytic activity* can be stimulated *in vivo* by stress, heavy muscular work, and the injection of adrenaline. It is markedly increased in anaphylactic shock.

DISTINGUISHING FEATURES OF PREMORTEM THROMBI AND POSTMORTEM CLOTS.

Premortem Thrombi	Postmortem Clots
Firmly attached to vessel wall	Weakly attached to vessel wall
Fibrin threads and cellular components produce laminar lines of Zahn	Homogeneous; non-laminated
Friable	Rubbery
Variegated coloration (Note: propagated tail is a soft red clot)	Firm and yellow ("chicken-fat") or soft and red ("current-jelly")

deposits must, however, be removed. As a matter of fact the phenomenon of fibrinolysis was first observed in 1846, although the name was not used until 1893. As in the case of coagulation, the process is dependent on a balance of activating and inhibiting agents (Astrup). *Plasmin* (fibrinolysin), a fibrin-splitting proteolytic enzyme, is produced from a precursor, *plasminogen*, in the blood. Two mechanisms seem to be available for producing fibrinolytic activity: (1) An interaction between plasminogen and an activator released from injured tissue. This activator is bound to the insoluble tissue proteins, so that the activation is mainly of local significance. (2) A pro-activator in the blood is changed into an activator of plasminogen. As this activator is soluble, it is carried with the blood stream to all the organs of the body. In the normal living organism there exists an equilibrium between the fibrin-producing process of blood coagulation and the fibrin-dissolving process. A shifting in the balance between these two physiological processes can lead to pathological changes, as we shall see (Astrup).

Fibrinolysis appears to play a part in a number of disease processes. Some of these have already been considered. Others will be discussed later and will merely be mentioned here.

Thrombolysis.—It is evident that anticoagulant drugs do not provide the answer to the important problem of thromboembolism, for they do not remove clots which have already formed. "The organism is left to its own devices in dealing with this occlusive mass" (Moser). The first fibrinolytic agent to attract attention was streptokinase, an enzyme obtained from filtrates of cultures of beta-hemolytic streptococci (Tillett and Garner). This had no direct action on fibrin, but it was an activator of plasminogen which produced the active lytic enzyme fibrinolysin (plasmin). Plasminogen (profibrinolysin) can now be isolated from the globulin fraction of plasma proteins and activated to fibrinolysin by small amounts of streptokinase, which is adsorbed by fibrin. While dissolving experimentally produced arterial and venous thrombi, it does not hinder coagulation, so that in clinical use, which at present is only in its infancy, it must be combined with anticoagulant drugs to prevent recurring thrombosis. Rapid resolution of signs and symptoms has been observed in patients treated within a few days of the apparent clinical onset of thrombosis. Fibrinolysin therapy was ineffective when started one week or more after the first manifestations of thrombosis (Sokal *et al.*). It does, however, appear to be the most promising fibrinolytic agent for lysing intravenous thrombi.

Wound Healing.—In our study of the healing of a healthy wound we have seen that the fibrin is replaced by invading fibroblasts and vascular endothelium, with the formation of granulation tissue which is presently converted into connective tissue or scar. Removal of the fibrin depends, at least in part, on the process of fibrinolysis. If the fibrinolytic system is of low potency, the fibrin deposits are not removed at normal speed, there is an increased ingrowth of fibroblasts and excessive formation of connective tissue, with the possible development of *keloid*. If, on the other hand, the potency of the system is too high, fibrin is broken down too quickly and the healing of the wound is delayed. "The activity of the fibrinolytic enzyme system in the body is a main factor in the regulation of connective tissue formation in tissue repair" (Astrup).

Spread of Infection.—In a previous chapter we have seen that the ease with which bacteria spread through the tissues depends to a marked degree on their power to produce hyaluronidase which acts on the acid mucopolysaccharides. It is also believed that the ability of streptococci to spread in the body is due in part to a breaking down of barriers of fibrin by fibrinolytic *streptokinase* produced by some streptococci. The more local effects of staphylococci are said to be caused by clotting principle (*coagulase*) produced by some strains. Other strains produce a fibrinolytic agent (*staphylokinase*), which permits them to spread readily.

Atherosclerosis.—Reference has already been made to Duguid's stimulating ideas regarding the relationship of mural thrombosis in arteries to atherosclerosis. According to this concept, originally suggested by Rokitansky over 100 years ago, in very many cases atherosclerosis is a result, not a cause, of mural thrombosis. We know that small amounts of fibrin are being continually deposited on the walls of arteries, especially where strain causes tissue damage with local release of thromboplastic agents. Normally these deposits are speedily removed, but when the fibrinolytic system is unbalanced the film of fibrin soon becomes covered by vascular endothelium, and acts as a barrier to the diffusion of oxygen and nutriments from the lumen to the underlying intima, with resulting degeneration and the picture we know as atherosclerosis. The question of the relationship of mural thrombosis to the pathogenesis of atherosclerosis will be discussed further in connection with the latter condition in Chapter 22. Atherosclerosis is not seen in veins, nor does it accompany venous thrombosis, perhaps because the vasa vasorum of veins penetrate to the intima, and venous blood has a higher fibrinolytic activity than has arterial blood.

Hemorrhagic Diatheses.—A diathesis is a predisposition toward a pathological condition. The hemorrhagic diatheses will be discussed in the chapter on diseases of the blood, but it may be mentioned here that some members of the group seem to be caused by circulating fibrinolytic agents. Two types may be distinguished. The first is *acute*, with sudden onset of the bleeding and usually a fatal termination. It is seen particularly in obstetrical cases, including fatal amniotic fluid embolism (see below), and indicates shock. The fibrinolytic activity in blood is very high, being caused by a plasminogen activator. The second type is *protracted*, with petechial hemorrhages. The fibrinolytic activity is usually much lower.

Clinical Effects.—*The effects of thrombosis depend on the site of the thrombus, the type of vessel involved, and the degree of occlusion.* In an artery the most serious effect is ischemia, while in a vein or the heart it is the threat of embolism.

1. *No serious effects.* When pure thrombosis is completely successful in its function it is clinically silent. When complicated by clotting it may or may not become clinically manifest.

2. *Edema of a limb,* occurring when venous

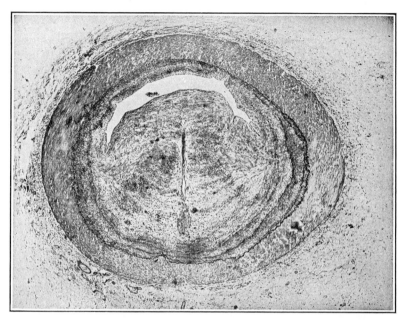

Fig. 68.—Thrombus in artery occluding most of the lumen, and becoming vascularized and organized.
× 30.

thrombosis is complicated by perivenous lymphangitis.

3. *Post-thrombotic ulceration* of the lower extremity due to a state of ambulatory local venous hypertension following canalization of the deep venous system. This is the result of impairment of the normal "venous heart" of the legs, owing to destruction of the valves of the deep venous system (Linton).

4. *Gangrene of a limb* caused by *thrombosis* of a main artery or occlusion by *embolism* from a thrombus in the heart or aorta.

5. *Gangrene of the bowel* due to thrombosis of the mesenteric artery or vein or to arterial embolism.

6. *Infarction* of the myocardium, retina, *etc.*, due to arterial thrombosis.

7. Finally the thrombus or a portion of it may become detached from the vein or the heart in which it is formed and be carried into the general circulation where it constitutes an *embolus*.

Subsequent Fate of the Thrombus.— Much depends on the presence and degree of infection. If the thrombus becomes septic, *i.e.*, if it is infected with pyogenic bacteria, it will become softened and disintegrated, and may even be converted into an abscess.

It is evident that in such a case the patient will be exposed to all the risks of pyemia. As a rule, however, the course is aseptic. *Contraction* of the thrombus occurs owing to the fibrin which it contains. The clot may shrink from the wall of the vein, leaving a space. *Absorption* of part of the thrombus may take place due to the activity of leukocytes. *Organization* of the thrombus may occur, commencing at the point where the thrombus is attached to the vessel wall (Fig. 68). This process, which is characteristic of arterial as opposed to venous thrombosis, must be distinguished from organization of a fibrinous exudate or the healing of a wound. In those cases the exudate or blood is converted into dense scar tissue, with the formation of a minimum of new vessels designed to keep the tissue alive. In an arterial thrombus the bands of fibrin and platelets become condensed into masses, which are quickly covered by endothelium, so that new vascular channels are formed which serve to establish a new thorough circulation (Fig. 69). This canalization of the clot may be accompanied by shrinkage of the thrombus from the wall of the vessel, leaving a space which is similarly relined. Dible points out that we now

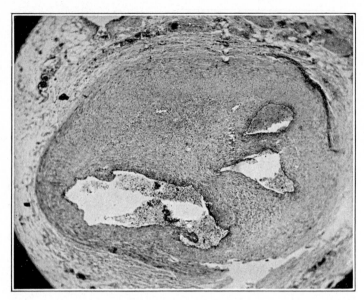

FIG. 69.—Canalization of an organized thrombus in an artery. × 30.

have two sets of vascular channels separated by the internal elastic lamina: (1) the vasa vasorum running in a radial fashion in the muscle coat; (2) new vessels running in a longitudinal direction through the thrombus. In the case of a vein calcium salts may be deposited in the thrombus to form a *phlebolith*.

When we come to study the pathogenesis of atherosclerosis in Chapter 22, we shall see that the incorporation of a thrombus with the arterial intima may play an important part in the process.

EMBOLISM

An embolus is a foreign body which is transported from one part of the circulatory system to another where it becomes impacted. The process is known as embolism. The usual form of embolus is a thrombus which has formed either in the heart or in the blood vessels and has become detached from the wall (thromboembolism). Other forms of emboli are fat, air, tumor, bone marrow, amniotic fluid, atheromatous material and clumps of bacteria. These will be discussed separately. In addition to blood vessel embolism, some consideration must be given to lymphatic embolism. Embolism is of

interest for two reasons: (1) it is the means by which solid material is transported from one part of the body to the other, and is thus of great importance in the dissemination of tumors, bacterial infection, etc., (2) emboli may produce serious effects at their point of impaction. It is of historical interst to note that it was in 1846 that Virchow for the first time introduced the concept of thromboembolism. Before that date when at autopsy a clot was found in a vein in the leg and a similar clot was seen to occlude the pulmonary artery, it was believed (and taught) that both were formed in situ and bore no relation to one another. Similarly, when a cancer was found in the rectum and other cancers of similar structure were present in the liver, all of the tumors were presumed to be primary in origin and unrelated to one another. The enormous importance of the "new" concept will be apparent to the reader.

The source of the embolus depends on the site of the thrombus from which it arises. In the heart there are three sites: (1) the auricle and auricular appendix, (2) a cardiac infarct in the left ventricle, (3) inflamed valves (the vegetations of endocarditis). The *veins* are of even greater importance. Postoperative thrombosis is of special danger,

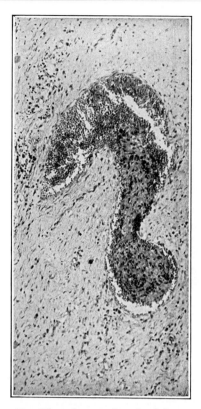

FIG. 70.—Thrombus at site of pelvic operation. Part became detached and caused fatal pulmonary embolism. × 125.

and will be referred to presently in discussing pulmonary embolism. (Fig. 70). The common sites of venous thrombosis have already been described in the previous section. In embolism following abdominal and pelvic operations the femoral veins must be carefully examined for thrombi. Thrombi in the right and left auricles, particularly in the auricular appendages, are not infrequently the source of emboli. An unusual form is the thrombus which is developed on an *atheromatous ulcer* in the aorta, and is then carried further into the arterial tree.

Infarction.—When an embolus (*embolos,* a plug) is impacted in an artery the effect is the same as if the vessel were suddenly closed by a clamp or ligature. This effect may be studied experimentally either by the use of artificial emboli such as seeds injected into the circulation or by clamping or tying the artery supplying the part. Everything depends on the *collateral circulation,* which in turn depends on the anastomosis between the affected vessel and the neighboring arterioles. In most parts of the body anastomoses are abundant so that when even a large artery is blocked an efficient collateral circulation is soon established; the palmar arch is an example of perfect collateral circulation. Ligature of the brachial artery is at first followed by blanching of the limb which becomes numb and cold. The anastomotic arteries undergo active dilatation, and blood finds its way into the ischemic tissue before any permanent damage is done. The collateral circulation must be maintained, *i. e.,* the dilatation is permanent. The walls of the dilated arteries become thickened to accommodate the increased pressure. It is evident that the *efficiency* of the collateral circulation will depend on *two factors:* (1) the state of the vessels, and (2) the strength of the heart. In an old person whose vessels are diseased owing to arteriosclerosis and whose heart is weak, the collateral circulation may be inadequate and gangrene will result. What has been said of ligature of an artery is equally true of obstruction from embolism.

An *infarct* is an area of coagulation necrosis resulting from a sudden arrest of circulation in the artery supplying an area without adequate collateral circulation. The word means a stuffing of blood (*infarcire,* to stuff), but this is not an essential feature of the process, depending on the collateral circulation and the looseness of texture of the part. It is only in the lung and the bowel that the part is stuffed with blood. In most of the viscera the anastomoses are less abundant than in the limbs.

After a transient initial period of hyperemia the infarct becomes ischemic and pale. The area is wedge-shaped owing to the fanlike distribution of the vessels. The collateral circulation endeavors to pour blood into the part, and owing to dilatation of the capillaries a hemorrhagic border is formed around the infarcted area. If this border is wide enough the entire area becomes hemorrhagic and stuffed with blood. An infarct may therefore be *pale* or *red,* the difference depending on the excellence of the collateral circulation. Infarcts of the kidney and heart

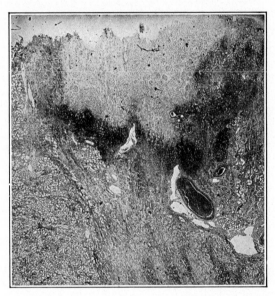

Fig. 71.—Infarct of kidney. The infarcted area is necrotic and is surrounded by a dark zone of congestion. Note the plugged artery. × 8.

tend to remain pale, those of the spleen tend to become red, while in the lung they are always red.

The redness is due to dilatation of the anastomotic vessels. Blood is forced into the collapsed vessels of the ischemic area, so that the part becomes stuffed with red cells. The overdistended vessels may give way, so that hemorrhage occurs. This is most marked in poorly supported capillaries such as those of the lungs and to a lesser degree in the spleen. In about two hours the red cells become fused together into a homogeneous mass in which their outline can no longer be distinguished.

The tissues in the ischemic area undergo necrosis and die, and within forty-eight hours the infarct of the kidney is completely necrotic. (Fig. 71). The necrosis is coagulative in type, so that dim outlines of the tubules and glomeruli may remain for a long time. The area is evidently kidney, but it is a city of the dead from which all life and activity have long since vanished. In sections the whole infarcted area stains diffusely with eosin, but at the margin nuclear remains may be seen, and the phenomenon of karyorrhexis is often very well marked. The nuclear fragments are apt to be mistaken for the nuclei of polymorphonuclear leukocytes. At the margin there is an extreme degree of hyperemia, and the hyperemic zone may be of considerable width. The hyperemia may be attributed to the irritation produced by the dead tissue. In old-standing cases a zone of fibrous tissue may be formed around the infarct.

The gross appearance of an *infarct of kidney* is very characteristic. (Fig. 72.) An irregular area is observed on the surface, often slightly depressed and surrounded by a pink zone of hyperemia. The cut surface shows an area which may be wedge-shaped or irregular involving the whole width of the cortex and some of the medulla, pale in color and surrounded by a pink border.

In the *spleen* the process is very similar, but the collateral circulation is better, so that the infarct may be either red or pale. Old infarcts, however, are always pale, for the hemoglobin is gradually removed, the red cells disappear, and decolorization takes place.

Infarction of the heart is the result of thrombosis of one or more of the coronary arteries; only in very rare instances is it due to embolism. It constitutes one of the most important forms of heart disease, and is considered

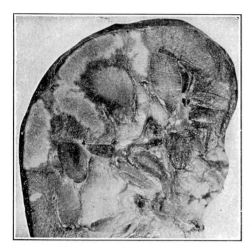

FIG. 72.—Infarct of kidney. There are several pale areas of infarction in the cortex.

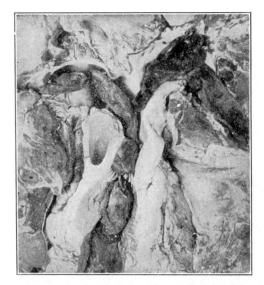

FIG. 73.—Pulmonary embolism. A twisted embolus occludes the pulmonary artery and its two main branches. The patient died in the course of a few minutes.

in detail in connection with diseases of that organ.

Pulmonary Embolism and Infarction.— Thromboembolism involving the pulmonary artery is of such paramount importance that it demands separate consideration. The condition used to be regarded as essentially a post-operative complication. "The operation is abdominal, and the more serene the events during and following the operation, the more likelihood there is of venous thrombosis and resulting embolism. Convalescence is peculiarly uneventful. Suddenly, almost out of a clear sky, there is strange restlessness, rapidly ensuing shock with substernal distress, air hunger and collapse, and death usually in two to fifteen minutes. The horror of the patient's relatives is echoed by the poignant distress and shock of the attending surgeon, colleagues and nurses" (Robertson). In one large surgical clinic it was estimated that 7 per cent of the postoperative deaths over a series of years were due to this cause. It is necessary to distinguish between pulmonary *embolism* and *infarction*. There may be: (1) embolism without infarction, and (2) infarction without embolism. (1) A large embolus may occlude the pulmonary artery or one of its main branches (Fig. 73), and the patient dies of shock in a few minutes; in such a case there is no time for an infarct to develop. Death seems to be due to constriction of the pul-

monary arterioles, as section of the sympathetic in animals prevents it. In a case of suspected pulmonary embolism special care must be taken with the autopsy. The pulmonary artery must be opened with the heart *in situ*, else the embolus is apt to be dislodged. The heart and lungs are then removed *en masse* and the branches of the artery carefully opened. A postmortem clot may be mistaken for an embolus. The embolus is more dry and brittle than the clot, and often shows a twisted, bent, or curled appearance which is very characteristic. In an embalmed body the clot may be as dry as an embolus, but microscopic examination will show the more complex structure of a true thrombus (fused platelets, etc.). (2) On the other hand an infarcted area, an area stuffed with blood, may be produced by thrombosis of one of the pulmonary veins quite apart from embolism. Postoperative emboli may be divided into three groups: (1) Large emboli which occlude a main artery and cause death with acute respiratory distress in the course of a few minutes. (2) Medium-sized emboli which produce the physical signs of an infarct. (3) Small emboli which give rise to characteristic symptoms (sudden pain in the side, spitting of blood) but no physical signs. The accident usually occurs in the second week of convalescence, but may occur during the first two or three days. Pulmonary embolism may take place in the puerperium.

No thrombus may be found in the veins of the leg, even though the clinical history may have suggested its presence. In such a case the thrombus may be represented entirely by the embolus in the pulmonary artery. The gun has been discharged, but not yet reloaded. Pulmonary emboli are frequently *multiple*, but it is common in fatal cases to find that the final episode has been preceded by minor attacks. It is in these cases that the use of anticoagulants and antithrombotics such as heparin and Dicumarol may be considered, or even, in the view of some surgeons, ligation of the femoral veins.

The concluding remarks of DeBakey's searching evaluation of the problem of thromboembolism in surgical practice are worthy of consideration. "There can be no doubt of the confusion which prevails and, for that matter, which has prevailed with no less intensity for more than fifty years in our understanding of the problem. It is evident, too, that many factors have contributed to this confusion, including particularly the lack of precise knowledge concerning the etiology and pathogenesis of the condition, and the absence of an accurate test or method of diagnosis."

We now know that fatal pulmonary embolism with its preceding phlebothrombosis is more common in medical (60 per cent) than in surgical (40 per cent) cases, which might well be expected when the factors involved in the pathogenesis of phlebothrombosis such as myocardial and respiratory failure are kept in mind. Here again the site of the thrombosis is the veins of the leg. Unfortunately venous thrombosis is usually a silent process. On an obstetrical and gynecological service the pulmonary emboli are found to come from the pelvic veins. Less than half the cases of pulmonary embolism are correctly diagnosed, being frequently mistaken for severe coronary thrombosis. A sense of apprehension is a marked feature. A triangular area of atelectasis (collapse) with its base at the lung periphery in the X-ray film, associated with localized pain on

respiration and a friction rub on auscultation complete the classical picture, which unfortunately is seldom complete and classical, for pulmonary embolism is a great masquerader which delights to mimic other clinical conditions.

Many aspects of the thromboembolism problem are singularly baffling. In one hospital series 85 per cent of the fatal cases had premonitory signs before the fatal episode, whilst in another institution 85 per cent did not, even though the staff was "embolism conscious." There has been no change in the total incidence during the past fifty years, but there is a confusing marked seasonal and annual variation, with irregular wave-like periodicity. There may be an extraordinary fluctuation in incidence in the same institution. *These facts must be borne in mind before the clinician can claim credit for some special form of therapy such as the use of anticoagulant drugs.*

The dramatic *clinical sequelae* of pulmonary embolism have always been an enigma. The general effects of embolism often far exceed those that might be expected from the size of the embolus, for even a small embolus may produce marked circulatory collapse and a sense of impending death. It is now believed that the causal factor may be the release of *5-hydroxytryptamine* (5-H.T.) or *serotonin* from platelets at the site of embolism (Smith and Smith). This humoral agent is produced by malignant carcinoid or argentaffin tumors of the alimentary tract, and may give rise to circulatory symptoms resembling those of pulmonary embolism. The intravenous injection of fragments of blood clot are found to produce vascular phenomena similar to those following injection of 5-H.T.

Infarcts of the lung are always red because the organ has a double blood supply. The bronchial artery supplies blood for nutrition at systemic pressure, whereas the pulmonary artery supplies blood for oxygenation at one-third of that pressure. The bronchial artery serves the important function of filling both circulatory beds with blood beyond an embolus. The collateral circulation is therefore abundant. Two results follow from this: (1) Occlusion of a pulmonary artery in a *healthy lung* is not followed by infarction,

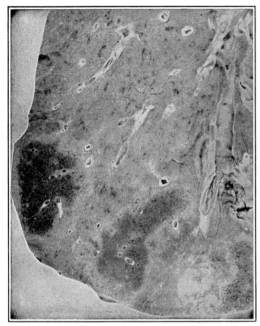

Fig. 74.—Infarcts of lung. Two infarcts are seen at the surface of the lower part of the lung. The artery passing to the lower infarct is filled by a pale embolus.

level and feels firm to the touch. The raised appearance is due to collapse of the surrounding lung when the chest is opened; if the chest is roentgen-rayed before being opened, the infarct will be seen to be depressed, not raised (Castleman). The cut surface is quite dry. The extent of the infarct varies enormously, often quite small, but sometimes involving the greater part of a lobe. *Microscopically* the alveoli are stuffed with blood, and their outlines are no longer visible, owing to necrosis of the alveolar walls. The presence of blood in the sputum is thus easy to understand.

Should the embolus be septic the element of infarction is obscured by the development of abscesses, usually multiple. The infected emboli may reach the right side of the heart *via* the superior vena cava (septic thrombosis of the lateral sinus and jugular vein, etc.), or *via* the inferior vena cava (septic thrombosis in the puerperal uterus, etc.).

Embolism of the mesenteric artery leads to infarction of the bowel and constitutes one of the acute abdominal catastrophes. The superior mesenteric is the vessel usually involved. The sudden loss of the blood supply of the bowel wall is followed by gangrene and other consequences which are described in Chapter 27.

Cerebral embolism leads to infarction of the brain and subsequent cerebral softening. Necrosis is followed by liquefaction, so that a cyst may be formed. This subject is discussed in connection with strokes in Chapter 42.

Embolism of the central artery of the retina results in sudden blindness with necrosis of the retina.

Paradoxical Embolism.—This term is applied to the case where an embolus arises in a vein but lodges in a systemic artery instead of in the pulmonary artery. The occurrence is rare, but an important example of the so-called "crossed" embolism is cerebral embolism with hemiplegia following puerperal thrombosis of the pelvic and femoral veins. The usual explanation given is that the embolus has passed through a patent foramen ovale. If the foramen is really large this is possible, (Fig. 75), but in many of the cases the foramen is small or completely closed. In these cases the following possibilities may

because of the abundant anastomosis. If the circulation in the lung is impaired, as in chronic venous congestion, embolism readily results in infarction. In postoperative cases, particularly when the abdomen has been opened, there is always such impairment owing to interference with the respiratory movements and to the patient lying on his back. (2) The infarct is hemorrhagic and remains red. In course of time the infarct will disappear, but if the lung is inflated and careful search be made, small peripheral scars will often indicate the site of previous infarcts. Castleman has shown that these lesions can be detected in roentgen-ray films as fine white lines, whilst microscopically they can be recognized by the presence of irregular elastic fibers presenting a bizarre curley-cue arrangement. The infarct appears as a firm bright red, wedge-shaped area; the base of the wedge is at the surface and covered by a thin pleural exudate. (Fig. 74.) The pleurisy is the cause of the characteristic pain in the side and the friction rub. The infarct is raised above the surrounding

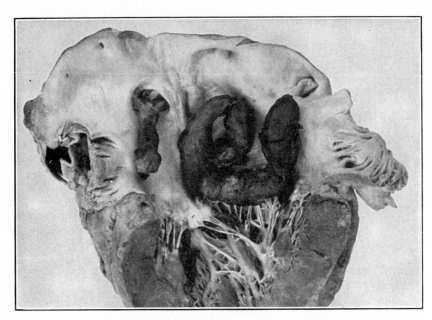

Fig. 75.—Paradoxical embolism. The embolus is passing through a large foramen ovale into the left auricle.

occur: (1) Clumps of bacteria may pass through the pulmonary capillaries and lodge in the cerebral vessels where they set up thrombosis with resulting softening of the brain and hemiplegia.   (2) Infarction of the lung which is so common in puerperal thrombosis may cause thrombosis of the pulmonary vessels, and from this an embolus may arise which may pass to the brain.   (3) An endocarditis on the left side of the heart may complicate puerperal sepsis, and the vegetations may form emboli which lodge in the brain.

Fat Embolism.—At first sight the subject of fat embolism appears to be childishly simple, and yet it has been a subject of heated debate since the first case, that of a crushed railroad worker, was reported by Zenker in 1862. The controversy regarding fat embolism relates to: (1) *its importance as a cause of death*, and (2) *the origin of the fat*. It has long been recognized that patients with recent fractures may suddenly become worse from one to several days after entering the hospital, passing into a state of severe shock which may prove fatal. When thick frozen sections of the lungs are examined the capillaries are seen to be filled with great numbers of fat globules. These are also pres-

ent in smaller numbers in the brain, kidneys, and other organs. Of particular significance is the fact that bone marrow emboli may also occasionally be observed. The same thing may happen after crushing injuries of fat tissue, operations on stout people, and manipulation of fractures. I have seen it cause death as the result of forcible loosening of an ankylosed knee joint, the bones of which had become extremely rarefied as the result of long disuse. The explanation would appear to be simple. Fat cells in the *bone marrow* or the *fat depots in soft tissue* are ruptured by the trauma and broken into smaller globules which are sucked into the torn veins, the rigid bony tissue holding the veins open. The fat is carried to the lungs where it is arrested, so that globules and cylinders of fat are found in the pulmonary capillaries, but unless frozen sections (which should be thick to prevent loss of emboli) and fat stains are employed, the fat will not be detected. (Fig. 76). Small globules may pass through the pulmonary capillaries or bypass the lungs *via* a patent foramen ovale and lodge in the brain, the renal glomeruli, etc. In the kidney the fat globules may be recognized as clear spaces in paraffin sections stained by ordinary methods. (Fig. 77). Fat often appears

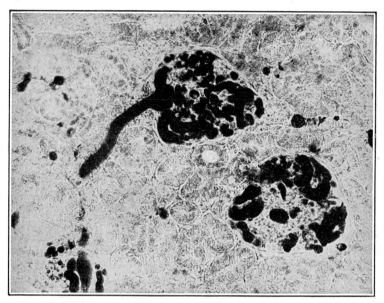

FIG. 76.—Fat emboli in kidney. Frozen section stained for fat. × 100.

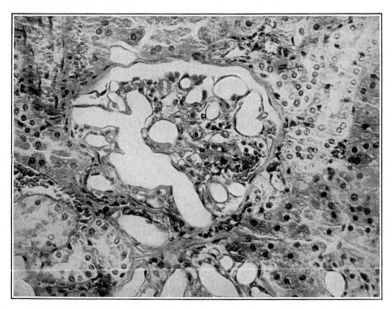

FIG. 77.—Fat emboli in kidney. Paraffin section. The spaces represent fat which has been dissolved out. × 200.

10

in the urine, and can be demonstrated even more regularly in the sputum.

The matter of fat embolism may appear quite simple from the above account, but this is far from being the case. In many instances in which there was no question of trauma, fat has been found in the pulmonary and other capillaries. In most of these cases there has been a shock-like picture similar to that associated with trauma to fatty tissue, but not in all. What is the source of this fat? In some cases it may be a *fatty liver*, in which the hepatic cells are transformed into fat cysts, which may rupture the walls of venules. Fat embolism is common in chronic alcoholics, in whom a profound degree of fatty degeneration of the liver is of common occurrence. Chronic alcoholics may go to bed with a severe headache and a choking feeling, only to be found dead in the morning. Mulitple fat emboli can be demonstrated in the brain, sometimes as many as 35 being counted in 1 sq. cm. of tissue (Lynch *et al.*). It has been suggested that repeated fat embolism may be one cause of alcoholic psychosis, with associated lesions such as patchy loss of neurons, focal degenerative lesions, atrophy, and proliferation of astrocytes (Lynch *et al.*).

It has also been suggested that one source of the fat is the *circulating blood*, the fat normally present becoming aggregated into larger particles because of a change in the chemical and physical character of the blood. In this connection it is of great interest to learn that sheaf-like masses of acicular crystals, best seen with crossed Nicol prisms because of their birefringence, are incorporated in the fat "emboli." These crystals give a positive Schultz test for cholesterol and cholesterol ester (LeQuire *et al.*). As it is necessary for fat to contain 10 per cent of cholesterol before the test is positive, and as depot (including marrow) fat contains only 1 per cent, the obvious source which could account for this amount of cholesterol is the circulating blood. A change in the emulsification of blood lipids may occur as a result of shock or tissue injury.

In view of these varied findings perhaps the wise course is to say that in some cases the source of the emboli is bone marrow or depot fat liberated as the result of trauma,

in others it is a fatty liver, particularly in chronic alcoholics, while in still others the fat may represent an aggregation of blood lipids following shock or trauma.

The *clinical picture* may be of two quite distinct types; these are the pulmonary and the cerebral. The *pulmonary type* manifests itself in the first two days after injury, and is marked by violent dyspnea with cyanosis and pulmonary edema due to widespread obstruction of the capillaries and arterioles of the lungs by fat emboli. The *cerebral type* is marked by symptoms of cerebral irritation followed by stupor deepening into coma. Death is likely to occur from 2 to 7 days after receipt of the injury. Petechial hemorrhages may appear in the skin of the upper chest, shoulder and neck; these are attributed to fat embolism of the small arteries. Reference has already been made to the presence of fat droplets in the sputum and urine.

A final point of dissention is the *relation of the fat in the vessels to the clinical symptoms* or the fatal outcome. Fat emboli in the pulmonary capillaries can frequently be demonstrated at autopsy if proper technique is used, not only in traumatic cases but in death from other causes. In 1000 consecutive battle casualties Wilson and Salisbury found only 8 cases of *clinical* fat embolism. Indeed Whitson considers that the autopsy findings described in pulmonary fat embolism are the same as those of shock, and that the presence of fat globules at autopsy indicates an anoxemic death. The symptoms are certainly those of surgical shock with pulmonary edema. A large amount of blood volume may be lost into the tissues at the site of a fracture, causing shock or impending shock.

These varied and divergent views are presented, not with the object of confusing the student, but to show that there are two (or more) sides to the challenging question of fat embolism.

Air Embolism.—Air may enter the veins as the result of operations on the neck, lobectomy for cancer of the lung, artificial pneumothorax, etc. Many cases are due to injection of air, with or without fluid, into the uterus in the production of criminal abortion. Air embolism may occur as the result of a blood transfusion, air being sucked into the vein after all the blood has been drawn from the flask. It is when a vein is only partially severed, thus preventing collapse, that there is danger of air embolism. This is particularly true in the large veins of the neck where there is marked negative venous pressure. The first sign is a hissing sound in the wound, the so-called "sifflement," as air is sucked in. The result is dyspnea, cyanosis, coma, and finally death. The air converts the blood in the heart into a froth which makes proper cardiac contraction impossible, or bubbles of air may reach the brain. In opening the heart at autopsy in a case of suspected air embolism special precautions must be taken. All vessels entering the heart must be tied before it is removed, and it must be held under water when the chambers are incised, so that any bubbles of escaping air may be detected.

Amniotic Fluid Embolism.—This condition, first described by Steiner and Lushbaugh in 1941, is perhaps the most common cause of obstetrical death during labor and the first few hours of the puerperium. In a case which I studied death occurred within ten minutes of delivery. The *emboli* consist of keratotic squames, lanugo hairs, and mucin. The two major components, namely squames and mucin, can be conveniently demonstrated in one section by combining alcian-green staining for mucin with phloxin staining for squames. The alcian-phloxin stain reveals much more embolic material than is seen with hematoxylin and eosin (Attwood). The condition appears to be the result of entrapped amniotic fluid with accompanying debris passing through a rent in the fetal membranes into the uterine venous sinuses. It has been difficult to explain the disastrous clinical consequences as a result of the rather trivial embolic findings. It now appears that the clinical course and death may be due to intravascular clotting with resultant defibrination and hemorrhage (Reid *et al.*). The amniotic fluid contains a substance which acts like thromboplastin. The extreme intravascular clotting results in an *afibrinogenemia*, which may be responsible for delayed death in a few hours time from postpartum hemorrhage. When thromboplastin is infused rapidly into an animal it

causes rapid death, but when given more slowly the result is defibrination. These concepts have given rise to the suggestion that it would be more realistic to speak of *amniotic fluid infusion* rather than embolism. The *symptoms* are those of shock, which may be so sudden in onset and course as to suggest an element of anaphylaxis, a question which has been touched on in connection with autoimmunity in Chapter 5. The first indication of impending disaster is sudden respiratory distress, usually during the first stage of labor.

REFERENCES

ASTRUP, T.: Lancet, 1956, *2*, 565. (Biological significance of fibrinolysis).

ATTWOOD, H. D.: J. Path. and Bact., 1958, *76*, 211. (Histology of amniotic fluid embolism.)

BIGGS, ROSEMARY and MACFARLANE, R. G.: *Human Blood Coagulation and its Disorders*, 2nd. ed., Oxford, 1957.

CASTLEMAN, B. and HAMPTON, A. O.: J. Tech. Methods, 1941, *21*, 5. (Pulmonary infarction).

DECAMP P. T., LANDRY, R. M., OCHSNER, A. and DEBAKEY, M. E.: Surgery, 1952, *31*, 43. (Spontaneous thrombophlebitis).

DEBAKEY, M. E.: Surg., Gynec. and Obst., International Abstracts of Surgery, 1954, *98*, 1. (Thromboembolism).

DIBLE, J. H.: J. Path. and Bact., 1958, *75*, 1. (Canalization in arterial thrombosis).

DUGUID, J. B.: Brit. Med. Bull., 1955, *11*, 36. (Mural thrombosis in arteries).

FLORY, C. M.: Am. J. Path., 1945, *21*, 549. (Embolism from aortic atheromatous plaques).

FRYKHOLM, R.: Surg., Gynec. and Obst., 1940, *71*, 307. (Thromboembolism).

LINTON, R. R.: Ann. Surg., 1953, *138*, 415. (Results of thrombosis).

LYNCH, M. J. G., RAPHAEL, S. S. and DIXON, T. P.: Arch Path., 1959, *67*, 68. (Fat embolism in chronic alcoholism).

LEQUIRE, V. S. *et al.*: Am. J. Path., 1959, *35*, 999. (Fat embolism).

MACFARLANE, R. G.: Brit. Med. Bull., 1955, *11*, 1. (Blood coagulation and thrombosis).

McGOVERN, V. J.: J. Path. and Bact., 1955, *69*, 283. (Pathogenesis of thrombosis).

McLACHLIN, J. and PATERSON, J. C.: Surg., Gynec. and Obst., 1951, *93*, 1; 1954, *98*, 96. (Venous thrombosis).

MOSER, K. M.: J.A.M.A., 1958, *167*, 1695. (Fibrinolysis for thromboembolism).

REID, D. E., WEINER, A. E. and ROBY, C. C.: Am. J. Obst. and Gynec., 1953, *66*, 465. (Amniotic fluid embolism).

SAMUELS, P. B., and WEBSTER, D. R.: Ann. Surg., 1952, *136*, 422. (Venous thrombosis).

The Internal Enviro
INTRACELLULAR F
INTERSTITIAL FLU
INTRAVASCULAR F
REGULATORS OF
ANCE
**Pathology of the In
vironment**
SODIUM
Depletion
Retention
POTASSIUM
Depletion
Retention
BODY TEMPERAT
Fever

THE INTE

THERE is go
began as a un
mordial sea.
sea was very d
ocean, which
evaporation an
from the land l
over countless
animals to lea
exchange for
their cells ha
solved the pro
ment with the
external envi
lived, salt wat
without whicl
exist. Gamb
ment of an er
regarded as t
evolution of
organism (th
in a kind of h
of external c
not subject
pendent. .
however var
object, that
ditions of lif
This famous

Smith, G. a~
Obst., 195
5-hydroxy
Sokal, J. E.
J.A.M.A.
Steiner, P.
1941, 117,
Thurlbeck,
J. Med.,
to kidney

homeostatic orchestra is the kidney, but the endocrine glands, especially the posterior pituitary (antidiuretic hormone), the adrenal cortex (aldosterone), and the thyroid all play their part. It is this mechanism which serves to maintain the constancy of the acid-base balance, the osmotic pressure, the concentration of the individual solutes or of ions, the blood sugar no matter how much glucose is consumed or how much is ingested, the body temperature despite changes in the outside temperature, and the blood volume even after severe hemorrhage or copious intravenous fluid infusion. When the mechanism breaks down we see the clinical picture that we call disease, a breakdown which if sufficiently profound and prolonged results in death.

The salt water which the first multicellular organisms took with them on leaving the sea is contained in three compartments, separated from one another by membranes freely permeable to water and of enormous extent. These compartments are the cells, the interstitial tissue and the blood vessels, and their contents constitute the intracellular fluid, the interstitial fluid and the blood plasma. The interstitial fluid and the blood plasma together comprise the extracellular fluid. The partitions which separate the three compartments are the walls of the capillaries and the membranes of the cells, and as these are freely permeable an interchange of fluid between the various compartments occurs continuously and in great volume (Fig. 79). These interchanges, involving water, electrolytes, nutrients and metabolites, are of course designed solely for the benefit of the cell, the fundamental unit of life, for which the internal environment exists.

Intracellular Fluid.—This makes up about 40 per cent of the body weight, the bulk of it being contained in muscle. The water content of the cells must be kept constant. When it is lowered, the deficit is at once made up from the interstitial compartment. This is accomplished by lowering of the osmotic tension, which depends on the concentration of sodium ions, this in turn being determined by excretion by the kidneys.

Interstitial Fluid.—This member of the

Relationships between Plasma, Interstitial Fluid, and Intracellular Fluid

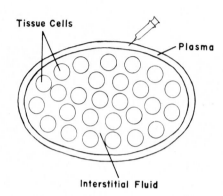

Fig. 78.—*Relationships between plasma, interstitial fluid, and intracellular fluid.* The cells are islands in the interstitial sea. Oxygen, electrolytes, and nutrients must traverse the capillary membrane, the interstitial fluid, and the cell membrane to maintain normal cellular activity and composition. The intracellular fluid volume is composed of an infinite number of minute cellular compartments separated from each other by interstitial fluid. (Hardy, *Fluid Therapy*, Lea & Febiger.)

extracellular pair comprises the real internal environment. Including the lymph, it constitutes 15 per cent of weight and measures 11 liters in a man weighing 150 pounds. The difference in the physical appearance between youth and age, between health and severe illness, is largely a matter of the amount of interstitial fluid. It is the adjustable element in the total water content of the body. Its volume and the solutes it contains are regulated by the kidneys, lungs, endocrine glands, and are influenced by the sweat glands and gastrointestinal tract. These regulators are connected with the interstitial fluid by the blood stream, the plasma being in equilibrium with the fluid in the interstitial compartment.

Intravascular Fluid.—The intravascular compartment contains the blood plasma and blood cells. The plasma constitutes 5 per cent of the body weight and 5 liters of fluid. The plasma together with the cells determine the *blood volume*, which amounts to 5 liters in a man of average size. The volume may be reduced or increased. *Reduction in volume* is by far the more serious, and may be caused by (1) hemorrhage, or (2) dilatation of the vascular bed, which results in a relative decrease in blood volume that may lead to the state of shock, an important subject discussed later in this chapter. *Increase in volume* is most likely to be due to congestive heart failure. A rare cause is a marked increase in the number of red blood cells, the condition known as polycythemia vera. The normal volume is dependent on the condition of the vascular endothelium which prevents the passage of colloids into the interstitial compartment. When the capillary wall is damaged by inflammation, allergic reactions, and other conditions we have already studied, the permability is increased to such a degree that colloid-rich fluid pours from the one compartment into the other.

Regulators of Water Balance.—Regulation of the water balance of the body is in essence regulation of the amount and content of the interstitial fluid, because it acts as the medium of exchange between the fluids in the vascular and intracellular compartments. Both of the latter contain abundant protein, but in the interstitial compartment the protein content is very low, as it would serve no useful purpose there. Water balance is for the most part regulated by *water loss*, which averages about 2500 cc. in the adult, although much more proportionately in children, whose surface area is large in proportion to their weight. This takes place by four routes: (1) 100 cc. from the intestine; (2) 300 to 600 cc. from the lungs in expired air; (3) 300 to 600 cc. from the skin; (4) 1200 to 1800 cc. from the kidneys. The first three are relatively constant, the kidneys removing any excess fluid. It must be added, however, that loss of water from the skin may vary enormously, depending on the temperature of the air, exercise, fever, etc. At least 500 cc. of water must be excreted by the kidneys to carry the solids which have to be eliminated. The kidney, therefore, is the organ most concerned with the volume and composition of the body fluids, its activities involving tubular reabsorption as well as

glomerular excretion, matters which will be considered in detail in the chapter on the kidney. It is well to recall that the kidneys filter water out of the blood at a rate of nearly 48 gallons a day, yet we lose only some 3 pints of water by this route. About 85 per cent of the glomerular filtrate is absorbed automatically by the proximal tubules. The fate of the remaining 15 per cent depends on reabsorption or excretion in the distal tubules, which is under the control of the anti-diuretic hormone of the pituitary, loss of which results in diabetes insipidus. The intestine also plays an important part in water balance, about 8,000 cc. of electrolyte-containing fluid being secreted daily into the bowel by way of the gastric juice, bile, etc., of which all but 100 cc. are reabsorbed. Diarrhea naturally leads to rapid dehydration, with corresponding disturbance in the electrolyte balance. Water lost in expired air is known as *insensible water* and is free of electrolytes. Moderate sweating, on the other hand, produces a fluid containing from 30 to 85 mEq./L of sodium and chloride and 5 mEq./L potassium.

The *movement of water* has already been referred to. The body fluids in the three great compartments are not only free to move, but they do move ceaselessly and in great volume like the currents of the ocean. The two main factors responsible for this continuous movement are (1) the hydrostatic pressure within the vessels and (2) the osmotic pressure of electrolytes and proteins. The hydrostatic pressure drives fluid out of the capillaries, while the osmotic pressure of the plasma protein pulls it back. The resultant of these forces determines the end result. At the arterial end of a capillary the hydrostatic pressure exceeds the osmotic pressure of the plasma protein, so that water and electrolytes pass from the vascular to the interstitial compartment. At the venous end of the capillary the conditions are reversed, and the flow is naturally also reversed. It is evident how great and constant a flow of fluid must result from such a dynamic mechanism. Changes in electrolytes, by altering the osmotic pressure, lead to a shift of water from the intracellular to the extracellular compartment, whilst the flow of lymph contributes still further to the movement of fluid.

Although the cell membranes and the capillary walls are both entirely permeable to water, they differ greatly in their permeability to electrolytes, the wall of the capillary being completely permeable, whilst the membrane of the cell is relatively impermeable. The result is that the composition of the intracellular and extracellular fluids differ profoundly from one another. Most of the sodium and chlorine of the body are in the extracellular fluid (the internal environment), while most of the potassium, magnesium and phosphate are in the intracellular fluid. When the osmotic pressure in the extracellular compartment is altered by a change either in its electrolyte or its water content, the osmotic equilibrium which is so essential to health is maintained by the passage of water from or into the intracellular compartment. Such a shift of water will of course change the volume of the two compartments. As the capillary wall presents no barrier to the passage of inorganic ions, although denying passage to the macromolecules of plasma protein, it follows that the two divisions of extracellular water are practically identical in inorganic content, the only chemical difference being the high protein content of the plasma.

The copious fluids of the gastrointestinal tract are similar in character to the plasma, except for the partial replacement of sodium ions by hydrogen ions in the gastric juice, and the higher content of bicarbonate ions in the intestinal and pancreatic juices. It follows that when these fluids are lost to the outside, either from vomiting, diarrhea, fistulæ or continuous drainage, the body is losing not only water but electrolytes as well.

PATHOLOGY OF
THE INTERNAL ENVIRONMENT

The major elements of the internal environment are water and electrolytes. Disturbances of fluid balance, which may be either in the direction of too little or too much, are discussed in the next section. Of the electrolytes, those substances which when placed in water become dissociated into electrically charged particles called *ions*, the two which demand our attention are sodium and potassium. Here again there may be too little or too much. The concentration in extracellular and intracellular fluid is strikingly reversed in the case of the two electrolytes. For sodium the higher levels for extracellular fluid in milliequivalents per liter are 150, but only 5 for intracellular fluid, whereas in the case of potassium the corresponding figures are 5 and 110. The volume and distribution of the body fluids is controlled largely by the sodium ions of the extracellular fluid and the potassium ions of the intracellular fluid. It has been well said that "the electrolytes form the chemical framework on which rests the stability of the physical properties of the extracellular fluid" (Gamble).

Sodium.—We have just seen that sodium is the paramount electrolyte of the extracellular fluid, just as potassium plays a similar part in the intracellular fluid. It would appear as if the crude primitive cells afloat in a sodium-salt prehistoric sea incorporated a few potassium ions into their substance, but kept sodium out, which they have continued to do ever since. It is true that in potassium depletion sodium may replace it in the cells, but with disastrous results, for the change in electrolyte balance injures the intracellular enzyme mechanism and initiates necrobiosis, an effect particularly noticeable in cardiac muscle.

Sodium Depletion.—The salt content of the body may be reduced, with secondary reduction in the water content. Salt deficiency may develop as the result of two very different mechanisms.

(1) *Direct loss of salt from the body*, mainly in gastrointestinal juices, as occurs in prolonged vomiting, diarrhea, and intestinal fistula. The most serious effects are seen in infants, whose kidneys are less able to reabsorb sodium, and in children. When salt and water are both lost, but only water is replaced, as in severe sweating accompanied by copious drinking of unsalted water, the salt depletion may be quite severe.

(2) *Loss of the power to retain salt*, as occurs in renal disease and in Addison's disease (lack of aldosterone), may cause severe salt depletion. In water depletion there is a loss of

intracellular fluid, but in salt depletion there is an excess of this fluid, since water passes into the cells in order to lower their osmotic pressure to that of the extracellular fluid. The patient, therefore, is not thirsty. The net result of the combined loss of water into the cells and from the kidneys is a reduction in the volume of the extracellular fluid, including the vascular compartment, with, it may be, oligemic shock and circulatory collapse. Such a picture may develop in untreated Addison's disease.

Sodium Retention.—Sodium is the chief component of the extracellular fluid on the basic side. Sodium concentration is regulated by its reabsorption from the glomerular filtrate as it passes along the renal tubules. If this reabsorption, which is controlled by aldosterone, is increased, sodium is retained, and the volume of extracellular fluid must increase if osmotic equilibrium is to be maintained. This means edema in the interstitial compartment, which may be obvious clinically, or may remain subclinical, although betrayed by increase in weight. In our future studies we shall encounter various examples of sodium retention.

Potassium.—During the last few years we have rather suddenly come to realize the great importance of potassium. This is largely due to the use of the flame photometer, with the aid of which quantitative estimations of potassium deficits and surfeits in body fluids and tissues can be made quickly, easily and economically. Moreover the advent of radioactive isotopes has made it possible to follow the movement of potassium atoms through biological structures. We have already noted the curious distribution of this electrolyte between the intracellular and extracellular fluids, 98 per cent being located in the cells, mainly those of the muscles. It is, indeed, the chief basic ion of the body cells. There is a curious inverse relationship between potassium and sodium. Any change in either the sodium or the potassium of the extracellular fluid is attended by an inversely proportional change in its counterpart, and the same is true of the intracellular fluid. The kidney seems to be designed to retain sodium by tubular reabsorption and to excrete potassium. The two contrasting mechanisms in the kidney

seem to be under the control of aldosterone, which stimulates reabsorption of sodium and excretion of potassium.

Potassium Depletion.—Hypopotassemia (*hypokalemia*) is much more common than potassium retention. It may develop from a variety of causes, some of which are as follows. (1) *Stress*, usually the result of surgical trauma, is perhaps the leading cause. The cells of the postoperative patient are leaking potassium into the extracellular fluid and thence at once into the urine. The factor responsible seems to be aldosterone liberated as part of the adrenal cortical reaction to stress. (2) *Potassium-losing nephritis* associated with *primary aldosteronism*, a condition which will be described in due course. (3) *Vomiting and diarrhea* when severe and prolonged. In the diarrhea of children the potassium contents of the intestinal fluid may be markedly raised. For some reason in tumors of the large bowel the intestinal fluid may be very rich in potassium. The prolonged and excessive use of laxatives may result in loss of potassium. Indeed loss by the bowel is one of the chief causes of hypopotassemia. (4) *Familial periodic paralysis*, a rare disorder of skeletal muscle in which the onset of the attack of paralysis is usually associated with a sharp and marked decrease in the serum potassium. (5) *Iatrogenic deficiency*, that is to say deficiency caused by therapy, is probably as common as that caused by disease. The part played by surgical stress has already been mentioned. The continued intravenous administration of salt and glucose solutions may lower the serum potassium level to a dangerous degree with the eventual production of an intracellular deficit, and the same is true of the parenteral control of acidosis or alkalosis if potassium be omitted.

The *clinical effects* of hypopotassemia begin to develop when the concentration in the serum falls below the normal level of 3.5 to 4.5 mEq/L, that level being maintained at the expense of the intracellular potassium. As the bulk of the potassium is within muscle cells, it is the muscles which suffer most. There is lack of muscular tone, flabbiness, weakness, and finally paralysis, which is attributed to blocking of nerve impulses to the muscles. Intestinal atony with abdominal distension in the postoperative patient are due to potassium depletion. Myocardial failure and cardiac dilatation with marked electrocardiographic changes are amongst the most serious of the sequelæ.

Potassium Retention.—This is much less common than potassium deficiency, because of the thoroughness with which the kidneys excrete the electrolyte. The major cause of hyperpotassemia is inadequate excretion of potassium by the kidneys. Indeed in the anuria of acute glomerulonephritis it may be the immediate cause of death. Lack of aldosterone in Addison's disease and the injudicious intravenous administration of potassium may also be responsible. The general *clinical picture* is again one of muscular weakness and listlessness, but the main effect is on the myocardium, with bradycardia due to interference with the conduction system.

Body Temperature.—One of the essential requirements of the internal environment is that the body temperature should be maintained within normal limits. This presented no problem to our oceanic ancestors, but when animals chose to leave water and live on land they had to face this problem. The living body is an engine which is continually producing heat. There is a constant production of heat by the metabolic processes, especially in the great glandular organs such as the liver; this represents the basal metabolism of the body at rest. The chief source of heat is the muscles. During muscular exercise the heat production may be increased from 200 to 300 per cent, whereas in fever it is only increased from 20 to 30 per cent, yet in the former the temperature remains normal, while in the latter it is raised. The regulation of the temperature is effected by maintaining a balance between heat production and heat loss. Of these the latter is the more important.

Heat production is largely regulated by muscular movement. When an animal is cold it shivers, and the fibrillary movement of the muscles increases the heat production. If this is not enough the animal moves about. Finally the muscular tone is increased. In cold weather the metabolic processes are increased and more heat is produced by oxidation. Most heat is produced by the oxidation of fat, protein gives less, and carbohydrate the least.

Heat loss in man is effected mainly through the skin and partly through the lungs. Heat is lost from the skin by conduction and radiation and by the evaporation of sweat. The normal regulation of the temperature in the skin is by means of peripheral vasoconstriction and vasodilatation. As more heat is produced in the body the vessels in the skin dilate and a large amount of additional heat is lost from the surface. If this is not sufficient to keep the temperature down, sweat is secreted, the evaporation of which cools the surface. In exophthalmic goiter the heat production may be 80 per cent above normal, yet the temperature of the body is not raised, for the skin is flushed and moist. Two accessory factors are of importance in heat loss; these are the humidity and the movement of the air. The higher the humidity, the less is the evaporation from the skin, so that with a high humidity heat stroke is more likely to occur. The conduction of heat from the surface is greatly facilitated by the movement of air, so that an electric fan may make heat supportable which otherwise would be unbearable. The importance of loose clothing is self-evident.

The *thermoregulator mechanism* lies in the hypothalamus and brain stem. Experimental puncture of this region or injury from hemorrhage may be followed by a marked rise in temperature. The anterior hypothalamus is involved when the temperature is rising, and the posterior hypothalamus when it is falling. The temperature of the blood bathing the hypothalamus activates the mechanism. As we have just seen, the response to a demand for increased heat loss is vasodilatation in the skin and an increased production of sweat.

Fever.—We have already learned that the body constant, temperature, may be upset in two ways: an undue strain may be thrown on the mechanism, or the mechanism itself may be interfered with. When a person is exposed to an extremely high temperature, especially when associated with high humidity, the mechanism breaks down and the temperature of the body rises. This is described under Heat Stroke in Chapter 17, and may conveniently be called hyperthermia. Exposure to undue cold is followed by a fall of the body temperature or hypothermia.

Fever or pyrexia is due to a disturbance of the regulating mechanism, probably the center in the brain. There may be an *increased production of heat*, but this is not necessary, nor is it ever so great as in non-febrile conditions such as hyperthyroidism and muscular exercise. Pyrexia may be produced by injury to the brain, by certain poisons, and by the intravenous injection of foreign proteins; in none of these is there any reason to think that heat production is increased. *Diminution of heat loss* is the chief factor, and at the beginning of a fever the patient does everything in his power to minimize this loss by huddling under the blankets.

The *causation of fever* is a complex and difficult subject. That simple yet delicate instrument of precision, the clinical thermometer, reveals a rise in temperature in a great variety of conditions. Something tunes the heat-regulating mechanism to a higher key, just as the regulator of a thermostat may be moved up a few degrees so as to keep a room at a higher temperature. The balance between heat production and heat loss is adjusted to a higher level. This is first effected by diminution of heat loss; later there is increase in heat production.

At the risk of being guilty of oversimplification we may say that fever is an accompaniment of tissue injury. This may be due to many causes. (1) All *infections*, whether bacterial, rickettsial, viral or protozoal, may cause fever. This has been blamed on the action of toxins on the heat-regulating centers in the brain. We shall return to the question of bacterial pyrogens in the next paragraph. (2) *Mechanical injury*, such as severe crushing and extensive surgical operations, is followed by fever for a few days. (3) *Vascular accidents* leading to ischemic necrosis and infarction are accompanied by fever, as is well seen in myocardial infarction. (4) *Diseases due to immune mechanisms*, as in at least some of the so-called collagen diseases, are marked by fever. (5) *Neoplasms* constitute the most puzzling group. The majority of malignant tumors may cause fever, although usually they do not. One of the best examples is renal carcinoma or hypernephroma. I know of a nurse who had a hypernephroma with no symptoms except daily fever and chills, as a result of which she spent one wasted year in a tuberculosis sanatorium. Carcinoma of the stomach or pancreas with liver metastases is often accompanied by fever. So is Hodgkin's disease and lymphosarcoma, in which fever may be the earliest symptom. The pyrogen is presumably some product of protein destruction.

For the student who is going to be a practising doctor the cause of fever of the greatest importance is of course that of bacterial and other infections. For long it has been believed, only naturally, that the fever was due to *the action of toxins on the thermoregulatory centers of the brain*. Many bacteria, more especially gram-negative bacteria, possess powerful endotoxins which, when injected intravenously, cause fever. They are mostly high-molecular-weight polysaccharides, relatively heat stable. As Barry Wood remarks, these are only too well known to the clinician as troublesome pyrogens which may contaminate glassware, needles, rubber tubing, and even intravenous fluids, being responsible for the chills and fever which so often complicate intravenous injections. They are characterized by a relatively long latent period, prompt leukopenia and then leukocytosis. One of the peculiar features of these bacterial endotoxins is that repeated injections at daily intervals produce a nonspecific immunity, so that the host is tolerant or refractory to other bacterial endotoxins as well as to the one being employed.

At first sight it would appear that here was the answer to the problem of fever in bacterial infections. We now know that saline *extracts of polymorphonuclear leukocytes contain a pyrogen* with very different properties, as shown in the accompanying table taken from Barry Wood's Shattuck Lecture on fever.

A glance at this table will show that these pyrogens are profoundly different, and that the leukocytic pyrogen produces the picture seen in the fever of bacterial infections. Bennett has demonstrated that the peritoneal exudate of experimental pneumococcal peritonitis contains a heat-labile substance with properties identical with those of leukocytic pyrogen, and that this substance is also present in the lymph of the thoracic dust. Later it was shown that this pyrogen is present in the blood, and that it acts directly

COMPARISON OF PROPERITIES OF LEUKOCYTIC PYROGEN WITH THOSE OF BACTERIAL ENDOTOXIN

Property	Leukocytic Pyrogen	Bacterial Endotoxin
Inactivated by heat	Yes	No
Length of latent period	Short	Long
Postinjection leukopenia	Slight or none	Marked
Activity in tolerant recipients	Unaffected	Depressed
Production of tolerance	No	Yes

on the thermoregulatory centers of the brain (King and Wood).

The relation of the bacterial endotoxin to the leukocytic pyrogen is apparently as follows. It would appear that when bacterial endotoxin and leukocytes are brought together in salt solution the luekocytes are injured by the endotoxin, and discharge their own pyrogen into the medium. If this happens in the circulating blood the pyrogen will be carried to the thermoregulatory centers of the brain, and there excite the production of fever.

The polymorphonuclear leukocyte seems to play an integral part in the pathogenesis of the fever of acute bacterial infections. This still leaves us with the problem of fever in agranulocytosis, viral infections and granulomatous diseases in which polymorphonuclears play a relatively insignificant role. There is also the question of the cause of fever in infarctions, neoplasms, and other conditions already mentioned. It has long been known that polysaccharide pyrogens can be extracted from normal tissue. Possibly these play some part in the production of fever, but of this there is absolutely no proof at the present time.

The *clinical picture of fever* is fairly characteristic. At the outset of a fever the skin is pale and dry. The pallor is due to vasoconstriction, the dryness to suppression of sweat. Loss of heat from the skin is reduced to a minimum, and the patient feels cold and may experience *chills*. It is difficult to explain the feeling of cold, as the skin may be hot, but it is probably due to the great difference in temperature between the interior and exterior of the body. In severe fevers there may be *rigors*. These are fine fibrillary contractions of the muscles, as a result of which much work is done and heat production is greatly increased. Metabolism is accelerated, particularly that of proteins and fats, so that the fire in the interior of the body becomes hotter. There is then less need for heat conservation, and the skin may become moist and flushed. It is when the fever suddenly abates that the skin becomes drenched with perspiration in an endeavor to bring the temperature down to the new level set by the heat-regulating mechanism.

The question of the possible *function of fever* is an important but still unanswered question. "*What is the meaning of fever?* Is it harmful or beneficent?" A very high temperature or hyperpyrexia (107° or 108° F.) is certainly harmful, and if long-continued will result in death through injury to the nerve cells. But there is no reason to think that a moderate degree of fever is harmful, so that it is unnecessary to attack it with antipyretic drugs. It probably plays some part in the defense mechanism against infection just as does inflammation. The heat does not injure the bacteria, but up to a certain point (105° F.) there appears to be an increase of phagocytosis and a more rapid production of antibodies and agglutinins. Above this point the cell protoplasm begins to suffer. The high and low limits of temperature recorded in patients who have recovered are 114° and 75° F. Very low temperatures are much less harmful than very high ones.

DISTURBANCE OF FLUID BALANCE

Dehydration.—In dehydration, as the name indicates, there is a decrease in the water content of the body. The deficiency may be due to an *intake* of water which is too little, or to a *loss* via the skin, lung, kidneys or gastrointestinal tract which is too great. A lessened intake may be due to dysphagia (difficulty in swallowing), to great weakness or to coma. Excessive loss of water (and salt) occurs through the skin in high fever. Vomiting, diarrhea and long-continued loss of fluid through a fistulous opening lead to marked dehydration, which in children can attain an alarming degree in a short time. A patient suffering from Asiatic cholera may become completely dehydrated in the space of 24 hours. Renal loss of water (diuresis) and of electrolytes (chiefly salt) may be due to destruction of the absorptive tubular epithelium—we have already seen that of 48 gallons of water filtered by the glomeruli we lose only 3 pints in the urine—or to lack of antidiuretic hormone from the pituitary or salt-retaining aldosterone from the adrenal.

Decrease of body water from whatever cause is naturally first seen in the intravascular compartment with a reduction in blood volume. The regulating mechanism we have already discussed comes into play, withdrawing fluid from the interstitial compartment, and finally the intracellular fluid. It is this which really counts, for cellular dehydration creates thirst that may become so intense as to be unendurable, and it interferes with cellular enzymes to a degree which may prove fatal.

EDEMA

Edema.—Edema is an abnormal accumulation of fluid in the tissue spaces and serous cavities. This accumulation may be *local* or *general*, a distinction of great importance; in the former the causal factor is local, in the latter it is general (anasarca). When water collects in the tissue it may be in free or combined form. When *combined* it is united with the protoplasm of the tissue elements. When *free* it lies between these elements and can be moved from one place to another. For this reason a pit is left when an edematous part is pressed on; this is known clinically as "pitting on pressure." Sometimes there is a *solid edema*, in which case there is no pitting on pressure. The water is taken up mainly by the connective tissue of the

muscles and skin, or rather the subcutaneous tissue. An initial accumulation of water cannot be detected clinically. Indeed it is only when 5 or 6 liters have collected in these water depots that edema becomes evident. But this invisible accumulation of fluid is indicated by a steady increase in weight.

Edematous fluid closely resembles lymph; the one is normal, the other abnormal, interstitial fluid. It contains less proteins, and the specific gravity is lower—1.006 to 1.012. It does not readily coagulate when removed from the body, but sometimes a thin clot may form. No clotting occurs within the body (*e. g.*, in the serous cavities). At the same time it must be recognized that the composition varies with the mode of production and the etiological agent. A distinction may be drawn between a transudate and an exudate. A *transudate* is ordinary edematous fluid; the specific gravity is below 1.015 and the protein below 3 per cent. An *exudate* is the fluid of an inflammatory edema: the specific gravity is above 1.018 and the protein above 4 per cent. Clotting is more marked when the fluid is removed from the body, and may occur within the serous cavities. It is evident that an exudate more closely resembles blood plasma than does a transudate, because of the increased permeability of the vessel wall induced by the inflammation.

Tissue Changes.—An edematous tissue has a pale watery appearance. Subcutaneous tissue may come to resemble jelly. In the lung where edema of the alveoli is very common, the affected part may feel solid, but fluid pours from the cut surface. The brain acquires a characteristically wet appearance. Under the microscope the tissue elements are widely separated by watery material which can be best demonstrated if the tissue is fixed in boiling formalin so that the fluid does not escape. In well-fixed specimens the fluid appears as fine granules. The fluid of edema is not always intercellular. Cells and fibrin may become edematous and swollen; this change is similar to hydropic degeneration.

Varieties of Edema.—Fluid may collect in the tissues under a variety of conditions which bear no relation to one another. Edema may be *local* or *general*. Of course, in general edema the condition may be more pronounced in one locality, but the etiological agent acts generally. The main forms of edema are *inflammatory, obstructive, cardiac*, and *renal*. Inflammatory and obstructive edemas are local, cardiac and renal edemas are general. To these must be added *angioneurotic* and allied forms of edema; also the edema of *chronic starvation* and that variety of it known as *war edema*. Instead of taking these up *seriatim* it will be better to consider the various factors which may cause edema, and then return to the special forms of the condition.

Causes of Edema.—There are three main causes of general edema, and a fourth factor which comes into play in local edema. In addition to these there are a number of secondary factors which will have to be considered. The primary factors in general edema are: (1) Increased permeability of the capillary wall, (2) decrease of the colloid osmotic pressure of the plasma proteins, and (3) increase of the hydrostatic pressure of the blood. The additional factor in local edema is (4) lymphatic obstruction.

1. INCREASED PERMEABILITY OF THE CAPILLARY WALL.—The normal capillary wall is a semipermeable membrane through which water and salts can pass in either direction with the greatest ease. Much has been written about increased permeability of the vessel wall as a cause of edema, especially in inflammation. The endothelial wall cannot become more permeable to water and crystalloids, because it already is completely permeable. Moreover, the rate of passage of these materials and their amount is independent of the condition of the capillary wall, being determined entirely by forces on either side of the wall, either in the blood or in the tissues. But the outward passage of colloids is intimately related to the condition of the vessel wall. Under normal conditions protein is prevented almost completely from passing from the blood into the tissues, but when the vessels are injured by toxins, lack of oxygen, etc., they become readily permeable to protein, as is seen in inflammatory edema. In the kidney this causes albuminuria, while elsewhere there is what Eppinger has called "albuminuria into the tissues." The passage of the large protein molecules is favored by dilatation of the capillaries, due

in turn to relaxation of the branching Rouget cells, and Krogh believes that this is one of the major factors responsible for the great escape of protein in the edema of inflammation.

The escape of protein is of the greatest importance in the production of edema, for it lowers the colloid osmotic pressure of the blood and raises that of the tissues, as a result of which water readily passes out through the capillary wall. The increased permeability to protein is thus a major factor in the production of edema.

2. DECREASE OF THE COLLOID OSMOTIC PRESSURE OF THE PLASMA PROTEINS.—We have seen that the water of the blood can escape with the greatest ease into the tissues. The force which holds it back is the colloid osmotic pressure of the proteins. If an animal is bled repeatedly but kept alive by reinjection of the red blood cells, the plasma proteins will fall to a low level and marked edema will develop. A fall of plasma protein below 5 per cent will cause edema. For this reason long-continued anemia is apt to be associated with edema. Marked ascites, when the fluid is rich in protein, as in malignant disease of the peritoneum, may lead to generalized edema (anasarca) owing to the severe plasma-protein loss. The different proteins of the plasma have different colloid osmotic pressures, albumin being about four times stronger than globulin. It follows that when there is a great loss of albumin from the blood, as in the albuminuria of subacute glomerulonephritis and the nephrotic syndrome with a reversal of the normal albumin-globulin ratio (3 to 1), edema will result. The colloid osmotic pressure depends therefore partly on the total amount of plasma proteins, partly on their relative proportion.

3. INCREASED HYDROSTATIC PRESSURE OF THE BLOOD.—The pressure in the capillaries is the force which overcomes the colloid osmotic pressure of the plasma and enables the normal passage of nutritive fluid into the tissues. If it is increased, edema will result. The pressure in the capillaries depends upon the venous blood pressure and not upon the arterial pressure. In cardiac failure the venous pressure rises markedly, and the increased capillary pressure leads to edema. The stretching and dilatation of the capil-

laries also renders them more permeable. The edema which follows thrombosis of the main vein of a limb is largely due to an increase in the capillary blood pressure. It must not be thought, however, that fluid can only leave the blood through the capillaries. In the case of the skin the permeability of the vessels to a slowly diffusible vital dye is much greater in the venules than in the capillaries. There is a mounting grade of permeability along the capillaries, being lowest at the arterial and highest at the venous end.

4. LYMPHATIC OBSTRUCTION.—This is an important factor in the production of local but not general edema. Much of the intercellular fluid in the tissues escapes by way of the lymphatics, so that obstruction to outflow through these channels will cause local edema. The obstruction may be due to inflammation, to the presence of tumor cells within the lumen, or filariasis caused by Filaria bancrofti, a parasitic worm which may block the channel. Pressure from without produces the same effect. This pressure may be due to a tumor or to collection of fluid. As the fluid increases the lymphatic obstruction becomes more marked, so that a vicious circle is formed. For this reason removal of part of an effusion in a serous sac is often followed by disappearance of the remainder, for reduction of the pressure allows the lymph channels to be opened up and the fluid to be drained away. Examples of lymphatic edema are the swelling of the arm which may develop in cancer of the breast; *elephantiasis* or swelling of the legs, scrotum, etc., seen in most marked form in obstruction due to filaria; *chylous ascites* and chylothorax, effusions of chylous fluid in the abdominal and pleural cavities due to obstruction of the thoracic duct by filaria, tumors, enlarged glands, etc. *Non-parasitic elephantiasis* is an edema of the leg occurring mostly in young women, due apparently to chronic lymphangitis of unknown origin. *Milroy's disease*, or hereditary edema, is also probably lymphatic in origin.

Secondary Factors.—In addition to the four primary factors just enumerated there are at least two secondary factors. These are the osmotic pressure in the tissues and chloride retention due to renal insufficiency.

It is evident that if the protein of the plasma escapes through the capillary wall the *colloid osmotic pressure of the tissue* will rise, and on that account water will pass out of the vessels. *Chloride retention* is a secondary but not a primary factor; it aggravates and continues an already existing edema, but does not initiate the condition. But although salt retention is not a primary factor in the production of edema, yet once the condition of edema is established and the chlorides pass into the tissues with the water, the greater the amount of salt available, the more water will be retained in the tissues because of the increase of the osmotic pressure there. That there is a real relation between salt retention and edema is shown by the fact that in renal edema the withdrawal of salt from the food is often followed by rapid disappearance of the edema and a corresponding increase in the flow of urine.

With these additional facts in mind we may briefly review some of the various forms of edema which have already been mentioned.

Inflammatory Edema.—The swelling which is one of the cardinal signs of inflammation is largely due to edema. Owing to the action of the irritant the permeability of the capillaries is increased and fluid pours out into the intercellular spaces. This fluid is rich in protein. Owing perhaps to the formation of a network of fibrin the fluid cannot be moved about through the tissues as in other forms of edema, nor is it influenced by gravity. There are other factors beside injury to the vessel walls, but these and other matters connected with the edema of inflammation have already been discussed in detail in Chapter 2. If the inflammation involves the pleura, pericardium, or peritoneum these serous sacs are filled with fluid from which fibrin is deposited on the surface.

Cardiac Edema.—This might better be called congestive edema, for it is apt to develop in any long-standing condition of venous congestion, though usually due to progressive cardiac failure. The obstructive edema seen when a large vein becomes thrombosed belongs to the same group. The fluid is loose in the tissues and readily changes its position under the action of gravity, so that it first appears in the dependent parts.

The serous sacs become filled with fluid. For some reason the effusion is much commoner in the right pleural sac than in the left. Several factors are probably at work. Owing to the failing circulation there is an increase of pressure in the veins and capillaries. For the same reason there is back pressure in the lymphatics. The capillary walls are stretched and rendered more permeable. Oxygenation is poor and the vascular endothelium suffers in consequence and fails to hold back the water, but this factor is probably not of much importance, else the proteins would come through in large amounts.

Pulmonary edema is a variety of cardiac edema. As the left side of the heart fails, blood accumulates in the lungs and fluid passes from the distended capillaries into the alveoli. The condition is most marked in the dependent parts of the lung. The changes are described in the section on the Lungs.

Renal Edema.—This resembles cardiac edema except that the fluid is less influenced by gravity. Nor are the serous sacs involved so soon. The protein content and specific gravity are much lower than in cardiac edema, indeed lower than in any of the edemas. Blood examination will at once differentiate the two, for in edema due to chronic nephritis the blood cholesterol is markedly raised, while in cardiac edema it is normal. Renal edema is seen in acute nephritis, in the subacute or wet stage, and in the condition known as nephrosis, which is probably merely a variant of true nephritis. In all of these the edema is associated with marked albuminuria but not with a high blood pressure. Indeed as the blood pressure goes up the edema tends to disappear. A number of factors appear to be responsible. In wet nephritis and nephrosis there is a fall in the blood proteins and a reversal of the normal (3 to 1) albumin-globulin ratio; both of these reduce the osmotic pressure in the blood so that water passes into the tissues. Crystalloids, especially sodium chloride, are retained in the tissues and raise the osmotic pressure there, so that when water is drunk it passes into the tissues instead of into the urine, what Fishberg calls a prerenal deviation of water.

CACHECTIC EDEMA.—In many wasting diseases and anemias edema develops in the later stages, affecting the feet and legs particularly. Several causal factors may be at work. There is likely to be cardiac exhaustion and circulatory failure, the nutrition of the vessel walls is interfered with, the blood proteins especially in anemia are lowered and the osmotic pressure falls.

FAMINE EDEMA.—In prolonged undernutrition and chronic starvation edema may develop. This was common among prisoners on the Continent during the First World War. The blood proteins are very low owing to absence of proteins from the diet, so that the osmotic pressure falls and fluid leaves the blood vessels. It is probable that absence of vitamin A has something to do with it, because in many cases there develops the ulceration of the cornea (xerophthalmia) characteristic of deficiency of that vitamin.

HEREDITARY EDEMA. MILROY'S DISEASE.—This is a chronic edema without any evident cause or constitutional disturbance. It is markedly hereditary. Milroy observed 22 cases in a family of 97 individuals (six generations). It is confined to the lower limbs, affecting one or both legs. The leg may be very greatly swollen. The condition should be distinguished from the non-parasitic form of elephantiasis, a condition which is usually confined to women, whereas Milroy's disease is equally common in both sexes.

A summary of the principal types of edema is given in the following table.

PRINCIPAL TYPES OF EDEMA

Local		Generalized	Miscellaneous

Obstructive	Venous
	Lymphatic
		Cardiac
		Renal
		  1. Acute glomerulonephritis
		  2. Nephrotic syndrome
		Nutritional (Famine)
		Hepatic (Cirrhosis)
			Angioneurotic
			Myxedema
			Milroy's Disease
			Toxic (local or
			general)

Capillary damage	Inflammation Allergy		

DISTURBANCE OF BLOOD VOLUME

Arterial and Capillary Hyperemia.—Active hyperemia is a dilatation of the arterioles and capillaries, which may be dilated together or singly. It may be regarded as a physiological response to a call of the tissue for more blood. It must be realized that the capillary bed of an organ at rest is never all in operation at one time. In a healthy kidney only a limited number of glomeruli are working at any given moment, and it is only through capillaries of these glomeruli that an active circulation is going on. The remainder remain collapsed. (Fig. 79). Whenever there is a call for more work the latent capillary bed becomes opened up. The same difference is observed between a muscle which has been actively contracting and one which is at rest. The active organ shows an active hyperemia. It has always been difficult to understand why in an organ of uniform structure, such as the liver, a blood-borne toxin tends to produce focal rather than diffuse lesions. The explanation appears to depend on the fact that some parts of the organ are relatively ischemic and therefore protected for a time from the injurious agent, while others are flooded with blood and thus exposed to damage.

Extremely active hyperemia of arterioles and capillaries is seen in inflammation. A comparison between the capillary bed in a normal and an inflamed omentum will soon prove the truth of this statement. In the early stages of pneumonia the vessels in the walls of the alveoli show an extreme degree of hyperemia. Inflammatory hyperemia is due to the direct action of toxins on the walls of the vessels, because it occurs when all the nerves to the part are cut, and yet nervous influence does exert some influence upon it. Active hyperemia may largely disappear after death.

Venous Congestion.—Venous congestion or passive hyperemia is a condition in which the blood accumulates on the venous side of the vascular tree. The congestion may be general or local. Both of these may be acute or chronic. Of these various forms chronic general venous congestion is by far the most important.

General Venous Congestion.—*Causes.*—As

11

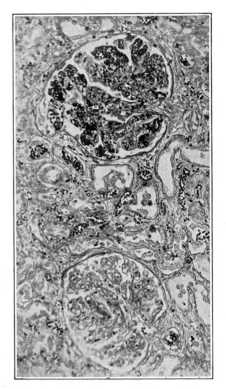

Fig. 79.—The upper glomerulus is full of blood and active; the lower one is ischemic and resting. × 200.

the condition is general the cause must be central. There are only two organs through which all the blood in the body must pass. These are the heart and the lungs. Obstruction to the circulation through either of these organs will give rise to general venous congestion. As the obstruction is usually chronic in type the congestion will be chronic. In the *heart* the common cause is mitral stenosis, but mitral incompetence and aortic valvular disease will lead in the end to the same result. Chronic myocardial failure from whatever cause is also associated with chronic venous congestion. Speaking generally, failure of the right ventricle is likely to lead to so-called "backward failure" in which the systemic veins become overloaded, whilst failure of the left ventricle results in "forward failure" with congestion of the pulmonary veins, as the failing left ventricle does not manage to pump out from the lungs all the blood pumped into them by the right ventricle.

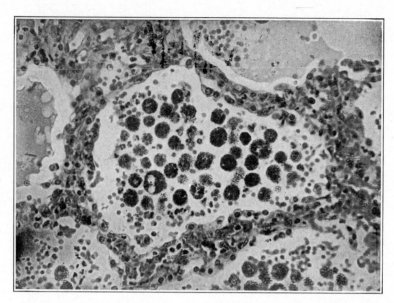

Fig. 80.—Heart failure cells in the lung. The alveolar walls are greatly thickened. × 250.

In actual practice both forms of failure are usually combined.

In the *lungs* the chief causes of obstruction are emphysema and fibrosis. In emphysema there is great distention of the alveoli with destruction of the alveolar walls and narrowing of the capillaries in those which remain. The result is a marked obstruction to the pulmonary circulation with distention of the right side of the heart and accumulation of blood in the veins. Fibrosis of the lungs as the result of tuberculosis or other chronic infections also leads to obliteration of the pulmonary capillaries with resulting venous congestion.

These forms of congestion are of the chronic type. If cardiac failure is more acute, usually left ventricular in type, the venous congestion will also be acute. This type of failure often develops as a terminal phenomenon, and as the lungs are the first to suffer, it is seldom that autopsy fails to reveal some degree of pulmonary congestion.

Clinical Effects of Venous Congestion.— These are both general and local. The *general effects* are due to insufficient oxygenation. Owing to accumulation of blood in the dilated veins the speed of the circulation is slowed down and the blood is not sufficiently aerated in the lungs. Moreover the edema of the lungs which so commonly develops still further prevents a proper interchange of gases. Owing to the resulting anoxemia there will be a varying degree of *dyspnea* or shortness of breath. As the blood remains unduly long in the venules and capillaries, there is a marked increase in the amount of reduced hemoglobin, the blood becomes more venous in type, and the patient manifests *cyanosis*, a blueness or lividity of the skin and mucous membranes, well seen in the ears and lips. Cyanosis is seen in other conditions in which the blood is imperfectly oxygenated, especially in pulmonary disease and in congenital heart disease where an abnormal communication exists between the right and left sides of the heart. Owing to the general congestion the walls of the veins are injured and fluid escapes from the vessels into the tissues causing *edema*, especially in dependent parts such as the feet. Fluid may also pass into the serous cavities with the production of ascites, pleural effusion, etc.

The *local effects* are described in connection with the individual organs, but the changes in the lung and the liver are so common that they may be outlined here.

In the *lungs* chronic venous congestion in its most marked form is caused by mitral stenosis due to rheumatic heart disease.

Both lungs are dark brown in color and of tough consistence, so that the condition is described as *brown induration*. Microscopically the vessels in the alveolar walls are dilated, varicose, and in section may give the wall a beaded appearance. The walls themselves are thickened. But the most characteristic finding is the presence in the alveoli of large phagocytic cells filled with yellow blood pigment which gives the reaction for iron. (Fig. 80). These cells are known as *heart failure cells*, but their presence does not necessarily indicate that the heart is failing—merely that there is some central obstruction to the free flow of blood. The pigment is derived from the red blood cells often seen lying within the alveoli and due to hemorrhage from the distended vessels. It is carried by the phagocytes into the lymphatics and is distributed throughout the framework of the lung, where it excites a certain amount of fibrosis. The pigment is therefore responsible for the "brown induration." Pulmonary edema is naturally a common accompaniment of venous congestion of the lungs.

The *liver* is involved early owing to its anatomical position. When the right ventricle fails the liver becomes enlarged and tender, both of which features may disappear with appropriate therapy. The gross appearance is described by the old-fashioned term *nutmeg liver*, the cut surface showing a mottled appearance of dark brown and light yellow areas. (Fig. 81). The term is a reminder of the days when pathologists developed a mania for applying the names of pleasant articles of diet to very unpleasant specimens of morbid anatomy, to secretions, and even to excretions. The dark areas represent the congested center of each lobule, the light areas being the fatty peripheral part. Microscopically, the sinusoids at the center of the lobule are distended with blood, and the liver cells are degenerated and atrophic, probably as the result of oxygen deficiency (anoxia), whilst at the periphery the cells are normal or merely show fatty degeneration. In very chronic cases there may be collapse of the lobules and fibrous thickening of the walls of the central veins with extension of fibrous tissue into surrounding lobules. This condition has been called cardiac cirrhosis, or better, *cardiac sclerosis*.

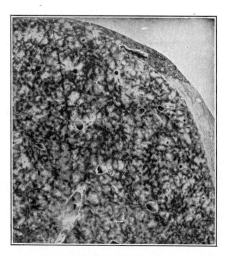

FIG. 81.—Nutmeg liver. The cut surface has a mottled appearance.

Local Venous Congestion.—When the main vein from a region or an organ is obstructed a condition of local venous congestion is produced. The obstruction may be acute or chronic. *Acute obstruction* is usually due to thrombosis in the vein, but may also be caused by sudden pressure on the vein, as in strangulation of a loop of bowel, twisting of the pedicle of an ovarian cyst, etc. The result is very similar to the production of a hemorrhagic infarct. There is no time for a collateral circulation to be set up, so that there is intense engorgement of the venules and capillaries; many of these rupture, and there is hemorrhage into the part which becomes dark purple. Under the microscope the tissues are seen to be stuffed with blood. The condition is best observed in strangulation of the bowel, but may also occasionally be seen in the spleen, kidney, and other organs.

In *chronic obstruction* due to the pressure of tumors, enlarged glands, aneurysm, etc., a collateral circulation is gradually established, so that the results are less severe. If the veins of the collateral circulation are superficial they can readily be seen and offer useful help in making a correct diagnosis. Even when they cannot be seen with the unaided eye, they can be made visible by photographing the area using infrared films. In obstruction of the superior vena cava these distended superficial veins are seen coursing over the clavicle and the upper part of the chest, while in the case of the inferior vena cava they pass upward on the abdominal wall. An important form of chronic local venous congestion is that due to obstruction of the portal vein, usually the result of cirrhosis of the liver. In *portal obstruction* the radicles of the portal vein become distended and varicose. Important varicosities are formed at the lower end of the esophagus and the lower end of the rectum. The latter form hemorrhoids or piles, and the former may rupture, causing hemorrhage into the stomach which may prove fatal. Just as coughing of blood (*hemoptysis*) is a sign of pulmonary congestion, so vomiting of blood (*hematemesis*) is a sign of portal congestion. Fluid may pass from the branches of the portal vein into the peritoneal cavity causing *ascites*.

Ischemia.—Ischemia is a local anemia, a cutting-off of the arterial blood supply to a part. It may be sudden or gradual. *Sudden obstruction* is, of course, produced when a vessel is ligatured, but in disease the usual causes are thrombosis and embolism. The result depends on the question of collateral circulation. If this can be established rapidly and adequately, blood reaches the part by other channels, and no serious damage is done. If such a circulation cannot be established, part or the whole of the area affected will quickly die. This change which is well seen in the heart, spleen, kidney, and brain, is the process of *infarction*, which has already been studied in relation to the effects of embolism.

Gradual obstruction is usually due to arteriosclerosis in which thickening of the intima leads to narrowing of the lumen. The area supplied atrophies, the parenchymatous tissue undergoes necrosis, disappears, and is replaced by fibrous tissue. This change is well seen in the kidney and the myocardium (ischemic necrosis). In the brain it leads to softening. Gradual obstruction of the arteries may also be produced by pressure from without, but this is of little importance apart from the pressure of splints and the formation of bed sores. Ischemia may be caused by prolonged arterial spasm in ergot poisoning and in Raynaud's disease, in both of

which conditions gangrene of the extremities may develop.

Anoxia.—The cells of the body suffer from anoxia when they are unable to obtain sufficient oxygen or are unable to use it. Its effect is not only to stop the machinery but often to wreck the machine. The following varieties may be distinguished: (1) *Stagnant anoxia* due to reduction in the flow of well-oxygenated blood. This is seen in ischemia, cardiac failure, and shock due to vasomotor collapse. (2) *Anoxic anoxia* due to insufficient oxygenation of the blood as it passes through the lungs, as seen in pneumonia and other widespread pulmonary lesions. (3) *Anemic anoxia* due either to reduction in the amount of hemoglobin or interference with its capacity to combine with oxygen, as in carbon monoxide poisoning. (4) *Histotoxic anoxia* due to inability of the cells to utilize oxygen, owing to the action of such poisons as alcohol, narcotics and cyanide.

HEMORRHAGE

Hemorrhage or the escape of blood from a vessel may occur from a variety of causes, some of which are simple, while others are obscure and indeed unknown. The hemorrhage may be due to a break in the wall of the vessel either from trauma or disease. In other cases there seems to be no distinct rupture of the wall, the red cells escaping out by a process of diapedesis. It is probable that many tiny hemorrhages occur in this way. The smallest hemorrhages, often no larger than a pin's head in size, are called *petechiæ*, while larger extravasations are called *ecchymoses*. When a hemorrhage of some size occurs into the tissue it may form a tumor-like swelling known as a *hematoma*.

Spontaneous massive hemorrhage is due to rupture of a vessel. The rupture may be caused by a local dilatation of the lumen with thinning of the wall (aneurysm formation). A second class of case is the septicemias, in which petechial hemorrhages, particularly in the serous membranes, are of frequent occurrence. Here the probable cause is injury of the capillary endothelium by the bacterial toxins, although this is difficult to prove. In some instances (bacterial endocarditis, typhoid fever) clumps of bacteria may lodge in the capillaries and cause hemorrhage. A third group is that of the bleeding diseases which will be discussed in the chapter on the Blood. Some of the chief of these are pernicious anemia, leukemia, and purpura. In the last-named there is a great decrease in the number of blood platelets, but in none of them can it be said that we really know the cause of the hemorrhage.

Changes in the Extravasated Blood.— When the hemorrhage is very small, *i. e.*, petechial in type, the red cells may be removed by phagocytes. When it is of any considerable size the red cells are broken down so that hemoglobin is liberated, and this stains the surrounding tissues. The coloring matter of the hemoglobin is disintegrated into two moieties; one is iron-free and called *hematoidin*, the other contains iron and is therefore called *hemosiderin*. The hematoidin may be deposited in the form of granules or rhombic crystals which are seen around old cerebral hemorrhages, but some of it is converted into bilirubin which is soluble and therefore carried away and excreted in the bile. Large hemorrhages such as that of a ruptured tubal pregnancy may therefore be accompanied by jaundice. The hemosiderin is taken up by phagocytic cells, and these give the Prussian blue reaction for iron. When the hemorrhage takes place into the tissue the vital iron is saved and can be used again for building red blood cells, but when the hemorrhage is internal or into the gastrointestinal tract the iron is lost for ever.

The Arrest of Hemorrhage.—This can best be studied in a vessel which has been divided. There is first temporary arrest of the hemorrhage by the formation of a blood clot, followed by permanent arrest due to the formation of an inflammatory exudate which becomes organized and seals the vessel.

The *temporary clot* is produced by the coagulation of the blood, a process which has already been considered in the previous chapter. The temporary clot is of two varieties, the red and the white. The *red clot* is composed of fibrin containing red cells in its meshes. The *white clot*, which is a thrombus, consists almost entirely of platelets, which form a sticky mass that adheres to the cut edges and serves to plug the hole in the ves-

sel wall. The temporary clot is like a nail, the head of which is formed by the white clot and closes the cut end of the vessel, while the stem is formed by the red clot which extends along the vessel for some distance.

The *permanent clot* results from the organization of the temporary clot. As the result of the injury an inflammatory exudate is formed around the latter, new capillaries and fibroblasts grow in, the clot is vascularized and fibrosed, and the opening in the vessel is finally plugged by a mass of fibrous tissue firmly adherent to the edges of the hole.

This process of healing only occurs properly in the absence of infection. If sepsis is present the formation of the permanent clot is interfered with, the temporary clot may be softened by the bacterial ferments, and *secondary hemorrhage* may occur one or two weeks after an operation. Before the days of asepsis such an accident was a common occurrence.

SHOCK

The basis of shock is essentially a circulatory disturbance, so that it may be considered here. This mysterious and sinister condition is liable to develop after: (1) extensive operations, particularly those involving handling of the abdominal viscera; (2) acute abdominal catastrophes (perforation of stomach or bowel, strangulated hernia, acute pancreatitis); (3) severe injuries; (4) extensive hemorrhage. The condition has continually to be guarded against by the surgeon, and is of special importance in war injuries.

Shock is a clinical state resulting from an upset of the normal physiological balance or homeostasis. The term was originally applied to the physical impact or shock produced by a bullet. Long ago it was defined as "an expression of sympathy of the whole frame with a part suddenly subjected to serious injury," a definition which fits in remarkably well with present day concepts. The trouble is that the expressions of sympathy may be so overpowering that they do more harm than good.

A distinction is often drawn between primary and secondary shock. These terms are regrettable and unnecessary. The only true shock is so-called secondary shock, which comes on after a delay of a variable number of hours, and which appears to be hormonal in origin. So-called *primary shock* is neurogenic or sometimes even psychic in origin, nervous stimuli leading to widespread capillary paralysis, with vasodilatation of the splanchnic vessels and pooling of blood, resulting in cerebral ischemia and unconsciousness. It is a *transient neurovascular collapse*, really a severe form of fainting or syncope, which may result from the sight of blood, from pain, even from the fear of imminent pain as in the case of a person awaiting his turn for a hypodermic inoculation. *Secondary shock* is in essence the result of a disparity between the volume of blood and the volume-capacity of the vascular system. The disparity may be due to a decrease in the blood volume, an increase in the volume-capacity of the vascular system, or a combination of these.

Etiology.—(1) *Reduction in Blood Volume.*—This may be due to blood loss, which may be traced to (*a*) blood lost *from* the injured part or (*b*) fluid lost *into* the injured part. The obvious example of the former is severe external or internal hemorrhage. The patient suffering from acute massive hemorrhage presents a picture of shock in its purest form. It is not merely the fluid loss which matters, but loss of the red blood cells (Moore). These are simply enormous in size by comparison with the albumin molecules, and for this reason they are an important space-occupying factor. Whole blood transfusion is therefore better than plasma and plasma substitutes, and not merely on account of the oxygen-carrying power of the red cells. As Moore puts it: "For once it is true that the bigger the better, and the erythrocyte is the biggest and best." The best examples of fluid loss into an injured part are offered by burns and by crushing injury to a limb. These are prime examples of the transfer of fluid from the vascular to the interstitial compartment. In both, unbelievable amounts of plasma may collect in the tissues (traumatic edema) and reduce the blood volume. Marked general fluid loss will result from persistent vomiting, as in upper gastrointestinal tract obstruction, and from severe diarrhea, especially in children. Acute deficiency in fluid or electrolytes may cause decrease in the blood volume. This

may occur in severe dehydration and in acute sodium deficiency, the classical example of the latter being pyloric stenosis.

(2) *Increase in the Vascular Bed.*—When the tone of the peripheral vascular system is lost and the walls of the vessels relax, the over-all capacity of that system is vastly increased. This may be brought about by a number of factors. (*a*) *Neurogenic stimuli.* Vascular tone is lost as a result of painful stimuli and a state of anxiety. As these are natural accompaniments of wounds, they are certain to increase the disparity between space and contents. (*b*) The release of *toxic metabolic products* and bacterial toxins may result in vasodilatation. (*c*) *Anoxia*, which is always present in shock, may act in the same way.

(3) *Acute Circulatory Failure.*—Sudden failure of the pump which keeps the circulation going will have a similar effect to reduction in blood volume and increase in the vascular bed. Such conditions as acute heart failure from myocardial infarction, paroxymal tachycardia and cardiac tamponade will quickly produce a state of shock.

Accessory factors undoubtedly play a part in the production of shock. Thus cold, exhaustion, depression, and general anesthesia predispose to its development. It has been said, with what truth it is difficult to determine, that shock is more common after a lost battle than after a victory.

PATHOGENESIS.—To enumerate a number of etiological agents which may precipitate a state of shock is one thing, but to elucidate their mechanism of action is another and more difficult one. Perhaps the greatest problem is to explain not merely the starting process but its continuation. The master word appears to be ischemia. Temporary ischemia of minor degree with its accompanying anoxia need cause no concern, but when it is severe and persistent it may lead to an anaerobic form of tissue metabolism that may result in the setting up of a vicious circle which perpetuates the process. The tissues vary greatly in their response to anoxia. The skin is resistant, the kidney is sensitive, but in shock the most serious effects are in the liver, the organ which is so susceptible to anoxia because two thirds of the oxygen normally used by that organ comes in the venous blood of the portal vein.

The observations of Zweifach and Chambers on the exteriorized mesoappendix and mesentery of the living animal show that the blood from the arterioles passes along what they term *preferential channels, i.e.*, specialized arterioles and capillaries the openings of which are guarded by a sphincteric mechanism. These constitute the main thoroughfare. Normally the vast majority of the capillaries of the part are empty, the blood flowing along the preferential channels past the tightly closed precapillary sphincters. According to Krogh the volume of blood in the active muscles of a guinea pig may be 275 times as great as when the muscles are at rest, and if the entire capillary bed were opened up there would be 750 times as much blood. The preferential channels are seen to display rhythmic contraction and relaxation of muscle, a vasomotion which is the essence of peripheral vascular tone and which disappears when that tone is lost. It is under humoral, not nervous, control. Epinephrine causes constriction of the precapillary sphincters. In the experimental animal the sphincters can be made more or less sensitive to epinephrine as the result of stress, and the changes in the vessels can be observed directly by this technique.

In the early stages of shock, the alarm reaction of Selye, vasoconstriction compensates for the loss of fluid, so that the relation of vessel volume to contents remains unchanged and the blood pressure is unaffected. The vasoconstriction involves first the less vital structures, thereby saving the more vital ones, then the kidney begins to suffer. Even when the kidney is reduced to a minimum of blood, the stage of kidney debacle, to use Van Slyke's vivid phrase, the liver still has a relatively good blood supply. When a point of maximum vasoconstriction is reached, vascular decompensation follows, the vast capillary bed of the body is opened up, and the blood disappears into it as if sucked up by a sponge. The patient may be said to bleed into his own capillaries. With this final step the blood pressure falls sharply, the rate of the heart rises, and the condition is completely irreversible.

The mechanism by which these successive steps are regulated is suggested by the experimental work of Shorr and his associates on specific *humoral vasotropic factors*. They have demonstrated the presence of a *vasoexcitor material* (V.E.M.) in the *kidney* and a *vasodepressor material* (V.D.M.) in the *liver* and *muscle* in the shocked animal. V.D.M. appears to be ferritin, the iron normally stored in the liver. Both are products of anaerobic metabolism resulting from ischemia. Their presence can be demonstrated in the circulating blood and their effect observed directly on the exteriorized mesoappendix of the rat. In the early period of stress the production of V.E.M. by the renal cortex rises and the power of the normal kidney to destroy this material is lost. When the anoxia involves the liver and induces anaerobic metabolism in that organ, the production of V.D.M. rises and the power of the healthy liver to destroy this material is lost. The effect of the V.D.M. now completely overshadows that of the V.E.M. Its vasodepressor action can be shown by its power to neutralize the vasoconstriction produced by epinephrine on the rat's mesoappendix. The depressant action of the V.D.M. on the preferential vascular channels finally opens the flood gates and the stage of irreversibility supervenes. In two cases of hemochromatosis studied by Taylor at the Vancouver General Hospital death was due to irreversible shock accompanied by acute abdominal pain. This may have been due to sudden release of the large amount of ferritin stored in the liver in hemochromatosis. During the hyperactive stage the abdominal viscera are pale and firm. In the hypoactive stage the bowel becomes congested and hemorrhage may occur. Later the liver is engorged and bleeds readily when cut. Finally hepatoportal resistance seems to develop, and the blood is diverted to the splanchnic viscera.

This would appear to be a story of the hemodynamic effect of agents of tissue origin resulting from anaerobiosis. While primary traumatic shock may be neurogenic, secondary shock seems to be humoral in origin. This concept has replaced the earlier view of Bayliss and Starling at the time of the first World War, that traumatic shock was due to the absorption of a toxic histamine-like substance liberated from the bruised muscles into the blood stream. The adrenal does not appear to play a leading role, at least in the later stages. It is true that a person with adrenal insufficiency, *e.g.*, Addison's disease, has poor resistance to stress, yet the administration of adrenal corticoid to a patient in shock is without proven benefit.

The part which *bacterial infections* may play in experimental shock is emphasized by Fine, who is of the opinion that some at least of the vasoparalysis may be due to the toxic products of intestinal bacteria which flourish under the anaerobic conditions of shock. There is certainly a diminished resistance to infection in shock, and it is of interest to note that in dogs bled to induce a state of shock there is a marked fall in the properdin level within two hours. In war injuries there is naturally frequent infection of wounds with anaerobic bacteria, the signs of which may be obscured by stress.

The experimental observations of Ochsner and his associates on Texan goats are of great interest in this respect. It has long been recognized that extensive soft-tissue injury, in particular large lacerations of the muscles of the thigh and buttocks with extensive crushing of the pelvis were almost certain to result in irreversible shock, no matter how energetic the surgical treatment. In the case of goats subjected to these injuries the injection of penicillin and other antibiotics increased the survival time more than did blood transfusion, although the best results were obtained by a combination of the two. The local application of ice to the wounds and early amputation both improved the recovery rate to a marked degree. These observations suggest that some toxic factor may be liberated in the injured tissues, and that bacterial infection confined to the damaged tissue may be an element of importance in the development of irreversible shock, particularly in the case of war wounds.

CLINICAL PICTURE.—The classic description of a person in profound shock is well known. He lies perfectly still and pays no attention to what is going on around him. The face is overspread by an ashen-grey pallor, large drops of sweat hang from the eyebrows, the eyes are weary, lusterless, and deeply sunken in their sockets, the cheeks hollow, the brows furrowed with anxiety, the skin cold and clammy. Four of the vital processes are notably depressed: (1) the *temperature* is sub-normal; (2) the *pulse* is extremely feeble, running and irregular; (3) the *respirations* are shallow and sighing; and, most important of all, (4) the *blood pressure* falls very low. Renal failure and traumatic anuria develop as the result of secondary changes in the kidney.

It is easy to recognize such a picture, just as it is easy to recognize the terminal stage of general peritonitis or carcinoma of the breast, when it is too late. This is the *decompensated* stage of shock, in which all attempts to preserve vasomotor tone have been frustrated. In the earlier or *compensated* stage the loss of blood volume is balanced by changes in the vessels. The compensated and decompensated stages may be compared with the two phases of Selye's alarm reaction, shock and countershock. Complete recovery is possible, either spontaneously or as the result of blood transfusion. When recovery occurs the shock is said to be *reversible*, when it fails to occur in spite of adequate blood transfusion the shock is *irreversible*. Shock may be regarded as a step towards the grave, but as long as the condition is reversible it is a step which can be retraced in the course of a few hours. It should be realized that the present concept of irreversibility may have to be changed at any time owing to new advances. Before the days of blood transfusion very many cases now regarded as reversible were then irreversible.

The signs and symptoms enumerated above are really those of an acute circulatory failure, which is the result of a decreased effective volume of circulating blood. This decreased volume is accompanied by decreased filling of the great veins, diminished return of blood to the right side of the heart, and, in consequence, decreased cardiac output and a fall in blood pressure. In compensated cases the fall in blood pressure stimulates the carotid and aortic arch reflexes with resulting vasoconstriction and cardiac acceleration which are adequate to maintain the circulation. In uncompensated cases the response is inadequate, the blood pressure continues to fall, and the resulting tissue anoxia leads to further capillary dilatation and transudation of plasma into the tissues, so that the volume of circulating blood is still further reduced. In this way a vicious circle is set up which it is difficult to break. In irreversible shock the tone of the smaller arterioles and and capillaries is completely lost, so that plasma passes freely into the intersitial tissues. This is the final step to the grave.

BIOCHEMICAL CHANGES.—Profound biochemical and physiological changes are observed during shock. Some of these, such as the reduction in blood volume and the dehydration, are inherent in the production of the condition. Others, such as the upset of electrolyte balance, acidosis and protein break-down are dependent on the lesions in the kidney and liver. The fluid of the body is contained in three compartments: (1) in the vessels, (2) in the interstitial tissues, (3) in the cells. In rapid dehydration due to massive hemorrhage, acute intestinal obstruction, etc., it is the plasma and the interstitial water that is lost. When dehydration is slow water is pulled out of all three compartments proportionately.

It will be realized that the collapse of shock with its accompanying hypothermia and hypotension may be regarded as protective devices calculated to slow down the metabolic fire. When carried to an extreme, however, they may become lethal. What Cannon has called "the wisdom of the body" may then become its folly.

LESIONS.—The lesions found at autopsy, as might be expected, are those of anoxia and increased capillary permeability. The *lungs* are dark and filled with blood and fluid. Microscopically the capillaries are widely dilated and the alveoli show marked edema. The *heart muscle* is the site of fatty degeneration in about 50 per cent of cases of severe shock. This may safely be attributed to the accompanying anoxia. In the *liver* fatty degeneration is again a leading feature, commencing in the central zone and extending to the capillaries. The sinusoids are of course dilated and engorged. The *adrenals* show marked cortical changes. If death occurs very early the cortex is widened and bright yellow in color due to an excess of lipids. This is soon followed by lipid depletion, with shrinking and pallor of the cortex. Microscopically the cortical cells lose their normal foamy appearance owing to loss of cholesterol, and small foci of focal necrosis may leave defects in the cortex.

The *kidney changes* are the most important. They present a picture of severe tubular degeneration which has been called the *"shock kidney."* This is the condition to which Lucké gave the name of *lower nephron nephrosis*, because the distal convoluted tubules, being farthest removed from the blood supply, are likely to be first involved. In the ordinary case seen at autopsy in the hospital both sets of convoluted tubules are likely to be equally involved, so that the name is liable to give a wrong impression. It would be better called *ischemic nephrosis*. Pigment is likely to be present in the tubules. This may be large in amount in shock due to transfusion with incompatible blood, massive hemorrhage in the interstitial tissues, and severe muscle trauma. Such cases may justify the term hemoglobinuric nephrosis applied to cases of war injury. In the Korean war renal failure appeared to be responsible for death in 15 per cent of injuries, while oliguria and other evidence of renal failure developed in over 30 per cent. We shall have to return to the question of nephrosis in our consideration of diseases of the kidney.

BURNS

Burns are coming to assume an ever-increasing importance for the student who is going to become a doctor by reason of the industrial age in which we live with its great furnaces, domestic heating with highly inflammable agents, automobile and airplane accidents, and, last but not least, atomic and hydrogen bombs. Over 80 per cent of the casualties at Nagasaki and Hiroshima suffered from burns. Burns constitute the most complex form of tissue injury. They present two very different features: (1) the *local lesions*, and (2) the *physiological disturbances*, which are essentially those of shock and may result in a fatal outcome. Two factors have to be considered in the local lesions: (1) tissue damage and (2) infection.

LOCAL LESIONS.—The effects of a burn

depend on two factors: (1) its severity, and
(2) its extent. An extensive burn of moderate severity may produce greater physiological disturbance than a more severe but
localized burn. Burns are classified in three
grades or degrees according to the depth of
the necrosis. In burns of the *first degree*
there is merely *hyperemia* and *slight edema*
of the epidermis. There may be necrosis of
the superficial layers of epithelium, but these
are desquamated in a few days and replaced
from the basal layers, so that there is no
scarring. In burns of the *second degree* the
entire thickness of the epidermis is destroyed,
and blebs or vesicles are formed between the
separating epidermis and the dermis. *Vesic-
ulation is the hallmark of the second degree
burn.* There is some degree of destruction
of the dermis. This may be (*a*) mild, (*b*)
severe. (*a*) In the mild cases enough epithelium is left in the hair follicles and dermal
glands to provide new cells for resurfacing
the burnt area. (*b*) In the severe cases not
enough epithelium remains, and grafting of
the burnt area is necessary. In burns of the
third degree there is *complete destruction of
the dermis*, including the sensory nerves.
Grafting must be done to cover the area.

Vascular changes of great importance occur
in the wounded area. There is an increased
flow of blood to the part owing to dilatation
of the small vessels, which in turn may be
due to direct injury to the vessel walls and
to the local liberation of histamine. This
increased flow is not followed by stasis as in
the usual forms of inflammation. *Capillary
permeability* is greatly increased, and through
the injured walls plasma rich in protein pours
in large amount and continually (Fig. 82).
It is the extent of the burned area rather
than its depth which determines the amount
of loss of this vital fluid. The exudate from
partial thickness burns begins to dry in
twelve to twenty-four hours, and in forty-
eight to seventy-two hours it forms a dry
brown crust which protects the wound. In
superficial burns this crust separates in one
or two weeks, but in deeper burns it will take
longer.

Infection is likely to occur, although at the
moment of burning the skin is sterilized. In
first degree burns the intact epidermis will
exclude infection. When the injury is deeper

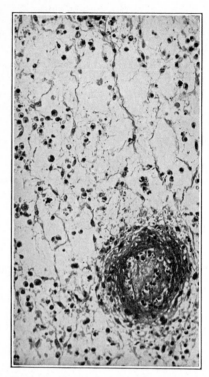

Fig. 82.—Severe burn of skin. Showing
great edema and thrombosed vessel. × 175.

the crust which forms will protect the raw
surface for a time. If this is broken, virulent
streptococci may enter and flourish in the
partially anaerobic necrotic tissue. The anemia, plasma loss and general malnutrition
in extensive burns severely handicap the
defense against infection.

PATHOLOGICAL PHYSIOLOGY.—The vascular damage leads to changes in the circulating
blood similar to those we have already studied in shock. This is indeed *burn shock*. The
local outpouring of fluid in the burned area
results in a remarkable concentration of the
blood as shown by hemoglobin estimation,
and this leads in turn to circulatory failure
and oxygen starvation of the tissues. The
hemoconcentration sends up the red cell
count, sometimes as high as 8,000,000. It
is evident that the severity of the general
reaction will depend on the extent rather
than on the local intensity of the damage.
The intense heat leads to destruction of red
blood cells and hemolysis, which in severe
cases may be massive and accompanied by

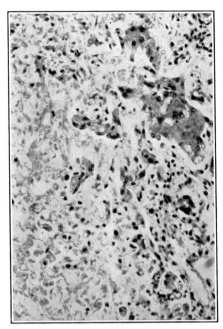

FIG. 83.—Necrosis of the liver in a case of burns treated with tannic acid. × 120.

at least to the writer. A feature of great interest is the fact that the most extreme necrosis was seen in the days when treatment with tannic acid was universal. (Fig. 83). Wells and his associates produced identical and fatal liver lesions in animals by the sub-cutaneous injection of tannic acid, and Erb, Morgan and Farmer of the Hospital for Sick Children, Toronto, found liver necrosis in the majority of fatal cases of burns which had been tanned, but in none of an untanned group. What more striking example of an iatrogenic injury (*iatros*, physician) could be found? Other lesions are those which we associate with shock. A large amount of blood pigment may be deposited in the collecting tubules of the *kidney* as the result of hemolysis. The *adrenals* are at first somewhat enlarged, deeply congested, and reddish-brown in color, indicating their response to stress. In severe burns there may be petechial hemorrhages and small areas of focal necrosis. I have seen bilateral necrosis of the adrenal cortex due to thrombosis. In cases where death ensues some days after the accident, the adrenals may be shrunken with extensive cytolysis, necrosis and hemorrhage. Ulcers of the *duodenum* and upper *jejunum*, the so-called *Curling's ulcer*, used to be more common before the days of modern therapy.

hemoglobinuria. These varied factors result in ischemia of important organs, in particular the liver and kidney, so that acidosis and uremia develop which may in themselves prove fatal. Much has been written about the so-called toxic symptoms of burns, such as fever, delirium, vomiting, bloody diarrhea and circulatory failure. It is possible that toxic material is absorbed from the burnt area into the general circulation, but it seems probable that bacterial infection which develops in the anerobic conditions of the dead tissue plays a more important part. Reference has already been made to this question in the general discussion of shock. It is obvious that every effort must be made to prevent infection from occurring. This problem was *apparently* solved with great satisfaction in the past by tanning the burnt area with tannic acid; the results of this treatment we shall see in the next paragraph.

POSTMORTEM CHANGES.—The *liver* may show areas of focal necrosis, and in the necrotic areas the cells may contain intranuclear inclusions and Councilman bodies similar to those seen in yellow fever. The significance of these inclusions is not clear—

REFERENCES

BERNARD, C.: *An Introduction to the Study of Experimental Medicine,* 1865. Translated by H. C. Greene, New York, 1927.

BEESON, P. B.: J. Clin. Investig., 1948, *27,* 524. (Leukocytic pyrogens).

BENNETT, I. L., JR.: Bull. Johns Hopkins Hosp., 1956, *98,* 216. (Leukocytic pyrogens).

CANNON, W. B.: *The Wisdom of the Body,* New York, 1932.

DAHL, L. K.: New Eng. J. Med., 1958, *258,* 1152. (Salt intake and salt need).

ERB, I. H., MORGAN, E. M. and FARMER, A. W.: Ann. Surg., 1943, *117,* 234. (Tannic acid lesions in burns).

FINE, J.: New Eng. J. Med., 1954, *250,* 889. Am. J. Gastroenterol., 1958, *29,* 596. (Relation of bacterial infection to shock.)

GAMBLE, J. L.: *Chemical Anatomy, Physiology and Pathology of Extracellular Fluid.* Cambridge, Mass., 1947. (The bible of the subject).

KING, M. K. and WOOD, W. B., JR.: J. Exper. Med., 1958, *107,* 279. (Leukocytic pyrogens).

MOON, V. H.: *Shock and Related Capillary Phenomena,* New York, 1938.

MOORE, F. E.: Ann. Surg., 1952, *135*, 143. (Shock).

OCHSNER, E. W. A., JACOB, S. W. and MANSBERGER, A. R.: Surgery, 1958, *43*, 703. (Experimental shock).

SHORR, E., ZWEIFACH, B. W., FURCHGOTT, R. F. and BAEZ, S.: Circulation, 1951, *3*, 42. (Pathogenesis of shock).

TAYLOR, H. E.: Am. J. Clin. Path., 1951, *21*, 530. (Shock in hemochromatosis).

WELLS, D. B., HUMPHREY, H. D. and COLL, J. J.: New Eng. J. Med., 1942, *226*, 629. (Liver lesions due to tannic acid).

WOOD, W. B., JR.: New Eng J. Med., 1958, *258*, 1023. (Cause of fever).

ZWEIFACH, B. W. and CHAMBERS, R.: Am. J. Anat., 1944, *75*, 173. (Pathogenesis of shock).

Chapter 8

Neoplasia: General Pathology

Introduction
The Nature of Neoplasia
The Neoplastic Cell
  LIGHT MICROSCOPE
    Mitosis
  ELECTRON MICROSCOPE
  METABOLISM OF THE CANCER
    CELL
Carcinogenesis
  CHEMICAL CARCINOGENS
  IONIZING RADIATION
  VIRUSES
  HORMONES
  ENVIRONMENT AND OCCUPATION
    Geography of Tumors

CO-CARCINOGENS
  Diet
  Age
  Heredity
  Chronic Irritation
  Trauma
Tumor Immunity
  HETEROLOGOUS TRANSPLANTA-
    TION
  SPONTANEOUS REGRESSION
Characteristics of Malignancy
  GRADING OF TUMORS
Precancerous Conditions
  CARCINOMA IN SITU
Spread of Tumors

DISTRIBUTION OF METASTASES
Laboratory Diagnosis
  HISTOLOGICAL EXAMINATION
  EXFOLIATIVE CYTOLOGY
  CANCER CELLS IN THE BLOOD
Cancer Therapy
Radiation of Tumors
  EFFECT ON THE CELLS
  EFFECT ON THE INTERCELLULAR
    TISSUES
  RADIOSENSITIVITY
  RADIATION SEQUELAE
The Relative Frequency of Tumors
Prognosis in Cancer
Is Cancer Increasing?

INTRODUCTION

OF all the processes which the student of pathology is privileged to study none is so intriguing, so fascinating, and so perplexing as that of neoplasia. The very name of the process gives a hint of the difficulties which lie ahead. Neoplasia means new growth. The regeneration of epithelium and the formation of granulation tissue are also examples of new growth, but these serve a useful purpose. When that purpose is served the new growth ceases, and the process obeys the normal laws of growth or rather the laws of normal growth. The term neoplasia is restricted in pathology to tumor growth, a process which serves no useful purpose, which continues unchecked, and which is not controlled by the laws of normal growth, although undoubtedly controlled in ways which remain to be discovered.

We shall have to study two varieties of tumors known as *benign* or innocent and *malignant*. The differentiation between these two types is all-important from the clinical standpoint of diagnosis, treatment and prognosis, but we shall defer a discussion of these differences until later in this chapter. Both are manifestations of neoplasia, but in actual practice the term neoplasm has come to be synonymous with the malignant type, commonly called cancer, and it is to the cancer

process that we shall now turn our attention. Many varieties of benign or malignant tumors arise from the different tissues of the body, but a consideration of these specific types will be reserved for the next chapter.

A lot of nonsense is talked about "the dark mystery of cancer," "the impenetrable veil" which clothes that mystery, and so on. In this respect it may be salutary to compare our knowledge of neoplasia with that of inflammation. Both are processes, not things. In both instances we are familiar with many etiological agents and classes of agents which may initiate the process. In the case of inflammation we have already seen that these agents are known as irritants, which may be bacteria, viruses, protozoa, animal parasites, heat, radiation, etc. An irritant by definition is something which causes inflammation, and we do not think of looking for one single cause. Neoplasia, as we shall see, may also be caused by a variety of agents known as *carcinogens*, which may be chemicals of various kinds, viruses, hormones, and ionizing radiation. Over the course of 100 years we have discovered the cause of most forms of inflammation, but some remain unknown. In the case of human cancer we know the cause in a few instances, but in most cases this still remains to be determined. We do not know how irritants cause inflammation, but we are beginning to make a good guess as to the mechanism by means of which carcinogens initiate and perpetuate the process of neoplasia. Inflammation may kill the patient, but recovery is the rule, whereas cancer if untreated will kill the patient, but in rare cases there may be spontaneous regression and recovery.

A final point may be made before leaving this comparison between inflammation and neoplasia. Inflammation may be initiated by a bacterial infection which hits a target organ, and when the bacteria are killed or die out the inflammation subsides, unless the infection persists as in tuberculosis or syphilis. Occasionally, however, a promoting factor seems to operate to continue the process as in glomerulonephritis, disseminated lupus, and other diseases which we shall study in the second part of this book. We have already seen that this continuing factor may be auto-immunity. In neoplasia an exciting agent such as a chemical carcinogen or radiation may initiate the process in the target organ and then be withdrawn, yet the neoplasia continues. Here the target organ itself, *i.e.*, the cell, has become the continuing agent, as we shall see shortly. In other cases the constant action of some continuing agent such as a hormone may be required, at least for a time.

The object of this comparison between the processes of neoplasia and inflammation is to suggest that perhaps neoplasia is not so much more mysterious and insoluble a problem than inflammation, as is generally believed, although its consequences are far more grave. We should also bear in mind the significant title of a paper by C. P. Rhoads: "The soluble puzzle of cancer control."

THE NATURE OF NEOPLASIA

The tumor cell is a modified normal cell. This modification comprises loss of the more specialized functions involved in differentiation plus acquisition of increased growth function, with resulting invasion and the formation of metastases. The more rapid the growth, the more primitive is the cell in structure and specialized function. The two great characteristics of cancer are *anaplasia* (a turning backward in form) and *autonomy*. The autonomy is only relative, for growth of

the neoplasm may be under hormonal and other influences. In the experimental animal growth of the tumor may actually exceed that of the host, which, as in the case of the human subject, actually loses weight. It is evident that the tumor diverts a disproportionate amount of the available food stuffs.

It would appear that the metabolic superiority of the tumor cell is largely due to its *enhanced amino-acid concentrating power* (Wiseman and Ghadially). The normal and neoplastic cells share a common volume of extracellular fluid and compete with each other for the available metabolites. The atrophy and necrosis of normal cells which is such a feature at the edge of a rapidly growing tumor is commonly attributed to pressure, but if this were correct would not the tumor cells also undergo necrosis? It seems more reasonable to suppose that the downfall of the normal cells is due to local competition for the available amino-acids in the extracellular fluid. One of the tissues to suffer early in this metabolic competition is the small intestine, with its enormous turnover rate, which in the rat may represent a replacement of the entire mucosa in one and a half days (Leblond and Stevens). This may account in part for the anorexia and cachexia so characteristic of the later stages of cancer, the damaged intestine being no longer able to replenish the metabolic pool with amino-acids from the diet. The matter of cachexia is discussed again on page 101.

We are now faced with the question as to the explanation of this profound difference between the neoplastic and the normal cell. It is becoming more and more evident that the basic biochemical lesion in a malignant cell concerns *desoxyribonucleic acid* (DNA), the substance which imparts basophilia to the chromosomal network of the nucleus and which is responsible for the Feulgen reaction. Cancer cells contain more nucleic acid, as shown by their greater basophilia, and it is of interest to note that nitrogen mustard, the first cancer chemotherapeutic agent to be used, destroys nucleic acid in cancer cells in dilutions so great as to have no effect on normal cells, while ionizing radiation depolymerizes nucleic acid, leading to death of the cell. DNA is a giant molecule present in the 46 human chromosomes, which are strings of genes in incalculable numbers per chromosome. This giant molecule has a helical or spiral-staircase structure. X-ray diffraction photographs reveal the structure to be actually a double helix, with two spirally rising chains of linked atomic groups and a series of horizontal members, like steps, connecting the two spirals. The two spirals are made of five-carbon sugar molecules (desoxyribose), alternating with phosphate groups. The steps connecting the two spirals are made of four bases, adenine and thymine, guanine and cytosine, linked in pairs.

DNA is not only the governing force controlling the life of the cell, but it also controls the genetics of the organism by virtue of the genes which are in essence composed of DNA. As the double-helix DNA molecules are thousands of turns long and are arranged by thousands in each chromosome, it is evident that a structure of such complexity may well become damaged, and it is believed that carcinogens such as certain polycyclic hydrocarbons, ionizing radiation, and viruses may bring about such a derangement. Many viruses are aggregates of DNA molecules wrapped in a coat of protein. When the virus infects a living cell, it leaves its coat outside and the DNA takes charge. We know that loose DNA can penetrate certain bacteria, changing them permanently into a new strain, and the same seems to be true of cells. C^{14} labelled adenine when given to patients with lymphatic leukemia has been recovered from the DNA of the leukemic cells as long as a year later, showing that it must have been transmitted in the large molecules during duplication.

It is known that the phosphoric acid groups arranged along the double helix of the DNA molecule carry negative electrical charges, and it now appears that this pattern of negative charges is closely associated with the overall activity of the nucleus, and in particular with protein synthesis. Indeed, if the DNA is replaced by other forms of nucleic acid or even simple synthetic substances, as long as their molecular structure is characterized by long-chain length and many repeating negative electrical charges, the function of the nuclei can be restored. Substances carrying positive electrical charges inhibit synthetic processes in the nucleus. The nucleus normally contains positively charged histones, which presumably serve to control nuclear activity. Indeed it has been found that the addition of histones to the isolated nucleus inhibits protein synthesis. This suggests the possibility of the use of positively charged material such as histones or even a synthetic substance in the control of malignant neoplasia.

One view of carcinogenesis is the *somatic cell mutation hypothesis*, a term which implies that cancer is a naturally occurring *spontaneous* mutation, involving a gene in one of the chromosomes of a somatic cell. While this possibility cannot be denied in some instances, it does not explain the fact that while mutation is an instantaneous reaction, carcinogenesis is one of the slowest biological processes known. It seems much more reasonable to suppose that some carcinogenic agent, either external in origin or produced within the body, has acted upon the cell, or rather on the nuclear DNA, to bring about this insidious change.

THE NEOPLASTIC CELL

As cancer is a disorder of cell growth, it is natural that we should turn to the neoplastic cell and compare it with the normal cell in our search for information on the nature of the process. The true comparison, however, should not be between the cancer cell and the normal adult cell but between the cancer cell and the embryonic cell, in both of which rapid growth is characteristic, in the former permanent, in the latter reversible. This must be due to a difference in enzymes. The living cell looks quiescent enough under the microscope, but we know that it is boiling with chemical action under enzymatic control.

Of the two main functions of the cell, work and reproduction, the former depends on the activity of the cytoplasm, the latter on that of the nucleus. Cancer cells are changed in character, so that they spend most of their energies on growth and little on function. As neoplasia is a disorder of cell reproduction, we should naturally look first at the nucleus. The cell may be examined histologically by the light microscope with staining of the sections or by the electron microscope using

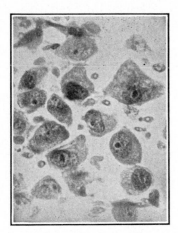

FIG. 84.—Smear of cancer of breast showing irregular cells and large nucleus and nucleolus. × 500.

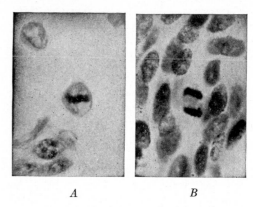

A   *B*

FIG. 85.—Mitotic figures. *A*, shows the monaster stage (metaphase) and *B*, the diaster stage (anaphase). × 700.

ultra-thin sections. The former gives us more information about the nucleus, the latter about the cytoplasm. It will be convenient to consider these two pictures separately.

Light Microscope.—The *nucleus* of the cancer cell is likely to be large in relation to the cytoplasm, although sometimes this relative difference is due to shrinkage of the cytoplasm rather than to increase in the size of the nucleus. The nucleus is hyperchromatic owing to an increased content of nucleoprotein, staining intensely with hematoxylin and basic aniline dyes, with coarsening of the chromatin network. The nucleolus is large in proportion to the size of the nucleus, an important feature which may be more evident in frozen sections of the unfixed tissue or in wet films (Fig. 84).

Mitosis.—This is so fundamental a process in cell growth that it may be well for us to refresh our memory regarding the rather confusing and meaningless names of the various steps in the process. After the resting stage or *interphase* comes the *prophase*, in which the dispersed chromatin granules of the nucleus become organized into a darkly staining spireme thread (*mitos*, thread), which undergoes segmental division into chromosomes and longitudinal splitting into two longitudinal halves or chromatids. At the same time the two centrioles of the centrosome in the cytoplasm separate and migrate to opposite poles of the cell, where they give off rays to form the achromatic spindle.

In the *metaphase* (*meta*, after) the chromatids of each pair separate and line up in two parallel bands across the center of the cell and become attached to the threads of the spindle. This is called the *monaster*, because it suggests a star when viewed endways. In the anaphase (*ana*, up) the two sets of new chromosomes separate and move to the opposite poles forming a *diaster*. In the end stage or *telophase*, (*telos*, end) the cytoplasm becomes constricted in the middle of the cell until division is complete, whilst the chromosomes take on their original granular appearance, which probably represents the intact genes.

The presence of numerous mitotic figures is suggestive of neoplasia, although it must be borne in mind that they are also seen in granulation tissue and in other rapidly regenerating cells (see Fig. 35, p. 69), so that they are no *proof* of malignancy. The more rapid the growth, the more numerous the mitoses. The nucleus may be represented by a dark mass of chromatin, or the chromatin may be collected as a bar across the center of the cell in the metaphase or monaster stage, the usual appearance (Fig. 85), or in two separate masses, one at each pole, in the anaphase or diaster stage (Fig. 85B). In highly malignant tumors multicentric division and other forms of atypical mitosis may sometimes be seen (Fig. 86). Colchicine has a remarkable power of arresting the mitotic process and preventing its comple-

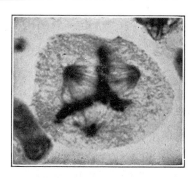

Fig. 86.—Atypical mitosis. The chromosomes have divided into three groups in the center. Three centrosomes and attraction spheres are also seen. × 1500.

tion, apparently by interfering with the formation of the spindle from the centrosomes. This fact is of interest in two respects. (1) The arrest of the process midway makes available large numbers of chromosomes for study. The addition of a hypotonic solution to a collection of dividing cells leads to swelling and rupture of the cells with spreading of the chromosomes, a process which can be intensified by placing a coverglass over the cells and squashing them with the thumb, followed by staining with orcein in acetic acid. The chromosomes in a neoplastic cell vary in number, but in no malignant tumor examined has their number been normal (Fig. 87). (2) As it is during mitotic division that the cell is most readily damaged by radiation, it is possible that the use of colchicine may find a place in the radiotherapy of cancer.

In *summary* we may say that the chief characteristics of the neoplastic cell as revealed by the light microscope are nuclear and chromosomal aberrations, decreased cytoplasmic-nuclear ratio, a coarse irregular chromatin network, and larger nucleoli than normal. "The structural pattern of a malignant tumor cell is sufficiently distinct from the normal cell to be identified in most instances even when viewed as an individual cell" (Sproul). Indeed this is the basis of the method of exfoliative cytology, which, as its name suggests, consists of the examination of separate exfoliated cells to determine the presence of cancer, as is described on page 215.

Globulin-Fluorescein Staining, a combination of chemical and histological technique,

may give the pathologist a powerful weapon in his task of deciding on difficult cases of neoplasia (King, Hughes and Louis). The results of the technique confirm the idea that the malignant cell differs from the normal in the loss of some cellular protein constituent. At first King and his associates used rabbit gamma globulin prepared by injecting homogenates of rat tissue. This globulin reacted with normal rat tissue but not with the cells of a malignant tumor of the same organ. The reaction was demonstrated visually by the use of a globulin-fluorescein complex which fluoresced in ultraviolet light. That this was not an antigen-antibody reaction was shown by the fact that the same result was obtained when the globulin originated from an animal which had not been injected. Nor is the reaction species-specific, for an equally marked effect is obtained with globulin from a dozen different animals, including man. As might be expected, the epithelium of a benign tumor such as a fibroadenoma of the breast behaves like normal tissue. Hitherto the pathologist has had to depend mainly on changes in general architecture for his diagnosis of malignancy, but now we appear to have evidence of the loss of a basic protein by which even an individual cancer cell can be distinguished from its normal neighbours (Figs. 88 and 89).

Electron Microscope.—It is in the field of the cytoplasm rather than of the nucleus that the electron microscope has made a real contribution. In general terms it may be said that the entire organized structure of the cytoplasm is highly deficient. The cytoplasmic constituents are of three main types: (1) large particles or mitochondria, (2) small particles or microsomes, ergastoplasm, (3) soluble constituents.

Mitochondria (*mitos*, a thread) are organized structures of the size and shape of bacteria. They present a complex internal structure being covered by a double-layered membrane, infoldings of the inner layer known as "cristæ" extending inward for a varying but often almost complete distance. In experimentally produced tumors the mitochondria are much reduced in number, it may be to one-quarter the normal cell complement, they vary considerably in size, the cristæ are irregular, and degenerating mito-

12

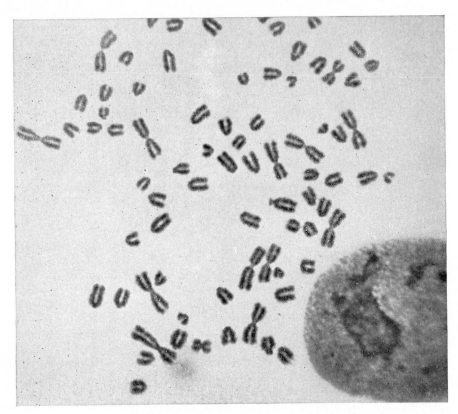

FIG. 87.—Chemically induced mouse sarcoma in tissue culture, showing 85 chromosomes instead of the normal 40. × 2000. (Kindness of Dr. A. A. Axelrad.)

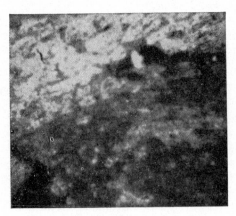

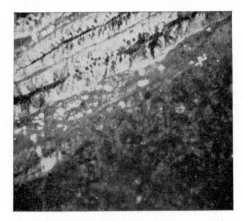

FIG. 88.—Photomicrograph (with ultraviolet light) of a frozen section of margin of a chemically induced *rat* hepatoma showing fluorescence of cytoplasm of normal cells and absence of fluorescence of cytoplasm of neoplastic cells. Stain—fluorescein-fowl globulin complex. (King, Hughes and Louis, courtesy of British J. Cancer.)

FIG. 89.—Photomicrograph of a frozen section of the margin of spheroidal cell carcinoma of the stomach (*man*) showing fluorescence of the cytoplasm of normal cells and absence of fluorescence of the neoplastic cells. Stain—fluorescein-dog globulin complex. (King, Hughes and Louis, courtesy of British J. Cancer.)

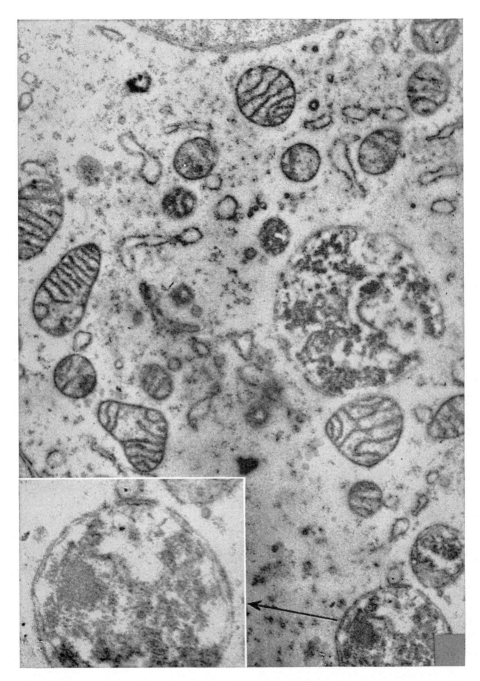

Fig. 90.—Electron micrography of hepatoma. × 24,000. Mitochondria show prominent cristae and some are degenerated (right middle). Insert represents a magnification of 39,800, and shows a degenerating mitochondrion with double limiting membrane still preserved. (Howatson and Ham, courtesy of Cancer Research).

chondria may be prominent (Howatson and Ham). (Fig. 90). The membranes are studded with large granules which contain respiratory enzyme systems, predominantly those of the Krebs citric acid cycle, but also those of the oxidative phosphorylative synthesis of adenosine triphosphate with its store of high-energy phosphate bonds for various anabolic activities of cell. These constituents of the cytoplasm necessary for the active functioning of the cell are largely depressed or lost in neoplasia.

Ergastoplasm is also known as endoplasmic reticulum, but perhaps the best name is *membranous vesicles* or sacs. These sacs are covered with minute granules, which are also found between the sacs. The granules consist of RNA, which is responsible for the basophilia of the ergastoplasm. In normal cells the membranous vesicles are numerous and flattened, being particularly numerous in cells developed to synthesize specialized protein secretions, *e.g.*, cells of the pancreas and salivary glands, osteoblasts, and plasma cells. The mechanism is evidently designed for function rather than for growth. In malignant cells, as might be expected, the membranous vesicles are reduced in number and are distended, indicating loss of function.

Virus-like particles may be seen in tumor cells, particularly in the Rous chicken sarcoma and in the mouse mammary cancer of a milk-factor strain, subjects which will be discussed in connection with carcinogenesis. These particles are few in number and are not seen in non-filterable tumors.

To correlate the morphological changes outlined above with corresponding physiological disturbances is not possible in any great degree at this early stage of our knowledge. It may be said, however, that the site of greatest activity in the neoplastic cell seems to have shifted from the mitochondria and ergastoplasm to the small granules and soluble fraction. The oxidative enzymes are less abundant and the steps of the Krebs cycle are less active. As a result the normal restoration of adenosine triphosphate is impaired, and therefore the production of energy and synthetic materials, while growth and cellular reproduction are less restrained.

Metabolism of the Cancer Cell.—We have seen that the nuclear and cytoplasmic components of the cancer cell differ materially from those of the normal cell. It might therefore be supposed that the new colony of cells which constitute a neoplasm would differ materially in function from the normal. Were this so we might have in our hands an instrument which would enable us to differentiate in the patient the neoplastic from the normal. Unfortunately at the present time this hope has not been realized. The essential feature of the change is that in the neoplasm, *the capacity for growth has supplanted that for function.* In the cancer cell there is a tendency to converge towards a common enzymatic pattern of activity, whereas the cells of normal organs and tissues possess specific chemical characteristics (Greenstein). Certain chemical functions are lost in the transformation of normal to neoplastic, and this restriction in capacity for function corresponds with the structural change of cellular anaplasia and loss of differentiation. We may consider this change under the headings of (1) energy, (2) function, and (3) competitive struggle.

1. *Sources of Energy.*—In the struggle which is being waged to control cancer there are several possible lines of chemical attack, such as inactivation of the carcinogenic agent, interference with the mitotic process, and inhibition of the metabolism of the cancer cell. The analogy of the successful control of bacterial infection by antibiotics would seem to point to the possibility of altering metabolism in the case of neoplasia. For this reason it becomes very important to know if the cancer cell with its changed behavior has developed an altered metabolism which would allow a chemical agent to differentiate between the neoplastic and the normal, wrecking the one and leaving the other unimpaired.

It was thirty years ago that Warburg demonstrated the first great generalization concerning tumor growth. The carbohydrate metabolism of a normal cell consists of two processes, glycolysis (splitting of the sugar molecule) and respiration (utilization of oxygen for further breakdown into CO_2 and water). Glycolysis may be anaerobic or aerobic, in the latter case much lactic acid being produced. Warburg, using slices of tissue, showed that the cancer cell derives its energy from anaerobic and to a lesser extent from aerobic glycolysis rather than from respiration; that is to say the metabolism of the cancer cell is mainly glycolytic and anaerobic in type, whereas the metabolism of the normal cell depends mainly on oxidation. He stated that neoplasia results from a shift from oxidation to glycolytic sources of energy, as a result of an irreversible injury to the oxidative cellular mechanism of normal cells. Normal cells "breathe" while cancer cells do not breathe but ferment. If tumor growth depends largely on energy derived from anaerobic glucose breakdown, its control might be effected by inhibition of the process of glycolysis or of the enzymes involved.

Unfortunately Warburg's generalization, while true for some tumors, proved to be an oversimplification. It is now known that a high rate of aerobic and anaerobic glycolysis is not confined to tumor tissue, so that it cannot be regarded as a distinctive characteristic of cancer, being shared by many normal tissues, more particularly the retina. Moreover, anaerobic glycolysis is absent in some tumors. It would appear that a neoplastic cell has a full complement of oxidative enzymes, but a reduced capacity for oxidation, much lower than that of the liver, kidney, heart or brain. No new pathways of metabolism in tumors are discernable, and no new enzymes or coenzymes are present. In *summary* it may be said that the interrelation between the enzyme systems present differs from that of many normal tissues with a dominance of anaerobic energy-yielding mechanisms over the aerobic, and that the general enzyme pattern tends to be more uniform than in normal tissue, so that we may speak of a common cancer enzymatic pattern. This might be regarded as the physiological counterpart of the anaplasia or lack of differentiation which is so characteristic a morphological feature of the neoplastic process.

2. *The Enzyme-Substrate Systems.*—A normal cell is more concerned with function, involving energy-releasing catabolism than with growth, involving anabolic energy. Tumor cells are concerned primarily with growth, not with function. The specific functional enzyme-substrate systems therefore become superfluous in comparison with those required for the anabolic processes of growth and cell division. Normal cells possess diversified metabolic activities, whereas in tumor cells there is much greater biochemical uniformity, as we have just seen.

3. *Competitive Struggle.*—A cancer, given sufficient time, will kill its host. It may do this by distorting important anatomical relationships, as when it closes the lower end of the esophagus or the urethra. But scar tissue may do the same. It may lead to death by causing ulceration of a mucous surface with resulting fatal hemorrhage or sepsis. But so may an inflammatory process. There remains the possibility of a much more subtle process, that represented by what may be termed the competitive struggle or *nitrogen trap* (Mider). Any growing tissue requires a source of material from which it may build its protoplasm and a supply of energy for that purpose. A large neoplasm acquires nitrogenous building blocks from the body stores to satisfy the continual demand for protein synthesis, but the supply of these blocks is not unlimited. Cancer cells appear to exercise priority over the demands of normal tissues for amino acids, thus constituting a nitrogen trap. That this is true can be shown by feeding isotopically marked amino acids to animals with rapidly growing transplanted tumor. When a normal diet was substituted and still more when food was withheld the radioactivity of the tumor protein continued to rise, whilst that of the liver and kidney steadily decreased (Greenless and LePage). It is this trap which accounts for the wasting and cachexia that are often so characteristic a feature of the later stages of malignancy.

One of the most perplexing puzzles presented by neoplasia is the occasional occurrence of *carcinomatous neuromyopathies*, that is to say the development of neuromuscular symptoms in cases of visceral carcinoma without metastatic involvement of the nervous or muscular systems (Brain). This is far more frequent in carcinoma of the lung than in cancer of other organs. In one case there was evidence of severe sensory neuropathy and myopathy for three and a half years before clinical recognition of the tumor in the lung (Dyck *et al.*). In this case there

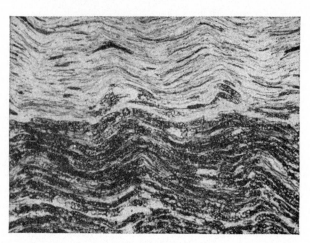

Fig. 91.—Severe demyelination of posterior spinal root fibers (upper) with relative sparing of anterior root fibers (lower) in a case of a small bronchogenic carcinoma. × 120. (Dyck, Bailey and Olszewski, courtesy of Canad. Med. Assn. Jour.)

was marked degeneration of the posterior roots of the spinal nerves (Fig. 91). Denny-Brown has reported degeneration of the posterior root ganglia in this type of case. No satisfactory explanation of this strange association is at present available. It has been suggested that a virus may be responsible, or that a disorder of metabolism may be involved. There is, however, no correlation between the size of the tumor and the severity of the neurological disorder.

CARCINOGENESIS

Cancer is in essence a change in cell metabolism. We have already seen that the regulator of the complex machinery of intracellular enzymal activity, the governor of the engine, is nucleic acid with its conjugated proteins.

The infinitely intricate and delicately balanced regulating mechanism of chromosomal genes and enzymes which controls metabolism and cellular reproduction can be upset in various ways. The interference may lead to permanent changes or mutations in the genes. If these mutations are sufficiently serious they may be lethal and the cell will die. If the change is such as to permanently speed up the mitotic rate the result will be cancer.

There is no reason to suppose that there is a single over-riding cause of cancer any more than there is to presume that inflammation has a single cause. There are manifold physical and chemical agents which can act as cancer-producers or carcinogens, and these may be presumed to operate by diverse biochemical routes, at least initially. The varied routes may well lead to a common kind of end result, possibly a somatic mutation by loss, involving the deletion of enzyme or protein systems with regulatory function, and so converting the normal cell from a state of nutritional dependence to one of self-sufficiency and unimpeded growth.

Knowledge that the regulatory mechanism of a cell can be tampered with offers a potent weapon for research both in the production and the control of malignant neoplasia. Just as the regulator of a watch may be moved to fast or slow, so may the mitotic rate be permanently accelerated by carcinogens or retarded by radiation and colchicine. As one cell will produce 60,000 daughter cells after sixteen divisions, it is apparent that even a slight increase in the rate and rhythm of cell division will soon produce a tumor. It is possible to prepare a synthetic substitute for the purine adenine, 2, 6-diaminopurine, which the cell will accept but which it will find poisonous instead of nutritious. This technique has already proved successful in the control of transplanted animal tumors in tissue cultures of malignant tumors, both animal and human.

It is perhaps justifiable at the present time to speak of exogenous and endogenous carcinogenic agents. Most of our knowledge of external agents naturally comes from observations on laboratory animals. In a few instances we can speak of external or *exogenous agents* causing human cancer, examples being irradiation, the occasional occupational cancer, excessive cigarette smoking, etc. In the vast majority of human cancers we are unable even to suggest an external agent. Under such circumstances it is natural to presume the presence of some internal or *endogenous agent*, and the first of these to suggest itself is one or more of the sex hormones. Both laboratory and bedside observation support this view. Cancer of the breast will not develop if the ovaries have been removed early in life, and the same is true of cancer of the prostate in relation to the testes. This does not mean, however, that the hormone is necessarily the *primary* etiological agent.

At the present stage of our ignorance it seems justifiable to speak of *initiating* and *promoting agents*. The initiating agent starts the process, while the promoting agent carries it on to maturity. The initiating agent is believed to produce an instantaneous change in the cell, a somatic mutation, which, however, does not manifest itself as neoplasia until the long-continued action of the promoting agent renders the condition irreversible. Urethane when applied to the skin of a mouse will not produce evident neoplasia, but when this is followed by the repeated application of croton oil a neoplasm develops. The croton oil is harmless unless the process has been initiated by urethane, for it does promote the process. It may well be that hormones act as promoters rather than as originators. The very term "hormone-dependent tumor" carries the suggestion of a promoting or continuing action. Chemical carcinogens and radiation must be regarded as initiators, with brief or instantaneous action. A virus, on the other hand, may possibly be regarded not only as an initiator but also as a promoter by reason of its ability to multiply within the cell and to enter the daughter cells.

There is, of course, no one cause of cancer, just as there is no one cause of inflammation.

Inflammation signifies a flame, a fire, but cancer is also a fire which burns continuously. There are many methods of starting a fire, some physical, some chemical. So also must there be many methods of starting different kinds of cancer and cancer of different organs. Moreover, a fire does not necessarily start at one spot; a match may be applied in several different places. This is true also of cancer. There is no need to think of it starting in one cell; it may originate in a number of adjoining areas. This is known as the wide field or origin, and is well illustrated in Fig. 107, p. 206. Under the heading of carcinogens we shall consider chemical compounds, ionizing radiation, viruses, and hormones.

Chemical Carcinogens.—The first observation on chemical carcinogenic agents was that of Sir Percival Pott in 1775, who noticed that cancer of the skin was especially common in men who worked with *tar* and he offered the suggestion that the tar acted in some manner as a causal agent. This may be linked with the observation that cancer of the lip is especially common among fishermen on the west coast of Scotland, who, in mending their nets, put the bone needle threaded with tarred twine between their lips. In 1915, that is to say one hundred and forty years after Pott's paper, Yamagiwa in Japan put this idea to the test by painting tar on a rabbit's ear every day for six months, and succeeded in producing cancer of the skin. This was an epoch-making discovery, because for the first time it was possible to produce a malignant tumor at will. Subsequent work has shown the mouse to be a much more suitable animal than the rabbit.

Tar is a highly complex substance containing a great variety of chemical agents. The next step was to determine the active agent or agents present in tar which were responsible for producing the cancer. This step was taken by Kennaway and Cook in 1932, when they succeeded in isolating the hydrocarbon benzpyrene from tar and showed that it possessed a high degree of carcinogenic activity. It was then noticed that benzpyrene gave a spectrum with fluorescent light very similar to that of a group of synthesized hydrocarbons, of which one of the important members is 1:2:5:6 dibenzanthracene. On following up this lead it was at once found that the latter substance was powerfully carcinogenic, and as it had the advantage of being a chemically pure substance of known composition, it has become the most popular agent in the experimental production of cancer. Many other members of this group of polycyclic aromatic hydrocarbons with a benzene or aromatic six-membered ring structure proved to be carcinogenic. The carcinogenic hydrocarbons must possess at least three condensed carbon rings to be active, and most of them have four. The fluorescence spectrum was the single golden thread that led through all this labyrinth. It is interesting to note that 1:2 benzanthracene has practically no carcinogenic activity, but the attachment of a new benzene ring in the 5:6 position gives it great carcinogenic power. A very slight change in the chemical structure of a substance may convert it from a non-carcinogenic into a carcinogenic agent. Methylcholanthrene is another actively carcinogenic hydrocarbon which deserves mention because it is an artificial compound prepared from cholic acid, an organic substance occurring *naturally* in the body, thus suggesting the possibility of an endogenous chemical carcinogen.

Any of these agents can produce either carcinoma or sarcoma at the site of application. If applied to an epithelial surface carcinoma develops, if injected subcutaneously sarcoma is the result. By this means it has been possible to produce carcinoma of the skin, kidney, liver, testis, bladder, and uterus, as well as sarcoma of the subcutaneous tissue and peritoneum. Brain tumors (gliomas) can be produced by the intracerebral implantation of pellets of methylcholanthrene. When fibroblasts from the rat or mouse are grown in tissue culture in a medium containing a powerful carcinogenic chemical, such as methylcholanthrene, they are changed into cells which are similar to the cells in cultures of sarcoma induced by injection of the carcinogen into subcutaneous tissue (Earle and Voegtlin).

A carcinogenic agent of extraordinary potency was discovered by accident in the course of testing the toxicity of a new insecticide, acetyl acetaminofluorine. This substance when implanted in the tissues causes neither inflammation nor tumors, but when given by mouth to rats it produces cancer of the liver, pancreas, breast, bladder, lung and salivary glands, as well as sarcoma and leukemias (Bielschowsky).

It may well be asked what all this has to do with the problem of human cancer with which the surgeon has to deal. What have these products of the chemist's ingenuity to do with "the cause of cancer," the search for which has become like the quest for the philosopher's stone? One answer to this question is that the work has demonstrated that many causes for cancer are already known. It is true that we do not understand how these agents act, but no more do we understand how irritants produce inflammation. As Willis remarks: "When we say that 'the tubercle bacillus is the cause of tuberculosis' we state only a part of a truth, and that the smaller part. The tubercle bacillus does not cause tuberculosis in a test tube, or in some species of animals, or even in some human beings. . . . The intrinsic properties of the tissues which render them susceptible and determine their reaction are as yet unknown. In this sense, then, the tuberculous reaction is no less 'mysterious' than the neoplastic reaction." We now have some keys which will open the door, so that it would be well to stop talking about the insoluble mystery of cancer. Other keys will be found. It is perhaps a little disturbing to learn that the processes by which the chemist changes a non-carcinogenic hydrocarbon into a carcinogen involve the use of high temperatures which are comparable with the temperatures used for cooking the hydrocarbons of food by frying, as well as other forms of cooking.

Another answer to our question is the *similarity which the molecular structure of the synthetic carcinogenic hydrocarbons bears to that of substances naturally occurring in the body*. While the work on the carcinogenic hydrocarbons was going on, organic chemists were investigating bile acids, the sterols such as cholesterol, and the sex hormones, and soon it became evident that the basic structure of these very different substances was fundamentally similar (Fig. 92). All of them possess the condensed-carbon-ring skeleton known as the phenanthrene nucleus, and the nucleus is also present in the benzpyrene,

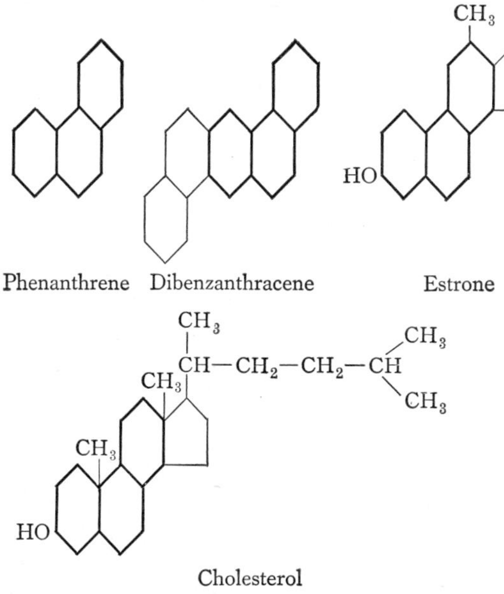

Phenanthrene   Dibenzanthracene   Estrone

Cholesterol

FIG. 92.—Similar chemical structure of carcinogenic hydrocarbons, estrone, and cholesterol. The phenanthrene nucleus is common to all. (Boyd's *Pathology for the Surgeon*, courtesy of W. B. Saunders Company).

benzanthracene and cholanthrene groups of carcinogenic hydrocarbons. At first it seemed as if the phenanthrene nucleus might be the key to carcinogenesis, but later, as has always happened with the cancer problem, this delightfully simple idea had to be abandoned. We have already seen that methylcholanthrene, which from its structure is seen to belong to the sterols, can be produced from bile acid by a series of processes which might well occur in the body. It becomes evident, then, that there is a structural relationship between the chemical carcinogenic compounds and the normal constitutents of the body, and we must admit that it is theoretically possible for carcinogenic agents to be produced within the body as the result of disordered metabolism affecting the sterols, bile acids or sex hormones.

The *carcinogenic azo compounds* have been overshadowed by the carcinogenic hydrocarbons, but they provide valuable tools of research, for their chemical structure is much simpler, and their metabolic products can be isolated and identified. They have a hydrogen atom link in place of a carbon atom link. Their carcinogenic property came to light as the result of an investigation into the action of scarlet red, an azo dye, as a stimulant of wound healing. They act at a distance and only on the liver, the main organ of metabolism in the body. Perhaps the most intriguing feature of this form of induced liver cancer is that it is influenced profoundly by diet. The carcinogenic action on the liver of paradimethylaminoazobenzene, the azo dye known as butter yellow, is only manifested when there is a deficiency in riboflavin. The ability of the liver to destroy the dye in vitro by an enzyme action needs the presence of riboflavin, which acts as a co-enzyme. In this sense the vitamin is anti-carcinogenic.

Alkylating agents must be added to the list of active chemical carcinogens (Haddow). These are reactive intermediates of nitrogen mustards, *e.g.*, ethyleneimenes, epoxides, and dimesyl compounds. Chromosome breakage is a prominent feature in the experimental animal, perhaps due to failure of synthesis. These agents are "radiomimetic," producing results similar to those of ionizing radiation. The tumors induced show a high percentage of nuclear abnormalities. Of course these gross alterations may merely be changes associated with a much more elusive essential alteration, perhaps on a molecular level.

When we turn to *cancer in man* we find much evidence in support of known external carcinogens, some of which are chemical and others physical.

Workers who come in contact with *tar products*, *oils* and *petroleum* are liable to develop *skin cancer*. *Aniline dye workers* get *cancer of the bladder*. The active agent is *beta naphthylamine*. which causes cancer of the bladder in the dog as well as in man, but not in the mouse and rat, because the metabolic product excreted in the urine by the latter is non-carcinogenic. This illustrates one of the pitfalls of experimental cancer work, because what may be harmless for man may be carcinogenic for the animal and vice versa. Other carcinogens which might be either chemical or physical are the chotta and the kangri. The *chotta* is a cigar which is smoked in southern India with the lighted end in the mouth. Addicts have a high incidence of cancer of the mouth. The natives of Kashmir wear a hot basket of charcoal, the *kangri*, under their clothes for purposes of warmth, and cancer of the abdominal wall is common among them, whereas it is almost unknown amongst other races. Most authorities believe that statistical evidence shows that heavy *cigarette smoking* bears a causal connection to cancer of the lung. *Circumcision* seems to prevent the development of cancer of the penis, by eliminating an accumulation of oily smegma under the foreskin which apparently acts as a carcinogen.

Ionizing Radiation.—Of the physical carcinogens the most striking is ionizing radiation in its various forms. Whole body radiation to the rat is a potent carcinogenic agent (Koletsky and Gustafson). Even a single dose of 660 r is followed by a wide variety of benign and malignant tumors of the skin, connective tissue and viscera in nearly half the animals, the malignant tumors being about evenly divided between sarcoma and carcinoma. The early workers with *x-rays* developed cancer of the skin of the hand after many years. Multicentric carcinoma of the breast developed in a patient irradiated ten years previously for Hodgkin's disease of the chest (Lisa *et al.*). Leukemia, a malignant condition of the blood-forming organs, is an occupational disease of radiologists, and the survivors of the Hiroshima and Nagasaki atomic blasts show a ten-fold increase in leukemia in the heavily exposed group, as well as other radiation-induced neoplasms. *Radium* produces the same effect. Girls in Newark, New Jersey, who painted the dials of watches with luminous radioactive paint developed bone sarcoma owing to the deposit of radioactive material in the bones. Carcinoma of the thyroid gland in children has frequently proved to be a sequel to irradiation of the thymus in infancy, at one time a favorite form of therapy for enlarged thymus, but now abandoned. Anyone who is continually exposed to radiations, whether he be a shoe salesman or a dweller near an atomic pile, is in danger of radiation cancer. As mankind is crossing the threshold into the atomic age, there is need for awareness of fresh dangers. It is possible that radiations may act by producing chemical changes with the formation of hydroxyl radicles from decomposition of water with depolymerization of the nucleic acid molecule and resultant chromosomal damage. The miners in Schneeberg and Joachimsthal for centuries have suffered from a high incidence of cancer of the lung; this is now known to be due to radioactive uranium. *Actinic light radiation* is also carcinogenic, thus explaining the high incidence of cancer of the skin and lip amongst field workers in the white population of the tropics, Australia, and the southern United States. This form of cancer is very rare in the negro, who is protected by the high melanin content of his skin.

An interesting example of an apparent relationship between sunlight and carcinogenesis is afforded by *xeroderma pigmentosum*. This is a rare congenital disease characterized by extreme hypersensitivity to light, with the development of solar dermatitis in early childhood. In a high proportion of these unfortunate persons skin cancer develops before the age of twenty years.

Viruses.—We now come to one of the most exciting of the more modern aspects of carcinogenesis, namely the part played by viruses. The concept of viruses being connected with neoplasia is of course very far from new, for it was in 1911 that *Peyton Rous* published his epoch-making observa-

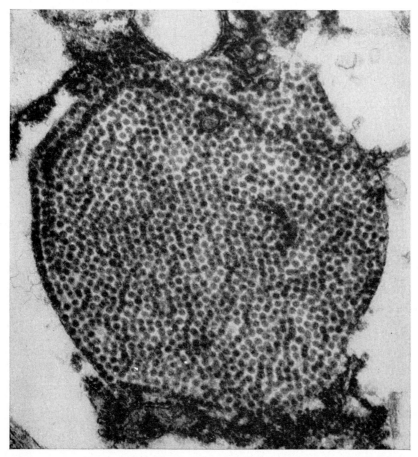

Fig. 93.—Polyoma virus. The nuclear material of a cell from the kidney of an infected hamster has been almost completely replaced by virus. × 60,000. (Kindness of Dr. A. F. Howatson.)

tions that a cell-free filtrate of a fowl sarcoma could produce a new tumor when inoculated into another fowl of the same Plymouth Rock breed, thus anticipating by four years the discovery of chemical carcinogenesis. Other tumors caused by filter-passing agents were soon described, but as these were confined to birds, no widespread enthusiasm was aroused. Then in 1932 *Shope* demonstrated that a papilloma of the skin in the wild cotton-tail rabbit was of a similar character, and that when the viral agent was injected into the domestic rabbit a more aggressive lesion was produced, which presently developed into a true cancer. When this stage was reached the active agent could no longer be isolated from the malignant lesion, a fact perhaps of great significance. In 1936 *Bitt-*

ner made the important discovery that cancer of the breast in mice can be transmitted to the newborn by an agent in the mother's milk, a subject which is discussed more fully below.

In 1951 *Gross* showed that cell-free extracts of leukemic tissue of mice of a high (spontaneous) leukemic strain when injected into new-born mice of a low strain would induce the development of leukemia some months later. This was shortly followed by the demonstration by *Sarah Stewart* that some of the mice so injected developed carcinoma of the parotid gland or fibrosarcoma of connective tissue. Still more startling was the discovery by Stewart and her associates that when the same leukemic agent was grown in tissue culture and a cell-free extract was injected into new-born mice, the animals developed a broad spectrum of more than a dozen apparently unrelated tumors. For this reason the agent was named the *polyoma* (PY) *virus* and the SE (Stewart-Eddy) virus (Fig. 93). The virus can no longer be found in the tumor at the end of one week, which may be related to the absence of virus in human cancer.

Finally, in this list of historic advances in the virology of neoplasia must be mentioned the great forward step in 1960 represented by the ability to produce true *neoplastic development of a mammalian cancer in cellular culture* (Vogt and Dulbecco), although this had been done previously with fowl virus. This technical achievement with the polyoma virus gave workers the opportunity to study two types of virus-cell reaction: (1) a *cytocidal interaction*, leading to extensive virus synthesis with cellular degeneration and destruction, the type of reaction we are familiar with in poliomyelitis and other human viral infections; (2) a *moderate interaction* leading to transformation of the cells of the culture into neoplastic cells, which are unable to produce detectable virus and are resistant to superinfection with the same virus. The cytocidal interaction is most frequent in mouse cultures, the moderate (neoplastic) interaction in hamster cultures. In the new-born mouse the virus produces extensive cellular degeneration, and only several months later do tumors develop. In the new-born hamster the virus produces few degenerative changes, but within a few weeks the formation of tumors becomes evident.

At the present time the production of malignant tumors of a variety of types by cell-free filtrates in laboratory animals has become commonplace. It seems only natural that a virus, which like an enzyme is a self-perpetuating nucleoprotein, could produce tumors by disrupting the normal regulating mechanism. The virus may be DNA or RNA in type. The former, being related to genes, may affect the genetic mechanism, so that the cells behave as mutants, the virus becoming invisible as it combines with the genetic material. Genes are linked together in the chromosomes, members of a community working for the common good. A virus is a detached solitary particle of nucleic acid, an outlaw or lone wolf, essentially anti-social in its effect, a parasite living on the wealth accumulated by the genes. RNA controls the synthesis of proteins, and hence is responsible for growth, so that the cell may be destroyed, but the virus may be visible with the electron microscope. The viruses responsible for the common viral infections are of this type. It must be understood, however, that carcinogenic viruses may be either of the DNA type (polyoma virus) or the RNA type (Rous chicken sarcoma virus).

In many of the virus-induced tumors in experimental animals characteristic particles can be seen with the electron microscope within the cytoplasm and in spaces between cells. These have a dense central body surrounded by a less dense zone and bounded by a dense membrane, being similar in appearance to well known viruses such as vaccinia and herpes simplex. The number of virus particles is related to the degree of differentiation of the cells, being much more numerous in highly differentiated tumors than in undifferentiated anaplastic tumors. It looks as if in rapidly growing tumors cell growth may outstrip virus growth, or the virus may be in a form not visible to the electron microscope.

It is now recognized that many viruses formerly undreamed of may course through the body and persist in the cells of the host for generations without damage. It seems highly probable that viruses may be latent more often than overt, just as saprophytic bacteria are far more numerous than pathogenic ones. A latent virus, however, may mutate to an active state, and this change may be brought about by a variety of agents. The idea of a virus living in symbiotic harmony with its host is not as fantastic as it may sound. The virus of herpes simplex is acquired in early life, when it may cause an acute stomatitis in the child. It then passes into a latent state from which it may be awakened at any time by changes in temperature or by various bacterial infections. Psittacosis may be changed from a latent infection in pigeons producing no pathological change into a fatal illness with tissue necrosis simply by withholding thiamine from the diet. If we knew nothing about the psittacosis virus we should say that thiamine deficiency was the true cause of psittacosis in pigeons. The mouse may acquire the virus of lymphocytic choriomeningitis *in utero*, but it appears to go underground, and in some strains every individual in the colony may harbor the virus in the brain without any clinical evidence of disease. Alterations in the host-parasite relationship may make a virus either necrotizing or carcinogenic, and in the course of adaptation to altered environment the malignant cell may be born.

Bittner's transmissible milk factor in breast cancer in mice appears to be a virus which has been isolated both from the milk and from the mammary tumor. In 1936 Bittner found that when newborn mice of a high mammary cancer strain were fostered by mothers of a low cancer strain the tumor incidence was greatly reduced. Conversely newborn mice of a low strain when fostered by mothers of a high strain showed an increased incidence of breast cancer, the tumor developing when the animal reached early adult life. Mouse mammary cancer is, then, a disease of the adult female acquired in infancy through an "agent" transmitted in the mother's milk. The factor responsible is evidently extrachromosomal in character, being transmitted not by the germ plasm but by the milk. What was apparently a hereditary trait turns out to be a transmissible infection. The infected female may or may not become cancerous, but she can transfer the agent in the milk to her progeny. Strange to say the male can also transmit the virus, probably in the sperm. For the development of the cancer three factors seem to be necessary: (1) genetic susceptibility, (2) hormonal stimuli, and (3) the virus. The applicability of this work to the problem of cancer of the human breast has not yet been determined. The Bittner and Rous viruses are not confined to the tumor which they produce, but are widely distributed throughout the tissues, whereas the Shope virus is only present in the local lesion through the papilloma-to-carcinoma sequence and is not found in the metastases.

Spherical particles, approximately 100 millimicrons in diameter, have been isolated by means of the ultracentrifuge from the milk of high cancer strain mice and also from the tumor (Fig. 94). These particles can readily be photographed with the electron microscope, and when injected into the young of a low cancer strain they cause the development of tumors in adult life. Similar particles have also been found in large numbers in human milk in cases where there is a marked history of cancer in the family, especially breast cancer. Where there is no cancer history they are present in only small numbers.

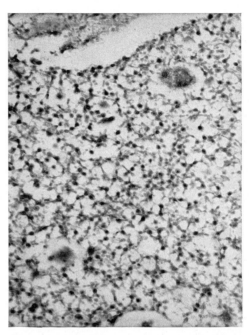

FIG. 94.—Bittner milk factor virus. × 18,000. (Dmochowski *et al*, courtesy of Genetics and Cancer, Texas, 1959).

A major advance in our thinking on the subject of the viral origin of cancer is represented by Gross's concept of *vertical transmission*. Every communicable disease with which we are familiar, whether bacterial or viral in nature, spreads from one host to another within the same generation. This may be termed "horizontal transmission." As the interval between viral spread and the appearance of clinical manifestations is only a matter of days or at most of a few weeks, it is usually easy to trace the transfer between donor and recipient, as for instance in small pox or measles. This is not true of viral neoplasia in animals. A chicken with leukemia or a mouse with an ulcerating mammary carcinoma can spend all its days in intimate contact with its fellows, yet the disease will never be transmitted to them.

Leukemia in mice is an example of a latent

virus infection which produces a neoplastic disease that develops spontaneously in an inbred strain when they reach early adult life. Gross has shown that the carcinogenic agent is transmitted vertically, that is to say from one generation to another, through the germinal cells. In the case of the mouse mammary gland carcinoma the virus is transmitted through the mother's milk. The agent may remain latent throughout the life-span of the host, which remains healthy, and yet carries and transmits the seeds of disease. That the seeds are there can be shown by inoculating cell-free filtrates into newborn mice of a low-leukemic strain (who would not develop the disease spontaneously) with the production of leukemia. A pure strain of mice can be produced by inbreeding in which from 80 to 90 per cent of individuals will develop leukemia in adult life. In a low-incidence strain, as we have just seen, the disease can be produced by inoculation of a cell-free filtrate containing the infective agent, but this must be done in newborn animals less than sixteen hours old.

In a *high-incidence strain* of mouse cancer the disease occurs "spontaneously," the carcinogen being evidently both initiating and promoting in character. In a *low-incidence strain* the virus is present in latent and harmless form, but it can be triggered into activity either by extrinsic agents such as chemical poisons or ionizing radiation, or by intrinsic agents either metabolic or hormonal in character. The leukemic agent can then be isolated from the tissues of the low-strain animal, and its presence demonstrated by inoculation of the newborn. Of course the skeptical pathologist may say that the triggering agent simply acts on the genetic mechanism of the nucleus, and that it is not necessary to suppose the presence of a virus.

It will be noticed that in the various experimental tumors referred to above the viral material was injected into the new-born animal. This is a point of fundamental importance, depending on the fact, already discussed in connection with auto-immunity in Chapter 5, that the fetus is unable to make antibodies against antigens to which it is exposed, an inability which persists in many species for a few hours or days after birth. When the virus of leukemia or the Bittner milk virus are inoculated later in life

they are destroyed by antibodies so that no carcinoma develops. This suggests the thought that a virus present in the body at birth may live in the cells for years until some promoting factor combines with it to turn it into a true carcinogen. A potentially carcinogenic virus seems to be able to live in the adult animal without doing any damage until the immunity mechanism of the host is broken down by radiation, cortisone, or other means. We must realize that *viruses are perhaps not really living organisms*, but chemicals made of the same material as the genes of the chromosomes. Viruses reproduce because they use the chemical machinery of the cell for their reproduction. Indeed it would be more accurate to say that the cells reproduce the viruses which they harbor. Furthermore, the virus may well interfere with the genetic nucleoproteins concerned with cellular reproduction, so that changes in the genes and chromosomes in neoplasia may not be due to so-called spontaneous mutation, but to virus interference (Ham). As is the case with bacterial infections, it may be that inability to resist the virus may be more important than the presence of the virus.

One of the most remarkable facts to emerge from the inoculation of newborn mice with the leukemic agent is that in a susceptible strain about two-thirds of the animals develop leukemia, whilst the remaining one-third develop bilateral carcinoma of the parotid gland or, more rarely, fibrosarcoma of subcutaneous tissue (Stewart). When the mice are from one to fourteen days old, only leukemia, never parotid tumors, develops as the result of inoculation. This suggests the possibility that we may be dealing with two separate viruses, one of which produces leukemia and the other parotid tumors.

Are these various tumors caused by a single virus or a number of different viruses? This question cannot be answered at the present time, although some of the evidence given above suggests the latter alternative. A granuloma may be caused by a wide variety of infective agents, and scarlet fever and measles used to be mistaken for one another clinically but are now known to be caused by two widely different agents, a streptococcus and a virus. If cancer is due to a viral infection there is no reason to suppose that only one type of virus is involved.

It is evident that the vertical transmission of a viral carcinogen is a challenging concept. It must not be confused with inheritance of disease, in which only genetic factors are involved. Vertical transmission presupposes an acquired infection, although it may have become acquired hundreds of years ago, with perfect adaptation of the parasite to the host. The occasional occurrence of several cases of leukemia in the children of one family can be explained on this basis.

In leaving the general subject of the carcinogenic action of viruses it is evident that these agents are coming to assume an ever-increasing importance. They can certainly cause the development of leukemia and a number of malignant neoplasms in animals. They may be changed from a latent to an active carcinogenic form by chemical poisons, ionizing radiation and possibly by hormones. Persons developing clinical manifestations of tumors or leukemia may well represent only a very small proportion of those carrying the seeds of the disease.

Numerous investigators are ready to accept viruses as etiological agents for cancers in animals, but deny them that role in *human cancer*. Pathologists in particular have been reluctant to accept a virus as a cause of the infinite variety of tumors with which they are familiar. They point out that so far no virus has been isolated from a human cancer, although they are known to be capable of causing cell multiplication, as is seen in vaccinia, fowl-pox and warts. It must be realized, however, that viruses may be highly specific, so specific indeed that a virus will infect and cause disease only in one kind of cell and in one kind of animal. A virus long adapted to human cells could hardly be expected to grow readily in most animal cells, and it is by such growth either by inoculation of the animal itself or by employing a living culture of the animal's cells that the etiological role of viruses in animal neoplasms has been demonstrated. The only known human neoplastic virus, that of the common wart, can be transmitted to human volunteers, but not to laboratory animals, nor can it be grown in tissue culture of human cells.

A noteworthy recent (1960) break in the species barrier seems to be provided by the work of Grace and his associates at Roswell Park, Buffalo. Extracts of human tumors were inoculated into a variety of established tissue cultures, and fluid from the cultures injected into mice and hamsters. No tumors resulted. Similar extracts of human cancers both with and without prior filtration, through a bacterial filter, were injected into newborn animals, and tumors developed in many of these animals after a latent period of from three to nine months, a relatively long period in the life span of such an animal. Most of the animal tumors were carcinoma of the breast, and the incidence of breast cancer was highest in pregnant mice, showing the importance of a conditioning hormonal factor. It may well be that the recently acquired power of growing human cells in tissue culture may provide a valuable experimental approach to the cancer problem in man. Microbiologists, who are intimately concerned with the behaviour of viruses even if not with the complexities of human cancer, find it easy to accept the viral concept of cancer. Their position has been forcibly stated by Wendell Stanley, himself a Nobel Prize winner in the field of viral disease of plants, in the following words: "It is difficult to escape the conclusion that viruses may be the etiological agents for most, if not all, cancer, including cancer in man, and that this represents by far the most intellectually satisfying working hypothesis which is consistent with all presently known facts."

Hormones.—We have already seen that cancerogenic agents may be initiating with immediate action or promoting needing long-continued action. Specific carcinogens initiate an irreversible change in cells which determines the site and nature of the tumor, whereas developing and promoting agents, which by themselves are unable to cause a tumor, determine the time of development and may be necessary for continued growth. Hormones, particularly sex hormones, seem to participate in both of these activities. Approximately 25 per cent of lethal human cancers arise in four organs, the growth and function of which are controlled by trophic hormones, namely breast, uterus, ovary and prostate. In general hormones differ from other carcinogens, (1) in that most frequently they induce tumors only in specific organs and usually in those organs upon which the hormone has a physiological effect, and (2) in that prolonged exposure of the susceptible tissue is required to incite a carcinogenic effect. It has been stated flatly that "prolonged stimulation of target cells by their trophic hormones is one of the causes of cancer" (Crile). In the experimental animl there is first hypertrophy of the target organ, then the formation of benign nodules, and finally development of cancer. At first the cancer may be dependent for continued growth on persistence of the endocrine imbalance which initiated the process, but if the imbalance persists an autonomous cancer develops and grows in an animal in whom there is no longer imbalance; it will indeed grow when injected into a normal animal. Thus when thiouracil is fed to rats the output of thyroid hormone is suppressed, the pituitary output of thyrotrophic hormone is accordingly increased, and the sequence of thyroid hyperplasia, benign nodule formation, and eventually carcinoma is put into action.

The *sex hormones* provide the most striking example of a carcinogenic action. From the structural resemblances between the carcinogenic hydrocarbons and the female sex hormones it might be deduced that their physiological activities are also similar. Such indeed proves to be the case. Certain of the hydrocarbons, such as benzpyrene, are able to replace the female sex hormones, while the administration of estrogen may result in cancer. Thus carcinogenic substances can be estrogenic, and estrogenic substances can be carcinogenic. Estrogens are inactivated by the liver. It is therefore perhaps only natural that in the African Bantu, in whom hepatic insufficiency is common owing to dietary insufficiency, gynecomastia, uterine fibromyoma and cancer of the male breast are notably frequent.

Estrogens frequently require the cooperation of one or more additional agencies or *co-carcinogens*. They are only one of the essential factors in tumor production, and will induce tumors only in favorable circumstances, in special situations and in animals with a special tendency to tumor formation. The most essential factor is heredity. The incidence of spontaneous mammary cancer is almost nil in some strains of mice and nearly 100 per cent in others. It is interest-

ing to note that spontaneous mammary cancer does not occur in the rat, but can be induced by estrogens. In this animal the tumor remains *hormonal-dependent*, whereas in the mouse it becomes *hormone-independent*. There are two kinds of inherited agents, the genic and the non-genic. The genic factor is much less significant than the non-genic. The non-genic is the Bittner milk factor which is viral in nature. Lacassagne showed that when estrogen is injected from birth onwards into a strain of mice which have a natural tendency to develop mammary cancer, the incidence of that tumor is very greatly increased, and even in male mice of the same strain mammary cancer can be produced, although the natural occurrence of this tumor in the male mouse is almost unknown. Even when the hormone is painted on the skin it produces its characteristic effect on the breast. If mice of a non-cancerous strain are used, the hormone is powerless to produce cancer. Removal of the ovaries at an early age in mice of a high cancer strain will prevent the occurrence of spontaneous mammary cancer, but hormonal administration will cause cancer to develop. Experimental carcinoma of the cervix has also been produced by the prolonged administration of estrogen

In the *breast* carcinoma can be produced both in male and female mice and rats of the right strain by means of estrogens. In women the obvious source of the hormone is the ovaries. In men it may come from the testes or the adrenals.

In the *prostate* there seems to be little doubt that an endocrine dysfunction is an etiological factor in the production of cancer in man. The hormones may be gonadal or adrenal in origin. The serum acid phosphatase and the urinary 17-ketosteroid levels can be used respectively as indicators of activity of malignant prostatic cells and of androgen secretion. Prostatic cancer cells do not appear to be as completely autonomous as other cancer cells, for they are controlled to some degree by the same hormonal mechanism which controls the normal cells of the prostate, as is shown by the remarkable effects of castration and the administration of estrogens.

Other hormones demand brief consideration in relation to cancer of the breast in women and cancer of the prostate in men. The *adrenal cortex* produces both androgens and estrogens. The estrogens appear to be more abundant in postmenopausal than in premenopausal women, and their activity is increased by ovariectomy. It is for this reason that adrenalectomy is of greater benefit for cancer of the breast after than before the menopause. The adrenals, indeed, may be regarded as the gonads of elderly women, and they may be the culprits which sustain the growth of breast cancer.

The *pituitary* exercises control over the output of sex hormones of the gonads and adrenals, and hypophysectomy reduces this output to low levels, and therefore indirectly influences hormone-dependent tumors. The remarkable and gratifying regression of cancer of the prostate after estrogen therapy seems to be the result of suppression of pituitary gonadotrophin with secondary depression of androgen produced by the testes. On the other hand in some strains of mice interstitial cell tumors of the testes appear when estrogens are given. It is assumed that the estrogens act upon the pituitary gland, which in turn stimulates the interstitial cells. Topical application of estrogen to the testes does not increase the incidence of interstitial cell tumors, indicating that there has been no direct action on the testes.

The subject of hormonal-dependent tumors has come to assume great clinical importance in relation to the treatment of cancer of the breast in women and of the prostate in men by means of the administration of estrogens, of adrenalectomy, or as a last resort of hypophysectomy. It is evident that benefit from hormone therapy or removal of endocrines can only be expected when the tumor is still hormone-dependent. In the experimental animal it can be shown that hormones may have an inhibitory effect on neoplasia. Whether this is due to direct interference with the reproductive mechanism of the neoplastic cell or whether it is caused by action on the pituitary with inhibition of some hormone it is not possible at present to say. It may be recalled in this connection that some chemical carcinogens may be cancer-destroying as well as cancer-producing. The role of hormones in the control of cancer may be attributed to the following mechanisms: (1) hormones may

directly inhibit neoplastic proliferation; (2) they may induce tissue differentiation that will either excite the defense mechanisms of the body or restore the normal mechanisms that limit cellular proliferation; (3) hormones may limit a modified production of specific requirements for the growth of the tumor, thus inhibiting the growth (Gardner). It is of interest to note that clinically the control of cancer of the prostate by the oral administration of estrogen is the one example of effective systemic therapy of human cancer, yet almost nothing is known of the factors concerned in the induction of prostatic cancer in man, nor has the disease yet been produced experimentally. For further information on the relation of estrogens to neoplasia the reader is referred to the monograph of Burrows and Horning, and on the hormonal regulation of tumor growth to the review by Noble with 456 references.

Environment and Occupation.—In many forms of cancer, although the exact causal agent may not be known, there is reason to believe that it is related to environment or occupation. Some forms of occupation bear a striking relation to cancer in particular sites. This is a subject of increasing importance in the industrial age in which we now live. Some idea of the terrifyingly long list of potential hazards may be gathered from the book and articles on occupational tumors by W. C. Hueper. Mere mention may be made of workers with coal tar and petroleum distillates, aniline dyes, x-rays and radioactive material, nickel, chromium compounds, arsenicals, asbestos, and many, many other raw materials and products. Several insecticides and food dyes when tested for toxicity were found to be carcinogenic, which is fortunate for us. The truth is that throughout life we seem to swim in a sea of carcinogens, and it is more by good fortune than good management that some of us escape to die from other causes. The contentious subject of cancer of the lung will be discussed in Chapter 24. Suffice it to say here that the disease began to show an increased incidence after the turn of the century, an increase which has greatly gained in momentum in recent years, more particularly in highly industrialized communities. In Norway the incidence of lung cancer rose in two decades (1930 to 1948) from 20 to 157.

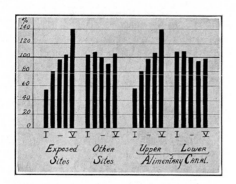

Fig. 95.—Cancer mortality by social classes. (Registrar-General's Decennial Suppl. England and Wales, 1921.)

It is of course all too easy to mistake for causal relations what are merely coincidental statistical relations to environmental agents. What has been called the social grading of cancer, *i.e.*, variations in incidence with different economic levels, is observed particularly in those organs which might be exposed to an external carcinogen (Fig. 95). This grading is very marked in the alimentary canal, but only above the pylorus. Cancer of the cervix in women and of the lung in men is much more prevalent amongst the poorer classes in Copenhagen. The Survey of Cancer in London, published by the British Empire Cancer Campaign in 1952, shows a significant excess of cancer of the lip and mouth in general and dock laborers, of cancer of the pharynx and esophagus in publicans and barmen, of cancer of the skin in workers in chemicals, pitch and tar, of cancer of the larynx in singers, actors and clergymen.

Geographic Cancer.—This is a part of the general subject of geographic pathology or the geography of disease, a fascinating topic in which the student might well develop a life-long interest. Unfortunately it is a subject bristling with pitfalls. Certain it is that the incidence of different forms of cancer varies greatly in different countries and even in different parts of the same country. Sometimes we know the reason for this, but in most instances we do not. In every case, however, there must be a reason, and when this is discovered it may give us a new lead on carcinogenesis. *Cancer of the urinary*

bladder is very common amongst Egyptian farmers. This is related to the high incidence of Schistosoma hematobium infection, although how the presence of the ova of the parasite in the bladder mucosa causes the cancer we do not know. We have already seen that *cancer of the skin* is common in white-skinned persons living in the tropics, because of actinic light radiation. On the other hand *cancer of the penis* is very rare in Israel, because circumcision soon after birth prevents the development of this neoplasm. *Cancer of the nasopharynx* is very common in the people of South China, which has been attributed, rightly or wrongly, to dietary deficiency in childhood. *Cancer of the oropharynx* is more frequent in the women of Northern Sweden than elsewhere. These women frequently suffer from chronic oropharyngitis with anemia (the Plummer-Vinson syndrome), which is said to be related to deficiency of vitamin B complex in the diet.

Cancer of the liver, a rare disease elsewhere, is common in Algeria, Senegal, the Sudan, Java, and Indonesia, indeed in a primary liver cancer belt stretching from Africa through Indonesia, into China and Japan. In the Bantu it is commonly met with in young patients, in some areas although not in others being associated with hepatic cirrhosis and therefore possibly connected with dietary deficiency in childhood. The total cancer mortality rates are identical in England and Sweden, but the proportion of *cancer of the stomach* in the two countries is 23 to 60; the incidence in Holland is the same as in Sweden. In Honolulu, which by reason of its isolation and its remarkable mixture of races may be regarded as a human laboratory for the study of cancer, gastric cancer is far more common amongst the Japanese than amongst the general population. Apart from cancer of individual organs, the *general cancer rate* in the United States varies from 79 in Arkansas to 150 in New York State. The high rate in the northeastern states of the U.S., particularly striking in the case of lung cancer, may be related to the fact that these represent highly industrialized regions. A remarkable instance of the geographic pathology of cancer is seen in two halves of a small compact community in West Devon, who for generations have intermarried and eaten the same food, but show a wide difference in the incidence of cancer. (Allen-Price). Those prone to cancer have a water supply from an entirely different geological formation. Some of the differences in the sex incidence of cancer may really be due to differences in occupation and environment; cancer of the lung is seven times more common in men and cancer of the esophagus ten times more common. From these statistics taken largely at random it will be evident how many traps await the unwary who draw rash conclusions, but it will also be evident that the problems presented are both fascinating and challenging.

Cancer in Africa provides one of the most exciting and challenging examples of the geographic pathology of cancer. It is challenging because the pattern of cancer in that continent differs profoundly from that in Europe and North America. There must be good reasons for these differences, but with a few exceptions we are ignorant of the reasons. They are presumably related to differences in environment, because the pattern changes with change in the social and economic conditions. Especially noteworthy is the fact that the pattern is quite different in the American Negro. Parasites apparently play a part of little importance.

Skin cancer is very common in tropical Africa, where it forms about 13 per cent of all tumors, with enormous preponderance arising in the legs in a scar of "tropical ulcer," a very chronic lesion of unknown etiology. On the other hand in Johannesburg in South Africa the proportion of squamous carcinoma is only about 4 per cent. *Malignant melanoma* of the foot is also very common, nearly always on the sole. *Kaposi sarcoma*, an angioma-like tumor of vascular tissue, is a rarity in Europe and North America, but is frequently encountered in tropical Africa. *Cancer of the liver* is common in all parts of the continent, but particularly in Central Africa. The relation to cirrhosis is a matter of debate. *Cancer of the stomach, colon, rectum* and *female breast*, so common elsewhere, are rare in Africa. *Cancer of the nasal sinuses*, infrequent elsewhere, is prevalent in rural areas, where the use of aloe snuffs containing carcinogens (3:4 benzpyrene) is habitual. *Cancer of the esophagus* is common, indeed in some areas fantastically so, possibly due to copious draughts of a home-made beer brewed in metal drums formerly containing asphalt, these drums being lined by soluble carcinogens. The incidence of carcinoma of the *penis* is very high; indeed, in Uganda it is the second commonest form of carcinoma. Perhaps the most fantastic abnormal pattern is that of *tumors of the jaws*, adamantinoma being common in adults, and in children a *multicentric* sarcoma of peculiar and unique character. If the student does not wish to become interested in these intriguing and challenging neoplasms he should on no account look at the Chapter on Cancer in Africa by Davies, professor of pathology in Kampala, Uganda, in Collins' *Modern Trends in Pathology*, where he will see fantastic illustrations, both clinical and pathological, of these extraordinary tumors.

Co-carcinogens.—To determine the cause of an occurrence is not the simple matter which at first sight it may appear. The philosopher tells us that scientifically the cause of anything is the total assemblage of the conditions which precede its appearance. This is particularly true of cancer, and a full realization of this fact will show how futile it is to speak about "*the* cause of cancer." A match may start a fire, but the material must first be inflammable, and a breeze will fan the flame to fierce activity. The other factors which come into play and without which the original carcinogen is likely to be powerless are called co-carcinogens. Included in this group are the "promoting" and "conditioning" agents to which reference has already been made.

The combination of two carcinogens such as a hydrocarbon and a virus may accelerate the process of carcinogenesis. Thus if the Shope papilloma virus is injected intravenously into a rabbit the skin of which has been tarred for some time, a rapidly growing carcinoma will quickly develop in the tarred area. The two carcinogens seem to act in unison. We have already seen that three conditions are necessary for the development of the mouse mammary carcinoma, namely the Bittner milk virus, the ovarian hormone, and a hereditary factor governing sensitivity to the virus. The carcinogenic hydrocarbons may only set the stage for the activation of a latent virus-like agent. Duran-Reynals showed that methylcholanthrene activated latent fowl-pox infection which appeared only in the painted region. On continuing the painting papillomas and epidermoid carcinoma developed. A hormone may act as a co-carcinogen to a hydrocarbon, and more than one hormone may be needed. Thus injections of estrogen followed by painting of the skin with methylcholanthrene will cause almost no mammary mouse tumors, whereas the addition of progesterone results in a high incidence of carcinoma. It is not only the sex organs which are involved, for removal of the thyroid protects the liver against the carcinogenic action of 2-acetyl-aminofluorene.

Cancer can be produced by the combined action of a chemical carcinogen too weak to produce a tumor and a co-carcinogen such as croton oil. Urethane of itself will not produce skin tumors in any dosage or length of time. It is not a carcinogen and causes no detectable histological changes in the skin. As we have already seen, however, when it is followed by an application of croton oil, cancer soon develops in the skin.

Among the agents which may play a part as co-carcinogens are diet, age and heredity. We shall also take a look at the subjects of chronic irritation and trauma.

Dietary Factors.—Very little is known about this subject, but one or two factors may be significant. When dimethylamino-azobenzene, an azo dye known as butter yellow because of its color, is given by mouth to rats fed on a diet of rice, cancer of the liver regularly develops. If, however, yeast or members of the vitamin B complex are added to the rice diet, no cancer occurs (Sugiura and Rhoads). This is the first instance in which experimental cancer has been prevented by a dietary constituent, deficiency of which acted as a conditioning factor. It would seem that the carcinogenic chemical took the place of the vitamin in the cell, thereby upsetting the regulatory mechanism. Choline deficiency in rats over a prolonged period may result in cancer (Copeland and Salmon). In 40 per cent of such animals carcinoma of the liver developed and in 38 per cent carcinoma of the lung. In those

peoples (Bantus, Javanese, Chinese) with a high incidence of cancer of the liver, the diet is very low in vitamins. It is possible that the cooking of fats at high temperatures may confer on them carcinogenic properties, for the higher the temperatures used in the fractionation of tar, the more highly carcinogenic are the products.

Age.—The age incidence of cancer is striking, for it occurs at the two ends of life. Perhaps the frequency in old age may be attributed to the long period of action required by carcinogens or the development of endocrine imbalance and other co-carcinogenic conditions with the passage of the years. In Western countries at least 50 per cent of the cases occur after the age of sixty-five, although the old age group constitutes only about 8 per cent of the total population. It is evident that even a small increase in the average age will result in a strikingly large increase in the over-all incidence of cancer. In backward countries the cancer incidence may be only one-tenth or less than that of more advanced countries, a decrease not due to the absence of carcinogens but to the fact that the average life expectancy may be only thirty years. To this must be added a low degree of accuracy in diagnosis, owing to lack of such aids as *x*-rays, biopsy, and autopsy. In families with a marked cancer predisposition the age of onset is much earlier, as in the family where a mother and three daughters died of cancer of the breast at the age of twenty-two, twenty-one, nineteen and fourteen years respectively. At the other end of life there is a group of tumors which appear to be congenital, being present at birth or developing in early childhood. Amongst these may be mentioned retinoblastoma of the eye, neuroblastoma of the adrenal medulla, and Wilms' tumor of the kidney. Other malignant conditions such as glioma of the brain, sarcoma of bone and leukemia may develop either in childhood or adult life.

Heredity.—In the experimental animal the genetic constitution may be a factor of supreme importance. Pure strains of animals of known heredity are as essential for cancer research as pure chemicals are for the chemist. The ease with which a tumor may be induced experimentally depends on the genetic make-up of the animal. There is no primary gene for cancer in general. The normal growth of each tissue and organ is under separate genetic control. So also each tissue is separately controlled in its tissue susceptibility to cancer. It is not possible to apply the results of breeding experiments in mice to man, but a few human tumors show so marked a familial tendency that every member of the family may die of the disease if he lives long enough. Such tumors are neuroblastoma of the retina and malignant papilloma of the large bowel. If both parents have suffered from cancer it is probable that at least some of the children will develop the disease. In one family cited by Warthin a cancerous mother and a cancerous father had six children; all died of cancer, as did the only grandchild. Thus the entire family of nine members in three generations died of cancer. The historic example of a familial tendency is that of Napoleon, who died at St. Helena from cancer of the stomach. His father, Charles Buonaparte, his grandfather Joseph Buonaparte, his brother Lucien, and his three sisters Pauline, Caroline and Eliza all died of cancer of the stomach.

Chronic Irritation.—In the past there has been no bogey-man of cancer against which more stones have been thrown than that of chronic irritation. The term is so vague that it is not easy to discuss it. There is the occasional instance in which cancer is preceded by and associated with the presence of a chronic irritant. Two examples which deserve mention are gall stones and cancer of the gallbladder on the one hand and the ova of schistosoma and cancer of the urinary bladder on the other. It is inconceivable that these inert objects could "irritate" the epithelium so as to make it neoplastic. An irritant causes inflammation, not cancer, but prolonged destruction of tissue demands constant replacement of parts, and it is possible that when this is continued over an extended period the regulating mechanism may become upset with resulting neoplasia. Such constant destruction and repair with consequent unstable cellular equilibrium may occur in ulcers of the mouth, the tongue and the stomach.

Trauma.—The relation of a single trauma to the development of cancer is very impor-tant from the point of veiw of compensation, but it presents an almost insuperable problem. When a tumor develops the patient often recalls having received a blow on that part not long before. This, of course, is no proof. It is not really possible ever to prove that trauma is the cause of a tumor, because it is impossible to be certain that the tumor was not there before. Only the experimental production of a tumor in an animal by a single trauma would constitute proof, and this has never been done. When a tumor appears shortly after the part has been traumatized it means that the patient's attention has been directed to the part by the injury, or that hemorrhage into the tumor has caused an increase in the size of the tumor. At the same time it should not be denied that injury may cause cell destruction followed by regeneration, and this may serve as a promoter where an initiating carcinogen has already produced a condition of latent cancer. The most likely instances where this may occur are sarcoma of bone and gliomas of the brain. Finally, wishful thinking cannot be excluded, even though there be no conscious desire to mislead the doctor. It is surely significant that the vast majority of instances of cancer supposedly due to trauma have been workmen's compensation or insurance cases.

TUMOR IMMUNITY

In recent years great interest has been aroused in the subject of tumor immunity particularly in the experimental animal, but it is a subject in which it is very difficult to think clearly. At least that is what I have found. In spite of that, it may prove to be a field of profound clinical importance in the fight to control, and, even better, to prevent cancer.

The idea of an immunological concept of cancer originated at the beginning of this century by the observation that mice in whom tumor transplants regressed spontaneously were immune to subsequent transplants of the same tumor. The experiments were performed at a time when we knew nothing about the difference between auto-immunity and iso-immunity, and were not aware of the importance of using pure bred strains. Much of the immunological reaction was against the tissue of the foreign animal rather than against the tumor. Now that pure inbred strains of mice are available there has been a keen reawakening of interest.

With the use of these inbred strains (mating of brother to sister) which have the same normal genetic and antigenic constitution it is becoming apparent that immunological differences between normal and malignant cells really do exist. The idea has arisen that malignancy may consist in the *loss* of cellular components which are supposed to control normal cell multiplication, although in virus tumors it is possible that additional components may be added. It has been found that prior immunization of one strain with normal tissue from another identical animal may protect the host from otherwise fatal tumor grafts from the partner strain. There is an apparent loss of iso-antigens by tumors in the course of serial transplantations.

Applying Burnet's concept of individual "self markers" by which a cell is recognized by its neighbours, Green has suggested an antigenic theory of cancer, which seeks to explain the ability of cancer cells to infiltrate the surrounding tissue by failure of the antigenic mechanism of the body to "recognize" the cell once it has lost certain marker antigens. Loss of a series of such marker antigens, one by one, may confer an increasing independence upon a cell, so that finally it will infiltrate beyond the normal physiological boundaries without arousing an adequate defense reaction.

A number of widely diverse observations support the concept of the development of some form of immunity against cancer cells. An "immunity" develops towards further tumor implants in experimental animals undergoing chemotherapy or other forms of treatment that result in complete regression of the tumor. Complement-fixing antibodies have been demonstrated in patients, most of whom had primary lesions which responded favorably to irradiation or which could be completely removed (Graham and Graham).

The injection of human cancer into animals has been reported to excite the production of specific antibodies against cancer cells but not against normal cells, due evidently to a difference in protein composition (Witeb-

sky). It would appear that the passive transfer of a tumor-inhibiting agent is possible by serum injections from resistant rats immunized by repeated implantations of tumor in susceptible tumor-bearers. The possibilities of applying such techniques to the treatment of human cancer is being actively pursued at the present time.

So far we have confined our discussion to the behaviour of cancer cells implanted into laboratory animals. *Human tumor transplants into human subjects* have been made in a group of volunteers among convicts at the Ohio State Penitentiary, Columbus, Ohio. The implantation was made into normal healthy subjects and also into men suffering from cancer (Southam *et al.*). In the *healthy volunteers* the implants excited an inflammatory reaction, and when the lesions were excised one week later they were found to consist of inflammatory tissue with no cancer cells or in the occasional case only a few moribund ones. The destructive action was even more rapid when a second implantation was made. In 13 out of 15 *cancer patients* on whom the implantation was made, the tumors continued to grow until they were removed in the course of from one to six weeks. The only factor associated with immunity in which cancer patients were demonstrated to be deficient in comparison with persons who were well was *properdin*, the natural defense agent in the blood which has already been discussed on page 98. Is it possible that the clinical cases of cancer which we see are those in which a natural immunological defense has failed?

Heterologous Transplantation.—All the early experimental work on cancer was done on the transplantation of tumors which occurred spontaneously in animals. With the discovery of the chemical carcinogens by means of which new tumors could be induced in the experimental animal, interest in transplantability languished. In the past it was only possible to transplant a tumor to another member of the same species (homo-transplantability), and because of this strict specificity heterotransplantability with human material was not possible. The demonstration that human cancer can be transferred to such animals as the rat, guinea pig and rabbit and maintained over successive generations has reawakened interest in the subject. The obstacle of specificity was overcome in three different ways: (1) Greene took the first step when he grew human cancer in the anterior chamber of the eye of the guinea pig and rabbit. The brain can also be used for the same purpose. (2) Tissue resistance can be overcome by preliminary radiation of the animal. This destroys the lymphoid tissue, which seems to play some part in the immunity mechanism. (3) Strict specificity can be broken down by the administration of cortisone, so that transfer of cancer could be made from rat to mouse and from man to mouse (Green and Whiteley, Toolan). The cortisone appears to depress antibody production to heterologous antigens in the transplanted tumor. This may be due to the great reduction in the number of lymphocytes which are known to produce antibodies. The ability to grow human cancer in the laboratory animal is a great step forward, which must prove of marked value in the experimental study of the restraint of malignant growth by chemotherapy and in the large-scale screening of new chemical agents against the disease.

Greene considers that the work on heterotransplantation demonstrates that "cancer is not a sudden transformation of normal cells but, on the contrary, represents a final step in a developmental process. Throughout the process, the tumor may remain static morphologically, but it does undergo profound biological changes. The most dramatic of these occurs near the end of its course, and consists of the attainment of the ability to metastasize. Coincidentally, the tumor attains the ability to grow on heterologous transfer." If this concept is accepted, heterologous transplantability and the power to metastasize go hand in hand.

Most instances of success in heterologous transplantation have occurred in animals (1) whose defense mechanisms have not been fully established, or (2) have been weakened by cortisone or radiation, or (3) at sites of inoculation such as the eye, brain or cheek pouch of the hamster where the defense mechanisms are at their lowest.

Heterologous transplantation is not possible with benign tumors nor even with preinvasive cancer, the latter fact recalling Green's ideas about the relationship of antigenic properties to invasion. In this connection we must note that the property of heterotransplantability is also shared by embryonic tissue. This brings up the concept of "self" or "recognition" already discussed in relation to auto-immunity in Chapter 5. The identity of reaction to foreign tissue shown by both embryonic and neoplastic tissue certainly suggests some common factor. It would appear that the step from embryonic tissue to cancer is a relatively short one, and probably concerned with the process of differentiation.

The acceptance of cancer transplants from another animal may be called immunological tolerance. Such tolerance may be acquired before or soon after birth at a period when antibody production has not yet begun. If cancer cells of a tumor which is resistant to transplantation be implanted in embryonic mice, and the same resistant tumor is implanted in the animal some time later, it will now grow well, because it encounters no defense mechanism.

Spontaneous Regression of Cancer.—We are apt to think of a cancer as growing continuously, progressively and at a uniform rate. This is true of a tissue culture of cancer cells, but it is not true of neoplasia either in the experimental animal or in man. Even though the growth potential of the cancer cells may remain uniform, the condition of the environment may change with consequent damage to the viability of the cells. When the blood supply is inadequate, the cancer cells will die, and it is common knowledge that malignant tumors often present large areas of necrosis for this reason. The extensive fibrosis seen in some cancers of the breast and of the stomach represents areas of repair where the balance has been turned against the malignant cells.

The metabolic balance may be upset in other and more subtle ways. A long period of quiescence may be followed by one of rapid growth. This is far more likely to be due to a change in the environment than a change in the tumor. The accelerated growth of breast cancer during pregnancy has long been recognized. The controlling effect of a variety of hormones on the growth of certain tumors has already been discussed

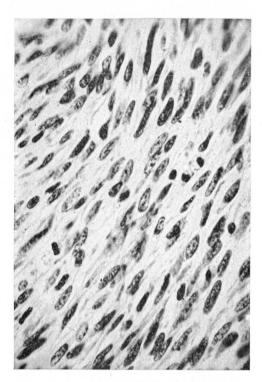

Fig. 96.—Myosarcoma of thigh showing several mitotic figures. This biopsy was taken when the patient was two-and-half months old. The neoplasm underwent spontaneous regression and the patient was alive and well thirteen years later. (Kindness of D. W. Penner.)

in relation to carcinogenesis. This knowledge has been put to therapeutic use in the control of cancer of the breast and prostate by the administration of estrogens and androgens, by castration, by adrenalectomy, and even by hypophysectomy. These measures are often followed by marked objective as well as subjective improvement, the metastases disappearing, the pathological fractures healing, the bones becoming recalcified.

In addition to these examples of therapeutic regression we must recognize the possibility of *spontaneous* regression. It is not uncommon for the rate of growth of a tumor to slow down, sometimes to a marked degree, and in rare cases the growth may stop completely, and the neoplasm, both primary and secondary, may resolve and eventually disappear. A number of such cases have been reported in the literature over the years. I

have collected and reported a series. A boy aged two and one half months was found to have a tumor of the thigh. Biopsy showed this to be a myosarcoma with numerous mitotic figures (Fig. 96). There was radiographic evidence of erosion of the femur by the tumor. Treatment was refused by the parents. The boy was seen again five years later, at which time he was in perfect health with no evidence of tumor (Penner). In many of these cases there has been partial surgical removal, palliative radiation therapy, or the occurrence of some acute bacterial infection. In all of these instances there seems to have been some change in the immunological relationship between the tumor and the host, activated possibly by some change in the protein complexes of the malignant cells. It may be regarded as the converse of the depression of immunological resistance induced by the use of cortisone. One particularly remarkable and suggestive example is reported by Stewart. The patient was a woman with an extensive inoperable myosarcoma of the uterus which had spread throughout the pelvis. The lesion was treated by means of radium bomb, but without any effect. Just before completion of the treatment a sudden and dramatic change occurred almost in the matter of a few hours. The patient developed a high fever, an urticarial rash, and a marked eosinophilia, all symptoms of an allergic reaction, at the same time losing several kilograms of tumor and ascitic fluid in the course of a few days. The tumor disappeared completely, and the patient was alive and well ten years later. Stewart suggests that some alteration took place in the tumor protein, that the patient became sensitized to this protein, and thus developed an intense immune reaction of the Shwartzman phenomenon type.

Some of the most striking examples of spontaneous regression are afforded by neuroblastoma, a highly malignant tumor of the adrenal medulla occurring in early childhood. In one case which I studied an adrenal neuroblastoma was removed in part from a child aged nine months at the Hospital for Sick Children, Toronto, but the remainder had to be left in the abdomen, yet the child, now seventeen years of age, is as active and well as her twin sister. In other cases distant metastases as well as the primary tumor have regressed and disappeared (Bodian). Sometimes surgical removal of the primary tumor is followed by the disappearance of secondary growths. This is perhaps best seen in carcinoma of the thyroid and in ovarian cancer with peritoneal metastases.

The object of the foregoing discussion is to indicate that the cancer problem is perhaps not quite so hopeless as it is customary to believe, that the body can develop some degree of immunity, either general or local, and that in the not distant future it may be possible by means of some chemical or hormonal agent, perhaps different for each variety of cancer, to so influence either the cancer cells or the environment in which they exist that the balance in favor of the body is restored and recovery becomes possible.

CHARACTERISTICS OF MALIGNANCY

In deciding the all-important question of the malignancy of a tumor it is necessary to consider both the *histology*, that is to say the *arrangement* of the tumor cells and their relation to the surrounding normal tissue, and the *cytology*, that is to say the character of the tumor cells and especially the *character* of their nucleus and nucleolus. Malignancy has two main functional qualities, invasion and the formation of metastases, and one main structural quality, anaplasia. Unfortunately none of the eight characteristics enumerated below is invariable, so that any one of them may be absent in a given malignant tumor. This will be better appreciated when we consider the specific forms of tumors in the next chapter, and even more in our study of the tumors of individual organs in the second part of the book.

1. *Invasion.*—A malignant tumor infiltrates the surrounding tissue. It sends claws into it like a crab. Indeed cancer is derived from the Latin word, *cancrum*, meaning a crab. An innocent tumor grows by expansion like a balloon, and is usually separated from surrounding structures by a capsule of compressed tissue. But a benign glioma blends imperceptibly with its surroundings, and an angioma infiltrates without being malignant. Conversely, a malignant tumor in its initial stage may be a non-invasive carcinoma or carcinoma in situ.

2. *Recurrence.*—This clinical term indicates that the tumor has reappeared after removal or radiotherapy. It does not mean that a new tumor has originated, but rather that some of the cancer cells have escaped injury and have multiplied to form another mass. Cancer cells may remain dormant for many years and then begin to grow again. The proof of this fact will be seen when the question of the spread of tumors is considered. There is always the possibility of the development of another tumor. Thus a cancer of the lip may be removed completely, but a second cancer may arise in another part of the lip some years later.

3. *Metastases.*—A malignant growth sooner or later sets up secondary growths or metastases in the lymph nodes which drain the part and in distant organs. Even here there are exceptions, for malignant gliomas do not behave in this way. The formation and distribution of metastases are considered in detail in relation to the spread of tumors.

4. *Rapidity of Growth.*—Rapid growth is characteristic of malignant in contrast to benign tumors, but to this there are many exceptions. Some cancers, especially in old people, are of very slow growth. If a benign tumor should start to grow quickly it should arouse suspicion of a malignant change. The presence of numerous *mitotic figures* is suggestive of malignancy. The more rapid the growth, the more numerous the mitoses.

5. *Nuclear Changes.*—The reproduction of a cell is governed by the nucleus, and in particular by the nucleoproteins of the chromatin. Ultraviolet spectroscopy shows that there is intense activity of this mechanism in cancer cells. For this reason the pathologist pays special attention to the nucleus in determining the question of malignancy of a tumor. The nucleus of a cancer cell is likely to be large and hyperchromatic, so that it stains intensely with hematoxylin, or the chromatin network may be coarse (Fig. 105). The nucleus varies much in size and shape, and the cells themselves show similar variation. The nucleolus is large in proportion to the size of the nucleus, an important feature which may be more evi-

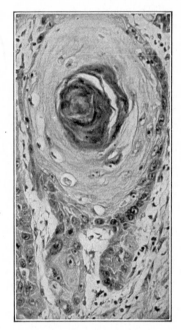

Fig. 97, Grade 1.

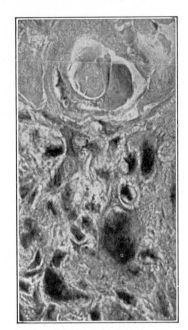

Fig. 98, Grade 2.

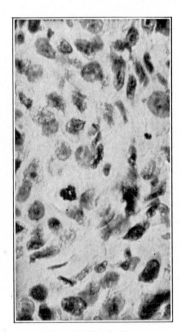

Fig. 99, Grade 3.

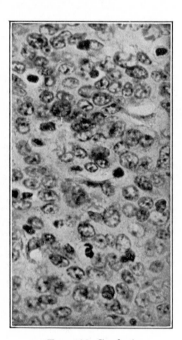

Fig. 100, Grade 4.

Figs. 97 to 100.—The four grades of epidermoid carcinoma.
Differentiation is complete in Fig. 97; Fig. 99 is extremely anaplastic with many mitotic figures. Fig. 97, × 200; Figs. 98 to 100, × 500.

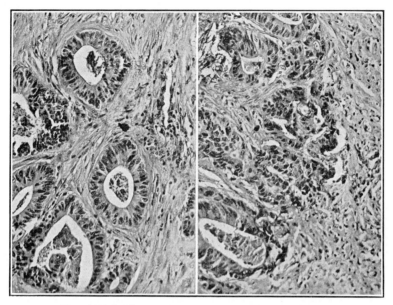

FIG. 101, Grade 1.   FIG. 102, Grade 2.

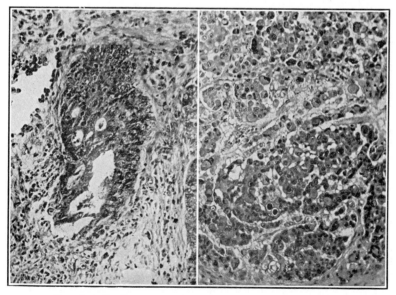

FIG. 103, Grade 3.   FIG. 104, Grade 4.

FIGS. 101 to 104.—The four grades of adenocarcinoma. × 125.

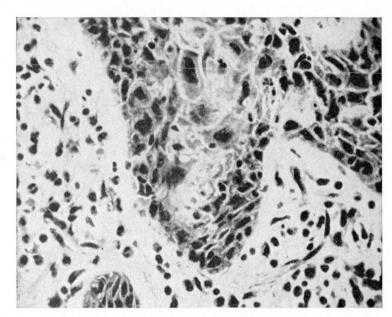

FIG. 105.—Highly malignant epidermoid carcinoma of skin. The cells are irregular
in size and shape, and the nuclei are intensely hyperchomatic. × 420.

dent in frozen sections of the unfixed tissue or in wet films (Fig. 84, p. 176). Micro-incineration shows an increased inorganic content of the nucleus.

6. *Anaplasia.*—A malignant tumor fails to reproduce the structure of the tissue from which it grows, whereas an innocent tumor may reproduce it perfectly. This lack of differentiation is called anaplasia, a concept first introduced by Hansemann in 1893. The more anaplastic the tumor, the more malignant it is likely to be.

7. *Loss of Polarity.*—Epithelial cells which are arranged in sheets show a regular polarity, by which is meant the arrangement of the cells with their long axis perpendicular to the surface of the sheet. One of the early signs of a malignant change is loss of the normal polarity, so that the cells now present what may be termed a jumbled arrangement in relation to the surface.

8. *Fatal Outcome.*—A malignant tumor, as its name implies, tends to kill the patient wherever it grows, even in the hand or foot. An innocent tumor will only cause death if it happens to grow in a vital organ.

Grading of Tumors.—The degree of malignancy depends mainly on loss of differentia-

tion (anaplasia), coupled with such features as hyperchromatism and the number of mitotic figures. On this basis it has become the practice in some laboratories to divide some of the carcinomas into four groups according to their microscopic appearance, group 1 being the most differentiated and benign, grade 4 the most anaplastic and malignant (Broders). Epidermoid carcinoma (Figs. 96–99) and adenocarcinoma (Figs. 100–103) are the types of cancer which lend themselves best to grading. The chief value of grading is that it serves to indicate those cases (grades 3 and 4) which may be expected to respond well to radiotherapy. The method has severe limitations, and generalizations based on it are dangerous, for a tumor may not show a uniform structure, and some parts may be much more differentiated than others, so that a biopsy may be misleading. The clinician must not take grading too seriously in determining the prognosis of a malignant tumor, but must consider the age of the patient, the extent of the disease, its duration, its rate of growth, and, most important of all, involvement of the regional lymph nodes.

DIFFERENTIAL CHARACTERISTICS OF BENIGN AND MALIGNANT TUMORS

Characteristics	Malignant	Benign
Nuclear changes.	Large; hyperchromatic (DNA); much variation in size and shape; nucleolus much enlarged.	Appearance more similar to normal cells in tissue of origin.
Cytoplasmic changes.	Variation in cell size; decreased cytoplasmic-nuclear ratio (RNA).	Less apparent or absent.
Differentiation.	Varying degrees of anaplasia.	Well differentiated.
Polarity.	Lost.	Maintained.
Rate of growth.	Rapid; mitotic figures.	Slow; no mitoses.
Method of growth.	Invasion and infiltration.	Expansion; usually encapsulated.
Metastatic spread.	Usual.	Never.
Recurrence after excision.	Not infrequent.	Rare.
Prognosis.	Frequently poor.	Uniformly good.

PRECANCEROUS CONDITIONS

The term precancerous is used in two senses, one clinical, the other pathological, the latter being known as carcinoma in situ. By precancerous the surgeon indicates that in his experience the lesion, at present benign, may become malignant. Long-continued chronic irritation comes into this category, and such conditions as gall stones, leukoplakia of the mouth, syphilitic glossitis, etc. come to mind. In these conditions a co-carcinogen may be at work. Certain benign tumors have a marked tendency to become malignant and might therefore be regarded as precancerous. Familiar examples are pigmented nevus of the foot and papillary tumors of the large bowel and bladder. Lockhart-Mummery has drawn attention to the three stages through which the mucous membrane of the rectum may pass. First, there are localized patches of hyperplasia, invisible to the naked eye, affecting an extensive area of the bowel. Secondly, a crop of adenomata appear over this area of hyperplasia. Thirdly, the development of carci-

noma in one of these adenomata. (These changes are well illustrated in Fig. 121, page 228).

Carcinoma in Situ.—An important step in the fight against cancer is the recognition by the pathologist of the very earliest beginnings of the malignant process. When metastases have occurred it is too late. When invasion of the deeper tissues can be recognized it may be too late. But when the malignant change is still cytological rather than histological the disease is curable. This state of affairs is known as carcinoma in situ or preinvasive carcinoma. The three cytological features which indicate this condition are *nuclear change, anaplasia,* and *loss of cellular polarity* (Fig. 106). The picture at once strikes the observer as being atypical and bizarre. The cells appear to be becoming restless. My associate in Toronto, Dr. W. Anderson, suggested to me the graphic metaphor of a number of wild horses running around in a coral looking for a way to get out. The question, is, must they get out in the long run? Is the condition irreversible, going on in-

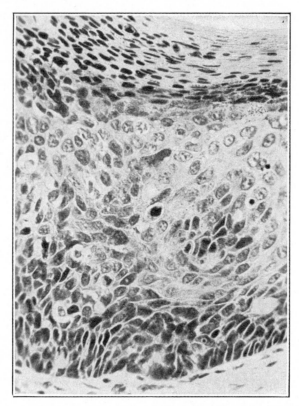

FIG. 106.—Preinvasive carcinoma (carcinoma in situ) of the skin. Note the hyperchromatic nuclei, jumbled arrangement of the cells (loss of polarity), mitoses, and impression of restlessness. There is lack of keratinization in the stratum corneum with abnormal preservation of nuclei. × 375.

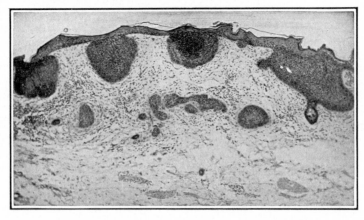

FIG. 107.—Multiple foci of independent growth in a rodent ulcer. × 45.

thoracic duct explains those cases in which cancer of the gastrointestinal tract is associated with pulmonary metastases whilst the liver remains clear. Involvement of the supraclavicular nodes on the left side of the neck is occasionally due to massive growth of tumor throughout the length of the duct, but usually to tumor emboli from the cisterna chyli lodging behind the valves at the termination of the duct, with extension along the lymphatics to the nodes.

The importance of the thoracic duct in the spread of malignant disease was first recognized by Virchow, and indeed the supraclavicular group of nodes goes by his name. The frequency of involvement of the duct is only revealed when the entire duct together with Virchow's nodes is dissected out and removed at autopsy, as has been done by Young (Fig. 110). In carcinoma the duct was found to be involved in over 40 per cent of cases, and in malignant lymphoma in 62 per cent. Most of the involved nodes were not palpable.

3. **Blood Spread.**—Cancer cells may reach the blood either by way of the thoracic duct or by direct invasion of the blood vessels. The veins are invaded with great readiness, but the arteries very rarely. The chief reason for this striking difference appears to be the fact that lymphatics frequently penetrate the walls of the larger veins and form a plexus reaching to the sub-endothelial region; this is not true of the arteries (Figs. 111A and 111B). A thrombus forms over the eroded endothelium, and this is invaded by tumor cells. It is this combination of thrombus and tumor which becomes detached and forms the tumor emboli that are likely to result in metastases. Clumps of tumor cells unconnected with thrombus may form pure emboli, but they may not give rise to metastases owing to inability to become colonized at the site of impaction. Tumor cells may be demonstrated in the peripheral blood, a matter which is discussed more fully in a later section.

The motility of the part may favor the formation of metastases. The continual contraction and expansion of organs such as the stomach and lung tend to squeeze tumor cells into the capillaries. In the appendix the tumor known as carcinoid occurs in old

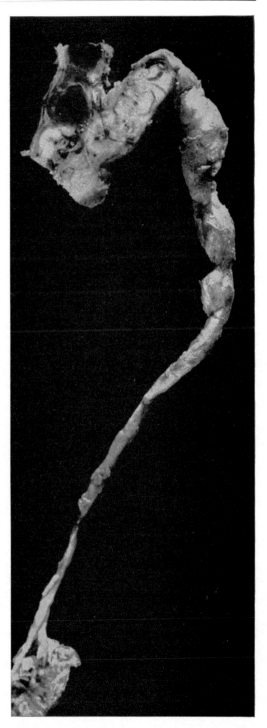

FIG. 110.—Spread of bronchogenic carcinoma along the thoracic duct. The Tumor has extended into the jugular and innominate veins where thrombosis has occurred. (Young, courtesy of Am. Jour. Path.)

14

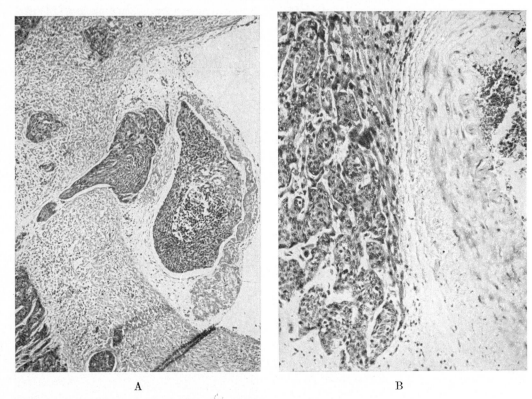

A   B

Fig. 111.—*A*, Tumor invading wall of vein via a lymphatic and surrounded by a thrombus. The darker material is the tumor. × 70. *B*, The same tumor failing to penetrate wall of artery. × 325.

scarred tissue in which there is no movement, and it remains localized, but in the motile small intestine it metastasizes to the liver.

The site of metastases is governed largely although not entirely by the anatomical distribution of blood vessels, especially veins. Cancers of organs drained by the portal circulation will metastasize for the most part to the liver. Cancers of the kidney, uterus and limbs, parts drained by the systemic veins, metastasize as a rule to the lungs.

Unfortunately it not infrequently happens that tumors do not behave according to rule and metastases occur in unexpected places. A few illustrations will suffice.

Four groups of veins may be invaded, the portal, pulmonary, systemic and vertebral groups. The consequences in each case will be different.

The *portal system of veins* is invaded by tumors of the gastrointestinal tract and pancreas. Secondary tumors of the liver are

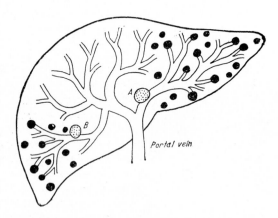

Fig. 112.—Diagram of intrahepatic metastasis. At *A* an initial metastatic (or primary) growth has invaded a main branch of the portal vein and produced daughter metastases throughout the corresponding lobe. At *B* an initial metastasis has invaded a peripheral branch vein and produced daughter metastases in a correspondingly restricted region of liver. (Willis, R. A.: *The Spread of Tumors in the Human Body*, courtesy of Butterworth & Co., Ltd.)

therefore very common. This does not, however, explain the incredible number of metastases which are often found in that organ compared, for instance, with the kidney or spleen. The explanation depends on the fact that the numerous branches of the portal vein are readily invaded by cells from the metastases and that the arterial distribution of the portal vein results in widespread dissemination of these cells with the formation of further metastases (Fig. 112). In this way successive generations of fresh tumors are born. The hepatic veins may also be invaded, with resulting metastatic tumor formation in the lungs.

The *pulmonary veins* provide another method of dissemination. Not only a primary bronchogenic carcinoma but also metastatic growths in the lung may penetrate the wall of a pulmonary vein and thus reach the left side of the heart and the systemic circulation. It can be shown experimentally that tumor cells readily traverse the pulmonary capillaries, but it is tumor emboli rather than individual tumor cells which set up metastases. The filter of the lung is likely to hold up emboli, so that the lungs share with the liver pride of place as regards frequency of secondary growths. Tumor emboli, however, are not synonymous with metastases. Tumor emboli in the lungs often die out, as M. B. Schmidt showed many years ago.

The *vertebral system of veins*, figured by Vesalius in 1543, adequately described by Breschet in 1828, but its clinical significance first clearly demonstrated by Batson in 1940, serves to explain many enigmas of tumor spread, particularly with regard to the very common involvement of the lumbar region of the spine in cancer of the prostate. These veins pass up inside the spinal canal and anastomose with sacral, lumbar, abdominal and thoracic veins, as well as with veins penetrating the vertebral bodies and cranial bones (Fig. 113). There are frequent reversals of flow in this vast intercommunicating system, the result of coughing, straining and increase of intra-abdominal pressure, for these veins are without valves. During these reversals a pathway up and down the spine exists which does not involve the heart and lungs, a system which is more a lagoon with occasional ebb and flow than a channel

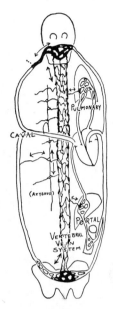

Fig. 113.—Vertebral system of veins and its connections. (Batson, courtesy of Ann. Surg.)

of streaming blood. Flow takes place into the system during coughing, serving to explain the high incidence of cerebral metastases in cancer of the lung and of cerebral abscess secondary to lung abscess. When cancer cells are injected into the femoral vein of rats or rabbits the resulting tumors are confined to the lungs. If, however, the abdominal pressure is momentarily elevated, tumors in the lung are rare, but common in the spine, the tumor cells being present in the lumen of the vertebral veins (Coman and de Long).

There has been marked difference of opinion as to whether large clumps of cells or individual tumor cells are responsible for setting up pulmonary metastases. When tumor cells are injected into a systemic vein, clumps of cells appear more likely to colonize in the pulmonary vessels than single cells. A truer picture is given by *spontaneous* blood-borne metastases in laboratory animals. When a subcutaneous transplant of an anaplastic carcinoma is made in the mouse, the tumor emboli are found to consist of single cells or at most of half-a-dozen cells (Baserga and Saffiotti). The cells lodge in the pulmonary vessels by adhering to the endothelium of the arterioles (Fig. 114), of the

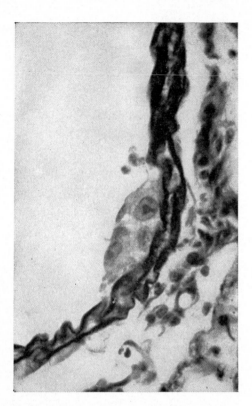

Fig. 114.—Tumor cell embolus adhering to the wall of a pulmonary artery; Weigert and Van Gieson stains; × 600. (Baserga and Saffiotti, courtesy of Arch. Pathology.)

capillaries. The tumor cells seem to have a thromboplastic property, and the thrombus which forms around them appears to act as a good medium for their growth. Metastases arise more frequently from tumor emboli lodged in the capillaries than those arrested in the arterioles. The process of metastasis formation has actually been observed *in vivo* through a window in a rabbit's ear following the slow injection of cancer cells stained with trypan blue into an arteriole (Wood). It would appear that the most decisive feature in the production of metastases is not the diameter of the capillaries, but the ability of the embolic cells to adhere securely · to the vascular endothelium (Wood *et al.*). Adhesion to the capillary endothelium is quickly followed by intracapillary thrombosis around the cancer cells, and in a few hours the vessel wall is invaded. It should be added that the vast majority of the cells die, approximately

4,000 being required to produce a metastasis in the lung.

4. **Spread by Natural Passages.**—Tumor cells may be carried along such passages as the bronchus, bowel and ureter, and it is conceivable that they might become implanted on an epithelial surface and form a new growth. This might explain the simultaneous occurrence of the same type of tumor in the renal pelvis and the bladder. It is more probable, however, that the cells have passed down lymphatics in the wall of the tube, or that two independent tumors have developed at the same time.

5. **Spread Through Serous Cavities.**—This method, known as transcelomic spread, is the explanation given for the frequent transfer of cancer cells from the stomach to the ovaries, rectal serosa, etc. Small implantations on the peritoneum can often be traced between stomach and ovary. There is nothing inherently improbable about this concept, but to the writer the arguments in favor of spread along lymphatics carry greater weight. One place where the passive transfer and implantation of tumor cells can be accepted without reserve is the cranial cavity, where there are no lymphatics. Malignant glial tumors shed cells into the ventricles and subarachnoid space, throughout which they may be carried by the cerebrospinal fluid and form multiple secondary growths.

6. **Inoculation.**—Every surgeon knows the possible danger of transferring tumor cells by inoculation into the surrounding tissue in the course of an operation for cancer. Instruments and gloves which may have become contaminated by cutting into the tumor to obtain tissue for a biopsy are not used again. Even the basin of water in which the surgeon dips his gloved hands may carry cells, which can be seen in a centrifuged specimen. In one case a carcinoma of the breast was removed and a skin flap was taken from the thigh to close the large gap. A few months later a nodule having the same structure as the breast cancer developed in the scar in the thigh. Everything had been changed between the two incisions with the exception of the contents of the basin which contamined the fresh gloves (Brandes *et al.*).

Distribution of Metastases.—From what

has been said about methods of spread the reader may think that the spread of tumors is well understood. This is far from the case. Every week the pathologist in a large hospital encounters examples which he cannot explain. Three carcinomas of the stomach seem alike in every respect, yet the first will remain localized apart from involvement of a few regional lymph nodes, in the second case the liver may be riddled with tumors, whilst in the third the liver may escape but the brain and other viscera may be the site of metastases. Endless examples could be given. There is certainly no relation between the size of the primary tumor and the occurrence of metastases. Nor is there any necessary relation between the number of tumor emboli and the number of metastases. Others as well as myself have observed the occasional case where the viscera are filled with innumerable emboli but secondary growths have not developed. The fate of the emboli may depend on chemical and metabolic factors. The *soil* must be considered as well as the *seed*, a truth which is self-evident in the case of transplanted tumors in the experimental animal. In the words of Coman, whose contributions to the subject are so noteworthy, the distribution of metastases is a problem which has been stared at rather than investigated.

The immunity of skeletal muscle to metastases is remarkable. And yet when a suspension of carcinoma cells is injected into the femoral artery of an animal there is massive involvement of the muscles of the leg (Eisenberg). Injection of the same material into the femoral vein results in massive tumors only in the lungs. Malignant gliomas spread only by infiltration and implantation; they do not metastasize. This is probably due to non-invasion of the blood vessels and to lack of any connection between the perivascular lymph spaces and extra-cranial lymphatics, because when gliomas are implanted intraperitoneally or into subcutaneous tissue they grow rapidly (Zimmermann).

Tumor emboli may develop quickly, as in the liver, or they may die out, as in the muscles, or they may remain after removal of the primary tumor and only begin to multiply many years later. The best example of a prolonged latent period is that of melanoma of the eye; metastases may develop in the liver twenty years after the primary tumor has been removed. Hadfield's expressive term, the *dormant cancer cell*, gives a good picture of the state of affairs during the latent period. Dormant cells are "malignant cells which, although remaining alive in the tissues for relatively long periods show no evidence of multiplication during this time, yet retain their former and vigorous capacity to multiply." Hadfield kept a mouse sarcoma for nearly five years at a temperature of $-70°$ C., yet six days after grafting into a mouse it formed a large mass. In such cases there must be a temporary mitotic arrest, surely a striking example of dormancy or hibernation.

Metastasis of cancer to cancer, although in itself a great rarity, provides some support for the soil hypothesis. For some obscure reason about two-thirds of the cases have been examples of bronchogenic carcinoma metastasizing to renal carcinoma. I have seen only two examples of the condition, one in Toronto, the other in Vancouver, and in both of these a bronchogenic carcinoma metastasized to a renal carcinoma (Fig. 115). Of 5 examples reported by Rabson and his associates in 1954, 4 were to renal carcinoma, 2 coming from the lung and 2 from the prostate. The first case reported in 1902 was to renal carcinoma. This would suggest that the soil in the renal tumor was particularly favorable to the growth of metastases, especially those coming from the lung.

The subject of the spread of tumors is obviously one of great importance to the surgeon. It has endless ramifications which cannot be discussed further here. For a full account of this fascinating subject the reader is referred to that mine of information, *The Spread of Tumors in the Human Body* by Willis.

As we shall see in the next section, cancer cells can be demonstrated in the peripheral blood stream in many cases even on sporadic examination. Indeed it seems possible that all cancers, including those with good prognosis, spread early by the venous blood. If this is true, it is evident that the soil is of equal importance with the seed. One of the most striking demonstrations of this fact is provided by the work of Fisher and Fisher.

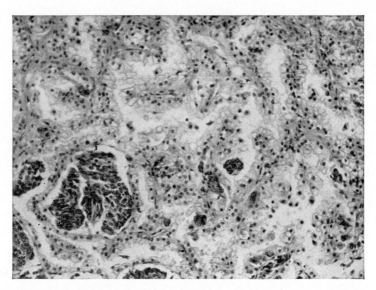

Fig. 115.—Bronchogenic carcinoma metastasizing to carcinoma of the kidney. × 134.
(Boyd's *Pathology for the Surgeon*, courtesy of W. B. Saunders Company).

These investigators showed that when 250 Walker tumor cells are injected into the mesenteric vein of the rat the number of hepatic metastases (20 per cent) was no greater after eight weeks than at the end of two weeks. After laparotomy and manipulation of the liver at the end of two weeks, however, in the course of twenty-one days 84 per cent of the animals developed tumors in the liver. Even the subcutaneous injection of chloroform in mineral oil raised the incidence to 60 per cent. With repeated laparotomy and manipulation of the liver there were liver metastases in almost 100 per cent of cases. It would appear that tumor cells may remain dormant (latent) for long periods, eventually to be triggered into growth by trauma, a rather sobering thought for the surgeon. It is evident that cancer cells can be converted from a state of "peaceful coexistence" to one of active growth by changed conditions.

LABORATORY DIAGNOSIS

Histological Examination.—When a tumor is removed by the surgeon in the operating room it is sent to the laboratory, where it is fixed, embedded in paraffin, sectioned and stained. It is on the examination of these sections that the final diagnosis is made as to whether or not the lesion is a malignant one. The pathologist studies the sections, paying special attention to (1) the cytological appearance of the tumor cells, and (2) the relation of these cells to the surrounding tissue, especially as regards the invasion of this tissue by the tumor cells. The pathologist should be supplied by the surgeon with a few pertinent clinical notes. For instance, when he examines the cervix it may make all the difference to his judgment of a section if he knows that the patient is pregnant, for the changes produced by hormonal stimulation may simulate those of early neoplasia.

The Biopsy.—Under some circumstances, particularly in the case of breast and intra-abdominal tumors, it may be highly desirable for the surgeon to have a report on the nature of the lesion *during the course of the operation*, so that he may determine the extent of his subsequent procedure. For this purpose the *frozen section* on unfixed tissue stained with polychrome methylene blue enables a "rush diagnosis" to be made in the course of a very few minutes. Some pathologists prefer to fix the tissue momentarily in hot formalin, stain the frozen section with hematoxylin and eosin, then dehydrate, clear and mount as with the customary paraffin technique.

The biopsy method of frozen section is invaluable, particularly in the case of breast tumors. It has, however, limitations which should be recognized, particularly by the surgeon. The frozen sections are twice the thickness of those of the paraffin method, so that fine cytological detail is less distinct. The examination of several blocks from different parts of the tumor is seldom possible in the rushed atmosphere of the operating room. Finally, some tissues do not lend themselves readily to this technique. If frozen sections of a bone lesion in the leg are of an ambiguous character, and the word of the pathologist is going to influence the surgeon as to whether he should merely excise the lesion or should perform a hind-quarter amputation, speed of diagnosis should be sacrificed, and twenty-four hours should be allowed to elapse so that the pathologist can give the most reliable opinion on multiple paraffin sections. The surgeon and the pathologist would both agree with this judgment if the lesion were in his own leg.

It must not be supposed from what has been said that frozen sections of unfixed tissue made *under ideal conditions* necessarily suffer from the disadvantages indicated above. What can be done with the method in the hands of a master may be judged from the illustrations in Dockerty's article, but it is from this article that the phrase "under ideal conditions" is taken. Very valuable practical suggestions regarding technique will be found in that paper.

Exfoliative Cytology.—Cancer cells lose the stickiness or adhesiveness characteristic of normal cells, so that they tend to be cast off or exfoliated from a surface very early in the disease, even in the preinvasive stage. The cells are found in exudates, secretions, washings and scrapings. The material may be examined in smears by the method which Papanicolaou introduced for the study of vaginal secretion, or it may be coagulated into a block, embedded in paraffin, and sectioned as a tissue.

This diagnostic method, often referred to loosely and inaccurately as cytology, has opened up new vistas in the early diagnosis of cancer. Its greatest value at present is in cancer of the cervix and bronchus, where it is possible to obtain fresh cells which do not show the misleading changes that develop so soon after exfoliation. The balloon technique in the stomach serves the same purpose. The method is of limited value in suspected cancer of the bladder, kidney and prostate. It has been used for the study of pleural and peritoneal effusions long before the present vogue for cytological examination. The errors are false negatives and false positives, but these cannot be discussed here.

Exfoliative cytology has its greatest value in very early cancers where the lesion is readily overlooked with ordinary methods of investigation. Where the cancer is advanced the test may be negative, because the surface material has become necrotic and therefore unrecognizable. Such a mistake is not likely to be serious because the advanced lesion can be recognized in other ways. No reference is made here to the contentious subject of the periodic "screening" of healthy persons for possible early cancer either in the cervix or elsewhere. A useful and conservative review of the whole subject of exfoliative cytological diagnosis will be found in a paper by Magner.

When screening is deemed desirable, the most suitable technical method is the use of *fluorescent microscopy* with acridine orange, a rapid and easy procedure (Bertalanffy, Dale). The technique gives a highly polychromatic picture, and serves to differentiate the DNA of the nucleus from the RNA of the cytoplasm, the RNA staining a flaming red or orange compared with DNA, which gives a green to yellow fluorescence. The malignant cells stain mainly red or orange, and the normal cells yellow or green, a distinction which is readily recognized with the low power of the microscope. It would appear that changes in the cytoplasmic RNA content may be an earlier sign of malignant transformation than the changes in the nucleus to which we are accustomed to pay so much attention. The method is not only of very great value in the diagnosis of uterine cancer, but also in suspected cancer of the gastrointestinal, urogenital, and more particularly the respiratory tract, the cells of which are apt to present difficulties with

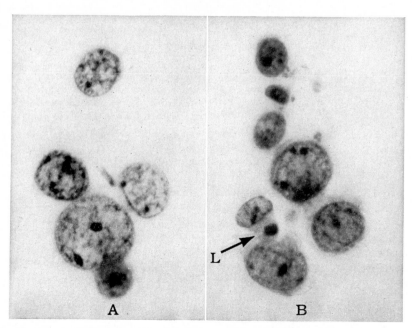

F IG. 116.—Carcinoma of the breast (Papanicolaou stain, × 1100) (a) Malignant cells from a direct smear of the resected tumor. (b) Malignant cells isolated from peripheral blood (anti-cubital vein) during the skin preparation incident to operation. The similarity of the groups is striking and would appear to leave no doubt that the cells obtained from the systemic vein are malignant. L=lymphocyte. (Cole, W. H., et al., Bull. New York Acad. Med.)

conventional cytodiagnostic methods. Malignant cells in the sputum and bronchial secretions show intense fluorescence.

Demonstration of Cancer Cells in the Blood.—It has long been known that in exceptional cases an occasional cancer cell can be detected in the peripheral blood, but the employment of various specialized techniques including the use of 10 cc. of blood has greatly enhanced the importance of this finding. In cases with a favorable prognosis few or no cells may be evident, but in 105 cases of advanced adenocarcinoma of the lung, stomach and colon with metastases 45 were positive and 60 were negative on a single examination (Sandberg and Moore). The number of positives is greatly increased by manipulation during operation. Tumor cells and clumps of cells are found much more frequently in blood taken by a plastic catheter from veins draining the tumor than in the peripheral blood. The cells may bear a striking resemblance to malignant cells from a direct smear of the resected tumor

(Cole *et al.*) (Fig. 116). Great care must be taken not to mistake megakaryocytes for tumor cells.

Appreciation of the fact, previously suspected, that surgical manipulation of a tumor tends to dislodge cancer cells into the circulation and thus increase the danger of metastases has suggested the possibility of attacking these cells in transit by chemoprophylaxis. Triethylene thiophosphoramide (thio TEPA) and other substances related to nitrogen mustard have been used in the treatment of advanced cancer. It has been found that the use of thio TEPA before and after the intravenous injection of malignant cells into laboratory animals greatly reduced the number of pulmonary metastases (Kramer *et al.*). Its effectiveness in preventing the establishment of metastases increases to a maximum in the forty-eight hours after tumor inoculation, and then decreases. It remains to be seen to what extent, if any, this idea can be applied to the surgical treatment of cancer in man. A consideration of the facts relative to cancer cells in the blood stream may impress on the student the importance of handling all tumors very gently, and, should he become a surgeon, the equal need to exercise great care in manipulating a tumor during removal.

Chemical Tests.—An enormous amount of time and labor has been devoted to the search for a chemical test of the blood serum or secretions which would indicate in general that neoplasia was in progress. The results have been uniformly disappointing, although in individual cases the tests may give results of clinical value. Thus the epithelium of the prostate normally elaborates acid phosphatase, and when this epithelium is greatly increased in amount, as in the frequent massive metastatic involvement of the bones in prostatic carcinoma, the serum acid phosphatase is likely to be raised to a significant degree. Cancers of placental tissue may be detected by the presence of chorionic gonadotropic hormone in the urine, just as occurs in pregnancy. Reference has already been made to the demonstration by the Grahams of complement-fixing antibodies in cancer of the uterus. The sum total of positive results is profoundly disappointing by comparison with the intensive search for some test or tests which would be of clinical value in the early detection of cancer.

CANCER THERAPY

At the present time cancer can be treated effectively by surgical removal or by radiotherapy (x-rays or radium) or both, and in some cases palliatively by chemotherapy. But this is only possible if the tumor is still localized when the patient is first seen by the doctor. Moreover it is impossible to avoid the destruction of normal tissue both by the surgeon's knife and by the even more lethal weapon of radiation. The ideal therapeutic agent would be one with a selective action on and affinity for malignant cells while leaving normal cells untouched. This may seem to be a vain hope, but the same could have been said of the chemotherapy of bacteria in the tissues before the introduction of the sulphonamides and the antibiotics.

As regards *chemotherapy* we are familiar with the fact that carcinogenic substances which upset the delicate chromosomal nucleoprotein mechanism may also be made to be carcinolethal. The best known example is radiations which may both cause and cure cancer, but it is also true of chemical agents and of viruses, which are radiomimetic in that they have this double action. What is potent for evil may also be made powerful for good. The carcinogenic hydrocarbons and certain vesicants such as mustard gas and nitrogen mustard may inhibit both normal and malignant growth. We have already seen that an abnormal precursor of nucleic acid, 2:6-diaminopurine, can cause selective injury to cancer cells both in tissue culture and in transplanted tumors in the experimental animal. Many other analogues of adenine have been prepared, and it is not too much to hope that future progress in the chemotherapy of malignant disease may follow the same fruitful line as has been seen in the chemotherapy of bacterial infection. We shall refer to antimetabolites, folic acid antagonists such as aminopterin and 6-mercaptopurine in particular, when we come to the subject of leukemia. A rather recent development is *regional chemotherapy*, which involves the isolation of a limb or organ from the general circulation followed by the injection of nitrogen mustard into the main artery of the limb in a concentration 15 or 20 times greater than can be used in ordinary intravenous therapy because of its action on the blood-forming organs. The best results have been obtained in malignant melanoma of a limb.

RADIATION OF TUMORS

No aspect of the study of tumors is of more practical importance than the effect of ionizing irradiation, whether by roentgen-rays or the gamma rays of radium. These radiations ionize the materials which absorb the rays, with resulting chemical and biological reactions. Only the general principles can be indicated here, but each kind of tumor and indeed tumors of each individual organ have to be studied separately. The *chief methods* used are: (1) external radiation (roentgen rays and radium), (2) surface application (radium), and (3) interstitial radiation (radium). For widespread malignant processes such as lymphosarcoma and leukemia roentgen rays provide the more practical method. The use of properly screened gamma rays avoids necrosis, but permits the specific selective action of the rays on the tumor cells. The aim of all modern radiotherapy is to eliminate this indiscriminate caustic action, and by adequate filtration and graduated exposure to administer such doses as shall have the maximum destructive effect upon the neoplastic cells with the minimum of danger to normal tissues. The effects of radiation depend partly on the action on the tumor cells, partly on the action on the tissues. The comparative sensitivity of various normal cells and tissues is shown in the Table on page 421 in the chapter on Ionizing Radiation.

1. **Effect on the Cells.**—The effect may be studied in tissue culture or in tumors in the experimental animal. This effect is twofold: (1) arrest of mitosis, and (2) degeneration and destruction of cells. Actively growing and dividing normal cells such as those of hemopoietic tissue and the testis are much more sensitive than ordinary cells, and the same is even more true of tumor cells. This is expressed in the "Law of Bergonié and Tribondeau" that the radio-sensitivity of any tissue depends on its reproductive activity. The more numerous the mitoses, the more sensitive is the tissue. There is chromosome breakage and inhibition and disruption of mitotic division. It follows that granulation tissue, embryonic tissue, and undifferentiated rapidly dividing cancer are most radio-sensitive. Partial or complete degeneration of the cell occurs. The nucleus breaks up and undergoes chromatolysis, the cytoplasm becomes granular and vacuolated, the cell dies and disappears. Ionizing radiation interferes with the metabolism of the nucleoproteins and inactivates the nuclear enzymes. Many of the cells die a sudden death, and in moving pictures they can be seen actually to "explode." The degree of sensitiveness depends on the position of the cell in the mitotic cycle, the most sensitive period being just before the commencement of mitosis. All the cells in the culture are never killed, even though the dose largely exceeds the therapeutic limit, but the lethal effect is much greater than would at first

sight appear. When subcultures are made of the irradiated culture it is found that the remaining cells have lost their power of reproduction, although this loss may not become apparent until the culture has passed through a dozen generations. As a result of this delayed effect all the cells ultimately die. In addition to its destructive action, ionizing radiation may cause gene mutations, thus conferring on the cell different hereditary characteristics. It will also induce the differentiation of previously undifferentiated cells.

The effect on mitotic division is the basis of the principle of fractionated dosage over a prolonged period as compared with a single application. By fractionation of dose the likelihood of irradiating more cells at the most sensitive phase of their mitotic cycle increases. This is well illustrated by radiation of the rabbit's testis. If this is given in small doses over a sufficiently long time to affect all the cells in mitosis, sterilization is the result, but not if a single massive dose is used.

Shields Warren and his associates have introduced a technique for the preparation of sections, which consists of freezing and drying the tissue followed by dry cutting and mounting. As chemical fixatives and aqueous solutions are not used, there is no diffusion of water-soluble compounds. By this method there is a more delicate preservation of nuclear details such as is seen in living cells under the phase-contrast microscope. When tumors of rats and mice are examined five minutes after contact with radioactive isotopes and three hours after external radiation, cytologic changes are seen which are not demonstrable by the usual method of preparation. These changes serve to distinguish the radio-sensitive from the radio-resistant cells. In the radio-sensitive cell there is a striking production of large intranuclear vacuoles which may rupture the nuclear membrane. Most of the nuclear membranes are irregular and wrinkled. The radio-resistant cells show a very slight degree of similar changes, so that the difference is quantitative rather than qualitative. The Feulgen reaction shows the desoxyribonucleic acid in the nucleus to be decreased in proportion to the degree of vacuolization.

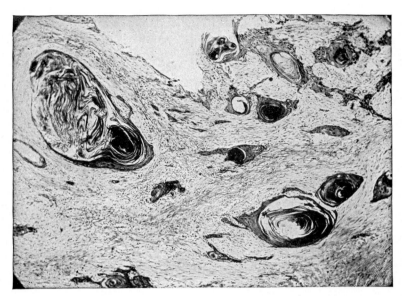

Fig. 117.—Secondary deposits of a squamous carcinoma in a lymph node, showing a considerable degree of necrosis as the result of radiation, together with marked fibrosis. (Boyd's *Pathology for the Surgeon*, courtesy of W. B. Saunders Company.)

Radiomimetic chemicals such as aminopterin which are lethal to tumor cells fail to produce vacuolization, but colchicine causes the same changes as radiation and is, therefore, truly mimetic.

Two types of effect may be obtained, depending on the method used. (1) *Autolytic degeneration* and softening. This is best seen in anaplastic undifferentiated tumors such as lymphosarcoma and Ewing's tumor of bone, but by using appropriate screening a similar effect may be produced in cancer of the mouth, tongue, tonsil, and cervix uteri (Fig. 117). (2) *Growth restraint.* Resistant tumors such as osteogenic sarcoma of bone when radiated over a long period may cease to grow, though failing to disappear. They have become quiescent, their malignancy is greatly diminished, and they can then be removed surgically with greater safety.

Effect on the Intercellular Tissues.—The effect of irradiation of the intercellular constituents of the normal tissue surrounding the tumor is of extreme importance, especially as emphasizing the need for as much protection of this material as possible. Acute inflammatory reaction, with an exudate consisting of serum and cells, the latter polymorphonuclears at first, followed later by lymphocytes, plasma cells and eosinophils. This is followed by a thickening of the collagenous and elastic fibers, and perhaps by marked fibrosis. These changes progress slowly, and may only become apparent some years after completion of the therapy. To make matters worse, there are accompanying changes in the smaller blood vessels as well as the lymphatics. The vascular endothelium is destroyed, the muscle disintegrates, and a proliferative endarteritis narrows and even closes the lumen. Thrombosis is common. The action of radiation on cells may be reversible, but the effect on intercellular tissue is progressive. As sclerotic tissue presents a barrier to radiation it is obvious that previous treatment with this agent will contraindicate irradiation therapy on a subsequent occasion. Heavy infection of the tumor bed is an important contraindication for treatment by radiation, as the resistance of the normal tissue is seriously impaired, and radiation may cause severe and fatal sloughing. This is particularly dangerous in the case of a hollow viscus such as the rectum.

Radiosensitivity.—Tumors vary in their

sensitivity to radiation. The variation is mainly an intrinsic factor, with characteristic radiosensitivity as a property of each type of tumor cell. As Ralston Paterson remarks, intrinsic sensitivity is a characteristic of each "species"—squamous cell carcinoma, basal cell carcinoma, adenocarcinoma, lymphosarcoma, melanoma, etc. The sensitivity remains relatively constant within each species. The purpose of the histological grading of tumors is an indication of the degree of malignancy, not an index of radiosensitivity. Thus a highly differentiated squamous cell carcinoma will respond as completely as a highly anaplastic one. It is true that the more differentiated the cells and adult the type of tissue, the more radio-resistant is the tumor, and vice versa, but the rate of regression is not a reliable indication of the actual sensitivity of the tumor *as a whole*.

Malignant tumors may be divided according to their radiosensitivity into three main groups: (1) *highly radiosensitive:* lymphosarcoma, multiple myeloma, lymphoephilthelioma (transitional-cell carcinoma), embryonal carcinoma; (2) *moderately radiosensitive:* epidermoid carcinoma, carcinoma simplex; (3) *highly radioresistant:* fibrosarcoma, osteosarcoma, neurosarcoma, melanoma, glioma, adenocarcinoma (except adenocarcinoma of the thyroid).

As Glucksmann points out, radiosensitivity as measured by the rate of macroscopic shrinkage bears no close relationship to radiocurability, with the single exception of basal-cell carcinoma of the skin. "Radiosensitive tumors are the 'miracles' of radiation, the source of conceit in the inexperienced radiotherapist, and the greatest source of disappointment when apparently brilliant successes become in due course dismal failures" (Sir Stanford Cade). Radiosensitivity depends largely on the preponderance of short-lived undifferentiated cells and is therefore linked with anaplasia. Radiocurability is related rather to differentiation. Even in normal tissues such as the cervix uteri radiation may change the extent and type of differentiation. In malignant tumors the promotion of differentiation and with it the sterilization of the tumor cells is of great importance.

A subject which is beginning to attract attention is the relationship of the degree of oxygenation to radiosensitivity. Oxygenated cells and tissues are about 3 times more sensitive to radiation than they are in the anoxic state. This is true both of tumor cells and of normal tissue. Areas of necrosis are common in human cancer, and the tumor cells adjacent to such areas must be 3 times more radioresistant than their well-oxygenated fellows. The radiosensitivity can be increased by having the subject breathe a high percentage of oxygen. Conversely, anoxia of normal tissue, which can be induced in a limb by pressure and other means, results in increased radioresistance or that a higher dose of radiation can be used. The speed with which this change takes place is quite remarkable. The bones of the growing mouse tail become fully radioresistant in four seconds after compression, and the resistance of the thymus glands of young mice is increased 3 times after ten or twenty seconds of breathing nitrogen. The reader will find a summary of recent work (up to 1958) on this subject in a Lancet Editorial, November 22, 1958, page 1107.

Radiation Sequelæ.—Radiation can be more injurious to the tissues than the surgeon's knife, although the damage is more insidious and long-delayed. Thus fibrotic changes in the bowel wall may progress relentlessly and lead to fatal complications many years after irradiation. Moreover fibrotic lesions are also less resistant to mechanical injury and infection, so that minor trauma may induce serious and even disastrous complications many years later. Unfortunately patients as well as tumors differ in their sensitivity to radiation. With *skilled treatment*, however, it is only the occasional case which develops the sequelæ outlined in this section. It is another matter when the treatment is unskilled.

When the *skin* has been heavily irradiated the result is first *acute* and later *chronic radiation dermatitis*. Telangiectasis may occur a year or more afterwards. This is accompanied by a varying amount of fibrosis and atrophy of the normal structures. Minor injury to such damaged skin may result in localized areas of necrosis which simulate malignant disease in appearance. These

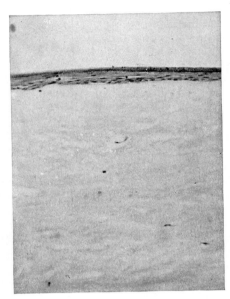

FIG. 118.—Radiation dermatitis, showing ironing out of epidermis and disappearance of dermal appendages. × 150. (Boyd's *Pathology for the Surgeon*, courtesy of W. B. Saunders Company.)

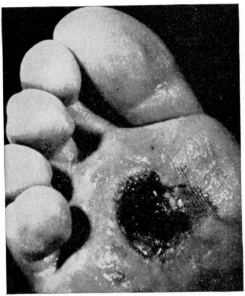

A

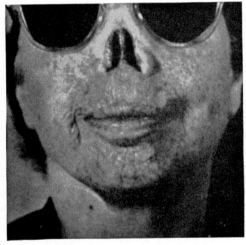

B

FIG. 119.—*A*, Extremely painful ulcer in a twenty-six year old man two years after a single x-ray treatment for a plantar wart.

B, Multicentric basal-cell and squamous-cell carcinoma of the face twenty-seven years after irradiation for acne. All surgical efforts were unsuccessful. (Cannon, Randolph and Murray, courtesy of New Eng. J. Med.)

skin lesions invariably heal, but they may take months to do so. The microscopic picture of the late stages of radiation dermatitis varies greatly. Common changes are thinning of the epidermis with loss of the rete pegs, sclerosis of the dermis with absence of hair follicles and sweat and sebaceous glands, and fragmentation of the elastic tissue which may be collected in clumps (Fig. 118). The possibility of chronic radiation dermatitis developing into low grade epidermoid carcinoma must be borne in mind.

In *bone* the effect of low and medium volt radiation is considerably increased by the greater absorption associated with the high calcium content. This reduces the bone tolerance on account of the greater damage to the small vessels in the Haversian canals. This devitalization of bone may not cause clinical symptoms until minor injuries or infections lead to signs of bone necrosis.

The *lung* will develop a variable degree of fibrosis at the apex following irradiation of the axilla and supraclavicular areas in cases of carcinoma of the breast. This change can be clearly seen in the x-ray film as a uniform density in the upper part of the lung field. It is without symptoms.

In *carcinoma of the cervix* adequate radiation may be followed by an inflammatory reaction in the anterior wall of the rectum in some 2 per cent of cases. The lesion develops about a year after completion of the course of treatment in these hypersensitive persons, the most frequent complaint being the passage of blood and mucus per rectum. The damage is usually minor in degree, but in some cases a large mass develops, which on healing leaves extensive scarring with stricture of the rectum.

Radiation necrosis is the term applied to necrosis of the healthy tissue produced by overdosage. If the dose is very large, there is immediate necrosis with sloughing, and the resultant defect will never heal. If the dose is smaller, the greater part of the lesion will heal, but a small area of necrosis may remain. If the overdosage is only slight, healing will be complete, but the tissue may readily break down again as the result of infection or trauma, for the resistance of radiated tissue is seriously impaired owing to progressive endarteritis. I have seen tissues break down as long as eight years after radiation. Correct estimation of dose is therefore all-important in radiation therapy.

Cannon and his associates sum up this very serious subject by saying that "irradiation for benign conditions may produce tissue changes more disabling than the original condition for which the *x*-rays were administered. Those who administer the irradiation may be unaware of the late consequences." Carcinoma, of either epidermoid or basal-cell type, developed in 22 per cent of their 165 cases (Fig. 119). In 5 cases the interval between *x*-ray exposure and the establishment of a diagnosis of cancer was over 40 years.

THE RELATIVE FREQUENCY OF TUMORS

Like so many of the other aspects of the cancer problem, the question of relative frequency is far less simple than might first appear. I have found it impossible to obtain reliable data as to the frequency of *all* malignant growths. What is true of one country, even of one part of that country, is not necessarily true of another. Cancer statistics are notoriously unreliable. The figures of the radiotherapist, the surgeon, the internist, the gynecologist, and the pathologist in the autopsy room naturally differ profoundly. Cancer of the skin is very seldom seen on the post-mortem table, whereas cancer of the lung is seen continually. This does not mean that cancer of the lung is more common than cancer of the skin; it merely means that it is more lethal. Conclusions drawn from mortality as opposed to morbidity records will differ not only as to frequency of the disease, but also as to the tissues or organs involved. Cancer statistics are naturally based on information in death certificates, and these contain many fallacies. Unless the figures are taken from autopsy material, the margin of error in diagnosis is enormous. Willis in his classic volume *The Pathology of Tumors* found in a study of nearly 1000 autopsies on cases of cancer that the clinical diagnosis was wrong in over 30 per cent.

The *sex incidence of cancer* is essentially the same, but there is a marked difference as to site of origin in the two sexes. In females nearly one-half of all cancer originates in the reproductive organs (breast, uterus, ovary), whilst among males only one cancer in eight originates in the reproductive organs. Nearly all forms of cancer other than cancer of the reproductive organs are more common in the male, the largest excess being in cancer of the lung and even more in laryngeal cancer.

The *age incidence* of cancer merits more than a passing thought. We think of cancer as a disease of advancing years, so that it is disconcerting to learn that the disease is the second most frequent cause of death in children between the age of five and fourteen years, being exceeded only by accidents. Carcinoma, however, is very rare in the child. Sarcoma is by far the most frequent form of cancer in children, being followed by embryomas and mixed tumors. When we come later to the study of disease in the various organs we shall find that the type of tumor which occurs in a given organ in the child may be quite different from that which occurs in the adult. This is particularly true of tumors which appear to have a genetic basis, such as the Wilms' tumor of the kidney and the neuroblastoma of the adrenal medulla, both of which are neoplasms peculiar to the child.

Cancer morbidity surveys were carried

out by the United States National Cancer Institute in 1937 and again in 1947. The reported cancer incidence rate in 1947 was 319 per 100,00 population; this is 30 per cent higher than in 1937. More than 500,000 new cases of cancer are being diagnosed in the United States every year. Under present conditions 32 out of every 100 newborn children may be expected to develop cancer at some time during their lives. In 1953 the cancer deaths in Canada were as follows: stomach, 3,006; large intestine, 2,339; lung, 1,776; breast, 1,752; male genitalia (prostate, *etc.*), 998; leukemia, 777; cervix uteri, 599; other sites, 7,873. It is well for the student to know that half of all forms of cancer originate in organs accessible to direct examination by the physician in his own office, and yet, exclusive of skin cancer, only 50 per cent of cancer developing in accessible sites is being diagnosed while it is still localized at the site of origin (Heller *et al.*).

The *incidence of multiple cancer* occurring in the same person at different times is a question regarding which very different opinions have been expressed. Does a cancer patient have the same, more or less chance of developing a second cancer? Does the fact that a person has had one cancer confer on him some immunity to a new primary malignant tumor, does it predispose him toward a second cancer, or does he have exactly the same chance as normal people of the same age have of developing a first cancer? A correct answer to this question is naturally of primary importance to the person concerned, and to his doctor. A careful analysis of the statistical material seems to indicate that the incidence of two or more primary malignant tumors does not differ from the ordinary incidence rate of cancer in a normal population (Watson).

In concluding this discussion of the relative frequency of tumors, a word may be devoted to the *zoological distribution of cancer*. All vertebrates suffer from spontaneous tumors, but the distribution varies widely. The disease is almost as common in the dog as in man. In the cat it is much lower, 0.5 to 6 per cent; in the horse 0.1 to 0.2 per cent; in cattle still lower; very low in the pig, goat and sheep. In the fowl, on the other hand, the incidence is high, especially for leukemia.

In random-bred laboratory animals cancer is very common in the mouse, less so in the rat, and infrequent in the guniea pig and rabbit.

PROGNOSIS IN CANCER

It is obviously impossible in such a work as this to enter into a detailed discussion of the prognosis of cancer. For one thing methods of treatment, both by surgery and radiation, are so continually improving that what may be said today is out of date to-morrow. The important thing for the student to realize is that the prognosis in malignant disease no longer presents the dark picture it used to. Over-all figures are of little value, because the outlook varies so enormously in different forms of cancer. In each group there are exceptions. Thus the prognosis in cancer of the parotid gland is bad, but in 1948 the author developed this lesion, which the moment it was diagnosed was treated by surgical removal followed by the implantation of radium needles, and at the present time he is alive and well. Cancer of the skin is a readily curable disease, whereas in some other forms the prognosis is very bad. The prognosis of individual tumors wil be discussed when they are considered in the second part of the book.

The figures of a cancer clinic in Ontario between the years 1936 and 1945 (McCormick) may be of interest. In this clinic 38 per cent of all patients seen with cancer were alive and seemingly well five or more years later. Of the patients treated for cure rather than merely for palliation (58 per cent) there was a 69.4 per cent five-year survival.

IS CANCER INCREASING?

This question, so often asked, is not easy to answer without giving a false impression. Undoubtedly there are many more deaths from cancer than there used to be. In Canada in 1901 the cancer death rate was 46.8 per 100,000; in 1921 it had risen to 75 per 100,000, an increase of 62 per cent. But in deciding whether the increase is real or apparent, such factors as the general age of the population have to be borne in mind.

The larger the proportion of old people, the higher will the cancer rate be. The truth appears to be that cancer is increasing both actually and relatively because of the great saving of life in the early years. It may also be said that the cancer rate is an index of the public health organization of a country; cancer is the legacy of preventive medicine. In the Vision of Mirza Addison describes the masses of mankind crossing the bridge of life which spans the river of death and falling into the dark flood below. In the bridge there are many trapdoors—infantile mortality, typhoid, malaria, smallpox— through which the unwary traveller may drop, but these seldom open now. So large numbers approach the end of the bridge and drop through a small number of wide doors, such as apoplexy, coronary occlusion and, above all, cancer.

In concluding this chapter the opening sentence may be recalled, and the student will perhaps agree that if the problem of neoplasia is intriguing and even fascinating, it is certainly most perplexing.

REFERENCES

ALLEN-PRICE, E. D.: Lancet, 1960, *1*, 1235. (Geographic pathology of cancer).

BASERGA, R. and SAFFIOTTI, W.: Arch. Path., 1955, *59*, 26. (Blood spread of metastases).

BATSON, O. V.: Ann. Surg., 1940, *112*, 138. (Spread of cancer by vertebral system of veins).

————.: Am. J. Roent., Rad. Therapy and Nuclear Med., 1957, *78*, 195. (The vertebral vein system).

BITTNER, J. J.: Science, 1936, *84*, 162. (Milk factor in mammary mouse cancer).

BLACK, M. M., KERPE, S. and SPEER, F. D.: Am. J. Path., 1953, *29*, 505. (Spread of cancer to lymph nodes).

BODIAN, M.: Brit. Emp. Cancer Campaign Rep., 1954, p. 198. (Spontaneous regression of neuroblastoma).

BOYD, W.: J. Canad. Ass. Radiol., 1957, *8*, 45, 63; Surg. Gynec. and Obst., 1921, *32*, 306. (Spontaneous regression of cancer).

————.: Can. Med. Ass. J., 1934, *31*, 273. (Benign epithelial invasion).

BRAIN, W. R.: Lancet. 1958, *2*, 971. (Neurological syndromes associated with carcinoma).

BRANDES, W. W., WHITE, W. C. and SUTTON, J. B.: Surg. Gynec. and Obst., 1946, *82*, 212. (Spread of cancer by inoculation).

BRODERS, A. C.: Arch. Path., 1926, *2*, 376. Surg. Clin. North America, 1941, *21*, 947. (Grading of tumors).

BURROWS, H. and HORNING, E. S.: *Oestrogens and Neoplasia*, Springfield, Ill., 1952.

CADE, STANFORD Sir.: *Malignant Disease and its Treatment by Radium*, Bristol, 1940.

CANNON, B., RANDOLPH, J. G. and MURRAY, J. E.: New Engl. J. Med., 1959, *260*, 197. (Malignant irradiation for benign conditions).

COLE, W. H. *et al.*: Bull. New York Acad. Med., 1958, *34*, 163. (Demonstration of cancer cells in blood stream).

COMAN, D. R.: Cancer Research, 1953, *13*, 397. (Spread of tumors).

COMAN, D. R. and DE LONG, R. P.: Cancer, 1951, *4*, 610. (Vertebral vein metastases).

COPELAND, D. H. and SALMON, W. D.: Am. J. Path., 1946, *22*, 1059. (Choline deficiency and cancer of liver).

CRILE, G. JR.: J. Nat. Cancer Inst., 1958, *20*, 229. (Endocrine imbalance in the genesis of cancer).

DAVIES, J. N. P.; in COLLINS, D. H., Ed.: *Modern Trends in Pathology*, London, 1959. (Cancer in Africa).

DENNY-BROWN, D.: J. Neurol., Neurosurg. and Psychiat., 1948, *11*, 73. (Carcinomatous neuromyopathies).

DES LIGNERIS, M. J. A.: Am. J. Cancer, 1940, *40*, 1. (Irritation as a co-carcinogen).

DOCKERTY, M. B.: Surg. Gynec. and Obst., 1953, *97*, 113. (The frozen section biopsy).

DYCK, P. J., BAILEY, A. A. and OLSZEWSKI, J.: Can. Med. Ass. J., 1958, *79*, 913. (Carcinomatous neuromyopathy in bronchogenic carcinoma).

EISENBERG, R. B.: Am. J. Path., 1949, *25*, 802. (Distribution of metastases).

FIDLER, H. K.: Am. J. Cancer, 1935, *25*, 772. (Cytology of cancer).

FISHER, B. and FISHER, E. R.: Ann. Surg., 1959, *150*, 731. (Spread of tumors).

GARDNER, W. U.: Can Cancer Conference, 1957, Vol. 2, 207. (Hormones and carcinogenesis).

GLUCKSMANN, A.: Brit. J. Radiol., 1948, *21*, 559; 1952, *25*, 38. (Radiosensitivity of tumors).

GRACE, J. T. JR., MIRAND, E. A. and MOUNT, D. T.: Arch. Int. Med., 1960, *105*, 482. (Viruses and human cancer).

GRAHAM, J. B. and GRAHAM, R. M.: Cancer, 1955, *8*, 408. (Production of antibodies in human cancer).

GREEN, H. N. and WHITELEY, H. J.: Brit. Med. J., 1952, *2*, 538. (Transplantation of tumors).

GREENE, H. S. N.: J. Exper. Med., 1940, *71*, 305. Cancer Research, 1953, *13*, 422. Ann. New York Acad. Sci., 1957, *69*, 812. (Heterotransplantation of tumors).

GREENLEES, J. and LEPAGE, G. A.: Cancer Res., 1955, *15*, 256. (The competitive struggle for nitrogen).

GREENSTEIN, J. P.: *Biochemistry of Cancer*, 2nd ed., Academic Press, New York, 1954.

GROSS, L.: Cancer Res., 1958, *18*, 371. Brit. Med. J., 1958, *2*, 1. (Vertical transmission of cancer).

HADDOW, A.: Canad. Cancer Conference, 1957, Vol. 2, 361. (Alkylating agents as carcinogens).

HADFIELD, G.: Brit. Med. J., 1954, *2*, 607. (The dormant cancer cell).

HELLER, J. R., CUTLER, S. J. and HAENSZEL, W. M.: J.A.M.A., 1955, *159*, 1628. (Epidemiology of cancer in the United States).

HIGGINS, G. K., and PACK, G. P.: Virus Therapy in Treatment of Tumors, Bull. Hosp. Joint Dis. *12*, 379, 1951. (Carcinolethal action of viruses.)

HOWATSON, A. F. and HAM, A. W.: Cancer Research, 1955, *15*, 62. (Electron microscope study of rat liver tumors).

HUEPER, W. C.: *Occupational Tumors and Allied Diseases*, Springfield, Ill., 1942. Arch. Path., 1954, *58*, 360. (Environmental cancer).

KOLETSKY, S. and GUSTAFSON, G. E.: Am. J. Path., 1953, *29*, 606. (Whole body radiation).

KING, E. S. J., HUGHES, P. E. and LOUIS, C. J.: Brit. J. Cancer, 1958, *12*, 5. (Globulin-fluorescein staining in neoplasia).

KRAMER, W. M., ECK, R. V. and SMITH, R. R.: Surg., Gynec. and Obst., 1958, *106*, 459. (Chemoprophylaxis spread of cancer).

LEBLOND, C. P. and STEVENS, C. E.: Anat. Rec., 1948, *100*, 357. (Turnover of cells in intestinal mucosa).

LISA, J. R., PACK, G. T. and GIOIA, J. D.: Am. J. Roentgen, Radium Therapy and Nuclear Med., 1952, *68*, 452. (Radiations as carcinogens.)

LOCKHART-MUMMERY, J. P. and DUKES, C.: Surg. Gynec. and Obst., 1928, *46*, 591. (Precancerous lesions).

MAGNER, D.: Canad. M.A.J., 1950, *63*, 103. (Exfoliative cytology).

MIDER, G. B.: Canad. Cancer Conference, 1955, *1*, 120. (Nitrogen trap).

NOBLE, R. L.: Pharmacolog. Rev., 1957, *9*, 367. (Hormonal regulation of tumor growth).

PATERSON, RALSTON: *The Treatment of Malignant Disease by Radium or X-rays.* London, 1948.

PENNER, D. W.: Cancer, 1953, *6*, 776. (Spontaneous regression of cancer).

RABSON, S. M., STIER, P. L., BAUMGARTNER, J. C. and ROSENBAUM, D.: Am. J. Clin. Path., 1954, *24*, 572. (Metastases of cancer to cancer).

RHOADS, C. P.: Ann. Roy. Coll. Surg. of England, 1957, *20*, 139. (The soluble puzzle of cancer control).

ROUS, P.: J. Exper. Med., 1911, *56*, 198. (Viral etiology of cancer in birds).

SANDBERG, A. A. and MOORE, R. E.: J. Nat. Cancer Inst., 1957, *19*, 1. (Demonstration of cancer cells in blood stream).

SHOPE, R. E.: J. Exper. Med., 1932, *56*, 793. (Viral etiology of cancer in the rabbit).

SOUTHAM, C. M., MOORE, A. E. and RHOADS, C. P.: Science, 1957, *125*, 158. (Homotransplantation of human cancer cells.)

SPROUL, E. E.: Lab. Investig., 1956, *5*, 194. (Particulate components of cytoplasm).

STANLEY, W. M.: Ca., 1957, *7*, 97. (Virus etiology of cancer).

STEWART, SARAH E. *et al.*: Virology, 1957, *3*, 380. (Viral production of cancer).

STEWART, F. W.: Texas Rep. Biol. and Med., 1952, *10*, 239. (Spontaneous regression of cancer).

SUGIURA, K. and RHOADS, C. P.: Cancer Research, 1941, *1*, 3. (Butter yellow and cancer of liver).

TOOLAN, H. W.: Cancer Research, 1953, *13*, 389. (Transplantation of tumors).

VOGT, MARGUERITE and DULBECCO, R.: Microbiology, 1960, *46*, 365. (Neoplastic growth in tissue culture).

WARBURG, O.: *The Metabolism of Tumors*, English Translation, London, 1930. Science, 1956, *123*, 309.

WARTHIN, A. S.: J. Cancer Research, 1928, *12*, 249. (Heredity in cancer).

WATSON, T. A.: Cancer, 1953, *6*, 365. (Incidence of multiple cancer).

WILLIS, R. A.: *Pathology of Tumors*, 2nd edit., London, 1953.

————.: *The Spread of Tumors*, London, 1954.

WISEMAN, G. and GHADIALLY, F. N.: Brit. Med. J., 1958, *2*, 18. (Protein synthesis from aminoacids in neoplasia).

WITEBSKY, E., ROSE, N. R. and SHULMAN, S.: Cancer Research, 1956, *16*, 831. (Immunity in cancer).

WOOD, S. JR.: Arch. Path., 1958, *66*, 550. (Metastasis observed in vivo).

WOOD, S., JR., HOLYOKE, E. D. and YARDLEY, J. H.: Canad. Cancer Conference. In Press. New York. (Mechanisms of metastasis production.)

YAMAGIWA, K. and ICHIKAWA, K.: J. Cancer Res., 1918, *3*, 1. (The experimental production of cancer by tar).

YOUNG, J. M.: Am. J. Path., 1956, *32*, 253. (Spread of cancer by the thoracic duct).

YOUNG, J. S.: J. Path. and Bact., 1959, *77*, 321. (Malignant invasion).

ZEIDMAN, I. and BUSS, J. M.: Cancer Res., 1954, *14*, 403. (Lymph node barrier to embolic tumor cells).

ZIMMERMAN, H. M.: Am. J. Path., 1955, *31*, 1. (Growth of gliomas outside the cranial cavity).

15

Chapter 9

Neoplasia II: Specific Tumors

Classification
Epithelial Tumors
Connective-Tissue Tumors
Muscle-Tissue Tumors

Tumors of Vessels
Tumors of Lymphoid and Hemo-
  poietic Tissue
Nervous-Tissue Tumors

Pigmented Tumors
Chorionic Tumors
Teratomas

CLASSIFICATION OF TUMORS

MUCH has been written regarding the classification of tumors and many classifications have been suggested. The most useful working method is to try to determine the tissue, the type cell, from which the tumor arises. This way may be easy or it may be difficult or impossible. The more undifferentiated and anaplastic the tumor, the more difficult is it to recognize the type cell. In the description of the various forms of tumors some will only be referred to; these are more conveniently considered in connection with the organs from which they grow.

If tumors are arranged in a series, at one end we have a group characterized by excessive proliferation of cells with resulting expansile growth but none of the stigmata of malignancy; they are essentially *benign*. At the other end the proliferating cells invade the tissues, metastasize locally and at a distance, and destroy the host. These are, of course, *malignant*. Between these two extremes there is a group called by Morehead *intermediate* in type, and marked by localized excessive growth of cells with invasion of surrounding tissue and sometimes local and even distant metastases, but without the progressive destruction of the host which is the hall mark of the true malignant neoplasm. Some of the best examples of this intermediate group are seen in the parotid and other salivary glands. Other examples are basal cell carcinoma, "metastasizing thyroid adenoma", carcinoid tumor of the appendix, bronchial adenoma, and mucoepidermoid tumors of the parotid. These tumors seem to hesitate between the

(226)

benign and the malignant, to dwell in the borderland dim between vice and virtue.

The following classification is based on the tissue of origin, and on the benign or malignant character of the tumor. It is, of course, not to be memorized. It will be seen that the general principle is to add the suffix "oma" to the name of the tissue of origin. Malignant tumors of epithelial origin are known as carcinoma, those of connective tissue origin as sarcoma. It will be observed that in some instances the only known tumors are malignant, no benign examples having been recorded.

EPITHELIAL TUMORS

Epithelium may assume one of two patterns; it may be surface or secretory. *Surface epithelium* covers the skin and tongue and lines the vagina and bladder. The tumors which grow from it are papilloma and squamous carcinoma. *Secretory epithelium* is met with in mucous membranes, and in such glandular structures are the breast, liver and kidney. The tumors which grow from this type of epithelium are adenoma and adenocarcinoma. Duct epithelium occupies an intermediate position both in structure and in function; it forms the lining of a tube and yet it is not secretory. Epithelial tumors like epithelial cells present certain features which distinguish them from connective tissue cells and tumors. The cells lie in apposition with one another to form groups. The groups are separated from each other by connective tissue, giving what is called an alveolar arrangement, but there is no con-

HISTOLOGICAL CLASSIFICATION OF TUMORS

Tissue of Origin	Benign Tumor	Malignant Tumor
Epithelial Tissues		
Surface epithelium	Papilloma	Squamous carcinoma
Glandular epithelium	Adenoma	Adenocarcinoma
Connective Tissues		
Fibroblast	Fibroma	Fibrosarcoma
Cartilage	Chondroma	Chondrosarcoma
Bone	Osteoma	Osteogenic sarcoma
Fat	Lipoma	Liposarcoma
Muscle Tissue		
Smooth muscle	Leiomyoma	Leiomyosarcoma
Striated muscle	Rhabdomyoma	Rhabdomyosarcoma
Vascular Tissue		
Blood vessel	Hemangioma	Hemangiosarcoma
Lymph vessel	Lymphangioma	Lymphangiosarcoma
Lymphoid and Hemopoietic Tissue		
Lymphocytes		Lymphosarcoma
		Lymphatic leukemia
Myeloid cells		Multiple myeloma
		Myeloid leukemia
Nervous Tissue		
Neuroglia	Astrocytoma	Glioblastoma
Medullary epithelium		Medulloblastoma
Pigment-forming Tissue		
Melanoblast	Benign melanoma (nevus)	Malignant melanoma
Chorionic Epithelium		
Trophoblast	Hydatidiform mole	Chorioncarcinoma
Embryonic Tissues		Teratoma

nective tissue between the cells of the alveolus.

BENIGN EPITHELIAL TUMORS

Papilloma.—A papilloma is a benign epithelial tumor in which the cells cover finger-like processes of stroma. It grows from a surface, either internal or external. The term is usually not applied to malignant tumors when they grow in this way, but sometimes it is (malignant papilloma). A papilloma may become malignant, but this is only common in one or two situations, *e. g.*, bladder and rectum. Papillomata may be squamous or mucous, depending on whether they grow from a squamous or mucous surface.

SQUAMOUS PAPILLOMA.—This tumor is commonest in the skin (Fig. 120), but may occur in the mouth, larynx, and any other cavity lined by stratified epithelium. The base may be narrow or broad.

A true papilloma shows proliferation of the squamous epithelium. The epidermis may be thickened and blunt processes may project down into the corium. The term *acanthosis* is applied to a proliferation of the cells of the Malpighian layer, whether neoplastic or otherwise, whilst *hyperkeratosis* signifies thickening of the stratum corneum. The so-called *plantar wart* is a flat papilloma with excessive epidermal thickening and very marked cornification of the surface layers. The thickened epithelium presses on the sensory nerve endings and causes pain on pressure just as does a corn. A corn is simply an excessive surface cornification. Every papilloma has a fibrous core, and in some

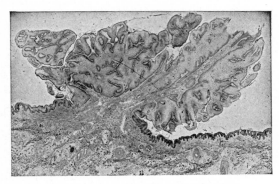

FIG. 120.—Squamous papilloma growing from skin. × 7.

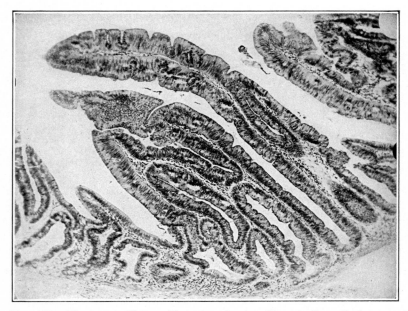

FIG. 121.—Mucous papilloma of large bowel. A malignant change had occurred
in an adjacent part of the tumor. × 60.

cases there seems to be more overgrowth of fibrous tissue than of epithelium, which may be of normal thickness.

MUCOUS PAPILLOMA.—This is commonest in the large intestine, but it may grow from any mucous membrane. In the stomach, intestine, etc., a papilloma is commonly called a *polypus*. Such a polypus is really more of an adenoma than a papilloma, for it is composed of proliferated glands. Gastrointestinal polypi are often multiple, and in the large bowel there may be hundreds. Mucous polypi in the large intestine and bladder are of great importance because they show a marked tendency to malignant change (Fig. 121).

Adenoma.—An adenoma is an innocent epithelial tumor of glandular structure which closely approximates that of the gland from which it arises. Unfortunately the matter is not quite so simple as it sounds. Many so-called adenomas are not true tumors, but merely examples of localized compensatory hyperplasia. When a portion of the liver is destroyed a mass of new tissue is formed which may project on the surface and be mistaken for an adenoma. A true adenoma is encapsulated, but it is doubtful if the

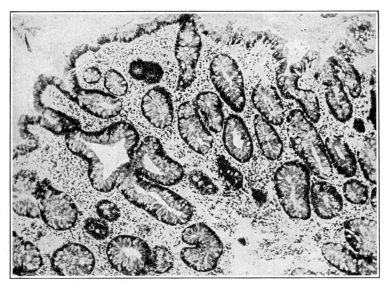

Fig. 122.—Adenoma of rectum. The new glandular acini are quite regular. × 90.

common encapsulated glandular nodules in the thyroid commonly called adenomas are really true tumors. Again an adenoma of the breast may contain more fibrous tissue than epithelium; such a tumor is a fibro-adenoma rather than a pure adenoma.

No general description of an adenoma is possible. It is a circumscribed encapsulated nodule which may resemble the gland from which it arises so closely that the microscopic picture of the two may be identical. It consists of gland-like spaces (breast, stomach, bowel, pancreas), or solid cords (liver, adrenal). The glands may be lined by more than one layer of cells, but the acini are perfectly regular, and there is no invasion of the deeper tissue (Fig. 122).

In the stomach and large intestine the adenoma commonly develops a stalk owing to contractions of the muscular wall, so that it hangs into the lumen as a polypus. Such a polypus is often called a papilloma, but polypoid adenoma or adenomatous polypus is a more correct name. The frequent development of malignancy in the adenomas of the large bowel has already been alluded to.

The secretion of the cells lining the glandular spaces of an adenoma may lead to distention of these spaces with the formation of cysts. Such a condition is called a cyst-adenoma. It is best seen in the ovary, where the cysts are lined by tall columnar epithelium which secretes a mucoid material. The cells lining such cysts may become flattened from pressure, or they may proliferate and project as papillary processes into the cysts, a condition known as papillary cystadenoma.

CARCINOMA

A carcinoma is a malignant epithelial tumor which tends to invade the lymph spaces of the surrounding connective tissue. It is the commonest of all malignant tumors, very much commoner than sarcoma. The cells show the characteristic epithelial arrangement; they are collected into groups or alveoli, with fibrous stroma between the groups but not between the cells of the group. The stroma varies greatly in amount, and largely determines the physical character of the tumor. When the primary tumor is sectioned it may appear to be made up of a large number of separate masses. These are really extensions of the central mass which on section give a fictitious appearance of multiplicity. A wax model would reveal the essential continuity of the tumor.

Spread.—Carcinoma may extend in four different ways. (1) *Invasion of the tissue spaces.* This is the fundamental method of

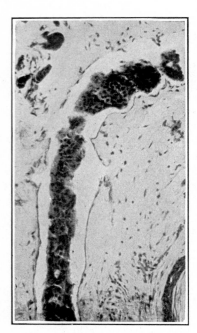

FIG. 123.—Lymphatic permeation by carcinoma.
× 125.

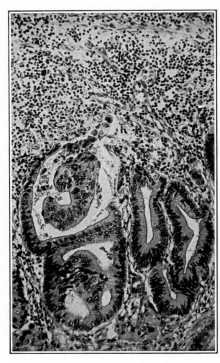

FIG. 124.—Glandular cancer in lymph node. × 150.

spread. The words cancer and carcinoma mean a crab, and these extensions are the claws of the animal. (2) *Lymphatic permeation*. The cancer cells invade the lymphatics and grow along them (Fig. 123.) Spread along perineural lymphatics is of importance in some tumors, particularly carcinoma of the prostate. (3) By *lymphatic embolism* tumor cells are carried to the regional lymph nodes and sometimes to more distant nodes. The nearer nodes may also be reached by permeation. (4) *Blood spread* carries the tumor cells to distant organs.

Carcinoma spreads primarily by the lymph spaces and lymphatic vessels. Lymph node involvement is therefore the rule (Fig. 124.) A lymph node may contain cancer cells and may yet appear normal to the naked eye and show no enlargement, a point of great surgical importance. Suspected early involvement of lymph nodes may be attacked by radiation. As the process becomes more advanced the gland is enlarged, and the cut surface shows a small opaque white nodule. Later the entire gland is occupied by the tumor. In that form of cancer known as squamous cell or epidermoid carcinoma of the skin, tongue, etc., spread is almost entirely by the lymphatics, although in the last stages the blood vessels may be invaded.

Spread by the blood stream is common, though not nearly so common as lymph spread (Fig. 125.) In cancer of the gastrointestinal canal and pancreas the tumor emboli are carried by the portal vein to the liver to form metastases. In carcinoma of other organs (breast, etc.) the lung is the commonest seat of secondary growths. The bones are frequently the site of metastases in carcinoma of the prostate, breast, lung, kidney (hypernephroma) and thyroid. Skeletal metastases may occasionally occur from other carcinomas.

Squamous Cell Carcinoma.—This is usually called *epidermoid carcinoma* and used to be known as *epithelioma*. It occurs wherever squamous or transitional epithelium is found, particularly in skin, mouth, tongue, larynx, cervix, uteri, and urinary bladder. Epidermoid carcinoma may develop in the edge of a chronic ulcer which refuses to heal. In rare cases it may arise from epithelium which has

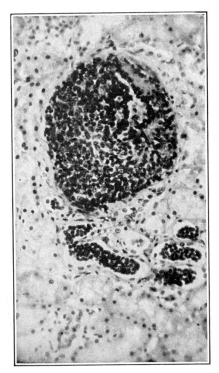

FIG. 125.—Metastasis from carcinoma of lung in glomerulus and renal tubules. × 175.

been changed from the columnar to the squamous stratified type owing to an irritation metaplasia. This is seen in the gallbladder and in a bronchiectatic cavity in the lung. Most of the skin cancers are on the face and neck; the lower lip is the commonest site. They develop at a point where there has been chronic irritation (fissure, ulcer, local thickening). The tumor begins as a slight thickening or small nodule. At this stage the disease is easily curable. Later an ulcer forms which refuses to heal; the edges are characteristically thickened and indurated. Epidermoid carcinoma spreads by the lymphatics, so that the regional lymph nodes become infected and enlarged. Blood spread is unusual, and only occurs late in the disease.

Microscopic Appearance.—Columns of epithelial cells grow down into the dermis (Fig. 126). The growth is therefore the reverse of that seen in papilloma. The lower parts of the columns often appear as masses separated from the rest of the growth by the obliquity of the section. In the center of these masses the same process of cornification goes on as occurs normally on the surface.

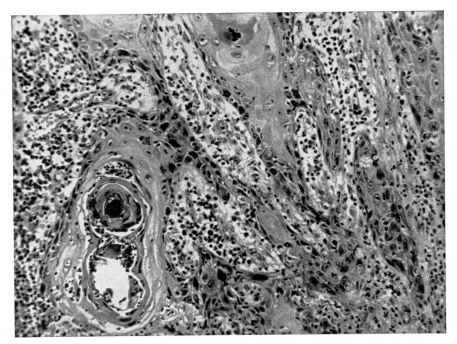

FIG. 126.—Epidermoid carcinoma showing downgrowths of epithelium, cornification and round cell infiltration in the dermis. × 150. (Boyd's *Pathology for the Surgeon*, courtesy of W. B. Saunders Company.)

Granules appear in the cytoplasm, and the cells become converted into hyaline structureless masses of keratin which stain brightly with eosin and are identical with the horny material on the surface of the skin. Such a general picture is well named an epidermoid carcinoma. The cornified masses are known as *cell nests* or *epithelial pearls*. The outer cells of the pearls are often arranged in a concentric manner. The unchanged cells show the "prickle-cell" appearance characteristic of epidermal carcinoma. Cell nests and cornification are absent in rapidly-growing tumors, as they are a sign of differentiation. They are best seen in skin cancers; sometimes they are found in cancer of the tongue and esophagus, but they seldom occur in cancer of the bladder or cancer of the cervix. The down-growing masses are often surrounded by masses of lymphocytes, especially in tumors of low grade.

Basal Cell Carcinoma.—This tumor, usually known as rodent ulcer, is a variety of epidermoid carcinoma which is confined to the skin. The most characteristic feature is the presence of a distinctive basal cell layer surrounding each group of tumor cells. In spite of its name it does not arise from the basal layer of the epidermis, but from non-keratinizing tissue, namely one of the skin appendages. Although it destroys the surrounding tissue, and thus merits the name of rodent ulcer, it has a singular inability to spread either by the lymph or the blood stream, so that it is one of the least dangerous of malignant tumors. As basal cell carcinoma is confined to the skin, it is described more fully in Chapter 46.

Lympho-epithelioma.—A cancer of distinctive individuality, both clinical and pathological, grows from the epithelium covering lymphoid tissue in the mouth and pharynx, *i. e.*, tonsil, wall of pharynx, nasal passages, and nasopharyngeal sinuses, in which areas the epithelium tends to be transitional between squamous and simple. Its chief characteristic is that the primary growth remains small and often undetected, whereas early dissemination gives rise to marked enlargement of the glands of the neck. The correct diagnosis of these nasopharyngeal tumors is

often missed for a long time. Visceral involvement (lungs, liver) may occur at a later date. *Microscopically* the cells are large and pale with indefinite outlines, and are arranged in sheets. There is usually a marked intermingling of epithelial cells and lymphocytes derived from the underlying lymphoid tissue (Fig. 127). When the tumor is purely epithelial in type it is referred to as *transitional cell carcinoma*. Mitoses are numerous. There may be a tendency toward differentiation with squamous characters ap-

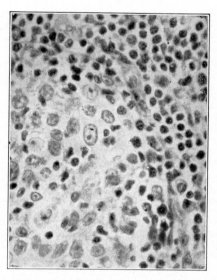

FIG. 127.—Lympho-epithelioma showing intermingling of epithelial and lymphoid cells. × 340.

pearing, or toward anaplasia so that the tumor in the lymph nodes may be mistaken for a lymphosarcoma. The tumor is markedly radiosensitive, in distinction to epidermoid carcinoma, and is more suitably treated by radiation than by surgery. In essence it is an anaplastic carcinoma of the throat.

Adenocarcinoma.—This is a columnar-cell carcinoma with formation of glandular spaces. The common sites are the stomach, large intestine, gallbladder, pancreas, uterus, and prostate. It may occur in the breast and other glandular organs. Spread occurs both

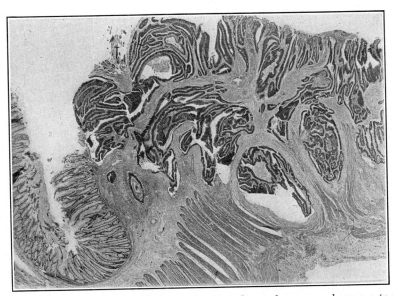

FIG. 128.—Adenocarcinoma, showing the sudden change from normal mucosa to the dark, irregular, infiltrating gland spaces on the right. × 10.

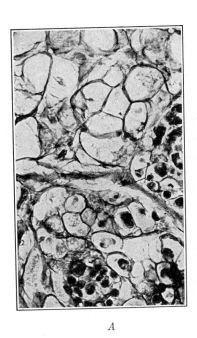

A

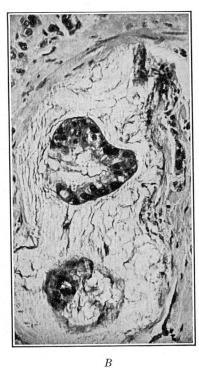

B

FIG. 129.—Mucoid carcinoma. *A*, The tumor cells are greatly distended with mucin. × 150. *B*, Secondary form of mucoid carcinoma. × 200.

by the lymphatics and the blood stream. The gastrointestinal tumors usually form bulky masses which project into the lumen, but they may be sessile or infiltrating. The change from the normal mucous membrane of the bowel to the irregular glands of the tumor is very sudden. The neoplastic glands are highly atypical with branching processes and darkly-staining cells which contrast strongly with the pale mucinous cells of the normal glands (Fig. 128). The lining cells are several layers in depth, and are not limited by the basement membrane, but invade the surrounding tissue. Mitoses are numerous. Most characteristic of all, new glands are found in abnormal positions, *e. g.*, deep to the muscularis mucosæ. Sometimes, particularly in the stomach, the glandular formation is lost, and the tumor assumes a scirrhous form with abundant stroma.

Mucoid carcinoma, formerly called colloid carcinoma, occurs principally in the large bowel, stomach, breast and bronchi. Two different forms may be distinguished: (1) *primary mucoid carcinoma* arising as a tumor of mucus-secreting cells; (2) a *secondary form* which is merely a mucoid degeneration of a preëxisting adenocarcinoma. Only 15 per cent of cases belong to the true primary form, which is characterized by bulky gelatinous masses, loss of glandular arrangement (also seen in the metastases), large signet-ring cells showing abundant evidence of proliferation, and a high mortality. Many of the cells are greatly distended with mucin (Fig. 129*A*), and large numbers of them disappear completely. In the secondary form the glandular arrangement is preserved with mucus in the acini (Fig. 129*B*), the picture is one of advanced degeneration with little evidence of proliferation, and the malignancy is roughly proportional to the degree of mucus formation.

Muco-epidermoid carcinoma is a peculiar form of tumor in which a tendency to a two-fold differentiation is apparent, in some places the tendency being toward epidermoid carcinoma, whilst in others it resembles adenocarcinoma with mucus-secreting cells producing much mucus. The usual site is the parotid and other salivary glands, but it may occur in the oral and nasal cavities, esophagus, bronchus, urinary bladder and

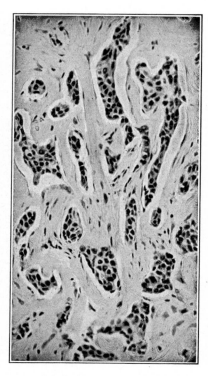

Fig. 130.—Scirrhous carcinoma of the breast. The compressed groups of tumor cells are separated by a dense stroma. × 175.

anus (Hamperl and Hellwig). The tumor is described in greater detail in Chapter 25.

An *undifferentiated adenocarcinoma*, which used to be known as carcinoma simplex, includes the well-known scirrhous and medullary forms. As a rule, it grows from the cubical epithelium of solid glands, particularly the breast. The cells are spheroidal or polyhedral, and are arranged in solid masses or columns. In *scirrhous carcinoma* the stroma is dense, the cell groups are small and often present a single column of cells, and the cells are compressed and stain darkly (Fig. 130.) Mitotic figures are not numerous, for the tumor is not of rapid growth. The dense stroma makes the tumor very hard. Most cancers of the breast are of the scirrhous type.

In the *medullary* or *encephaloid* form of carcinoma simplex the proportion of cells to stroma is reversed (Fig. 131). The cells are collected in large masses, are actively growing, and show many mitotic figures.

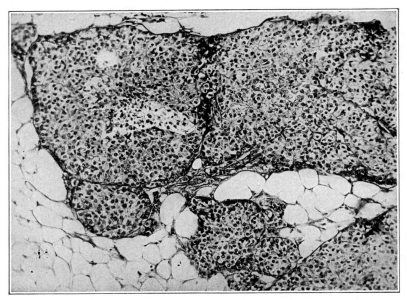

FIG. 131.—Medullary carcinoma of breast, highly cellular. × 110.

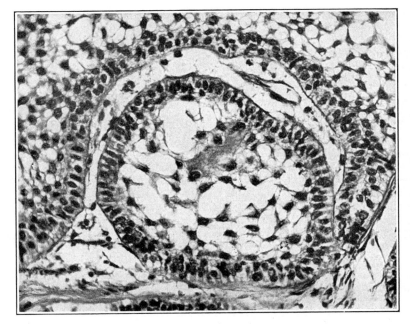

FIG. 132.—Adamantinoma showing palisade of enameloblasts and vacuolated cells. × 220.

The stroma is scanty, so that the tumor is soft (*encephaloid*, brain-like). Degeneration and necrosis is common. As one part of a tumor may show a scirrhous picture under the microscope and another a medullary picture, and as the primary tumor may be scirrhous while the metastases may be medullary, it is evident that the distinction between the two forms is in no way fundamental.

ADAMANTINOMA.—This is a rare epithelial tumor of the jaw which is one variety of *odontoma*. There are various views as to its origin, but it seems probable that it arises from the group of embryonal cells which comprise the outer epithelial layer of the enamel organ (Zegarelli), so that it may be called an *enameloblastoma*. It is composed of masses of epithelial cells which may become hollowed so as to give a glandular or cystic appearance. There is no constant microscopic picture. The cell type is the basal cell, but there may be all degrees of differentiation of the enamel organ. When differentiation is marked there may be an outer palisade layer of columnar cells, the enameloblasts, and a central core of "star cells" with large vacuoles and connecting cytoplasmic bridges (Fig. 132). Or there may be strands of epithelium of epidermoid type which branch and form a fantastic network. The undifferentiated forms consist entirely of basal cells. The tumor grows slowly and causes expansion of the jaw until a mere shell of bone is left. Cyst formation may occur. The tumor is usually innocent, but there may be invasion and, in rare cases, metastases.

Similar tumors are found in the stalk of the pituitary, where they are known as suprasellar tumors, and in the tibia. The pituitary stalk arises as an invagination of the oral epithelium, and as the enamel organ has a similar origin it is easy to understand why epithelial cells which retain their embryonic character should give rise to similar tumors in two different sites. The very rare tumors of the tibia are more of a puzzle, but may possibly be explained on a basis of abnormal embryonic epithelial invaginations.

CONNECTIVE-TISSUE TUMORS

INNOCENT CONNECTIVE-TISSUE TUMORS

Fibroma.—The type cell of the fibroma is the fibroblast. It is composed of fibrous tissue. The proportion of cells to collagen fibers varies greatly. *Hard* fibromas are acellular with abundant collagen. *Soft* fi-

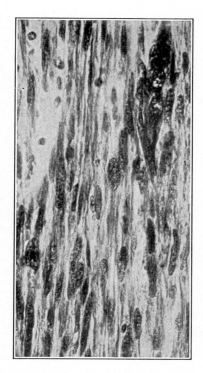

FIG. 133.—Fibroma showing fibroblasts and fibers. × 400.

bromas are highly cellular. Of course, there are all grades. The more highly cellular the tumor, the nearer does it approach to malignancy. It might be thought that the fibroma would be a common tumor. On the contrary, it is quite rare in a pure form.

Gross Appearance.—The gross appearance is that of an encapsulated rounded tumor, firm, white in color, the cut surface being flat and intersected with glistening bands. *Microscopically* it presents intersecting bundles of fibers between which are a varying number of fusiform cells (Fig. 133).

SITES.—In the *skin* there may be hard or soft fibromas. As the latter arise from cutaneous nerves they will be considered in connection with neurofibromas. Fibromas of *mucous membranes* are found in the submucous coat of the stomach and intestines. They often project into the lumen and become pedunculated. *Visceral* fibromas occur in the ovary, kidney, and other organs, usually remaining quite small. Fibromas growing from the nasopharynx may attain a large size and threaten the life of the patient.

Fibroma of the *abdominal wall* is called a *desmoid tumor* (*desmos*, band or fiber). It grows from the sheath of the rectus abdominis, and may attain a considerable size and invade the muscle. The muscle fibers enclosed in the tumor undergo a peculiar change with the formation of multinucleated masses like foreign body giant cells. About 80 per cent of the cases occur in women who have borne children. In the remaining cases there is usually a history of trauma to the abdominal wall.

Fibroma of *nerve* may be divided into cutaneous neurofibroma and neurofibroma of the subcutaneous and deeper nerve trunks. (1) The *cutaneous neurofibroma* may be single, forming a firm and often very tender nodule in the skin. The tumor arises from the connective-tissue sheath of the nerve.

Multiple neurofibromata constitute the condition known as von Recklinghausen's disease, or molluscum fibrosum. There may be hundreds of tumors. They usually grow from cutaneous nerves and form soft nodules in the skin, but they may grow from the deep nerves and cranial nerves. The skin is often pigmented in patches. Death is not uncommonly due to sarcomatous change in one of the tumors.

(2) *Neurofibroma of the deeper nerves* grows from the subcutaneous nerves and the deeper trunks. It is much less common than the cutaneous form, but is of importance in that it has a strong tendency to become malignant. The condition is described more fully under the heading of Neurosarcoma or Neurogenic Sarcoma. A *plexiform neuroma* is a diffuse over-growth of the endoneurium of the nerves in the subcutaneous tissue. It is made up of coiled and thickened nerve trunks, many of which can be dissected out. The usual site is the head and neck.

Xanthoma.—As its name indicates, a xanthoma is a yellow tumor (*xanthos*, yellow), and has the general structure of a fibroma. At least three distinct forms can be distinguished.

1. *Xanthelasma*, by far the commonest variety, is not a real tumor but a degeneration of the muscle of the eyelid. It occurs as small yellow nodules on the eyelid in elderly persons.

2. *Xanthoma multiplex*, also known as X. dia-beticorum, in which groups of yellow nodules are scattered over the surface of the body. It is associated with a high blood cholesterol (the yellow color is due to cholesterol), and is therefore found in diabetes and obstructive jaundice.

3. *Large xanthomas* are rare tumors which occur in connection with tendon sheaths, and which may resemble giant cell tumors.

All of the tumors are of a bright yellow color. They consist of connective-tissue cells greatly distended with lipoid droplets (cholesterol ester) so that the cell has a pale and foamy appearance. In addition to these "xanthoma cells" there are fibroblasts and foreign body giant cells. The latter are especially numerous in the single large tumors, and these tumors often contain much blood pigment. In some cases a striking feature is the so-called *Touton giant cells*, which are characterized by a remarkable ring of nuclei right around the periphery of the cell. They may be very numerous. I have not met with them in any other condition.

In some forms of xanthoma the basis of the condition may be a general disturbance of lipid metabolism associated with hypercholesterolemia. In others the defect may be intracellular, involving certain cells of the reticuloendothelial system.

Myxoma.—A myxoma is a connective-tissue tumor with the structure of umbilical cord. It very rarely occurs as a pure tumor, but mucoid or myxomatous degeneration is common in connective-tissue tumors, both innocent and malignant. The appearance of myxomatous degeneration in what appears to be an innocent connective-tissue tumor is always suggestive of a malignant change. A definite sarcoma showing myxomatous tissue is called a *myxosarcoma*. The *microscopic* appearance is that of Wharton's jelly in the umbilical cord. Branched connective-tissue cells are scattered through a jelly-like or mucoid matrix. This material can be stained with mucicarmine.

Chondroma.—A chondroma is a tumor composed of cartilage. It is hard, bluish-gray in color, and translucent like normal hyaline cartilage. This, and the fact that is is well lobulated and so encapsulated that it is readily shelled out, make recognition easy. Microscopically it differs from normal hyaline cartilage in that the cells are arranged singly instead of in groups (Fig. 134). Being non-vascular it is very liable to myxomatous degeneration. It often becomes calcified. It grows from the ends of long bones

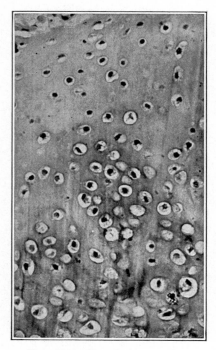

Fig. 134.—Chondroma. × 240.

in young persons, originating from the epiphyseal cartilage. When the bone stops growing, the tumor also ceases to grow and becomes calcified or ossified. These tumors also grow from the bones of the hands and feet, and from flat bones like the sternum and pelvis. The latter may attain a great size, and sarcomatous change is common.

Cartilage is found in developmental tumors (embryomas) of the testicle and in mixed tumors of the salivary glands. These should not be called chondromas. Multiple chondromas (multiple cartilaginous exostoses) will be considered in relation to diseases of bone.

Osteoma.—New formations of bone are common (callus of fractures, exostoses, and other forms), but true osteomas, like true fibromas, are comparatively rare. The *cancellous osteoma* is made up of cancellous bone. It originates from the epiphyseal cartilage as a chondroma, and though converted into bone a cap of cartilage covers the growing tip. As the bone grows in length the tumor becomes separated from the epiphyseal line. A *subungual exostosis* is a cancellous osteoma

which grows from the dorsal surface of the terminal phalanx of the big toe. It forces the nail up and causes much pain. A *compact osteoma,* also called an ivory exostosis because of its hardness, grows from the vault of the skull. It is a sessile tumor which may press on the brain or invade the orbit.

Lipoma.—A lipoma is a tumor composed of fat. It is a common tumor, occurring mainly in the subcutaneous tissue of the neck, shoulders, back, and buttocks. Occasionally it grows from the mesenteric and retroperitoneal fat, and still more rarely from the submucous coat of the stomach and intestine where it may form a polypoid mass. The "diffuse lipoma" of the neck is not a neoplasm but a lipomatosis. A lipoma does not waste when the rest of the fat wastes in cachectic diseases.

A lipoma is a soft circumscribed, lobulated, encapsulated tumor, easily shelled out. It is not attached to the deep fascia, but the overlying skin is often dimpled, owing to fibrous bands passing between it and the tumor. The lipoma is a very innocent tumor, but retroperitoneal and perirenal lipomas may rarely contain embryonic portions which grow rapidly and infiltrate. These tumors are called liposarcomas.

Hibernoma, as the name suggests, used to be regarded as a tumor arising from brown fat similar in nature to that seen in the so-called hibernating gland of some animals. The usual site is the interscapular region, but it has been reported in the axilla and the thigh. The large cells are filled with small fat vacuoles, giving them a characteristic appearance. The name is still acceptable, if only from a historical point of view, but it seems probable that the tumor is merely a lipoma developing in immature adipose tissue (Cox).

MALIGNANT
CONNECTIVE-TISSUE TUMORS

Sarcoma.—A sarcoma is a malignant tumor of connective tissue. It forms a large heterogeneous group, the limits of which should be greatly narrowed. Many tumors are called sarcoma although they are not connective-tissue tumors nor do they behave like them. Such are lymphosarcomas, melanotic sarcoma, myosarcoma. None of these will be considered here, and where possible the names should be changed. It is not always realized by the student commencing the study of pathology that carcinoma is an infinitely more common malignant tumor than sarcoma.

The malignancy of sarcoma varies enormously. This adds to the difficulties of microscopic diagnosis. The more malignant forms are easily recognized as such, but as we approach the dividing line we encounter a picture which on the one hand may resemble a cellular fibroma and on the other hand granulation tissue. Only long experience will give the pathologist the feeling that a lesion is malignant, a feeling which he may find difficult to justify in words. With repeated removal of a recurring tumor the histological picture may alter markedly for the worse.

Gross Appearance.—The sarcomas vary so greatly that no general description can cover the group, but they have certain points in common. A typical sarcoma has a fleshy appearance (*sark*, flesh). It forms a bulky mass which is more sharply demarcated from the surrounding tissue than is a carcinoma. The more cellular forms may resemble the white matter of the brain. The tumor varies much in consistence, but it is often soft like the brain. The cut surface is homogeneous, and this is one of its chief characteristics. But degenerations are common, and these may interfere with the homogeneous character of the tumor. The growth of the tumor may outstrip its blood supply, with the result that a species of infarction occurs. Necrosis, mucoid or myxomatous softening, and actual liquefaction are frequent. The most common of these changes is hemorrhage from the abundant and very thin-walled blood vessels.

Microscopic Appearance.—The less differentiated forms are highly cellular and the stroma may be so scanty as to be indistinguishable. The greater the differentiation, the more abundant and characteristic does the stroma become. Thus in the osteosarcoma there is osteoid tissue or bone between the cells. The general histological arrangement of a sarcoma differs fundamentally from that of a carcinoma in the same way that connective tissue differs from epithelium.

The cells of a carcinoma are arranged in groups separated by a stroma, but the stroma does not penetrate between the individual cells of the group. This is called an alveolar arrangement, and resembles that of the epithelium from which the tumor arises. In a sarcoma, on the other hand, there is no alveolar grouping; the cells are uniformly distributed, and are separated by a stroma. This may be very abundant as in bone sarcoma, or it may be so fine that it requires special staining methods to bring it out. Sarcoma cells have other mesoblastic characteristics. They tend to have poorly defined borders compared with carcinoma cells, and extensions of the cytoplasm form an intercellular matrix. Numerous blood vessels, often mere capillaries or sinusoids, penetrate the tumor, whereas in carcinoma the vessels are confined to the regular stroma which separates the groups of cells. Thus necrosis is more apt to occur in carcinoma, as the growth of cells outstrips that of the vessels. Sarcoma grows expansively on this vascular framework, and it is small wonder that hemorrhages are frequent. Carcinoma tends to grow rather by infiltration. Mitotic figures are significant in mesenchymal tumors, but much less so in epithelial tumors; they are often seen in inflamed and irritated epidermis.

The type cell may be the fibroblast, the osteoblast, the cartilage cell, etc. In the most undifferentiated forms the type cell cannot be recognized. Many of these tumors are polymorphic, showing a variety of cells. Mitotic figures are very numerous in the rapidly growing sarcomas, scanty in the slowly growing ones. Their presence is of great value in the differentiation from a cellular fibroma, but it must be remembered that mitotic figures may be present in rapidly growing granulation tissue. Tumor giant cells form a feature of some highly malignant sarcomas. If the tumor becomes infected the giant cells may phagocytose many of the leukocytes, a rare occurrence (Fig. 135).

SPREAD.—A sarcoma grows *expansively* so as to form a bulky mass, but it also *infiltrates* the surrounding tissue. The rate of growth varies greatly. Unsuccessful (incomplete) operative interference is often followed by a great increase in the rate of growth. A rapidly growing sarcoma may sometimes out-

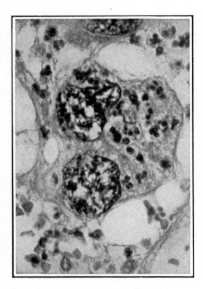

FIG. 135.—Phagocytic tumor giant cell. × 600.

strip its blood supply, so that the tumor may
halt and even retrogress. Infiltration of the
surrounding tissue occurs. The tumor cells
creep along the fascial plane, between the
muscle fibers, through the Haversian canals
of bone, etc. Owing to this tendency removal is likely to be incomplete and recurrence is very common.

Distant spread takes place by the blood
vessels. The vessels are so abundant and so
thin-walled, and the sarcoma cells so readily
invade them that early blood dissemination
is inevitable. Metastases are first formed in
the lungs, but the tumor cells may pass
through the lungs to any of the viscera.
Owing to this early spread the lungs should
be roentgen-rayed for metastases even in
what appear to be the most operable of
sarcomas. Spread by lymph stream is uncommon, but may occur in from 5 to 10 per
cent of cases.

The *sites* of a sarcoma are varied, since
connective tissue occurs in every part of the
body. They are especially common in bone,
subcutaneous tissue, fascia, and muscle.

Two methods may be used in the classification of the sarcoma. The first is cytological,
the second histological. In the first the tissue
is named according to the form of cell which
predominates, so that we have a round cell

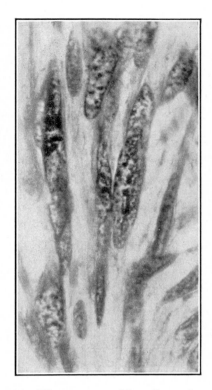

FIG. 136.—Fibrosarcoma. The cells are large and
fusiform. × 1000.

(small and large) sarcoma, a spindle cell
(small and large) sarcoma, a mixed cell sarcoma, and a giant cell sarcoma. This method is the refuge of the destitute, and should
be avoided to the utmost of one's ability. In
the second or histological method the tumor
is named according to the type of connective
tissue from which it arises, so that we have
a fibrosarcoma, osteosarcoma, chondrosarcoma, etc. This is the only satisfactory
method, but if differentiation has not gone
sufficiently far it may not be possible. The
interstitial tissue is often more characteristic
than the cells of the tumor, *i. e.*, it may be
osseous, cartilaginous, collagenous, etc.

HISTOLOGICAL TYPES OF SARCOMA.—1. *Fibrosarcoma.*—This is a spindle cell sarcoma,
the type cell being the fibroblast. (Fig. 136.)
It is not really a common tumor, as used to
be thought. Many malignant connective-
tissue tumors formerly regarded as fibrosa-
comas are now known to be neurogenic in
origin, arising from peripheral nerves. The

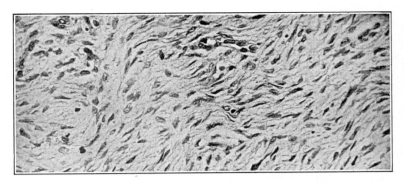

FIG. 137.—Neurogenic sarcoma, showing the fasciculated arrangement. × 300.

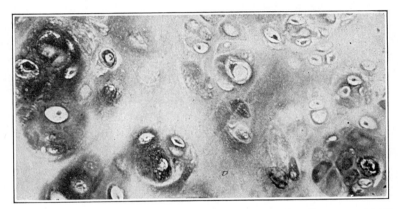

FIG. 138.—Chondrosarcoma. Great irregularity in size of cells. Compare with Fig. 134 which has same magnification. ×240.

cells are fusiform, and may be small or large, the latter being the more malignant type. Both the gross and the microscopic features vary much, depending on the degree of anaplasia. In the anaplastic forms the tumor may be very soft, and the cells may be so slightly fusiform that the non-committal name of round-cell sarcoma is applied. The stroma varies. It may be very scanty, or abundant fibrils may be formed so that it may be difficult to distingusih the tumor from a soft fibroma. The presence of mitotic figures is one of the most valuable points. Its behavior is that of a sarcoma of varying degrees of malignancy.

2. *Neurosarcoma (Neurogenic Sarcoma).*— The term *neurogenic sarcoma* was introduced by Ewing to designate a type of spindle-cell tumor which was supposed to arise from deeply situated peripheral nerves. This con-

cept has become generally accepted to such a degree that the great majority of fibrosarcomas are now regarded as of neurogenic origin. This concept has been vigorously attacked by Stout, who points out that no proof exists of the origin of these tumors from nerve fibers, a view with which the writer is in agreement. The histological feature which is taken as an indication of neurogenic origin is a tendency for the tumor cells to run in interlacing bundles or fasciculi.

At first the neurogenic sarcoma is localized, but with continued growth and especially on recurring it infiltrates the surrounding tissue. The *microscopic appearance* is in general that of a fibrosarcoma, but the elongated cells are arranged in characteristic intertwining bundles, fasciculi and whorls (Fig. 137). The appearance suggests the neurogenic origin, but it may be very difficult to determine the

16

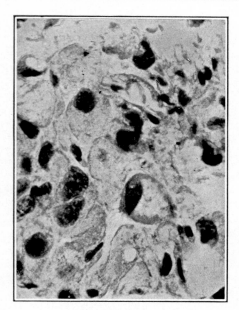

FIG. 139.—Liposarcoma. Some cells have granular cytoplasm, others are filled with fat. × 510.

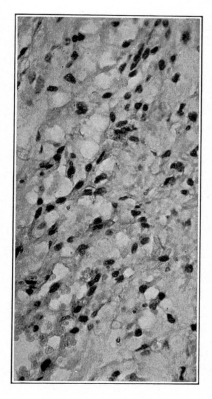

FIG. 140.—Myxosarcoma. × 350.

question of malignancy. It is highly radio-resistant, a point of some value in differential diagnosis.

3. *Osteosarcoma (Osteogenic Sarcoma).*—This is one of the most important and common forms of sarcoma. The type cell is the osteoblast, but it is by the intercellular substance (bone, cartilage) that it is most readily recognized. It is considered together with other bone tumors in Chapter 43.

4. *Chondrosarcoma.*—A chondroma may show evidence of malignancy (rapid growth, irregularity in the size and shape of the cells, mitoses), and is then known as a chondrosarcoma (Fig. 138). It arises from a bone, often the sternum or pelvis, may attain a huge size, and invades the blood vessels causing pulmonary metastases. The distinction between a chondroma and chondrosarcoma may be very difficult, and the pathologist may have to depend on the clinical course and the gross appearance (invasion, etc.) rather than on the microscopic picture. Myxomatous degeneration should arouse suspicion.

5. *Liposarcoma.*—This tumor is by no means so rare as is commonly supposed; it is easily missed, especially if fat stains are not used. It may occur wherever there is fat, but is commonest in intermuscular tissue, around joints, and in the retroperitoneal and perirenal regions. At first encapsulated, it tends to recur after removal and then becomes infiltrating, so that the prognosis is bad. The *microscopic picture* varies in different cases, and there may be a most confusing variation in a single tumor. The common cells are spindle cells and large polyhedral cells; the cytoplasm is granular and may or may not contain fat, best shown, of course, by means of fat stains. The pale, swollen, polyhedral cells may resemble epithelial cells (Fig. 139) and thus suggest secondary renal carcinoma (hypernephroma), a mistake especially likely to occur when the tumor is in bone. Cells resembling fetal fat cells may be present, and tumor giant cells are not uncommon.

6. *Myxosarcoma.*—This is not a real group, but merely a mucoid or myxomatous degeneration of a sarcoma (Fig. 140). The term is useful if it serves to suggest the ominous

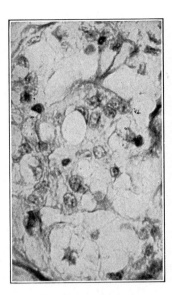

FIG. 141.—Chordoma. The clear vacuolated appearance of the cells is characteristic.

character of myxomatous change in a connective-tissue tumor.

CHORDOMA.—This tumor arises from remnants of the notochord, a structure of hypoblastic origin. It occurs at the upper and lower ends of the vertebral column, because the notochord is enclosed in the bodies of the permanent vertebræ. At the upper end it grows between the pituitary fossa and the foramen magnum, while at the lower end it occurs in the sacro-coccygeal region. It is a very rare tumor of rather low malignancy which spreads by infiltration, and only in the end stages does it form metastases. The tumor, which may reach a large size, is elastic in consistence, and shows numerous areas of translucent chordal tissue separated by patches of hemorrhage. *Microscopically* it consists of large clear cells closely packed together without any intercellular substance. The cells are distended with mucinous material, so that the tumor may be mistaken for a mucoid carcinoma. The cytoplasm, however, has a vacuolated appearance which is very characteristic (Fig. 141).

MUSCLE-TISSUE TUMORS

Just as there are two types of muscle, plain and striated, so there are two forms of myoma or tumors arising from muscle cells. These are the leiomyoma and the rhabdo-

myoma. To these a third form, the myoblastoma, must be added.

Leiomyoma.—The leiomyoma (*leios*, smooth) is an innocent tumor of plain muscle. It is extremely common in the uterus, so much so as to constitute the commonest tumor in the body. The special characters of myomata of the uterus will be considered in connection with diseases of that organ. Leiomyomata are curiously rare in other parts of the body which contain plain muscle. They may occur in the ovary, tubes, and broad ligament, in the alimentary canal where they often form polypoid masses which project into the lumen, and in the bladder and ureters. The muscular walls of the blood vessels are immune.

The *gross appearance* resembles that of a fibroma. The tumor may be of any size, from the very small to the very large. It is hard or at least firm, well encapsulated and easily removed. The cut surface presents a characteristically whorled appearance, due to interlacing bundles of fibers cut in various planes. Degenerative changes are common, such as hyaline and mucoid degeneration, softening, and sometimes complete calcification so that the tumor is converted into a mass of stone.

Microscopically the leiomyoma consists of interlacing bundles of plain muscle fibers, separated by a varying amount of fibrous tissue. The cells may be distinguished from those of a spindle cell sarcoma by the long rod-like nuclei and the absence of mitoses (Fig. 142).

Occasionally a part of the tumor may become malignant, and is then called a *malignant myoma* or *leiomyosarcoma*. The nuclei are larger, the cells more active-looking, and mitotic figures can be seen. These tumors seldom give rise to metastases, and may not recur after removal, so that they are usually not highly malignant.

Rhabdomyoma.—The rhabdomyoma is a tumor of striated muscle (*rhabdos*, a stripe). It is curiously rare, indeed extremely so. Nor is it found where it might be expected, *i. e.*, in voluntary muscle. A pure rhabdomyoma is the rarest of all, being practically confined to the heart. Striated muscle is found in embryonal tumors of the kidney, of the vagina of children, and of the testicle.

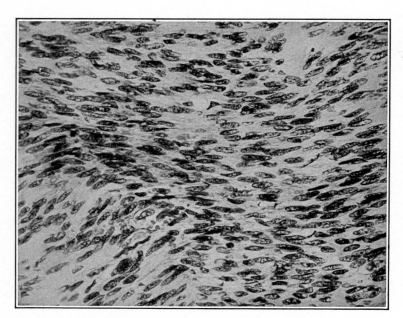

FIG. 142.—Leiomyoma showing plain muscle cells.   × 300.

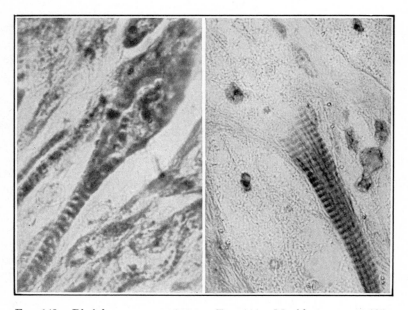

FIG. 143.—Rhabdomyoma.   × 940.   FIG. 144.—Myoblastoma.   × 625.

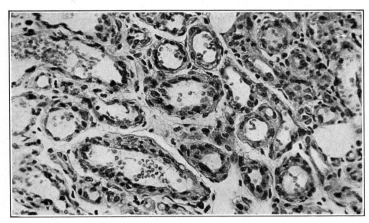

Fig. 145.—Capillary angioma. In addition to many new vessels there is a solid mass of endothelial cells in the upper right hand corner. × 225.

In these tumors the muscle is mingled with other tissues. Only some of the cells are cross-striated. These mixed tumors are highly malignant and metastasize by the blood stream (Fig. 143).

Myoblastoma.—This tumor of striated muscle was first described in 1926, but 50 cases were reported in the next eight years. The common sites are the tongue, larynx and skin, but it has also been found in the lip, upper part of esophagus, and leg. It consists of polygonal cells with characteristic highly granular cytoplasm. In addition there may be ribbon-like syncytial masses with granular cytoplasm. No cross-striations are seen. It is open to doubt if these tumors really arise from primitive myoblasts, as is generally believed, for they may occur in sites devoid of striated muscle. Moreover they are essentially benign, whereas true differentiated rhabdomyoblastomas are highly malignant. Fust and Custer present evidence suggesting that these tumors are derived from nerves and not from skeletal muscle. The lesions contain concentric masses of granular tumor cells arranged around bundles of axis cylinders with what appears to be frayed nerve sheaths at the periphery (Fig. 144).

VASCULAR TUMORS

An angioma is a tumor composed either of blood vessels or lymphatics. The former is called a hemangioma, the latter a lymph-angioma. The hemangioma is much the more common, and is commonly referred to as an angioma, the term lymphangioma being reserved for the lymphatic type.

Hemangioma.—A hemangioma is a new formation of blood vessels. It may be difficult to distinguish this from telangiectasis, which is merely a dilatation of previously existing vessels. Two types are encountered, the capillary and the cavernous. The former is much the commoner.

Capillary Angioma.—This consists of a network of new-formed capillaries filled with blood. (Fig. 145.) The neoplasm affects only one segment of a vessel, from which buds of endothelium grow out and form new vessels. There is therefore a more or less closed system of vessels, not a dilatation of all the vessels of the part. The capillaries appear to arise from a rudiment destined to form blood vessels, and thus form a mass which is to some extent withdrawn from the general circulation, so that any hemorrhage which may occur from it is not necessarily severe.

Cavernous Angiomas.—This form is less common. It has the same structure as erectile tissue, being composed of large blood-spaces or sinusoids lined by endothelium. The commonest site is the liver, where it forms a small dark-red tumor which is discovered accidentally at autopsy. These tumors in the liver may be multiple, but they seldom become large. The cavernous angi-

oma occurs in other positions, *e.g.*, lips, subcutaneous tissue, and muscle. It is not encapsulated, and may infiltrate the surrounding
tissue like a malignant tumor. In rare cases
metastases are formed in the lungs.

Other types of blood vessel tumors are
discussed more appropriately in relation to
diseases of the arteries in Chapter 22.

Lymphangioma.—This is much less common than an hemangioma. Like the hemangioma it is congenital. It may be localized or
diffuse. The vessels may be small or cavernous, and they contain lymph instead of blood,
so that the tumor lacks the characteristic
color of the hemangioma. Lymphangioma
of the tongue causes a diffuse enlargement,
known as *macroglossia* (big tongue); a similar
swelling of the lip is *macrocheilia* (big lip).
Cystic hygroma is a large soft swelling in the
neck of children which may be mistaken for
a cold abscess. More rarely it occurs in the
axilla or the side of the thorax. It may be
present at birth and tends to become smaller
or disappear as the child grows up.

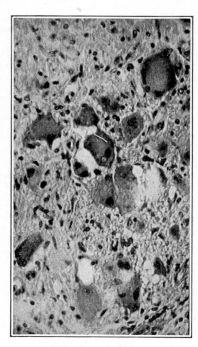

Fig. 146.—Ganglioneuroma. × 300.

OTHER TUMORS

Carcinoma and sarcoma may occur anywhere in the body where there is epithelium
or connective tissue. Other tumors are confined to one organ or system, and these are
more conveniently considered in the later
part of this book than in this discussion of
the general pathology of tumors. Only a
word or two will be devoted to these tumors
of special parts in this chapter.

Tumors of Hemopoietic Tissue.—This
group includes tumors of the lymphoid tissue
and bone marrow. The principal members
of the group are lymphosarcoma, reticulum-
cell sarcoma, Hodgkin's disease, leukemia,
and multiple myeloma. They arise in blood-
forming organs, and will be considered in
connection with diseases of these organs.

Nervous-tissue Tumors.—Although the
central nervous system is ectodermal in origin, it becomes divided into parenchymatous
tissue (nerve cells and fibers) and supporting
tissue (neuroglia). Tumors of the parenchymatous tissue are very rare, tumors of the
neuroglia are very common.

The two main tumors are glioma and neuroblastoma. *Gliomas* constitute the important
group of brain tumors and are considered in
connection with diseases of the nervous system. Neuroblastoma is a tumor of neuroblasts, usually occurring in the adrenal medulla, but occasionally in connection with
other parts of the sympathetic nervous system. It is described in the section on Diseases
of the Adrenal Glands.

Retinoblastoma.—This tumor has been
called glioma of the retina, neuroblastoma,
and neuro-epithelioma. It is composed of
cells which started from the anlage of the
retina in the embryo and were not developed
into functioning cells. It seems best, therefore, to use the term retinoblastoma. It is
an uncommon tumor, and presents three
striking clinical characteristics: (1) it is bilateral in at least 20 per cent of the cases;
(2) over 90 per cent of the cases occur before
the fourth year, in this resembling neuroblastoma of the adrenal; (3) it shows an
extraordinary familial tendency. In a family
of 16 children 10 died of retinoblastoma.
The tumor is locally destructive, but later it
may form metastases in the lymph nodes and
internal organs. *Microscopically* it is composed of small round cells with practically no

cytoplasm and no fibrils. The chief characteristic is the presence of circles or ' rosettes" of columnar cells, which, however, may be absent. They probably represent inclusions of cells which normally develop into rods and cones.

GANGLIONEUROMA.—A very rare tumor composed of adult nerve cells and fibers (Fig. 146). It is commoner in peripheral ganglia than in the central nervous system. The condition is benign.

Pigment-forming Tumors.—The benign member of this group is the nevus or pigmented mole, a very common lesion of the skin. The malignant member, known as the melanoma or malignant melanoma, formerly as melanotic sarcoma, arises from the nevus, which is sometimes called a benign melanoma. As the subject of the origin of the nevus, whether from the epithelium of the epidermis (epidermal theory) or from nerve elements of the skin (neurogenic theory), is a highly contentious one, we shall defer a discussion of the nevus and melanoma until tumors of the skin are considered in Chapter 46.

Chorionic Epithelium Tumors.—From the trophoblast of the chorionic villi which constitute the fetal portion of the placenta may arise either a benign tumor known as a hydatidiform mole, or a malignant tumor, the chorionepithelioma or choriocarcinoma. In about 30 per cent of cases the malignant lesion is preceded by the benign one. The tumors are described in connection with diseases of the female reproductive system.

TERATOMAS

A teratoma is a composite mass derived from more than one germinal layer. In some there are representatives of all three layers. It is not a tumor in the strict sense of the word, but rather an attempted formation of a new individual within the tissues of the patient. A malignant growth may develop in a teratoma and may be carcinomatous or sarcomatous in type.

Every grade of complexity may be met with in a teratoma. At one end of the series is the parasistic fetus, an acardiac monster attached to a normal child. Or a jumbled mass of structures may be attached externally either to the upper jaw (*epignatus*) or in the sacral region (*sacral teratoma*). Or again such a mass may develop within the body, usually in the genital glands.

The structure may be simpler, comprising only one or two tissues as in the embryoma (teratoma) of the kidney. Finally there may be inclusions of the surface (inclusion dermoids), which may cause tumor-like swellings.

In the early stage of the developing and segmenting ovum the first blastomeres are totipotent; they have the capacity of forming a new individual as shown by the occasional development of identical twins from the one ovum. The later blastomeres are multipotent, *i. e.*, they can form all of the three germinal layers. In the segmenting ovum primitive sex cells (germinal cells) are separated from the somatic cells and migrate finally to the testicle and ovary, where they develop into spermatozoa or ova. Theoretically it is quite possible for one of the primitive germ cells to be segregated either in the sex glands or in some other part of the body, where, if it could be stimulated to divide, it may form a teratoma which is an abortive attempt at the production of a new individual even to the extent of forming chorionic membranes, for the chorionic epithelium is merely a modification of the fetal ectoderm. A blastomere may also be segregated, and if it is stimulated to grow it will form structures derived from the three germinal layers, a confused jumble of tissues, but not including fetal membranes. MacCallum suggests that the teratomas may be divided into two main classes, the first representing the development of a primitive *germinal* cell, the second being derived from a segregated *somatic* blastomere. These two forms belong to different generations, the first being analogous to a true offspring, the second to a twin brother.

Jacques Loeb, as is well known, succeeded in inducing parthenogenesis in the unfertilized ova of sea-urchins and even frogs by employing various physical and chemical stimuli. The resulting animals were apparently normal except that they possessed no sex cells. In 1926 Bosaeus published an account of some extraordinarily interesting experiments on the parthenogenetic formation of teratomas. He removed an ovum from a frog's ovary, pricked it with a needle, and reimplanted the stimulated ovum into the body of the same frog. As the result of parthenogenesis a teratoma developed which was similar in type to some of the teratomas occurring in man. When the ovum was placed in the body of another frog it failed to develop.

A new possibility is provided by advances in experimental embryology. It is now known that differentiation depends on two factors: (1) chemical organizers, (2) susceptibility or "competence" of the cells to the action of the organizers. Both of these change as development proceeds. Thus there are primary, secondary and tertiary organ-

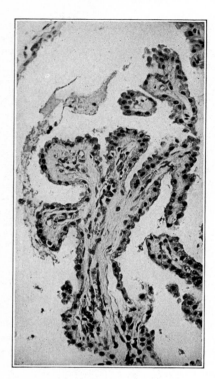

Fig. 147.—Choroid plexus in teratoma (chorionepithelioma) of testicle. × 175.

izers, and the susceptibility of the cells alters with
the course of development. When there is perfect
balance between organizers and susceptibility,
differentiation proceeds normally, but if organizers are produced too abundantly or too early
or if susceptibility persists beyond the period at
which it is normally lost, the result may be uncontrolled differentiation with the production of a
jumble of structures so characteristic of teratomas.

Perhaps the most varied structures are encountered in teratomas of the genital gland. In the
dermoid cyst of the ovary are found skin, hair,
sebaceous material, teeth, bone, brain, thyroid,
etc. In teratoma of the testicle, glands, cartilage,
muscle, brain, and even choroid plexus may occur
(Fig. 147).

INCLUSION DERMOIDS.—Although these have
the same name as the congenital tumors occurring
in the genital glands, their origin is quite different.
They may be divided into congenital and implantation dermoids; in both cases there is inclusion
of dermal and epidermal structures.

Congenital Dermoids.—Congenital dermoids are
inclusions of dermal tissue along the line of the
embryonic fissures. Dermal tissue, it may be with
hair and cyst formation, is found in the middle
line of the abdomen and chest (mediastinal dermoid), in the skull (line of attachment of dura
mater to tentorium cerebelli), in the line of the
thyroglossal duct and the duct leading from
pharynx to pituitary, and at the site of the
branchial clefts, particularly the second.

Implantation Dermoids.—Implantation dermoids are the result of a small piece of skin being
implanted in the deeper tissues, usually as the
result of trauma with a pointed instrument. A
small cyst lined by epidermis is formed. These
cysts are most common on the hands of manual
laborers.

REFERENCES

Cox, A. J.: Am. J. Path., 1954, *68*, 511. (Hiber-
    noma).
HAMPERL, H. and HELLWIG, G.: Cancer, 1957, *10*,
    1187. (Muco-epidermoid tumors).
MacCallum, W. G.: *Textbook of Pathology*, Phila-
    delphia, 1932, Chap. 72. (Teratoma).

Chapter 10

Growth and its Disorders

General Considerations
Metaplasia
    Epithelial Metaplasia
    Connective-tissue Meta-
        plasia
Atrophy

Hypertrophy and Hyperplasia
    Hypotrophy
        Compensatory Hypertrophy
    Hyperplasia
Malformations
    Monsters

GENERAL CONSIDERATIONS

Growth is the most fundamental of all physiological functions. It is brought about by multiplication of cells, not by increase in their size. There is little difference in size between the cells of a mouse and the cells of an elephant; the difference is one of number. In the same way the cells of a cancer may be actually smaller than those of the tissue from which it arises. The cells of any given species of animal have a strictly limited power of multiplication. When this limit is reached the growth of the animal ceases. This it is which determines the size of animals, so that all members of one species are of approximately the same size, no matter how the external condition may vary. To this rule the fish offer an exception, for the members of a species, such as trout, may greatly increase in size when placed in a more suitable environment. Growth is brought about by the change of non-living into living material. All dead matter is potentially living, and we see the transformation of dead into living matter going on ceaselessly. ' The molecules of the dead world are waiting to be delivered from the bonds of death, ' as Lorrain Smith remarks in a delightful monograph which should be consulted by anyone interested in the subject of growth. He points out that theoretically the whole inorganic substance of the material world might be converted into living substance by the substance already living.

Cells not only grow (multiply); they also differentiate. Now differentiation and growth are mutually antagonistic, and this is a profound biological principle. Differentiation depends on environment. Unless cells are compelled by their environment to differentiate they will feed, grow and multiply forever without doing any work, thus resembling human beings. Division and function are not possible at the same time. The more highly differentiated a cell becomes, the more does it lose its power of reproduction, and therefore its ability to give rise to tumor formation; this is seen in the case of striated muscle, nerve cells, red blood cells, etc. Cancer cells fail to differentiate; instead they continue to grow. As Lorrain Smith says, they do not fall into the normal procession. They fall out. They do not keep step; the procession is moving slowly and they move fast.

METAPLASIA

Metaplasia is the transformation of one type of tissue into another type. This process has definite limits. An epiblastic tissue can only produce another epiblastic tissue, mesoblast can only produce mesoblast. Metaplasia is best seen in the closely-related connective tissues, as when cartilage is converted into bone. *Anaplasia*, or reversionary atrophy, must not be confused with true metaplasia. *Anaplasia is merely the reversion of a more highly to a less highly differentiated form.*

Epithelial Metaplasia.—True metaplasia occurs in response to a call for altered function or at least as the result of altered environment. If the prolapsed uterus becomes everted the columnar epithelium is changed into a squamous stratified form

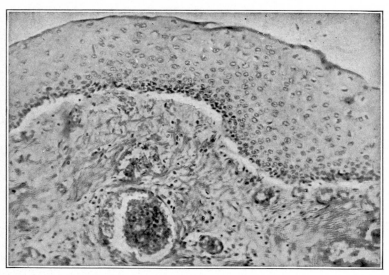

FIG. 148.—Remarkable metaplasia of epithelium lining a bronchiectatic cavity. The single layer of columnar cells is converted into typical stratified squamous epithelium. × 150.

better fitted to withstand friction. As the result of continued irritation, *e. g.*, from gall-stones, the columnar epithelium of the gall-bladder may also become squamous, and from this altered epithelium a squamous cell carcinoma may arise. The bronchial epithelium in a bronchiectatic cavity may undergo the same change and come to resemble the epidermis (Fig. 148). The more highly specialized glandular epithelia (liver, kidney, etc.) appear to be incapable of true metaplasia.

Connective-tissue Metaplasia.—Examples of this are of common occurrence. Fibrous tissue, myxomatous tissue, cartilage, and bone are all closely related, and one may become changed into the other. The commonest change is that of cartilage into bone. In old age ossification of the laryngeal and tracheal cartilages is common enough. This is certainly not due to altered function, but may be connected with altered environment. Bone may be formed in the walls of degenerated arteries, the seat of arteriosclerosis, or in an eye which is destroyed and functionless. It may be encountered in the edges of a wound in the abdominal wall. Apparently the connective-tissue cells become converted into bone-forming cells. In *myositis ossificans* bone is formed in the voluntary mus-

cles and may replace them to a large extent; this bone is probably formed from the connective tissue between the muscle fibers. Many examples of metaplasia are seen in connective-tissue tumors; thus the cells of an osteogenic sarcoma of bone may form fibrous tissue, mucoid tissue, cartilage or bone.

Endothelial Metaplasia.—When serosal endothelium such as that lining the pleura or peritoneum is irritated either experimentally or by disease it may undergo marked metaplastic changes. In place of being flattened it may become cubical, columnar, or even stratified. The cubical and columnar cells may surround spaces so as to give a glandular appearance.

ATROPHY

Atrophy is a diminution in size, a shrinking of cells or fibers which have reached their full development. Hypoplasia indicates a failure of full development. Atrophy may occur under a great variety of different conditions. Some of the most important of these are old age, lack of nourishment, disuse, the action of toxins, pressure and interference with nerve supply. As *age* advances there is a general tendency towards atrophy, best seen in the uterus, ovary, breast, lymphoid tissue, and bone marrow. Chronic *starvation* causes wasting of adipose tissue and muscles; atrophy also follows decreased blood supply due to arteriosclerosis. *Disuse* of a structure results in atrophy, as is seen in the anterior horn of the spinal cord after amputation of a limb. *Pressure* atrophy is seen in the erosion of bone by an aneurysm or the atrophy of liver cells in amyloid disease. *Neurotrophic* atrophy is due to loss of trophic impulses when a motor nerve is injured, but it is difficult to be sure how much of this is due to disuse.

HYPERTROPHY AND HYPERPLASIA

Hypertrophy.—Hypertrophy is an increase in the size of individual cells or fibers as a result of which the organ may become enlarged. Enlargement of an organ from any other cause should not be called hypertrophy. There is no increase in the number of the individual elements; such an increase is covered by the term *hyperplasia*. True hypertrophy never occurs as the result of irritation, but always in response to some demand for increased function. It is convenient to recognize three varieties of hypertrophy—physiological, adaptive, and compensatory—although the dividing lines cannot be drawn too sharply.

PHYSIOLOGICAL HYPERTROPHY.—Physiological hypertrophy occurs apart altogether from disease. The best example is the pregnant uterus. At the end of pregnancy the muscle fibers are ten times as long and four times as broad as in the non-pregnant uterus. The hypertrophy of muscles which follows hard work (the blacksmith's arm) may be placed in this group or in the next.

ADAPTIVE HYPERTROPHY.—Adaptive hypertrophy is best seen in hollow muscular organs when the outlet is partially obstructed. The wall of the organ becomes thickened owing to an increase in the size of the muscle fibers. As examples may be mentioned the left ventricle in stenosis of the aortic valve or high blood pressure with its increased peripheral resistance (Fig. 149), the stomach in pyloric obstruction, the bowel in chronic intestinal obstruction, and the bladder in stricture of the urethra. The hypertrophy

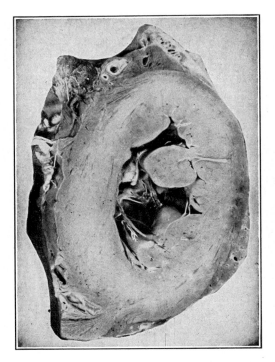

FIG. 149.—Concentric hypertrophy of the left ventricle in aortic stenosis.

of voluntary muscle as the result of exercise may be placed in this group or in the preceding one.

COMPENSATORY HYPERTROPHY. — Compensatory hypertrophy is an increase in size to compensate for loss of tissue. It is best seen in paired organs. When one kidney is removed or atrophies because of disease the remaining kidney does the work of the two and becomes correspondingly enlarged (Fig. 150). There is no formation of new elements, but merely an increase in the size of the existing tubules and glomeruli. When a portion of the liver or thyroid is removed the organ is restored to its original size, a process often spoken of as compensatory hypertrophy, but this is a hyperplasia rather than a hypertrophy.

Hyperplasia.—By hyperplasia is meant an increase in the number of the cells of a part. Its limits are more shadowy than those of hypertrophy, and it gradually merges into the process of neoplasia or tumor formation. Hyperplasia, unlike hypertrophy, is often the result of irritation, although it may

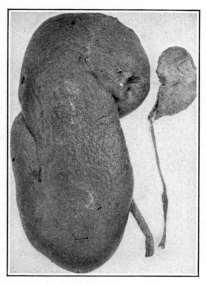

Fig. 150.—Compensatory hypertrophy
of one kidney.

also be compensatory or adaptive. Lymphoid tissue readily undergoes hyperplasia as the result of local irritation. Compensatory hyperplasia is seen in the bone marrow which so readily becomes hyperplastic when there is a demand for more blood. When a portion of the thyroid gland is removed the remaining tissue undergoes marked hyperplasia so as to compensate for the loss. The liver also has remarkable powers of compensatory hyperplasia.

MALFORMATIONS

The subject of malformations, maldevelopment, and monsters is an extremely large one, involving as it does a study of all the possible errors which may occur during the complex process of development. The scope of this work, not to mention the lack of knowledge of the writer, makes any attempt to cover the subject out of the question. All that will be attempted will be to give a catalogue of the principal conditions, so that the student will at least become familiar with their names. For convenience the subject may be divided into: (1) maldevelopments, inclusions, etc.; (2) local malformation; (3) double monsters.

When we seek for an explanation of developmental malformations and monstrosities we are inevitably groping in the dark, like the blind man looking for a black cat in an unlighted room. A few rays of light, however, begin to penetrate the darkness. We now know that if a pregnant woman suffers an attack of rubella (German measles) in the first three months of her pregnancy, there is a likelihood that her child may suffer from congenital heart disease. The laboratory approach to the problem of congenital malformations in the human embryo has illuminated the subject still more. It now becomes evident that environmental factors may affect embryonic development adversely. Fish embryos in particular permit direct visualization of the embryo subjected to stress, hypoxia in particular (Ingalls and Philbrook). With respect to monstrosities, embryonic development may be permanently altered by profound metabolic and hypoxic distress. The result of experimentally induced hypoxia may be *ectromelia* (congenital absence of limbs or parts of a limb), anophthalmia, cyclopia, or conjoined twins, conditions which are referred to below. The stage of development of the embryo at the time when the hypoxic stress originated is naturally a factor of prime importance in the resulting deformity.

MALDEVELOPMENTS.—Many minor errors of development are compatible with life and even with health. Most of these will be described when diseases of the individual organs are discussed. There may be too few digits or too many (supernumerary). Two or more of the fingers or toes may be fused together, a condition of *syndactyly*. The kidneys may be fused at the upper or the lower pole, the horseshoe kidney. Remnants of fetal structures which normally disappear may remain, *e.g.*, Meckel's diverticulum, Wolffian ducts, thyroglossal duct, ductus arteriosus, *etc.* The congenital anomalies of the heart form a subject in itself. In the course of development portions of an organ may become detached and included in another organ. Thus inclusions or "rests" of adrenal cortex may be found in the kidney and the pelvic organs, pancreatic tissue occurs in the wall of the stomach and duodenum, thyroid tissue at the base of the tongue and elsewhere in the neck. This displacement of tissue is called *heterotopia*. Along the normal lines of closure of developmental clefts dermal tissues may be infolded and included in the underlying structures. The included tissue may start to grow, forming an *inclusion dermoid*. There lesions are commonest in the face and the middle line of the body both anteriorly and posteriorly. It is possible that certain tumors of mixed structure may arise from these inclusions.

LOCAL MALFORMATIONS.—During normal development a number of grooves and fissures must be accurately closed. If any of these remain open either wholly or in part grave malformations may result. These may be reviewed briefly.

Neural Groove.—The entire groove may remain open, but usually the deficiency is only partial. If the cranial part is open the condition is called *cranioschisis*; if the spinal part is unclosed it is called *rhachioschisis*. In cranioschisis the brain may be absent save for an amorphous mass of tissue on the floor of the cranial cavity, a condition of *anencephaly* or *acrania*; the child is an anencephalic monster. The frontal part of the cranium may be closed, while the occipital part remains open and the brain hangs out at the back. When the patency is more limited in extent there may merely be some prolapse of the meninges or the brain covered by skin—meningocele or encephalocele. In the spinal canal by far the commonest defect is *spina bifida*, the lowest part of the canal remaining unclosed. Here also there may be meningocele or meningomyelocele.

Sternal Fissure.—If the patency is at all marked extra-uterine life is impossible, for the lungs are unable to expand. The heart may protrude through the opening, a condition of *ectopia cordis*.

Abdominal Fissure.—The two halves of the abdominal wall may fail to close. There will then be eventration or protrusion of the viscera.

Urogenital Fissure.—The bladder may be extruded or it itself may fail to close, a condition of *ectopia vesicæ*. If the urethra does not close it is represented by a groove on the dorsal surface of the penis or clitoris, a condition of *epispadias*.

Facial Clefts.—If there is gross failure of the various facial clefts to close, the fetus will be a monster. Very much commoner is *harelip* and the often associated *cleft palate*. The maxillary process fails to unite with the intermaxillary bone and the defect may be limited to the lip or may extend back into the hard and even the soft palate. The lesion may be unilateral or bilateral. If the intermaxillary bone is absent there will be a median cleft palate.

Branchial Clefts.—The branchial clefts below the first (which forms the Eustachian tube) may remain open. The third is the most frequently involved. The entire cleft may remain open, constituting a *branchial fistula* which connects the pharynx with the skin surface of the neck. The outer end may remain open; this is a *branchial sinus*. The commonest lesion is a *branchial cyst*, in which both ends are closed, but the intermediate portion remains open.

Rectal Malformations.—There may be a *persistent cloaca*, in which the rectum fails to be separated from the external genitalia. If partial separation occurs a *fistula* is formed, the rectum communicating by a passage with vagina, bladder or urethra. The septum which separates the skin from the hind gut may not be broken down as normally occurs; this is a condition of *imperforate anus*.

DOUBLE MONSTERS.—Monsters may be single or double. Instances of single monsters have already been given, although of course it is not always easy to say when a defect is sufficiently severe to justify the use of the word monster. One form has not yet been mentioned. The two eyes may be fused so that there is a single eye in the center of the forehead. The condition is known as *cyclops*, named of course after Polyphemus in the *Odyssey*. Double monsters are an anomaly of twin formation. They may be symmetrical or asymmetrical.

Symmetrical Monsters.—In these, two individuals are joined together. The union may be in the head region, in the thoracic region, or in the sacral region. (1) *Craniopagus* is fusion in the head region. The fusion often only involves the scalp and cranium. There may be two faces looking in opposite directions. Or there may be a single head, the two bodies remaining separate. The position may be reversed, the bodies being fused into one, while the heads remain separate. There is then a two-headed monster or dicephalus. (2) *Thoracopagus* is fusion in the thoracic region, the remainder of the two bodies remaining separate. There may be a common thoracic cavity with a double set of viscera. Sometimes there is only union between the ensiform cartilages and the surrounding soft parts. Such a condition is quite compatible with life, and it was in this way that the Siamese twins who lived to the age of sixty-three years were united. (3) *Ischiopagus* is fusion in the pelvic region. The head, thorax, and spinal column of each individual remain separate, but there is union below the umbilicus and a pelvic ring in common. In the above description only the main types of symmetrical double monsters have been mentioned. There are endless variations.

Asymmetrical Monsters. — 1. *Unequal Twins.*—As a rule, both twins develop equally. But one may die and be converted into an amorphous lump of flesh. In other cases the fetus is fairly well developed, but the heart is poorly developed or rudimentary. This is an *acardiac fetus*. In such cases the course of the circulation has been reversed; the acardiac fetus is nourished by the blood of the other twin, so that the heart, having little to do, does not develop.

2. *Parasitic Fetus.*—This is an example of a double monster in which the development of one of the twins is arrested. This twin does not die as in the case of unequal twins, because it is united with the other twin upon which it lives as a parasite. The parasite may be attached in the cranial, thoracic, or pelvic region, giving a *parasitic craniopagus*, *parasitic thoracopagus*, or *parasitic ischiopagus*. The parasite may be fairly well developed or may be a mere jumble of tissues. When such a rudimentary mass is attached to the mandible it is called an *epignathus*. It may be attached to the sacrum, forming a *sacral teratoma*.

3. *Congenital Teratomata.*—As already indicated, the parasitic mass may be unrecognizable as a separate individual, consisting merely of a confused mass of tissues such as brain, bone, cartilage, teeth, skin, hair, and glands. This may be attached to the exterior of the body, most often in the sacral region, or it may be included in the body cavity (mediastinum, ovary, testicle, *etc.*). These are congenital teratomata or dermoids, so-called because they contain dermal structures. They are to be distinguished from the teratomata which develop in adult life, usually in the ovary, more rarely in the testicle, and which are probably derived from segregation of one of the blastomeres of the developing ovum.

REFERENCES

BOYD, W.: Can. Med. Assn. J., 1934, *31*, 124. (Growth).

INGALLS, T. H. and PHILBROOK, F. R.: New Eng. J. Med., 1958, *259*, 558. (Monstrosities induced by hypoxia).

SMITH, J. LORRAIN: *Growth*, Edinburgh, 1932.

Chapter 11

Bacterial Infections

General Considerations
  Biological Activity
  Pathogenicity and Virulence
  The Struggle for Survival
  The Production of Toxins
  The Changing Picture of
    Infection
  Spread of Infection
  Tissue Changes
  Host Defense
  Clinical Picture
  Classification
Staphylococcal Infections
Streptococcal Infections
  Streptococcus Pyogenes
    Erysipelas
    Scarlet Fever
    Rheumatic Fever
  Streptococcus Viridans
Pneumococcal Infections
Meningococcal Infections

Gonococcal Infections
Coliform Bacteria
  E. Coli
Bacteroides
Typhoid Fever
  Other Salmonella Infections
  Food Poisoning
Bacillary Dysentery
Cholera
Friedländer's Bacillus
Diphtheria
Glanders
Tuberculosis
  Tuberculoid Lesions
  Chromogenic Acid-fast Bacil-
    lary Infections
  Sarcoidosis
Leprosy
Syphilis
  Yaws
  Pinta

Bejel
Spirochetal Fevers
  Relapsing Fever
  Weil's Disease
Hemophilus Bacilli
  Influenza
  Whooping Cough
  Chancroid
Brucellosis
  Undulant Fever
Pasteurella Infections
  Tularemia
  Plague
Anthrax
Anaerobic Spore Bearers.
  Clostridia
  Tetanus
  Gas Gangrene
  Botulism
Bartonella
  Oroya Fever

GENERAL CONSIDERATIONS

In this chapter we shall consider some of the diseases produced by pathogenic microörganisms. Many of these will be described fully in the section on Special Pathology in connection with the organs principally affected (pneumonia, dysentery, etc.). In such cases the condition will only be mentioned here in passing. In others the lesions affect many organs (tuberculosis), or the infection may be general rather than localized (the infectious fevers). These conditions will be considered here more fully. No attempt is made to give bacteriological detail, as that would merely usurp the function of a text on bacteriology, but a few of the principal features of the microörganisms will be mentioned in order to recall them to the student's mind.

Biological Activity.—When we speak of bacterial infection the picture suggested is that of a hostile invader attacking a relatively defenseless host. As biologists, however, we might do well for a few moments to think of the situation from the viewpoint of the bacterium. Bacteria are living cells which have to maintain life. Many can do

so in an external environment such as the soil. Others prefer the living body of animals or man, where they flourish as non-pathogenic commensals, living on the skin, or in the mouth or the intestinal tract, feeding on what they find, but doing no harm to the host. A few invade the tissues, and compete with the host for nourishment, with resulting injury to structure and function. These, from the viewpoint of the host, we describe as pathogens, because the host becomes "ill." A microbe must be a parasite to cause disease, that is to say it must depend on its host for nutriment, but a parasite does not necessarily cause disease.

When a microörganism invades the tissues of a host, one of three things may happen. First, and most likely, the invader may die. Second, it may survive without giving rise to what we call disease, but often causing a host immune reaction which may prevent reinfection. Third, and only exceptionally, it may survive and produce clinical disease, which in rare cases may prove fatal, not only to the host, but probably also to the invader.

Bacteria obtain their energy by breaking down complex compounds into simpler substances by means of respiratory enzymes

(255)

similar to those of the animal cell. They do this in various ways. (1) *Fermentation of carbohydrates*, as a result of which acid and gas (CO_2 and H_2) are produced. This production of acid and gas is utilized by the bacteriologist for identifying certain bacteria, and by the industrialist for the manufacture of alcohol, vinegar, cheese, etc. (2) *Proteolysis*, resulting in putrefaction, which is accomplished by the complex system of enzymes possessed by many anaerobic bacteria. (3) *Lipases*, which are used in the making of butter and cheese. (4) *Pigment production*, seen in growth of *Staphylococcus aureus* and of chromobacteria. It is well for us to realize that none of the higher animals and plants could survive without bacterial activity, which ensures the decay of their bodies after death, with a return to the soil of the elements of which they are composed and which were originally derived from the soil.

Even the gram stain, which is so invaluable in the differentiation and classification of bacteria, is dependent on their chemical structure. It was in 1884 that Christian Gram introduced his gentian violet (or methyl violet) and iodine method of staining. Gram-positive bacteria resist decolorization by alcohol, gram-negative bacteria do not and have to be demonstrated by a counterstain. The dye-retaining material in gram-positive organisms is a complex of magnesium ribonucleate and basic protein, which can be removed with ribonuclease. Gram-negative organisms do not contain this substance. The nucleic acid extracted from gram-positive bacteria is entirely of the ribose variety, but it does not give the reaction unless united with protein. Organisms so treated can reabsorb magnesium ribonucleate and again become gram-positive. It is natural that methyl violet should be much more bactericidal to gram-positive than to gram-negative bacteria, and it is of interest to note that the same is true of the sulfonamides and antibiotics. We shall see presently that the biological activity of gram-positive bacteria is very different from that of gram-negative bacteria, a difference of profound significance to the host.

Pathogenicity and Virulence.—The terms pathogenicity and virulence are often used interchangeably. It seems preferable to use pathogenicity for a class of microörganism and to reserve virulence for a particular strain in that class. Streptococci as a class are pathogens, but the virulence of different strains varies markedly. Pathogenicity as well as virulence may depend as much on the host as on the invader. If the microörganisms enter in larger numbers sufficient to overcome resistance, they alone may cause the disease. When in smaller numbers, other conditions become necessary, especially depressed vitality, either local or general. A bacterium may survive only in one animal, as we see in the case of leprosy, the causal agents of which flourish abundantly in man, but die when transferred to a laboratory animal. Others live mainly in the lower animals, where they may or may not cause disease but at any time may be transmitted to man, as we see in the case of typhus, tularemia, brucellosis and glanders. Some microörganisms are selective not only for the host, but for some particular tissue of that host. Thus the meningococcus prefers the meninges and the gonococcus the mucous membrane of the genital tract. Some, such as the bacillus of tetanus, live by preference outside the body and therefore do not deserve to be classed as parasites; most choose the tissue ground substance as their abode; whilst a special group, the rickettsiæ and viruses, settle down within the cells themselves.

Virulence may be *increased by passage*. This is well recognized in the laboratory, where an infection may be transferred from animal to animal with steady heightening of the virulence. It may also be observed in man. Thus in the days before antibiotic therapy if a pathologist pricked his finger at an autopsy on a case of fatal streptococcal infection, the effect might be almost as vicious as that produced by the bite of a cobra. He was now infected with microörganisms which had been multiplying continuously in the tissues of the patient, even after death, and had therefore learned how to live in a human environment.

We cannot state with certainty the mechanism by which bacteria may acquire *resistance to antibiotics*. It may be that in a mixture of strains those which are sensitive are killed off, whilst the resistant members survive and multiply. In some cases a long-term genetic change may give rise to the development of a mutant resistant strain. There may be a change in the bacterial enzymes, with corresponding loss of their affinity for the drugs. There may even be increased destruction of the antibiotic by the microörganism (the drug by the bug), the best example being the production of penicillinase by staphylococci.

The narrow-spectrum antibiotics inhibit biochemical reactions in a limited number of bacteria, whilst broad-spectrum antibiotics inhibit these reactions in a much larger number. They may well have a similar action on a correspondingly wide variety of cells, and this may explain the more marked toxic properties of the wide-spectrum antibiotics.

The Struggle for Survival.—We have already seen that it is unjust to regard a bacterium as an invader with hostile intent. It is merely a colonist striving to survive in a new country. Unfortunately for the host the colonist both demands nourishment and excretes products of metabolism which may interfere with the normal functioning of the host's cells, and which we therefore label as poisons or toxins. The pathogenic effects of the invaders may be due to either of these two processes.

The demand for nutriment may be either at the expense of the food stuffs or of the tissues of the host. A bacterium is a packet of enzymes with actions which have already been indicated. Many gram-negative organisms possess enzymes which can attack a variety of amino acids, whereas gram-positive bacteria have a very limited ability to break down these acids. The bacterium multiplies at an astronomical rate, and parasitism is merely an example of the universal law of eat or be eaten. From this we can appreciate the truth of the statement that "infectious disease is no more and no less than part of that eternal struggle in which every living organism strives to convert all the available foodstuffs in its universe into living organisms of its own species" (Burnet). Practically all animals live at the expense of some other organism, and in this sense, of course, man himself is a parasite.

The Production of Toxins.—Some bacteria produce metabolic products which are poisonous to living cells; these are *exotoxins*. Good examples are the diphtheria bacillus and the *Clostridia* group Other bacteria liberate toxins when they die and disintegrate; these are *endotoxins*. Examples are the gram-negative enteric group. Still others produce no demonstrable toxins. The gram-positive spore-bearing bacilli, the *Clostridia*, provide an interesting example of variation in exotoxin production and action. The three pathogenic members of the group are the organisms of tetanus, gas gangrene and botulism. Tetanus bacilli grow under anaerobic conditions in dead tissue and there produce an exotoxin which causes no local inflammatory reaction, but passes along the course of the peripheral nerves to the central nervous system with catastrophic results. The organisms of gas gangrene, on the other hand, cause local death of tissue by means of enzymes such as lecithinase which destroys the lecithin of cell membranes, thus allowing the bacteria to spread freely and produce ever-widening destruction Finally the bacilli of botulism do not need to live in the tissues of the host, but proliferate in insufficiently sterilized canned goods, where they elaborate one of the most powerful poisons known, which when ingested quickly kills the recipient.

The Changing Picture of Infection.—Even under normal conditions life in the bacterial world is a constant intense competition for survival. The main function of bacterial enzymes is to produce the protein needed for growth of the bacteria The multiplicity of these enzymes evolved over countless centuries has insured the survival of at least some strains. If the local environment becomes unfavorable, the power to mutate or to bring latent enzyme systems into play becomes apparent. Modern conditions, and particularly the widespread and often unnecessary use of antibiotics, has greatly exaggerated this tendency. As we have already seen so frequently, what is potent for good can be powerful for evil, and the wonder drugs may become harbingers of death.

Antibiotics are made by fungi in the soil, so it is only natural that bacterial pathogens should have developed powers of resistance to one or more of the antibiotics This is seen in most striking degree in the case of *Staphylococcus aureus* in relation to penicillin, a few strains of *Streptococcus hemolyticus* in relation to tetracyclines, and the tubercle bacillus. In the latter instance resistance to streptomycin can be overcome by the addition of para-aminosalicylic acid and isoniazid. In the Toronto General Hospital resistant strains of the Staphylococcus aureus rose from 6 per cent in 1947 to 60 per cent four years later. Similar or even more depressing figures are reported from other institutions. We are now faced with the situation that our hospitals are filled with carriers of antibiotic-resistant strains of staphylococci in the nose and throat of both patients and staff, and the distance between the nose of a surgeon and an operation wound is very short. Moreover, the published reports of epidemics are almost certainly comparable to the visible part of an iceberg, of which the greater portion remains undisclosed. We have been given the invaluable gift of the wonder drugs, but, as Colebrook remarks, it is sad that all too often triumph has been tinged with tragedy.

There has been a dramatic shift in the nature of life-threatening infections in the past twenty years. The majority of fatal infections used to be produced by streptococci, staphylococci and tubercle bacilli, originating in healthy persons outside a hospital. Now the common culprits are gram-negative bacilli, staphylococci, viruses and fungi. Nature likes to maintain a biological balance, and this is true of the bacteriological field. A chemotherapeutic substance, however, can displace the normal flora of the throat, with resulting invasion by coliform organisms, so that the secretion may resemble a culture from the intestine. Serious infections and invasion of the blood stream now occur with intestinal bacteria which have hitherto been regarded as relatively harmless, among the worst offenders being the Aerobacter, Proteus and Pseudomonas organisms (Finland *et al.*). It is indeed a tragic paradox that the more an antibiotic is used (or abused) in a hospital community, the less valuable does it become. The practice of operating under a prophylactic antibiotic umbrella is all too often asking for trouble, for the umbrella is apt to turn into a sieve. The incidence of penicillin-resistant staphylococci is much higher in hospital in-patients than out-patients, it is still lower in the general population, and in the latter it is related to previous treatment with penicillin or to hospitalization (Finland).

Steroid therapy may be responsible in some cases for the changing picture of infection, although not to a degree comparable with the emergence of antibiotic-resistant bacteria. Some antibiotics kill the bacteria. Members of the broad spectrum group are merely bacteriostatic, not bactericidal, but neither the antibiotics nor the sulfonamides arrest the inflammatory reaction. The corticosteroid hormones and ACTH have no antibacterial action, but they do reduce inflammation to a marked degree and induce a striking feeling of well-being. Judicious hormone therapy may prevent the serious vascular collapse of severe infection, especially that due to the gram-negative bacteria. These hormones, however, reduce the effectiveness of antibiotics, interfere to some degree with defense mechanisms, and may activate peptic ulcers. The good must be balanced against the bad.

Viruses preying on bacteria can change the heredity of their victims and therefore their virulence in relation to a host. In this process of *transduction* a virus invades a bacterium and breaks it up, reorganizing its material into hundreds of new virus particles. If these particles in their turn infect another bacterium and it survives, they sometimes change it into a new strain. The virus seems to take hereditary material from the first bacterium and transfer it to the second.

We must not suppose that this changing pattern of bacterial disease is a new thing. Dubos in a thoughtful and arresting address on this subject gives some dramatic and almost unbelievable examples of similar changes in the past. The incidence, character and severity of microbic diseases may change from one generation to another. Leprosy practically disappeared in England during the 16th century. Of London children born between 1762 and 1771 (in the century called the Age of Reason) two-thirds died before the age of five years. Queen Anne had 17 pregnancies, but not one child survived—an example of effort unrewarded

In 1863, one hundred years later, of every million children born in Liverpool, 27,000 died of scarlet fever before the age of five years. Long before the modern era of chemotherapy syphilis had changed its character profoundly, and the mortality from tuberculosis had steadily fallen. There may be a change in resistance due to repeated exposure to small doses, as well as change in the virulence of the infecting agent. A genetic change may play a part, for the susceptible breeds in an isolated community (*e. g.* an island) may be killed off, the survivors being genetically resistant. All human beings are infected with a host of viruses, bacteria, fungi and parasites which are potentially pathogenic, but usually remain latent or silent. The incidence of latent infections is likely to increase with chemotherapy, but a state of biological equilibrium can be disturbed by any change in internal or external environment, such as sudden change in weather, mental stress or overwork, nutritional deficiency, etc. "It is folly to speak of the *conquest of disease*. Health is an expression of perfect fitness to the environment. As man and his environment change continuously, fitness is never permanent, so that disease will continue to recur" (Dubos).

Spread of Infection.—With very few exceptions the organisms of disease are spread from another person or animal, who may be sick (patient) or well (carrier). There are 4 principal methods of spread: (1) physical contact, (2) air, (3) food, and (4) insects.

Physical Contact.—The venereal diseases furnish the classic example of spread of infection by *direct contact*. The life both of the gonococcus and the *Treponema pallidum* outside the body is extremely short.

Indirect contact through *fomites, i. e.* clothing, eating utensils, and other possessions of the patient, is seen in a variety of infections caused by pathogens which exist for a time outside the body. The water of swimming pools deserves special mention in this regard.

Air-borne Infection.—Bacterial and viral diseases of the respiratory tract are retransmitted through the air either by dust or droplets. *Dust infection* comes from bacteria in dried sputum which become attached to dust particles, seen particularly well in the case of tuberculosis. Such dust is harmless as long as it remains on the floor, but when it is swept into the air by the energetic housewife or ward maid, the results may well be imagined. *Droplet infection* is the basis of epidemics of upper respiratory disease. It is estimated that 20,000 droplets containing possible pathogens may be expelled by one sneeze, and that droplets of 1 mm. in diameter may pass over a distance of 15 feet. Still more dangerous are the tiny droplets which evaporate before they fall, their infected centers remaining suspended in the air and pass around a room with every air current. With such facts as these in mind the wonder is that anyone remains free from respiratory infection.

Food-borne Infection.—This is too large a subject to discuss here. The possibility of infection by food or water must be considered in every major epidemic of intestinal disease. The method of transmission does not need to be direct, for the feet of fecal-feeding flies may foul the food. Food-borne infection is seen particularly in typhoid fever and dysentery. The milk of animals may convey infection, as in Malta fever.

Insect-borne Infection.—This again is a vast subject in itself. It is seen with viruses, as in the spread of yellow fever by mosquitoes; with the Rickettsiæ, as in the spread of typhus by lice; in bacterial disease, as in the spread of plague from rat to man by the rat-flea; and even in the case of the protozoa, as in the spread of malaria by the mosquito. It has been said that swords and lances, arrows, machine guns, and even high explosives have had far less power over the fates of the nations than the typhus louse, the plague flea, and the yellow fever mosquito.

Tissue Changes.—Different bacterial pathogens produce widely differing lesions. Some are focal, others diffuse, some are suppurative, others granulomatous, and so on. A general idea of the type of agent may be gathered from a consideration of the character and histological appearance of the lesion, but absolute certainty can only come from such bacteriological techniques as staining the organisms in smears or tissue, growing them in culture, reproducing the disease in an animal, or demonstrating the presence of immune bodies by appropriate serological

methods. We may indulge in a few histological generalizations, but they will be of
little real value to the student.

Suppurative lesions are produced in the
great majority of cases by one or other of
the pyogenic cocci, *i.e. Staphylococcus aureus,
Streptococcus hemolyticus*, pneumococcus and
gonococcus, although gram-negative organisms such as the colon bacillus may also be
responsible. When the suppuration remains
localized, as so often happens with Staphylococcus aureus, the lesion takes the form of
an abscess, with necrosis of tissue and collections of polymorphonuclear leukocytes. *Diffuse* suppuration spreading through the
interstitial tissue without abscess formation
is more likely to be caused by hemolytic
streptococci. *Interstitial inflammation without suppuration* characterized by a mixture
of polymorphonuclears, lymphocytes, plasma
cells and histiocytes without frank necrosis
or abscess formation, is likely to be caused
by exotoxin-producers such as the diphtheria
bacillus, some of the *Clostridia*, and beta
hemolytic streptococci. The *Treponema pallidum* produces the same type of lesion.
Granulomatous inflammation is characterized
by a histiocytic reaction without the partici-
pation of cells from the blood, the lesions
often terminating in fibrosis with healing.
It is the antithesis of pyogenic inflammation.
The classic example is, of course, tuberculosis, but other pathogens, both known and
unknown (as in sarcoidosis) may excite a
similar histological response. It will be evident that the ultimate diagnosis of the nature
of a granuloma cannot be determined by a
histological examination, although an educated guess of undoubted value can be given.

Host Defense.—Parasitism in general and
bacterial infection in particular necessarily
involve a host as well as an invader. From
what has already been said here as well as
in the chapters dealing with inflammation
and immunity it is obvious that the part
which the host plays in infection is as important as the part which the medium plays
in bacterial cultures. To repeat these discussions would be absurd. Suffice it to say
that what determines whether or not a person will fall prey to an infection seems to
depend on: (1) The natural protective qualities of the tissues, including the elements of

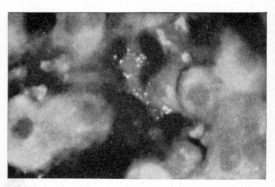

Fig. 151.—Pasteurella tularensis in Kupffer cells
in sinusoids of liver, stained with fluorescent antibody technique. (Kindness of Dr. George P. Blun-
dell, Fort Detrick, Maryland).

the reticuloendothelial system; (2) the presence of natural immune mechanisms in the
serum; (3) the development of specific immune antibodies as the result of previous
infection by the invading organism; (4) the
general health of the patient; (5) the possible
displacement of normal commensals by antibiotic therapy. Amongst the natural immune mechanisms of the serum must be
included the *properdin system*, a bactericidal
mechanism effective over a wide range of
bacteria and viruses which does not require
specific immunization for its activity. Its
components are: (1) properdin, a globulin
of high molecular weight, (2) complement,
and (3) magnesium ions.

The fact that specific immune antibodies
are produced is the basis of the fluorescein-
labeled antibody technique of Coons applied
to the demonstration of microörganisms in
bacterial mixtures, smears, and even within
leukocytes. A globulin antibody against a
particular antigen is labelled with fluorescein
isocyanate; it can then be used to demonstrate the presence of the corresponding
antigen with which it produces a bluish-green
fluorescence (Fig. 151).

Clinical Picture.—The general clinical picture of infection is only too well known to
everyone. Apart from local lesions, the
symptoms and signs are the result of toxemia
caused either by exotoxins or endotoxins.
These are malaise, a feeling of tiredness of
varying degree, vague aches and pains in the
limbs, fever, chills, loss of weight, and in
severe cases prostration. The loss of weight

is the result of heightened catabolism due to the fever, with increased loss of nitrogen in the urine. A shift of fluid from the vascular to the interstitial compartment is responsible for the prostration.

Classification.—There is no ideal and perfect method of classifying bacterial infections at the present time. The arrangement given below is intended to convey to the student the most important groups of pathogens coupled with a few distinctive features such as staining reactions and conditions of growth. The diseases caused by some will be discussed in the pages which follow, whilst in the case of others it will be more convenient to consider the main aspects of disease in relation to the organs principally involved in the second part of this book.

Gram-positive pyogenic cocci. Staphylococcus, streptococcus, pneumococcus.

Gram-negative cocci (Neisseria). Meningococcus, gonococcus.

Intestinal gram-negative bacilli. E. coli, Bacteroides, Salmonella (typhoid, paratyphoid), Shingella (dysentery), Vibrio choleræ, Friedlander's bacillus.

Cornyebacteria. Diphtheria.

Malleomyces mallei. Glanders.

Mycobacteria. Tuberculosis, leprosy.

Spirochetes. Treponema pallidum, pertenue, recurrentis.

Leptospira. Ictero-hemorrhagiæ, canicola.

Hemophilis bacilli. H. influenzæ, pertussis, ducreyi.

Brucella. Undulant fever.

Pasteurella. Tularemia, plague.

Aerobic spore-bearers. Anthrax.

Anaerobic spore-bearers. Clostridia. Cl. tetani, Welchii, botulinum.

Bartonella. Oroya fever.

It is unavoidable that bacteria should be named and classified according to their shape, their method of staining and their way of growth in artificial culture. Sometimes, indeed, they are known by the names of their discoverers. All of these devices can be recognized in the classification given above. It is of course very much more important to know what bacteria *do* than what they *look* like. In the following pages we shall concern ourselves more with their activities than with their appearance.

In *summary* of these general considerations of the bacteriological aspects of infections we may say that an immediate diagnosis of the nature of the infective agent is of prime importance so that appropriate antibiotic therapy may be commenced at the earliest possible moment. The first step is gram-staining of smears, which allows a preliminary classification before the final culture and sensitivity tests become available. It may be said in general terms, of the gram-positive organisms, the staphylococcus responds best to erythromycin, organisms other than staphylococci to penicillin. For gram-negative organisms such as the enteric group, streptomycin and chloramphenicol seem to be best. The worst type of infection to deal with is that caused by a combination of gram-positive and gram-negative organisms. Bacteria lodged in pus, an empyema, etc. cannot be reached by antibiotics, so that drainage is essential. An *exact* bacteriological diagnosis is far more necessary now than formerly, because of the fact that micro-örganisms respond so differently to different chemotherapeutic agents.

STAPHYLOCOCCAL INFECTIONS

The staphylococcus is a gram-positive pyogenic organism, and its action as a pus producer has already been described in connection with inflammation and suppuration. It occurs normally on the skin, and is prone to produce skin infections, entering through cracks, abrasions, or even by way of the hair follicles. In staphylococcal lesions of deeper organs (kidney, bone) an active skin infection (boil) or one which has recently healed can usually be found. In human blood there are natural agglutinins to the staphylococcus, so that when the tissues are invaded the organisms tend to adhere together and to the surrounding structures. For this reason staphylococcal lesions are more likely to be localized than diffuse. Some staphylococci produce a coagulase, which causes a marked formation of fibrin from the fibrinogen of the plasma. These *coagulase-positive* organisms are more dangerous, because the film of fibrin protects them from the action of antibodies and antibiotics. The presence of this enzyme is the most reliable criterion of virulence. It must be admitted that the fibrin tends to limit the spread by blocking paths of dissemination, as shown by the fact that when a dye is injected it does not spread along the lymphatics. In all of these respects staphylococci differ from streptococci, which tend to invade mucous membranes, and produce a fibrinolysin that breaks down the defense barrier. Some strains of staphylococci produce a soluble "spreading factor" which markedly increases the permeability of the tissues (Duran-Reynals' phenomenon). Under appropriate environmental conditions, of which the hydrogen-ion concentration is one of the most important, certain strains have the power of forming an extremely *powerful exotoxin in culture*. Broth filtrates are found to produce three effects which may be called the hemolytic, the necrotizing, and the killing. Injection of a small amount of toxin into the skin of the animal results in marked necrosis. The killing power of the toxin is its most striking characteristic; an extremely small quantity injected intravenously leads to death in a few minutes. The tragedy at Bundaberg in Queensland, when 12 out of 21 children, injected with diphtheria toxin-antitoxin mixture, died in the course of a few hours was due to contamination of the mixture with a toxigenic strain of staphylococci. The toxin can be detoxicated by the addition of formalin; the resulting product is called toxoid, and this still retains its antigenic property. Superficial staphylococcal infections apparently do not provide an adequate antigenic stimulus, for persons with repeated boils may show no increase of antitoxin in the blood.

Staphylococci can survive dried in dust for many months. We have already seen that resistance to antibiotics is readily acquired, more especially in hospitals. Penicillin-resistant strains always produce penicillinase. In man staphylococcal infection manifests itself in three principal forms. (1) *Circumscribed purulent lesions*, which usually remain localized, but may be associated with a bacteremia, transient or persistent. At times this bacteremia may be virulent or even overwhelming. (2) *Widespread membranous lesions*, particularly in the respiratory passages and in the intestinal tract. It is when the normal commensals of the bowel have been replaced by pathogenic staphylo-

cocci as the result of injudicious antibiotic therapy that the danger arises of a severe and sometimes fatal inflammation. This condition, known as *pseudomembranous enterocolitis*, which was recognized even before the antibiotic era, is described on page 746. (3) The severe *shock-like syndrome* which was seen so dramatically in the Bundaberg disaster.

Observations on *experimental staphylococcal infections* in laboratory animals have brought some interesting facts to light, although it does not follow that all of these are applicable to the human subject. They concern in the main host factors rather than virulence of special strains. When staphylococci are injected into the animal they are quickly ingested by leukocytes to a degree seldom seen in the case of other pathogens. Virulent coagulase-positive staphylococci survive within the leukocytes for a prolonged period, whereas coagulase-negative strains do not. They seem to be protected against antibiotics and the natural substances in the extracellular fluids which ordinarily destroy them. From 50 to 200 times the amount of penicillin and streptomycin are needed to destroy intracellular compared with extracellular organisms. In this respect they resemble Brucella and tubercle bacilli. When staphylococci are injected into the blood of a laboratory animal they are sequestrated in the spleen and liver, after which they multiply rapidly in the kidney, where they persist for many months. It is this behavior in the kidney which determines the outcome of the infection.

The hallmark of staphylococcal disease, the *focal abscess*, may of itself play an important part in the nature of the infection. Enormous numbers of organisms, ranging from several millions up to one billion, may be present in a single lesion. These are not destroyed by antibiotics, regardless of the degree of *in vitro* sensitivity. It is for this reason that evacuation of the abscess is so important. The inadequacy of chemotherapy is not due to inability of the drug to penetrate into the interior of the abscess, but to the excessive crowding of the bacterial population with resulting sluggish metabolic activity.

Antibodies are not demonstrated during

active infection in the experimental animal, and humoral immunity appears to be of little importance in recovery, although antibodies are formed if the infection becomes disseminated. Fibrin films are believed to limit the movement of antigens. In any case antigens are unable to pass through the abscess wall. This is certainly true of a dye such as trypan blue when injected into an abscess cavity, nor does typhoid vaccine introduced into the abscess produce the characteristic fever seen in a control animal.

In man an absence or a breakdown of resistance on the part of the host is often the determining factor. Thus staphylococcal infections are particularly liable to occur in newborn infants, and in such debilitating conditions as leukemia, diabetes, renal failure, and after surgical procedures, steroid therapy, and the use of broad-spectrum antibiotics. The staphylococci, in common with certain enteric bacilli and fungi, are normal inhabitants of normal persons, so that, in the words of a noteworthy paper by Rogers which summarizes this subject: "these microbes might be considered the jackals of the microbial parasite world; unable to mount an attack against normal humans, they commonly invade in other disease states where host resistance appears crippled or compromised."

STREPTOCOCCAL INFECTIONS

Streptococci, which resemble staphylococci so closely in appearance and staining character, differ sharply from their cousins in many biological respects. Actually they form a large and heterogeneous collection, the common characteristic of which is to grow in chains. Their power of hemolyzing blood provides one of the most convenient methods of differentiation and classification. When they are grown on blood agar there may be: (1) Complete hemolysis, with a clear transparent zone around the colonies; this is known as beta-hemolysis, and the organisms form the group of *beta-hemolytic streptococci*, usually called hemolytic streptococci, the most virulent of these pathogens. (2) An incomplete or alpha-hemolysis, with the production of a green pigment, an iron-containing derivative of hemoglobin within the red blood cells, so that the organism is known as *Streptococcus viridans*. (3) The blood in the culture medium may be unchanged, these organisms, known as *non-hemolytic streptococci*, occurring in feces, water, etc. The hemolytic streptococcic are nearly always potentially pathogenic, whereas the non-hemolytic strains are seldom pathogenic.

Streptococcus Pyogenes.—Some 12 groups of streptococci have been identified by Lancefield, using precipitin reactions with appropriate sera which identify specific polysaccharide haptens in the organisms. These are designated by the letters of the alphabet. *Streptococcus pyogenes*, the pus-producer which concerns us most as it includes the majority of the strains pathogenic to man, belongs to Lancefield Group A.

Streptococcus pyogenes used to be one of the most dreaded of the pathogens, and it is still a formidable foe. It is responsible for most cases of scarlet fever, erysipelas, puerperal sepsis, and acute tonsillitis. Its most striking characteristic is its ability to travel through the tissues, rather than to create localized focal lesions as does the staphylococcus. This power of infiltration seems to depend largely on the power to produce fibrinolysin and hyaluronidase. *Fibrinolysin* prevents the formation of fibrin and tends to dissolve any that has formed, thus eliminating the fibrin barrier to the spread of infection. *Hyaluronidase* is the enzyme which digests hyaluronic acid, the mucopolysaccharide of the ground substance which forms a natural obstacle in the interstitial compartment. Transmission of streptococcal infection is a matter of direct spread from an infected individual to a healthy person, the most effective transmitter being a person incubating the infection, with tonsillectomized children providing great numbers of such dangerous carriers.

The principal sites of the lesions produced by the streptococcus pyogenes have already been mentioned. Acute tonsillitis is the commonest result. The organisms may spread outwards, producing a peritonsillar abscess, to which the old-fashioned name of *quinsy* or severe sore throat is still applied. Occasionally the infection may involve the floor of the mouth, the neck, and the pharynx and larynx, a condition known as *Ludwig's angina*. (Here angina is used to indicate a sense of choking and strangulation, which was the original meaning of the word in the term angina pectoris). In most cases of severe streptococcal sore throat the regional lymph nodes will be enlarged and tender, and more distant spread of the infection may involve the mastoid cells, the dural venous sinuses, and even the meninges. It is obvious that spread by the blood stream may set up secondary suppurative lesions in any part of the body.

Two manifestations of streptococcal infection, namely erysipelas and scarlet fever, are of so special a character that they merit separate description. Two others, namely rheumatic fever and glomerulonephritis, are sequelæ not caused by the streptococcus pyogenes directly, but representing an immunological response to hypersensitivity byproducts. The former will be described here, the latter in connection with diseases of the kidney.

Erysipelas.—This is an acute inflammation of the lymphatics of the skin caused by hemolytic streptococci with marked erythrogenic (rash-producing) power, which enter through some break in the surface, often very minute. The face or scalp is the usual site, and it is probable that the starting-point is often a latent infection of the nose or nasal sinuses. The common idea that erysipelas is an extremely infectious condition is wrong. Unless there is a discharge from the skin there is no danger of infection. From the site of inoculation the infection spreads outward, producing a bright red indurated area with a characteristically sharp margin. Just beyond this margin the lymph spaces are crowded with streptococci. There is a curious absence of suppuration, the inflammatory cells which crowd the tissue being almost all lymphocytes or mononuclears. In the more severe cases the deeper tissues may may be involved, with thrombosis, cellulitis, and suppuration. General constitutional symptoms such as high fever and leukocytosis are not due to a blood invasion by the streptococci, but to the absorption of the erythrogenic toxin produced locally.

Scarlet Fever.—Scarlet fever or scarlatina is an acute streptococcal fever characterized by a high fever, sore throat, and widespread rash, which may be followed by nephritis, otitis media, and suppuration of the cervical lymph nodes. The characteristic clinical features, the fever and rash, are the result of the erythrogenic toxin produced by streptococci in the inflamed tonsils. The mucous membrane of the tongue shows a similar dilatation of capillaries so that it has a strawberry appearance known as the *strawberry tongue*. It is the *susceptibility or immunity of the individual to the erythrogenic toxin* which determines whether infection with streptococcus pyogenes manifests itself as scarlet fever or merely as acute tonsillitis. No special strain of streptococcus is involved, as used to be thought. The question of immunity can be determined by the *Dick test*, which consists of the intradermal injection of a test dose of erythrogenic toxin. Most persons are immune by reason of possessing a specific antitoxin. If the test is positive the toxin produces a localized erythema due to capillary dilatation. *Glomerulonephritis* is a common complication of convalescence, coming on in the third week or later. It is an immunological phenomenon due to an antigen-antibody reaction, which will be discussed in connection with diseases of the kidney.

Rheumatic Fever.—Rheumatic fever is a complication of streptococcal throat infection, characterized by a widespread inflammatory reaction of the fibrous tissue of the joints, the heart, and other organs. In spite of its name, suggesting an acute arthritis flitting from joint to joint, it is now recognized that it is the heart rather than the joints which is first affected. It has been wittily said that rheumatism is a disease which licks the joints, but bites the heart.

The disease pursues a somewhat different course in children from what it does in the adult. In children the joint pains may never appear. The child suffers from tonsillitis and sore throat, these are replaced by chorea (St. Vitus' dance), and finally a heart murmur is discovered. In the adult the intensely painful swelling of the joints is much more characteristic, fever is higher and skin lesions are much rarer. It must be emphasized, however, that rheumatic fever is principally a disease of childhood; about 75 per cent of the cases occur before the age of twenty years. Conversely, about 95 per cent of heart disease in children is rheumatic.

The *etiology* of rheumatic fever has been a matter of confusion and difference of opinion for many years. A relationship with streptococcal infection was early recognized, but these organisms could never be demonstrated in the cardiac or joint lesions with any regularity or in any appreciable numbers. The answer to the conundrum is supplied by immunology and the action of host factors. Group A hemolytic streptococci in the throat are believed to sensitize the tissues of the heart, joints, etc., the prosthetic groups in the organisms uniting with connective tissue protein to create an antigen. This in turn excites the formation of specific antibodies, the reaction of the two resulting in a focal allergic necrosis accompanied by a characteristic cellular response. This is the type of interaction which we have already studied in the discussion of immune and anti-immune phenomena in Chapter 5. The allergic reaction would link rheumatic fever with the collagen diseases.

In support of a streptococcal etiology of acute rheumatism three sets of facts may be mentioned. (1) The demonstration of elevated titers of streptococcal antibodies, such as antistreptolysin and antistreptokinase, in patients with rheumatic fever, indicating recent contact with streptococci. (2) The effect of the treatment of acute streptococcal infections with antibiotics and sulfonamides in reducing the incidence of rheumatic fever. (3) The fact that acute streptococcal infections in children are not infrequently followed by an attack of rheumatic fever, and that persons who have had one attack are likely to have exacerbations after subsequent streptococcal infections.

The invariable presence of *C-reactive protein* in the serum in acute rheumatic fever whilst the reaction is completely negative in normal persons provides a valuable laboratory test, but it is of course in no way specific for rheumatic disease. The name comes from the fact that the blood of patients with pneumococcal pneumonia contains a protein which reacts with the carbohydrate (hence the *C*) of the pneumonoccus to form a precipitate. The test, which is indicative of an inflammatory or tissue-destroying process, is particularly useful in doubtful cases of acute rheumatic fever (Roantree and Rantz).

We have to face the fact that, fortunately, only a few individuals show the rheumatic response to streptococcal infection. There can be little doubt that accessory factors play an important part in the etiology. Reference has already been made to the influence of geography. Rheumatic fever is a disease of poverty. This may be explained in part by overcrowding which encourages the spread of infection, in part by food deficiency, especially vitamin C (Rinehart). As rheumatic fever is one of the collagen diseases, it is possible that the response of the tissues may be under the influence of hormones, particularly the adrenal corticoids.

Coburn points out that the incidence of rheumatic fever parallels in a striking manner the incidence of hemolytic streptococci in the throat and also the incidence of streptococcal diseases such as scarlet fever in which the primary infection is in the upper part of the respiratory tract. This incidence is affected to a marked degree by climate. Both are common in cold, damp climates, but are rare in many parts of the tropics. Both are common in the children of the poor, but rare in the children of the wealthy. A child who suffers from recurring attacks of rheumatic fever and streptococcal sore throat in the slums of New York remains well when transported to South America. In the western part of the United States rheumatic heart disease is about ten times commoner in school children living in regions near the Canadian border than in those from regions near the Mexican border. From these observations Coburn concludes that the infectious agent which *initiates* the rheumatic process is *Streptococcus hemolyticus*, but that some other factor as yet elusive is required to complete the picture. This factor may be a vitamin or other food deficiency.

1. The *lesions* involve fibrous tissues and certain serous membranes. A characteristic lesion is produced known as the Aschoff body. This corresponds to the miliary tubercle of tuberculosis. It is a proliferative lesion. Even earlier, as Klinge pointed out, is so-called *fibrinoid degeneration* or *necrosis*, regarded by him as a change

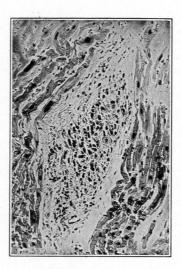

Fig. 152.—Aschoff body in myocardium. The oval body separates the heart muscle fibers.

There are four components of the Aschoff nodule. (1) A center of fibrinoid necrosis, often quite small in amount. (2) Aschoff cells. These form the characteristic feature. They are large cells of the epithelioid type, usually multinucleated. They are probably derived from the histiocytes, members of the reticuloendothelial system. Many are really giant cells, but they have seldom more than six or seven vesicular nuclei, and resemble the giant cells of Hodgkin's disease rather than those of tuberculosis. (3) Lymphocytes and plasma cells, with an occasional polymorphonuclear leukocyte. (4) Proliferation of fibroblasts with subsequent fibrosis. Edema, thrombosis, and swelling of the endothelium of the small vessels may also be present. Gross and Ehrlich have described what they call the life cycle of the Aschoff body, showing that a progressive series of changes can be recognized. Swelling of the collagen is a conspicuous feature of the earliest lesion. So also is the formation of a network of argentophilic reticulum fibers, as first pointed out by Klinge. For the details of the life cycle the original paper should be consulted.

The special rheumatic lesions of the *heart* will be considered in connection with Diseases of the Heart. There is a pancarditis (myocarditis, endocarditis, pericarditis), and these "bites" in the heart are by far the most important part of the disease. Rheumatic fever is the chief cause of chronic valvular disease.

The *pharynx* may be regarded as the site of the primary lesion from which the rest of the body is infected. A sore throat frequently precedes or is associated with the onset of an attack of rheumatic fever. Rheumatic nodules have been described in the pharyngeal tissues during an acute attack. Similar nodules were present in the neighborhood of the tonsils, in the lingual and laryngeal tonsils, and in the upper deep cervical lymph nodes.

In the *skin* the rheumatic lesion is known as the *subcutaneous nodule*. It occurs in the deep fascia, especially over bony prominences, and is composed of a group of Aschoff bodies. The general structure is the same, though the outline is more indefinite.

In the *joints* the lesion is exudative, and

in the ground substance and collagen as a result of which the connective tissue assumes a lattice-like appearance with some of the staining characteristics of fibrin. More recent work suggests that fibrinoid represents a constituent of the plasma, a matter which has already been discussed on page 86. This change is best seen in the subcutaneous nodules, not in the cardiac lesions. In addition there is an exudative lesion, an outpouring of serum, most marked in the joints. The remarkable effect of salicylates on the symptoms of rheumatic fever are well known. The salicylates interfere with the spreading effect of hyaluronidase, just as does cortisone. It is possible that they act through the anterior lobe of the pituitary and the adrenal cortex, for they are without effect on hyaluronidase after adrenalectomy or hypophysectomy.

The *Aschoff body* is seen in most typical form in the interstitial tissue of the myocardium (Fig. 152.) It is the result mainly of proliferation, but the exudative element is also present. It may be just visible to the naked eye, but is often invisible. In the heart it is oval or lemon-shaped. It is paravascular in distribution, being situated in relation to the adventitia of the small arteries, but it is at one side of the vessel and does not surround it.

it is to the sudden exudation in a tissue supplied so abundantly with small sensory nerves that the pain is due. Proliferative and vascular changes are also found in the synovial membrane, the capsule and the periarticular fibrous tissue. It is possible that the infective form of chronic arthritis may prove to be related to rheumatic fever. At least it appears to be a joint manifestation of a low-grade streptococcal infection.

The *brain* may be affected and the patient suffers from chorea (St. Vitus' dance). The lesions are in no way distinctive. There are perivascular collections of round cells, thrombosis, and endothelial proliferation in the meninges, cerebral cortex, and corpus striatum. The condition is a rheumatic meningo-encephalitis.

Rheumatic pneumonia is seen in patients dying in the acute stage, the lung having a peculiar India rubber consistence. There may be true Aschoff nodules in the fibrous septa, an interstitial infiltration of large, often multinucleated, cells, or areas of acute focal necrosis. (Gouley and Eiman.) *Pleural lesions* have been described. In many of the fatal cases there is a pleurisy, at first dry and later with effusion. There is metaplasia of the endothelium and inflammation in the subpleural layers.

STREPTOCOCCUS VIRIDANS.—This variety of streptococcus, which produces a green color on blood agar, is always present as a commensal in the mouth and throat. Under ordinary circumstances these organisms are only very slightly pathogenic, but when the resistance of the tissue is weakened they come on the scene as jackals, and may set up a pathological process which may eventually cost the patient his life. After the extraction of teeth they often cause chronic inflammation in the tooth socket, but their greatest threat is when they establish themselves on heart valves which have been damaged by previous rheumatic fever or some congenital malformation. The result is the condition known as *subacute bacterial endocarditis*, which used to be almost invariably fatal. The bacteria lie deep within the avascular granulations on the valves, where many of them are dormant and are therefore not killed by penicillin, which acts only on dividing bacteria. The bacteriostatic (broad-spectrum) antibiotics are useless, because the organisms cannot be reached by the body's defense mechanisms. Very large doses of penicillin must be given daily, together with ordinary doses of streptomycin.

Over 90 per cent of cases of subacute bacterial endocarditis are due to *Streptococcus viridans*. The remainder are caused by *Str. fecalis* or other non-hemolytic streptococci. The morbid anatomy and clinical features of the disease are discussed in the chapter on The Heart.

PNEUMOCOCCAL INFECTIONS

The principal disease caused by the pneumococcus is lobar pneumonia. This is described in connection with diseases of the lungs. The pneumococcus is a pyogenic organism with a polysaccharide capsule which may prevent the formation of the coating of body protein that is necessary if phagocytosis is to occur. It also has a marked ability to excite the formation of fibrin. The pulmonary alveoli are therefore filled with an inflammatory exudate composed mainly of pus cells and fibrin. Pleurisy is an invariable and empyema a less common accompaniment of lobar pneumonia.

Other lesions caused by pneumococci are endocarditis, pericarditis, peritonitis (especially in children), arthritis, meningitis, middle-ear suppuration, infection of the nasal sinuses, etc. These conditions will be described in their proper place.

MENINGOCOCCAL INFECTIONS

We now turn from the gram-positive to the gram-negative cocci, that is to say the *Neisseria* group, and we shall encounter some rather startling differences. Most of the *Neisseria* are commensals in the nasopharynx. Indeed the non-pathogenic *Neisseria*, together with *N. catarrhalis* and *Str. viridans*, form the basic normal flora of the throat. The members of the group resemble one another morphologically as closely as the proverbial two peas. In addition to being gram-negative, they are bean-shaped diplococci with the convex surfaces opposed. The two pathogenic members, the meningococcus and the gonococcus, are found in large numbers within the polymorphonuclears of the pus, an environment in which they seem to flourish.

The *meningococcus* or diplococcus intracellularis meningitidis of Weichselbaum, to use its somewhat grandiloguent cognomen, has a singularly intriguing natural history by reason of the clearness with which we can follow its progress and the extremely varied possibilities which this presents. It is a normal inhabitant of the nasopharynx, and in times of epidemic up to 90 per cent of persons in a crowded army camp may carry the germ. Under these circumstances it is natural that severe epidemics should break out, with occasional sporadic cases in the endemic interval. Depending on differences of antigenic structure, a number of groups can be distinguished by serological technique. Most of the epidemic strains belong to Group I, whilst in sporadic cases and carriers the organisms belong to Group II. No exotoxin is formed, although an endotoxin can be extracted. The meninococcus is extremely sensitive to sulfonamides and a wide range of antibiotics, and it is pleasant to learn that acquired resistance is unknown. It does not grow at all readily on culture media.

Possible Course of the Infection.—There are three pathogenic possibilities open to a meningococcus living in a person's throat. (1) It may set up a *nasopharyngitis* which remains localized and causes little or no discomfort.

(2) It may invade the blood vessels, which it does with great readiness, setting up either a bacteremia without clinical disturbance, or a *meningococcemia*. The latter may be an *acute* fulminating disease, with high fever and the development of a widespead petechial or ecchymotic rash, the character of which has given this form of the infection the name of "spotted fever." The basis for the rash is an acute vasculitis of the small vessels, leading to minute hemorrhages, often with tiny foci of suppurative necrosis. The character of the disease may become still more fulminating through the development of what is called the *Waterhouse-Friderichsen syndrome*, a combination of acute meningococcemia and hemorrhage into the medulla of the adrenal glands owing to vascular damage, often with complete

destruction of both adrenals. The combination of severe toxemia and acute adrenal insufficiency is usally sufficient to kill the patient within 24 hours. In exceptional cases a *chronic meningococcemia* may develop in place of an acute one. The presence of circulating meningococci in the blood is only manifested by occasional attacks of mild fever, perhaps with a few petechial skin lesions, but with no suggestion of a severe infection.

(3) *Acute meningococcal meningitis* is the third possibility, which gives the organism its name. This suppurative meningitis may be the result of a meningococcemia, or the infection may reach the meninges from the nasopharynx by passing along the sheath of the olfactory nerves. *Diagnosis* is made by examination of the cerebrospinal fluid obtained by lumbar puncture. This shows a polymorphonuclear leukocytosis, increased pressure, a reduced sugar content, and the presence of meningococci which may be intracellular or extracellular. Modern chemotherapy has entirely altered the prognosis of the disease. The lesions and clinical features of meningococcal meningitis are described in the chapter on the Nervous System.

GONOCOCCAL INFECTIONS

In physical appearance and staining characters the gonococcus or *Neisseria gonorrheæ* is the split image of the meningococcus, but in its biological behaviour it is very different. It is still harder to grow than the meningococcus, and the dried organisms die within one hour. It is an example of the complete parasite living on a human host. It produces no exotoxin, but on dying it releases a powerful pyogenic endotoxin. Unlike the meningococcus it does not live in the body as a harmless commensal.

With two exceptions to be mentioned below it is essentially a venereal disease, being transmitted through sexual intercourse. The initial site of infection is the mucous membrane of the male and female genital tract, namely the anterior urethra in the male and the urethra, vulvovaginal glands and cervix in the female. Stratified squamous epithelium is highly resistant, so that the adult vaginal canal remains unaffected.

The initial process is an acute suppuration developing from two days to a week after exposure to infection. There is a copious discharge of pus loaded with gram-negative organisms, many of them intracellular. If prompt and effective treatment is instituted, the discharge disappears like magic and the infection clears up.

In the *untreated* case, or if treatment is not effective, the process ceases to be acute, but the infection spreads upward causing chronic suppuration followed by fibrosis, often with serious consequences. In the male there is spread to the posterior urethra, the prostate, seminal vesicles and epididymis, with the threat of stricture of the urethra or sterility. In the female the endometrium is singularly resistent, but the Fallopian tubes are seriously damaged, the fimbriated ends becoming closed by adhesions so that the lumen is distended to form a bag of pus, with sterility as an inevitable result. Before the sealing of the tubes the infection has spread to the peritoneum causing pelvic peritonitis followed by extensive adhesions involving the bowel and other structures. The result may be chronic invalidism.

Hematogenous spread is a rare occurrence, in contrast with meningococcal infection. Acute endocarditis is an occasional result. *Arthritis* is a much more common complication, but although the cocci have been isolated from the synovial fluid it is believed that the condition is allergic in character rather than a direct infection.

The infection may be non-venereal in origin. This is the case in *ophthalmia neonatorum*, a gonococcal conjunctivitis of the new born where the infection is conveyed from the mother to the child at the time of delivery. This used to be an important cause of blindness before the days of the local application of penicillin and silver compounds. *Epidemic vulvo-vaginitis* spreads by non-venereal contact in girls' institutions. The vaginal epithelium does not become keratinized until the age of puberty, so that the gonococcus can gain a ready hold at this period of life.

The *treatment* of gonorrhea is still an important public health problem. When the sulfonamides were first introduced the gonococcus proved to be so susceptible that it seemed as if the disease might be completely eliminated, especially in view of the fact that the organism is unable to live outside the body. Soon, however, most strains became resistant. Penicillin took the place of the sulfonamides with complete success, a single dose curing 90 per cent of cases, but again the sad story of resistant strains was repeated (King). Then came streptomycin, but the cocci proved as resourceful as ever. Yet they had now again become sensitive to the sulfonamides. And so the battle of attack and defense continues with varying fortune.

The pathological lesions of gonorrhea are described in connection with diseases of the male and female reproductive systems.

COLIFORM BACTERIA

We now leave the gram-negative cocci, the *Neisseria*, and pass to the gram-negative bacilli of the intestine. It is important for us, in thinking of the intestinal bacteria, to realize that "the teeming myriads normally present are harmless saprophytes," to quote from that compressed gold mine of information, Whitby and Hynes' *Medical Bacteriology*. Many, indeed, are not only harmless, but serve a useful purpose, such as synthesizing vitamin K and members of the B complex, so that we must beware of banishing them too completely through ultra-modern chemotherapy. In addition to the harmless saprophytes, some, such as *E. coli* and *Clostridia*, cause disease when implanted in tissue with diminished resistance, whilst still others, such as the *Salmonella* and *Shigella* groups and the *cholera vibrio*, are dangerous pathogens, which invade the intestine in contaminated food and water, and set up violent inflammation in the wall of the bowel. With the exception of the cholera vibrio these various gram-negative bacilli are indistinguishable from one another morphologically, but the coliform organisms are lactose-fermenters, whilst the majority of the pathogens are not, a simple means of differentiation. In the duodenum and upper jejunum there are very few bacteria, a tribute to the sterilizing power of the acid gastric juice, in the lower small bowel we meet coliforms and staphylococci, whilst in the colon the bacteria are mostly anerobes.

E. Coli.—*Echerichia coli, Bacterium coli,* or the colon bacillus, a gram-negative, motile bacillus producing acid and gas in lactose, is generally a harmless inhabitant of the bowel, but it is a common cause of acute and chronic inflammation elsewhere, especially when accompanied by other organisms. By virtue of a fairly potent endotoxin it may be responsible for acute inflammation in the appendix and gall-bladder, and in the pelvis of the kidney and the urinary bladder in cases of obstruction from stone or an enlarged prostate. It is in children and the aged that infection with *E. coli* is most to be feared, in the former because immunity has not developed, in the latter because of poor resistance. The presence of *E. coli* in drinking water is strong evidence of pollution.

Proteus and *Pseudomonas* are two groups of gram-negative motile intestinal bacilli, which have come to assume increased importance because of their extreme resistance to antibiotics, so that they tend to supplant other bacteria in the alimentary tract when such therapy is long-continued. The proteus group ferments carbohydrates, the pseudomonas group does not, but produces distinctive pigments. *Proteus vulgaris*, as its name implies, is the common species of the proteus group, whilst the clinically important variety of the pseudomonas group is *Ps. aeruginosa*, generally called *Bacillus pyocyaneus*, the "bacillus of blue-green pus." Both of these organisms belong to the jackal tribe, for in health they are harmless inhabitants of the intestine, but when resistance is lowered or tissue damaged they become dangerous invaders, proteus producing acute abscesses and Pseudomonas thrombosis of small arteries with infarction. The *urinary tract* is most frequently involved, with a resulting pyelonephritis, but there may also be infection of the middle ear and mastoid, the eye owing to implantation on abrasions of the cornea causing severe ulceration, and the skin due to infection of burns and decubitus ulcers.

Bacteremia has a tendency to develop in infections with gram-negative intestinal bacilli. This is most frequently seen in the case of *E. coli* and *B. pyocyaneus*. The site of origin is usually the genitourinary tract (60 per cent) and the gastro intestinal tract (25 per cent) (Spittel *et al.*). In about 50 per cent of cases operative procedures, generally on the genitourinary tract, preceded the bacteremia. Invasion of the blood is marked by fever, often with pronounced spiking of the temperature, chills, and sometimes sudden vascular collapse (see below). In occasional cases metastatic abscesses develop.

Traumatic Shock may be related to the endotoxins of coliform bacteria (Fine). Over 80 per cent of experimental animals recover from traumatic shock if the lost blood is returned within ninety minutes, but not if an interval of four hours or more is allowed to elapse. In such a case the animal dies with hemorrhagic necrosis of the wall of the intestine and focal intestinal hemorrhage. Similar lesions are seen in animals killed with a known endotoxin such as that of *E. coli*. Moreover, the animal dies when transfused within the safety time limit with blood from an animal dying of hemorrhagic shock. A normal dog is not affected by even 1 liter of shock blood, whereas as little as 100 ml. of this blood will kill an animal already in shock. The source of the endotoxin is believed to be such gram-negative organisms as may be present in the animal's tissues together with endotoxins normally present in the gastrointestinal tract, which appear to enter the circulation at a steady rate, though in minute amounts. These endotoxins should be neutralized by the reticuloendothelial system, but this potential is destroyed in shock, allowing the toxins to paralyze the flow of blood in the peripheral circulation, with necrosis of the walls of the small vessels. If this hypothesis should prove correct it may have a bearing on traumatic shock in the human.

BACTEROIDES

We now come to a group of organisms with a most peculiar history. They are small, gram-negative bacilli resembling *E. coli* and outnumbering that organism in the colon, but differing from it sharply in being strictly anaerobic and difficult to grow in culture, requiring enrichment with serum or even blood. It differs from the anaerobic *Clostridia* in not producing spores. Gas is formed in culture, but not in the tissues.

Bacteriology.—There are many members of the group, but it was only in 1919 that these were collected into a genus, to which the name *Bacteroides* was applied. The history of these organisms, however, goes back a long way. In 1884 Loeffler isolated one member of the group in calf diphtheria. This he called *Bacillus necrophorus*, as it produced necrotic lesions in mice on subcutaneous inoculation. Necrobacillosis is a term in common use in Great Britain at the present time (Alston). In 1896 Vincent described a fusiform bacillus of the same group in ulcerative lesions of the throat (Vincent's angina), whilst in 1898 others were found in appendicitis and also in the female genital tract. In spite of these discoveries the group aroused almost no interest until recent years, when it began to be realized that this was a common infection commonly overlooked, and that necrotic lesions in many farm animals are caused by these organisms. Even in 1952 a review of the subject opens with these words. "There is probably no subject in modern medicine more neglected than that of *Bacteroides*-caused infections. Recent textbooks of internal medicine, surgery, obstetrics, urology, otolaryngology, and even bacteriology scarcely mention this condition" (McVay and Sprunt). It will be noticed that pathology has been omitted from this list, perhaps through inadvertance. And again in 1958: "Recent textbooks on general medicine and its various specialties scarcely mention *bacteroides* although it is a common genus" (Rubin and Boyd).

Undoubtedly the chief reason for the oversight has been the strict anaerobic requirement of the organism. A *smear* of intestinal contents, or of pus from intra-abdominal lesions may show great numbers of gram-negative bacilli and streptococci. Thus in one series of 111 consecutive specimens of pus from lesions in the abdomen, *Bacteroides* were present and numerous being associated with *E. coli*, and aerobic and anaerobic streptococci (Gillespie and Guy). In aerobic *cultures* it is seen that the bacilli are *E. coli*,

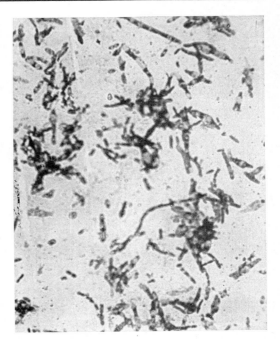

Fig. 153.—Bacteroides funduliformis, showing the bizarre and varied morphology.

but is not realized that these have been outnumbered by Bacteroides which failed to grow. The slow growth of *Bacteroides* even under anaerobic conditions is a further factor in the general neglect. What we do not know we do not see. The universal use (or abuse) of antibiotics has brought these organisms to the fore, for they are resistant to penicillin, streptomycin, bacitracin and neomycin, although quite sensitive to tetracyclines and chloramphenicol.

The names of the different members of the genus are more remarkable for their sonorousness than for their descriptive quality. Thus the alternative name for *Fusiformis necrophorus*, the cause of calf diphtheria, is *Bacteroides funduliformis*. We shall limit our consideration to two, *Bact. funduliformis* and *Bact. fragilis*. (1) *Bact. funduliformis* (*fundulus*, a sausage) is so-named because of its tendency during one phase of its growth in culture to appear as ball-like forms with spherical bodies from which daughter forms arise. The organisms tend to be large, but are very varied and often bizarre in appearance (Fig. 153). The necrophorus bacilli are probably identical with funduliformis. The pus is thick, greenish yellow, and somewhat foul, although not putrid. Metastatic abscesses are common and the mortality is high. Organisms are present in the smears in large numbers. (2) *Bact. fragilis* are less numerous, smaller, cocco-bacillary forms.

Pathogenesis.—The organisms are normal saprophytes, their areas of predilection being the throat, colon, female genital tract and middle ear. They are, however, facultative jackals, and become pyogenic in tissues with depressed resistance and in association with other invaders. They are found in the pus in acute appendicitis, in abscesses of the liver and lung due to blood spread, in brain abscess and acute meningitis, generally spreading from chronic otitis media. They may be associated with chronic ulcerative colitis, especially during acute exacerbations, and with carcinoma of the colon. There is a tendency to thrombosis, and infection spreading from the appendix to the liver may be associated with pylephlebitis and jaundice. The lesions are granulomatous abscesses, developing into putrid and gangrenous lesions in the lungs, with thick, foul-smelling pus (empyema) in the pleural cavities. The diagnosis of *Bacteriodes* infection is suggested by a peculiar odor, like that of over-ripe Camembert cheese. If *bacteremia* develops the prognosis is much more grave, with the danger of metastatic abscesses. The patient now presents a markedly toxic appearance, with high fever, chills, great weakness and exhaustion. It is naturally very much easier to obtain a pure culture from the blood or from a metastatic abscess, than from a primary lesion, where infection is sure to be mixed. A bacteriological diagnosis is made from a smear of pus stained with Gram's method, followed by a culture planted as soon as possible, because the bacteria quickly die under aerobic conditions.

Reference has already been made to the efficacy of tetracyclines and chloramphenicol, especially in cases with bacteremia. Surgical drainage and removal of necrotic debris to correct anaerobic conditions is obviously indicated. Combined medical and surgical treatment has quite changed the prognosis in *Bacteroides* infections.

TYPHOID FEVER

Salmonellæ are gram-negative, motile bacilli, identical morphologically with *E. coli*, but remarkably different in biological activity. They are non-lactose fermenters, and, although powerful pathogens, they are nearly always non-pyogenic in action, indeed suppressing the polymorphonuclear leukocytes which are the hall mark of suppuration. They possess a number of antigens that excite the formation of the antibodies which are so useful in laboratory diagnosis. Of these we need only mention the H or flagellar and the O or somatic antigens. The initials come from the German *hauch* (breath, film, ectoplasm, *i.e.* from flagella) and *ohne hauch*, *i.e.* from the body of the bacillus. An antigen in such an organism can be identified with confidence by agglutination with an appropriate serum.

Salmonella typhosa is so much the most important member of the group from the point of view of human pathology that our discussion will be confined mainly to the disease which it causes, namely typhoid or enteric fever. The term enteric fever comes to us from the days when it was believed that the condition was just a disease of the intestine. We now know that although two of the most serious of the clinical complications, namely intestinal hemorrhage and perforation, are due to lesions of the bowel, in essence it is a generalized infection; that is why it is discussed in this place. The meaning of the word typhoid we shall see presently.

INFECTION.—The source of fresh infection is always human, either a patient suffering from the disease or a healthy carrier. The infection is alimentary, and is conveyed by infected water, milk or food, or by direct contagion. Epidemics can usually be traced to either water or milk infection. The bacilli do not multiply to any degree in water, but they multiply rapidly in milk, so that a milk-borne epidemic is more violent and explosive due to the massive infection. Food and milk may be infected by the contaminated fingers of a carrier (cook, dairyman) or of a nurse who has been looking after a typhoid patient. Flies may convey the infection from uncovered dejecta to uncovered food. Water

infection is usually due to sewage contamination.

One of the chief sources of danger is the
chronic carrier. A patient who recovers from
the disease may continue to harbor the
bacilli in his body, which are discharged for
years usually in the stools, sometimes in the
urine. A carrier is only dangerous when his
occupation entails the handling of food or
milk or if the excreta are not properly disposed of (camp life, armies in the field, *etc.*).

The bacilli must be swallowed in large
numbers to ensure passage past the watch-
dog of the acid gastric juice. In the intestine
they are taken up by mononuclear phagocytes and carried to lymphoid tissue, in
particular the Peyer's patches of the lower
ileum and the mesenteric lymph nodes as
well as the spleen and liver. Here they
proliferate in enormous numbers during the
incubation period of ten days or so, throughout which time there is great hyperplasia of
the lymphoid structures and the spleen.
At the end of this period or even sooner the
bacilli pass along the thoracic duct and
enter the blood, setting up a bacteremia
which may last a number of weeks. At the
same time many of the bacilli are broken
down with release of powerful endotoxins
which are responsible for the general symptoms and most of the lesions.

LESIONS.—Typhoid fever is primarily an
infection of the hemopoietic tissue, and in
particular the lymphoid tissue of the intestine, the abdominal lymph nodes, the spleen,
and the bone marrow. As there is always a
bacteremia any organ may be involved, but
the most important lesion to add to the
above is infection of the gallbladder. The
typhoid bacillus excites a peculiar cellular
reaction which is quite characteristic, and
unlike the suppurative reaction produced by
its pyogenic cousins, the colon bacillus and
the dysentery bacillus. There is an almost
complete absence of polymorphonuclear
leukocytes, their place being taken by large
mononuclear phagocytes of the reticuloendothelial system (Fig. 154). These phagocytes may contain lymphocytes, red blood
cells, and bacteria. Erythrophagocytosis is
is a most distinctive feature. The bacilli
within the phagocytes seem to be protected
against the action of antibodies. The lesion

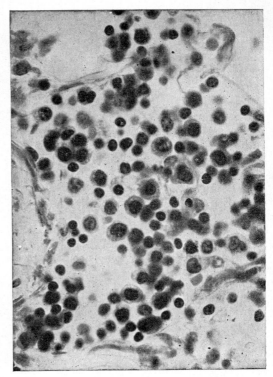

FIG. 154.—Typhoid fever. Sinus in a lymph node
packed with mononuclear cells. × 600. (Boyd,
Pathology for the Physician.)

is productive rather than exudative in type.
The red marrow is filled with these cells, to
the exclusion of the polymorphonuclear and
eosinophil leukocytes, thus explaining the
leukopenia and the disappearance of polymorphonuclears and eosinophils.

The *intestinal lesions,* which are confined to
the lymphoid tissue, are most marked in the
lower part of the ileum, but may involve the
greater part of the small intestine and also
the colon. The Peyer's patches and the
solitary follicles are crowded with the large
mononuclear phagocytes, so that the lymphoid masses project above the surface. By
the end of the first week these lesions
become necrotic, the overlying mucosa forms
a slough, and when this separates it leaves
an ulcer (Fig. 155). The ulcers are round
or irregularly oval with the long axis in the
long axis of the bowel, since that is the
direction of the Peyer's patches. In the
cecum and colon the ulcers are smaller,
owing to the smaller size of the solitary

18

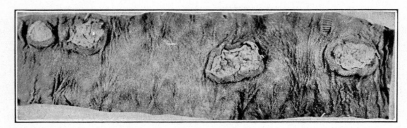

Fig. 155.—Typhoid ulcers of the bowel. A necrotic slough occupies the center of each lesion.

follicles. Many are quite shallow, but the submucosa is often perforated, so that the floor of the ulcer is formed by the muscularis or even the peritoneum. There may be no ulcers, for the patient may die of toxemia before ulceration has time to take place. The number and size of the ulcers bear no relation to the severity of the disease. But the ulcers are accountable for the two complications which are responsible for a majority of the deaths, namely, *hemorrhage* and *perforation*. As the patient may have a deep ulcer and yet be only slightly ill, it follows that every case of typhoid must be treated with the greatest care. The ulcers heal with the formation of little or no scar tissue. The ulcer is covered by a simple type of epithelium without the formation of new glands.

The *lymph nodes* of the mesentery are always involved, especially those which drain the lower ileum. Their sinuses are distended with large mononuclear phagocytes, and the nodes are therefore swollen and soft.

The *spleen* shows acute splenic swelling. It is moderately enlarged, usually weighing about 500 grams, deep red in color and very soft. *Microscopically* the usual collections of large mononuclear cells are seen with small areas of necrosis, but the most striking lesion is a crowding of the pulp with enormous numbers of red blood cells, so that it may seem to contain little but blood. The reason for this extreme congestion is not clear, for it is not seen in the other lesions; possibly the masses of mononuclears obstruct the outflow from the sinuses so that they become overfilled with blood.

In the *liver* the typhoid lesion is focal necrosis. The lesion is really a combination of mononuclear proliferation and necrosis. The large mononuclears block the sinusoids

and the liver cells become necrosed. The lesions are quite small and resemble miliary tubercles.

The *gallbladder* is always infected, although the lesions may be negligible. The bacilli live in the bile and pass down into the bowel, where they are most numerous in the duodenum. Most of the bacilli in the stools come from the gallbladder, not from the ulcers in the bowel. They may continue to live in the gallbladder after recovery and are excreted in the stools. Such a person is a typhoid carrier.

The *kidneys* show cloudy swelling and clumps of bacilli, so that bacilli often appear in the urine. A urinary carrier continues to discharge bacilli long after recovery.

The *lungs* may show bronchitis in the early stage and pneumonia (lobar or bronchopneumonic) later. The pneumonia is usually pneumococcal, but it is sometimes due to the typhoid bacillus.

The *heart* muscle is soft and swollen, and the blood pressure low. The pulse is characteristically slow, and the pulse often dicrotic.

The *veins* are often thrombosed, especially the femoral and saphenous veins and the cerebral sinuses.

The *muscles* may show *Zenker's degeneration*, a hyaline change in which the fibers lose their transverse striations and are broken up into swollen hyaline masses (Fig. 156). The chief sites are the lower part of the rectus abdominis, the diaphragm, and the thigh muscles. Rupture of the muscle may occur with hemorrhage. The condition, which is due to the toxins, may also occur in other infections.

The *bones* may show a chronic suppurative lesion, either abscess or periostitis, which

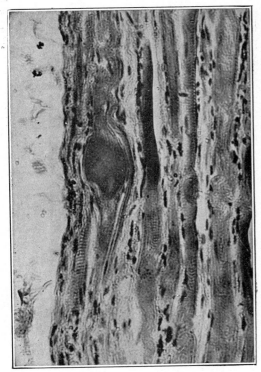

FIG. 156.—Zenker's degeneration of muscle in typhoid fever. The affected parts of the fibers have lost their transverse striations and are dark and swollen. (Boyd, *Pathology for the Physician*.)

may come on months or years later. The common sites are the tibia, sternum, ribs, and spine. In extra-abdominal lesions the bacilli appear to acquire a pyogenic property. The pus often contains living typhoid bacilli.

The *blood* shows a marked leukopenia (2000 to 5000 per c.mm.), with decrease in the polymorphonuclears and eosinophils (these may vanish) and an increase of large mononuclear cells.

LABORATORY AIDS IN DIAGNOSIS.—The four most valuable laboratory tests are: (1) blood culture, (2) the Widal test, (3) the demonstration of bacilli in the feces and the urine, and (4) the leukocyte count. *Blood culture* is positive at the beginning of the disease (the period of bacteremia) and during the first week. After that more and more bacilli are destroyed so that it becomes increasingly difficult to get a positive culture. The *Widal test* has a great reputation, but it has very real limitations and is less valuable

now than formerly for the two reasons that many persons who have been inoculated against typhoid give a positive agglutination reaction, and many cases of typhoid do not give a reaction until late in the disease, by which time the diagnosis is self-evident. After recovery the agglutinins persist for months, sometimes for years, while the agglutinins due to inoculation usually disappear in a few months, although they may reappear after a number of years as the result of some non-typhoid disease (*anamnestic reaction*). The Widal test is frequently negative in carriers.

Efforts have been made to overcome the difficulty of the persistently negative case. The typhoid bacillus contains two antigens, which give rise to two different kinds of agglutinins, termed respectively "O" and "H". In most cases of typhoid the "O" agglutinin appears earlier than the "H" agglutinin. On the other hand nearly all test cultures consists of "H" forms only. Thus the early appearing "O" agglutinin is entirely missed in the ordinary Widal test. The agglutinins which appear in a previously inoculated person as the result of a subsequent non-typhoid infection (anamnestic reaction) are of the "H" and not of the "O" type. If, therefore, the "O" type can be demonstrated in the blood it is proof that the infection belongs to the typhoid group, and that the reaction is not due to a previous inoculation. Bacterial suspensions of both "H" and "O" types are now available. It is obvious that the "O" type is to be preferred in performing the Widal test. With the macroscopic method the "O" type gives a small flaking reaction, while the "H" type gives a large flaking reaction.

Bacilli in the stools are found more readily in carriers than in the active disease. They are most numerous in the third week, as by that time the bile is loaded with bacilli. The *urine* may contain bacilli in the third week. The *diazo reaction* in the urine is negatively pathognomonic, as it is present in practically every case, but is also found in other infective fevers, especially miliary tuberculosis, which may simulate typhoid. Culture of the *bile* obtained by *duodenal drainage* is one of the best methods of detecting a carrier. The peculiarities of the *leukocyte count* have already been described. For making an early diagnosis the two most valuable tests are blood culture and the leukocyte count. In the first week blood culture, in the second the agglutination test, and in the third week culture of the stool may be expected to be positive.

Relation of Symptoms to Lesions.—The symptoms are partly general, partly intestinal, and partly hemopoietic. The general symptoms such as fever, headache, lethargy, and a clouding of the mind which gives the name to the disease (*typhos*, a cloud). They are due to the endotoxins which are liberated when the bacilli are broken down in the blood stream. The rose spots are caused by bacterial emboli in the skin capillaries. The enlargement of the spleen which forms one of the chief clinical pictures is due to the great accumulation of cells in the splenic pulp. The *intestinal symptoms* including hemorrhage and perforation are the result of the ulcers. The *blood changes* (leukopenia, disappearance of polymorphonuclears and eosinophils) are the direct result of the lesions in the bone marrow. The carrier state is an indication that the constant infection of the gallbladder has become chronic instead of clearing up. Were we asked what were the *most significant lesions* of the disease, we would answer those of the lymphoid tissues, of the bone marrow, and of the gallbladder. In respect to the occurrence of *complications*, the intestinal lesions take first place.

Other Salmonella Infections.—Enteric fever may occasionally be caused by other members of the Salmonella group, more particularly *Salm. paratyphi A* and *B*, the former being prevalent in Asia, the latter in Britain and North America. *Paratyphoid B infection* is usually due to milk, ice cream, and other dairy products. As the dose necessary for infection is much higher than for typhoid, water-borne epidemics are rare. In keeping with the name, the clinical picture resembles that of typhoid, but is usually milder.

Food Poisoning.—This term denotes an acute gastroenteritis caused by bacterial contamination of food or drink. The condition is a toxemia rather than a bacterial

invasion. There are two distinct forms of different origin but with a similar clinical picture. These are the *infection type*, in which bacteria in the contaminated food multiply and produce their toxins in the bowel, and the *toxin type*, in which toxins are produced in the food before ingestion, the responsible bacteria not multiplying in the body. Both forms are marked by violent vomiting and diarrhea accompanied by severe or even profound prostration. The symptoms come on from 6 to 12 hours after eating the infected food, being naturally earlier in the toxin type, later in the infection type.

Infection Type.—The infection is usually caused by one of the Salmonella group, occasionally by a Shigella *Salm. typhimurium* (*Bact. aertryeke*) and *Salm. enteritidis* (*Gaertner's bacillus*) are perhaps the commonest. The food has usually stood for two or three days in warm weather, but it does not smell nor does it look bad. The infection may come from animals or game birds, or the food may be contaminated from the feces of infected mice or rats in the house. The outbreak is likely to involve all the members of a family. Larger outbreaks will follow such social gatherings as church picnics, where large numbers of persons partake of a common food supply, probably imperfectly cooked. Complete recovery is usual in the course of a week, but there is a mortality of about 1 per cent.

Toxin Type.—Here the toxin, usually powerful in type and violent in action, is formed in the food before it is eaten. As is natural, symptoms of poisoning soon make their appearance, sometimes within an hour. The bacteriology is obscure. It is known that some strains of *Staphylococcus aureus* produce a powerful enterotoxin. Some *Proteus* strains may produce a similar type of enterotoxin in decomposing meat. Apart from these, little is known, although a variety of organisms may be grown from the infected food.

BACILLARY DYSENTERY

Dysentery is an acute colitis characterized by *diarrhea*. Two entirely different diseases go by this name as the result of ancient usage. These are bacillary dysentery and amebic dysentery, only the first of which will be considered here. In bacillary dysentery the responsible bacteria remain in the bowel which they damage by their toxins, so that blood culture is useless. In amebic dysentery the parasite first damages the wall of the bowel, and then enters the mesenteric veins, to be carried by the portal veins to the liver, where it sets up multiple amebic abscesses.

The *Shigella group* of bacteria which are responsible for bacillary dysentery are intestinal parasites peculiar to man. They are gram-negative bacilli identical morphologically with the coliform and Salmonella groups already considered, but, unlike the others, they are non-motile. There are many members of the group, only a few of which are pathogens. The best known of these are *Sh. shigæ*, also known as Type I and Shiga bacillus, *Sh. flexneri* (Flexner group), and *Sh. sonnei*, (Sonne bacillus). Shiga's bacillus causes a much more severe disease than the other members, associated with toxemia and even collapse. This may be because it is the only one which produces a soluble exotoxin. Flexner's bacillus is the commonest cause of dysentery. Sonne's bacillus often gives rise to an acute gastroenteritis rather than a true dysentery, which is essentially a colitis.

Bacillary dysentery is very common in tropical countries, but is also found in the temperate zone, especially where men are crowded together under poor hygienic conditions. It is thus a great destroyer of armies in the field, it appears in large mental hospitals in both endemic and epidemic form, and it is the chief cause of the acute enteritis of children associated with the passage of pus and blood. In ordinary practice the disease may be of any grade of severity, varying from the prostrating and fatal case to one so mild as to escape clinical detection. In any epidemic the proportion of mild and symptomless cases is high, so it is easy to understand how the infection may spread widely. The disease is likely to be spread in two ways: (1) by hands, food or utensils of symptomless patients; (2) by the feet of flies flying from feces to food. These two methods were combined in the statement of my professor of medicine at Edinburgi that typhoid was caused by "the fouling of food with fingers and the feet of fecal-feeding flies." Transference by true carriers is probably rare.

Lesions.—Bacillary dysentery resembles diphtheria in that the bacilli remain localized, do not penetrate the tissues at first nor invade the blood stream, and produce local necrosis and distant damage by the means of their exotoxins. When an ulcer has been produced the bacilli may penetrate into the deeper parts of the wall. The disease is an acute colitis, but the lower part of the ileum may also be involved. The toxins cause an acute inflammation of the wall of the bowel, patches of the mucous membrane become necrotic, are converted into sloughs, and when these separate, ulcers are formed. The surface of the ulcer may become covered by an inflammatory exudate consisting of fibrin and polymorphonuclear leukocytes which together with the necrotic material, may form a false membrane (diphtheritic inflammation). The ulcers seldom penetrate the muscularis mucosa, but sometimes they may reach the serous coat and perforate. The ulcers are clear-cut, and have not the undermined edges seen in the amebic form. There may be many small ulcers, or they may coalesce to form a few very large ones. The mucosa between the ulcers may become papillomatous.

Microscopically the wall of the bowel is infiltrated with polymorphonuclear leukocytes (Fig. 157). This is in marked contrast to the mononuclear type of inflammation seen in typhoid fever. There is marked edema and thickening of the submucosa. Large numbers of gram-negative bacilli are present in the floor of the ulcer. *Healing* takes place by the formation of granulation tissue which becomes covered by a simple epithelium without glands. If the ulceration is superficial there is little scarring, but when deep there may be much scar formation with the production of marked stenosis of the bowel.

Relation of Symptoms to Lesions.—Dysentery, which means bowel trouble, was described by the father of medicine as a diarrhea characterized by the presence of

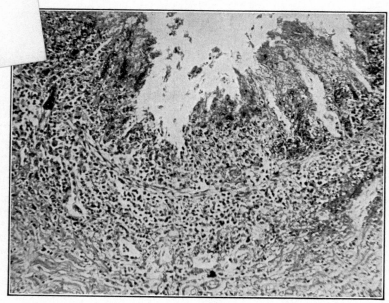

Fig. 157.—Bacillary dysentery. The mucosa is necrotic and densely infiltrated with inflammatory cells. ×100. (Boyd, *Pathology for the Physician*).

blood and pus in the stools (a "bloody flux") and accompanied by straining and tenesmus. This clinical definition of Hippocrates cannot be bettered at the present day. The infection is an acute one, although of varying severity, lasting for several weeks, but the condition may become chronic or there may be periodic recurrences. In addition to the local symptoms the patient may show evidence of the action of a powerful diffusible toxin and die of toxemia.

The pain, tenesmus, and diarrhea are due to the acute inflammation of the large bowel. The pus and blood in the stools are the result of the ulceration. Mucus may be abundant, especially in the chronic cases. As the disease is a local one there are no signs of septicemia, such as acute splenic swelling. The toxins may act on the nervous system, producing a peripheral neuritis, and on the joints causing a painful effusion. Liver abscesses are very rare (*cf.* Amebic dysentery). The organisms are insensitive to penicillin and erythromycin, but the sulfonamides, streptomycin, chloramphenicol and tetracyclines are fully effective.

CHOLERA

Asiatic cholera is an extremely acute inflammatory disease of the intestine due to a motile, gram-negative bacillus shaped like a comma. It was therefore called the comma bacillus by Koch, its discoverer, but is now known as a vibrio. *Vibrio choleræ* releases a powerful endotoxin on dying. It also contains a mucinase, which may be responsible for the *extreme cellular desquamation* of mucosal epithelium that is so characteristic a feature. The endotoxin causes intense dilatation of the capillaries along the length of the small and large bowel, with the result that huge quantities of watery fluid pour into the lumen, converting the contents into something like thin barley soup, which when passed constitutes the "rice-water stool." The vibrios find this a medium so much to their liking that they proliferate at an enormous rate as if they were in a test tube, giving a practically pure culture of the organism. The result of this pouring of fluid from the blood into the bowel is a degree of *dehydration* so profound that it kills the patient in 75 per cent of untreated cases. Treatment consists in restoring fluid and electrolytes to the blood at the earliest possible moment. Antibiotics may kill the organisms, but they do nothing to neutralize the endotoxin.

The principal *lesions* are as follows. The entire length of the intestinal mucous membrane is intensely congested, being deep red in color. Hemorrhages are common. Unlike typhoid and dysentery there is no ulceration, but the epithelium covering the mucosa is shed off so that a raw surface is left, although the mucosa itself is not destroyed. The lymph follicles are swollen, and the mesenteric nodes may be necrotic. A striking feature of the dead body is the extraordinary degree of rigor mortis, the arms and legs being as stiff as iron rods.

The *epidemiology* of this remarkable disease is of singular interest. It is called Asiatic cholera because the lower basin of the Ganges is the one area where the disease is endemic and from which fearful epidemics would spread across the world. In 1831 some 50,000 persons died of cholera in England. Now it is unknown. This triumph of preventive medicine was the result of the simple discovery that infection was due to drinking polluted water from wells or streams. The wise Chinese are the only Orientals who do not suffer from cholera; they use boiled water and cooked food, they drink tea and eat hot rice. When there is danger of exposure to infection vaccination against the disease is of great value. The cholera vibrio is singularly susceptible to a bacteriophage which rapidly destroys it, and in the past this phage has been used with success in limiting the spread of epidemics by reducing the infectivity of the discharges.

Friedländer's Bacillus.—This gram-negative bacillus which differs from E. coli in being non-motile and possessing a prominent capsule (hence its name *B. mucosus capsulatus*), is present in the feces of 5 per cent of people, but it is more common in the respiratory tract, where it is a harmless commensal, known also as the pneumobacillus. It may, however, act as a secondary invader in bronchiectasis, tuberculosis, influenza and other diseases of the lung. Finally, for some obscure reason, in about 2 per cent of bacterial pneumonias it is responsible for an infection with a high mortality and a characteristic mucoid type of exudate.

DIPHTHERIA

We now pass from the gram-negative to the gram-positive group of bacilli. It is interesting to compare diphtheria with cholera. In both cases the offending organism remains localized and produce a powerful toxin, but in the case of cholera this is an endotoxin which acts on the bowel wall, wheras the diphtheria bacillus produces an exotoxin which passes into the blood and excites the formation of an antitoxin with resulting immunity. Virulent diphtheria bacilli are often found in the throats of healthy (immune) persons, but the presence of cholera vibrios in the stools spells the disease cholera. Both conditions provide us with remarkable examples of triumphs in the prevention of infectious disease, but the methods by which this was achieved bear no resemblance to one another.

Bacteriology.—The Klebs-Loeffler bacillus belongs to the genus, *Corynebacterium*, so-called because the members tend to assume a club-like shape due to the presence of metachromatic granules at the poles. The genus contains many species, and the species *C. diphtheriæ* consists of three types, known as gravis, intermedius and mitis, which have different staining, cultural and biochemical properties. As the names signify, the *gravis* type is the most virulent, the *intermedius* type less so, whilst the *mitis* gives rise to only a mild form of infection. As we have already seen, the most virulent forms may live in the throat of healthy persons who have established a complete immunity.

The bacilli produce an exotoxin which causes necrosis and inflammation locally, and when absorbed into the blood may damage the myocardium, and act on the nervous system with resulting paralysis of groups of muscles. Diphtheria toxin is used for the preparation of antitoxin used for passive immunization, for toxoid used for active immunization, and for testing susceptibility in the Schick test. Toxoid is merely toxin which has been deprived of its toxicity by treatment with dilute formalin, but which retains its antigenic power so that it stimulates the formation of antitoxin and thus induces immunity. In the Schick test a very weak solution of toxin is injected into the skin. If enough antitoxin is present in the blood, the toxin is neutralized and the test is negative, indicating immunity. If the subject is not immune the toxin damages the cells of the skin, and a deep red patch of inflammation develops. Children with a negative Schick test practically never develop diphtheria.

Lesions.—The disease usually involves the pharynx, nose and larynx, but occasionally there may occur infection of open wounds, vulva or conjunctiva. Sometimes it starts in the larynx or even the trachea. The toxin kills the surface cells, and the bacilli grow in the necrotic tissue with no phagocytes to molest them. There they produce more toxin, which leaks into the blood stream. In the Schick-negative child the first toxin produced is at once neutralized by antitoxin, so that bacilli have no dead tissue to grow in and are killed by the phagocytes which soon arrive on the scene. In the severe inflammation produced by the gravis and intermedius types the exudate is intensely fibrinous, and this coagulated material combined with the abundant necrotic cells forms a dirty, pseudomembrane or *"false membrane,"* which can be recognized at a glance by the physician. It is naturally adherent, and when forcibly removed leaves a raw surface. Under the membrane there is a neutrophilic infiltration varying in severity with the type of infection. The membrane may extend to the larynx, where it may seriously embarrass respiration, even to the point of suffocation. The infection may start in the larynx. For some reason laryngeal diphtheria is usually due to the mitis type of organism.

Toxic lesions due to the exotoxin are best seen in heart (diphtheritic myocarditis), where, before the days of the prevention and successful treatment of diphtheria, they were a frequent cause of fatal cardiac failure. The muscle fibers undergo an acute degeneration, being swollen, granular, and losing their striations. A secondary cellular inflammatory reaction develops around the necrotic foci. *Diphtheritic polyneuritis* is a degenerative demyelination involving the nerve roots and the proximal portion of the nerves. As a result of the affinity of the diphtheria toxin for nervous tissue there may be paralysis of the palate, of the extra-ocular muscles of the eye, sometimes followed later by paralysis of the proximal

muscles and the muscles of respiration. There may of course be degeneration of the cells of the various parenchymatous organs, and Zenker's hyaline degeneration of striated muscle may be encountered.

Clinical Picture.—In an unprotected population diphtheria is likely to be seen between the age of two and five years, being rare after the age of fifteen years, immunity being established by then through repeated subclinical attacks of low virulence. The disease is spread by droplet infection from carriers, occasionally from infected dust. The onset is marked by fever, chills and malaise, together with a sore throat. In the untreated case, and in the olden days when diphtheria was so dreaded a disease of childhood, the formation of a false membrane in the larynx and trachea would lead to acute respiratory embarrassment and finally suffocation. Death may occur from myocardial failure about a week after the development of the throat symptoms. Electrocardiographic changes are present in about 75 per cent of cases of the disease. There is a curious lag in the development of the neurological symptoms, which do not become apparent for some weeks after the acute phase has subsided. The picture outlined above has become a rarity at the present day owing to the almost unbelievable success of preventive immunization and treatment.

GLANDERS

Glanders, a disease of horses and donkeys and very occasionally transmitted to man, is caused by an organism of the genus *Pfeifferella*, considered to be intermediate between actinomyces and mycobacterium. It is known as *Pfeiferella mallei* and also as *Malleomyces mallei*. The name comes from the club-ends resembling a mallet which may develop in culture. The organism is negative in all respects; it is non-motile, has no capsule or spores, is gram-negative, non-acid-fast, and is relatively inert biochemically, but it can produce a devastatingly acute form of disease. Glanders is essentially a disease of equines, but grooms, veterinary surgeons, *etc.* also suffer in countries where infected animals are not destroyed. Cattle and pigs are absolutely resistant, but the disease can be transmitted to laboratory animals, and laboratory workers are readily infected. Infection from a glandered animal is usually through the intact skin, but the organisms may be inhaled from nasal discharges or implanted on the conjunctiva. The disease, whether in animals or man, may be acute or chronic.

Acute Glanders.—This may take the form of an overwhelming septicemia and pyemia. After an incubation period of a few hours or days there is an abrupt onset of fever, chills, aches and pains, and prostration. The local lesion is an abscess of the skin, with speedy spread along the lymphatics, abscesses of the lymph nodes, invasion of the blood stream, and metastatic abscess formation in the lungs, bones, meninges, and elsewhere. Up to 90 per cent of the cases die in a week or two.

Chronic Glanders.—This variety, which is less common, takes the form of a chronic granuloma, with the development of inflammatory swellings involving the skin, lymph nodes, liver and spleen. The term *farcy* is applied to ulcerated lesions in the horse involving the skin, together with enlargement and induration of the lymphatics (farcy pipes) and lymph nodes (farcy buds). The *microscopic appearance* is that of an infective granuloma but without caseation. Giant cells are rare, and unless the bacilli can be demonstrated a correct diagnosis may be very difficult. The infection may persist in a remitting form over many months or even years, but in the end over 50 per cent of the cases die of the disease.

The *Strauss reaction* is useful for diagnosis. The suspected material is injected into the peritoneal cavity of a male guinea-pig, and within twenty-four hours an acute inflammation develops in the tunica vaginalis. The fluid from the tunica is implanted on potato, and a yellow honey-like culture is obtained. Unfortunately the reaction is not entirely specific, being given by *Brucellæ* and a few other organisms.

TUBERCULOSIS

So far we have been considering infections which are essentially acute in character, of limited duration, and with a corresponding type of inflammatory and cellular response. Now we turn to the supreme example, at least in the adult, of a chronic and long-drawn-out infection, in which the response of the body is entirely different. Tuberculosis presents more intriguing problems, some of which have been solved whilst others remain to be solved, than perhaps any other infectious disease.

Bacteriology.—The tubercle bacillus belong to the genus of Mycobacteria, of which there are many saprophytic species. The only one of the non-pathogens which deserves mention here is *Mycobacterium smegmatis*, commonly found in the smegma both of men and women. The presence of the smegma bacillus in the urine may lead to a mistaken diagnosis of tuberculosis. The only two pathogens, those of tuberculosis and leprosy, are strict parasites. The mycobacteria resist decolorization with acid after being stained intensely with hot carbolfuchsin (*acid-fastness*), and they are stained by dyes that fluoresce in ultraviolet light, so that they appear as luminous rods on a dark background (*fluorescent microscopy*). Robert Koch's discovery of the tubercle bacillus in 1882 is one of the masterpieces of bacteriological research, for in the course of one year he found the organism, invented a culture medium on which it could be grown, and reproduced the disease in animals.

Mycobacterium tuberculosis is very inactive compared with the organisms of typhoid fever and diphtheria. Ordinary bacteria grow to double their size and divide into two every 30 minutes if supplied with suitable food, whereas the tubercle bacillus takes a day to pass through the same cycle. It is natural, therefore, that the rate of production of symptoms should be correspondingly slow, and the course chronic. Although it grows slowly, it is hard to kill, and it resists drying for long periods. It neither produces an exotoxin like the diphtheria bacillus nor liberates an endotoxin on disintegrating like the typhoid bacillus. Nevertheless, as we know only too well, it is far from harmless. Much of its pathogenicity is related to its antigenic activity, and this in turn depends on its chemical composition. It consists of lipid, protein and carbohydrate.

The *lipid fraction*, which constitutes approximately 50 per cent of the organism, forms a waxy sheath around the bacillus, or is interspersed throughout its substance. It is responsible for the following special features: (1) It makes the organism more difficult to stain, so that heat and a mordant are required, and it is responsible for its acid-fastness. (2) It renders the bacilli more resistant to therapeutic agents. (3) It protects them against digestion when taken up by phagocytes, in whose interior they can live for long periods. (4) It is less irritating to the tissues than the surface of rapidly multiplying bacteria, so that the type of cellular response is less acute. (5) The lipid seems to be responsible for transforming the mononuclears and macrophages of the exudate into the epithelioid type of cell, and thus for the formation of the tubercle which gives the disease its name.

The *protein fraction* was originally extracted by Koch, who named it tuberculin. Tuberculoprotein, as we shall see, is the active antigen responsible for producing the state of hypersensitivity of the tissues which alters the whole course of the disease. It is rather curious that tuberculoprotein of itself does not have this power when injected into an animal. It is only the protein within the bacillus which can produce this effect. The destructive power of the tubercle bacillus is dependent on the *acquired sensitivity* of the tissues, which takes from ten to fourteen days to develop. The hypersensitivity (allergic) reaction takes the place of the damaging exotoxins and endotoxins of other micro-organisms.

The *carbohydrate fraction*, a polysaccharide, when injected excites a speedy accumulation of polymorphonuclear leukocytes at the site of injection. This, it may be noted, is the first response of the tissues to invasion by the tubercle bacillus.

Human and Bovine Infection.—Tuberculosis may be caused by two types of bacilli, human and bovine. Under modern conditions of life the human type is the only one of importance in man, but before the days of the testing of cows for tuberculosis and the pasteurization of milk bovine infection was extremely common. Both are equally pathogenic for man. The bovine type of bacillus is primarily a parasite of cattle, so that it is of great importance in veterinary pathology. It is mainly responsible for tuberculosis of lymph nodes and bones in children who acquire the infection through drinking unpasteurized milk from tuberculous cows. The primary lesion is in the lymphoid tissue of the nasopharynx with involvement of the cervical nodes, or in the intestinal mucosa with extension to the mesenteric nodes. The danger is greater in the country where the child may be exposed to repeated massive infection from one ailing cow than in the city where the contaminated milk is diluted by the milk from a hundred healthy animals. The disease caused by the bovine bacillus is not highly fatal, nor can the infection be conveyed to other persons because the lungs are not involved. The rabbit is very susceptible to the bovine but not to the human type of infection, whereas the guinea pig is equally susceptible to both, a fact which is used for differentiating the two types. Living bovine bacilli rendered avirulent are used in the B.C.G. method of vaccination against the human disease (see below).

Methods of Infection.—Infection with the human type is *air-borne* from patients with open pulmonary tuberculosis. This is mostly due to tiny droplets of sputum loaded with bacilli and expelled during coughing. The threat to a susceptible person living in the same house and room with a patient who does not observe such elementary hygienic precautions as shielding his mouth with a handkerchief is obvious. It is true that pathogenic bacilli may survive for months when dried, but the danger of dust from dried sputum is not as great as used to be believed. Infection is commonest under the age of 5 years, at which period it is apt to be rapidly progressive and fatal. Then it declines until late adolescence, reaching its maximum in women between twenty and twenty-five, in men between forty and fifty years of age, more especially in alcoholics. In the adult the disease is much more chronic. Infection through the *alimentary tract* used to be of major importance when a glass of milk was likely to contain many tubercle bacilli, but it has now become a rarity in most quarters. Infection through *the skin* is occasionally seen in the hand of a nurse, hospital orderly, or a pathologist (verruca necrogenica) handling infected material. Such infection may spread to the regional lymph nodes, but seldom goes farther. *Congenital infection* through the placenta is extremely rare, but I know of one case, the child of a tuberculous mother, in which the baby developed a lesion of the umbilicus at the age of one week, and died of generalized tuberculosis within the space of a month, the lesions swarming with bacilli, a condition reminiscent of congenital syphilis.

Methods of Spread.—The tubercle bacillus is non-motile, but it can be transported in the bodies of phagocytic cells. There are four chief methods of spread:

(1) By *direct extension*, the phagocytes carrying the bacilli into the lymph spaces of the surrounding tissue. (2) By the *lymphatics*. Tuberculosis is primarily an infection of lymphoid tissue. The bacilli may be detained by the lymph follicles of the mucosa (pharynx, bronchi, intestine) or by the regional lymph nodes. If they succeed in passing the Scylla of the lymph follicles and the Charybdis of the lymph nodes, they set out upon an Odyssey which may carry them far and wide, but always toward the lungs, for they pass by the thoracic duct to the venous blood stream and eventually the lungs and it may be the systemic circulation. (3) By the *blood stream*. Tuberculous bacillemia is a natural accompaniment of tuberculous infection, because of the drainage of the lymphatics into the venous system. This explains the occurrence of isolated lesions in almost any organ in the body. A bacillemia must be distinguished from a *general miliary tuberculosis*, where enormous numbers of bacilli are poured into the blood stream. This may be due to heavy infection via the lymphatic-venous route, or a caseous lesion may ulcerate through the wall of a vein and flood the circulation with bacilli. The result is an acute toxic infection which may terminate in death in the course of a few weeks. Tiny miliary tubercles are found in every organ of the body, though these may hardly be visible to the naked eye. Generalized acute miliary tuberculosis used to be as rapid in meningitis. Streptomycin and isoniazid

(isonicotinic acid hydrazide) have greatly lessened the gloom of the picture. Untreated miliary tuberculosis is not necessarily acutely fatal. A chronic miliary form is compatible with years of life and with recovery. Healed tubercles are found not only in the lungs, but also in the spleen, liver and other organs. (4) By the *natural passages*. Infection may spread along the bronchi, ureter and vas deferens. In these cases, however, it is difficult to be certain that the bacilli have not been carried along the lymphatics in the submucosa.

The Tissue Reaction.—The reaction of the body to the tubercle bacillus varies considerably, depending on the following factors: (1) the species of animals, (2) the size of dose, (3) the question of whether the animal is tuberculosis-free or has already been infected. The influence of these factors will be discussed as we proceed. In spite of possible variations there is a standard type of reaction caused by a moderate dose of bacilli of unattenuated virulence in a susceptible species of animal which is infected for the first time. *Polymorphonuclear leukocytes* are the first to arrive in response to an injection of tubercle bacilli. They are actively phagocytic, but are unable to damage the bacilli which they engulf. They play a useful part, however, in focalizing the infection by preventing to some extent the drift of bacilli through the tissues. The response of the polymorphonuclears is very much more marked in a reinfection, *i.e.*, in the allergic inflammation of an already tuberculous animal. Their appearance is transitory, and within twenty-four hours they are replaced by *mononuclear phagocytes* or *histiocytes*.

These cells represent the essential reaction of the body to the tubercle bacillus, but it is to the fatty envelope of the bacillus that the response is made, for the same effect is obtained by the injection of lipid extracted from the bodies of the bacilli. In some of the experimental work they have been the first cells to arrive. Thus Fried found that the intratracheal injection of bacilli in the rabbit caused an amazingly rapid appearance of mononuclears. When the animal was killed one minute after the injection the cells had begun to appear and in the course of five minutes a definite primitive tubercle has been formed within the alveoli. The mononuclears are highly phagocytic members of the reticuloendothelial system. The bacilli and also the polymorphonuclears containing bacilli are phagocytosed by the mononuclears, by which they are gradually broken down with dispersion of the lipid throughout the cytoplasm. This dispersion results in the transformation of the mononuclear into the *epithelioid cell* (epithelial-like), which is the most characteristic single feature of the tuberculous reaction. It is a large, pale cell with rather indistinct margins, the nucleus is large and vesicular, and the abundant cytoplasm often presents processes which pass from one cell to another to form an epithelioid reticulum. The epithelioid cell, then, may be regarded as a large mononuclear which has partially digested tubercle bacilli, and its distinctive cytoplasmic state seems to be the result of destruction of many bacilli with progressive emulsification of their lipid. The epithelioid cell is particularly rich in ascorbic acid (vitamin C), and it seems probable that this substance is connected with the enzyme activity of the principal reactive cells. The lymphocytes of the tubercle do not contain any demonstrable ascorbic acid. It is evident that by the time the mononuclears have become transformed into epithelioid cells the bacilli have undergone extensive destruction. This explains the difficulty which is experienced in demonstrating bacilli in the ordinary type of lesion in man, in which they are few and far between and may only be found after prolonged search, although in acute fulminating lesions such as tuberculous caseous pneumonia they may be present in enormous numbers. The mononuclears do not always have the power of destroying the bacilli which they engulf. Thus in the rat the bacilli thrive and multiply within the phagocytes, and the latter also multiply with the remorselessness of a malignant growth, until finally the animal succumbs to the cellular accumulation.

Giant cells are formed by fusion of a number of epithelioid cells. They may attain a great size, and contain large numbers of nuclei, usually arranged either around the periphery or at one or both poles. These are the typical *Langhans' giant cells*, the center of which appears to be necrotic. Ordinary foreign body giant cells with small nuclei scattered throughout the cytoplasm may also be present. Giant cells are not formed until necrosis has occurred. They are found in small caseous areas or at the edge of larger areas. They often contain tubercle bacilli, and their function is to digest and remove dead tissue. They are foreign body giant cells, and indicate that an active resistance is going on. Giant cells are very characteristic of tuberculosis, but they occur in other chronic inflammations (syphilis, actinomycosis), and they may be absent in the acuter forms of tuberculosis where resistance is low (tuberculous meningitis, *etc.*).

By the end of a week *lymphocytes* appear, and form a ring around the periphery of the lesion. They are small cells with dark nuclei, identical with the lymphocytes of the blood, but they are probably derived from the cells of the perivascular lymph sheath or other lymphoid structures. The lymphocytes are one of the principal sources of the gamma globulins which constitute the immune bodies.

The Tubercle.—The small mass of newly-formed or newly-arrived cells constitutes a tiny translucent nodule visible to the naked eye and known as a *tubercle* or *miliary tubercle* (Fig. 158), since it is at first about the size of a millet seed, although it increases in size and several tubercles may fuse to form a larger mass. It is avascular, so that when the vessels of a tuberculous organ such as the lung are injected with a colored medium the tubercles stand out unstained. By the end of the second week *caseation* begins. This is a form of coagulation necrosis caused by the liberated protein fraction of the bacilli, and the intensity of the necrosis varies with the size of dose. The term caseation really really means cheese-like, and was originally applied to the gross appearance of the lesion. Massive infection is likely to be accompanied by extensive caseation, as in acute tuberculous pneumonia. In the center of the tubercle the cells lose their outline, the nuclei disappear, and all structure is lost (Fig. 159). The tubercule bacillus grows and multiplies best in a rather high oxygen

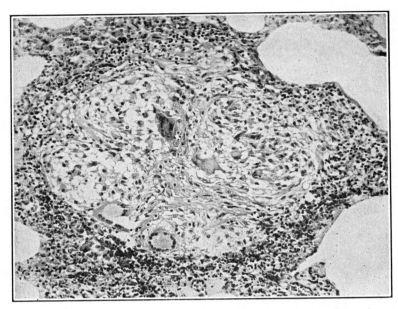

FIG. 158.—A miliary tubercule in the lung, showing epithelioid cells, Langhans giant cells, and peripheral lymphocytes. × 150.

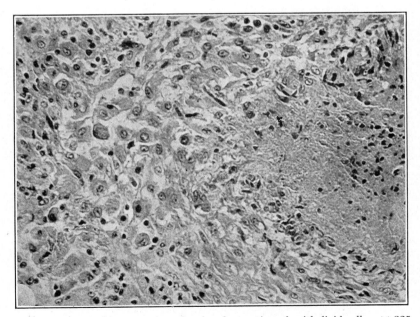

FIG. 159.—Tuberculous caseation, showing destruction of epithelioid cells. × 325.

tension, and only slowly when the oxygen tension is reduced. In the avascular center of the caseous area bacterial growth is at a minimum. Fatty acids, which are released in caseous tissue, further inhibit reproduction and may even destroy the organisms, so that it is small wonder that bacilli cannot be found in the center of such an area and must be looked for at the extending periphery of the lesion. The tubercle now presents a homogeneous caseous center staining red with eosin, a periphery of pale epithelioid cells with one or more giant cells, and an outer zone of dark blue lymphocytes. Caseation is the most characteristic single feature of the tuberculous lesion, and one should be reluctant to make the diagnosis unless caseation is present.

There is a tendency for caseation to be followed by *softening and liquefaction*, although this need not necessarily occur. Long points out that softening of the caseous tubercles is the key problem in tuberculosis, for were it not for softening the disease would be self-limited. It is the escape of the liquefied material which is responsible for the formation of the tuberculous cavity. When softening is associated with discharge of the material on to a surface such as that of a bronchus an extraordinary multiplication of bacilli occurs owing to the raised oxygen tension. From this it follows that acute fresh cavities discharging soft yellow lumps in the sputum are highly infective, while old chronic cavities are not an important source of infection.

Modern chemotherapy, more particularly the combined use of streptomycin, isoniazid, and para-aminosalicylic acid over a prolonged period, has a profound effect on the progress of the disease. This effect is most readily seen in surface lesions. Ulcers of the larynx, bronchial tract and intestine heal quickly. The contents of a cavity in the lung become inspissated, and later invaded by large numbers of neutrophils with resulting liquefaction and the formation of a cyst lined by squamous epithelium or fibrous tissue. Tubercle bacilli may still be demonstrated by staining, but not by culture nor animal inoculation.

The microscopic picture in tuberculosis is characteristic and readily recognized, but it must be borne in mind that a *histological diagnosis of the disease is only presumptive*. Other conditions may present a similar or even identical microscopic picture, for example sarcoidosis, coccidioidomycosis, histoplasmosis, brucellosis, and syphilis. In some of these (coccidioidomycosis, histoplasmosis) the etiologic agent can be found in the tissue, in others (brucellosis, syphilis) serologic tests are of value. Finally the sections may show only a picture of chronic inflammation with none of the features characteristic of tuberculosis, yet tubercle bacilli may be found on culture.

The *future history of the tubercle* varies greatly. (1) The experimental tubercle may resolve, disappear completely, and leave no trace. It is difficult to know if this occurs in man, but it probably does. The peritoneum may be found studded with tubercles, and yet if the abdomen is opened a year later the membrane may be smooth and normal. (2) A very common occurrence is for the caseous area to be surrounded by fibroblasts which form a fibrous capsule for the tubercle. Lime salts are deposited, and the calcified tubercle is said to be *healed*, but even in this quiescent lesion living bacilli may still lurk and can be demonstrated by animal inoculation. Reticulum may be present in tubercles composed entirely of epithelioid cells, and as reticulum is formed before connective tissue it is possible that the one may develop into the other, and that the mononuclears may take some part in the formation of collagen. (3) There may be a low-grade inflammation with the formation of *tuberculous granulation tissue* with many tubercles but little or no caseation. This is due to low virulence or high resistance, and is a rare form of the disease. This hyperplastic form is seen in the synovial membrane of joints and occasionally in lymph nodes. (4) There may be *spread* of the infection, the bacilli being carried by phagocytes through the tissues giving rise to the formation of new tubercles which fuse together until large caseous areas are formed. (5) There may be an *acute inflammatory reaction* when the infection is virulent or massive, as seen in tuberculous meningitis and acute tuberculous pneumonia. This reaction, in place of being mainly productive, is essentially exudative in type and is characterized by a great outpouring of polymorphonuclear leukocytes and serum with, it may be, an abundant formation of fibrin. It is, however, not in first infections but in reinfections, sometimes called secondary infections, that the acute inflammatory reaction is seen to best advantage, and we may now turn to a consideration of the lesions which develop in the already tuberculous or allergic animal or man.

Immunity and Hypersensitivity.—We now come to the heart of the problem of tuberculosis. How is it that an organism with very limited powers of multiplication in comparison with other bacteria, non-motile, and unable to produce exotoxin or endotoxin, can be the greatest killer in the entire realm of bacterial infections (the Captain of the Men of Death), or merely cause an infection so slight that it remains entirely subclinical and terminates in complete healing? The answer to this question appears to be intimately bound up with the development of immunity or resistance and hypersensitivity or allergy. The resistance referred to here is acquired resistance, which must be differentiated from native resistance to be discussed presently. Both resistance and hypersensitivity are the result of the action of tuberculoproteins on the tissues. There has been a prolonged controversy as to the relationship of the two processes. Is hypersensitivity the cause of the increased resistance, or is it merely an associated phenomenon, a two-edged sword which may be more harmful than protective? There is still room for difference of opinion, but the evidence seems to favor the view that the two processes are quite distinct. Although they are invariably associated and develop about the same time, it is now possible to separate than by experimental methods. The reader with leisure will find a full discussion of the problem in Rich's monumental monograph, *The Pathogenesis of Tuberculosis.*

Our knowledge of the subject dates back to the observation by Robert Koch that there is a fundamental distinction between the reaction to the tubercle bacillus in a healthy animal and in one already suffering from tuberculosis. This is the difference between a primary and a secondary infection.

In the *primary infection* the injection of a pure culture of tubercle bacilli into the skin of a healthy guinea pig is attended by no visible reaction for ten to fourteen days. At the end of that period a nodule develops, which breaks down with the formation of an ulcer that never heals, for the guinea pig, unlike man, has no natural resistance. The regional lymph nodes become enlarged and caseous, for the bacilli are not retained at the site of inoculation. Indeed their spread is facilitated by the accelerated lymph flow which accompanies the reaction. The entire process is a manifestation of allergic hypersensitivity which develops after the lapse of two weeks. It is comparable to the tuberculosis of childhood in the human subject, although, as we shall see presently, healing of the lesions is the rule in the child.

In *secondary infection* the sequence of events is quite different. The injection is now made into an animal which has been made tuberculous by an injection some weeks or months previously. Next day the site of inoculation is found to be indurated and dark, the reaction spreading till it involves an area from 0.5 to 1.0 cm. in diameter. This area breaks down and forms a shallow ulcer, but the ulcer quickly heals, and the regional lymph nodes do not become enlarged. The animal is able to fix the second invasion of bacilli at the point of entry and then destroy them. This is known as the *Koch phenomenon*, and is an indication of resistance or immunity.

The *microscopic* changes can be observed by injecting a culture of bacilli into the skin of a group of normal and hypersensitive animals, and removing the sites for histological study at intervals. Within an hour both the normal and hypersensitive animals show some inflammatory outpouring of fluid and polymorphonuclear leukocytes. In the course of a few hours a great difference can be observed, the site in the hypersensitive animals swarming with leukocytes, in contrast to a very moderate emigration in the controls. The same difference can be observed in the mononuclear cells. Necrosis now becomes apparent, reaching a maximum between forty-five and seventy-two hours, after which time the necrotic area may slough, leaving an ulcer. The mononuclear cells form sheets and definite tubercles. Finally the ulcers heal. In the controls the lesions enlarge progressively until, with the establishment of hypersensitivity, the inflammation becomes more intense, with necrosis, sloughing, and the formation of ulcers which refuse to heal.

There are two respects in which the lesion of reinfection differs from the primary lesion: (1) there is much more destruction of tissue; (2) the infection tends to remain localized. The two are dependent on two different mechanisms, for the destructiveness of the lesion of reinfection is due to allergic inflammation, whereas the localization of the bacilli seems to be due to the action of immune bodies such as agglutinins and opsonins.

It would appear that the reactions observed in the Koch phenomenon represent a combination of resistance and hypersensitivity. Perhaps the allergic factor speeds up the accumulation of phagocytes, whilst the immune factor enables the phagocytes to destroy the bacilli which they have engulphed. Acquired resistance, however, is not necessarily dependent on hypersensitivity, as may be seen from the following considerations. (1) There is no relation between the degree of resistance and hypersensitivity. (2) Acquired resistance inhibits the spread of infection and destroys the bacilli in the complete absence of allergic inflammation. (3) Hypersensitivity can be abolished, without at the same time destroying specific acquired immunity in previously immunized hypersensitive animals. (4) The resistance of an immunized hypersensitive animal can be passively transferred without transference of the hypersensitivity. (5) Acquired resistance remains intact after hypersensitivity has spontaneously disappeared, and also after it has been abolished by desensitization.

It is remarkable on what good terms tubercle bacilli may live with tissue cells if hypersensitivity is not set up. Great numbers of living bacilli can be injected intravenously into normal animals without toxic effect until hypersensitivity has been established. Living tissue culture cells are not damaged by virulent proliferating bacilli. Tubercle bacilli can live and multiply in macrophages without hurting them, these cells laden with bacilli wandering through a culture for days without suffering injury. Contrast this with other microorganisms, even non-pathogenic saprophytes, that may contaminate a tissue culture and rapidly prove fatal to the living cells.

Childhood and Adult Tuberculosis.—So far we have confined our discussion to tuberculosis in the experimental animal, and in particular to the guinea pig, which is completely lacking in resistance. When we turn our attention to the human subject with a natural native immunity and seek to differentiate between primary and secondary infection we are on far less certain ground, for we cannot be sure of the time and place of infection nor of the size of dose. It has been customary to speak of childhood or primary infection and adult or secondary infection. This distinction is no longer as valid as formerly. The *primary complex*, as it is called, that is to say the reaction in tissues not sensitized to tuberculoprotein, used to develop in nearly every child, but now in many places not more than 10 or 15 per cent of children develop the infection as shown by the tuberculin test. More primary infection develops in adults than in children, and it is equally harmless in the great majority of children. In spite of these facts it is still convenient to consider the two types of infection under the headings of childhood and adult.

The distinction between primary and secondary infection can be seen in the lungs. Using the regional lymph node involvement as an indicator of the *primary lesion*, Ghon was able by careful dissection to demonstrate a primary lung lesion in over 90 per cent of children. This lesion, often called the *Ghon lesion* (Fig. 160), is a small caseous focus not more than 1 cm. in diameter, usually single, and situated in any part of the lung, but generally just under the pleura, and limited by a fibrous capsule. There is a larger caseous focus in the lymph nodes draining this area. It is of interest to note that Ghon's work was published in 1912 but the lesion known by his name was described in every detail in 1898 by a Paris physician, George Küss, who wrote a monograph on the subject which has been completely neglected. Very many of these

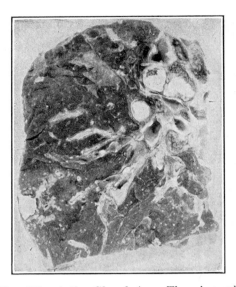

Fig. 160.—Active Ghon lesion. There is a sub-pleural caseous lesion in the lower lobe. The lymph nodes at the hilus are enlarged and caseous. Miliary tubercles are scattered through the lung, especially in the lower lobe. Some of the upper lobe has been removed. Death was due to general miliary tuberculosis.

lesions are healed, not only calcified but ossified. They seldom contain viable tubercle bacilli, as shown by culture and guinea-pig inoculation. If healing does not occur the child becomes allergic, the caseous lesions break down, and a rapidly spreading tuberculous pneumonia is apt to develop, often due to a caseous node ulcerating into a bronchus. The younger the child, the greater is the danger, for he has not had time to become immunized by repeated minimal infections. Therefore tuberculosis is especially dangerous in the first year of life. The child with primary infection either recovers or dies; he does not develop the chronic thick-walled cavities so characteristic of the disease in the adult.

A period of latency separates the primary and secondary types. The years from four to fourteen are almost free from fatal pulmonary tuberculosis.

When an adult develops pulmonary tuberculosis he has already been infected in childhood. At least that used to be the case. The one lesion is not necessarily a develop-

ment of the other, but the result of a fresh infection from without, massive enough to break down the immunity produced by the primary lesion. In other cases a few bacilli may remain dormant in a primary scar, but reawaken to activity at the time of adolescence, the scar breaking down and releasing many organisms. As the adult lesion is of the *secondary type* it will become caseous and break down with the formation of a cavity. If the immunity due to the primary lesion has disappeared, reinfection will be of the nature of a first infection, and the patient may die of acute tuberculous pneumonia as in the first year of life. Owing to the greatly decreased incidence of childhood tuberculosis, primary tuberculosis in the adult is becoming increasingly common. The majority of resistance may be native or acquired.

In general terms it may be said that in man a primary infection with the tubercle bacillus causes a minimal reaction, represented by a little spot in the lung with involvement of the regional lymph nodes, usually going on to healing, and without symptoms. Most or all of the organisms are destroyed, but in the process tuberculoprotein is liberated. This is an antigen, which excites the formation of an antibody that is taken up by nearly all the cells of the body, although it is hardly detectable in the blood. It appears probable that in reality two types of antibody are formed, one a *protective antibody*, possibly a circulating one, the other a *sensitizing (fixed) antibody*. If an animal or human acquires resistance to tuberculosis, he is always allergic to an intradermal injection of tuberculin. In this respect the allergic state is an index of immunity, and may indeed be part of the immune state. It would appear that hypersensitivity may be an advantage, leading to fixation of the bacilli at the point of entry, or it may be a hindrance, owing to the tissue damage which accompanies it. The *Schick reaction* (intradermal injection of tuberculin) is a test for immunity, not for hypersensitivity. The same is true of the *patch test*, which consists in the application to the skin of tuberculoprotein on a piece of gauze. In man the allergic state, as shown by the tuberculin reaction, is an index of immunity and may be part of the immune

19

state. It has been found that tuberculosis is more likely to develop in hospital nurses who are tuberculin-negative than in those who are tuberculin-positive.

From this somewhat confused account it becomes evident that immunity or resistance is the master word in tuberculosis. It is more to be desired than freedom from infection, for the latter is an unattainable ideal, and the rarer the infection, the more dangerous does it become.

Native Resistance.—It is natural that different animals and men should vary widely in their natural resistance to infection with the tubercle bacillus. This variation is true for species, races, and individuals. *Species* vary widely. Many species are completely immune. The guinea pig has no resistance, whereas the rabbit is nearly immune to human but extremely susceptible to bovine infection. *Human racial immunity* also shows wide variations. In the United States the mortality rate from tuberculosis in Negroes is 4 times, and in North American Indians 10 times as high as amongst the white population. At least these figures used to be correct. Of course other factors such as overcrowding and poor hygiene must be taken into account. When the disease is introduced into a primitive community previously free from infection the result is disastrous, but here the lack of previously acquired resistance plays an important part. *Individual immunity* seems to be largely genetic in character. The chance of developing tuberculosis increases in proportion to the degree of blood relationship with an affected individual. Thus it is known that the chance of developing the disease is more than 3 times as high in twins when the relation is uniovular (identical) rather than binovular. Other factors are intercurrent infections, occupation and age. Respiratory tract infections such as whooping cough and measles tend to scatter the exudate of a latent infection and may possibly depress the immunity, although it is obviously not possible to be certain of the latter. Occupations involving the inhalation of silica dust are certainly dangerous in this respect. Chronic debilitating diseases especially in old persons may awaken latent infection to activity. It has been noted that alcoholics are much more prone to develop tuberculosis than those of more temperate habits.

Decreasing Incidence.—In the middle of the 19th century tuberculosis was the most important cause of death. Now the death rate is only one-fifth of what it used to be. At the beginning of the present century almost the entire adult population of large cities were positive to the tuberculin test, indicating that at one time they had become infected. Now it is commonplace to find adults who are tuberculin negative.

What is the explanation for this remarkable change? In the absence of any startling discovery in the realm of therapy we naturally look to the bacillus and the host. There is no proof that the tubercle bacillus is losing its virulence, although in some cases the evidence is at least suggestive. In 1958 tuberculosis killed about 200,000 persons in Pakistan. The per capita death rate in that country is 30 times that of the United States. The general decline in incidence is not due to segregation of the infective cases, because the change began before the inception of the sanitarium era, although such segregation was undoubtedly of the greatest value. We must therefore look to host factors.

Resistance of the body to tuberculous infection depends on such factors as nutrition, strain, fatigue from overwork, *etc.* Poor housing, overcrowding and faulty hygiene are calculated to ensure that young children receive maximum doses of infection. The remarkable increase in the incidence of tuberculosis in the Scandinavian countries, Belgium, and Holland during the years of occupation in the Second World War offers striking evidence of the importance of privation as a factor in the pathogenesis of tuberculosis. Another factor was the intense weeding out of persons with an inheritable tendency of the disease in the earlier part of the 19th century. Such persons died before they could have children. A similar weeding out of weak stock in the North American Indians took over 100 years.

Extrapulmonary Tuberculosis.—Tuberculosis is primarily an infection of the lungs. The lesions of pulmonary tuberculosis are described in the chapter on Diseases of the

Respiratory System. As the blood stream is often invaded from the pulmonary lesions, infection of other organs must be of frequent occurrence. Most of the resulting lesions heal spontaneously, presumably by reason of local resistance. The chief exceptions are the kidney and bones. Others of less frequent occurrence are the adrenals, epididymis, Fallopian tubes, and the brain and meninges. The lesions and the disturbance of function resulting from these lesions will be described in the appropriate sections of the book. Here we are only concerned with the general biological process of tuberculous infection.

Treatment and Prevention.—Reference has already been made to the modern treatment of tuberculosis by a combination of streptomycin, isoniazid and para-aminosalicylic acid. The great value of isoniazid is that it penetrates the macrophages within which the bacilli lurk, and it crosses the blood-brain barrier, so that it is invaluable in the treatment of tuberculous meningitis, which used to be so extremely fatal. The bacilli early acquire resistance to the individual drugs, so that resistant strains easily emerge in the course of treatment and may spread to the general population. This tendency can be overcome by varying the proportions of the drugs used. Mention must also be made of surgical methods such as resection of localized or "coin" lesions, but these were much more in vogue before the introduction of chemotherapy, although they still have their place. The same is even more true of artificial pneumothorax designed to put the affected lung at rest.

Prevention rather than treatment is of course the ideal method of controlling tuberculosis. Endless attempts have been made in the past to immunize persons against infection with the tubercle bacillus, but without success. At the present time the most promising method is vaccination with B.C.G. or Bacille-Calmette-Guérin, which is a bovine strain of tubercle bacillus rendered avirulent by prolonged subculture on special media. The bacilli, which are living, have lost all power of producing disease on injection into animals, but still have an immunizing power against infection with a virulent culture. It is a remarkable fact that the method was introduced as long ago as 1922 by the French bacteriologist Calmette as a means of protecting infants born into tuberculous families. The method did not gain general favor by reason of the fear of the physician for injecting a live culture, but since 1946 enthusiasm has been growing, and great numbers of children and of nurses and hospital employees exposed to the risk of infection have been immunized by this means, with marked reduction both in the incidence and mortality of the disease.

TUBERCULOID LESIONS

Granulomatous lesions are not infrequently encountered which bear a resemblance to tuberculosis or sarcoidosis histologically, but which are not manifestations of these general disorders. Such lesions may be called tuberculoids. A sarcoid which is not associated with the generalized disease may also be regarded as a tuberculoid. A *foreign body*, a metal, a *fungus*, or an *antigen* liberated by disintegrating cells may excite histiocytic proliferation with the formation of epithelioid and giant cells, so that a non-caseating granuloma results.

The *talc granuloma of the peritoneum* due to the presence of crystals of magnesium silicate in the dusting powder of a surgeon's gloves is an example of a reaction to a foreign body. *Beryllium granuloma* is an example of a metal producing a similar reaction. *Fungi* such as coccidioides immitis and histoplasma capsulatum may cause lesions identical with those of sarcoidosis. Tuberculoid (sarcoid-like) lesions may occur in lymph nodes draining the seat of a primary carcinoma (Symmers). In such a case the granulomatous reaction may result from the presence of irritant products released as the result of necrosis or of the action of radiotherapeutic agents on the tumor. Sarcoid lesions may be seen in lymph nodes draining the lesions of *Crohn's disease* and even in the wall of the ileum. Giant cell granulomas in *Riedel's struma* of the thyroid which represent a reaction to liberated colloid may be mistaken for tuberculosis. Even a virus may excite a similar tissue response, as is seen in lymphogranuloma venereum. Many other examples of such tuberculoid reactions could be given.

From all this it becomes apparent that the diagnosis of tuberculosis on purely histological evidence is not as simple a matter as one might think, and this is even more true of sarcoidosis. McDonald and Weed point out that tubercle bacilli may be obtained by culture or animal inoculation from tissues on which a histological diagnosis of Hodgkin's disease and sarcoidosis has been made, and conversely that a biopsy diagnosis of tuberculosis may be reversed by the bacteriologist's subsequent report of brucellosis, histoplasmosis, or coccidioidomycosis.

Chromogenic Acid-fast Bacillary Infections.—In addition to the tuberculosis-like lesions produced by inanimate material, we are now encountering diseases caused by acid-fast bacilli which are not tubercle bacilli, although easily taken for those organisms. More and more such cases are being reported (Hensler). The disease produced by these "atypical" organisms is entirely similar in clinical and pathological manifestations to the disease caused by M. tuberculosis, except that the symptoms are milder and the progress slower. The bacilli grow at room temperature on egg media, they produce yellow pigment (chromogenic), they are longer and broader than tubercle bacilli with more prominent beading, and above all, they do not grow in the guinea pig. Moreover, the chromogens are resistant to two or more of the three major anti-tuberculous drugs, namely streptomycin, para-aminosalicylic acid, and isoniazid. The infections produced by these chromogenic organisms are discussed further in connection with disease of the lung.

SARCOIDOSIS

It is difficult to known where an account of the condition known as sarcoidosis or Boeck's sarcoid should be included, for the simple reason that we know nothing of its etiology. We have no proof, indeed, that it is of bacterial origin. The granulomatous lesions, however, are in many respects so similar to those produced by the mycobacteria, and particularly to those of tuber-

culosis, that it seems not unreasonable to introduce the subject in this place.

The condition was first described by Jonathan Hutchison in 1869, but it has masqueraded under such a variety of names that it is only in recent years that it has come to command general attention. Perhaps the best descriptive name is that of *benign lymphogranuloma*, for clinically the lesions may simulate those of Hodgkin's disease, (a form of lymphoblastoma), whilst histologically it may mimic tuberculosis. Sarcoid is certainly a misleading name. There is usually an astonishing absence of symptoms, the disease is seldom fatal, and autopsy reports are correspondingly rare. The condition appears to be particularly common in Scandinavian countries.

Lesions.—The diversity of lesions, or rather of organs involved, is remarkable. The chief tissues affected are the skin and lymph nodes, both superficial and deep, but there may be splenomegaly, hepatomegaly, and lesions of the lung, myocardium, pancreas, testis, tonsil, digits, parotid and lachrymal glands, and uveal tract of the eye. The mediastinal and thoracic nodes are involved in some 75 per cent of cases, and are often visible in the x-ray film. I have seen a sarcoid lesion in the hypothalamus which caused diabetes insipidus, and two cases of myocardial sarcoidosis. To make matters more confusing, lesions may be confined to the skin or lymph nodes or bones or the eye. The bone lesions are practically limited to the phalanges of the fingers and toes. The disease lasts for months or years, with a tendency to fibrosis and healing. Healed lesions are represented by scars. In the lungs this scarring is of particular importance, because there can be little doubt that many cases which in the past have been considered as healed miliary tuberculosis are in reality examples of healed sarcoidosis. There may be quite generalized interstitial pulmonary fibrosis causing dyspnea and cyanosis due to failure of the right ventricle. Radiologically the bones show a peculiar reticulated rarefaction in the early stages; later there are small punched-out areas. There is a remarkable *alteration in the plasma proteins*, consisting of an increase in the globulin fraction, usually with a pro-

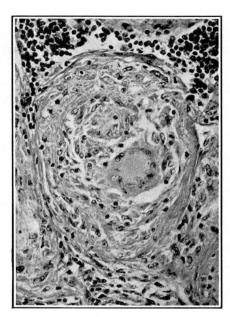

FIG. 161.—Sarcoidosis. × 160.

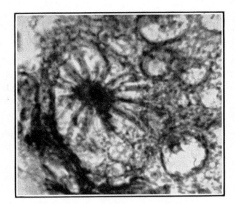

FIG. 162.—Asteroid in giant cell in sarcoidosis.
× 1240.

nounced elevation in the total plasma protein. In this respect the disease resembles multiple myeloma, kala-azar and lymphogranuloma venereum, in all of which elevation of the plasma globulin is a distinctive feature.

The *microscopic appearance* is that of rounded, circumscribed masses resembling miliary tubercles, the chief component of which is epithelioid cells, together with macrophages, giant cells, and occasional eosinophils. It may be difficult to decide between sarcoidosis and tuberculosis, particularly in a lymph node, but the peculiarly clean-cut, almost diagrammatic, character of the sarcoid lesions help the observer in his decision. The giant cells are larger than those of tuberculosis and contain more nuclei (Fig. 161). Inclusion bodies, both *"asteroids"* and the spherical *Schaumann bodies* with calcified concentric laminations, may be a striking feature of the giant cells. Neither of these, however, is pathognomonic of sarcoidosis. The asteroid inclusions consist of clear areas containing a dark central body from which radiate delicate spinous processes giving an appearance of a starfish (Fig. 162). They may be derived from lipids which are no longer soluble in fat solvents or may represent protein deposits on former lipid crystals. Excellent illustrations of the various inclusions will be found in Engle's paper. There is a striking and characteristic absence of caseation, and there is generally no surrounding lymphocytic infiltration. Fibrosis increases with the age of the lesion. Silver stains show a delicate reticulum which is absent owing to destruction in tuberculosis. In the later stages of the disease the lesions undergo a hyaline transformation. Teilum suggests that this is due to the precipitation of a homogeneous substance (?globulin) in the reticuloendothelial cells. This substance, which he refers to as paraamyloid because of its resemblance to amyloid, seems to be related to the hyperglobulinemia and may be a product of the plasma cells. The process may represent an antigen-antibody reaction. The difficulty is to name the antigen.

It is now possible to grow sarcoid tissue in tissue culture. Patchy degeneration of the outgrowing fibroblasts is associated with large eosinophilic inclusion bodies in these changed areas. These features are apparently restricted to sarcoid tissue.

A fresh outlook on the natural history of the disease is suggested by Barrie and Bogoch. From an examination of a large amount of material they believe that granuloma formation is preceded by a diffuse mononuclear cell proliferation and infiltration in all the sites where granulomas are found, *i.e.*, the lymphatic and filter systems (nodes, spleen, marrow).

A similar infiltration is found in the lungs, liver, heart, salivary glands, and central nervous system. These lesions are prominent only in early biopsies or when death has occurred early in the disease. It would appear that a foreign agent may be taken up by the mononuclear phagocytes, which react by proliferation and are changed into mononuclear cells, the granuloma representing a stabilization of the phagocytic process, the purpose being to isolate the foreign agent. The granuloma then disappears or may be followed by fibrosis. There may be widespread fibrosis of the lungs, which may explain some of the cases of so-called idiopathic pulmonary fibrosis.

The *etiology* of the condition has been a matter of endless debate, and is no nearer settlement. A fundamental and challenging question first demands answer: Is sarcoidosis a specific disease, a true entity? There are some who would answer this question in the negative, regarding the condition merely as a type of histological response to a variety of agents—bacterial, viral, fungal, protozoal and mineral. In this respect it is of prime importance to distinguish a solitary sarcoid from systemic sarcoidosis. A *sarcoid reaction* may be observed in tuberculosis, histoplasmosis, beryllium poisoning, and even in lymph nodes adjacent to a neoplasm. The pathologist must be careful not to commit himself and his clinical colleague to a diagnosis of sarcoidosis from the examination of a single section showing a sarcoid reaction. There is a danger of the diagnosis of sarcoidosis becoming a refuge of the destitute. *Systemic sarcoidosis* should show, in addition to epithelioid tubercles in the biopsy specimen and a negative tuberculin reaction, hyperglobulinemia, hypercalcemia, and involvement of one or more of the following sites: superficial and mediastinal lymph nodes, eyes, skin, bones of hands and feet, liver and spleen, lacrimal and parotid glands, the heart and pituitary. Bone changes in the hands and feet are found in some 17 per cent of cases, changes which are quite rare in other granulomas (Israel and Sones). It has been suggested that the disease is an atypical form of tuberculosis without caseation, or an atypical reaction to the tubercle bacillus, but it seems more probable that it is a chronic granuloma produced by some hitherto undiscovered agent or agents.

An etiological agent which has come to light recently is *pine pollen* (Cummings and Hudgins). Attention has been drawn to this agent by the realization that the disease (or syndrome) is prevalent in endemic areas. These areas correspond with pine forest distribution in the United States. The chief foci of the condition are the United States, Scandinavia, France, Germany and Switzerland, countries where pine forests are common. Pine pollen has acid-fast staining characteristics similar to those of tubercle bacilli, and contains acid-fast lipid. The material is capable of evoking epithelioid granulomata in normal animals.

The *Kveim test* for sarcoidosis was introduced in 1941. It is an immunological reaction, the antigen being made from cutaneous sarcoids, and the result being expressed either as a gross nodule or as a microscopic sarcoid lesion. It is therefore similar to the lepromin test for leprosy. The test originated in Norway, where the disease is particularly prevalent, and Scandinavian observers in general have been strong supporters of its value. Some American workers consider that the test is not specific, being often positive in tuberculosis and often negative in sarcoidosis. It is generally regarded as a worthwhile diagnostic procedure in patients who do not have skin lesions or palpable lymph nodes accessible for biopsy, although an attitude of reserved caution is desirable.

A *gastrocnemius muscle biopsy* specimen selected at random has proved extremely useful in the diagnosis of systemic sarcoidosis, as muscle granuloma is very rare in tuberculosis and other conditions which may be confused with sarcoidosis. In the past liver biopsy has been used in cases where there are no local lesions which may be examined.

In *summary* of the foregoing rather confused and sometimes contradictory statements we may say that: (1) the diagnosis of sarcoidosis must be based on the correlation of clinical, radiological, immunological and laboratory data plus the histological picture; (2) the keystone of diagnosis rests on a widespread organ involvement with few or mild constitutional manifestations, there being few diseases with such protean patterns;

(3) the exclusion of all other possibilities; (4) the classic microscopic picture is "a diffuse infiltration of an organ by uniform discrete non-caseating epithelioid granulomas with central multinucleated giant cells of either a foreign body or Langhans. type, with or without inclusions (asteroid or Schaumann bodies)" (Talbot *et al.*).

LEPROSY

Leprosy is caused by *Mycobacterium lepræ*, an acid-fast organism discovered by Hansen as long ago as 1874, and often called Hansen's bacillus. It is more easily stained and decolorized (less acid-fast) than the tubercle bacillus. Until recently it had never been grown in culture, nor had the disease been transferred to an animal, so that leprosy was a purely human disease, a fact which was a great handicap to the investigator. Now Binford has succeeded in producing granulomatous lesions in the golden hamster, lesions which resemble those of human lepromatous leprosy in histological pattern, number of intracellular acid-fast bacilli, and the presence of bacilli within nerves. Negative results were obtained with albino hamsters, white mice, white rats, hairless mice, and white guinea pigs. Bacteria from the lesions grow slowly in Lowenstein's medium.

It is instructive and intriguing to compare the biology of leprosy with that of tuberculosis. The infectivity and virulence of the lepra bacillus is very low. A tissue may be teeming with myriads of bacilli and yet show no obvious clinical change. The hypersensitivity which we have seen to be so striking a feature of the reaction of the tissues to the tubercle bacillus seems to be conspicuous by its absence. Infection is believed to occur in childhood or early life, yet the disease may remain latent for 20 years suggesting a remarkable resistance on the part of the tissues. Leprosy was once spread over the entire known world, and was a universally dreaded disease. The leprous patient was given a bell which he had to ring as a warning as he passed through a village. In English churches one can still see the hagioscope (*hagios*, holy) or squint,

the oblique opening in the massive wall through which the leper was allowed to watch the sacrament at the altar. Yet its infectivity appears to be remarkably low, and it is now largely confined to hot moist climates, more than 1 per cent of the population of central Africa and of the West coast of India suffering from the disease. Infection seems to come from nasal discharges and from ulcerating lesions. Intimate and long-continued contact is necessary for infection to occur. Nurses and doctors in charge of leper colonies are very seldom infected if they take proper precautions. As already mentioned, the incubation period is long and the exact time is unknown. In spite of the sluggish character of the infection, the bacilli become very widely distributed throughout the body, and few organs may escape. From the clinical point of view the most important structures to suffer are the skin, the peripheral nerves, and the kidneys.

Two main forms are recognized, the tuberculoid or maculoanesthetic and the lepromatous or nodular. The two forms are frequently combined.

The *Lepromatous* form is characterized by the development of nodules or masses formed in the skin, particularly of the face, hands, and feet (Fig. 163); in the latter there are anesthetic patches on the skin. A cellular granulation tissue is formed. This is composed mainly of large mononuclear cells known as *lepra cells*. These usually have a pale foamy appearance owing to a high lipid content. They may be crowded with acid-fast bacilli, the source of the lipid (Fig. 164). Some of the cells attain a large size and may be called giant cells, but they are quite different from the multinucleated giant cells of tuberculosis. The new granulation tissue is diffuse, and does not show the grouping of the cells into follicles so characteristic of tuberculosis. Nor is there any caseation, but ulceration of the superficial lesion is common, so that there may be great destruction of the fingers, nose, ears, *etc.*, with terrible disfigurement. Leprous lesions are found in the liver, spleen, and other organs. The nodular lesions (lepromas) of the face together with wrinkling of the skin may give to the sufferer what has been described as a leonine expression. In

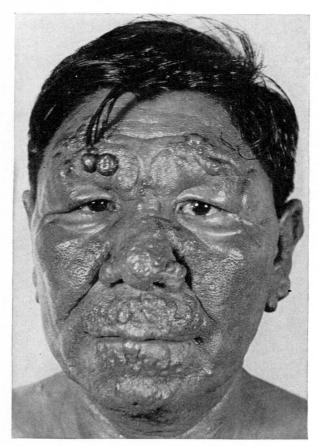

Fig. 163.—Leprosy. A striking example of the lepromatous form, with multiple nodules in the skin. (Kindness of Dr. Goerge L. Fite, Carville, La.)

the final stages of the disease there may be autoamputation of the fingers and toes.

The *Tuberculoid* lesions begin as skin macules with an indurated border. This is followed by an extension of the infection to the peripheral nerve trunks. There is a perineuritis, and the thickened nerves can be felt as cords under the skin of the arm and leg. The bacilli penetrate between the nerve bundles, and there is first a formation of loose granulation tissue and later fibrosis (Fig. 165). The nerve fibers are destroyed, so that anesthetic areas are produced, followed later by motor and trophic disorders. The destructive lesions already mentioned may be partly trophic, but in part they are due to loss of sensation with subsequent injury. As we have seen with the lepromatous form, there is no caseation, and few

or no bacilli can be demonstrated. What it means it is hard to say. Perhaps the tuberculoid form develops in those with a high native resistance, the organisms dying out in the burnt-out lesions in the course of time.

The autopsy picture is well presented by Powell and Swan in a study of 50 cases at the United States National Leprosarium, at Carville, La., although they are careful to point out that the pattern of leprosy in other parts of the world may be quite different. Of these 50 cases, 48 were of the lepromatous type and only 2 of the tuberculoid. In 68 per cent of the cases bacilli were demonstrated in the skin, peripheral nerves, testes, liver, kidney, adrenal, lymphoid tissue, bone marrow, eye, or nasal mucosa. *Secondary amyloidosis* was present in almost 50 per cent of cases, usually in the kidneys, and the commonest

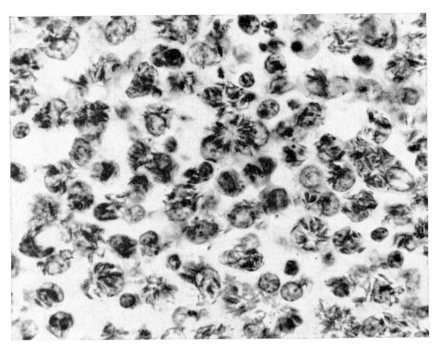

FIG. 164.—Lepromatous lesion at the height of activity, with bacilli forming small bundles radiating away from the nucleus, typical of the most active growth phase of the organism. (Kindness of Dr. George L. Fite, Carville, La.)

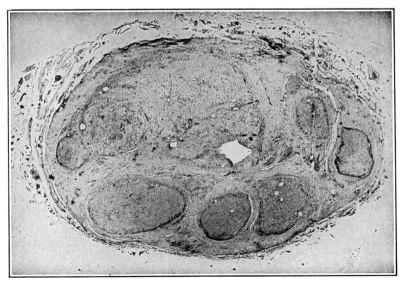

FIG. 165.—Nerve lesion in leprosy. Nerve bundles bound together by fibrous tissue. × 18.

cause of death was renal insufficiency from this lesion. Leprosy was usually the predisposing rather than the immediate cause of death.

The *lepromin test* corresponds to the tuberculin test for tuberculosis. It consists of the intracutaneous injection of an extract of lepra bacilli obtained by mincing up a leprosy lesion. A positive reaction is shown by the development of a nodule in the course of two weeks, and is obtained in normal persons and in the tuberculoid, while a negative result is obtained in the lepromatous form. This of course is very different from the tuberculin test in tuberculosis, and again no ready explanation can be offered on an immunological basis. It seems to be an indication of relative immunity.

The *clinical diagnosis* may be very difficult before nodular lesions and anesthetic patches are well developed, but in doubtful cases the acid-fast bacilli may be demonstrated in the discharge from the nose and the skin lesions, or a section of skin can be removed and stained for lepra bacilli. In active cases of the cutaneous type myriads of bacilli may be found in smears of serum made from a small incision in any part of the skin, even though it may appear quite normal. In the nerve lesions, on the other hand, bacilli can seldom be detected.

When we seek for an explanation of the tremendous decrease in incidence of the disease over the centuries, we are again at a loss. Possibly improved hygiene and the segregation of infective cases may play a part. Or there may have been a decline in the virulence of the organism since the days of the bell and the hagioscope. Modern treatment with sulfones and thiosemicarbazones make the open cases non-infective in the course of two years, but this is a recent innovation.

SYPHILIS

Syphilis, tuberculosis and leprosy form a trio of infectious granulomata which have many features in common, so that it is convenient to consider the first of these here, even though the causal agent is not remotely related to the mycobacteria. Syphilis shares with the others the distinction of presenting some of the most perplexing immunological puzzles in relation to resistance and hypersensitivity in the whole realm of infectious disease. The disease seems to have lost much of its virulence since it was first introduced into Europe by the sailors of Christopher Columbus returning from the New World. At that time it swept through Italy like a pestilence, so that it came to be called lues (a plague), the name by which it is still known at the present day. Perhaps leprosy has changed in similar manner.

Bacteriology.—The problems of the etiology and treatment of syphilis have engaged the attention of investigators for hundreds of years, but the fundamental contributions to our present knowledge were all crowded into the first decade of the twentieth century. In 1903 Metchnikoff and Roux succeeded in inoculating a chimpanzee with syphilis, in 1905 Schaudinn and Hoffman discovered the causal organism, in 1906 Wassermann published his complement fixation test, and in 1910 Ehrlich introduced the arsenical treatment ("606"), which marked the birth of chemotherapy, although it has in turn been replaced by penicillin. In the knowledge of no other disease have such extraordinary advances been made in so short a time. One of the most remarkable chapters in the history of syphilis is the story of how John Hunter inoculated himself on the glans and prepuce with the discharge from a venereal sore, and proceeded to observe and record with the detachment of the scientist the lesions as they appeared and disappeared over a period of three years. He experimented with various forms of mercurial treatment, but always stopped when there appeared to be danger of curing the disease!

Syphilis is caused by *Treponema pallidum*, which belongs to the species of spirochetes, and used to be known as *Spirocheta pallida*. The pale spirochete is a delicate spiral, thin enough to pass through a bacterial filter. In fresh preparations it moves actively by virtue of flagella-like structures revealed by the electron microscope. The spirochete cannot be stained with ordinary aniline dyes, but in dried films it is shown by Giemsa's stain, whilst for sections of tissue the silver impregnation method of Levaditi is invaluable. Dark-ground illumination is the best method for fresh material.

Trep. pallidum cannot be cultivated, and it is extremely susceptible to drying, so that it cannot survive outside the body, as well as to heat. The disease can be reproduced in the chimpanzee, and the spirochete will grow in the anterior chamber of the eye, or testis of the rabbit.

Immunology.—A patient suffering from syphilis is immune to reinfection. This immunity, which becomes established as soon as the primary lesion develops, is associated with the appearance of two distinct antibodies in the serum, namely syphilitic reagin and treponema-immobilizing antibody. *Reagin* is a substance normally present in the plasma in small amount associated with gamma globulin. It reacts like antibody with certain extracts of normal tissues. In syphilis reagin is very greatly increased in amount, and this forms the basis of the complement fixation (Wassermann) and the precipitin (Kahn) reactions. The *complement fixation test* is a method for demonstrating a pathological increase of reagin, using an antigen-like substance present in bovine heart muscle and other tissues. It will be seen that the Wassermann is in no sense a specific test for syphilis, but fortunately it works in practice. The *Kahn precipitation test* is also non-specific, depending on the production of a precipitate by the interaction of an increased amount of reagin with a tissue antigen. Precipitation tests are more sensitive in treated cases, so that the Kahn test may be positive when the Wassermann reaction has become negative. Both tests usually become positive within two weeks of the appearance of the primary lesion, which itself does not develop for three or four weeks after infection, they are invariably positive during the secondary active stage, but in the tertiary stage without active lesions they are negative in some 25 per cent of cases.

The *treponema-immobilization test*, unlike the Wassermann and Kahn reactions, is a specific test for a true syphilitic antibody. Living spirochetes from the testis of a rabbit are immobilized and finally killed by serum from a patient with syphilis as shown by dark-field microscopy. The test is considerably more reliable than the ordinary reagin reactions. It is useful in the differentiation of latent syphilis and biological false-positive reactions. In patients with late manifestations it is positive, even though the reagin tests have become negative. Unfortunately at the present time the test is not a practicable routine procedure, but a rather highly specialized one.

Natural History of the Disease.—Until recently syphilis was one of the most common and important diseases in the world. It was more common than measles, twice as common as tuberculosis, and was responsilbe for 10 per cent of all cases of insanity. It has now fallen from its high estate because of treatment with antibiotics, and the late manifestations, particularly those due to involvement of the central nervous system, are rapidly becoming a thing of the past. For this reason the following account will be greatly abbreviated from that of earlier editions. At the same time it must not be thought that syphilis is no longer to be feared. Every organ may be infected, and nearly every disease may be simulated by syphilis. Of all diseases it is the most subtle. It is a master of disguise. It is hardly an exaggeration to say that there is no symptom which it cannot cause, no syndrome for which it may not be responsible.

In the vast majority of cases infection is acquired during sexual intercourse. The spirochetes may be present in recent lesions on the genital organs, or they may be transmitted in the semen many years after the original infection. There may be extragenital infection on the lips (kissing), mouth, tongue, fingers, or nipple (nursing an infected child). The spirochetes may penetrate an unbroken mucous membrane, but it is unlikely that they can enter the skin unless there is some crack or abrasion.

Syphilis is a general systemic infection in the course of which certain local lesions are produced which are sufficiently striking to attract clinical attention. Long before the first lesion (chancre) appears the spirochetes have infected the entire body. When an infected needle is passed through a rabbit's testicle and the testicle removed in forty-eight hours, in a week's time the blood is so heavily infected with spirochetes that 0.5 cc. will transmit the disease.

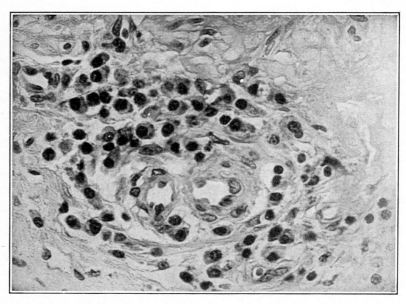

FIG. 166.—Syphilitic reaction. Lymphocytes and plasma cells collected around two small vessels with swollen endothelium. × 500.

When the spirochetes penetrate the surface they invade the perivascular lymph spaces, multiply exceedingly, and pour into the regional lymphatics and the blood stream. It is evident that no treatment of the local lesion, which only develops after general infection has occurred, can have any effect on that infection. The disease is divided clinically into three stages. These stages indicate that different sets of tissues are developing a hypersensitivity which causes them to react to the irritant sufficiently violently to produce the symptoms of disease. The organs vary in the time they take to develop this hypersensitivity, some are early, others late. The stages are separated by curious latent intervals. These stages and intervals have nothing to do with the spread of the infection, for that has already taken place.

The spirochetes in the perivascular lymph spaces excite the syphilitic reaction. This consists of an accumulation of mononuclear cells, chiefly lymphocytes and plasma cells (Fig. 166). The plasma cell is the characteristic cell of syphilis; in tuberculosis it is not at all prominent, but in non-specific inflammations it is sometimes present in large numbers.

The new tissue is highly vascular in comparison with the avascular lesion of tuberculosis. Swelling of the endothelium lining the capillaries may cause narrowing of the lumen or obstruction. Fibroblasts are stimulated to proliferate, and when healing sets in there may be marked fibrosis. In late lesions (tertiary stage) necrosis is frequent (*gumma formation*) and is associated with the presence of giant cells, but these are far less numerous than in tuberculosis.

As the result of the inflammatory reaction the spirochetes die out locally, and healing occurs with replacement of the inflammatory cells by fibrous tissue. But unfortunately clinical healing does not correspond with cure, and some of the spirochetes may survive. In the course of time the tissue immunity wears off, and then the spirochetes revive, multiply again, and cause a relapse. This sequence of events may take place in any part of the body, although it is least likely to occur in the primary lesion where the local reaction has been most violent. The testicles may appear normal clinically, but virulent spirochetes may be discharged in the semen years after the Wassermann reaction has become negative and all gross signs

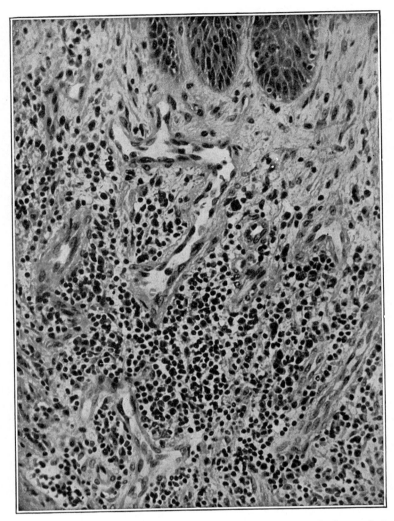

Fig. 167.—Primary syphilitic lesion showing surface epithelium, marked vascularity, swelling of vascular endothelium, and dense round cell infiltration. × 250.

of the disease have disappeared. It is evident that clinical healing is not synonymous with the cure of the disease.

The Primary Lesion.—The primary lesion appears at the site of inoculation. This is usually on the genitalia, but it may be extragenital (lip, fingers, etc.). The common genital sites are the penis in the male and the cervix in the female; the cervical chancre is highly infective on account of the moist character of its surroundings and it is easily overlooked owing to its hidden nature and freedom from pain and discharge. The primary lesion is generally single but may be multiple. It usually develops in from three to four weeks after infection, but this latent period may be as short as two or as long as six weeks. It first takes the form of a hard nodule, but the surface tends to become ulcerated and a "hard sore" or *chancre* is formed from the surface of which enormous numbers of spirochetes are discharged. These are most readily detected by means of the dark-field method. The chancre is the earliest clinical manifestation, but from the pathological standpoint the chancre is really a late affair, as we have already seen. The hardness is due to dense cellular infiltration, but does not appear for the first few days. Later it is caused by a marked degree of fibroplasia. The floor of the ulcer is a dull red, but later it becomes glazed and coppery. It is characteristically insensitive. In the course of a few weeks healing occurs. Whether or not a scar is left depends on the amount of tissue destruction.

The microsopic appearance is that of all syphilitic lesions but lacking in "late" features; there is a dense accumulation of lymphocytes and plasma cells especially around the small vessels, and fibroblasts multiply and lay down collagen fibrils (Fig. 167). Syphilis in some respects may be regarded as a disease of small arteries. Destruction of tissue is seldom marked, but the surface epithelium is usually lost. If the section is stained by the Levaditi method an incredible number of spirochetes are brought to view (Fig. 169). The regional lymph nodes (inguinal, submental, *etc.*) are enlarged in the primary stage. These nodes are hard and shotty, but not painful or tender. They thus resemble the chancre in all respects. Microscopically the nodes usually merely show a diffuse hyperplasia. Puncture of the nodes will show spirochetes in the dark-field, and sections stained by the Levaditi method contain great numbers of spirochetes.

The Secondary Lesions.—After the appearance of the primary lesion there is a latent period during which apparently all is well. If the patient has not received adequate treatment at the end of from two to three months after infection the tissues of ectodermal origin develop the power to react and lesions appear in the skin, mucous membranes, and central nervous system. These persist for a period of months and then disappear. There is no destruction of tissue (necrosis) at this stage, so that no scars are left, but there may be some coppery pigmentation.

Secondary lymphadenitis is one of the earliest changes. The nodes all over the body are enlarged in distinction to the regional involvement of the primary stage. The enlargement is never great, but it may persist for months or years. Swelling of the

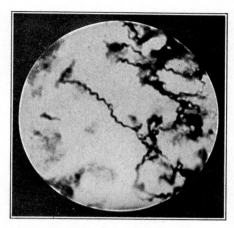

Fig. 168.—Spirochetes in tissue stained by the Levaditi method. × 2500.

epitrochlear and posterior cervical nodes is specially characteristic.

The *lesions of the skin* are of great variety, but they are symmetrical in distribution (tertiary lesions are asymmetrical), they are polymorphous in type, *i.e.*, present several varieties of lesion at the same time, they possess a copper tinge, and their outline is that of the segment of a circle. Like other secondary lesions they do not destroy tissue. The lesions may be macular, papular or pustular. A *condyloma* is a large flat papule occurring in moist situations, *i.e.*, between the vulva, around the anus, *etc.* These are swarming with spirochetes and are highly infectious. There may be *mucous patches* of the mouth, pharynx, and vagina. These are flat superficial lesions which have been appropriately likened to the track left by a snail. They also swarm with spirochetes and are highly infectious.

The Tertiary Lesions.—The subsidence of the secondary lesions is followed by another latent interval during which all is quiet. In a year or not for many years a third set of lesions appears with something of the inevitability of a Greek tragedy. These are not symmetrical, they affect deep as well as superficial structures, and they show a tendency to necrosis and destruction. They are only slightly infective, for they contain only a few spirochetes. These are not easy to demonstrate in silver preparations.

Two main types of tertiary lesion may occur. The one is gross and localized (the gumma), the other is microscopic and diffuse. The *gumma* is a necrotic, localized, yellowish homogeneous mass of rubbery consistence composed of the usual mononuclear cells. It used to be so common that it had to be considered in the differential diagnosis of any mass of obscure character. Now it is hardly ever seen. In the center of the lesion necrosis and caseation occur with the formation of a peculiar gummy material, but there is not the same complete wiping out of structure as in tuberculous caseation. A few giant cells may be seen at the margin.

Gummata of the skin, mouth, tongue and nose may lead to extensive ulceration. The liver may show one or several masses (Fig. 169) which heal with fibrosis so that deep scars are formed, producing a peculiar lobed appearance known as *hepar lobatum*. In the testicle the gumma forms a hard mass which may be mistaken for a tumor; there is characteristic loss of testicular sensation on palpation. Gummata in the bones, the brain and other places used to be confused with tumors of these organs.

In the *diffuse lesions* the spirochetes are widely distributed and set up a diffuse chronic inflammatory reaction with lymphocytes and plasma cells, tissue destruction, but no caseation. The principal sites are the thoracic aorta and testicle. In the thoracic aorta a frequent result is the development of an *aneurysm* of that vessel. The most serious of all the late lesions, sometimes called quaternary because they develop after all evidence of active infection has disappeared, are those of the *central nervous system* which may come on many years after the original infection, especially when treatment has been inadequate. These may affect chiefly the meninges, the brain (*general paresis*), and the spinal cord (*tabes dorsalis*).

Natural History Reviewed.—Now that we have traced the extraordinary natural history of syphilitic infection we may ask ourselves what it all means. We have spoken in casual fashion about hypersensitivity and immunity, but when we try to visualize what is actually going on we are at a complete loss. First, the spirochetes invade the superficial tissue, but some four weeks

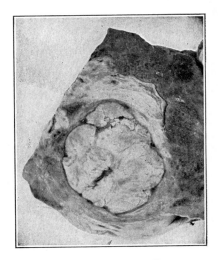

Fig. 169.—Gumma of liver.

elapse before signs of an inflammatory reaction appear. It seems reasonable to presume that these lesions are allergic in nature, and the primary sore is shown by dark-field examination to be teeming with spirochetes. This lesion may be comparable to that of primary infection in tuberculosis. The chancre heals, and nothing happens for a number of months, although the spirochetes have been widely distributed throughout the body. Suddenly, without reinfection as in tuberculosis, a fresh lot of entirely different lesions flare up in the skin and mucous membranes, which may be presumed to have become sensitized in the interval. Again these are swarming with spirochetes. Once more things clear up, and after a deceptive calm of a few years, gummata develop in the liver and elsewhere, and an aneurysm of the thoracic aorta makes its appearance. The formation of gummata suggests still another type of reaction of tissue to invader. Finally, when everything has been forgotten or when evidence of previous disease has been minimal, active lesions develop in the central nervous system, which send the patient to end his days in a mental hospital. How can we reconcile this unique sequence of events without concepts of immunity and hypersensitivity as affecting the reaction of the tissues to the invader? Perhaps some reader of these pages may furnish the answer.

Congenital Syphilis.—Syphilis may be transmitted from the father or the mother, but in all cases the mother is infected, although often she shows no evidence of the disease. There are three possibilities. (1) The child may be born dead, usually showing well-marked evidence of syphilis. Syphilis is an important cause of still-birth. (2) The child may be born alive with external evidence of syphilis. (3) The child may appear healthy, but lesions develop later.

When the child is born dead the appearance is usually characteristic. There is no primary lesion, as infection takes place through the placenta. The child is usually premature and undersized. The skin may be macerated. If not, it usually shows bullæ. The spleen is enlarged, and often the liver. Syphilitic epiphysitis is one of the commonest and most diagnostic features. It is best seen at the knee by splitting open the lower end of the femur or upper end of the tibia. In place of the normal thin, regular, white epiphyseal line there is a broad irregular somewhat yellow line which is highly characteristic.

The chief *microscopic* change at this stage is an interstitial round cell infiltration of many of the internal organs combined with a varying degree of fibrosis. In the liver this produces a fine form of intercellular cirrhosis. Levaditi preparations of the liver, heart, adrenals, *etc.*, show enormous numbers of spirochetes. It is evident how infectious such a body must be, and great care is necessary in performing an autopsy.

If the child is born alive the skin may show the varied lesions already described in the acquired form. Common sites for the lesions are the buttocks, anus, angles of the mouth, and the palms of the hands and soles of the feet. Radiating scars are formed at the angles of the mouth which are very characteristic. The skin is often wrinkled, so that the child has a dried-up, wizened appearance. Enlargement of the spleen is very constant. The liver and other organs show the changes already described. The mucous membranes show the same lesions as in the acquired form. In the nose there is ulceration and destruction, so that the bridge of the nose may fall in giving the characteristic *"saddle nose"* of congenital

syphilis. One of the most useful aids to diagnosis is roentgenographic evidence of epiphysitis and periostitis in the long bones.

In the late type lesions develop over a period of years which stamp the patient as being a congenital syphilitic. The permanent teeth show the appearance known as *"Hutchinson's teeth"*; these are small, widely-spaced, peg-shaped (narrow at the apex), and the central incisors are notched. The molars are pitted and honey-combed. An interstitial keratitis develops at the time of puberty producing a ground-glass opacity in the cornea. Nerve deafness is common. The scars at the angles of the mouth known as *rhagades* have already been mentioned. Gummata develop in the bones, or a diffuse thickening affecting especially the tibia (*"saber tibia"*). There may be involvement of the central nervous system similar to that seen in the acquired form (juvenile paresis and juvenile tabes).

Syphilis is the disease due to treponemal infection with which I and most of my readers are acquainted. There are, however, three other conditions due to treponemata, which resemble syphilis in many ways and which are of major importance in some parts of the world, but are *non-venereal* in origin. These are yaws, junta, and bejel.

Y AWS.—Yaws or *frambesia* is another non-venereal spirochetal disease closely resembling syphilis in many respects. It is caused by *Trep. pertenue*, and is a disease of the tropics, being prevalent in the South Pacific islands, the Philippines, India, Africa, and in some areas of South America and the West Indies.

Infection is acquired from open sores by direct contact, usually in early childhood. As in the case of syphilis the disease passes through a primary, a secondary, and a tertiary stage. The *primary lesion*, corresponding to the chancre of syphilis, is known as the "mother yaw," and forms a strawberry-like red mass on the skin, giving the disease its name of frambesia (strawberry). The *secondary lesions*, as in syphilis, involve the skin and mucous membranes, and are associated with a bacteremia. Unlike syphilis, they tend to form granulomatous masses resembling the mother yaw, leaving scars on healing. The *tertiary lesions*, which come on after one or several years, are confined to the skin and bones. They take the form of strawberry-like masses or of subcutaneous gummata. These often occur on the soles of the feet, where they break down due to trauma, forming painful ulcers. Unlike syphilis, visceral gummata and involvement of the cardiovascular and central nervous systems are extremely rare.

The *microscopic lesions* resemble those of syphilis, with particular involvement of the small blood vessels. Spirochetes abound both in the mother yaw and in the secondary lesions.

In its well-developed form the disease is easily recognized. Tertiary lesions of the skin and of the bones of the face produce mutilating deformities, whilst the painful plantar lesions are responsible for a peculiar waddling, crab-like gait which is so characteristic that this stage of the disease is known as *"crab yaws."*

PINTA.—This is the second of the diseases caused by Treponema, *T. carateum*, which resembles syphilis in many respects, but is non-venereal in origin, and has got a very different prognosis. The disease is endemic in some parts of South America and Central America, as well as Africa. It differs from syphilis in that the infection occurs through the open skin, and it attacks children as well as young adults.

As in the case of syphilis, three stages may be recognized. The *primary stage*, which develops after an incubation period of two to three weeks, is marked by the development of the primary papule, which progresses to ulceration, and may attain a great size. Microscopically, there is epidermal thickening with an exudate of mononuclears in the dermis. The really characteristic lesion is an increase in the number of melanophores in the dermis, and increased pigmentation in the basal layers of the epidermis. This gives the hyperpigmented skin lesion, the *pintid*, (Spanish, painted), to which the disease owes its name. Treponemata in great numbers are discharged from the ulcerated lesion. Later there is depigmentation with scarring. The *secondary stage*, which develops in the course of a year, is again characterized by pigmented cutaneous lesions, a maculopapular rash which varies in color, from pink due to increased vascularity to brown or even black from melanin accumulation. Here again there is gradual depigmentation. In the *tertiary stage*, which may last for many years, there is a varying piebald picture, with areas of depigmentation alternating with areas of hyperpigmentation. Very occasionally there may be mesaortitis and cardiovascular lesions recalling those of syphilis.

BEJEL.—This remarkable condition appears to be a non-venereal form of syphilis which is prevalent amongst the Bedouin Arabs. About 75 per cent of the Bedouins show evidence of infection, although there is no gonorrhea amongst them, and sexual promiscuity is unknown. It is a disease of the whole community, like measles, and is acquired in childhood, the infection being contracted from some other child in the acute stage, probably by means of drinking vessels. The earliest lesions are gray patches about the mouth, followed by a papular eruption on moist areas. In about a year, the lesions vanish, and the child appears healthy. They may never recur, but frequently gummata of bones, skin and pharynx appear many years later. The cardiovascular and nervous systems are not attacked. The Wassermann and Kahn reactions are positive.

SPIROCHETAL FEVERS

Relapsing Fever.—This is a disease of tropical countries, though some cases have been reported in the United States. It is characterized by a peculiarly recurring type of fever. The febrile attacks last a few days and are separated by short periods during which the patient feels quite well. The disease is caused by several closely related species of spirochetes, of which *Treponema recurrentis obermeieri* was the first described and is the best known. During the febrile attacks the spirochetes are present in the blood in great numbers, where they are readily seen in a stained film, but during the afebrile intervals they vanish. The infection is conveyed by lice and ticks. These do not inject the organisms directly into the blood, but when the body of the louse is crushed on the surface by scratching, the spirochetes are liberated and penetrate through the skin abrasions. The mortality is not high. The postmortem *lesions* are those of septicemia, particularly enlargement of the spleen, cloudy swelling of the internal organs, and hemorrhages in the serous and mucous membranes.

Weil's Disease.—This is also known by the more academic term, *leptospirosis ictero-hemorrhagiæ*, because the condition is caused by a leptospira (with much finer and more closely-wound spirals than the treponemata), and is characterized by icterus and hemorrhage. The organism is a common parasite of rats, which suffer no ill effects, but the kidneys become infected, and the leptospiræ are excreted in the urine and infect water, where they can survive for several days. The organisms probably enter the human body through cracks in the skin infected by

20

the contaminated water. The resulting disease is discussed in connection with infectious jaundice in Chapter 28.

HEMOPHILUS BACILLI

Hemophilus Influenzæ.—It is regrettable that this organism has retained the name of influenza bacillus, first given to it when it was thought to be the cause of influenza. It is also called *Pfeiffer's bacillus*, a much better name. *H. influenzæ* is a small, gram-negative cocco-bacillus, which requires hemoglobin for its growth. It is a common inhabitant of the nasopharynx, and when resistance is lowered by virus infections such as influenza and measles, it invades the lung and cause a secondary *bronchopneumonia*. In epidemics of influenza it may be found in almost pure culture in the lungs of fatal cases. It is also an important pathogen in chronic bronchitis and bronchiectasis. In all of these conditions the organism plays the part of a jackal, ready to take advantage of a situation already created.

H. influenzæ can act as a primary pathogen for two tissues, the conjunctiva and the meninges. It is the commonest cause of *infective conjunctivitis* or "pink eye", being found in great numbers in the mucopurulent discharge. It may be noted that the organism of acute conjunctivitis used to be known as the Koch-Weeks bacillus. *Influenzal meningitis* is not caused by the influenza virus, but by Pfeiffer's bacillus. The disease is commonest in infancy and in early childhood. The clinical picture resembles that of meningococcal meningitis, and we must beware of confusing *H. influenzæ* with the meningococcus, both being gram-negative, and the influenza bacillus is often intracellular.

Whooping Cough.—Whooping cough or *pertussis* is an acute infectious disease of the respiratory tract, as a result of which there are spasmodic attacks of coughing with a prolonged inspiration known as a "whoop". The disease consists of a catarrhal stage of one or two weeks' duration marked by a hard dry cough (this is the infectious period), and a paroxysmal stage of four to eight weeks' duration marked by severe paroxysms of coughing and whooping, and by attacks of vomiting. Common *complications* are bronchopneumonia, atelectasis, emphysema and convulsions. One attack of the disease confers immunity for life. In Great Britain whooping cough causes more deaths in childhood than any other specific fever, because of the secondary bronchopneumonia which may follow (Whitley and Hynes). For this reason immunization by vaccination is of particular importance in preventing the relatively fatal attacks of whooping cough in the first year of life.

The *etiological agent* is *H. pertussis* of Bordet and Gengou, a minute gram-negative hemophilic bacillus, which is found in great masses entangled in the cilia of the bronchial mucosa. Rich and his associates have shown that in chimpanzees the oral inoculation of pure cultures of Bordet-Gengou bacilli resulted in a condition similar in all respects to whooping cough, and characterized by coryza followed by a protracted paroxysmal cough, associated with lymphocytosis and a positive complement fixation toward the Bordet-Gengou bacillus.

CHANCROID.—This *acute* venereal disease, also known a *soft chancre* or soft sore, is caused by *H. ducreyi*, a gram-negative hemophilic bacillus. The organism is a normal parasite of the vaginal canal, and the lesions appear on the penis and labia. The disease is common in the Orient, the West Indies, and Africa. In the United States most cases occur in the Negro. The *lesions* appear within two weeks of infection, but they lack the induration of syphilis, being suppurative in character, giving rise to ulcers which heal spontaneously. The regional lymph nodes become inflamed, enlarged and very tender (*cf.* syphilis), with suppuration and abscess formation. There are none of the sequelae which make syphilis so serious a disease.

BRUCELLOSIS

The Brucella group of microorganism are named after Sir David Bruce, who first isolated then in 1886 in Malta fever. They are essentially pathogens of animals which may be transmitted to man. Brucellosis, indeed, is the most common illness conveyed to humans from animals (Brande and Spink). There are several varieties of Brucella. *Br. melitensis* occurs in goats and sheep,

Br. abortus in cows, and *Br. suis* in pigs. The disease causes great loss in dairy products and the death of many animals intended for food. All three forms may infect man and cause undulant fever. Unfortunately there is evidence that cross infection is occurring between the different classes of animals.

Undulant Fever.—This disease was originally known as *Malta fever*, an infectious condition of goats in the Mediterranean countries and conveyed to man in goat's milk. Later it was realized that the organism was closely related to *Br. abortus*, the cause of contagious abortion in cattle, an extraordinarily common condition in farm stock; 90 per cent of the herds in Connecticut being infected. This is far the commonest cause of undulant fever in man, being responsible for 80 per cent of cases. It should be noted that though the cows have a tendency to abort, and pass large quantities of the bacilli in the milk, they show no evidence of disease. The goats also suffer no inconvenience from melitensis infection. It was not until 1918 that an intimate relationship was demonstrated by Evans to exist between *Brucella melitensis* of Malta fever and *Brucella abortus* of contagious abortion. The two are closely related but not identical. The most important step was the last, when in 1924 Keefer showed that *Brucella abortus* was infective for man. The various forms are best included under the name of undulant fever, of which there is a melitensis type and an abortus type. The abortus infection may come from swine (porcine form) or cows (bovine form). The abortus infection is not so pathogenic for man as the melitensis form. Most of the persons who drink infected cow's milk show no evidence of the disease, though they may have agglutinins in the blood. Thus the morbidity for the human subject is low.

Infection is acquired via the alimentary tract, usually by drinking unpasteurized cow's milk, so that most human cases in temperate countries are examples of abortus infection. In view of the fact that this is a milk infection it is curious that the disease is rare in children. Laboratory infections may be acquired through cracks in the skin, the scratch of an infected needle, *etc.* Contact infection may also occur in workers in packing houses, farmers, veterinarians, and others who come in contact with infected material. The method by which infection passes from one animal to another is not certainly known. Undulant fever used to be regarded as a rarity. It is undoubtedly very much commoner than was formerly thought. Many fevers of remittent type, pyrexias of unknown origin (P.U.O.) as they are known in the Services, are examples of brucellosis. It should enter into the differential diagnosis of every long-continued fever when such conditions as typhoid, tuberculosis and subacute bacterial endocarditis are being ruled out. The mortality is low, less than 2 per cent. Brucella infection may not give rise to typical undulant fever, but merely to persistent malaise and indisposition with some irregular fever. In endemic areas a certain proportion of the population suffers from a latent infection, so that the blood gives a positive reaction to the agglutination test. Women with latent infection may show a tendency to abortion.

The disease begins insidiously with an evening rise of temperature, and the patient may be ill for some time without knowing that he has any fever. The *clinical picture* is so varied as to defy brief description. Persistent weakness, muscle pain, low back pain, arthritis, and marked perspiration with a peculiar sweet sickly odor to the sweat are some of the common features of a disease which may easily pass unrecognized. Orchitis is an occasional symptom. The fever may come in waves, hence the name undulant fever, though this is not common, and the infection may last for months and even years. Three months is an average duration. There is a remarkable absence of positive physical signs, owing to the general rather than the local character of the infection. Many of these unfortunate people are diagnosed as neurasthenia. The spleen is palpable in more than a third of the cases. The lymph nodes may be enlarged. A blood culture may be obtained at the height of the fever, but it is often negative and has to be kept at least a week before any growth is apparent. The culture should be kept for five weeks before being discarded as negative. The organisms are often excreted in the urine, and a culture may be obtained from a catheterized specimen. Agglutination is the most reliable means of diagnosis. Agglutination with a titer of 1 in 300 or over in the presence of fever and the other clinical symptoms indicates active infection. A titer of 1 in 100 in the absence of clinical symptoms indicates latent infection. A titer of 1 in 80 and under in the absence of clinical symptoms indicates a past infection. Correct interpretation of the lower titers is difficult and apt to be misleading. The brucellin skin test is similar to the tuberculin test and of no greater value. Occasionally active cases fail to give agglutination, but this is uncommon. A source of confusion is a cross-agglutination with *P. tularense* which sometimes occurs.

Lesions.—Very few studies of the autopsy findings in undulant fever have been recorded owing to the low mortality of the disease. The spleen is enlarged, averaging 500 grams, and there is a general swelling of the mesenteric lymph nodes. Inflammatory masses may involve the soft tissues, the bones or the viscera. In the spine, destruction of bone and intervertebral discs may cause one form of spondylitis. These show a nonspecific chronic inflammatory cell reaction with granulomatous formation, necrosis, and epithelioid and giant cells. Involvement of the *reticuloendothelial system* is a marked feature, in particular the liver, spleen, lymph nodes and bone marrow. There is a tendency to attack the heart valves, especially the aortic valve, and this may be responsible for some cases of aortic stenosis (see page 486). The usual cause of death is endocarditis, and this may be associated with myocardial lesions resembling Aschoff bodies, which raises the questions of the accuracy of the pathological diagnosis in some cases of supposed rheumatic aortic valve disease (Peery and Belter). The parasites are often intracellular, an appearance referred to as parasitization of the reticuloendothelial cells. In the often extremely difficult task of making a correct clinical diagnosis biopsy of a lymph node or bone marrow may be of value, but the microscopic picture may present a confusing resemblance to sarcoidosis or tuberculosis. Caseation, however, is absent. The biopsy

material should always be cultured. Blood culture is usually positive in the febrile stage of *Br. melitensis* and *Br. suis* infections, but in only 10 or 20 per cent of *Br. abortus* infections.

The most satisfactory antibiotic treatment is with cathomycin, which seems to be specific for undulant fever, preventing relapses (Gost). Chronic brucellosis of the glandular type may be suggestive of Hodgkin's disease.

PASTEURELLA INFECTIONS

The Pasteurella are tiny, gram-negative, highly pleomorphic cocco-bacilli, which may take a coccal or a bacillary form. Two strains are responsible for two widespread diseases in man and infections in animals, *P. pestis* causing the dreaded bubonic plague and *P. tularensis* causing tularemia. Both inhabit animal reservoirs, from which they pass to man, either directly or through the medium of insect vectors. Both produce powerful necrotizing toxins, which destroy the tissue at the site of infection. Both are extremely invasive. The prognosis, however, is very different, untreated plague being fatal in 50 to 90 per cent of cases, whereas tularemia is only fatal in about 4 per cent.

Tularemia.—Tularemia, due to *Pasteurella tularensis*, bears a remarkable biological resemblance to plague, the next disease to be discussed. Like plague it is primarily a disease of animals, which may be incidentally transmitted to man.

In animals it has the virulence and septicemic qualities of plague, but in man the infection is milder and recovery is the rule. In spite of this greater resistance man is extraordinarily susceptible to the infection. Although related to plague, the *symptoms* in man *may closely simulate typhoid fever*, and the *lesions may as closely resemble those of tuberculosis*. The disease was first observed as an acute epidemic infection among ground squirrels in Tulare County, California, and took its name from the county. Later it was found that the infection could be conveyed to man. At first it was thought that tularemia was a disease peculiar to the United States. Its problems have been worked out by American bacteriologists, and by Francis in particular. It is now known that it is world-wide in distribution. It is transmitted to men from a rodent, not from another man. The great reservoir of the disease is the ground squirrel and the jack-rabbit, but many other rodents are now known to harbor the infection. The domestic rabbit does not suffer from the disease. Infection is carried in three ways: (1) by biting flies, particularly the deer-fly, *Chrysops discalis*; (2) by ticks; (3) by contact with the skins or internal organs of infected rabbits. It therefore occurs in farmers, hunters, market men, butchers, housewives, and cooks. The microörganisms enter through cracks in the skin or through the eye. Laboratory workers handling and performing autopsies on infected animals are extremely liable to infection, even though alive to the danger.

Two types of the disease may be recognized in man, the glandular and the typhoid.

Glandular Type.—This resembles a mild form of bubonic plague, except that a local lesion develops at the site of inoculation. After an incubation period of a few days there is a sudden onset with pains, prostration and fever. The regional lymph nodes draining the site of infection become enlarged, inflamed, and tender. If the portal of infection is the eye the preauricular, submaxillary, and cervical glands are involved. Not until twenty-four hours later does a papule appear at the site of infection. Both the primary lesion and the lymph nodes undergo necrosis, suppuration, and ulceration. The bacteria have not been demonstrated in the tissues, but a bacteremia occurs early, and a positive blood culture can be obtained during the first week. By the end of the second week agglutinins appear and reach their height in the third week. After that they decline, but persist in small amounts for several years. Cross-agglutination occurs with *Brucella melitensis*, so that the disease may be confused with undulant fever. Recovery is the rule, but convalescence may take some months.

Typhoid Type.—Here there is no obvious primary lesion and therefore no glandular involvement. The portal of entry is unknown, but it is probably the unbroken skin, for the bacilli can penetrate the skin of the guinea pig and set up a septicemia.

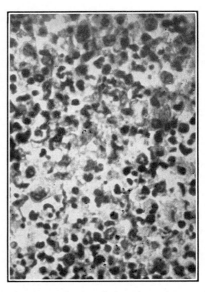

Fig. 170.—Focal necrosis in tularemia. × 490.

The typhoid type is usually due to laboratory infection.

Lesions.—In man the lesions may be of two types, acute and chronic. The *acute* lesions are characterized by focal necrosis and suppuration (Fig. 170). These changes are seen in the primary lesions and the regional lymph nodes, and to a lesser extent in many of the internal organs (spleen, liver, lung). The *chronic* lesions resemble those of tuberculosis for which they are easily mistaken. They are focal in type with central necrosis, epithelioid cells and giant cells.

Diagnosis.—The disease is apt to be mistaken for typhoid fever (when no primary lesion is present), for undulant fever (because of cross-agglutination), and for tuberculosis (a mistake made by the pathologist). When the physician thinks of tularemia on account of the primary lesion, the regional lymph node enlargement, and the history of having dressed a wild rabbit or of being bitten by a tick or fly, he can confirm his diagnosis in two ways: (1) agglutination of *P. tularensis* by the blood serum in the second week, and (2) isolation of *P. tularensis* from guinea pigs inoculated with material taken from the primary lesion or enlarged glands or with the patient's blood. The guinea pig will die in a week and show enlarged caseous lymph nodes and a spleen studded with tiny foci of necrosis. Smears and cultures taken from the patient are useless.

Plague.—Plague holds a place of singular interest among the bacterial infections for two main reasons. (1) Although responsible for the most devastating of epidemics, as its name implies, plague is primarily a disease of rodents, man only being involved incidently. "The great plagues of history were biologically unimportant accidents, the result of human entanglement with a self-contained triangular interaction of rodent, flea and plague bacillus" (Burnett). (2) No infection gives such an overwhelming septicemia in so short a time, the multiplication of the bacilli in the body recalling that seen in cholera in the lumen of the bowel.

Pasteurella pestis is a small, gram-negative, extremely pleomorphic bacillus, showing characteristic bipolar staining. It cannot exist outside the body except in the stomach of the flea. The wild rat forms the reservoir of infection, which is usually mild, but flares at times into epidemic proportions when the rat world becomes overcrowded. In the laboratory the white mouse and guinea pig are killed in two or three days by the infection. It is only in rodents, not in man, that the septicemia becomes so intense that the flea becomes infected through sucking the blood. Many of the bacilli become impacted in the throat of the flea, and when the insect in search of its next meal bites a new host it regurgitates some of the new blood ingested and with it the lurking bacilli. When a rat dies the infected fleas leave the cooling body to seek a new supply of food. If man is available, the flea will bite and infect him. The problem of plague control is in essence the problem of the deadly triangle of the rat, the flea, and the man. The flea is to plague what the louse is to typhus. The bacilli occasionally enter through cuts and abrasions, as well as by inhalation of infected droplets of sputum in the pneumonic form.

The disease occurs in an endemic and an epidemic form. A human epidemic is accompanied or preceded by a rat epidemic. The great scourges of the middle ages originated in the East and swept across Europe with the rat. One of the most historic was the Black Death (1348), which started in Southern Russia and coincided with an invasion of black rats from India which replaced the indigenous rats, each supporting a colony of fleas with a taste for human blood as well as that of the rat. About one-quarter of the population of England died, mostly adult males. It devastated Florence, but it gave us the *Decameron* of Boccacio in return. The next wave was the Great Plague of 1665, to which we are indebted for Defoe's *Journal of the Plague*. Not long afterward the periodic attacks ceased, due, apparently, to the black rat being supplanted by the brown, great hordes of which swam the Volga in 1729. Fortunately the fleas of the brown rat do not prefer the rat to man. The disease remains prevalent in the East and in India, from which continually sail ships carrying their cargo of rats and fleas. It is obvious that the prevention of plague rests largely with harbor authorities, who must eliminate the rat population, prevent rats leaving the ship and kill the fleas with insecticides.

Bubonic Plague.—Two forms of plague are encountered, bubonic and pneumonic, depending on the method of infection. In the bubonic form the bacilli spread from the flea bite to the regional axillary or inguinal lymph nodes, which become much enlarged, suppurate, and form the *bubos* which give the disease its name. The nodes at first show ordinary inflammatory hyperplasia, but abscess formation and hemorrhage follow. The bacilli invade the blood stream and are found in enormous numbers in the internal organs, where they produce necrosis, abscesses, and toxic changes. The patient dies of an overwhelming septicemia before there is time for very marked lesions to develop.

Pneumonic Form.—In bubonic plague some changes are always found in the lung such as small patches of consolidation and great engorgement with large numbers of bacilli in the alveoli. Sometimes the epidemic takes a pneumonic form, in which infection is spread by tiny droplets of sputum. There are no buboes, and the patient is overwhelmed by one of the most deadly and rapidly fatal of all infections with a mortality without treatment of 100 per cent. There is not time for any extensive pneumonic consolidation, so that here also the changes are a patchy consolidation with intense congestion and alveoli crowded with plague bacilli. The rest of the body shows evidence of an overwhelming septicemia.

The infection is completely resistant to penicillin, but is sensitive to the sulfonamides, streptomycin, chloramphenicol and tetracyclines. Early treatment with streptomycin has greatly altered the prognosis.

ANTHRAX

Anthrax is another of the diseases transmitted from animals to man, but the causal agent is very different from those causing undulant fever, tularemia and plague. It is very prevalent in European animals, especially cattle and sheep, but is much less common in North America, so that human infection is comparatively rare there. *Bacillus anthracis* is a large, gram-positive, aerobic sporebearer, in contrast to the anaerobic sporebearers about to be considered. The spores, which are only formed outside the body, are extremely resistant, withstanding boiling for 10 minutes, so that infected wool, hides, *etc.* may remain a source of danger outside the body, it is illegal in Britain to perform a postmortem examination on an animal suspected of anthrax. A smear of blood from the ear of the dead animal is usually sufficient for demonstration of the bacilli. A small inoculation is sufficient to kill guinea pigs and white mice in a couple of days, yet the organisms are highly sensitive to most antibiotics. Cattle and sheep are usually infected by feeding on pasture contaminated by spores, a fact originally discovered by Pasteur. It is indeed remarkable that more than a hundred years ago the father of bacteriology immunized sheep against anthrax by means of a vaccine consisting of bacilli attenuated by culture at a raised temperature. The non-pathogenic *B. subtilis* must not be mistaken for the anthrax bacillus, which it closely resembles except that it is motile by virtue of flagella.

Infection is nearly always conveyed through the skin, rarely by inhaling infected material (wool-sorter's disease) or by swallowing it. The latter is the common method by which animals are infected, so that in them the lesions are usually intestinal. In man the lesions are nearly always in the skin; pulmonary and intestinal lesions are very rare. Infection is conveyed from the wool and hides of diseased animals, so that butchers, tanners, wool-sorters, *etc.*, are the chief sufferers. The bristles of a new shaving brush may carry the infection. It is said that biting flies may convey infection from animals to man, but this seems open to doubt.

The *skin lesion* is the *malignant pustule*. It commences as a pimple on an exposed part of the skin (face, hands). This soon develops into a vesicle (not a pustule) containing clear serous or blood-stained fluid swarming with anthrax bacilli. The diagnosis is readily made by staining a smear of this fluid. When the vesicle bursts a black eschar is formed, around which a fresh row of vesicles develops; further out there is a brawny induration. The microscopic picture is one of acute inflammation. The rare *pulmonary* and *intestinal lesions* are similar in nature, *i.e.*, they show an acute hemorrhagic inflammation.

At any stage the bacilli may enter the blood stream causing an *anthrax septicemia* with infection of all the organs. This is constantly seen in highly susceptible animals such as the mouse and guinea pig. The postmortem findings are those of a hemorrhagic septicemia, with enlargement of the spleen, *etc.* From what has already been said, it will be obvious that extreme care must be taken at the autopsy to prevent the formation of spores.

ANAEROBIC SPORE-BEARERS.
CLOSTRIDIA.

The genus *Clostridium* is composed of many members which live in the soil, active in the process of putrefaction, so that they are readily ingested in vegetables, and establish themselves in the colon. They are strict anaerobes, so that they are unable to multiply in living tissue, confining themselves to dead tissue, in which, however, they can manufacture lethal toxins. Some of these toxins are of extraordinary potency.

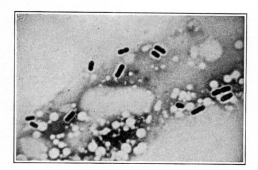

Fig. 171.—*Welchii*, showing capsules. × 1000.

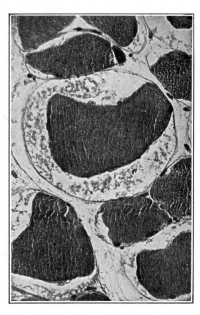

Fig. 172.—Gas gangrene. A muscle fiber separated from its sheath and from its blood supply by gas and fluid. × 250.

It is estimated that 0.008 mg. of pure botulinum toxin is enough to kill a man. All the organisms are gram-positive bacilli, all produce spores either readily or with reluctance, and all except *Cl. welchii* are motile, though they move with "a slow and stately motion." The spores can survive in dry earth for years, and are extremely resistant to heat and antiseptics. The bacilli themselves are sensitive to the sulfonamides and antibiotics, with the exception of streptomycin. The pathogenic members of the genus are: (1) the gas-producing anaerobes, *Cl. welchii*, *Cl. septicum* and *Cl. oedematiens*, (2) *Cl. tetani*, and (3) *Cl. botulinum*.

Gas Gangrene.—The common cause of gas gangrene is *Cl. welchii*; *Cl. septicum* comes in second and *Cl. oedematiens* third in frequency. All three may be present in a given case. It is in the dead tissue of war wounds that these organisms assume supreme importance. All are saccharolytic, not attacking proteins if carbohydrates are available, and they grow best in tissues containing an abundance of carbohydrate, *i.e.*, muscle and liver. *Cl. welchii*, a non-motile thick rod, is not only the commonest invader but the chief gas producer. As well as producing gas gangrene it is the cause of postmortem gas formation with its characteristic foul smell. Except when grown in special media it does not form spores, but in tissue fluids it has a well-marked capsule (Fig. 171). The other organisms readily form spores.

These bacteria are putrefactive. They are unable to gain a footing in living tissue until it has been devitalized. They are ordinarily saprophytes. Thus *Cl. welchii* was found in 80 per cent of wounds in the First World War, yet less than 10 per cent of these developed gas gangrene. Trauma and other organisms fail to activate it, but soil and dead muscle act as a spark which lights the fire. As the organisms feed on muscle sugar, it follows that early excision of dead muscle is the best prophylactic. Gas gangrene is a disease of muscle, which is at first a dull red and then becomes green or black. Bubbles of foul-smelling gas and blood-stained fluid can be pressed up and down the length of the muscle. The bacilli spread up and down the muscle in the interstitial tissue, and the muscle fibers are separated from their sheaths by toxic fluid, as a result of which they are killed and are then invaded by the putrefactive bacteria (Fig. 172).

The following vivid description of the wounded man who has developed gas gangrene is taken from the paper by MacFarlane and MacLennan. "The patient lies collapsed and obviously desperately ill. He has a livid pallor, the extremities are cold, and sometimes the veins cannot be filled sufficiently to make venipuncture possible. . . .

Mentally the patient is unusually alert and clear, anxious, even terrified, and apparently fully aware of his danger. Sometimes he lapses into coma or delirium before death, but more often he dies suddenly, particularly during some disturbance, such as being moved or anaesthetized. Death appears to be due to circulatory failure."

It would appear that many of the effects of the toxin of *Cl. welchii*, such as edema, hemorrhage, local necrosis and shock, are probably due to the action of a lecithinase on capillary permeability and on the permeability of cell membranes, leading to leakage of material from the damaged cells, as well as to hemolysis (Elder and Miles).

Tetanus.—Tetanus is a disease caused by wound infection with an anaerobic bacillus, *Cl. tetani*, but it differs entirely from the group of anaerobic infections just described, for there are no local symptoms. The bacillus develops a terminal spore, which gives it the familiar drumstick appearance. The organisms can be seen in the pus from infected wounds. The disease is an infection of septic wounds, not merely a wound infection. Its growth is favored by the presence of aerobic bacteria, so that it is never found in pure culture in a wound. The bacillus is a normal inhabitant of the intestine of the horse and other animals, and is therefore found in ground which has been manured. Wounds contaminated with garden soil, or the dirt of streets, are therefore always liable to infection by tetanus. Civilians with wounds of this character and all wounded soldiers must be protected by a prophylactic injection of antitetanic serum. Active immunization can be produced by inoculation with formol toxoid.

The *incubation period* varies greatly, averaging from ten days to a fortnight. In the case of face wounds it may be only three or four days. If the spores are surrounded by scar tissue they may remain quiescent for months. A subsequent operation, as for removal of a foreign body, may activate the spores, so that a second injection of serum should be given before such an operation.

The bacilli remain in the wound, where they produce a toxin which acts on the central nervous system. The tetanus toxin is one of the most powerful toxins known.

In this respect it is comparable with the botulinum toxin, both of which are infinitely more potent than the toxin of *Cl. welchii*. It used to be thought that the toxin was absorbed from the motor end-plates, passing along the axis cylinders to reach the spinal cord. The concept of an axonal spread may be acceptable in the case of viral infections, but the relatively rapid rate of travel of the tetanus toxin, sometimes less than twenty-four hours from a peripheral nerve to the lumbar cord, is quite incompatible with diffusion of such large protein molecules. The axon is highly viscous in texture, almost semi-solid, but a large proportion of the space inside the epineurium of the motor trunks, at least in the rabbit, is occupied by interstitial fluid. It seems likely that currents of this fluid generated by the high intramuscular pressures created during contraction are responsible for centripetal spread of the toxin (Payling Wright). In support of this view is the fact that injection of a sclerosing solution into a large motor nerve, with resulting fibrosis, blocks the absorption of tetanus toxin although not the transmission of nerves impulses, and that the toxin is not absorbed when a limb is immobilized. The phenomenon of "local tetanus," which may develop in the wounded part long before the general symptoms manifest themselves, may be due to a direct action of toxin on neuromuscular junctions. When the toxin reaches the cord and brain stem it becomes so firmly anchored to the motor nerve cells that it cannot be dislodged.

The symptoms are the result of an extreme hypersensitiveness of the motor nervous system produced by the action of the toxin on the motor nerve cells. As the result of this the most trivial sensory stimuli produce a series of terrible clonic and tonic spasms, and the patient dies exhausted by his convulsions or asphyxiated by tonic spasm of the respiratory muscles. The earliest symptom is usually spasm of the masseter muscles, producing the "lock-jaw" which gives the disease its common name. As the condition is purely toxic and not inflammatory, no characteristic lesions are found at autopsy.

Postoperative tetanus is fortunately rare. It is usually due to catgut infection with the spores of tetanus. When the catgut is absorbed in the wound the spores are set free and develop into bacilli. Not every case is due to the catgut. The dressings, dusting powder, *etc.*, may be infected. Finally it must be remembered that the patient may be an intestinal carrier of tetanus bacilli which may reach the tissues through an operation wound involving the bowel.

Botulism.—We have already seen that in gas gangrene the organisms spread through the tissues they have killed by their toxins, whilst in tetanus the organisms remain at their point of entry, where they elaborate their fatal poison. In botulism, the third member of the group of diseases caused by pathogenic clostridia, the conditions are again entirely different, for here the bacteria never enter the body, but produce their unbelievably potent poison in contaminated food, with resulting food poisoning.

Cl. botulinum is essentially a soil-bacterium, but is also found in the intestine of domestic animals. The spores, which cannot germinate without anaerobic conditions, can resist boiling for hours, but the toxin they produce is destroyed by boiling for 10 minutes. They develop in improperly cooked food stuffs, (*botulus*, a sausage), especially those preserved in tins for long period without adequate refrigeration. In the United States, where the disease is commoner, the foods are likely to be home-canned vegetables and tinned asparagus, whilst in Great Britain meat pies or meat and fish pastes are often responsible. Unfortunately the food may not appear to be spoiled, as there is no smell or production of gas, but sometimes it may be obviously affected owing to contamination by other bacteria. Most outbreaks are the result of eating tinned food which has not been recooked, conditions likely to occur at school or church picnics. The toxin is extraordinarily powerful, as minute an amount as 0.000,01 ml. of a filtrate killing a mouse in the course of a day. All who eat the food suffer, generally within twenty-four hours, sometimes as soon as two hours, occasionally not for two weeks.

The *symptoms* are due to the action of the toxin on the peripheral nerves. The toxins of botulism and tetanus are both strict neurotoxins, the main distinction being in the site of action. Botulinus toxin acts ex-

clusively on cholinergic nerve endings of peripheral somatic and autonomic fibers, whereas tetanus toxin acts only on nerve cells in the cerebrospinal axis. Possibly both clostridial toxins inflict similar biochemical lesions, but on different nervous elements. The clinical picture is characterized by vomiting, diarrhea, paralysis of the muscles of the orbit, pharynx, larynx and respiration, together with thirst and the production of thick, viscid sputum. The mortality is about 50 per cent. No treatment is of any value. As might be expected, the lesions are negligible, merely some hyperemia and thrombosis of small vessels. How different from the picture of gas gangrene.

BARTONELLA INFECTIONS

OROYA FEVER.—This is a disease occurring in Peru characterized by intermittent fever and a severe rapidly progressive anemia, ending fatally in a large number of cases. The red blood corpuscles contain minute rod-like motile organisms first described by Barton in 1909 and known as Bartonella bacilliformis. A large proportion

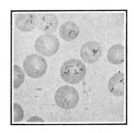

FIG. 173.—Bartonella muris.
(McCluskie and Niven.)

of the erythrocytes may be affected. The organism first invades the endothelium of the arterioles and the cells of the reticuloendothelial system, from which it attacks the erythrocytes. It is now known that the fatal cases are those which are complicated by paratyphoid B infection. In cases in which paratyphoid infection has not occurred the prognosis is good, no matter how great the destruction of red blood cells.

Certain strains of rats may become infected with another type of Bartonella,

Bartonella muris. The infection remains latent, no organisms are found in the red blood cells, but a few days after splenectomy severe and fatal anemia rapidly develops, due to invasion of the red blood cells by the Bartonella (Fig. 173), just as in Oroya fever. The latency appears to be due to the inhibitory action of the reticuloendothelial elements in the spleen.

REFERENCES

ALSTON, J. M.: Brit. Med. Jour., 1955, 2, 1524. (Necrobacillosis).

BARRIE, H. J. and BOGOCH, A.: Am. J. Path., 1953, 29, 451. (Sarcoidosis).

BINFORD, C. H.: Lab. Investig., 1959, 8, 901. (Transfer of leprosy to golden hamster).

BRAUDE, A. I. and SPINK, W. W.: Advances in Internal Med, 1950, 4, 163. (Brucellosis).

BURNET, F. M.: Natural History of Infectious Disease, 2nd ed., Cambridge, 1953. (A fascinating account of infection and parasitism).

COBURN, A. F. and PAULI, R. H.: J. Exper. Med., 1932, 56, 609. (Rheumatic fever).

COLEBROOK, L.: Lancet, 1955, 2, 885. (Hospital infections).

CUMMINGS, M. M. and HUDGINS, P. C.: Am. J. Med. Sci., 1958, 236, 311. (Pine pollen and sarcoidosis).

DUBOS, R. J.: Can. Med. Assn. J., 1958, 79, 445. (Historical evolution of infectious diseases).

ELDER, J. M. and MILES, A. A.: J. Path. and Bact., 1957, 74, 133. (Action of lecithinase in gas gangrene).

ENGEL, R. L., JR.: Am. J. Path., 1953, 29, 53. (Cell inclusions in sarcoidosis).

FINE J., et al.: New England J. Med., 1959, 260, 214. (The bacterial factor in traumatic shock).

FINLAND, M.: New Eng. J. Med., 1955, 253, 909. (Antibiotic-resistant bacteria).

FINLAND, M., JONES, W. F., JR. and BARNES, M. W.: J.A.M.A., 1959, 170, 2188. (Serious bacterial infections since the introduction of antibiotic agents).

FRANCIS, E.: Medicine, 1928, 7, 411. (Tularemia).

FRIED, B. M.: Arch. Path., 1931, 12, 689. (Cellular reaction in tuberculosis).

GILLESPIE, W. A. and GUY, J.: Lancet, 1956, 1, 1039. (Bacteroides in abdominal sepsis).

GOST, J. T.: Lancet, 1958, 1, 191. (Treatment of brucellosis).

GOULEY, B. A.and EIMAN, J.: Am. J. Med. Sci., 1932, 183, 359. (Rheumatic pneumonia).

GROSS, L. and EHRLICH, J. C.: Am. J. Path., 1934, 10, 489. (Life cycle of the Aschoff body).

HENSLER, N. M., FLANAGAN, P. and SPRAGUE, E. M.: Am. J. Med., 1959, 26, 376. (Chromogenic acid-fast bacilli).

ISRAEL, H. L. and SONES, M.: Ann. Int. Med., 1955, 43, 1269. (Sarcoidosis).

KING, A.: Lancet, 1958, 1, 651. (The varying incidence of venereal diseases).

KLINGE, F.: Virchow's Arch. Path. Anat., 1932, 286, 344. (Pathology of rheumatic fever).

LONG, E. R. and FAUST, R.: Am. J. Path., 1941, 17, 697. (Spread of tuberculosis).

MacFARLANE, R. G. andMacLENNAN, J. D.: Lancet, 1945, 2, 328. (Gas gangrene).

McDONALD, J. R. and WEED, L. A.: Am. J. Clin. Path., 1951, 21, 223. (Tuberculoid granulomas).

McVAY, L. V. and SPRUNT, D. H.: Ann. Int. Med., 1952, 36, 56. (Bacteroides infections).

PEERY, T. M. and BELTER, L. F.: Am. J. Path., 1960, 36, 673. (Brucellosis and heart disease).

POWELL, C. S. and SWAN, L. L.: Am. J. Path., 1955, 31, 1131. (Lesions of leprosy).

RICH, A. R.: The Pathogenesis of Tuberculosis, Springfield, Ill., 1944.

RINEHART, J. F., et al.: Arch. Int. Med., 1938, 61, 552. (Rheumatic fever).

ROANTREE, R. J. and RANTZ, L. A.: Arch. Int. Med., 1955, 96, 674. (C-reactive protein test).

ROGERS, D. E.: Bull. New York Acad. Med., 1959, 35, 25. (The nature of staphylococcal infections).

RUBIN, S. H. and BOYD, L. J.: Amer. J. Gastroenterology, 1958, 29, 131. (Bacteroides infections in gastroenterology).

SPITTEL, J. A. JR., MARTIN, W. J. and NICHOLS, D. R.: Ann. Int. Med., 1956, 44, 302. (Bacteremia due to gram-negative bacilli).

SYMMERS, W. ST. C.: Am. J. Path., 1951, 27, 493. (Tuberculoid granulomas).

TALBOT, F. J., KATZ, S. and MATTHEWS, M. J.: Am. J. Med., 1959, 26, 340. (Diagnosis of sarcoidosis).

TEILUM, G.: Am. J. Path., 1948, 24, 490. (Sarcoidosis).

WHITBY, SIR L. and HYNES, M.: Medical Bacteriology, 6th ed., London, 1956.

WRIGHT, G. PAYLING: Proc. Roy. Soc. Med., 1953, 46, 319. (Pathways of ascent of tetanus toxin).

Chapter 12

Fungus Infections

General Considerations
Actinomycosis
   Botryomycosis
   Nocardiosis
Blastomycosis
   South American Blasto-
     mycosis

Cryptococcosis (Torulosis)
Coccidioidomycosis
Histoplasmosis
   Primary
   Progressive
Moniliasis (Candidiasis)

Aspergillosis
Mucormycosis
Sporotrichosis
Rhinosporidiosis

GENERAL CONSIDERATIONS

Fungi are plants, although higher in the scale of life than bacteria. Unlike algæ, they lack chlorophyll, so that they cannot manufacture their own food. They are therefore either saprophytic or parasitic. Fungi are extremely common and are widespread in distribution, but fortunately only a few of them are pathogenic. For growth they require a high humidity, warmth, and a free supply of oxygen. The warmth and humidity of the tropics are particularly favorable for their multiplication. The line which separates them from the bacteria is tenuous in some instances, as in the case of actinomyces, which is sometimes included in the one class, sometimes in the other. They are more resistant than bacteria to drying, alcohol and the action of antibiotics, which after all are derived primarily from fungi. The lower forms reproduce only by budding, but in the higher types repeated budding with failure to separate gives rise to long filamentous branching hyphæ which form cotton-wool colonies or "molds."

Systemic mycotic infections may fall into one of three categories: (1) *Primary infections*, the incidence of some infections varying greatly with the geographic distribution. (2) *Secondary infections*, which develop during the treatment of bacterial or viral infections with broad-spectrum antibiotics; this is particularly true of moniliasis. (3) *Complicating infections*, which are complications of chronic debilitating illnesses, especially when treated with corticosteroids or antibiotics. In these cases death is often the

result of invasion of the tissues by the fungus rather than due to the primary disease. The majority of pathogenic fungi can be isolated directly from the patient's exudates, and grown on suitable culture media in the course of a few days. Culture of gastric aspirated material of patients suspected of having pulmonary mycotic infection is especially valuable.

The subject of fungi and fungus diseases is a highly specialized one with a distinctly forbidding terminology. Here we shall consider only the more important members of the group producing lesions in man, excluding those limited to the skin. For more detailed information the reader is referred to *Manual of Clinical Mycology* by Conant *et al.* or other larger works. The damage to the tissues is not caused by toxins, but is the result of allergic necrosis due to sensitization to the proteins of the fungi. Skin tests for hypersensitivity to these foreign antigens are of marked value in many instances, as we shall see. The McManus periodic acid-Schiff stain, together with recent modifications, has proved of great value for the demonstration of fungi in tissue.

The subject of fungus infections is rapidly acquiring a new importance by reason of the use and abuse of multiple antibiotics. These wipe out the harmless bacteria with which the fungi are accustomed to live, and which serve to restrain their growth. With elimination of the bacteria the fungi come to occupy the field, to multiply without restraint, and to assume the role of pathogens. Those diseases which we shall discuss, as well as the less important mycoses such as chromoblastomycosis and epidermophytosis may come to present a new threat to the health of the patient. The student may find it convenient to refer to the table summarizing the principal granulomatous inflammations on page 63.

Fungal infections may be divided into two groups: superficial and systemic. The fungi that cause *superficial infections* spread from animals to man. In *systemic infections* the fungi seem to come from the soil, bird droppings and vegetation. Pathogenic fungi become established in the body in a very insidious manner and it is often difficult and sometime impossible to distinguish the clinical picture from that caused by other infective agents.

ACTINOMYCOSIS

This is the commonest of the mycoses in man, that is to say a granuloma characterized by chronic suppuration, probably allergic in nature. The disease is much commoner in domestic animals, such as horses, cattle and pigs. It is world-wide in distribution, as indicated by the statement: "Wherever there is a microscope and a laboratory, the fungus has been found to be the cause of disease" (Cope).

The disease is caused by Actinomyces bovis or ray fungus, so-called because of the radiate arrangement of threads at the edge of the colonies. The fungus is a streptothrix which forms little yellow clumps in the tissue known as "sulfur granules." These clumps are composed of a felted mass of filaments with spores and club-shaped bodies at the periphery. The filaments are gram-positive and the clubs gram-negative. There are several types of actinomyces, some *aerobic*, others *anaerobic*. *The great majority of human and animal infections are due to strict anaerobes.* This is the probable reason why the fungus is not found in draining lesions.

The method of infection is still uncertain. There is no evidence that it is conveyed directly from animals to man, but it is much commoner in farmers and other country-dwellers. Ears of grain have been found embedded in the mouth lesions, and the

usual view is that infection is carried by grain which has been chewed, but the Actinomyces bovis has never been found in grains or grasses in a state of Nature. The fungus probably becomes an inhabitant of the mouth or intestine in country-dwellers, and enters the tissues through some break in the surface, the root of a carious tooth, etc. Secondary invasion by pyogenic organisms is common, and the resulting suppuration may reduce the oxygen tension in the tissues and favor even more the growth of anaerobic actinomyces. Once penetration of the surface has occurred the wound heals promptly, and the pathological process works outward from the mouth, intestine or rectum as the case may be.

Spread.—The spread is different from that of such infectious granulomata as tuberculosis and syphilis, for the lymph vessels and nodes are not involved, a valuable point in diagnosis. The infection starts in the subcutaneous or submucous tissue and spreads by direct continuity. The lesion may rupture into a blood vessel, and there may be blood spread to the liver, brain, and heart, but this is not common.

Lesions.—The lesions occur in four chief sites: (1) head and neck (60 per cent), (2) ileocecal region and appendix (20 per cent), (3) lungs (15 per cent), and (4) skin (5 per cent). The three groups which are of interest to us are the cervicofacial, the thoracic and the abdominal. In these the fungus presumably enters the tissue as the result of an injury in the mouth, the respiratory tract, or the ileocecal region.

Cervicofacial actinomycosis is the common form, and fortunately has the best prognosis. Entry may be by way of the tonsils or carious teeth, or may follow the extraction of a tooth. A firm mass develops, usually under the lower jaw, followed by a brawny induration of the neck. After a time the mass breaks down and becomes riddled with abscesses and sinuses. These multiple sinuses perforating the skin are characteristic of actinomycosis (Fig. 174). There is progressive destruction of connective tissue, muscle, and bone. The pus contains the tiny yellow *sulfur granules* from which the diagnosis can most readily be made (Fig. 175). These should be looked for whenever

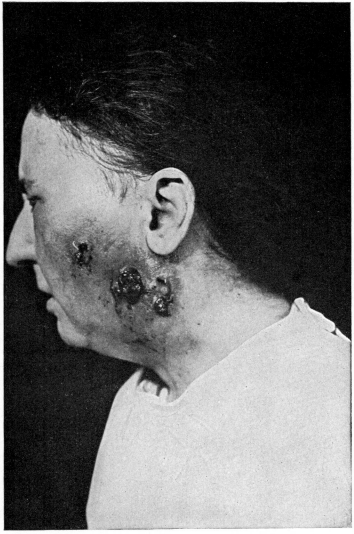

Fig. 174.—Actinomycosis of the face. Note swelling of subcutaneous tissues and multiple sinus formation. (Conant *et al.*, *Manual of Clinical Mycology*, courtesy of W. B. Saunders Company.)

the abscess is opened, as they may disappear later.

Abdominal actinomycosis develops in the cecum, or appendix owing to the actinomyces in the mouth being swallowed in the saliva and invading the intestinal mucosa. A firm mass is formed which is easily mistaken for carcinoma, although the earliest symptoms may suggest acute or subacute appendicitis. The further progress is similar to that of the cervicofacial form, with perforation of the bowel, and the formation of sinuses in the abdominal wall. Spread to the liver is frequent, with resulting abscesses which may honeycomb the organ, or the infection may penetrate the diaphragm and reach the lungs.

Thoracic actinomycosis is usually due to aspiration of the fungus from the mouth, but it may extend through the diaphragm from abdominal or hepatic lesions. The early symptoms suggest pneumonia, but later the condition is apt to be mistaken for tuberculosis or even for a neoplasm when the

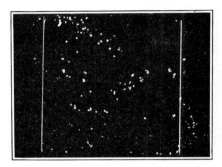

FIG. 175.—Sulfur granules, photographed on slide with black background.

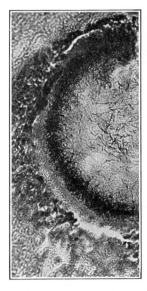

FIG. 176.—Colony of fungus in actinomycosis. Many mycelial threads can be seen in addition to the dense feltwork at the periphery. × 275.

x-ray picture shows massive consolidation in the region of the hilus. The subsequent course is just what we might expect, namely spread throughout the lung, invasion of the pleura with the formation of pleural adhesions and exudate, and frequent involvement of the ribs.

Microscopic Appearance. — The microscopic appearance is that of a granuloma with the addition of suppuration (Fig. 176). There are chronic inflammatory cells, fibroblasts, and giant cells. If suppuration is marked the picture approaches that of acute inflammation. It is uncommon to find colonies of the fungus in viable tissue (Fig. 177); these are much more easily demonstrated in the discharge. It is evident that the histological appearance is not at all characteristic, and that not much need be expected from biopsy examination.

Antibiotic therapy with penicillin has changed actinomycosis from a chronic disease with a high mortality rate, especially in the thoracic and abdominal forms, to one in which the prognosis is excellent.

Botryomycosis.—This misleading name was given in 1884 to a chronic, suppurative, granulomatous lesion under the impression that it was due to a true fungus. The specific feature is the presence of fungus-like grains or granules (*botrys*, grape) within the suppurative foci (Winslow). The granules used to be mistaken for fungi, but they are now known to consist of non-branching bacteria, usually staphylococci or gram-negative bacilli, sometimes one of the proteus group. Either the skin or the viscera may be involved. The lesions are apt to be very misleading, being granulomatous in type, and containing many epithelioid cells and giant cells. Sometimes they simulate actinomycosis very closely, so that the name staphylococcic actinophytosis has been applied. Little is known of the factors which cause certain bacteria to produce lesions of this type. Probably there is a decrease in virulence and an increase in resistance, resulting in a delicate balance between the infecting agent and the host.

Nocardiosis.—This is an acute or chronic infection that may closely resemble other suppurative conditions. It is caused by Nocardia asteroides, which belongs to the actinomyces family, but, unlike Actinomyces bovis, it is aerobic and usually weakly acid-fast. The cattle studied by Nocard in 1888 suffered from multiple abscesses, draining sinuses, and pulmonary involvement. The condition is frequently misdiagnosed as actinomycosis. The fungus is invisible in a hematoxylin and eosin preparation, but is readily shown by Gram's stain and also by an acid-fast (Ziehl-Neelson) stain. In the latter case there is the danger of mistaking the condition for tuberculosis.

Unlike actinomycosis, the main lesions are pulmonary (Weed *et al.*). They take the

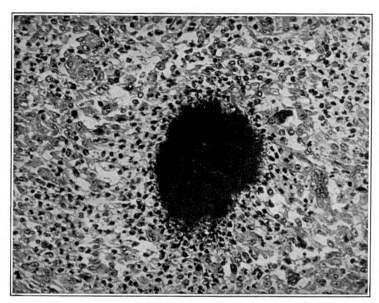

FIG. 177.—Actinomycosis showing suppuration immediately around central mass of ray fungus, and granulomatous lesion farther out. × 200.

form of abscesses, generally multiple and often confluent, and without the extensive fibrosis, burrowing and sinus formation which characterize actinomycosis. Secondary lesions in the central nervous system are common.

Mycetoma is a localized form of the disease more likely to occur in the tropics. It is a unilateral infection of the extremities usually the foot and leg, rarely the hand and arm, following injury and the introduction into the tissues of the aerobic, saprophytic but potentially pathogenic nocardia. There is a remarkably long latent period before a nodule appears, which develops into an abscess, and finally discharges as a sinus. Eventually a series of abscesses and interlocking sinuses involve the bones, resulting in extreme deformity.

As early correct diagnosis is important, because the condition responds readily to sulfonamide therapy, although not to antibiotics. The latter feature serves to distinguish it from lesions caused by pyogenic cocci.

BLASTOMYCOSIS

This is a chronic granuloma caused by a yeast-like fungus known as blastomyces.

The organisms are spherical, two or three times the diameter of a red blood corpuscle, and show two *characteristic features:* (1) a clear double contour, and (2) budding like yeast cells. The blastomyces are beautifully demonstrated by the periodic acid-Schiff stain (Fig. 178). The method of infection may be through a break or wound in the skin or by inhalation. The disease occurs in two forms, cutaneous and systemic.

Cutaneous Form.—The cutaneous form is known as blastomycetic dermatitis. The lesions are commonest on the face, the back of the hand, and the front of the leg. At first they are papules, but they undergo suppuration and ulcerate. The disease spreads over the surface, so that a large area may be involved. The microscopic picture is similar to that of actinomycosis, *i.e.*, a granuloma (lymphocytes, mononuclears, giant cells) with suppuration added. At the edge of the ulcer there may be very marked epithelial hyperplasia *which may closely simulate the appearance of epidermoid carcinoma.* The spherical fungi are seen in sections of the tissue or in smears of the discharge.

Systemic Form.—The systemic form is much less common. The lungs are most

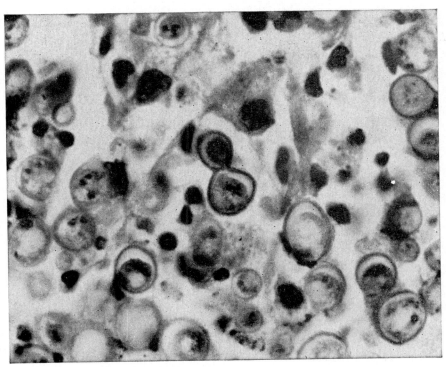

Fig. 178.—Blastomycosis of lung. Section of tissue showing budding forms. Periodic acid-Schiff stain. × 1500. (Dr. Norman F. Conant *et al.*, *Manual of Clinical Mycology*, courtesy of W. B. Saunders Company.)

often involved, but any organ may be affected. Infection is spread by the blood stream. The pulmonary lesions are nodules and abscesses and are very liable to be mistaken for tuberculosis. The fungi are very numerous in the tissues in the systemic form. This form used to be nearly always fatal, but the cutaneous form is seldom fatal and may last for many years. The various lesions are well illustrated in Baker's paper, and in that by Starrs and Klotz.

South American Blastomycosis.—This is a chronic granulomatous disease of the skin, mucous membranes, lymph nodes and viscera caused by Blastomyces brasiliensis. It is commonest in Brazil, but has been reported from most of the South American countries. The most characteristic clinical feature is enlargement of the lymph nodes, particularly those of the neck, which is present in practically all cases. The fungus is much larger than the North American variety, with a thick wall and numerous buds. The disease may present itself in (1) a *cutaneous form*,

with lesions of the skin and mucous membranes, particularly in the region of the mouth and nose, with early involvement of the regional nodes; (2) a *lymphangitic form*, most marked in the cervical, supraclavicular and axillary regions; (3) a *visceral* form, with involvement of the liver, spleen, pancreas and other abdominal organs. The lesions are of the same nature as those of North American blastomycosis.

CRYPTOCOCCOSIS (TORULOSIS)

Cryptococcosis or torulosis is a subacute or chronic infection caused by Cryptococcus neoformans (Torula histolytica), which may involve the lungs, skin and other parts, but has a special predilection for the meninges and brain, so that it is always potentially very dangerous. The causal organism is a blastomyces, a parasitic yeast although a saprophyte in nature, and the disease is also known as European blastomycosis, to distinguish it from the North and South

21

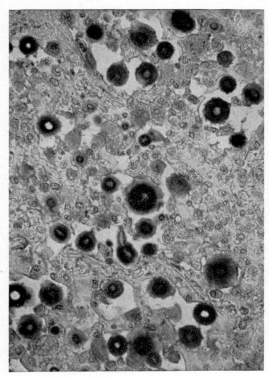

FIG. 179.—Cryptococcosis neoformans. The thick capsules of the organisms have been preserved by mounting in glycerin-jelly, omitting dehydration. Alcian blue stain. (Kindness of Dr. R. W. Mowry in Boyd, *Pathology for the Physician*.)

American forms. This is unfortunate, because the disease has been reported from every quarter of the world where laboratory facilities are available. The cryptococcus resembles the other blastomyces, but it is characterized by a heavy gelatinous capsule, which in sections is seen as a clear space around the organism. This is brought out clearly by the use of India ink, but the capsule is stained beautifully with the PAS technique, and still better with Alcian blue (Fig. 179). In lesions where the organisms are very sparse the fluorescent labelled antibody technique is of value.

The organism has been isolated from the milk of apparently healthy cows, and has been found in the soil. There is no evidence of the passage of infection from man to man or from animal to man. It seems probable that infection may enter the body through the respiratory tract, the skin or the intestine. There is frequently a curious association with other diseases such as sarcoidosis, Hodgkin's disease, etc.

The *lesions* are granulomatous in character, but are not marked by the intense tissue destruction and cellular exudation seen in blastomycosis. The two principal sites of infection are the lungs and the meninges, but the fungi may be scattered far and wide by the blood stream. *Pulmonary cryptococcosis* may present rounded, solid lesions, sometimes as large as an orange. The smaller lesions are easily mistaken for tubercles, but the characteristic organisms make differentiation easy. *Meningeal cryptococcosis* is the real threat which gives its distinctive mark to the disease, and serves to distinguish it from other fungous infections. Once the yeast has broken through the blood-brain barrier and entered the cerebrospinal fluid, it is quickly seeded over the central nervous system, where it finds nutrients for growth and develops a big capsule which increases its resistance to antibiotics (Littman). Even in fatal cases the meninges and brain may appear grossly normal, so uniform is the dispersal of the organisms in the subarachnoid space, with scarcely a suggestion of cloudiness. The cut surface of the brain may show small cystic spaces.

Microscopically, there may be masses of fungi in the subarachnoid spaces, whilst in other cases there is a marked granulomatous reaction. The small cysts in the surface layers of the brain are due to invasion of the perivascular spaces, the microcysts being filled with organisms and their mucoid secretions. The cerebrospinal fluid shows the increase of protein and cells and the decrease of sugar which is found in tuberculous meningitis, but the cryptococcus can be identified in smears or by culture. The symptoms such as headache of increasing severity, dizziness, and stiffness of the neck, are likely to suggest the possibility of tuberculous meningitis.

COCCIDIOIDOMYCOSIS

This uncommon disease was originally thought to be confined to the San Joaquin Valley, California, so that it came to be known as the "California disease." It is

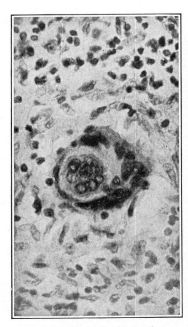

FIG. 180.—Coccidioides in tissues.

now known to be distributed all over the United States. It is an infective granuloma closely resembling tuberculosis, but caused by *Coccidioides immitis*, a yeast-like fungus. This is a spherical body with a double contoured highly refractile capsule. It resembles the blastomyces, but can be differentiated by the fact that it multiplies by the formation of endospores, the blastomyces by budding. The coccidioides are much larger and may measure 50 microns (Fig. 180). *Clinically* the disease is easily mistaken for tuberculosis, syphilis and blastomycosis, and many cases of supposed tuberculosis are probably examples of this disease. Infection is due to the inhalation of dust containing the fungus. There is no passage of the infection from man to man. The morbidity is relatively low. The infection has also been found in cattle. The disease can be reproduced in the guinea-pig, the characteristic lesion being a suppurative orchitis.

Dissemination of the infection follows failure of the body to "focalize" the disease at its primary site. It is an endogenous reinfection and comes on shortly after the primary infection of which it is a continua-

tion. Dissemination involves every body tissue, with the exception of the intestinal tract. Multiple abscesses, spread widely throughout the body and are frequent, meningitis somewhat less so. The prognosis is grave, because the mortality is at least 50 to 60 per cent. Therapeutic agents of some value are now becoming available.

The *lesions* are usually in the lungs, bones and skin, but any organ may be involved. They are in the form of granulomatous masses and abscesses (Fig. 181). They cannot be distinguished from those of tuberculosis with the naked eye, but it may be said that in the lungs there is less cavitation than is usual with tuberculosis, and in the bones the lesions are more extensive. The microscopic appearance also resembles that of tuberculosis; tubercle formation, epithelioid cells and giant cells are common (Fig. 182). The pathognomonic feature is the presence of the double-contoured highly refractile coccidioides filled with spores. The PAS stain shows up parasites which may be overlooked in sections stained with hematoxylin and eosin. The parasites are also found in pus from the lesions.

The work of Dickson has shed new light on the disease. He has shown that the condition begins as a mild infection of the respiratory tract often accompanied by erythema nodosum. The great majority recover promptly in the course of a few weeks, but in a few cases the mild attack is followed by the chronic granulomatous disease known as *coccidioidal granuloma*. Dickson suggests the term coccidioidomycosis to cover both forms.

Cultures of the hyphæ are extremely infective to the laboratory worker, so that extreme caution must be exercised in transferring or examining cultures. The fungus should not be grown in petri dishes, lest the cultures become dry, powdery, and disseminated into the air of the laboratory.

HISTOPLASMOSIS

Histoplasmosis has had a remarkable, indeed extraordinary, history. It was first described in 1906 by Darling who demonstrated an organism which he called Histoplasma capsulatum, in the bodies of three

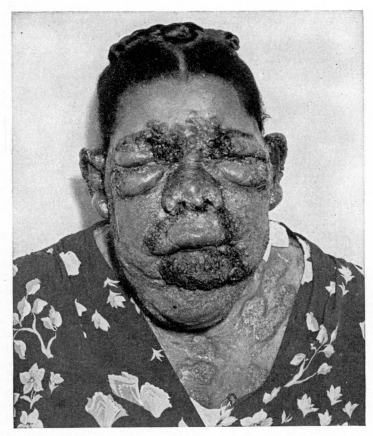

Fig. 181.—Coccidioidomycosis. Multiple granulomatous lesions; some show ulceration. (Kindness, Dr. M. A. Gifford, in *Manual of Clinical Mycology*, courtesy of W. B. Saunders Company.)

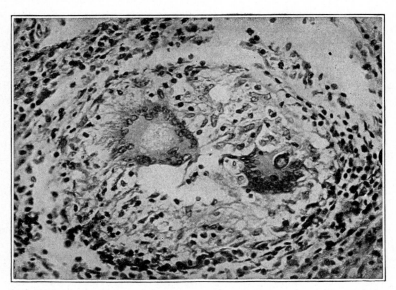

Fig. 182.—Coccidioidal granuloma. Tubercle-like lesion, the right hand giant cell containing coccidioides. × 200.

patients in the Panama Canal zone, This organism was of about the same size and appearance as the Leishman-Donovan bodies of kala-azar, so it was natural that Darling took it to be a protozoon. The disease was regarded as a very rare tropical malady, invariably fatal. Nothing more was heard of the condition until 1926, when another fatal case was reported in Minnesota. In 1934 DeMonbreum of Nashville, Tennessee, isolated and cultured the organism, demonstrating that it was a fungus.

The next and most important step was the introduction of a sensitivity test, the histoplasmin skin reaction, using culture of H. capsulatum as an antigen, although skin tests must be interpreted with care because of cross reactions with other mycoses such as blastomycosis and coccidioidomycosis. This was followed by the use of a complement fixation test. These procedures proved to be revolutionary, for they showed that infection with the fungus was extremely prevalent in the northeastern and central part of the United States, the central Mississippi Valley in particular, and that in much lesser degree it was world-wide in distribution. The disease is more prevalent in rural than in urban areas, and in some rural regions more than in others (Christie). It also soon became apparent that there were two very different forms of the disease, one mild, localized and common, the other severe, disseminated and fatal. Large numbers of persons, up to 75 per cent of the population in the endemic areas, were infected by the fungus as shown by laboratory tests, but showed no evidence of disease. It is now known that several million people in the United States have been infected, with few or no clinical consequences.

H. capulatum appears in a sporulating mycelial phase in the soil and in laboratory cultures, and in a yeast cell form in the body. The infection does not appear to be transmitted directly from person to person, but to be inhaled in dust from the soil, where the fungus can be demonstrated. In this it resembles coccidioidomycosis, which, as we have seen, has a very definite geographic distribution. Many domestic animals are susceptible to infection, and several epidemics have been associated with contamination of the soil by animal excreta, especially that of pigeons and chickens. The two forms already mentioned, forms which the disease may take, may be called primary and progressive.

Primary Histoplasmosis.—This is a relatively benign inhalation infection of the lungs. It is fortunate that histoplasmosis is usually a benign and self-limiting disease, for, although many agents have been tried, no one method of therapy has proved of value. At least 95 per cent of the cases of primary histoplasmosis are asymptomatic. It is startling to find roentgenographic evidence of extensive localized infiltration in the lungs with no symptoms or physical signs. The hilar lymph nodes are nearly always enlarged. A few patients have cough, fever and loss of strength. Even if there is sputum, it is seldom that the organism can be recovered. Healing is curiously slow. A few of the infiltrations undergo complete resolution, some densely calcified. The calcified areas as seen in x-ray film are much more rounded than those of tuberculosis.

Progressive Histoplasmosis.—Probably less than 0.1 per cent of cases of primary infection develop into the progressive and nearly always fatal form of the disease. The primary lesion is often extrapulmonary in the lips, mouth, pharynx or intestine. Severe disease is commonest in young children and in elderly persons suffering from some debilitating disease. Acute disseminated histoplasmosis is generally the result of a heavy infection with the fungus or poor resistance in young children and debilitated persons.

The *clinical manifestations* are extremely varied. Fever, enlargement of the spleen and liver, cough, and loss of weight are the common symptoms, but there may be diarrhea and other evidence of gastroenteritis. About half the cases have ulcerative and granulomatous lesions of the skin and mucous membranes. Purpuric manifestations in the skin in children due to involvement of the bone marrow are of evil omen. Young children rarely live more than a few weeks after the onset of the infection. In adults the disease runs a more chronic course for a number of months, with occasional recovery. Complement-fixing antibodies ap-

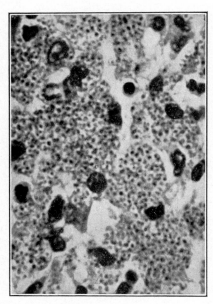

FIG. 183.—Reticuloendothelial cells of lymph node packed with Histoplasma capsulatum. × 510. (From a section by Dr. W. A. D. Anderson.)

pear in the blood about three weeks after the acute onset of the disease. Massive progressive histoplasmosis may suppress antibody formation, and at the same time the skin-test sensitivity may be reduced or even disappear. The bone marrow is infected in nearly all cases, with corresponding changes in the blood picture. Histoplasma may be demonstrated in blood smears. The organism can be cultured successfully from many sites, but bone marrow and blood are preferred.

The *lesions* are of the nature and distribution already indicated. Tubercle-like nodules and necrotic foci are found in the lungs, liver, spleen and kidneys, together with ulcerating lesions of the mouth, larynx and intestine in many cases. Enlargement of the liver and spleen may be the only gross abnormality observed. *Microscopically* the reticuloendothelial cells are particularly involved, and they may be crowded with the organisms (Fig. 183). These are best demonstrated by means of the McManus PAS stain.

An extensive and very well illustrated review dealing with all aspects of this intriguing subject will be found in the paper by Silverman *et al.*

MONILIASIS

This condition is caused by the fungus Candida (Monilia) albicans, so that an alternative name is *candidiasis*. It is also known as *thrush* when it occurs in the mouth. Moniliasis is an excellent example of the truth that infection depends not only on the virulence of the invader, but also on diminished resistance of the host. As the fungus is found in the throat, vagina and stools of healthy persons, its order of virulence is evidently very low. It is natural, therefore, that infection should be seen in infants or in those whose resistence has been lowered by malnutrition, diabetes and other wasting diseases. The continued administration of antibiotics also favors growth of the fungus in the body, possibly by replacing bacteria which have a restraining effect on fungal growth. Conditions of moisture also favor growth, so that the common sites of infection are the mouth, vagina, urinary tract, and axillary folds. The local humidity may be occupational in origin, as is seen in the hands of housewives, bakers, waiters, bartenders and fruit pickers whose skin is macerated by frequent contact with water.

The *lesions* involve the skin and mucous membranes. They consist of white patches made up of growing mycelia, which penetrate into the underlying tissue. When the white membrane is removed the surface is red and looks inflamed, but microscopically there is only a minimal inflammatory reaction. The lung may show focal granulomata resembling tuberculosis, and in rare instances there may be dissemination by the blood stream and mycotic endocarditis has been reported in drug addicts. The fungus consists of branching mycelial filaments with budding yeast-like cells with thin walls, very different from the thick capsule so characteristic of the cryptococcus (Fig. 184). One must be wary of diagnosing moniliasis merely from the presence of Candida albicans, because the fungus is a frequent saprophytic commensal in the sputum of patients with tuberculosis, lung abscess, and other pulmonary conditions.

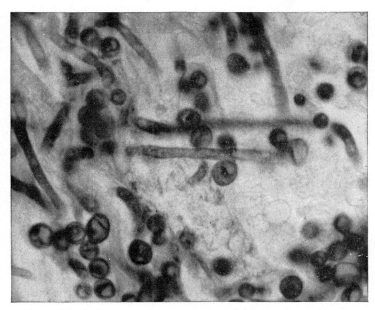

Fig. 184.—Candidiasis of brain. Growth of *Candida albicans* in ventricle in fatal meningitis. Periodic acid-Schiff stain. × 1200. (Conant *et al., Manual of Clinical Mycology*, courtesy of W. B. Saunders Co.)

ASPERGILLOSIS

This infection is caused by *Aspergillus fumigatus*, a filamentous fungus with a basal stem and a stalk supporting a spore-bearing head. As in the case of moniliasis, the infection has become more common and serious since the widespread use of antibiotics and sulfonamides, and fatalities are occurring in patients receiving antibiotic therapy. As the fungus often contaminates grain, the disease occurs amongst bird fanciers, pigeon stuffers, agricultural workers, and other grain handlers. The *lesions* are similar to those of tuberculosis, with necrosis and cavitation. Mats of mycelial threads may be seen in some areas.

MUCORMYCOSIS

Mucormycosis appears to be a new disease (Baker). The first report of the cerebral form appeared in 1943, the pulmonary form in 1948. Cases have now been observed in all parts of the United States, Canada and England, and the disease is probably worldwide. It is caused by certain fungi, especially Rhizopus, that are common contaminants of laboratory cultures and are not ordinarily pathogenic. The increasing frequency of the disease is probably due to the use of antibiotics, which reduce the number of bacterial infections but permit fungus invasion. Cortisone, ACTH, and antileukemic drugs favor the development of the mycosis, as do diabetes and leukemia. In the diabetic patient mucormycosis is a rapidly fatal disease which may take the form of a pneumonia or of meningoencephalitis.

The fungus enters the nose and leads to sinusitis, orbital cellulitis and meningoencephalitis. It grows rapidly, and is characterized by broad, branching, non-septate hyphæ known as rhizoids. A unique feature in the infection is a great affinity for arteries, the fungus penetrating the tough muscular walls and growing in the lumen, where it incites thrombosis with resulting infarction (Fig. 185). Thrombosis of the ophthalmic and internal carotid arteries leads to cerebral softening. The organisms extend deeply into the brain, producing a mycotic encephalitis. They may also spread in the bronchi and alveoli, producing mycotic bronchitis and pneumonia. The patients have been of all ages, from six months to sixty-five years.

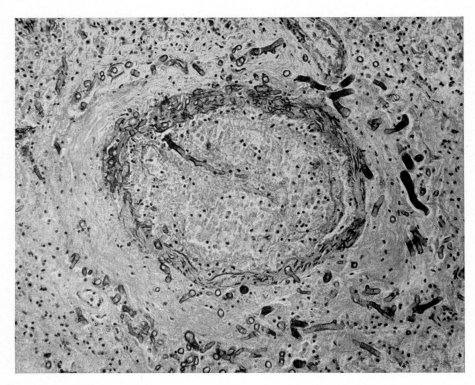

FIG. 185.—Mucormycosis invading cerebral vessels and occupying the lumen (Kindness of Dr. Roger D. Baker, in Conant *et al.*, *Manual of Clinical Mycology*, courtesy of W. B. Saunders Company.)

The duration of the fatal encephalitis may be as short as one day, an astonishing fact considering that the infecting agent used to be regarded as nonpathogenic.

SPOROTRICHOSIS

This is a chronic infection caused by the fungus Sporotrichium. In many respects it closely resembles blastomycosis, but the fungus is demonstrated by culture, not in smears. Like blastomycosis it is usually confined to the skin, but occasionally the internal organs are involved. The skin lesions are, as a rule, on the hand or forearm. They take the form of nodules which later break down and suppurate. The infection advances along the lymphatics, so that a line of nodules is formed along the arm, an appearance always suggestive of sporotrichosis.

The *microscopic* picture is that of tuberculosis and fungous granulomata, namely caseous necrosis with macrophages, giant cells and some polymorphonuclear leukocytes. The absence of visible organisms in sections or smears is highly suggestive of sporotrichosis. In all of the other fungus diseases the causative fungus can be readily seen when the material is suitably stained.

RHINOSPORIDIOSIS

This is a local inflammatory condition of the anterior nares, fairly common in India but extremely rare elsewhere, the only other cases reported coming from the Argentine and the United States. It is rare in the female. The lesions takes the form of a polypoid growth in the nose composed of granulation tissue and presenting an extraordinary and characteristic microscopic picture, for the tissue is crowded with the huge parasitic cysts, each a single organism, which constitute the etiological agent. This is a fungus known as Rhinosporidium seeberi (first described by Seeber), which commences its life cycle as a parasite meas-

Principal Pathogenic Fungi

Disease	*Causative Agent*
Actinomycosis	Actinomyces bovis (ray fungus; gram-positive filaments with gram-negative clubs; most pathogens anaerobic)
Nocardiosis	Nocardia asteroides (aerobic, weakly acid fast)
Blastomycosis	Blastomyces dermatididis (budding of double-contoured yeast-like cells)
South American Blastomycosis	Blastomyces brasiliensis (larger cells with thick walls and numerous buds)
Crytococcosis (Torulosis) (European Blastomycosis)	Cryptococcus neoformans (Torula histolytica) (budding cells with thick capsule)
Coccidioidomycosis	Coccidioides immitis (yeast-like cells with double-contoured refractile capsule and endospores)
Histoplasmosis	Histoplasma capsulatum (yeast forms in body; sporulating mycelial forms in soil and cultures)
Moniliasis (candidiasis)	Candida (monilia) albicans (branching filaments with budding yeast-like cells)
Mucormycosis	Rhizopus (broad branching non-septate hyphæ rhizoids)
Sporotrichosis	Sporotrichium (resembles blastomycosis but demonstrated by cultures and not by smears)
Rhinosporidiosis	Rhinosporidium seeberi (tissues crowded with huge parasitic cysts)

uring 8 microns, but grows by nuclear division until it reaches a size of 200 to 300 microns and contains over 4000 nuclei which form 16,000 spores. The mature parasite, now called a sporangium, presents a double-contoured chitinous envelope with a germinal pore, through which the spores are discharged. The mode of infection and transmission is unknown.

REFERENCES

BAKER, R. D.: Am. J. Path., 1942, *18*, 479 (Blastomycosis).

————: J.A.M.A., 1957, *163*, 805. (Cerebral mucormycosis).

————: Am. J. Path., 1956, *32*, 287. (Pulmonary mucormycosis.)

CHRISTIE, A.: Ann. Int. Med., 1958, *49*, 544. (Disease spectrum of human histoplasmosis).

CONANT, N.F., et al.: Manual of Clinical Mycology, 2nd ed., Philadelphia, 1954.

COPE, V. Z.: Actinomycosis, London, 1938.

DICKSON, E. C.: J.A.M.A., 1938, *111*, 1362. (Coccidioidal granuloma).

LITTMAN, M. L.: Am. J. Med., 1959, *27*, 976. (Cryptococcosis).

LITTMAN, M. L. and ZIMMERMAN, L. E.: Cryptococcosis, New York, 1956.

SILVERMAN, F. N., SCHWARZ, J., LAKEY, M. E. and CARSON, R. P.: Am. J. Med., 1955, *19*, 410. (Histoplasmosis).

WEED, L. A., ANDERSEN, H. A., GOOD, C. A., and BAGGENSTOSS, A. H.: (Nocardiosis).

WINSLOW, D. J.: Am. J. Path., 1959, *35*, 153. (Botryomycosis).

Chapter 13

Viral and Rickettsial Infections

VIRUSES
General Considerations
  NATURE
  CELLULAR CHANGES
  IMMUNITY
  REPRODUCTION OF THE VIRUS
  SPREAD OF INFECTION
  CLASSIFICATION
Skin Infections
  SMALLPOX (VARIOLA)
  VACCINIA
  CHICKENPOX (VARICELLA)
  HERPES ZOSTER
  HERPES SIMPLEX
  MEASLES (RUBEOLA)

GERMAN MEASLES (RUBELLA)
MOLLUSCUM CONTAGIOSUM
WARTS
Respiratory Tract
  THE COMMON COLD
  INFLUENZA
  ADENOVIRUSES
  PSITTACOSIS
Nervous System
  POLIOMYELITIS
  RABIES
Viscerotropic
  YELLOW FEVER
  INFECTIVE HEPATITIS
    Serum Hepatitis

Miscellaneous
  MUMPS
  LYMPHOGRANULOMA VENEREUM
  CAT SCRATCH DISEASE
  CYTOMEGALIC INCLUSION
    DISEASE
  EPIDEMIC HEMORRHAGIC FEVER
RICKETTSIAL DISEASES
Typhus Fever
  TSUTSUGAMUSHI FEVER
  ROCKY MOUNTAIN SPOTTED
    FEVER
  TRENCH FEVER
  RICKETTSIAL POX
  Q FEVER

VIRUS DISEASES

GENERAL CONSIDERATIONS

It is not possible to give a concise and satisfying definition of a virus. It represents a most minute and primitive form of life. Even this statement may be questioned, for the virus seems to exist in the dim border-land between living things and chemical compounds. It is a submicroscopic unit containing nucleic acid and protein. Unlike bacteria, viruses are not capable of supporting life on their own owing to a lack of enzymes. In order to exist and multiply they must occupy living cells, which provide them with the necessary material and energy. For this purpose culture in the developing chick embryo (hen's egg) or in some tissue from that embryo is particularly suitable. It is evident that a virus is a perfect example of a parasite. Some viruses have a host-specificity, attacking only man, as in the case of measles and mumps, or only other animals or birds. Many also show a striking tissue-specificity, some being *neurotropic*, as in poliomyelitis, some *dermotropic*, as in smallpox, and some *viscerotropic*, as in hepatitis. The true nature of a virus is naturally a matter of opinion. Some regard a virus as an isolated gene, some as a mutant of a bacterium which has lost certain enzyme

(330)

systems, and some as representing the earliest and lowest form of life, which originally would require it to be saprophytic. The reader can take his choice.

Viruses may cause disease not only in man, but also in other mammals, birds, amphibia, fish, insects, plants and bacteria. We have already seen that they are capable of producing cancer in a number of laboratory animals and birds. The development and wide-spread use of antibiotics for the successful control of bacterial infections has served to bring those due to viruses into vivid prominence. Although Jenner long ago devised a prophylaxis against smallpox and Pasteur one against rabies, the existence of a *virus was first demonstrated* in 1892 by the Russian botanist Iwanowski, *in the case of tobacco mosaic*, a mottling of tobacco leaves. The *first demonstration of an animal viral disease* in 1898 was *foot-and-mouth* disease of cattle. This was quickly followed in 1901 by proof of the first virus disease in man, namely yellow fever. In 1918 came the greatest outbreak of infectious disease in the history of mankind, epidemic influenza, with an estimated 500 million cases of infection, 15 million of whom died. It was not until 1931, however, that the virus of influenza was isolated.

A quarter of a century ago medical virology was an academic subject, with few diagnostic tests which could only be done in a handful of centers. Since that time the most startling progress has been made, comparable with the advances made in bacteriology in the latter part of the 19th century, when nearly every year a new germ was discovered. A curious difficulty has arisen in that there are now more viruses than diseases. It used to be a matter of disease in search of a virus, as in the case of influenza. The situation is now reversed, and it is a case of viruses in search of a disease. Viruses in this forlorn condition are known as "orphan" viruses, a term to which we shall return presently. There are some 50 known viral diseases of man, but at least 150 different viruses have been recovered from man.

These advances, as so often happens, are due to the introduction of new methods of technique. A great impetus to the subject was given in 1930 by the demonstration of the viral etiology of influenza, but it was in the late 1940's that a new era dawned with two discoveries of extreme practical importance. (1) The demonstration in Albany, New York, that viruses would grow when inoculated into newborn mice, although not in mice more than a few days old, uncovered a whole new field of human pathogenic viruses, the so-called Coxsacki group, now known to cause several important and common diseases. (2) The discovery by Enders and his associates in Boston that the virus of poliomyelitis could be grown *in vitro* in tissue culture, whereas previously it could only be propagated in the brain of a live monkey. The most suitable medium proved to be epithelial cells of monkey kidney. The virus not only grows luxuriantly in these cells, but is also present in large quantity in the supernatant fluid. Moreover, the virus in the cells causes them to degenerate, a change which can readily be seen under the microscope. This is known as the *cytopathogenic effect*, and its great importance in offering a simple and rapid diagnostic method for detecting the presence of a virus will be at once apparent. The effect is inhibited by specific antiserum, so that antibody levels in the patient's blood can be measured by this technique. The tissue culture technique of Enders is also used for the development of vaccines, especially for

poliomyelitis and the adenoviruses. Many of the new viruses revealed by these recent culture methods appear to cause common diseases whose cause has hitherto remained obscure, such illnesses as conjunctivitis, febrile catarrh, sore throat, summer diarrhea, aseptic meningitis, *etc*. "This is indeed the golden age of virology, an age of exciting advances and stimulating challanges" (Rhodes).

Nature.—Viruses differ from bacteria not only in size. As a matter of fact they vary in size to a enormous degree, the largest approaching the dimensions of the smallest bacteria, while the smallest are little larger than the largest molecules. We used to refer to viruses as ultramicroscopic and filter-passing. Both of these terms are out-of-date. With the electron microscope one can now determine the shape of a virus and measure its exact size (Fig. 186). The filter-passing term was a crude expression of size, but some bacteria such as spirilla can also pass through the pores of a fine filter. Their outstanding characteristic is their inability to multiply unless they are within living cells. They are devoid of enzymes, so that they are dependent on the substance and energy of living cells for their reproduction. Unlike bacteria, they are unable to live and multiply on lifeless material like gelatin and agar. Their intracellular position makes them singularly difficult to attack, and the antibiotics and sulfonamides which are so effective against invading bacteria are valueless against the viruses.

All purified viruses are composed of a core of nucleic acid and a coating of protein, with the addition of lipids and carbohydrates in the case of animal viruses. Nucleic acid is the heart of the virus, it can attack and enter a cell and multiply there, but its activity is enormously increased by combination with protein.

When the nucleic acid component enters a bacterial cell it leaves its protein overcoat outside, and breaks into smaller units which are replicated a hundred times or so, acquiring a new protein overcoat from the cell before leaving its shelter. Apparently the same process is repeated in plant and animal viruses. Small wonder, then, that the multiplication of a virus is explosive in

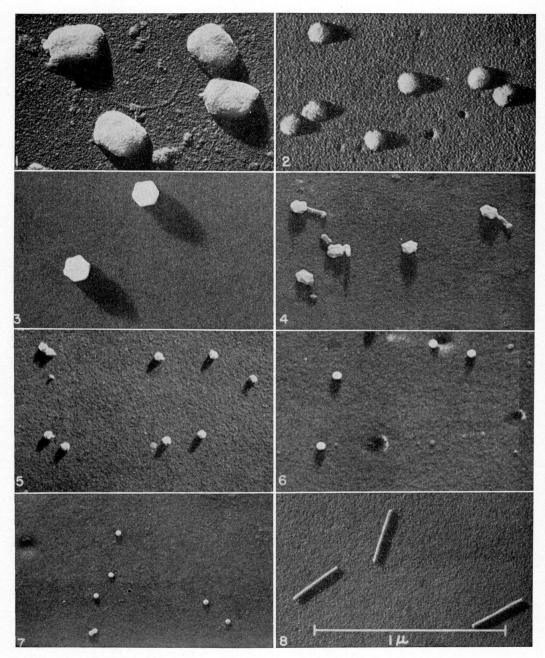

Fig. 186.—Electron micrographs of 8 viruses shown at the same magnification. × 50,000. 1, vaccinia virus; 2, PR8 influenza virus; 3, cytoplasmic virus of *Lipula* poludosa (R. C. Williams and K. M. Smith, unpublished); 4, T₄ bacteriophage; 5, T₃ bacteriophage; 6, Shope papilloma virus; 7, poliomyelitis virus 8, tobacco mosaic virus. Micrographs 3 to 7 shown frozen-dried preparations. (Micrographs by R. C. Williams, unpublished; virus preparation (1) by R. C. W.; (2), (6) and (8), by C. A. Knight; (4) and (5) by D. Fraser; (2) by C. E. Scheverdt and F. L. Schaffer, all of the Virus Laboratory, University of California, Berkeley. Rivers and Horsfall, *Viral and Rickettsial Diseases of Man*, courtesy of J. B. Lippincott Co.)

suddenness and rapidity. The virus of tobacco mosaic disease was first isolated by Stanley as crystallisable nucleoprotein which retained the properties of a virus, and since then many other viruses of plants, bacteria, animals and man have been isolated in chemically pure form, several in crystalline form, including the poliomyelitis and Coxsackie viruses.

Cellular Changes.—A virus may enter a cell and produce no change in structure or disturbance in function. This is seen in the enteric viruses and the adenoviruses; in both instances the agent may be demonstrated in apparently healthy persons, who therefore act as carriers. At the other extreme we have the explosive effects in the liver cells in yellow fever and in the anterior horn cells of the spinal cord in acute poliomyelitis. In some diseases there are *intracellular inclusion bodies* that are highly characteristic of virus infection. These bodies may be regarded as the fingerprints of a special and limited group of viruses, for viruses, like burglars, may act without leaving fingerprints. It is doubtful if all intracytoplasmic inclusions are necessarily an indication of virus infection. The inclusions may be cytoplasmic or intranuclear; sometimes both forms are present. In some diseases, such as fowl-pox, vaccinia and psittacosis, cytoplasmic inclusions consist of aggregates of virus particles, which when dispersed are known as *elementary bodies*. In other diseases, such as rabies and yellow fever, the status of the inclusion body is uncertain. Some "inclusions," particularly intranuclear ones, may represent products of degeneration. Inclusions represent the intracellular pathology of the virus diseases. The best-known examples are the Guarnieri bodies of smallpox (Fig. 187), the Negri bodies of rabies, the Lipschütz bodies of herpes, and the molluscum bodies of molluscum contagiosum They are also found in yellow fever, poliomyelitis, and psittacosis. The inclusion bodies were known long before filterable viruses were dreamt of, for the molluscum bodies were described in 1841.

Immunity.—Immunity to viral infections is extremely variable. Thus in smallpox, measles and chicken pox immunity is prolonged or permanent, whereas in the common

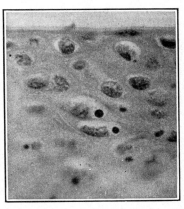

Fig. 187.—Inclusion bodies. The Guarnieri bodies of smallpox. (Kindness of Dr. J. Craigie.)

cold, influenza and herpes simplex the immunity is transitory, and the patient is liable to recurring attacks. The duration probably depends on the behaviour of the virus within the cells. If it produces rapid destruction of the cells, the virus is liberated into the blood stream in enormous numbers, and there is every opportunity for abundant antibody formation. If on the other hand growth in the cell extends over a prolonged period, antibody formation is inadequate. This seems likely in view of the fact that the virus persists in psittacosis, lymphogranuloma venereum and herpes simplex, yet there is a tendency to relapse and recurrences after physiological insults. In some cases of transient immunity, as with influenza and the common cold, the virus may actually be eliminated, for these are surface cell infections. The fact that antibodies to viruses are produced is utilized in the fluorescent labelled antibody technique of Coons, already mentioned in relation to bacterial and fungus infections. By this means the localization of the virus antigen in the target organ can be determined in some cases, *e.g.* the parotid gland in mumps, the respiratory epithelium in influenza, and the nerve cells in poliomyelitis.

Prolonged immunity is seen in smallpox and measles, where there is generalized infection and viremia, with overflow of the virus into the blood stream and secondary localization in the skin with production of the typical rash. In yellow fever and equine encephalitis, both of which are due to insect inoculation, the virus has to reach the liver and brain respectively by the blood stream, with the opportunity for antibody formation. Vaccination against smallpox, yellow fever and measles is effective, because the gamma globulins produced block the transport of any virus which may gain entrance to the blood.

Transient immunity may be due to a number of factors. In the case of influenza and the common cold the virus is localized in the ciliated cells of the respiratory epithelium which are essentially outside the vascular system, so that the virus does not enter the blood. Moreover, in respiratory virus infections we are dealing with multiple immunologic types, and several strains within each type. Even if immunity is developed, it is of no avail when the victim is exposed to infection by another strain of virus.

Reproduction of the Virus.—Reference has already been made to the question of the multiplication of virus. The matter is well illustrated by yellow fever, the first human disease to be recognized as viral in nature, for here the mosquito acts as an assistant investigator (Horsfall). The original observers, Walter Reed and J. Carroll, noticed in 1902 that mosquitoes were infective when they had sucked blood from human volunteers during the first 3 days of the disease, but not if they bit early in the incubation period or late in the disease. Moreover they did not become infective until a lapse of 12 days after biting, and they then remained infective for life. These findings were a mystery at that time, but their explanation has become simple. When an infected mosquito bites, naturally a very small amount of virus is introduced into the blood of the volunteer. This small amount promptly disappears, and does not reappear in the blood until just before the disease develops. During the incubation period the virus is multiplying in the cells of the liver, but it has disappeared from the blood, so that the mosquito itself does not become infected during the incubation period. When great numbers of liver cells are destroyed, clinical evidence of the disease develops, and

at the same time virus is poured in quantity into the blood, so that the mosquito becomes infected. After about the fourth day of the disease, neutralizing antibodies begin to appear in the blood, the virus begins to disappear, and when it has gone the biting mosquito no longer becomes infected.

The same series of events take place in the body of the mosquito. After the blood is swallowed the virus multiplies in the cells of the stomach and elsewhere. This process takes about 12 days, and it is only at the end of that period that the enormously multiplied virus reaches the salivary glands and so for the first time becomes infective for man. The mosquito does not develop neutralizing antibodies, so that it cannot rid itself of the virus and therefore remains infective for life. Moreover, in spite of the extensive reproduction of the virus, the tissues are not damaged and the mosquito remains in good health. Thus the puzzling though accurate observations made by Reed and Carroll in 1902 become readily understandable in the light of present-day knowledge.

The *incubation period* depends on two variables: (1) the number of cells initially infected, and (2) the rate of virus reproduction. The larger the number of cells initially infected, the shorter will be the incubation period, whilst the slower the rate of reproduction, the longer will be the period. The concentration of virus particles increases in infected tissue at a logarithmic rate, and reaches a high level before clinical evidence of infection becomes apparent.

The biochemical events which result in the synthesis of new virus particles have been investigated particularly in the case of bacterial viruses, with rather startling results. Bacteriophage particles are now known to resemble tiny sperms, with both a head and a tail-like structure. The shell of the head and tail are composed largely of protein, whilst inside the head there is nucleic acid, in this case entirely of the desoxyribose type. The tail penetrates the bacterial wall, and serves for the introduction of nucleic acid from the head, but the shell of the head and part of the tail are left outside. The phage-particle therefore disintegrates, merely adding nucleic acid to the bacterium. The latter soon stops synthesizing its own components and starts to manufacture nucleic acid and protein for the phage. Then heads without tails appear in the bacterial cytoplasm. Finally the entire phage is assembled, with the addition of the tail, and the introduction of nucleic acid into the head. It is evident that the bacterial virus toils not neither does it spin, for it has learned the art of living at someone else's expense. In participating in this remarkable process, however, the bacterium commits suicide.

There are undoubtedly some differences between the reproduction of animal viruses and that of bacterial viruses. Animal viruses are tiny spheres with no tails, and their nucleic acid may be either of the ribose (RNA) or desoxyribose (DNA) type, sometimes both. More important than these differences is the fact that reproduction of many animal viruses does not result in destruction of the cell, whereas with bacterial phage it does. The number of new particles released from the cell varies from a few to more than 1000, with the possibility of infecting 1000 other cells in the neighbourhood or at a distance. It is small wonder that viral hepatitis is diffuse, involving the entire liver, whereas bacterial lesions of the liver are localized.

The various stages of the cycle of infection have received descriptive and appropriate names. First there is *attachment* of the virus to the prospective host cell. During this phase the protein coat is shed. (2) Very soon *penetration* occurs through the cell wall. We have seen that in the case of bacteriophage the tail of the virus plays the part of a syringe through which the nucleic acid is injected. The *eclipse* phase in which the virus vanishes develops immediately after penetration due to the separation of protein and nucleic acid, so that no mature particles are seen immediately after infection. Two possible courses are now open. (1) There may be a *productive response*, with multiplication of the building materials provided by the cell, the formation of new particles, maturation of the virus, destruction of the cell, and liberation of 100 or 200 new virus particles. This is the action of a *virulent virus*. (2) There may be a *reductive response*, the nucleic acid becoming part of the bacterial

chromosomes, with no vegetative reproduction, so that the cell survives, although the genetic mechanism may be altered. This is what happens in the case of a *latent* or *temperate virus*.

It becomes evident, as Horsfall points out in his Mayo Foundation Lecture on this subject, that there is a world of difference between *viral infection* and *viral disease*. In viral infection multiplication proceeds without damage to the cell. In viral disease the cytopathic effect becomes evident, usually in the form of degeneration, occasionally as cell stimulation to abnormal growth in the case of tumor-inducing viruses. Viral infection is very much commoner than viral disease—indeed it may be universal. Thus poliovirus infection is many hundred times commoner than the disease, and adenovirus infection of the tonsils is present in about 90 per cent of normal persons, although disease caused by these viruses occurs in a very small percentage.

In viral infection a virus may sojourn indefinitely in the comfortable surroundings of the cell. It is more than a boarder, for it has become one of the family, and it can live with the family for generations without causing trouble. Various internal or external agents may upset the harmony and convert the latent virus into a virulent one, which usurps the cell's biosynthetic machinery for the production, almost exclusively, of viral progeny (Swartz and Littlefield). Such factors as age, genetic make-up, nutrition or hormonal balance may be responsible. So may bacterial infection, one of the best examples being the well-known relation between herpes simplex ("cold sore" on the lip) and pneumococcal pneumonia. Influenza is believed with reason to predispose the patient to respiratory tract bacterial infection, but it is also possible that such an infection may precipitate an attack of influenza through the conversion of a latent into an active virus.

It is now known that a protein is produced by virus-treated cells in tissue culture which is capable of inhibiting or interfering with the growth of many other viruses. This material has been named *interferon*, and it seems to have many of the properties of a viral antibiotic, so that we may hear more of it in the future (Isaacs and Burke). Recovery, as opposed to immunity, does not depend on the production of antibodies. The factors responsible for recovery are at present unknown.

The practical importance of the theoretical considerations which have just been outlined lies in the fact that as viral disease is dependent on viral reproduction, and as viral reproduction is dependent on biochemical processes, it may be possible to interfere with these processes and thus inhibit reproduction by chemical compounds. First steps in this direction have already been taken, but we have to face the unfortunate fact that by the time signs and symptoms of disease are apparent, reproduction of the virus is far advanced. It is evident that the control of viral diseases presents the same formidable obstacles as the control of cancer and for the same reason, namely that we are dealing with a disorder within the cell itself.

Spread of Infection.—Viral infection may reach the human subject in a variety of ways, which depend on the virus involved. Spread may be by *direct contact*, as in molluscum contagiosum, or by coitus, as in lymphogranuloma venereum. It may be due to *inhalation* of droplets, as in the common cold, influenza, and measles, or of dust from fomites, or from dried feces, as in psittacosis. *Bites* of animals, as in rabies, or of insects, as in yellow fever, may be responsible. Entry may be through *mucous membranes*, for instance the conjunctiva, as in trachoma, the mouth, as in mumps, the nasopharynx, as in measles and the common cold, the respiratory tract, as in influenza and psittacosis, the genital tract, as in lymphogranuloma venereum.

Having gained entrance, the virus may affect cells at the point of entry, or it may travel to susceptible cells by the blood, as in yellow fever, by the lymphatics, as in lymphogranuloma venereum, by the nerves as in herpes, poliomyelitis and rabies. It may cause hyperplasia of the infected cells, as in warts, or necrosis, as in yellow fever and poliomyelitis. Finally, it may produce cancer in a variety of animals.

Classification of Viruses.—Bacteria are classified by their shape (cocci, bacilli, spirilla), by their staining properties (gram-negative or positive), by their growth demands (aerobic or anaerobic), and so forth. The classification of viruses is much more difficult.

An obvious method of grouping is according to the target organ or tissue, coupled with similarity of action. The following system, with slight modification, is taken from Whitby and Britton's "Medical Bacteriology." I. *The Pox Group.* 1. Vaccinia, 2. Smallpox. II. *Neurotropic Viruses.* 1. Poliomyelitis. 2. Rabies. 3. Anthropod-transmitted encephalitis: (*a*) St. Louis encephalitis (*b*) Japanese encephalitis (*c*) Equine encephalitis (*d*) Aseptic meningitis. III. *Viscerotropic Viruses.* 1. Yellow fever. 2. Infectious hepatitis 3. Homologous serum hepatitis. IV. *The Herpes Group.* 1. Herpes simplex 2. Other members. V. *Varicella and Herpes Zoster.* VI. *The Myxoviruses Group (myxo* meaning mucus). 1. Mumps. 2. Influenza. 3. Newcastle disease of chickens. VII. *The Lymphogranuloma-Psittacosis Group.* 1. Lymphogranumola venereum. 2. Psittacosis. 3. Primary atypical pneumonia. 4. Trachoma. VIII. *Miscellaneous Viruses.* 1. Measles. 2. Rubella (German measles). 3. Coxsackie viruses. 4. Adenoviruses. 5. The common cold. 6. Warts. 7. Molluscum contagiosum. IX. *Bacteriophage.*

Before closing this discussion on classification brief reference may be made to some terms which have come into common usage, to indicate the large numbers of hitherto undescribed viruses which have been isolated from human material, largely as the result of the newer techniques such as tissue culture and the use of suckling mice. A fuller consideration of the subject will be found in the account of the various diseases caused by these agents in the second part of the book, but a word may not be out of place with reference to the meaning of some of the more unusual terms.

Adenoviruses.—At the end of 1953 a number of strains of viruses were isolated from adenoids removed surgically from children. This was followed immediately by the report of the cultivation of similar viruses from cases of acute respiratory disease. At least 18 serotypes are now known to cause catarrhal inflammation of the mucous membrane of the respiratory and ocular systems, with follicular enlargement of the submucous and regional lymphoid tissues. The varied illnesses which result are known by such descriptive names as *acute febrile pharyngitis, pharyngo-conjunctival fever, acute respiratory disease* (ARD), and some forms of *atypical pneumonia*.

Enteroviruses.—This is a large group of viruses cultured from the stools of infected persons. They include 3 forms of poliomyelitis virus, 20 ECHO viruses, and the Coxsackie viruses.

ECHO Viruses.—This strange-looking term is made up of the first letter of the four words, enteric, cytopathogenic, human and orphan. *Enteric* signifies the intestinal site of the infection. *Cytopathogenic* indicates that degenerative changes are observed in the cells of tissue cultures. *Human* simply tells us that these are infectious of man. *Orphan* is the expression referred to earlier as denoting that at one time these viruses seemed to be orphans looking for a disease by which they might become adopted. This group gives rise to transitory infections of the alimentary canal, particularly in children, which are not comparable to infections with the enteric bacteria that may be lifelong residents of the intestinal tract.

Coxsackie Viruses.—These constitue a large family including 30 distinct types. They are named for the village on the Hudson River in New York State where the virus was first isolated by Dalldorf in 1947 from a patient with poliomyelitis. The main biological character of these viruses is that they are pathogenic for *suckling mice*, not for older animals nor for monkeys.

The *Coxsackie family of viruses*, best isolated from the stools, can be divided into two main groups, A and B. These viruses appear to play an important role in the causation of such diversified human diseases as aseptic meningitis, epidemic pleurodynia (Bornholm disease), acute benign pericarditis, acute myocarditis (especially in newborn infants), herpangina, polio-like illnesses, and vague flu-like conditions. These varied maladies are discussed in Chapter 42 in reference to diseases of the nervous system. Like poliomyelitis, these virus diseases occur mainly during the late summer and early fall months (July to October, with the peak incidence in August and September). In an epidemic area there is a high attack rate and a high family incidence.

Reference has already been made to the phenomenon of *virus interference*, the presence of one virus disease in a community preventing or modifying disease caused by other viruses. In 1931 there occurred in Sweden a large epidemic of pleurodynia, believed to be due to Coxsackie B virus infection. During the same year the incidence of severe or fatal poliomyelitis was the lowest recorded for a 20-year period. In the laboratory, infection with the same virus prevents or delays muscle paralysis in mice inoculated with the poliomyelitis virus.

The student who has not the leisure to peruse the special treatises devoted to viral diseases will find an excellent account of recent work in a symposium on viruses and viral infections in Modern Medicine, October, 1958, pages 67 to 123.

We may now turn to a consideration of some of the principal examples of virus diseases. These will be discussed under the headings of the principal tissue involved, namely (1) skin, (2) respiratory tract, (3) nervous system, (4) liver, and (5) miscellaneous.

SKIN

The *pox group* of viruses are large, chemically complex organisms, with a primary affinity for the skin, in which they produce a vesico-pustular eruption. In the Middle Ages, when diseases began to be named, there were four types of pox or pocks. These were known as the Great Pox (syphilis), the Small Pox (Variola), Cow Pox (vaccinia —from *vacca*, a cow), and Chicken Pox (varicella), so-called because the chicken typified something gentle and mild. But when the virus of chickenpox attacks the nervous system with resulting herpes zoster and in rare cases encephalitis, it is far from chicken-like. In addition to the human poxes (variola and varicella), there are a number of animal poxes. The viruses grow readily in the developing chick embryo (chorioallantoic membrane), producing well-developed pocks, and the vaccinia virus was one of the first to be grown in tissue culture. The pox viruses develop in epithelial cells into large intracytoplasmic eosinophilic inclusions, the *Guarnieri bodies* (Fig. 187). The chickenpox virus does not belong to this group. It cannot be transmitted to animals, it does not grow in the chicken embryo, and inclusion bodies are intranuclear rather than cytoplasmic.

Smallpox.—Smallpox or *variola* is an acute infectious fever characterized by the formation of "pocks" or pustules in the skin. Headache and persistent pain in the back are characteristic symptoms. After an incubation period of ten to twelve days the skin lesions appear and slowly develop. At first they are papules, in the course of a few days these become vesicles, and the vesicles are converted into pustules, over which scabs are formed. Healing occurs under the scabs or crusts, but when these are cast off a scar may be left. The depth of the scar depends on whether or not the destructive process has reached the cutis vera. The disease is extraordinarily contagious, the infection being conveyed by the discharge from the lesions and by the crusts. This may happen from personal contact, from contact with clothing or possessions of the patient, or by air transmission, the virus being carried on particles of dust from the scabs. Before the introduction of vaccination the disease used to be as common as measles. It was seen mostly in children, because a previous attack bestowed on adults a permanent immunity. Macaulay with characteristic rhetoric speaking of 17th Century England paints this picture: "The small pox was always present, filling the church yards with corpses, tormenting with constant fears all whom it had not yet stricken, leaving on those whose lives it spared the hideous traces of its power, turning the babe into a changeling at which the mother shuddered, and making the eyes and cheeks of the betrothed maiden objects of horror to the lover." The student may be interested to know that Gray of *Gray's Anatomy* was killed by smallpox in England at the age of 34, one hundred years ago.

Alastrim is a form of smallpox met with principally in South America. It differs from smallpox in having a very low mortality,

but is probably a variant of that disease due to the same cause.

Lesions.—Only some of the lesions of smallpox are specific, *i.e.*, are due to the virus itself. The others are due to the secondary streptococcal infection which seems to occur in every case. The streptococci are responsible for the pustular lesions, and usually for the death of the patient. The specific lesions are the papules and vesicles of the skin. The virus is epitheliotropic and multiplies in the epidermis. There is a peculiar degeneration of the epithelial cells which become swollen (ballooning) and undergo liquefaction. The change is more marked at the periphery of the lesion, so that the edges are raised, giving the center a sunken or umbilicated appearance. There is a fluid exudate in the vesicular stage, but this is clear and almost free of cells. When suppuration occurs it is crowded with pus cells. In the vesicular stage there are abundant plasma cells in the tissues, but in the pustular stage these are replaced by polymorphonuclear leukocytes. The Guarnieri bodies have already been described. The mucous membranes of the mouth and nose show the same lesions as the skin. In the internal organs there are lesions of focal necrosis (liver, kidney, heart) due to the secondary infection. Inflammatory necrotic nodules in the testicle are common. Death is often due to bronchopneumonia.

Vaccinia.—As the name implies this is a condition caused by a virus originally derived from cowpox (*vacca*, a cow), and now maintained by alternate passage from the calf to the rabbit. The live virus is used for immunization against smallpox, as even the most massive doses of killed or inactivated viruses of the pox group are ineffective.

Vaccination of the non-immune with the vaccine lymph is followed in the course of 4 days by the appearance of a papule which becomes vesicular on the next day. By the eighth day the vesicle becomes a pustule, the surrounding skin being red and hot, and the regional lymph nodes enlarged and tender. The inflammation begins to subside on the tenth day, and by the end of three weeks healing is complete with scarring.

Generalized vaccinia is fortunately rare,

although the virus always circulates in the blood. Usually the constitutional disturbance is mild, with a few scattered vesicles, but in the rare and tragic case it is fatal, resembling fulminating smallpox. In such a case the child evidently has no natural resistance, and there is a complete absence of the circulating antibody which should develop after successful vaccination giving immunity. *Post-vaccinal encephalitis* is another rare but often fatal complication. It is a form of post-infection encephalitis, and will be discussed in relation to diseases of the nervous system.

Chickenpox (Varicella).—This is a mild but extremely infectious viral disease of childhood. Immunity is life-long. The vesicles frequently do not develop into pustules. In spite of the name, the virus is not related to the pox group but is identical with the virus of herpes zoster. Indeed it has become customary to speak of the varicella-zoster group, and to regard the clinical syndromes as merely two phases in the activity of a single virus. Adults have acquired herpes zoster a few days after exposure to children with varicella, and the occasional person develops varicella following exposure to a patient with herpes. It is suggested that a person may become only partially immune to the virus by virtue of a previous attack of chickenpox, and develop herpes zoster on reexposure in later life. The primary lesion in varicella is in the upper respiratory tract, where elementary bodies can be seen in the early stages. The vesicles appear in successive groups over the same area of skin, so that lesions of different ages are found in the same area. The lesions are more marked over the trunk, than on the face and limbs, differing in that respect from smallpox. Acidophilic intranuclear inclusions develop at an early stage, with ballooning and degeneration of the cells. Encephalitis is a rare complication. Death is very rare, in spite of the development of complications.

Herpes Zoster.—As we have just seen, the virus causing this condition is closely related to or the same as that of varicella. The disease is marked by severe nerve-root pains usually passing in zonal fashion around the trunk (hence the name), and by the development of vesicles similar to those of varicella along the course of the nerves, the condition known as *shingles*. The primary lesion seems to be in the dorsal root ganglia of the spinal nerves, but the virus is also present in the vesicles. The ganglia are infiltrated with mononuclear cells, the nerve cells degenerate and disappear, with myelin degeneration of the sensory nerve fibers, whilst intranuclear inclusions similar to those of varicella may be seen in the vesicles.

Herpes Simplex.—The virus responsible for this condition is one of the most widely distributed in the general population. The reason for this is that after the initial attack the virus continues to be harbored in the cells in a latent stage. It often escapes from the buccal mucosa of healthy persons into the saliva, and the infection is transmitted by close contact, as in kissing.

The characteristic lesions are on the skin and mucous membranes, particularly the mucocutaneous junctions such as the lips. The primary infection may be without symptoms, but in childhood there are usually marked lesions in the mouth and a considerable general reaction. In adults the primary infection may resemble mild smallpox. As a result of the primary infection, neutralizing antibodies appear in the blood and persist during life. The virus continues to multiply in the epithelial cells without causing symptoms, but if the resistance is lowered by other infections secondary attacks of herpes may occur from the latent virus, with the production of crops of herpetic vesicles at the mucocutaneous border. An interesting commentary on the relation between some debilitating influence and activation of the virus is the use of the common names "cold sore" and "fever blister" for the herpetic vesicles.

As with the other viruses we have been considering, a viral encephalitis may occasionally be caused by the virus of herpes simplex.

Measles (Rubeola).—Measles because of its extreme contagiousness is one of the commonest diseases in the world. A second attack is extremely rare. Contagion is due to direct exposure to a case of the disease with inhalation of infected material. The experimental injection of infected blood into human volunteers and monkeys has been

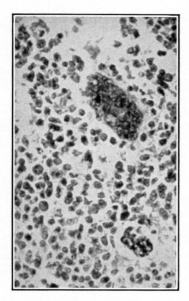

FIG. 188.—Tonsil in measles. × 360.   FIG. 189.—Appendix in measles. × 360.

successful in producing the disease. It must be noted, however, that many monkeys possess measles neutralizing antibody, so that inoculation with the virus may not produce symptoms. Monkeys brought direct from the forests of Malaya and the Philippines develop symptoms of measles on inoculation. It would appear that natural dissemination of the virus from man to monkey and from animal to animal occurs during collection, transportation and acclimatization.

The immunity following an attack of measles is associated with the presence of immune bodies in the serum, and these can be used as a means of treatment and prevention. Measles is an outstanding example of a virus disease, which can be controlled by immune serum therapy. The immune serum may prevent or modify an attack. Prevention can be even better achieved by the use of live attentuated vaccine (Katz *et al.*) As measles kills twice as many children in the United States as does poliomyelitis, the importance of prevention is self-evident.

The chief *symptoms* are fever, the characteristic rash (macular lesions which later become maculo-papular), and evidence of an acute catarrhal infection of the upper res-

piratory tract and eyes. The commonest complication is bronchopneumonia.

In the *skin* the chief change is a round-cell infiltration about the blood vessels, hair follicles, and sweat glands. In the deeper layers of the epidermis there are areas of colloid degeneration of the epithelial cells passing into coagulation necrosis. These areas are surrounded by fibrin and leukocytes, and are probably due to the direct action of the virus on the epithelium.

The *mucous membrane* of the mouth and upper respiratory tract shows catarrhal inflammation. In the mouth the epithelium is thickened and in places shows foci of fatty degeneration, giving rise to the white dot which forms the center of the *Koplik spots*, the pathognomonic sign of measles.

The *lungs* of fatal cases nearly always show bronchopneumonia. This should be regarded as a complication rather than as an essential lesion. If the patient recovers from the bronchopneumonia he may develop an acute form of pulmonary tuberculosis due to the lowered resistance produced by the virus.

The *lymph nodes* and *spleen* may be swollen, but never to any great extent. A peculiar *giant-cell formation* may occur in lymphoid tissue. This has been observed in the *tonsils* (Fig. 188) and in the *appendix* (Fig. 189) in the prodromal stage, probably about seven days before the rash. The multinucleated giant cells seem to correspond to the inclusion bodies of other virus diseases, and may be regarded as a specific response to the virus of measles. They are found in the lymphoid tissue throughout the body in the prodromal phase of the disease (Roberts and Bain). Monkeys injected with blood from measles patients show giant cells in the lymph nodes (Gordon and Knighton). The spleen is seldom palpable. The *liver* often shows areas of focal necrosis. The *brain* may be the seat of a meningo-encephalitis, a lesion which will be described in connection with that disease. The *blood* shows a characteristic *leukopenia*, a frequent manifestation of viral diseases, due to a diminution in the number of polymorphonuclear leukocytes. This forms a striking contrast to the leukocytosis of scarlet fever.

In the *giant-cell pneumonia* of infants and young children, which is an interstitial pneumonitis characterized by multinucleated giant cells containing intranuclear and intracytoplasmic inclusions, measles virus has been demonstrated by means of human renal-cell culture (Enders *et al.*). In these cases there are no signs or symptoms of measles. It is known that pneumonitis may follow the subsidence of the clinical evidence of measles, the virus being found at autopsy. The interest of the observations on giant-cell pneumonia lies in the demonstration that a virus may persist and be the cause of severe and progressive illness for considerable periods after the initial infection, perhaps as the result of depression of antibody formation.

German Measles (Rubella). — German measles or rubella is an extremely mild infection marked by a slight degree of fever, a rash resembling that of measles, and a characteristic enlargement of the lymph nodes. The disease is less common than measles in children, with the result that persons in early adult life are more likely to be infected.

Although the constitutional disturbances are apparently so trivial, rubella in a young woman during the first trimester of pregnancy may have far from trivial results for

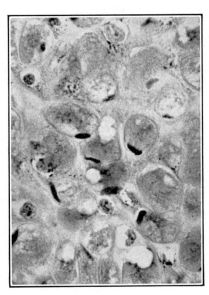

FIG. 190.—Molluscum bodies.   × 500.

the offspring who often exhibit congenital malformations. In some series the incidence has been as high as 90 per cent. The principal lesions are *cardiac malformations*, *microcephaly, deafness* and *cataract*. From the point of view of the pathologist the all-important fact is that *a very real relationship exists between congenital heart disease in the child and the occurrence of rubella in the mother during the first three months of pregnancy*. It must also be borne in mind that in those cases of congenital heart disease in which no history of maternal rubella can be elicited, the infection may have been present in subclinical form or not diagnosed. How the virus produces these effects on the developing fetus is quite unknown.

It is evident that a woman in the first trimester of pregnancy must be carefully guarded against infection. Unfortunately the recognition of rubella apart from an epidemic may be far from easy, because of the trivial character of the illness in a child with whom the pregnant woman may come in contact, for there may be no fever, and the rash may be the first evidence that the child is sick. Indeed rubella is a unique example of a viral disease in which it might be well to ensure that young girls are exposed to the infection before they reach the child-bearing age.

Molluscum Contagiosum.—This is a contagious viral lesion of the skin marked by the development of small, white nodules chiefly in children. The prickle cells of the skin are greatly enlarged and contain hyaline inclusion bodies known as *molluscum bodies* (Fig. 190). These represent masses of elementary bodies. The condition is described in connection with diseaases of the skin.

Warts.—These transient skin lesions are believed to be caused by a virus, as the condition can be transmitted by filtrates. The lesion provides an example of pure hyperplasia unmodified by necrosis.

RESPIRATORY TRACT

A large number of viruses may attack various parts of the respiratory tract. Many of these will be considered in detail in Chapter 24. A few will be referred to here.

The Common Cold.—Common colds seem to be caused by a number of viruses, or at any rate by a number of strains. The infection can be transmitted to volunteers by means of filtrates of nose and throat washings from patients. The virus can be grown on tissue of human and monkey embryo kidney, in which it produces recognizable degenerative changes, a technical advance of the first importance (Tyrrell *et al.*). No animal is susceptible. Immunity is remarkably transient, and reinfection with the same virus can take place within three weeks after recovery. Contributory factors such as chilling of the body or sitting in a draught are of course of major importance, but none of these can produce a cold in the absence of the virus. The lesions of the common cold are described on page 623.

Influenza.—Influenza is the most puzzling of all the infectious diseases. It is usually the mildest of infections, lightly referred to as "a touch of the flu." At long intervals it suddenly assumes a virulent form, and like "a blast from the stars" great epidemics and pandemics sweep across the world killing millions of people. At such times, as in the 1918–1919 pandemic, it seems that "the

Angel of Death is abroad in the land; you can almost hear the beating of his wings." During that pandemic 500,000,000 were attacked and 15,000,000 were killed, more than were killed amongst all the combatants in World War I.

Etiology.—At the end of the great pandemic of 1889–1892 Pfeiffer found a minute gram-negative hemophilic bacillus in the sputum and bronchial passages of influenzal patients, and concluded that this must be the cause of the disease, so that it became known as Bacillus influenzæ. It has now been established that epidemic influenza is caused by a virus, or rather by at least two A and B, of which A is by far the commoner; B has only been found in small isolated outbreaks. The two viruses are perfectly distinct, as shown by neutralization tests with immune serum. None of the ordinary laboratory animals are susceptible to direct inoculation from man, but in 1933 Smith, Andrewes and Laidlaw showed that ferrets are susceptible and also swine. After passage through the ferret white mice can be infected by instillation into the nostrils. Ferret infection is contagious whereas mouse infection is not. The explanation of the difference is simple; the ferret sneezes and the mouse does not. Pneumonia only occurs after either anesthesia or after repeated passage through ferrets. The solid lung is bacteriologically sterile, but rich in virus. The virus responsible for the great 1918 pandemic can no longer be isolated from man. It has vanished. It used to be believed that the virus passed into swine, causing the swine influenza which appeared in 1918, and that it survives in swine though dying out in man. Unfortunately this pretty theory has now had to be abandoned.

Both A and B viruses can be grown in tissue cultures and also on the chick embryo (fertile egg), which they kill within three days, the virus being increased one million times in the course of two days. Suspensions of the virus are highly toxic to mice, apparently due to an endotoxic-like action. It seems probable that the profound prostration of severe epidemic influenza, from which some of us have suffered, is due to a similar action. The virus, which is strictly limited to the respiratory epithelium, does not penetrate any deeper nor enter the blood stream.

Hemagglutination of the red cells of the fowl, man, and the guinea pig is produced by dilute suspensions of the virus, whereas the red cells of the mouse, rabbit, sheep and ox are relatively insusceptible. The virus particles attach themselves to specific receptor groups of two or more red cells, and so bring them together in agglutination. Hemagglutination is inhibited by a known antiserum, and the hemagglutination inhibition test is sharply specific in differentiating between closely related strains.

The part which other organisms may play in association with a virus is well illustrated by Shope's work on swine influenza. This disease can be produced experimentally in pigs by means of a filterable virus acting in conjunction with Hemophilus influenzæ suis, a small hemophilic organism which is present in the natural disease, but is quite unable to induce the disease by itself when inoculated intranasally. The virus alone was unable to produce the typical disease, but did cause an exceedingly mild infection which was contagious. The combination of the comparatively innocent virus and a culture of H. suis produced severe and typical lesions, so that it appeared as if the virus conferred powers of invasion on H. suis. Some such coordinated mechanism may be at work in human influenza.

Lesions.—The lesions of fatal cases of influenza will be described in connection with diseases of the respiratory system. It may be said here that in all cases the essential lesion seems to be an acute inflammation of the upper respiratory tract, commencing in the nasopharynx, affecting the sphenoidal and other air sinuses, and passing down to cause a tracheobronchitis. Patches of interstitial pneumonia with mononuclear collections in the bronchial walls similar to those in measles form a characteristic feature. The influenzal pneumonia with great hemorrhagic edema in the pulmonary alveoli which is so frequently seen at autopsy is probably due to secondary invaders.

Attempts at the prevention and treatment of influenza have been singularly disappointing and frustrating. Vaccines of killed virus have been used in large-scale trials. These have temporarily raised the antibody level in the circulating blood, but of what value is this against a virus which never penetrates below the surface layers of cells and is never exposed to contact with the blood stream? Antibiotics and chemotherapeutic agents are without effect on the virus, although they may be life-saving by destroying secondary invaders.

A point of academic, although not at present of practical, interest is the *inhibitory action of brain ganglioside* on the neurotoxic (convulsive) effect of influenza viruses on the mouse brain (Bogoch *et al.*). It also suppresses the development of hemagglutinins in tissue culture. The inhibition of the neurotoxic effect may be a competitive one, the other competitor for the virus being the brain ganglioside in the nerve cells. As might be expected, once the virus has penetrated the cell, the added brain ganglioside can no longer compete.

Adenoviruses.—The new and rather bewildering group of viruses originally removed from excised adenoids and later found to be responsible for common infections in the upper respiratory tract and conjunctiva has been referred to on page 336. Perhaps a more descriptive and inclusive term is the *adenoidal-pharyngeal-conjunctival group.*

Psittacosis.—This is a viral disease of South American parrots and parakeets (*psittakos*, parrot), often known as parrot fever, which may be transmitted to man. When a pandemic occurs among the birds, small epidemics are certain to appear in the countries to which the parrots are exported. Canaries and finches in contact with parrots may acquire the infection. Ducks, chickens, turkeys and pigeons may be infected with similar viruses. Viral disease in birds other than parrots is known as *orinthosis* (*ornis*, bird). Unfortunately birds may carry the virus and be infective without showing any evidence of disease. Man to man infection may occur, but is not common. The last notable epidemic occurerd in 1929–1930 in many parts of Europe and America, but even in epidemic periods the disease is really rare. It is extremely infective for laboratory workers investigating the disease, even though they have not come in actual contact with diseased birds. The virus is present in the nasal discharge and feces of infected birds, contaminates the air in the vicinity of the cages, and is inhaled by persons in the vicinity.

The virus grows well in tissue culture and in the chick embryo. It thrives in reticulo-endothelial or epithelial cells. When an elementary body enters a cell the body quickly becomes enlarged, and soon begins to divide into a large number of particles which form a large aggregated mass or inclusion body filling most of the cytoplasm. Rupture of the cell results in the discharge of enormous numbers of elementary bodies. The condition is accompanied by viremia, so that lesions are found in the reticulo-endothelial cells of several of the viscera.

Lesions.—The chief lesions are in the lungs. There is patchy pneumonia, but with very little fibrin in the exudate and no fibrinous pleurisy. The really character-istic lesion, however, is a remarkable swelling of the epithelium lining the alveoli and a proliferation of the cells as indicated by numerous mitotic figures. The proliferated cells may become desquamated and form characteristic clumps and plugs in the alveoli. Apart from this the human lesions are not characteristic, for they are very varied, due probably to secondary infections. In inoculated mice foci of necrosis are found in the spleen and liver. The bronchioles are filled with an exudate which blocks the lumen and causes areas of collapse to be formed. Elementary body inclusions have been described in the endothelial cells of the lung, liver and spleen in parrots which have died of the disease. Other lesions in the body are a moderate degree of enlargement of the spleen and congestion of the internal organs.

NERVOUS SYSTEM

There is a large and rather indefinite group of *neurotropic viruses* which produce encephalitis, meningoencephalitis, and en-cephalomyelitis, that is to say, inflammation of the brain, meninges and spinal cord. The infection is confined to the central nervous system. Two diseases of the nervous system, however, stand out clearly from the view-point of virology. These are poliomyelitis and rabies.

Poliomyelitis.—The name suggests that this is an infection of the gray matter (*polios*, grey) of the spinal cord. The usual result of infection with the virus, however, is either a symptomless carrier state or a mild and transient infection with fever and symptoms pointing to the upper respiratory or the gastrointestinal tracts. Or these symptoms may be followed in a few days by meningism and changes in the spinal fluid indicative of inflammation. This is called *non-paralytic poliomyelitis.* In a few, per-haps less than 1 per cent of all cases of infection, the condition progresses to frank paralysis, indicating invasion and destruc-tion of the motor nerve cells in the anterior horn of the spinal cord.

The virus grows readily in culture of both human and monkey tissues. One of the best culture media is the HeLa strain of epithelial cells, so-called because they were originally derived from a cervical carcinoma in a woman with this abreviated name, Helen La. In these cells the virus produces a cyto-pathogenic effect. This effect is neutralized by specific immune sera, thus providing a method of typing unknown strains. The virus does not grow in the chick embryo.

The poliomyelitis virus may belong to one of three types, which differ antigenically. These are named the *Brunhilde type* or Type I, which comprises the majority of epidemic strains and can be transmitted only to the monkey; the *Lansing type* or Type 2, which is present in sporadic cases and can be transmitted to mice as well as to the monkey; the *Leon type* or Type 3, of minor importance, capable of being trans-mitted to the monkey, but differing anti-genically from the Brunhilde type.

Mode of Infection.—The virus is present both in the nasopharynx and in the feces of patients and also of contacts. It is evident, therefore, that infection may be acquired either by inhalation or ingestion. For long it was taught that the virus reached the central nervous system by way of peri-pheral nerves and along the olfactory tract. It has been shown, however, that a viremia precedes invasion of the nervous system in monkeys and it now appears probable that infection usually spreads to the spinal cord by the blood stream. The heavy infection of the feces supports this view, an infection which is present in varying degree in contacts. Sewage is therefore readily infected, and in this material the virus may survive for several months.

As infection with the virus is so common, and as the viremia which accompanies it gives rise to the production of neutralizing antibodies, it follows that the serum of most adults contains such antibodies. Human gamma globulin has therefore been used in prophylaxis in individual cases. Much more effective, of course, is inoculation with the *Salk vaccine*, made by growing the virus in tissue culture of monkey kidney, followed by killing with formol. The oral administration of attenuated live virus may prove to give even better immunization.

Rabies.— Rabies or hydrophobia is a disease affecting animals (carnivora, *e.g.*, dog, wolf) and man. The infection is transmitted to man by the bites of rabid animals, the infective agent being excreted in the saliva. The incubation period is fortunately remarkably long, usually over two months, and in rare cases as long as a year. This gives time for preventive treatment. The length of the incubation period depends on the position of the bite, being very much shorter in bites of the face and head than in bites of the leg, for a reason that will be apparent shortly. The principal symptoms are cerebral irritation, pharyngeal spasm especially at the sight of water so that the patient is unable to drink, (hence the name, *hydrophobia*), and generalized convulsions. *Rabies has the worst reputation of any virus*, and the disease is invariably fatal unless preventive treatment is employed. There is no proved instance of recovery.

Etiology.—Rabies is caused by a filterpassing agent which is neurotropic, so that the true lesion is in the nerve cells of the brain. The virus is also present in salivary and other glands. The disease can be produced by inoculating an emulsion of the brain of a rabid animal into the subcutaneous tissue of another animal. It may, if wished, first be passed through a Berkefeld filter. As the symptoms are cerebral it is evident that the virus must pass from the site of inoculation to the brain along the peripheral nerves. It is for this reason that the incubation period is long for bites on the foot, short for bites on the head; it is all a question of how far the virus has to travel. Once the virus reaches the central nervous system it is rapidly disseminated throughout the brain and spinal cord.

Lesions.—There are no naked eye changes apart from congestion of the gray matter of the brain and cord. Microscopically there is cell degeneration, phagocytosis of the degenerating cells, and collars of inflammatory cells (lymphocytes and plasma cells) around the small blood vessels. The pathognomonic feature is the presence of *Negri bodies*. These are inclusion bodies varying much in size found in the cytoplasm of the ganglion cells in the hippocampus major as well as in the cells of the medulla, cerebellum, *etc*. They are acidophilic bodies with a blue center. The basophilic material probably represents virus, whilst the outer acidophilic material may be a host-tissue product. When a dog suspected of rabies has bitten a person, the dog's brain must be examined for Negri bodies. The most rapid method is to take a cover-glass impression of the cut surface of the hippocampus major, but a more certain method is to stain sections. When Negri bodies are not found in the dog's brain, some of the tissue should be injected intracerebrally into white mice before concluding that the dog was not rabid.

Preventive Inoculation.—It is rather strange that the modern treatment of rabies is that introduced by Pasteur who had never heard of filterable viruses or Negri bodies. Pasteur found that the spinal cord of animals infected with the disease was rich in the virus, as shown by the results of animal inoculation. He also found that he could lower the virulence of the virus by the simple expedient of hanging up the cord and allowing it to dry. By drying a series of cords for varying lengths of time he obtained a series of viruses of varying virulence. Treatment is of no use once the symptoms have manifested themselves, but Pasteur availed himself of the very long incubation period which is so striking a feature of the disease. He found that if inoculation with attenuated virus was commenced within five days of receiving the bite it was successful in nearly 100 per cent of the cases, that is to say there was complete prevention. This is surely an extraordinary *tour de force* for the earliest days of modern bacteriology.

VISCEROTROPIC

Yellow Fever.—Yellow fever is primarily a disease of monkeys and other jungle animals, but it is readily transmitted to man. It is an acute infection with high fever, acute nephritis, hemorrhages in the skin and from the stomach and bowels, and jaundice. It occurs in certain endemic centers in Central and South America and in West Africa which in the past have served as starting-points of epidemics. The American centers have been almost completely controlled, but that is far from being true of West Africa, where both Stokes and Noguchi died of yellow fever while investigating the disease. Of course we must remember that the airplane can carry mosquitoes as well as passengers. The mortality is above 60 per cent, but if recovery takes place a permanent immunity is established. The virus is transmitted from one person to another by a mosquito, *Stegomyia fasciata* (Aedes aegypti). Twelve days must elapse before the mosquito becomes infective for another person. The story of the Reed Commission which worked out the method of transmission, and of General Gorgas who waged war on the stegomyia and cleansed Havana and Panama of yellow fever after they had been infested for centuries, is one of the romances of medicine.

The virus can be grown in tissue culture containing mouse embryonic tissue. Infection is naturally readily conveyed to the monkey. Before this was known, human volunteers had to be used by the Reed Commission in order to prove that the mosquito was the carrier of the infection. Lazear, one of the volunteers, died as the result of the experiment. Young mice are also easily infected by any route, but adult mice can only be infected by the intracerebral or intranasal route. In both young and adult mice the virus will only multiply in nervous tissue. Rats and rabbits are completely resistant. No killed vaccine confers immunity, but a living virus highly attenuated and rendered neurotropic by repeated passage through the brains of mice is effective. Diagnosis of the disease in man can be made by intracerebral inoculation of the serum into mice. If the mouse dies of encephalitis, the test is positive.

Lesions.—These serve to explain very completely the clinical symptoms. The virus attacks the capillaries, the liver, and the kidneys, so that there are hemorrhages, jaundice, and marked urinary disturbances. There is hemorrhage into the stomach, thus giving the "black vomit" which is so characteristic of the later stages. The intestine may be full of blood. There are hemorrhages in the myocardium, endocardium and epicardium. The most characteristic of all the lesions is the *Councilman body* of the liver. This is a non-inflammatory hyaline necrosis affecting many liver cells and forming a dense acidophilic mass in the cytoplasm. As the condition advances areas of necrosis are produced and the bile passages are ruptured with escape of the bile into the blood, but it is the early discrete lesion which is really characteristic. Intranuclear acidophilic inclusion bodies have been described in the liver cells in both the human and the experimental disease (Hoffmann). There is an extensive necrosis of the renal epithelium, so that the convoluted tubules are blocked with necrotic cells; the marked albuminuria, abundant casts, and final anuria are natural sequelae, and they are among the worst prognostic signs. The spleen is of normal size, but shows a striking loss of lymphocytes. Congestion and hemorrhages in the lungs are common.

Infective Hepatitis.—This common epidemic disease is now known to be viral in nature, and the virus has now been cultivated on tissue culture (Rightsel *et al.*). It is present in the blood and feces during the acute phase of the disease, as has been shown by administering infective material to human volunteers by feeding and intravenous injection. Neutralizing antibodies to the virus can be shown to be present in great numbers of the general population, showing that subclinical infection must be widespread.

Serum Hepatitis.—This is a viral liver disturbance similar to that which we have just considered, but transmitted by blood transfusions, the injection of plasma, or even the use of an inadequately sterilized needle in a doctor's or dentist's office. It is believed that in some 1 per cent of apparently healthy individuals the virus responsible for this form of hepatitis circulates in the blood, unable to do harm because of the immunity which has developed. If, however, contaminated whole blood or plasma is injected into a non-immune person, hepatitis results. The infection may be conveyed by a needle which has been used first on a carrier and then on a virus-free non-immune individual, if the needle has not been sufficiently sterilized, *which is by no means easy.* The danger of using blood from a large pool is self-evident. The virus is not the same as the virus of infectious hepatitis, for there is no cross-immunity between the two diseases, and the incubation period of serum hepatitis is from sixty to one hundred and twenty days, compared with that of infectious hepatitis, which is ten to forty days.

The lesions, symptoms and possible sequelæ of viral hepatitis are discussed in Chapter 28.

MISCELLANEOUS

Mumps.—Mumps or epidemic parotitis is caused by a virus which can be demonstrated in the saliva. The lesions produced by the virus are epithelial necrosis and round cell infiltration of the interstitial tissue of the parotid gland and occasionally of other salivary glands. Inflammation of the testis (orchitis) occurs occasionally, and rare complications are acute pancreatitis and meningo-encephalitis. Aseptic meningitis may be the only manifestation of mumps. The involvement of organs other than the parotid gland is much more frequent in adults.

The virus can be grown in the developing chick embryo. The disease can be reproduced in the monkey by injection of a filtrate of saliva from human cases into Stenson's duct. The suckling mouse is the only other susceptible animal. Agglutination of red blood cells by the virus is similar to the hemagglutination already described in connection with the influenza virus. Antibodies to mumps can be demonstrated and estimated by the hemagglutination inhibition test.

Lymphogranuloma Venereum.—This venereal disease is commonly known as *lymphogranuloma inguinale,* but as that name is continually confused with granuloma inguinale, lymphogranuloma venereum is to be preferred. It is a contagious venereal disease caused by a filterable virus, which can be transferred to the monkey, rabbit and guinea-pig. The infection may, however, be non-venereal in children, doctors, nurses, and research workers. The virus is present in the primary lesion, regional lymph nodes, urethral and vaginal discharges, pelvic abscesses, blood stream, and spinal fluid. It has been demonstrated forty years after the original infection. The *initial lesion* is on the glans or vulva; it is small and indurated, heals quickly, and may never be noticed. Several weeks later the inguinal nodes become enlarged, indurated, matted together and painful, the overlying skin assumes a bluish-red color, fluctuation develops, and a purulent fluid is discharged, leaving a chronic ulcer of the skin with sinuses; these lesions may be extremely slow in healing. The *microscopic picture* is the same in the primary lesion and the lymph nodes. The basic lesion is a focal proliferation of large mononuclear cells which form aggregates. These cells accumulate around vessels, invade their walls, and finally obliterate their lumen. This obliteration is not associated with endothelial proliferation or thrombosis. The result is the formation of small solid granulomatous nodules. Ischemic necrosis follows, with invasion by polymorphonuclears and the formation of stellate abscesses. After necrosis occurs intracytoplasmic inclusions (*Gamma bodies*) may be seen in the mononuclears. These represent phagocytozed cellular débris.

When sterilized purulent fluid from one of the nodes is injected intracutaneously in a person suffering from the disease, it produces a marked allergic skin reaction. This is known as the intradermal test of Frei and Hoffmann, and the skin allergy on which it depends persists throughout life. When the virus is injected into the brain of monkeys or mice a meningo-encephalitis is produced, and brain emulsion makes a stable antigen for the Frei reaction which is preferable to using material from an infected person.

Marked increase in the plasma protein is common.

The disease is commoner in the negro but it often occurs in the white. Cole saw 52 cases in one year in Cleveland. Rectal stricture is a common complication, and in the past has been incorrectly attributed to syphilis. Most authors agree that rectal lesions are much commoner in women, but Mathewson reports 74 cases in San Francisco, of whom 60 were men and only 14 women. The site of the primary lesion and not the sex determines the incidence of secondary lesions in the inguinal nodes or the rectal nodes. Owing to lymph drainage, infection of the glans and prepuce in the male and the clitoris and vulva of the female lead to inguinal lesions, whereas infection of the posterior urethra in the male and the vagina in the female are responsible for inflammatory lesions and subsequent stricture of the rectum. On these grounds rectal lesions might be expected to be more frequent in the female. The Frei-Hoffmann test is particularly useful in these cases of rectal stricture in the female with no external evidence of the disease. Lymphogranuloma venereum must not be confused with granuloma inguinale. In the former the essential lesions are in the lymph nodes with secondary involvement of the skin, while the latter is primarily a disease of the skin. The presence of the Frei-Hoffmann test and the absence of Donovan bodies serve to characterize lymphogranuloma venereum.

Cat Scratch Disease.—This disease, although only recognized in 1951, appears to be of wide distribution. It is probably caused by a virus.

There is always a history of an association with cats, but, in spite of the name, there is not necessarily evidence of a scratch or bite. There may be an initial skin lesion, or there may be enlargement of regional lymph nodes without any evident primary lesion. The microscopic picture is a nonspecific granuloma with a very occasional giant cell resembling that of tularemia and lymphogranuloma venereum (Fig. 191). The infection nearly always pursues a benign course with recovery in a few weeks, but in rare cases it may cause a fatal encephalitis. The clinical problem which the patient presents

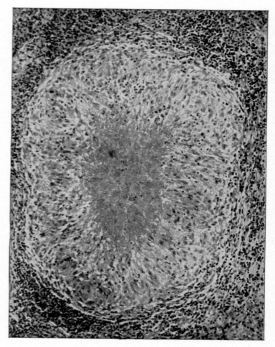

Fig. 191.—Cat scratch disease showing characteristic granulomatous reaction. (Kindness of Dr. J. L. Blaisdell.)

is one of localized lymph node enlargement, and he is likely to consult his doctor because of this condition. An intradermal skin reaction similar to the Frei test for lymphogranuloma venereum is of diagnostic value, using an antigen prepared from infected human tissue.

Cytomegalic Inclusion Disease.—This condition is also known as inclusion disease and generalized salivary gland virus infection. The occurrence of inclusions in the salivary gland of the newborn, infants and young children has long been recognized. The inclusions may be intranuclear or cytoplasmic. The former may occur alone, the latter never in the absence of the former. The intranuclear body is a large dense mass which is acidophilic or may be purplish with hematoxylin and eosin (Fig. 192). The cytoplasmic bodies are small and basophilic. The infection appears to be primary in the salivary glands, and the lesions are identical with those of salivary gland virus disease of rodents. The human disease, however, is not transmissible to animals nor does growth take place on eggs or tissue culture, so that the evidence in favor of a virus is merely by analogy. In rodents the infec-

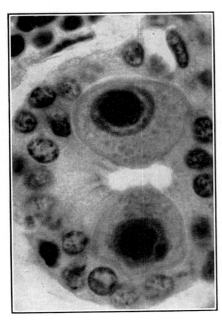

Fig. 192.—Salivary gland inclusion disease.
(Kindness of Dr. W. L. Donohue.)

tion is confined to the salivary glands, but in the child it may become generalized and cause death. A great variety of organs may be affected, but the liver, kidneys, pancreas (islets of Langerhans) and lungs (interstitial pneumonia) deserve special mention.

EPIDEMIC HEMORRHAGIC FEVER.—This disease has been endemic in the Far East for many years and has been reported by Russian and Japanese observers in Manchuria and Siberia. It has been brought to the attention of Western medicine by the occurrence of many cases amongst the United Nations' forces in the war in Korea (Mayer; Hullinghorst and Steer). It is believed to be a virus or rickettsial disease, the infective agent being carried by small rodents such as the field mouse and mole, with a mite as the insect vector, but none of this has so far been proved. The portal of entry is not known. The agent is extremely virulent, must multiply rapidly, and appears to produce a diffusible capillary "toxin" which gives rise to widespread hemorrhages. The condition is different from any other known hemorrhagic disease. The chief *clinical features* are oliguria, anuria, uremia, shock-like episodes, severe hemorrhage, and pulmonary edema. The hemorrhage appears to be in the nature of a diapedesis of red cells resulting from vasoparalysis rather than an extravasation due to rupture of vessels. There is a striking absence of jaundice,

perhaps related to the fact that the red cells in the tissues do not undergo hemolysis. The course is fulminating, over half the fatal cases dying in eight days or less, some within two days. Death seems to be due to shock and renal failure.

The *principal lesions* are: (1) widespread capillary hemorrhage, but without apparent capillary damage or thrombosis; (2) a peculiar type of coagulation necrosis suggestive of infarction, but without vascular occlusion; (3) a cellular infiltrate consisting mainly of mononuclear macrophages seen principally in the myocardium, pancreas, spleen and liver. The cellular infiltrate is not related to the necrosis nor the hemorrhage. The hemorrhage is most severe in the gastrointestinal tract and the kidneys. The necrosis is best seen in the kidneys, pituitary and adrenals.

The *kidneys* present a dramatic picture to which the Russians have given the name of renal apoplexy. The organs are enlarged, the average weight being over 500 grams. Perirenal hemorrhage is frequent. The cortex is pale, but the medulla is deep red in color. Pale areas of necrosis may be detected in the pyramids and papillæ. Microscopically the hemorrhage may be so severe that the collecting tubules seem to be floating in a pool of blood. The picture suggests that the "toxic agent" is concentrated in the renal medulla, being excreted in the tubules. Nephrotic lesions and numerous pigment casts in the tubules may be attributed to the accompanying shock. Marked hemorrhage in the renal pelvis is a common feature. The *pituitary* is nearly always soft and hemorrhagic, and infarct-like areas of necrosis are present in the anterior lobe. In one-third of the cases the entire anterior lobe is destroyed. There may be hemorrhage but no necrosis in the posterior lobe and hypothalamus. The *adrenals* present hemorrhage in half the cases, and often large areas of necrosis. In the *heart* a distinctive feature is severe subendocardial and subepicardial hemorrhage frequently limited to the right auricle. The left auricle is less often hemorrhagic, but mononuclear infiltration is more common, and this may involve the adjoining ventricle. The entire *gastrointestinal tract* is deep red from hemorrhage, but this is most marked in the lower part of the small intestine.

RICKETTSIAL DISEASES

In 1909 H. T. Ricketts described minute bodies in the blood of patients suffering from Rocky Mountain fever and in the tick which carries the disease. In 1910 Ricketts and Wilder found the same minute bodies in the intestinal canal of lice which had fed on typhus patients. These are now known as Rickettsia bodies or simply Rickettsiæ.

Rickettsiæ are minute bacterium-like organisms just visible with the light microscope. They might well be considered with the bacterial diseases, but they do not grow on artificial culture media, demanding the presence of living cells in tissue culture or the developing chick embryo. Like the viruses they are obligate intracellular, multiplying only within living cells, apparently lacking enzyme systems which must be supplied by the cells in which they live. In these fundamental respects they resemble viruses more than bacteria, and for this reason they are discussed in this chapter. Viruses, however, multiply most rapidly when the cells which they inhabit are growing actively, whereas rickettsiæ grow best when cellular activity is at a minimum. Certain chemotherapeutic agents that are effective against bacteria are also active against rickettsiæ, because the latter undergo a period of extracellular growth in the intestinal tract of their arthropod vectors, whereas no clinically effective antiviral agent is at present available. We may straddle the fence and regard the rickettsiæ as representing the borderline between bacterium and virus. They are primarily intestinal parasites of blood-sucking arthropods such as lice, rat-fleas, mites and ticks. These are the vectors which spread the disease to man, just as the virus of yellow fever is carried by the mosquito. In man they live only in the mesothelial cells of the vascular and reticuloendothelial systems. They cause a cutaneous rash, and nervous and mental symptoms. The serum of patients contains agglutinins for the Proteus group of bacteria. They develop in the gut of the arthropod host, multiply there, and are discharged in enormous numbers in the dejecta. Six are known to be pathologic for man, causing typhus, tsutsugamushi fever, Rocky Mountain spotted fever, trench fever, rickettsial pox and Q-fever.

TYPHUS FEVER.—Typhus is an acute infectious fever which used to be one of the great scourges of man. Being carried by the body louse, it is seldom seen in ordinary life, but was fearfully prevalent during the First World War, especially in the Balkan States.

No disease has been more fatal to the men who have investigated it. Ricketts, Prowazek, Bacot, and many others are among its distinguished victims. It is caused by Rickettsia prowazeki, which is found both in the human patient and in the lice which have been feeding on him.

Zinsser, in his delightful and entertaining *Rats, Lice and History*, remarks that "louse transmission was the great discovery made by Nicolle, which furnished the first powerful weapon for a counter-attack against the disease. It explained the manner in which epidemics are propagated. It removed all mystery from the historic association of typhus epidemics with wars, famines, and wretchedness. But it left unanswered the problem of the smouldering embers of the virus in interepidemic periods." For the human louse soon dies on being infected with typhus. The secret reservoir of infection was found to be the domestic rat, transmission from animal to animal being through the agency of the rat flea. If the rat dies and the rat flea is hard put to it to find a new host he may bite man. This is the sporadic case. If the victim is lousy and lives in a lousy community, the result is an epidemic. Zinsser points out that "the louse shares with us the misfortune of being prey to the typhus virus. . . . For the host may survive, but the ill-starred louse that imbibes the loathsome virus with his nourishment is doomed beyond succor. . . . His tiny body turns red with blood extravasated from his bowel, and he gives up his little ghost. . . . To the louse, *we* are the dreaded emissaries of death."

The onset of the disease is acute, with high fever, great weakness and prostration, tracheobronchitis with bronchopneumonia, and a macular rash which is often characteristically hemorrhagic. There is great mental apathy, which may pass into stupor. There may be necrosis of the skin.

Lesions.—The gross pathological changes are not characteristic. There is acute splenic swelling and cloudiness of the organs. The *microscopic changes* are quite characteristic, taking the form of proliferative and thrombotic lesions in the vessels of the skin, the skeletal muscles, the heart, and the central nervous system. It is these which are responsible for the hemorrhagic rash and the occasional necrotic lesions. There is a swelling and proliferation of the vascular endothelium, and at the site of this swelling thrombosis is liable to occur. In Giemsa preparations the swollen endothelial cells may sometimes be seen to be crowded with rickettsiæ. Only the cytoplasm of the vascular endothelium is invaded, not the nuclei, as is the case in spotted fever. Perivascular accumulations of mononuclear and polymorphonuclear cells are common, and in addition tubercle-like nodules are scattered through the central nervous system. These are produced by neuroglial proliferation, and provide another example of the proliferation which is so characteristic a feature of the microscopic lesions.

In man the rickettsiæ are found in the endothelial cells. In the louse they are confined to the lining epithelium of the gut, where they multiply prodigiously. Beautiful illustrations of the lesions and the rickettsiæ will be found in Wolbach's monograph. Infection is carried by the body louse, which does not become infective until seven days after feeding. The infection is not necessarily caused by bites, for the excreta of the louse are swarming with rickettsiæ, and these, when deposited on the skin, may enter through scratches and abrasions. Bacot died of typhus although he was never bitten. Rickettsia are present in the blood, in the leukocytes and in the blood platelets. The disease can be transmitted to monkeys and also to guinea-pigs by the subcutaneous injection of infected blood and by the bites of infected lice.

The *Weil-Felix reaction* is a curious example of heterologous antibody action. The blood of typhus patients gives a marked agglutination with many coliform organisms, and particularly with the Proteus group. This Bacillus proteus reaction is positive by the fifth day in 50 per cent of cases, and soon becomes positive in over 90 per cent of cases. It is therefore of great diagnostic value. Though described by Weil and Felix in 1916 it was previously described by Wilson of Belfast in 1910.

TSUTSUGAMUSHI FEVER.—This typhus-like infection, also known as *scrub typhus*, is endemic in Japan, Malaya and the East Indies. It is caused by *rickettsia orientalis*, and the disease is transmitted by the bite of an infected larva of certain mites. The habitat of the mite is in rotting vegetation and tall grass, hence the name scrub typhus. Indeed it would be better called mite typhus, just as we may distinguish louse-borne typhus (ordinary typhus), tick-borne typhus (Rocky Mountain spotted fever), and flea-borne typhus. Only in louse-borne typhus is the infection transmitted directly from man to man. A characteristic ulcer usually develops at the site of entry of the infection, associated with local and general lymphadenopathy (Allen-Spitz).

ROCKY MOUNTAIN SPOTTED FEVER.—Rocky Mountain fever or *spotted fever* bears a remarkable resemblance to typhus fever in regard to symptoms, lesions, and bacteriology. It is an acute infection with headache, continued fever, pains in the muscles, and a macular eruption which often becomes hemorrhagic ("spotted fever"), and sometimes necrosis of the skin. It used to be thought that the disease was confined to the northwestern part of the United States (Rocky Mountain region), but it is now known that the infection may be acquired over a considerable part of the United States, east as well as west, and in southern Canada. There is some difference between the lesions in the eastern and western forms of the disease.

The disease is caused by one of the rickettsia group, and is therefore conveyed by an arthropod, this time a wood tick, Dermacentor venustus. The disease is confined to regions and seasons (spring and early summer) in which wood ticks abound. As in the case of typhus, laboratory workers may acquire the disease without being bitten by the tick. In such cases the infected material must get on the skin and penetrate through cracks and scratches. The infection can be transmitted to the monkey, rabbit, and guinea-pig. In the guinea-pig the disease is much more severe than when the animal is infected with the rickettsia of typhus, and there is often necrosis of the external genitals. The organism has never been cultivated on artificial media, nor is it filterable. It is always intracellular in the tick. Unlike Rickettsia prowazeki, it can be transmitted from one generation of ticks to another without the intervention of man. Washed red and white blood cells can transmit the disease to an animal, although rickettsiæ are almost never seen within these cells, suggesting that the organism may assume a form in which it cannot be demonstrated at present. A vaccine has been prepared from an emulsion of infected ticks. By its use (dose = 4 ticks) the mortality in the Bitterroot Valley, Montana, has been reduced from 90 per cent to 9 per cent.

Lesions.—These are very similar to those of

THE PRINCIPAL RICKETTSIAL DISEASES

Condition		Causative Agent	Mode of Transmission to Man
Typhus Fever	Epidemic & Brill's Disease	Rickettsia Prowazekii	Louse (infected feces)
Tsutsugamushi Fever (Scrub Typhus)		Rickettsia Orientalis	Mite (bite)
Rocky Mountain Spotted Fever		Rickettsia Rickettsii	Wood tick (bite)
Trench Fever		Rickettsia Quintana	Body louse (infected feces)
Rickettsial Pox		Rickettsia Akari	Mite (bite)
Q Fever		Rickettsia Burneti	Ticks (inhalation of infected material)

typhus fever. The spleen is enlarged, and there may be hemorrhage in the ovaries and testes, but the only characteristic lesions are microscopic. There is the same proliferative arteritis combined with thrombosis. The endothelial cells lining the vessels become greatly swollen and undergo division. Thrombosis, both mural and occluding, occurs on the swollen endothelium. The result of the vascular occlusion is seen in the hemorrhagic rash and the necrotic areas on the skin. In the eastern form of the disease focal brain lesions consisting of axonal swelling and degeneration, together with a proliferative gliosis, are very characteristic; they are never found in the western form.

TRENCH FEVER.—This is the third of the rickettsial diseases, but differs from typhus fever and Rocky Mountain spotted fever in having a mortality so low that nothing is known of the lesions in man. The infection is carried by the body louse, so that the disease affects troops under conditions of trench warfare. It was the commonest of all the diseases affecting the troops in France during World War I. It is an acute febrile disease characterized by great prostration, severe pain in the muscles and bones ("shin bone fever"), and recurring attacks of fever often at intervals of five or six days ("intermittent fever," "five-day fever"). Pain in the muscles is severe and very characteristic. In many cases there is a red macular rash. It will be seen that the symptoms are not unlike those of typhus and Rocky Mountain spotted fever. A striking feature is the long period during which the patient harbors the infection. Lice have been infected from a patient more than a year after the onset of the disease. The recurrences which sometimes occur many months after the inital attack are thus easy to understand.

Infection can be transmitted from one person to another by the injection of whole blood or of washed red or white corpuscles, but not by the use of serum. The infection is therefore carried in the cells. The rickettsiæ are found in lice which have fed on trench fever patients. The organisms are present in enormous numbers in the excreta of the louse. Infection is due either to bites or to excreta being rubbed into scratches and abrasions.

RICKETTSIAL POX.—A new rickettsial disease was recognized in 1946 in New York. Because of an eruption not unlike that of chickenpox it was named rickettsialpox. The prognosis is uniformly favorable. The initial lesion due to the bite of a tick is a dark red papule. There is mild fever of about one week's duration, a papulovesicular rash, sore throat, and in some cases enlargement of lymph nodes and spleen. Knowledge of the lesions is dependent on biopsy material (Dolgopol). The initial lesion resembles that of scrub typhus. The rash is similar microscopically to that of other rickettsial diseases; there is the same cellular infiltration and vascular change. In the lymph nodes the necrosis characteristic of scrub typhus is absent.

Q-fever will be described in relation to diseases of the lungs, page 643.

REFERENCES

ALLEN, A. C., and SPITZ, S.: Am. J. Path., 1945, *21*, 603 (Tsutsugamushi fever).

BOGOCH, S., LYNCH, P. and LEVINE, A. S.: Virology, 1959, *7*, 161 (Brain ganglioside and influenza virus).

COLE, H. N.: J.A.M.A., 1933, *101*, 1069 (Lymphogranuloma venereum).

DOLGOPOL, V. B.: Am. J. Path., 1948, *24*, 119 (Rickettsial pox).

ENDERS, J. F., *et al.*: New Eng. J. Med., 1959, *261*, 875, 882 (Measles virus in giant-cell pneumonia).

GORDON, H. and KNIGHTON, H. T.: Am. J. Path., 1941, *17*, 165 (Giant cells in lesions of measles).

HORSFALL JR., F. L.: Can. Med. Ass. J., 1955, *73*, 778, (Virus reproduction and spread). Proc. Staff Meet. Mayo Clinic, 1960, *35*, 269 (Viral infection and viral disease in man).

HULLINGHORST, R. L. and STEER, A.: Ann. Int. Med., 1953, *38*, 77 (Epidemic hemorrhagic fever).

ISAACS, A. and BURKE, D. C.: Brit. Med. Bull., 1959, *15*, 185 (Interferon).

KATZ, S. L. *et al.*: New Eng. J. Med., 1960, *263*, 181 (Live attenuated measles virus vaccine).

MAYER, C. F.: Lab. Investig., 1952, *1*, 290 (Epidemic hemorrhagic fever).

RHODES, A. J.: Modern Medicine (of Canada), 1958, Oct., p. 69.

RHODES, A. J. and VAN ROOYAN, C. E.: *Textbook of Virology*, 3rd ed., Baltimore, 1958.

RIGHTSEL, W. A. *et al.*: J.A.M.A., 1961, *177*, 671 Virus Hepatitis).

RIVERS, T. M. and HORSFALL, JR., F. L.: *Viral and Rickettsial Infections of Man*, 3rd ed., Philadelphia, 1959.

ROBERTS, G. B. S. and BAIN, A. D.: J. Path. and Bact., 1958, *76*, 111 (Pathology of measles).

SHOPE, R. E.: J. Exper. Med., 1931, *54*, 349, 373 (Swine influenza).

SWARTZ, M. N. and LITTLEFIELD, J. W.: New Eng. J. Med., 1960, *262*, 287 (Biochemistry of viral infections).

TYRRELL, D. A. J., *et al.*: Lancet, 1960, *1*, 235 (Culture of common cold virus).

WHITBY, SIR L. E. and HYNES, M.: *Medical Bacteriology*, 6th ed., London, 1956.

WOLBACH, S. B., TODD, J. L. and PALFREY, F. W.: *The Etiology and Pathology of Typhus*, Cambridge, Mass., 1922.

ZINSSER, H.: *Rats, Lice and History*, Boston, 1935.

Chapter 14

Animal Parasite Infections

General Considerations
Protozoa
  Entamoeba Histolytica
    Balantidium Coli
  Plasmodium Malariae
  Trypanosomiasis
    Nagana
    Sleeping Sickness
    Chagas' Disease
  Leishmaniasis
    Kala-azar
  Toxoplasmosis

Nematodes or Round Worms
  Ankylostoma Duodenale:
    Hookworm
  Ascaris Lumbricoides:
    Roundworm
  Enterobius Vermicularis:
    Pinworm
  Trichinella Spiralis:
    Muscleworm
  Tricocephalus Trichiurus:
    Whipworm
  Filaria:
    Blood worm
  Dracunculus Medinensis:
    Guinea worm

Cestodes or Tapeworms
  Taenia Saginata:
    Beef tapeworm
  Taenia Solium:
    Pork tapeworm
  Diphyllobothrium Latum:
    Fish tapeworm
  Taenia Echinococcus:
    Hydatid tapeworm
    Echinococcus Alveolaris
Trematodes or Flukes
  Schistosomiasis
External Parasites: Arthropods
Arthropods as Carriers of Disease

GENERAL CONSIDERATIONS

Pathogenic parasites are of common occurrence even in temperate countries, and when the tropical parasites are included we meet some of the most widespread diseases of mankind. Many of the parasites pass through a complicated life cycle, which adds to the interest (and the difficulty) of the subject. Very few parasites pass their life cycle in only one host. The eggs produced in the body of a man or animal do not develop in the same body. They may develop into larvæ in the soil, or they may be ingested by another host and develop there. The *definitive host* is the host of the adult parasite (sexual cycle), and the *intermediate host* is the host of the embryo (asexual cycle). Thus man is the definitive host of the common tapeworms, but the intermediate host of the malarial parasite. A *vector* is a means of conveying parasites to a new host; vectors may be vegetable or animal foodstuffs or insects. An insect vector may also be a host. A knowledge of the life history of the parasite outside as well as inside the patient is essential if the disease is to be attacked rationally and successfully.

Parasitism is a specialized type of life. When an animal decides to adopt this way of life, it must be prepared to make certain sacrifices, including freedom. As Cameron points out in *Parasites and Parasitism*: "organs of locomotion are reduced or atrophied, organs of special sense required for hunting prey or avoiding enemies disappear, and the central nervous system often becomes reduced. Organs of feeding become more specialized and better adapted for their purpose." On account of the fact that the life cycle is not completed in the same host, the hazards of survival become much greater. In the course of evolution the number of offspring produced has been adjusted to meet the probable death-rate, the latter being governed by the chances of reaching a host. The egg output of some parasites is simply astronomical. Thus the fish tapeworm of man lays several million eggs *daily* and lives for several years, while Haemonchus, the stomach worm of sheep, lays an egg every ten to twenty *seconds*. The problem of reproduction is also simplified in some species by the sexes being brought together more or less permanently, in some cases the young adult male later becoming a female. This is said to be a specially efficient technique in cestodes, whilst in others the male is dispensed with entirely, a somewhat disturbing thought.

Parasitism, whether animal or bacterial, is not necessarily a matter of invader and defender. The point of view of the parasite must also be considered. The host provides the parasite with all the comforts of life. It is really a biological accident if some metabolic incompatibility between host and parasite should lead to the manifestations of disease. When a parasite invades a host there are 4 possibilities: (1) the parasite may die at once; (2) it may survive without causing symptoms; (3) it may survive and cause disease; (4) it may kill the host. Of these, the first is probably the most common, because when the parasite is taken in by the wrong host it cannot survive. The second is also very common—much more so than the third or fourth. The successful parasite is the one which does not jeopardize the survival of the host, because in so doing it jeopardizes its own survival.

The teacher of pathology commonly finds that the student experiences great difficulty in mastering the subject of the animal parasites, for which he is apt to acquire a marked distaste. This is because he is overwhelmed by the number of parasites and the need of learning the exact dimensions of the male and female of each species. For this reason only a limited number of parasites will be described here, and emphasis will be laid on their biological behavior and the disturbances they produce in man rather than on their structural detail. The latter can be obtained in any book on parasitology.

The subject will appear less vast and confusing if the beginner will realize the following facts. Disease-producing parasites belong to two great groups, protozoa (unicellular organisms) and worms. There are four important protozoal parasites, causing malaria, Leishmaniasis, trypanosomiasis, and and amebic dysentery. The worms are divided into flukes, tapeworms and round worms. Of these one fluke will be considered, four tapeworms, and six round worms. A wealth of information and superb illustrations will be found in the *Atlas of Pathology of Tropical Diseases* by Ash and Spitz.

PROTOZOA

Entamœba Histolytica.—This is the cause of amebic dysentery, which is considered in connection with diseases of the intestine. The ameba is a single cell from 20 to 30 microns in diameter, with an outer hyaline

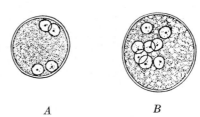

A   *B*

Fig. 193.—*A*, Cyst of E. histolytica stained with iodine, showing 4 nuclei; *B*, cyst of E. coli with 8 nuclei. (Blacklock and Southwell, *Human Parasitology*, H. K. Lewis & Co.)

ectoplasm and an inner granular endoplasm. Movement is effected by an outflowing of the outer hyaline zone in the form of pseudopodia into which flows the granular endoplasm. The parasite is recognized by its mobility, which can be studied in an absolutely fresh specimen of feces on the warm stage of the microscope. Differentiation from the harmless Entamœba coli, which also occurs in the stools, is difficult; Entamœba histolytica frequently contains red blood cells and vacuoles, whereas Entamœba coli does not. In chronic cases, such as are seen in temperate countries, there are often no mobile forms, for under unfavorable conditions the ameba becomes globular, shrinks in size and is converted into a cyst measuring 10 to 15 microns and having an outer capsular layer. The cystic forms of Entamœba histolytica and Entamœba coli are much more easily differentiated than the active forms, for the former cysts have four nuclei when fully developed, the latter have eight nuclei (Fig. 193). The cysts are the infective form of the parasite, for the active form is killed by the gastric juice as it passes through the stomach. Multiplication is by direct division; there is no sexual stage.

The cysts may live outside the body for weeks or months in moisture and shade. The active form is detected by direct microscopic examination of a warm stool preparation, but the encysted form is shown up best when such a preparation is stained with a mixture of iodine and eosin. The cysts do not occur in the tissues, nor are they passed in any numbers in the acute diarrheal stage of dysentery; they are generally found only in semisolid or formed stools. For doubtful encysted forms a fixed smear should be stained with iron hematoxylin. In acute cases, therefore, the stool contains the active form, while in chronic cases and carriers the encysted form is to be expected.

The ameba is arrested in the colon, where it may invade the mucosa and set up the acute inflammation of dysentery. From the intestine it may invade the radicles of the portal vein, be carried to the liver, and there give rise to amebic abscesses. The disease is spread from person to person and by flies. While fly injection must be guarded against in the country, in the city the chief danger is from food handlers who are chronic carriers, and in whose stools the cysts may be found. Amebic dysentery is endemic in the tropics, but isolated cases and occasional epidemics occur in England, the United States, Canada, *etc.* These can usually be traced to food carriers. It is commonly stated and believed that 10 per cent of the population of the United States harbor Entamœba histolytica in the intestine. Actually, the over-all incidence in the United States and Canada is probably less than 1 per cent (Magath). We must distinguish between amebiasis and dysentery. As Lynch remarks: "Amebic dysentery is the comparatively uncommon acute phase or end-result of intestinal amebiasis." It is not known what upsets the usual balance between parasite and host.

The lesions and clinical features of amebic dysentery are described in Chapter 27.

BALANTIDIUM COLI.—This is a ciliated protozoön parasite which, like *Entamœba histolytica*, occurs in the bowel in an active or trophozoite form and in an encysted form. The cysts are passed in the stools and are infective, while the active form dies outside the body. In the intestine the encysted parasites develop into trophozoites, which invade the mucous membrane and produce ulcers, chiefly in the large intestine, but occasionally in the lower part of the small intestine. The ulcers resemble those of amebic dysentery, and the symptoms are dysenteric in type.

Plasmodium Malariæ.—The malarial parasite was discovered by Laveran in 1880, and in 1895 Ronald Ross showed that the disease was transmitted by the anopheles mosquito. These are the two great landmarks in the fight against one of the most important diseases which afflict man. The word malaria is of interest. It means bad

---

EXPLANATION OF PLATE III[1]

Partly schematic. Drawn and rearranged by Williams, partly from Muir and Ritchie, partly from Kolle and Hetsch and partly original. Giemsa's stain.

The asexual forms show cycle of the organism in the red blood cells of the human host. They show schematically the time of fever and the day of segmentation.

Tertian type.

FIG. 1.—Segmented organism.

FIG. 2.—Young ring form in cell and a young form on surface.

FIG. 3.—Growing schizont; irregular form due to great motility; beginning pigment formation; red blood cell becoming paler.

FIG. 4—Larger schizont. Red cells pale and stippled (Schüffner's dots).

FIG. 5.—Nucleus divided into four clumps.

FIG. 6.—Further division of chromatin and formation of irregular rosette. Pigment finely granular in center.

FIG. 7.—Segmentation. Note 18 merozoites (usually 16).

Quartan type. Shows following differences from tertian: Slightly larger, fewer segments (usually 8), and more regular. Pigment coarse. Red blood cells unaltered. Segmentation every seventy-two hours.

Malignant tertian type. Shows following differential points: Merozoites smaller and more numerous (32); organism less motile with less pigment. Red blood cells smaller and greenish color (in fresh cells).

Sexual forms. Show cycle of development in mosquito.

FIG. 1 (*A* to *E*).—Male ($\male$) and female ($\female$) forms of tertian type formed in human blood; *F*, flagellation of male type in stomach of mosquito; *G, H*, changes in female type and fertilization in stomach of mosquito.

FIG. 2.—Development of sporocyst within mosquito. Liberation of sporozoites which find their way to the salivary gland.

FIG. 3.—Sexual forms of malignant tertian type found in human blood, showing development of sickle-shaped bodies.

[1]From Park and Williams: Pathogenic Microörganisms.

PLATE III

A. PLASMODIUM VIVAX

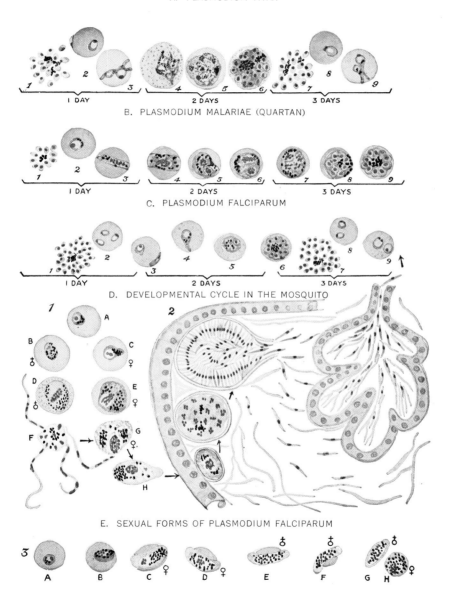

1 DAY   2 DAYS   3 DAYS

B. PLASMODIUM MALARIAE (QUARTAN)

1 DAY   2 DAYS   3 DAYS

C. PLASMODIUM FALCIPARUM

I DAY   2 DAYS   3 DAYS

D. DEVELOPMENTAL CYCLE IN THE MOSQUITO

E. SEXUAL FORMS OF PLASMODIUM FALCIPARUM

air (*malo*, bad; *aria*, air), and is a reminder of the days when the disease was thought to be transmitted by the miasmic vapors of marshes. It was the mosquitoes, not the miasmas, that lived in the marshes. Among all tropical diseases malaria is supreme. It is the most persistent, the most destructive, the most widespread, and the most difficult to control. Osler, indeed, has called it the greatest single destroyer of the human race. Malaria afflicts some 350,000 persons a year, with an average mortality of perhaps 1 per cent. Those peoples touched by the shaking finger of malaria have undergone a gradual decadence, as may be seen in the history of Greece and Rome.

There are three forms of malaria: *benign tertian* caused by *Plasmodium vivax*, *quartan* caused by *Plasmodium malariæ*, and *malignant tertian* or subtertian caused by *Plasmodium falciparum*. The third form is also known as *estivo-autumnal*, because in subtropical countries it occurs principally in the later summer and autumn. In benign tertian the characteristic chill or attack of fever occurs every forty-eight hours (every other day) and lasts only two or three hours, in quartan it occurs every seventy-two hours (every third day), and in the malignant tertian it occurs every forty-eight hours, but is prolonged for several hours with a plateau rise of temperature making the attacks seem closer together. The distribution is as wide as that of the anopheles mosquito; it embraces the tropics, the southern United States, and many parts of Italy, Greece, the Balkans, *etc.* The disease may recur after one or several years, for the parasites hide in the spleen and bone marrow, and come out when the patient goes to a cold climate. The parasite passes an asexual stage of its life cycle in man and a sexual stage in the mosquito (See Plate III).

Asexual Stage.—The *tertian*, the commonest form, will be taken as an example. When an infected mosquito bites a man it injects a large number of rod-shaped parasites known as *sporozoites* or spores into the blood stream. One sporozoite attaches itself to an erythrocyte, penetrates it, becomes rounded, and enters on the stage of asexual development. A multitude of names have

been given to the various steps of the process by zoölogists, but these will be omitted for the most part. The parasite, being a cell, consists of a nucleus and cytoplasm. It forms a rounded body within the red blood corpuscle, the nuclear chromatin staining red with Wright's stain and the cytoplasm blue. The parasite often assumes a signet-ring form, with red nucleus at one side of the ring. The parasite grows rapidly at the expense of the hemoglobin, so that the red cell becomes pale and swollen. Electron microscopy of the erythrocyte shows that the parasite engulfs large portions of host cytoplasm into food vacuoles by invagination of its cell membrane. The phagocyte is therefore an intracellular phagotroph. The parasite contains dark brown granules of pigment derived from the hemoglobin and commonly called *malarial pigment*. The pigment is manufactured by the parasite, and does not give the reaction for hemosiderin. The cytoplasm of the erythrocyte shows a fine red stippling (*Schüffner's dots*) which is not seen in the quartan and estivo-autumnal forms (see colored plate). Asexual division then occurs. The nuclear chromatin divides into 18 or 20 fragments (in the tertian type), and the cytoplasm is divided so as to surround each of these. The new bodies are arranged around the periphery of the erythrocyte to form a *rosette*. The rosette breaks up into a number of new individuals or *merozoites*, and at the end of forty-eight hours these are discharged from the ghostly remains of the erythrocyte into the blood stream. This process is repeated in all the infected erythrocytes at practically the same time, and it is the sudden outpouring of foreign protein into the blood which is the cause of the chill and fever. Each merozoite now becomes attached to and enters a fresh erythrocyte, and the whole process is repeated. It is evident that a profound anemia may be produced in this way.

Sexual Stages.—Some of the merozoites develop into parent sexual cells or *gametocytes* which are set apart for sexual reproduction. In the malignant tertian type these have a characteristic crescentic form. If the gametocytes are taken into the stomach of the female anopheles mosquito they enter upon the sexual stage of the life cycle. The gametocytes are male and female. From the male gametocytes are protruded a number of whip-like bodies resembling spermatozoa. These are detached and form the *male gametes*. The female gametocyte loses some nuclear chromatin and becomes the *female gamete*. One male gamete then enters a female gamete and conjugation takes place. The impregnated cell is called a *zygote*. The zygote burrows through the epithelium of the gut and forms a cyst within which the nucleus divides into hundreds of rod-like bodies, the *sporozoites*. The entire process occupies about twelve days. The sporozoites make their way to the salivary glands, and when the mosquito bites a person they are injected into the blood stream, where the asexual cycle is once more repeated.

The sexual cycle is needed for the rejuvenation and continued existence of the parasites. But without the assistance of this phase they may live in the internal organs (chiefly the spleen) of the patient for months or even years without giving rise to symptoms. He may move to a temperate country where there are no mosquitoes, quite unconscious that he is still a sufferer from the disease. Then an exposure to cold or some lowering of the vitality may bring on a typical pyrexial attack with numerous parasites in the peripheral blood stream.

Morbid Anatomy.—At autopsy the two most striking changes are a slate-colored or blackish pigmentation of the abdominal organs and great enlargement of the spleen. The discoloration is due to malarial pigment which resembles melanin in color. It contains iron but does not give the Prussian blue reaction. The spleen is very large, and in acute cases it is extremely soft and diffluent, but in chronic cases it becomes very hard. *Microscopically* the parasites are seen in the capillaries and there are great deposits both of malarial pigment and hemosiderin. In the occasional *acutely fatal case* the capillaries are stuffed with parasites. This is best seen in the brain, where the condition may be responsible for coma. *Microscopically* there is widespread vascular injury, evidenced by fatty degeneration of the endothelium, ring hemorrhages in the brain, and hemorrhagic necrotizing lesions in the myo-

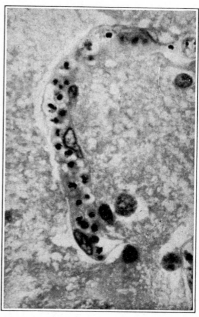

FIG. 194.—Parasitized red cells in capillaries of the brain. × 1000.

cardium, adrenals, *etc.* The capillaries of the brain are stuffed with parasitized red corpuscles (Fig. 194), a condition which may result in coma. A fundamental feature of the acute disease is a marked slowing of the capillary circulation, especially in the brain. This is due to an altered physical quality of the parasitized red corpuscles, which, particularly in the malignant tertian form, become sticky and adhere to the vessel walls. As a result of this the red cells become agglutinated and form capillary thrombi. There is moreover "blocking" of the reticuloendothelial system by the liberated pigment. The pigment deposits are most marked in the spleen, liver, and bone-marrow, much of the pigment being within the swollen reticuloendothelial cells of these organs. In the late stages the spleen may be greatly fibrosed. The enlarged spleen may be ruptured even by slight trauma, a point of medico-legal importance, as this used to be a favorite method of assassination in the crowded bazaars of the Orient.

BLACKWATER FEVER.—Blackwater fever is a complication of malignant tertian malaria characterized by the passage of red or almost black

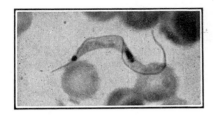

Fig. 195.—Trypanosoma gambiense. × 1500.

urine. In severe cases death is the rule. There is a rapid and massive destruction of red blood cells, which may fall as much as 2,000,000 in number in twenty-four hours. The result is hemoglobinemia, hemoglobinuria, intense jaundice, anuria, and frequently death. Methemoglobin is responsible for the very dark color of the urine. The spleen is greatly enlarged, bright red and velvety. The administration of quinine may precipitate an attack. Blackwater fever appears to be an *allergic response to reinfecion with the parasite of malignant tertian*. Most people develop a certain degree of immunity, but a few become allergic. Injection of a suspension of ground-up parasites into the skin of such persons produces an allergic reaction. Quinine liberates the allergen from the parasites. The acute manifestations are in the nature of anaphylactic attacks.

Trypanosomes. — Trypanosomes are spindle-shaped protozoan parasites characterized by a macronucleus and a micronucleus, an undulating membrane, and a flagellum (Fig. 195). They therefore belong to the group of the flagellates, and vary in length from 10 to 30 microns. The macronucleus is in the center of the parasite, while the micronucleus is a small mass of chromatin at one end. The undulating membrane is a wavy structure which runs like a fin along the length of the parasite. The flagellum arises from the micronucleus, passes along the undulting membrane, and is prolonged as a free structure which waves about so that the parasites are actively motile. Sexual development occurs in an invertebrate host, the *tsetse fly*, which transmits the infection from one person to another. Asexual reproduction is by means of longitudinal division in the blood of the intermediate host, *i.e.*, man and many wild animals. There are many varieties of trypanosomes and many tsetse flies, but only two are concerned in the production of serious disease. Trypanosomiasis, the disease caused by trypanosomes, is confined to tropical Africa.

Animal Trypanosomiasis (Nagana).—This is caused by *Trypanosoma brucei* (named after Sir David Bruce who discovered it), and the intermediate host is the tsetse fly, *Glossina morsitans*. The wild animals (deer, *etc.*) act as a reservoir for the infection, although they suffer no symptoms, but when domestic animals (horses, cattle) are taken into the fly belt they are at once infected and the disease is extremely fatal.

Human Trypanosomiasis (African Sleeping Sickness).—The human disease is caused by *Trypanosoma gambiense* (called after the Gambia River in which district the fever is prevalent), and is carried by the tsetse fly, *Glossina palpalis*. The trypanosomes live in the blood, causing fever, weakness, emaciation, and enlargement of the cervical and other lymph nodes. It is only later that they invade the central nervous system and cause true sleeping sickness with its characteristic lethargy and coma. The trypanosomes are found in the blood during attacks of fever, in the lymph nodes at any time, and in the cerebrospinal fluid when symptoms of sleeping sickness have developed. The brain lesions are foci of round-cell perivascular infiltration much like those of general paresis of the insane.

Chagas' Disease.—Chagas' disease is a form of trypanosomiasis occurring in South America. Unlike the African form these trypanosomes (*Trypanosoma cruzi*) penetrate the tissue cells, lose their flagellum, and develop into round leishmania-like bodies about 4 microns in diameter which divide repeatedly and fill the cell. After this intracellular multiplication the rounded bodies develop a flagellum and emerge in the circulation. Various bugs constitute the definitive host. The symptoms of Chagas' disease depend upon the organs the cells of which are penetrated by the parasites, *e.g.*, heart, brain (neuroglia cells), kidney, adrenal, thyroid. The general symptoms include anemia, enlarged lymph nodes, and fever.

Leishmaniasis.—This tropical disease is caused by the Leishmania group of flagel-

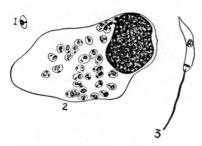

FIG. 196.—Leishmania. 1, Individual parasite; 2, mass of parasites in a macrophage; 3, flagellate form. (Blacklock and Southwell, *Human Parasitology*, H. K. Lewis & Co.)

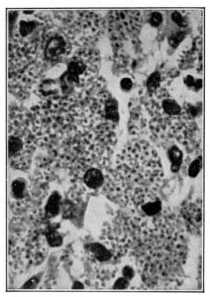

FIG. 197.—Reticuloendothelial cells of lymph node packed with histoplasma capsulatum. × 510. (From a section of Dr. W. A. D. Anderson.)

lates, *i.e.*, a parasite which may lose its flagellum and develop into a small, round or oval body about one-half the size of a red blood cell, containing two nuclear bodies, one much smaller than the other, which stain red with the Leishman and other Romanowsky stains (Fig. 196). Only the leishmania form occurs in man, the flagellate form being found in the gut of certain insects which have fed on an infected patient, or in culture of his infected blood. Leishmaniasis occurs in two clinical forms, visceral and cutaneous.

Toxoplasmosis.—This disease is caused by a protozoan parasite, *Toxoplasma gondi*, so-called because it was first found in the gondi, a small North African rodent. It is crescentic in shape, measuring 7 microns in length and from 2 to 4 microns in width, although in sections of fixed tissue they may be considerably smaller. In such sections they are seen as masses lying in mononuclear and endothelial cells. The growth requirements of the parasite are apparently easily satisfied, for it has a wide distribution in animals, occurring in the dog, mouse, rat, rabbit, *etc.*, as well as in birds. Human infection also appears to be very common, although relative few cases of disease have been reported, and the condition has only been recognized in recent years. It is said that from 10 to 50 per cent of adults show evidence of previous infection, so it is apparent that in the vast majority of instances the infection is symptomless. Yet in fatal cases almost every tissue may be involved. This, together with the intracellular character of the parasite, recalls the similar state of affairs in histoplasmosis. In

spite of the apparent harmlessness of the parasite, it may wreck the life of the newborn and kill the adult with an acute typhus-like fever. It is these extreme and at present inexplicable variations that make the infection such an interesting one.

The *mode of infection* is unknown. It is possible that children may acquire the parasite from sick pets. It is certain that a pregnant woman who becomes infected can transmit the infection to the fetus. Subsequent children, however, are immune.

The *clinical picture* varies to a remarkable degree, being influenced by the age of the patient. The *newborn infant* may be suffering from an acute infection, with fever, leukocytosis, rash, and evidence of meningoencephalitis, as well as hepatitis, pneumonitis and myocarditis (Callahan *et al.*). Hepatomegaly and splenomegaly are present. The parasites can be demonstrated in the cerebrospinal fluid. In such a case the mother has acquired the infection during pregnancy, although it has remained asymptomatic. In other cases the picture is more chronic, with hydrocephalus, microcephaly, chorioretinitis with macular lesions in the retina, and mental retardation. One of the most characteristic after effects is *cerebral calcification*, which is readily recognized in the *x*-ray film. The child is more likely to show a picture of glandular fever (infectious mononucleosis, with enlargement of the lymph nodes, but with a negative heterophile (Paul-Bunnell) reaction which is so characteristic of the latter condition. In the adult the condition is also likely to simulate infectious mononucleosis. Occasionally the adult may develop a very fatal acute fever with a rash like that of typhus fever, the parasites being demonstrated in skin biopsy. From this brief outline it will be evident that toxoplasmosis is indeed an infection with an incredible wide range of possibilities.

The *lesions*, as might be expected, are almost entirely microscopic. In the infant, however, there may be cysts in the brain, and a thickening of the choroidal lining which may be the basis of the hydrocephalus. The toxoplasma can only multiply within living cells, with a special predilection for those of the reticuloendothelial system. They are also well seen within nerve cells (Fig. 198). As multiplication proceeds the cells become distended, rupture, and release the parasites into the tissue fluids. As immunity develops the cells do not rupture, but form pseudocysts. During the acute stage small granulomata are formed, consisting of macrophages, lymphocytes, plasma cells, and fibroblasts. These lesions may heal with fibrosis and finally calcification. In the adult there is often a well-marked interstitial pneumonia, resembling a virus pneumonia.

Laboratory tests may be of value if the index of suspicion is sufficiently high, which is unlikely. Toxoplasma has been grown from the saliva, the blood, the cerebrospinal fluid, in an excised lymph node, whilst intracellular protozoa can be demonstrated in a biopsy from the skin rash. Skin tests of toxoplasma are positive, but this is no proof of an active infection, as is also the case with histoplasmosis. The same is true of the *dye test*. The parasites mixed with normal serum stain well with methylene blue, but not if the serum contains specific antibodies. Unfortunately this is the case in about 50 per cent of normal adults. The complement fixation test is positive in 10

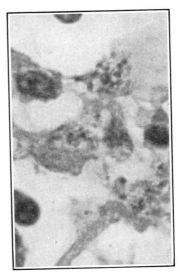

Fig. 198.—Cerebral toxoplasmosis.

per cent of normal adults. These facts serve to show how widespread the infection appears to be, and what an important part acquired immunity plays in the picture.

NEMATODES OR ROUNDWORMS

We now leave the protozoa and come to the metazoa. The metazoal parasites which infect the tissues are the *helminths* or worms, some of which are very long, whilst others are minute. The parasitic worms can be classified into three main divisions: (1) nematodes or roundworms, (2) cestodes or tapeworms, and (3) trematodes or flukes. Only the more important of the disease-producing worms will be considered. Eosinophilia in the peripheral blood is often present in helminth infections, a point of value in diagnosis. The eosinophilia appears to be part of an allergic reaction to the foreign protein of the worm. The largest group is that of the nematodes or roundworms with which we shall commence. They are differentiated into male and female forms, of which the female is always the larger. With a few exceptions no intermediate host is required for completion of the life cycle. This is in striking contrast to some of the protozoa and many of the other helminths. A large variety of roundworms may be

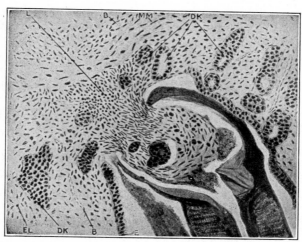

Fig. 199.—Section through human intestine, showing method of attachment of hookworm to the wall. (After Oudendal, in *Transactions of Biennial Congress of Far Eastern Association*, courtesy of John Bale Sons & Danielsson, Ltd., London.)

parasitic for man both in tropical and temperate climates. Some of these are pathogenic, others are not. Only six will be considered here.

Ankylostoma Duodenale.—(*Hookworm*).—Ankylostomiasis or hookworm disease, like malaria, is one of the most prevalent diseases in the world. It has been said that as a world producer of death, incapacity and misery it is second only to malaria. The Rockefeller Commission estimated that there were some 900,000,000 cases. The hookworm belt extends 'round the world on either side of the equator. The American variety of the worm is slightly different and is called *Necator americanus*. It is also found in temperate climates where the conditions are such that the soil is moist and warm as in deep mines, in long tunnels, as in the one between Italy and Switzerland, *etc.*, so that hookworm disease is known locally as miners' anemia, tunnel disease, *etc.*, and the skin manifestations are known as ground itch. The reason for all this will be apparent shortly.

The worm, as its name implies, lives in the upper part of the small intestine, although more in the jejunum than the duodenum. Large numbers, even hundreds, are found hanging firmly attached to the intestinal mucous membrane. It is said that as many as 10,000 have been found in one person. The worm is quite small, from 1 to 2 cm. in length, and is furnished with four teeth (*ankylos*, hooked), and a muscular esophagus by means of which the intestinal mucosa is drawn into the mouth (Fig. 199). The patient develops a profound anemia as the result of this heavy infection. This is due to the peculiar feeding habits of the hookworm, which draws blood from the mucosa of the bowel, pumps it through the alimentary tract, and forces it out from the anal orifice, a process which can be watched in the experimental animal. By means of such a mechanism 10,000 worms can soon remove a lot of blood. There is marked eosinophilia, a common manifestation of worm infections. The patient becomes weak, apathetic, and unable to work. There is marked evidence of anemia, including edema of the face.

The *mode of infection* provides one of those romances which makes the study of parasitology so interesting. The worms may live for six or seven years in the bowel, but they cannot multiply there. The eggs, of which 10,000,000 may be laid at one time, are passed in the feces, and if deposited in warm moist soil they develop into active embryos. These may be swallowed by another person, but the usual route is quite different and much more remarkable. In

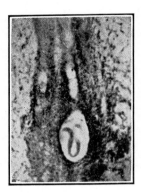

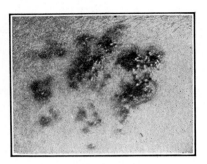

FIG. 201.—Hookworm dermatitis.
(Dove, Am. J. Hygiene.)

FIG. 200.—Hookworm larva (coiled) penetrating
the skin. (Stumberg, Am. J. Hygiene.)

1901 Looss, working in Egypt, showed that the hookworm sets forth on a veritable Odyssey in its effort to reach the small intestine. If wet mud containing the larvæ is rubbed on the skin a burning and itching is soon experienced, and by the time the mud is dry the active larvæ have disappeared through the skin leaving their own skins behind them. Looss followed their course in a leg about to be amputated. The larvæ are found to penetrate the hair follicle (Fig. 200), and from there they bore their way into the lymphatics by which they are carried to the venous blood stream or they may penetrate the veins directly. They are carried by the venous blood to the right heart and thence *via* the pulmonary artery to the lungs. When large numbers of larvæ enter the lungs it is common to find bronchitis and transient bronchopneumonia. In experiments on dogs it was found that the larvæ are filtered out of the circulation in the lungs, being unable to pass through the pulmonary capillaries. They burrow into the air vesicles, enter the bronchi, and crawl up the trachea. Having reached the glottis they climb over the epiglottis and down the esophagus. The further passage through the stomach and into the duodenum is plain sailing. In the small intestine they develop into adult worms. How long the larvæ take to complete their Odyssey it is difficult to say, but as long as ten weeks has elapsed between the skin infection and the appearance of the eggs in the feces.

Ashford has added an important chapter to the story of the hookworm cycle by describing what he calls the larval stage of uncinariasis. He points out that the majority of the larvæ which penetrate the skin never reach the intestine, but die soon after invasion, as shown by the fact that the highest leukocytosis and eosinophilia occur at the beginning of the infection. Many other larvæ stray from the direct path and get hopelessly lost, remaining wanderers in the tissue until they perish. At the end of three months there is a second rise in the leukocyte count, due to the end of the natural term of life of the larvæ. During the larval stage there may be no adult worms in the bowel, but the patient suffers from marked lassitude, while his blood shows an eosinophilia. The latter, which may reach 60 per cent, appears to be due to disintegration of the larvæ and absorption of the foreign protein. Ashford's paper will be found extraordinarily interesting reading.

It is evident that coolies in coffee plantations, natives working in the mud on the banks of the Nile, miners in deep mines, tunnel-workers, *etc.*, are peculiarly liable to the disease once the ground is heavily infected. The "ground itch," an eczematous skin eruption which affects those who walk in infected water with bare feet (Fig. 201) is merely an indication that the larvæ are invading the skin. When native workmen in hookworm areas are compelled to wear shoes the incidence of the disease shows a marked falling off. Proper disposal of excreta is another factor of prime importance in prevention of the disease. The diagnosis is made from the anemia, the eosinophilia and the presence of ova in the stools.

Ascaris Lumbricoides.—(*Roundworm*).—This is the common roundworm which resembles the earthworm, being from 6 to 16 inches long, with tapering pointed ends and a pearly-white appearance. It is a common inhabitant of the small intestine, especially in children in whom it may produce reflex nervous disturbances; possibly a toxic element may also play a part. The worms, of which there are usually several, appear in the mouth. They lie free in the lumen of the bowel, and are not attached to the wall. Occasionally they are present in enormous numbers and may form masses which cause intestinal obstruction.

Although the ascaris is so different from the hookworm, yet parts of their life history are not dissimilar. Indeed, the behavior of the ascaris is even more strange. The ova develop into embryos in moist soil. The freshly passed eggs are not infective, and ten days or more must elapse before they are capable of causing infection. The capacity of the uterus has been estimated at about 27,000,000 eggs, and the average daily output for each female at 200,000. Infection is due to the ingestion of developing eggs on uncooked vegetables, *etc*. When the eggs are ingested they hatch into larvæ in the intestine. But here we come to the strange part. The larvæ are apparently unable to undergo complete development in the intestine until they have undertaken an extra-intestinal migration. They penetrate the wall of the intestine and are carried to the right side of the heart either by the lymph and blood stream or by the mesenteric veins and inferior vena cava. They are filtered out by the lungs, and pass up the trachea and down the esophagus into the intestine just as in the case of the hookworm. This strange migration occupies about ten days. In the intestine they develop into maturity if they have been derived from a human source, but not from the pig. In the latter case they are passed out of the body.

In the pig, on which animal most of the experimental observations have been made, large numbers of larvæ can be seen in sections of the lungs, as well as foci of hemorrhage and inflammation. In man the experimental ingestion of mature eggs has been followed in a few days by the development of the clinical picture of pneumonia. Koins swallowed approximately 2000 eggs; six days later he developed fever, chills, headache, malaise, rapid respirations, and a productive cough with blood and larvæ (178 in one day) in the sputum. There was dullness over the chest and crackling râles. In clinical practice only a few eggs are likely to be taken at any one time, so that as a rule there are no physical signs. Ashford suggests that, as in ankylostomiasis, the larvæ may become lost and wander through the tissues, and that the presence of larvæ in the meninges may be responsible for the convulsions and nervous disorders in young children.

Enterobius Vermicularis.—(*Oxyuris vermicularis, pinworm*).—The pinworm or seatworm is a very common intestinal parasite, especially in children. It is only about 5 mm. long, and when passed in the stools resembles a motile piece of white thread. It lives in the lower part of the small intestine and the large intestine. The worms may pass out *per anum* and cause intense irritation and itching around the anus and in the vagina, owing to the nocturnal wanderings of the gravid female worm. A simple diagnostic method is to make a smear from the perianal region and examine it for ova, which adhere to the hairs in large numbers. In the bowel they usually cause no symptoms, but in weakly children they excite reflex nervous disturbances such as convulsions and enuresis. Masses of pinworms may occupy the lumen of the appendix. Their presence in ulcerative lesions of the small and large intestine is merely a fortuitous association. Even in acute appendicitis they are not a significant cause of the inflammation, as was at one time thought. In rare cases, however, they seem to be responsible for a symptomless *oxyuris granuloma*, which is found incidentally at operation or autopsy (Symmers). The reported cases, with one or two exceptions, have been confined to the Fallopian tubes and the female pelvic peritoneum. These lesions seem to be caused by worms that have strayed from their usual haunts and died. There is no intermediate host, and infection is direct from contaminated vegetables, fruit, *etc.*, with none of the complicated life cycles which a number of the other nematodes have evolved. Massive reinfection may occur from the child's contaminated fingers.

Trichinella Spiralis.—(*Muscle worm*).— The disease trichinosis is caused by a tiny round worm, the life history of which presents some very interesting features. It passes its complete life cycle in the body of one animal, but unless the host be eaten by another animal the embryos will all die. Surely a curious arrangement to have been evolved by a worm, but apparently a satisfactory one.

The parasite infects a variety of animals, in particular the rat, the pig, and man. Man becomes infected by eating the pig, and the pig is infected by eating the rat. Thus the life cycle is continued, but it comes to an end with man. Epidemics occur, particularly in Germany, from eating imperfectly cooked pork in sausages, *etc.* The embryos ingested in the infected pork develop into adult male and female worms in the intestine. These are very tiny, from 1 to 3 mm. long. After copulation the males die and the females burrow into the intestinal villi. The ova develop into embryos within the uterus of the worm, and the embryos are then discharged into the lymphatics. One female may discharge from 1000 to 1500 embryos in this way. The embryos enter the blood stream, and as their diameter is smaller than that of a red blood cell (6 microns broad though 100 microns long), they pass through the lungs and are carried to all parts of the body. During the stage of invasion they can be found in the blood if it is laked and in the cerebrospinal fluid. They are actively motile, and penetrate the capillaries to invade the various organs. But they can only develop in the voluntary muscles and die out elsewhere. Every muscle in the body may be infected. Even the heart is infected at the beginning as indicated by the frequent presence of inflammatory foci, but the young embryos are apparently killed and disappear at an early stage.

Each embryo now enters a muscle fiber and undergoes partial development toward an adult worm, but full development is not possible unless the parasite finds itself in the

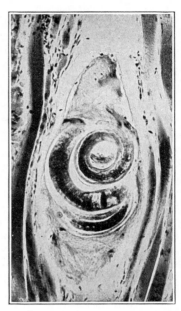

FIG. 202.—Trichinella spiralis in muscle. × 175.

digestive canal of another animal. The muscle fiber degenerates and loses its transverse striations. The embryos are found in the muscles as early as the ninth day after infection. They set up an acute myositis with infiltration of polymorphonuclears, eosinophils, lymphocytes, and giant cells. At first the long axis of the embryo is parallel to that of the muscle fiber, but by the end of the second week it becomes coiled up, encysted, and surrounds itself with a thick hyaline capsule (Fig. 202). Later this may become calcified. The encysted embryos are lemon-shaped, with the long axis in the direction of the muscle fibers. The embryos may remain alive for years awaiting the chance to complete their development in another animal. The life cycle is exactly the same in the pig. When the encysted embryos are swallowed by man the capsule is dissolved by the digestive juices, the embryos are liberated, and may attain maturity in a couple of days, when the whole process is repeated.

It has been found that a dose of 15,000 r filtered x-ray to meat infected with trichina larvæ will render it non-infective to the rat. This suggests a method of sterilizing commercial quantities of pork.

Symptoms.—The symptoms of trichinosis occur during the period of invasion and are partly due to the irritation in the intestine, partly to the acute myositis. The muscles are hard and swollen and often extremely painful. Edema is usually present and is often marked in the face. Fever is a common symptom and may last for days or weeks. The severe cases are easily mistaken for typhoid fever, especially when there is diarrhea, but the leukocytes are increased in number and there is a marked and *very characteristic eosinophilia*, sometimes over 50 per cent. The eosinophilia usually disappears, but may persist for years. Convalescence sets in about the sixth week, but death may occur earlier from paralysis of the respiratory muscles. Many cases die in the early stage of the infection, apparently from the intense irritation in the wall of the intestine. The intradermal injection of a saline extract of trichina larvæ gives a positive reaction in about 90 per cent of cases after several weeks of infection. A positive reaction may still be obtained several years after the acute attack.

Tricocephalus Trichiurus.—(*Whipworm*).—This worm, known as the *whipworm* is one of the commonest intestinal parasites, living in the cecum and appendix, and sometimes associated with acute appendicitis. The worm is only a few centimeters long. The posterior end of the male is coiled on itself, but most characteristic are the barrel-shaped eggs with a knob at each end (Fig. 203). The whipworms are attached only lightly to the intestinal mucosa and as a rule cause little or no disturbance to the unwitting host.

Filaria.—Filariasis is an infection by a nematode worm in which the adult worm lives in the lymphatics while the larvæ travel in the blood. It is a disease of tropical countries. There are several varieties of filaria, the most important being *Filaria bancrofti*, the larval or microfilarial form of which is known as Filaria *sanguinis hominis*. This parasite is of great historical interest, because it was in connection with it that Manson showed for the first time the part which the mosquito plays in the transmission of disease. It was Manson's work which suggested to Ross that malaria might also

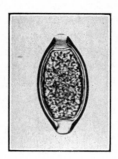

Fig. 203.—Egg of tricocephalus trichiurus. (Kindness of Dr. J. C. Colbeck.)

be conveyed by a mosquito, even though the infecting agents were so very different—the one a nematode worm, the other a protozoan parasite.

The life history and habits of the filaria are remarkable even for an animal parasite. The adult worm lives in the lymphatics, especially those of the groin and pelvis. It is from 0.5 to 1 cm. in length and extremely thin. The male and female live together, and the ova develop in the uterus of the female into active larvæ. These are little eel-like bodies with a diameter no greater than that of a red blood corpuscle, so that they can pass through the smallest capillaries. Their most extraordinary characteristic is their periodicity, for they only appear in the peripheral circulation at night, hiding in the vessels of the lung and the large thoracic vessels during the day. Their appearance synchronizes with the evening appearance of the mosquitoes, for they can only attain maturity in the body of that insect, and if they spent the night in the lung they would never meet a mosquito. One wonders how such an arrangement was first started. If the patient sleeps during the day and is kept awake during the night the larvæ are deceived and come out by day, so that the mosquitoes are disappointed. The larvæ do the patient no harm. This nocturnal periodicity may go on for years, the larvæ patiently awaiting the coming of the mosquito.

Lane points out that the usual explanation of filarial periodicity is not to be lightly accepted, for the hiding place of the larvæ by day has never been demonstrated, and it seems unlikely that they can maintain them-

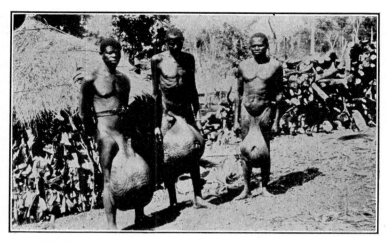

FIG. 204.—Extreme degree of elephantiasis of scrotum in African negroes.

selves in position in the large vessels of the thorax against the strong current of blood. He suggests that there may be a daily cyclical parturition by the females, and that the microfilariæ perish rapidly. This view is supported by the observations of O'Connor who made serial sections of lymphatic tissue containing worms excised at operation. One extraordinary fact was brought to light. When the worms were removed before midday the turgid female was found to be crammed with microfilariæ, but after 2 P.M. the females were collapsed and empty. All the living female worms from the same patient showed the same stage of development of the sex cycle. In a volunteer 720,000 microfilariæ were injected into the blood stream; all were gone in the space of two hours. Destruction apparently takes place chiefly in the lymph nodes.

The *mosquito*, usually a member of the genus culex, bites an infected person, and the larvæ pass with the blood into its stomach. They penetrate the stomach wall and lodge in the thoracic muscles. Here they develop into young worms which make their way to the base of the proboscis and await injection into man, where sexual development may be attained and reproduction take place. The parasite is not actually injected by the mosquito but is deposited close to the hole in the skin made by the proboscis, and through this hole it penetrates the skin. It is said that the worms often

pass out in pairs—probably male and female. They pass to the lymphatics, become mature, larvæ are liberated into the blood, and the cycle is complete.

Pathological Effects.—There may be none, though the patient may have larvæ in his blood for years. The adult worms are apt to produce *lymphatic obstruction*, especially if they are present in masses, and above all if they die and disintegrate. The obstruction causes varicosity of the superficial vessels and lymphatic edema. The regional lymph nodes are enlarged, their sinuses being distended with lymph. *Elephantiasis* may develop. This is a condition in which the tissues become enormously thickened and indurated. The legs and scrotum are the parts commonly affected (Fig. 204). It is probable that lymphatic obstruction alone will not give rise to elephantiasis, but that infection and lymphangitis must be superadded. The abdominal lymphatics may rupture, especially if there is obstruction of the thoracic duct, and lymph escapes into the peritoneal cavity giving chylous ascites. If the renal or vesical lymphatics are obstructed there may be *chyluria*. The patient may show small subcutaneous nodules not necessarily associated with edema. These represent an inflammatory reaction around a coiled-up worm. I have seen such a nodule removed from the arm under the impression that it was a thrombosed vein (Fig. 205).

Dracunculus Medinensis.—(*Filaria med-*

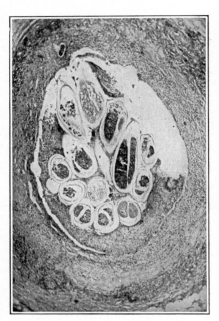

FIG. 205.—Filaria in a small vessel.   × 40.

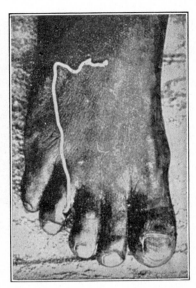

FIG. 206.—Guinea worm partially removed from a ruptured eschar of the fourth toe. (After Castellani and Chalmers, *Tropical Medicine*.)

inensis, Guinea Worm).—This parasite of tropical countries, commonly known as the guinea worm, is surpassed by none of its relatives in peculiarity of behavior. As usual the male is insignificant, but the female is long and very thin; the average length is 50 to 80 cm., but it may reach 1½ meters. The intestinal canal is atrophic and the anus absent, but the uterus, crowded with larvæ, runs almost the entire length of the worm. The larvæ have to be discharged into water, and the female finds the necessary water with a certainty which a water-diviner might envy. The worm works its way through the tissues until it reaches a surface. As the natives go bare-footed, the worm usually makes its appearance on the sole of the foot, but it appears in the upper extremities of Europeans, where water is more often in contact with the hands and arms, and on the backs of water-carriers whose water-skin is slung over that part. The passage down the leg may take as much as eighteen months. The head of the worm pierces the surface with the formation of a small blister, and when water is poured on the skin enormous numbers of larvæ are discharged from the greatly distended uterus

so that the fluid becomes milky. The larvæ are taken up by a fresh-water crustacean belonging to the genus Cyclops, in which they pass through a necessary stage of development before being ingested by man. It is for this reason that the worm has to make for water, however long the journey may be.

If the worm dies or if the larvæ are liberated into the tissues as the result of injudicious attempts at removal, there may be severe inflammation and abscess formation. The natives have an ingenious method of persuading the worm to leave its habitat. They pour water on the foot, and in the resulting effort of parturition the worm is induced to emerge on the surface. The protruding part is wound round a small stick and the treatment is repeated at intervals, the stick being given an additional twist on each occasion. By this simple means as the result of patience and perseverance the worm can finally be completely removed (Fig. 206). It has been suggested that these worms were the "fiery serpents" which afflicted the Children of Israel in the migration from Egypt, and that Moses was the first in history to demonstrate the classical method or removal by winding the "serpent" on a rod, gradually drawing it out. He made a model in brass of the procedure.

CESTODES OR TAPEWORMS

There are four tapeworms of importance in human pathology. All are hermaphrodite, and require the interposition of an intermediate host for the completion of their life cycle.

Three of these pass an adult stage in the intestine of man and a cystic stage in an intermediate host. They are known as the beef tapeworm (Taenia saginata), the pork tapeworm (Taenia solium), and the fish tapeworm (Diphyllobothrium latum). The fourth (Taenia echinococcus) passes the cystic stage in man (the intermediate host) and the adult stage in the dog; this is the one which causes hydatid disease, and is the only really dangerous member of the group.

Taenia Saginata.—(*Taenia mediocanellata. Beef tapeworm*).—The beef tapeworm is the common tapeworm of the United States and Canada. It is the largest tapeworm and it has the largest intermediate host. It consists of a tiny head or scolex and segments or proglottides (Fig. 207). The head is 2 mm. in diameter and possesses four suckers by which it adheres to the intestinal mucosa. It has no hooks. The worm may be 30 feet long and possess some 2000 proglottides. The proglottides are crowded with eggs, and as these become mature the segments break off and are discharged in the feces. When taken up by cattle the ova develop into embryos which migrate to the muscles and there develop into cysticerci. If the beef from an infected cow is eaten imperfectly cooked or in a raw state human infection will result. The diagnosis is made by finding the segments in the feces. The worm, which is usually single, causes wonderfully little disturbance in spite of its great length.

Taenia Solium.—(*Pork Tapeworm*).—The pork tapeworm is much rarer than Taenia saginata. It is usually under 10 feet in length and resembles Taenia saginata. The head, however, is armed with a double row of hooks. Generally only one worm is found (*solium* means single), but in a few instances there may be two or three. The pig is the

24

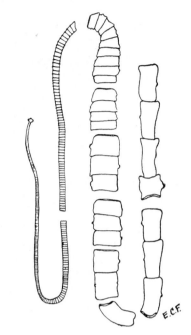

Fig. 207.—Strobila of *Taenia saginata*, Two-thirds natural size. (After Leuckart, *Parasiten des Menschen.*)

intermediate host, its muscles contain large numbers of cysticercus cellulosæ, and man is infected by eating imperfectly cooked "measly" pork. The eggs may be swallowed owing to self-infection and occasionally the embryos invade the body and develop into the larval cystic form, man thus acting as the intermediate host. This does not occur with Taenia saginata. The *cysticercus cellulosæ* thus formed may be present in large numbers in the brain, meninges, eye, muscles, and other organs. The larval worm is inverted and the epithelium of the highly tortuous canal of the body becomes continuous with the epidermis covering the outside of the cyst (Fig. 208). MacArthur has shown that many soldiers who develop idiopathic epilepsy some years after serving in the tropics are really sufferers from cerebral cysticercosis. In the Millbank Military Hospital in London there were 20 cases in one year. The parasites may be present for years before symptoms develop, for they are tolerated while alive, but act as foreign irritants when they die. They become calcified, and can be seen in radiographs of

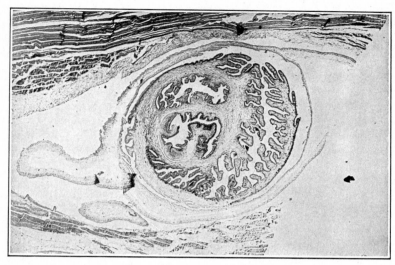

FIG. 208.—Cysticercus cellulosæ showing continuity of epithelium on surface and that lining body canal. × 22.

the muscles. As a rule there is no history of intestinal infection in these cases of cerebral cysticercosis cellulosæ.

Diphyllobothrium Latum.—*Fish Tapeworm*).—The fish tapeworm has from 3000 to 4000 segments filled with eggs. The eggs are discharged from the ripe proglottides, but only empty and shrivelled segments are shed, in this respect differing from the other two tapeworms. It follows that in stool examinations the presence of ripe segments indicates Taenia saginata or Taenia solium, the presence of eggs indicates Diphyllobothrium latum. The average output of eggs in the stool per day is 1,000,000. The tiny head is flattened and does not possess suckers or hooks but is provided with two longitudinal suctorial grooves. When the ova are discharged they develop into free-swimming larvæ and these are taken up by small water crustaceæ which are in turn devoured by some of the larger fish (pike, perch, *etc.*), where they invade the muscles and pass into the cysticercus stage.

The geographical distribution is important. It used to be found principally among the fish-eating peoples in the Scandinavian countries, Russia, and in parts of Asia, but lately it has been imported into the United States and Canada, and is now indigenous in the districts around the Great Lakes and Lake Winnipeg. The fish in these lakes are probably infected from dogs, who also harbor the parasite. If the fish are properly cooked there is no danger.

A large number of the worms may be found in one person. In 999 out of 1000 infectioned persons it is a harmless parasite,

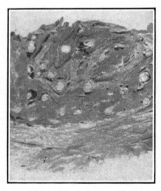

FIG. 209.—Taenia solium cysts in measly pork. (Kindness of Dr. J. C. Colbeck).

provided that the patient is unaware of its presence, although a mild hemolytic anemia is common. In very exceptional cases the patient may develop a severe anemia identical in type with pernicious anemia, but this is seldom seen even in fish-eating communities

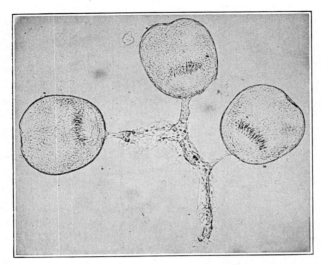

FIG. 210.—Stalked scolices of hydatid cyst showing hooklets. × 200.

where the infection is extremely prevalent; only in Finland is the anemia at all common.

Taenia Echinococcus.—This tapeworm is entirely different from the others. It is extremely small, measuring only 5 mm. in length, and possesses only 3 proglottides The cystic stage is passed in man and many other animals and the adult stage in the intestine of the dog, where there may be hundreds of worms. Man therefore serves as the intermediate host. Human infection is usually due to eating unboiled vegetables soiled by the excreta of dogs. The dogs are infected by eating the flesh of infected sheep. Hydatid disease, as the human infection is termed, is most prevalent in Australia, South America, and other great sheep-raising countries, where dogs and men come into very close contact. Syria has perhaps the largest incidence. Iceland used to be a hot-bed of the disease, but during recent years it has been nearly eradicated by hygienic measures.

When the eggs are swallowed by man they develop into embryos which penetrate the wall of the bowel and are carried in the portal vein to the liver and through the liver to any other part of the body. The embryos form larval cysts (hydatid cysts) which are naturally most common in the liver and mesentery. The cyst consists of two layers. The outer layer or ectocyst is white and presents a characteristic lam-

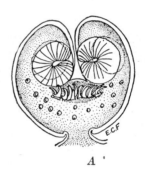

A

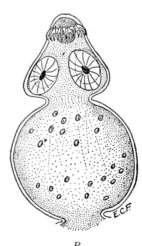

B

FIG. 211.—Scolex of hydatid cyst. *A*, Invaginated in cyst membrane; *B*, with evaginated hooklets and suckers. × 400. (Faust.)

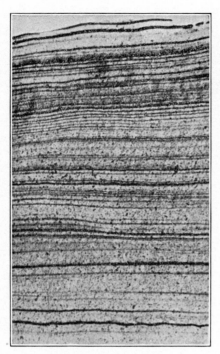

FIG. 212.—Laminated membrane of hydatid cyst. × 200.

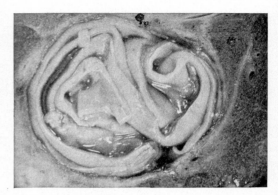

FIG. 213.—Echinococcus cyst of liver showing characteristic lining.

inated structure like the coats of an onion (Fig. 212). The inner or germinal layer is granular and it is in this material that fluid collects so that a cyst is formed (Fig. 213). At various points along the germinal layer buds arise which become hollowed to form brood capsules in which little clusters of new scolices on stalks are produced (Fig. 210). Some of the buds develop into daughter cysts which become detached and float in the cavity of the mother cyst. From the lining of the daughter cyst new buds may arise which in turn produce new scolices. Each scolex is provided with 4 suckers and a crown of 30 to 50 hooklets. The scolex becomes invaginated into its own body in order to preserve the hooklets from injury, so that the suckers and hooklets face inward (Fig. 211). When the infected material (in the sheep or other intermediate host) is eaten by a dog the head is evaginated, and the scolices become attached to the intestinal wall by their hooklets and suckers, proceed to form proglottides, and develop into the mature worm.

The cysts may attain a great size and cause marked enlargement of the liver, form masses in the mesentery, *etc.* The fluid is clear and sterile, but contains a toxic substance which may cause attacks of urticaria or produce toxic effects if the cysts are ruptured during removal. The blood may give a complement-fixation reaction against this substance. Intradermal injection of the fluid is said to give a specific reaction in cases of hydatid disease. Identification of the cysts is made by finding the characteristic hooklets, or by cutting sections of the wall and demonstrating the laminated structure of the ectocyst (Fig. 212).

Echinococcus Alveolaris.—There are two forms of echinococcus: E. hydatidosus, which has just been described, and E. alveolaris or multilocularis, a much rarer form. The hydatid echinococcus forms large cysts filled with fluid, but the alveolar echinococcus cysts are entirely different, being extremely numerous, varying in size from the microscopic to that of a grain of seed or a pea, and containing gelatinous material but as a rule no scolices. They cause great enlargement of the liver, which at autopsy may be mistaken for mucoid carcinoma or congenital cystic liver. Necrosis may develop with the formation of large ragged abscess cavities. The microscopic appearance may closely simulate tuberculosis with necrosis, epithelioid cells and giant cells. The disease is fairly common in Bavaria, Switzerland, and Russia, but is practically unknown in the great hydatid countries such as Australia, South America, and Iceland.

TREMATODES OR FLUKES

The flukes are small, flat, leaf-shaped, unsegmented worms. Liver flukes are common parasites of sheep and cattle, living in the bile ducts and producing inflammation of the liver. Infestation of the liver in man is very prevalent in China, where it is caused by *Clonorchis sinensis* (Chinese liver fluke) (Fig. 214). *Fasciola hepatica* (sheep liver fluke) is met with in sheep-raising countries. The lung fluke (*Distomum pulmonis*) is a common parasite in China and Japan, where it is an important cause of hemoptysis; the ova are found in the blood-stained sputum. The life cycle of trematodes cannot continue without an intermediate host, which is a water snail.

Schistosomiasis.—This is the most common and most important of the diseases caused by flukes. Three of the flukes are pathogenic to man: *Schistosoma mansoni* and *S. japonicum* involving chiefly the liver and intestine, and *S. hematobium*, often known as *Bilharzia hematobia*, involving the bladder. *S. mansoni* is distributed widely throughout the northern part of South America and also in Africa, *S. japonicum* in Japan and the East Indies, and *S. hematobium* in Africa, particularly along the Mediterranean coast. The ova are discharged into water and taken up by a water snail, the intermediate host, from which escape large numbers of active embryos or cercariæ. These penetrate the skin of persons while bathing. The cercariæ of non-pathogenic flukes may penetrate the skin, causing an intense inflammatory reaction known as *swimmer's itch.*

The cercariæ enter the venous circulation, and reach their final habitat, the mesenteric veins in the case of *S. mansoni* and *S. japonicum*, the vesical plexus in the case of *S. hematobium*. During the period of migration through the lungs there may be asthma, transient infiltrations in the lungs radiologically, and eosinophilia in the blood. The embryos develop into adult flukes about 1 cm. in length in the aforementioned veins, where they may live for years, continually

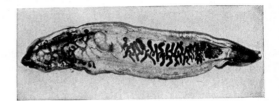

FIG. 214.—Clonorchis sinensis.

producing new ova. It is these ova which are responsible for the symptoms, dysentery in *S. mansoni* and *S. japonicum* infections, hematuria in *S. hematobium* infections. Moreover it is from the ova that identification of the species is made. *S. mansoni* has a prominent lateral spine, *S. japonicum* a rudimentary lateral spine, and *S. hematobium* a long terminal spine. The severity of the disease is conditioned by the daily output of ova. In the case of *S. japonicum* this is 50 to 30, in *S. hematobium* it is 20 to 30, and in *S. mansoni* it is only 1 to 4.

The ova of *S. mansoni* and *S. japonicum* are deposited in the intestine, where they produce an inflammatory reaction with polypoid overgrowths and dysenteric symptoms. Carcinoma of the colon is a late sequel. Rectal biopsy, and in particular examination of the second valve of Houston, is of greater value than the search for ova in the stools. *Microscopically* the response is at first leukocytic and eosinophilic, but later the lesions take the form of pseudotubercles with epithelioid cells and giant cells surrounding the necrotic ovum, and final fibrosis. The ova pass readily in the portal circulation to the liver, where they cause the development of portal cirrhosis, rapid in the case of *S. japonicum*, slow in *S. mansoni* on account of the smaller number of ova.

S. hematobium (bilharzia) causes widespread disease in Egypt and other parts of northern Africa. The population of Egypt is 25,000,000; 6,000,000 of these used to be infected, and 1,000,000 bedridden owing to the disease. The flukes live in the pelvic and vesical veins, and the ova are laid in the wall of the bladder and rectum, where the sharp terminal spine produces an intense reaction. Chronic cystitis and hematuria result. Polypoid masses are formed in the bladder, and these may become the starting-

point of carcinoma. In Egypt carcinoma of
the bladder is said to be 10 times commoner
in those suffering from schistosomiasis. Pulmonary lesions are found in some 33 per
cent of cases (Shaw and Gharceb). The ova
become impacted in the pulmonary arterioles,
causing an acute necrotizing arteriolitis, as
a result of which the ova escape into the
lung and produce a parenchymatous tubercle.
In the great majority of cases only a few
ova reach the lungs, and only a few tubercles
are formed. When the infestation is heavy
there may be an obliterative arteriolitis,
which in rare cases gives a clinical picture of
death from congestive heart failure.

EXTERNAL PARASITES: ARTHROPODS

A few of the more common parasitic
arthropods which, as their name implies, are
distinguished by having jointed legs, will be
merely mentioned. For detailed description
the reader is referred to works on skin diseases
and parasitology. A few of the external
parasites are of importance not only because
of the irritation they produce but because
of the much more serious diseases which
they may be the means of carrying. The
commonest skin parasites are "itch insect"
causing scabies, lice and fleas.

The bites of arthropods are unpleasant
and to be avoided if possible, for they (1)
always itch, (2) may be poisonous, and
(3) may transmit disease. *Itching* is due to
the development of hypersensitivity to the
saliva which is deposited at the site of the
bite. At first the bites do not itch, but they
do so in the course of a few days, and finally
hypersensitivity may be so extreme that the
itching becomes almost intolerable. It is
relieved by antihistamine drugs. Over a
long period sensitivity is replaced by resistance, as is seen in natives in tropical countries. *Poisons* may be injected with the
stings of wasps and the bites of ants. The
most striking example is *tick paralysis*. The
saliva of the pregnant wood tick contains a
powerful neurotoxin that induces an ascending paralysis in the host, which in children
may result in fatal respiratory paralysis.
Transmission of infection by arthropods has
been discussed repeatedly in the previous

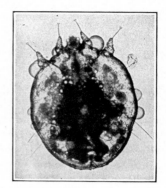

FIG. 215.—Acarus scabiei.   × 75.

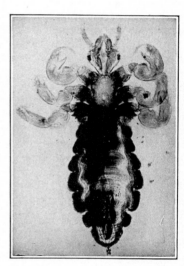

FIG. 216.—Pediculus capitis.   × 30.

chapters. The subject is summarized at
the end of the present chapter.

Acarus Scabiei.—The "itch insect" which
causes scabies is shaped like a turtle and is
about 0.5 mm. long (Fig. 215). The impregnated female bores a tunnel into the
skin, laying her eggs at the end of the tunnel
where the young are hatched. These in
turn bore new tunnels. The male remains
quietly on the surface and causes no trouble.
The symptoms of scabies depend on the
irritation produced by the burrowing female.
The burrows take the form of curved dark
lines, and are most common between the
fingers, at the wrists, in the axillæ, *etc.*
Vesicles may form at the entrance to the

SOME HUMAN DISEASES TRANSMITTED BY ARTHROPODS

Disease	Type of Microorganism	Vector	Reservoir
Plague	Bacterium (Pasteurella pestis)	Flea	Rat or other rodents
Tularemia	Bacterium (Pasteurella tularensis)	Tick	Wild rodents
Relapsing fever	Spirochete (Borrelia recurrentis, etc.)	Louse	Man
Typhus	Rickettsia (R. prowazeki, mosseri, and tsutsugamushi)	Louse	Man
Rocky Mountin spotted fever	Rickettsia (R. rickettsi)	Tick	Wild rodents
Yellow fever	Virus	Mosquito	Man, monkey
Malaria	Protozoan (Plasmodium malariæ, etc.)	Mosquito	Man
Trypanosomiasis (African Sleeping Sickness.)	Protozoan (Trypanosoma gambiense)	Tsetse fly	Man, wild mammals
Kala-azar	Protozoan (Leishmania donovani)	Sand fly	Man
Filariasis	Nematode (Filaria bancrofti, etc.)	Mosquito	Man

burrows and these are often infected by the scratching induced by the intense itching.

Pediculi.—A variety of pediculi or lice may infest the body. *Pediculus capitis*, the head louse, lives on the scalp (Fig. 216). The ova or "nits" are minute white bodies which can be seen attached to the hairs. They hatch out in about a week. *P. corporis*, the body louse, lives on the surface of the skin and breeds in the clothing. By its bites it causes great irritation of the skin, and the itching causes scratching with subsequent infection. The body louse is responsible for carrying the infection of typhus fever, relapsing fever, and trench fever. It does this in the same way as the mosquito, *i.e.*, by biting first a sick man and then a healthy person. *P. pubis* is found especially in the pubic region.

Fleas.—*Pulex irritans* is the common flea, a wingless insect 2 to 4 mm. long. *P. cheopis*, the rat flea, is of importance because it conveys plague not only from one rat to another but also from rat to man.

Flies.—The body tissues or cavities may be infected with the larvæ (maggots) of certain flies, a condition known as *myiasis*. The eggs may be laid in the nasal cavities, wounds, *etc.*, where they develop into maggots. One type of larva tunnels about in the skin, causing the condition called "creeping eruption." This condition may, however, be produced in other ways. In the southern

United States probably the commonest cause is the larva of Ankylostoma braziliense.

ARTHROPODS AS DISEASE CARRIERS

In the course of our study of infection, whether due to bacteria, rickettsiæ, viruses or protozoa, we have seen that an arthropod vector or conveyer, usually an insect, is necessary in many instances for the continuation of the infection. A vector may be mechanical or biological. The *mechanical vector* merely picks up the infecting agent from the body or excreta and deposits it on exposed food (house flies in relation to typhoid, bacillary and amebic dysentery, *etc.*), or conveys infection through contamination of the biting organ (flies and mosquitoes in relation to anthrax and virus encephalitis). The *biological vector* plays an essential part in the completion of the life cycle of the pathogen rather than merely offering it a free ride. The pathogen may undergo cyclic changes (filariasis) or multiplication (plague) or both (malaria) during its sojourn in the vector. The internal arrangements of the arthropod might be specially designed for the conveyance of infection, consisting as they do for the most part of a large blood-filled space, with a complete digestive tract lying alongside it. In many instances it is only the female that transmits disease, an illustration of the old saying that the female of the species is more deadly than the male. In the case of the pathogenic worms the place of the vector is taken by the intermediate host. Global air travel has complicated the picture, for now disease-carrying vectors can themselves be carried in a few hours from an area where disease is endemic to another area where it is unknown. Some of the principal human diseases transmitted by arthropods are given in the table on page 375.

The reader who thinks that he knows something about animal parasites from a perusal of the preceding pages has only to open *Clinical Parasitology* by Faust and Russell to be quickly disillusioned. The size of the subject has become overwhelming, and it seems incredible that any living thing can escape these universal invaders, aided so ably by their insect vectors.

REFERENCES

ASH, J. E. and SPITZ, S.: *Pathology of Tropical Diseases, an Atlas*, Philadelphia, 1945.

ASHFORD, B. K., PAYNE, G. C. and PAYNE, F. K.: J.A.M.A., 1933, *101*, 843. (Ankylostoma duodenale).

BLACKLOCK, D. B. and SOUTHWELL, T.: *A Guide to Human Parasitology for Medical Practitioners*, 4th ed., Baltimore, 1940.

CALLAHAN, W. P., RUSSELL, W. O. and SMITH, M. G.: Medicine, 1946, *25*, 343. (Toxoplasmosis).

CAMERON, T. W. M.: *Parasites and Parasitism*, London, 1956.

FAUST, E. C.: *Human Helminthology*. Philadelphia, 1939.

FAUST, E. C. and RUSSELL, P. F.: *Clinical Parasitology*, 6th ed., Philadelphia, 1957.

LANE, C.: Lancet, 1933, *2*, 399. (Filariasis).

LYNCH, K. M.: *Protozoan Parasitism of the Alimentary Tract*, New York, 1930.

MACARTHUR, W. P.: Trans. Roy. Soc. Trop. Med. and Hyg., 1934, *27*, 343 (Cysticercosis and epilepsy).

MAGATH, T. B.: Am. J. Clin. Path., 1960, *33*, 441. (Incidence of Entamoeba histolytica).

O'CONNOR, F. W. and HULSE, C. R.: Lancet, 1933, *2*, 404. (Filariasis).

SYMMERS, W. St. C.: Arch. Path., 1950, *50*, 475. (Pathology of oxyuriasis).

Chapter 15

Deficiency Diseases

General Considerations
KWASHIORKOR
Fat-Soluble Vitamins
VITAMIN A
Hypervitaminosis A
VITAMIN D
Rickets

Osteomalacia
Hypervitaminosis D
VITAMIN E
VITAMIN K
Water-Soluble Vitamins
VITAMIN C
Scurvy

VITAMIN B COMPLEX
Thiamine. Vitamin B₁
Beriberi
Riboflavin. Vitamin B₂
Nicotinic Acid. Niacin
Pellagra
Vitamin B₁₂
Folic Acid

GENERAL CONSIDERATIONS

THE term deficiency disease connotes a nutritional deficiency. We are not thinking of the total deficiency of starvation. Nor of an insufficiency of dietary protein which in the form of *Kwashiorkor* is the most widespread and important dietary disease in the world to-day (Brock). It is encountered particularly in East and Central Africa, the cinoma in the adult), kwashiorkor is described in connection with diseases of the liver in Chapter 28. The effect which a food intake high in carbohydrate and refined fats but low in protein is demonstrated in a striking manner by Figure 217, which shows a rat that was fed the nutritional equivalent of the diet used by a seven-year-old boy whose skeletal development was retarded by nearly two years (Spies *et al.*).

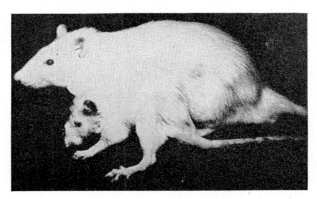

FIG. 217.—Small rat, restricted to deficient diet eaten by child, contrasted to larger rat, a litter mate which was given test diet plus milk supplement. (Spies, courtesy of Jour. Am. Med. Assn.)

West Indies, and some parts of South America, regions where there has been a replacement of protein (animal) food by starchy foods due to the development of agriculture. Protein requirements are greatest in the first years of life due to rapid growth, and evidence of deficiency develops soon after the child is weaned. As the chief lesions involve the liver (extreme infiltration with fat in the child, probably related cirrhosis and car- Our cells are never static, and in time they must be replaced in varying degrees by the nutrients obtained from food. While it is obvious that a marked deficiency of any of the food stuffs used by the body must have deleterious effects, it is only the nutrients known as accessory food substances and present in minute amounts which concern us here, and we shall confine our discussion to the group called the vitamins. There is

(377)

really little justification for these food constituents sharing a common name, as they differ from one another in chemical structure, physiological action, and natural distribution. It is true that they make possible the more efficient utilization of other food factors, but so do essential amino-acids and other organic compounds present in very small amount and essential for the normal functioning of tissue. Custom, however, now decrees that they shall be known as vitamins. Vitamins are organic catalysts of exogenous origin, which are intimately related to the enzyme systems. They play a part as co-enzymes in the chemical mechanism of the cell by which the true food stuffs are metabolized. In many respects they resemble the hormones, which also act through the enzymes, the chief distinction being that hormones are endogenous in origin, whereas vitamins are exogenous, the body being unable to synthesize them. Vitamins do not play a part in the production of energy, nor are they built into the structure of the cell.

Vitamin deficiency or avitaminosis may be due to two very different conditions. (1) The supply of the food factor may be inadequate. This is known as *primary* or *simple deficiency*, and is exogenous in origin. It is of decreasing importance in developed countries, except among food faddists and other health cranks, but it is widely prevalent in undeveloped countries, particularly Africa and the Orient. (2) The supply is adequate, but for various reasons it cannot be used properly. This is *secondary* or *conditioned deficiency*. The following conditions may prevent the vitamin from being utilized (1) *Reduced intake*, as may occur in prolonged vomiting, esophageal obstruction, painful lesions of the mouth, and loss of appetite. (2) *Malabsorption*, occurring in chronic pancreatitis and in chronic enteritis. In Chapter 27 we shall have to consider the condition called the *malabsorption syndrome*. It is obvious that in such cases if the vitamin is administered it must not be given by the mouth but parenterally. (3) *Excessive demand*, seen especially in infancy and puberty, but also during pregnancy and lactation, and as the result of continued fever, hyperthyroidism, and other conditions

which fan the metabolic fire. (4) *Reduced storage facilities*, the best example of which is diffuse disease of the liver such as cirrhosis. The chronic alcoholic with liver disease is a likely subject for vitamin deficiency, not only because of the widespread damage to his liver cells, but also because the alcohol takes the place of food stuffs.

Most of the vitamins are of plant origin, so that they are ingested in plant or animal food—unless they happen to be bought at the corner drug store. Unlike other substances, it is only deficiency which is harmful. With the exception of vitamins D and A, apparently you can't have too much of a good thing. It is customary to divide the vitamins into two groups, the fat-soluble and the water-soluble. The fat-soluble members are less easily absorbed than the water-soluble, so that they are more readily affected by conditioning factors. The *fat-soluble vitamins* are A, D, E and K, the *water-soluble* being C and B. It is true that the latter pair are more readily absorbed, but this advantage is off-set by the fact that there may be an inadequate supply of C, whilst in the case of B the body stores are limited and only small amounts are available in food, so that deficiency of a simple exogenous variety may develop. Moreover, on account of being soluble in water they are more readily lost as the result of cooking or the modern processing of food.

Although clinical evidence of vitamin deficiency was first recognized in the human subject, much of our knowledge is due to the vast amount of work carried out on the experimental animal. It must be remembered that malnutrition is often not the result of absence of any one vitamin, that man seldom shows the picture of pure deficiency seen in the experimental animal, and that the administration of a single vitamin in a chemically pure state may not serve to correct the condition. We now know enough, however, to prevent the *five major vitamin-deficiency diseases*, namely *beriberi*, *pellagra*, *scurvy*, *rickets*, and *keratomalacia*. It may be added that a number of congenital anomalies in mammals have been shown experimentally to be due to maternal dietary deficiencies. It is possible that some day this knowledge may have a human application.

For more detailed information on the subject of vitamin deficiencies the reader is referred to *the Pathology of Nutritional Disease* by Follis and *The Vitamins* (in 3 volumes) by Sebrell and Harris. Full details on the food content of the various vitamins will be found in *Nutrition in Health and Disease* by Cooper, Barber, Mitchell and Rynbergen.

VITAMIN A

Physiology.—Vitamin A as such occurs in bright yellow animal foods such as butter and the yolk of eggs. Various plants such as corn and sweet potatoes contain precursors of the vitamin which are converted into active vitamin A by animal tissues. Being fat-soluble, it is stored in the fat of animals, and it is present in greatest abundance in cod-liver oil (although much is lost in the process of refining), but fresh milk contains an adequate supply for the growing child, especially when combined with yolk of eggs. Animals can synthesize it in the liver from the vegetable pigment carotene, so that it may be given directly as cod-liver oil or indirectly as vegetables. The conversion takes place in the liver through the action of an enzyme. The vitamin has been isolated in chemically pure form, and has been synthesized.

Vitamin A gives a *green fluorescence* in ultraviolet light, which disappears rapidly. Popper points out that similar fluorescence, presumably due to vitamin A, can be seen in frozen sections of certain tissues. It is most marked in the liver, adrenal cortex, and corpus luteum. In hypervitaminosis A the amount is increased.

Vitamin A deficiency is essentially a conditioned deficiency. Such enormous quantities are stored in the liver that it is only in the experimental animal that a deficiency is likely to be caused by insufficient intake. The fat-soluble vitamin is absorbed in the small intestine and carried to the liver. It follows that vitamin deficiency may develop in disease of the biliary tract, in pancreatic dysfunction, and in such disorders of fat absorption as sprue and the malabsorption syndrome. Diffuse hepatic disease may produce a similar result, but several years may have to elapse before the supplies in the liver are exhausted.

The chief functions of vitamin A are to preserve the visual purple in the rod cells of the retina, to maintain the epithelial surfaces of the body in a normal state, and to regulate the growth of bone in the young animal.

Pathology.—The basic lesion of vitamin A deficiency is atrophy of columnar epithelium and a substitution of stratified keratinizing epithelium due to proliferation of the basal cells, *i.e.*, a *keratinizing metaplasia*, which may be regarded as an attempt at repair following atrophy (Wolbach and Howe, Wolbach and Berry). In the human infant this occurs in the conjunctiva, nasal mucosa, accessory nasal sinuses, salivary glands, trachea, bronchi, pancreas, renal pelvis, ureters, and uterus. The commonest and earliest change is in the *trachea* and *bronchi*, and death is often due to pneumonia. The lumen of the ducts is blocked by desquamated keratinized cells so that cysts are formed in glands, bronchiectatic cavities in the lungs, *etc.* In the *eye* a late effect is *xerophthalmia*. The cornea dries up (*xero*, dry) and becomes ulcerated and infected. This is due to involvement of the lacrimal glands, as a result of which the tears are no longer produced and the cornea is not bathed with fluid as it should be. The infected cornea becomes softened and may finally undergo perforation. These corneal changes are known as *keratomalacia*. The salivary glands also become dried up. Xerophthalmia is rarely seen in Europe and America, but in Japan and other eastern countries poorly nourished children not infrequently develop the condition. The characteristic *skin* lesion is *follicular hyperkeratosis*. Multiple tiny papules giving a "toad skin" appearance develop in various parts, most often on the arms and thighs. These are caused by the formation of keratin plugs in the sebaceous glands. Bacterial infections are common in the affected organs, but this seems to be due to the structural change rather than to the loss of any specific anti-infective property of the vitamin.

Night-blindness (hemeralopia, more correctly *nyctalopia*) has long been known to be benefited by cod-liver oil. Hippocrates recommended ox liver dipped in honey for a cure, and in Newfoundland cod's liver is a popular remedy. Any source of vitamin A will effect a cure. Night-blindness is due to exhaustion of the visual purple after prolonged exposure to brilliant sunlight, and lack of vitamin A interferes with regeneration of the visual purple.

Bone growth in young animals is retarded by deficiency of vitamin A. The effect seems to be due to interference with the growth of epiphyseal bone. When large doses of the vitamin are given the rate of growth is enormously accelerated in the experimental animal. A similar effect has not been observed in the human child, probably due to the abundant supply of milk which it receives.

Hypervitaminosis A.—Vitamin A is a two-edged sword, even though the two edges are not equally sharp, for it is possible, though rare, to have too much as well as too little of the vitamin. This is likely to come about through self-medication by the patient, as in one case where a young woman consumed 500,000 units of the vitamin over a period of eight years with the object of improving a skin condition (Gerber *et al.*).

The *clinical manifestations* of chronic vitamin A toxicity are reflected in the nervous system, the skeleton and the skin. *Neurological* disturbances comprise persistent severe headache with disorder of vision, but without localizing signs. These are the result of increased intracranial pressure, itself due to excessive production or decreased absorption of cerebrospinal fluid, so that an intracranial tumor may be suspected. *Bone pains* are usually present. These seem to be due to calcification in the pericapsular, tendinous and subperiosteal tissues, and the condition may be mistaken for chronic infective or rheumatoid arthritis. *Skin involvement* may take the form of pruritus, fissuring and soreness at the corners of the mouth, coarsening of the hair, and pigmentation. Rapid clinical improvement occurs upon stopping excess vitamin A intake.

VITAMIN D

Physiology.—Like vitamin A, vitamin D is a fat-soluble vitamin, which is contained in milk, egg-yolk, and other fats, but far the most abundant supply is cod-liver oil. It has the same chemical formula as ergosterol, and appears to be an isomer of that substance, being formed from it by the action of ultraviolet light. It is now recognized that the vitamin can be represented by (1) activated ergosterol (calciforol), or (2) activated cholesterol. Both of these are used in therapy.

The *clinical manifestation* of vitamin D deficiency is *rickets in the child, osteomalacia in the adult.* The reason for this is that vitamin D controls calcium metabolism and indirectly phosphorus metabolism. Rickets has been recognized clinically from the earliest times, but it was only in 1918 that it was realized that the condition was due to deficiency of an accessory factor in the diet. Even later it was recognized that accessory factors, particularly sunlight which activates the pro-vitamin in the skin, plays a part in the pathogenesis. It is easy to understand why rickets is unknown in countries bathed in sunshine.

As in the case of vitamin A, vitamin D is absorbed from the intestine, so that *deficiency* may be produced by an inadequate supply of bile salts, pancreatic insufficiency, and the malabsorption syndrome, as well as by an inadequate production of the vitamin. Its chief store-house is the liver, so that diffuse liver disease may result in vitamin deficiency. These factors are more likely to play a part in the osteomalacia of adults. The rickets of infants and children is due to a primary deficiency of the vitamin. Vitamin D regulates the absorption of calcium and, to a lesser extent, phosphorus from the intestine. The raised level of calcium in the serum depresses parathyroid activity, with resulting increased tubular reabsorption of phosphorus. When the vitamin is deficient all this is reversed, so that there is an insufficiency of calcium and phosphorus.

Pathology. — Rickets. — The essence of rickets is interference with the calcification of the proliferating cartilage at the epiphyses. This must be distinguished from ossification, which consists in the replacement of the calcified cartilage by true bone and bone marrow. In vitamin C deficiency (scurvy) the bone disorder is one of ossification. The manifestations of rickets in the skeleton may

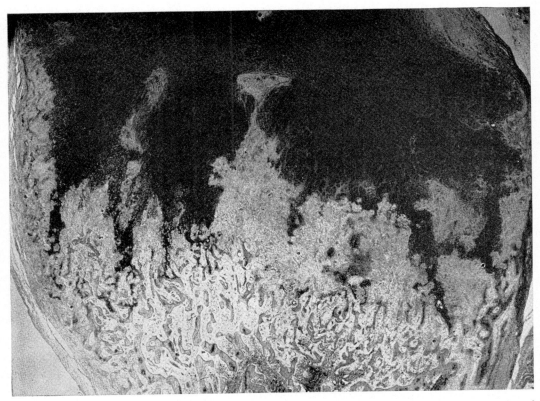

FIG. 218.—Rib. Severe Rickets. Costochondral junction from a seven-months-old colored male dying of unexplained fever and diarrhea; he had been sick for one month. There is extreme swelling in the region of the cartilage shaft junction. Note the increase in width of the zone of mature cartilage cells and the irregularities in calcification. There is complete disorganization in this region due to collapse of the cartilage and trabeculæ, many of which are composed of osteoid. H. and E., × 15. (Follis, *The Pathology of Nutritional Disease*, 1948, courtesy of Charles C Thomas.)

be produced by a deficiency of calcium, phosphorus or vitamin D, singly or together. There is failure of lime salts to be deposited in the cartilaginous matrix, and failure of the cartilage cells to undergo degeneration. At the same time the zone of mature cartilage cells becomes increased in width. The result is a broad zone between the multiplying cartilage cells and the shaft, composed of tongues of cartilage extending toward the shaft (Fig. 218). True rickets occurs chiefly in the first two years of life, and is influenced very largely by the amount of sunlight available, so that it is unknown in the tropics, no matter how inadequate the supply of milk and egg-yolk may be, not to mention cod-liver oil.

Osteomalacia.—This condition, as we have seen, is the adult counterpart of rickets. It is very uncommon in North America as a purely nutritional condition. In China, on the other hand, it is very prevalent, particularly in child-bearing women. This is due to a combination of poor diet and insufficient sunlight during pregnancy and lactation, particularly in North China. In the United States it is seen as a result of chronic renal insufficiency, resulting in the deranged calcium and phosphorus metabolism which characterizes chronic nephritis.

Development of the teeth is interfered with both in the experimental animal and in the child. When the diet contains an abundance of vitamin D (milk, egg-yolk, *etc.*), the teeth are even, bright, shiny, and well formed. With a diet poor in vitamin D,

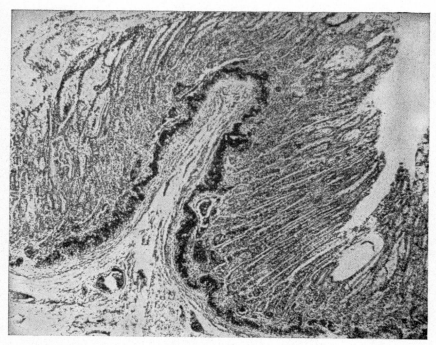

FIG. 219.—Stomach in hypervitaminosis D. Note the extensive calcification in the mucosa. **Von Kossa** stain. × 80. (Kent *et al.*, courtesy of Am. J. Pathology.)

especially if it is rich in cereals, the teeth are uneven, poorly calcified, dull, and discolored. *Caries* is a disease of poorly developed and poorly calcified teeth, but there is no general agreement as to the relationship between avitaminosis and the development of human caries.

Hypervitaminosis D.—This condition can readily be induced in the experimental animal, and it may even occur in the child through some error, although there is no danger of this with ordinary therapeutic doses. When large overdoses of vitamin D (irradiated ergosterol) are given there is hypercalcemia and hyperphosphatemia. If, on the other hand, the diet is rich in calcium the bones are much less affected, but there are calcareous deposits in many of the tissues, being most marked in the renal tubules and the walls of the arteries. Renal insufficiency favors calcification of the soft tissues, for it interferes with the excretion of phosphorus, and high serum phosphorus is even more important than high serum calcium in promoting calcification of soft parts.

An interesting involuntary experiment resulting in hypervitaminosis D is reported by Kent and his associates. Due to an error on the part of a manufacturer of monkey food an entire colony of monkeys received excessive amounts of calcium, phosphorus and vitamin D over a period of 3 months. The result was extensive deposits of calcium, particularly in the kidneys, lungs, salivary glands, and gastric mucous membrane (Fig. 219).

VITAMIN E

This fat-soluble vitamin represents a group of tocopherols. It is more abundant in an ordinary diet than any of the other vitamins. As a consequence, little or nothing is known about deficiency of vitamin E in the human, but a large amount of work has been done on the experimental animal. It has been called the antisterility vitamin. Deficiency of the vitamin produces different lesions in the two sexes. In the male animal the spermatozoa are destroyed, and there is finally degeneration of the entire seminiferous epithelium. In the female the ovaries do not appear to be injured, fertilization of the ovum occurs, and gestation commences, but about the eighth day in the rat pathological changes develop in the placenta and the fetus dies and is absorbed. In addition to its effect on the reproductive function, vitamin E is a necessary factor for the preservation of the integrity of skeletal muscle. When female mice are maintained on a vitamin E low diet but are given a single dose of vitamin to ensure the birth of living young, the offspring show marked necrosis of skeletal muscle in 20 per cent of cases with early calcification (Pappenheimer).

VITAMIN K

Physiology.—This, the fourth of the fat-soluble vitamins, is of very much greater clinical significance than vitamin E on account of its relationship to bleeding. In 1930 Dam, of Copenhagen, noticed that chicks fed on a deficient diet developed hemorrhages owing to the loss of coagulating power of the blood, and that this was prevented by giving alfalfa. The coagulation factor in the alfalfa was extracted, crystallized and finally synthesized. It was called Koagulations-vitamin or vitamin K. The vitamin is necessary for the manufacture of prothrombin, so that when the vitamin is deficient the prothrombin in the blood is low, a condition of *hypoprothrombinemia*. Estimation of the plasma prothrombin thus affords a simple method of determining if there is a deficiency of vitamin K. Such deficiency in man is probably never due to lack of the vitamin in the food. In addition to the supply in the food, the vitamin is also manufactured by the normal bacteria of the bowel. As we have already seen in the case of fat-soluble vitamins A and D, it is a conditioned deficiency rather than a deficient supply of the vitamin which is the threat.

Pathology.—The three groups of conditions which may bring about vitamin K deficiency are: (1) biliary obstruction; (2) malabsorption of fat in celiac disease, pancreatic disease, sprue, hypermotility of the bowel, *etc.*; (3) failure of bacterial synthesis of the vitamin due to the action of antibiotics. The two major clinical conditions in which there is a dangerous degree of vitamin K deficiency are obstructive jaundice and hemorrhagic disease of the newborn. Unless bile is present in the bowel vitamin K is not absorbed, prothrombin is not formed in sufficient amount, and hemorrhage occurs. In *obstructive jaundice* bile is prevented from entering the bowel. This explains the marked tendency to bleeding after operations on jaundiced patients. The bleeding can be prevented by the administration of bile and vitamin K, or by giving the synthetic vitamin by mouth (the synthetic product is absorbed without the assistance of bile), or intravenously. If the liver is severely damaged (cirrhosis, amyloid, *etc.*) the administration of vitamin K is of no avail, because it is in the liver that the prothrombin is produced which is essential to coagulation. The explanation of *bleeding in the newborn* is that vitamin K is produced by the action of intestinal bacteria, and these are absent during the first few days of life. A contributing factor is the failure of the liver to produce bile during this period. At birth the baby has sufficient prothrombin from the maternal blood, but this rapidly falls, and there may be severe and even fatal hemorrhage, particularly intracranial. This is now prevented by giving the mother vitamin K before delivery. Bleeding due to vitamin K deficiency is of particular importance following operations for the relief of obstructive jaundice. In addition to bleeding from severed vessels, there may be hemorrhages in the skin and mucous membranes, particularly that of the bowel.

VITAMIN C. ASCORBIC ACID

We come now to the *water-soluble vitamins*, namely vitamin C and the B complex. Being soluble in water they are rapidly and readily absorbed from the small intestine, but for the same reason they are largely removed from food by the ordinary methods of cooking. The vitamin deficiency will therefore be of the primary type due to lack of the vitamin in the food, and not secondary to or conditioned by loss of power of absorption or storage of the vitamin.

Physiology.—Vitamin C is identical with ascorbic acid, and it has been both crystallized and synthesized. This vitamin is present in all fresh fruits and vegetables, being particularly abundant in tomato, orange, lemon, and grape-fruit. It is present in smaller amount in fresh meat and milk. Steffanson maintained himself in the Arctic on a diet of fresh meat alone without developing scurvy. The vitamin is easily destroyed by heat, so that boiled or pasteurized milk may be completely lacking in it. It is the duration of heating rather than the actual temperature which seems to matter. The drying of fruits also destroys the vitamin. It is rapidly absorbed from the bowel, and is stored in a great variety of tissues, most abundantly in the adrenal cortex. Ascorbic acid is necessary for the health of the ground substance of mesenchymal structures such as collagen, osteoid, the cement of capillary walls, and dentine. When it is deficient these structures all suffer. It is probably the mucopolysaccharides of the ground substances which are influenced. In health the tissues should be saturated with the vitamin. The main difficulty of vitamin C deficient tissue seems to be its inability to oxidize the side chain of tyrosine.

Our knowledge of avitaminosis C comes from two sources, the study of scurvy or scorbutus in man and deficiencies produced in the laboratory animal. The human disease has been observed and described throughout the ages, and in the 18th century it was recognized by Lind that the juice of citrus fruits contains a substance which protects against scurvy. In the experimental animal we encounter a curious species difference with respect to the effect of the deficiency. This can be produced and observed in the guinea pig, monkey and man, but the mouse, rabbit, rat and dog do not need an exogenous source of the vitamin so that no dietary deficiency is possible. In consequence nearly all the experimental work has been done on the guinea pig. A notable exception is afforded by the observations of Crandon, who put himself on a vitamin C deficient diet. The long interval of time which elapsed before evidence of scorbutus appeared is an indication of the abundant store of the vitamin in the tissues. The plasma ascorbic acid level fell to zero in 41 days, but by the end of 3 months an incision healed normally, and it was not until 182 days had elapsed that healing no longer occurred.

Pathology.—*Scurvy* or *Scorbutus.*—Scurvy is the result of a deficiency of vitamin C in the food. Once the scourge of sailors and explorers who were unable to carry supplies of fresh fruit and vegetables, it is now seldom seen in the adult since it was found that lime juice would act as an excellent preventive. The reason for the prophylactic power of the lime juice is, of course, a modern discovery. In war, in beleaguered cities, *etc.*, scurvy may still prove a menace. In some countries the potato is the chief antiscorbutic article of diet during the winter months. In such a country as Ireland a potato famine has often been accompanied by an outbreak of scurvy. But it is in children that the disease is most likely to be seen at the present day, for modern methods tend to destroy the vitamin in the child's natural food. Scurvy is practically never met with in breast-fed children, but it may develop in bottle-fed babies, for the sterilization of the milk (boiling or pasteurization) destroys the antiscorbutic vitamin. Even keeping the milk instead of using it fresh lessens the vitamin content. The addition of orange juice to sterilized milk restores to the full its antiscorbutic power.

The *lesions* and the *clinical manifestations* of scurvy can conveniently be arranged in 4 groups, but the basis of each of these is the fundamental defect of metabolism of mesenchymal ground substance described under the heading of physiology. This defect may be reflected in: (1) delayed healing of wounds, (2) defective bone formation, (3) interference with the formation of teeth in the experimental animal, and (4) a hemorrhagic diathesis.

Wound Healing.—The now classical studies of Wolbach and Howe in 1926 showed that the failure of skin incisions to heal in the scorbutic animal was due to the lack of formation of collagen. Fibroblasts proliferated in normal fashion, but they failed to lay down collagen in a pink-staining fluid-like substance which represented the

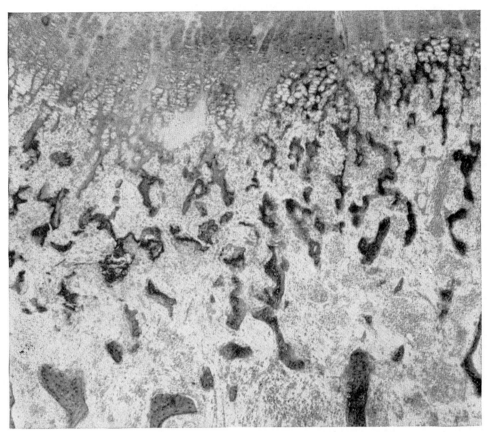

Fig. 220.—Costochondral junction of rib in scurvy. Note numerous fractures with spicules of calcified cartilaginous matrix material scattered in all directions. Although there is an abundance of fibroblast-like cells they seem quite impotent of forming collagen or osteoid. Changes in the cartilage, such as defects in calcification and irregularity in lining up of the cells, are due to mechanical factors. H. and E., × 60. (Follis, *The Pathology of Nutritional Disease*, 1948, courtesy of Charles C Thomas.)

ground substance. Similar results were observed in man in the experiments conducted by Crandon on himself. Even when the wound does eventually heal it is lacking in tensile strength, so that it tends to break down under strain.

Bone Formation.—The changes are most evident at the epiphyseal ends of a growing bone. It will be remembered that normally the cartilage cells of the epiphyseal plate multiply and are arranged in rows, lime salts are deposited in the matrix between these cells, osteoid tissue formed by osteoblasts replaces this lime salt matrix, and is immediately converted into bone by the deposition of calcium and phosphorus. In scurvy the osteoblasts fail to form osteoid,

the calcified cartilage is not replaced. The result is a wide area of calcified cartilage under the epiphyseal plate, with spicules of this material extending downward to form what has been called a "scorbutic lattice," but without true bone formation (Fig. 220). It will be seen that this is not a disturbance of calcification, as in rickets, but of ossification. The normal narrow line of ossification is broadened and dense, giving a pathognomonic picture in the roentgen-ray film. When a proper diet is given, osteogenesis is rapidly resumed. The x-ray picture is highly characteristic. This poor substitute for true bone easily gives way under strain, so that fractures are common. The capillaries in this tissue are readily ruptured with resulting hemorrhage, which is most extensive and evident under the loosely attached periosteum.

Teeth.—Lesions of the teeth are not observed in man, but in the young experimental animal there is marked interference with the development first of the dentin and then of the enamel organ. Rarifaction of the alveolar bone leads to undue mobility and loss of the power to withstand the mechanical stresses of chewing. In human subjects great stress has been laid in the past on gingivitis. The gums are soft, spongy and bleed readily, but this may have been due to poor oral hygiene rather than to ascorbic acid deficiency.

Hemorrhagic Diathesis.—A marked tendency to bleeding is characteristic of scurvy. This may be presumed to be due to deficiency of the intercellular cement which holds together the cells of the capillary endothelium, although this cannot be demonstrated by present microscopic methods. Hemorrhage is most marked in the subcutaneous and subperiosteal tissue, and into the gums, joints and muscles of the leg. Much blood may be lost from the nose, the bowel, and in the urine.

Infantile Scurvy (Barlow's Disease).—Infantile scurvy is similar to adult scurvy, but the symptoms due to the bone lesions dominate the picture. The legs are so tender that the child screams if they are even touched. This tenderness is due to subperiosteal hemorrhages. Growth of the bones is naturally in abeyance. The gums may be tender and bleeding. The disease usually appears in the second half of the first year. After the second year it is seldom seen in an acute form as the diet is more varied, but there may be minor manifestations which are often unrecognized.

The *diagnosis* of scurvy in doubtful cases can be made from the evidence of absence of osteogenesis in the x-ray picture, the low level of plasma ascorbic acid, and the demonstration of increased capillary fragility by the development of petechial hemorrhages when a tourniquet is applied to the arm.

VITAMIN B COMPLEX

What was originally called vitamin B is now known to be a group of substances of different chemical composition and different physiological action. For this reason the term vitamin B complex is in common use. The complex may be defined as the collection of vitamins present in the yeast cell. The principal members in relation to human disease are thiamine or vitamin B_1, riboflavin or vitamin B_2, niacin, folic acid, and B_{12}. Like vitamin C, these are all water-soluble, therefore readily absorbed. This group of vitamins is one of the most widely distributed, being present in all natural foodstuffs, but much of it is lost in the process of refining and of converting natural into artificial foods, as in the case of white bread, polished rice, *etc.* At least three of the vitamins—thiamine, riboflavin and niacin—are required as coenzymes in the Krebs citric acid cycle of energy-transfer reactions in cell respiration.

Thiamine. Vitamin B_1.—Thiamine is known as the anti-neuritic or anti-beriberi factor. It was in 1897 that Eijkman, a Dutch physician in Java, noticed that the poultry at the prison hospital fed on scraps of polished rice thrown out from the prison tables developed symptoms similar to those of his patients suffering from beriberi, but recovered when fed with other food. This was one of the most profound observations in the science of nutrition. The missing material is vitamin B_1 or thiamine, which is stored in the body in the form of thiamine pyrophosphate. It is not stored in large amount, however, and as there is a constant daily demand, it follows that a relatively short period of deficiency may result in clinical disturbances. This is the opposite to what we observed in the case of vitamin C. Thiamine is widely distributed in a large variety of animal and vegetable tissues, but with the striking exception of pork there are few foods in which it occurs in abundance. For this reason bread and cereals are now enriched so as to make it easier for the average person to meet his requirement economically. The vitamin is an essential factor in enzyme systems concerned with carbohydrate metabolism, more particularly that involving the nervous system. When rice is polished the skin and the embryo are removed, and it is these which contain the vitamin. Birds fed on polished rice develop an avitaminosis known as the polyneuritis of birds or rice disease.

Pathology.—It is not too easy to correlate the clinical and pathological findings of thiamine deficiency, nor the manifestations of the deficiency in the experimental animal and man. The polyneuritis of birds fed on polished rice is characterized by extreme ataxia followed by paresis due to peripheral neuritis, together with anemia, lymphopenia and hyperglycemia. In detailed observations on pigs Follis and his associates found focal and diffuse myocardial necrosis associated with marked cardiac dilatation in animals dying of thiamine deficiency. Thiamine deficiency is involved in the neuritis recurring in chronic alcoholism, pregnancy and diabetes. Mild forms of thiamine deficiency, which may be due to the use of a diet composed largely of white bread, are not uncommon. They are characterized by symptoms suggesting myocardial disease, such as tachycardia, dyspnea, edema, and enlargement of the heart, symptoms which may be associated with numbness and tingling of the hands and feet.

In the *experimental animal* thiamine deficiency results in lesions in the myocardium and nervous system. The *myocardium* at autopsy shows patchy necrosis of the muscle fibers, together with collections of leukocytes. These lesions are present both in the auricles and ventricles, but are more marked in the auricles and sometimes confined to those structures. It may be noted that the oxygen consumption of the auricles is significantly lower in thiamine deficient rats than in the normal animal. Corresponding with these lesions the principal clinical findings are bradycardia, extensive electrocardiographic changes such as a prolonged P–R interval and abnormalities in the P wave, auricular fibrillation, and finally complete block. The *nervous lesions* are more controversial than those of the myocardium. We have such a statement as: "The most constant and striking findings of thiamine deficiency arise from chemical alterations which lead ultimately to degenerative changes in the nervous system—Changes in the posterior root ganglion and anterior horn cells have been noted—Degeneration is most severe in the sciatic nerve and its branches, but

degenerative changes may be found in any of the peripheral nerves" (Spies and Butt). Others consider that there is not sufficient justification for calling thiamine the antineuritic vitamin, and that the polyneuritis of birds is due to deficiency of several nutrients rather than a single one.

Beriberi.—Beriberi has been recognized as a human disease in the Orient for centuries, but our first real understanding of the condition came with Eijkman's already mentioned classic observation on the relationship between deficiency disease in pigeons and human beriberi. The disease is endemic in such countries as South China, where the staple article of diet is rice which has been polished and therefore deprived of its thiamine content. It may also occur in modified form in Western countries among low income groups, food faddists, and chronic alcoholics in whom alcohol takes the place of food. The *principal features* are peripheral neuritis, edema, and myocardial weakness, a triad of symptoms which is found in perhaps no other disease. The disease differs in some respects from the experimental rice disease of birds. In both there is polyneuritis, but the birds do not show the edema and cardiac failure, while the beriberi patients do not show the anemia, lymphopenia, and hyperglycemia characteristic of the experimental disease. Vitamin B deficiency is an essential factor in the production of beriberi, but it is rarely so complete as to be the sole agent.

Three main general types of the disease are recognized, dry, wet, and cardiac. *Dry beriberi* is marked by weakness, paresthesias, sensory loss, *etc.*, symptoms which are referable to the neuromuscular system. *Wet beriberi* is characterized by generalized edema. *Cardiac beriberi* is recognized by evidence of cardiac failure, dilatation of the heart, elevated venous pressure, and electrocardiographic changes similar to those already described in the experimental animal. Death is due to cardiac failure. As one might expect, these three types are often mixed.

Autopsy findings are edema of the legs, fluid in the serous sacs, and marked enlargement (both hypertrophy and dilatation) of the right side of the heart. Thiamine deficiency myocarditis is seen in chronic

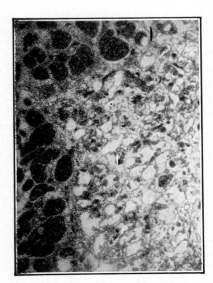

Fig. 221.—Beriberi heart. (Boyd's *Pathology for the Physician*.)

alcoholics in North America (Weiss and Wilkins). The heart may appear normal, or it may be dilated and hypertrophied and overweight. Microscopically there is often hydropic degeneration and vacuolation of the myocardial fibers, including those of the subendocardial conduction system (Fig. 221). The onset of symptoms of myocardial failure in an alcohol addict may be sudden or gradual. The condition is relieved by the administration of thiamine. Electrocardiographic changes develop in healthy volunteers on a thiamine deficiency diet.

The *nervous lesions* involve the peripheral nerves (*polyneuritis*), both motor and sensory, the spinal cord, and the brain stem. The most marked changes are seen in the sciatic nerve. There is first fatty degeneration of the myelin sheaths, followed later by fragmentation of the axis cylinders (Fig. 222). In severe cases there may be an ascending polyneuritis. The production of the nerve lesions does not appear to be due to thiamine deficiency alone.

Wernicke's encephalopathy is a cerebral form of beriberi due to thiamine deficiency. This rare condition is marked clinically by paralysis of the eye muscles, stupor or excitement, and usually death in a few days. The lesions are curiously restricted. The corpora mammillaria are constantly affected; in addition there may be lesions in the hypothalamus, thalamus, and periaqueductal gray matter. The characteristic microscopic lesion is vacuolation and disintegration of the intercellular tissue with preservation of the nerve cells. The condition is described in more detail in Chapter 42.

Riboflavin.   Vitamin B₂.— *Physiology.*— *Riboflavin* has been called the *tissue respiratory vitamin*. It is a yellow-green fluorescent pigment with properties similar to those of a "yellow respiratory enzyme" which had already been isolated. The term flavin is derived from the yellow color (*flavus*, yellow). The vitamin is widely distributed in plant and animal foods. It is required for normal cellular respiration, taking part in the transfer of oxygen from the plasma to the cells of the tissues. Like the other water-soluble vitamins it is rapidly absorbed from the bowel and widely stored in the tissues, more particularly the liver.

Pathology.— In growing animals aribo-flavinosis is characterized by atrophy of the epidermis and raggedness of the skin, corneal degeneration and vascularization, the latter often quite intense, and degeneration of the myelin sheath of nerves.

In man the *lesions* of riboflavin deficiency show a curious distribution confined to the structures of the head and face. The significant foursome are: (1) *cheilosis*, the early development of cracks and fissures at the angle of the mouth (Fig. 223); (2) *glossitis*, the tongue becoming smooth and of a striking magenta color, with atrophy of the mucosa, and projection of small bulbs of fungiform papillæ, giving the organ a pebbly, or cobblestone appearance; (3) *interstitial keratitis*; (4) *scaling dermatitis*, beginning in the nasolabial folds and extending to the cheeks, with a butterfly distribution. The most serious disturbances are those involving the eye. In those whose occupation exposes them to bright light (including workers with the microscope) there may be photophobia, eye fatigue, redness of the conjunctiva and lower lids. The earliest and most common sign is circumcorneal injection, best revealed by the slit lamp. In more advanced cases there is invasion of the cornea

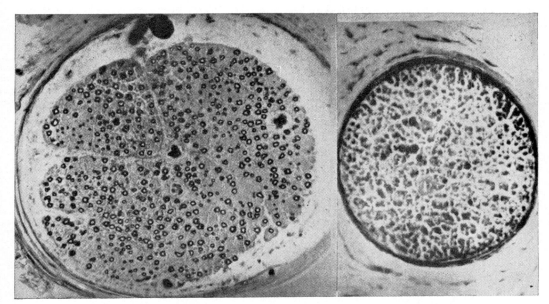

FIG. 222.—Beriberi. On the left is the section of nerve from a control and on the right the section from the patient. Both were stained with osmic acid. Note the disappearance of the sheaths of Schwann, which is characteristic of vitamin B₁ deficiency and which supports the clinical impression of beriberi, in the nerve from the patient suspected of having beriberi. (Spies, *et al.*, courtesy of Postgraduate Medicine.)

by capillaries arising from the limbic plexus with final corneal opacity and keratitis.

The lesions of riboflavin deficiency are common and severe in the Orient. Mild forms of the condition are not uncommon among the undernourished, chronic alcoholics, and those who subsist on absurdly inadequate diets with the object of supposedly improving their figures. Severe eye lesions used to be seen in the Southern states of America in the low economic groups. The condition has been eliminated in areas adopting successful nutritional programs, particularly the enrichment of bread and flour with B₁, B₂ and niacin.

Nicotinic Acid (Niacin).—*Physiology.*—Nicotinic acid or niacin is a water-soluble vitamin which enters into the formation of two coenzymes, I and II. These in turn form an essential part of the respiratory enzyme system of cells. The vitamin is widely distributed in a variety of foods, such as meats, vegetables, and whole grain cereals. Deficiency is seen particularly in maize-eating countries, such as Italy and the Southern United States. After being absorbed, the vitamin is transformed into the

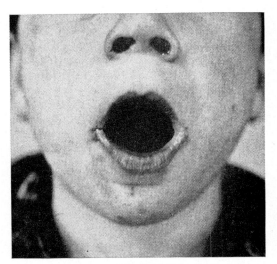

FIG. 223.—Bilateral cheilosis which disappeared following riboflavin therapy. (Spies, courtesy of J. Med. Assn. State of Alabama.)

amide of nicotinic acid, which is then utilized to form the respiratory coenzymes.

Pathology.—*Pellagra.*—Niacin deficiency is believed to give rise to the condition known as pellagra, which literally means rough skin (*pelle*, skin, *agra*, rough). In the dog the corresponding condition is known as "black tongue." The disease is probably not an example of a pure avitaminosis, but is apparently due to protein deficiency in addition. In experimental *pure* niacin deficiency in man there are few if any of the symptoms described below and none of the morphological changes. In addition to the all-important dietary deficiency, there may be such endogenous factors as chronic alcoholism, gastrointestinal disturbances, the extra demands of pregnancy and hyperthyroidism, *etc.*, which we have already encountered in the other water-soluble vitamin deficiencies. The *clinical picture* has been summed up as consisting of dermatitis, diarrhea and dementia. There are corresponding lesions of the skin, the alimentary tract, and the central nervous system.

The *skin* becomes reddened, thickened and *hyperkeratotic* owing to interference with the normal metabolism of the epidermis. There is a curiously symmetrical pigmentation and erythema, followed by desquamation of the exposed parts of the body, especially the face and the back of the hands. Factors such as strong sunlight and trauma undoubtedly play a part in the distribution, which is well described by the term *gauntlet* or *glove dermatitis*. *Microscopically*, in addition to the marked hyperkeratosis of the epidermis there is edema and congestion in the dermis, with some round cell infiltration in the superficial layers. In the *alimentary canal* lesions similar in character develop in the mouth and over the tongue and esophagus, with complete disappearance of the lining epithelium and the formation of ulcers teeming with bacteria. Similar extensive lesions are found in the colon. In the experimental animal, particularly the dog, the onset of oral lesions may be very acute, giving a hyperemic and smooth tongue (*bald tongue*), whilst in the chronic stage it has been likened to raw meat, with fissures and crevases. The *nervous system* lesions are represented by degeneration of ganglion cells in the cerebral cortex (dementia), and myelin degeneration of the same tracts in the spinal cord which are involved in pernicious anemia, a matter which is discussed in Chapter 42.

Gillman and Gillman, by means of repeated liver puncture on South African negroes suffering from pellagra, have shown that fundamentally important changes take place in the liver in the course of the disease. The first change is extensive fatty degeneration. This is followed by a massive accumulation of iron pigment in the liver cells, necrosis of these cells, and finally cirrhosis. This of course is the picture of hemochromatosis. According to Gillman and Gillman 20 per cent of pellagrins in South Africa show evidence of incipient or frank cirrhosis of the liver.

It is well to remember that pellagra, beriberi, and riboflavin deficiency in man frequent coexist (Spies *et al.*). All three involve water-soluble vitamins, and it is only natural that a diet which is deficient in one may well be deficient in several. The subclinical deficiencies of the water-soluble vitamins are often labelled as manifestations of neurasthenia, on account of such complaints as poor appetite, nervousness, "crying spells," "heartburn," and so on.

Vitamin B_{12} and Folic Acid.—Vitamin B_{12} and folic acid are growth factors in the maturation of red blood cells in the bone marrow. B_{12} is derived from food, and it is absorbed from the intestine only in the presence of the intrinsic factor (hemopoietin) secreted by the stomach. Pernicious anemia and other megaloblastic anemias develop because the stomach no longer secretes the intrinsic factor, so that the vitamin cannot be transported across the intestinal mucous membrane, a perfect example of poverty in the midst of plenty. The megaloblastic anemia which develops after total gastrectomy has a similar explanation. There is an abundant supply of vitamin B_{12} in the tissues, which is used up very slowly, so that it may be several years after gastrectomy that the anemia develops. The vitamin B_{12} of the food is associated with animal protein, having been detected in only one or two vegetable foods, such as groundnuts. Vegetarians might therefore be expected to develop pernicious anemia after a lapse of years, but such is not the case. The reason is that the vegetarian does actually consume a lot of protein in the form of milk, butter, cheese, and other dairy products. In this way the British vegetarian gets as much animal protein in his diet as the ordinary Greek or Italian, and much more than most people in India. A small and select group known as vegans have eliminated all dairy products from their food, nor do they touch even groundnuts. After a number of years these enthusiasts (fanatics?) are found to develop such symptoms of megaloblastic anemia as sore tongue, paresthesias, and other nervous symptoms (Wokes *et al.*). Failure of growth in children is said to be benefitted by B_{12}, which is also a growth factor to bacteria in unbelievably small amounts.

The various disturbances which result from vitamin deficiency are summarized in the following table.

In concluding this discussion on deficiency disease it may be well to point out that the laboratory worker naturally concentrates on producing a single deficiency in the experimental animal. In man many of the deficiency diseases are multiple deficiencies, for dietary deficiency is rarely confined to a single factor, at least in this country. For this reason the administration of pure vitamins is rarely sufficient for a cure, and is never a substitute for a good general diet.

TABLE OF HUMAN VITAMIN DEFICIENCY DISEASES

Vitamin **A**	Night blindness, xerophthalmia, keratomalacia, epithelial keratinizing metaplasia.
Vitamin D	Rickets, osteomalacia.
Vitamin K	Hypoprothrombinemia, hemorrhagic diathesis.
Vitamin C	Scurvy.
Thiamine (B_1)	Beriberi, polyneuritis.
Riboflavin (B_2)	Cheilosis, glossitis, eye lesions.
Niacin (Nicotinic Acid)	Pellagra (skin, alimentary canal, central nervous system)
B_{12} and Folic Acid	Pernicious and other macrocytic anemias.

Folic acid, which is pteroylglutamic acid, is useful in some macrocytic anemias, and is specific for the nutritional anemia of tropical sprue. Its disadvantage is that it does not prevent involvement of the central nervous system, which is so serious a feature of pernicious anemia, whereas this complication is prevented by B_{12}. Vegetables contain relatively large amounts of folic acid, and, since folic acid is known to precipitate the onset of neurological symptoms in classical pernicious anemia, it is possible that the folic acid in the vegetable diet may have a similar effect in vegans who have become really deficient in vitamin B_{12}. The deficiency symptoms are less marked in Dutch vegans, and practically absent in the American group. This may well be because the British vegans have the lowest protein intake.

In 1939 over \$86,000,000 were spent by the United States public in buying vitamins, and at the present time the figure must be very much higher. It is better and infinitely cheaper to get one's vitamins from the grocery store, where they have been manufactured by Nature, than from the drug store where they have been manufactured by man.

REFERENCES

BROCK, J. P.: Lancet, 1959, *2*, 859, 923. (Nutritional disease).

COOPER, L. F., BARBER, E. M., MITCHELL, H. S. and RYNBERGEN, H. J.: *Nutrition in Health and Disease*, 13th ed., Philadelphia, 1958.

CRANDON, J. H., LUND, C. C. and DILL, D. B.: New Eng. J. Med., 1940, *223*, 333 (Experimental human scurvy).

FOLLIS, R. H., JR.: *The Pathology of Nutritional Disease*, Springfield, Ill., 2nd ed., 1958.

FOLLIS, R. H., JR., *et al.*:   Am. J. Path., 1943, *19*, 341 (Thiamin deficiency).

GERBER, A., RAAB, A. P. and SOBEL, A. E.:   Am. J. Med., 1954, *16*, 729. (Vitamin A poisoning).

GILLMAN, J. and GILLMAN, T.:   Arch. Path., 1945, *40*, 239 (Pellagra).

KENT, S. P., *et al.*:   Am. J. Path., 1958, *34*, 37. (Hypervitaminosis D in monkeys).

PAPPENHEIMER, A. M.:   Am. J. Path., 1942, *18*, 169 (Vitamin E deficiency).

POPPER, H.:   Arch. Path., 1941, *31*, 766. (Vitamin A fluorescence).

SEBRELL, N. H., JR., and HARRIS, R. S.:   *The Vitamins: Chemistry, Physiology, Pathology*, New York, 1954.

SPIES, T. D. and BUTT, A. R.:   *Vitamins and Avitaminosis in Diseases of Metabolism*, ed. by Duncan, G. G., Philadelphia, 1942.

SPIES, T. D.:   J.A.M.A., 1958, *167*, 675. (Recent advances in nutrition).

SPIES, T. D., VILTER, R. W. and ASHE, W. F.:   J.A.M.A., 1939, *113*, 931.   (Water-soluble vitamin deficiencies).

WEISS, S. and WILKINS, R. W.:   Ann. Int. Med., 1937, *11*, 104. (Thiamine deficiency myocarditis).

WOKES, F., BADENOCH, J. and SINCLAIR, H. M.:   Amer. J. Clin. Nutrition, 1955, *3*, 375 (Vitamin B_{12} deficiency).

WOLBACH, S. B. and BESSY, O. A.:   Physiol. Rev., 1942, *22*, 233. (Deficiency of vitamin A and other vitamins).

WOLBACH, S. B. and HOWE, P. R.:   Arch. Path., 1926, *1*, 1. (Intercellular substances in experimental scurvy).

————.:   Arch. Path., 1928, *5*, 239 (Vitamin A deficiency).

Chapter 16

Pigments and Pigmentation

Hemoglobin
   Hematoidin
   Absorption of Iron
   Hemosiderosis
    Transfusional Hemosiderosis
   Hemochromatosis
    Siderosis of the Globus Pallidus

Bilirubin
   Jaundice
Porphyrins and Porphyria
   Congenital Erythropoietic
     Porphyria
   Intermittent Acute Porphy-
    ria

Porphyria Cutanea Tarda
Melanin
   Melanosis
    Melanosis Coli
   Ochronosis
Lipochromes
Exogenous Pigments

The pigments are not only the most beautiful but some of the most vital substances in the body. Life on earth depends almost entirely on the process of photosynthesis in green plants. Light energy from the sun is transformed into a chemical energy which can be stored and made available for the animal as well as the plant world. In addition this process liberates the oxygen required for cellular respiration. It is chlorophyll, a green pyrrole pigment, which plays a decisive role in photosynthesis, while hemoglobin plays a similar role in energy exchange (Lemberg and Legge). These are *endogenous pigments*, synthesized in the plant and in the body respectively. In connection with hemoglobin we shall also consider the hemoglobin derivatives, bile pigments and porphyrins. Other endogenous pigments not related to hemoglobin are lipochromes and melanin. The *exogenous pigments* are introduced into the body from without through the respiratory tract, the alimentary canal, or the skin.

HEMOGLOBIN

Hemoglobin belongs to the group of chromoproteins. It consists of a protein, *globin*, united with a pyrrole pigment, *heme* or *hematin*, which belongs to the group of porphyrins (*porphyra*, purple). The porphyrin nucleus consists of four pyrrole rings linked by carbon atoms. Two types of arrangement are encountered. (1) In the porphyrins, and in hematin and chlorophyll compounds, the system of four pyrrole rings is kept together by four single carbon atoms in the form of a *closed ring system*. In bile pigments, on the other hand one of these carbon atoms is missing, *giving* an *open ring system*, which is less rigid, so that greater variation is possible.

If a metal such as iron is introduced into the porphyrin molecule, a metalloporphyrin is formed. This is *protoporphyrin*, which, as the name indicates, is the prototype of the various naturally occurring porphyrins. Protoporphyrin is the basic pigment of hemoglobin, and is really synonymous with heme or hematin. It is the non-protein, insoluble, iron constituent of hemoglobin. It will be seen that hemoglobin is composed of three constituents joined together, globin—iron—porphyrin. If the metal is magnesium, the result of the combination is chlorophyll.

Hematoporphyrin is of great historical interest, but of no biological importance. It was in 1871 that Hoppe-Seyler first obtained a purple pigment from hemoglobin by the action of concentrated sulfuric acid. This he called hematoporphyrin because of its origin and its color. It was an *iron-free* or pure porphyrin, the protoporphyrin (hematin) of the hemoglobin having lost its iron atom owing to action of the strong acid. Hematoporphyrin, however, is only a laboratory porphyrin, as it does not occur in the natural state. Although hemoglobin contains iron, it does not give an iron reaction with the ordinary tests, because the iron is bound to globin. When hemoglobin is broken down under ordinary conditions two moieties are formed: the one, *hematoidin*, is iron-free, corresponding to the artificially produced hematoporphyrin, while the other, *hemosiderin*, contains iron and gives the iron reaction. (It will be recalled that *hematin* or heme, the substance with the confusingly similar name, is the *iron-containing pigment* bound to globin in the hemoglobin molecule). The *iron-free portion* is converted into *bilirubin*, and excreted in the bile, but the iron of the hemosiderin is too valuable to be lost and is retained within the body to be built up again into hemoglobin.

Hematoidin.—Hematoidin may assume the form of yellowish-brown rhombic crystals or of amorphous granules seen in the neighborhood of any old hemorrhage. The granules are usually extracellular, but may also be found within phagocytic cells. They constitute the brown granules in the familiar *heart failure cells*, the phagocytes which occupy the pulmonary alveoli in cases of congestive heart failure in which there is hemorrhage into the alveoli from the over-distended pulmonary capillaries. Hematoidin is closely related chemically with bilirubin, and is excreted as such in the bile. In conditions of increased hemolysis there is therefore an increased formation of bilirubin; this may accumulate in the blood and stain the tissues yellow, giving rise to that form of jaundice known as hemolytic jaundice. When the van den Bergh test for bilirubin is applied to local and not too recent extravasations of blood, a positive reaction is obtained. It is only when the hemorrhage is large and absorption is imperfect that the pigment is deposited in solid form. In small hemorrhages the pigments are soluble and stain the surrounding tissue with the familiar color of a bruise.

Absorption of Iron.—We may leave the subject of hematogenous pigmentation for a few moments in order to consider the question of the absorption of iron. The absorption of iron takes place chiefly in the duodenal region, where the relatively low pH prevents the readily absorbed ferrous iron from being converted into ferric hydroxide. A certain amount of absorption may, however, take place all along the gastrointestinal tract. Once the iron is absorbed, practically none of it is lost. As a result of this rather unique property, the absorption of iron is regulated by the demand for this substance. The intestinal mucosa has a very active aerobic metabolism, so that the iron is absorbed into the mucosal cells in ferrous form, but it is stored in ferric form as *ferritin*. A decrease in the oxygen supply in the blood will lead to an increased amount of the ferric being converted into the ferrous form, which then diffuses into the blood and is finally used for the manufacture of hemoglobin and red cells. Any block in the intestinal absorptive mechanism will result in anemia. If, on the other hand, the gate for the entry of iron is opened too wide, the storage of iron is carried beyond normal limits and hemosiderosis results. A single large dose of oral iron inhibits or blocks the absorption of iron for a period of several days. A "mucosal block" seems to have been set up. When the "acceptor" in the intestinal mucosa, namely ferritin, is saturated, no more iron can pass through the mucosal cells until the surplus has been removed and transported to the depots. In post-hemorrhagic states, however, where there has been blood loss, transfusional hemosiderosis ordinarily does not occur, even with this number of transfusions.

HEMOSIDEROSIS.—Hemosiderin, the iron-containing pigment, gives the Prussian blue reaction for iron with potassium ferrocyanide and hydrochloric acid. This test may be applied either to microscopic sections or to the gross specimen. The pigment takes the form of fine yellowish-brown crystals which are usually contained within cells. Hemosiderin, therefore, is chiefly intracellular, hematoidin chiefly extracellular. The hemosiderin may be formed as the result of hemorrhage or of general hemolysis. In the former the hemosiderosis is local, in the latter it is widespread. The reticuloendothelial system is intimately connected with hemosiderosis in three different ways: (1) The pigment-filled cells which surround an old hemorrhage are histiocytes belonging to this group. (2) Certain hemolytic diseases, *e.g.*, hemolytic jaundice, are dependent on the activity of the reticuloendothelial system; the hemolysis is followed by the deposition of hemosiderin. (3) General hemolysis may be due to some extraneous source such as snake venom, but again hemosiderin is found within the reticuloendothelial cells.

Hemolysis from whatever cause is therefore likely to be followed by hemosiderosis. The pigment is not only found in the reticulo-endothelial cells, but also in the epithelial cells of the liver and kidney. A marked Prussian blue reaction is obtained in those cells in pernicious anemia. Hemolysis is always accompanied by an increased formation of bilirubin. When this is marked it can readily be detected in the blood; it stains the tissues, but does not escape in the urine. In the curious condition of paroxysmal hemoglobinuria there is marked hemosiderosis of the liver and the cells of the convoluted tubules of the kidney as the result of the increased destruction of blood.

There may be an increase in the iron content of certain tissues, and yet the iron may not be demonstrable by ordinary histological methods. This invisible iron can now be demonstrated microscopically (Popoff). It is readily detached from the erythrocytes, and is rapidly taken up by mesenchymal and epithelial cells. Siderosis due to this cause is seen in hemolytic and other conditions, but it is especially striking in congestive heart failure, in which practically all the septal cells of the lung may be seen to be loaded with iron granules instead of a mere sprinkling of phagocytes containing hemosiderin.

Transfusional Hemosiderosis.—The limited degree of siderosis which accompanies the hemolytic anemias is not of functional significance, for it does not give rise to fibrosis. The siderosis which accompanies repeated blood transfusions is another story. When iron is introduced into the body parenterally it is gradually laid down in various reticuloendothelial storage depots, because there is no adequate mechanism for its excretion. When the depots become overfilled the parenchymatous cells take up the excess with resulting fibrosis (Schwartz and Blumenthal). This is in contrast to hemochromatosis, where the parenchyma is primarily affected.

As a rule over 100 transfusions are needed to produce the picture of hemochromatosis. For some reason the total iron in the transfused blood does not seem to account for the total amount of the iron overload as indicated by the degree of fibrosis, for in some cases hemosiderosis has developed after only a dozen transfusions (Dubin). Moreover the quantities of iron in the tissues, even in the liver alone, may be greater than the amount in the transfused blood. This may be due to an increased absorption of iron from a normal duodenal mucosa in response to a greater demand added to the amount in the transfused blood. The normal total body iron is 4 to 5 gm. and the content of iron in the plasma is roughly 120 to 140 mg. per cent.

Hemochromatosis. This rare disease, first described by Trousseau and formerly known as *bronzed diabetes*, is an inborn error of metabolism as a result of which iron is absorbed from the bowel in excessive amount and slowly accumulates in the body over a period of years. Its chief features are cirrhosis of the liver, diabetes mellitus, pigmentation of the skin, and testicular atrophy with resulting loss of libido and gynecomastia. Before the introduction of insulin the patient used to die of diabetic coma. Now he survives to die of hepatic coma, or of hepatoma in older patients or cardiac failure in younger ones. One of the most striking features of the disease is the sex incidence, which is nearly exclusively male. Whether this is related to the monthly loss of blood in women is an open question. It is sometimes spoken of as endogenous or primary hemochromatosis in distinction to the exogenous or secondary hemochromatosis of transfusion hemosiderosis (Schwartz and Blumenthal). The exogenous form has been called the illegitimate offspring of the endogenous, but the resemblance to the parent is so strong that it may be allowed to bear the family name (Schwartz). As a matter of fact, it is only the secondary form which truly deserves its name, as in it the iron is hematogenous in origin, whereas in endogenous hemochromatosis it is not related to the blood, and the condition should rather be called cytosiderosis.

The essence of the condition is a weakening of the duodenal mucosal block. A very small difference in the amount of absorption of iron a day will make a vast difference over a period of thirty or forty years, and we must remember that the defect in the block probably dates from birth. When a test dose of radioactive ferrous iron is given by mouth, the patient with hemochromatosis may retain 20 per cent or more compared with the normal person who retains only 2 per cent. It is natural, therefore, that elevation of the plasma iron should be the best presumptive test for endogenous homochromatosis, particularly in the early stage when the increased absorption is most marked and the iron level may be 200 gm. per cent instead of the normal 120 to 140 mg. A normal mucosal block may be weakened if it is strained unduly. Thus the person who from early childhood continues to take large daily doses of medicinal iron in ferrous form over many years may well increase his supply of storage iron. In pellagra amongst the South African Bantu repeated needle biopsies have shown a series of changes in the liver cells beginning with fatty degeneration and ending with massive accumulations of iron (Gillman and Gillman). Hemochromatosis appears to be a common sequel of pellagra in these natives.

The *lesions* are due to deposits of iron. The normal amount of iron in the entire body is only about 2.5 gm., but in this disease the liver alone may contain 30 or 40 gm. The liver cells slowly undergo necrosis, and a finely nodular cirrhosis of the Laennec type develops which may be mild or extreme in degree. It is rather curious that in spite of the very widespread parenchymal involvement, there is usually no clinical evidence of this, and seldom any marked laboratory evidence, nor are signs of portal hypertension at all striking. From this it will be evident that needle biopsy of the liver is the best way of confirming the diagnosis. Deposits of iron also occur in the pancreas where both the acinar tissue and the islets of Langerhans are destroyed and to a much lesser degree in the kidneys, adrenals, spleen, heart and voluntary muscles, thyroid, skin and abdominal lymph nodes. The affected organs give a vivid Prussian blue reaction for iron. The pigmentary cirrhosis is not due entirely to hemosiderin, for *hemofuscin*, a dark brown or blackish pigment which does not give an iron reaction, is also present. It seems to be related to melanin, and either it or melanin are responsible for the pigmentation of the skin. *It is therefore useless to do a biopsy in order to*

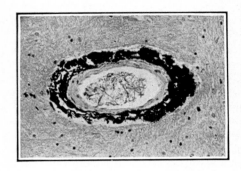

Fig. 224.—Iron in vessel wall in lenticular nucleus. × 150.

test the skin for iron, at least in the early stages when doubt exists. Primary carcinoma of the liver develops in about 20 per cent of cases. Further information on hemochromatosis will be found in Sheldon's monograph.

In closing this discussion on hemochromatosis and hemosiderosis we may include both conditions under the common term, *iron-storage disease*, which may be primary or secondary. The *primary form* is represented by hemochromatosis, an inborn error in metabolism which permits unduly large absorption of iron. The *secondary form* or hemosiderosis may be due to (1) repeated blood transfusions, (2) undue hemolysis as in hemolytic anemias, (3) refractory anemias with resulting increased absorption of iron from the bowel, and (4) prolonged administration of medicinal iron or the high iron, low phosphate diet of the Bantu.

SIDEROSIS OF THE GLOBUS PALLIDUS.—The globus pallidus of the lenticular nucleus usually gives a marked iron reaction, due to the presence of iron in the walls of the vessels in this region of the brain. The condition has been mistaken by many workers for calcification owing to the dark blue staining with hematoxylin (Fig. 224). The walls of the vessels are infiltrated with iron salts which appear to be derived from the nucleus itself. The iron is seemingly not hematogenous in origin, and there is no increase in conditions of undue hemolysis. Pallidal siderosis appears to be the expression of a slow involutionary atrophy affecting the lenticular nucleus in at least 60 per cent of persons over the age of thirty years. It appears to predispose to the acute bilateral necrosis of the lenticular nuclei which is so often seen in carbon monoxide poisoning.

BILIRUBIN

Bilirubin is formed from the hemoglobin of broken-down red blood cells by the cells of the reticuloendothelial system, principally those of the bone marrow and spleen. Rudolf Virchow in 1847 showed that hematoidin, the orange pigment found at the site of old blood extravasations, was similar to or, as he thought at the time, identical with bilirubin. It may be remarked here that Virchow, the father of modern pathology, was the first to demonstrate the real meaning of so many of the pathological phenomena which today we accept as commonplace knowledge.

Jaundice.—Jaundice or icterus is the familiar yellow pigmentation of the skin, mucous membranes and internal organs which is associated with increased bile pigment concentrations in the plasma. It may be the result of either *excessive production* or *inadequate removal* of the pigment. Oxidative rupture of the closed porphyrin ring of hemoglobin occurs before separation of the prosthetic group from iron and globin. Biliverdin is probably first formed in an intermediate stage, and this is reduced to bilirubin. (It is biliverdin which is responsible for the greenish color of a bruise before the yellow stage develops).

With increased hemolysis, the bilirubin content will rise. The bile acids are synthesized only by the liver. The bilirubin thus formed is carried to the liver. We can picture a hepatic cell as flanked on one side by a sinusoid and on the other by a bile canaliculus, the bilirubin passing from one to the other through the parenchymal elements, and escaping along the bile duct into the intestine. In the large bowel it is reduced by bacterial action to colorless fecal urobilinogen. The greater part of the stercobilinogen is excreted in the feces, but part is reabsorbed into the portal circulation and passes again to the liver. Most of this fraction is once more excreted by the hepatic cells, but a small part passes on into the general circulation and is excreted as urobilinogen in the urine. When the liver is diffusely damaged it fails to excrete the reabsorbed urobilinogen again, so that it passes into the systemic circulation and thence through the kidneys into the urine in increased amount.

The bilirubin in the liver sinusoids is different from the bilirubin in the bile canaliculi. This was shown by van den Bergh in 1918 by means of Ehrlich's well-known diazo reagent (diazotized sulfanilic acid), which gives an immediate red color with bile or with the icteric serum of obstructive jaundice; this is known as the *direct van den Bergh reaction.* When the serum of a patient with hemolytic jaundice is added to the diazotized sulfanilic acid reagent, an immediate reaction is obtained *only* on the addition of alcohol; this is therefore called the *indirect van den Bergh reaction.* The two types of bilirubin are known as *direct-reaction bilirubin*, which has passed through the liver cells, and *indirect-reaction bilirubin* which has not, or, more conveniently, as *cholebilirubin* and *hemobilirubin* (Harrison), although the latter terms are not yet of general acceptance. In hemolytic jaundice a positive reaction is obtained even without the use of alcohol after a delay of ten minutes; this is the *delayed direct* reaction. If the color develops at once in the absence of alcohol but deepens on standing, we have a combination of the two types, known as a *biphasic* reaction, which indicates the presence both of hemobilirubin and of cholebilirubin.

The significance of the two main types of van den Bergh reaction, the direct and the indirect, has long been a subject of debate. That the indirect-reacting pigment, the hemobilirubin, was soluble in alcohol but not in water whilst the direct-reacting pigment, the cholebilirubin was soluble in water seemed to be established. Partition chromatography has served to demonstrate quite unequivocally that *the direct and indirect pigments are separate entities.* Bilirubin is *conjugated with glucuronic acid* in its passage through the liver cells, and the resulting glucuronide is far more soluble in water than is unconjugated bilirubin. This may be the explanation of the fact that cholebilirubin readily passes the renal filter whereas hemobilirubin is held back. The glomeruli, indeed, are as efficient at distinguishing between the two types of bilirubin as is the van den Bergh qualitative reaction. During the passage through the liver cells the bilirubin seems to be combined with sodium, and it is the sodium bilirubinate thus formed which is responsible for the direct reaction.

For practical purposes the refinements of the van den Bergh reaction, with direct, immediate, indirect, delayed and biphasic variations have been replaced by *prompt direct* and *total bilirubin* estimations, the amount of the indirect-reacting factor being the difference between the total and the direct-reacting factor (Watson). It is the bilirubin of the bile, of course, which gives the prompt direct reaction.

The most rational classification of the disturbances of bilirubin which constitute jaundice takes the liver cell as its pivotal point. The jaundice may originate *before*, *in*, or *after* the liver cell; that is to say, it may be prehepatic, hepatic (hepatocellular), or posthepatic. From what has already been said it will be obvious that prehepatic (hemolytic) jaundice is concerned with hemobilirubin (indirect bilirubin), whilst posthepatic (obstructive) jaundice is concerned with cholebilirubin, which has already passed through and been modified by the hepatic cells.

The various forms of jaundice are discussed in connection with diseases of the liver and the biliary passages in Chapter 28.

PORPHYRINS AND PORPHYRIA

The porphyrins are among the most important of the natural pigments. Although they have been known for almost a century, they have come into prominence in recent years, because of certain rather rare genetic disturbances of porphyrin metabolism occurring both in man and animals, and characterized by the excessive production of these pigments in the body. They may occur free or as complexes with metals. The iron complex constitutes the heme of hemoglobin, as we have already seen. Iron porphyrin complexes combined with proteins constitute *cytochromes*, the respiratory catalysts in every living cell which utilize oxygen. The porphyrins give an intense red fluorescence with ultra-violet light, a reaction so delicate that it may be given with an incredibly high dilution of the solvent. The bony skeleton of most animals contains porphyrin,

although too little to be seen with the naked eye, but the bones of the ground squirrel and some other rodents have a distinctly brownish tint, and they give a brilliant red fluorescence under ultra-violet light, which is particularly marked in the teeth. The very bright and beautiful color of the wings of the turacos, African birds allied to the cuckoo, is due to a high content of porphyrin.

Reference has already been made in the discussion on hemoglobin earlier in this chapter to the very characteristic four-pyrrole ring structure of the porphyrin nucleus, the rings being linked by methene bridges. Each porphyrin has a number of stereoisomers, the ones which concern us being uroporphyrin types I and III and coproporphyrin types I and III. Coproporphyrin and uroporphyrin are really one and the same compound and may be found in either the urine or the stool. It may be mentioned that chlorophyll is a magnesium-porphyrin compound.

The *terminology of the porphyrins* is apt to be a little confusing to someone making their acquaintance for the first time. A few words of explanation may therefore be in order. Porphyrin is the name (*porphyra*, purple) first given to the iron-free compound which appears when blood is treated with concentrated sulfuric acid. *Protoporphyrin*, as its name suggests, is the prototype of the naturally occurring porphyrins, being the basic pigment in combination with iron, of the heme of hemoglobin. It is, therefore, the most important of the porphyrins physiologically. It is not present in the urine. The amount of fecal protoporphyrin is related to the amount of blood in the gastrointestinal tract, and the rate of liberation of the porphyrin from hemoglobin by fecal bacteria. *Porphobilinogen* is the colorless precursor of the three porphyrins, uroporphyrin, coproporphyrin and protoporphyrin. On standing it becomes changed into uroporphyrin, and it is intermediate in the formation of coproporphyrin and protoporphyrin. *Coproporphyrin* is the porphyrin excreted under normal conditions mainly by liver into the bile and feces (*kopros*, dung). *Coproporphyrinuria* may occur in lead poisoning, poliomyelitis, liver disease, hemolytic anemia, and Hodgkin's disease. This is secondary coproporphyrinuria, merely an interesting accompaniment of these conditions, whereas the primary form constitutes an essential part of porphyria. *Uroporphyrin* is normally excreted by the kidney but is present in the urine in only trace amount. It is increased in lead poisoning and greatly increased in porphyria. *Porphyria* signifies a group of diseases with peculiar clinical features, together with the excessive formation and excretion of uroporphyrin and coproporphyrin and/or porphyrin precursors such as porphobilinogen in the urine (Watson). The laboratory diagnosis of porphyria is made by the demonstration of one of the uroporphyrins or of the colorless chromogen, porphobilinogen, shown by the Ehrlich aldehyde reagent, in the urine. *Porphyuria* is merely the presence of excessive secretions of porphyrins in the urine. This excess may be (primary) or may not be (secondary) related to porphyria.

Classification.—We have seen that porphyria is a group of disease states rather than a single one. Both the classification and the nomenclature are somewhat varied. It is labor-saving but not entirely accurate to speak of *congenital, acute* and *chronic types.* The acute form is characterized by acute attacks separated by remissions, so that a more accurate term is acute intermittent. The chronic form is marked by pigmentation and a long delayed appearance of symptoms, so that it is appropriately named the cutanea tarda type. It is probable that all three types represent an inborn error in porphyrin synthesis which is recessive in the congenital form, dominant in the acute, and indeterminate in the cutanea tarda. Finally there is a so-called *mixed* type, which combines the features of some of the other three varieties. Perhaps a more fundamental classification on the basis of pathogenesis is into (1) the *erythropoietic* or congenital type and (2) the *hepatic* type, which includes the acute intermittent and the cutanea tarda. In the erythropoietic type the error of metabolism is in the bone marrow, in the hepatic type the error appears to be in the liver. It seems probable that uroporphyrin type I is responsible for the photosensitivity lesions of the skin which characterize the congenital type, whilst porphobilinogen is responsible

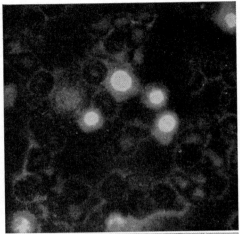
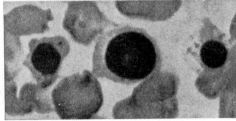

FIG. 225.—Erythropoietic porphyria. *Above,* unstained preparation of bone marrow, photographed in the fluorescence microscope under ultraviolet light; the white areas represent red fluorescence. *Below,* Wright-stained bone marrow preparation, central normoblast showing hemoglobin inclusion. (Kindness of Dr. Watson, *Advances in Internal Medicine,* The Year Book Publishers, 1954.)

for the abdominal and nervous symptoms of the acute form.

Congenital Erythropoietic Porphyria.—Congenital porphyria, which fortunately is much the rarest of the forms, is a genetically determined abnormality of the normal enzymatic conversion of porphobilinogen to type I and III porphyrins in the bone marrow (Gray). Excessive quantities of the porphyrins are synthesized in the marrow. Normally this conversion results in great predominance of type III porphyrins which are used in the synthesis of heme-proteins, together with a very small amount of type I. In congenital porphyria, on the other hand, the amount of type I is very great. This is useless for the prosthetic groups, it is not degraded to bile pigments, and it is therefore excreted in excess or is deposited in the tissues. It is this deposition which is the cause of the photosensitivity that is so characteristic a feature of the disease, this being due to the release of histamine. Similarly the presence of uroporphyrin I in the erythrocytes may lead to a photo-sensitized hemolysis of these cells in the form of hemolytic episodes, and to fluorescence of the normoblasts of the bone marrow with ultraviolet light (Fig. 225).

The condition, which is present at birth or develops in infancy, is characterized by marked hypersensitivity to light owing to the deposition of porphyrin in the tissues, and a red-colored urine. The extreme photosensitivity is evidenced by the development of *blisters on the face and hands*, with scarring of these parts and eventual mutilation, such as loss of the fingers and of parts of the nose and ears. The development of hemolytic anemia is associated with splenomegaly. The concentration of porphyrin in the *teeth* may give them a *pink* or *lavender color*. In cattle the condition is known as "pink tooth," and it is possible to breed cattle with pink tooth. Even if the teeth are not colored, they will at least fluoresce bright red with ultraviolet light, the whole tooth glowing and not merely the surface. The phalanges may also fluoresce. *Hirsutism* is common. There are large amounts of uroporphyrin and coproporphyrin in the normoblasts of the bone marrow, and it is these pigments that give the pink or red color to the urine, which, it may be noted, contains no porphobilinogen. The condition is slowly progressive, death being due to intercurrent infection or hemolytic anemia. Splenectomy may benefit the anemia, the photosensitivity, and the porphyrin excretion. At autopsy the bones may be red, whilst the marrow shows erythroid hyperplasia.

Intermittent Acute Porphyria.—This member of the hepatic group is the commonest, the most dramatic, and the most puzzling of the three main types of porphyria. Its most arresting feature is its intermittent character. It is inherited as a dominant character, and the siblings of the patient may have *latent porphyria*, as shown by the presence of porphobilinogen in the urine. The acute condition develops in young adults or in middle age. There is a complete

absence of the photosensitivity which is so characteristic of the congenital form because of the absence of free porphyrins. The clinical course is extraordinarily varied, the most striking manifestations being acute abdominal crises, neurological disturbances, and the presence of porphobilinogen in the urine. In addition to porphobilinogen the urine may also contain excessive amounts of uroporphyrin and to a lesser extent coproporphyrin types I and III.

The *abdominal crises* are in the nature of acute attacks of colic, which may simulate any of the acute abdominal emergencies as evidenced by the silent testimony of multiple surgical scars. The characteristic symptom is intense abdominal pain, which may be associated with vomiting and obstinate constipation. The acute attack is easily mistaken for renal colic, because of the character of the pain and the red color of the urine on standing. In the intermissions between attacks the patient is free from symptoms. The mechanism by which the latent disease is converted into the acute form is quite unknown, although barbiturates and other chemicals may precipitate an attack. The *nervous symptoms* may take the form of delirium, convulsions, emotional disturbances and psychoses. The more acute attacks may be preceded by years of nervousness, neurasthenia and mild hysteria. Pain in the limbs is often the first symptom, and there may be an ascending paralysis of the Landry type. Perhaps the crampy abdominal pains may also be neurological in origin, being caused by interference with normal motor innervation and resulting disturbed motility of the bowel. The transient hypertension which is often seen may be due to spasm of the neuromuscular bed.

It is well to realize that mild attacks are much commoner than the acute ones, and and that the picture is often one of chronic neuromuscular rather than fulminating disease. "Bedeviled as they are by their disease, the victims of porphyria go from doctor to doctor seeking a diagnosis or a cure for their disorder" (Kark).

The urine, when freshly passed, is colorless, but it contains large quantities of *porphobilinogen*, a colorless non-fluorescent substance, which becomes converted into colored porphyrins on standing owing to oxidation, so that it may develop a Burgandy or port-wine color. During remissions it is present in reduced amount or may actually be absent, and it appears to be fundamentally related to the abdominal and nervous symptoms. The diagnosis of acute porphyria depends on the demonstration of porphobilinogen in the urine. This is done conveniently by the Watson-Schwartz modification of the Ehrlich aldehyde reaction (para-dimethylaminobenzaldehyde).

Both porphobilinogen and urobilinogen give a red color with the Ehrlich reagent, but Watson and Schwartz showed that when chloroform is added the porphobilinogen, being insoluble in chloroform, remains in the aqueous upper layer of the tube, so that that layer is red, whereas urobilinogen, being soluble in chloroform, is found in the lower layer. The test is positive in acute porphyria, but negative in the congenital erythropoietic and cutanea tarda forms.

The *lesions* in a case dying during the acute stage are entirely microscopic. Porphobilinogen is present in the liver in large amount, and to a lesser degree in the kidney and the blood, whereas the bone marrow shows neither porphobilinogen nor excess porphyrins. The peripheral and autonomic nerves and the white matter of the spinal cord and brain may show a patchy demyelination, with relatively minor involvement of the axis cylinders, over the nerve cells of the posterior root ganglia and the anterior horn of the spinal cord (Hierons).

The *biochemical lesion* evidently concerns porphobilinogen, which is present in the liver in such large amounts, and is then excreted in the urine. This might be due either (1) to a block in the conversion of porphobilinogen to porphyrins in the liver, or (2) to an excessive production of this chromogen by the body. In porphyria produced by sedormid in the experimental animal there is a fall in the liver catalase, which is a heme-protein. Unfortunately in the human disease no fall in liver catalase can be demonstrated, so there may be a production of porphobilinogen (by the liver?) in excess of that required for normal heme synthesis. It is evident that the seat of the trouble is in the liver, just as it is in the bone marrow in the congenital erythropoietic form of the disease.

Porphyria Cutanea Tarda.—This chronic form of porphyria has been classed with the hepatic type, and Kark calls it cutaneohepatic porphyria because of the frequent association with liver disease and frank cirrhosis, which may precede the development of skin lesions. It will soon be evident, however, that it has much in common with the erythropoietic type. Rimington, indeed, considers that cutanea tarda is entirely distinct from the acute intermittent form. The most pronounced feature is the late development of photosensitivity in the third and fourth decades. The skin lesions resemble those of the congenital variety, but with less mutilation. There are no acute abdominal nor nervous system symptoms. The liver porphyrins are high, but those of the marrow are normal.

Porphyrins are produced in excessive amount, but they are eliminated in the feces, and do not raise the urinary porphyrin level much above normal except during severe transient exacerbations. The urine, therefore, may or may not be red.

The so-called *mixed type of porphyria* combines cutaneous, abdominal and nervous symptoms. It will not be discussed here. We have just seen that the cutanea tarda type also provides us with a mixed picture.

The accompanying table shows some of the principal features of the various forms of porphyria. The stated facts only represent averages, to which there are many exceptions. Thus, there may be attacks of colic in cutanea tarda, and the freshly passed urine of the acute intermittent form is occasionally red.

We may close this discussion of the complex problem of the porphyrias with the eloquent opening of Kark's account of the clinical aspects of the subject. "Clinicians with an eye for color have long been fascinated with the lavender teeth of congenital porphyria, with the port-wine urine excreted by some patients with intermittent porphyria, and with the brilliant red fluorescence of the porphyrin pigments when they are exposed to ultraviolet light. Unfortunately the clinical course and management of disorders associated with gross porphyrinuria

THE PORPHYRIAS

	Congenital	Acute Intermittent	Cutanea Tarda
Inheritance	Recessive	Dominant	Negative
Photosensitivity	Very early	Negative	Late
Abdominal colic	Negative	Positive	Negative
Nervous symptoms	Negative	Positive	Negative
Skin pigmentation	Negative	Occasional	Positive
Fresh urine	Red	May be normal	Red?
Porphobilinogenuria	Negative	Positive	Negative
Uroporphyrinuria	Type I very marked	Types I and III	Types I and III
Marrow porphyrin	Much increased	Normal	Normal
Liver porphyrin	Slight	Much increased	Much increased
Fluorescence	Positive	Negative	Positive

and porphyrinorrhea must still be painted in somewhat somber hues."

MELANIN

Melanin, its name derived from the Greek *melas*, meaning black, is the coloring matter of the skin, hair, iris, choroid coat of the eye, and certain parts of the central nervous system. The pigment is in the form of granules which vary in color from light brown to black. Melanin is formed from the amino acid tyrosine by the action of the enzyme tyrosinase, a copper-protein complex. The presence of copper ions is necessary for the activity of the enzyme. Tyrosinase was demonstrated in mushrooms as long ago as 1896, and is known to be present in plants, insects and marine animals. Indeed it is found in greatest abundance in the cells lining the ink-sac of the cuttlefish. It was more than half a century later that Lerner and Fitzpatrick succeeded in showing that tyrosinase is also present in mammalian tissue, including human skin. This can be done by incubating sections of tissue in a buffered solution of tyrosine which acts as the substrate. The formation of melanin indicates the presence of tyrosinase.

A similar reaction, the *dopa reaction*, was introduced previously by Bloch. Dopa is a contraction for dihydroxyphenylalanine, an amino acid which reacts with tyrosinase to produce melanin. Tyrosinase has the ability to catalyze the oxidase of both tyrosine and dopa with the formation of melanin, but in normal mammalian skin the ability to catalyze tyrosine oxidase is absent or rather inhibited, while the ability to catalyze dopa is present. This is true also of the nevus, a benign tumor of melanin-forming cells. In malignant melanoma, the malignant variety of these cells, both tyrosine and dopa are catalyzed by tyrosinase.

The cells which form the pigment are peculiar branched cells derived from the neural crest and intercalated among the basal cells of the Malpighian layer of the skin. They may or may not contain pigment granules. These cells are known as *melanocytes* to the biologist, the person fundamentally concerned with the problems of pigment in the animal kingdom, but the pathologist calls them *melanoblasts,* a term reserved by the biologist for the immature pigment cell during its migration from the neural crest. A macrophage which takes up melanin discharged from the melanocytes is known to the biologist as a *melanophage*, to the pathologist as a *melanophore* (*phoreo*, I carry). The terminology of the biologist has been recommended for general use, but old names are hard to relinquish. Applying the dopa reaction to these various cells, it is obvious that the melanoblasts (melanocytes) and the tumor cells arising from them will be dopa-positive, while the melanophores will be dopa-negative.

Inhibitors of melanin formation demand brief consideration. The removal of copper ions and the action of ascorbic acid both inhibit tyrosinase. Copper is essential for the activation of the enzyme and for normal pigmentation in mammals. Copper-deficient diets result in depigmentation of the skin of the experimental animal. Sulfur-containing compounds, such as thiouracil, remove the copper by combining with it. Thiouracil administered to a black rat causes depigmentation, and in a patient with malignant melanoma and melanuria it has been known to change the urine from black to a normal color.

It would appear that in the skin of white persons sulfydryl groups may bind the copper and inhibit activation of the tyrosinase, so that little or no melanin is formed even though tyrosin and tyrosinase are both present. Ultraviolet energy activates the system, probably by decreasing the concentration of the sulfydryl groups, so that melanin appears in the melanoblasts (melanocytes) and in their long dendritic processes. This is the mechanism of sun-tanning and serves to explain the melanosis of those living under a tropical sun. Temperature also influences the reaction, which is the probable reason why the pigmentation of Addison's disease is marked not only in those parts exposed to the light but also in creases and folds of the skin covered by clothes.

Melanosis.—In man the normal amount of melanin in the skin is very small. It is much greater in the Negro than in the white man, but even in the Negro the entire skin does not contain more than one gram of pigment. In the malignant melanoma as much as 300 grams of melanin have been removed from the liver alone, so that under some conditions the pigment-forming power of the body is greatly increased. As the result of inflammation of the skin the melanin may become mobilized and transported by melanophages to the regional lymph nodes, where the microscopic picture may simulate that of a melanotic tumor.

In man the function of melanin appears to be to serve as a protection against strong actinic light. In cold-blooded vertebrates the behavior of pigment in response to stimuli is of much greater importance. This response consists in the dispersion of melanin granules in the long dendritic melanocytes, so that the pigment may seem to ebb and flow in the skin. Changes in temperature and environment and the use of certain drugs activate these changes in the frog and in fish, but only when the animal has an intact pituitary. It would appear that at least in the frog the pituitary controls the movement and possibly the production of melanin. A *melanocyte-stimulating hormone*, MSH, has been obtained from the pituitary. When MSH is injected into the hypophysectomized frog it causes melanin dispersion, and even does so when incubated with a piece of isolated skin.

The part which MSH plays in the *control of pigment movement* has been proved in the frog, but not yet in man. A number of clinical facts suggest that in man also the pituitary may exercise an important influence over melanin. Conditions believed to be associated with *increased pituitary activity*, such as pregnancy, Addison's disease and acromegaly, often show a marked increase of melanin pigmentation. In the third trimester of pregnancy the serum copper is increased, MSH is present in the urine in large amount, and pigmentation of the skin occurs in areas exposed to sunlight, a triad to which the name of *melasma* has been applied. The same is true of Addison's disease, in which decreased adrenal cortical activity seems to be compensated for by overactivity of the pituitary and a great increase in the formation of melanin. The presence of MSH in the urine in pregnancy can be demonstrated by an increase of melanin in the frog's skin when the urine is applied topically. When the *activity of the pituitary is decreased*, as in panhypopituitarism, there is a disappearance of pigment from the skin. Copper seems to play a part in this mechanism. Administration of MSH causes the serum copper to rise, and this is accompanied by increase in melanin formation.

It is possible that the *pigmentation of Addison's disease*, in which both adrenals are destroyed, may be more directly dependent on adrenal hormones. If these control the concentration of sulfydryl groups at the site of melanin formation, loss of the hormones would result in decrease of sulfydryl concentration and the melanin-forming enzyme system would no longer be inhibited. Another suggestion depends on the fact that epinephrin and melanin are derived from the same precursor. If the adrenals do not use this substance for the manufacture of epinephrin, it may accumulate and be converted into melanin. It must be admitted, however, that the mechanism responsible for the pigmentation in Addison's disease is not yet fully understood.

Estrogenic hormones may also play a part in the control of pigmentation. Estrogens given orally induce pigmentation in the nipples and areolæ in man, and local unilateral application to the nipple produces the same result in the guinea pig.

Under pathological conditions too much melanin may be formed or too little. The chief examples of too much pigmentation are the melanotic tumors, Addison's disease, melanosis coli, and chloasma. Ochronosis is related to melanosis. Diminished formation of melanin is seen in albinism and leukoderma. When too much melanin is formed it is excreted in the urine. In Addison's disease and melanotic tumors the kidneys often contain much melanin in the epithelial cells of the loop of Henle and the collecting tubules. Here, as in other positions, it may be necessary to differentiate between melanin and hemosiderin granules, both of which are yellowish brown when thinly distributed. Hemosiderin can be stained a bright blue with the Prussian blue reaction and melanin deep black by the Fontana silver technique.

For further information on the behavior of melanin in health and disease the excellent review by Lerner and Fitzpatrick should be consulted.

Melanosis coli is a condition in which a black pigment, either melanin or closely related to melanin, is deposited in the mucous membrane of the large intestine and appendix. Like so many other pathological states, it was first described by Virchow. The extreme grades are comparatively rare, but if the slighter forms are included the incidence is fairly high. Stewart and Hickman found it in 11.2 per cent of 600 autopsies. The incidence is higher in those over middle age, and much higher in carcinoma of the colon. Melanosis of the appendix may occur apart from any pigmentation of the colon; it may be seen in appendices removed at operation. The coloration which varies from gray to inky black can be seen through the intestinal wall, and is sharply limited by the ileocecal valve. In advanced cases there may be metastases of pigment to the submucosa and the mesocolic lymph nodes. The granules of pigment are found within large mononuclear cells in the stroma of the mucous membrane; the epithelium is not affected. The condition is often associated with chronic intestinal stasis either from organic obstruction or simple constipation. The pigmented cells are "dopa"-negative, and are, therefore, melanophores that have taken up pigment which has either been ingested in the food or synthesized in the bowel.

Other examples of melanosis or pigmentation in which a melanin-like substance is formed can only be mentioned. *Chloasma* is a condition in which brown patches appear in the skin of the face and elsewhere. They are seen in pregnancy and diseases of the uterus and ovaries, tuberculosis, Graves' disease, and following the application of heat (hot-water bottles). In *cachexia* the skin often shows patches of pigmentation. If such a patch be excised it will be found to give a marked "dopa" reaction. The *body louse* injects a fluid which produces a black spot of melanin in the deepest layers of the epidermis. An emulsion of the insect's salivary glands has the same effect when injected.

Absence of melanin is much rarer than excess of the pigment. *Albinism* is a congenital absence of melanin, which may be partial or complete. In *leukoderma* there are white patches of skin, as the name implies, due usually to a process of depigmentation; a section of such a patch is negative to the "dopa" reaction, suggesting that the cells are lacking in the specific ferment. White patches of skin are found in leprosy, due apparently to interference with the nerve supply. The whitening of hair is due to a loss of melanin. The white winter fur of arctic animals contains no melanin.

For further information on the behavior of melanin in health and disease the excellent reviews by Lerner and Fitzpatrick and by Lerner should be consulted.

OCHRONOSIS.—This very rare condition was given its name by Virchow because of the ochre color which the nose and ears may present (*ochros*, sallow). It is one of the inborn errors of metabolism, with a genetic enzymatic defect in the intermediary metabolism of tryosine. The pigment is either melanin or closely related to that substance. A rather similar condition of abnormal pigment deposition results from the prolonged administration of phenol-containing compounds, so that the pigmentation was seen more frequently in the days when carbolic acid dressings were in vogue. There is nearly always marked *alkaptonuria*, but this is not a disease *per se*, but merely an early manifestation of hereditary ochronosis.

There is a blackish discoloration of the cartilages, and sometimes of connective tissue, sclerae, muscles, and epithelial cells. When the cartilages are subcutaneous (nose, ear), the color may shine through the skin. The pigment may be deposited in the kidneys. In the only case which I have seen, the pyramids of the kidneys and the choroid plexus of the lateral ventricles were a startling black color. The skin of this patient was a peculiar gray, as if it had been black-leaded. Ochronosis results in a more or less disabling arthritis and ankylosing spondylitis of a specific nature (Lichtenstein and Kaplan). It is the cartilage rather than the bone in which pigment is deposited and which undergoes degeneration. The intervertebral discs are heavily impregnated with pigment and become remarkably radio opaque.

LIPOCHROMES

The colored fats form a loose group regarding which little is known. They are yellowish granules found in the heart muscle, nerve cells, seminal vesicles, adrenal cortex, corpus luteum, and interstitial cells of the testis. They have been called "wear and tear" pigments, being apparently produced from the cytoplasm in the process of wasting of the myocardial fibers seen in old age and cachectic disease conditions, and accompanied by a great collection of brown granules in the muscle fibers at either pole of the nucleus. These granules, which are normally present in small amount, stain red with Sudan. Similar granules are seen in the nerve cells, especially the large cells of the cerebral cortex, in senile and mental conditions. Some of these pigments may belong to the group of *plant pigments* (carotin and xanthophyll) found in carrots and other vegetables, egg-yolk, *etc*. If a person eats too many carrots he may develop *carotinemia*, with bright yellow coloration of the blood serum, the palms of the hands, and the nasolabial folds. The condition is sometimes seen in diabetes.

EXOGENOUS PIGMENTS

Pigments may be introduced from without and be deposited in the body. This introduction may occur through the respiratory tract, the alimentary canal, and the skin.

Through the *respiratory tract* dusts may be inhaled and deposited in the lungs, where they cause varing degrees of chronic irritation, a condition known as *pneumokoniosis*. Of these dusts the only two of importance are silica (in gold miners and stone masons) causing silicosis, and coal dust (in coal miners) causing anthracosis. These diseases are considered in the chapter on the Lungs.

Alimentary canal pigmentation is of much less importance. The two most important examples are silver and lead. Long-continued administration of silver salts may give rise to a condition of *argyria*. The silver is deposited as an insoluble albuminate in the form of fine granules. The skin and conjunctiva may assume an ashen-gray color, and there is pigmentation of the internal organs. The pigment causes no disturbance, but the importance of the condition lies in the fact that the coloration of the skin is permanent, so that the face has an ashen appearance for the rest of the patient's life. The pigment is not intracellular, but seems to lie in the cement substance. In the skin it is found in the corium just under the epithelium and around the sweat and sebaceous glands. In the kidney it is chiefly in the glomeruli and outside the epithelium of the tubules. In other organs the distribution is similar.

Lead poisoning or *plumbism* is considered in the section on the Action of Poisons. Pigmentation of the gums is a common sign. The lead is absorbed from the alimentary canal or may pass through the skin. It circulates in the form of a soluble salt, and when this comes in contact with hydrogen sulfide formed from decomposing food around diseased teeth, lead sulfide is formed and deposited in the gum where it gives a characteristic "blue line."

Pigment is introduced through *the skin* in the process of tattooing. It is taken up by histiocytes and is lodged permanently in the connective-tissue spaces. None is found in the epithelium. Some of the pigment is carried by phagocytes to the lymph nodes where it is deposited.

REFERENCES

DUBIN, I. N.: Am. J. Clin. Path., 1955, *25*, 514. (Transfusion hemosiderosis).

GILLMAN, J. and GILLAMN, T.: Arch. Path., 1945, *40*, 239. (Nutritional hemochromatosis).

GRAY, C. H., in R. H. S. THOMPSON and E. J. KING: *Biochemical Disorders in Human Disease*, London, 1957.

HARRISON, G. A.: *Chemical Methods in Clinical Medicine*, London, 1947.

HIERONS, R.: Brain, 1957, *80*, 176. (Nervous lesions in acute prophyria).

KARK, R. M.: Med. Clin. N. Amer., 1955, p. 11. (Clinical aspects of the porphyrias).

LEMBERG, R. and LEGGE, J. W.: *Hematin Compounds and Bile Pigments*, New York, 1949.

LERNER, A. B.: Am. J. Med., 1955, *19*, 902. (Melanin pigmentation).

LERNER, A. B. and FITZPATRICK, T. B.: Physiol. Rev., 1950, *30*, 91. (Melanosis).

LICHTENSTEIN, L. and KAPLAN, L.: Am. J. Path., 1954, *30*, 99. (Hereditary ochronosis).

POPOFF, N. W. and POPOFF, A.: Yale J. Biol. and Med., 1943, *16*, 197. (Invisible iron).

RIMINGTON, C.: Acta. Med. Scand., 1952, *143*, 161, 177. (Hemes and porphyrins in health and disease).

SCHWARTZ, S. O. and BLUMENTHAL, S. A.: Blood, 1948, *3*, 617. (Transfusional hemosiderosis).

SCHWARTZ, S. O.: Am. J. Clin. Path., 1956, *26*, 744. (Exogenous hemochromatosis).

SHELDON, J. H.: *Hemochromatosis*, London, 1935.

STEWART, M. J. and HICKMAN, E. M.: J. Path. and Bact., 1931, *34*, 61. (Melanosis coli).

WATSON, C. J.: Blood, 1946, *1*, 99. (Natural derivatives of hemoglobin).

———: Can. M.A.J., 1949, *61*, 483, J.A.M.A., 1940, *114*, 2427. (Retention and regurgitation jaundice).

———: Advances in Internal Medicine, 1954, *46*, 235. (Porphyria).

WYATT, J. P.: Arch. Path., 1956, *61*, 42, 56. (Pathology of iron storage).

Chapter 17

Physical Irritants

Heat
  (BURNS)
  HEAT STROKE
Cold
  DEATH FROM FREEZING

FROSTBITE
Light
Electricity
  LIGHTNING
(**Ionizing Radiation**)

Trauma
Increased Atmospheric Pressure
  CAISSON DISEASE

HEAT

Burns.—The very important subject of burns has already been considered in the chapter on Derangements of Body Fluids. It is true that the local lesions are very painful and demand treatment, but the real threat to health and it may be to life is the disturbance in the body fluids. There is an enormous flow of lymph from the burnt surface, and fluid is drawn from the intravascular to the extravascular compartment. When the burn is at all extensive, marked hemoconcentration develops with the production of shock, which may be severe or even fatal if not adequately treated. There is great loss of potassium in the urine, which must be replaced. The lesions and pathological physiology are discussed on page 169.

Heat Stroke.—This is essentially a paralysis of the heat-regulating mechanism caused by exposure to excessive heat. The actual temperature required depends on the humidity and varies with different persons. Heat loss is largely regulated by sweating, and some people can perspire very little. Complete saturation of the air with water vapor when the temperature is 90° F. causes an uncontrollable rise of body temperature. When the air temperature exceeds the body temperature all loss of heat by radiation ceases, and regulation of temperature is entirely dependent on sweating. A distinction is often drawn between heat exhaustion and heat stroke. It is doubtful if they differ other than in degree. In *heat exhaustion* the heat-regulating mechanism is severely strained, and the patient manifests weakness, pallor, stupor, and low blood pressure. The temperature may be slightly raised, but

on the other hand it may be subnormal. In *heat stroke* the heat-regulating mechanism is overwhelmed, and the temperature may rise 10° or more. One case is on record in which the temperature reached 117° F. It should be noted that the rectal temperature may be much higher than the temperature in the mouth or the axilla.

Heat stroke may be caused by direct exposure to the sun, the condition known as sun stroke. The ultraviolet rays have no relation to the condition. But the same effect is produced by exposure to any great heat, especially when combined with marked humidity. Men in steel works, engine rooms, *etc.*, often suffer in this way.

In the condition of heat stroke the patient may die with startling suddenness. He may fall down unconscious, a condition known as *heat apoplexy*, not uncommon in soldiers on forced marches in tropical countries. Even in the less sudden cases the patient may soon become unconscious. In heat exhaustion the skin may be moist, but in heat stroke it is usually dry and burning; the patient appears unable to perspire. The temperature may rise to great heights, but not in every case.

The *pathological lesions* are very indefinite. The chief autopsy findings are petechial hemorrhages in the skin and mucous membranes, hyperemia or actual hemorrhages in the brain, cerebral and pulmonary edema, enlargement of the spleen, and cloudy swelling of the liver, kidneys and heart. The water content of the brain is high. Patients with a temperature of 110° F. have recovered, but such a temperature can only be endured for a short time, for it has been shown experimentally that a temperature of 108° F. if long continued will cause coagulation of the

(407)

globulin of the nerve cells. After death from heat stroke the body shows very rapid and very marked rigor mortis. Postmortem decomposition also sets in very quickly.

COLD

Death from Freezing.—When a person inadequately protected is exposed to severe and long-continued cold, the blood is driven from the surface into the interior of the body. The temperature gradually falls, metabolism slows down, and the patient is overcome by the irresistible and fatal desire to sleep, so well known to mountaineers caught by bad weather at high altitudes. When the temperature reaches 70° F. the heart stops.

Frostbite.—The action of extreme cold on exposed parts of the body (nose, ears, hands, and even feet), especially when combined with the rapid loss of heat caused by wind, is to produce frostbite. As in the case of burns there are various degrees. In mild frostbite the part, which is at first white and bloodless, becomes red, swollen, and very painful during the process of thawing out. In more marked cases there is some necrosis of the epidermis, with formation of blisters and subsequent desquamation. In the severe cases there is necrosis of the entire part and gangrene. If the cold is sufficiently great the fluid of the cells is crystallized, and the cells are torn to pieces by the ice crystals. In ordinary cases the major factor in the production of the gangrene is the ischemia due to extreme contraction of the blood vessels, together with damage to the capillaries with the formation of hyaline thrombi.

An important element in the production of ischemia and anoxia is the process of *stasis*, which occurs quite early in frostbite (Kreyberg). As a result of severe injury to the vessel wall there is exudation of the fluid elements of the blood, so that the red cells become agglutinated into a jelly-like column which blocks the lumen effectively with resulting necrosis. This condition is known as sludging of the blood. The process is reversible if treatment be not delayed too long, even though the tissues have been frozen solid. The word stasis is here used in the European sense, rather than in its usual connotation of slowing the blood stream.

High altitude frostbite in aviators may present a special problem. In an airplane at great altitude the face can be exposed to severe cold for several hours, but under similar conditions the fingers suffer to such an extent that gangrene may result. Intense reflex vasospasm of the peripheral arterioles causes ischemia and local anoxia. The constriction, which is almost instantaneous, occurs chiefly at the terminal end of the arterioles. This is followed by damage to the endothelium of the terminal capillary loops, with increased permeability of the loops or thrombosis at the arteriolar-capillary junction. If extravasation of fluid occurs before thrombosis, the hand may become dropsical owing to accumulation of fluid between dermis and epidermis, or blistering may occur. In cases where amputation of the fingers has been necessary, later the arteries may show a remarkable fibrous thickening of the intima apparently unrelated to previous thrombosis.

Cold is now used for the production of *hypothermia* during operations on the cardiovascular system. Lowering of temperature is known to reduce the metabolism of cells *in vitro*, producing slowing of the heart beat, decrease in the respiration rate, fall in blood pressure, and reduction in oxygen consumption. In this state of "suspended animation" the requirements of the cells are reduced to a minimum by cooling, thus eliminating the need of an extra-corporeal circulation by means of pumps and oxygenators in operations involving the opening of the heart or the great vessels. This is obviously a tremendous technical advance, but we must bear in mind that exposure of dogs to cold not beyond the "ideal surgical stage" is followed by serious histochemical changes in the liver, kidneys and adrenals, more particularly a marked accumulation of fat in these organs, together with vacuolation of the granular cells of the zona reticularis of the adrenal cortex, adrenal changes similar to those described by Selye as the bodily reactions to stress (Knocker).

LIGHT

Light is a form of energy and may act as an irritant just as does heat. It is made up of vibrations of very varying wave length. The shorter the wave length, the less is the penetrating power and the more are the rays arrested in the skin where they excite irritation. The rays beyond the short wave end of the visible spectrum (ultraviolet) create most irritation, while those beyond the long wave end (infrared) are most penetrating and cause least irritation. Light may affect the body in the following ways:

1. Ultraviolet light produces the condition known as *sunburn*. This is independent of heat, for climbers on high snow peaks may be severely burned. The greater the altitude the more severe is the effect, for the short wave rays are no longer filtered out by a thick layer of atmosphere. Direct sunlight is not necessary, for the most severe burn I have ever experienced was on a day of thick mist in the Alps. The sensitivity of the skin varies much in different persons, depending on the amount of melanin it contains. Blondes burn much more readily than brunettes. The process of tanning (not burning) consists in a deposition of melanin in the more superficial layers.

The pathology of sunburn is the same as that of a first degree burn. There is intense hyperemia, a varying degree of edema, and some emigration of leukocytes. The edema may be so great as to raise the skin in blisters. Marked desquamation may follow the burn.

2. Those whose occupation exposes them for long periods to bright sunshine, *e. g.*, farmers and sailors past middle age, often develop thickened patches or *keratoses* on the skin of the face and back of the hands. The importance of these keratoses is that not infrequently they form the starting-point of carcinoma.

Probably related to this condition is the rare but remarkably interesting disease known as *xeroderma pigmentosum*. This appears to be a congenital hypersensitiveness to the action of light. In young children following prolonged exposure to sunlight there appear patches of erythema which go on to pigmentation. These patches then become rough and scaly, warty elevations appear (keratoses), and many of these become cancerous, so that the disease is usually fatal before the twentieth year. Metastases

are rare both in this disease and in carcinoma following senile keratoses. There may be several cases in one family, but it is limited either to the males or the females.

3. A *hypersensitiveness to light* may be present. This has already been discussed in relation to *congenital porphyria* in the previous chapter. Even more remarkable is the sensitization which follows the experimental injection of hematoporphyrin. When an animal is treated in this way it becomes as sensitive to ordinary white light from which the ultraviolet rays are excluded by red glass as is a normal animal to ultraviolet rays. The hematoporphyrin appears to act as a sensitizer in the photographic sense. When the sensitized tissues are exposed to ordinary light, there is a complete stasis in the vessels followed by necrosis. Exposure to intense light is followed by acute general effects, *i.e.*, excitement, convulsions, and death in the course of a short time.

4. Ultraviolet light exerts a *photochemical action on the lipids of the skin*. The cholesterol of the skin seems to be activated by ultraviolet light and converted into vitamin D. Sunlight or the ultraviolet light from a mercury-vapor lamp is as efficacious in the treatment of a vitamin D deficiency disease like rickets as is the administration of cod-liver oil.

ELECTRICITY

The passage of an electric current through the body may cause burns of varying severity or may result in death; the latter condition is known as electrocution.

The *local effects* are those of a burn. The current enters the body at one spot and leaves it at another. It is at these points where resistance is encountered that evidence of the burn is most marked. At the point of exit the lesion is particularly severe, as in a gunshot wound, the tissues sometimes showing radiating tears. The point of exit is often on the feet, as the current leaves the body there to pass into the ground. The burn may be of any degree of severity. It usually does not look as bad as it really is. At first it is dry and bloodless, but in the course of thirty-six hours marked hyperemia and edema have developed. Little cavities may be found in the epidermis, supposed to be caused by the sudden generation of steam. A slough separates, and the ulcer thus formed is singularly slow to heal, usually taking two or three times as long as in the case of an ordinary burn.

The *general effects* resemble those of any severe burn. In fatal cases the viscera are congested, the serous membranes show petechial hemorrhages, the lungs are edematous, and the right ventricle is full of dark fluid blood. Death is probably due to respiratory rather than to cardiac failure, for the patient may sometimes be resuscitated by prolonged artificial respiration. The muscles are flaccid, although during life they may be in a state of severe tetanic spasm. There may be chromatolysis and degeneration of the nerve cells. The blood vessels are severely injured for they serve as good conductors of the current, so that thrombosis and severe hemorrhages are common. In judicial electrocution the current is applied to the central nervous system and death is instantaneous, so that most of the above changes are not found.

Lightning.—The results produced by lightning are very similar. There may be all kinds of skin wounds—puncture wounds, lacerations and bruises. Bands of scorched skin may pass from the point of entry (usually the head) down the body to the point of exit. The most characteristic feature is the so-called current markings or lightning figures, peculiar arborescent red lines on the skin which are probably caused by the current being split up in dendriform fashion within the body.

IONIZING RADIATION

The most powerful of all physical irritants is ionizing radiation, for it injures not only organs and cells, but the very molecules and atoms of which cells are composed. We have long been familiar with the effects produced by X-rays and radium, but in the atomic age we have to face other sources of radiation. The subject of ionizing radiation has come to assume a position of such outstanding importance that it is considered in a separate chapter instead of in the present one as formerly.

TRAUMA

The commonest of physical irritants is trauma, so common indeed that were the subject to be considered fully it would necessitate a discussion of injuries of every organ in the body. A few of its effects may be considered here. The most readily recognized result of trauma is *bruising*, due to tearing of minute vessels in the subcutaneous or deeper tissues. The resulting extravasation of blood may be diffuse or localized depending on the looseness or density of the tissue. The kaleidoscopic procession of colors in bruising of the tissues is well known; first red, then bluish-green, and finally fading away into yellow, as the hemoglobin is converted into bilirubin and then gradually removed. Signs of inflammation are also present especially when the injury is severe, due to liberation of histamine by the lacerated tissues. If there is great destruction of tissue, the histamine passing into the circulation may produce a condition of shock. There may be *rupture of viscera* such as liver, spleen or bowel. It must be noted that serious internal injuries may be produced without bruising of the skin, even though the trauma be quite severe. Traumatic head injuries, with or without fracture of the skull, are considered in Chapter 42.

Many other instances of the effect of trauma will be encountered in the sections dealing with Special Pathology; the examples given above are merely chosen as characteristic of the varied reactions which it may produce in the tissues. A full account of the various lesions which may be caused by trauma will be found in Moritz's monograph, *Pathology of Trauma*.

INCREASED ATMOSPHERIC PRESSURE

Caisson Disease.—Caisson disease or diver's palsy is the result of a sudden alteration in the atmospheric pressure. A caisson is a cylinder containing air under high pressure used for sinking piers in the construction of bridges. Caisson workers, tunnel workers (under rivers), and divers are subjected to high air pressures. If they are "decompressed" too quickly or return to a normal atmosphere too suddenly they develop headache, vertigo, dyspnea, pains all over the body called "the bends," and it may be paralysis. While the person is under high pressure a large amount of air, particularly nitrogen, is dissolved in the blood plasma. As the result of sudden decompression this gas is released as bubbles in the blood, and these form emboli particularly in the brain and spinal cord. Numerous small infarcts of the central nervous system are produced in this way and are responsible for most of the symptoms. Bubbles of gas may also be liberated in the nervous tissue and cause disintegration.

REFERENCES

KNOCKER, P.: Lancet, 1955, *2*, 837. (Effects of hypothermia on vital organs).

KREYBERG, L.: Lancet, 1946, *1*, 338. (Tissue damage due to cold).

MORITZ, A. R.: *The Pathology of Trauma,* 2nd ed., Philadelphia, 1954.

Chapter 18

Ionizing Radiation

General Principles
 The Atom
 Radioactivity
  Particulate Radiation
  Electromagnetic Radiation
  Ionization
   Sources of ionizing radiation
   Radioactive isotopes
Biological Reactions
 Target Effect
 Toxic Effect
 Nuclear Lesions

Cytoplasmic Lesions
Comparative Radiosensitivity
 Radiosensitive
 Radioresponsive
 Radioresistant
Neoplastic Cells
Specific Tissues
 Skin
 Lymphoid Tissue
 Hematopoietic Tissue
 Gastrointestinal Tract
 Germ Cells

 Bone
 Lung
 Diagnostic Radiation Hazards
Genetic Hazards
Atomic Bomb Radiation
 Acute Radiation Syndrome
Radiation Carcinogenesis
Protection Against Radiation
 Injury
Chronology

GENERAL PRINCIPLES

The fundamental feature of physical ionization is the *detachment of an electron from an atom*. All living matter is continuously exposed to "background" ionizing radiation, but only in minute amount. Now that the atomic age has arrived, with nuclear energy producing electricity, propelling ships and submarines, and providing the warheads of long-range ballistic missiles, everybody concerned with practical medicine is compelled to acquaint himself with the effects of ionizing radiation in man (Gerstner).

Although the atomic age was born on July 16, 1945, with the explosion of the first atomic bomb at Alamogordo, New Mexico, in the United States, it was conceived a long time ago. Becquerel in 1896 showed that uranium emitted rays which fogged a shielded photographic plate. This was followed by Roentgen's demonstration of the *x*-rays from a cathode vacuum tube, and the isolation of radium from pitchblende by Marie and Pierre Curie. In 1911 came the fundamental discovery by Rutherford of the atomic nucleus. A list of the names, dates and countries of the men and women responsible for the atomic age being conceived and finally born is given at the end of this chapter.

The Atom. The atom consists of (1) a *nucleus* made up of *protons* with a positive charge and *neutrons* without charge, and (2) negatively charged *electrons* which circulate in orbit around the nucleus. The number of electrons equals the number of protons, so that the electric charges balance, with resulting neutrality. The electron, as its name implies, may be regarded as an electric charge with a mass so small that it may be ignored; the proton is a mass with an electric charge, and the neutron a still larger mass without charge. The atomic number indicates the sum of the protons, while the atomic weight indicates the sum of the protons and neutrons, *i.e.* the total number of particles. It follows that the higher the atomic number the greater will be the number of electrons, so that we may speak of a cloud of electrons. If the nucleus contains an excess of either neutrons or protons it is radioactive, because there is redistribution of the particles with emission of energy in the form of radiation. An *isotope* is formed by varying the atomic weight by the addition of neutrons. It is possible to produce an isotope of any element by driving extra neutrons into its nucleus. A natural element is generally a mixture of isotopes. Some isotopes are stable, whilst the rest are radioactive, decaying as the result of beta emission.

The *basic particles of the atom* are held together by extremely powerful forces in the nucleus; these nuclear forces can be released and used. The atom is largely void space consisting of widely separated particles, so that it may be compared with the solar system. As Sears puts it in his delightfully simple book, if the cloud of electrons was lacking, a man could walk through a stone wall without serious injury either to himself or to the wall. The hydrogen nucleus consists of a single proton, but no neutron. The neutron is the instrument of nuclear fission, because its neutrality endows it with great permeability. For the same reason it can inflict serious biological injury.

Radioactivity.—"High energy radiation can be defined as a stream of energy carried by very small particles travelling at high speeds" (Hoyt). These particles escape from the atomic nucleus. It is the energy emitted from a physically unstable atom, the nucleus of which reacts until stability is attained over a period of time known as the half-life. Atomic energy is the source of 99 per cent of all energy known to man, both stored in fuels as previous energy from the sun or streaming continuously in solar radiations. It is the energy of motion, and escapes from the atom as: (1) *charged particles*, which may be negative *beta particles* (electrons), positive *alpha particles* (helium nuclei); (2) *uncharged particles* or neutrons; (3) *photons* or *waves*, which may be light (infrared, visible or ultraviolet) or *X*- and *gamma rays*. The gamma ray is similar to a high-energy *x*-ray, the only difference being one of length, the gamma rays being shorter and therefore having more energy. The only ionizing waves are *x*- and gamma rays. *Cosmic rays* from outer space disrupt the atomic nuclei which they encounter in the atmosphere, releasing energies which are expressed in billions of electron volts, and against which complete shielding is impracticable. The energy released by nuclear transformations are infinitely greater than those of chemical reactions because there is a change in total mass, and energy (E) and mass (M) are related according to the theory of relativity by Einstein's famous equation: $E = Mc^2$, where c is the velocity of light in centimeters per second, *i.e.*, 30 billions. There are thus two forms of radiation energy: (1) particulate radiation, and (2) electromagnetic wave radiation.

Particulate Radiation.—When radiation particles collide like bullets with an atom, energy is lost by the particle and gained by the atom. The particles concerned are alpha particles or rays, neutrons and protons.

Alpha particles, which are helium nuclei, have a greater mass than any of the other particles, consisting of 2 neutrons and 2 protons, so that they have a positive charge. They have great kinetic energy but little penetrating power owing to their large mass and positive charge. They collide very early with atoms which they encounter, and only penetrate for a fraction of a millimeter. This is fortunate, because they produce devastating injury. Alpha particles are liberated from disintegrating thorium. *Beta rays* are electrons released from many radioactive elements, as well as from cathode-ray tubes. They are of course smaller and more penetrating than alpha particles, extending into the tissues for 2 or more millimeters, depending on their energy, but they have less ionizing power. A colliding electron, however, may not displace the electron of the atom which it encounters, but be incorporated into the atom, imparting energy to it. In this way hydrogen peroxide may be formed from the abundant water in the cell as the result of ionization, producing very important toxic effects which are described below. *Neutrons* are present in all atoms with a weight above that of hydrogen. They are discharged in great amount from uranium and plutonium in atomic piles reactors and bombs. As they carry no electrostatic charge they can penetrate the electron cloud of the atom and reach the nucleus. They may be "captured" by the nuclei, which then give off more potent forms of radiation.

Electromagnetic Radiation.—These radiations form a continuous spectrum with wave lengths varying from many thousands of meters in the case of long electrical waves, through infrared, visible and ultraviolet light, to *X*- and gamma rays with a wave length of one ten-millionth of a millimeter. Only the latter two have the power, by virtue of their short wave lengths, of detaching an electron from the atom on which they impinge, with resulting ionization. The detached electrons, as we have already seen, constitute beta radiation, which in turn produces further biological effects. Electromagnetic radiations of short wave length are immensely more penetrating than particulate radiations, and may affect cells many centimeters below the surface. It

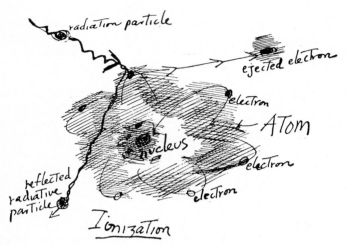

FIG. 226.—(Rosalee C. Hoyt, courtesy of Bulletin of the Atomic Scientists).

will be evident that alpha and gamma rays are at the opposite extremes of penetrating power.

Ultraviolet light is an example of non-ionizing radiation. It hardly penetrates the skin, but it produces severe sun burn and, with continued exposure, a tendency to the late development of skin cancer. If, however, the irradiated objects are extremely small, as in the case of bacteria and viruses, ultra violet light penetrates fully, and is an effective mode of killing such objects.

The *latent period* which elapses before the effects of electromagnetic radiation become apparent varies with the wave length. As the length becomes shorter, the energy of the wave increases, and the latent period corresponds with the position of the energy along the electromagnetic spectrum. Thus infrared rays burn the skin immediately, ultraviolet rays produce sunburn after several hours, and the effect of x-rays is not evident for two or three days.

Ionization.—Ionizing radiations produce electrically charged particles—ions—on their passage through any matter, living or non-living. When an electron is ejected from an atom, it leaves the electrically unbalanced residue of the atom as a positively charged ion. This is the essence of ionizing radiation. The detached electron may become attached to some other atom, which also loses its electric neutrality, and thus becomes charged,

ionized or "excited" (Figs. 226 and 227). Thus it is as difficult for some atoms as for some countries to remain neutral when exposed to hostile influences. Either the loss or the gain of an electron may alter the chemical behavior of the molecule affected.

Sources of Ionizing Radiation.—These sources are as follows: (1) *Cosmic rays,* (2) *Radioactive materials occurring in nature,* such as uranium and radium. (3) *X-rays* for therapeutic and diagnostic machines. (4) *Istopes,* which are elements having the same atomic number but different atomic weights, and therefore unstable. Thus an isotope of hydrogen with one neutron as well as one proton forms deuterium (heavy hydrogen or heavy water). Tritium has 2 neutrons, but still only one proton and one electron, so that it is unstable and therefore radioactive. Isotopes may occur in nature or may be made in an atomic pile reactor through bombardment with neutrons. It is evident that ionizing radiation may be (1) *natural* (cosmic rays, radioactive materials occurring in nature), also known as *background radiation,* or (2) *man-made* (x-ray machines, artificial isotopes, atomic pile reactor, atomic bomb) (Tabershaw).

Radioactive Isotopes.—These have proved of value in medicine in two very different ways. They may be used either as "tracers" or in therapy. *Isotopes as tracers* depend on the fact that a radioactive isotope of an

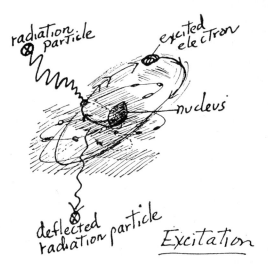

Fig. 227.—(Rosalee C. Hoyt, courtesy of Bulletin
of the Atomic Scientists.)

element is *chemically* identical with the non-radioactive form, and can therefore be substituted for it in a chemical compound. This is known as "tagging." The presence of radioactive atoms can be demonstrated by means of a Geiger counter. The tagged molecules can now be followed through complex chemical and metabolic processes. This has been done for sodium, phosphorus, carbon, iodine, and other elements. It is even possible to tag vitamins, hormones and antibodies by supplying animals and plants with radioactive nutrients. This technique has placed a powerful weapon in the hands of the physiologist.

Isotopes in therapy are used in much larger doses. The method depends on the selective concentration of an element in a particular organ or tissue. The best example is the use of radioactive iodine in hyperplasia and cancer of the thyroid gland, since any iodine administered is concentrated to an overwhelming degree in the thyroid. Phosphorus is concentrated in the bones, so that radioactive phosphorus is used in the treatment of diseases of the cells of the bone marrow, such as leukemia and polycythemia vera. Finally radioactive isotopes of long half-life may be inclosed in needles and used in the same way as radium. Cobalt-60, a radioactive isotope of cobalt made in the atomic pile reactor, has proved of particular

value in place of the much more expensive natural radium. It is used in a teletherapy unit.

Dosage and Half-life.—Electromagnetic radiations were first derived by Roentgen from the vacuum cathode tube, and they are naturally measured as roentgens or r. In estimating dosage, however, it must be remembered that effect is proportional to the amount absorbed, not to the amount delivered. Alpha particles because of their size and electric charge have little power of penetration, so that they act primarily on the skin. The energy of beta particles varies widely, and so does their penetrating power. Gamma rays on the other hand, penetrate deeply, and have much less action on the skin, although they may cause redness, swelling and loss of hair.

The *half-life* of a radioactive element is the time required to lose 50 per cent of its radioactive atoms which have broken down. The difference in the half-life of various materials is simply fantastic. Thus in the case of uranium the time is 4 billion years, with radium 226 it is 1,590 years, with strontium-90 twenty-eight years, and with iodine-138 only six seconds. A consideration of these facts will show that whilst man still lives in an environment of minimal (natural) radioactivity, in the dark backward and abysm of time the exposure must have been much higher. It is interesting to speculate on what effect this may have had on the mutation rate which made evolution possible. It is evident that for clinical use the half-life must be short, otherwise permanent radiation injury would result.

BIOLOGICAL REACTIONS

"All matter is composed of elements, all elements are composed of atoms. All atoms are composed of the basic particles of physics. Living forms use atoms to build biologic structure for chemical molecules. Radiation disrupts and destroys these molecules and hence destroys life" (Sears). Chemical molecules are held together by interactions between the outer orbital electrons of the atoms. Damage to living cells is effected by a transfer of energy from the radioactive agent to the cells by the process of ionization, which, as we have already seen, is the loss or the acquisition of an electron by an atom.

The complex subject of the biological effects of ionizing radiation may be considered from the point of view of the target and poison or toxic theories, of injury to nucleus and cytoplasm, of the action on somatic and germinal cells, of the varying radiosensitivity and resistance of different tissues, of immediate and after-effects, and of local as opposed to whole body radiation. In general biological terms we may say that the effect may be *mutation, inactivation* (as of a virus), or *death of the cell*. From the viewpoint of pathology there may be one or all of four processes: (1) *necrosis*, (2) *hemorrhage*, (3) *infection* and (4) *neoplasia*. Necrosis is a primary type of reaction to radiation injury, and so perhaps is neoplasia, whereas hemorrhage and infection are secondary results of injuries which we shall study later.

Target Effect.—The cell contains many particulate structures. In the nucleus there are the 46 chromosomes with their thousands of genes, and in the cytoplasm there are the various organelles, such as the mitochondria carrying enzymes on their surface and the centrosomes which carry the spindle of mitosis. Any of these may be hit by the electron bullets. The devastating effects are due to the high energies delivered to small volumes of the cell, much as a high velocity bullet may inflict only localized but fatal damage. If the target is small, as in the case of an enzyme molecule attached to a mitochondrion, the biological result will be small, because there are many more similar molecules to carry on the function, but if it is large, as in the case of a gene, the effect may be serious, resulting in a mutation. An average single cell in human tissue contains about a hundred thousand billion molecules, which might suggest undue crowding, yet to an approaching electron the material would appear mostly as open space. A dose of 1000 roentgens of whole body radiation, which would kill a man in a few days, results in the ionization of only about one molecule out of every hundred million in the body. These facts suggest the thought that the target theory may not be as adequate in

explaining the ill effects of radiation as might appear at first sight.

Toxic Effect.—Water constitutes a large part of every cell, and disruption of the molecules of water may lead to the formation of free hydrogen and hydroxyl radicles, and then hydrogen peroxide from the dissolved oxygen. This and other toxic substances lead to diffuse biochemical poisoning, which is probably responsible for the immediate effects known clinically as acute radiation poisoning. We have spoken above of the target and toxic theories, but it is evident that they are in no way exclusive, and that both may operate, although in different degree in different cases.

Nuclear Lesions.—The effects of ionizing radiation on the nucleus are most evident during mitosis, and it is in the early prophase that the nucleus is most sensitive owing to the formation of discrete targets, the chromosomes. These changes are best studied in pure tissue cultures of cells. During the prophase two threads, the chromatids, appear, which in the metaphase become attached to the mitotic spindle. The *visible changes* produced by ionizing radiation are rupture of the chromosomes and chromatids with fragmentation. The two halves of different chromosomes may fuse before being divided into chromatids, this being known as *interchange of chromosomes*, or there may be reunion between broken chromatids of two different chromosomes, *i.e. interchange of chromatids*. Thus there may be repair of chromosomes with restitution of the original pattern, or they may remain fragmented, or finally the fragments may unite to form new combinations. Many new configurations may result from the fusion of non-homologous chromosomes and chromatids. Since chromosomes carry the genes, it is evident that mutations may result. The number of fractures (and mutations) increases with the square of the dose. At low dosages mutations are very rare. At least two breaks must occur in order to permit the rearrangement necessary for mutation. If these rearrangements involve germinal cells, the result may be serious or disastrous.

A small dose of radiation may arrest mitosis, followed by increased mitosis. A higher dose arrests mitosis permanently with cell death. Finally, long continued exposure to sublethal doses of irradiation may result in neoplasia. *Abnormal mitosis* may be evident in tissue cultures. Thus there may be *tripolar division*, so that three or even four cells may be formed instead of two. The cell may fail to divide, so that a giant cell is formed with more than one nucleus, a condition known as *endomitosis*. It must be realized that these varied changes in the cell may be produced by other agents than ionizing radiation. Thus the administration of colchicine leads to mitotic arrest, followed by abnormal division of cells, and the same is true of nitrogen mustard.

Cytoplasmic Lesions.—Changes of the organelles of the cytoplasm comparable to the breaks in the chromosomes can not be demonstrated, but there is no doubt of the importance of the role of the cytoplasm in the cellular change. The purely mechanical interpretation of chromosomal breakage can no longer be maintained. "The impact of an ionizing particle with a chromosome can not be compared with the snapping of a telephone wire by a bullet" (Bacq and Alexander). Nuclei freed of cytoplasm are remarkably radioresistant; indeed no lesion may be produced after exposure to a dose as high as 30,000 r. If an incredibly minute amount of the cytoplasm of a cell which has been irradiated several days previously is injected into the cytoplasm of a normal cell, the latter shows all the changes characteristic of radiation lesions within one or two hours. A biochemical as well as a mechanical mechanism seems to be involved in the production of the nuclear effects of radiation. It has indeed been suggested that *radiation damage* to the cell may consist of three phases: (1) primary physical or radiochemical changes in the cytoplasm; (2) chemical metabolic processes which allow protoplasmic nuclear toxins to accumulate in the cytoplasm; (3) transmission of these toxic substances into the nucleus (Duryee).

COMPARATIVE RADIOSENSITIVITY

So far we have been considering the changes produced in cells by ionizing radiation in an impersonal manner, as if the character of the cell was of no importance.

Nothing, of course, could be farther from the truth. Different tissues vary widely in their their sensitivity to radiation. Different kinds of animals also vary in a similar and, at present, quite inexplicable manner. LD-50-30 signifies the lethal dose of irradiation necessary to kill 50 per cent of a group of animals over a period of thirty days. The wide variation in sensitivity is indicated by the figures which for the pig is 275 r, the mouse 600, the rat 900, man 400–500, the tortoise 1500, and E. coli 5600. E. coli may escape easily because of its small size, which does not permit absorption of all the energy. Cold-blooded animals are less sensitive than mammals.

Radiosensitivity in general parallels the rate of mitotic division, which is only natural in view of the preceding discussion. It is only in the early prophase of mitosis that the cells are hypersensitive. When mitosis is arrested in metaphase the cells have the same resistance as resting cells. As long ago as 1904 Bergonié and Tribondeau formulated a "law" which may be called the biological foundation for radium and roentgen-ray treatment. This *law of Bergonié and Tribondeau* is as follows: "Immature cells and cells in an active state of division are more sensitive to irradiation than are those that have acquired adult morphological and physiological characteristics." To this, however, there are some notable exceptions. When a piece of liver is removed there is extremely rapid regeneration, yet the great numbers of dividing cells apparently remain as relatively insensitive as before. The small lymphocyte, which rarely is seen dividing, is one of the cells most susceptible to radiation. This may well be related to the enormous metabolic activity of the lymphocyte, which, together with its close relative the plasma cell, is the factory for the production of antibodies. The inactive polymorphonuclear leukocyte is very resistant to radiation. There must, therefore, be other explanations of the differing sensitivity of various tissues, but what these are remains for the present unknown.

In general terms it may be said that those cells are especially radiosensitive which normally continue to multiply throughout life, owing to their own short life span. Such

27

are the cells of the hematopoietic and lymphatic systems, the epithelial cells of the gastrointestinal tract and skin, and the germinal cells of the gonads. We would expect a lymphocyte, with its life span of a few hours, to be more sensitive to radiation than a nerve cell which never divides. It is convenient to divide the tissues of the body into three main groups: radiosensitive, radioresponsive, and radioresistant (Shields Warren).

Radiosensitive.—A dose of 2,500 r or less kills or seriously injures many cells. Examples are lymphocytes and lymphoblasts, bone marrow blast cells, epithelial cells of the stomach and intestine, and germ cells of the ovary and testis. It must be realized, however, that although many lymphocytes in a node may be affected by a dose of 100 r, many times that dose can be given without destroying every lymphocyte in the node.

Radioresponsive.—The dose is 2,500 to 5,000 r. This group includes the epithelium of the skin and its appendages, vascular endothelium, salivary glands, growing bone and cartilage, the tissues of the eye, and collagen and elastic tissue.

Radioresistant.—A dose of over 5,000 r is necessary. This group includes viscera, mature bone and cartilage, muscle, brain and other nervous tissue. It will be seen that except in very large doses radiation does not cause serious damage to vital organs such as the heart and brain; such injury would be immediately fatal.

Cancer Cells.—The cells of a neoplasm, like the normal cells from which they originate, may be sensitive, responsive or resistant to irradiation. Here again undifferentiated, rapidly growing cells of embryonic type and showing numerous mitoses may be expected to respond well. But the radiotherapist must beware of generalizations and know the peculiarities of individual tumors. Thus such tumors as malignant melanoma and osteogenic sarcoma may be teeming with mitoses and yet be quite radioresistant. Lymphocytes which have a very short life and have therefore to be continually renewed are amongst the most radiosensitive of cells, and the same is even more true of lymphosarcoma, which may melt away like a snowball before the fire. Unfortunately even the most radiosensitive of tumors have often a small proportion of cells which survive, and these cells transmit the property of resistance to their progeny, so that eventually the entire mass may be radioresistant. This is comparable with the behavior of many bacteria to antibiotics. *There is a profound difference between radiosensitivity and radiocurability.* To repeat the quotation from Sir Stanford Cade which I have already used in Chapter 8: "Radiosensitive tumors are the 'miracles' of radiation, the source of conceit in the inexperienced radiotherapist, and the greatest source of disappointment when apparently brilliant successes become in due course dismal failures." This must not be taken to suggest that the treatment of malignant tumors by ionizing radiation is not of great value. When the neoplastic cells are exposed to irradiation adequately and for sufficient time all the cells may be killed either directly or in combination with ischemia resulting from vascular changes and perhaps an immunological response on the part of the cells of the stroma. In practice it is found that the tumors which are curable by radiation are of moderate radiosensitivity, neither very sensitive nor very resistant. The general subject of the treatment of malignant tumors by ionizing radiation has already been discussed on page 217, so that it will not be considered farther here.

Radiation Lesions of Specific Tissues.—Lesions of various tissues may occur as the result of radiotherapy, undue and careless exposure to radiation as in the case of the early roentgenologists, leakage from commercial atomic power installations, and finally the total body irradiation of an atomic explosion. The lesions may therefore be local or general, in both cases the injury being of the same character. In addition to local or general lesions there may be systemic effects, which demand separate consideration. The flux of neutrons is particularly liable to produce *cataract of the lens* owing to their greater mass. Severe cataracts have developed as a late effect in cyclotron workers who may have had occasional serious over-exposure to the eyes. The cataracts which developed in the total body radiation of the Japanese bomb explosions were slight in character and usually caused no disability.

Skin.—The skin does not belong to the radiosensitive group of tissues, but it is the structure most frequently involved, because all external radiations, whether therapeutic or accidental, must pass through the skin. *Acute radiodermatitis* is really a burn of the skin. The lesions do not appear at once, but only after a latent period of a few days to two weeks. The skin becomes reddened, giving an appearance of sunburn, with swelling and falling-out of the hair. In severe cases blisters form, and a necrotic slough separates leaving an ulcer. The burned skin may become like parchment and may not separate for a considerable time. Healing is likely to be very slow, and scarring may go on for many months, causing marked deformity. At any time fresh ulceration may develop in the affected area, more particularly if the part is again exposed to radiation. Repair indeed is never complete. It has been well said that a healed roentgen-ray burn is not a cured roentgen-ray burn.

Chronic radiodermatitis is likely to be the result of frequent small doses. It was a common lesion on the hands of radiologists before efficient screening was practiced. Telangiectasis may develop one or more years after exposure, a good example of the delayed character of many radiation lesions. This is accompanied by thinning of the epidermis with loss of the rete pegs together with sclerosis of the dermis and absence of hair follicles and sweat and sebaceous glands (Fig. 228). Such skin is devitalized, so that minor injury may result in localized areas of necrosis, which often take months to heal. In cases of long standing the epidermis may show marked signs of proliferation, with downgrowths of epithelial cells into the corium. It is in such lesions that carcinoma is apt to develop, often after an interval of many years since the last exposure to radiation. Vascular changes are always present. Reference has already been made to the telangiectases caused by capillary dilatation. In the arteries, and to a lesser degree in the veins, there is a remarkable thickening of the subendothelial coat producing extreme narrowing of the lumen and in many cases complete occlusion. This is a main reason for proper healing being impos-

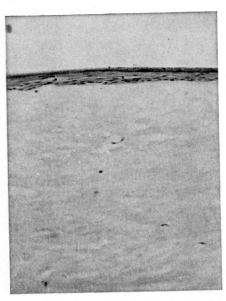

Fig. 228.—Radiation dermatitis, showing ironing out of epidermis and disappearance of dermal appendages. × 150. (Boyd's *Pathology for the Surgeon*, courtesy of W. B. Saunders Company.)

sible and for the frequent breaking-down of the scar.

Lymphoid Tissue.—Reference has already been made to the extreme radiosensitivity of lymphoid tissues, including the spleen. Both the nucleus and the cytoplasm of the lymphocytes show marked degenerative changes terminating in necrosis of the cells. As the life span of the lymphocyte is only a few hours, extensive injury to lymphoid tissues is immediately followed by a marked drop in the number of lymphocytes in the circulating blood.

Hematopoietic Tissue. — Hematopoietic cells are even more sensitive to radiation than those of lymphoid tissue, both the granulocytes and the thrombocytes of the bone marrow being either killed or so damaged that they are unable to mature and proliferate. There is thus a striking drop in the numbers of circulating granular leukocytes and blood platelets. The fall is not so abrupt as in the case of lymphocytes, because the survival time of granulocytes and platelets is several days longer than that of the lymphocyte, the maximal effect being seen about the end of the first week of total

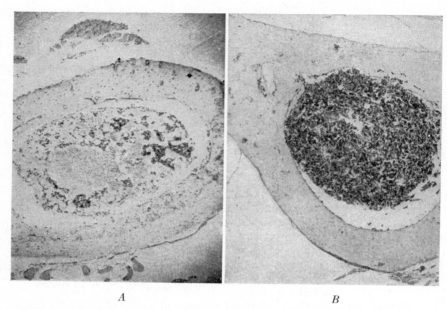

A   B

FIG. 229.—*A*, Shaft of femur of a mouse ten days after irradiation with 600 r *x*-rays. *B*, Shaft of femur of control mouse. (Mole, courtesy of Société de Chemie Physique).

body irradiation. By that time the bone marrow is almost acellular, consisting of little more than loose connective tissue (Fig. 229). Should the patient survive, regeneration of the few remaining cells may eventually result in a hyperplastic marrow, although this may not be reflected in the circulating blood picture for many weeks or even months, owing presumably to failure of the proliferating marrow cells to mature properly. The persistent granulopenia is responsible for the recurring infections which constitute such a serious feature of total body irradiation, and which serves as an index of the severity of the damage. Similarly the lack of platelets are connected with the frequent hemorrhages in these cases. The occasional subsequent marrow hyperplasia may be related to the leukemia frequently seen in radiologists exposed to repeated minimal doses of ionizing radiation as well as in patients receiving long-continued heavy radiation therapy for ankylosing spondylitis. In the latter cases the incidence rises progressively, so that with the highest doses it is nearly 40 times that of controls. Leukemia is said to be unduly frequent in children who have been subjected to irradia-

tion before birth by reason of *x*-ray pelvic examination of the mother. As the red cells have a life span of some 6 weeks in the circulating blood, anemia does not develop for several weeks after severe exposure.

Gastrointestinal Tract.—The epithelium of the stomach and intestine belongs to the radiosensitive class, as it is being constantly desquamated and as continually replaced, but the deep location of these structures tends to shield them from external radiation. As we shall see presently, ulcerative lesions of the intestine, especially the small intestine, constitute a serious feature of severe total body radiation. When radium is implanted for the treatment of carcinoma of the cervix or other pelvic neoplasms, the mucosa of the rectum and colon may be seriously injured. Degeneration is followed by ulceration and atrophy of the bowel comparable with what we have already studied in the case of the skin. In about 2 per cent of presumably hypersensitive persons inflammatory lesions may develop in the anterior wall of the rectum from 6 months to several years after completion of the course of treatment. Painful chronic ulcers are formed, the most frequent complaint being the passage of blood and mucus per rectum. Distressing fistulous connections may be formed between the rectum, bladder and vagina. Even if the lesions heal there may be extensive scarring with stricture of the rectum.

Germ Cells.—The germinal cells of the ovary and testis are in the radiosensitive group, so that these structures have to be shielded with particular care in persons liable to be exposed to radiation. If the

as calcium is, and over a period of many years it may make its presence felt.

Lungs.—When the chest has been repeatedly radiated, the lungs may develop a *radiation pneumonitis.* The lungs are pale, dry and rubbery, with thick alveolar walls often lined by a hyaline membrane.

The following table summarizes some of the important facts concerning radiosensitivity.

COMPARATIVE RADIOSENSITIVITIES

Radiosensitive	Radioresponsive	Radioresistant
(Requires less than 2,500r to kill or seriously injure).	(Requires 2,500 to 5,000 r to kill or seriously injure.)	(Requires more than 5,000 r to kill or seriously injure.)
Hematopoietic and lymphoid tissues. Epithelium of G.I. tract. Germ cells.	Epithelium of skin. Vascular endothelium. Growing bone and cartilage. Salivary glands. Lens, cornea, and conjunctiva. Collagen and elastic tissues.	Liver, thyroid, parathyroids, pituitary, kidneys, pancreas, adrenals, mature bone and cartilage, smooth and striated muscle. Nervous tissues.

cells are killed, sterility is the result. If, on the other hand, one of the chromosomes or even one of its genes is damaged, the result may be a mutation which becomes hereditary, a subject which is discussed below in relation to genetic hazards.

Bone.—The growing epiphyses of children may easily be injured by radiation. We have come to realize the insidious danger of fluoroscope installations in shoe stores, which give such a fascinating view of the bones of a child's foot in the shoe being fitted, but which are liable to innocent abuse. Mature bone is very much more resistant, but the resistance breaks down if radioactive material is deposited in its interior. A classic example was the necrosis of the mandible which occurred in girls engaged in painting the luminous dials of watches, the camel hair brushes carrying radioactive paint material being continually given a finer point by their lips. Some of the girls who survived developed sarcoma of bone many years later. Radioactive strontium, which is present in large amount in the fall-out of atomic explosions, is deposited in bone just

Diagnostic Radiation Hazards.—We have been discussing the harmful effects which may accompany or follow radiation therapy, and we shall have to consider the radiation effect on the general population of atomic bomb explosions. In addition to these there is the recently aroused awareness of the possible dangers of diagnostic radiation. Formerly it was the radiotherapist who was the victim, but with adequate precautions this hazard has been removed, and the patient has come to occupy the foreground. Nothing is more difficult than to determine whether or not ordinary diagnostic procedures involving the use of x-rays constitute a hazard to health, but it may be of interest to quote the conclusions of a physicist attached to the radiation department of a large general hospital. "The hazards of diagnostic radiography to the patient, even by the most pessimistic standards, are small. They are low enough to be outweighed by the expectation of a small potential benefit. The somewhat larger genetic hazards of most examinations are surpassed by those accruing from wearing a radium-dial wrist watch, and, apparently, from wearing trousers" (which raise the local temperature 3.3° C.) (Webster).

GENETIC HAZARDS

Genetic information is transmitted from one generation to another through the chemical medium of the desoxyribosenucleic acid of the chromosomes. A *mutation* is some alteration in this material which, when the chromosomes reproduce themselves, is itself replicated. Mutations may be spontaneous or induced, and by far the most potent agent of induction is ionizing radiation. Mutations are not confined to the *reproductive cells*, for they can involve the genes on the chromosomes of *somatic cells*. In the case of somatic cells the mutation is transmitted from one cell to its daughter cells, as may occur in cancer, where radiation may so upset a well balanced, smoothly running genetic system as to evoke abnormal types of growth. Most if not all genes are concerned with specific enzymes, each of which governs one chemical step in a metabolic pattern which cannot be altered with impunity. When germinal cells are involved the mutation is transmitted to future generations, unless the mutation is lethal and dominant.

It was in 1927 that H. J. Muller, then at the University of Texas, discovered that radiation with x-rays produced a large increase in the number of mutations in *Drosophila*, the fruit fly. Not one of the dozens of animals and plants which since that time have been exposed to radiation has failed to produce more mutations. Indeed the mutation rate is 15 times greater in the mouse than in *Drosophila*. The number of mutations is strictly proportional to the total amount of radiation reaching the germinal cells during a reproductive lifetime. Each dose, however small, carries a risk. There is no such thing as a harmless dose, for the effect is cumulative, so that many small doses have the same effect as one large one. The hereditary changes induced by radiation depend on the loss of a part of the genetic material, a loss which cannot be made good. In Drosophila one-quarter of all mutations are lethal, 15 to 20 per cent

producing sterility in one or both sexes. Most mutations are recessive, affecting only one of the two alleles of a gene, but they are transmitted from one generation to another, with results which can well be imagined.

It is not possible to speak at the present time with any certainty about the exact genetic hazards of ionizing radiation to man. Studies on the children of the survivors of Hiroshima and Nagasaki have been inconclusive. Speaking from the viewpoint of the geneticist Crow states that from observations over many years on Drosophila we may conclude "that the most frequent mutants in man are not those leading to freaks or obvious hereditary diseases, but those causing minor impairments leading to higher embryonic death rates, lowered life expectancy, increase in disease, or decreased fertility." If the mutation is recessive, requiring a double dose to become evident, hundreds of generations may intervene before the damage occurs. This is one of the many reasons why it has not been possible to draw definite conclusions from the Japanese experience. International commissions have fixed a "maximum permissable dose" of 0.3 r per week. With this dose the danger of carcinogenic action to the individual is nil, but it amounts to 400r in 26 years, the course of active sexual life, which is 5 times the dose that, according to geneticists, doubles the incidence of spontaneous mutations. It may be noted in passing that a complete radioscopic and radiographic examination of the stomach subjects a patient to a dose of about 30r. Male germ cells are much more radiosensitive and easily killed than those of the female. On the other hand any dose received by the germ cells less than a lethal dose could result in chromosome mutations which are transmitted to future generations. This is still more true of the female.

We have already seen that radiation may be (1) background or (2) man-made. With respect to man-made radiation we are particularly concerned in this regard with the total body radiation produced by fall-out.

Background radiation comes to some extent from cosmic rays, but to a much greater degree from soil and rock. This varies greatly from one locality to another. Thus in Trevancor in southern India the population lives on highly radioactive sand. It is natural that the figure for safe background radiation is being continually revised.

Fall-out radiation is at the present time most likely to come from atomic bomb explosions, which are discussed below. The present rates of fall-out seem to add only a small fraction, less than 5 per cent, perhaps only 1 per cent, to natural irradiations. So far we may say that "the mutations induced by bomb-bursts are only a small fraction of radiation-induced mutations, and a still smaller number of all mutations" (Crow). In the near future we shall be faced with the genetic hazards of the peaceful application of atomic energy. It is said that a 100 megawatt heat reactor will produce annually the same quantity of long-lived fission products as the detonation of a 1-megaton fission bomb (Anderson *et al.*). By 1965 Great Britain expects to be producing 6000 megawatts of atomic energy, and within twenty years the United States may be producing from 20,000 to 40,000 megawatts. The problem of the ultimate disposal of the waste material from such sources will be a future headache of the first magnitude, for "if even 1 per cent of long-lived fission products produced at a 20,000 megawatt annual level of atomic power were to be released by leakage or accident, the effect would be equivalent to the radiation from 100 bombs of the Hiroshima size" (Glass).

ATOM BOMB RADIATION

An *atomic explosion* depends on the fission of atomic nuclei by neutrons, which can readily penetrate the nuclei by reason of their neutral electric charge. A *chain reaction* will result if fission is attended by the simultaneous emission of extra neutrons from an element the unstable nuclei of which contain this additional number. In elements of high atomic weight nuclear stability calls for a great excess of neutrons over protons, so that many neutrons will be freed if fission occurs. Thus the nuclei of uranium–235 contain 143 neutrons and only 92 protons. U-238, which constitutes 99 per cent of pure uranium, will not of itself sustain a chain

reaction, because the neutrons are captured without fission, building the U-238 up to U-239. The half-life of U-238 is 4.5 billion years, whereas that of U-239 with its captured neutron is only 23.5 minutes. U-238 is only fissioned by fast neutrons, but U-235 can be fissioned by low-energy slow neutrons, with the release of energy several million times greater than is represented in the fissioning neutron, together with the release of two additional fast neutrons. This reaction provides use for the abundant U-238 in the bomb.

Critical mass or size determines explosion of U-235. A chain reaction is obviously impossible if too many neutrons are lost through the surface of the uranium mass. As a sphere enlarges, its exposed surface grows relatively smaller, so that finally enough neutrons are retained in the mass for a chain reaction to occur. *An atom bomb is merely a trigger mechanism for the rapid assembly of subcritical masses.*

Total body irradiation may be the result of exposure to radiations from atomic (or hydrogen) bomb bursts in war, from atomic weapon tests, or from accidental leakage from atomic energy installations. Two bomb bursts killed 100,000 men, women and children out of a population of 500,000 in the Japanese cities of Hiroshima and Nagasaki. In the present connection it is important to remember that the great majority of the deaths were due to burns or blast. From 15,000 to 20,000 deaths were due to ionizing radiations, which produced early or delayed effects, by reason of the great flux of neutrons thrown out by the nuclear explosion. The average lethal dose appeared to be about 500 roentgens. A dose of 400 r over the total body surface is believed to be enough to kill half of a given human population. The problem of dealing with these cases may be realized in part when we learn that in Hiroshima 90 per cent of the physicians were casualties, of 1,780 nurses some 1,650 were killed or injured, and the hospitals were destroyed.

In an *airburst* the problem of residual radiation is not of immediate medical importance, but *radioactive strontium* (Sr^{90}) with a long half-life of 25 years and formed in abundance as a fission product of uranium and plutonium may be disseminated by stratospheric winds, and it is readily taken up from the soil by plants and animals which may be eaten by man. Its close chemical similarity to calcium, which leads to its deposition in the bones in large amount make it the single most dangerous component of the fall-out. Sr^{89}, with a half-life of only 54 days, is of little danger to the adult, but it presents a hazard to the unborn child, as the growing fetal skeleton reflects the diet of the mother, and the fast-growing fetus is especially vulnerable to damage from radiation. If the explosion is at a low altitude, the expanding fireball with a million degree temperature vaporizes 20,000 tons of surface rock and soil, which become radioactive from the intense neutron irradiation during detonation. The immediate threat of radiation becomes serious in *underwater explosions*. Here the water, again rendered radioactive by the flux of neutrons and other fission products, is raised into the sky, converted into cloud, and descends as rain.

A *hydrogen bomb explosion* is a very different matter from that of an atomic bomb. The fall-out may cover thousands of square miles and deposit radioactive material sufficient to cause the acute radiation syndrome (see below), without thermal or blast effects. This, of course, is the reverse picture to that seen at Hiroshima and Nagasaki. The "fireball," the luminous sphere of hot gasses is 8000 feet in diameter, compared with 200 feet in the case of the atomic bomb. What may happen under these circumstances is vividly illustrated in the case of the hydrogen device exploded at the Bikini atoll on the morning of March 1, 1954. A Japanese fishing boat, rather ironically named the Lucky Dragon, was 100 miles from Bikini at that moment. In the early morning some members of the crew looking for the sunrise saw a faint red light in the western sky. Seven minutes later they heard a dull noise, and three hours later they observed fleecy clouds in the blue sky, and a white substance fell on the deck for a period of five hours. A few hours later the sailors began to experience fatigue, headache, drowsiness, loss of appetite, nausea and vomiting. All symptoms disappeared by the fourth day and the men remained well for two weeks, but by the end of one month after exposure they were all in hospital with severe depression of the bone marrow. As a result of active treatment the great majority recovered.

Acute Radiation Syndrome.—This syndrome, due to whole body radiation, must be distinguished from *radiation sickness*, the result of intensive local radiotherapy. The latter is characterized by anorexia and nausea, but rarely vomiting, and seems to be due to the absorption of protein-split products from the local lesion.

The acute effects of total body irradiation may be thought of in terms of simple cell depletion, involving cells which renew themselves by continual division and maturation. This applies particularly to the intestine, the bone marrow and the testes, but with a marked difference in the time element. After a single small exposure the maximum damage to the small bowel occurs within a few days, to the granulocytes in three to five weeks, while the human sperm count takes nearly one year to reach its minimum.

In the true acute radiation syndrome there are two deciding factors: (1) *dose*, and (2) *individual susceptibility*. There is a wide variation in individual susceptibility, both in the experimental animal and in man. The explanation for this is unknown.

The *relation of dose to effect* can be observed in animals exposed to whole body irradiation. The mean survival time curve shows three distinct steps in relation to dose, with involvement of different pathogenic mechanisms (Gerstner). In the *low-dose range* (100 r) death is caused by depression of the hematopoietic mechanism; in the *middle-dose range* (500 r) it is due to gastrointestinal denudation and inflammation; in the *high-dose range* (2000 r) it is the result of failure of the central nervous system. These differences are shown in the accompanying table taken from Gerstner's paper. The corresponding data for man are largely unknown, but are probably similar. It is the latter two which are the major hazards.

1. Within two hours of exposure there is a sudden onset of anorexia, nausea, fatigue, malaise and drowsiness. These are the symptoms manifested by the Japanese fishermen. Perhaps they should not be regarded

as the true radiation syndrome, but rather its prodromal phase. By the third day the patient feels well.

2. Some three weeks later there is a sudden onset of chills, fever, malaise and dyspnea, followed in a day or two by purpura, hemorrhages, severe mouth infections, diarrhea and other evidence of ulceration of the colon. The purpura and hemorrhage are due to destruction of the megakaryocytes with consequent loss of platelets. The granulocytes also disappear. The mechanism for producing antibodies is damaged, and this may well be an important factor in the development of infection. Severe anemia develops after several weeks as the result of hypoplasia of the erythroblastic tissue.

Such reports are naturally inclined to overlook the fact that leukemia, cataract and cancer are common afflictions of mankind.

RADIATION CARCINOGENESIS

Although irradiation is an invaluable weapon in the treatment of cancer, it can also cause cancer; as we have so often seen already, what is powerful for good can be potent for evil. Carcinogenesis is in essence the mutation of cells with a well balanced genetic mechanism to cells with an unbalanced one. Ionizing radiation is an instrument which might have been designed to produce mutations. It is small wonder, then, that exposure to prolonged radiation may

THE ACUTE RADIATION SYNDROME

	Hematopoietic Form	Gastrointestinal Form	Cerebral Form
Threshold dose	100 r	500 r	2,000 r
Characteristic signs and symptoms	Leukopenia; purpura; hemorrhage; infection	Diarrhea; fever; disturbance of electrolyte balance	Convulsions; tremor; ataxia; lethargy
Time of death	Within two months	Within two weeks	Within two days

A moving account of the development of the acute radiation syndrome in an entire community representing the last survivors in the world of a war fought with atomic weapons will be found in Nevil Shute's novel, *On the Beach.*

It should be emphasized that the facts available do not justify too fatalistic and pessimistic an approach to the subject of the acute radiation syndrome. Over a wide dose range man can overcome the condition by appropriate therapy and return to a useful life. "There exists no account of the many thousands of survivors of Hiroshima and Nagasaki who resumed their previous occupation with full vigor, while there are several reports relating each case of leukemia, cataract, or neoplasm" (Gerstner).

result in cancer. This matter has already been discussed in Chapter 8.

PROTECTION AGAINST IRRADIATION INJURY

This vital subject is still in its infancy. The one fact that is known with certainty is that injury is much greater when the local oxygen tension is high, and much lower under nearly anoxic conditions. The difficulty is to reproduce this state in the living body. Reducing substances such as cysteine and glutathione have been tried out with the object of inactivating the oxidizing radicles which result from ionization of the abundant water in the cells. So far the results have been encouraging for laboratory animals, but this has not proved to be the case with humans. There is, of course, another line of approach. If very many of the deaths caused by total body radiation are due to destruction of blood-forming elements, what can be done to rectify this situation and tide the patient over for a sufficient time to allow his bone marrow to recover? The obvious answer is to supply bone marrow material from normal persons. The difficulty is that here we encounter the distinction between tissues that are "you" and "not-you", a matter which has already been discussed in Chapter 5. Foreign material from another person, unless it be an identical twin, acts as an antigen which excites the formation of antibodies that destroy the antigen. The antibody-forming material, however, is for the most part the reticuloendothelial tissue of the marrow. This tissue has largely been inactivated for the time being by radiation. In the future some way may be found to utilize this fact, by virtue of which a short-lived substitute for the patient's destroyed hematopoietic tissue may be used. This has already proved possible in a few cases of scientists exposed to lethal doses of ionizing radiation in the course of their work. The bone marrow of patients about to receive intensive radiation treatment for cancer can be removed, stored in a frozen state, and reinjected later.

CHRONOLOGY

It may be of interest to recall some of the more important events and dates in our knowledge of the atom and the radiation which may be released from it, together with the countries in which the fundamental work was done. The following data are taken from the table in *Radioactive Isotopes in Clinical Practice* by Quimby, Feitelberg and Silver.

ATOMIC TIME TABLE

1808 John Dalton (England) presented experimental basis for atomic hypothesis.

1811 Amadeo Avogadro (Italy) distinguished between atoms and molecules.

1895 Wilhelm Roentgen (Germany) discovered x-rays.

1896 Henri Becquerel (France) discovered radioactivity of radium.

1897 J. J. Thompson (England) showed electrons present in all atoms.

1898 Marie and Pierre Curie (France) discovered radium.

1905 Albert Einstein (Switzerland) suggested equivalence of mass and energy.

1911 Ernest Rutherford (England) discovered the atomic nucleus.

1919 Ernest Rutherford (England) produced nuclear transmutation.

1932 James Chadwick (England) discovered the neutron.

1939 O. Hahn and F. Strassman (Germany) discovered nuclear fission (U-235).

1939 Enrico Fermi (Italy) suggested possibility of chain reaction in nuclear fission.

1942 (USA) Nuclear chain reaction in a uranium-graphite "pile."

1945 Atomic bomb exploded July 16 in New Mexico, U.S.A., August 6 and 11th over Hiroshima and Nagasaki, Japan.

For further information on the comparatively new and vitally important subject of ionizing radiation in relation to man the student reader is referred to the monographs and papers at the end of this chapter and to the special number of the Bulletin of Atomic Scientists, January, 1958, entitled Radiation and Man.

REFERENCES

BACQ, Z. M. and ALEXANDER, P.: *Fundamentals of Radiobiology*, London, 1955.

CADE, STANFORD SIR: *Malignant Disease and its Treatment by Radium*, Bristol, 1940.

CANNON, B., RANDOLPH, J. G. and MURRAY, J. E.: New Eng. J. Med., 1959, *260*, 197. (Malignant irradiation for benign conditions).

CROW, J. F.: Bull. of the Atomic Scientists, 1958, *14*, 19. (Genetic effects of radiation).

DURYEE, W. R.: J. Nat. Cancer Inst., 1949, *10*, 735. (Radiation damage to cell nuclei).

GERSTNER, H. B.: United States Armed Forces Med. J., 1958, *9*, 313. (Acute radiation syndrome).

GLASS, B.: Science, 1957, *126*, 241. (Genetic hazards of nuclear radiations).

HOYT, R. C.: Bull. of the Atomic Scientists, 1958, *14*, 9. (What is radiation?).

QUIMBY, E. H., FEITELBERG, S. and SILVER, S.: *Radioactive Isotopes in Clinical Practice*, Philadelphia, 1958.

SEARS, T. P.: *The Physician in Atomic Defense*, Chicago, 1953.

TABERSHAW, J. R.: J. Chr. Diseases, 1959, *9*, 134. (Industrial hazards of ionizing radiation).

WARREN, S.: Arch. Path., 1943, *34*, 443, 562, 749, 917, 1070; 1943, *35*, 121, 304. (Effects of radiation of normal tissues).

WEBSTER, E. W.: Radiology, 1959, *72*, 493. (Hazards of diagnostic radiology).

Chapter 19

Chemical Poisons

CORROSIVE ACIDS
CAUSTIC ALKALIS
CARBOLIC ACID
BICHLORIDE OF MERCURY
ARSENIC

PHOSPHORUS
LEAD
PRUSSIC ACID
ALKALOIDS
METHYL ALCOHOL

ETHYL ALCOHOL
CHLOROFORM
CARBON MONOXIDE
BOTULISM

THE subject of the action of chemical poisons on the body is a very large one, and is adequately treated in textbooks of toxicology and forensic medicine. But the medical practitioner may at any time have to perform an autopsy on a case of suspected poisoning, and it is desirable that he be familiar with the pathological findings caused by some of the more common poisons and the precautions which should be observed in collecting the material for chemical analysis.

Poisoning may be suicidal, homicidal or accidental. In a case of suspected poisoning which may assume medico-legal importance extreme care must be taken in performing the autopsy. The external appearances should be noted. Everything should be recorded in writing and nothing left to the memory. The stomach and bowel must be kept. When there is a question of diffusible toxins such as arsenic and strychnine, it is well to keep all the internal organs and much of the muscles. These various specimens are sent to the chemist for chemical analysis. They must be put into clean glass jars, which are then stoppered, sealed, and labelled. No preservative of any kind should be added.

In the description which follows only the commoner and everyday exogenous poisons are discussed. The endogenous poisons produced as the result of abnormal metabolism and bacterial poisons (toxins) are not considered.

CORROSIVE ACIDS.—The strong acids most likely to be taken for suicidal purposes are sulfuric, nitric, and hydrochloric. They are similar in action, and produce burns not only in the stomach, but also in the mouth, pharynx, and esophagus. The lesions of the lips must not be overlooked. The stomach is contracted as the result of irritation and thrown into folds. Patches of necrosis are scattered over the folds, and if the patient lives long enough the slough separates and leaves a raw surface. Similar changes are seen with all corrosive poisons. The acids vary as regards the color of the burns. With sulfuric acid the burnt tissue is brownish-red or black, with nitric acid it is yellow, and with hydrochloric acid white. The microscopic appearance is one of necrotic tissue on the surface with intense inflammation of the surrounding tissue. The acid removes water from the cells and dissolves epithelium and connective tissue. Nitric acid poisoning is common in munition works where smokeless powder is made from nitrocellulose obtained by treating cotton with strong nitric acid. If the fumes of the acid are inhaled severe inflammation of the larynx and trachea is produced.

CAUSTIC ALKALIS.—The strong alkalis (caustic soda, caustic potash, and lime) are also corrosive in their action. They dehydrate the cells and saponify the fats. The common form of alkali poisoning is by commercial lye taken either for suicidal purposes or accidentally by children. The lesions are similar to those of the corrosive acids. There is severe burning of the lips, mouth, throat, esophagus, and stomach, with acute inflammation and softening of tissue. Should the patient recover, cicatricial stricture of the esophagus often develops and sometimes stricture of the pylorus.

CARBOLIC ACID.—Strong carbolic acid is so easily obtained that it is commonly used for suicidal purposes. The picture differs in several ways from that of poisoning by other strong acids. The burns on the lips and in the mouth, throat, and stomach have a peculiar opaque, dead-white appearance. The stomach is contracted, and the dead patches are seen on the summit of the folds. Phenol is not a corrosive acid. It is an excellent fixative, so that the tissue instead of being de-

stroyed is perfectly fixed. It follows that although the gross appearance is so abnormal, the
microscopic picture is actually more normal than
usual, because the customary postmortem changes
in the stomach are absent. If the patient survives
for some time the dead tissue will become detached with separation of a slough. The effect
of dilute carbolic acid is rather different. The
tissue is not killed and fixed so completely, and
an intense hemorrhagic inflammation is the result
of the irritation. When the stomach is opened in
carbolic acid poisoning the characteristic color of
phenol can be recognized.

BICHLORIDE OF MERCURY.—Corrosive sublimate is a favorite with suicides. When bichloride
of mercury is taken in the form of a concentrated
solution and in large quantity it fixes the tissue
in the same way as does phenol. Grayish-white
patches of coagulation necrosis are surrounded
by an area of intense inflammation. When, as
often happens, tablets are swallowed, they produce severe local necrosis with deep ulceration.
After a few days a second set of symptoms develops connected with the colon and the kidney.
By whatever route mercury enters the body,
through the skin and mucous membrane (vaginal
douches) as well as by the mouth, it is excreted
into the large bowel, where it produces an intense
hemorrhagic colitis. It is also excreted by the
kidney. The cells of the convoluted tubules show
extensive necrosis, and there is marked suppression of urine and sometimes anuria. In the course
of a week or less there occurs an "acute calcification" of the renal lesion, calcium salts being
deposited in the masses of necrotic cells, many
of which lie free in the lumen of the tubules. This
very rapid calcification is a remarkable phenomenon which is difficult to explain.

ARSENIC.—Arsenical poisoning may be acute
or chronic. The acute form is usually suicidal,
Paris green, rat poison, etc., being easily obtained.
Chronic arsenical poisoning may be homicidal.
Many of the famous murders in history have been
accomplished by the continued administration of
small doses of arsenic. Fashions change, however, and more violent methods are now in vogue.
Arsenic is an intense irritant, so that in acute
poisoning there is severe hemorrhagic inflammation of the entire gastrointestinal canal. The
poison is excreted into the bowel, giving an enteritis as well as a colitis. Paris green or crystals
of arsenic may be seen in the folds of the stomach.
In chronic poisoning the lesions are mainly in the
skin and the nervous system. There is pigmentation and extreme keratinization of the skin. The
nervous changes are mental disorders and paralysis of the peripheral nerves due to neuritis.
Arsenical poisoning may be the result of the

careless administration of arsphenamine and other
arsenical preparations. In these cases the chief
changes are optic atrophy with blindness and
extensive necrosis of the liver. The latter lesion
is often fatal.

PHOSPHORUS.—This is likely to be taken in the
form of rat poison or the phosphorus may be
obtained from the heads of matches. Phosphorus
poisoning may be acute or chronic. In the *acute
form* there is a hemorrhagic inflammation of the
stomach. The characteristic smell of phosphorus
may be detected when the stomach is opened.
After an interval of some days there is acute
necrsois of the liver with a picture of acute yellow
atrophy, accompanied by intense jaundice and
widespread hemorrhages. Phosphorus is one of
the most potent causes of fatty degeneration, and
this change is present in marked degree in the
liver, kidneys, heart, and even the voluntary
muscles. *Chronic poisoning* is due to exposure to
phosphorus vapor, and is an occupational disease.
Apart from fatty degeneration the chief lesion is
necrosis of the jaws (phossy jaw) with destruction
of bone and loss of the teeth. The process is
dependent on bacterial infection, commencing
around the roots of carious teeth. In this and
other respects it closely resembles the lesion of
industrial radium poisoning.

LEAD.—Lead poisoning (plumbism) differs from
those already described in being chronic in type;
acute lead poisoning is of no importance. Plumbism is usually an occupational disease, the lead
being inhaled in the form of dust or fumes or
absorbed through the skin. White-lead workers
and pottery workers are liable, and painters unless
they wash their hands well before eating. A
severe anemia develops, of which the characteristic feature is an extreme degree of basophilic
granular degeneration (stippling) of the red cells.
In no other disease is this change so marked. A
blue line (lead line) of lead sulfide appears at
the junction of the gum and the teeth, owing to
the action of sulfuretted hydrogen on the lead.
Constipation is a marked feature, and there may
be painful colic. Peripheral neuritis affecting particularly the musculospiral and peroneal nerves
may lead to drop-wrist and drop-foot. There
may be depression, delirium, convulsions, and
mental changes, with degenerative changes in the
cerebral cortex like those of general paralysis.

Lead poisoning in children, a fairly common but
usually unrecognized disease, presents many
points of special interest. It is often mistaken
for poliomyelitis. The incidence is highest in
infants and young children with erupting teeth,
who put painted objects containing lead (yellow
paint is specially dangerous) into their mouths.
Many suffer from perversion of appetite (pica),

and lick the paint off their cribs and the furniture. The child may drink water containing lead or inhale fumes from storage battery casings used in the stove for fuel. In Japan congenital plumbism is common, owing to the pregnant mother covering her face and neck with cosmetics containing lead. Gastrointestinal symptoms (vomiting, colic, constipation) and anemia may be marked, but the most striking symptoms are those of *lead encephalitis*, i. e., a change in the mental state, visual disturbances, convulsions and coma. The blood pressure may be raised, there may be choked disc, and even separation of the cranial sutures. The actual cerebral lesions are merely minute hemorrhages and cellular infiltrations; the symptoms are caused by rapid increase of the intracranial pressure due to intense cerebral edema, as a result of which the brain is swollen, the convolutions flattened, and the medulla pressed into the foramen magnum. The cerebrospinal fluid pressure may be as high as 700 mm. of water (normal 120 mm.). Peripheral neuritis is rare. The lead line on the gums is seldom seen in children (no doubt owing to the healthy condition of the mouth) and stippling of the red cells may be absent. One of the most useful signs is a lead line in the bones in the roentgen-ray film; there are zones of increased density at the growing ends of the long bones, where lead is deposited in place of calcium. This line is rarely absent, even in mild cases.

Much of the lead is stored in the bones. Parathyroid extract, with its well-known effect on calcium metabolism, causes both calcium and lead to be mobilized, removed from the bones, and excreted in the urine. There is a corresponding rise in the blood calcium. Much of the lead can be rapidly removed in this way, but the remainder is firmly united to the bone and is only excreted slowly. Acid-fast intranuclear inclusions may be found in the liver and kidney at autopsy. These inclusions may be of diagnostic value in difficult cases.

PRUSSIC ACID.—Hydrocyanic acid and the cyanides are suitable for suicidal purposes because they are so rapidly fatal. The poison is not corrosive, but the gastric mucosa has a bright chestnut-brown color. The blood remains fluid. The poison kills by acting on the nervous system and the heart, and there are no special postmortem lesions, but the characteristic peach-kernel smell can often be detected when the stomach is opened.

AKLALOIDS.—The poisonous alkaloids such as opium (morphine), strychnine, cocaine, atropine, etc., produce no characteristic postmortem changes. Their detection therefore depends on chemical analysis.

ALCOHOL.—METHYL ALCOHOL.—Methyl alcohol, so common an ingredient in bootleg liquor, and used for "denaturing" ethyl alcohol, is highly toxic. The deaths which follow the drinking of "canned heat," etc., are due to methyl alcohol poisoning. In these cases there is nothing to be found at autopsy apart from severe gastritis and a smell of alcohol in the stomach, lungs, and brain. After a few hours this smell may disappear. If the patient recovers he may be blind from optic atrophy.

ETHYL ALCOHOL.—Ethyl alcohol may also produce death in a few hours if taken in sufficient quantity and concentration. The postmortem findings are the same as those of acute methyl alcohol poisoning. If the patient has lived a few days there may be marked edema of the brain. The effects of *chronic alcoholism* are very debatable. Undoubtedly resistance to infection is lowered, so that the patient may die of pneumonia, etc. Many degenerative lesions are attributed to chronic alcoholism. Among these are cirrhosis of the liver, chronic gastritis, chronic nephritis, and arteriosclerosis. The direct relation of any of these to alcohol is more than doubtful but it may well act as a contributory cause.

CHLOROFORM.—A person may die while under chloroform anesthesia, or may die an acute death after swallowing the liquid. In these cases there are no characteristic postmortem changes apart from the odor of chloroform. The patient may die later of "delayed chloroform poisoning," and autopsy will reveal profound fatty degeneration of the liver, heart, and kidneys. These changes were seen in the days when chloroform was the common anesthetic.

CARBON MONOXIDE.—In carbon monoxide poisoning the gas may come from illuminating gas, from stoves or furnaces, from the products of explosions in coal mines, but the most important source at the present day is the exhaust from automobiles. A car running in a small closed garage will generate enough gas in a few minutes to kill a person. Garage workers breathing a smaller concentration may suffer from a train of symptoms such as headache, vertigo, and weakness. Traffic policemen directing very heavy automobile traffic in large cities may suffer from minor forms of poisoning.

The carbon monoxide combines with the hemoglobin, replacing the oxygen and forming carboxyhemoglobin. The patient therefore dies of asphyxia. But in addition there seems to be a direct poisonous action on the vital centers, for the patient may become unconscious with extraordinary suddenness. It is this rapidity of action which constitutes the great danger of the gas in concentrated form. As the carboxyhemoglobin is of a bright color, the face, the blood, and the viscera become cherry-red. This and a markedly fluid blood constitute the chief portmortem changes. If the patient should live for some days a remarkable bilateral necrosis is found in the lenticular nucleus of the brain, being most marked in or confined to the globus pallidus. It is the iron of the hemoglobin with which the carbon monoxide unites. It is therefore possible that the gas may combine with the iron in the walls of the vessels of the globus pallidus, the iron content being higher than in any other vessels of the body. The necrosis is probably due to ischemia, which in turn is probably caused by thrombosis of these small vessels.

BOTULISM.—Although botulism is caused by a bacterial poison it may for convenience be considered here. The toxin is formed by the Bacillus botulinus (*botulus*, a sausage) which grows in spoiled sausages, preserved meat, canned vegetables, fruit, ripe olives, etc., especially those preserved by home canning in which the temperature employed is insufficient to insure sterilization.

Thus the poison is ingested ready-made, and is not manufactured inside the body. It is easily destroyed by heat, so that cooking renders the food harmless. It is extremely powerful, and even small amounts may cause death. Like the tetanus toxin it does not act at the point of absorption, for there is never any evidence of gastrointestinal irritation. The symptoms are entirely cerebral, and are apt to be mistaken for those of epidemic encephalitis. Indeed, the first cases of the latter disease which appeared in England were thought to be examples of botulism. The most characteristic symptoms are ophthalmoplegias (squint, double vision), ptosis, and difficulty in swallowing and in speech. All of these are due to cranial nerve palsies. The postmortem findings are merely those of toxemia—cloudy swelling, petechial hemorrhages, etc.

REFERENCES

HAMILTON, A. and HARDY, H. L.: *Industrial Toxicology*, 2nd ed., New York, 1949.

Chapter 20

Genetic Factors in Disease

HEREDITY IN DISEASE
General Principles
  MUTATION
The Inheritance of Disease
  AUTOSOMAL
  AUTOSOMAL DOMINANT INHERIT-
    ANCE
  AUTOSOMAL RECESSIVE INHERIT-
    ANCE

MODIFIED INHERITANCE
SEX-LINKED INHERITANCE
  Sex Chromatin
Hereditary Defects and Diseases
  BLOOD DISEASES
  METABOLIC DISORDERS
  SKELETAL DEFECTS
  NEUROMUSCULAR DISORDERS
  SKIN DISORDERS

EYE DISEASES
MENTAL DISEASES
SUSCEPTIBILITY TO INFECTION
HEREDITY IN CANCER
Genetic Hazards of Radiation
Twins
CONSTITUTION IN DISEASE
  HABITUS
  INFLUENCE OF SEX

HEREDITY IN DISEASE

General Principles

WE close this discussion of General Pathology, which is in essence the Principles of Pathology, with a chapter dealing with one of the most intricate and exciting aspects of the subject, namely the relation of genetics to disease. Perhaps such a chapter should be among the first. On the other hand it might well be the last one in the book, because some familiarity with a large variety of diseases is requisite for full appreciation of the discussion. The present arrangement is a compromise between these two extremes. It is of interest to recall the penetrating words of that great surgeon and pathologist, Sir James Paget, in 1882, regarding malformations: "We ought not to set them aside with idle thoughts or idle words about 'curiosities' or 'chances.' Not one of them is without meaning; not one that might not become the beginning of an excellent knowledge. If only we could answer the question —why is this rare?—or, being rare, why did it in this instance happen?" We shall see that a beginning of this "excellent knowledge" has now been made.

In the causation of disease two great factors always demand consideration; these are environment and heredity. So far we have been concerned for the most part with the environmental diseases, those caused by bacteria, animal parasites, trauma, physical irritants, chemical poisons, and so forth. For the last century or more, medicine has concerned itself with these extrinsic agencies which are more readily studied and for which more can be done than in the case of hereditary defects of the germ plasm. Far reaching and profound observations have been made in the past, above all by the Austrian monk Gregor Mendel in 1866. Mendel did his work in a garden plot 30 by 7 feet in a small country town. He crossed a red and a white pea. In the second generation four plants bore red flowers, but in the third generation three were red while one was white. Mendel enunciated the concept of a dominant (red) and a recessive (white) character, the latter being hidden but present in the second generation. This marked the birth of the science of genetics, but Mendel's paper attracted absolutely no attention until it was brought to light, by three investigators working independently. The modern era dawned in 1907 when T. H. Morgan began his work on *Drosophila*, the fruit fly, which has proved the ideal animal for investigation with its short and concentrated reproductive life span and the large size of its chromosomes, particularly those of the salivary gland. The studies of Mendel and Morgan, although carried out on the pea and on fruit flies, have served to show, were the proof needed, that men are not created free and equal, but handicapped from the beginning.

A distinction is sometimes drawn between *familial* and *hereditary* disease. This distinction is entirely imaginary, for familial diseases are always hereditary. When both parents must transmit the defect before it

(431)

becomes recognizable we have the so-called familial cases, but this is merely an example of a recessive character. The parents need not and generally do not exhibit the defect themselves. A "familial disease" is one in which it is dominant. A recessive character may be transmitted indefinitely in the germ plasm without coming to light until it meets a similar recessive from another strain. Disease factors in man are generally dominant, but they may be recessive or sex-linked. A disease, *e.g.*, diabetes mellitus, may in one family appear to be hereditary and in another familial, depending on the distribution of the genes for diabetes in the chromosomes. A *congenital* defect is one which is present at birth, although it may only develop later to a sufficient degree to be detected clinically, *e.g.*, congenital cystic kidney, congenital cerebral aneurysm. *This defect may be hereditary, but frequently it is acquired in utero*; congenital syphilis, for instance, should not be called hereditary syphilis, for it is not transmitted by the germ plasm. It is now recognized that viral infections of the mother during pregnancy may result in congenital defects, either evident at birth or developing later. The chief offender is *rubella* (German measles), which seems to inflict its most severe damage on whichever tissues happen to be developing fastest when the infection strikes. Rubella causes cataracts in the 6th week, deafness in the 9th, congenital cardiac defects in the 5th to the 10th weeks, and dental deformities in the 6th to the 9th weeks. Mumps appears to be next in line as a crippler *in utero*. In none of these congenital defects is the genetic mechanism involved.

In the study of human genetics the method of statistical summation is a standard, widely applied. "Clearly, it is best suited to the investigation of characters which are at the same time fairly obvious to an untrained observer, relatively uncommon, unlikely to lead to death prematurely, and yet make their appearance early in life" (Payling Wright). Although we shall confine our attention to human genetics, it will be obvious that it is much easier to study the pedigree of domestic and laboratory animals than the family tree of a man or a woman.

The masterword of heredity, the key to genetics, is nucleic acid, D N A in the nucleus, R N A in the cytoplasm. The *chromosomes* consist of D N A. They are 46 in number, 44 somatic, known as *autosomes*, and 2 *sex chromosomes*. If the nucleic acids are to convey genetic information they must be so constructed as to form a chemical code. As we have already seen in the chapter on the Cell, the chromosomes are long-chain polymers with a purine or pyrimidine base forming connecting links in the chain. These nitrogenous bases are of four different kinds, adenine with thymine and guanine with cytosine, they are the only variable constituents, and they are probably arranged in a definite sequence which constitutes the genetic code. Indeed the nuclei of the reproductive cells contain a genetic "instruction code" which determines the development of the future organism, a code which consists of four letters, so that the genetic language is written in a four-letter alphabet on an immensely long scroll. A mutation is perhaps a change in a single nucleotide. Thus it is known that sickle-cell anemia represents the substitution of a single amino acid in the hemoglobin molecule. Chromosomes under the microscope appear short and thick, because they are tightly coiled, like spiral springs (Fig. 230). They are really long filaments along which the genes are arranged.

The *genes* appear to be chemical particles of D N A located along the chromosomes. The gene acts as a biochemical carrier of biological information from one generation to the next. As in the case of the chromosomes, the genes are in pairs known as *allelomorphs* or *alleles* (*Allelon*, one another), one member of the pair being maternal, the other paternal in origin. Allelic genes from father and mother are situated at the same spot or *locus* on the two members of the pair of homologous chromosomes. Each gene is a mold or template according to which pattern the individual synthesizes a molecule or a specific structure. Fundamentally genes control enzymes, and enzymes control the chemistry of life. Indeed we are now trying to identify specific genes relative to specific enzyme defects and the disease resulting from these defects. If any mutation takes place in the structure of a

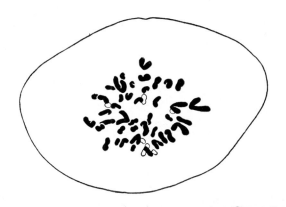

FIG. 230.—*Above*: The chromosomes in a human cell. × 3000 (Koller). *Below*: The human chromosomes arranged in pairs; a drawing based upon thirteen male nuclei. (From Evans and Swezy's *Chromosomes of Man.*)

These drawings show the chromosomes as relatively short, thick bodies, which is characteristic of the stage just preceding cell-division, during which they can be counted and their individual appearance discerned. At an earlier stage they are long, thin filaments. (J. A. Fraser Roberts, *An Introduction to Medical Genetics*, courtesy of Oxford University Press.)

gene, there will be a corresponding modification of the gene product, and this in turn will result in a functional disturbance somewhere in the body. This is the basis of the concept of *hereditary molecular diseases*. The abnormal protein that is formed may be an enzyme, a hemoglobin, or an essential component of the renal transport system. Some of these genetic anomalies and disorders we have already encountered. Others we shall meet in our future studies.

It is evident that the information from the genes in the nucleus must be transmitted to the cytoplasm. This is apparently done through the R N A, which is synthesized in the nucleus, receives its instructional patterns, and then migrates to the cytoplasm, where it imprints its patterns on the enzymes and other proteins synthesized there. This concept of an imprinted pattern is known as the *template hypothesis*.

Genes are of differing grades of potency, the more powerful being known as *dominant*, and the weaker as *recessive*. Both genes of a pair occupying the same locus on the homo-logous chromosomes may be dominant or both recessive, a *homozygous* condition, or *one may be dominant and the other recessive*, the resultant being *heterozygous*. If the gene is dominant, the individual will show the corresponding characteristic, whether the arrangement is homozygous or heterozygous, because the strong gene does not need to be reinforced. If, however, it is weaker (recessive), the gene has to be duplicated (homozygous) before it can make itself apparent. We shall see presently that there is a difference between what may be called a single (heterozygous) dose and a double (homozygous) dose, and that it is easier to alter a single-dose effect through the influence of other genes than the effect of a double dose. In human anomalies and diseases, if the gene is dominant the person is nearly always heterozygous. When the gene is recessive, the corresponding character is not evident and the individual plays the part of a passive carrier. Only when both genes of the pair (homozygous) are recessive does the character become apparent. The single recessive

28

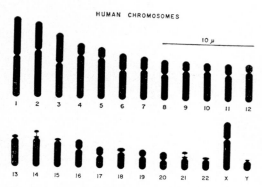

HUMAN CHROMOSOMES

10 μ

1 2 3 4 5 6 7 8 9 10 11 12

13 14 15 16 17 18 19 20 21 22 X Y

Fig. 231.—Idiogram of Human Chromosomes.
(D. Yi-Yung Hsea, courtesy of New Engl. J. Med.)

gene holds its place on the chromosome, biding its time in obscurity. It may have to wait for many generations (in the case of humans, for hundreds of years) before it gets its chance by being free of suppression by a dominant gene. It is small wonder that some hereditary diseases are not recognized as such.

As the *chromosomes* constitute the essential machinery of heredity, an increasing amount of attention is being focussed on these structures. It is now possible to study and count the individual chromosomes in man by using tissue cultures of aspirated bone marrow, and preventing the formation of the mitotic spindle by the administration of colchicine so that the chromosomes are widely separated, not closely aggregated on the spindle as in a normal metaphase. If it is not yet possible to name the individual chromosomes, we can at least arrange them as an idiogram in order of length and give them numbers (Fig. 231). The X-chromosome pair is the seventh in order of length among the 23 pairs, the Y-chromosome being much smaller, indeed comparable in size to the smallest of the autosomes.

We now speak of *chromosomal diseases*, abnormal conditions in which there is variation from the normal number. This is known as *heteroploidy*, which may take the form of *polyploidy*, where somatic cells contain an exact multiple of the normal haploid complement (one-half the diploid number of paired chromosomes) of the germ cells, or *aneuploidy*, where the count is other than

an exact multiple of the haploid number. A case of a malformation syndrome associated with triploidy has been reported in which the chromosomes in cell culture numbered 69 (Böök and Santesson). Aneuploidy is encountered much more frequently than heteroploidy. The principal examples are Klinefelter's syndrome, Turner's syndrome, mongolism, and a few unclassified cases of mental deficiency. (1) In *Klinefelter's syndrome* (seminiferous tubule dysgenesis) the individual develops as a somatic male, but the chromatin pattern is female or chromatin-positive. There are 47 chromosomes, the extrachromosome being contributed by an XXY-sex chromosome complex. (2) In *Turner's syndrome* (gonadal dysgenesis) the individual is apparently a female, but the nuclei have a male or chromatin-negative pattern. There are the usual 44 autosomes, but the X-chromosome is unpaired with either another X-chromosome for a female sex chromosome complex or a Y-chromosome for a male sex chromosome complex, so that the total number is 45. The two syndromes and the subjects of nuclear sex, intersexuality and sex reversal are discussed more fully in Chapter 32. (3) A third possibility is the *super-female*, in whom there are 44 autosomes and 3 X-chromosomes, a total of 47 (Jacobs *et al.*). Cells from the buccal mucosa and the blood contain 2 sex chromatin bodies. (4) In *mongolian idiocy* there is an additional small autosome, and it would seem that the cause of the disease is a developmental imbalance resulting from this excess of genetic material. The extra "mongol" chromosome is the second smallest chromosome pair.

The exciting new advances in our knowledge of human chromosomes in general and the sex chromosomes in particular together with the relation of chromosome variations to sex reversal, mongolism, and other hitherto impenetrable mysteries are considered in Chapter 32, which deals with disorders of the male reproductive system.

So far the genetic anomalies we have been considering have been of a gross and structural character. Much more subtle and important are *diseases of enzymatic defect* due to an abnormal or malfunctioning gene. It was in 1908 that Garrod made the profound suggestion, at a time when biochemistry and genetics were in their infancy, that a small group of diseased conditions represented genetically transmitted biochemical defects in which there was deficiency of enzymes necessary to normal metabolism. To this group Garrod gave the now famous name of the *inborn errors of metabolism*. The original group has become enormously enlarged, and includes genetic alterations in the metabolism of carbohydrates, proteins, lipids, nucleic acids, porphyrins and pigments. In albinism, for instance, the most obvious feature is the absence of melanin. Various examples of these metabolic disorders are given on page 439.

Mutation.—The genes are remarkably stable, but as each gene is made up of millions of atoms, it is natural that occasionally a rearrangement of the atoms may occur, giving the gene fresh properties. Such a change is called a mutation. Mutation is one of the great driving forces of evolution which creates new variations in living, for living conditions never remain the same for very long periods, without mutation there could be no variety, and life would never have evolved beyond its first primitive forms. Yet the majority of new mutants are harmful or even lethal, because in a delicately balanced system like the gene complex almost any change is likely to be for the worse, just as one cannot make a random interchange of parts in a Rolls-Royce engine and expect nothing unpleasant to happen.

Mutations may involve color, shape, and many other characters. Color mutations play a major role in horticulture and in fancy breeding of animals, for mutants are inherited just as are normal genes. Animals with protective coloration owe their protection to a helpful mutation. The black sheep of a white flock may blame its color on mutation, and the same might be said of the black sheep of a human family. The Siamese cat owes its distinction to the mutation of white hair to black on the most exposed parts of the body. In man even the white forelock and male baldness are examples of the inheritance of mutant genes.

When we come to the study of the *sex-linked recessive* we shall encounter the only example of a mutation which behaves as a recessive in one sex and as if dominant in the other. The X-chromosome carries many genes, some connected with sex determination, while others are not. The Y-chromosome carries very few genes, and no partner genes to the sex-linked genes on the X-chromosome. Therefore a man, who alone provides a Y-chromosome in addition to an X, receives sex-linked genes from both parents. The effect will always be manifest in the male, whether the gene is dominant or recessive.

THE INHERITANCE OF DISEASE

Unit characters may be transmitted from parents to offspring, and their characters, depending on whether they are dominant or recessive, will appear in the first or second generation *provided the breeding is controlled*. In addition to such characters as color, shape, size, fertility, vigor, length of life, *etc.*, definite defects may also be transmitted, and these constitute hereditary disease in man. It is at once evident that the study of these defects is a very different matter from the investigation of the mode of transmission in peas and guinea pigs, for in the case of man breeding is a matter of chance beyond control. Many of the hereditary diseases are relatively rare. For these reasons there has been a tendency on the part of the medical profession to minimize the importance of heredity and that of environment. That tendency has now been reversed, and we have come to realize that all the inborn errors of metabolism, the problem of the blood groups and the Rh factor, such diseases of the blood as sickle cell anemia and thalassemia, sex-linked blood disorders such as hemophilia, many chronic progressive diseases of the nervous and neuromuscular systems, many of the so-called degenerative phenomena, and a host of anomalies and malformations of the skeleton have a firm genetic foundation, that is to say, they are due to gene mutations. Of particular importance, although more difficult to demonstrate, is the concept that a genetic constitution (specific genotype) may condition the susceptibility of the host to environmental insult. *Mutation in bac-*

teria is well recognized; in the process of *transduction* there appears to be a transfer of genes from one strain of bacterium to a second strain by the mediation of a bacterio-phage.

Autosomal Dominant Inheritance.—This is the easiest type to recognize. Each affected individual has an affected parent and grand-parent. The character can be transmitted by a parent of either sex to a child of either sex. If one parent has the dominant gene, two out of four children will inherit this gene, and although the condition is heterozygous, they will show the trait. The other two children did not receive the dominant gene and are homozygous for the recessive gene, so that they will appear normal. If two heterozygous cousins mate in the third generation, three out of four children will show the trait. The heredity is not sex-linked. Examples are brachydactyly (short fingers and toes), multiple cartilaginous exostoses, progressive pseudohypertrophic polyneuritis, Huntington's chorea, multiple polyposis of colon and rectum, sickle cell anemia, diabetes insipidus and angioneurotic edema. All of these diseases are commoner in the male, and are often transmitted by the male. In one family there were 23 cases of diabetes insipidus among 91 members in 4 generations.

Autosomal Recessive Inheritance.—This type of inheritance is much more difficult to recognize. The defect is only obvious in a homozygous individual, one in whom both allelic genes (double dose) determine the same defect. It must therefore have been inherited from both heterozygous parents, neither of whom exhibited it, merely acting as carriers. The condition may thus remain unsuspected for many generations, until a homozygous mating brings two recessive genes together. This is most likely to happen with a marriage of first cousins, or in isolated communities where consanguinous marriages are inevitable. A moving account of such a happening will be found in H. G. Wells' short story, *The Valley of the Blind*, written many years ago. Normality is nearly always dominant to defectiveness. That is one of the blessings of a recessive character. A lethal gene may be paired with a normal (dominant) gene, but its possessor goes through life unconscious of the fact that genetically he is half dead. The parents of children with amaurotic (blind) family idiocy, the disease with the tragically descriptive name, are always normal, although both carrying the gene. No affected person ever grows up to be a parent, as the disease is fatal in early life. Examples of recessive inheritance in man are amaurotic family idiocy, retinitis pigmentosa, Fried-reich's ataxia, alkaptonuria, xeroderma pig-mentosum, and albinism. An albino will usually marry someone who does not carry that particular gene; all the children will be heterozygous carriers. If he marries a heterozygote, half the children will be albinos, and half unaffected heterozygotes. If two albinos marry, all the children will be albinos.

The five possible results of mating dom-inant with recessive autosomal genes are shown in the following table, where D represents a dominant gene and d a recessive one.

1. $D D \times D D = D D$
2. $d d \times d d = d d$
3. $D D \times d d = D d$
4. $D D \times D d = \frac{1}{2} D D + \frac{1}{2} Dd$
5. $Dd \times Dd = \frac{1}{4} DD + \frac{1}{2} Dd + \frac{1}{4} dd$

Modified Inheritance.—A character or trait may be neither typically dominant nor recessive. Dominance is not a fixed property of a gene, but can be modified by the pres-ence or absence of other genes, converting a heterozygote into a dominant or a recessive one (Allison and Blumberg). The effect may depend on whether there is a single or double dose of gene. There may be all stages be-tween dominance and absence of dominance. When Mendel crossed a pure-breeding red-flowered pea and a pure-breeding white-flowered pea, the progeny resembled the red-flowered plant, but whiteness reappeared in subsequent generations. This is an ex-ample of pure dominance and recessiveness. There are all stages between dominance and absence of dominance. It is not a matter of all or nothing, black or white. When a red snapdragon is crossed with a white one, all the first generation is pink. In this case there is no complete expression of either the red or the white gene.

The word *penetrance* is used in connection

with the expression or non-expression of genes. If penetrance is *complete*, the gene is expressed in single dose, if dominant, in double dose if recessive. When the gene is not always expressed, penetrance is *partial*. It would now appear that a single-dose expression of an abnormal gene can be increased by the presence of *modifiers* at other loci. This becomes understandable when we recall that most genes probably act by the production of enzymes which may modify the action of neighboring genes. The opposite effect, namely diminution of a single-dose expression by modifiers, converting the character into a recessive one, is much more common.

The best examples of the effects of mutant human genes in single and double dose are conditions associated with abnormal hemoglobins. Thus some cases of the form of anemia known as thalassemia are mild, whilst others are severe; the former are probably heterozygous, the latter homozygous, for the thalassemia gene. In the case of sickle cell anemia, if the gene is heterozygous (single dose) the person only manifests what is known as the sickle cell trait, that is to say the red blood cells become sickle-shaped when the blood is deoxygenated in the laboratory. The person (? patient) remains in perfect health unless he is exposed to low oxygen tension, as in flying at high altitude in an unpressurized aircraft, when the red cells may become sickled with resulting splenic infarction. If the gene is homozygous (double dose), the individual is a true patient suffering from hemolytic disease. Other examples of the difference between the effect of single dose (mild) and double dose (severe) are afforded by brachyphalangy (short fingers and toes), telangiectasia, chondrodystrophy, psoriasis and still other unusual conditions.

A particularly striking example of a single gene modifying the heterozygous expression of another gene is provided by the abnormal hemoglobins of sickle cell anemia and thalassemia. In a person heterozygous for the sickle cell gene (sickle cell trait) only from one-quarter to one-half of the hemoglobin is of the sickle cell type, the remainder being of the normal type; in the sickle cell homozygote the great bulk of the hemoglobin is

of the sickle cell type; but in a person heterozygous for both the sickle cell and thalassemia genes there is almost no normal hemoglobin, so that the thalassemia gene appears to assist the heterozygous sickle cell gene so that it behaves like a sickle cell zygote.

Sex-linked Inheritance.—Each of the 44 chromosomes (autosomes) contributed by a male gamete is homologous with a corresponding chromosome contributed by a female gamete. In addition there are two chromosomes which determine the sex of the individual; these are known as the X and Y sex chromosomes. In the female there are two homologous X-chromosomes, whereas in the male the arrangement is heterologous, with one X- and one Y-chromosome. These can be distinguished in the case of the large chromosomes of the salivary gland of the fruit fly by the larger size of the X-chromosome and the peculiar shape of the Y. In the reduction division which precedes the formation of a gamete there will be two kinds of spermatozoa, one set with one X-chromosome, which on fertilization will result in a female offspring, the other with one Y-chromosome, will result in a male. The father passes on the Y-chromosomes received from his father to all his sons, and the X-chromosomes received from his mother to all his daughters. Both of the sex chromosomes carry additional non-sexual genes, which are known as sex-linked genes. As the female has 2 X-chromosomes she will be heterozygous and therefore a mere carrier for a mutant gene in a single X-chromosome, whereas the male with a single X-chromosome will be homozygous for the mutant gene, so that the trait will become apparent. The gene in question may be passed from father to daughter and from mother to son, but if it is recessive it is only in the male, in which it is unmasked, that it will become apparent. The abnormality is thus confined to the male, but transmitted by the female (Fig. 232). In the female the recessive gene (X) will be masked by the dominant normal gene on the other X-chromosome. This explains what is at first sight the peculiar sex distribution of hemophilia, the finest example of a sex-linked inherited disease in which an extreme tendency to hemorrhage is due to deficiency in

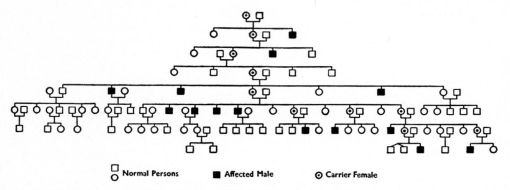

Fig. 232.—Pedigree of a family with hemophilia showing its transmission through eight generations. (G. Payling Wright, *Introduction to Pathology*, courtesy of Longmans, Green & Co.)

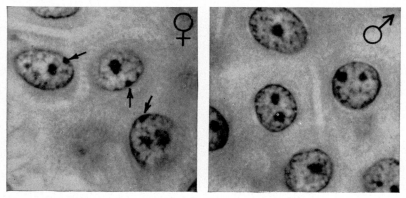

Fig. 232A.—Female and male cells showing presence or absence of sex chromatin. (Kindness of Dr. Murray L. Barr.)

the clotting power of the plasma. Only the male is affected and only the female transmits the disease. The reason why, as a rule, only half the sons inherit the disease and half the daughters become carriers is that in the heterozygous female only one X-chromosome carries the taint, and there is an even chance that this is the one which may be lost in the maturation of the ovum. In the male there is no dominant normal gene to inhibit the mutant gene, as there is no other male X-chromosome in the fertilized ovum. In the past most hemophilic boys have died of hemorrhage before attaining maturity, but in the extremely unlikely event of a hemophilic father marrying a carrier mother, a daughter as well as a son may be a hemophiliac. In addition to hemophilia other examples of sex-linked inheritance of disease are color blindness,

night blindness, progressive muscular dystrophy, and Leber's hereditary optic atrophy.

Sex Chromatin.—It was in 1949 that Barr and Bertram first demonstrated that female somatic cells could be differentiated from corresponding cells in the male by the presence of a tiny aggregation of chromatin known as sex chromatin at the periphery of the nucleus (Fig. 232A). This chromatin body is visible in most cells of chromosomal females, but very rarely in the nuclei of males. Its apparent origin is from particles of the 2 X-chromosomes of the female, but not from the single X-chromosome of the male. The sex chromatin was originally observed in the nerve cells of the cat, then in skin biopsies, and now oral smears of the buccal mucosa serve to determine the genetic sex as opposed to the apparent sex of an individual. Thus what a few years ago was a purely academic observation has provided the basis of a highly valuable practical test in doubtful cases of intersex. In the investigation of sterility, if the chromatin test reveals a discrepancy between apparent sex and chromosomal sex, the chances of fertility are almost nil. The question of intersex is discussed more fully in Chapter 32.

HEREDITARY DEFECTS AND DISEASES

A very large number of diseases, for the most part rare, are now believed to have their origin in some hereditary defect in the germ plasm, although, for reasons already discussed, the physician may find it impossible to establish the hereditary factor in an isolated case. These defects depend on specific genes in the chromosomes of the germ cells. In addition to well established hereditary traits, new mutations may arise owing to a sudden change in the genes. Mutations may be spontaneous or they may be induced experimentally in animals and plants by chemical mutagens or ionizing radiation. A good idea of the number of diseases in which heredity may play a part can be obtained by consulting the list in Madge Macklin's article or in Crew's monograph.

Blood Diseases.—The most important of these are hemophilia, pernicious anemia and sickle cell anemia. *Hemophilia*, a perfect example of a sex-linked recessive character, has already been considered. *Pernicious anemia* usually gives little or no evidence of a hereditary tendency unless a very full family tree can be drawn up, but several cases of achylis gastrica may be found in the same family, and this condition undoubtedly precedes the onset of pernicious anemia. It looks as if the achylia were a hereditary character, the operation of some extraneous factor occasionally precipitating in such persons an attack of the disease. *Sickle cell anemia* behaves as a dominant. *Eosinophilia* may be familial. I have studied two brothers, in one of whom the eosinophils averaged 80 per cent and in the other around 20 per cent. *Hemorrhagic telangiectasia*, a condition characterized by spontaneous bleeding from dilated vessels in the nose and mouth and the appearance of red spots in the skin commencing about the time of puberty, behaves as a dominant. *Favism* has been known for centuries as a disease affecting the red blood cells in persons living in the Mediterranean basin, particularly the islands of Sardinia and Sicily. The disease is due to sensitivity to the ingestion of the broad bean (*Vicia faba*) or to inhalation of the pollen. There is marked hemoglobinuria, the urine varying in color from red to black, intense jaundice, and very severe hemolytic anemia. We now know that the basis of the condition is a familial deficiency in the red cells which makes them allergic to the protein of the broad bean, a deficiency in the enzyme, glucose-6-phosphate dehydrogenase. The defective red cells can be detected by laboratory tests. One of the most striking examples of human heredity is afforded by the *blood groups*, the agglutinogens acting as dominants. The A and B group genes are dominant to the O gene. Genes for abnormal hemoglobins produce distinct single and double dose effects, the effect of an abnormal double dose being naturally much more severe than that of a single dose.

Metabolic Disorders.—We have already referred to the group called by Garrod "the inborn errors of metabolism," a name which itself indicates the hereditary origin, although recessive in character. The "error" is the result of an enzymatic defect, which may involve proteins, carbohydrates, lipids, or pigments. The lipid storage diseases (Gaucher's disease, Niemann-Pick disease, *etc.*), hepato-lenticular degeneration (Wilson's disease), and abnormal glycogen accumulation (von Gierke's disease) have an enzyme genetic basis. A deficiency or absence of an enzyme may lead to an accumulation of substances that normally are intermediates in the metabolic process. *Phenylketonuria*, a disorder of protein metabolism, was the first of the inborn errors in which Garrod's triad of criteria—gene, enzyme, and clinical abnormality—was convincingly demonstrated. The basis is deficiency of a hepatic enzyme, phenylalanine hydroxylase, which normally converts phenylalanine to tyrosine. The most striking clinical feature is severe mental retardation, to which may be added a variety of neurological disturbances. The defect is transmitted as a recessive trait by a single autosomal gene. The parents are apparently normal, but each is heterozygous, carrying one abnormal gene.

Another type of metabolic disorder is dependent on the *absence of enzyme systems that normally regulate renal tubular transport*. The defect may show itself as excessive urinary loss of an essential metabolite due to failure of tubular reabsorption, as is seen in *cystinuria*, where there is marked loss of cystine with recurrent formation of renal stones; or there may be excessive tubular reabsorption with accumulation of a catabolic substance in body fluids, as occurs with uric acid in *gout*, a disease in which heredity is usually strongly marked. Numerous other metabolic disorders are now known to be of genetic origin, among which may be mentioned diabetes insipidus, alkaptonuria, and porphyria, which is an enzymatic defect of pigment metabolism associated with the excretion of excess porphyrins.

Skeletal Defects.—The skeleton is often the site of hereditary defects. *Multiple cartilaginous exostoses* is also known as hereditary deforming chondrodysplasia, a name which announces the inherited nature of the defect. *Brachydactyly*, or short fingers, the first example of Mendelian inheritance demonstrated in man, is a simple dominant. The fingers have only two phalanges, the second and third being fused owing to absence of an epiphysis in the former. A similar type of defect in the hand has been transmitted from one of Henry the Sixth's nobles in the 15th century to descendants living at the present day; the recently exhumed skeleton of the original earl showed the same bony change. A particularly striking example of a hereditary malformation traceable to one gene is that of the Dionne quintuplets, all developed from a single fertilized ovum, and all showing a webbing between the second and third toes of each foot. *Fragilitas ossium*, a condition characterized by multiple fractures and sometimes associated with blue sclerotics, may show a very marked familial tendency, nearly always dominant. Males and females are about equally affected, transmission taking place equally through both sexes.

Neuromuscular Disorders.—The nervous and neuromuscular systems furnish a large variety of hereditary diseases. Progressive muscular atrophy, pseudohypertrophic muscular dystrophy (dominant or recessive or sex-linked), Friedreich's ataxia (dominant or recessive), peroneal atrophy, amyotonia congenita, myotonia congenita and many others are familial in character due to inherited defects in the germ plasm. Muscular tremor may be markedly hereditary, and is usually dominant.

Skin Disorders.—The skin and its appendages show a variety of inherited defects. Mention may be made here of *baldness*, which is markedly hereditary in character. It is much commoner in men than in women, being dominant in males, but recessive in females. The male may inherit it from father or mother, but the mother, being heterozygous, is not bald. *Xeroderma pigmentosum*, a disease of the skin occurring in childhood and characterized by the occurrence of inflammation when exposed to the sun with subsequent development of multiple cutaneous carcinomata, is recessive in all cases. *Von Recklinghausen's disease*, or multiple neurofibromatosis, is always dominant, but in some cases pigmented areas take the place of tumors, so that the dominant character is apt to be overlooked.

Eye Diseases.—These constitute one of the largest groups and serve to fill the blind asylums. Chief among these may be mentioned *retinitis pigmentosa* and *hereditary optic atrophy* (*Leber's disease*), the latter offering an excellent example of a sex-linked disease, being confined to the male but transmitted through the female. *Blue sclerotics* is an ocular manifestation of a defect of connective tissues in general, including the bones (fragilitas ossium). The blue color is due to the underlying choroid shining through the thin sclera. The condition is a good example of a dominant nonsex-linked defect. It is not transmitted by those not affected, it appears in both males and females, it is transmitted from fathers to sons and daughters and from mothers to sons and daughters. The defect is of course not carried in the sex chromosome. *Colorblindness* and some forms of night-blindness (the patient becoming blind at dusk owing to lack of the visual purple in the rods of the retina) are both sex-linked. *Coloboma of the iris* and its extreme form, known as *aniridia* or absence of the iris causing blindness, are markedly hereditary. Risley records an extraordinary and tragic family history in which one blind man had 13 children who were all blind, 61 blind grandchildren out of 63 and 39 great grandchildren out of 42, a total of 113 blind offspring out of 118. A strong argument for eugenics! *Retinoblastoma*, a neoplasm which is fatal unless removed early, often shows a marked hereditary tendency. In a family of 16, 10 died of this tumor. It is always recessive. There is a marked hereditary tendency in all varieties of *cataract*, and in *amaurotic family idiocy*. Strabismus is dominant in some families, recessive in others.

Mental Diseases.—Disorders of the mind are often due to a defect in the germ plasm. *Dementia præcox* offers a good example. *Huntington's chorea* is an example of a simple dominant autosomal character. One family from Long Island has furnished practically 1000 cases of this disease. Some types of feeble-mindedness are inherited as simple recessives. Matings of feeble-minded persons with each other gave only 6 normal children out of 482 from 144 such unions. The 6 normals may have been a mistake, as in the case of two feeble-minded white parents who had 10 feeble-minded and 2 normal children, but the two normals were black! Amaurotic family idiocy and Mongolian idiocy are always recessive.

Susceptibility to Infection.—In addition to the defects, anomalies and diseases known to have a genetic basis, there is the question of inherited susceptibility or resistance to specific infectious disease, either bacterial or viral. This is naturally a matter on which it is extremely difficult to make definite statements, but animal experiments and to a much lesser degree observations on human disease point to the conclusion that in some cases at least the hereditary factor may be the deciding one. Selective breeding of laboratory animals such as mice can create populations which are susceptible or resistant to one particular infection, so much so indeed that epidemics may arise in the susceptible groups. Susceptibility to tuberculosis in the laboratory animal can be shown

to have a definite hereditary basis, and this appears possible also in man. Susceptibility to the virus of poliomyelitis seems to be dependent on a simple non-sex-linked recessive gene, and the same seems to be true of rheumatic fever.

Heredity in Cancer.—This matter has already been discussed in connection with neoplasia, so it will only be touched on here. The part played by heredity in the development of cancer is easily demonstrated in the pure-bred laboratory animal, but it is far from easy when we come to man.

People do not know what their grandparents and great aunts died of, and if they did, the diagnosis would be as often wrong as right. Moreover, an hereditary character may be transmitted through a son incapable of showing that character, *e.g.*, a bull is valuable because it comes of a famous milk-producing strain. A woman with cancer of the uterus may transmit that gene to her son, but it cannot manifest itself; it may be transmitted in the same way to a grandson, and the fatal character may finally appear in his daughter. In such a case it is natural that the hereditary tendency should be completely lost sight of. One of the neoplasms in which the influence of heredity is best seen is polyposis of the rectum and colon with its marked tendency to become malignant. Dukes records the case of a man who died of rectal cancer at the age of forty-two years. He had 9 children, 7 of whom developed rectal cancer; 5 were already dead, 1 at the age of twenty-seven years. The disease also appeared in the next generation. It is impossible to believe that in such a case as this there was not some hereditary defect in the germ plasm which acted as a determiner for cancer of the rectum. A man and his wife had cancer of the stomach, and 6 of their 7 children died of the disease. The seventh was killed at the age of twenty-eight years in an accident. In the experimental work on mice the incidence of cancer, its site and its character were all influenced by heredity. It is worthy of note that the larval stage of *Drosophila* suffers from a sex-linked entodermal tumor, which kills one-quarter of the males and is transmitted by the unaffected females.

GENETIC HAZARDS OF RADIATION

In all organisms ionizing radiation produces gene mutations and chromosome breaks. This genetic hazard has already been discussed in Chapter 18, to which the reader is referred. Most of the work has been done on *Drosophila* and on the mouse. The dominant visible mutations are the rarest, so that they need not be expected in the children of parents whose gonads have been irradiated. Nor will the vast majority of x-ray induced recessive mutations be apparent in the children, as it is extremely unlikely that a spermatozoon will carry the same newly mutated gene as the ovum it fertilizes. When a child who carries a new recessive gene has children of its own, half of these will inherit the new gene, which may become apparent in the fulness of time. It will be evident that the popular idea that a person whose gonads have been exposed to powerful ionizing radiation will produce children with all sorts of monstrosities is entirely wrong.

It must be obvious that any prediction as to the genetic effects of ionizing radiation can be only an informed guess. The *radiation* may be *natural, diagnostic, therapeutic,* or due to "*fall-out.*" About 4 per cent of all individuals born will suffer at some time in their lives from hereditary defects due to naturally occurring mutations. Present day (1959) opinion on the effect of radiation, whether natural, diagnostic, therapeutic or due to "fall-out," is illustrated by the following summary by the head of the Biology Board, Atomic Energy of Canada: "The frequency of the conditions which are mutation-maintained will increase with any rise in the level of ionizing radiation. Present levels of exposure resulting from the medical uses of x-rays average about 3 roentgens per generation per person in the population, and might eventually increase the load of hereditary defects by as much as 10 per cent. The genetic effect of "fall-out" from nuclear weapon testing is probably about one-thirtieth of this" (Newcombe and James).

TWINS

Twins provide a singular opportunity to study the effect of heredity and constitution

on disease. In the case of identical (monozygotic) twins, one serves as a control animal for the other. It is as if we were watching one individual leading two physical existences. Margolis and Eisenstein give the following examples of disease developing more or less simultaneously in both twins: (1) *Tumors.* Twins developed retinoblastoma of the left eye within a few months of each other. Cancer of the right testicle appeared in both at the same time. (2) *Nervous and mental disease.* Dementia præcox, paranoia, and other mental disorders have developed at the same time. (3) *Non-infectious systemic disease.* At the age of sixty twin brothers developed diabetes characterized by the same set of symptoms, and both died within a few months of each other. Twin sisters in New York and San Francisco developed diabetes at the age of fifty-two and died within a short time of each other. Other diseases which have developed simultaneously in twins are lymphatic leukemia, nephritis, asthma, bronchiectasis, cataract, and Hodgkin's disease. (4) *Infections.* Twin sisters developed tuberculosis of the right kidney within seven months of each other. Many other similar examples could be given illustrating the profound influence which origin from a common germ plasm has on the development of disease.

CONSTITUTION IN DISEASE

The subject of constitution is bound up with that of heredity. It has become the custom rather to smile at our medical forefathers when they talk in their writings of the weak constitution of the patient, but the central doctrine of Greek medicine was that of temperaments and constitutions, and the conceptions of Hippocrates are worthy of consideration even at the present day. Constitution, according to Draper, whose monograph on the subject should be consulted, is "that aggregate of hereditarial characters, influenced more or less by environment, which determines the individual's reaction, successful or unsuccessful, to the stress of environment." It is a summation of all inherited characters. John Hunter, Addison, and other great clinical observers of that period believed firmly that the habitus or physical form of the individual bears an important relationship to disease. This physical form is the anatomical aspect of constitution, and although by no means the only aspect it is the one which has been most carefully studied and the only one which will be considered here. "The anatomic features of an individual form one of a set of basic unit characters, predetermined by heredity, and influenced to some extent by environment, which together make up the constitution" (Draper). The anatomical aspect is related to the physiological, psychological and immunological aspects, and it was a recognition of this fact which formed the basis of the marvellous unconscious skill of the older physicians. The three basic elements of the disease problem are Man, the lesion, and the environmental stress, and we are so much engaged with the two latter that the first is apt to be forgotten.

The capacity of an individual to react to the environmental stress is a constitutional quality, just as specific as body size and capable of being transmitted to his offspring. Longevity, which is the result and expression of a good constitution, is certainly inherited; everyone knows of families, the majority of whose members reach the late seventies or eighties, no matter what kind of life they may have led. We have already seen that this is the case with resistance to infection. Sex, which is considered below, has a profound influence on disease reactions, and this is determined by the presence or absence of the extra X-chromosome. In some way this must be linked with the commonness of gallbladder disease and the comparative rarity of chronic peptic ulcer in the female. Size of body has been shown in animals to be a unit character. The entire skeleton may be altered by a defect in a single gene, and the person may be a giant or a dwarf. In this instance the determiner appears to act through an endocrine gland (pituitary). Race may play a part in predisposition to a disease. Thus certain diseases are peculiar to the Hebrew race. Amaurotic family idiocy is practically confined to Jewish children, while Gaucher's disease and Niemann-Pick's disease are much commoner in these children; Buerger's disease, diabetes

mellitus, and pentosuria are commoner among Jews.

Habitus.—The habitus or general build of the body is a resultant of a combination of height and weight. On this basis it is possible to divide persons into the sthenic and asthenic groups. The *sthenic* individual is short and stout, with a wide costal angle and deep chest, inclined to be florid, of cheerful sanguine disposition, liable to gallbladder disease, arterial hypertension and likely to die of arteriosclerosis, apoplexy or coronary occlusion owing to defects in his germ plasm at the time of conception. The *asthenic* individual is tall and thin, with a narrow costal angle, a pallid countenance, easily fatigued and inclined to be melancholy; he has a long, drooping stomach which empties poorly and intestines which sag, so that his melancholy may be aggravated by dyspepsia and constipation. He is a likely subject for peptic ulcer. He seldom has heart or arterial disease and is likely to be long-lived if he escapes tuberculosis in youth. The gall-stone man seldom has ulcer; the ulcer man seldom has gall stones. The pages of Shakespeare and Dickens are filled with immortal characterizations of these types.

Influence of Sex.—The question of sex has already been considered in connection with sex determination and the sex-linked inheritance of disease. We have now to consider sex from the standpoint of human constitution, *i.e.*, the manner in which it influences the reaction of the individual to the stress of environment. In such a discussion the organs peculiar to either sex must be excluded, only those common to both being considered. When this is done the surprising fact emerges that very few serious organic diseases are commoner in the female. Most diseases of the gastrointestinal tract, respiratory tract, blood vessels, heart, bones, joints and urinary tract are commoner in males than in females. Some diseases such as thromboangiitis obliterans are almost confined to the male, while others such as angina pectoris, coronary occlusion, peripheral arteriosclerosis, pernicious anemia, leukemia, lymphosarcoma, *etc.*, are more frequent in that sex. The gallbladder is a notable exception to the general rule, and to a lesser degree mitral stenosis. Functional disorders, on the other hand, such as Raynaud's disease, hypertension, migraine, hysteria and chronic nervous exhaustion are commoner in the female. There is a higher mortality for the male throughout all the periods of life. This cannot be explained away, as is commonly done, by reference to overwork, industrial hazards, abuse of alcohol and tobacco, venery, *etc.*, for the difference in the sex mortality is most striking in intrauterine life and during the first few years of childhood. There appears to be an inherent weakness in the male, a sex-linked inferiority, so that by comparison with the female he is a weakling at all periods of life from conception to death. This holds true throughout the animal kingdom, the males being shorter-lived. As Allen remarks, the price of maleness is weakness, and woman is far from being "the weaker vessel." Only a few organic diseases, such as those of the gall-bladder and thyroid, are commoner in females.

REFERENCES

ALISON, A. C. and BLUMBERG, B. S.: Am. J. Med., 1958, *25*, 933. (Dominance and recessivity in medical genetics.)

ALLEN, E. V.: Ann. Int. Med., 1934, *7*, 1000. (Sex and disease.)

BARR, M. L.: Science, 1959, *130*, 679. (Sex chromatin and sex anomalies).

BÖÖK, J. A. and SANTESSON, B.: Lancet, 1960, *2*, 858. (Malformation associated with triploidy.)

CREW, F. A. E.: *Genetics in Relation to Clinical Medicine*, Edinburgh, 1947.

DRAPER, G., DUPERTIUS, C. W. and CAUGHEY, J. L., JR.: *Human Constitution in Clinical Medicine*, New York, 1944.

HSIA, D. Y-Y.: New Eng. J. Med., 1960, *262*, 1172. (Medical genetics.)

JACOBS, PATRICIA, A. *et al.*: Lancet, 1959, *2*, 423; 1960, *1*, 1213. (Super-female.)

MACKLIN, M. T.: Medicine, 1935, *14*, 1. (The role of heredity in disease.)

MARGOLIS, H. M. and EISENSTEIN, V. W.: Ann. Int. Med., 1933, *6*, 1489.

NEWCOMBE, H. B. and JAMES, A. P.: Can. J. Pub. Health, 1959, *50*, 140 (Genetic effect of radiation).

PAGET, J.: Lancet, 1882, *2*, 1017. (Hereditary malformations.)

ROBERTS, J. A. F.: *An Introduction to Medical Genetics*, 2nd ed., London, 1959.

SORSBY, A.: *Clinical Genetics*, St. Louis, 1958.

STERN, C.: *Prinicples of Human Genetics*, San Francisco, 1949.

WRIGHT, G. PAYLING: *An Introduction to Pathology*, 3rd ed., p. 38, London, 1958.

Part II. Regional Pathology

Chapter 21

Diseases of the Heart

General Considerations
STRUCTURE
Conducting System
Blood Supply
FUNCTION
Rhythmicity
Expansibility
Cardiac Reserve
Cardiac Pain
Transaminase
Glycogen
HEART DISEASE
Rheumatic Heart Disease
VALVULAR LESIONS
MYOCARDIAL LESIONS
PERICARDIAL LESIONS
Aortic Lesions
RHEUMATOID HEART DISEASE
Rheumatoid Arthritis
Ankylosing Spondylitis
Bacterial Endocarditis
SUBACUTE BACTERIAL ENDO-
CARDITIS
ACUTE BACTERIAL ENDO-
CARDITIS
Coronary Artery Disease

CORONARY OCCLUSION
ANGINA PECTORIS
ARTERIOSCLEROTIC HEART
DISEASE
SUDDEN CARDIAC DEATH
Sudden Death
HEART BLOCK
Hypertensive Heart Disease
Congenital Heart Disease
ATRIAL SEPTAL DEFECTS
Lutembacher's Disease
VENTRICULAR SEPTAL DEFECTS
Tetralogy of Fallot
Eisenmenger Complex
Pure Pulmonary Stenosis
PATENT DUCTUS ARTERIOSUS
COARCTATION OF THE AORTA
ENDOCARDIAL FIBROELASTOSIS
MISCELLANEOUS CONDITIONS
Endocardial Lesions
THROMBOTIC NON-BACTERIAL
ENDOCARDITIS
CARCINOID CARDIOVASCULAR
DISEASE
Chronic Valvular Disease
MITRAL STENOSIS

MITRAL INSUFFICIENCY
AORTIC INSUFFICIENCY
AORTIC STENOSIS
Tricuspid Stenosis
Pulmonary Stenosis
Myocardial Lesions
MYOCARDITIS
Isolated (Fiedler's) Myocarditis
Granulomatous Myocarditis
TOXIC MYOCARDITIS
MYOCARDIAL DEGENERATIONS
DEFICIENCY DISEASES
TRAUMA
TUMORS
Pericardial Lesions
PERICARDITIS
Acute Idiopathic Pericarditis
Tuberculous Pericarditis
Chronic Constrictive Peri-
carditis
Uremic Pericarditis
Cholesterol Pericarditis
HEMOPERICARDIUM
HYDROPERICARDIUM
Heart Failure

GENERAL CONSIDERATIONS

FROM the earliest of times our ancestors have realized the importance of the heart to life itself. Our language testifies to this fact, particularly the languages of the poets. We say that a man is broken-hearted, or wounded to the heart, or that he wears his heart on his sleeve, or that it is in his throat or in his boots. The heart beats 100,000 times a day, and yet it rests (during diastole) twice as long as it works. Our knowledge of the anatomy and physiology of the heart has advanced to an incredible degree. We can pass catheters into its cavities, record the electrical changes in its muscle, and estimate its enzymes. But we still do not understand how it is that one man may have extensive myocardial fibrosis without suffering unduly, while in another who dies apparently of sudden heart failure, no adequate explana-

tion can be found at autopsy. Before embarking on a study of the various forms of heart disease it will be helpful if we recall a few facts relating to normal structure and function, so that these may be compared later with the changes which result from disease.

Structure.—When we examine the heart at autopsy we pay attention to the pericardium, pericardial cavity, the size and weight of the heart, the myocardium, atria, ventricles, endocardium, valve cusps, valvular openings and coronary arteries. The *pericardial cavity* normally contains from 10 to 30 cc. of clear, straw-colored fluid. The *visceral pericardium* is smooth, shiny, thin and translucent. The *size* can only be learned by frequent observation of the normal. It may be enlarged by reason of hypertrophy of the wall or dilatation of the cavities. The average *weight* is 300 grams in the male, 250 grams in the female, but these figures will be considerably exceeded in a big muscular laborer or reduced in a tiny fragile woman. In animals the weight varies with the size of the animal; thus in one sperm whale the weight was 256 pounds; (the animal weighed 47,700 pounds). The weight is largely dependent on the thickness of the left ventricle. The wall of the *left ventricle* measures from 10 to 15 mm., that of the *right ventricle* about 5 mm. Both undergo hypertrophy when they have increased work to do, the left ventricle in arterial hypertension and aortic stenosis, the right ventricle in mitral stenosis with accompanying pulmonary hypertension. The *endocardium* lining the cavities is smooth, shiny and translucent, so that the underlying muscle should be visible. The smoothness of the endocardium reduces friction and a tendency to clotting. Damage to this smooth surface by infection, infarction or stasis may lead to intracardiac thrombosis with subsequent embolism. Fibrosis and opacity of the left atrium is seen in rheumatic heart disease, and a similar condition of the left ventricle in coronary artery disease, hypertension, disease of the aortic valve, and cor pulmonale. The *valve cusps* should be as thin and smooth as fine silk. The commissures of the aortic valve, *i.e.*, the points where the cusps are joined together, have no appreciable thickness; any widening of these commissures is an indication of disease, nearly always syphilis. As regards the *valvular openings*, the mitral measures about 10 cm. in circumference, the tricuspid 12 cm., the aortic 7.5 cm., and the pulmonary 8.5 cm. The *skeleton of the heart* consists of dense fibrous rings around the atrio-ventricular openings, which prevent these outlets from becoming dilated and are connected with similar rings that surround the origin of the aorta and the pulmonary artery.

Microscopically, the features of interest to us are the arrangement of the muscle and the conducting system. The *muscle fibers* are grouped in four main bundles, which are spirally arranged to encircle the ventricles, being fixed at each end to the fibrous skeleton. The result of this spiral arrangement is that when the bundles contract they expel blood from the ventricles like the wringing of a wet cloth. Damage caused by an infarct will of course interfere with this mechanism.

Similar but more delicate bundles of muscle are present in the atria.

Conducting System.—The conducting system serves to carry the impulse to contract to the right place at the right time. This system, sometimes known as the Purkinje system, consists of (1) the sino-atrial node, (2) the atrio-ventricular node of Tawara, and (3) the bundle of His. (Fig. 233). It is made necessary by the fibrous skeleton of the heart, which separates the artia from the ventricles and prevents the passage of electrical activity between the two sets of chambers. It is responsible for the initiation and propagation of the electrical activity which stimulates the heart beat. The *sino-atrial node*, which initiates the normal beat and is therefore called the *pacemaker of the heart*, is situated between the right atrium and the superior vena cava. Delicate strands of specialized conducting muscle extend upwards on the vena cava and down over the walls of the atria. The *atrio-ventricular node* lies between the mouth of the coronary sinus and the septal cusp of the tricuspid valve. From it the atrio-ventricular bundle of His pierces the fibrous rings of the skeleton of the heart to reach the interventricular septum, where it divides into left and right branches The importance of the conducting system will become apparent when we come to the subject of heart block and of sudden death (page 472 and 473).

Blood Supply.—The blood supply to the myocardium is all-important. In the most primitive vertebrates, such as the lamprey, and also in the amphibian, there are no coronary vessels, the highly spongy myocardium being supplied with blood from within its cavities. The question is now being asked as to whether it is possible to turn the mammalian heart back over eons of time into a primitive heart capable of surviving in a primitive way without coronary arteries. When the epicardium of the left ventricle in a laboratory animal is removed and a thin layer of avalon sponge is placed directly on the bared myocardium, blood vessels from the fibrous pericardium grow through the sponge into the heart muscle (Vineberg *et al.*). This seems to open up long-forgotten sinusoidal channels, and nutrition reaches the muscle both from the outside and from inside the ventricular cav-

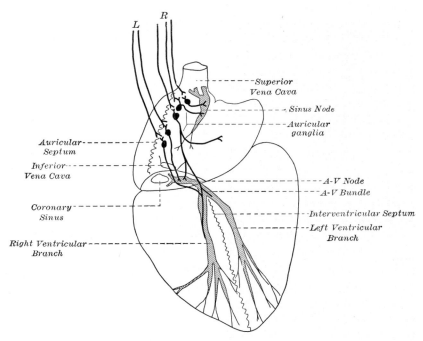

Fig. 233.—Schematic figure showing relations of S–A node, A–V node, A–V bundle, His-Tawara branches as well as probable connections of ganglion cells and extrinsic nerve fibers. R, Right vagus; L, Left vagus. (Wiggers, *Physiology in Health and Disease.*)

ity. The possible importance of this concept in relation to the treatment of the myocardial ischemia resulting from coronary occlusion is self-evident. In the mammalian heart the capillaries of the coronary arteries are the most essential vessels. There is an average of 3342 capillaries per sq. mm. (Roberts). This concentration naturally falls with hypertrophy of the myocardium, with resulting loss of efficiency. This loss may be of particular significance in relation to surgery for such a condition as mitral stenosis, a large heart being much more unfavorable than a small one. Most of the posterior surface of the heart is supplied by the right coronary artery, the remainder drawing its blood from the left.

The question of *anastomotic connections* between the two sets of coronary arteries is one of the most important from the point of view of coronary artery disease to be considered presently. It is a curious fact that wide divergencies on this fundamental and apparently simple matter have been expressed over the years. As Gregg puts it in his monograph on the coronary circulation

in 1950: "In no field of the circulation have our views changed more frequently than in the interpretation of the coronary circulation." At first it was presumed that a free collateral circulation existed between the two vessels. Then in 1881 they came to be regarded as end-arteries. Using new techniques of injection and examination Schlesinger in 1938 came to the conclusion that functionally important anastomoses developed only in response to disease, that is to say, when and where they were needed. This provided authoritative support for the idea that the coronary arteries in normal hearts are true end-arteries, without functional and anatomical connection. Anastomoses between the two sets of arteries were supposed to be minimal in youth, although some connections did open up with advancing years and arteriosclerotic narrowing of the main vessels, so that complete occlusion of one of the main arteries could be endured without infarction occurring.

In 1958 an investigation by Laurie and Woods of Natal on the heart of the Bantu seems to completely reverse this concept.

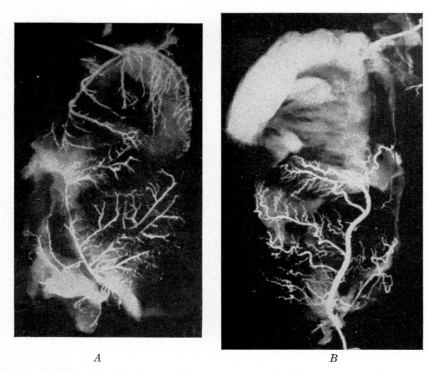

A   B

Fig. 234.—A, Heart from healthy infant aged nine months, showing complete anastomoses on one side from perfused material in the other coronary artery.

B, Heart from patient with chronic ischemic disease but with no anastomosis. (Laurie and Woods, courtesy of Lancet.)

Using a radioopaque mass to perfuse only one artery in normal and diseased hearts hearts they find functionally significant anastomoses in 75 per cent of normal hearts from the earliest years, but in only 23 per cent of patients with chronic ischemic heart disease. (Fig. 234). As the myocardium when deprived of its blood supply can only survive for twenty minutes, the practical importance of this concept is self-evident. The difference between these two arrangements appears to be determined on a genetic basis, which probably accounts for the difference of familial and sex distribution of coronary heart disease. In the words of Laurie and Woods: "Disease does not produce coronary anastomosis, but appears despite, or because of lack of, a normal pre-existing anastomosis. This would explain why some people are naturally endowed with a high resistance."

If both arteries become markedly nar-

rowed, extracardial anastomoses may be established with other branches from the aorta. Luminal vessels from the cavities of the heart may also supply blood to the ischemic myocardium.

Function.—The heart is a double-cylinder pump, and it is therefore endowed with the two primary features of a pump, namely: (1) rhythmic propulsive power and (2) intake (atrio-ventricular) and exhaust (aortic and pulmonary) valves of the flap type. If something goes wrong with either of these, the result will be heart disease. The myocardium is unique among muscles in that it can never rest for a period of time. If the pump ceases to work, life ends. Coronary sinus catheterization now enables us to look into the physiology of the myocardium and cardiac metabolism in a way never before possible. Physiologists have even begun to explore the electric activity of single heart muscle cells by inserting a microelectrode

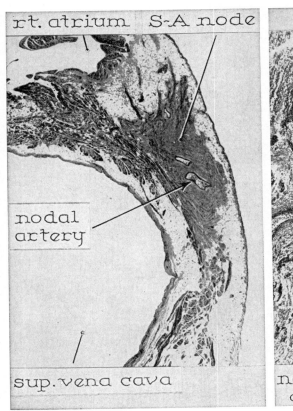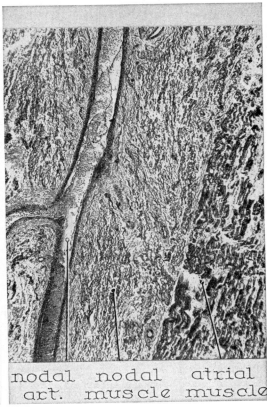

FIG. 235.—(*Left*) Low-power cross section of the right wall of the superior vena cava at its junction with the right atrium, cutting through the sinu-atrial node. (*Right*) Low-power longitudinal section of the sinu-atrial node, showing the fine muscle fibers of the node, in contrast with the larger darker-staining atrial muscle. Note the nodal artery running through the center of the node. (Preparation by J. Duckworth.) (Ham, *Histology*, courtesy of J. B. Lippincott Company.)

into the interior of a cell (Bing *et al.*). Normal cardiac metabolism is almost entirely aerobic, with a marked preference for glucose. When carbohydrate is not available, fatty acids become a major source of oxidative energy. A decrease in the work load of the normal heart reduces its energy requirements and thus its metabolism. In congestive heart failure, however, the energy produced remains normal despite the decrease in the mechanical work, indicating an inefficiency on the part of the contractile proteins in the utilization of available energy. Digitalis, that oldest of cardiac drugs, seems to improve this inefficiency without causing an alteration in metabolism.

From the point of view of what we term disease, which is merely disturbed function,

we are interested in such matters as rhythmicity, expansibility, cardiac reserve, and cardiac pain.

Rhythmicity.—The heart muscle is unique in its rhythmic contractibility. The rhythm originates in the pacemaker, the sino-atrial node, which starts each beat. How it does this is not known, presumably as the result of cyclic chemical changes. The initiation of the impulse corresponds with the P wave of the electrocardiogram. The passage of the wave of excitation is associated with a changing electrical potential along the fiber, whether specialized conducting fiber or ordinary cardiac muscle. The particular site over which the wave is passing is negatively charged in relation to the other parts of the fiber. The impulse passes to the node of

29

Tawara, along the bundle of His and its two branches to the subendocardial plexus, and thence to the muscle of the ventricle, where it inscribes the Q R S complex on the electrocardiogram (Fig. 235). Heart muscle is subject to the "all or none" law. When subjected to a stimulus of sufficient intensity it contracts to the maximum, otherwise it does not contract at all, in this respect differing diametrically from voluntary muscle. Moreover, a property of *refractoriness* prevents the muscle from responding until an interval of time has elapsed. If the refractory period becomes excessive, the result is *heart block*. Other fibers also have the power of initiating rhythmic contraction, so that if the sino-atrial node fails the pacemaker may be shifted to atrial muscle, the atrio-ventricular node or bundle, or even the ordinary muscle fibers. The mechanism now has become less efficient, and the normal sino-atrial rhythm is replaced by an arrhythmia.

When blocks of tissue are taken to include the atrio-ventricular node and bundle, lesions will frequently be found which correspond closely to electrocardiographic changes observed during life and also in cases of sudden cardiac death (Lumb and Shacklett). These lesions have included those of (1) ischemia (including infarction), fibrosis and calcification; (2) inflammation, including myocarditis, abscess, and rheumatic fever; (3) hemorrhage; (4) amyloidosis; (5) fibroelastosis. The conduction mechanism does indeed appear to be the critical weak spot, the Achilles heel, of the heart.

Expansibility.—Contraction of the ventricles is followed by expansion, which restores the heart to its normal volume. This seems to be brought about by a rearrangement of the molecules in the muscle fibers in the biochemical cycle of the heart beat. If the power of expansion is lost, the result is heart failure. Expansibility may be limited by cardiac tamponade (blood or fluid in the pericardial cavity), pericardial constriction especially when accompanied by calcification, and compression by tumors, deformities of the chest, etc.

Cardiac Reserve.—This term denotes the quite remarkable capacity of the heart muscle to meet extra demands placed upon it. As disease of the heart advances, the reserve is progressively reduced and finally lost. Hypertrophy in itself may be harmful, as we have already seen, and there may be good reserve until hypertrophy sets in. It may be noted that hypertrophy is due to an increase in the size of the individual fibers, not to the formation of new fibers.

Cardiac Pain.—Pain is due to myocardial ischemia. The lack of oxygen, combined with failure of the local circulation to remove lactic acid and other products of metabolism, leads to an accumulation of these products, with pain as a result. The pain may be felt in the precordium, or may be referred to a distance, as in the pain of angina pectoris which radiates down the left arm.

Transaminase.—Glutamic oxaloacetic transaminase (G.O.T.) removes an amino group from glutamic acid, which is then transferred to oxaloacetic acid with the formation of aspartic acid. The enzyme is widely distributed in the body, but the content is greatest in the heart, although high also in the liver, and to a lesser extent in voluntary muscle and the kidney. The normal serum level is low, from 4 to 40 units. In myocardial infarction a large amount is released into the blood, so that the serum level is a sensitive and very valuable index of recent necrosis of the myocardium. We shall return to the subject of myocardial transaminase in the discussion of coronary artery occlusion and myocardial infarction. Transaminase levels are determined either by paper chromatography or by the faster and more accurate spectrophotometric method.

Glycogen.—We have already seen the all-important part which glucose plays in myocardial metabolism. The normal myocardium is rich in glycogen during life. The amount of glycogen, as shown by the periodic acid-Schiff reaction with diastase digestion, varies widely in infants, often approaching that seen in glycogen-storage disease, and large amounts are frequently present in diabetes (Mowry and Bangle). The practical importance of the subject is that loss of glycogen is the earliest histological or histochemical change that has been demonstrated in myocardial ischemia. In dogs an almost complete loss of glycogen can be demonstrated in the ischemic area a few minutes after ligation of a coronary artery (Kent and

Riseker). The hope that this would prove a valuable method for demonstrating the earliest changes in human myocardial infarction proved illusory when it was found that glycogen is lost from the myocardium after death unless the body is refrigerated very promptly and at a very low temperature. The next earliest change is the appearance of a PAS-positive diastase-resistant material in the sarcoplasm of the muscle fibers in the area of ischemia. This material is not glycogen, and it becomes evident within four hours after the onset of ischemia. Glycogen depletion is not considered to be a mere post-mortem phenomenon, for experiments in the rat indicate that it may be initiated by agonal cardiovascular failure and completed during the process of dying (Wittels and Reiner).

Heart Disease. — Heart disease has become the commonest cause of disability and death in modern developed countries. If we include involvement of the kidneys and peripheral vessels under the convenient term cardio-vasculo-renal disease, it is no exaggeration to say that about one-half of all deaths are due to this cause. The statistics of the Metropolitan Life Insurance Company show that 600,000 people die of heart disease in the United States every year, and that 1 out of every 3 of the population living at the age of ten years will succumb to organic disease of the heart. The incidence of heart disease, as indicated by mortality statistics, has been steadily rising. One reason for this is the increased life span. The average duration of human life in the United States in 1790 was about thirty years, whereas in 1947 it was sixty-five years for white men and seventy-and-a-half years for white women (White). As we grow older our coronary arteries get narrower, just as our hair grows gray or even white. These are perhaps natural processes, jsut as death is a natural process, a fact which it might be well at times for the physician to admit.

It might appear rational to discuss diseases of the heart in relation to the three main anatomical elements of which the heart consists, namely the endocardium, the myocardium, and the pericardium. There are, however, five main organic diseases which demand attention, and which do not neces-

sarily respect anatomical boundaries. These are: (1) *rheumatic heart disease*, (2) *bacterial endocarditis*, (3) *coronary artery occlusion*, (4) *hypertensive heart disease*, and (5) *congenital heart disease*. Of these much the commonest are hypertensive heart disease and coronary artery occlusion; then comes rheumatic heart disease; very much less common are bacterial endocarditis and congenital heart disease. I have not given actual figures, because these vary so widely in different countries and even in different parts of the same country, as can be seen from the table on page 276 in Paul White's book. Syphilis used to be ranked with the important causes of heart disease, but modern therapy has completely changed the picture. When the big five have been discussed, we shall turn to miscellaneous lesions of the endocardium, myocardium and pericardium.

We have been speaking of organic heart disease. It must be remembered, however, that no organ is influenced to so marked a degree by nervous stimuli and what are commonly referred to as the emotions. As my colleague, Dr. Allen Walters, has pointed out, the simple every day words of our language testify to the truth of this statement. We say that a person is heavy-hearted, hard-hearted, heartless, good-hearted, that his heart aches with loneliness, flutters with alarm, or stops with fear. Although cardiac symptoms may have an emotional rather than an organic basis, we are concerned in this place primarily with structural changes.

RHEUMATIC DISEASE OF THE HEART

The etiology and the general pathology of rheumatic fever have already been discussed in the chapter on Bacterial Infections (p. 264). There we saw that the causal agent is Group A hemolytic streptococci which sensitize the fibrous tissues in many parts of the body, uniting with connective tissue protein to form an antigen. This in turn excites the formation of specific antibodies, and the ensuing antigen-antibody reaction results in the focal allergic necrosis with accompanying cellular response characteristic of the collagen diseases, which have been discussed in the chapter on the Intercellular Substance and its Reactions. Rheumatic fever is therefore not a simple streptococcal disease like scarlet fever, because usually no bacteria can be demonstrated in the blood or the lesions, and an interval of from ten to fourteen days elapses between the initial throat infection and the development of rheumatic fever. It is an allergic response to the streptococcus and its products. This response is accompanied by changes in the plasma proteins, particularly hyperglobulinemia, first of the alpha and later of the gamma globulins. The C-reactive protein which precipitates with the carbohydrate of pneumococci is contained in the alpha globulin, and is high in the acute stage, a feature of great diagnostic value.

The heart is a pump, and as impairment of the valves of a pump will wreck its efficiency, it is natural that attention should have been focussed on rheumatic disease of the valves. Rheumatism, however, is a pancarditis, an infection of the fibrous tissue of all parts of the heart (endocardium, myocardium, and pericardium), nor does the aorta escape. The characteristic pathological lesion, the Aschoff nodule, is seen in most typical forms in the myocardium, but lesions sufficiently distinctive to be recognized occur in the cardiac valves, pericardium, synovial membrane, periarticular tissues, skin, etc. The damage is primarily to the supporting tissues, *i.e.*, collagen and elastic tissue. The first change is fibrinoid degeneration, followed later by actual necrosis. The fibrinoid material of this and other collagen diseases appears to be, at least in part, fibrin deposited from the blood, as can be shown by the use of fluorescein-labelled anti-serum against human fibrin (see Fig. 44, page 87). Exudation characterizes the early stages, proliferation the later, and finally fibrosis. In the valves this leads to postinflammatory adhesions and contraction with accompanying stenosis or incompetence, in the myocardium it leads to scarring, and in the pericardium to adhesions. Rheumatism may lick the joints, especially in children, but it certainly bites the whole heart. It is the valvular rather than the myocardial damage which is the chief threat to the patient.

Rheumatic heart disease is predominantly a disease of childhood and youth. Probably more than 70 per cent of the cases occur before the age of twenty, the peak of onset being between the ages of five and ten. Acute rheumatic fever may also be seen in the *adult*, about 50 per cent of such cases occurring in the third decade (Pader and Elster). Acute migratory polyarthritis is more frequent in the adult than acute carditis. As the disease has a decided tendency to recur, there may (or may not) be a history of previous attacks in childhood. A correct diagnosis is more difficult in the adult, because the condition may be confused with other forms of arthritis, such as early rheumatoid arthritis and acute gout. A raised C-reactive protein in the serum, although non-specific, is of great diagnostic help. An estimation of the antistreptolysin-O titer is valuable in differentiating rheumatic fever from other arthritides, as a raised titer demonstrates an antecedent streptococcal infection.

Rheumatic fever is an acute disease with a decided tendency to recur. The patient may die from heart failure: (1) during the first acute phase, (2) during a relapse, or (3) as a result of the effects of the infection on the valves. The great majority of cases recover.

Valvular Lesions.—By far the commonest valvular defect resulting from rheumatic fever is mitral stenosis. In the aortic valve there may be a moderate degree of incompetence (never so complete as in the syphilitic form) or, more rarely, stenosis which years later may take the form of so-called calcific sclerosis. The lesions of the valves on the left side are more extreme owing to the greater strain on those valves. The mitral valve suffers more frequently in women, the aortic valve in men. The reason for this is not known. If the valve ring, to which the cusps are attached and which is really the proximal part of the valve, be examined microscopically, all four valves will be found to be involved in most cases (Gross and Friedberg). In the mitral and aortic valves the process is usually progressive, less often in the tricuspid, and least in the pulmonary, so that in the two latter gross lesions are correspondingly rare. Infection seems to begin in the valve rings, although the pri-

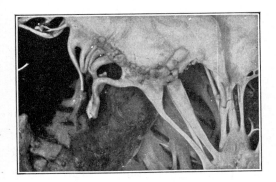

FIG. 236.—Rheumatic endocarditis. A bead-like row of vegetations runs along the line of contact of a cusp of the mitral valve.

mary focus in the case of the mitral is probably the wall of the auricle, and in the case of the aortic the root of the aorta. Infection may readily spread between the mitral, aortic and tricuspid rings by way of the intervalvular fibrosa and the septum fibrosum. The close proximity of a fibrous pericardial wedge to most of the valve rings favors spread of infection from pericardium to valves. It must be understood that the rings may show microscopic lesions although the cusps remain free.

The essential lesion in rheumatic endocarditis is the presence of rheumatic nodules in the endocardium of the valves. The condition, however, is a valvulitis, not merely an endocarditis. This leads to a diffuse thickening of the cusps. An additional although not essential feature is the formation of rheumatic vegetations. These are tiny bead-like warty (verrucose) nodules arranged in a row along the margin of contact (not the free margin) of the cusps, and therefore on their proximal aspect. (Fig. 236.) They consist of platelet thrombi deposited on the raw surface which results from trauma to the endothelium of the valve along the line of contact. This trauma is greatest on the left side of the heart where pressure is highest, but when mitral incompetence develops the pressure on the right side also rises, so that if the infection recurs vegetations will be formed on the tricuspid valve. They are firm and adherent, so that they are not detached by the heart's action. For this reason embolic phenomena are not seen in rheuma-

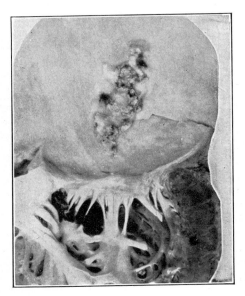

FIG. 237.—Healed rheumatic lesion in auricle. (Boyd, *Pathology for the Physician.*)

tic endocarditis. When they are rubbed off, the underlying surface is raw. The mural endocardium may also be involved. On the posterior wall of the left auricle just above the mitral valve there may be a rough thickened patch which becomes scarred later, and may form a nidus for Streptococcus viridans in subacute bacterial endocarditis. This is often called the *MacCallum patch*, (Fig. 237).

The *microscopic picture* is that of a valvulitis as well as an endocarditis. Many new vessels have been formed in the thickened valve, and inflammatory cells are grouped in relation to these vessels. These are the same cells which constitute the Aschoff nodule, of which the most characteristic is the large multinucleated Aschoff cell, but the arrangement is more diffuse and less distinctive than it is in the myocardium. In the early cases the lesion may take the form of a palisade of cells set at right angles to the surface along the contact edge of the valve. Edema, a marked feature of the inflammatory lesion, accounts for much of the swelling of the valve. There is fibroblastic proliferation, followed later by the production of fibrous tissue. Meanwhile the endothelium covering the cusps degenerates, particularly along the the line of closure, and is soon lost. Platelets are deposited on the raw surface together with a certain amount of fibrin, and it is these which form the vegetations. Fibroblasts and capillaries invade the vegetations, and these become converted into granulation tissue and organized, so that finally they blend with the thickened valve and become indistinguishable. The inflammation is not confined to the valves, for the endocardial lining of the left auricle may show the same type of lesion. In the acute stage there is roughening and in the chronic stage thickening of the surface lining. The chordæ tendineæ may contain Aschoff nodules, and the subsequent fibrosis causes shortening of these cords which is so marked a feature of mitral stenosis. In old lesions of the mitral valve the cusps show gross vascularity, the principal vessels being small thick-walled arteries or arterioles of musculo-elastic type. This vascularity may be regarded as one of the stigmata of rheumatic fever.

The consequences of all this are fatal to the health and efficiency of the valve. During the acute stage the inflamed edges of the cusps adhere together, and with the onset of fibrosis these adhesions become very firm, so that the cusps cannot open as they should, and there is narrowing or stenosis of the valves, both mitral and aortic. The new fibrous tissue makes the cusps rigid, and its contraction both in the cusps and in the chordæ tendineæ still further aggravates the stenosis so that the mitral opening may appear as a mere slit or button hole, or as a rigid funnel when viewed from the auricular aspect. It may be said with reasonable assurance that every case of true mitral stenosis is rheumatic in origin. Calcification of the injured cusps is common. It attains its most extreme form in the aortic valve of men over middle age in the lesion known as *calcified nodular aortic stenosis*.

Myocardial Lesions.—The typical myocardial lesion is the *Aschoff nodule*, which is fully described in Chapter 12. There is little to be seen in the gross appearance of the muscle in an acute case except a dilatation of the left ventricle, but tiny white specks may be seen under the endocardium of the left ventricle and left auricle. These are the Aschoff bodies. They are scattered through the fibrous tissue of the myocardium, most

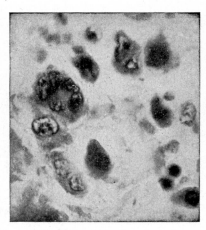

Fig. 238.—Large multinucleated Aschoff cells. × 1100

abundant at the base of the interventricular septum, numerous in the left auricle, not so common on the right side. They are submiliary in size, oval or lemon-shaped, and consist of a central necrotic, reticulated area, lymphocytes, plasma cells, and the characteristic large multinucleated *Aschoff cells*. (Fig. 238). They are usually found in the adventitial coat of medium-sized arteries. The so-called *Anitschkow myocyte* is often found in large numbers in the cardiac lesions although not in rheumatic lesions elsewhere. It is a cardiac histiocyte which in inflammation shows increased cytoplasm, a highly characteristic serrated bar of chromatin in the center of the nucleus, and fibrils radiating from the bar to the periphery. (Fig. 240). For a detailed account of the finer features of the Aschoff body the paper by Gross and Ehrlich should be consulted, in which will be found a description of the various stages of the life cycle through which the lesion passes. Fibroblasts are abundant and lay down collagen fibers, which replace the inflammatory lesion when the infection has died down. This may not happen for a long time, and Aschoff bodies have been found a number of years after the attack of rheumatic fever. As a result of the inflammation there is a varying degree of myocardial destruction, sometimes very great. The end-result is scarring. As the Aschoff lesion usually lies alongside a blood vessel, so the rheumatic

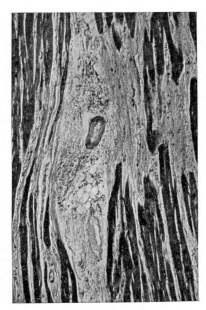

Fig. 239.—Healed Aschoff body. × 50.

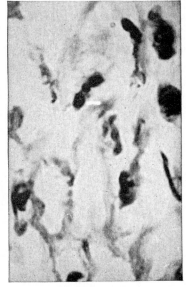

Fig. 240.—Anitschkow cells. × 750. (Boyd, *Pathology for the Physician.*)

scar often is at the side of or surrounds a small artery. (Fig. 239).

Aschoff nodules may not be found, for they are present in only about 80 per cent of cases. There may be a diffuse type of lesion instead of the circumscribed nodule. This is especially common in the wall of the left auricle, and the damage it causes may be responsible for subsequent auricular fibrillation. Moreover the Aschoff nodule is merely the productive feature of rheumatic pathology. The exudative feature, though less marked in the myocardium than in the joints, is also important. The inflammatory edema, which is transient, no doubt interferes temporarily with the conduction bundle, and is responsible for the temporary functional disturbances which electrocardiographic studies show to be present in over 90 per cent of cases of rheumatic fever.

Interest in the Aschoff lesions of the myocardium has been reawakened by the opportunity provided by the removal of biopsy specimens from the left atrial appendage in the course of operations on the mitral valve. The proportion of active lesions varies considerably in the reports of different workers. Clark and Anderson in 78 cases operated on in the Toronto General Hospital found Aschoff granulomas in 50 per cent of cases,

and basophilia (metachromasia with methylene blue) probably due to sulfated mucopolysaccharides, even more frequently. In 10 of the cases no lesions were found. The average age of the patients was thirty-six years, the incidence of the granulomas varying inversely with the age.

What is the significance of active rheumatic lesions in the absence of all clinical and laboratory evidence of activity? Two possibilities suggest themselves. (1) The rheumatic process may have been continuously active in the tissues, although subclinical. (2) The lesions may be due to recrudescences of the process dependent on periodic reinfection, such recrudescences becoming less frequent with the advancing years. In view of the fact that in one series of biopsies half the cases had no history of rheumatic fever, yet active lesions in all stages of development were present in 64 per cent of cases, it would seem that "rheumatic carditis is mainly subclinical, and that acute attacks of rheumatic fever are rare episodes in the course of the disease." (Lannigan). When the frequency of occurrence of Aschoff bodies in the left atrial appendage obtained at the time of commissurotomy is compared with the nature and length of the clinical course before operation, it becomes apparent that the presence of Aschoff bodies is an indication of a progressive and acute course of rheumatic heart disease, just as atrial fibrillation is, in general, a reflection of the chronicity of severe rheumatic heart disease (Dalldorf and Murphy).

Pericardial Lesions.—Rheumatic fever is the commonest cause of acute pericarditis. The acute stage presents little that is characteristic; it is merely an acute serofibrinous inflammation of a serous membrane. The fluid exudate is small in amount, only a few ounces, and is serous, never purulent. The chief element is the fibrin which is deposited on both surfaces of the pericardium giving it a shaggy or "bread-and-butter" appearance, as if two slices of buttered bread had been stuck together and then pulled apart. Even where no fibrin can be seen the natural gloss of the membrane is lost, but this may have to be looked for carefully.

In the *microscopic* picture any rheumatic lesions are apt to be hidden by the acute inflammatory reaction, but an occasional Aschoff body may be found in the subendothelial tissue. The surface endothelium is cast off, successive layers of fibrin are laid down, and this becomes organized by the invasion of new vessels and fibroblasts. The inflammatory cells are mostly lymphocytes and plasma cells with only an occasional polymorphonuclear leukocyte. The inflammation extends through the subpericardial fat down to the heart muscle. From this it may be realized how widespread and continuous are the lesions in rheumatic carditis; they may be traced from the pericardium to the myocardium, to the papillary muscles, and along the chordæ tendineæ to the valves themselves.

The *after-effects* vary. There may be merely one or two opaque white patches of thickened epicardium known as *milk spots*. If absorption of the exudate is less complete there may be numerous adhesions. Finally there may be a completely *adherent pericardium*. Calcification of the lesions may occur, so that stony plates are formed on the heart. It is not, however, the intrapericardial adhesions which are of supreme importance to the future welfare of the heart, but those which are extrapericardial in nature, adhesions, that is, of the parietal pericardium to the mediastinal tissues and the chest wall.

These are always associated with intrapericardial adhesions, and it is they which endanger the functional power of the heart.

Aortic Lesions.—The fibrous tissue of the aorta suffers in common with the fibrous tissue of the heart, so that Aschoff bodies or more diffuse lesions may be found in the adventitia. Although scars of the media have been described it is doubtful if these lesions ever weaken the wall sufficiently to produce an aneurysm, thus differing from the similar but more extensive and destructive lesions of syphilis.

Relation of Symptoms to Lesions.—The *endocardial* symptoms or rather signs of rheumatic heart disease are the cardiac murmurs. The *mitral systolic murmur* is due to mitral regurgitation, which in turn is due to myocardial weakness and dilatation of the auriculo-ventricular ring. The *mitral diastolic murmur*, on the other hand, is valvular in origin, and is due to the stiffness of the cusps and the stenosis of the opening. The intensity of the murmur depends on the power of contraction of the auricle, and as this becomes weaker in the late stages, so the murmur may grow faint. Other features of the clinical picture of mitral stenosis are discussed on page 483. *Aortic incompetence* with its *diastolic murmur* is due to retraction of the cusps and not to myocardial weakness, thus differing from mitral incompetence. Aortic stenosis due to rheumatism is uncommon. The symptoms of cardiac failure are due in the main to valvular disease. The *myocardial* effects may be acute or chronic. In the acute stage there may be death due to ventricular failure. In the chronic stage auricular fibrillation develops, owing to the degenerative lesion blocking the path of the impulse so that it goes around in a circle, and the pulse becomes totally irregular. The chief *pericardial* symptom is pain, just as the chief sign is a friction rub. *Pain* is often absent, though friction may be well marked. The *friction rub* is due to the rough surfaces rubbing together, but it is probable that some degree of tension and stretching is necessary before pain is produced, as is the case with pleural pain.

Rheumatoid Heart Disease.—Before leaving rheumatic heart disease, a few words may be devoted to what has been called rheumatoid lesions of the heart, including the aorta. This is a difficult and confused subject. It may be considered under two not necessarily related headings: (1) cardiac lesions of rheumatoid arthritis, and (2) carditis and aortitis of ankylosing spondylitis.

Rheumatoid Arthritis.—In a considerable number of cases of rheumatoid arthritis granulomatous and fibrinoid necrotic lesions may be found in the pericardium, myocardium, valves, and even in the coronary arteries (Handforth and Woodbury). Coalescence of a number of these granulomas may give a picture which may be mistaken for the lesions of rheumatic fever, but there is an absence of the Aschoff bodies and other hall marks of that disease. The lesions present a necrotic center surrounded by a zone of cellular collagenous tissue with a strong tendency to a radial arrangement, the cells being mostly of large mesechymal type, together with fibroblasts, lymphocytes and plasma cells (Cruickshank). There may be large non-bacterial vegetations on the valves. Both rheumatic fever and rheumatoid arthritis may be regarded as allergic reactions in connective tissue, the former specific in character, the latter probably non-specific. The clinical picture in rheumatoid disease may be one of pericarditis, of heart block due to a lesion of the conduction system, and so on.

Ankylosing Spondylitis.—Much rarer and more puzzling is the carditis and aortitis which may complicate ankylosing spondylitis, also known as rheumatoid spondylitis or Marie-Strümpell disease. This is a rheumatoid condition of the joints of the vertebral column and sacroiliac joints ending up with ankylosis (page 1282). Its relation to characteristic lesions of the aortic valve and aorta has only been recognized in recent years. The chief clinical feature is aortic regurgitation, but in addition there may be cardiac enlargement, interference with conduction due to atrioventricular block, substernal pain, and finally congestive heart failure. The changes are concentrated at the root of the aorta (Fig. 743, p. 1284). The *principal lesions* are: (1) dilated incompetent aortic valve; (2) shortened, thickened aortic valve cusps with rounded margins; (3) a dilated aorta with the intima wrinkled, thickened and covered with pale plaques; (4) patchy destruction of the elastica of the media with replacement of fibrous tissue; (5) endarteritis obliterans of the vasa vasorum of the tunica externa; (6) absence of any significant damage to the other valves (Toone *et al.*). All of these features without exception are also characteristic of syphilitic aortitis and valvulitis, yet in none of the reported cases has there been any suggestion of syphilis.

Smythe points out that two distinct fibrous rings can be distinguished at the root of the aorta: (1) a "superior ring" of the aortic valve, from which are suspended the valve cusps and the walls of the sinuses of Valsalva; (2) the annulus fibrosus of the valve, which lies at a lower level and forms a sleeve surrounding the attachment of the cusps. Of the three major causes of insufficiency of the aortic valve, in syphilis there is an aortitis which spreads down to and destroys the superior ring, leaving the annulus fibrosus little affected; in ankylosing spondylitis it is the region below the superior ring which is affected, with dilatation of the sinuses of Valsalva and the annulus fibrosus; in rheumatic heart disease the aortic insufficiency is due to destruction of the cusps themselves. The lesion in spondylitis is nearly always sharply localized to the root of the aorta, in this respect differing fundamentally from syphilitic aortitis; very occasionally it may be more diffuse.

BACTERIAL ENDOCARDITIS

In the continually changing picture of disease it would be difficult to name a condition which has altered its appearance more completely in recent years than bacterial endocarditis. It used to be a malady in which the heart was beating muffled marches to the grave, in quick time in the acute form, with a slower but just as deadly rhythm in the subacute variety. Now, thanks to antibiotics, it has become a curable disease, although with provisos and reservations, which will be discussed later. Early cases can be aborted, later ones controlled or cured. This as Maxwell Finland remarks, is one of the great triumphs of antibiotic and chemotherapy.

The disease, although frequently, indeed usually, preceded by rheumatic heart disease, presents a curious contrast to that condition. The etiology is obvious and not open to debate. The infecting micro-örganisms are present in enormous numbers, the lesions are primarily in the valves without diffuse involvement of the heart and other tissues as in rheumatic infection, the vegetations are strikingly different in the two conditions, whilst embolism is all-important in the one but not the other.

A sharp distinction has been drawn in the past between the acute and subacute forms of bacterial endocarditis. The importance of this distinction has rather faded, and more emphasis is laid on the infecting agent. It is, however, still convenient to speak of acute and subacute varieties.

Subacute Bacterial Endocarditis.—The subacute is more important than the acute form because it is considerably commoner, it is more insidious in onset and therefore more difficult to recognize in time to prevent irreparable damage, and it is a continual threat to valves previously damaged by rheumatic infection.

Etiology.—As a rule the infection attacks previously damaged valves. An active or healed rheumatic lesion is present in from 75 per cent (Gross and Fried) to 90 per cent of cases. A congenital bicuspid aortic valve is a predisposing condition. In a minority of cases the valves were previously healthy.

In about 95 per cent of cases the infecting organism is *Streptococcus viridans*, so that the condition is sometimes called streptococcus viridans endocarditis. The organism is of low virulence for animals; *the fatal issue seems to be due to the failure of the immunological forces rather than to the virulence of the germ.*

The probable *source of infection* is the mouth and throat. Transient bacteriemia, mostly with *S. viridans*, is common after tooth extraction and tonsillectomy, especially when the gums are infected. Even biting on hard candies will cause an immediate blood infection in cases of pyorrhea. It is easy to understand how a valve damaged by rheumatism or by a congenital defect may be attacked by these circulating organisms. They grow on and destroy the valve because there is no adequate defence, for the blood cells rush past like water from a bath tap.

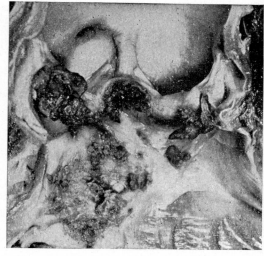

FIG. 241.—Subacute bacterial endocarditis. The friable vegetations, the mural spread, and the old thickening of the aortic cusps are all very characteristic.

There are no capillaries through which the blood can trickle slowly, with the leukocytes sticking to the walls and passing into the tissues. This is how it is that a relatively harmless organism can grow in a situation exposed to the full force of the blood, and yet remain unharmed, going on to kill the patient.

Lesions.—The lesions may be divided into three groups: (1) cardiac, (2) embolic, and (3) general.

1. The *cardiac lesions* are mainly *valvular;* myocardial and pericardial lesions do not play a prominent part as they do in rheumatic disease of the heart. It seems probable that the infection is implanted on the surface of the injured valve, rather than carried into its substance by newly formed vessels. The mitral valve is most often involved, the aortic valve coming next. Infection of the pulmonary valve is very rare.

The lesions are proliferative rather than destructive, but occasionally large portions of the cusps are destroyed as in the acute ulcerative form. The characteristic lesion takes the form of large friable, polypoid vegetations, very different from the tiny firm vegetations of rheumatic endocarditis. (Fig. 241.) They originate along the line of contact (proximal aspect of the cusp), but may

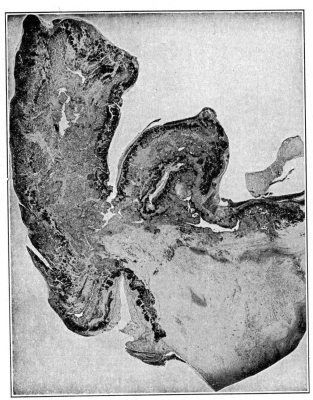

Fig. 242.—Subacute bacterial endocarditis. Large vegetation on thickened valve with masses of bacteria on the surface. × 6.6.

cover the valve. At autopsy part of the valvular lesion may be calcified, showing that there have been attempts at healing. A highly characteristic feature is a tendency for the vegetations to spread on to the mural endocardium. This may be from the mitral valve to the wall of the left auricle or the chordæ tendineæ which may be weakened and rupture, or from the aortic valve to the wall of the ventricle. The distribution of the vegetations on the left auricle corresponds with that of the rheumatic lesion (MacCallum patch) in that region.

Microscopically the vegetations are amorphous masses consisting of fused platelets and fibrin. (Fig. 242.) A striking feature is the presence of masses of bacteria on the surface of the vegetations. They are best shown by Gram's stain (Fig. 243), but are quite evident in hematoxylin and eosin preparations. In some cases they are buried beneath a mass of platelets and fibrin; in such cases the blood culture may be negative.

The valve itself is infiltrated by mononuclear cells, which are most numerous at the attachment of the vegetation to the cusp. Larger multinucleated cells not unlike Aschoff cells may be present. There is a remarkable absence of polymorphonuclear leukocytes. No bacteria are found in the substance of the valve where the cells are, and there are no cells among the bacteria. That is the weakness of the situation from the immunological standpoint. Fibroblasts are present in the deeper parts of the lesion, and calcification is not uncommon. There is thus a distinct tendency to repair.

As the plasma is rich in specific antibodies, only those bacteria which are protected by a covering layer of fibrin are able to proliferate. Emboli are sterilized when they break off from the vegetation, and the subsequent infarct is not infected. In the *acute* form of the disease the humoral defence mechanisms are not effective, the bacterial colonies grow apace without any protecting "fibrin um-

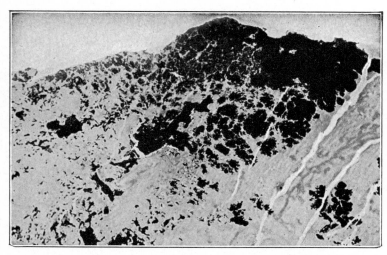

Fig. 243.—Subacute bacterial endocarditis. Bacteria stained black on surface of lesion. In this type of case the blood culture would probably be positive. × 50.

brella," and the embolic lesions are frequently infected.

Myocardial lesions are not common. There may be *Bracht-Wächter lesions*—little collections of polymorphonuclear leukocytes around necrotic material, practically tiny abscesses. In other cases Aschoff bodies may be present. In the *pericardium* petechial hemorrhages are common, but pericarditis is rare.

2. *Embolic lesions* are very common, as the vegetations are friable and easily detached. They are non-suppurative, in contrast to the suppurative embolic lesions of acute ulcerative endocarditis. The petechial hemorrhages in the *skin* and the Osler nodes are usually regarded as embolic in origin, but there is no proof of this. It is more likely that they represent a perivascular reaction to the endotoxin, possibly allergic in nature. Large infarcts due to blocking of medium-sized vessels are seen in the enlarged *spleen* and in the *kidneys*. Many of the more minute lesions appear to be due to toxic necrosis of vessel walls rather than to emboli, although the name embolic is still retained. This is particularly true of the so-called *focal embolic glomerulonephritis* originally described by Löhlein and known as the Löhlein lesion. Only a few glomeruli are involved and usually only a part of a glomerulus. A few loops of the tuft are blocked with an accompanying acute reaction, as a result of which red blood cells appear in the capsular space and pass out into the urine. Although these lesions were commonly believed to be embolic it appears more probable that the blocking of the loops is due to capillary thrombosis and necrosis. Healing occurs owing to the ready access of cells to the irritant, and a homogeneous mass of organized tissue is formed in one segment of the tuft, giving an appearance which is pathognomonic of this disease. In the acute stage small red spots are seen on the surface when the capsule is stripped off, an appearance known as the *"flea-bitten kidney."* Occasionally there is a diffuse glomerulonephritis with renal insufficiency terminating in uremia. In the *central nervous system* there may be *cerebral embolism* and softening in the internal capsule with a resulting hemiplegia, or tiny inflammatory lesions may be scattered through the brain. The *retina* may show pathognomonic transient "canoe-shaped" elliptical hemorrhagic spots with a pale center. *Mycotic aneurysms* may be produced in the cerebral, superior mesenteric, and other arteries.

3. The *general lesions* are of less importance. Some are due to cardiac failure, some to toxemia. Among the latter are cloudy swelling and fatty degeneration of the liver and kidneys, enlargement of the spleen, a

secondary anemia, and in rare cases degenerative lesions of the spinal cord like those of subacute combined degeneration.

The *relationship to rheumatic heart disease* has been investigated by a number of workers. Although bacteria are so abundant in the one disease and lacking in the other, the feeling is that in many cases of subacute bacterial endocarditis the bacterial lesion is superimposed on a heart which is at the time of infection the site of active rheumatic carditis, and that the two diseases are etiologically similar although differing in their tissue response to the infecting agent.

Healing.—Even before the days of chemotherapy and antibiotics it was evident that the tissues made a determined attempt at healing, but the attempt was frustrated by the favored position of the invaders which has been outlined above. Fibroblasts can be seen proliferating in the deeper parts of the lesion and extending towards the zone of bacteria (Fig. 244). There is no reason to doubt that in exceptional cases the bacteria were eradicated and the process of healing successfully completed. There is strong clinical evidence in support of this view. Healing of nonbacterial thrombotic endocardiosis with subsequent calcification before bacterial infection had occurred must have been frequent, and it has even been suggested that some cases of calcific aortic stenosis may have been produced in this manner.

With the advent of modern effective control of the infection and the production of typical lesions in the experimental animal, it has become possible to trace the course of events as they develop. Acute endocarditis itself can now be prevented through sterilization of septic foci, and in both the acute and subacute forms early cases can be aborted, and later cases controlled or even cured. The bacteria disappear, a mass of granulation tissue and hyaline connective tissue surrounds a central core of eosinophilic material, finally becoming converted into a pale hard mass of dense connective tissue, frequently calcified, and covered by a layer of endothelium (Geiger and Durlacher). It is but natural that as a result of effective treatment the incidence and appearance of vegetations on the valves has changed to a striking degree, with a decrease in the

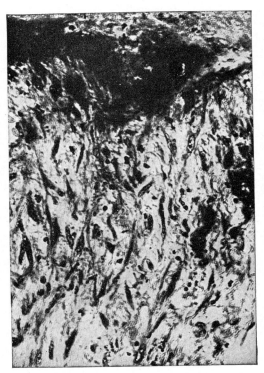

FIG. 244.—Subacute bacterial endocarditis. Fibroblastic proliferation in the deeper part of the lesion. × 350. (Boyd, *Pathology for the Physician.*)

classical type of picture and an increase of nonbacterial thrombotic endocardiosis.

Relation of Symptoms to Lesions.—The four most common findings, present in over 50 per cent of cases, in their order of frequency are cardiac murmurs, fever, anemia and a positive blood culture. Less common, under 50 per cent, are a palpable spleen, petechiae, embolic phenomena, microscopic hematuria, clubbing of the fingers, and Osler's nodes (Newman *et al.*).

As a cause of *continued fever* the disease should be classed with tuberculosis, typhoid fever, sepsis, and undulant fever. If a patient with a history of previous rheumatic fever or the physical signs of mitral stenosis or aortic stenosis or incompetence develops persistent evidence of toxemia such as malaise, weakness and fever, subacute bacterial endocarditis may be diagnosed even in the absence of embolic phenomena and a positive blood culture. The *embolic phenomena* are very varied: there may be crops of petechial hemorrhages in the skin, painful cutaneous nodules (Osler nodes), hemiplegia (cerebral vessels), sudden blindness in one eye (retinal artery), petechial hemorrhages in the retina, each with a white center (Roth's spots), pain in the splenic region, blood in the urine, diarrhea, and vomiting (mesenteric vessels). *Skin petechiae*, often in crops which fade in a few hours, are perhaps not embolic but rather in the nature of a toxic vascular reaction. They are of particular diagnostic value, and the whole body should be searched for them on more than one occasion. The *blood* may show a progressive anemia and a moderate leukocytosis, but often there is leukopenia with relative lymphocytosis.

The *cardiac signs* (murmurs) are due to the vegetations and the valvular destruction. But at first there may be no murmurs, and of course murmurs are no proof of an active endocarditis. Later in the disease the valvular insufficiency leads to cardiac decompensation and enlargement of the heart. Cardiac pain is not uncommon. I know no explanation of this. Death is usually due to cardiac failure, cerebral embolism, uremia, or some intercurrent infection.

The *embolic phenomena* are readily explained by the friable nature of the large soft vegetations. The blood in the urine which is so characteristic a feature is due to the thrombotic glomerular lesions. It is better to speak of red blood cells rather than blood, for the microscope is generally needed for their detection, and as they are not present every day the examination may have to be repeated a number of times. The occasional occurrence of renal insufficiency and uremia is due to a rather uncommon diffuse glomerulonephritis.

Formerly the *prognosis* in fully developed cases was practically hopeless. The heart was indeed beating muffled marches to the grave. The advent of penicillin therapy greatly altered this outlook. When antibiotics are used sufficiently long and in sufficiently large doses the results are remarkably good. In many cases the blood rapidly becomes bacteria-free and the course of the disease is arrested. Much depends on the sensitivity of the strain of infecting streptococci to penicillin. With modern thera-

peutic resources early diagnosis is essential, and this may be a task of great difficulty, so gradual, insidious and sneaking is the development of the disease in many cases. In one series over 60 per cent of cases had evidently been infected for more than 6 months before a correct diagnosis was made (Christie). Even when all the bacteria are finally killed, the patient may be left with badly damaged valves, and he may suffer from congestive heart failure and other cardiac complications.

Acute Bacterial Endocarditis.—This is a group, a good deal less common than the preceding form, in which an acute destructive process is caused by pyogenic cocci which produce suppurative lesions not only in the valves but also in the organs where emboli lodge. As the name implies, the course of the disease can be measured in weeks, while that of the subacute form before the days of antibiotic therapy was a matter of many months or even a year or two. The chief bacteria responsible are *Staphylococcus aurens*, *Streptococcus haemolyticus*, pneumococcus, and occasionally gonococcus. Staphylococcal endocarditis has become much commoner of late, and it carries a very high mortality owing to the resistance of the organism to antibiotic therapy.

The two chief *gross features* of the valvular lesions are the very large, exuberant, friable vegetations and the marked destruction, so that a cusp may be perforated or largely ulcerated away and the chordae tendinae destroyed. The mitral and aortic valves are affected with equal frequency, and the tricuspid often suffers. Endocarditis of the tricuspid alone occurs in heroin addicts who develop staphylococcal septicemia from contaminated intravenous injection of the drug. In recent years abscesses of the valve rings have been found in a high percentage of cases (Shelden and Golden). They appear to arise from mycotic aneurysms in the valve rings, and often represent the only persistent focus of infection. Antibacterial agents which control the infection on the valves do not penetrate to the valve ring abscess. Two or even three valves may show the lesions of acute endocarditis, owing to spread of infection from one ring to another (Fig. 245). The *microscopic picture* of the lesions of the valve

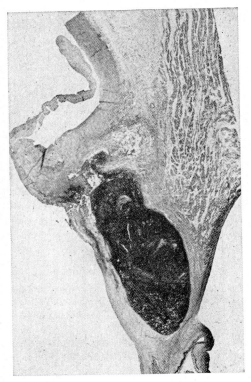

Fig. 245.—Abscess involving both aortic and mitral rings partly filled with laminated thrombus. The abscess has ruptured through mural endocardium beneath aortic leaflet (left center) Phloxine-methylene blue, $\times$ 6.5. (Sheldon and Golden, courresy of Circulation.)

is one of acute suppuration, the cusps being crowded with polymorphonuclear leukocytes.

As the infecting bacteria are pyogenic, it follows that the embolic lesions are suppurative in character, and before the days of antibiotics multiple abscesses were found in the skin, myocardium, brain and kidneys. These lesions are becoming only of historic interest as the result of modern therapy, although unfortunately history has a habit of repeating itself, as we are seeing in the case of staphylococcal infections.

CORONARY ARTERY DISEASE

The convenient but somewhat ambiguous term coronary artery disease really connotes disease or malfunction of the myocardium due to an insufficient supply of blood from the coronary arteries, *i.e.* myocardial ischemia, which may be absolute or relative. This may give rise to the clinical syndromes of (1) *coronary occlusion*, or (2) *acute coronary insufficiency* with its accompanying *angina pectoris*. In addition to these two acute events there may be (3) *arteriosclerotic heart disease*, a chronic slowly progressive condition presenting a very different clinical picture.

Coronary Occlusion.—The term occlusion signifies a sudden complete stoppage of the blood flow in a main coronary artery or one of its branches. Although the final block is sudden, the way has usually been paved by processes of a more gradual character. Coronary occlusion is one of the most important and challenging processes which the medical student has to study. It is important, because many of us are certain to suffer from the condition, and it is challenging because of the various problems which, as we shall presently see, still remain to be solved.

Pathogenesis.—Three things may happen when one of the larger branches of the coronary arteries is occluded: (1) The patient may die immediately. By far the commonest cause of sudden death is cardiac failure; indeed it is the only thing which will kill a person *instantaneously*. The commonest cause of sudden cardiac failure is coronary occlusion. (2) He may linger for a few hours or days. (3) In many cases he recovers, at least for a time. Death from coronary occlusion is common among doctors and other professional men. Deaths from coronary disease appear to be increasing in frequency. The figures in round numbers for the United States were 28, 000 in 1930, 101,000 in 1940, 114,000 in 1942, and 333,757 in 1949. The corresponding figures for England and Wales were 1,900 in 1926, 25,000 in 1945, and 33,000 in 1947.

Complete occlusion of a coronary artery may be produced in a variety of ways. (1) *Atherosclerotic narrowing* of the vessel with complete obstruction of the lumen. (2) *Hemorrhage into an atheromatous plaque.* (3) *Rupture of such a plaque* into the lumen. (4) *Thrombosis* in an already atheromatous artery. Patients with ischemic heart disease are known to have *hypercoagulability of the blood.* Rare causes are (5) syphilitic aortitis sealing the mouths of the coronaries and (6) an embolus from a vegetation on the aortic valve. When an embolus blocks a main coronary artery, death occurs with dramatic suddenness. Occasionally syphilitic arteritis of the coronary artery may cause occlusion. At the site of the atheromatous plaque numerous lymphocytes are sometimes present in the adventitia. This appearance must not be mistaken for the perivascular cellular infiltration characteristic of syphilis. Of these various causes by far the most important is atherosclerosis, with or without an added thrombosis. The coronary arteries share in the general atherosclerosis of old age. As Paul White remarks, one of our difficulties is to decide when the natural process of aging stops and disease begins. In young adults, however, the coronaries may be the only vessels affected, the condition being much more common in men than in women. Dock points out that the intima of the coronaries lying in the epicardium is much thicker than that of any artery of similar caliber elsewhere in the body, and that this is much more pronounced in the male, being present even in infants. This anatomical peculiarity may have some etiological significance. Up to the menopause, women develop coronary thrombosis far less often than men, but later in life the incidence becomes similar, suggesting some sex hormone influence.

Atheroscolerosis.—Atherosclerosis or atheroma is a slow degenerative process, which will be considered in detail in the following chapter in relation to diseases of the arteries. The commonest site is the coronary system of vessels. For our present purpose we may say that the lesion, which is curiously patchy in character, consists of a central soft, pultaceous, lipoid material in the intima of the vessel surrounded by fibrous tissue, the latter representing the "sclerosis." The lipid is the same as that found in the blood plasma, namely cholesterol, cholesterol esters, phospholipid and neutral fat, and in the same ratio. The lesions are most marked in (1) the main stem of the left coronary artery and the first part of its anterior descending branch, (2) the first portion of the right coronary, and (3) the begining of the circumflex branch of the left artery.

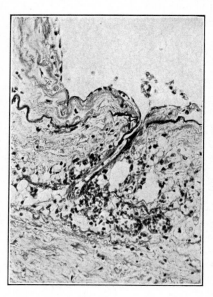

FIG. 246.—Coronary capillary passing from lumen into wall. × 160. (Kindness of Dr. J. C. Paterson).

Heredity.—In some cases heredity seems to play a prominent part in the pathogenesis. The occasional marked familial character of the condition certainly points to the operation of a genetic factor.

Vascularization.—Penetration of the atheromatous lesion by new capillaries can be demonstrated in a large proportion of the cases. These new vessels may come from the lumen of the vessel or from the adventitial and periadvential vessels. There is a marked difference of opinion as to the relative frequency of these two sources, and, as we shall see presently, the question is not merely an academic one. Paterson, to whom we are indebted for first drawing attention to the subject and its significance, considers that the new capillaries come mainly from the lumen, (Fig. 246), while Wartman traces them in large part from the adventitial vessels.

Hemorrhage into an Atheromatous Plaque.—That hemorrhage into the lesion from new capillaries can occur was first demonstrated by Paterson and later by Winternitz. The hemorrhage may result (1) in complete occlusion of the lumen by expansion of the atheroma, or (2) in rupture of the atheroma and subsequent thrombus formation (Fig.

PLATE IV

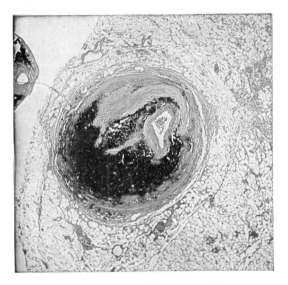

Old Hemorrhage into Atheromatous Plaque.
The hemosiderin is stained intensely with the Prussian blue method.

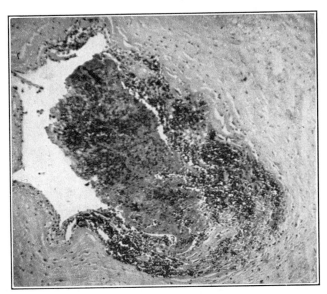

Fig. 247.—Internal hemorrhage and thrombosis of a coronary artery. The thrombus is deposited in close relationship to the hemorrhage. (McManus, *Progress in Fundamental Medicine*, Lea & Febiger.)

247). There is, unfortunately, marked difference of opinion as to the frequency with which intimal hemorrhage is the cause of occlusion of the lumen, either directly or by precipitating thrombus formation. Paterson maintains that this is the cause in 90 per cent of the cases, Wartman in 50 per cent, and Hamilton in 25 per cent. When the coronary arteries of adults who die suddenly are examined by means of preliminary perfusion and fixation followed by dehydration and clearing, hemorrhages are found with remarkable frequency (Durlacher *et al.*). These are nearly always multiple, and vary in age from fresh extravasations to areas of iron-containing pigmentation (Plate IV). Thrombi are more frequently associated with older hemorrhages than with fresh ones. Those who wish to follow up this important subject farther may consult the editorial in the British Medical Journal, April 11, 1959.

Transformation of Organizing Thrombi into Atheromatous Plaques.—This change has been shown by Duguid to occur in many instances. The fibrin of the thrombus is converted into fibrous patches which fuse with the intima and become covered with endothelium. When the thrombus contains large numbers of red blood cells, fatty degeneration occurs,

and this gives a picture indistinguishable from that of the plaque of atherosclerosis. Moreover, vascularization is part of the processes of organization of the thrombus, and hemorrhage may occur from these new capillaries, still further adding to the lipid content of the lesion. There is often clear evidence that the thrombus occluding the coronary artery has been built up slowly, at least in the earlier stages of the process. This matter is discussed more fully in relation to the pathogenesis of atheroma (page 514).

Effort and Stress.—These have been incriminated in the pathogenesis of coronary occlusion, but this is another matter on which there is marked difference of opinion. From the clinical standpoint it is true that *sudden and unwonted exertion* especially in cold weather (shovelling snow, etc.) may be followed by sudden death. Unfortunately in these cases an autopsy is seldom considered necessary, as the patient is assumed to have died of "a coronary." The obvious explanation is the occurrence of intimal hemorrhage owing to the sudden rise in blood pressure. This might be expected if the new capillaries came from minute vessels in the adventitia. Perhaps of greater importance is the demand made by the myocardium for additional

30

blood supply. In the normal heart this demand can readily be met, but when the coronary arteries are markedly narrowed, the call goes unanswered. The question of an ordinary degree of effort is quite another matter. The point is not merely one of academic interest, for compensation is being awarded to so many workmen who have developed coronary thrombosis at work that employers are refusing to hire those in an age category in which this disease might well occur, even though the man was sitting at home or asleep in bed (Hamilton). The *stress* of modern life is frequently blamed for the increasing incidence of coronary occlusion. A woman whom I knew developed a fatal heart attack at the wedding reception of her only daughter. The condition certainly seems to be more common in those exposed to continued tension, such as business executives and surgeons; it is much less common in pathologists.

The question of the relation of coronary heart disease to *moderate* continued physical activity is a different matter. It has been shown to the satisfaction of statisticians that work involving physical exercise may be beneficial rather than harmful, and that Government clerks more often suffer from fatal cardiac infarction than do postmen. "Physical activity of work is a protection against coronary (ischemic) heart disease. Men in physically active jobs have less coronary heart disease during middle age, what disease they have is less severe, and they develop it later than men in physically inactive jobs" (Marris and Crawford).

The question is often asked, but never answered to everyone's satisfaction, as to why atherosclerosis is so much more common in the coronary arteries than in other vessels of similar size. We must remember that with every systole and diastole there is a change in length of the coronaries. To meet this stress we find intimal supports of longitudinal muscle lying in a matrix of connective tissue. These supports are more developed in males than in females, they are the site of lipid accumulation, and they have been blamed for the bad name which the coronary arteries enjoy.

Trauma.—The relation of *trauma* to coronary thrombosis may present a knotty prob-

lem in compensation cases. Many cases have been reported in which a blow over the heart has been followed almost at once by symptoms of thrombosis and infarction. The time sequence in some of these cases has been too striking for it to be purely coincidental. Hemorrhage into an atheromatous intima may be the starting point of thrombosis, and it is reasonable to suppose that a severe blow to the precordia may cause hemorrhage into a weakened intima and thus precipitate thrombosis and infarction.

Mast Cells.—For some time investigators have been interested in the relation, if any, between heparin and mast cells on the one hand and thrombosis and atherosclerosis on the other. Mast cells, which are present in the adventitia of arteries, secrete heparin, which in turn inhibits thrombosis. It is believed that an increase in blood coagulability promoted by deficiency of heparin may be an important factor in the thrombotic tendency of persons with atheroma. Heparin also seems to discourage the development of atheroma. The rabbit, in whom atherosclerosis can readily be induced by feeding cholesterol, has practically no mast cells in the aorta, whereas the rat, which is completely resistant to the production of atheroma by cholesterol feeding, has an abundance of mast cells. From these facts it might be expected that in coronary thrombosis the arteries would be deficient in mast cells. The reverse has proved the case, for instead of a deficiency there is a constant and considerable excess, the highest counts being found in those segments of arteries which were the sites of fresh thrombi (Pomerance). The increase of mast cells is not a reaction to the presence of thrombus, for it is not seen when the thrombus is not of local origin, as in the case of embolus or propagated thrombus. Pomerance considers that the increase in mast cells precedes the thrombosis and is a factor in its pathogenesis. She suggests that there is an inhibition of the normal mechanism of heparin release, and that this accounts for the increase in the number of mast cells. Further work may provide different answers to this difficult question.

Dietary Factors.—The question of the relationship of diet, particularly the lipid elements, to the occurrence of atherosclerosis is

PLATE V

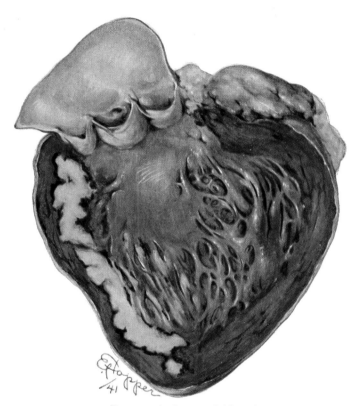

Recent Infarct of Heart

The yellow necrotic tissue in wall of left ventricle is edged by a narrow dark red border.

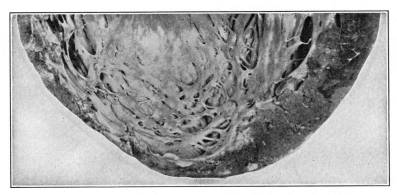

Fig. 248.—Myocardial fibrosis following infarct. The wall of the ventricle at one side and at the apex is markedly thinned.

discussed in connection with the disease in arteries in general. Myocardial infarction due to coronary artery thrombosis and atherosclerosis has been induced in the Rhesus monkey by feeding with a diet high in butter fat and cholesterol (Taylor *et al.*). Many persons have denied themselves butter, eggs, and other pleasant features of the breakfast table for fear of developing coronary occlusion. Such action would appear rather premature at the present time.

Gallbladder Infection.—Myocardial degeneration is often associated with cholecystitis and calculi. Coronary sclerosis and gall stones were both present in the autopsy of John Hunter, who suffered from recurring attacks of angina pectoris. Patients with gallbladder disease may show symptoms of angina or cardiac failure. We do not understand what this means, although we refer vaguely to "referred pain."

Summary.—From this discussion of pathogenesis the truth of the opening statement that the problem of coronary occlusion is a perplexing and challenging one becomes very evident. We may say that acute occlusion is usually due to a combination of coronary atherosclerosis and thrombosis in a person with a genetic predisposition; that the atherosclerosis is caused by a number of factors discussed in the next chapter; that thrombosis is dependent on local factors, one of which may be the presence of mast cells in the adventitia; that hemorrhage from new capillaries into an atherosclerotic patch in the intima is an important factor in the pro-duction of thrombosis in a goodly number of cases; and that the effect of the occlusion on the myocardium will depend largely on the presence or absence of a functionally efficient inherited coronary anastomotic blood supply.

Lesions.—The occlusion is usually in the anterior descending branch of the left coronary about 2 cm. from the commencement. Distal to the occlusion there may or may not be a thrombus. The atheromatous patch may block the lumen so completely that not even the finest probe can be passed along it. The result of acute occlusion, most readily understood when thrombosis completes the occlusion, is the production of a *myocardial infarct*. Of course, if the occlusion causes sudden death there will not be time for an infarct to be produced.

The *area involved* includes the anterior part of the interventricular septum, the apex, and the anterior part of the wall of the left ventricle. The papillary muscles suffer most severely. When the right coronary is occluded the infarct includes the posterior half of the interventricular septum and the posterior part of the wall of the left ventricle, with little or no involvement of the right ventricle. The immunity of the right ventricle to infarction may be due to the fact that the Thebesian vessels open almost entirely into that chamber, so that the wall of the right ventricle can receive blood from this collateral source. The areas are irregular in shape, yellow in color, and often surrounded by a red zone. (Plate V.) The larger areas may undergo softening

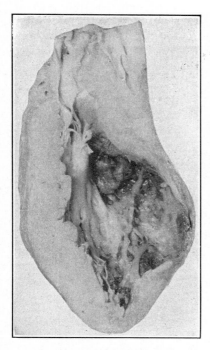

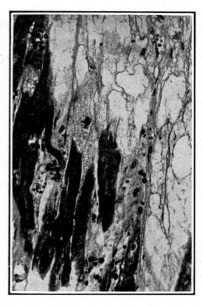

Fig. 250.—Infarct of heart, early stage. The dark material represents normal muscle fibers, the pale areas are degenerated fibers. × 200.

Fig. 249.—Aneurysm of heart showing bulging and thinning of ventricular wall.

(myomalacia cordis), and this may lead to *rupture of the heart*. If the endocardial surface is involved a *mural thrombus* will be formed on the necrotic area, and if the pericardial surface is involved there will be a patch of *pericarditis*. The area of pericarditis is more extensive than the apparent area of infarction. *Embolism*, sometimes fatal, may occur as a result of the mural thrombus becoming detached. There is a double threat of embolism in myocardial infarction, systemic from the mural thrombus and pulmonary from venous thrombosis in the leg which may result from circulatory failure and confinement to bed. Gradually the infarct becomes replaced by fibrous tissue, so that it is represented by a white patch of scar visible both on the endocardial and on the cut surface with corresponding thinning of the wall of the ventricle. Should the patient survive for some time the weakened area will give way and bulge outward, so that an *aneurysm of the heart* is formed with marked thinning of the wall (Fig. 249). This usually involves the anterior wall of the left

ventricle near the apex. In course of time this aneurysm may rupture, causing sudden death. Rupture of the heart may, therefore, be the result of a recent infarct or of a cardiac aneurysm. This is the only way in which a person may die of a broken heart. Sometimes a thrombus will form on an area of scarring, even though there is no recent necrosis. A heart which is the site of an old infarct is usually hypertrophied; in many cases this hypertrophy is not related to hypertension. *Cardiac hypertrophy may be caused by anoxia of the myocardium.* In transposition of the great vessels the coronary arteries arise from the pulmonary artery with resulting myocardial anoxia and marked hypertrophy of the left ventricle.

The *microscopic appearance* of the infarct depends on its age. The sequence of events was determined in the experimental animal by Karsner and Dwyer in 1916, and more recently in the human subject by Kenneth Mallory and his associates. Necrosis is not evident till the end of six hours, when the muscle fibers become hyaline and stain a deeper red with acid dyes. The striations are indistinct and finally lost, the clear out-

PLATE VI

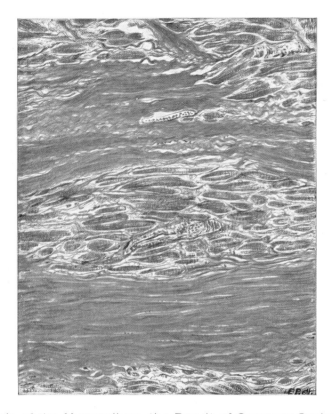

Fibrosis of the Myocardium, the Result of Coronary Occlusion.

The heart muscle is red, the fibrous tissue blue. (Mallory's connective tissue stain.)

line of the fibers are now smudged, the spaces between the fibers are filled with granular debris, and the nuclei disappear. Some of the fibers may become swollen and vacuolated before disintegrating (Fig. 250). In the *first week* there is slight polymorphonuclear infiltration of the necrosed area at the end of twenty-four hours, and by the fourth day this has become marked. Removal of the necrosed tissue begins. In the *second week* this removal is carried out by great numbers of pigment-filled macrophages, which replace the polymorphonuclears. The pigment is partly muscle pigment and partly blood pigment resulting from hemorrhage from greatly distended vessels. New capillaries and fibroblasts grow into the infarcted area. In the *third week* removal of the dead muscle may be completed in small infarcts, though much delayed in large lesions. The fibroblasts begin to form collagen. From the *fourth* to the *sixth week* collagen formation is marked (Plate VI). By the *end of the second month* the process is complete and the infarct is healed. All the dead muscle is replaced by dense scar tissue, and only a few cells and granules of blood pigment remain. (Fig. 251.) The speed of the process varies with the size of the infarct and the state of the remaining circulation.

This is the classical concept, which pictures the infarct as being replaced by granulation tissue and finally by a collagenous scar. Barrie and Urback have called this concept in question. They point out that below a certain critical size the stroma of the infarct does not undergo necrosis, the dead muscle being removed by macrophages without the intervention of polymorphonuclear leukocytes. The original stroma is condensed without a hint of granulation tissue and scar formation. A similar sequence of events is seen at the margin of larger infarcts. In the subendocardial zone a narrow band of myocardial fibers is usually spared from necrosis owing to diffusion of oxygen from the cavity of the ventricle. In this way the conducting fibers are spared, and the likelihood of thrombosis on the surface of the endocardium is much diminished. The central portion of the infarct is invaded by polymorphonuclear leukocytes, but the dead muscle seems to be removed solely by macro-

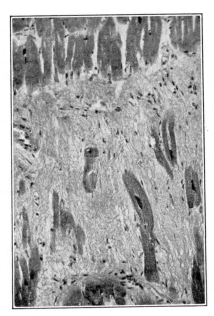

Fig. 251.—Healed infarct of heart. × 140.

phages, and is not replaced by granulation tissue. The entire process seems designed to maintain the status quo of the heart while it continues to function. If this is correct, prolonged bed rest, based on the concept of a slow replacement of the infarct by granulation tissue, may not be as necessary as has been supposed. In any case it would appear as if clinical assessment of cardiac function is of much greater importance in determining the optimum period of rest than are the histological changes.

Disturbance in the chemistry of the muscle cells can be demonstrated before the ordinary histological changes become evident. Thus *succinic dehydrogenase*, one of the most important enzymes in biological oxidation and particularly abundant in the heart, may be reduced in the future infarct as early as two hours after the onset of acute symptoms, and is soon lost completely (Wachstein and Meisel). *Transaminases* are enzymes which transfer amino groups from one amino acid to another. *Glutamic oxaloacetic transaminase* is concentrated to a greater degree in normal heart muscle than in any other tissue. It is therefore of interest to learn that serum transaminase activity in a series of cases of myocardial infarction rose from 2 to 20 times the normal within twenty-four hours, returning to normal levels in from three to six days (LaDue *et al.*). *Loss of glycogen* is the earliest demonstrable microscopic change, which may be apparent in the experimental animal in the course of thirty minutes, long before any recognizable change by routine histological methods (Kent and Diseker). Even as little as 5 per cent total infarction can cause increased activity (Conrad).

The long delay in the recognition of the relation of coronary artery disease to cardiac infarction and to the accompanying clinical picture is one of the mysteries of medical history. Even those great masters of morbid anatomy in the first half of the nineteenth century, Virchow in Berlin and Rokitansky in Vienna, failed to recognize the connection, regarding the myocardial fibrosis and aneurysmal bulging as the result of inflammation. Acute infarcts were considered to be examples of fatty degeneration of the myocardium. Although some of the leaders of German pathology clearly demonstrated the relationship as early as 1880—1882, the profession at large failed to accept this demonstration, now so obvious to everyone. It was not until the early years of the twentieth century that the papers of Herrick (1912) and others finally carried conviction. Now any medical student can recognize the relationship at a glance. Goethe might have used this as an illustration of his great aphorism: "Was man weiss, sieht man." There must be many other relationships which we could see if only we could first know.

In rare cases there may be *infarction without coronary occlusion*. These cases, which are very puzzling, must be attributed to *relative* myocardial ischemia, which may be only temporary. In most of the cases hypertension has been present, a condition in which vasoconstrictor phenomena are common, and in which there is myocardial hypertrophy with a correspondingly increased demand for blood. There may be a temporary fall of the intra-aortic blood-pressure, or failure of the mechanism regulating compensatory dilatation of the coronaries. Finally, the pathologist may have failed to demonstrate occlusion of one of the smaller arteries.

Relation of Symptoms to Lesions.—Parkinson remarks that when a man of advancing years is seized while at rest with severe pain across the sternum, which continues for hours and which is accompanied by shock, you may diagnose coronary occlusion. The chief incidence is between forty-five and sixty years of age. After sixty years the disease is not so common because of increasing anastomoses and vascularity in the myocardium of the left ventricle. Sudden death from extreme atheromatous occlusion of the coronary arteries may occur in the early twenties and thirties, as illustrated by the report of French and Dock on 80 cases in soldiers between the ages of twenty and thirty-six. The *pain* is abrupt in onset; the patient is well one minute and in agony the next. It is usually precordial but may be epigastric, and as there is often slight fever and a moderate leukocytosis, an acute abdominal condition is apt to be diagnosed. Newspaper accounts of death from acute indigestion are examples of coronary occlusion. Sometimes there is no pain. *Dyspnea* is the most constant symptom. The face is ashy pale and bathed in sweat. *Shock* is present, but is not to be explained by any of the current theories for traumatic shock. It is a manifestation of heart failure. There may be *angor animi*, a feeling of impending dissolution. Weak heart sounds, acute pulmonary edema, enlargement of the liver, and albuminuria are common features. There is an *increase in the sedimentation rate*, usually about the fourth or fifth day. A *pericardial friction rub* which is characteristically fleeting is often present. The *prognosis* varies. About one-half die suddenly. Of the remainder about one-half make a complete functional recovery and are able to resume work. The other half develop congestive heart failure or anginal attacks.

The sudden pain, distress, dyspnea, angor animi are due to the heart having received a sudden trauma from the cutting-off of the blood supply to part of the muscle. When any muscle is suddenly deprived of its blood supply as by embolism it goes into a painful spasm. An ordinary muscle can be rested, but the heart cannot afford to stop and rest. Sudden death is generally due to disturbance of the conduction system with ventricular fibrillation or heart block. The leukocytosis is due to the formation of what is practically an aseptic abscess in the heart. The fever is probably in the nature of a protein reaction from the dead tissue. The pericardial friction rub is due to the presence of a patch of aseptic inflammation caused by necrosis of the muscle on the surface of the left ventricle. It is not heard in occlusion of the right coronary artery, as the affected area is on the posterior surface of the heart.

Like the erythrocyte sedimentation rate, the C-reactive protein determination and other nonspecific means of detecting tissue damage, the measurement of the *level of serum transaminase* is merely a method of demonstrating tissue breakdown. Nevertheless this simple spectrophotometric blood test promises to be one of the most useful recent developments in the diagnosis of acute heart attacks, especially in the differentiation of recent infarction from such conditions as pulmonary embolism and infarction. Marked *reduction in the stainable glycogen* occurs within one hour of coronary occlusion in the experimental animal (Yokoyama *et al.*).

Angina Pectoris.—Angina pectoris or sudden pain in the chest is a clinical rather than a pathological entity, the result of *acute coronary insufficiency* which reduces the supply of oxygenated blood to the myocardium to the danger point. The acute insufficiency may be manifested by sudden death, sudden cardiac failure, or angina pectoris. Angina in its typical form differs sharply from the clinical picture of acute coronary occlusion, for the pain in angina comes on as the result of sudden exertion or emotional excitement and goes off when this has passed, it tends to pass down the arms, particularly the left, and there is none of the fever and leukocytosis of infarction of the heart. In many cases, however, the pictures come closer together, and a person may have a number of attacks of angina pectoris and finally die of coronary occlusion. The patient may die in the first attack, or he may have many attacks as did John Hunter, who described one of these in the following vivid words: "As I was walking about the room I cast my eyes on a looking-glass and observed my countenance pale, my lips white, and I had the appearance of a dead man looking at himself."

Two types of pain must be recognized:

(1) The retrosternal pain felt at the cardio-aortic starting-point; (2) the peripheral radiations. If the starting-point of the pain is still open to doubt, the subsequent course of the sensory impressions is perfectly clear. From the heart or the aorta they pass to the cardiac plexus, giving rise to the retrosternal pain. Thence they are carried by the sympathetic fibers through the inferior cervical ganglion to reach the eighth cervical and first and second dorsal segments of the cord, the transmission occurring chiefly on the left side. The pain radiates to the periphery along the nerves arising from these segments. If the excitation is intense the stimulus may pass across the cord and down the right side.

It is generally believed that the pain is due to temporary myocardial ischemia, the attack being brought on by physical exertion or emotional excitement which throw an additional strain on the heart. The ischemia is relative, and may be caused not only by coronary atheroma, syphilitic aortitis, aortic stenosis, etc., but also by cardiac hypertrophy without a corresponding increase in the coronary circulation. It is evident that anginal attacks may finally terminate in cardiac infarction.

Arteriosclerotic Heart Disease.—This is the chronic manifestation of coronary artery disease. Arteriosclerosis is a vascular degeneration characteristic of the later years of life. It appears, indeed to be part of the aging process, although it may also develop in younger age groups. The gradual narrowing of the coronary arteries leads to two changes in the myocardium: (1) atrophy of the muscle fibers, and (2) increase of the fibrous tissue framework. Broad streaks of fibrous tissue may (or may not) be seen running through the muscle. Some writers are of the opinion that the valves share in this process, more particularly the aortic valve, leading to the condition known as *calcific aortic stenosis*. The nature of this lesion, which is regarded by most workers as rheumatic in origin, is discussed on page 486.

The *effect on cardiac function* will depend on the degree of narrowing of the arteries, as well as on the tempo of the process. There may be good compensation for years, and if death occurs from other causes there may never be cardiac symptoms. Sooner or later, however, decompensation may set in, and symptoms of heart failure develop. This is more likely to happen if there is an associated arterial hypertension, as is often the case at this age. At any stage complete occlusion may develop owing to thrombosis or some of the other factors already discussed. An adequate collateral circulation may succeed in compensating for the occlusion, whilst in other cases the result may be a myocardial infarct or sudden death from myocardial ischemia.

Sudden Cardiac Death.—When a person dies suddenly of heart failure (instantaneously or in the course of a few minutes or hours), the cause may lie in the myocardium, the coronary arteries, or the aorta. (1) There may be rupture of the *heart* due either to softening of an infarct or to the formation of an aneurysm of the heart at the site of a scar. Sudden death on exertion may follow the myocardial degeneration of diphtheria. The quickest way to make the heart stop beating is to block the conduction system. (2) *Coronary occlusion* is the commonest cause of sudden cardiac death. The occlusion may be at the mouth of the artery as in syphilitic aortitis, or in the course of the artery as in atheroma. (3) In the *aortic group* may be placed rupture of an aortic aneurysm, some cases of angina pectoris, and aortic incompetence. Finally there remains a group of cases in which the patient dies of sudden heart failure, but no satisfactory cause can be found at autopsy. Such cases may be put down to shock, status lymphaticus, or a visitation from God.

Sudden Death.—A brief note may be allowed here on the subject of sudden death, *i.e.*, death occurring unexpectedly in the course of a few minutes. When called upon to perform an autopsy on such a case it is well to bear seven possibilities in mind: (1) cardiac, (2) pulmonary, (3) abdominal hemorrhage, (4) cerebral hemorrhage, (5) traumatic shock, (6) poisons, and (7) status lymphaticus. Sudden *cardiac* death has just been discussed. Sudden *pulmonary* death may be caused by pulmonary embolism, edema of the glottis, laryngeal diphtheria, and foreign bodies in the pharynx and larynx. Spasm of the glottis is a frequent cause of asphyxia in drowning. In children inhalation of stomach contents may cause fatal spasm of the glottis. The rare cases of death from anaphylaxis may be placed in this group. Fatal *abdominal hemorrhage* may occur into the stomach from a gastric ulcer or a varicose vein at the lower end of the esophagus, or into the adrenals especially in children. In the latter case death is due to acute adrenal insufficiency rather than to loss of blood. Ruptured tubal pregnancy and ruptured abdominal aneurysm may be included here. *Cerebral hemorrhage* may be rapidly fatal if massive enough (into the ventricles or a cerebral tumor) or if into a vital center (medulla). Sudden death may occasionally follow epileptiform seizures. *Traumatic shock* may cause death at once or after a few minutes; the heart stops beating. *Poisons* must be borne in mind if no cause of death can be found. The odor of the gastric contents may indicate acute alcoholism or prussic acid (smell of bitter almonds). The contents of the stomach should be placed in a jar and sealed. *Status lymphaticus* is considered in Chapter 41. Of these varied causes by far the commonest are trauma and cardiac failure. It is they which are likely to result in really sudden death. The others (hemorrhage, etc.) are more apt to bring about death in the course of some hours. In one group of cases of *instantaneous* death, *i.e.*, death in a matter of seconds, not minutes or hours, no lesions may be found in vital organs other than those which in other persons are compatible with good functional capacity. Such cases are probably examples of fatal syncope due to increased irritability of nerve endings and hyperactivity of the reflexes, a physiological state which may be caused by transient undetectable factors (chemical, emotional, etc.) as well as by organic lesions. Most of these cases may be put down to vagal inhibition with sudden cessation of the heart's action.

The *clinical picture* is the natural result of the lesion in the conducting system cutting off the normal impulses from the sino-auricular node, so that the ventricle beats with its own slow rhythm. The pulse accordingly drops to about one-half its usual rate, a condition of *bradycardia*. The chief effect is felt by the *brain*. The mildest form of cerebral disturbance is *dizziness*. In more severe cases there may be attacks of *syncope*, attacks which are fleeting but in which the loss of consciousness is complete. Finally we have the full fledged picture of the *Stokes-Adams syndrome*, with convulsions added to the syncopy, a seizure in which the patient may die. These varied disturbances are all due to cerebral anoxia from ischemia, and there is danger that the cardiac origin of the condition may be overlooked unless the possibility is kept in mind.

Heart Block. — Reference has already been made to the conducting system under General Considerations. Any lesion which interferes with this system in any part of its course may result in heart block. Complete heart block may be caused by inflammatory, vascular, degenerative, neoplastic, traumatic and congenital lesions. In 12 cases where sudden death seemed to be due to a lesion of the conducting tissue, in 3 there was massive myocardial calcification, in 3 myocarditis, in 2 primary cardiac amyloidosis, and in 1 hemorrhage into the atrio-ventricular node (Lumb and Shacklett). A not infrequent cause is extension of an inflammatory or an atheromatous condition of the aortic valve to the bundle in the close neighborhood.

HYPERTENSIVE HEART DISEASE

The four principal forms of heart disease are those due to rheumatic fever, bacterial endocarditis, coronary artery occlusion, and arterial hypertension. The last of these is the commonest. A person with hypertension may live for many years without showing any symptoms. During this time the heart is accommodating itself to the increased work it has to do. As the patient gets older, as the coronary arteries become narrowed, and particularly if the blood pressure continues to rise, the day will come when the myocardium is no longer equal to the strain, and congestive heart failure develops.

The most striking feature is marked *hypertrophy of the left ventricle*, so that when the heart is grasped it feels like a closed fist. The walls are rigid, the heart maintaining its curved form when laid on the table. In the late stages dilatation may be added to the hypertrophy. Strands or patches of fibrous tissue are often scattered through the wall of the left ventricle.

Apart from this fibrosis, which may be minimal in degree, the heart muscle appears normal. The individual fibers are healthy and show no suggestion of degeneration. Why they should fail remains a mystery. "Looking at the heart, one would surmise it to be a more powerful muscular organ, capable of more than a normal amount of sustained work. Actually it has failed to do its work well enough to maintain a circulation capable of sustaining life. Viewed with the fluoroscope after the condition has developed, this powerful-appearing heart may be seen to be contracting with a diminished vigor; the palpating hand may feel a non-forceful tapping impulse in lieu of the expected powerful thrust" (Christian). What seems to be powerful muscle is unable to expel the blood from the heart with any vigor. The pathologist has to accept the fact that in the myocardium morphological appearance does not necessarily correspond with functional capacity.

It is important to realize that hypertension and left cardiac hypertrophy are not necessarily, though usually, associated. The heart may be of normal size with a systolic blood pressure well over 150 mm. ,and on the other hand the left ventricle may be hypertrophied in the absence both of valvular lesions and of hypertension. The probable explanation of the first anomaly is that the increase of pressure has been so gradual that it has thrown no sudden strain on the muscle fibers, whilst in the second case it is possible that the hypertrophy is due to a previous hypertension which was no longer evident at the time of the final illness. And yet perhaps it would be better to speak of *idiopathic cardiac hypertrophy*, thus confessing our ignorance, rather than to invoke a hypertension which has come and gone. Cases are on record where the heart has weighed as much as 800 gm. without evident hypertension or valvular disease.

CONGENITAL HEART DISEASE

A great variety of congenital abnormalities of the heart may occur, some very rare, others incompatible with life, *e.g.*, absence of the heart, ectopia cordis, displacement of the heart in the neck or the abdomen, etc. There may be minor defects such as a lacunar fenestration of the semilunar valves, which are of no functional significance. Only the commoner conditions will be touched on here. For a fuller account the writings of Maude Abbott and the book of Helen Taussig should be consulted.

Etiology.—Until recently nothing was known about the causation of congenital cardiac defects. Whatever goes wrong, it must be before the end of the third month of gestation, because the heart is completely developed by that time. It is now certain that in a certain number of cases the defects are due to infection of the mother with the *virus of German measles*, which can apparently pass through the placental barrier and interfere with early somatic fetal development. The earlier the pregnant woman develops the infection, the more liable is the child to have congenital cardiac defects. In the third month the chances are about 50 per cent, but much higher in an early period. This of course suggests the possibility that other viral infections during the time the fetal heart is developing may produce similar results. Vitamin and other nutritional deficiencies, especially riboflavin and vitamin D, to which the mother may be subjected are also worthy of consideration. When one considers that the heart develops from a simple tube in the course of three weeks of fetal life, that from this tube two separate but communicating systems are evolved by the formation of septa, and that one defect such as pulmonary stenosis may give rise to others, perhaps the wonder is that a normal heart is so common.

The key to most of the defects lies in variations in the formation of the septum which divides the heart into a right and left side. The primitive heart consists of three chambers, auricle, ventricle, and aortic bulb. Separate septa are formed which divide these chambers longitudinally into right and left sides, and subsequently fuse. If anything goes wrong with this fusion, congenital defects will result.

While the septum which divides the aortic bulb into aorta and pulmonary artery is being formed, a spiral twisting occurs so that the pulmonary artery moves forward and to the right, the aorta backward and to the left. If this twisting does not take place the aorta will rise from the right ventricle and the pulmonary artery from the left. This condition is known as *transposition of the great vessels.*

Much commoner is a *deviation of the septum*, nearly always to the right, so that the pulmonary artery is narrower and the aorta wider than normal. In this way pulmonary stenosis is produced. The bulbar septum is now unable to fuse with the ventricular septum, and the root of the aorta is astride the latter so as to arise partly from the left and partly from the right ventricle. A gap remains in the upper or membranous part of the interventricular septum.

Even if the deviation of the bulbar septum is not sufficient to bring the aortic opening astride the ventricular septum, the upper part of that septum will still tend to remain open, for the narrowing of the pulmonary opening raises the pressure within the right ventricle so that the blood tends to flow from it into the left ventricle, thus interfering with the closure of the opening in the interventricular septum. The same holds true for closure of the interatrial septum and the ductus arteriosus which connects the pulmonary artery with the aorta in intrauterine life. It is for this reason that pulmonary stenosis is so often associated with other congenital cardiac defects. Deviation of the septum to the left will cause stenosis of the aortic opening, a much rarer condition.

The all-important feature of congenital heart disease is the possibility of an *intermingling of the blood in the systemic and pulmonary circulations as the result of an arteriovenous shunt*, as can be shown by cardiac catheterization, angiocardiography, and even the use of a radioactive gas. The three common causes of left-to-right shunts are patent ductus arteriosus, atrial septal defect and ventricular septal defect. In all of these the lungs become overloaded with blood. An equally important clinical distinction is between *cases with cyanosis and without cyanosis.* Cyanosis will be caused by a right-to-left venous-arterial shunt, because venous blood then enters the systemic circulation. As the pressure on the left side is normally higher than on the right, special complicating conditions are necessary for the flow to be reversed. By far the most important of these is pulmonary stenosis, in which too little venous blood goes to the lungs and too much goes to the left side of the heart. The flow through a septal defect may originally be from left to right, but when the left ventricle begins to fail the direction of flow may be reversed. It is, therefore, important to differentiate between cyanosis which has been present since birth (blue baby) and cyanosis which has developed only when cardiac failure has set in. Apart from cardiac failure, even the most extreme degree of cyanosis is not associated with edema, a highly characteristic feature.

Congenital defects are points of weakness against bacterial infection. Not infrequently the patient with congenital heart disease dies of subacute bacterial endocarditis. The vegetations may be found on a bicuspid aortic valve, a stenosed pulmonary valve, or at the site of coarctation of the aorta.

At least 90 per cent of the patients with congenital disease of the heart and great vessels fall into one of four groups. These are, in their order of frequency: septal defects, coarctation of the aorta, patent ductus arteriosus, and the tetralogy of Fallot. All of these are amenable to surgical treatment.

Atrial Septal Defects.—Patency of the foramen ovale is the commonest and the least important of all congenital cardiac anomalies. The foramen remains patent in about 25 per cent of normal persons, but, as the opening is usually very small and oblique or valvular, little blood can pass from one side to the other.

A true septal defect due to failure of development is quite another matter. The opening may be very large. I have seen one 5 cm. in diameter in a middle-aged woman, and in such cases there may be a trilocular heart with what amounts to one auricle and two ventricles. The proportion of females to males is four to one. Blood passes so readily from the left side of the heart to the right that both the right auricle and the right ventricle become greatly dilated and hypertrophied. The large volume of blood which is pumped so continuously into the pulmonary artery leads to a remarkable degree of dilatation of that vessel, and atherosclerosis may be marked in it and in its branches. The aorta is small and hypoplastic. Twice as much blood may pass through the pulmonary as through the systemic circulation. For this reason there will be no cyanosis until cardiac failure sets it, and the patient may live from thirty to fifty years. Paradoxical embolism may occur through the large opening in the septum (Fig. 75, page 144). The diagnosis can be made with accuracy from the loud pulmonary systolic murmur caused by blood rushing into the dilated pulmonary artery, the large pulmonary artery shadow and the small aortic shadow in the x-ray film, and marked right axis deviation in a person in fairly good health except for dyspnea.

Lutembacher's Disease.—This is the combination of an *atrial septal defect* with *mitral stenosis.* The latter may be due to a congenital defective development of the valve or to acquired rheumatic heart disease. The combined effect of the two lesions is strikingly different from that produced by either singly. Instead of the distended left atrium of mitral stenosis, it remains small, whereas the right atrium becomes greatly enlarged due to the extra blood it receives from the left atrium. *Dilatation of the pulmonary artery* is invariably present. The septal defect acts as a safety valve for the mitral stenosis, relieving somewhat the burden on the pulmonary circulation. One woman with this disease lived to the age of seventy-four years, having successfully passed through 11 pregnancies and 3 abortions. Such cases must be exceptional, because of the burden which the extra blood throws on the right heart.

Ventricular Septal Defects.—An uncomplicated defect of the ventricular septum is known as *Roger's disease.* The opening is usually small, situated in the membranous part of the septum, and causes little disturbance. It may, however, be much larger (Fig. 252) and in some cases there is complete absence of the septum, so that the heart has one ventricle and two auricles. Right ventricular hypertrophy, dilatation and failure will result, but here again cyanosis will be absent except as a terminal phenomenon. Both ventricles become enlarged, so that the

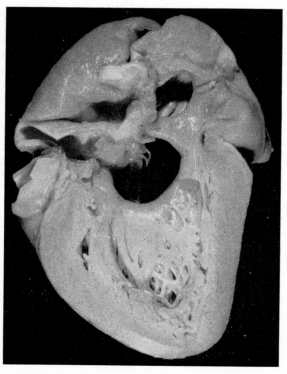

FIG. 252.—Large interventricular septal defect in colored boy, who suffered from 3 attacks diagnosed as pneumonia. There was a loud apical systolic murmur. Higher up there is a large interauricular opening at the site of the fossa ovalis.

heart assumes a characteristic globular form. When the defect is small, as is usually the case, the characteristic physical sign is a loud systolic murmur, described as a *machinery murmur*, usually accompanied by a thrill. Bacterial endocarditis occurs in many cases (possibly 40 per cent), so that surgical closure of the defect is indicated. The membranous part of the interventricular septum is a downgrowth from the partition which divides the bulbus arteriosus into a pulmonary artery and aorta, so that septal defects may readily be combined with defective development of these vessels and their valves. When associated with pulmonary stenosis, as in the tetralogy of Fallot, cyanosis will be the dominant feature, because now the shunt will be from right to left.

TETRALOGY OF FALLOT.—This is the most important congenital lesion of the heart, and it is the most common of the lesions causing cyanosis. About 70 per cent of the "blue babies" seen clinically are examples of the tetralogy of Fallot. The condition is essentially a ventricular septal defect associated with other cardiac anomalies, and is dependent primarily on maldevelopment of the membranous septum which divides the truncus arteriosus into the pulmonary artery and aorta and becomes continuous with the interventricular septum. As the name indicates, there are four defects in the complex: (1) a high ventricular septal defect, (2) pulmonary stenosis, (3) dextraposed overriding aorta, and (4) right ventricular hypertrophy (Fig. 253).

The dextraposition is perhaps the basic change, leading to narrowing of the pulmonary opening. The stenosis is mainly of the infundibular type, with muscular hypertrophy and narrowing of the subpulmonary tract. The valve may also be involved, with thick and fleshy leaflets fused to form a diaphragm. The aorta is wide and thick-walled

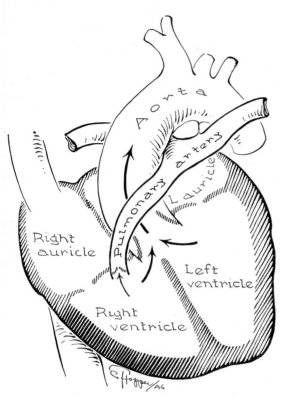

FIG. 253.—Tetralogy of Fallot showing pulmonary stenosis, wide aorta, hypertrophied right ventricle and defect in interventricular septum. (Boyd, *Pathology for the Surgeon*, courtesy of W. B. Saunders Co.)

compared with the pulmonary artery which is narrow and hypoplastic. The aorta overrides the septal defect in the upper part of the interventricular septum, so that it receives blood from the right as well as the left ventricle. If the pulmonary stenosis is extreme or complete, the ductus arteriosus must remain open if blood is to reach the lungs. In such cases, early closure of the ductus is incompatible with life, unless an adequate collateral circulation can be established with the bronchial arteries. In those patients who survive for many years, there is a balance between the degree of stenosis of the pulmonary opening and the patency of the ductus. Widespread thrombosis of the smallest pulmonary vessels is very common, and this may well add to the decrease of oxygenation (Rich).

The principle of the Blalock-Taussig op-

eration is to by-pass the obstruction by making an *artificial ductus* through which an adequate supply of blood is poured from the systemic into the pulmonary circulation. The most suitable cases are those with a small or closed ductus. The operation increases the flow of blood through the lungs to the left heart, raising the pressure in the left ventricle, abolishing the right to left shunt, and often relieving the cyanosis and dyspnea to a miraculous degree. In many cases the results are dramatic in the extreme. The blue baby becomes pink, the polycythemia disappears, the dyspnea is a thing of the past, and the child for the first time is able to develop along normal lines. The right ventricle, however, will continue to pump some venous blood into the systemic circulation because the aorta is overriding. This may cause little if any clinical cyanosis but the oxygen saturation of the arterial blood will be found in the neighborhood of 85 per cent instead of the normal 100 per cent.

The clinical manifestations of the condition are discussed at the end of this section in relation to the lesions responsible for them.

Eisenmenger Complex.—This condition is a rare variation of the tetralogy of Fallot *without pulmonary stenosis*. The aorta overrides a high septal defect, so that the blood from the left ventricle pours directly into the pulmonary artery. Pulmonary hypertension is therefore a characteristic feature, the pulmonary artery segment is dilated, and atherosclerosis is observed in the main artery and muscular hyperplasia and necrotizing arteritis in its small branches (Old and Russell). Radiographically, the lung fields are dense. As the shunt is left-to-right, cyanosis is only a late feature due to cardiac failure.

Pure Pulmonary Stenosis.—Stenosis with no defect in the interventricular septum is rare. It is a stenosis involving the cusps, which become fused. As there is no intermingling of the blood streams, there is no cyanosis throughout most of the illness. A heavy load is thrown on the right ventricle, which becomes enormously hypertrophied, but eventually fails slowly or suddenly. This is not a lesion which can be by-passed surgically, as in the case of the tetralogy of Fallot, for obvious reasons, but the stenotic valve can be incised and dilated.

Patent Ductus Arteriosus.—The ductus arteriosus is the channel by which in intra-uterine life the blood passes from the right heart into the aorta without passing through the lungs. It arises at the bifurcation of the pulmonary artery and ends in the aorta beyond the opening of the left subclavian artery. It is patent at birth, but becomes obliterated during the third and fourth weeks of extra-uterine life. It often remains open as the result of other congenital defects.

When the ductus remains patent, a condition which is twice as common in females as in males, the blood flows from the aorta into the pulmonary artery. In uncomplicated cases, therefore, there is no cyanosis. There may, however, be a temporary reversal of flow owing to heightened pulmonary pressure, as in prolonged crying, violent physical exertion, or terminal heart failure, with resulting cyanosis. If the ductus is acting as a compensatory mechanism to other congenital cardiac anomalies, cyanosis may be present even under resting conditions. There may be a rumbling systolic murmur and thrill in the pulmonary area. By means of cardiac catheterization the pressure effect of the flow of arterial blood into the pulmonary artery can be demonstrated and the increased oxygen content of the blood can be confirmed with absolute certainty.

Although the condition is compatible with a long and active life, in the great majority of cases life expectation is considerably shortened. The great danger is the development of Streptococcus viridans endarteritis. This threat can now be averted by ligation of the ductus, or even better, by complete division.

Coarctation of the Aorta.—This is a condition of narrowing of the aorta (*coarctare*, to press together) in the region where it is joined by the ductus arteriosus. Two forms are recognized, the infantile and adult, depending on the relation of the constriction to the ductus. In the *infantile type* the constriction is proximal to the ductus, between it and the subclavian artery, and the ductus remains widely patent. Other cardiac anomalies are common in this form. In the *adult type* the constriction is at or just distal to the ductus, which is obliterated. Other anomalies are rare, but subacute bacterial endocarditis is a

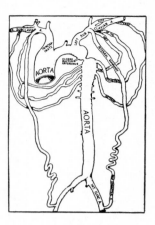

Fig. 254.—Coarctation of aorta with collateral circulation. (Maude Abbott and Dawson, International Clinics, courtesy of J. B. Lippincott Co.)

common cause of death. The infantile form is not compatible with continued life, and is found in the stillborn and young infants. The narrowing may be so great that the opening may barely admit a probe. In the adult form the blood makes its way to the lower part of the body by means of *greatly dilated collateral vessels*, the subscapular and internal mammary arteries from the subclavian anastomosing with the intercostals and epigastrics respectively. (Fig. 254). This collateral circulation fails to develop in the infantile type, as the blood from the patent ductus enters the aorta beyond the obstruction. The *clinical picture* is characteristic, *i.e.*, arterial hypertension in the upper part of the body, large pulse volume in the arm and small in the leg, palpable or visible vessels along the dorsal border and angle of the scapula (subscapular collaterals), and a grooving of the ribs in the roentgen-ray film (internal mammary and intercostals).

The two most distinctive signs are a relative weakness and delay (lag) in the pulse of the lower limbs compared with that in the arms, and evidence of the anastomotic vessels.

Mild forms of coarctation are compatible with a comparatively long life, but the average span of life is greatly reduced. As a rule there are few symptoms in childhood. The *hazards* which must be borne in mind are: (1) severe hypertension in the upper part of the body with resulting cardiac failure, cerebral hemorrhage, etc.; (2) bacterial endoarteritis at the site of the coarctation; (3) aneurysm formation immediately above or below the coarctation owing to faulty development of the wall of the aorta; (4) development of a dissecting aneurysm; (5) rupture of the aorta. In view of this sinister catalogue it is fortunate that modern surgery can offer a prospect of cure. Aided by the collateral circulation the surgeon is able to clamp and divide the aorta above and below the constriction, and then suture the divided ends or replace the resected portion with a plastic tube. Occasionally, however, the repair is in a sense too successful, for when the full force of the high blood pressure hits the portion of the arterial tree distal to the narrowing, the result may be widespread necrosis of the branches of the abdominal aorta with gangrene of the small intestine (Benson and Sealy). The academic interest of this catastrophe is that it serves to confirm the view that hypertensive arterial necrosis is a direct result of excessive filling tension.

Endocardial Fibroelastosis.—As the name indicates, this is a thickening of the fibrous and elastic tissue of the endocardium lining one or more of the cavities, usually the left ventricle. It is generally diffuse, but may be focal. In addition to a thickening of the entire mural endocardium, most marked just below the aortic valve, the valves may also be thickened producing stenosis, due probably to an extension of the process to the cusps. The heart is markedly hypertrophied, frequently to two or three times the normal weight. Microscopically, the endothelium may be swollen, but is often normal. Beneath the endothelium there is a broad collagenous region containing parallel elastic fibers (Fig. 255). Interlacing fibrous strands may penetrate and surround degenerated areas of subendocardial myocardium.

When examined with the electron microscope the surface layers of the thickened endocardium are found to consist of fibers morphologically indistinguishable from fibrin and entirely different from those of collagen. This suggests that the incorporation of fibrin is an important factor in the thickening of the endocardium.

At least the majority of cases should be

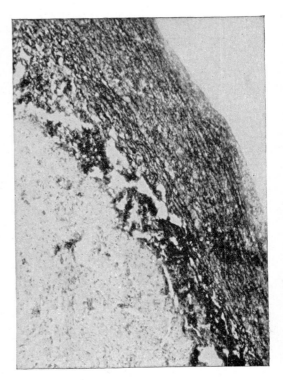

Fig. 255.—Endocardial fibroelastosis. Great thickening of endocardium by elastic and fibrous tissue. (Boyd, *Pathology for the Physician.*)

regarded as congenital in nature, that is to say they are intrauterine in origin. Rare cases are familial and therefore genetic in nature, due apparently to a lethal gene, a genetic mutant. Most of the cases develop cardiac symptoms in infancy or childhood, and it is often fatal during the first few months of life. Occasionally clinical evidence is delayed until childhood is past.

The *etiology* is in doubt. It seems reasonable to blame anoxia, for the condition develops in association with malformations which could produce endocardial anoxia (Johnson). The most striking of these malformations are anomalous origin of the left coronary artery from the pulmonary artery, premature closure of the foramen ovale which prevents the normally oxygenated blood from the umbilical vein flowing into the right atrium from reaching the left atrium, and valvular atresia with resulting stagnation.

The *clinical picture* is not easy to explain. In infancy, there may be a sudden or gradual onset of heart failure, and death usually occurs within the first six months of life. Older children may die suddenly, without any history of previous symptoms. Adult victims usually have a history of congestive heart failure. It has been suggested that the greatly thickened endocardium interferes with the normal contractions of the myocardium in the same way as these are interfered with in constrictive pericarditis. The sudden end may be due to impairment of the normal conduction of contraction impulses, thus explaining the frequent occurrence of arrhythmias and delayed conduction.

Other forms of fibrosis of the endocardium are encountered in a variety of cardiac diseases. The thickening which occurs over myocardial infarcts can be attributed to anoxia. A similar change is observed in the beriberi heart. A particularly interesting form is that known as *East African endomyocardial fibrosis*. In this condition, the lesion is very similar to that just described, and it is one of the commonest causes of congestive heart failure in East African natives (Davies). A rather similar condition has been reported as a common form of heart disease in West Africa, the chief features being fibrosis of the left ventricle, collections of cells like Aschoff nodules, and a raised antistreptolysin-O titer during the active phase (Abrahams). All of these conditions must be regarded as different in character from the endocardial fibroelastosis of infants and children.

Miscellaneous Conditions.—*Transposition of the Great Vessels.*—This unusual anomaly is more common in the male than the female in the ratio of 4:1. In its pure form it is of course incompatible with life, but when associated with a septal defect a partial correction takes place. This defect is usually a patent foramen ovale, but in some cases there is also an interventricular septal defect or a patent ductus arteriosus. Death from heart failure usually occurs before adult life is reached. The right ventricle, which carries the main load, is much hypertrophied. It is now possible to correct the disability to some extent by making an atrial septal defect or an anastomosis between the subclavian and right pulmonary arteries as is done for the tetralogy of Fallot.

Right Aortic Arch.—In rare cases the aorta arches over the right instead of the left bronchus, an arrangement which is normal in birds. Shortly after the 13 mm. stage of fetal life the left dorsal aorta may be obliterated. If this occurs before atrophy of the distal part of the right dorsal aorta, the latter is kept open by the pressure of blood. The condition usually occurs alone, but it may be associated with an obliterated left arch, and sometimes even with a patent left arch. In uncomplicated cases it is not likely to interfere with health. The condition can be diagnosed with certainty during life by roentgen-ray examination. When viewed with the fluoroscope, barium in the esophagus is seen to be diverted sharply to the left at the level of the aortic arch. In a diagonal view the arch of the aorta is seen to pass over the right bronchus.

Aortic Valve Lesions.—Aortic stenosis is much less common than pulmonary stenosis. Apart from stenosis there may be an abnormal number of cusps, two or four. A bicuspid aortic valve is peculiarly liable to suffer from subacute bacterial endocarditis. If a bicuspid aortic valve is really congenital in nature it will be associated with other developmental cardiac defects; such cases are usually seen in children. In adults the condition is usually acquired in nature, rheumatic in origin, and not associated with other defects.

Relation of Symptoms to Lesions.—The introduction of cardiac catheterization and angiocardiography has greatly increased the accuracy of localization of lesions, but it is well to remember that a satisfactory appreciation of the situation can still be attained by the long-established and time-honored methods of clinical examination.

Cardiac catheterization reveals the pressure and oxygen content in the various chambers and great vessels. Normally there is little difference in the oxygen content in the superior vena cava, the right atrium and ventricle and the pulmonary artery. With a defect in the atrial septum, the oxygen content of the blood in the right atrium will naturally be higher than that in the vena cava. Similarly, in patent ductus arteriosus the oxygen content in the pulmonary artery will be higher than in the right ventricle. Moreover, the volume of blood flowing through the shunts can be calculated from the oxygen content. The overall cardiac shunt represents the difference between systemic and pulmonary artery blood flow, and this governs the direction of the shunt. Other things being equal, the flow will be from left to right, but with obstruction in the pulmonary artery, as in the tetralogy of Fallot, the flow will be right to left. There is also the possibility that the flow may become reversed owing to a building up of pulmonary artery flow as in patent ductus arteriosus. Although the intracardiac hemodynamics are reflected with beautiful accuracy by catheterization technique, it will be realized that the presence or absence of cyanosis is a reliable clinical indicator of the direction and magnitude of any shunt which may exist.

In those defects associated with excessive blood flow through the pulmonary vessels, the three common examples of which are atrial septal defects, ventricular septal defects, and patent ductus arteriosus, cardiac catheterization reveals an interesting difference in the level of the pressure in the pulmonary artery. The pressure is approximately normal in atrial septal defects, often raised in patent ductus and raised even more frequently in ventricular septal defects (Swan *et al.*). The maintenance of a high pulmonary resistance is essential for survival in many cases of ventricular septal defects and patent ductus. It is possible that the pulmonary hypertension may be due to the ejection of blood from a high to a low pressure system, as occurs in ventricular septal defects and patent ductus, but not in atrial septal defects. These kinetic energy factors may then lead to degenerative occlusive changes in the small pulmonary arteries, changes which maintain and intensify the hypertension.

Angiocardiography provides visualization of the chambers of the heart, the aorta and the pulmonary artery. It can be useful in right-to-left shunts, but the intravenous use of a radiopaque substance is not without danger.

Electrocardiography is of limited value. It is normal in uncomplicated patent ductus arteriosus, and is seldom abnormal when the increased work of both ventricles is equal. The most frequent abnormality is right ventricular preponderance, which might be expected in such conditions as the tetralogy of Fallot, isolated pulmonary stenosis, atrial septal defects, and the Eisenmenger and Lutembacher complexes. Left ventricular preponderance is naturally present in coarctation of the aorta and tricuspid atresia.

Cyanosis is the most characteristic symptom of congenital heart disease, which may be present from the moment the blue baby makes it appearance in the world, but usually develops later. Sometimes it is only terminal, owing to a reversal of a left-to-right shunt or to congestive failure. Cyanosis is due to a shunt of at least 30 per cent of venous blood into the systemic circulation, or to insufficient oxygenation of blood in the lungs, which may occur in atrial septal defects with overloading of the pulmonary circulation, or to pulmonary arteriosclerosis which may develop as the result of hypertension in the lesser circulation. At least 5 gm. of hemoglobin must be present in order to have evident cyanosis.

Dyspnea on exertion is equally common, but is of all grades from the slightest to the most severe. In atrial septal defects, it is due to overloading of the pulmonary circulation, and in right-to-left shunts to the amount of unoxygenated blood shunted into the systemic circulation. Cough, hemoptysis and repeated attacks of pulmonary infection are associated with congestion of the lesser circulation.

Polycythemia, which is compensatory in nature, serves for a time to offset the deficiency of oxygen. The size of the erythrocytes is increased, a compensatory macrocytosis. Weakness goes with the lack of oxygenation, and is no doubt related to the frequent squatting during short walks which is characteristic of the blue baby, especially one with the tetralogy of Fallot. Growth is often arrested, and the patients may be short and puny.

Clubbing of the fingers is due to a disturbance of nutrition of the tissues which affects both the terminal phalanges and the nails, the latter being thickened and curved. The bone of the digits shows no change.

Cerebral symptoms are frequent owing to the anoxia and occasionally to cerebral thrombosis associated with the polycythemia. Faintness, dizziness, syncope, even convulsions and coma may occur, particularly in the cyanotic group. Metastatic brain abscess is an occasional complication, usually occurring in the tetralogy of Fallot.

31

The abscess is nearly always single. The septal defect apparently permits a short-circuiting of the circulation through the lungs, so that organisms may reach the cerebral circulation, although why abscess formation should be limited to the brain and to only one spot in the brain remains a mystery.

With these general facts in mind, and deciding whether the condition involves a right-left shunt as in the tetralogy of Fallot or a left-right shunt as in patent ductus arteriosus, it is not difficult for the student to work out for himself the signs, symptoms and laboratory data which may be expected in the various conditions we have been discussing. By reversing this process in his future practice he will arrive at a correct diagnosis.

The following table will serve to summarize some special features of the more important malformations of the heart.

ENDOCARDIAL LESIONS

Having considered what may be called the Big Five in cardiac pathology, we now turn to other regional lesions of endocardium, myocardium, and pericardium. The two most important endocardial lesions, those of rheumatic disease and bacterial endocarditis have already been discussed.

Thrombotic Non-Bacterial Endocarditis. —It has long been known that in many chronic diseases (nephritis, diabetes, cancer) small nodules may be found on the valves at autopsy, a condition known as *terminal* or *marantic endocarditis* (*marasmos*, wasting), although wasting is not a necessary antecedent. The basic lesion here, and probably in all other forms of endocarditis, is a degeneration and swelling of the valvular collagen with depolymerization of the mucopolysaccharides of the ground substance and a

IMPORTANT FEATURES OF THE PRINCIPAL CONGENITAL HEART LESIONS

Condition	Major Alterations	Cyanosis
Atrial septal defect	Failure of interauricular septum to develop	Mild to moderate
Lutembacher's disease	Atrial septal defect, mitral stenosis, dilatation of pulmonary artery	Mild to moderate
Roger's disease	Ventricular septal defect	Absent initially
Tetralogy of Fallot (four defects; common)	(1) High ventricular septal defect. (2) pulmonary stenosis, (3) dextraposed overriding aorta, (4) right ventricular hypertrophy	Marked
Eisenmenger complex (rare)	Same as tetralogy of Fallot without pulmonary stenosis	A late feature
Pulmonary stenosis	Fusion of valve cusps	Usually absent
Patent ductus arteriosus	Absence of normal obliteration of ductus	Absent
Coarctation of aorta	(1) Infantile type; constriction proximal to open ductus. (2) Adult type; constriction distal to closed ductus	Absent
Endocardial fibroelastosis	Associated malformations causing endocardial anoxia	Present if cardiac complications develop
Transposition of the great vessels	Associated septal defects allow temporary survival	Marked
Aortic valve lesions	(1) Stenosis rare (2) Bicuspid valve prone to bacterial endocarditis	Absent

tendency to necrosis. This is a *degenerative endocardosis* rather than a true endocarditis (Allen and Sirota). The reactivity of the collagen is probably controlled by such factors as endocrine function, reaction to stress, and the state of nutrition. If the destructive process is more severe, platelets are deposited on the damaged valve and true thrombotic verrucae are formed. This is the condition called thrombotic non-bacterial endocarditis (Gross and Friedberg). Occasionally it is a source of multiple emboli. If infection supervenes, subacute or acute bacterial endocarditis will result, depending on the type of infecting organism. It seems probable that all forms of bacterial endocarditis develop in this manner.

The incidence of the different forms of endocarditis encountered at autopsy has changed remarkably since the advent of chemotherapy and antibiotics (Angrist and Marquiss). There has been a marked decrease in bacterial endocarditis and a corresponding increase in the non-bacterial forms of the disease. Transitional forms between the non-bacterial and bacterial types and between the acute and subacute varieties are now seen much more frequently, as are healing phases of the latter forms. The "atypical verrucous endocarditis" described originally by Libman and Sacks in disseminated lupus erythematosus is a variant of the non-bacterial form.

Carcinoid Cardiovascular Disease.—The fantastic combination of *carcinoid tumor of the small bowel* metastasizing to the liver and *stenosis of the valves on the right side of the heart* was naturally regarded as a pure coincidence when it was first reported. Then it was realized that these patients often showed a particular type of telangiectasia of the face with episodic cutaneous vasomotor phenomena, in particular flushing and a patchy cyanosis. The dramatic changes in the skin have been described as "resembling in clinical miniature the fickle phantasmagory of the Aurora Borealis" (Bean *et al.*). Hyperperistalsis and bronchiolar constriction with corresponding clinical disturbance may also develop. Some of these sufferers were no doubt regarded as examples of what the British term the Baron von Munchausen syndrome, because the affected persons

travel widely from hospital to hospital telling dramatic tales of symptoms which are regarded as purely fictitious (McKusick). But fact can be stranger than fiction.

The subject of malignant carcinoid of the intestine is considered in detail in connection with tumors of the bowel. Suffice it to say here that the strange story opens with the demonstration by Pierre Masson 40 years ago that the enterochromaffin cells are of endocrine nature, and that the so-called carcinoid tumors of these cells have endocrine function. The amine 5-hydroxytryptamine, 5-HT, known as *serotonin*, can be isolated from carcinoid tumors. It is manufactured from the amino acid tryptophane, is adsorbed selectively by the blood platelets which act as circulating reservoirs, and is excreted in the urine as 5-hydroxyindoleacetic acid. Large amounts can be demonstrated in the urine by a simple colorimetric test when there are massive metastases in the liver. Serotonin is inactivated by passage through the lungs and through the liver. This explains why the valves on the left side of the heart are not involved unless there is a right-to-left shunt through an interatrial defect or a large patent foramen ovale, why a primary carcinoid tumor in the bowel is not associated with cardiac lesions, and why secondary growths in the liver or in the ovary (the latter by-passing the portal circulation) are responsible for the changes in the valves.

Cardiac Lesions.—It seems that 5-HT in concentrated form produces a sclerosing effect, so that when it is poured directly from liver metastases into the right side of the heart it produces an increase in the ground substance of the tricuspid and pulmonary valves with fibrous thickening of the cusps and eventual stenosis. Serotonin causes spasm of the plain muscle, which in the respiratory system results in asthmatic attacks and in the digestive system in temporary obstruction or loose and watery diarrhea.

CHRONIC VALVULAR DISEASE

Mitral Stenosis.—The normal average circumference of the mitral opening is 10 cm. Anything less than 7 cm. must be regarded as stenosis. Most, if not all, cases of mitral stenosis are rheumatic in origin. It is pos-

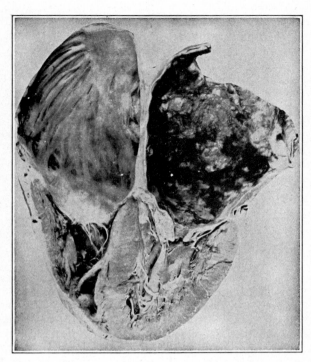

FIG. 256.—Mitral stenosis. Small left ventricle, narrowing of mitral opening, great dilation of left auricle and right side of heart.

sible that mild forms of subacute bacterial endocarditis may end in healing with adhesion of the cusps. It is much commoner in women than in men. The left atrium and the right side of the heart are greatly dilated owing to the obstruction, but the left ventricle is normal in size or even smaller than normal (Fig. 256). When a the heart is opened the left atrium is seen to be enormous. It may contain as much as 500 cc. instead of the ordinary 30 or 40 cc. The valve looks like a deep funnel, the walls of which are formed by the fused cusps. The blood rushing through this rigid funnel causes a vibration of its walls which is responsible for the diastolic murmur and thrill with or without presystolic accentuation. The opening may be a mere button-hole which will hardly admit the tip of the little finger. (Fig. 257.) The thickened and sclerosed cusps may become calcified, so that the valve can neither open nor shut, a combined condition of stenosis and incompetence. The chordæ tendineæ may be so thickened and shortened

that the papillary muscles seem to be implanted on the valve. There may be *thrombus formation* in the *dilated left atrium*, particularly in the atrial appendix. This is very important, because the clot may become detached and give rise to cerebral embolism. Moreover a thrombus often forms in the right atrium, and this may cause pulmonary embolism, especially when auricular fibrillation sets in. Thus, though in rheumatic endocarditis there are no friable vegetations which can become detached, yet embolism is a common complication of mitral stenosis. *Angiocardiography* is of great value in demonstrating the presence of atrial thrombi, of differentiating these from intracardiac tumors, and of indicating the possibility of surgical intervention and the advisability of preliminary prophylactic anticoagulant therapy before operation is undertaken. In rare cases a ball thrombus may be present, a large globular mass lying free in the auricle.

The *general effects* of mitral stenosis are those of chronic venous congestion, which

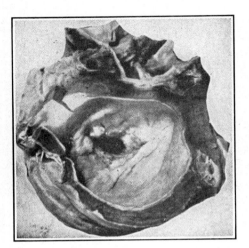

Fig. 257.—Mitral stenosis. The thickened cusps have fused so as to cause extreme narrowing of the opening.

has already been described in Chapter 7. This is most marked in the lungs and liver. The distended pulmonary capillaries may rupture into the alveoli causing hemoptysis. Mitral stenosis is the commonest cause of hemoptysis or the coughing up of blood. The common explanation for this is the distended condition of the pulmonary capillaries, but it seems more probable from the observations of Ferguson and his associates that the hemorrhage takes place from varicosities in the submucous bronchial veins. These workers by means of injection methods showed that there is a free communication between the main pulmonary veins and the bronchial veins, and that in mitral stenosis the latter veins become dilated and varicose. Areas of hemorrhage and infarction are common in the lungs, and there are great numbers of heart failure cells in the alveoli. Owing to extravasation of blood there is fibrosis of the septa, and the lung becomes brown and firm, a condition known as *brown induration*. The pulmonary artery and its branches often show marked atheroma owing to the continued strain though the aorta may be normal. The pulmonary arterioles may show a hyperplastic sclerosis and necrosis similar to that seen in the renal arterioles in malignant hypertension. These arterioles become greatly narrowed. As a consequence two stenoses are present in the lesser circulation,

one at the mitral orifice, the other in the lung, and of these the latter may become the more serious, nor can it be relieved by the skill of the surgeon. Parker and Weiss point out that in severe cases of mitral stenosis there may be great thickening of the basement membrane supporting both the alveolar epithelium and the vascular endothelium, and that the space between them may become widened by edema, so that the alveolar tissue may be twenty times thicker than normal. As a result there is a grave interference with gaseous exchange, the blood being separated from the alveolar air by so thick a partition. This explains why it is that intense cyanosis may persist in spite of myocardial improvement. The liver shows marked congestion and may become indurated. The other organs are congested to a lesser degree.

The surgical treatment of mitral stenosis by valvotomy (commissurotomy) and reconstruction of the valve has made necessary a reassessment of the patient in the past, in other words the natural history of the disease before the days of cardiac surgery. In an excellent study published by Oleson from Denmark on a follow-up of 351 cases of mitral stenosis, some 70 per cent of the patients with dyspnea on mild exertion and normal sinus rhythm survived for twenty years, and of these 40 per cent were still in the same state as at the beginning. These facts must be taken into consideration in assessing the effect of mitral valvulotomy on survival. They also serve to show that although rheumatic heart disease may develop silently and progress with equal silence, it may not progress at all.

Mitral Insufficiency.—The organic as opposed to the functional form of mitral incompetence is due either to sclerosis and contraction of the cusps or to dilatation of the ring. The common cause is rheumatic endocarditis. Subacute bacterial endocarditis will also cause incompetence because of the large vegetations, the sclerosis, and the occasional destruction of the cusps. In old age the cusps may undergo degeneration and calcification which will interfere with their efficiency. The condition of the heart is similar to that of mitral stenosis except that the left ventricle is also much dilated owing to the increased amount of blood which it has to accommodate. In the end-stages the heart is greatly enlarged.

Aortic Insufficiency.—Insufficiency or incompetence of the aortic valve may be due to endocarditis of the valve cusps or to dilatation of the aorta and the aortic ring. The two principal causes of aortic insufficiency are *rheumatic endocarditis* and *syphilitic aortitis*. Two additional causes are *subacute bacterial endocarditis* and the aortitis associated with ankylosing or *rheumatoid spondylitis*. Incompetence due to endocarditis is caused by adhesions, thickening, and retraction of the cusps. It may be combined with stenosis, and is seldom so extreme as the incompetence caused by syphilis. In the syphilitic form the incompetence may be due to one or more of three factors: (1) dilatation of the aortic ring caused by destruction of the elastic tissue; (2) widening of the commissures; and (3) retraction of the cusps and a characteristic cord-like thickening of their free edge. The dilatation may be so great that the valve becomes useless though the cusps may be healthy, and the incompetence is complete. High blood pressure and severe physical strain naturally aggravate the condition. It is doubtful if atheromatous degeneration alone can cause incompetence, but the possibility cannot be denied.

The condition of the heart is the opposite of that of mitral stenosis. Here the heart is all left ventricle. It is extremely enlarged and globular in outline, the *cor bovinum*. The left ventricle is greatly hypertrophied as well as dilated. The regurgitant stream of blood escaping through the incompetent valve impinges on the wall of the ventricle, and may lead to the formation of crescentic thickenings of the endocardium. These thickenings may develop into miniature leaflets with shallow pockets directed towards the jet. These are known as the *pockets of Zahn*.

The *clinical picture* is highly characteristic, but is much more extreme in the syphilitic form. The symptoms and signs are due to the escape of blood from the aorta back through the incompetent valve. The arteries thus contain too much blood during systole and too little during diastole. This accounts

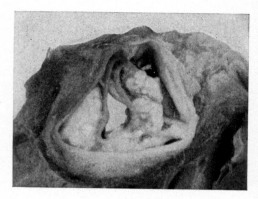

Fig. 258.—Calcific aortic stenosis.

for the leaping peripheral vessels ("the dance of the arteries"), the capillary pulsation, the water-hammer pulse (Corrigan pulse), the low diastolic pressure, and the high pulse-pressure, the giddiness and attacks of syncope due to cerebral anemia. The diastolic murmur which is the most characteristic physical sign is due to the blood escaping back into the ventricle.

Aortic Stenosis.—This is quite uncommon in a pure form, although in the rheumatic variety of aortic incompetence the rigid and adherent cusps may be unable to open fully so that a relative degree of stenosis is produced. Pure aortic stenosis usually occurs in men over fifty years of age, and is of the *calcified nodular type*, best called *calcific aortic stenosis*. The cusps adhere together to form a kind of diaphragm as in mitral stenosis, but the most striking feature is the presence of warty calcified masses which may cover the cusps or be confined to the base. (Fig. 258.) The entire valve is incredibly hard and rigid. The calcification can be seen in roentgen-ray films. There is much difference of opinion as to whether the lesion is a manifestation of arteriosclerosis or is an end result of rheumatic infection. The general opinion is that in the great majority of cases, perhaps in every case, the lesion is rheumatic in origin (Hall and Ichioka, Karsner). On the other hand there is evidence to suggest that in some, perhaps in many cases, the lesion may be the result of endocarditis caused by *Brucella abortus* (Peery). Mitral stenosis is

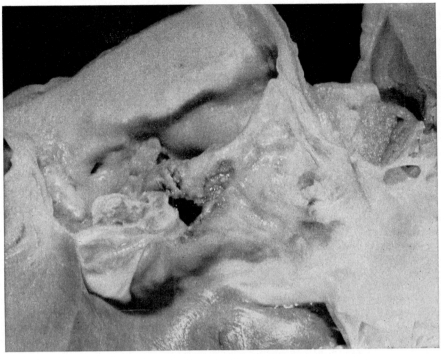

Fig. 259.—Aortic stenosis. The heart weighed 750 gm., due chiefly to hypertrophy of the left ventricle. The cusps of the valve are fused, calcified and ulcerated, with thickening of the commissures. The orifice of the valve is a small irregular hole. Note the smooth lining of the aorta.

predominantly a disease of women and develops in the earlier period of life, whereas calcific aortic stenosis is a disease of men over middle age. The usual cause of death during brucellosis is endocarditis. The disease chiefly affects the aortic valve, especially in *Brucella abortus* infections, the strain most often encountered in the United States. Fatal Brucella endocarditis is essentially a chronic disease, with a particular tendency to fibrosis and calcification. Most patients die from valvular deformity with congestive heart failure. Lesions resembling Aschoff bodies are commonly found in the myocardium. It is possible, therefore, that many cases heretofore labelled as rheumatic fever are really examples of brucellosis (Peery and Belter). The prevalence of the disease in males may be attributed to the fact that serious brucellar lesions of the heart are usually the result of heavy, recurrent occupational exposure, as in farmers, meat packers and veterinarians.

The heart shows a perfect example of pure or concentric hypertrophy of the left ventricle, although toward the end it may undergo dilatation. The average weight is about 650 grams, and in one of Christian's cases it weighed over 1000 grams. The aorta is remarkably smooth and free from atherosclerosis for patients over middle age, and it almost seems as if the vessel wall has been protected by the stenosis (Fig. 259). As so little blood enters the aorta the pulse is small and fainting attacks are common. The *pulse tracing* with its slanting upstroke and rounded camel's hump speaks eloquently of the resistance at the aortic opening. The most characteristic physical sign is a *rough rasping systolic murmur and thrill* at the aortic area. If incompetence is also present, a diastolic murmur will be added. The clinical diagnosis of aortic stenosis used to be merely of academic interest. Now that cardiac surgery promises relief with a reasonable degree of safety, recognition of the lesion has become a matter of importance. If the condition is unchecked, cardiac hypertrophy will be followed by dilatation and eventually congestive failure, with the additional threat of subacute bacterial endocarditis. The diagnosis should be made long before the clinical physical signs become marked, which is when the circumference of the valve has been reduced from the normal 7 or 8 cm. to 5 cm. or less. The x-ray demonstration of calcification in the area of the aortic valve may serve to confirm the diagnosis.

TRICUSPID STENOSIS.—Rheumatic infection may spread from the mitral to the tricuspid valve ring, and the subsequent endocarditis may cause the leaflets to be glued together, with resulting stenosis.

PULMONARY STENOSIS.—In most instances this lesion is congenital (developmental) in origin. The rare acquired cases are due to rheumatism.

MYOCARDIAL LESIONS

The myocardium is the pump without which the circulation of the blood is impossible. The pathology of the myocardium must therefore be a subject of the greatest importance, and yet it is a subject of which it is singularly difficult to give a clear and coherent account for the student. Two of the most important lesions, those of rheumatic fever and coronary occlusion, have already been described. The remaining lesions may be arranged in four main groups: (1) myocarditis, (2) degenerations, (3) deficiencies, and (4) tumors. Overlapping is inevitable, more particularly with the second and third groups.

Myocarditis.—Inflammation of the myocardium may be caused by bacteria, viruses, animal parasites, and toxins. The inflammation is sometimes referred to as secondary and primary. *Secondary* infections are complications of infections in other sites, and these are so numerous that nothing would be gained by listing them here. These are for the most part acute infections. Mention may, however, be made of the association of myocarditis with acute nasopharyngitis and acute tonsillitis (Gore and Saphir). In many of these cases heart disease was not suspected clinically, and death was often quite unex-

pected. In addition to acute myocarditis there are chronic or granulomatous inflammations to which brief reference will be made. A peculiar form of chronic myocarditis is prevalent in South American countries, more particularly Venezuela. Both ventricles are hypertrophied and all chambers are dilated, yet the myocardium is flabby. The condition may be a manifestation of Chagas' disease (trypanosomiasis). *Primary* or idiopathic inflammations are those in which the cause is not apparent, the outstanding example being the condition known as isolated myocarditis.

Isolated Myocarditis.—Many different names have been given to this rare and obscure condition, such as *Fiedler's myocarditis*, granulomatous myocarditis, and idiopathic myocarditis, names which are a silent tribute to our lack of understanding of the subject. The term "isolated" indicates that the lesions are confined to the myocardium, and do not spread, as in other infections, to the endocardium and pericardium. In 1899 Fiedler reported a small series of cases of rapidly progressive heart failure with diffuse interstitial cellular infiltration of the myocardium. Death may be sudden and completely unexpected. In 1402 cases of myocarditis analyzed at the Armed Forces Institue of Pathology, Washington, during World War II there were 43 of such cases with unknown etiology (Gore and Saphir). It is probable that they represent a heterogeneous collection and not a definite entity. The inflammatory cells are for the most part lymphocytes, plasma cells, and macrophages (Fig. 260). Giant cells may be present, often associated with necrosis of muscle fibers. Magner reports a case from my laboratory in which the patient had previously been in good health, and died unexpectedly after the removal of a non-toxic goiter. Many small foci of subacute inflammation were scattered throughout the myocardium; in these areas the muscle fibers had disappeared, there were many mononuclear inflammatory cells, and multinucleated giant cells were a prominent feature.

A good review of this confusing subject is given by Saphir. It seems possible that in many instances the causal agent is a virus,

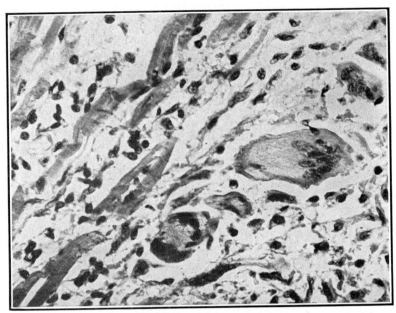

Fig. 260.—Fiedler's myocarditis showing characteristic pleomorphic cellular picture and giant cells. × 300. (Boyd, *Pathology for the Physician.*)

in which case the condition should be called a *viral myocarditis*. The Coxsackie virus, and other viruses such as those of poliomyelitis, measles, mumps, viral hepatitis, and infectious mononucleosis are known to produce similar myocardial lesions. Identical lesions due to a virus occur in the anthropoid ape (Schmidt). All of these, of course, would belong to the secondary group, whereas Fiedler's myocarditis represents the primary group.

GRANULOMATOUS MYOCARDITIS.—It is an interesting fact that whilst the infective granulomata represent serious infections in nearly every other organ, they are of little or no importance in the myocardium. *Tuberculous myocarditis* is very rare. There may be miliary tubercles scattered through the myocardium. Still more rarely there are large yellow caseous lesions of the myocardium unlike anything else found in the heart. *Syphilitic myocarditis*, apart from congenital syphilis, in which the myocardium may be swarming with spirochetes, and the extremely rare gumma of the interventricular septum, is so doubtful an entity that it will be passed by.

TOXIC MYOCARDITIS.—This is a degenerative condition rather than an inflammatory one. *Diphtheria* offers a good example. There is an acute degeneration of the muscle followed later by a secondary cellular inflammatory reaction. The muscle fibers are swollen and granular and have lost their striations. In septicemia and toxemia, even though no microscopic changes may be evident, the heart is often so flabby and lacking in tone that it flops down on the autopsy table. The *sulfonamide drugs* may cause an acute interstitial myocarditis both in man and in experimental animals. The exudate is rich in eosinophils.

MYOCARDIAL DEGENERATIONS.—The various degenerations which may affect either cells or intercellular substance, including those of the myocardium, have already been described and illustrated in Chapters 1 and 4. *Fatty degeneration* is caused by the usual factors responsible for fatty degeneration of which severe anemia, especially the pernicious form, is the chief. In the gross the heart shows the characteristic mottled "thrush-breast" appearance, best seen under the endocardium covering the papillary muscles of the left ventricle (Fig. 261). The yellow spots represent areas of fatty change. Microscopically rows of fat droplets are seen in the muscle fibers in frozen sections; they can be stained red with the usual stains for fat. *Fatty infiltration* is a lipomatosis of the heart, with deposits of fat under the pericardium and in the interstitial tissue. It is merely part of a general adiposity. The

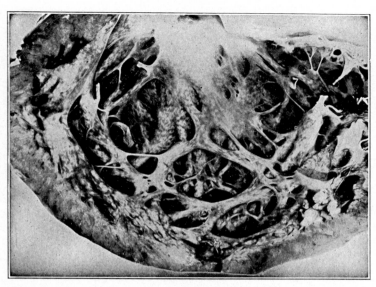

FIG. 261.—Fatty degeneration of the heart. The "thrush breast" appearance is well shown. From a case of profound anemia.

muscle fibers may suffer from pressure, and if the infiltration is very marked there may be interference with the heart's action. *Amyloidosis* of the myocardium may occur in any of the forms of systemic amyloidosis, but in primary amyloidosis the lesions may be confined to the heart. Such lesions are not uncommon in old persons, but they are of little clinical significance. *Brown atrophy* is the name given to a heart in which there is such a large collection of lipochrome pigment in the muscle fibers that the wasted organ is of a brown color. The muscle fibers are small, and at each pole of the nucleus there is a collection of yellow pigment, which must not be mistaken for hemosiderin. The condition is seen in long-continued wasting diseases and in old age.

Deficiency Diseases.—Vitamin deficiency may lead to myocardial failure associated with lesions in the heart muscle, a condition often loosely referred to as *deficiency myocarditis*. *Beriberi*, the oriental disease due to lack of vitamin B (thiamine) from eating polished rice, is marked by nervous and cardiovascular manifestations. It is coming to be recognized that an occidental form also exists, caused again by thamine deficiency due, as a rule, to chronic alcoholism (Weiss and Wilkins). Other factors, at present unrecognized, must be necessary, for chronic alcoholism is very common, whilst beri-beri

is rare. The condition of the heart varies to a bewildering degree. The heart may appear normal or may be dilated or hypertrophied and overweight. There may be no microscopic changes, but usually there is "hydropic" degeneration and vacuolation of the myocardial fibers including those of the subendocardial conduction system, (Fig. 262), edema of the interstitial tissue, and fibrosis in the later stages. The onset of symptoms of myocardial failure in an alcoholic addict may be sudden or gradual. The condition is relieved by the administration of thiamine. It may be noted that electrocardiographic changes develop in healthy volunteers on a thiamine deficient diet.

It sometimes happens that a person without any obvious history of vitamin deficiency dies with all the symptoms of chronic heart failure, but with no evidence of valvular disease, hypertension or coronary occlusion. The heart is greatly enlarged, being often double the normal weight. Here also there is evidence to suggest that some of these cases are due to dietary deficiency, possibly thiamine or some other member of the vitamin B complex (Dock). A striking feature may be great thickening of the endocardium with or without mural thrombosis. It is well

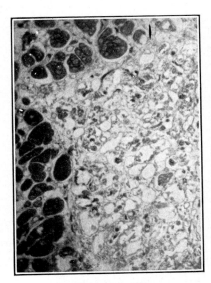

FIG. 262.—Beriberi heart.

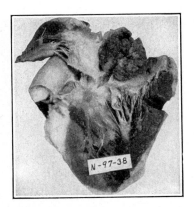

FIG. 263.—Myxoma of heart growing from wall of left auricle.

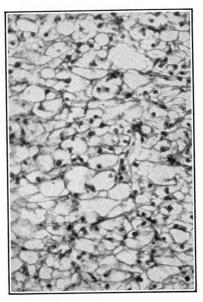

FIG. 264.—Congenital rhabdomyoma of heart. × 165.

known that the cardiac failure of beri-beri is associated with great hypertrophy and dilation of the heart, the so-called beriberi heart.

Potassium deficiency induced both in man and the experimental animal by a prolonged potassium depletion regimen is associated with histological changes in heart muscle, which have been loosely labelled myocarditis. Similar lesions are seen in severe potassium deficiency induced by chronic diarrhea and after excessive desoxycorticosterone therapy in Addison's disease. The individual muscle fibers lose their striations, the nuclei undergo pyknosis and lysis, and the necrotic area is infiltrated first by polymorphonuclear and later by mononuclear phagocytes, with eventual replacement by fibrous tissue. The potassium content of the heart muscle in the experimental animal is 35 per cent lower than in controls. It is of interest to note that the myocardial lesions bear a striking resemblance to those of poliomyelitis, suggesting that in the latter condition the lesions might be due in part to potassium deficiency.

TRAUMATIC INJURY.—Nonpenetrating injuries to the heart may result in a variety of lesions. There may be partial or complete laceration of the myocardium. In the former case rupture may occur some days later. The trauma may produce infarction due either to coronary angio-

spasm or to hemorrhage into an atheromatous patch in the intima of a coronary artery with consequent thrombosis. Pericardial effusion may occur, and even subsequent constrictive pericarditis has been reported. In occasional cases a blow to the chest has resulted in death, although autopsy failed to reveal any structural damage to the heart. The importance of the subject from the medicolegal and compensation standpoint is obvious.

TUMORS OF THE HEART.—*Primary tumors* of the heart are very rare, and need only be men-

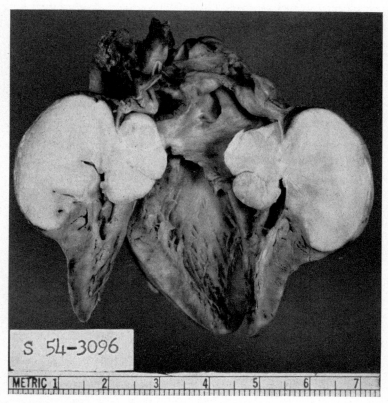

Fig. 265.—Congenital rhabdomyoma of heart in left ventricle of a girl, aged two weeks.
(Kindness of Dr. Robert W. Mowry.)

tioned. *Myxoma,* the commonest of these rare tumors, is a soft pedunculated tumor growing from the wall of the left auricle at the site of the closed foramen ovale (Fig. 263). The surface may be papillary in character. The microscopic picture is myxomatous, but may suggest that the tumor is really an endothelioma. Myxoma has come to assume clinical importance, because by reason of its site and the fact that it may attain a large size, it may narrow the atrioventricular opening and mimic the clinical picture of mitral stenosis. It may thus be encountered by the surgeon operating for that condition, and be excised with satisfactory results. Fibroma, angioma, and rhabdomyoma have been described. *Congenital rhabdomyoma* is also known as *congenital glycogenic tumor* of the heart (Batchelor and Maun). It presents a characteristic vacuolated appearance due to great accumulation of water-soluble material in the tumor cells (Fig. 264). This material in alcohol-fixed tissue is strongly PAS-positive, so that it is presumably polysaccharide, but at the present time we have

no proof that it is ordinary glycogen (Beaird *et al.*) These tumors are seen chiefly in infants and the newborn (Fig. 265). They are really developmental tumors, and are often associated with tuberous sclerosis of the brain and developmental defects in the kidneys. *Secondary tumors* are of more frequent occurrence than primary ones. They often give rise to unexplained arrhythmias, from which they can be diagnosed correctly and sometimes removed surgically. There are three possible mechanisms for the arrhythmia, all involving the atrial wall. These are: (1) involvement of atrial sympathetic fibers, (2) invasion of atrial coronary artery, (3) invasion of atrial myocardium. In one case of bronchogenic carcinoma all three of these were involved (James and Carrera).

PERICARDIAL LESIONS

Pericarditis.—It used to be easy to speak about the *causes* of inflammation of the peri-

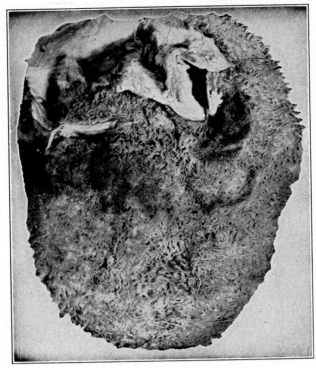

Fig. 266.—Acute pericarditis. The shaggy nature of the exudate is well shown.

cardium with regard to frequency. By far the most common was *rheumatic fever*, the pericardial lesion forming part of a rheumatic carditis. Next came the *pneumococcus*, spreading from a pneumonic lung to the pericardium by way of the lymphatics. Pericarditis may complicate any of the *infectious fevers*. The *tubercle bacillus* may be the infecting agent. Finally it may be a terminal condition in the uremia of Bright's disease (*uremic pericarditis*). At the present time *acute idiopathic pericarditis*, probably *viral* in origin in most cases, has come to dominate the picture.

Lesions.—The pericardium shows the usual characteristics of inflammation of a serous membrane. A thick fibrinous deposit is laid down on both the visceral and parietal layers, giving the heart a shaggy appearance. (Fig. 266). Its gross and microscopic characters have already been described in connection with rheumatic heart disease. There is a varying amount of serous exudate, scanty in the rheumatic form but abundant and sometimes purulent in pneumococcal and other infections. The fluid collects first at the base of the heart. The fibrinous exudate may be largely absorbed, but some of it may be organized by the ingrowth of fibroblasts, and opaque white patches or *milk-spots* are left usually on the anterior surface of the right ventricle. Organization of the exudate may lead to the formation of adhesions between the two surfaces, and these may involve the whole heart, a condition known as adherent pericardium. Calcification may occur in the organized tissue with the formation of stony plates on the surface of the heart.

Acute Idiopathic Pericarditis.—This condition, known by a variety of names such as acute non-specific benign pericarditis, is perhaps the commonest form of pericardial inflammation at the present time. It is characterized by the sudden development of substernal pain aggravated by movement in a patient with a relatively mild respiratory infection, and as the attack is often severe it

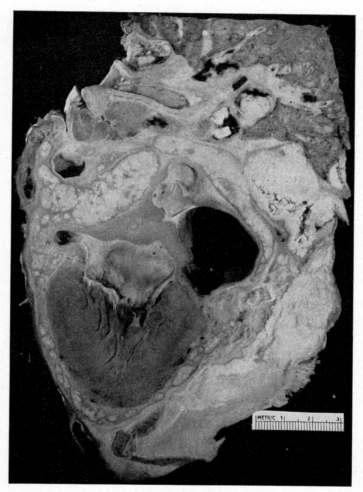

Fig. 267.—Tuberculous pericarditis, showing caseous foci in the pericardium
and the mediastinal lymph nodes.

may simulate myocardial infarction (Parker and Cooper). It pursues a benign course, however, although recurrences are common. For obvious reasons, the morbid anatomy is not known. It seems probable that many of these cases are examples of *viral pericarditis*, usually due to the Coxsackie group of viruses, sometimes to the Echo group. The evidence in the past has been only indirect. The Coxsackie cases are often associated with an epidemic of Coxsackie infection in the community, there are cases of epidemic pleuropneumonia and aseptic meningitis in the district at the same time, Coxsackie B5 (group B, type 5) virus is excreted in the stools, and there are elevated antibody titers in the serum against Coxsackie B5 virus (McLean *et al.*). The virus itself has now been isolated from the pericardial fluid.

TUBERCULOUS PERICARDITIS. —The heart is usually covered with a fibrinous caseous exudate which completely conceals the tubercles (Fig. 267.) The effusion is generally very abundant and purulent. If a pericardial sac is distended with pus, the condition is likely to be tuberculous or pneumococcal. Hemorrhage is common. A bloody exudate should suggest either tuberculosis or malignant disease. Microscopically the characteristic tubercles are seen under the fibrinous exudate.

CHRONIC CONSTRICTIVE PERICARDITIS.—

In this uncommon condition the heart is compressed by a layer of dense tough fibrous tissue which envelops the organ. There is great uncertainty as to the cause of the dense envelope. Rheumatism can be ruled out. The thick, dense envelope may present large cavities containing inspissated caseous material. The tissue is hyalinized, any collagen fibers are huge, calcification is common, and tissue destruction is marked. It seems probable that most cases are tuberculous, although complete healing may have occurred.

The compression prevents the normal diastolic filling of the auricles, so that there is great distention of the jugular veins, marked enlargement of the liver and recurring ascites. The heart, although profoundly disabled, is characteristically small and quiet, because it is unable to dilate or hypertrophy. The liver and spleen may be coated with a layer at first fibrinous and later fibrous, the so-called sugar-icing (Zuckerguss). This is apparently due to the long-standing ascites. The pleura may be similarly involved. This polyserositis has been called *Pick's disease*. Resection of the thickened and constricting pericardium has given excellent results in many cases.

Uremic Pericarditis.—In persons dying of uremia a thin layer of fibrinous material may cover the pericardial surface. This contains urea crystals, as can be demonstrated in the autopsy room by means of the xanthydrol reaction. The condition is of pathological rather than clinical interest.

Cholesterol Pericarditis.—Pericardial effusion with a high cholesterol content is usually associated with myxedema, but it may occur without obvious cause and give rise to chronic constrictive pericarditis (Creech *et al.*). Microscopic examination of the resected pericardium shows what are apparently cholesterol clefts in dense fibrous tissue, a few foreign body giant cells, and many foam cells. Experimental evidence suggests that lipids in high concentration within the pericardial sac may produce constrictive pericarditis.

Relation of Symptoms to Lesions.—The chief clinical features of pericarditis are *fever*, *precordial pain*, and a *friction rub* which at first may be soft like the rustling of silk, but later is rough and rasping like the creaking of leather. No acute infection may be more insidious in onset than pericarditis, and there may be no fever, no pain, no friction. Often the condition is discovered for the first time at autopsy, to the great surprise of the clinician. The most characteristic physical sign, the friction rub, is due to the two roughened surfaces rubbing against one another. If fluid accumulates to any extent the surfaces may be separated and the friction disappears. If the fluid is very abundant the heart sounds will be faint and distant. The pain is due to the same cause as the friction, the rubbing together of the inflamed surfaces. It may be slight or absent, and disappears as the fluid accumulates.

Hemopericardium.—Hemorrhage into the pericardial sac may be due to rupture of the heart, wounds of the heart, or rupture of an aneurysm of the first part of the thoracic aorta. If the hemorrhage is rapid it will compress the auricles so that they cannot be filled, and death occurs from heart failure. If the hemorrhage is only a slow leak the heart may accommodate itself to the pressure. Blood is often found in the fluid exudate in tuberculous pericarditis and in effusion due to secondary tumors of the pericardium. Petechial hemorrhages in the serous membrane are common in septicemic and anemic conditions.

Hydropericardium.—This is a dropsy of the pericardial sac, usually part of a general dropsy due to cardiac or renal disease. The sac may be greatly distended with clear watery fluid, which may interfere seriously with the heart's action.

HEART FAILURE

The most common cause of death is failure of the heart. This may be sudden or slow. Sudden failure has already been considered in relation to coronary artery occlusion and angina pectoris. The three great causes of gradual failure are *valvular disease, arteriosclerotic narrowing of the coronary arteries*, and *arterial hypertension*. We may therefore speak of valvular heart disease, arteriosclerotic heart disease, and hypertensive heart disease. Hypertensive heart disease is probably the commonest of these.

Failure may develop under the following

conditions. (1) Not enough blood is supplied to the heart. This is seen in peripheral circulatory failure, where there is a decrease in the inflow load. This is what Harrison terms the hypokinetic syndrome, in contradistinction to the dyskinetic syndrome of congestive heart failure. (2) Too much blood may be supplied, so that the inflow load is greater than the heart can stand. This is seen in the primary increase of inflow load in the overactive heart of thyrotoxicosis, or when too much intravenous fluid has been given, or in the excessive sodium and water retention associated with injudicious adrenal steroid or ACTH therapy. If there is adequate systolic emptying, there is no danger of failure developing. (3) The arterial load may be excessive, as in arterial hypertension and aortic stenosis. (4) There may be myocardial failure. Such failure may be primary due to structural changes in the myocardium, as in infarction, but in most cases these are absent, the failure being secondary to fatigue of the muscle. A convenient summary of the cause of heart failure is that suggested by McMichael: (1) *Valvular* (obstructive and backflow lesions); (2) *Myogenic* (destruction of cardiac muscle by ischemia, inflammation, etc.); (3) *Mechanical* (pericardial disease); (4) *Extrinsic* (a) physical—systemic or pulmonary hypertension, Paget's disease of bone, salt and water retention; (b) metabolic —beriberi, hyperthyroidism, uremia, cholemia.

In congestive heart failure due to chronic valvular disease in which we are primarily interested, perhaps the most striking clinical manifestation is edema. The relationship between the failure and the edema has long been a subject of controversy, crystalized into the two expressions "backward failure" and "forward failure."

The concept of *backward failure* dates from James Hope, who in 1842 compared the circulatory situation to the back pressure behind a failing pump. Blood is dammed back in the pulmonary and systemic veins; there is an increase in venous pressure, which in turn leads to a rise in the capillary pressure, to increased transudation of fluid, and therefore to an accumulation of fluid in the extracellular compartment, which finally manifests itself clinically as edema.

In the concept of *forward failure*, the clinical picture of congestive heart failure with edema is due primarily not to back pressure in the veins but to decreased cardiac output and diminished flow of blood to the tissues, the kidney in particular, as the result of cardiac decompensation, the edema being due to retention of sodium with associated anions and enough water to yield an isotonic extracellular fluid. According to this view, the increased venous pressure may be the result, not the cause, of the edema.

It is evident that the crux of the situation is the retention of sodium and water. A decrease in the glomerular filtration rate in the presence of normal tubular function (reabsorption) results in the retention of sodium and water. Indeed almost complete tubular reabsorption occurs when the filtration rate falls to a moderate degree. Moreover, when the cardiac output is inadequate for the body's metabolic needs, other mechanisms may affect the tubular activity directly. The increased stress of acute heart failure or intensification of chronic failure causes increased discharge of aldosterone from the adrenal cortex with retention of water and electrolytes due to increased reabsorption. There may also be increased production of the antidiuretic hormone by the posterior pituitary, causing water retention without retention of sodium.

One of the basic phenomena of congestive heart failure is inadequate emptying of the ventricle during systole. In the early stage, dilatation of the ventricle during systole results in an increased systolic output to satisfy the needs of the tissues in conformance with the so-called "Starling's law of the heart", which states that when the myocardial fibers are stretched, the heart contracts with greater force. Up to a certain point, this law remains true, but when the fibers are stretched beyond that point or are stretched too often, the overdilated ventricle responds with decreased stroke volume and decrease in the cardiac output.

Forward and backward failure are not mutually exclusive. Both mechanisms may operate, either separately or together. Failure of the two ventricles will now be considered separately, although with the progress of the disease they will become combined.

1. **Left Ventricular Failure.**—This may be brought about either by increase of the work which the ventricle has to do (aortic valvular disease, arterial hypertension) or from disease of the heart muscle, usually due to narrowing of the left coronary artery. The symptoms and signs are those of increased tension in the pulmonary circulation with normal pressure in the systemic veins. The outstanding symptom is dyspnea, often in the form of cardiac asthma. The pulmonary second sound is louder than the aortic, thus reversing the normal state of affairs, an infallible indication of hypertension of the lesser circulation. There may be acute pulmonary edema, often associated with acute left ventricular failure and characterized by abundant, pink, frothy sputum. This phase may last for years, but right ventricular failure is generally soon superadded; when this occurs the dyspnea is greatly relieved, the pulmonary hypertension subsides, and the liver and feet begin to swell.

2. **Right Ventricular Failure.**—The commonest cause of right heart failure is left heart failure. The commonest cause of *pure* right failure or cor pulmonale is emphysema. In emphysema the obstruction is in the arterioles, not in the capillaries.

It is now known that anoxia may produce this rise in pressure. Inhalation of a low oxygen content may at once double the pressure in the pulmonary artery, suggesting that some functional change has occurred, possibly constriction of the pulmonary arterioles (Motley *et al.*). Poor pulmonary ventilation causing a vasoconstrictor reaction may be the key to many forms of pulmonary heart disease, such as is seen in emphysema, kyphoscoliosis with limited movement of the thoracic cage and strangling of the bronchioles by peribronchial lymphatic carcinomatosis (McMichael).

In a pure obstructive lesion such as aortic stenosis the chamber proximal to the obstruction will undergo a *work hypertrophy*, the muscle fibers becoming larger but not more numerous. The best example is seen in the so-called *concentric hypertrophy* of the left ventricle in arterial hypertension, whether of the primary "essential" type or secondary to chronic nephritis. In arteriosclerotic heart disease there may or may not be hypertrophy, depending on whether there is or is not an associated hypertension.

In course of time *dilatation* is added to hypertrophy. This may be compensatory or may be due to failure. Compensatory dilatation is seen in aortic incompetence. During diastole the blood regurgitates from the aorta through the incompetent valve into the ventricle in addition to that entering it from the auricle. If venous congestion is to be avoided the ventricle must dilate. At the same time it hypertrophies in order to cope with the increased amount of blood it has to expel with each contraction.

Dilatation from failure is likely to be the end of every cardiac lesion if the patient lives long enough. For a time hypertrophy can look after the increased load, but there comes a time when the effort fails, the muscle becomes exhausted, and the cavity dilates. This is more apt to occur when the myocardium itself is not healthy, as from fatty degeneration or myocardial scarring. A healthy heart may be acutely dilated as the result of very great and sudden exertion. The cavities will gradually return to normal size with rest in bed, but there may be functional cardiac disability for some time

Whatever be the pathogenesis of the failure, the systemic veins are engorged, the liver is large and tender, and the legs are swollen with edema. Cyanosis is much more intense than dyspnea, although the latter is also present. A compensatory polycythemia is a natural accompaniment. The fully fledged picture is that of congestive heart failure.

REFERENCE

ABBOT, MAUDE E.: *Atlas of Congenital Cardiac Disease*, New York, 1936.

ABRAHAMS, D. G.: Lancet, 1959, *2*, 111. (Heart disease in West Africa).

ALLEN, A. C. and SIROTA, J. H.: Am. J. Path., 1944, *20*, 1025. (Thrombotic non-bacterial endocarditis).

ANGRIST, A. and MARQUISS, J.: Am. J. Path., 1953, *29*, 594. (Thrombotic non-bacterial endocarditis).

BARRIE, H. J. and URBACK, J. G.: Can. Med. Assn. 1957, *77*, 100. (Histology of myocardial infarcts).

BEAN, W. B., OLCH, D. and WEINBERG, H. B.: Circulation, 1955, *12*, 1. (Carcinoid heart disease).

BEAIRD, J., MOWRY, R. W., and CUNNINGHAM, J. A.: Cancer, 1955, *8*, 916. (Congenital rhabdomyoma of heart.)

BENSON, W. A., and SEALEY, W. C.: Lab. Investig., 1956, *5*, 360. (Coarctation and arterial necrosis.)

BING, R. J., DANFORTH, W. H., and BALLARD, F. B.: J.A.M.A., 1960, *172*, 438. (Physiology of the myocardium.)

CHRISTIAN, H. C.: *The Diagnosis and Treatment of Diseases of the Heart*, New York, 1935.

CHRISTIE, R. V.: Brit. Med. J., 1948, *1*, 1. (Bacterial endocarditis.)

CLARK, R. M. and ANDERSON, W.: Am. J. Path., 1955, *31*, 809. (Aschoff bodies in auricular appendages).

CREECH, O., JR., *et al.*: Circulation, 1955, *12*, 193. (Pericarditis.)

CRUICKSHANK, B.: J. Path. and Bact., 1958, *76*, 223. (Heart lesions in rheumatoid disease).

DALLDORF, F. G. and MURPHY, G. E.: Am. J. Path., 1960, *37*, 507. (Relation of Aschoff bodies to natural history of rheumatic heart disease).

DAVIES, J. M. P. and BALL, J. D.: Brit. Heart J., 1955, *17*, 337. (Endomyocardial fibrosis.)

DOCK, W.: Trans. Ass. Am. Phys., 1940, *55*, 61. (Deficiency myocarditis.)

DUGUID, J. B.: J. Path. and Bact., 1946, *58*, 207. (Pathogenesis of coronary atherosclerosis.)

DURLACHER, S. H., FISK, A. J. and FISHER, R.: Am. J. Path., 1953, *29*, 558. (Coronary artery lesions in sudden death.)

FERGUSON, F. C., KOBILAK, R. E. and DEITRICK, J. E.: Am. Heart J., 1944, *28*, 445. (Pulmonary hemorrhage in mitral stenosis.)

GEIGER, A. J. and DURLACHER, S. H.: Am. J. Path., 1947, *23*, 1023. (Bacterial endocarditis.)

GORE, I. and SAPHIR, O.: Am. Heart J., 1947, *34*, 831. (Association of myocarditis with acute throat infections.)

GOULD, S. E.: *Pathology of the Heart*, Springfield, Ill., 2nd ed., 1960. An encyclopedic work, covering all aspects of the subject.

GREGG, D. E.: *Coronary Circulation in Health and Disease*, Philadelphia, 1950.

GROSS, L. and FRIEDBERG, C. K.: Am. J. Path., 1936, *12*, 855. (Rheumatic heart disease.)

GROSS, L. and FRIEDBERG, C. K.: Arch. Int. Med., 1936, *58*, 620. (Thrombotic non-bacterial endocarditis.)

HALL, E. M. and ICHIOKA, T.: Am. J. Path., 1940, *16*, 761. (Aortic stenosis.)

HANDFORTH, C. P. and WOODBURY, J. F. L.: Can. Med. Ass. J., 1959, *80*, 86. (Cardiovascular manifestations of rheumatoid arthritis.)

HARRISON, L. V. and WOOD, P.: Brit. Heart J., 1949, *11*, 205. (Relation of hypertension to ischemic heart disease.)

HARRISON, T. R.: *Failure of the Circulation*, 2nd ed., 1938.

HERRICK, J. B.: J.A.M.A., 1912, *59*, 2015. (Coronary occlusion.)

JAMES, T. N. and CARRERA, G. M.: New Eng. J. Med., 1959, *260*, 869. (Arrhythmias due to cardiac metastases.)

KARSNER, H. T. and KOLETSKY, S.: Trans. Ass. Am. Phys., 1940, *55*, 188. (Aortic stenosis.)

KENT, S. P. and DISEKER, M.: Lab. Investig., 1955, *4*, 398. (Glycogen loss in early myocardial ischemia.)

LANNIGAN, R.: J. Path. and Bact., 1959, *77*, 49. (Rheumatic lesions in atrial appendage.)

LAURIE, W. and WOODS, J. W.: Lancet, 1958, *2*, 812. (Anastomosis in the coronary circulation.)

LUMB, G. and SHACKLETT, R. S.: Am. J. Path., 1960, *36*, 411. (Lesions of the conduction system.)

MAGNER, D.: Am. J. Med. Sci., 1939, *198*, 246. (Fiedler's myocarditis.)

McKUSICK, V. A.: Bull. Johns Hopkins Hosp., 1956, *98*, 13. (Carcinoid heart disease.)

McLEAN, D. M., WALKER, S. J., and BAIN, H. W.: Can. Med. Ass. J., 1958, *79*, 789. (Coxsackie virus pericarditis.)

McMICHAEL, J.: Brit. Med. J., 1952, *2*, 525. (Congestive heart failure.)

MORRIS, J. N., and CRAWFORD, M. D.: Brit. Med. J., 1958, *2*, 1485. (Coronary heart disease and physical activity of work.)

MOTLEY, H. L., *et al.*: Am. J. Physiol., 1947, *150*, 315. (Pulmonary heart disease.)

MOWRY, R. W. and BANGLE, R.: Am. J. Path., 1951, *27*, 611. (Histological demonstrable glycogen in human heart.)

OLD, J. W. and RUSSELL, W. O.: Am. J. Path., 1950, *26*, 789. (Eisenmenger complex.)

PADER, E. and ELSTER, S. K.: Am. J. Med., 1959, *26*, 424. (Acute rheumatic fever in the adult.)

PARKER, F., JR. and WEISS, S.: Am. J. Path., 1936, *12*, 573. (Pulmonary lesions in mitral stenosis.)

PARKER, R. C., JR., and COOPER, H. R.: J.A.M.A., 1951, *147*, 835. (Acute idiopathic pericarditis.)

PATERSON, J. C. in *Progress in Fundamental Medicine*, Edited by J. F. A. McManus, Philadelphia, 1952.

————.: Arch. Path., 1938, *25*, 474. (Hemorrhage into coronary artery wall.)

PEERY, T. M.: J.A.M.A., 1958, *166*, 1123. (Brucellosis and calcific aortic stenosis.)

PEERY, T. M., and BELTER, L. F.: Am. J. Path., 1960, *36*, 673. (Brucellosis and heart disease.)

POMERANCE, A.: J. Path. and Bact., 1958, *76*, 55. (Relation of mast cells to coronary thrombosis.)

RICH, A. R.: Bull. Johns Hopkins Hosp., 1948, *82*, 389. (Pulmonary vessels in congenital heart disease.)

ROBERTS, J. T. in SODEMAN, W. A.: *Pathologic Physiology*, 5th ed., 1949, Philadelphia. (Conduction of impulses.)

SAPHIR, O.: Am. Heart J., 1942, *24*, 167. (Isolated myocarditis.)

SCHILDER, D. P., HARVEY, P. and HUFMAGEL, C. A.: New Eng. J. Med., 1956, *255*, 11. (Rheumatoid spondylitis and aortic insufficiency.)

SCHLESINGER, M. J.: Arch. Path., 1940, *30*, 403. (Coronary artery anastomoses.)

SCHMIDT, E. C. H.: Am. J. Path., 1948, *24*, 97. (Isolated myocarditis.)

SHELDEN, W. H. and GOLDEN, A.: Circulation, 1951, *4*, 1. (Abscesses of valve rings in endocarditis.)

SMYTHE, H. A.: *In Press.* (Pathology of spondylitis heart disease.)

TAUSSIG, H. B.: *Congenital Malformations of the Heart*, Cambridge, Mass., 1960.

TAYLOR, C. B., *et al.*: Am. J. Path., 1959, *35*, 674. (Myocardial infarction produced by diet.)

TOONE, E. C., PIERCE, E. L. and HENNIGAR, G. R.: Am. J. Med., 1959, *26*, 255. (Aortitis of rheumatoid spondylitis.)

VINEBERG, A., DELIYANNIS, T., and PABLO, G.: Can. Med. Ass. J., 1959, *80*, 948. (Myocardial nutrition after avalon sponge operation.)

WARTMAN, W. B.: Am. Heart J., 1938, *15*, 459. (Hemorrhage into coronary artery wall.)

WEISS, S.: New Eng. J. Med., 1940, *223*, 793. (Sudden death.)

WEISS, S. and WILKINS, R. W.: Ann. Int. Med., 1937, *11*, 104. (Deficiency myocarditis.)

WHITE, P. D.: *Heart Disease*, 4th ed., New York, 1951.

WINTERNITZ, M. C., THOMAS, R. M. and LE COMPTE, P. M.: *The Biology of Arteriosclerosis*, Springfield, Ill., 1938.

WITTELS, B., and REINER, L.: Am. J. Path., 1960, *36*, 55. (Glycogen in human myocardium.)

Chapter 22

Diseases of the Blood Vessels

THE ARTERIES
General Considerations
Arteriosclerosis
  ATHEROSCLEROSIS
    Pathogenesis
      Blood Lipids
      The Vessel Wall
      Mural Thrombosis
      Other Elements: stress, hypertension, intimal hemorrhage, age, heredity.
      Accessory Factors: enzymes, hormones.
  MÖNCKEBERG'S SCLEROSIS
    Medionecrosis of the Aorta
  ARTERIOLOSCLEROSIS
Arterial Hypertension
  RENAL HYPERTENSION
  ENDOCRINE HYPERTENSION
  VASCULAR HYPERTENSION
  ESSENTIAL HYPERTENSION
  HYPERTENSIVE ARTERIOLAR
    LESIONS
  Benign
  Malignant

Polyarteritis Nodosa
  TEMPORAL (GIANT-CELL)
    ARTERITIS
  AORTIC ARCH (TAKAYASHU)
    SYNDROME
  WEGENER'S GRANULOMATOSIS
Disseminated Lupus Erythematosus
Thromboangiitis Obliterans
Bacterial Arteritis
  ACUTE PERIARTERITIS
  ACUTE ENDARTERITIS
  SYPHILITIC AORTITIS
  SYPHILITIC ARTERITIS
    Rheumatic Arteritis
    Rheumatoid Aortitis
    Aortitis of Undetermined Origin
Aneurysms
  ANEURYSM OF THE AORTA
    Atheromatous Aneurysm
    Syphilitic Aneurysm
    Dissecting Aneurysm
    Aneurysm of Sinus of Valsalva
  ARTERIOVENOUS ANEURYSM
  ARTERIOVENOUS FISTULA

Angiospastic Diseases
  RAYNAUD'S DISEASE
THE VEINS
Phlebitis and Thrombosis
  THROMBOPHLEBITIS
  PHLEBOTHROMBOSIS
  THROMBOPHLEBITIS MIGRANS
    Chiari Syndrome
Phlebosclerosis
Varicose Veins
  HEMANGIOMA
    Capillary
    Cavernous
  SCLEROSING HEMANGIOMA
  HEMANGIOENDOTHELIOMA
    Benign
    Malignant
  HEMANGIOPERICYTOMA
  KAPOSI'S SARCOMA
  GLOMANGIOMA

THE ARTERIES

GENERAL CONSIDERATIONS

THE heart may be the most important organ in the body for the preservation of life in general, but the arteries are of equal importance for the preservation of life in individual organs and tissues. Just as the heart can never rest, so the arteries are under the continual strain of the pressure of blood. Moreover, as we shall see presently, their capillary blood supply operates under difficulties. It is small wonder, then, that degenerative changes are more common in the arteries than anywhere else in the body, and that these degenerations are amongst the most important of all causes of disease and death.

We are apt to think of arteries as passive tubes for the conduction of the blood. Holman (1959) points out that the artery should be regarded as an organ, with the functions of such a structure. The electron microscope reveals a metabolic machinery in the form of mitochondria and Golgi apparatus. This machinery is capable of great activity. It burns sugar, consumes oxygen, and liberates carbon dioxide. Moreover, it synthesizes cholesterol, phospholipids, triglyderides, mucopolysaccharides and proteins. We shall return to these activities when we come to the question of the pathogenesis of atherosclerosis.

It is convenient to divide the arteries into three main groups: (1) the large or elastic arteries, (2) the medium-sized distributing or muscular arteries, (radial, renal, superior mesenteric, etc.), and (3) the small arteries and arterioles. The distinction is valuable, because in the elastic type atherosclerosis is the common degenerative lesion, in the muscular type medial calcific sclerosis is frequent, while in the arterioles the sclerosis is of the diffuse hyperplastic type. All of these are varieties of arteriosclerosis. Exceptions to this generalization will be encountered, such as atherosclerosis in small vessels like the coronaries and the cerebrals, but the generalization is useful nevertheless.

Elastic Arteries.—These are represented by the aorta and its main branches. They are the only vessels the walls of which consist mainly of elastic tissue. Their function is to maintain the blood pressure within the arterial system during cardiac diastole, and they do this by virtue of their elastic tissue, which serves to cushion the force of the cardiac pump. When the elastic tissue degenerates owing to disease or ageing the arteries may become dilated, and if the degeneration is localized, the result may be aneurysm formation. Loss of the elastic tissue will interfere with the ability of the vessel to expand during systole, the effect of which may be a gradual rise in the blood pressure.

Distributing Arteries.—These carry the blood from the main trunks to the various organs and tissues. The different parts of the body require different amounts of blood under differing conditions, and the supply is regulated mainly by the distributing arteries. For this reason their walls consist for the most part of plain muscle, which serves to control the size of the lumen and the amount of blood which passes along it. The elastic tissue is concentrated in two layers, the internal elastic lamina between the intima and media, and the external elastic lamina, less sharply defined, between the media and adventitia.

In the fetus *cushion-like thickenings* composed of longitudinal muscle and elastic tissue occur in the walls of some arteries, particularly at their mouths. These cushions are best developed in the coronary, popliteal and lower brachial arteries. It seems probable that their function is to buffer the stresses produced by the anchoring effect of the branch on the systolic elongation of the parent vessel. They become exaggerated in the first two decades, most of all in the coronaries, that is to say in vessels where pulsation is most marked. Their effect is to narrow the lumen of the artery. The reason that these fetal cushions are mentioned here is that they mark the site of future atherosclerotic plaques, and represent one of the mechanical factors which determine the localization of patches of atheroma (Robertson). Many of the smooth muscle cells observed in atherosclerotic plaques undergoing fibrosis represent ingrowth in this muscle.

Arterioles.—These and the small arteries extend between the ends of the distributing arteries and the capillary beds. Their overall diameter is 100μ or less, the ratio of thickness of wall to diameter of lumen in a normal vessel averaging 1:2. The wall gradually loses its two elastic laminae, so that the three coats merge as the vessels become smaller. The degree of pressure in the arterial system is regulated largely by the tonus of the smooth muscle of the arterioles. They act as pressure reduction valves that protect the capillaries from rupturing owing to the high pressure, or as the nozzle on a garden hose, allowing the blood to be sprayed gently into the capillary bed. Any disease of the walls of the different classes of arteries may interfere with one of the various functions just enumerated.

It must be remembered that the post-mortem appearance does not necessarily represent the true condition of the artery during life. The small lumen and deeply folded intima and internal elastic lamina are due to contraction of the media after death, and will naturally vary with the amount of contraction. These artefacts introduce a fallacy which invalidates much of the work of measuring arterial walls and lumina.

Blood Supply.—The blood supply to the wall of the artery presents a special problem. Ordinary capillaries are supplied with blood under very low pressure owing to the valve-like action of the arterioles. Such capillaries would collapse in the intima of a large artery by reason of the high pressure in the lumen of that vessel. The intima, therefore, is lacking in low-pressure capillaries, being supplied by diffusion of blood from the lumen. It is obvious that the deposition of substances in the intima, as occurs in arteriosclerosis, will interfere with this diffusion. The media is supplied with blood by capillaries from small vessels in the adventitia and peri-advential tissue. We have already had to consider this problem in relation to coronary artery disease.

The inner wall of the artery has no lymphatics, for they also would collapse because of their low pressure. As it is the lymphatics which drain off the colloids of tissue fluids which escape from the blood, these substances will tend over the years to accumulate in the intima. It is small wonder, then, that the degeneration of the wall and the accumulation of colloids which characterize atherosclerosis are of such frequent occurrence in the large arteries.

The main diseases of arteries are degenerations and inflammations. As the former group is by far the more important and common, it will be considered first. It includes arteriosclerosis and the effects of arterial hypertension. The inflammations may again be divided into two groups: (1) those of unknown etiology, including the diffuse collagen diseases and thromboangiitis obliterans, and (2) those due to bacteria, such as acute and syphilitis arteritis. Arterial disease may (1) *weaken the vessel wall*, with resulting aneurysm or rupture; (2) *narrow the lumen*, causing ischemia; and (3) *damage the endothelium*, with thrombosis as a result.

ARTERIOSCLEROSIS

Of all arterial lesions arteriosclerosis is the most common, the most important and the most obscure. The very name is enigmatic.

It seems best for the present to use arteriosclerosis in a broad sense to include a variety of non-inflammatory forms of arterial disease which may or may not have a common etiology. Three main forms may be distinguished, which differ sharply in microscopic appearance and in some degree in distribution. These are: (1) atherosclerosis, a patchy lipoidal degeneration of the intima, by far the commonest and most important of the three; (2) medial calcification, commonly called Mönckeberg's degeneration; and (3) diffuse arteriolar sclerosis, a degenerative thickening of the intima of the smaller visceral arteries which may assume more than one form. Medial fibrosis of the medium-sized arteries is common in persons over middle age. Collagenous thickening of the intima (endarteritis obliterans) may cause so marked a narrowing of the lumen of the smaller arteries of the extremities in the later period of life as to lead to gangrene.

1. **Atherosclerosis.**—Atherosclerosis or atheroma is a nodular type of arteriosclerosis which affects the large arteries, especially the aorta, and the small arteries, particularly the coronaries and cerebrals. It is the fact that these arteries supply the myocardium and the brain, and that this is the only form of arteriosclerosis which commonly predisposes to thrombosis, which lends to atheroma a sinister significance. The medium-sized arteries of the muscular type are not so liable to the disease. The term atherosclerosis is better reserved for the process, and atheroma for the nodular lesions, but the two are often used interchangeably. "While mental disease is our greatest socio-economic problem, cancer our greatest enigma, arthritis and rheumatism our greatest crippler, and accidents our greatest disgrace, atherosclerosis is by far our greatest killer" (Holman *et al.*). It kills by diminishing the blood supply to a vital organ, in particular the heart, the brain and the kidneys.

LESIONS.—The *gross appearance* is most readily studied in the aorta. The most severe changes are seen in the abdominal aorta, especially in elderly persons; they are more marked in the descending than the ascending thoracic aorta. Thus the distribution of the lesion is the reverse of that seen in syphilis. They are especially marked around the mouths of the intercostal and lumbar arteries. The earliest lesions may take one of three forms: (1) small yellow dots and streaks consisting of lipid and collections of foam cells; (2) gelatinous translucent elevations representing edematous swelling of the ground substance of the intima and infiltration with plasma; (3) thrombotic deposits which may be grossly invisible (Movat *et al.*) The fatty streaks may be seen in young people after an attack of one of the infectious fevers. In such persons it seems probable that the lipid deposits may be absorbed and that the lesions may never progress to true atheroma, so that a distinction may be drawn between the atheromatosis of youth and the atherosclerosis of advancing years. The intima over the fatty patch becomes raised and at the same time thickened, so that the yellow color of the underlying material is no longer visible and the plaque becomes pearly and looks as if a drop of wax had fallen on the lining of the aorta. The patch contains a soft, yellow, porridge-like material from which the disease takes it name (*athere*, gruel). The process of atheromatous softening may reach the surface, and the pultaceous material is then discharged

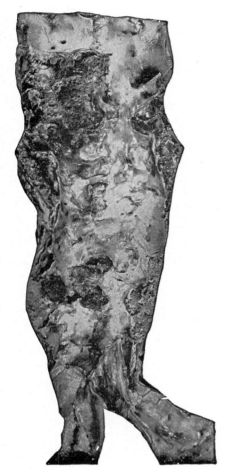

FIG. 268.—Atheroma of abdominal aorta. Thickened patches surround the openings of the lumbar arteries and there is much ulceration. (Boyd *Pathology for the Surgeon*, courtesy of W. B. Saunders Co.)

main features are: (1) *fatty streaks*, (2) *wax-like plaques* of heaped-up intima, (3) *atheromatous ulcers*, and (4) *calcification*.

In the small arteries such as the coronaries and cerebrals the chief characteristic of the lesions is their patchiness. Yellow nodules are seen both on the outer and inner surfaces of the arteries in the circle of Willis, etc. In these small vessels the nodules may cause serious narrowing or even complete occlusion of the lumen. This, for instance, is the chief cause of gradual coronary artery occlusion. The aorta is so wide that the nodules can have no appreciable effect on its lumen.

The *microscopic changes* are primarily in the intima, but lesions, usually regarded as later in development, may also be seen in the media. Without attempting at this stage to assess priority in the sequence of the lesions, a subject which will be discussed in relation to pathogenesis, it may be said that there is a swelling or increase of the mucinous ground substance of the intima, disintegration of the elastic fibers and deposition of the lipids in the deeper part of the lesion. The all-important changes in the mucopolysaccharides of the ground substance are shown by abundant metachromasia with such a dye as toluidin blue, and still more vividly by utilizing the affinity of this material for colloidal iron followed by the use of ferrocyanide, thus giving the Prussian blue reaction (Rinehart and Abul-Haj). It is of interest to note that Virchow, who stole the thunder of modern observers in so many fields, stated that the earliest change in atherosclerosis is a "gelatinous swelling" of the intima and that this "structureless, diaphenous, intercellular substance" resembles mucus both in structure and in chemical composition. This was in 1856, working with unstained tissues!

The lipids are lipoproteins containing cholesterol ester. Some of the lipid is taken up by macrophages, which become pale, swollen, vacuolated "lipid cells." The change gradually extends from the deeper part of the intima to the surface. At the same time there is a thickening of the connective tissue of the intima overlying the fatty area, *i.e.*, the sclerotic part of the atherosclerotic process. Cholesterol, like silica, may remain as an inert substance in the tissues and act as a chronic stimulant to

into the lumen of the vessel and an atheromatous ulcer is formed (Fig. 268). A thrombus may be formed on the surface of the ulcer, which sometimes is the starting-point of an embolus. Calcification of the lesion is very common, since lime salts are readily deposited in fatty material, and in advanced cases the wall of the aorta is converted into a calcareous tube which is cracked in places as readily as a shell. Blood may penetrate through these cracks and separate the layers of the wall. The more advanced the age of the patient, the more likely is there to be marked calcification, especially in the lower part of the abdominal aorta. To sum up, the

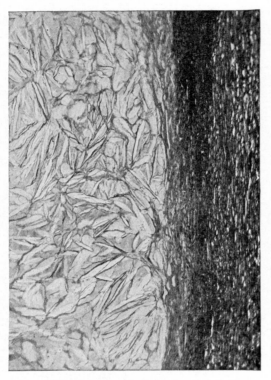

Fig. 269.—Acicular cholesterol crystals in an atheromatous patch. The dark layer is the media. × 75. (Boyd, *Pathology for the Physician.*)

fibroblasts. This new tissue becomes hyaline so that no cells can be seen in it. The deeper part of the lesion consists of a kind of pulp in which the cholesterol ester is broken up into crystals of cholesterol which appear in paraffin sections as needle-like clefts (Fig. 269). In frozen sections the lipid can be stained with Sudan and other stains for fat. Calcium salts are deposited in the fatty material and appear as fine granules stained dark blue with hematoxylin. The same change is seen in the small arteries, but here the internal elastic lamina tends to be broken up into strands, some of which pass superficial and some deep to the lesion, uniting on the far side.

The essential atheromatous lesion is the intimal plaque. In the aorta this has no appreciable effect on the lumen, but in small vessels such as the coronaries and the arteries at the base of the brain, the plaque may seem

to partially or almost wholly occlude the lumen (Fig. 270). When these small vessels are viewed from the outside the atheromatous area can readily be detected as hard yellow nodules which may give to the vessel a beaded appearance. This is particularly noticeable in the cerebral arteries, because in these vessels the elastic tissue is concentrated in the heavy internal elastic membrane, which is liable to rupture rather than disintegrate as the result of degeneration. The contents of the atheromatous lesions are therefore squeezed through these breaks into the media, where they are visible as yellow patches under the adventitia (Duff and McMillan).

Intimal hemorrhage is a common feature of atherosclerosis. Paterson first drew attention to it in the coronary arteries, and it has been found in the pulmonary, cerebral, carotid renal and femoral arteries. The hemorrhages, which are more frequent in hypertension, are often multiple, and that they may occur at intervals is indicated by the presence of old hemosiderin in the atheromatous lesions. The hemorrhage seems to be from intimal capillaries which develop in atherosclerosis and communicate with the lumen of the artery. These capillaries are illustrated in figure 271. The hemorrhage enlarges the atheromatous plaque, and may narrow or occlude the lumen of a small vessel such as a coronary or a cerebral artery. In a large artery such as the femoral this effect is negligible. The intimal hemorrhage may further add to and intensify the atherosclerotic process. Finally, it may rupture into the lumen of the artery and initiate thrombosis. Willis, who found intimal hemorrhage in the femoral and popliteal vessels in 55 cases in 152 routine autopsies, draws an interesting analogy between atherosclerosis and scurvy. In both of these the fundamental fault is in the ground substance of the vessels, new capillaries are formed, hemorrhage is common and thrombosis may be an accompaniment. Moreover in scorbutic guinea pigs Willis observed an abundant deposition of lipids in the ground substance of the aorta in from two to three weeks.

Hartroft has demonstrated in all the atheromatous aortas he has examined the

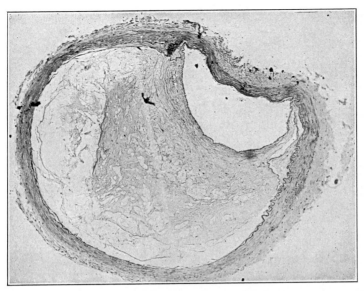

Fig. 270.—Extreme degree of atheroma in a cerebral vessel. The intima is greatly thickened owing to lipid deposits. The lumen is much narrowed, and this led to softening of the brain. × 60. (Boyd, *Pathology for the Physician.*)

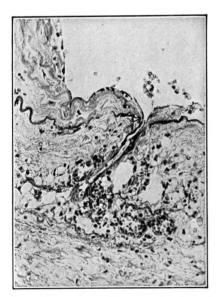

Fig. 271.—Coronary capillary passing from lumen into wall. × 160.

presence of a yellowish-brown pigment apparently identical with the *ceroid* found in the cirrhotic livers of choline-deficient rats. The striking feature of this substance is that it gives an intense staining with the Sudan stains for fat in paraffin sections, and yet is insoluble in alcohol, xylol and other fat solvents. It appears to be derived, at least in part, from red blood cells.

Holman points out that there are different stages in the development or *natural history of atherosclerosis.* These stages, which may well be caused by different factors, are as follows in early aortic lesions seen in New Orleans. (1) *Fatty streaks* (atheroma), probably reversible, which appear from the age of three years onward; (2) *fibrous plaques* (3) *complications of the lesions*; (4) the *clinical disease* (Fig. 272). The percentage of fatty streaks in the New Orleans case rose slowly until the age of eight years, at which time it began to rise sharply in the negro and five years later in the white. An interval of fifteen to twenty years elapses before some fatty streaks are converted into fibrous plaques. The rate of conversion varies in different geographic areas, and this probaby affects the frequency of myocardial infarction. The rapid rise in the lesions during the years of puberty suggests some relation to changing hormonal activity during that period rather than to dietary factors.

Pathogenesis.—Atherosclerosis is responsible for about 95 per cent of deaths from coronary artery disease, about 50 per cent

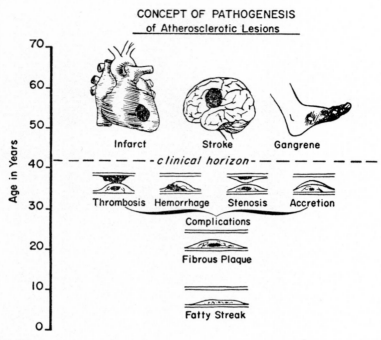

Fig. 272—Showing the various stages of the atherosclerotic lesion, together with some of the complications, and the ages at which they are likely to develop. (R. L. Holman *et al.*, courtesy of Am. J. Path.)

of deaths from diabetes, and about 50 per cent of those from cerebrovascular disease. The causation of the condition is therefore of prime importance if anything is to be done to prevent this common and crippling disease of declining years. It is better to speak of the pathogenesis of atherosclerosis, its mode of production, rather than the etiology, which suggests one causal agent. It is a complex process rather than a "disease" in which many agents may play a part, some being dominant in certain cases, others being important in other cases. As Page puts it in his stimulating review: "Atherosclerosis results from the collaboration of a variety of mechanisms." The amount of time and labor which has been devoted to the problem is vast, and the literature is overwhelming, as may be gathered from the 787 references in a book devoted only to the subject of nutrition and atherosclerosis (Katz, Stamler and Pick). And yet the answer still eludes us.

The most obvious fact to be explained, if possible, is the presence of cholesterol and other lipids in the early stage of the atheromatous lesion. Indeed, it is the character of this fatty material which gives the lesion its name. In the course of time there tends to be at least a partial replacement of the lipid by fibrosis, with the formation of a fibrous plaque. The term atherosclerosis indicates the double character of the process. But is this deposit of lipid a primary or a secondary phenomenon, a cause or an effect? It is as difficult to answer this question with confidence as it is to give a coherent, balanced and orderly account of the pathogenesis of atherosclerosis, because widely differing concepts are championed by workers convinced that theirs is the only correct view with a fanaticism which used to be reserved for religious discussions in a bygone age. Instead of joining with one or another of these groups I feel that it is preferable to allow the student to weigh the evidence and decide for himself. It may help us to keep our feet on the ground if we consider the subject of pathogenesis under three main headings: (1) *the blood lipids*, (2) *the vessel wall*, and (3) *mural thrombosis*. *Accessory factors* also demand consideration.

The Blood Lipids.—We have already seen

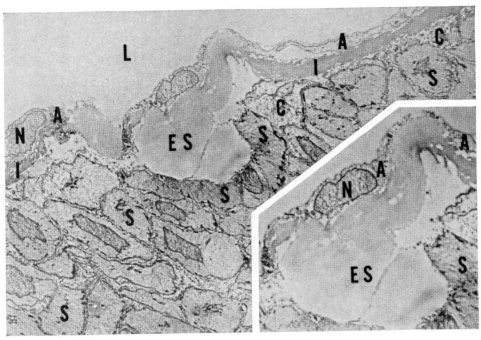

Fig. 273 Fig. 274

Fig. 273.—Normal-appearing internal elastic lamina (I) merges with an area which is characterized by a decrease in density, and there is bulging of the elastica interna with loss of its characteristic fibrillar nature. The initial elastic lesion is seen to cause the endothelial cell cytoplasm to protrude into the lumen. It also encroaches upon the smooth muscle cells (S). × 4000

Fig. 274.—The initial lesion pictured in Fig. 273, at higher magnification. × 6000. (Parker, courtesy of Am. J. Path.)

that one of the most obvious features of the atheromatous lesion is the presence of lipids, and more particularly cholesterol. At once we are faced with the question as to whether these lipids have been produced locally or have reached the intima from the blood stream. The experimental work points to the latter explanation. This work dates from 1913, when Anitschkoff succeeded in producing lesions in the rabbit's aorta which resembled those in man by means of a diet rich in cholesterol. Unfortunately in this respect the rabbit, a herbivorous animal, is in a class by itself. Duff pointed out that the rabbit is an unsatisfactory experimental subject, because its normal blood cholesterol is low and the excretion of cholesterol is poor, so that the concentration in the blood can be easily raised to fantastic limits by feeding. In recent years, however, successful results have been obtained with the chicken, an omnivorous creature more closely related in this respect to man, and in still other animals. Fatal myocardial infarction due to coronary artery atheroma has developed in the rhesus monkey with diet-induced hyper-cholesterolemia (Taylor et al.). Holman and his group point out that there is a primate which develops fat-containing arterial lesions on a low fat diet in its natural habitat, namely the African baboon (McGill et al.). Of 163 baboons, intimal lipid deposits were found in the aorta in 74 per cent of mature animals and in 14 per cent of immature. A few had fibrous plaques in addition to the fatty streaks.

Cold plays a part in the development of coronary atherosclerosis in the experimental animal (Sellers and Baker). Rats fed on commercial laboratory rations develop only very mild atherosclerosis after a long period. When the animals are exposed to cold (2° C.)

the incidence and intensity of the lesions is increased; and hyaline material containing blood elements and lipids collects in the sub-intimal tissue. Severe coronary lesions develop in old rats kept in the cold and fed a high fat, 2 per cent cholesterol diet for only six weeks. In some cases small dissecting aneurysms were apparent in these dogs, recalling the observations by Paterson of hemorrhage from newly formed capillaries in human atheromatous lesions. The rats exposed continuously to cold ate almost double the quantity of food consumed by the controls, so that the uptake of cholesterol was twice as great.

As might be expected, the *electron microscope* has been found to throw new light on the mechanism of hypercholesterolemic atherosclerosis in the experimental animal (Parker). Acute hypercholesterolemia was induced in rabbits by forced feeding with the stomach tube or intravenous injection; chronic lipemia was achieved by ordinary dietary means. With the electron microscope caps of dense material, believed to be lipoprotein, were seen overlying the inner surface of some of the endothelial cells of the coronary artery. Similar material was present in indentations of the plasma membrane, in dilated vesicles in the endoplasmic reticulum, and finally in the internal elastic lamina, which showed discrete defects in structure (Figs. 273 and 274). This picture, which developed in as short a space of time as 24 hours in acute lipemia, seems to correspond to the foam cells seen with the light microscope and to the picture in frozen sections stained for fat. The importance of the observations with the electron microscope is that they support the inhibition theory as originally suggested by Virchow rather than the view that the lipid is of endogenous origin, resulting from degeneration in the arterial wall.

Evidence obtained from the *human subject* is suggestive although by no means conclusive. There can be no doubt that long-sustained hyperlipemia aggravates the tendency to develop atherosclerosis, as is seen in diabetes, nephrosis, myxedema and xanthomatosis. On the other hand most patients who develop the disease have relatively normal blood cholesterol levels. In such cases, however, it is quite possible that the level may

have been raised months or years before the sample of blood was tested. The suckling baby is inbibing an abundance of cholesterol in the milk, so that the seeds of atherosclerosis may have been sown at a very early age.

The relationship of diet to serum cholesterol and atherosclerosis is one of the most contentious aspects of the subject. Modern so-called civilized man with increasing wealth consumes more food rich in animal fats and indulges in less physical activity, which he prefers to watch. It is an inexorable law that when energy intake exceeds energy expenditure, calories must be stored within the organism, usually as lipid. This subject of diet is of enormous practical importance not only with respect to prevention of the disease, but also to the dairy and food industries, the great bulk of the cholesterol in the diet coming from milk, eggs and their products, foods which are not partaken of in quantity by native races or by wild animals. Katz and his associates assert with confidence the undoubted relationship between diet, serum cholesterol and atherosclerosis. The present day North American diet is rich in cholesterol-lipids derived mainly from dairy products. This is a diet of civilization and is unknown to wild animals.

The prevalence of atheroma as evidenced by coronary artery disease in peoples living under different dietary conditions has been used as an argument. Thus in the Korean War 50 per cent of the American dead, of an average age of twenty-two years, showed grossly visible atheroma, and in 10 per cent of cases one coronary artery had its lumen reduced more than 50 per cent. The Korean and Chinese soldiers, on the other hand, with a negligible intake of milk products and a low consumption of eggs and meat, showed no coronary artery atheroma (Dock).

The fallacy in such statistics as these is that we are dealing with different races, in whom genetic factors may be more important than dietary differences. Much more convincing are observations made on Japanese living in Japan, Hawaii and California (Keys *et al.*). Of all countries with detailed vital statistics, Japan has the lowest mortality rate for coronary artery disease. This disease is very rare in Japan, fairly common in Hawaii, and the leading cause of death in the Los Angeles Japanese Hospital. The Japanese in Hawaii and California were not recent emigrants, but native born. As regards diet, fats provided less than 10 per cent of the total calories for farmers in Japan, 30 per cent in Hawaii, and almost 40 per cent in Los Angeles. Similar investigations in other parts of the world, particularly for the Bantu native and white man in South Africa, show a low incidence of atherosclerosis and of coronary artery disease and a low average level of cholesterol in the blood in populations subsisting on low-fat diets in comparison with populations on high-fat diets.

It may be added that the same type of diet which causes hypercholesterolemia also causes *increased blood coagulability* and hence a tendency to the deposition of thrombin. We shall return to this point presently.

We may say, then, that the dietary enthusiast regards atherosclerosis as a metabolic disease in which altered cholesterol-lipid-lipoprotein metabolism plays a critical role in persons with a habitually unbalanced diet, high in calories, total fats, unsaturated fatty acids, and cholesterol. It is only fair to the enthusiast to add that he does not regard atherosclerosis as purely and simply a dietary disease. Diet seems to be a decisive factor in a population, but not in an individual, in whom multiple factors come into play, just as we see in tuberculosis (Katz *et al.*).

The observations of Paterson and his associates are of interest from the point of view of the individual as opposed to a population. Serum cholesterol determinations were carried out at least once a year on 800 elderly ambulatory patients who were permanently confined to hospital. These determinations were begun in 1953, and by 1959 there were 191 deaths with autopsy. The results lent little support to the contention that the severity of atherosclerosis is related to the level of serum cholesterol, except perhaps when it exceeds 300 mg. per cent. The question of raised cholesterol levels in earlier years is another matter.

It would appear that the size and physical state of the lipid molecules may be more important than the level of serum lipid. Gofman and his associates have shown by measuring the flotation rate in the ultracentrifuge that several species of lipoproteins may exist in the human subject. The units used are called Svedberg flotation or S_f units. Two classes of lipoproteins are elevated significantly in patients with coronary artery disease, namely those between S_f 12 and S_f 20 (the S_f 12–20 class) and those between S_f 20 and S_f 100 (the S_f 20–100 class). As these two classes represent only 10 to 15 per cent of the total lipids of serum, it would seem that 85 to 90 per cent of serum lipoproteins are not related to atherosclerosis, so that estimations of total serum cholesterol are without value and indeed misleading. It is believed that the S_f 10–20 molecules bear a significant relationship to human atheroma, and that these macromolecules (giant molecules) may become entrapped between the overlying endothelium and the underlying elastica. When the neutral fats and fatty acids are absorbed the cholesterol and its esters are left behind. The significant S_f levels are raised in certain diseases, *e.g.*, diabetes, nephrosis, myxedema, hepatitis and xanthomatosis. The level is also raised in obesity, and it is not without interest to note that atheroma is ten times more common in the obese than in the lean. The administration of heparin has a remarkable influence in shifting the serum lipoprotein pattern toward normal. It clears a lipemic serum, apparently activating a plasma enzyme system, a lipoprotein enzyme.

It must not be forgotten that there is an endogenous production of cholesterol which exceeds the normal dietary intake of carniverous animals. All the cells of the body can produce cholesterol from acetate. The main factory of cholesterol synthesis is the liver, whence it passes into the bile to be reabsorbed from the bowel. The name cholesterol indicates, of course, the original source from which it was first isolated. The possibility of developing blocking agents which can prevent reabsorption of cholesterol from the bowel is being investigated. Vegetable sterols appear to be much more innocuous than animal sterols. Not only are corn germ and the *sitosterols* (plant sterols) not absorbed, but they inhibit hypercholesterolemia and atherogenesis in cholesterol-fed chicks and rabbits.

Before leaving the intriguing, even fascinating, subject of the relationship of blood lipids to atherosclerosis, brief reference may be made to the question: Are we sure that the lipids which are found in the atherosclerotic aorta, coronary arteries and circle of Willis are necessarily the same? It has been assumed that the composition of the lesions in the aorta and the coronary artery must be the same. Not it would appear that they may be different, the most striking difference being the high percentage of triglycerides in coronary artery lesions compared with those of the aorta. In the circle of Willis the triglycerides are the same as in the aorta, as also are the total lipids extracted, but the cholesterol esters are high and the free cholesterol is extremely low. It seems probable that there are other differences which are still unknown.

We may close this discussion of the relation of lipids to atherosclerosis by saying that the popular current concept regards atheroma as a local manifestation in the arterial wall of a general disturbance of lipid metabolism or transport, but it is not certain whether the lipid deposits are primary initiating events or merely secondary sequelae in the pathogenesis of the lesions (Hartroft and Thomas).

The Vessel Wall. — In their admirable review of the entire subject of atherosclerosis Duff and McMillan emphasize the importance of local factors in the vessel wall.. The lesion may be regarded as the resultant of an accumulation of substances filtered from the blood by the vessel wall and the reaction of the wall to these substances. Or again, it may be taken as the expression of a relationship between two opposing groups of dynamic processes concerned with the deposition and the removal of lipids from the intima. The walls of arteries may be regarded as filter beds, with material from the plasma continually passing through the intima to be picked up by the vessels and lymphatics of the adventitia. There is every reason to believe from experimental observations that normally a large movement of plasma constituents occurs through the vessel wall. Some of the filtered material, particularly the lipids, the only class of vital substances insoluble in water, may be held back due to

(1) changes in the filter, (2) abnormal size of the lipid particles. The lipid then becomes "foreign." When the cells of the intima from a human aorta are grown in tissue culture in human blood serum to which cholesterol is added, lipid is deposited in the cells in an amount proportional to the quantity of cholesterol added, the cells becoming enormously increased in size (Rutstein *et al.*). The deposition of lipid can be inhibited by an unsaturated fatty acid and potentiated by the corresponding saturated fatty acid.

In the section on General Considerations we have already seen that it is a mistake to regard the arterial wall as merely a passive filter (Holman). It seems unlikely on physical grounds that lipid molecules of such diversified size, shape, electrical charge and chemical configuration should be filtered through the wall at a uniform rate. The filtration theory does not explain the spotty distribution and the variable size and shape of the lesions. Nor the prolonged period of cholesterol feeding necessary to induce atherosclerotic lesions in laboratory animals in whom the blood cholesterol level begins to rise in the first week or two, but the lipid lesions do not develop for at least 3 months. Nor the fact certain hypercholesterolemias are not associated with atherosclerotic lesions, as in the alloxan-induced diabetes of rabbits. We must face the possibility that a local accumulation of lipids might be due to increased local formation or decreased local removal rather than to increased filtration. This does not mean that diet does not play a role in the genesis of atherosclerosis, but it may do so not by filtration, but by upsetting the control mechanism (? hormones, enzymes) which normally protect the wall.

In trying to form for ourselves a concept of the pathogenesis of atheroma it is well to distinguish between the parts played by ground substance, elastic tissue, fibrous tissue and lipid. The most fundamental of these may be the *ground substance*, the matrix from which elastic and fibrous tissue may be formed and to which they may return. It is, moreover, a prime factor in controlling tissue permeability. It consists mainly of the mucopolysaccharides hyaluronic acid and chondroitin sulfate, the latter being the sulfated form of the former. It stains metachromatically with toluidin blue and is beautifully demonstrated by the colloidal iron technique which stains it an intense blue, especially when it is increased in amount or altered in character as the result of disease (Rhinehart and Abul-Haj). In infancy the metachromatic substance is distributed evenly throughout the entire width of the wall of the aorta between the elastic fibers, but with advancing years the ground substance becomes condensed in focal masses of foamy metachromatic material especially in areas showing fragmentation of elastic fibers (Taylor). It may be that there is a relationship between increased metachromia and degeneration of the elastica, the highly polymerized mucopolysaccharides of elastic tissue being returned to the metachromatic pool. The process is seen in most striking form in medionecrosis of the aorta, and is not necessarily associated with atheromatous plaques. This medial degeneration is met with at all ages, but is most pronounced in later years and in cases of arterial hypertension. Destruction of the elastica may be due to overactivity of the enzyme elastase or to lack of the inhibitor of the enzyme which is present in normal serum.

Mural Thrombosis.—It was in 1852 that Rokitansky suggested his *incrustation hypothesis* in which atherosclerosis was traced to deposition of thrombotic material which became incorporated with the intima, with vascularization from the intima and adventitia, hemorrhage from the new vessels, and liberation of cholesterol from the erythrocytes. This seemed a very satisfying theory, remarkably modern in outlook. Only four years after Rokitansky's paper appeared, Virchow, his arch opponent with enormous authority, introduced the concept that atherosclerosis was due to an imbibition of plasma by a damaged intima with deposition of lipid in the ground substance of the intima. Rokitansky's thrombogenic theory was promptly dropped into the discard, but in 1926 it was revived by Duguid, more particularly with regard to the coronary arteries. Duguid concentrated attention on fibrin, which became the all-important element in the process, although why fibrin was not so clear. Duguid's concept, supported by Crawford and Levene and well reviewed by McLetchie, has gained in favor with the passing years. Experimental evidence in support of this hypothesis is not lacking (Williams). An organizing coronary thrombus covered by endothelium from the intima may be indistinguishable microscopically from an atheromatous lesion into which hemorrhage has occurred. According to the thrombogenic hypothesis, these lesions should not be regarded as occasional complications, but as an important factor in pathogenesis (Duguid et al., 1957). Many agents serve to maintain the delicate equilibrium between the formation and the removal of fibrin, with *fibrinolysis* acting as a critical factor. Small amounts of fibrin are believed to be continually deposited on the walls of the vessels because of the ubiquity of thromboplastic agents. Normally these deposits are removed by the fibrinolytic system, which consists of a fibrin-splitting proteolytic enzyme, plasmin, that is produced from a precursor, plasminogen. If, however, the person with the artery has an unbalanced fibrinolytic system, where lysis is delayed, the consequences may be serious (Astrup).

The observations of More and his associates on the development of atherosclerotic lesions of the aorta from an early to an advanced stage lend strong support to the idea that deposition of fibrin and platelets is an important factor in many cases. The fully developed lesion is a complex focal connective tissue thickening of variable composition, often rich in lipids which may be intracellular or extracellular. The early lesions were represented by white opaque plaques consisting of thrombus material, mainly fibrin, and pearly white plaques, which proved to be thrombi in various stages of organization. Many of these lesions were too small to be seen with the naked eye. Fibrin and platelets may be deposited on an intima which shows no morphological alteration (Fig. 275). suggesting that a disturbance in the clotting mechanism is responsible for the formation of the precursor thrombi. In other cases a protein-rich material is deposited in the intima, the type of lesion which has been termed serous inflammation. In this work the early lesions fell into three groups: (1) subendothelial accumulations of lipid-rich cells with some extracellular lipid; (2) a

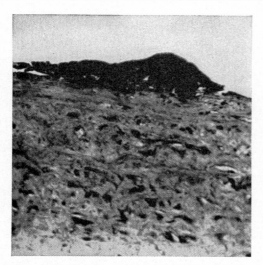

FIG. 275.—Small mural platelet-fibrin thrombus on the surface of unaltered intima. Trichrome stain. × 250. (Movat, Haust and Moore, Courtesy of Am. J. Path.)

serofibrinous exudate or edema; (3) surface deposits of platelet and fibrin thrombi. The later sclerotic lesions represent organization of the second or third of these three components. The cellular elements involved in the repair phase of many atherosclerotic lesions of the thrombotic type have morphological features characteristic of smooth muscle cells rather than fibroblasts, and are believed to be derived from endothelium which regenerates following damage in the atherosclerotic process (Haust, *et al.*).

The work of Mustard and his associates serves to bring together the thrombogenic and the dietary lipid aspects of the problem. A lipid source is necessary for blood coagulation. Normally this is provided by the release from the platelets of lipid material which is needed for thromboplastin formation. The presence of certain lipids free in the blood can replace the material from the platelets, and since this is already free it seems to accelerate the coagulation. In this respect the important phospholipid is phosphatidyl ethanolamine, which accelerates the clotting mechanism both *in vitro* and in the experimental animal, thus taking the place of platelets. The two common food sources of the phospholipid are butter and eggs, a fact perhaps better forgotten at the breakfast table. Margarine is without effect, but the addition of the phospholipid to margarine makes it as active as butter. Swine on a high fat diet with butter as the chief constituent show a marked increase in the incidence and severity of the atherosclerosis which they commonly present, whereas with margarine the increase is quite slight (Rowsell, Downie and Mustard). Coagulability of the blood is most active in butter-fed swine with the greatest degree of atherosclerosis, but there is no increase in the blood cholesterol. Rabbits on a similar diet develop marked hypercholesterolemia, but only one-third of the animals showed severe atherosclerosis. Men with clinical evidence of atherosclerosis or a positive family history have a more active clotting mechanism than do controls.

Factors which favor excessive deposition of platelets on the surface appear to be: (1) increased stickiness of the platelets, (2) changes in the blood flow due to local factors, and (3) damage to the vessel wall. *Increased stickiness* is characteristic of young, newly-formed platelets. Various conditions are known to cause the production of new platelets, but in this connection we are concerned with the increased stickiness which accompanies the administration of phospholipids in the diet. *Changes in the blood flow*, such as slowing or eddies, favor the deposition of platelets. This agrees with the localization of the plaques of atherosclerosis around areas where there are changes in the blood flow, such as the bifurcation or origin of vessels. *Damage to the vessel wall* has already been considered in the general discussion on coagulation and thrombosis in Chapter 6. It is well exemplified by the deposits of platelets and fibrin on an atheromatous ulcer.

From what has been said there appears to be a continuous thread running through and connecting hyperlipemia, increase in the adhesiveness of platelets, platelet deposits, early atherosclerosis, intimal hemorrhage and fibrin deposits, with possible final thrombosis and closure of the vessel. If the mural thrombogenic theory is correct it would support the use of anticoagulant therapy, which would prevent not only occlusion of the lumen by a thrombus but might interfere with the farther development of the atherosclerotic process.

A number of additional factors must be taken into account in any discussion of the pathogenesis of atherosclerosis.

Stress.—The ground substance of the intima may be affected by injury in the form of strain, with resulting deposition of lipids. This is seen in the localization of the lesions at the origin of branches or the bifurcation of arteries. At these points the lumen is normally dilated, and the effect of stress and tension varies directly with the radius of the lumen. Mechanical support may protect an artery from injury. Thus the portion of the internal carotid artery which lies within the carotid canal at the base of the skull rarely shows atheroma, whereas the parts proximal and distal to the canal are very prone to the condition (Willis). The coronary arteries are more frequently involved with atheroma and at an earlier age than any other artery. This may be related to their origin directly from the aorta, there being no opportunity to step down the high pressure they receive directly from the main arterial truuk. One of the most puzzling features of atherosclerosis is its segmental distribution. One artery is involved, whilst another is spared; one segment of an artery shows marked lesions, whilst an adjoining segment is apparently normal. The meaning of this is obscure, but it must be related to local factors, of which stress or injury in its various forms may be one.

Hypertension.—When two conditions are very common in the same age period it is always difficult to know if they are related causally. This is true of arterial hypertension. Different sites must be considered separately. I am convinced that the frequent association of hypertension and atherosclerosis of the coronary arteries is not entirely fortuitous, particularly in young persons, but there seems to be no connection between the two in the aorta. Hypertension may accelerate the atherosclerotic process by favoring the production of intimal hemorrhage (see below). The most convincing examples of correlation are afforded by local hypertension, for example the pulmonary arteries in the pulmonary hypertension of mitral stenosis, the aorta proximal to a coarctation, the dilated internal mammaries in a coarctation, etc.

Intimal Vascularization and Hemorrhage.—Paterson has shown that there is a well-marked relation between atherosclerosis and vascularization of the intima. We have already seen that hemorrhage into an atheromatous patch from these new capillaries is a frequent occurrence especially in the coronary arteries. It would appear that intimal hemorrhage, which is aggravated by hypertension, is a probable factor in at least the acceleration if not the initiation of the atherosclerotic process (Paterson). If the lipid content of the extravasated blood is high, more lipid will be deposited at the site of the hemorrhage. Vascularization of the intima may be an early rather than a late phenomenon in the course of atherosclerosis, perhaps even a precursor, for by means of the alkaline phosphatase technique for demonstrating endothelium, capillary structures can be seen in the superficial layers of the aortic intima in the earliest lesions (Paterson *et al.*).

Age.—Atherosclerosis is a degenerative process associated with advancing years, which in one way seems as natural as the graying of the hair. It is the end of a song that is first sung in the cradle, for, as we have seen, the beginnings of the process can be detected in the earliest years. As Clifford Allbutt put it many years ago in his own inimitable fashion: "It cannot be supposed that the stealthy hours carry away no qualities of tissue, no quantities of energy." The older the person, the more likely is there to be marked atheroma, a fact which is enshrined in the saying: "A man is as old as his arteries," but to this there may be notable exceptions, for in persons over eighty years of age the aorta may show hardly a trace of atheroma, whereas it may be quite marked in the young. These exceptions probably have a genetic basis, as discussed below. It is possible that it is the elastic fibers of the media which are damaged by the ageing process, and that the loss of elasticity may lead to degeneration of the intima. When a disease appears in the later years of life there is another possibility to be kept in mind, namely that the long span of years has merely given a mildly acting causal agent time to produce its effects. We have already seen this to be the case with regard to carcinogenesis. The slow accumulation of lipids in the intima of arteries may also occupy a long interval of time.

Heredity.—There can be no doubt that heredity plays a part in predisposing to atherosclerosis. Thus in one analysis of 300 cases of the disease a family history was present in 67.5 per cent, and many of the remainder did not know the cause of death of their ancestors. One patient, whose father died of apoplexy and mother of cardiovascular-renal disease, had 9 brothers and sisters all of whom had died of apoplexy, and he himself had already had a stroke. Other people seem to inherit arteries with an architecture so sturdy that the various atherogenic factors make no impression on it.

There are grounds for believing that genetic factors influence the serum lipid level, possibly by determining enzymatic chain reactions (Adlersberg and Schaefer). This belief is supported by the knowledge that such conditions as familial xanthomatosis and idiopathic hypercholesterolemia, which are certainly hereditary, are often associated with coronary artery disease. Finally, there is the fact that certain breeds of chickens develop atherosclerosis spontaneously, whereas another breed, kept under the same conditions of diet, housing and exercise, had almost no atherosclerosis. It is perhaps worthy of note that the serum lipid and cholesterol levels of the two sets of birds showed no significant difference, despite marked differences in the degree of atherosclerosis (Clarkson *et al.*).

Accessory Factors.—Among these may be mentioned enzymes and vitamins. *Enzymes,* more particularly *esterase,* may play a part in the disposal of any cholesterol which may be disposited in the intima of the artery. In this regard the observations of Constantinides on the *mast cells* in the rat are of interest. It is impossible to produce atherosclerosis in the rat by feeding cholesterol alone. Now the connective tissue of the rat is abundantly supplied with mast cells, whereas in the atherosclerotic-susceptible rabbit these cells are practically absent. The mast cell is believed to produce *heparin,* and the injection of this substance, which is related chemically to mucopolysaccharides, inhibits lipemia and retards atherogenesis in the cholesterol-fed rabbit. Women were found to have more mast cells than men except in a group with marked atheroma, and these cells were found to be fewer in atherosclerotic old persons than in non-atherosclerotic young adults. Other workers have failed to confirm a relation between mast cells and the degree of atherosclerosis, although there is a reduction in the number of these cells in cases with complications such as thrombosis and infarction (Paterson *et al.*).

Hormones.—Various hormones can play a part in determining the onset and progress of atherosclerosis (Oliver and Boyd). The importance of sex hormones is evident from the prevalence of the condition in the male and the relative immunity of the female up to but not beyond the menopause. The development of lesions in the coronary arteries in cholesterol-fed male chickens is prevented by the administration of estrogens, even though the blood cholesterol remains high, but this is not true of the aorta, suggesting a local effect on the ground substance of the intima rather than a generalized action on the plasma. It must be remembered, however, that the result of the administration of a certain hormone at a given dose level to one species gives little indication of the result which may be obtained in another species. Certain it is that the clinical syndrome of coronary heart disease is very distinctly increased in certain human endocrine disorders in which the blood lipid level is also elevated, more particularly myxedema, diabetes mellitus, and following bilateral ovariectomy. Indeed there seems to be an inverse relationship between endogenous estrogen secretion on the one hand and coronary disease, blood lipid level, and a tendency to fibrin formation owing to changes in blood coagulation and the fibrinolytic system, on the other.

The esterase mechanism may be under chemical or hormonal control. This is suggested by the fact that the cholesterolosis of the aorta produced in rabbits by feeding cholesterol is prevented by the administration not only of thyroid gland, but also of iodine. The incidence of atheroma in Iceland is remarkably low (Dungal), and it has been suggested that this may be due to the abundant iodine supply in the food, soil and air of that country. Atheroma is also very common in China, as are other conditions involving disturbance of lipid metabolism. The facts of geographic pathology are always of interest, but fact must be distinguished from theory, and it is wise not to let fancy run too free in suggesting explanations. Possibly the temporary lipid deposits in the intima which are met with in adolescence may be due to transient inhibition of esterase owing to hormonal imbalance.

Vitamin deficiency has been shown to play a part in atherosclerosis in the experimental animal. In the case of *Vitamin B₆ or pyridoxine deficiency* the character and distribution of the lesions in the deficient monkey are much more analogous to the atherosclerotic lesions of man than are those of the experimental cholesterolosis of rabbits. The initial change is a swelling of the mucinous ground substance of the intima followed later by the appearance of lipids. *Vitamin C or ascorbic acid deficiency* produces atherosclerosis in guinea pigs which closely resembles the human variety (Willis). Scurvy is essentially a disease of ground substance, and ascorbic acid appears to be essential for the health of the ground substance of the intima.

Summary.—A large volume of facts and ideas have been paraded before the reader regarding the causation of atherosclerosis. The length of the discussion is a testimony to our confusion of thought on the subject. When the answer is known it may perhaps be expressed in a sentence. The two most striking features of the lesions are the accumulation of lipids in the intima and the fibrosis or hyalinization of that structure. The explanation of these lesions has followed three main lines of thought. (1) *Imbibition of lipids*, cholesterol in particular, as the result of a high lipid level (at some time) in the blood stream, this in turn being due to a high fat content of the food. There is much epidemiological evidence to support this concept, but other factors must also be involved, for of every 4 or 5 persons living under identical conditions from the environmental and dietary viewpoint, only one will develop the disease. (2) *Changes in the vessel wall* may well determine the localization of the lesions. Degeneration of the mucopolysaccharides of the ground substance of the intima may pave the way for the deposition

of lipids. Capillary hemorrhage resulting from vascularization of the lesion will certainly provide an abundant supply of lipids. (3) *Thrombotic encrustation of the intima* with material derived from the blood, the platelets in the early stages with fibrin deposits later. The initial change in the platelets seem to be related to the amount and type of lipid content of the food. The lesions are superficial at first, but later become incorporated into the intima.

It may well be that these widely differing views may not be as mutually exclusive as might at first appear, and that all of them may play some part, depending on the conditions prevailing in the particular patient. Obviously other factors also come into play, such as heredity, age and sex, and whatever it is which determines the localization of the lesions.

Mönckeberg's Sclerosis.—This is the type of arteriosclerosis which is observed by the clinician when he feels the arteries, for it is the vessels of the limbs, arteries of the muscular type, which are affected. The pipestem radials, the tortuous and prominent temporals, belong to this class. The condition is a senile degenerative change with no relation to high blood pressure, although the long-continued administration of adrenalin in animals leads to calcification of the media. In these respects it resembles atheroma. The two lesions may both be present in the same artery. What relation, if any, it bears to atheroma it is not safe at present to say. The arteries most affected are the femoral, popliteal, the radial just above the wrist, and the parietal vessels such as the gluteal and pudendal. The visceral arteries (mesenteric, etc.) are seldom involved, but typical examples may be seen in the uterus and ovary in old persons.

LESIONS.—It is probable that the first change is fatty degeneration of the media. Calcium is then deposited in the degenerated tissue, and the vessel becomes hard and brittle.

The chief *microscopic* change is in the media (Fig. 276). The muscle fibers undergo fatty changes with degeneration, fragmentation, and the deposition of lime salts. These may be in the form of fine granules or large masses. Bone containing bone marrow has

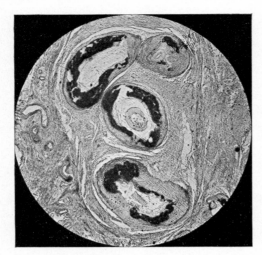

FIG. 276.—Mönckeberg's sclerosis of ovarian vessels. In the media of three of the arteries there is a large deposit and in the fourth a small deposit of lime salts. × 16.

sometimes been observed. The other coats are often normal, in which case there will be no narrowing of the lumen. Atheroma is often added, and this may produce marked occlusion, a change seen in senile and diabetic gangrene of the leg.

Medionecrosis of the Aorta.—With advancing years the aorta often develops a basophilic mucin-like substance in the interstitial tissue of the media which stains blue with hematoxylin, intensely blue with colloidal iron, and gives a polychromatic (violet) reaction with such basic aniline dyes as thionin and toluidin blue. This polychromatic material represents a change in the mucopolysaccharide (hyaluronic acid) of the ground substance. The chromatropic material presents a vacuolated and even bubbly appearance (Fig. 277), the elastic tissue may be largely replaced, and focal necrosis may develop, especially in the inner and middle thirds of the wall. Cyst formation may occur in these necrotic patches, the idiopathic cystic medionecrosis of the aorta first described by Erdheim. The result of these changes, which can only be appreciated if the sections are stained for elastic tissue and with a stain for mucopolysaccharide, is to weaken the wall of the aorta to such a degree that a dissecting aneurysm may develop or in rare cases spontaneous rupture of the

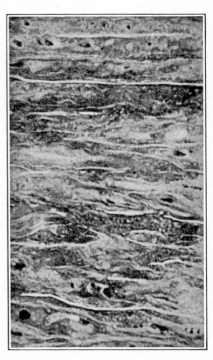

FIG. 277.—Medionecrosis of aorta, showing marked vacuolization of ground substance. × 400.

aorta. The pathologist sometimes encounters at autopsy cases of great cardiac hypertrophy with no obvious explanation such as arterial hypertension or aortic valvular disease. In a number of such instances I have seen marked medionecrosis with disappearance of elastic tissue and in one case a loud aortic diastolic murmur was heard, suggesting that the cardiac hypertrophy might be due to aortic insufficiency.

Arteriolosclerosis.—This form of arterial degeneration is also called diffuse hyperplastic sclerosis. The term arteriole is vague and not susceptible of strict definition. In the present connection it is used to indicate the smaller arteries of the viscera, the intimate vasculature, vessels 100 microns in diameter or less. The lesions are not all of one type, but in general they cause thickening of the wall and narrowing of the lumen. Arteriolar sclerosis may be widespread, but is most frequent in the spleen, pancreas, kidney and adrenal. The arteries involved are of a smaller order than the "small" arteries affected by atheroma, *e.g.*, coronary and cerebral vessels.

Hypertension and the *ageing process* seem to be the two principal etiological factors. That hypertension is a causal agent is indicated by the fact that identical lesions are found in the experimental hypertensive animal. On the other hand similar lesions, although usually less pronounced, may be present in persons without hypertension, especially in the aged. Hypertension appears to accentuate and speed up a normal wear-and-tear degenerative process. As arteriolosclerosis is so intimately associated with hypertension, the changes in the vessels will be considered in relation to that condition.

ARTERIAL HYPERTENSION

The blood pressure in a state of health is the resultant of a number of forces, among the chief of which are the contractions of the heart and the peripheral resistance provided by the arterioles, although the elastic recoil of the large arteries and the state of the capillary bed are also of importance. In spite of the fact that these varied factors are continually altering, so perfect is the coördination between the several parts of the circulatory system that under ordinary conditions any sudden change in pressure is rapidly restored to normal. Should the pressure be *continuously* below or above normal the condition is called respectively hypo- or hyper- tension. The systolic pressure alone may be increased, or both systolic and diastolic pressures may be elevated. From the standpoint of the patient systolic hypertension is of no importance. It appears to be dependent on the loss of elastic tissue in the large arteries which occurs with advancing years. Diastolic hypertension, on the other hand, is a true disease phenomenon. Hypertension is defined by the life insurace companies as any elevation of the systolic pressure above 140 mm. of mercury and of the diastolic pressure above 90 mm. of mercury. This may be statistically true for a community, but the figures must be much more elastic when applied to the individual, otherwise the physician will label as an invalid a person who is and who will remain in vigorous health for the normal span of life.

Arterial hypertension is at present divided into two forms, *primary* or *essential*, where the cause is unknown, and *secondary*, where there is some associated lesion such as chronic nephritis or adrenal cortical tumor, which is believed to be responsible for the raised blood pressure. Essential hypertension, which constitutes about 90 per cent of all cases of hypertension, may again be divided into so-called benign and malignant forms. The *benign form* is characterized by a gradual onset and a long-continued course, often of many years. The *malignant form*, very much less common, is frequently of abrupt onset, and runs a course measured in months rather than years. It often ends with renal failure (uremia), but not necessarily so. Hypertension is sometimes divided into two types, renal and extrarenal. One difficulty is that not only can renal disease, and in particular renal ischemia, produce hypertension, but hypertension, by inducing arteriolosclerosis in the kidney, can lead to renal ischemia. In childhood essential hypertension is extremely rare. When hypertension is encountered it is almost certain to be secondary in character, caused by coarctation and other conditions peculiar to children.

Some of the more important causes of hypertension are given below. Most of these will be discussed in later chapters, but a few may be considered here.

CLASSES AND CAUSES OF HYPERTENSION

ESSENTIAL HYPERTENSION
  Idiopathic
  Benign
  Malignant

SECONDARY HYPERTENSION
  Renal
    Glomerulonephritis
    Chronic pyelonephritis
    Polycystic kidney
    Renal vascular disease
    Renal amyloidosis
    Urinary tract obstruction
  Endocrine
    Pheochromocytoma
    Primary aldosteronism
    Cushing's syndrome
    Pituitary basophil adenoma
  Vascular
    Coarctation of the aorta
    Polyarteritis nodosa
  Toxemia of Pregnancy

Renal Hypertension.—The relationship of the kidney to hypertension is associated with the names of two men, although ninety years separate their work. It was Richard Bright who first recognized the relationship between chronic renal disease and elevated blood pressure as indicated by the hypertrophied heart of chronic nephritis. Nearly a century had to elapse until Harry Goldblatt provided experimental proof by producing hypertension by rendering both kidneys of the dog ischemic by means of clamps on the renal arteries which are slowly tightened over a considerable period. When the rat is used, *unilateral* renal ischemia causes persistent hypertension, together with the arterial lesions of malignant hypertension in the *opposite* kidney (Wilson and Byrom).

When we look for an explanation of these facts we find ourselves in difficulty. It would appear that the kidney has two opposing functions with regard to blood pressure both in the experimental animal and in man, the one function hypertensive, the other antihypertensive. It is believed that the ischemic kidney produces a pressor substance, probably the enzyme renin, which acts on a substrate, hypertensinogen, in the plasma to form hypertensin (angiotonin or angiotensin). The Goldblatt kidney is a renin-producer. This cannot be the complete explanation of the relation of the kidney to hypertension, because dogs in whom *both kidneys have been removed*, but who have been kept alive by peritoneal lavage or other similar means, develop sustained hypertension (Grollman *et al.*). This hypertension does not develop for some seventy-two hours, and it would appear to be due to the absence or failure of a *normal antihypertensive function of the kidney*. It has been suggested that the hypertension which develops in man as the result of widespread renal ischemia may be due to the destruction or inhibition of an antihypertension factor rather than to the liberation of a pressor agent by the kidney. Strongly against this view is the demonstration of both renin and hypertensin in the blood of the experimental animal as well as in man in renal ischemia.

Choline deficiency hypertension is a remarkable example of renal hypertension produced in the experimental animal by a dietary deficiency. Weanling rats kept on a diet deficient in choline for a mere five or six days developed a marked degree of hypertension on reaching the age of six or seven months, the weight of the heart being almost double that of the controls (Hartroft and Best). Subsequently it was found that within two weeks of the low-choline diet the glomeruli exhibit a progressive reduction of the capillary bed, with thickening of the basement membrane and proliferation of the glomerular epithelial cells (Ashworth and Grollman). There is no hypertension at this early stage. Later the glomeruli become extensively involved, with fibrous replacement of much of the glomerular capillary system. Hypertension is generally present at this stage.

Renal hypertension in man may be associated with: (1) *glomerulonephritis*, a diffuse glomerular capillary ischemia, in which hypertension may be present in both the acute and chronic stage; (2) *chronic pyelonephritis*, a much more common condition, in which removal of the affected kidney in the exceptional unilateral case may be followed by complete and permanent cure; (3) *stenosis of one or both of the main renal arteries*, due to atheroma in the elderly, to fibrous intimal proliferation (possibly developmental in origin) in the young, and very occasionally to occlusion of one branch of the renal artery by an embolus, with segmental infarction. In all of these instances renal ischemia is a dominant feature.

Endocrine Hypertension.—The *adrenals* seem to play a part in the regulation of blood pressure. One of the earliest advances in endocrine physiology was the discovery in 1890 that an active principle in the adrenal medulla (adrenalin, epinephrine) would cause marked elevation of the blood pressure through action on the sympathetic nerves supplying the arteries. The sustained or paroxysmal hypertension associated with *pheochromocytoma*, the chromaffin tissue tumor of the adrenal medulla, is due to a similar vasoconstrictor action. From these facts it might be supposed that the medulla of the adrenal is concerned with the normal regulation of blood pressure. All the evidence goes to show that the reverse is the case, and that control lies with the cortex. The administration of corticosteroids produces hypertension, especially in a unilaterally nephrectomized animal, but this effect is greatly enhanced if there is a liberal supply of *sodium* in the diet. The sodium content of the median and intimal coats of the renal arteries in human hypertensive patients is 22 per cent higher and the water content 17 per cent higher than in normotensive subjects (Tobian and Binion). If the same degree of water concentration were also present in the hypertensive arterioles, the decrease in the diameter of the lumen could increase flow resistance as much as 54 per cent, with resulting elevation of the pressure. This is the basis for the restriction of salt in the diet in the treatment of hypertensives. It may also explain the action of *chlorothiazide*, a valuable antihypertensive agent which is not only a powerful non-mercurial diuretic, but is also saluric in action, increasing the urinary excretion of sodium, potassium and chloride in addition to water. It can be used in conjunction with a ganglion-blocking agent such as hexamethonium or a centrally-active vasodepressor such as reserpine. Antihypertensive drugs may be life-saving in cases of malignant hypertension. In *primary aldosteronism* the salt-retaining hormone, produced in excess by a tumor of the adrenal cortex, is associated with hypertension as well as with severe urinary potassium loss and renal damage.

The *pituitary* may also be related to hypertension. Injection of posterior pituitary extract causes a rise of pressure far more sustained than that produced by adrenalin, but little is known of its physiological action. In Simmonds' disease, a manifestation of pure anterior pituitary insufficiency, the pressure is low. Basophil adenoma of the anterior lobe is always accompanied by hypertension, and the kidney often shows evidence of vascular nephritis (nephrosclerosis).

Vascular Hypertension.—Elevation of the blood pressure may be due primarily to narrowing of a main vessel, as in coarctation of the aorta, or to a generalized constriction of small arteries and arterioles, as in polyarteritis nodosa. *Coarctation of the aorta* has already been described in the preceding chapter. On account of the location of the obstruction, the effects of the hypertension are only apparent in the upper part of the body and the upper limbs. It is a principal cause of hypertension in childhood, of particular importance to recognize because of the possibility of successful surgical treatment. The lesions of *polyarteritis nodosa* are described on page 523. The very widespread inflammatory swelling of the small arteries and arterioles leads to marked narrowing of the lumen, with secondary hypertension developing in over 50 per cent of cases. The *arteriolar narrowing* of *age* may be related to the tendency of the blood pressure to rise with the passage of the years.

Essential Hypertension.—This form of hypertension has not been left to the last because of its rarity. It is, indeed, by far the commonest, and is, perhaps, the most frequent cause of death in the adult. Its name has even less meaning than the alternative terms, primary and idiopathic. They all indicate our lack of any real knowledge of the nature and cause of the condition. In view of the experimental work already referred to, there is a natural tendency to lay the blame on the kidney, but the numerous similarities between experimental hypertension in the animal and essential hypertension in man do not prove that they have a common pathogenesis. It is true that at autopsy varying degrees of arteriolosclerotic narrowing of the renal vessels will be found, but this may be minimal in degree. The degree of narrowing does not compare with that needed to produce hypertension in the experimental animal. It is difficult to believe that such insignificant lesions should be responsible for a hypertension which may have lasted for a number of years. It seems much more likely that the vascular sclerosis is the *effect rather than the cause* of the hypertension. It is true that in the *late stages* of essential hypertension the arteriolosclerosis may cause renal ischemia, which in turn may give rise to hypertension, so that a vicious circle may be established, but this does not mean that the primary lesion is a renal one.

A particularly interesting report is that of Castleman and Smithwick on 100 biopsies on the kidneys of hypertensive patients in the course of lumbar sympathectomy. In more than half the cases there was no significant degree of arteriolosclerosis in the renal vessels. It is true that only a very small area of kidney could be examined in this way, but the authors consider that the method gives fair sampling, and conclude that in 50 per cent of cases the hypertension was not preceded or caused by the vascular lesions.

If the part which the kidney plays in maintaining normal blood pressure is by inhibiting an extrarenal pressor mechanism, it seems reasonable to suppose that overactivity of that mechanism may overcome the normal restraining influence of the kidney. There are good reasons for suspecting that at least one extrarenal pressor agent is secreted by the adrenal cortex, and that it regulates arterial tone by controlling the distribution of electrolytes and sodium in particular. In animals with experimental hypertension total adrenalectomy is followed by a profound fall in blood pressure. This is restored to normal by substitution therapy with cortisone or desoxycorticosterone.

A penetrating analysis of the whole problem of the renal and extrarenal factors in relation to hypertension will be found in Clifford Wilson's Oliver-Sharpey lectures, which open with these significant words "The subject of these lectures is at present one of the most popular topics for research and one of the most controversial in clinical application."

Heredity plays a part in determining if a patient will develop essential hypertension. Indeed the condition has been described as an inherited tendency to develop high blood pressure in middle life. In one investigation in families where the parents had normal blood pressure the incidence of hypertension was only 3 per cent; where one parent suffered from hypertension the incidence in the children was 45 per cent. (Ayman). In 1956 a family was reported with three generations of hypertensive patients (Wear). All of the first generation died of stroke except one who died of "high blood pressure" at the age of sixty-two. All three of the sisters married men with moderate hypertension, and their three children, one of them a girl aged twelve years, all have blood pressure above normal. The hereditary tendency is generally transmitted as a Mendelian dominant.

Hypertensive Arteriolar Lesions.—Refer-

ence has already been made to the two varieties of hypertension, benign and malignant. The vascular lesions differ in the two forms, although the distinction between the two is not always as sharp as indicated here. In each form there may be two significant lesions.

Benign Arteriolosclerosis.—The characteristic lesions are hyaline degeneration and elastic hyperplasia. *Hyaline degeneration*, the commonest manifestation of arteriolosclerosis, is best seen in the smallest vessels, such as the afferent arterioles of the kidney, although not confined to these vessels. There is a sharply defined, smooth, acidophilic thickening of the subintimal tissue. In course of time the change may involve the entire thickness of the wall (Fig. 278), but some trace of nuclear structure usually remains. The appearance suggests an accumulation or deposition of hyaline material which leads to narrowing and in extreme cases to complete obliteration of the lumen. In the spleen hyaline arteriolosclerosis is so common as to have no pathological significance. In the kidney it is almost invariably associated with hypertension, whereas in non-hypertensives the kidney is one of the organs least frequently involved. In no other organ is there this constant relationship between arteriolosclerosis and hypertension, but in such organs the lesions are more frequent and more severe in persons with hypertension. Hypertension is, therefore, the most important causal factor, but, except in the case of the kidney, it is not an essential factor.

Elastic hyperplasia, sometimes called *elastosis*, is most marked in the larger arterioles and medium-sized arteries, but some degree of it can be seen even in the smallest vessels. The internal elastic lamina is split up into several layers, a process known as *reduplication* (Fig. 279). There may also be proliferation of endothelial cells which become intermingled with the new elastic fibers. At first the elastosis is confined to the intima, causing narrowing of the lumen, but as time goes on both intima and media are seen to be composed largely of elastic fibers in sections stained to show that tissue. The muscular type of artery has become converted into the elastic type characteristic of large arteries

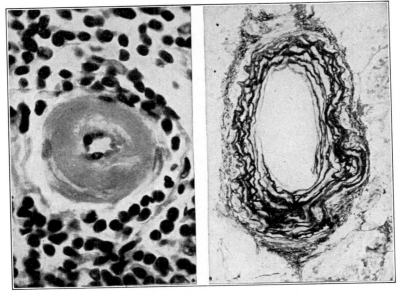

Benign

FIG. 278.—Hyaline degeneration.   FIG. 279.—Elastic hyperplasia.

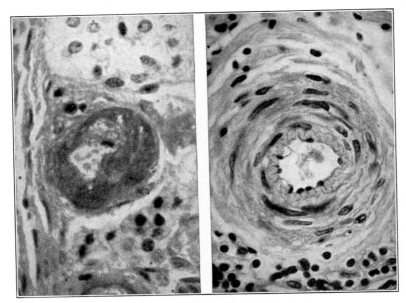

Malignant

FIG. 280.—Arteriolar necrosis.   FIG. 281.—Cellular hyperplasia.

FIGS. 278, 279, 280, 281.—ARTERIAL CHANGES IN HYPERTENSION.

such as the aorta which are designed to withstand great strain and are little more than passive conducting tubes. The amount of elastic tissue in the walls of an artery approximately corresponds to the pressure of blood within it.

Malignant Arteriolosclerosis.—In the malignant form of hypertension, in which the process has a quickened *tempo* and the vessels have less time to adapt themselves to increased strain, the characteristic lesions in their order of importance are arteriolar necrosis and cellular hyperplasia. In *arteriolar necrosis,* also called necrotizing arteriolitis, the whole thickness of the vessel wall becomes necrotic and structureless (Fig. 280). The affected area stains diffusely red with eosin, and its limits are fuzzy and indistinct, as if it had been freshly painted and someone had smeared it with his thumb. This is in sharp contrast to the clean-cut smooth appearance of hyaline degeneration, in which sharply defined nuclei often persist. A rapid rise in blood pressure is likely to lead to arteriolonecrosis due to the sudden and severe mechanical strain and extreme vasoconstriction. The lesion can be produced in the course of a few days in the experimental animal. The necrotic wall often becomes infiltrated with red cells, and hemorrhage is common, especially in the brain. Aneurysmal dilatation can occur. Arteriolonecrosis is commonly seen in hypertension complicated by renal failure (uremia). A renal factor may possibly aggravate the process in an already hypertensive person or animal, but it is not, as believed by some, a primary and essential element in the production of malignant arteriolosclerosis. *Cellular hyperplasia,* commonly called productive endarteritis and hyperplastic arteriolosclerosis, is a condition in which the walls of the arterioles are thickened by a concentric cellular proliferation, so that they may present an "onion-skin" appearance (Fig. 281). The proliferation may be mainly subintimal, so as to merit the term endarteritis, but often the hyperplasia is most marked in the media, a natural response to the increased intravascular pressure. Without an elastic tissue stain it may be impossible to distinguish the limits of the nucleated thickened intima and the hyperplastic media. When the process

is slower the nucleated appearance is lost and the new tissue becomes collagenous. Fatty degeneration may be marked in frozen sections. Elastic hyperplasia of the intima is not a special feature of the condition; such hyperplasia appears to be a reaction to gradually increasing and prolonged hypertension. It may, of course, be present in the medium-sized arteries of any one over middle age, but under these conditions it has no significance.

For the sake of convenience these four lesions have been described separately. They may, however, be combined and intermingled, for the slow (benign) form may have an acute (malignant) termination. Similar arteriolar lesions are seen in the hypertension of glomerulonephritis.

In *summary,* we may say that *essential hypertension is the end result of the interaction of certain unknown environmental variables and a genetic constitution.* Our review of secondary hypertension suggests that these varied factors may be *renal, adrenal, neural,* and *electrolyte.* The incidence of hypertension in the natives of East Africa is very low. In the American Negro the incidence is higher than in the white man. In the Bahamas almost 1 of every 2 Negro adults has hypertension, and the death rate from this cause is very high. There is no reason to think that transportation (from West, not East Africa, it is true) has changed the Negro's genetic constitution. It is much more probable that he is now exposed to new pathogenetic factors such as stress, electrolyte imbalance, etc. It may be noted that the salt content of the water in the Bahamas is very high, and that almost all food is fried in salt pork oil. With regard to neural vasoconstrictor stimuli passing from the brain via the autonomic system to the arteries it would almost appear as if in hypertension the thermostat were set at a higher level than normal. Sympathectomy is designed to lower that level. Very real advances have been made with regard to ganglion-blocking and other antihypertensive drugs, but we have to admit that we do not yet understand the workings of the carbureter of blood pressure, and have to content ourselves with putting a little sand in the fuel line to cut down the flow of gasoline.

Pulmonary hypertension is quite another matter with different problems. It is considered in Chapter 24.

POLYARTERITIS NODOSA

Polyarteritis nodosa, one of the group of the *diffuse collagen diseases* (see chapters 4 and 5), is also known as *periarteritis nodosa,* by reason of the periarterial inflammatory exudate which is often a prominent feature. It is now recognized that all the coats of the vessel wall are involved, and one of the most striking features is the widespread character of the lesions. For these reasons polyarteritis is to be preferred to periarteritis as a descriptive name, although the latter term is in common use.

Etiology.—Perhaps polyarteritis nodosa is the best example of a collagen disease in which there is excellent reason to accept a hypersensitivity factor. A preceding history of asthma is a feature of some cases, or asthma may develop during the course of the disease. The very widespread character of the lesions supports this idea, and also the fact that identical lesions have been found in a number of cases of serum sickness and hypersensitiveness to sulfonamides. Rich has reported a series of such cases, and has succeeded in producing diffuse polyarteritis nodosa experimentally by establishing in rabbits a condition analogous to serum sickness in man. The disease is apparently much commoner than it used to be, and this might be attributed to acquired sensitivity to the multitude of new drugs continually poured into the body by the physician or the patient.

LESIONS.—The principal vessels affected are those of the gastro-intestinal tract (mesenteric and celiac axis), the kidney and the heart, but the brain, lungs and skin may also be involved. The lesion is a panarteritis rather than a periarteritis, and in my experience most of the cases fail to show the "nodosa" feature. This term indicates the presence of small inflammatory nodules scattered along the artery like peas in a pod. There may be hundreds of these nodules on the mesenteric vessels. The fundamental *microscopic* change is increased permeability of the vessel wall (Pagel). The earliest change is edema and escape of fibrinogen into the

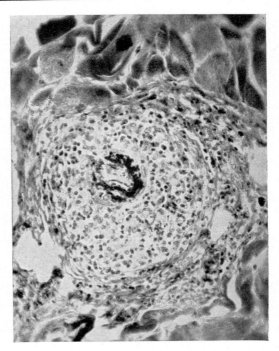

FIG. 282.—Polyarteritis nodosa. All the coats of the artery are infiltrated by inflammatory cells. Fibrinoid material is prominent in the intima. (Kindness of Dr. Henry Z. Movat.)

wall with the formation of fibrin or material which stains like fibrin. This is followed by fibrinoid necrosis, first of the media and later of the other coats. Fragmentation of the elastica is a prominent feature which explains the frequency of aneurysm formation. Inflammatory cell infiltration involves all the coats (Fig. 282). At first the cells are neutrophils and eosinophils; later these are replaced by more chronic types. Owing to involvement of the intima thrombosis is common, and small infarcts are produced in the heart, kidneys and other organs. Renal lesions are particularly common, occurring in 75 to 85 per cent of the cases (Davson *et al.*). In addition to multiple infarcts there may be diffuse changes in the renal parenchyma resembling those of glomerulonephritis. Hypertension may be associated with healed occlusive lesions of the branches of the renal artery.

Pearl Zeek draws a distinction between the typical or classical type of polyarteritis nodosa and what she calls *hypersensitivity angi-*

itis, which are those cases in which the lesions more closely resemble those seen in the experimental animal. In this type (1) the arterioles, venules and capillaries are affected, rather than the small and medium-sized arteries of muscular type as in the classical form, so that the lesions occur in the substance of the viscera; (2) the spleen and the lungs are most frequently involved; and (3) the condition is a fatal fulminant one, often with a history of recent exposure to some antigenic substance.

The Relation of Symptoms to Lesions.—The condition is commoner in males than females in the proportion of 3 or 4 to 1, in striking contrast to what is found in the closely related disseminated lupus erythematosus, which is almost exclusively a disease of the female. For this striking sex difference there must be a good reason, and one would very much like to know what it is. The disease usually runs an acute febrile course, often ending fatally in a few weeks. As the lesions are so varied and widespread the clinical picture may be equally varied, but there is a certain recognizable clinical pattern, the outstanding features being prolonged fever, weakness, quick pulse, limb pains suggesting rheumatism or neuritis, chest symptoms such as cardiac pain or asthma, abdominal pain, and finally albuminuria and hematuria. Hypertension develops in at least 50 per cent of cases. Blood examination reveals a constant leukocytosis, eosinophilia in about one-fifth of the cases, a high sedimentation rate, and a negative blood culture. This complex symptomatology, corresponding to no system disease, may itself suggest a correct diagnosis.

There may be *acute abdominal symptoms* due to involvement of the mesenteric arteries, *acute cardiac symptoms* from coronary artery involvement, *muscular pains* simulating myositis or trichinosis, *albumin and blood in the urine* due to involvement of renal arteries, etc. *Neuritic pains* are common; they are due to lesions of the peripheral nerves (Kernohan and Woltman). Death is often due to a ruptured aneurysm. In the healed stage the symptoms will be those of ischemic sclerotic lesions of the heart, kidneys, etc.

Temporal Arteritis.—This condition is a chronic inflammatory process involving the temporal arteries of elderly persons, but extending to the arteries of the scalp and face. The vessels can be felt as cord-like swellings. Cooke and his associates have shown that, while the name is conveniently descriptive, the lesions are by no means confined to the temporal arteries, and may involve also the aorta, radial, subclavian, femoral, coronary, renal, mesenteric, and retinal arteries. The inflammation appears to spread from the adventitia to the media. There is marked thickening of the intima due to the formation of a zone of loose cellular connective tissue. The walls of the involved vessels (the medium-sized muscular arteries) are thickened and thrombosis may occur. Foreign body giant cells formed in response to disintegration of the elastica is a striking feature of many cases. For this reason the name *giant cell arteritis* or *granulomatous giant cell arteritis* has been suggested instead of the misleading temporal arteritis which has become a misnomer (Gilmour). Unfortunately giant cells occur in other destructive lesions of arteries such as Buerger' disease. Eosinophils are sometimes present in considerable number.

The onset of the illness is marked by malaise, myalgia and arthralgia, anorexia, and loss of weight. After some months more localized symptoms appear, especially severe headache, mental confusion, and visual disturbance which may end in blindness. There may be symptoms suggesting generalized arterial disease. A variable degree of fever is often present. The disease is self-limited, but owing to its generalized nature it may end fatally.

The *etiology* is unknown. It will be seen that the condition bears a close resemblance to such generalized arterial disease as polyarteritis nodosa, in which the inflammation is most probably allergic in character. It occurs at an older age period than that disease.

THE AORTIC ARCH (TAKAYASHU) SYNDROME.—This very rare condition, first described by the Japanese ophthalmologist Takayashu, is also known as the *pulseless disease* or *syndrome*, owing to the frequent absence of the radial pulse. The condition has been called *"young female arteritis"* because it is predominantly a disease of young women in the reproductive years. The *lesions* consist of a thickening of the wall of the arch of the aorta and of the origins of the main vessels which arise from it, together with an associated thrombosis. Microscopically there is an arteritis suggestive of the lesion of temporal (giant-cell) arteritis, and the lesion is sometimes referred to as *giant cell aortitis*. On this account it has been suggested that the condition is hyperergic in character. It should be pointed out that the aortic arch syndrome is not strictly synonymous with the "young female arteritis" of Takayashu, for the term signifies involvement of the arch with a tendency to obliteration of the large vessels which arise from its convexity, a state of affairs which may be caused by syphilis and other pathological conditions such as severe atherosclerosis.

The *clinical picture* is striking. There is lack of pulses in the arms, neck and head, owing to stenosis of the branches of the aortic arches, with good pulsation in the legs, *the reverse of what is observed in coarctation of the aorta*. The cerebral manifestations are identical with those of thrombosis of the internal carotid artery. Vertigo, especially on rising from the horizontal positon, is the most common symptom, to which may be added very distressing headache, hemiplegia and loss of consciousness (Ross and McKusick).

WEGENER'S GRANULOMATOSIS.—This is perhaps the newest addition to the collagen disease family being first cousin to polyarteritis nodosa. It has been called *necrotizing respiratory granulomatosis*, the three most characteristic lesions being (1) *necrotizing giant cell granulomata of the respiratory tract*, (2) *generalized angiitis*, and (3) *necrotizing glomerulitis*. The condition probably represents a hypersensitivity antigen-antibody reaction, in some cases to streptomycin and other antibiotic agents.

Lesions.—The principal lesions are in the lungs, kidneys and arteries. A remarkably severe and destructive inflammation involves the upper respiratory tract, with sharply circumscribed granulomatous masses containing multinucleated giant cells in the lungs. In the kidneys there is a focal necrotizing glomerulitis generally limited to a single glomerular lobe, resembling the renal lesions of subacute bacterial endocarditis. There is widespread angiitis perhaps best seen in the spleen. This may involve the medium-sized arteries, and resemble the necrotizing lesions of classic periarteritis nodosa being visible to the naked eye, or the lesion may be confined to the arterioles. Cutaneous and subcutaneous nodules showing characteristic lesions are common, and biopsy examination of these lesions are of diagnostic value (Churg and Strauss).

The *symptoms* are likely to be mainly respiratory in the beginning. Evidence of renal damage such as albuminuria and hematuria are constant, and death may occur from uremia. The skin and the nervous system are often involved.

DISSEMINATED LUPUS ERYTHEMATOSUS

This member of the group of the diffuse collagen diseases, also known as *systemic lupus*, has already been discussed at length in Chapter 5. As the name suggests, the lesions are widely disseminated throughout the connective tissues and ground substance of the body, resulting in a correspondingly complex clinical picture. In this place we shall confine our attention to lesions of the arteries. These lesions are most common and severe in the kidneys, but they may be found in any organ, although not necessarily in the same case. The most striking feature is a fulminating fibrinoid necrosis, in response to which there may be a secondary exudation of inflammatory cells, mostly lymphocytes and plasma cells. This is the reverse of the typical picture in polyarteritis nodosa. Moreover arterioles and capillaries are likely to be involved, whereas in polyarteritis a larger order of vessels is affected. Another puzzling difference is that disseminated lupus is predominantly (over 90 per cent) a female disease, whereas polyarteritis nodosa is much commoner in the male. Both are believed to be examples of hyperergic reaction, possibly auto-immune in character. The demonstration of the L.E. cell reaction in the blood (page 119) is invaluable in diagnosis, and the presence of hematoxylin bodies in the tissue is said to be pathognomonic.

THROMBOANGIITIS OBLITERANS

This is in essence a thrombotic occlusion of the vessels of the legs in relatively young men with resulting gangrene of the toes and then the feet. It was originally described by von Winiwarter in 1879, but it was Buerger, at Mount Sinai Hospital, New York, who brought the condition to the attention of the medical profession in 1908, so that it became known as *Buerger's disease*. At that time he considered arterial thrombosis to be the primary event, but subsequently he changed that opinion in favor of a primary inflammation of the vessels with consequent thrombosis. There were supposed to be three stages: (1) acute inflammation, at first purulent, later with giant cell inflammatory foci; (2) a stage of healing; (3) thickening of the intima with sclerosis of the vessel wall. It is true that acute lesions were almost never found, but their absence was explained on the grounds that the material examined was from amputated lower limbs in which the inflammatory stage was long since past.

The *sex incidence* is striking, for the disease used to be practically confined to men, although cases in women are becoming more common. The race incidence, though less striking, is also pronounced. Buerger's original cases were practically all young Russian and Polish Jews, but this was perhaps natural in view of Buerger's hospital. It is now recognized that Gentiles may also suffer, and even Scotsmen are not immune. It is a disease of young adult life. The lesions are usually in the vessels of the legs, but the arms may also be affected.

Etiology.—For the past fifty years Buerger's disease has been regarded as a specific entity, and various infective agents have been suggested both by Buerger and by other workers, but none have been confirmed. The excessive use of tobacco, especially cigarettes, has long been added by clinical observers to such factors as sex, race and age. Certain it is that the disease is largely confined to heavy smokers, and that when the victim gives up smoking, which he is often loth to do, the symptoms are often relieved. This does not mean that the disease is a separate entity, for ischemic conditions caused by atherosclerosis, as, for instance, coronary artery heart disease, are aggravated by heavy smoking, probably because of the vasoconstriction which the use of tobacco produces.

At the present time opinon is beginning to swing away from Buerger's concept of thromboangiitis obliterans. Certain it is that *thrombosis* is the dominant feature of the

disease rather than inflammation, as is indicated by the name. It may well be that the basic disturbance is in the coagulative mechanism of the blood and not a lesion of the arterial wall, that the initial event is thrombotic occlusion of the small arteries and arterioles that are subject to vasospasm, that organization of these lesions accounts for all of the inflammatory features, and that the disease progresses by retrograde extension of the thrombus (Gore and Burrows). In support of this view is the fact that an intimal reaction of the arteries is the earliest change, with later involvement of the accompanying veins. Moreover in about 20 per cent of cases the superficial veins of the part show what Buerger calls a *migrating phlebitis*, evidenced by the presence of painful red spots which last for a week or so. It was from the study of excised portions of such vessels that the concept of an acute inflammatory stage originated.

Others regard Buerger's disease not as a distinct morbid process, but as a condition indistinguishable from atherosclerosis, systemic embolization, or peripheral thrombosis. For this reason the diagnosis is becoming increasingly rare. During the past ten years no case with this diagnosis has been seen at the Beth Israel Hospital, Boston (Wessler *et al.*). We have already seen that thrombosis is naturally a frequent accompaniment of atherosclerosis, and that it may represent the first step in the development of an atherosclerotic lesion, if we accept the "incrustation" theory of that disease.

Lesions.—The *acute lesions* to which reference has already been made are really those of an acute migrating thrombophlebitis, better called a phlebothrombosis. In the artery the only indication of a hypothetical previous acute inflammation is the occasional presence of giant cell foci, which may be seen in an organizing thrombus.

The *chronic lesions* are those seen when the leg is amputated for gangrene months or years later. All signs of active inflammation have disappeared, and artery, veins, and nerves are bound together in a dense mass of fibrous tissue. The clot has become organized and converted into fibrous tissue, and there is no sign of the original lumen (Fig. 283). New vascular channels lined by endo-

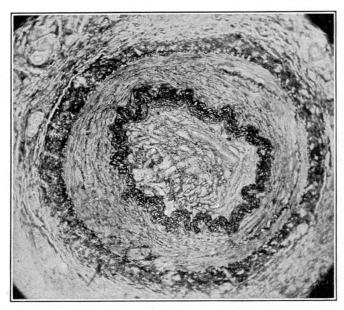

Fig. 283.—Thromboangiitis obliterans. The lumen is closed by fibrous tissue which is partially canalized. Hypertrophy of elastica. Elastic tissue stain. × 40.

thelium are formed in the fibrous mass, so that the lesion is often mistaken for a mere thickening of the intima, an endarteritis obliterans. Thickening of the elastic tissue, both internal and external is a striking feature, as is well seen in Fig. 285. There is no calcification, so that the vessel throws no shadow in the roentgen-ray picture.

Relation of Symptoms to Lesions.—The first symptoms are usually indefinite pains in one foot or cramp-like pains in the calf after walking a short distance, a condition known as intermittent claudication (*claudicare*, to limp). No pulse can be felt at the ankle. When the foot hangs down it becomes bright red (erythromelia) and throbs painfully. When the foot is raised it becomes more blanched than normally. Later in the disease trophic disturbances appear in the form of ulcers and gangrene of the feet. The formation of trophic ulcers is often accompanied by excruciating pain, and suicide is not an uncommon termination of this distressing condition.

The symptoms are due to loss of the peripheral blood supply or to disturbances of the collateral circulation which is set up. The prognosis depends on the extent to which the collateral circulation can be established, and modern methods of treatment are directed to the encouragement of this circulation. The *cramp-like pains in the muscles* are due to the painful spasm which accompanies an insufficient blood supply when the muscle is in a state of activity. The *flushing of the foot* when it hangs down and its blanching when elevated is due to loss of vasomotor control, the nerves in the periadventitial tissue being involved in the inflammatory and sclerotic process. The *trophic lesions* may be due to a similar cause, a view supported by the fact that when the affected segment of vessel is resected the trophic lesions may heal quickly and permanently.

BACTERIAL ARTERITIS

It is rather remarkable that we are so ignorant regarding the etiology of the various important forms of arteritis which have so far been considered, and it is a relief to turn to one or two in which the cause is better known.

Acute Periarteritis.—Acute inflammation may attack an artery from the outside or the inside. An artery which passes through a

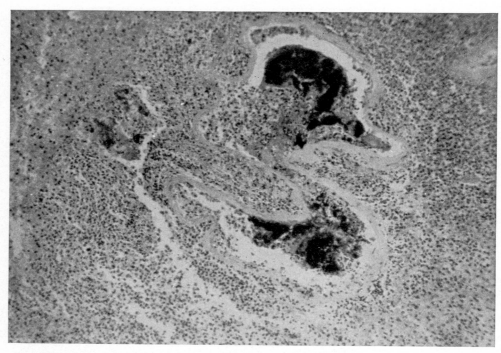

FIG. 284.—Acute arteritis in staphylococcal septicemia. Septic reaction in blood vessel of spleen.
(Kindness of Dr. A. J. Blanchard, Sunnybrook Hospital, Toronto.)

focus of suppuration such as an abscess should be very liable to infection, but on the contrary it is quite resistant. Sometimes, however, the bacteria penetrate the wall and produce an acute arteritis and periarteritis, the media and adventitia being filled with polymorphonuclear leukocytes. The wall may be so weakened that hemorrhage may occur. Before the days of asepsis *secondary hemorrhage* was very common in operation wounds and was due to an acute suppurative arteritis produced by the septic ligature which was buried in the lacerated wall of the vessel. After a number of days the destruction of the wall was so great that hemorrhage occurred into the wound, and this was often fatal.

Acute Endarteritis.—If an infected embolus from a septic thrombus in a vein or a vegetation of an acute endocarditis lodges in an artery it infects the vessel from within. Again the vessel wall becomes acutely inflamed. The results may be (1) septic thrombosis with breaking up of the thrombus and the formation of secondary metastatic ab-

scesses (Fig. 286); (2) the production, by weakening of the wall, of a small mycotic aneurysm. This may burst and lead to severe or fatal hemorrhage.

Syphilitic Aortitis.—Syphilis attacks two important sets of vessels: (1) the aorta and its large branches, and (2) the cerebral arteries. Other vessels may be affected, but the clinical effects are of relatively little importance compared with these two. Aortitis used to be one of the commonest and most important of syphilitic lesions, but modern antibiotic therapy has enormously decreased the incidence of the condition. It is usually found in males between the ages of thirty and fifty-five years. Symptoms seldom appear within five years of the primary lesion, although the perivascular lymphatics are probably infected from the very beginning of the disease.

Lesions.—The *gross appearance* is very characteristic unless it is obscured by the development of atheroma. The lesion begins in the aortic wall just distal to the aortic cusps, and spreads horizontally around the

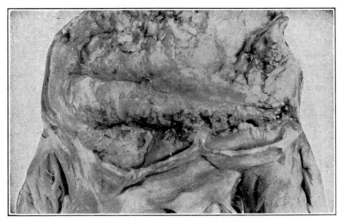

Fig. 285.—Syphilitic aortitis. The surface of the aorta is nodular, wrinkled, and scarred. There is widening of the commissure, and thickening of the free margin of the aortic cusps.

root of the aorta and distally as far as the mouths of the great vessels springing from the arch. This forms in many cases a zonal lesion picturesquely known as the *girdle of Venus*. Even more frequently the whole arch is diffusely involved. The probable reason why the suprasigmoid portion is the site of election is that it has such an abundant lymph supply, the spirochetes being carried in the perivascular lymphatics. The gross changes may be traced down as far as the diaphragm, where they suddenly stop, and as a rule the abdominal aorta is free from lesions.

In the affected area the intima is raised into patches, at first smooth and pearly, but later pitted and scarred. The intervening tissue is wrinkled like the bark of a tree. Longitudinal wrinkling is striking, but is not specific. It is the fine transverse wrinkling due to stellate scars which is highly characteristic of syphilis. The swelling of the intima may so narrow the openings of the coronary arteries that they are reduced to mere pin-points or one of them may be completely closed. In such a case there may be symptoms of coronary obstruction or the patient may suddenly drop dead. The disease does not spread along the coronary arteries. In a pure case the yellow fatty changes, calcification and ulceration of atheroma are absent, but it must be remembered that atherosclerosis often complicates syphilis. The adventitia is thickened, and the

vessel is often unduly adherent to the mediastinum. The cut edge shows thickening of the intima with a corresponding thinning and interruption of the media. Owing to destruction of the elastic tissue by the spirochetes there is a dilatation of the vessel and especially of the aortic ring. In this way an extreme degree of aortic incompetence may be produced, for the cusps are quite unable to come together.

The condition of the *aortic valve* deserves close attention. In some cases the cusps are quite normal, even though there is a marked degree of incompetence. In other cases a characteristic condition of *syphilitic endocarditis* is present. This never occurs apart from syphilitic aortitis, and is never seen in the mitral valve. There are two distinctive lesions (Fig. 285): (1) the cusps are sclerosed and contracted, and the free edge shows a peculiar *cord-like thickening* quite unlike that seen in any other form of endocarditis. (2) There is a *widening of the commissure*, i. e., a separation of the cusps at the point where normally they should meet, as if a wedge of tissue had been forced between each pair. The infection has evidently extended into the valve from the aortic wall, and the central part of the cusps is the least affected.

The *microscopic picture* is that of a periarteritis and mesaortitis with secondary changes in the intima. The earliest change is in the adventitia in the form of masses and linear streaks of lymphocytes and plasma

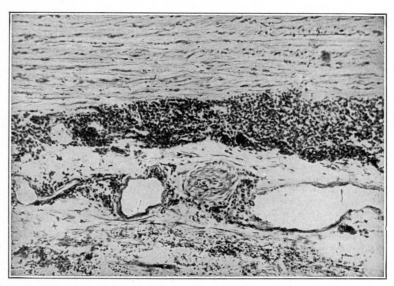

Fig. 286.—Syphilitic aortitis. A linear collection of inflammatory cells at the junction of media and adventitia. × 100.

cells (Fig. 286). These are collected around the vasa vasorum, owing to the distribution of the spirochetes in the perivascular lymphatics. The vasa vasorum normally penetrate only the outer third of the media but the inflammation stimulates them to grow and branch so that they invade the whole thickness of the media. This is associated with fibroblastic proliferation and marked fibrous overgrowth of the intima which later becomes hyaline. The infection spreads into the media where there are foci of inflammatory cells, necrosis, and extensive destruction of the elastic tissue. It is the mesaortitis which is the most serious part of the disease, because with destruction of the elastic tissue the aorta loses its resiliency and either undergoes a general dilatation or develops an aneurysm. New capillaries are formed which pass far into the media. The necrotic material is replaced by scar tissue. It is the contraction of this scar tissue which gives rise to the characteristic wrinkling seen on the inner surface, so that the wrinkling is naturally a late phenomenon.

Relation of Symptoms to Lesions.—The chief symptom is *substernal pain*. The pain is probably due to inflammation of the tissue at the root of the aorta. The destruction of elastic tissue and loss of elasticity may cause

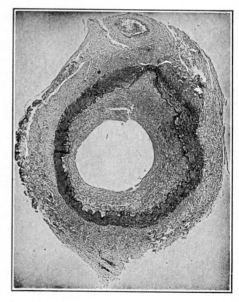

Fig. 287.—Syphilitic endarteritis of basilar artery, showing uniform thickening of the inner coat and thickened internal elastic lamina (elastic tissue stain).

either general dilatation of the thoracic aorta as shown in the roentgen-ray picture, or the local dilatation known as an aneurysm. Symptoms of coronary occlusion and even

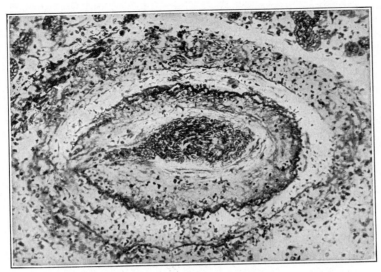

FIG. 288.—Vascular lesion in rheumatic fever. Great thickening of the inner coat, and infiltration of all the coats by inflammatory cells. × 200.

sudden death may be caused by closure of the openings of the coronary arteries by plaques of thickened intima. The three most dangerous *complications* of syphilitic aortitis are: (1) *aortic incompetence* (the commonest), (2) *stenosis of the coronaries*, and (3) *aneurysm*.

Syphilitic Arteritis.—This is best seen in the central nervous system in the small arteries of the meninges and the vessels at the base of the brain. The lesion is both a periarteritis and an endarteritis (Fig. 287). As the spirochetes are in the lymphatics of the adventitia, the vessel is surrounded by a mantle of lymphocytes and plasma cells. There is some atrophy of the media, but this is not an important lesion. The intima shows a marked uniform thickening with great narrowing of the lumen, an endarteritis obliterans, quite different from the patchy atheroma which often affects these vessels. The narrowing of the lumen is apt to lead to *thrombosis* and *cerebral softening*. As the infection dies out the arteries become sclerosed and stiff, and have been likened to macaroni.

RHEUMATIC ARTERITIS.—The visceral vessels may show very characteristic lesions first described by von Glahn and Pappenheimer. These lesions may occur in the arteries of the lung, kidney, pancreas, ovary and testicle. The lesion is a panarteritis, all the coats being involved (Fig. 288). The wall is filled with an inflammatory exudate containing much fibrin, so that it is greatly thickened. The most remarkable feature is the subsequent vascularization of the damaged wall; new capillaries are formed in the wall so that the original lumen is surrounded by spongy vascular tissue. There is no thrombosis, so that the lesions do not injure the parts supplied by the vessels involved. In rheumatic fever the coronary arteries may show a severe exudative and necrotizing arteritis involving all the coats.

RHEUMATOID AORTITIS.—It is now recognized that in rheumatoid arthritis and particularly in ankylosing spondylitis, lesions may develop at the root of the aorta which, both in gross and microscopic appearance, may resemble those of luetic aortitis. These have already been described on page 456. The chief clinical effect is aortic insufficiency.

Aortitis of Undetermined Etiology.—In the past it has been customary to accept as syphilitic any case of aortitis which presents the classical lesions of that disease. Perhaps the time has come to face the possibility that the end result of other etiological agents may cause similar or identical responses in the aortic wall. McGuire, Scott and Gall have reported 5 cases of chronic aortitis with severe and fatal aortic insufficiency in which the lesions were those associated with true

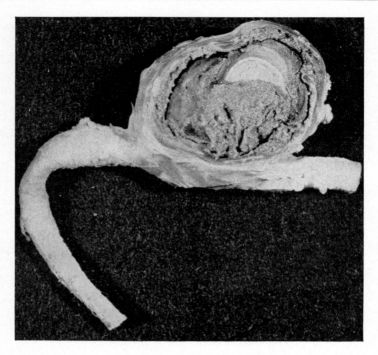

Fig. 289.—Saccular aneurysm of the femoral artery. The laminated character of the clot, due to its being formed at intervals, is unusually distinct.

syphilitic aortitis, but in which no evidence of syphilis nor any of the other causes of aortitis were present. One of the patients was a girl twenty-two years old, and another a boy of fifteen years.

ANEURYSMS

An aneurysm is a localized dilatation of an artery.

Causes.—Every aneurysm is caused by weakening of the arterial wall. As a rule, it is the media which is damaged. Syphilis used to be the most important cause of aneurysm of the large arteries. With the modern control of syphilis and with the increasing age of the population atheroma now rivals or indeed exceeds syphilis as a causal factor. Syphilis seldom or never leads to aneurysm formation in the small arteries, because in them the lesion is a diffuse thickening of the intima with little involvement of the media. An infected embolus will lead to suppuration of the vessel wall and destruction of the media, so that an infective or *mycotic aneurysm* is formed. Polyarteritis

nodosa may weaken the vessel and lead to the formation of multiple small aneurysms. Infection from an abscess or a tuberculous focus may form the starting-point of an aneurysm. Finally, congenital weakness of the media in the arteries at the base of the brain has been suggested as a cause of a *congenital aneurysm.*

Varieties.—A *true aneurysm* is one in which the sac is formed by the wall of the vessel. A *false aneurysm* is one in which the sac is formed by the surrounding tissues. It is caused by the rupture of a vessel, and is a hematoma rather than an aneurysm. A *fusiform aneurysm* is a dilatation of a segment of the vessel, and is seen in the aorta and its large branches. A *saccular aneurysm* is a pouching of the vessel at one point (Fig. 289). This is the usual form of aneurysm. A *traumatic aneurysm* is a false aneurysm, a hematoma, formed by laceration of the vessel wall. Other varieties of aneurysm are considered in detail below.

Aneurysm of the Aorta.—Aortic aneurysm is so much more common and important than the other forms that it will be considered

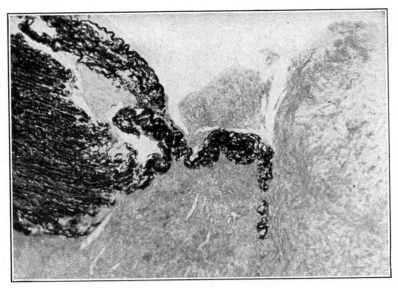

Fig. 290.—Edge of syphilitic aneurysm of aorta, showing how the elastic tissue (black) suddenly ceases. Elastic tissue stain. × 75.

separately. Syphilis, especially in the thoracic aorta, used to be far the commonest etiological factor, as it is a great destroyer of elastic tissue (Fig. 290). Syphilitic aortitis is now much less frequent, but atheroma of the abdominal aorta, which causes a more diffuse disintegration of elastic fibers, seems to be taking its place. Each time the aorta dilates it does not quite return to the normal size owing to destruction of the elastic tissue. A syphilitic aneurysm is more likely to be saccular, an atheromatous aneurysm to be fusiform.

Atheromatous Aneurysm.—Aneurysm due to atherosclerosis occurs at a later age than does the syphilitic form, it generally affects the abdominal aorta, and it usually causes diffuse dilatation of the vessel. The site of election is the lower part of the aorta below the origin of the renal arteries. This is singularly fortunate because it makes possible the replacement of the aneurysm by an aortic homograft or plastic tube, which may be a life-saving procedure, as most patients with aneurysm of the abdominal aorta survive less than one year after the onset of symptoms. Such an operation, however, is far from without risk in an elderly brittle patient, often hypertensive and with diseased coronary arteries.

Syphilitic Aneurysm.—A syphilitic aneurysm develops on an average ten years earlier than does an atheromatous aneurysm. The dilatation begins in the ascending aorta or the arch (Fig. 291). and decreases in frequency as we pass downwards.

Usually it is localized (saccular aneurysm), but sometimes it is more uniform (diffuse aneurysm). The mouth has a smooth rolled edge. The aneurysm may grow forward, eroding the sternum, or backward, eroding the bodies of the vertebræ (though not the intervertebral disks), causing great pain in the back. It may press on the trachea with difficulty in breathing, on the esophagus with difficulty in swallowing, on the left recurrent laryngeal nerve with hoarseness and aphonia. It may rupture on the surface, or into the trachea, bronchi, esophagus, pericardium, or pleural cavity.

The adjoining parts of the aorta show the characteristic wrinkling of syphilitic aortitis, but in the aneurysmal sac the direct evidence of syphilis is usually obscured by atheroma. Thrombosis occurs on the roughened lining, and layer after layer of clot is laid down and becomes incorporated with the wall of the sac. The clot therefore shows a characteristically laminated appearance. Microscopic examination of the wall of the sac shows that

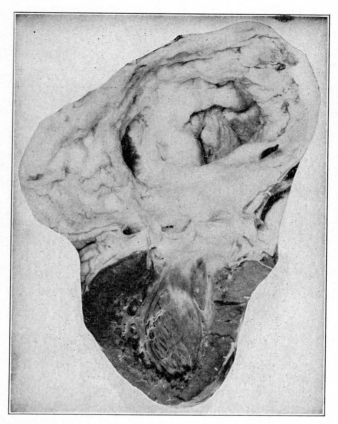

FIG. 291.—Aortic aneurysm. The rolled edge is well seen, as well as the characteristic nodular appearance of syphilitic aortitis. The aortic cusps are normal.

it consists only of adventitia; the intima and media have disappeared. Adjoining parts of the wall show the microscopic lesions of active syphilitic aortitis.

Dissecting Aneurysm.—A dissecting aneurysm is not a true aneurysm, *i. e.*, the vessel is not dilated. A hemorrhage occurs in the media of the aorta between the middle and outer thirds, commencing at the base and spreading along the vessel for a variable distance, splitting the media into two layers in its passage (Fig. 292). The blood tends to encircle the aorta, and may pass along its entire length to the bifurcation. In one of my cases the blood had dissected its way along the renal, splenic and superior mesenteric arteries causing gangrene of the bowel through pressure on the latter vessel. There may be ischemic necrosis of various tissues due to the blood in the wall of the aorta compressing the exit of arterial branches, as, for instance, in the case of the spinal arteries. On this account there may be a confusing multiplicity of symptoms. Usually the blood ruptures externally, with death to the patient, but it may rupture into the lumen. Should the patient survive, the blood may be absorbed, and two tubes are formed, one inside the other. Dissecting aneurysm is a disease of later life, and is rare before the age of fifty years. The *primary lesion* in the great majority of cases is marked *medionecrosis of the aorta* causing rupture of the vasa vasorum, but I have seen an occasional instance of blood entering the media through an atheromatous crack in the intima. As a rule a tear in the intima (especially at the spot where the latter is normal) is an effect rather than a cause of the condition. Syphilis is not a factor of any importance. There

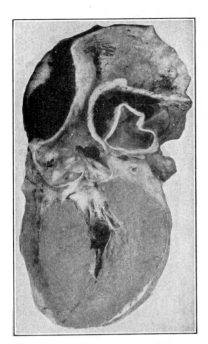

Fig. 292.—Dissecting aneurysm of the aorta. The media of the ascending aorta has been split into two layers. The dark mass between the layers is blood.

may be large collections of lymphocytes and plasma cells in the adventitia; this is not the result of syphilis, but is due, apparently, to irritation produced by the accumulation of red blood cells in the wall of the aorta.

Hypertension appears to be an important predisposing cause (Halpert and Brown). As a matter of curiosity it may be mentioned that dissecting aneurysm of the aorta is encountered in *Marfan's syndrome*, a congenital anomaly of mesenchymal tissue in general and the skeletal and cardiovascular systems in particular, and in *lathyrism* produced in young rats by feeding a diet containing 50 per cent of the seeds of Lathyrus Odoratus (sweet pea), which results in degeneration of the mucopolysaccharides of the ground substance and fragmentation of the elastic fibers (Ponseti and Baird; Backhuber and Lalick). Lathyrism has also been reported in man.

The *symptoms* are characteristic. The patient is seized by a sudden sharp or excruciating pain in the chest or the abdomen, accompanied by prostration. He often experiences what he describes as a tearing

sensation. The pain passes off, but in a typical case death occurs some days later from the bursting of the aneurysm into the pericardial sac, the chest, or the abdominal cavity. The symptoms may suggest disease of the heart, brain, kidney or bowel, owing to involvement of the arteries arising from the aorta and passing to these structures. For this reason the diagnosis is sometimes very difficult. It is particularly important to keep the possibility of dissecting aneurysm in mind, because immediate surgical intervention may save the life of the patient. The surgeon may imitate nature's corrective procedure by creating a second break in the intima, as close as possible to the primary rupture under hypothermia, thus providing re-entry into the true lumen of the aorta. Much more important, he can now replace the diseased segment of aorta with a portion of another aorta or a piece of plastic tubing, a feat undreamed of a few years ago.

So far we have spoken of dissecting aneurysm as if it were confined to the aorta. This is not so (Foord and Lewis). It is occasionally encountered both in other systemic vessels and in the pulmonary arteries. The renal arteries are most often involved, followed by the coronaries and intracranial vessels. Hypertension has been present in most cases, trauma in about one-quarter, but no specific changes in the media. The most likely result is narrowing of the lumen with infarction of the part supplied.

Aneurysm of Sinus of Valsalva.—The aortic sinuses or sinus of Valsalva are three small pouch-like dilatations in the wall of the aorta immediately above the cusps of the valve, two of them giving origin to the coronary arteries. Aneurysms of this structure are rare, but they have been recognized with increasing frequency since the classic paper of Jones and Longley in 1949. They may be congenital or acquired, the latter being more common. The *congenital* form may be associated with other developmental defects such as bicuspid aortic valve and coarctation of the aorta. The basic lesion is a lack of continuity between the aortic media and fibrous ring (the annulus fibrosus) of the aortic valve (Edwards and Burchell). At the site of the aneurysm the sinus wall is formed by the adjacent wall of the right

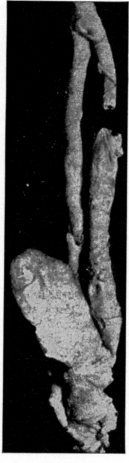

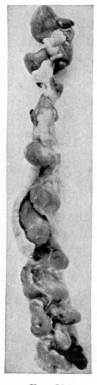

FIG. 293   FIG. 294

FIG. 293.—Arteriovenous aneurysm. The result of a gunshot wound injuring the external iliac artery and vein.

FIG. 294.—Varicose veins of the leg. (Boyd, *Pathology for the Surgeon*, courtesy of W. B. Saunders Co.)

atrium which has been forced by aortic pressure into an aneurysm that bulges into the atrium. The aneurysms are paper thin, and they tend to rupture into the right atrium of the heart with sudden dyspnea due to overloading of the right cardiac chambers. Bacterial endocarditis is a rather common complication. The *acquired* form is usually due to syphilis, occasionally to endocarditis. The diagnosis can now be made readily by means of angiocardiography. Aortic regurgitation is common, due to dilatation of the aortic ring.

Arteriovenous Aneurysm.—An arteriovenous aneurysm is an abnormal acquired communication between an artery and a vein, usually due to simultaneous laceration of an adjoining artery and vein. In war time the injury is likely to be produced by a bullet (Fig. 293), in civil life by a stab wound. The condition should be born in mind more particularly in the case of people given to stabbing one another. The blood passes from the artery into the vein, and produces a local distention of the vein which pulsates as forcibly as the artery. A marked thrill can be felt and a loud hum heard over the aneurysm.

Arteriovenous Fistula.—This is a *congenital* condition due to a defect in the development of the vascular system, a direct "shunt" between an artery and a vein without the interposition of capillaries. The blood passes forcibly into the vein, which becomes dilated (arteriovenous varix). The lesion is commonest in the leg, but may occur in the arm or the scalp; in the latter position, it forms a mass of dilated vessels known as a *cirsoid aneurysm*. The *clinical features* are striking and make recognition easy: (1) *higher blood-pressure and temperature* in the affected limb; (2) *increased circumference of the limb* and the presence of *bruits and thrills*; (3) *cardiac hypertrophy*; (4) *venous blood is redder* on the affected side (pathognomonic); (5) *roentgen-ray visualization of the fistula* after the injection of thorotrast (arteriography).

Arteriovenous fistula of the lung presents a special instance of the condition, of interest of itself and of importance because of the possibility of relief by surgical measures. The shunt of venous blood through the fistula, bypassing the lungs, causes cyanosis, polycythemia and hypertrophy of the right ventricle. A continuous murmur may be audible on auscultation over the lesion. There is radiographic evidence of an area of increased density usually near the hilus and rendered more opaque by the intravenous injection of diodrast. The condition is considered in greater detail in Chapter 24.

ANGIOSPASTIC DISEASES.—The muscular walls of the arterioles are supplied both with constrictor and dilator fibers. In inflammatory conditions of arteries such as Buerger's disease the lesion irritates the sensory sympathetic fibers and thus causes constriction of the anastomotic and terminal arteries. For this reason operative procedures designed to paralyze the sympathetic may be of great benefit by increasing the collateral circulation. Recent embolism and rapid thrombosis have a similar action on the sympathetic. In advanced non-inflammatory arterial occlusion (arteriosclerotic) there is inhibition of vasoconstrictor tonus, so that no benefit is obtained by paralyzing the sympathetic.

Raynaud's Disease.—*Raynaud's disease* is a condition of long-continued arterial spasm resulting in local asphyxia and symmetrical gangrene. It usually affects the fingers. Raynaud's disease is the reverse of Buerger's disease, for it is much more common in the female, the upper limbs are affected rather than the lower, and no organic lesions are found in the vessels to account for the bilateral local ischemia. It is generally believed that the essential cause is a disturbance of the vasomotor mechanism, although it has been suggested that there is some local fault in the periphery independent of the vasomotor mechanism. Mild cases of angiospasm ("dead fingers") are very common; they occur usually in women. Vasodilatation is the basis of *erythromelalgia* (*erythros*, red; *melos*, limb; *algos*, pain), a condition marked by a paroxysmal throbbing and burning pain usually in the feet, sometimes in the hands, accompanied by a dusky mottled redness of the parts.

THE VEINS

The veins are in such direct continuity with the arteries and are so similar in general structure and function that it might be assumed that the diseases of veins would be similar to those of arteries. Nothing could be farther from the truth. Pathological conditions in veins are very common, but there is none of the wealth of disease entities which we have just encountered in the arteries. Indeed they may be practically all included under the three headings of thrombophlebitis, venous thrombosis and varicose veins.

Veins differ from arteries as regards structure in three respects, all of which have a bearing on the development of disease: (1) they have *valves*, (2) they have *lymphatics*, and (3) they have *little* of the *elastic tissue* which is so abundant in the medium-sized and larger arteries. Failure of the valves is one of the important features of varicose veins. The presence of abundant lymphatics

and their absence in arteries accounts for the fact that malignant growths invade veins with the greatest ease, (Fig. 111, page 210), but seldom invade the walls of arteries. Bacteria from without can also readily penetrate the vein wall by way of the lymphatics. The lack of elastic tissue agrees with the absence of the localized dilatations which constitute arterial aneurysms.

Thrombophlebitis and venous thrombosis have already been discussed in Chapter 6 in connection with the general subject of thrombosis. Only a brief summary, therefore, will be given here.

PHLEBITIS AND THROMBOSIS

Phlebitis, or inflammation of the wall of a vein, and thrombosis are even more intimately associated than are arteritis and thrombosis. Inflammation of the vein wall is almost certain to be accompanied by thrombosis, and the presence of a thrombus in the lumen may incite an inflammatory reaction in the vein wall. The latter fact is apt to create confusion, for it may be difficult for the pathologist to be certain which was the primary and which the secondary event. Two main forms may be recognized: (1) thrombophlebitis, which, in spite of the confusing order in the name, is first a phlebitis and only secondarily a thrombosis, and (2) phlebothrombosis, which is primarily a thrombosis in a vein.

Thrombophlebitis.—As we have seen, thrombophlebitis should signify phlebitis, that is to say inflammation of the vein wall, with thrombosis as a secondary event, although the term is often used loosely and incorrectly for venous thrombosis. When I was a medical student it was a condition of great importance, for chemotherapy and antibiotics had not yet been introduced. Before the days of antisepsis and asepsis it was still more important, and it is of interest to recall that Virchow's first research was to check Cruveilhier's statement: "Phlebitis dominates all pathology." (Incidentally, every student of medicine should make himself familiar with Rudolf Virchow, the incredible man and his work). It was really a *suppurative phlebitis* involving a vein passing through an abscess or an area of cellulitis, and caused by pyogenic bacteria invading the wall of the vein from without via the lymphatics. The resulting thrombus become septic, underwent softening, and disintegrated into fragments which formed septic emboli, with resulting pyemic abscesses all over the body. The picture of disease certainly does change, especially at the present time.

Simple Thrombophlebitis is the term given to a condition which seems to be intermediate between acute septic phlebitis and phlebothrombosis. There are clinical signs of inflammation, such as tenderness, redness and swelling, but little to be seen under the microscope. There may be an associated lymphedema, giving the condition of *phlegmasia alba dolens* or "milk leg," which sometimes develop after childbirth.

Phlebothrombosis: Venous Thrombosis.— I prefer to speak of venous thrombosis rather than phlebothrombosis, simply because the latter is so easily confused with thrombophlebitis. Here emphasis is said on the element of thrombosis rather than that of phlebitis. Clinically it is a quiet process, often completely unsuspected, but it is the quietness of the submerged rock which may wreck the ship. The great danger of course is that of pulmonary embolism, for the thrombus is soft and easily dislodged. It is of interest to recall that Virchow was the first to demonstrate the origin of emboli, and that embolism is of very common occurrence. These matters are discussed in Chapter 6.

Thrombophlebitis Migrans.— At the present time migrating thrombophlebitis remains the engima of venous pathology. It has already been discussed on page 133, so it will be sufficient to recall that it is characterized by recurring attacks of thrombosis in widely separated short segments of vein, and that it may be associated with carcinoma of various organs, most frequently the pancreas. The great Trousseau observed and recorded this condition in himself when he was dying of carcinoma of the pancreas, so that the term *Trousseau's syndrome* has been fittingly applied to the association. It has been suggested that this may be due to release of trypsin, which has a thromboplastic action, from the disrupted tissue of the tumor bed (Gore). Even secondary tumors of the pancreas may produce this effect. In about 50 per cent of the cases the condition may be called primary or idiopathic, there being no associated tumor. These cases may be expected to recover. In both groups the etiology is unknown. Under these circumstances we may take shelter in that refuge of the destitute, an auto-immune hypersensitivity reaction.

Chiari Syndrome.—This rare condition is also known as the *Budd-Chiari syndrome*, being described by Budd in 1857 and by Chiari in 1899. The syndrome is a combination of (1) *thrombosis of the hepatic vein*, usually at its junction with the inferior vena cava, (2) the *rapid development of ascites* or an accumulation of fluid in the peritoneal cavity, and (3) a *large, tender liver*, purple in color. The thrombosis may be part of a thrombophlebitis migrans, or it may be caused by invasion of the vein wall by a malignant tumor. The condition must not be confused with the very much more common condition of the slowly developing ascites which is associated with thrombosis of the portal vein.

PHLEBOSCLEROSIS

The condition of phlebosclerosis or phlebofibrosis is not uncommon, although seldom recognized because seldom looked for. It does not appear to be related to arteriosclerosis, for it occurs at an earlier period of life, being commonest in young men between twenty and thirty years of age; it is not associated with fatty degeneration or calcification; and it bears no relation to hypertension. It affects chiefly the veins of the legs, where the affected vessels feel like hard mobile cords, which may be mistaken for tendons. There are no associated symptoms. It is a disseminated lesion affecting both superficial and deep veins and is always bilateral. It has been called endophlebitis and hyperplastic phlebitis, but it is a degenerative and not an inflammatory condition. The affected vein is thickened and the lumen narrowed. The chief microscopic change is a marked increase of the connective tissue of the media and corresponding atrophy of the muscle fibers, together with a lesser fibrosis of the intima. The innermost layers of the thickened intima are hyaline, and the endothelial lining is missing. The distinction between the coats of the vessel is largely lost. The exact nature of the condition is uncertain and the cause is quite unknown.

VARICOSE VEINS

A varix or varicose vein is one that is dilated, lengthened, and tortuous. The three common sites are: (1) The veins of the leg, especially the internal saphenous, (Fig. 294), (2) the hemorrhoidal veins (*hemorrhoids* or *piles*); (3) the pampiniform plexus of the spermatic cord (*varicocele*).

CAUSES.—These may be predisposing and exciting. An important *predisposing* cause appears to be a congenital and inherited weakness of the walls and valves of the veins. The condition may run in a family for generations, and the same vein may be affected each time. The *exciting* factor is an increase of pressure in the vein, and may be caused in the following ways: (1) Central obstruction to the venous return (mitral stenosis, emphysema, cirrhosis of the liver). (2) Pressure of a tumor, gravid uterus, or loaded rectum. (3) Prolonged standing. (4) Straining at stool and violent muscular effort; the former aggravates piles, while the latter explains the frequency of varicose veins of the legs in athletes.

LESIONS.—The essential lesion is a giving way of the valves, and the vein becomes dilated, elongated and tortuous. A phlebosclerosis develops. At first there is hypertrophy of the media from increased strain, followed later by atrophy and replacement fibrosis. The intima and adventitia also become fibrosed and thickened. The thickening is irregular, and pouching of the wall occurs in the intervals. Thrombosis in these pouches is very common.

EFFECTS.—The effects are felt by the veins and the tissues which they drain. Hemorrhage, phlebitis, and thrombosis are the important *venous complications*. Hemorrhage is commonest in the case of piles, where the veins are covered only by mucous membrane (hence the name hemorrhoids). There may be hemorrhage from the veins of the leg as the result of trauma or ulceration of the overlying tissue. The hemorrhage may be into the tissue or on the surface. The presence of ulceration naturally predisposes to infection and thrombosis.

The *tissues* suffer severely as the result of the varicosity. Because of the incompetency of the valves of the deep veins and of the communicating veins between the deep and superficial systems, the blood from the deep veins may flow into and down the superficial veins, so that the *normal direction of the blood stream is reversed*. The blood is picked up in the feet and returned by the superficial veins, and in this way a vicious circle is set up. The blood in varicose veins may have only two-thirds the normal oxygen content, and the carbon dioxide is correspondingly increased. There is chronic congestion and the circulation is greatly interfered with. Edema is apt to develop, probably as the result of an associated lymphangitis, the overlying skin becomes sodden and devitalized and atrophic from pressure, and a varicose ulcer may be formed, usually on the lower third of the leg. This type of ulcer is likely to be very chronic, and may heal and break down repeatedly, causing great disability and suffering to the patient. The skin of the lower part of the leg acquires a mahogany-brown color, due to pigmentation from repeated small hemorrhages into the tissues. When the effect of gravitation is overcome by strapping the ulcerated area and the leg with adhesive plaster of an elastic type, the results are often miraculous.

TUMORS OF BLOOD VESSELS

Tumors of blood vessels form one of the most confused chapters in the subject of oncology, as can be readily seen from the bewildering variety of names which are encountered in the literature. It is difficult to know if some of them should be regarded as true neoplasms, or merely as diffuse overgrowth or even dilatation of the vessels of the part. Perhaps the question is rather an academic one, because the latter lesions, although they may be diffuse and invasive, are very rarely malignant. In many cases it would be more correct to speak of an angiomatosis rather than an angioma. Many of the lesions are in the nature of congenital malformations. They involve the capillaries rather than well formed arteries and veins.

The wall of a *capillary* consists of (1) a continuous lining of flattened endothelial cells, (2) an investing sheath of reticular fibers best demonstrated by silver staining, and (3) certain cells scattered at intervals over this sheath known as the contractile cells of Rouget or the *pericytes* of Zimmermann. Without a silver stain it may not be possible to determine whether the cells of a tumor lie within (endothelial) or without (pericyte) the reticulin sheath. True neoplasms derived from blood vessels are therefore of two types; the one composed of endothelial cells, the *hemangioendothelioma*, the other composed of the pericytes of Zimmermann. The latter includes two variants of very different clinical significance: (1) the *glomus tumor*, a sharply circumscribed, superficial, completely benign but often intensely painful tumor; (2) the *hemangiopericytoma*, which may be benign or malignant, superficial or deep, painless but infiltrative (Stout). In addition there is the very much more common group of *hemangiomas*, in which the lesion consists of a group of new capillaries. We shall consider the following types of blood vessel tumors: (1) hemangioma, (2) sclerosing hemangioma, (3) hemangioendothelioma, (4) hemangiopericytoma, (5) glomus tumor, (6) Kaposi's sarcoma.

Hemangioma.—Two varieties of this tumor are recognized, the capillary and the cavernous. The distinction is convenient, but in no way fundamental.

Capillary hemangioma is a network of new-formed capillaries filled with blood. The neoplasm affects only one segment of a vessel, from which buds of endothelium grow out and form new vessels (Fig. 295.) The cells may proliferate to such an extent that they may obliterate the lumen.

The common site is the skin, but it may occur in the mucous membrane of the nose, lip, tongue, gum, or rectum, in which latter position it may occasion severe hemorrhage.

A cutaneous angioma is usually a bright red, sharply defined patch, not raised above the general level, but it may present a somewhat velvety surface. It is generally present at birth, and from a minute red spot it may spread to cover a large surface. The favorite position is the face or head, where it often

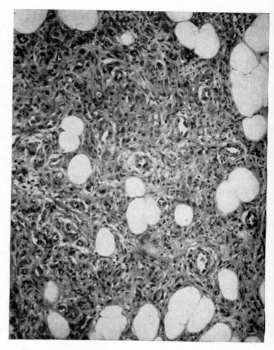

Fig. 295.—Capillary hemangioma invading adipose tissue. There is good differentiation of the capillaries and lack of intercapillary endothelial cells. × 125. (Kindness of Dr. H. J. Barrie.)

follows the distribution of the fifth nerve, and it is almost always strictly unilateral, stopping short of the middle line.

Cavernous hemangioma, which is very much less common, has the structure of erectile tissue. It consists of large blood spaces or sinuses lined with endothelium. The common site is the liver, where it may be multiple. It is also found in the skin in various regions, including the lip, where it forms a raised mass, often of distinctly higher temperature than the surrounding structures, the overlying skin generally shows a bluish tinge, and gentle pressure may succeed in emptying the tumor. It may infiltrate the subcutaneous tissue and underlying muscles, and I have seen the most alarming hemorrhage result from an ill-advised attempt at removal in such a case.

Sclerosing Hemangioma.—Here we come to a subject which at first sight is simple, but with deeper study becomes complex and confusing, with endless ramifications. There is no disputing the fact that certain capillary hemangiomas exhibit regressive changes marked principally by fibrosis (Gross and Wolbach). In these sclerosing hemangiomas the capillaries become partially or completely obliterated, while only segregated groups of endothelial cells remain. It may obviously be difficult or impossible to determine the vascular origin of such a lesion.

Microscopically three different elements may be present in varying proportion: (1) *spindle-shaped* cells arranged either in tight curlicues or grouped as fasciculi, the latter arrangement suggesting a neurofibroma (Fig. 296); (2) *foamy macrophages* filled with lipid; (3) *hemosiderin pigment* also contained for the most part within phagocytic cells. The pigment may be so abundant as to be mistaken for melanin, a very serious mistake on the part of the pathologist, which can readily be avoided by the use of a stain for iron. The histiocytes may fuse to form foreign body giant cells. Both the hemosiderin and the lipid may be presumed to be the result of hemorrhage from capillaries undergoing destruction.

Hemangioendothelioma.—We have seen that the common hemangiomas or angiomas are benign lesions which are usually more in the nature of a proliferation of blood channels than true tumors. The hemangioendothelioma is a true neoplasm of vascular endothelium. It may be benign or malignant.

Benign hemangioendothelioma occurs chiefly in the skin, but may occasionally be found in the viscera, especially the liver and spleen. It forms a well-circumscribed firm mass a few centimeters in diameter and reddish gray in color. *Microscopically*, it consists of masses and sheets of spindle-shaped endothelial cells, uniform in size and appearance, with large vascular spaces surrounded by these masses of cells.

Malignant hemangioendothelioma, more conveniently called *hemangioendotheliosarcoma*, may occur anywhere in the body. It is commoner in young people. It forms a large, pale, soft mass with ill-defined margins, and frequent central areas of necrotic softening and hemorrhage. *Microscopically*, it shows the familiar malignant picture of cellular pleomorphism, anaplasia, and numerous mitoses. In the more malignant forms no new formation of blood vessels may

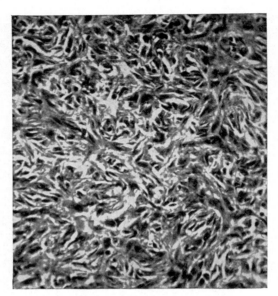

Fig. 296.—Sclerosing hemangioma. × 250.

be apparent, although this is not true of the better differentiated varieties. It will be appreciated that some of these tumors may easily be mistaken for fibrosarcoma. The tumor is locally invasive, and spread takes place by the blood stream, with the formation of distant metastases.

Hemangiopericytoma.—In this neoplasm the *tumor cells, derived from pericytes, lie outside the vascular sheath*, and are closely packed about the numerous capillary-sized vessels which are lined by normal endothelium. The relationship of tumor cells to vessels is best shown by a reticulin stain (Figs. 297 and 298). The neoplastic pericytes usually resemble epithelium, but if they become spindle-shaped, hemangiopericytoma may easily be mistaken for a vascular fibrosarcoma or leiomyosarcoma.

These soft tissue tumors occur most often in the extremities of either sex and at any age. They are usually slowly growing and painless, so that they are likely to be of large size before the patient seeks medical advice. The malignant possibilities of these tumors have been underestimated in the past. In a series of 20 cases reported by Fisher, there were metastases, either hematogenous or lymphogenous, in 45 per cent. It is extremely difficult, if not impossible, to dis-

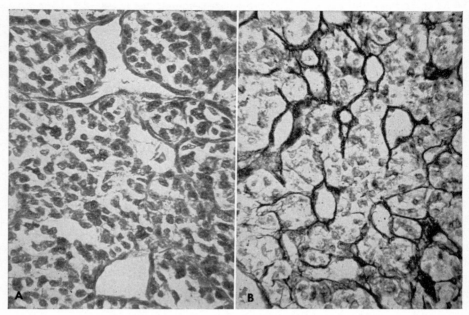

FIG. 297   FIG. 298

FIG. 297.—Hemangiopericytoma. The angular neoplastic cells are packed closely around blood vessels lined with normal endothelium. × 460.

FIG. 298.—A reticulin stain outlines distinctly the vascular sheath. There is proliferation of neoplastic cells outside the vascular sheath. Reticulin surrounds groups of cells. × 460. (Kennedy and Fisher, courtesy of J. Bone & Joint Surg.)

tinguish the metastasizing variety by means of the microscopic picture alone (Stout). Local excision is almost certain to be followed by recurrence. Radical removal results in apparently permanent cure in 50 per cent of cases (Fisher).

Kaposi's Sarcoma.—This very rare lesion is also known as *idiopathic multiple hemorrhagic sarcoma*, a highly descriptive name, although it cannot be said that the term "idiopathic" contributes much information. Multiple bluish-red patches occur in the skin and occasionally in the viscera. The disease is of long duration. At first the skin lesions may resemble capillary hemangiomas, but in the course of time they become more cellular, neoplastic and invasive. It is considered again with tumors of the skin in Chapter 46.

Glomangioma.—This lesion, commonly known as glomus tumor, is given last place in the tumors of blood vessels, not because of its lack of importance, especially if you happen to be the sufferer, but because it has

so little relation to other members of the series. It is purely a tumor of the skin, so that it will be described in connection with skin tumors in Chapter 46. It may be said here that the glomus is a specialized arteriovenous anastomosis surrounded by large pale cells (glomus cells) between which are numerous fine nerve fibers. It is most abundantly present in the region of the nailbed, the tips of the fingers and toes, and the palmar surface of the phalanges. The glomangioma is of similar structure. It never becomes large nor malignant, but its abundant supply of nerves and its position at points of pressure such as the nailbed are responsible for its highly characteristic single symptom. This consists of spasmodic attacks of agonizing radiating pain, which may be spontaneous or elicited by the slightest pressure. The pain is caused by the dilated glomus vessels pressing on the numerous nerve endings. Removal of the tumor is followed instantly by complete and permanent relief. No minor operation wins a greater share of the patient's gratitude.

REFERENCES

ADLERSBERG, D. and SCHAEFER, L. E.: Am. J. Med., 1959, 26, 1. (Interplay of heredity and environment in atherosclerosis.)

ASHWORTH, C. T. and GROLLMAN, A.: Arch. Path., 1959, 67, 375. (Hypertension in choline deficiency.)

ASTRUP, T.: Lancet, 1956, 2, 565. (Fibrinolysis in relation to the development of atherosclerosis.)

AYMAN, D.: Arch. Int. Med., 1934, 53, 792. (Hypertension and heredity.)

BACHHUBER, T. E. and LALECH, J. J.: Arch. Path., 1955, 59, 247. (Lathyrism in dissecting aneurysm).

CASTLEMAN, B. and SMITHWICK, R. H.: J.A.M.A., 1934, 121, 1256. (Relation of vascular disease to the hypertensive state.)

CHURG, J. and STRAUSS, L.: Am. J. Path., 1951, 27, 277. (Wegener's granulomatosis.)

CLARKSON, T. B. et al.: Am. J. Path., 1959, 35, 673. (Heredity in spontaneous atherosclerosis in pigeons.)

CONSTANTINIDES, P. and HARDER, F.: Arch. Path., 1953, 56, 36. (Mast cells and heparin in atherosclerosis.)

COOKE, W. T. et al.: Quart. J. Med., 1946, 15, 47. (Granulomatous giant-cell arteritis.)

CRAWFORD, T. and LEVENE, C. I.: J. Path. and Bact., 1952, 64, 523. (Mural thrombosis in atherosclerosis.)

DAVSON, J., BALL, J. and PLATT, R.: Quart. J. Med., 1948, 11, 175. (Polyarteritis nodosa.)

DOCK, W.: Ann. Int. Med., 1958, 49, 699. (Relation of diet to coronary artery atheroma.)

DUFF, G. L.: Arch. Path., 1935, 20, 81, and 259. (Pathogenesis of atherosclerosis.)

————: Can. Med. Ass. J., 1948, 58, 317. (Diffuse collagen disease.)

DUFF, G. L. and McMILLAN, G. C.: Am. J. Med., 1951, 11, 92. (Pathology of atherosclerosis.)

DUGUID, J. B.: Brit. Med. Bull., 1955, 11, 36. (Mural thrombosis in pathogenesis of atherosclerosis.)

DUNGAL, N. P.: Lancet, 1936, 1, 1354. (Atherosclerosis in Iceland.)

EDWARDS, J. E. and BURCHELL, H. B.: Proc. Staff. Meetings Mayo Clinic, 1956, 31, 407. (Aneurysm of sinus of Valsalva.)

FISHER, J. H.: Can. Med. Ass. J., 1960, 83, 1136. (Hemangiopericytoma.)

FOORD, A. G. and LEWIS, R. D.: Arch. Path., 1959, 68, 553. (Dissecting aneurysm of peripheral and pulmonary arteries.)

GILMOUR, J. R.: J. Path. and Bact., 1941, 53, 263. (Giant-cell arteritis.)

GOFMAN, J. W. et al.: Circulation, 1952, 5, 119. (Blood lipids in human atherosclerosis.)

GOLDBLATT, H.: Renal Origin of Hypertension, American Lecture Series, Springfield, Ill., 1948.

GORE, I.: Am. J. Path., 1953, 29, 613. (Trousseau's syndrome.)

GORE, I. and BURROWS, S.: Am. J. Clin. Path., 1958, 29, 319. (Thromboangiitis obliterans.)

GROLLMAN, A., MUIRHEAD, E. E. and VANATTA, J.: Am. J. Physiol., 1949, 157, 21. (The kidney and hypertension.)

GROSS, R. E. and WOLBACH, S. B.: Am. J. Path., 1943, 19, 533. (Sclerosing hemangioma.)

HALPERT, B. and BROWN, C. A.: Arch Path., 1955, 60, 378. (Dissecting aneurysm of aorta.)

HARTROFT, W. S.: Am. J. Path., 1952, 28, 526. (Ceroid in atherosclerosis.)

HARTROFT, W. S. and BEST, C. H.: Brit. Med. J., 1949, 1, 423. (Hypertension in choline deficiency.)

HARTROFT, W. S. and THOMAS, W. A.: J.A.M.A., 1957, 164, 1899. (The relation of lipids to atherosclerosis in man.)

HOLMAN, R. L. et al.: Am. J. Path., 1958, 34, 209. J. Louisana State Med. Soc., 1958, 110, 361. (Natural history of atherosclerosis.)

KATZ, L. N., STAMLER, J. and PICK, R.: Nutrition and Atherosclerosis, Philadelphia, 1958.

KERNOHAN, J. W. and WOLTMAN, H. W.: Arch. Neurol. and Psychiat., 1938, 39, 655. (Neuritis in polyarteritis nodosa.)

KEYS, A. et al.: Ann. Int. Med., 1958, 48, 83. (Relation of diet to atherosclerosis.)

KLEMPERER, P.: Am. J. Path., 1950, 26, 505. (Diffuse collagen disease.)

KLEMPERER, P., POLLACK, A. D. and BAEHR, G.: Arch. Path., 1941, 32, 569. J.A.M.A., 1942, 119, 331. (Diffuse collagen disease.)

LEARY, T.: Arch. Path., 1949, 47, 1. (Cholesterol in the pathogenesis of atherosclerosis.)

McGILL, H. C. JR., STRONG, J. P., HOLMAN, R. L. and GEER, J. C.: Fed. Proc., 1959, 18, 493. (Atherosclerosis in the African baboon.)

McGUIRE, J., SCOTT, R. C. and GALL, E. A.: Am. J. Med. Sci., 1958, 235, 394. (Aortitis of undetermined etiology.)

McLETCHIE, N. J. B.: Am. J. Path., 1952, 28, 413. (Mural thrombosis in atherosclerosis.)

MELLORS, R. C. et al.: J. Exper. Med., 1957, 106, 191.

MORE, R. H., MOVAT, H. Z. and HAUST, M. D.: Arch. Path., 1957, 63, 612. (Fibrin thrombi in genesis of atheromatous plaques.)

MOVAT, H. Z., HAUST, M. D. and MORE, R. H.: Am. J. Path., 1959, 35, 93. (The early lesions of atherosclerosis.)

MUSTARD, J. F., et al.: In the press. (Lipids, platelets and atherosclerosis.)

OLIVER, M. F. and BOYD, G. S.: Lancet, 1956, 2, 1273, Vitamins and hormones, 1958, 16, 148. (Endocrine factors in coronary heart disease.)

PAGE, I. H.: Circulation, 1954, 10, 1. (Pathogenesis of atherosclerosis.)

PARKER, F.: Am. J. Path., 1960, 36, 19. (Electron microscopic study of experimental atherosclerosis.)

PATERSON, J. C.: Arch. Path., 1936, 22, 313. (Intimal hemorrhage in atherosclerosis.)

PATERSON, J. C., MILLS, J. and MOFFATT, T.: Arch. Path., 1957, 64, 129. (Vascularization of early atherosclerotic plaques).

PATERSON, J. C., DYER, L., and ARMSTRONG, E. C.: Can. Med. Ass. J., 1960, 82, 6. (Serum cholesterol levels in human atherosclerosis.)

PATERSON, J. C. and MILLS, JEAN: Arch. Path., 1958, 66, 335. (Myocardial mast cell counts in coronary sclerosis.)

PONSETI, I. V. and BAIRD, W. A. Am. J. Path., 1952, 28, 1059. (Lathyrism in dissecting aneurysm.)

RICH, A. R.: Bull. Johns Hopkins Hosp., 1942, 71, 123. (Polyarteritis lesions in sickness).

RINEHART, J. F. and ABUL-HAJ, S. K.: Arch. Path., 1951, 52, 189. (Staining of ground substance in atherosclerosis).

ROBERTSON, J. H.: J. Clin. Path., 1960, 13, 199. (Mechanical factors in localization of atherosclerosis.)

ROSS, R. S. and McKUSICK, V. A.: Arch Int. Med., 1953, 92, 701. (Aortic arch syndrome.)

ROWSELL, H. C., DOWNIE, H. G. and MUSTARD, J. F.: Can. Med. Ass. J., 1958, 79, 647. (Atherosclerosis in swine fed on butter.)

SELLERS, E. A. and BAKER, D. G.: Can. Med. Ass. J., 1960, 83, 6. (Coronary atherosclerosis in relation to cold.)

STOUT, A. P.: Cancer, 1949, 2, 1027. Lab. Invest., 1956, 5, 217. (Hemangiopericytoma.)

TAYLOR, H. E.: Am. J. Path., 1953, 29, 871. (Mucopolysaccharides in atherosclerosis.)

TAYLOR, C. B., COX, G. E. and COUNTS, M.: Am. J. Path., 1959, 35, 674. (Coronary atheroma in rhesus monkey induced by high fat diet.)

TEILUM, G.: Am. J. Path., 1948, 24, 409. (Disseminated lupus erythemalosus.)

TOBIAN, L. JR. and BINION, J. T.: Circulation, 1952, 5, 754. J. Clin. Invest., 1954, 33, 1407. (Electrolyte content of arterial wall in hypertension.)

VON GLAHN, W. C. and PAPPENHEIMER, A. M.: Am. J. Path., 1926, 2, 235. (Rheumatic arteritis.)

WEAR, L. E.: Lancet, 1956, 1, 83. (Heredity in hypertension.)

WEGENER, F.: Beitr. Path. Anat., 1939, 102, 36. (Wegener's respiratory granulomatosis.)

WESSLER, S., et al.: New Eng. J. Med., 1960, 262, 1149. (The case against Buerger's disease.)

WILLIAMS, G.: J. Path. and Bact., 1955, 69, 199. (Experimental thrombosis in atherogenesis.)

WILLIS, G. C.: Can. Med. Ass. J., 1954, 70, 1. (Localizing factors in atherosclerosis.)

————: Can. Med. Ass. J., 1957, 77, 106. (Ascorbic deficiency and atherosclerosis.)

WILSON, C.: Lancet, 1953, 2, 579, 632. (The kidney and hypertension.)

WILSON, C. and BYRON, F. B.: Quart. J. Med., 1941, 10, 65. (Relation of the kidney to hypertension.)

ZEEK, P. M.: New Eng. J. Med., 1953, 248, 764. (Polyarteritis nodosa.)

Chapter 23

Diseases of the Kidney

General Considerations
STRUCTURE OF THE NEPHRON
  Electron Microscopy
FUNCTION
  Glomerulus
  Convoluted Tubules
  Tubular Enzymes
  Juxtaglomerular Apparatus
  Renal Function Tests
NEEDLE BIOPSY
Diseases of the Glomeruli
DIFFUSE GLOMERULONEPHRITIS
  Acute Stage
  Subacute Stage
  Chronic Stage
FOCAL GLOMERULITIS
RADIATION NEPHRITIS
CHRONIC GLOMERULAR
  NEPHROSES
  Lipoid Nephrosis (Membran-
  ous Glomerulonephritis)
  Amyloid Nephrosis
  Diabetic Glomerulosclerosis
  Wire-loop Glomerulonephrosis
  Renal Vein Thrombosis
  Nephrosis of Pregnancy
Diseases of the Tubules
ACUTE TUBULAR NEPHROSES
  Anoxic Nephrosis
    The Crush Syndrome
    Transfusion with Incom-
    patible Blood

Sulfonamide Poisoning
The Hepato-renal Syn-
  drome
  Toxic Nephrosis
VACUOLAR NEPHROPATHY
GLYCOGEN DEPOSITS
PIGMENT DEPOSITS
Diseases of the Interstitial Tissue
ACUTE DIFFUSE INTERSTITIAL
  NEPHRITIS
PYELONEPHRITIS
  Pyonephrosis
  Perinephritic Abscess
PAPILLITIS NECROTICANS
THE PYEMIC KIDNEY
TUBERCULOSIS
Diseases of the Blood Vessels
ARTERIOLAR NEPHROSCLEROSIS
  Benign Nephrosclerosis
  Malignant Nephrosclerosis
  Senile Nephrosclerosis
  Relation of the Kidney to
  Hypertension
INFARCTION
BILATERAL CORTICAL NECROSIS
Renal Failure
ACUTE
CHRONIC
  Uremia
The Kidney and Electrolyte
  Disorders
THE WATER-LOSING KIDNEY

THE SALT-LOSING KIDNEY
THE POTASSIUM-LOSING KIDNEY
  Conn's Syndrome
THE PHOSPHATE-LOSING KIDNEY
THE PHOSPHATE-RETAINING
  KIDNEY
  Renal Osteodystrophy
CALCIUM AND NEPHRO-
  CALCINOSIS
INNATE FUNCTIONAL TUBULAR
  DEFECTS
  Fanconi Syndrome
  Renal Tubular Acidosis
DIURETICS
Tumors
ADENOMA
CARCINOMA ("HYPER-
  NEPHROMA")
EMBRYOMA (WILMS' TUMOR)
OTHER TUMORS
Cysts
CONGENITAL POLYCYSTIC
  KIDNEY
SOLITARY CYST
Miscellaneous
OBSTRUCTION AND CALCULUS
  FORMATION
MYELOMA KIDNEY
CONGENITAL ANOMALIES
HEMATURIA
ORTHOSTATIC ALBUMINURIA

GENERAL CONSIDERATIONS

WE now come to the kidney, one of most intriguing and challenging organs to the pathologist, both as regards altered structure and disturbed function. In former editions of this book the kidneys were considered in the latter part of the volume. But the heart, the arteries and the kidneys form one physiological whole. The heart sends blood via the arteries to the kidneys to be purified and freed from the products of metabolism by excretion. When the heart fails, the kidneys also fail. Conversely, primary renal failure may be associated with arterial hypertension, which in turn, as we have already seen, results in arterial lesions and cardiac failure. For this reason it is better to consider the kidneys as part of a cardio-vascular-renal unit, disturbance of which results in cardio-vascular-renal disease. Although we have spoken of the kidneys as excretory organs, it is now recognized that the regulation of the acid-base balance of the body fluids and the maintainance of the normal concentrations of electrolytes, in other words the preservation of the internal environment, the milieu intérieur, of the organism, are functions of equal or even greater importance. The kidney, indeed, alters the internal environment to fit the organism, much as the nervous system modifies the behavior of the organism to fit the external environment. "The function of the kidney is to keep the volume and composition of the extracellular fluid within normal limits; it is also concerned with the maintenance of a normal blood pressure" (de Wardener). As Homer Smith puts it: "In the last analysis, the composi-

(545)

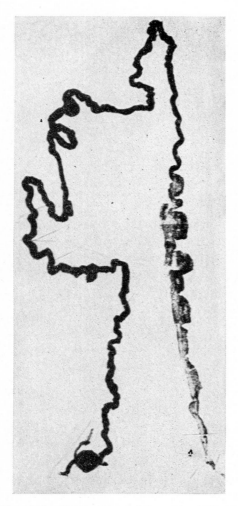

Fig. 299.—Photomicrographic montage of proximal convolution from human kidney in diabetes showing the storage of glycogen in the terminal segment; iron hematoxylin stain. × 28. (Oliver, courtesy of Harvey Lectures.)

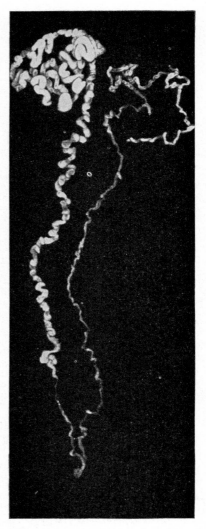

Fig. 300.—A hypertrophied nephron from chronic glomerular nephritis. × 15. (Oliver, *The Architecture of the Kidney in Chronic Bright's Disease*, Paul B. Hoeber-Harper Bros.)

tion of the plasma is determined not by what the body ingests but by what the kidneys retain and what they excrete. It may fairly be said that this regulatory function, so long overlooked, is just as important as the excretion of waste products of metabolism or of foreign substances, which hitherto has received nearly all the emphasis.'' The urine is, in truth, merely the by-product of these regulatory functions. The lower urinary tract, which serves the more humble function of storing the urine and conveying

it from the body, is considered in a later chapter.

Structure.—In the adult the normal weight of the kidney is about 150 grams and the normal thickness of the cortex from 1.2 to 1.5 cm. Each kidney contains over 1,000,000 units, the nephrons. Each nephron consists of four units which are different in structure and in function. These are the glomerulus, the proximal convoluted tube, the loop of Henle, and the distal convoluted tubule. In addition that curious structure, the juxtaglomerular apparatus, demands consideration. The collecting tubules which carry the urine to the bladder are mere conduits and are not included in the nephron complex. Our concept of the structure of the different units of the nephron has undergone violent revolution as the result of the introduction of electron microscopy, to which reference will be made. Microdissection of individual nephrons, an old technique modernized and developed into a fine art by Jean Oliver, has proved invaluable for the localization of individual functions in different parts of the nephron, more particularly in renal disease, as may be seen in Figures 299 and 300. Many of the theories of renal physiology have originated as explanations of the phenomena of disease rather than in animal experimentation, as is usual in other organs.

Glomerulus.—The structure of the glomerulus as well as that of the convoluted tubules is so familiar to every student that only those features will be mentioned which have a special functional significance or which are revealed by the electron microscope. The glomerulus is essentially a filtration mechanism, and it is constructed with this end in view. It consists of a tuft of capillaries which are unique in that they empty not into a vein but into an artery. The diameter of the efferent arteriole is only half that of the afferent one, which must materially raise the pressure in the glomerular capillaries and thus facilitate filtration. The glomerular fluid is the same as tissue fluid, such as develops in edema. The afferent arteriole divides into 3 or 4 branches, which give the tuft its somewhat lobulated appearance that may become accentuated in disease. There is a difference of opinion as to whether the capillaries arising from the afferent arteriole remain as separate loops or anastomose to form a network as capillaries do elsewhere. The basement membrane covering the capillaries, one of the most important constituents of the glomerulus from the stand-point of pathology, is continuous between the capillaries, but it does not enclose the entire circumference of any single capillary. The endothelial cells lining the capillaries form small groups in the areas between the capillary lumens, but of course within the basement membrane. These are known as *interluminal cell aggregates*. They occupy what used to be called the *intercapillary space*, and constitute the *mesangium* of the older terminology, which was pictured as a mesentery-like attachment of basement membrane and epithelium that the capillaries carry with them.

Electron microscopy of the glomerulus shows a startlingly new and unexpected picture (Mueller *et al.*, Pease). The *epithelium* covering the capillaries, which of course is the visceral layer of Bowman's capsule, presents countless delicate villous processes, which extend in orderly array to the capillary wall, where they terminate as feet, the soles of which are firmly planted on the basement membrane of the capillary, somewhat like the tentacles of an octopus (Fig. 301). For this reason the cells have been called *podocytes* (foot cells). The main body of the podocyte is lifted from the basement membrane by the processes, thus allowing filtration to occur without the fluid passing through the epithelial cell. When looking at Figure 301 it is of interest to remember that Bowman denied the existence of a glomerular epithelium! This illustrates the power of a new technique. The cytoplasm of the lining *endothelium* is seen to be riddled with pores, giving it a fenestrated or "chickenwire" appearance.

It becomes evident that the *basement membrane* is the only continuous barrier between the vascular and urinary spaces. What is seen under the light microscope as basement membrane is really a combination of endothelium, true basement membrane, and a portion of the foot processes of the epithelial cells. With the electron microscope various changes become evident in the true basement membrane under pathological conditions which are not so evident with the light microscope. This is particularly true of the Kimmelstiel-Wilson lesion in diabetic glomerulosclerosis (p. 573). It has been suggested that the massive proteinuria of the nephrotic syndrome is due to the development of gaps or pores in the membrane (Spiro), but the evidence in support of this view is not convincing.

Proximal Convoluted Tubule.—The tubules

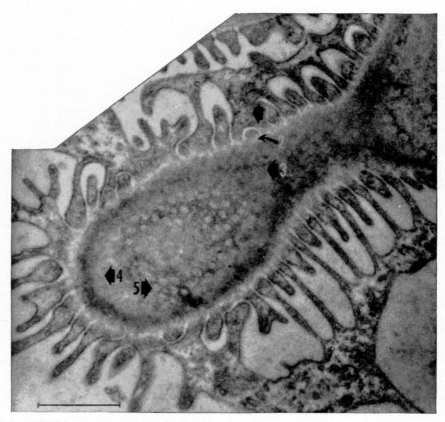

FIG. 301.—A high resolution micrograph of a glomerular capillary sectioned tangentially. All five layers can be identified without difficulty as indicated. The interdigitating epithelial processes show to particularly good advantage at the lower right. The homogenous character of the dense basement membrane is apparent. The closely spaced fenestrations of the endothelial sheet can be seen without difficulty, and their diameter determined to average a little over 0.1 μ. (Pease, courtesy of J. Histochem.)

are more fundamental than the glomeruli, although less spectacular, for some animals, such as primitive fishes, have tubules but no glomeruli, whereas none have glomeruli but no tubules. In development the tubules precede the glomeruli. Most of the tubules seen in a section of cortex belong to the proximal segment because of its greater length. The large size of the lining cells, the marked granularity of the cytoplasm due to numerous mitochondria, and the brush border are all familiar features which indicate great metabolic activity that will be referred to presently. The main function of the proximal tubule is absorption, and *electron microscopy* reveals a multitude of microvilli on the surface of the cells facing the lumen, thus increasing the absorptive surface to an enormous degree (Fig. 302). This arrangement, of course, suggests the structure of the small intestine, which is designed primarily for absorption. Moreover, infolding of the cell membrane may extend down into the cytoplasm and connect with large vesicles there.

Loop of Henle.—The wall of the bottom of the loop of Henle is as thin as that of a capillary, suggesting absorption of fluid and concentration of electrolytes. Only animals with loops of Henle can excrete urine that is hypertonic to blood.

Juxtaglomerular Apparatus.—The ascending limb of the loop of Henle returns to the glomerulus of that nephron where it becomes the distal convoluted tubule which bends in between the afferent and efferent arteriole

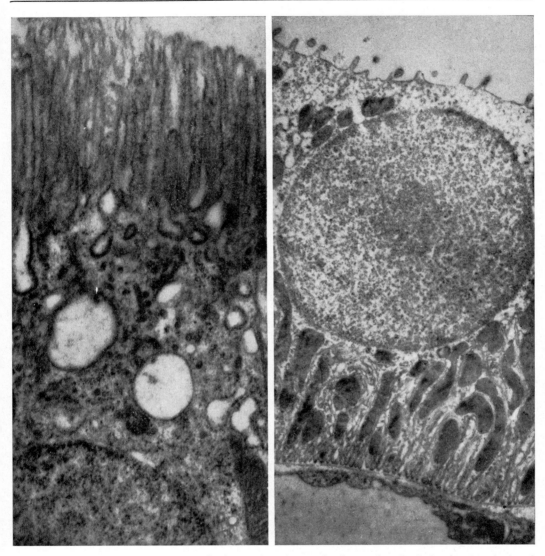

Fig. 302.—(*Left*) Electron micrograph of a section of a proximal convoluted tubule, showing the brush border of microvilli and tubules descending into the cytoplasm, as well as numerous RNA granules. (*Right*) A similar preparation of a section of a distal convoluted tubule. Note the infoldings of the cells membrane at the base of the cell and the many large mitochondria between them. (Pease, courtesy of J. Histochem.)

and takes part in the formation of the macula densa and the juxtaglomerular complex. This return of the tubule to the parent glomerulus is a truly remarkable anatomical arrangement that must have some deep functional significance, which so far eludes us. The term *macula densa* denotes a concentration of nuclei in the tubule, the cells of which are columnar and rich in acid mucopolysaccharide. Between the macula densa and the glomerulus proper there is a collection of small cells with pale nuclei to which the name polkissen has been attached. The cells of the media of the afferent arteriole in the glomerular root are markedly granular and have the character of epithelial rather than smooth muscle cells. These *juxtaglomerular cells* are absent from the adjoining efferent arteriole, surely a suggestive feature, although what it suggests remains obscure. Moreover the basement membrane which surrounds the nephron in its entire length is absent at the macula densa, so that the juxtaglomerular cells are in intimate contact with the cells of the tubule (McManus). It is surely a significant fact that the macula densa is found throughout the animal kingdom, so that it must be of very real functional value.

Distal Convoluted Tubule.—This section of the nephron which commences at the macula densa is concerned both with reabsorption and with excretion. It is shorter than the proximal tubules, so that fewer examples are seen in a cross section. Only a few poorly developed villi are visible on the surface of the cells, which agrees with their minor absorptive function. On the other hand there are highly developed infoldings of the cell membrane at the base of the cell, dividing this part of the cytoplasm into compartments. This area is also particularly rich in mitochondria (Fig. 302).

Function.—Passing reference has already been made to the functions of the various parts of the nephron. The enormous activity of the kidney is indicated by the fact that one-fifth of the total blood of the body circulates through the kidneys every minute. From this it is easy to understand how readily the kidney may be damaged by circulating toxic substances.

Every twenty-four hours some 170 liters of glomerular filtrate are emptied into the tubules, of which 169 liters are reabsorbed. Thus tubular reabsorption is just as important as glomerular filtration. The blood from the efferent arterioles has already lost 10 per cent of its fluid and crystalloid content into the glomerular spaces, so that its colloid content is increased. This naturally raises the osmotic pressure and thus facilitates absorption from the tubules with which this blood is in contact.

Glomerulus.—The glomerulus is the renal filter, an indiscriminating and apparently wasteful filter, for it allows a huge volume of water to leave the blood temporarily, as well as glucose, amino acids, chloride, sodium, potassium and calcium, all of which must be reabsorbed, because they are essential to the body. On the other hand the proteins of the blood are nearly completely retained in health, although in disease albumin may be lost in the urine in large amount. The explanation is that glomerular filtration is essentially a physical process, depending on such elements as the hydrostatic pressure in the capillaries, the pores in the endothelial cells, the arrangement of the podocytes, and the permeability of the basement membrane. When any of these becomes deranged because of disease, the result becomes evident in the urine. A fall in the hydrostatic pressure from shock or severe hemorrhage or a rise in the intrarenal pressure from obstruction will result in renal failure. Glomerular function is expressed in terms of *renal clearance*. This is a quantitative description of the rate at which the kidney excretes various substances relative to their concentration in the plasma. It gives the glomerular filtration rate or G.F.R. The rate of filtration is measured by the use of such a substance as inulin, which is neither secreted nor absorbed. It remains remarkably constant at 130 cc. per minute in spite of fluctuations of blood pressure unless shock supervenes. The filtrate is identical with blood plasma, except for protein and substances bound to protein.

Proximal Convoluted Tubule.—The *function of the tubules in general* is threefold: (1) reabsorption, (2) secretion, and (3) preservation of the acid-base balance. *Reabsorption* involves in particular water, glucose, chloride, phosphate, and also bicarbonate, sodium, potassium and calcium, as well as amino acids and probably albumin. *Secretion* comes into play in the case of exogenous creatinine and potassium, as well as diodrast in experimental work. *Regulation of the acid-base* balance is achieved by the formation of ammonia, and the exchange of hydrogen for sodium ions, which reduce the loss of fixed base in acid elimination. These functions are distributed along the various portions of the nephron, and when any part is injured by disease the corresponding function is apt to be affected. As we shall see later, some of these functions have a genetic basis, a subject to which we shall return in connection with innate functional tubular defects.

The function of the *proximal convoluted tubule* is *conservation through reabsorption*. Of the 99 per cent of glomerular filtrate which is reabsorbed before reaching the bladder, 80 to 85 per cent is absorbed in the proximal convoluted tubule. The microvilli with which this segment is so plentifully endowed enormously increase the absorptive surface and capacity. The reabsorption of water is a *passive* phenomenon due to changes in the hydrostatic and osmotic pressures in the peritubular capillaries of the efferent arterioles. It is this absorptive power which accounts for the great ease with which this portion of the tubule is damaged by a variety of poisons. The so-called *high threshold substances* are of value to the body, so that they are reabsorbed, and are therefore normally absent from the urine or only present in low concentration. Such are glucose, sodium, potassium, calcium, chloride, and some others. The reabsorption of these is *active*, being mediated by the energy of the cellular enzymes of the proximal tubule. If the tubules are extensively damaged, as from toxic injury, there may be renal glycosuria and excessive loss of salt. When the fluid in these tubules is rich in solutes, as in the glycosuria of diabetes, less water is reabsorbed so that polyuria follows the administration of sodium, potassium, *etc.*

Hyaline droplets may appear in the cells of the proximal tubules under pathological conditions. When the glomerular filter breaks down and a large amount of protein escapes, it is absorbed by the tubular epithelium and is seen as hyaline droplets.

Loop of Henle.—This short segment of the nephron appears to aid in maintaining the osmotic equilibrium of the urine before it enters the distal tubule. Under some conditions it is probable that a considerable amount of water may pass through the thin segment of the loop into the vasa recta with which it is in contact.

Distal Convoluted Tubule.—This final segment of the true nephron, which commences at the macula densa, is concerned both with reabsorption and with excretion. The distal tubule reabsorbs water and salt according to the need of the tissues, and under the control of the hypothalamus and posterior pituitary. This is the final governor of urinary volume, reducing the flow and raising the specific gravity to 1.020 or 1.030. Mercurial diurectics act by depressing over-all tubular reabsorption; less salt is absorbed and therefore less water.

Reabsorption of water in the distal tubule is known as *facultative*, because the water may be either saved or discarded. This contrasts with water reabsorption in the proximal tubule which is designated as *obligatory*, because it is not governed by extraneous influences. Reabsorption of water in the proximal tubule may be regarded as passive, that of the distal tubule as active. The amount reabsorbed by the distal segment is from 10 to 20 per cent of the total amount absorbed. Reabsorption of water in the distal tubule and possibly in the loop of Henle is under control of the *antidiuretic hormone* of the posterior lobe of the pituitary, which receives stimuli from the hypothalamic area, which in turn is influenced by such factors as pain, excitement, hypertoxicity of the extracellular fluid, *etc.*, all of which may affect the flow of urine. When reabsorption is active the urine is scanty and concentrated; when it is in abeyance the urine is abundant and of low specific gravity. In the total absence of the antidiuretic hormone, from 25 to 30 liters of urine a day will be passed, a condition of complete *diabetes insipidus*. It becomes evident that variations in the volume of reabsorbed fluid are of much greater importance in altering the flow of urine than are changes in the glomerular filtration rate.

It is generally believed that the antidiuretic hormone acts by increasing the permeability of the cells of the distal tubules. It now appears from the work of Ginetzinsky of Leningrad that the water may be reabsorbed not through the cytoplasm but through the cement substance of the intercellular lines and the basement membranes, with its high content of the mucopolysaccharide hyaluronic acid. The pituitary hormone stimulates the cells of the distal tubules and even the so-called collecting tubules to secrete hyaluronidase in the fashion of an apocrine gland. This enzyme depolymerizes the mucopolysaccharides of the cement substance, so that the membranes become permeable to water. Ginetzinsky had previously shown that the urine of all mammals under certain conditions contains hyaluronidase, although after water-loading none may be present. In hyper-hydration the cement becomes almost completely waterproof, allowing a hypotonic urine to be formed.

Reabsorption of electrolytes is also under hormonal control. The pituitary hormone inhibits the reabsorption of sodium and chloride while increasing the reabsorption of water. Adrenal hormones, on the other hand, are essential for the reabsorption of normal amounts of sodium and chloride. In Addison's disease, which is caused by adrenal insufficiency, loss of salt and water is an outstanding feature, but potassium is retained owing to increased reabsorption.

Tubular excretion is generally believed to be a function of the distal tubule. This portion of the nephron is responsible for *the preservation of acid-base balance* by (1) the formation of an acid urine and (2) the formation of ammonia by the lining cells of the distal tubule. (1) The kidney *makes the urine acid* partly by reversing the proportion of acid and alkaline phosphates. In the glomerular filtrate, as in the plasma, the ratio is $\dfrac{NaH_2PO_4}{Na_2HPO_4} = \dfrac{1}{5}$, but in the urine the ratio has become $\dfrac{NaH_2PO_4}{Na_2HPO_4} = \dfrac{9}{1}$. In highly acid urine the ratio may be 50:1. A large amount of base, chiefly sodium, has thus been conserved. Hydrogen ions arising from carbonic acid formed in the tubular epithelium are exchanged for alkali cations in the tubular urine. The coagulation of protein, which is the fundamental feature of the formation of casts, only occurs in an acid urine, and for this reason casts are confined to the distal convoluted and collecting tubules, although the Bence-Jones casts of multiple myeloma can also occur in the proximal segment. It is in the protein-losing kidney that casts are most abundant, and here they may produce tubular damage to which we shall return later. (2) The distal tubule also conserves base by *manufacturing ammonia*, which is combined with acid radicles so that they are excreted as ammonium salts. The ammonia is formed from amino groups by the action of enzymes in the tubular epithelium.

The view that acidification of the urine is essentially a function of the distal tubule is based on work on the frog, it being assumed that this holds true for all species of animals. This concept has been challenged by the observations of Nicholson, as well as other workers, which show that when the urine is markedly acid, the acid is produced at the brush border of the proximal tubules, but not when the urine is alkaline. Moreover, when the proximal tubule is damaged by the injection of racemic sodium tartrate into the renal artery, the intravenous injection of aldosterone or desoxycorticosterone, which would produce a marked drop in the sodium excretion from a normal kidney, has no effect on the damaged kidney. On the other hand, when the distal tubule is damaged by the injection of mercuric chloride into the ureter, adrenal hormones produce as great an effect on the damaged kidney as on the normal kidney (Nicholson). These observations certainly suggest that the facultative reabsorption of sodium under the control of the adrenal-cortex takes place in the proximal rather than in the distal tubule, as is generally believed.

Tubular Enzymes.—These constitute the dynamic force that brings about the functional changes which have been very briefly outlined, the most important of which are reabsorption, excretion, and the various chemical reactions. Of the enzymes which lend themselves to histological demonstration by special staining methods the most important to us are the esterases, including alkaline phosphatase, 5-nucleotidase, and succinic dehydrogenase. *Alkaline phosphatase* is the best known of the enzymes, and it can readily be demonstrated by special staining. It is concerned with the all-important reabsorption of glucose in the proximal tubule, and is concentrated in the brush border of the epithelium. It is decreased in glomerulonephritis and anoxic tubular nephrosis (McManus and Mowry). *5-Nucleotidase,* a phosphatase which acts on 5-nucleotide, itself a breakdown product of adenosine triphosphate, is also present in the proximal tubules. It is not diminished in those conditions which show a marked decrease in alkaline phosphatase, but there is a striking concentration of the enzyme in glomeruli undergoing obsolescence (McManus and Lupton). A full discussion of these and many other tubular enzymes together with striking illustrations will be found in Wachstein's papers.

The oxidative enzymes are located in the mitochondria of the tubular epithelium. Their presence can be shown by appropriate histochemical technique demonstrating dehydrogenase reactions (Hess). In experimental nephrosis produced by the administration of an aminocucleoside, resulting in the development of a disturbance marked by profound proteinuria, fluid retention, and other features of human nephrosis, changes in the activity of the enzymes are indicated by mitochondrial swelling, principally in the epithelium of the proximal convoluted tubules. The mitochondrial changes indicate profound alterations in the energy-yielding mechanism in the tubular cells. Proteinuria in this type of nephrosis seems to represent failure in the mechanism of tubular reabsorption, as albumin in the normal glomerular filtrate is reabsorbed by intact proximal tubular epithelium.

Juxtaglomerular Apparatus. — Reference has already been made to the structure of the curious collection of cells in close proximity to the glomerulus in the angle between the afferent and efferent arterioles, together with the specialized cells in the wall of the afferent arteriole. Granules are present in the epithelioid cells in the lower animals, but are very sparse in man except for such conditions as malignant hypertension, the crush kidney, cirrhosis of the liver, and Addison's disease. It has been suggested that the juxtaglomerular bodies regulate the blood flow through the glomeruli. Over twenty years ago Goormaghtigh proposed the theory that it was these cells which produced the pressor substance, renin, but there was no direct evidence in support of this idea.

The experimental work of Edelman and Phyllis Hartroft in particular, using fluorescein-labelled anti-renin and demonstrating correlations between juxtaglomerular granulation and renin assay (Pitcock and Hartroft), together with the contributions of other observers, now provides strong evidence that the site of elaboration of renin is the juxtaglomerular cell. When all the cortical and medullary tubules are rendered atrophic by constricting the renal artery in the rat or the rabbit, the juxtaglomerular cells show marked hyperplasia and increased granularity, and they contain 3 times the normal amount of renin (Demopoulos *et al.*). There is some evidence that renin may act as a trophic hormone for the zona glomerulosa of the adrenal cortex, thereby controlling the release of aldosterone, with its consequent effects on salt-retention and hypertension. In adrenalectomized animals there is a profound increase in the granules of the juxtaglomerular cells, and this is prevented or reversed by administration of desoxycorticosterone acetate (DCA) (Dunihue). Corresponding changes can be induced in the intact rat by salt restriction which increases the granulation, while an excessive intake of salt results in degranulation (Hartroft and Hartroft). In these animals changes were observed in the zona glomerulosa of the adrenal cortex, the zone responsible for the electrolyte-regulating function. It is the zona fasciculata which is stimulated by the ACTH of the pituitary. Increased granulation of the juxtaglomerular cells seems to be associated with increased activity of the adrenal cortex, and degranulation with suppressed activity.

Experimental hypertension produced by constriction of one renal artery is associated with degranulation in the contralateral kidney, and in human hypertension of the Goldblatt type the relatively normal contralateral kidney undergoes degranulation of the juxtaglomerular cells, so that the cytoplasm of these cells presents a clear appearance. Occlusion of one ureter results in severe hydronephrosis and elevation of the blood pressure, with persistence of the granules of the juxtaglomerular cells in the hydronephrotic kidney, but decrease in the contralateral one. There is evidently a relation between elevation of the blood pressure and degranulation of the juxtaglomerular cells (Hartroft).

Most of the work referred to above has been done on laboratory animals, more especially the rat. The granules in man are much fewer and more difficult to demonstrate. They are not apparent in hematoxylin and eosin preparations, and are best

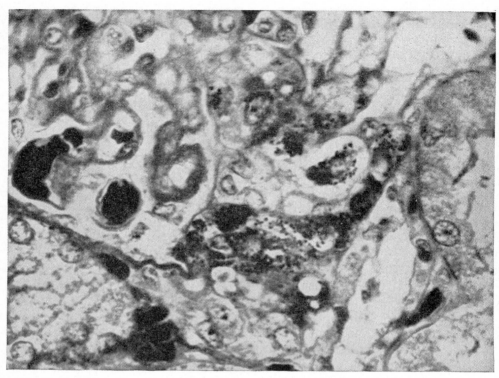

Fig. 303.—Section through a glomerular root, demonstrating advanced hypergranulation of the juxta-glomerular cells. Bowie stain. × 1000. (Pitcock and Hartroft, courtesy of Am. J. Pathology.)

demonstrated by a special stain such as the Bowie or the P A S technique (Fig. 303). As hyperplasia of the juxtaglomerular elements is usually associated with hyper-granulation, in hematoxylin and eosin preparations of human material hypercellularity may be taken to indicate hypergranularity and increased activity. In man the degree of granularity is inversely related to the levels of plasma sodium, but so far no significant relationship has been demonstrated between the level of blood pressure and the degree of juxtaglomerular granulation (Pitcock and Hartroft).

At the present time the evidence strongly suggests that this interesting structure in such close association with the glomerulus and also with the origin of the distal tubule controls the electrolyte balance, and also, in some obscure way, the blood pressure. Future work, perhaps by some reader of these words, may throw additional important light on this problem.

From this discussion of renal function it becomes apparent that the real work of the kidney is done by the tubules, which reabsorb $\frac{1}{2}$ lb. of glucose, $2\frac{1}{2}$ lbs. of salt, and 50 gallons of water in one day. The tubules deserve more attention than is generally paid to them by the student looking down the microscope, his eye naturally being attracted by the glomeruli, which play a relatively passive role in the production of urine, their energy for filtration coming from the heart.

Renal Function Tests.—Perhaps the best tests for renal function are as follows: for *glomerular function*, the *urea clearance test* (volume of blood cleared of urea in one minute's excretion of urine); for *tubular function*, the *diodrast clearance test for tubular excretion*, and the *urine concentration test for tubular absorption*. The urinometer, in the hands of one who knows how to use it, is in some ways a more potent weapon for estimating the functional capacity of the kidneys than the complex and expensive methods of blood chemistry.

Finally the remark of an old writer may be be borne in mind: "The good physician trusteth not the single witness of the water if better testimony be had. For reasons drawn from the urine alone are as brittle as the urinal."

Needle Biopsy.—In spite of the small amount of tissue obtained by introducing the Vim-Silverman needle into the kidney through the skin from behind, this method has proved of great value in the hands of Kark and others in the diagnosis of medical as opposed to surgical diseases of the kidney. By means of serial needle biopsies the natural history of renal disease can be followed, the steps can be traced by which a lesion such as glomerulonephritis may progress to a happy termination on the one hand or to an inexorable conclusion on the other, and the effect of treatment on the course of the disease can be determined. The illustrations of renal lesions in the paper by Muehrcke, Kark and Pirani are particularly striking and convincing. Biopsy has proved of value in revealing minimal lesions of chronic nephrosis at a stage when they were responsive to ACTH therapy. The procedure may of course give no information in localized lesions such as those of acute pyelonephritis, abscess, tuberculosis and neoplasm.

It is helpful to our thinking if we classify the diseases of the kidney according to the four main units of structure of which the organ is composed. These are the glomeruli, the tubules, the interstitial tissue and the blood vessels. It is unfortunately true that in the end stage of renal disease, the stage which is likely to meet the eye of the pathologist in the autopsy room or looking down a microscope, a disease process which *primarily* affects one of these four units may *ultimately* involve all four. This certainly does not make the task of the pathologist any easier when he tries to trace the course of any one renal disease. Percutaneous needle biopsy of the kidney has served to throw some much needed light on this problem. We shall begin with diseases of the glomerulus.

DIFFUSE GLOMERULONEPHRITIS

It was in 1827 that Richard Bright published his celebrated book entitled *Reports of Medical Cases selected with a view of Illustrating the Symptoms and Care of Diseases by a reference to Morbid Anatomy.* In this book he describes many patients with generalized edema or dropsy who had well marked lesions of the kidney, and in these cases the urine was coagulated by heat. Although some of the kidneys were large and pale, whilst others were small and contracted, and many other organs, such as the heart, were abnormal, Bright with the touch of the master laid his finger on the kidneys as the seat of the primary disease, and considered that it was the glomeruli which were involved. It is best to confine the term *Bright's disease* to glomerulonephritis, although in previous editions of this book it was applied to a variety of diffuse nonsuppurative lesions of the kidney. It should be pointed out that Bright is not only the father of renal pathology, but that he taught us how to investigate disease at the bedside, and, as may be gathered from the title of his book, he showed that the path to advance lay in a search for a correlation between clinical findings, morbid anatomy and histology, and biochemical observations. Without a blood pressure apparatus or modern biochemical methods he remarks that his patients with disease of the kidneys frequently had a pulse that was "full and hard," and that "nice analysis" of the blood serum will often detect a great deficiency of albumin, and sometimes the presence of urea! The student may be interested to know that Bright, Addison and Hodgkin were all on the staff of Guy's Hospital at the same time. With every justification they are known as "the great men of Guy's."

Diffuse glomerulonephritis is an inflammatory condition affecting the glomeruli primarily, but with secondary damage to the other parts of the nephron as well as the interstitial tissue later. It is the condition which should be understood when the word nephritis is used without qualification. The glomerulonephritis is diffuse in distinction to other less important forms of focal glomerulonephritis. The pathology and symptomatology of glomerulonephritis vary to such an extreme degree that three different forms have been described under the names acute nephritis, subacute or subchronic nephritis, and chronic nephritis. It has long been believed that these forms correspond to three stages of one disease. It is true that in most cases it is difficult or impossible to detect a transition from one stage to the other clinically, but it has been assumed that the second and third stages are preceded by subclinical acute attacks. Moreover, in the occasional case there is a well defined progression through the acute and subacute to the chronic stage.

The *acute stage* is characterized clinically by urinary evidence of acute inflammation, signs of acute renal insufficiency, edema, and a varying degree of hypertension. In the *intermediate stage*, also called *subacute* and *subchronic*, there is edema and albuminuria. The chief features of the *chronic stage* are hypertension and renal failure. Recovery is usual after the first stage, but repeated sub-infections may cause the kidney to pass through all three stages if the patient survives long enough.

The concept of Volhard and Fahr that glomerulonephritis is a single entity with varying manifestations and three stages has been challenged by Ellis and his associates at the London Hospital. This is the result of a study of the natural history of the disease in some 600 cases over a period of twenty years with postmortem examination of 200 of the cases. The conclusion reached is that there are two different kinds of glomerulonephritis, with different etiology, lesions, course and prognosis. These they call Type 1 and Type 2 nephritis. Needless to say, not all authorities agree with this view.

Type 1 corresponds with first stage or acute glomerulonephritis. It is identical in etiology, age incidence and lesions. There is gross hematuria of abrupt onset a week or two after an acute infection. About 85 per cent of cases make a complete recovery. In 10 per cent the albuminuria persists, and in the course of years hypertension and renal failure with contracted kidneys develop as in the usual concept, but without a picture of nephrosis.

Type 2 has a remarkably insidious onset with progressive edema and albuminuria but no history of an acute infection or gross hematuria. The etiology is unknown. The

progress is slow but remorseless, and at least 95 per cent of cases die either from infection resulting from loss of gamma globulin or from renal failure associated with hypertension. The basic lesion is a slow thickening of the capillary basement membrane with progressive hyalinization of the glomerular tufts. This matter is taken up again later in connection with membranous glomerulonephritis (p. 560).

A summary of the contrasting clinical features of the two types of glomerulonephritis is given above. below

Etiology.—Acute diffuse glomerulonephritis is an acute, non-suppurative, proliferative inflammation in which no bacteria can be demonstrated. It is a sequela of an acute infection with Group A hemolytic streptococci in the upper respiratory tract, otitis media or scarlet fever. Only certain

Ellis Type I	*Ellis Type II*
Mostly children and young adults.	Any age; frequently older adults.
Onset abrupt; usually following an acute streptococcal infection	Onset insidious; usually no history of an acute antecedent infection.
Hematuria marked.	Hematuria rare.
Edema present at onset, soon disappearing. 85–90% recover completely.	Edema progressive and persistent. 90–95% mortality.

strains of Group A streptococci are capable of initiating acute glomerulonephritis. Most of the nephritogenic strains belong to Lancefield's type 12, but types 4 and 25 may also produce this complication. In infectious disease hospitals it often follows scarlet fever in children after an interval of two or more weeks, and in throat infections there is often an interval. This latent period, together with the absence of bacteria and the peculiar proliferative type of lesion, strongly suggests that sensitization of the tissue is an essential feature and that the inflammation is allergic in character due to an antigen-antibody reaction in the glomerulus, perhaps the most vulnerable part of the whole vascular system. The fact

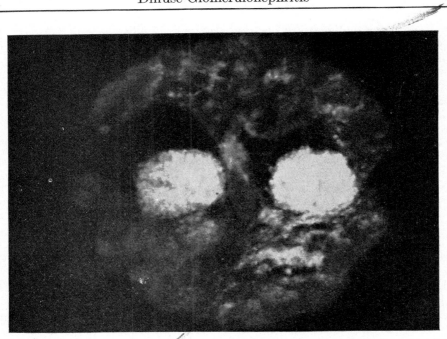

Fig. 304.—Kidney of a rabbit having proliferative glomerulitis. The fluorescence intensity of the glomeruli is much greater than that of the tubules. (Mellors, Arias-Stella, Siegel and Pressman, courtesy of Am. J. Pathology.)

that streptococci can convert nephrotoxic haptens to complete antigens in the experimental animal suggests that these organisms may initiate an auto-immune process in human glomerulonephritis.

Hypersensitivity is also the factor common to all types of experimental glomerulonephritis. This state may be induced by a variety of antigens, such as bacteria and their products and foreign proteins. The two methods most successful in reproducing the human type of lesions in animals have been the use of bovine serum gamma globulin (More and Waugh), and Masugi's so-called nephrotoxic serum, which is a specific antibody prepared by immunizing an animal of one species (rabbit) with a suspension of kidney tissue from another species (rat). When the glomeruli are separated from the other renal components, as can readily be done, and are used as antigen, a potent nephrotoxic serum is produced, whereas all other cortical components are without effect (Green and Krakower).

A powerful new weapon has been forged by combining microfluorescence with immunological technique as suggested by Coons and

Kaplan (Mellors). By this method gamma globulin antibodies have been localized in the glomerular basement membrane, not only in the experimental animal, but also in human glomerulonephritis, as well as in lipoid nephrosis, renal amyloidosis, and the vascular lesions of polyarteritis nodosa, and disseminated lupus erythematosus (Mellors and Ortega). Rabbit antisera against human globulins are coupled with fluorescent material, and the antibodies so labelled localize in the glomerular loops in frozen sections, indicating the presence of antigen, and confirming the view that these conditions have an immuno-allergic basis. The resulting appearance is very striking (Fig. 304).

The structural element of the glomerulus which is involved in the antigen-antibody reaction is the basement membrane which we have already studied. This can be shown both by the fixation of radioiodine-labelled antibody in the basement membrane after intravenous injection, and by the preparation of active antigens from the basement membranes after ultrasonic dissociation of isolated glomeruli (Krakower and Greenspon). Nephrotoxic antigens are not confined to the glomerular basement membrane, but are widely distributed throughout the body, including the heart muscle, lung, liver and alimentary canal. In spite of this wide distribution of antigen, the lesions that result from the injection of the antisera are confined to the glomeruli. This may be due to the extremely intimate contact between the circulating blood in the glomerulus and the underlying basement membrane that is permitted by the peculiar structure of the capillary endothelium revealed by electron microscopy.

The great difficulty is to correlate the mass of experimental work on laboratory animals with what probably happens in human glomerulonephritis. It would appear that antigenic substances, usually streptococcal in nature, localize in the glomerular basement membrane, that specific antibodies unite with the antigen exciting an Arthus type of reaction, or that soluble antigen-antibody complexes, which occur with antigen excess, are themselves responsible for the production of allergic lesions. Moreover it has been shown that an antigen may persist in the glomerulus for some time, and excite the development of antibodies produced at a remote site. This would explain both the latent period after a known infection and the continued manifestations of the disease.

In streptococcal and other infections, more particularly subacute bacterial endocarditis, it is not unusual at autopsy to find proliferation and swelling of the endothelium of the glomerular capillaries, causing narrowing but not occlusion of the lumen. Such cases may be regarded as examples of subclinical glomerulonephritis, in which there is no clinical evidence of renal disease during life. It would seem that acute glomerulonephritis is not a specific entity with one and only one etiological agent such as the typhoid bacillus, but rather an extreme degree of a common reaction of glomerular endothelium (Bell).

Having reviewed the problem of the pathogenesis of acute glomerulonephritis, we may return to the contentious subject of the relationship of the acute to the subacute form, of Ellis type I to Ellis type II. In an analysis of what he calls *nephrotic glomerulonephritis* Jones outlines the large number of differences between the two types, but adds that the evidence suggests they belong to the same family. Both possess circulating antiglomerular auto-antibodies. Antibody titers in both rise with activity and fall during remission. Human gamma globulin is bound to glomeruli in both types I and II, the gamma globulin being an antiglomerular auto-antibody. In type I a streptococcal infection triggers an auto-antibody production. Streptococcal products seem to combine with glomerular connective tissue to form an antigen which results in antibody production, together with an Arthus type of injury to the glomerulus. When the antibody level falls, the injury ceases. In type II no triggering mechanism can be demonstrated. The process is gradual, with remissions and exacerbations. And yet an auto-antibody formation similar to that of type I seems to be present, although the mechanism remains obscure.

Lesions.—*Acute Glomerulonephritis.*—In the first or acute stage (Ellis type I) the kidneys are usually swollen, and the capsule tense and stretched to such a degree that when it is incised the renal substance bulges through the opening. The surface is smooth and gray, and sometimes presents numerous red dots, corresponding to petechial hemorrhages into the capsular spaces.

Microscopically there is a combination of acute inflammatory exudate in the interstitial tissue or mesangium, edema of this tissue, and swelling of the endothelium of the capillary loops. These changes are best seen in the extremely thin sections made possible by the ultramicrotome designed for electron microscopy (Grishman and Churg). As the mesangium becomes widened the normal clover-leaf lobules become ballooned out into club-shaped structures with resulting compression of the capillaries and great ischemia of the glomerulus. The characteristic lesion of acute glomerulonephritis is the greatly increased cellularity of the tuft (Figs. 305 and 306), due in part to the cells in the interstitial space and not merely to proliferation of the vascular endothelium which is the usual view. These changes are beautifully illustrated in Jones' paper. An earlier but

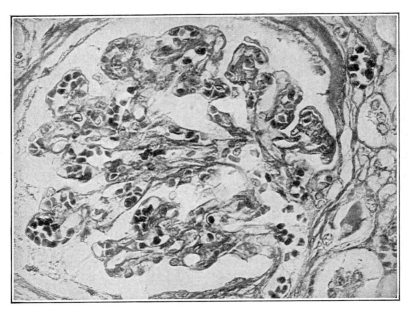

FIG. 305.—Normal glomerulus, showing individual units, the capillary loops of which the tuft is composed, widely separated. × 400.

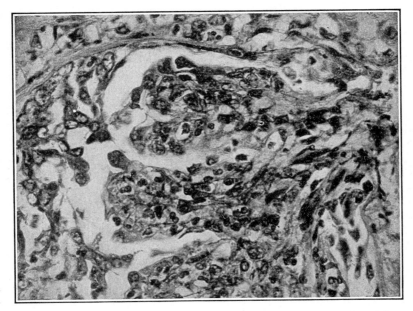

FIG. 306.—Glomerulonephritis, showing cellular proliferation and avascularity of the tuft. The case is in the intermediate stage; epithelial crescent to left. × 450.

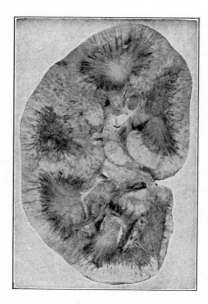

FIG. 307.—Kidney in the intermediate stage of glomerulonephritis; the "large white kidney."

less important change is swelling and multiplication of the epithelium of the tuft, so that the cells fill the spaces between the loops. Later they undergo degeneration and are cast off into the capsular space. Polymorphonuclear leukocytes collect in large numbers in the glomerular capillaries, and there is a varying amount of exudate (serum, fibrin, leukocytes and red cells) in the capsular space, which passes into the urine. The proliferating interstitial cells give rise to the formation of fibrils and later of connective tissue as healing proceeds. This causes an all-important obliteration of the capillary bed of the glomerulus, a process which may be aided by proliferation of the vascular endothelium.

As a result of the proliferative and inflammatory changes little or no blood flows through the glomerulus. The blood supply to the tubules passes through the glomeruli, so that the ischemia will lead to secondary tubular degeneration and in turn to increase of the interstitial fibrous tissue. These changes, however, are not seen in the first stage of nephritis.

The *further course* may be toward *healing* or *chronicity*. In the scarlatinal cases there is usually complete recovery, and if the patient dies some years later the glomeruli may show no trace of former lesions; in other cases a greater or less number of glomeruli are found to be obliterated. In other cases, especially those due to streptococcal infections of the throat, the kidney is exposed to repeated reinfection, so that the process advances to the second and finally the third stage of nephritis.

Subacute Glomerulonephritis.—The gross appearance is well described by the old term "large white kidney" (Fig. 307). The kidney is slightly or considerably enlarged, the capsule strips easily, and the exposed surface is smooth and pale. The cut surface shows marked swelling and pallor of the cortex, in comparison with which the pyramids appear unnaturally dark. The pallor is due chiefly to a great accumulation of lipid in the cells of the convoluted tubules, but in part to emptying of the capillaries from swelling of the parenchyma. There may be bright yellow streaks and patches in the cortex due to large deposits of lipid. The consistence is soft.

The *glomeruli* show an extreme cellularity which is highly characteristic. While both the epithelial and the endothelial cells of the tuft take part in the process, one or other of these may show the most proliferation. When the epithelial cells are principally involved the lesion is referred to as *extracapillary glomerulonephritis*. The epithelium of Bowman's capsule proliferates, so that large masses of cells occupy the capsular space. The whole circumference of the glomerulus is seldom involved, so that the cells form a semilunar mass in the capsular space which is known as the *epithelial crescent*, and provides the most easily recognized evidence of subacute glomerulonephritis (Fig. 308). The proliferating cells become thrown into folds which fuse together and may surround spaces resembling tubules. There is also a constant proliferation of the epithelium in the proximal convoluted tubules with the formation of "increscences" identical in structure with the crescents (García-Cáceres). Red blood cells, desquamated epithelium, and fibrin are present in the capsular space in varying amount. In course of time the crescents become fibrosed and fuse with the tuft which also undergoes hyalinization.

In the so-called *intracapillary form* there are few or no cells in the capsular space, but

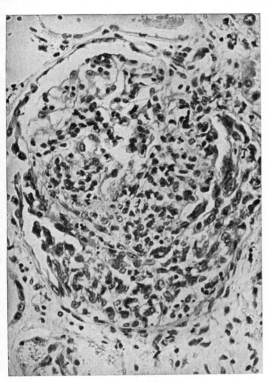

Fig. 308.—The epithelial crescent of glomerulo-nephritis. The space between the tuft and Bowman's capsule is occupied by proliferated epithelial cells.

a great proliferation of the endothelial cells gives the tuft a highly cellular appearance, and again contributes to ischemia.

We have left the *basement membrane* to the end, not because of its unimportance, but because the changes it shows in ordinary sections are to all appearance so insignificant. There is a diffuse, homogeneous thickening of the capillary basement membranes, the condition which Bell originally called *membranous glomerulonephritis*, and which Churg and Grishman term *membranous transformation* of the capillary wall because evidence of inflammation is often lacking. This condition will be considered separately in relation to nephrosis. The change in the basement membrane results in a remarkable increase of glomerular permeability, particularly to protein, as we shall see presently, and this forms the basis of the nephrotic syndrome.

The natural history and the subsequent course of glomerulonephritis, at any rate in the experimental animal, seems to depend

on what happens to the basement membrane (Hamilton and Fremes). Thus in glomerulonephritis produced in unilateral nephrectomized rabbits by repeated injections of foreign protein (horse serum), if the basement membrane remain intact although swollen, the other stigmata such as swelling and proliferation of glomerular endothelium and of the mesangium, subside and resolve in the course of 2 to 4 weeks. If, however, the basement membranes become fragmented and ruptured the proliferating epithelium of Bowman's capsule lays down collagen with ultimate periglomerular fibrosis and obliteration of the glomerulus, while the endothelial and epithelial cells of the glomerular loops become converted into hyaline material. These changes, of course, are irreversible.

The *tubules* show marked degenerative changes, which are most pronounced in the convoluted tubules. The epithelium of the convoluted tubules shows cloudy swelling, fatty degeneration or necrosis. The fat content may be very high. In addition to neutral fat the cells may contain large amounts of lipid material, chiefly cholesterol ester, which can be seen as bright anisotropic globules in frozen sections under crossed Nicol's prisms. As the tubular degeneration progresses, many of the epithelial cells are cast off and the tubules become atrophic.

Chronic Glomerulonephritis.—This is the *stage of scarring.* In an advanced case the kidney is small and shrivelled, its surface is covered with fine granules, and the capsule is so adherent that, when it is stripped off, portions of the cortex come away with it (decortication) (Fig. 309). The meaning of the granularity is shown by the microscopic examination. Sometimes the surface may be smooth even though the microscopic changes are marked. The cut surface shows extreme irregularity and atrophy of the cortex, which in places may be only 1 or 2 mm. in width. The irregularity corresponds with the granularity of the surface. The normal vertical markings of the cortex produced by the vasa recta are lost.

Microscopic examination reveals an organ which one can hardly recognize as being a kidney owing to the complete loss of the renal architecture. The parenchyma, which normally consists practically entirely of

36

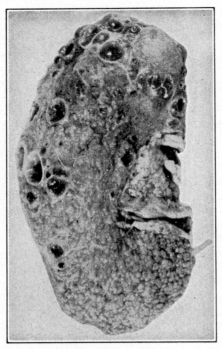

Fig. 309.—Chronic glomerulonephritis
(granular contracted kidney).

tubules with a few scattered glomeruli, has been replaced by the cheap substitute of fibrous tissue. It is this disappearance of tubules which strikes the observer most on first examining the section.

The *glomeruli* show hyalinization in its most extreme form. Owing to the disappearance of the tubules and the shrinkage of the cortex there may be large numbers of hyaline glomeruli in a low-power field (Fig. 310). Other glomeruli are atrophic and shrunken, but their capillaries still allow the passage of some blood. Still other glomeruli are greatly hypertrophied. It is these which carry on the work of the kidney and keep the patient alive. The hyaline glomeruli fade away and blend with the surrounding tissue until they can no longer be distinguished.

The *convoluted tubules* show an extreme degree of atrophy, and only their outline may be detected under the high power. Some of the tubules appear normal or more often are dilated and lined by a high epithelium with papillary buds projecting into the lumen, although when the dilatation is marked the cells become low or even flattened. These tubules, which are connected with hypertrophied glomeruli, may be regarded as showing evidence of compensatory or work hypertrophy. They are collected in little groups which stand out in striking contrast to the rest of the shrunken parenchyma, and it is these islands of tubules which, projecting above the surrounding surface, give rise to some of the granularity. Microdissection has shown that a hypertrophied tubule may be attached to a completely atrophied glomerulus, suggesting the condition found in the aglomerular kidney of certain fish where the tubule plays the part of the glomerulus (Oliver).

The *interstitial tissue* shows a very great increase, which is mostly apparent due to the concentration of tissue, but to some extent is real. Groups of small round cells may form a striking picture in the fibrosed cortex especially in the neighborhood of the hyalinized glomeruli.

The *arteries* supplying the fibrosed atrophic areas show the changes of disuse atrophy, the chief feature of which is marked fibrous thickening of the intima causing narrowing of the lumen. This is a form of endarteritis obliterans similar to the change which occurs when a vessel is ligated. If hypertension becomes marked, hypertensive vascular lesions may develop, some of which unfortunately may resemble those of disuse atrophy. The chief of these hypertensive vascular lesions is arteriolosclerosis with marked narrowing of the lumen. This may have two effects: (1) by causing renal ischemia it may accentuate the hypertension, which in turn leads to further arteriolosclerotic ischemia, so that a vicious circle is set up; (2) by depriving the remaining nephrons of their blood supply it may add the *coup de grâce* to the already faltering kidney and bring about its final downfall.

Relation of Symptoms to Lesions.—In some cases the patient may pass through the three stages of glomerulonephritis, although we have seen that this statement is open to question, in others he will die in the second stage, in still others symptoms of the first two stages may never be detected, and only those of the third stage are in evidence. *Acute glomerulonephritis* is characterized by

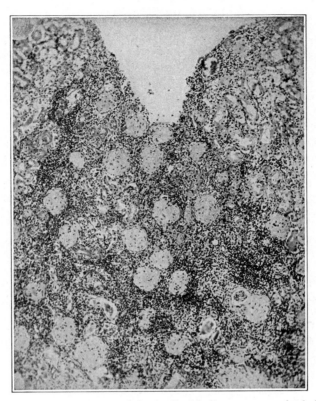

Fig. 310.—Complete hyalinization of glomeruli with disappearance of tubules in center of field and round cell infiltration.   × 60.

pain in the back, fever, edema, a rise in the blood pressure, and such urinary changes as oliguria, high coloration, high specific gravity, the presence of albumin, blood, and casts, and a low urea content, with a corresponding non-protein nitrogen retention in the blood. With the exception of the urinary changes almost any of these symptoms may be absent. *Subacute glomerulonephritis* is the stage of wet nephritis, nephritis with edema. The *chief symptom is edema*, which may be extreme. The *chief urinary finding is albuminuria*, which also may be very marked, but casts of various descriptions are also present. The renal function shows little sign of impairment, although the kidney is grossly diseased, a condition which has been described as compensated renal hypofunction. The blood changes are those commonly associated with nephrosis, namely high blood cholesterol, lowered serum albumin, and a reversal of the ordinary albumin-globulin ratio. There is no retention of urea or other nitrogenous substances. The basal metabolic rate is also below normal, because of the continued loss of protein bound iodine in the urine, and also the fact that the apparent weight of the patient is not his true weight, owing to the tissues being saturated with fluid. It is evident that this stage may be called the *nephrotic phase of glomerulonephritis*, for the clinical symptoms and the blood and urinary findings are identical with those of that somewhat misty entity. The patient is likely to die as the result of the edema or from some intercurrent infection. Owing to the compensation of the renal hypofunction, there is little danger of death from uremia.

The passage into *chronic glomerulonephritis* is evidenced by the *appearance of signs of renal failure*; it is preëminently the stage of renal insufficiency, or decompensated renal hypofunction, a functional rather than an anatomical division. Albumin and casts in small amount may be present, but these are of little significance. Just as loss of the power of concentrating the urine is the earliest evidence of impairment of renal function, so in the later stages when the specific gravity is fixed around 1.010 blood chemistry becomes the all-important instrument for estimating the degree of renal failure. An ever increasing degree of nitrogen-retention develops and the final picture is usually that of uremia. The edema, should any have been present, disappears, the blood pressure mounts steadily, the left ventricle becomes hypertrophied, and there may be hemorrhages in the retina and in the brain.

In chronic glomerulonephritis the filtration rate and the renal plasma flow are variably reduced. The most characteristic functional change is a reduction of the filtration rate, owing to the glomerular lesions. Late in the disease tubular excretion (Tm_D or the maximum tubular clearance of diodrast) is reduced to very low values, the remaining tubules being practically impotent. As Homer Smith remarks, in the overall functional picture it is not the aglomerular tubules which predominate but the atubular glomeruli.

It would be a vain task to take up one and all of the multitudinous symptoms of nephritis, many of which have not been included in the above catalogue, and attempt to give a rational explanation in each case, but a few of the most important will be selected for discussion.

Albuminuria.—The albuminuria is of glomerular origin, being due to damage to the renal filter, in particular damage to the basement membrane. This filter is a very delicate affair, which may be interfered with by processes which leave no anatomical trace. Thus mere clamping of the renal artery for thirty seconds will cause albuminuria due to temporary anoxia. Albuminuria is present in the acute stage, but it is most massive in the so-called second stage. Here it is commonly associated with ascites, the combination constituting the nephrotic syndrome.

Edema.—Renal edema may be divided into nephritic edema and nephrotic edema. *Nephritic edema* occurs in acute glomeru-

lonephritis. It is evidently due to an increased permeability of the capillaries, because the fluid in the tissues contains over 1 per cent of protein, a condition which Eppinger has called "albuminuria into the tissues." The capillaries of the subcutaneous tissue are probably injured, perhaps in the same way as are the capillaries of the glomeruli. It is therefore an inflammatory form of edema. *Nephrotic edema* occurs in so-called chronic nephrosis, in the nephrotic or second stage of glomerulonephritis (wet nephritis), and in the amyloid kidney. The protein content of the dropsical fluid here is less than 0.1 per cent, *i.e.*, one-tenth that of nephritic edema. It is evident that the mechanism of production of the edema must be quite different. Here there is great loss of plasma protein through the heavy albuminuria (Fig. 311) with particular loss of the albumin as shown by the reversed albumin-globulin ratio, the larger globulin molecules being still unable to pass through the damaged filter. The colloid osmotic pressure of the plasma is therefore diminished, and fluid is free to escape into the tissues.

It is a curious but easily explained fact that chronic renal edema varies inversely with the degree of impairment of renal function. As long as a patient with subacute glomerulonephritis shows little or no sign of renal insufficiency, the edema is marked. When renal insufficiency develops, the edema disappears. The reason is that obliteration of the leaking glomeruli stops the loss of albumin as well as paralyzes renal function, the blood proteins rise with an accompanying increase of the colloid osmotic pressure, and the fluid is drawn from the tissues back into the blood.

We must distinguish between edema which is renal and that which is cardiac in origin. Moreover the renal edema of the earlier stages of the illness may be replaced later by cardiac edema due to failure of the circulation. The distinction between the two is usually easy, as for instance by observing the effect of digitalis upon the edema. Renal edema is less dependent upon gravity than is the cardiac form, nor does it involve the serous cavities so frequently.

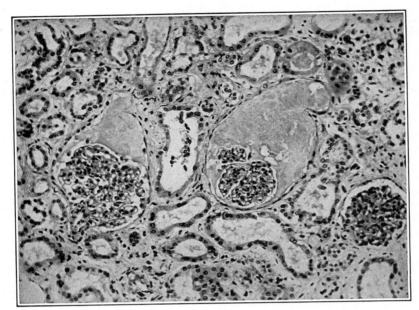

FIG. 311.—Albuminous fluid in the glomerular space in a case of nephrotic edema. × 150.

Hypertension.—A rise in blood pressure, moderate in degree, occurs in about one-third of the acute cases. It becomes much less and sometimes disappears entirely in the second stage. In the third stage it forms one of the dominating features, but seldom attains the extreme degree seen in essential hypertension, and usually remains under 200 mm. The relation of the kidney to hypertension is discussed on page 601.

High Non-protein Nitrogen.—The high level of non-protein nitrogen in the blood, which may be taken to indicate a retention of non-protein, is due to insufficiency on the part of the renal glomeruli. It is moderate in the first stage, disappears in the second stage, and may become extreme in the third stage. Its presence does not necessarily indicate the presence of nephritis, for it may be due to extrarenal causes such as the production of more urea than can be excreted (leukemia, etc.). Even when renal in origin there may be no nephritis, for in the stasis or cardiac kidney associated with a failing circulation the non-protein nitrogen may be raised.

Blood Cholesterol.—This is increased in nephritis with edema. It may be very high

in the nephrotic form. In acute nephritis the increase is moderate, while in the chronic stage it is normal or below normal. The meaning of the increase is not known. It is possibly due to some extrarenal disturbance of lipid metabolism. Although associated with edema it does not appear to be related to it. The distinction between nephritic and cardiac edema is sometimes quite difficult. Here the blood cholesterol is of great value, for while high in nephritic edema it is normal in the edema of heart failure.

Retinal Changes.—*Renal or albuminuric retinitis* is characterized by the formation of exudates and hemorrhages in the retina. The exudate appears as soft, white, "cotton-wool" patches which impair the local translucency, or as "star figures" which radiate in lines from the macula. Microscopically the exudate takes the form of an infiltration of the layers of the retina by a fine fibrinous meshwork, some of which is absorbed by large lipid-filled phagocytes, while the rest becomes hyalinized. The hemorrhages are flame-shaped, as are other retinal hemorrhages.

Uremia.—The subject of uremia is discussed in relation to renal failure from whatever cause (p. 606), so that it will not be considered here.

Anemia.—Anemia, first described by Bright, is one of the most characteristic features, and is evidenced by the increasing pallor of the patient. The degree of the anemia is relative to the azotemia, so that it is a good indication of the progress of the case. It may be due to interference with the building up of hemoglobin in the liver or to toxic arrest of the maturation of red blood cells. It is difficult to overemphasize the importance of anemia in assessing the progress of a case of uremia. Estimation of the hemoglobin level is an economic and convenient substitute for periodic determination of the non-protein nitrogen in chronic cases.

Urinary Changes.—The urine varies with the type of nephritis. In the acute form the characteristic finding is *red blood cells,* in addition to *albumin* and *casts,* the latter consisting of protein from the glomerulus with contributions of epithelium and granular and fatty detritus from the tubules. *Anisotropic, i.e., doubly-refractive bodies,* may be found in the urine in the second stage by means of Nicol's prisms. They consist of cholesterol ester, and are related to the deposits of cholesterol in the renal tubules. The *polyuria* is merely a compensatory mechanism whereby the failing kidney tries to excrete waste products. It has lost its concentrating power, and in order that the necessary amount of solids may be eliminated, a greatly increased quantity of fluid must be poured out. The *loss of concentrating power* is indicated by the *low and fixed specific gravity,* and is largely due to atrophy of the convoluted tubules whose essential function is absorption. This atrophy in turn is caused mainly by the loss of blood supply to the tubules.

Reference has already been made to the tests for renal function and renal failure on page 554.

Focal Glomerulitis.—This is or used to be a common renal complication of subacute bacterial endocarditis. It was for long called *focal embolic glomerulonephritis,* but this is a misnomer, for although the lesions are certainly focal, the condition is neither embolic nor a glomerulonephritis. The mistake is a natural one, because large infarcts caused by arterial emboli from the cardiac vegetations are a frequent finding, and it was reasonable to suppose that the tiny lesions involving one or two loops of the glomerular tuft were due to embolic blocking of the capillaries. No explanation could be offered for the absence of these lesions in acute bacterial endocarditis, a condition in which the vegetations are more friable and easily detached than in the subacute form. Nor was there any explanation for the strange distribution of hundreds of minute emboli in one pair of organs and no where else. Nor why fragments of bacterial vegetations are very seldom found in the glomerular lesions. A better name is *thrombotic glomerulonephritis.* It is now believed that, like so many other conditions involving the vessels of the kidney, the lesions represent a hypersensitivity reaction of the glomerular capillaries to the circulating bacteria. Now that the blood can be rendered free of bacteria by modern chemotherapy, this formerly commonplace lesion is threatening to become a rarity.

Scattered over the surface of both kidneys there are great numbers of tiny red spots, giving a picture of the "flea-bitten kidney." These represent small hemorrhages into the glomerular spaces. The glomerular lesions may be diffuse or focal. The chief diffuse lesions are proliferation of the capillary endothelium, so that the tuft has a more cellular appearance than normal, and thickening of the capillary basement membrane. The focal lesions are less common, but are much more striking, and indeed are pathognomonic. The lesion takes the form of a patch of coagulation necrosis in the tuft which is readily recognized (Fig. 312). The lumen of the glomerular capillaries is filled with hyaline thrombi, similar to the material which blocks the vessels in acute glomerulonephritis (Bell). Hemorrhage takes place into the glomerular space owing to necrosis of the capillary loops, but the blood is more readily seen in the tubules than in the space, for it is washed out by the flow of urine. If the necrotic part of the tuft comes in contact with the capsule there may be a localized proliferation of the capsular epithelium with the formation of a kind of

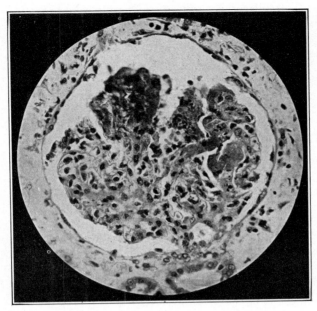

FIG. 312.—Glomerular lesion in subacute bacterial endocarditis. The upper part of the tuft is completely necrotic. $\times$ 300.

epithelial crescent. Or adhesions may form between the tuft and capsule. If the patient lives long enough there will be healing and fibrosis.

The only *symptom* is the presence of red blood cells in the urine. As so few glomeruli are involved there is no danger of renal insufficiency. In the exceptional case which may die of uremia it will be found that a true diffuse glomerulonephritis has been added.

Radiation Nephritis.—Exposure of both kidneys to radiation can result in serious and sometimes fatal damage. This can happen in irradiation of periaortic abdominal lymph nodes in cases of malignant tumors of the testis, of carcinoma of the ovary, of neuroblastoma of the adrenal, *etc.* Luxton reported the development of radiation nephritis in 27 of 137 patients treated for seminoma of the testis. It seems probable that many cases of radiation nephritis are not recognized as such owing to the latent period for the development of acute symptoms being from 6 months to a year (Cogan and Ritter). The condition seems to be more common in Britain, perhaps because British radiotherapists are accustomed to use more widespread irradiation than their

American confréres. Even at autopsy the kidney may show little or no change to the naked eye, although the capsule may be thickened. *Microscopically* the glomeruli are primarily affected, as shown by percutaneous biopsy, with thickening of the glomerular tufts and Bowman's capsule. Tubular atrophy and interstitial fibrosis appear to be secondary. Hypertension may develop, accompanied by arterial changes either of the benign or malignant type. Experimental irradiation of the kidneys of the rat produce two different biological effects, interstitial fibrosis and hypertension, which seem to be independent of one another (Wilson *et al.*). The hypertension itself may be responsible for some of the interstitial fibrosis owing to the vascular occlusion which develops, as we shall see when we come to study nephrosclerosis. Finally, to make things still more difficult, renal hypertension may develop in the absence of any recognizable structural lesion.

Chronic Glomerular Nephroses.—The term nephrosis has passed through many vicissitudes. It was first introduced by Friedrich Müller in 1905, his innocent intention being to indicate that the principal lesion in some damaged kidneys was tubular degeneration rather than glomerular inflammation. At a later date the clinician appropriated the word and applied it to a certain clinical picture characterized by marked edema and massive albuminuria, with in addition low plasma protein and high cholesterol, normal blood pressure and absence of signs of renal failure. If this condition is called the *nephrotic syndrome, i.e.*, a group of clinical features with no reference to tubular lesions, confusion can be avoided. Indeed, as will be seen presently, the basic lesion in such cases is glomerular rather than tubular.

Kimmelstiel has suggested a simple and valuable classification of the nephroses into glomerular nephrosis, in which the essential lesion is in the glomerulus, and tubular nephrosis, in which the lesion is in the tubules. It is valuable because it serves to clear up much of the confusion involved in the nomenclature. *Glomerular nephrosis* is likely to be associated with the nephrotic syndrome of edema and massive albuminuria due to damage to the glomerular filter, as a result of which protein leaks through from the capillaries of the tuft into the capsular space; *tubular nephrosis* is associated with oliguria or anuria and terminal azotemia due to damage to the tubular epithelium, as a result of which water and electrolytes leak from the tubules into the interstitial tissue of the kidney and fail to reach the bladder, a condition of unselective tubular reabsorption. *In glomerulonephritis oliguria is caused by too little excretion of water by the damaged glomeruli; in nephrosis it is caused by too much absorption of water by the damaged tubules.* Only the glomerular nephroses will be considered in this section dealing with glomerular lesions. The very different tubular nephroses will be discussed in relation to lesions of the tubules.

There remains one difficulty concerning nomenclature. The name nephrosis is apt to suggest a degenerative lesion. This is true for the tubular varieties, but in the glomerular form the lesion may be inflammatory (in the sense of reaction to injury) as in lipoid nephrosis, also called membranous glomerulonephritis and nephrotic glomerulonephritis, or it may be degenerative as in amyloid nephrosis, diabetic glomeruloscler-

osis, renal vein thrombosis, and the nephrosis of pregnancy. For this reason *it is best to accept nephrosis as a term with a clinical but not a pathological connotation*, a state of disordered physiology marked by massive proteinuria and edema, but which may be caused by a number of pathological processes, all of which apparently alter the permeability of the glomerular basement membrane.

Lipoid Nephrosis: Membranous Glomerulonephritis.—The name lipoid nephrosis is derived from the lipid deposits in the cells of the convoluted tubules, more especially the proximal tubule, and the presence of anisotropic lipids in the urine, but *the basic disturbance is hyperpermeability of the basement membrane of the glomerular capillaries for protein and lipids*, which pour from the plasma into the urine, with absorption into the tubules. We have already seen that the massive albuminuria and consequently the edema of subacute glomerulonephritis and of Ellis type II nephritis are associated with, indeed due to, increased permeability of the basement membrane. When this condition occurs divorced from the endothelial and epithelial hyperplasia of glomerulonephritis and the formation of an epithelial crescent, but associated with marked deposits of lipid in the proximal convoluted tubules, we find it tagged as lipoid nephrosis or pure lipoid nephrosis, although it might well be called a pure membranous glomerulonephritis or glomerulonephrosis. As might be expected, these patients do not have hematuria, azotemia or hypertension.

The great unanswered question is whether lipoid nephrosis is a separate entity or is merely a modification of the subacute stage of glomerulonephritis (Ellis type II) with the lesion limited strictly to the basement membrane. The condition, which is mainly seen in children, has the hallmarks of a hypersensitivity reaction, as also does glomerulonephritis. By means of renal needle biopsy and electron microscopic technique the nephrotic lesions, which at first tend to be patchy, may be traced into the diffuse lesions which characterize subacute glomerulonephritis. Cases are markedly benefitted by cortisone, which is of value in other supposedly allergic conditions. In the experimental animal

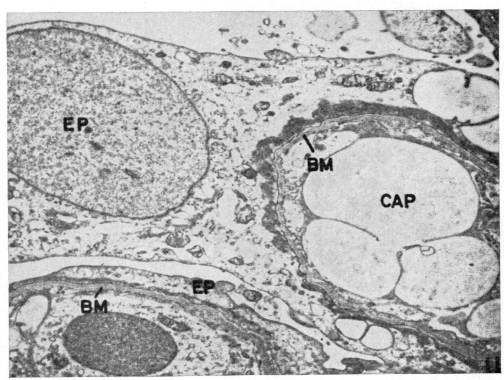

FIG. 313.—Glomerular loop in nephrosis as seen with the electron microscope. An epithelial cell (E.P.) completely covers and appears to clasp the surface of a capillary (CAP). Its cytoplasm is highly vacuolated and that portion which adjoins the basement membrane (BM) is unusally dense. Note the complete absence of foot processes. × 10,300. (Farquhar, Vernier and Good, courtesy of Am. Jour. Path.)

lesions similar to those of lipoid nephrosis can be produced by injections of anti-kidney serum. It would appear as if lipoid nephrosis, if not an unusual manifestation of subacute glomerulonephritis, is at least a close cousin of that condition, and that the one may pass into the other.

Lesions.—The *glomerular capillary basement membrane* is thickened, although this thickening may well be overlooked unless special connective tissue stains are used. In past years, indeed, the glomeruli used to be passed over as normal, with attention directed to the more obvious but functionally unimportant lesions in the tubules. It was not until Bell drew attention to the thickening of the basement membrane that lipoid nephrosis assumed its rightful place as a glomerular disease. The membranous thickening may involve the entire glomerulus (diffuse) or only single lobules (local). It is

now realized that severe glomerular structural changes may occur, which are invisible by conventional techniques but are easily detected by the electron microscope. Striking changes in the epithelial cells covering the glomerular loops have been demonstrated with the electron microscope in renal biopsies from children with nephrosis (Farquhar *et al.*). The foot processes are greatly reduced in number and in some areas are virtually absent, their place being taken by broad masses of epithelial cytoplasm which cover and envelope wide areas of the capillary loop (Fig. 313). This appearance should be compared with that of a normal glomerulus (Fig. 301, p. 548). Finally this technique showed that the thickening of the basement membrane, called by Allen *chronic membranous nephritis*, seems to be a sequel to the increased permeability of the membrane, as a result of which there is exudation and

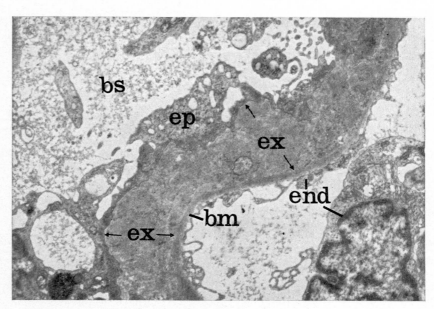

Fig. 314.—Segment of a capillary loop from a man with membranous glomerulonephritis. Protein exudate separates the basement membrane from the epithelium. This accounts for the apparent thickening of the basement membrane seen in the light microscope. The lamina densa is of normal thickness. The foot processes of epithelial cells are fused. end = endothelium; ep = epithelium; bm = basement membrane; bs = Bowman's space; ex = exudate. Protargol stain, × 12,000. (Kindness of Dr. Henry Z. Movat.)

precipitation of plasma protein, probably antigen-antibody complexes, between the basement membrane and the epithelial cells, as well as between the foot processes of the podocytes (Movat and MacGregor) (Fig. 314). Vacuoles and hyaline droplets probably representing swollen mitochondria are seen in the glomerular epithelium as well as in the proximal convoluted tubules.

In *summary*, our concept of the glomerular lesions of lipoid nephrosis may be said to have passed through 4 stages. (1) In the beginning the glomeruli were thought to be normal. (2) Improved staining technique and observation then showed a thickening of the basement membrane. (3) The electron microscope demonstrated changes in the epithelial elements, with loss of podocytes and spreading out of the cytoplasm. (4) Finally the precipitation of a protein-rich material between the basement membrane and the epithelial cells due to an increased permeability of the membrane was seen to be responsible for at least some of the apparent thickening of that membrane and the structural changes in the epithelium.

The changes in concept are illustrated in Figure 315.

The *tubular lesions* attract the eye, but do not appear to interfere with renal function. The epithelium is loaded with lipids, both neutral fats and cholesterol esters, and it presents a striking appearance in frozen sections stained with Scharlach R. The esters are best seen under crossed Nichol's prisms, the lipids appearing as bright doubly-refractive bodies. The tubular lesions are responsible for the *gross appearance*, which is that of the so-called "large white kidney" with pale swollen cortex presenting numerous yellow streaks and patches of lipids.

Relation of Symptoms to Lesions.—It is important to distingusih between the condition as it manifests itself in children and in adults. In children, in whom the onset of edema is often remarkably rapid, the disease generally pursues a relatively benign course with complete recovery in from one to three years in about 50 per cent of the cases. The remainder, however, tend to develop infections, such as peritonitis, against which they have little resistance owing to hypo-

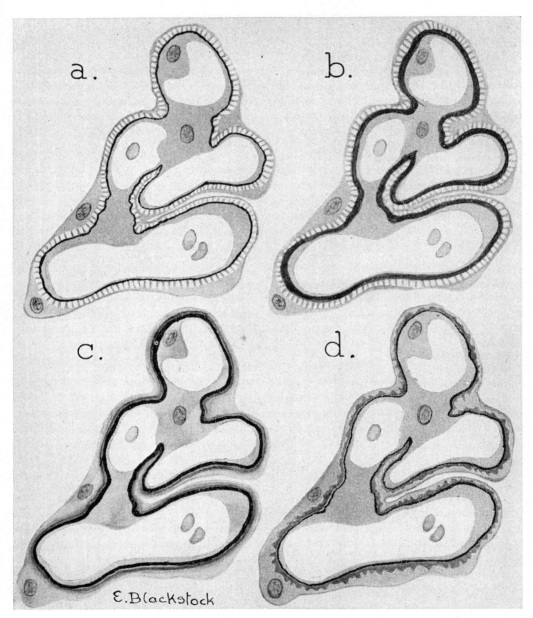

Fig. 315.—This diagram represents the various concepts of membranous glomerulonephritis: *a*, capillary loops of a normal glomerulus; *b*, thickening of the basement membrane (Bell); *c*, in children loss of foot processes and thickening of the basement membranes (Farquhar and associates) and *d*, in adults deposit of protein between the basement membrane and epithelium. (Movat and McGregor courtesy of Am. J. Clin. Path.)

gammaglobulinemia, caused by massive proteinuria, or they succumb to renal insufficiency. In adults the nephrotic syndrome is merely a stage in the relentless progressive course of chronic glomerulonephritis. To restate the question asked above: Are these two conditions separate entities, or are they manifestations of the same process modified to a marked degree by the age of the patient? The former may be called the dualistic, the latter the unitary concept.

The *clinical picture of nephrosis*, in other words the *nephrotic syndrome*, is based on a *massive albuminuria* with resulting *hypoproteinemia* of sufficient intensity to cause *edema*. *It is a syndrome with many causes, not a disease.* In a series of 98 cases of nephrosis in which percutaneous needle biopsy was done, Kark found the following examples of increased glomerular permeability to protein: 46 cases of glomerulonephritis, 18 of systemic lupus erythematosus, 15 of the glomerular lesions of diabetes mellitus, 11 of "pure" lipoid nephrosis, 3 of renal amyloidosis, and 4 of increased renal vein pressure. Percutaneous renal biopsy has indeed become one of the useful methods of investigation, especially if combined with dissection of nephrons and electron microscopy. *Edema* is the presenting symptom. As a result of the reduced colloid osmotic pressure attendant on the hypoproteinemia, water and salt pass into the interstitial tissue spaces. *Proteinuria* may arise in two ways: (1) *increased glomerular filtration* caused by damage to the capillary basement membrane; (2) *reduced tubular reabsorption* of protein. These two, of course, are not mutually exclusive. The loss of protein due to failure of tubular reabsorption may add up to a large amount when extended over days, months and even years. It is well known that when the tubules are poisoned with heavy metals, marked proteinuria is one result. The blood pattern as shown by paper chromatography is characteristic and indeed unique. The albumin is markedly decreased, and the gamma globulin is absent, both having passed into the urine. Alpha₂ globulin, on the other hand, is tremendously increased in the blood, but does not appear in the urine. *All depends on the molecular weight of the fractions, i.e.* the size of the molecules and their relation to the glomerular pores (Hardwicke). The albumin and gamma globulin molecules are small and pass readily, whereas those of alpha₂ globulin are large and are retained in the blood.

It must not be assumed that all the water and salt retention is due to the reduced colloid osmotic pressure caused by the hypoproteinemia. The extent of the edema, which in defiance of gravity appears first in the most distensible tissues such as the eyelids and external genitalia, bears no constant relation to the level of plasma protein nor the degree of albuminuria. The reduction in the circulating plasma volume may cause an increased secretion of aldosterone, and in consequence an increased tubular reabsorption of sodium with farther accumulation of interstitial fluid. In this way a vicious circle may be established. The urine of nephrotic children shows high sodium-retaining activity due to the presence of a sodium-retaining material which is similar to, if not identical with, aldosterone, the most powerful of the salt-retaining corticoids (Luetscher and Johnson). The most useful drugs in the treatment of nephrosis are the steroid hormones, both for their direct action on the glomeruli, and their indirect action whereby the secretions of the adrenals are suppressed. The return of the glomerular epithelial cells toward normal as the result of prednisone therapy has been observed in serial renal needle biopsies.

Nephrotic children and to a lesser extent adults have a *greatly lowered resistance to infection,* and are liable to succumb to peritonitis due to pneumococci, streptococci or E. coli. This lowered resistance is probably related to the loss of gamma globulin through the damaged glomerular filter giving a hypogammaglobulinemia, although the loss of plasma albumin is greater than the loss of globulin, a loss which may bring about a reversal of the normal albumin-globulin ratio in the blood.

The *basal metabolic rate* is low, and this seems to be due to deficiency in thyroxine caused by the loss of protein-bound iodine in the urine. *Anemia* is a characteristic symptom, and this is attributed to the loss of iron-binding proteins such as transferrin, with resulting low serum iron.

Amyloid Nephrosis.—Renal amyloidosis is considered briefly in this place, because it is likely to give a clinical picture of the nephrotic syndrome. Amyloid disease used to be nearly always secondary to tissue destruction with marked protein loss such as occurs in pulmonary tuberculosis and chronic suppuration. As the result of chemotherapy such destructive lesions are seldom seen at the present time, and many cases are of the so-called primary type without any very obvious cause, and are therefore labelled as idiopathic.

The kidneys are large and pale, and may closely resemble the "large white kidney" of subacute glomerulonephritis or nephrosis. But they are of firm consistence, and the cut surface has the characteristic translucent or waxy appearance of amyloid organs. When the iodine test is used the affected glomeruli stand out as dark-brown dots on the cut surface. If the progress of the disease is slow and the patient does not die of the original suppurative lesion, the kidneys may become contracted and granular.

Microscopically the amyloid is deposited in the glomeruli as well as in the arterioles and around the collecting tubules. The most striking lesions are in the glomeruli (Fig. 316). The deposit of amyloid is supposed to be limited to the region between the basement membrane of the loop and the vascular endothelium, but the electron microscope shows the material to be deposited on either side of the *intact* membrane, between the epithelium and the membrane as well as between the endothelium and the membrane. The epithelium is vacuolated and the foot processes are flattened or lost (Movat). Some of the loops remain open for a long time, and through these damaged loops large quantities of albumin escape into the urine. In time the glomeruli are converted into large bloodless structureless masses of amyloid. When the glomerulus is occluded the corresponding tubule undergoes atrophy and is replaced by fibrous tissue. In this way marked tubular atrophy, fibrosis, and shrinking of the kidney may occur. In the earlier stages the tubules show marked evidence of degeneration, and the epithelium is filled with fatty and hyaline droplets and may contain cholesterol ester. Large homo-

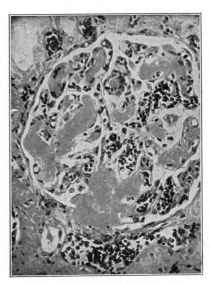

Fig. 316.—Amyloid disease of the kidney. The glomerulus is greatly enlarged by the amyloid, but the presence of blood cells (black) shows that the circulation is still going on. × 275.

geneous casts are formed in the tubules, and in the urine they are known as "colloid" casts. Much of the atrophy of the parenchyma is due not only to ischemia from glomerular atrophy but to pressure from the amyloid which gradually accumulates in the arteries and in the connective tissue around the tubules.

The *symptoms* are *nephrotic* in type, *i.e.*, massive albuminuria and edema, but if the patient lives long enough he may die of *uremia* with high non-protein nitrogen in the blood and hypertension. The nephrotic symptoms are based on hyperpermeable and still patent glomerular capillaries, while the terminal nephritic picture is that of the contracted ischemic kidney. Amyloid disease may last for many years. If the underlying cause can be arrested, the amyloid disease may also cease to progress and even retrogress. Experimental evidence shows that amyloid material may become absorbed, and perhaps this may occur in man.

Diabetic Glomerulosclerosis.—A peculiar and distinctive degenerative glomerular lesion was described in 1936 by Kimmelstiel and Wilson as *intercapillary glomerulosclerosis* occurring in long-standing cases of diabetes

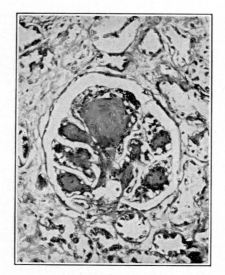

FIG. 317.—Intercapillary glomerulosclerosis.
× 120.

often associateed with hypertension, particularly in persons over forty years of age. Three forms have been described, the nodular, the diffuse and the exudative. The *nodular* form, which is the true *Kimmelstiel-Wilson lesion*, is specific for diabetes, but is found in less than a third of the cases. It is the most reliable criterion for the histological diagnosis of diabetes in persons over the age of forty. It must be borne in mind that clinical evidence of diabetes may disappear with the onset of the intercapillary sclerosis and the development of renal failure, so that the glomerular lesion may be found in those who are apparently not diabetic. A fact of interest is that the diabetes of hemochromatosis is not associated with the Kimmelstiel-Wilson lesion. In 62 examples of this condition Lonergan and Robbins found no case which showed nodular intercapillary glomerulosclerosis, although some of the cases had had diabetes for many years. Others have encountered both nodular and diffuse lesions in similar cases of long standing (Becker and Miller).

The nodular lesion is a localized exaggeration of the diffuse form. In the center of the tuft or in the center of one of the lobules, there is a sharply localized hyaline mass rather suggestive of amyloid (Fig. 317). This used to be regarded as a broadening of the intercapillary connective tissue, as indicated by the original name. Then opinion switched to a primary splitting of the capillary basement membrane (Bell). Examination of renal biopsy material with the electron microscope serves to confirm this opinion, showing fibrillation and great thickening of the basement membrane, accompanied by precipitation of a hyaline material in the cytoplasm of the glomerular endothelial cells (Bergstrand and Bucht) (Fig. 318). The thickening of the basement membrane corresponds to the diffuse lesions, while the enlargement of the endothelial hyaline deposits is responsible for the nodular lesions. Some workers believe that the hyaline deposits are extra cellular products of the glomerular endothelium lying between rather than in the endothelial cells (Farquhar *et al.*). The material appears to be a mucopolysaccharide with a low protein and a high carbohydrate content, which gives a strongly positive reaction with the periodic acid-Schiff stain, and is believed to be deposited from the blood in the glomerular intercapillary space (McManus).

Hartroft suggests from evidence he has obtained both in the experimental animai and in the human diabetic that fat emboll plugging the glomerular tufts may cause exudation of plasma into and between the capillary walls with the formation of fibrin and eventually the true Kimmelstiel-Wilson lesion. It is conceivable, therefore, that a chronic form of intermittent fat embolism from fat deposits in the liver may be related to the glomerular lesions in diabetes. It is evident that similar lesions due to fat emboli might occur apart from diabetes, and this idea is supported by the observations of Raphael and Lynch, who found identical lesions in necrotizing pancreatitis and in alcoholic fatty infiltration of the liver.

The *diffuse* form is non-specific for diabetes. It is a deposition of fibrillary and homogeneous hyaline material extending from the glomerular hilus to the periphery. We have already seen that it represents a generalized thickening of the glomerular basement membranes.

In addition to the classical Kimmelstiel-Wilson lesions, other glomerular changes, which may be called *exudative lesions*, are

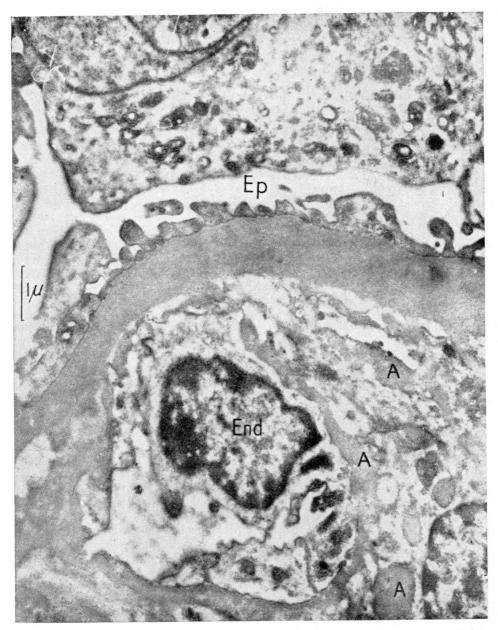

Fig. 318.—Intercapillary glomerulosclerosis. Detail of capillary wall. In the cytoplasm of the endo-thelial cell hyaline masses (A) are visible. Some of these are included in the cell cytoplasm and others are connected to the basement membrane proper. The foot processes (pedicles) are distinctly visible in the epithelial cell (EP) above. (Bergstrand and Bucht, courtesy of Jour. Path. & Bact.)

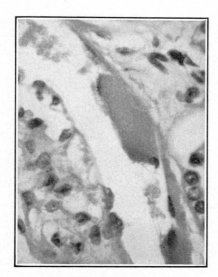

FIG. 319.—Capsular drop.

found in diabetics. Two of these are well illustrated in a paper by Barrie, Askanazy and Smith. The first they call the *fibrin cap*, a deposit of material giving the staining reactions for fibrin between the basement membrane and the tuft. The second they term the *capsular drop* (described in Kimmelstiel and Wilson's original paper), which is a drop-like formation of lipo-carbohydrate-protein beneath the parietal layer of epithelium (Fig. 319). It seems probable that fibrinogen and lipids escape from the diabetic blood and form these lesions. It should be emphasized that the renal lesions just described are not individually specific for diabetes, but a combination of two or more of these features are highly suggestive that diabetes was present.

Severe atheroma of the larger renal and intrarenal arteries is highly characteristic of diabetes. Indeed Hall believes that without these arterial lesions the glomerulosclerosis may be without clinical manifestations.

The *clinical picture* is likely to be nephrotic in type with *massive albuminuria* and *marked edema*; in mild cases there are no renal symptoms. A characteristic feature is the presence of *lipoid* or *fatty cells and casts in the urine*. They form a striking picture under the polarizing microscope, but are readily detected with ordinary light, and should at once suggest an investigation for diabetes.

Hypertension is usually present, but whether as cause or effect is uncertain. *Retinal microaneurysms* are of common occurrence, and these may lead to blindness. Although only recognized in 1936, diabetic glomerulosclerosis is now known to be more important numerically than chronic glomerulonephritis, and carries a constant threat to the diabetic of renal failure, hypertension, and blindness.

Wire-loop Glomerulonephrosis.—This is a renal manifestation of disseminated lupus erythematosus. There is a patchy thickening of the glomerular capillary membrane with the occasional development of a nephrotic picture. It has already been discussed in relation to disseminated lupus.

Renal Vein Thrombosis.—Thrombosis of the renal vein may give rise either to the nephrotic syndrome or to an acute picture with severe pain in the loins, hematuria, fever and leukocytosis. The thrombosis may extend from the vena cava, or it may be secondary to renal disease such as pyelonephritis and amyloidosis, and in rare cases it may be primary (Harrison). Sudden thrombosis will result in fatal uremia, but if the obstruction of the vein is gradual and there is time for the establishment of a collateral circulation a clinical picture of nephrosis develops, with very early proteinuria, and edema most marked in the legs and feet. The condition may be unilateral or bilateral. Bilateral renal vein thrombosis is generally secondary to renal disease, except in young children.

Serial needle biopsies of the kidney show the glomerular basement membrane to be thickened, whilst the tubules become progressively atrophied (Pollak, Kark *et al.*). The damage to the tubules is quite out of proportion to the glomerular damage, and is attributed to the rise of intrarenal pressure which accompanies the rise of pressure in the renal vein. Protein escapes through the weakened glomeruli and is not absorbed by the grossly damaged tubules, with the development of massive proteinuria and the nephrotic syndrome.

Nephrosis of Pregnancy.—*Eclampsia* is a complication of the latter part of pregnancy characterized by the *nephrotic syndrome combined with hypertension and convulsions*. In the absence of convulsions, which are probably secondary to the hypertension, the

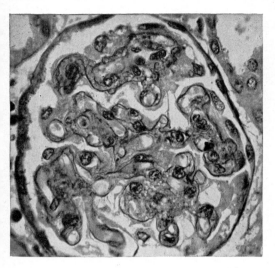

Fig. 320.—The glomerulus in eclampsia, with narrowing of the capillaries and general thickening of their walls, due primarily to reticulation and vacuolation of the intercapillary area. PAS with hematoxylin. (Kindness of Dr. J. A. McManus.)

condition is called preeclampsia or the toxemia of pregnancy. The general aspects of the subject are discussed in Chapter 33. Renal lesions are present in every case. These represent a true glomerulonephrosis. Even in hematoxylin and eosin sections the glomeruli are seen to present a peculiarly solid appearance, with great narrowing or actual occlusion of the tuft. There may be some swelling of capillary endothelium, but connective tissue stains show that the essential lesion is a thickening of the capillary basement membrane, said to be associated with thickening of the mesangium and widening of the intercapillary space, which becomes reticulated or vacuolated, at first by edema, so extreme in degree that a diagnosis of toxemia of pregnancy can be made from the renal picture (Govan) (Fig. 320). It will be realized that this lesion is similar in kind to that seen in lipoid nephrosis with the addition of narrowing or occlusion of the capillaries. The clinical picture is also that of the nephrotic syndrome with the all-important addition of arterial hypertension. The hypertension of toxemia usually disappears after delivery and removal of the placenta. This suggests that some hormonal pressor substance acting on the arteries is

37

produced by the placenta. The permanent hypertension which sometimes develops may be due to glomerular ischemia. In very rare cases there is the condition known as symmetrical necrosis of the renal cortex (see p. 603), in which complete cortical necrosis of both kidneys is associated with thrombosis of the small renal vessels with resulting uremia.

DISEASES OF THE TUBULES

Acute Tubular Nephroses.—Now we pass from conditions in which the primary and important lesion is a change, either inflammatory or degenerative, in the glomeruli to those in which the essential lesion is a degeneration, sometimes a frank necrosis, of the convoluted tubules. To these lesions the pathologist has attached the old name of nephrosis, which includes the so-called lower nephron nephrosis, while the clinician has appropriated the term chronic nephrosis to describe a clinical condition which is now known to be glomerular in origin. As Oliver remarks, nephrosis with its various connotations has become all things to all men. The situation reminds one of *Alice in Through the Looking Glass*, "When I use a word," Humpty-Dumpty said, in rather a scornful tone, "it means just what I choose it to mean—neither more nor less." "The question is," said Alice, "whether you *can* make words mean so many different things."

The most important function of the kidneys is to maintain a normal and constant internal environment. In performing this function selective absorption by the tubules is as essential as excretion by the glomeruli. Damage to the tubules such as occurs in tubular nephrosis must interfere with this function, but the most striking result is oliguria or anuria. These cases of anuria may be divided as regards causation into two groups: (1) a large and important group in which the pathogenesis is uncertain, but which is probably anoxic or ischemic in nature; (2) a smaller and simpler group due to exogenous poisons such as mercuric chloride. These two groups may be termed anoxic nephrosis and toxic nephrosis. These conditions are often referred to as *anoxic (ischemic) tubular necrosis* and *toxic tubular necrosis*, but this is inaccurate and misleading, because the lesions are in essence a degeneration which does not necessarily proceed to necrosis.

Anoxic Nephrosis.—Oliguria and anuria associated with tubular degeneration may develop in a bewildering variety of extrarenal conditions. Examples of such conditions are shock, burns, trauma, severe hemorrhage, the crush syndrome, intestinal obstruction, dehydration, incompatible blood transfusion and blackwater fever. This group may be subdivided into (*a*) those cases which may be confidently attributed to renal ischemia, and which have been called the "shock kidney," and (*b*) cases of uncertain and mixed etiology where both ischemia and toxic factors may play a part, *e.g.* the crush syndrome, incompatible blood transfusion, *etc*. The same pathological changes are present in both, so that no attempt will be made to differentiate them.

The *clinical picture* is striking and characteristic. The primary injury (and the same is true of the ingestion of a chemical poison) is followed by a brief initial period during which all seems to be well. There is then a rapid decrease in the excretion of urine, leading to *extreme oliguria* or even complete *anuria*. The kidneys have gone on strike. *Azotemia* soon develops, and within a week the full-fledged picture of uremia is evident, usually terminating in death. If recovery occurs it is heralded by marked diuresis, often sudden in onset with limitation of tubular function. The early danger is oliguria and uremia, but a *late danger* is *diuresis* with *excessive loss of electrolytes*. The structural and functional recovery of the tubules may take many weeks, during which time the immature regenerating epithelium is lacking in mitochondrial rodlets and the all-important enzymes which they contain. Loss of function of the proximal tubules is indicated by inability to concentrate urea and creatinine. *Electrolyte imbalance* is constantly associated with acute tubular degeneration. *Renal failure* becomes evident when interference with function is so great that the internal environment can no longer be maintained within normal limits. This upset may be reversible or irreversible. A *rise in serum potassium* is of

particular significance, because it may poison the myocardium, leading to death from cardiac failure. We have already seen that dangerous electrolyte loss may occur as the result of diuresis during recovery. As regard *prognosis*, in the ischemic type it is the number of damaged nephrons that count, whereas in the toxic cases it is the severity of the lesions. Both types of damage interfere with cellular respiration.

Traumatic tubular nephrosis or *necrosis* is the commonest cause of acute oliguric renal failure. In war time it is naturally due to wounds, but in civil life it is caused by accidents or severe surgical procedures. The prognosis is very much worse in traumatic tubular necrosis, where in some series the mortality has been as high as 70 per cent, than in the toxic variety, where the blood urea can be kept within safe limits by hemodialysis with the artificial kidney, a life-saving procedure during the period of complete anuria.

Lesions.—The kidneys are enlarged, the cortex pale from ischemia and swollen, and the medulla dark and engorged. The principal microscopic lesions are degeneration and necrosis of the tubules. For years a rather furious controversy has raged among pathologists as to the exact site of these tubular lesions. Large numbers of fatal cases of what Mallory called *hemoglobinuric nephrosis* following severe injury from wounds in the Second World War showed lesions in what appeared to be the distal part of the convoluted tubule and the loop of Henle, and the condition was therefore named *lower nephron nephrosis* (Lucké). This term, more euphonious than accurate, was taken up with remarkable enthusiasm by the clinician who was attracted by the pleasant sound and the suggestion of pin-pointing the lesion, but with much more reservation by the pathologist. The essential feature of acute renal failure is the nature of the lesion, not its location. In ischemia tubular nephrosis the lesions are scattered at random among the nephrons and may be found in any part of the nephron, whereas in toxic nephrosis the lesions involve every nephron, but are limited to the proximal tubules, because it is these which are functionally concerned with handling the poison. In ordinary hospital

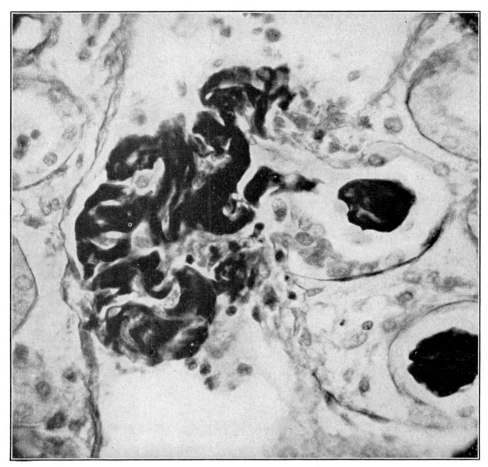

FIG. 321A.—Tubulovenous thrombosis. This photomicrograph shows the fashion in which the venous thrombi are produced. There is a rupture of a hyaline cast through a thin wall of the vein. The thrombus is laid down on top of this. (McManus, *Medical Diseases of the Kidney.*)

material where death has not occurred for a number of days the proximal and distal convoluted tubules may be equally involved, and indeed the changes may be more pronounced in the former. When the lesions are advanced it may not be possible to distinguish between the two sets of tubules. The lining epithelium is greatly swollen and undergoes complete necrosis. Between the tubules there are collections of inflammatory cells, mainly lymphocytes and plasma cells, with occasional polymorphonuclears and eosinophils.

The most characteristic lesion is a disruptive one known as *tubulorhexis*. It is best revealed by microdissection (Oliver *et al.*), which shows a solution of continuity of the wall of the tubule due to disruption of the basement membrane and disintegration of the epithelium, so that the lumen lies open to the intertubular tissue and its veins. With rupture of the necrotic tubules their contents become extruded, and a granulomatous type of reaction may develop around them. At this stage the inflammatory and reactive changes may dominate the picture, although these are entirely secondary. Intertubular edema is often a marked and important feature, especially in the boundary zone. Sometimes *tubulo-venous lesions* may be seen, due to herniation or actual rupture of the tubular contents into a vein with occasional thrombosis (Fig. 321A), so that blood may pass into the tubules with result-

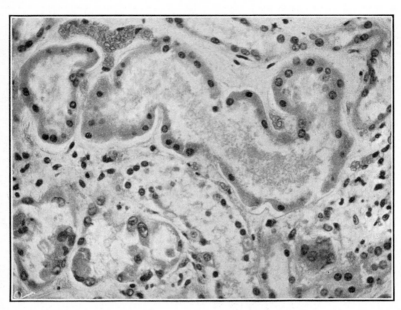

Fig. 321B.—Nephrotic degeneration of renal tubules. × 300. (Boyd, *Pathology for the Physician.*)

ing *hematuria. Casts* are a prominent feature, especially in the boundary zone and medulla. At first these are non-pigmented, but with the passage of time they acquire blood pigment, so that the condition has been given the misleading name of *pigment nephrosis.* In the crush syndrome the pigment is myohemoglobin. The casts may become overgrown by epithelium, or they may be extruded into the intertubular tissue where they excite a further inflammatory reaction. The condition of the first convoluted tubules varies. The lumen may be filled and lined by flattened epithelium (Fig. 321B). This striking dilatation suggests distension of the lumen by urinary secretion which has been unable to pass a barrier in the boundrary zone, where the tubules seem to be reduced in number owing to collapse of their walls. The vasa recta of the medulla are greatly congested and dilated, giving an impression of complete stagnation. In contrast to the devastation of the tubules, the glomeruli appear normal.

The above account reflects the popular view at the present time, namely that the acute renal failure of traumatic uremia indicated by the oliguria, azotemia, and disturbance in electrolytes, is due to the tubular lesions. That is only natural, but we must remember that association does not prove causality. The tubular concept is now being challenged (Sevitt). It is pointed out that there is a non-oliguric as well as an oliguric form, although it is naturally more readily overlooked. Azotemia may become marked in both forms, with a severe fall in the urea and creatinine clearance. Moreover traumatic uremia may occur without tubular necrosis. It is now stated that disturbance of glomerular function is primarily responsible for the clinical picture. The oliguria is explained by the low glomerular filtration rate, due in turn to renal ischemia caused by vasoconstriction of the renal vessels. "The rate of urine flow is determined by the balance between the reduced glomerular filtration rate and the reduced tubular reabsorption of water. Oliguria occurs when the decreased reabsorption is insufficient to balance the fall in the glomerular filtration rate, but, when a balance has been achieved, the flow of urine is adequate" (Sevitt).

The heart and lungs deserve mention. The *heart* is soft and flabby, perhaps as the result of potassium poisoning. The *lungs* are heavy and edematous because of the heart failure. The danger of increasing the

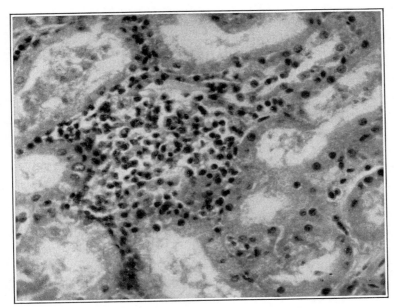

Fig. 322.—Sulfonamide nephritis. Note the focal interstitial nephritis and marked degeneration of tubular epithelium. × 240.

pulmonary edema by over-treatment with fluids in the vain hope of "washing out the kidneys" is self-evident.

The Crush Syndrome.—So-called crush nephrosis or nephritis, the *shock kidney*, the classic example of the ischemic type, occurring in persons buried under masonry and sustaining injuries to muscles as the result of air raids, was responsible for attracting attention to the relation between tubular necrosis and acute renal failure (Bywaters and Dible). The patient might appear in good condition when extricated, but in a few days time an ominous anuria developed, followed shortly by fatal uremia. It has been said that the commonest cause of acute renal failure is the crush or shock kidney. There is a characteristic patchy loss of alkaline phosphatase in the outer part of the cortex, not in the juxta-glomerular portion (McManus and Mowry).

Transfusion with Incompatible Blood.—This also belongs to the anoxic type of nephrosis. When a donor of the wrong group is used for blood transfusion, the patient shows marked hemoglobinuria, and may develop anuria and die of uremia. Hematin casts are found in the renal tubules, apparently depending on acidity of the urine. The presence of blood pigment casts in the tubules is valuable evidence that the blood used in the transfusion was incompatible.

Sulfonamide Poisoning.—Although generally referred to as sulfonamide nephritis, this is really a nephrosis. Again death is due to anuria and renal failure. In many cases this is due to a state of natural or induced hypersensitivity to the drug (Rich). The general subject of sulfonamide allergy is discussed in Chapter 5. The two striking renal lesions are a nephrotic degeneration of the epithelium of the convoluted tubules and a focal interstitial nephritis (Fig. 322). The anuria may be attributed to the tubular lesions, which are similar to those seen in incompatible blood transfusion and the crush syndrome. It is from the interstitial lesion that the pathological diagnosis can be made. There are small areas of focal necrosis, associated with which are collections of inflammatory cells, chiefly macrophages, plasma cells, and often large numbers of eosinophils, the latter always suggestive of an allergic lesion.

The Hepatorenal Syndrome.—This rather

nebulous entity is marked by necrotic cells both in the liver and kidney. There is tubular necrosis with bile staining of the necrotic cells, and focal areas of necrosis in the liver. The condition may develop as the result of crush injuries to the liver and operations on the gall bladder, or in cases of obstructive jaundice which have been subjected to severe abdominal operations. The toxic action of the bile may intensify the necrosis. In the kidney there is a striking absence of the interstitial inflammatory reaction so characteristic of true nephrosis.

Crowson and More point out that there is a close correlation between renal necrosis and such structural changes in the liver as necrosis and cirrhosis of varying degree, and they suggest that vasodepressor substances which are normally removed by the liver may accumulate in the blood during hepatic insufficiency and produce renal ischemia with resulting tubular degeneration and necrosis.

Pathogenesis of Anoxic Nephrosis.—The mechanism by which the lesions and the anuria are produced has long been a matter of debate. There seem to be good grounds for believing that the most constant etiological factor is diminution of the renal circulation. For this reason the name of *renal anoxia* has been suggested for the entire group (Maegraith *et al.*). When one kidney in the rabbit is removed and the renal artery of the remaining kidney is partially occluded temporarily, changes similar to those of human traumatic uremia are produced (Badenoch and Darmady). The first lesions occur in the loop of Henle, the part of the nephron which is the last to be supplied with blood and therefore most vulnerable to anoxia. Trueta and his associates have suggested that in shock and allied conditions the large efferent arterioles leading into the medulla from the juxtamedullary glomeruli can divert blood from the cortex and thus produce cortical ischemia. The evidence of this supposed "shunt" was derived from radiography and the injection of dyes into rabbits. Studies comparing renal blood flow with the volume of glomerular filtrate fail to confirm this theory of circulatory diversion, and no evidence has been brought forward to prove that it occurs in man. It is possible that a venous reflux by which the large veins in the medulla become filled may account for the appearance which has been attributed to a shunt.

There can be no question that the renal arteries respond to nervous and possibly hormonal stimuli by vasoconstriction. Reflex anuria, *i.e.*, the complete cessation of urinary output from both kidneys which follows obstruction of one ureter by a calculus, must be attributed to reflex vascular changes in the other kidney. The same mechanism operates in the shock kidney, the crush syndrome, and apparently in incompatible blood transfusion. The resulting renal ischemia causes necrosis in the tubules farthest removed from the blood supply. From this point onward the key concept, the master word, is increased intrarenal pressure, particularly in the boundary zone. A barrier or road block is built up across the base of each pyramid which obstructs both the tubules and the thin-walled vessels in the medulla. The chief elements in this block are (1) the interstitial edema due to leakage both from the tubules and blood vessels, (2) the inflammatory exudate which is excited in part by tubular rupture, (3) obstruction of the tubules by swollen epithelium, cellular débris and casts, and, as Barrie points out, (4) spasm of the calyceal muscle and its intrinsic component. Any obstruction increases the exudate from the ruptured tubules, and the exudate in turn still farther increases the intrarenal pressure. Thus a vicious circle is established. The most easily recognized sign of raised intrarenal pressure is the presence of the so-called tubulovenous thromboses (Barrie, personal communication). These are really herniations of renal substance into the veins, sometimes with secondary thrombosis. The dilated proximal tubules, the stasis of the vasa recta and to some extent the anuria may be attributed to the block in which raised intrarenal pressure is so important a factor.

It would be a mistake to think that the whole problem has been solved by the above discussion. The most baffling feature is the anuria, which may develop immediately after an incompatible blood transfusion and be accompanied by sudden pain in the loin. In such a case is the mechanism glomerular or tubular? If the patient dies in a very early

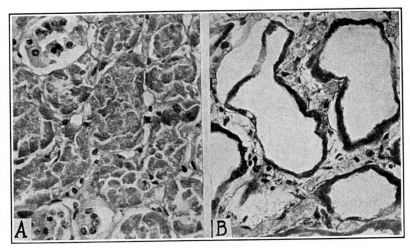

FIG. 323.—Mercuric chloride poisoning. *A*, early; *B*, late. × 250.

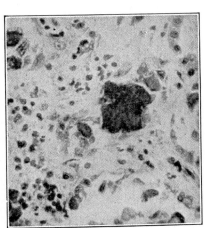

FIG. 324.—Mercuric chloride poisoning. Acute calcification of the epithelium of the renal tubules. The two dark masses represent calcified cells. × 300.

stage there may be no visible tubular degeneration nor intertubular exudate. The same is true in experimental ischemia earlier than the second day. It may be that there is an initial and transient glomerular shut down, or some humoral mechanism such as the pituitary antidiuretic hormone may allow fluid to pass through the walls of the tubules and be absorbed without any observable lesion in the tubular walls.

Toxic Nephrosis.—Here the problem is much simpler. An exogenous poison such as *mercuric chloride* (vaginal douching, at-

tempted suicide) or *carbon tetrachloride* is excreted by the kidney, concentrated in the tubules owing to reabsorption of water, and causes massive necrosis, most marked in the proximal convoluted tubule, the first part to encounter the concentrated poison. Anuria rapidly develops, the non-protein nitrogen in the blood rises, and death may occur from uremia. If the patient does not die at this stage the anuria is followed by diuresis, the first urine being of low specific gravity. When death take place after two or three days there is seen to be extensive necrosis of the tubular epithelium, the necrotic cells becoming detached and blocking the lumen of the tubules, thus accounting for the anuria (Fig. 323A). Acute calcification of the necrotic cells occurring in the course of a few days is not uncommon (Fig. 324). There is none of the tubulorhexis with extrusion of the contents of the tubules into the interstitial tissue and granulomatous reaction which is often so striking a feature of the necrotic lesions of anoxic nephrosis. By the end of a week the tubules may be clear, yet the anuria persists. Apparently the glomerular filtrate escapes back through the bare walls of the tubules into the interstitial tissue, so that none of it reaches the bladder. This mechanism can be watched in the living kidney of the frog poisoned with mercuric chloride. After the first week the tubules become relined with low, darkly-staining epithelium which is of little use for absorbing water and concentrating the urine (Fig. 323B). The new epithelium gradually develops into a fully formed and functioning lining of the tubules.

VACUOLAR NEPHROPATHY.—This indefinite term is a convenient description for the presence of clear well-defined vacuoles in the convoluted tubules, which may balloon out the cells and displace the nucleus to the base of the cell. They do not stain for either fat or glycogen, and may be presumed to be watery in character, a form of hydropic degeneration. Such vacuoles are seen after the intravenous administration of large quantities of glucose and particularly sucrose. A striking degree of vacuolization has been observed in chronic intestinal disease, more especially ulcerative colitis (Kulka et al.). Here the condition may be related to deficiency in potassium or other electrolytes.

GLYCOGEN DEPOSITS.—These occur in von Gierke's disease and also in severe cases of diabetes mellitus, although they are more rarely seen since the introduction of insulin. In diabetes the cells chiefly affected are those lining the loop of Henle. The affected cells are large and perfectly clear owing to the glycogen being dissolved out, so that the tubule has a very striking and characteristic appearance. It is probable that the glycogen is derived from the sugar in the urine.

Pigment Deposits.—*Blood pigment* may accumulate in the cells of the convoluted tubules when there is much blood destruction and the hemoglobin passes through the glomeruli and is concentrated in the tubules. This is well seen in pernicious anemia and paroxysmal hemoglobinuria. The granules of hemosiderin gives the Prussian blue reaction for iron. Casts of hematin granules are seen in the tubules as the result of hemoglobinuria from unsuitable blood transfusion. *Bile pigment* may accumulate as fine granules in the cells of the convoluted tubules in persistent jaundice. In severe cases of jaundice of the new-born the pigment may be deposited in the apices of the pyramids, a condition known as *bilirubin infarcts*. A much commoner condition seen in new-born children is *uric acid infarcts*. They take the form of yellow streaks at the apices of the pyramids, and consist of deposits of urates in the collecting tubules. It is probable that they soon disappear. When melanin is excreted it appears in the cells of the loop of Henle.

DISEASES OF THE INTERSTITIAL TISSUE

So far we have been considering diseases of the nephron involving primarily either the glomeruli or the tubules. We now come to conditions in which the lesions are primarily in the interstitial tissue, although sooner or later the nephrons will naturally be involved.

Acute Diffuse Interstitial Nephritis.—This rare condition occurs as a complication of the acute infectious fevers, especially scarlet fever and diphtheria. There is an acute diffuse inflammation of the interstitial tissue which is packed with lymphocytes, plasma cells, and a few polymorphonuclears. Yet the glomeruli and tubules remain intact. Kimmelstiel believes that the condition represents an allergic reaction to foreign proteins rather than a bacterial infection. As the glomeruli and tubules are not invaded there is no renal insufficiency so that the cases seldom come to autopsy. The urine merely shows a little albumin and a few lymphocytes and red blood cells.

Pyelonephritis.—Pyelonephritis, a localized as opposed to a diffuse inflammation, is the commonest form of renal disease, but it usually passes unrecognized. Less than 1 in 5 cases are diagnosed correctly before death (Schreiner). One of the reasons for this is that the disease is one of the great imitators, and it may manifest itself in different ways. It may be acute, chronic or healed; it may be bilateral or unilateral (rarely); it may be secondary to some obvious infection or it may be apparently primary. It is the most frequent cause of death from uremia. In the experience of Brod of Prague, whose paper should be consulted, fatal uremia occurred in 36 per cent of cases of chronic pyelonephritis, but in only 19 per cent of glomerulonephritis and 14 per cent of arteriolar nephrosclerosis. The disease which used to be regarded as the province of the urologist but is now very much the concern of the internist, is unique in renal disorders in that it may last for several decades, even as long as thirty or forty years. A long history of renal disease should at once suggest the possibility of chronic pyelonephritis.

Etiology and Pathogenesis.—Acute pyelonephritis is a focal suppurative inflammation of the interstitial tissue of the kidney and renal pelvis. A better name would be focal interstitial nephritis without any reference to the renal pelvis. The acute process usually clears up, but it may become chronic with acute exacerbations, the result being a gradual nibbling away of the kidney. By far the commonest invading organism is E. coli, which is present in about 50 per cent of cases. In other cases Aerobacter aerogenes, Proteus vulgaris, Pseudomonas pyocyaneus, coagulase-positive staphylococci, hemolytic streptococci, and enterococci may be responsible. Aerobactor aerogenes is coming to assume particular importance in infections of the lower urinary tract because of the development of antibiotic-resistant hospital strains as the result of quick mutation. But the problem is: How do the bacteria reach the kidney? There are two possibilities: (1) they may ascend from below, seeing that the lower urinary tract communicates with the exterior; (2) the infection may be hematogenous. Hot controversy has enveloped this question, but on calmer thought it is obvious that both methods of access are possible. Diabetes is a common predisposing factor, possibly on account of the high sugar content of the urine.

In autopsy material the obstructive form is 12 times as common as the non-obstructive (Bell). Low obstruction (below the bladder) is more important than high obstruction (above the bladder). An ascending infection is particularly common in infancy, pregnancy, and over the age of fifty years due to prostatic enlargement in men and cancer of the cervix as well as uterine prolapse in women. In children the ascending infection is commoner in girls, coming from the vagina, while in boys the cause is congenital anomalies, as yet undiscovered, of the lower urinary tract. In pregnancy there is dilatation of the ureters, as well as pressure on the ureters where they pass over the pelvic brim. More attention must be paid to the ureter than has been done in the past (Talbot). The ureter is not an inert tube, but an active muscular structure. Previous parenchymatous damage or ureteral obstruction may affect the wall of the tube and facilitate ascending infection. The subepithelial tissues of the bladder, ureter and renal pelvis provide a direct route of invasion which is continuous with the interstitial tissue of the kidney. Mechanical obstruction is an obvious factor in ascending infection, but *functional* obstruction may develop

as the result of inflammatory changes, obstruction which may not be obvious to the naked eye, but which can be inferred from serial x-ray studies. In acute cases the ureter is continuously infected from the site of obstruction up to the kidney.

The element of obstruction is of the greatest importance in determining the outcome. G. K. Mallory and his co-workers showed this by injecting colon bacilli intravenously into rabbits in which one ureter had been partially ligated; acute pyelonephritis developed in the obstructed kidney in 75 per cent of the animals, but never in the unobstructed kidney. Release of the obstruction after a few days induced healing of the pyelonephritic process. In man the question of whether a blood infection will cause unilateral or bilateral renal lesions is probably largely dependent on the presence or absence of obstruction. In ascending infection some element of obstruction in the urinary tract is likely to be present from the beginning. The lymphatics from the kidney drain directly into the thoracic duct, often with no intervening lymph nodes, so that infective material may reach the blood stream in quantity and give rise to pyrexia and chills.

There are still a number of puzzling features about the bacteriology of pyelonephritis, in particular the difficulty of correlating the bacterial findings in the urine with the clinical picture. Pyelonephritis may or may not be associated with *significant bacteriuria* when the patient presents himself. It is true that acute pyelonephritis and acute exacerbations of chronic pyelonephritis are accompanied by abundant evidence of urinary infection, but significant bacteriuria may be lacking in spite of widespread parenchymatous damage. Correct thinking has been handicapped in the past by failure to distinguish between infection (significant bacteriuria) and contamination. It is now recognized that very erroneous conclusions may be drawn from the bacteriological examination of urine collected by catheter even under the most sterile conditions. The distal one or two centimeters of the urethra, both male and female, contain an abundant microflora, which are often drug-resistant, especially in hospitals where cross infection is so common. The tip of the catheter inevitably becomes infected, and the bacteria thus collected grow readily in the urine which forms an excellent culture medium, whether in the bladder or in a flask.

Quantitative urine culture represents a great forward step in the study of pyelonephritis. The number of bacteria present in a properly collected specimen is fully as important as identification of the type of organism. This is done by means of a clean midstream voiding technique (discarding the first and last portions), followed by high dilution (10^{-3}) with sterile saline, prompt inoculation of culture plates, and counting the resulting colonies. Significant bacteriuria is present when there are 100,000 bacteria per ml. of urine. Not infrequently there are 1,000,000 microorganisms. At least 50 per cent of patients with significant bacteriuria are without clinical symptoms; they have "asymptomatic bacteriuria." This does not mean that they do not have pyelonephritis, but rather that they have "inapparent pyelonephritis," which provides a missing link between the clinically apparent acute and chronic forms of the disease. The over-all incidence of asymptomatic bacteriuria rather closely approaches the frequency with which morphological evidence of pyelonephritis is seen in the postmortem room, which exceeds the incidence of the clinically evident disease by as much as 5 times. For further information on this important aspect of a common disease the reader is referred to the comprehensive review by Kleeman and his associates.

Lesions.—The *gross appearance* varies extremely with the stage of the disease. As a rule both kidneys are involved, but the lesions are often much less advanced in one than in the other. They may be focal or diffuse. In the *acute stage* the kidney is swollen and congested, and the pelvis is of a bright red color and filled with pus. Under the capsule there are numerous yellow spots representing areas of suppuration, as well as irregular patches which form the base of wedge-shaped areas in the renal substance. The superficial lesions are often raised above the surface as small pustules. If healing occurs later they are represented by depressed U-shaped scars. The cut surface

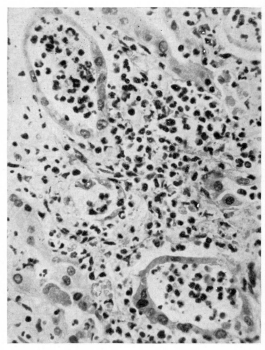

Fig. 325.—Acute pyelonephritis. Both the interstitial tissue and the tubules are filled with polymorphonuclear leukocytes. × 375.

shows patchy areas of suppuration which tend to be spherical in the cortex and linear in the pyramids. If suppuration is progressive, abscess cavities are formed with gradual destruction of renal tissue. The outline of the calyces is destroyed, and the resulting distortion seen in the x-ray film is an important feature in the clinical diagnosis.

The disease may develop in a more gradual and insidious manner with little frank suppuration. The inflammation, which is *subacute* or *chronic* in character, extends here and there in the kidney, destroying renal tissue, but being followed later by healing, fibrosis, and contraction. The result is a contracted kidney on the surface of which there are depressed scars. If these scars are of considerable size they are apt to be regarded as healed infarcts. When they are much smaller the effect is to give the kidney a granular appearance which may be hard to distinguish from that of chronic glomerulonephritis or arteriolar nephrosclerosis. This condition is called *pyelonephritic contracted*

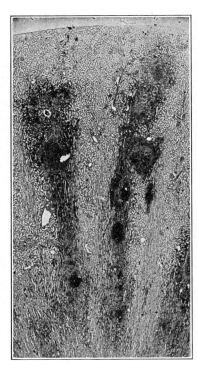

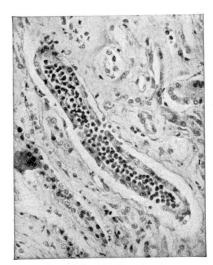

FIG. 327.—Pyelonephritis: pus cells in renal tubule. × 250. (Boyd, *Pathology for the Surgeon,* courtesy of W. B. Saunders Co.)

FIG. 326.—Pyelonephritis. The linear circumscribed lesions involve both cortex and medulla.

kidney, and in the past it has frequently been mistaken for the two diseases just mentioned. Chronic and healed pyelonephritis is a much commoner condition than used to be supposed. Weiss and Parker in their classic paper found it to be a more frequent cause of contracted kidney than glomerulonephritis. The surface of the kidney is finely granular in glomerulonephritis, more coarsely scarred in chronic pyelonephritis. The scars of nephrosclerosis are pale and on the cut surface are V-shaped like those of healed infarcts. The scars of pyelonephritis tend to be dark (due to vascularity) and saddle-shaped on the outer surface and U-shaped on the cut surface. In distinguishing between chronic pyelonephritis and other conditions with which it may be confused, attention should be paid to the renal pelvis (thickened), calyces, and ureter.

The *microscopic picture* varies with the stage as much as does the gross appearance. There may be many small abscesses and widespread interstitial infiltration with poly-

morphonuclear leukocytes. Much more usual, however, is a streaky linear round-cell infiltration with an admixture of polymorphonuclears (Fig. 326). In both cases there is destruction of the renal tubules, with gradual replacement by scar tissue which is more abundant and dense than in nephrosclerosis. Foam cells are often seen, and occasionally there are tubercle-like collections of these cells, especially in the pyramids. In rare cases there may be yellow lobulated granulomatous masses made up of epithelioid and giant cells, with foam cells between the granulomas. These lesions, which are possibly due to B. proteus infection, may naturally be mistaken for tuberculosis. Many tubules are filled with pus cells (Fig. 327). The process is characteristically patchy, and in the chronic cases the tubules in the intervening areas are either normal or dilated. A striking feature, especially in the scarred areas, is the presence of dilated tubules lined by flattened epithelium, and filled with dense, acidophilic *colloid-like material,* so that in places the tissue may resemble the thyroid gland (Fig. 328). *Periglomerular fibrosis* is a marked feature even when the glomeruli are intact (Fig. 329). In the renal pelvis there is round-cell infiltration or fibrosis, a valuable diagnostic feature for the

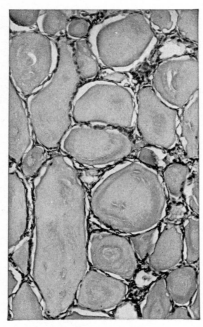

FIG. 328.—Pyelonephritis: colloid casts in tubules. × 120. (Boyd. *Pathology for the Surgeon*, courtesy W. B. Saunders Co.)

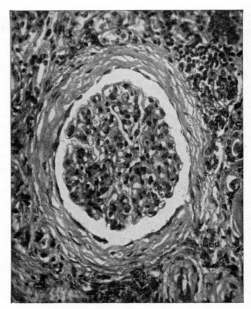

FIG. 329.—Periglomerular fibrosis in chronic pyelonephritis. × 384. (Boyd, *Pathology for the Physician*.)

pathologist in quiescent cases. The arteries in the affected areas show *endarteritis obliterans*, such as may occur in any area of chronic inflammation. Much of the arterial thickening represents disuse atrophy; it is an adjustment of the lumen to the decreased blood flow.

Relation of Symptoms to Lesions.—The clinical picture will naturally depend on the stage of the disease. In *acute cases* there is pain and tenderness over the kidneys, fever, leukocytosis, and pyuria. In *chronic cases* with extensive scarring the symptoms will be those of contracted kidney due to other causes, those, namely, of renal failure with or without hypertension.

The commonest complication is *hypertension*, and the longer the pyelonephritis has lasted, the more likely is hypertension to develop. It may give rise to diffuse nephrosclerosis, cardiovascular accidents, or cardiac failure. In the occasional case where the hypertension is due to unilateral pyelonephritis, nephrectomy may give excellent results. The hypertension is presumably due to renal ischemia, but the matter is not quite so simple as it seems, for of two patients with equally ischemic kidneys one may have marked hypertension whilst in the other the blood pressure is normal. In the pyelonephritis which is so common after the age of fifty, hypertension is a frequent accompaniment, but as both conditions are common at this period the element of coincidence cannot be eliminated. In the pyelonephritis of childhood, the late stage of which was first recognized by Longcope, this element does not need to be considered. In some of these cases hypertension has developed a number of years after the onset of the disease.

The clinical diagnosis is based on the dissociation between disturbances of glomerular and tubular functions and the dissociation between leukocytes and erythrocytes in the Addis count. The two best indications are: (1) the presence of a large excess of leukocytes in the urine, and (2) long-continued loss of renal concentrating power. Disorder of the distal tubules also results in decreased ability to save base (Na), decreased alkali reserve and acidosis. An important distinguishing feature from the other main renal disorders is the striking difference which may exist between the functional capacity of the two kidneys. Roentgenography shows structural asymmetry between the kidneys in some 70 per cent of cases. Undue reliance has perhaps been placed on the presence of pathogenic bacteria in the urine, a point which has already been discussed. These organisms were grown from the urine in only 81 per cent of chronic cases, whilst they were present in 50 per cent of cases of chronic glomerulonephritis (Brod). The sterile urine, even in the presence of marked pyuria without antibiotic therapy, is certainly a puzzle. It is possible that the microorganisms are locked in the interstitial tissue, and do not gain access to the urine. It is in such cases that percutaneous needle biopsy with bacteriological examination of the specimen may be of great value. *Bone changes* such as poor calcification in the growth period, and osteomalacia, osteitis fibrosa and osteosclerosis in the adult are sometimes encountered. The cause of these lesions is not obvious, possibly some change in the balance of electrolytes.

The *prognosis* in *acute* pyelonephritis is excellent, the attack usually lasting only one or two weeks, so that any form of treatment gives good results. *Chronic* pyelonephritis is a very different matter. It must be remembered that once a kidney has been damaged it becomes an easy prey to subsequent hematogenous infection, and that an abnormally functioning lower urinary tract predisposes to repeated ascending infections in the wall of the ureter.

Pyonephrosis.—In pyelonephritis, when obstruction is marked from the beginning the element of hydronephrosis enters the picture, hydronephrotic atrophy leading to destruction of the medulla and much of the cortex. The kidney becomes converted into a bag of pus, a condition known as *pyonephrosis* (Fig. 330). A pure hydronephrosis in an advanced stage may become infected. Such a kidney is much enlarged, the surface irregularly lobulated, and when it is opened it presents a picture of pyonephrosis in which a mere shell of kidney tissue is left.

Perinephritic Abscess.—This condition, also called perirenal abscess, is a localized suppuration in the perirenal tissue, usually due to *Staphylococcus aureus* from a boil or carbuncle in the skin. Occasionally a pyelo-

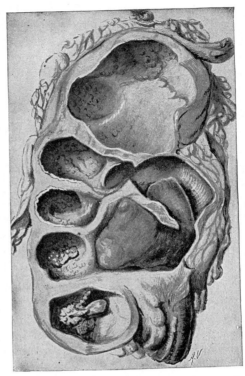

Fig. 330.—Kidney in a condition of pyonephrosis. The dilated pelvis is occupied by a large calculus. (Boyd, *Pathology for the Surgeon*, courtesy of W. B. Saunders Co.)

nephritis or a small localized focus of suppuration in the kidney is the evident source of infection, but in most cases the perirenal lesion has the appearance of being primary. As the result of experimental work on hematogenous infection in animals it is known that staphylococci may produce a minute lesion in the renal cortex, and then pass along cortical lymphatics through the capsule to the perirenal tissue. This is what probably happens in man, and an abscess is produced, usually behind the kidney.

Papillitis Necroticans.—Necrotizing papillitis is an uncommon but serious condition, for when bilateral it usually gives rise to acute and fatal renal failure. A number of papillæ are soft and yellowish, and because of their strategic position the ducts of Bellini are obstructed. The necrotic lesion resembles an infarct, pale yellow in color

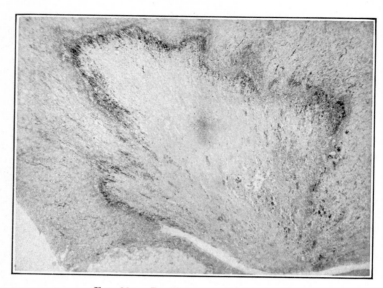

FIG. 331.—Papillitis necroticans. × 15.

with a red border of inflammatory reaction (Plate VII and Fig. 331). Indeed it is an ischemie infarction of the medullary pyramids often confined to the papillæ, and never involving the cortex or the interpyramidal medulla. The condition may occur as a complication of diabetes or as a result of ureteral obstruction. In the diabetic cases there is first a pyelonephritis due to the predisposition of diabetics to infection, and the interstitial inflammation leads to pressure necrosis of the papillæ. In nondiabetic persons with urinary obstruction this order is reversed; increased pressure leads to ischemic necrosis of the papillæ, with pyelonephritis as a secondary event. This belief is supported by the fact that experimental ligation of the ureter may result in necrosis of the renal papillæ (Muirhead *et al.*). In recent years there has been a marked increase in the incidence of papillary necrosis in Switzerland and Scandinavia following excessive use of phenacetin and phenacetin compounds in headache powders. The destruction of the papillæ which follows the necrosis can be demonstrated radiographically (Lindvall).

The *clinical picture* varies, depending on whether the condition is acute or subacute. Neither the incidence nor the severity of the necrosis seems to depend on the severity of the diabetes. In the *acute* cases there is evidence of the sudden onset of infection followed rapidly by pyuria, oliguria and uremia, with coma. There may be hematuria, usually scanty but sometimes massive. This is due to sequestration of the necrotic material, and it may be accompanied by renal colic due to the passage of blood clots and sequestrated tissue along the ureters. Sudden hematuria in a diabetic should suggest the possibility of papillary necrosis. Retrograde pyelography may show irregular filling defects and ring shadows in the calyces due to loss of one or more papillæ. The *subacute* form develops in a patient with previous evidence of acute pyelonephritis. It is likely to occur in non-diabetics with urinary obstruction. As the lesion is often unilateral, recovery may occur.

The Pyemic Kidney.—This is merely a renal manifestation of a general pyemia. Owing to a widespread blood infection pyemic abscesses are formed in various organs, including the kidneys. The infecting agent is usually *Staphylococcus aureus* or *Streptococcus hemolyticus*. When staphylococci are injected into the blood stream of a rabbit they are arrested by the glomeruli and produce multiple small abscesses. Small yellow abscesses surrounded by a red zone are scattered over the surface and throughout

PLATE VII

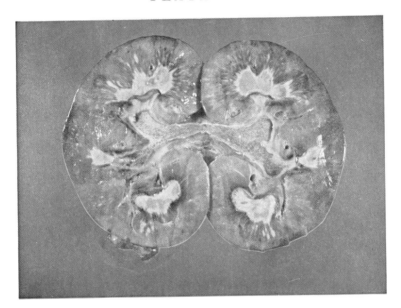

Papillitis Necroticans.
Several of the pyramids as well as the papillæ are yellow and necrotic.
From a case of diabetes mellitus.

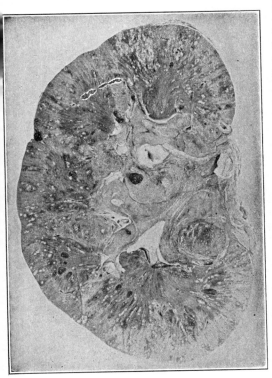

Fig. 332.—The pyemic kidney. Pyemic abscesess are scattered diffusely through both cortex and medulla.

the substance of both kidneys (Fig. 332). *Microscopically* they consist of circumscribed collections of polymorphonuclears, and often contain masses of cocci. The condition is a terminal one, and the patient dies of septicemia before there is time for any marked degree of renal destruction. Modern chemotherapy has changed the condition from a common one into a rarity.

Tuberculosis.—Tuberculosis of the kidney occurs in two forms: (1) acute miliary tuberculosis, and (2) chronic tuberculosis. *Miliary tuberculosis* is merely part of a general miliary infection, and is a postmortem finding. The kidney is studded with miliary tubercles, which on the surface may be mistaken for the abscesses of a pyemic kidney, but they show no border of congestion.

Chronic tuberculosis, also known as ulcero-caseous tuberculosis and surgical tuberculosis, is at first a local condition. The primary lesion is often in bone. The

bacilli are carried to the kidney by the blood. It used to be believed that tubercle bacilli could be excreted by healthy kidneys (excretory bacilluria). This is wrong. A lesion is always present in the kidney, although serial sections may be needed to demonstrate it. Band points out that the earliest lesions occur in the cortex in relation to the glomeruli, although they may only be seen in microscopic sections (he examined 2,000 sections from each half kidney). These minute primary lesions often heal. There are two positions in which gross lesions are likely to make their appearance: (1) in the boundary zone at the base of a pyramid; (2) in the apex of a papilla as it projects into the pelvis.

To have reached these positions the bacilli must either have traversed the glomerular capillaries and been carried downwards by the intertubular set of capillaries; or, what is more probable, they have been excreted into the capsular space, passed for some distance along the tubule, and there been arrested. Ulceration of the calyces develops from the lesion in the papilla, and in the *x*-ray picture (pyelogram) a characteristic distortion of the outline of the calyces and pelvis may be detected, which may allow a remarkably early diagnosis to be made.

The lesion at the apex of the pyramid is at first a localized nodule, but infection spreads up the lymphatics along the line of the collecting tubules, as well as down into the pelvis. In this way a *tuberculous pyelonephritis* is produced. In the tuberculous form there is a much greater tendency to destruction (*renal phthisis*), and large cavities with rough ragged walls are produced containing thick creamy odorless pus which is sterile on culture unless secondary infection has occurred. These communicate with the pelvis, so that a large amount of pus appears in the urine. The condition is now a *tuberculous pyonephrosis* (Fig. 333). Caseation, softening, and liquefaction may eventually lead to destruction of the entire kidney. The kidney may be considerably enlarged or may become shrunken. Much depends on whether tuberculous stricture of the ureter occurs. Such a stricture may prevent the pus from reaching the bladder, and thus mask the true nature of the con-

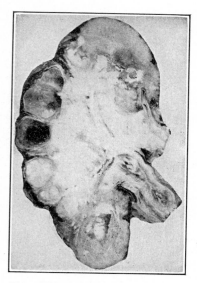

FIG. 333.—Tuberculous pyonephrosis. In the cortex of the lower part there are solid caseous areas; further up cavity formation has taken place; the ureter is considerably thickened.

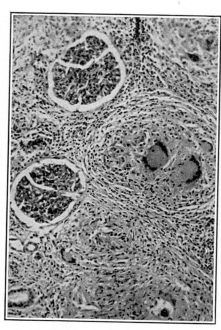

FIG. 334.—Renal tuberculosis. × 100.

dition. In the shrunken kidney the pus becomes inspissated and converted into a putty-like material in which lime salts may be deposited. In the roentgenogram these deposits may give an outline of the calcareo-caseous sac representing the kidney or merely spotty shadows. The *microscopic appearance* is that of tuberculosis in its various stages (Fig. 334).

The *spread of the disease* is of great importance. At first localized, the infection spreads very readily in the connective tissue of the submucosa of the renal pelvis. Infection spreads to the *ureter* with the formation of tubercles and tuberculous granulation tissue in the mucosa and ulceration of the surface. The chief lesions are in the upper and lower thirds. A stricture may develop, but more often the ureter is converted into a rigid, thickened, dilated tube. The *bladder* is infected early, and the chief symptoms— pain and frequency of micturition—are due to this infection. It begins at the opening of the ureter, where hyperemia and tubercles can be seen with the cystoscope and an early diagnosis established in this way. The infection spreads along the submucosa of the trigone, causing ulceration of the overlying

mucous membrane. It may extend to the prostate and seminal vesicles, and along the vas deferens to the epididymis, thus producing a *genitourinary tuberculosis*. There is a remarkable tendency for the bladder lesions to heal, and removal of the kidney may be followed by complete recovery. The *other kidney* tends to become infected sooner or later. This involvement is probably due to an ascending infection from the bladder. The alarmist picture painted in the foregoing account has been profoundly modified by modern chemotherapy.

Relation of Symptoms to Lesions.—The two chief symptoms are frequency of micturition and blood in the urine. These are early as well as common symptoms. The frequency is vesical and the hematuria renal in origin. The *frequency*, which is often associated with pain on urination, is due to lesions in the sensitive trigone of the bladder. It becomes more marked as the capacity of the bladder diminishes. There is often an associated *polyuria*. Renal pain is not an early or a prominent symptom, although there may be an aching in the loin aggravated by jolting. *Renal colic* may be caused by the release of blood along the ureter. The *hematuria* is caused by destruction of vessels in the renal calyces. *Pus in the urine* is a later development, depending on the amount of caseation and liquefaction. It is seldom as abundant as in pyelonephritis and pyonephrosis. Tubercle bacilli may be found with the microscope, or culture and guinea-pig inoculation may be necessary. There are usually no ordinary pyogenic bacteria. Death is usually due to uremia from renal failure, sometimes to general miliary tuberculosis. Again it must be stated that the above is a picture of an untreated case.

DISEASES OF THE BLOOD VESSELS

Arteriolar Nephrosclerosis.—There is no more perplexing subject in pathology, none more baffling and tantalizing, than the relationship between arterial and renal disease. This relationship is reciprocal, for as in glomerulonephritis we find arterial degeneration, so also in arterial degeneration we find glomerular changes.

The condition of essential hypertension may be accompanied by degenerative and fibrotic changes in the kidneys. These changes were originally included under the heading chronic interstitial nephritis, but when they came to be differentiated from chronic glomerulonephritis, they were given such names as the hypertensive kidney, the arteriolosclerotic kidney and arteriolar nephrosclerosis. The latter term describes a process, just as do glomerulonephritis and nephrosis, and therefore seems preferable. The condition has long been known as the primary contracted kidney, in contrast to the secondary contracted kidney of glomerulonephritis. Both were originally included under the term granular contracted kidney.

Essential hypertension may continue for twenty or thirty years without evidence of renal involvement, the patient usually dying of one of three causes dependent on the prolonged hypertension: (1) *congestive heart failure*, (2) *coronary sclerosis*, (3) *cerebral hemorrhage*. If he survives these accidents he may gradually develop symptoms of renal insufficiency and finally die of chronic uremia. Such cases are known as *benign hypertension* and the renal lesions are those of benign nephrosclerosis. In a younger group of

patients the hypertension may develop rapidly and pursue an acute and fatal course reckoned in months rather than years. This is the group of *malignant hypertension*, constituting about 10 per cent of the whole, and the renal lesions are those of malignant nephrosclerosis. The patient may or may not die of acute uremia. From a careful study of the kidney the pathologist should be able to form some opinion as to whether the patient did or did not suffer from essential hypertension, whether the hypertension was of the chronic or the acute type, and if the latter, whether or not death was due to acute renal failure.

The primary renal lesion, which we believe to be the result of the high blood pressure, is arteriolosclerosis (arteriolar sclerosis), causing ischemic atrophy of the glomeruli and tubules resembling that seen in chronic glomerulonephritis. The word arteriole is used in different senses by different workers. It is important to realize this, because it serves to explain the differences in the statistical results of different workers, such for instance as the frequency of renal arteriolosclerosis in hypertension. Some confine it to the afferent and efferent arterioles, whilst others include the distal portions of the interlobular arteries, that is to say, the vessels contained within the true cortex, as contrasted with the interlobular arteries in the medulla. Either system is justifiable, but for the discussion of arteriolosclerosis it is more convenient to use the word arteriole in the wider sense, *i.e.*, as synonymous with small arteries.

Hypertension and nephrosclerosis are not synonymous. Arteriolosclerosis of the afferent arterioles always indicates hypertension, but hypertension may be present without sclerosis of these vessels in 10 per cent of cases before renal insufficiency has developed. If the interlobular arteries and afferent arterioles are taken together, sclerosis is present in 100 per cent of hypertensives, but it is also present in many elderly persons without hypertension. In cases of hypertension with renal failure sclerosis of the afferent arterioles is always present. Benign hypertension and benign nephrosclerosis are therefore not necessarily related, but hypertension acts as an accelerating factor. On the other hand malignant hypertension and malignant nephrosclerosis show a definite correlation, so that malignant nephrosclerosis may be regarded as the renal end-stage of malignant hypertension.

BENIGN NEPHROSCLEROSIS.—The *gross appearance* of the kidney depends on the duration and intensity of the vascular lesions. The kidney may appear normal even though there are marked microscopic lesions. Bell and Clawson found smooth kidneys in 75 per cent of cases of essential hypertension, although hyaline arteriolosclerosis was present in 97 per cent. In cases of long standing the kidney may be small, hard, and granular; this is the *primary contracted kidney*, and it may be greatly shrunken. The surface is covered with little granules produced by an alternation of pale nodules and red depressed portions. The red color is due to atrophy of the cortex which allows the underlying vascular tissue to shine through. Small cysts of the surface are common. The cut surface shows irregular atrophy of the cortex and loss or distortion of the cortical vascular markings. The small arteries, especially those at the base of the pyramids, are thick-walled and gape. The gross appearance may closely resemble that of the granular contracted kidney of chronic glomerulonephritis, but in the latter condition the granules on the surface tend to be finer owing to the diffuseness of the lesions, and the arterial lesions are not so evident. Greater shrinkage is possible than in glomerulonephritis, because the remaining glomeruli, being normal, are able to carry on renal function and maintain life. Often the distinction is impossible.

The basic *microscopic lesion* is arterial and arteriolar sclerosis. The vascular changes of hypertension have already been described in detail on page 520. When the hypertension is of gradual development and long continued, the so-called benign form, two characteristic lesions develop in the renal vessels. These are hyaline degeneration and elastic hyperplasia. Similar changes are found in the arteries of other organs, but not to the same degree nor with the same frequency as in the kidney. *Hyaline degeneration* is best seen in the smallest vessels, such as the afferent and efferent arterioles. It is

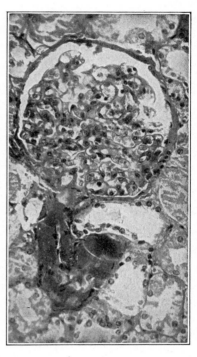

Fig. 335.—Hyaline thickening of afferent arteriole in benign nephrosclerosis with great narrowing of the lumen. × 225.

at first a smooth acidophilic thickening of the subintimal tissue, but in course of time it may involve the entire thickness of the arterial wall, leading to extreme or complete obliteration of the lumen (Fig. 335). Fat is deposited in the degenerated tissue, so that in frozen sections stained with Scarlet Red the arterioles may appear as thick red rings. The larger arteries are often the seat of atherosclerosis. *Elastic hyperplasia* or *elastosis* is most marked in the larger arteries, but some degree of it may be apparent in the arterioles. When the section is stained with an elastic tissue stain it is seen that the internal elastic lamina is split into a number of layers, and the greater part of the thickened intima is composed of elastic fibers, with resulting narrowing of the lumen (Fig. 336). Splitting of the elastica is not seen in an old glomerulonephritis, a point of value in the sometimes difficult task of differentiating that condition from the kidney of hypertension.

The vascular lesions may remain the only

PLATE VIII

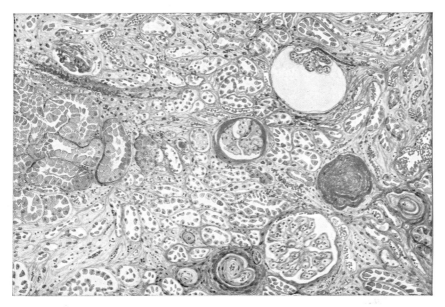

Arteriolar Nephrosclerosis.

Thickening and narrowing of the arterioles, atrophy and fibrosis of the glomeruli, degeneration of some tubules, and gradual atrophy of the remainder. One glomerulus is normal, one is shrunken, one is completely fibrosed, and one shows thickening of Bowman's capsule. (Azocarmine.)

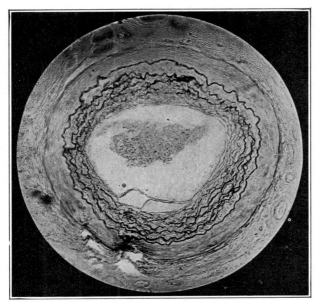

FIG. 336.—Elastic intimal thickening. Marked thickening of the inner coat with reduplication of the internal elastic lamina. (Elastic tissue stain.) × 125.

lesions for a considerable time if the lumen of the small arteries and arterioles, the really significant vessels, is not materially narrowed. When such narrowing occurs, ischemic changes follow. Lesions of afferent arterioles affect individual glomeruli whilst lesions of larger vessels affect groups of glomeruli and tubules.

The glomerular picture is very varied. The most characteristic lesion is a marked thickening and wrinkling of the capillary basement membrane of the tuft, a lesion which is best brought out by a special connective stain such as the periodic acid—Schiff reaction. Atrophy of the glomeruli is common, in some cases manifested by a general shrinkage of the tuft, in others by a breaking up of the tuft into a number of finger-like processes owing to collapse of many of the capillaries. The capillary loops in well-marked cases are completely bloodless. In the true granular kidney the glomeruli can only be injected partially and with great difficulty (Fig. 337A and B), whereas in the senile kidney injection is easy. Eventually the entire glomerular tuft bebecomes converted into a hyaline mass (Plate VIII). At the same time the connective

tissue of Bowman's capsule becomes markedly thickened, fusing with the hyaline tuft and obliterating the capsular space. The corresponding tubules atrophy owing both to disease and ischemia.

The end stage of glomerular damage, what has been called by McManus *glomerular obsolescence*, in arteriolar nephrosclerosis, as also in glomerulonephritis and pyelonephritis, is represented by scarred hyaline knots in the cortex, each of which represents the gravestone of a glomerulus. With hematoxylin and eosin these may be indistinguishable from one another, but with the alcian blue-periodic acid-Schiff stain details can be made out which allow differentiation. In *arteriolosclerosis* it is usually possible to distinguish a peripheral basement membrane, hyaline material filling the capsular space, and a compressed thickened glomerulus. In *chronic glomerulonephritis* the appearance is that of a hyaline knot surrounded by a halo of newly formed tubular structures, which have already been described (p. 560). The characteristic feature of *chronic pyelonephritis* is fibrosis extending into one segment of the glomerulus from a point of adhesions between the tuft and the capsule, eventually

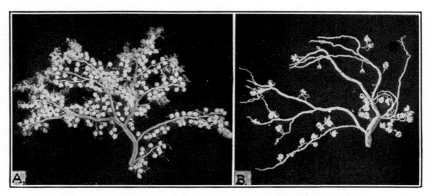

FIG. 337.—Neoprene casts of injected renal vessels (A) normal, (B) in prolonged hypertension. (Kindness of Professor G. Lyman Duff, McGill University.)

involving the entire glomerulus. Finally the Kimmelstiel-Wilson lesion of *intercapillary glomerulosclerosis* may be distinguished from the other hyaline glomeruli, all of which are ischemic, by the absence, as a rule, of any evidence of ischemia.

Ischemic obsolescence is the commonest way in which glomeruli cease to function. It is found at all ages, rarely absent in persons past early adult life (McManus and Lupton). The process begins with the wrinkling and thickening of the capillary basement membranes already mentioned, and these become compressed into a hyaline knot, which is hardly recognizable as a glomerulus with hematoxylin and eosin, but the tell-tale wrinkled membranes can be seen with the PAS method. At the same time the foot processes of the podocytes disappear. Bowman's space may become altered in one of two ways. (1) The more usual process is a filling of the capsular space with dense hyaline material, which stains deeply with the 5-nucleotidase histochemical method. Later this material becomes resorbed, the hyaline appearing to be dissolved away (Fig. 338). The source of the hyaline has not been determined. (2) The other pattern of change is for the capsular space to become enlarged, cystic, and filled with faintly PAS-positive granular material. This apparently represents the genesis of the common subcapsular cysts of the arteriolosclerotic kidney.

The feature common to the various conditions associated with glomerular obsolescence

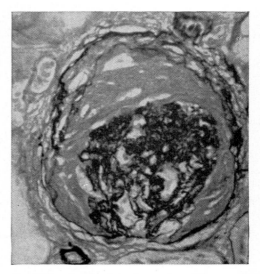

FIG. 338.—An obsolete glomerulus with preservation of detail and what seem to be open vascular channels in the glomerulus. Note the spaces left in the hyaline which fills the space of Bowman's capsule. These clefts are occupied by fibrocytic-like cells; the hyaline is rich in 5-nucleotidase. × 225. (McManus and Lupton, courtesy of Laboratory Investigation.)

is generalized or localized *renal ischemia*. The wrinkling of the basement membranes is probably the result of collapse due to the removal of intraluminal pressure. An arteriole-like structure generally remains in the middle of the shrunken obsolete glomerulus joining the original afferent and efferent arterioles. The progressive stages of ischemic obsolescence can be traced in Figure 339.

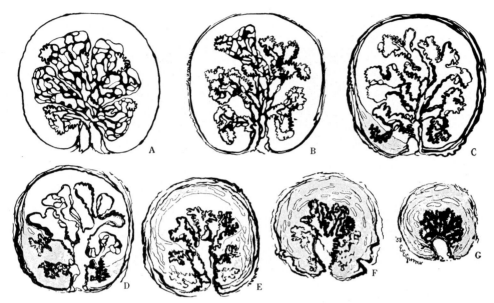

FIG. 339.—Progressive stages of ischemic obsolescence. Sequence (A–G) of patterns observed in ischemic obsolescence showing changes. (McManus and Lupton, courtesy of Laboratory Investigation.)

Hypertension is a very common accompaniment. It is important to realize that the obsolete glomeruli may be resorbed and disappear completely.

Closure of the arteries cuts off the blood supply to areas of cortex of varying size, so that wedge-shaped patches of atrophy are seen here and there (Fig. 340). In these areas both glomeruli and tubules have disappeared, whilst between them the tubules are normal or dilated and the epithelial lining hypertrophied. This hypertrophy and dilatation (compensatory) is especially marked when renal insufficiency has developed, and is always suggestive of that condition. The alternation of atrophic and hypertrophic areas is responsible for the sometimes coarse granularity of the surface.

MALIGNANT NEPHROSCLEROSIS: THE KIDNEY OF MALIGNANT HYPERTENSION.—In over 90 per cent of cases of essential hypertension there is no serious impairment of renal function, at least for a long time. If the patient escapes death from cerebral hemorrhage or cardiac failure he may eventually die of uremia. In these cases autopsy will reveal very extensive damage to the renal parenchyma, as might be expected. But there is another group of cases in which

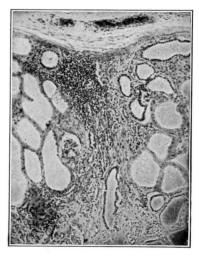

FIG. 340.—Benign nephrosclerosis, showing a patch of atrophy with dilated tubules on either side. × 60.

at a younger age period (usually in the thirties and forties, sometimes in the twenties) the patient develops an acute and progressive renal insufficiency. The blood pressure is very high, but death is likely to be due to uremia. In some cases the patient dies before the onset of uremia. Hyperten-

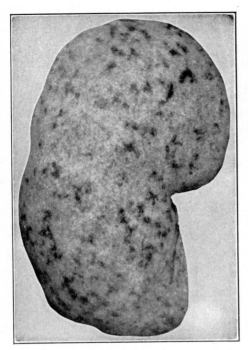

FIG. 341.—Malignant nephrosclerosis. The surface of the kidney is covered with blotchy hemorrhages.

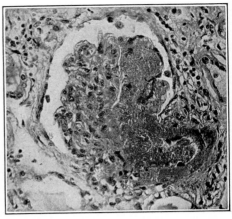

FIG. 342.—Arteriolar necrosis in malignant nephrosclerosis. The afferent arteriole and the right-hand side of the tuft show the smudgy necrotic appearance characteristic of this condition. × 225.

sive retinopathy, characterized by edema of the disc and retina and retinal exudates, also serves to distinguish malignant hypertension from benign hypertension with gradual renal failure. The clinical condition is one of malignant hypertension, and the corresponding renal lesions are those of malignant nephrosclerosis.

The *gross appearance* may be sufficiently characteristic to enable a diagnosis to be made with the naked eye. As a rule the kidney is of normal size and may even be enlarged whilst the surface is smooth; the *tempo* of the process has been too fast for atrophy to develop. Sometimes sufficient time has elapsed for it to become contracted and granular. Not infrequently the two kidneys differ markedly in size. The surface may be covered with hemorrhages, usually large and blotchy (Fig. 341), sometimes small and petechial.

Microscopically the significant lesions are again in the vessels, and again they are two in number, namely, cellular hyperplasia and arteriolar necrosis. *Cellular hyperplasia,*

also called productive endarteritis and hyperplastic arteriolosclerosis, is the hallmark of rapidly developing hypertension. The walls of the smaller arteries are thickened by a concentric cellular proliferation, so that they may present an "onion-skin" appearance (Fig. 281, p. 521). Fatty degeneration may be marked in frozen sections. Elastic hyperplasia is not a special feature. *Arteriolar necrosis,* also called necrotizing arteriolitis, is best seen in the afferent arterioles. Nuclear detail is lost, the elastica disappears, the wall stains brightly with eosin, and its limits become indistinct as if red paint had been smudged across it (Fig. 342). Aneurysmal dilatation may occur, the necrotic wall is infiltrated with red cells, and hemorrhage is common. Arteriolonecrosis is not nearly so common as productive endarteritis, and its significance is different. It is usually an indication of renal failure, although this is not invariably the case. It appears to be a product of rapid severe hypertension coupled with the action of toxic retention products.

The various forms of arterial change may not present the clean-cut picture of a textbook description; thus intimal and medial cellular proliferation may blend so that they cannot be distinguished separately. The important thing is to recognize hyperplastic small arteries and arterioles. In the chronic long-drawn-out cases (benign) the characteristic feature is hyalinization; in the more acute and rapid (malignant) forms the small arteries stand out prominently as thick-walled cellular structures with narrowed lumen.

The *renal parenchyma* does not show the advanced atrophy that is seen in the benign form owing to the quickened *tempo*. Two features may often be observed in cases marked by rapid renal failure. These are focal glomerulitis and tubular dilatation with hyperplasia of the lining cells. *Focal glomerulitis* is characterized by fusion and necrosis of the capillary loops, swelling, degeneration (fatty, hyaline droplets, or necrosis) of the epithelium covering the tuft, and the formation of fibrinous adhesions between the glomerular loops and the lining of Bowman's capsule. There may be patchy necrosis of the tuft with hemorrhage into the capsular space. *Tubular hyperplasia*, probably compensatory in character, when present in marked degree is excellent evidence of renal failure. It is most marked in chronic glomerulonephritis, is quite pronounced in malignant hypertension, and may be present in lesser degree in benign hypertension if the stage of renal failure is reached.

Other organs may show the characteristic hyperplastic arteriolosclerosis and arteriolonecrosis. These are most frequently seen in the fatty capsule of the adrenals or in the glands themselves, but they are also present in the pancreas, retina and brain. In the retina they may be responsible for the lesions of hypertensive retinopathy and in the brain for those of hypertensive encephalopathy.

The *retinal lesions* are of particular interest and importance to the physician, because they are the only ones which he himself can see during life, and which may enable him to make a correct estimate of the state of renal function and therefore the prognosis. There are three fundamental retinal lesions in hypertension. (1) *Retinal arteriolosclerosis* is the least significant of the three, for it does not necessarily indicate any renal insufficiency, the patients often living many years and dying eventually of cardiac failure, coronary occlusion, or cerebral hemorrhage. The arteries are sclerosed and show white lines, there may be some irregular constriction of the vessels, but there is complete absence of papilledema. Small hemorrhages may be present in the retina together with white spots of sharp outline ("hard" spots), some of which may form a star-shaped figure round the macula. (2) In *malignant hypertensive neuroretinitis* papilledema is usually the first change and is the distinguishing feature of the condition. The previously described retinal changes are again present, namely, hemorrhages and white spots, but the latter are of the "soft" or "cotton wool" variety, although hard spots may also be present. The arteries are always markedly narrowed owing to functional vasoconstriction, which appears to be responsible for the lesions. (3) *Choked disc* is the result of cerebral edema. The increased intracranial pressure thus produced may give rise to changes in the disc.

The main features by which, in characteristic cases, malignant hypertension can be distinguished from the benign form are as follows. In malignant hypertension a relatively young person develops an unusually high blood pressure (over 200 mm. Hg), papilledema is a constant feature, hematuria is common, and death is usually due to acute uremia. The kidneys are of normal size or only moderately contracted, and may show hemorrhages on the surface. The significant microscopic features are cellular hyperplasia, arteriolonecrosis, focal glomerulitis and tubular hyperplasia, the corresponding features in benign hypertension being elastic intimal hyperplasia, hyaline arteriolosclerosis and hyalinization of the glomeruli.

SENILE NEPHROSCLEROSIS.—In persons over the age of fifty in whom the aorta and its larger branches show atherosclerosis, the kidneys are often contracted and grossly scarred. The condition might be called the scarred contracted kidney. The scars appear on the surface as depressions and give an impression of old infarcts. If the vascular lesions are more diffuse the kidney may be coarsely granular. The renal artery is markedly atheromatous, with narrowing of the lumen of some of its branches.

The *microscopic picture* corresponds to the gross appearance. Owing to atheromatous

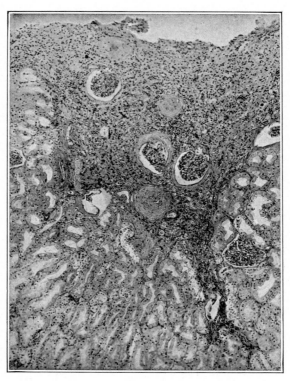

Fig. 343.—Wedge-shaped area of sclerosis in senile arteriosclerotic kidney. × 75.

narrowing of the larger branches of the renal artery there are wedge-shaped areas of fibrosis where the glomeruli are completely hyalinized, and the tubules have disappeared and been replaced by fibrous tissue. The wedge-shape is caused by the fan-like distribution of the vessels (Fig. 343). The condition has no relation to hypertension, so that the arteriolar lesions characteristic of that state are not seen. The intervening tissue between the sclerotic areas is normal.

Relation of Symptoms to Lesions.—In *senile nephrosclerosis* there is no hypertension and no renal insufficiency. The kidney is withered and scarred, but, as Clifford Allbutt puts it, it is "a starved but not a corrupt kidney, sufficient for the smaller life of an elderly man." It is not the result of essential hypertension, and as the remaining parenchyma is healthy, there is no danger of renal insufficiency.

In *benign nephrosclerosis* the patient may live for many years with no sign of renal involvement. Sooner or later there will be a lowering of the specific gravity of the urine, a loss of the concentrating power of the kidney owing to atrophy of the convoluted tubules from loss of their blood supply, and the appearance of small quantities of albumin and occasional granular and hyaline casts. Such a kidney will show sclerosis of many glomeruli and disappearance of the corresponding tubules, but the remaining parenchyma can still be whipped up to perform the work of excretion, as is indiated by hypertrophy of the residual parts, so that there is compensated renal hypofunction but no true insufficiency. As a matter of fact, obliteration of the glomerular capillaries may lead to direct communication between the afferent and efferent arterioles, thus supplying with blood tubules which may persist and hypertrophy. If the patient lives long enough the advancing nephrosclerosis will destroy the last remnants of parenchyma and true insufficiency will develop, but as a rule the overstrained vessels of the brain will burst, the laboring heart will suffer defeat, before symptoms of uremia have time to appear.

In *malignant nephrosclerosis* the patient may rapidly lose weight. Retinal lesions (edema, hemorrhage and patches of exudate) may be the first indication of the gravity of the condition. It is probable that arteriolar spasm, which may be observed directly in the retinal vessels, is a factor of primary importance in the production of many of the widespread lesions. As has already been pointed out in connection with eclampsia, spasm of an arterial segment is accompanied by dilatation of the segment immediately distal, and through the wall of the dilated segment diapedesis of red blood cells may occur and large quantities of plasma be poured out, giving rise to edema. This is the basis of the retinal lesions, and probably of the lesions responsible for such symptoms of hypertensive encephalopathy as transient paralysis, convulsions and finally coma. There is soon evidence of renal failure, the concentrating power of the kidney is lost, the specific gravity of the urine falls though never to the extreme low limits of chronic glomerulonephritis, being seldom below 1.010, albuminuria may be marked and casts are constantly present, there may be red blood cells in the urine, the nonprotein nitrogen is retained in the blood, and the patient dies of uremia. These lesions are due to the rapidly produced ischemic lesions of the glomeruli. The presence of the red cells in the urine is explained by the hemorrhage into the capsular spaces, which in turn is due to the necrotic lesions of the glomeruli and afferent arterioles.

Relation of the Kidney to Hypertension.— The subject which must now engage our attention is one of the most important and baffling in the whole realm of clinical medicine. If the reader should feel some doubt as to the truth of this statement, he would do well to consult the April, 1958, number of Circulation, in which some 200 pages are devoted to the basic mechanisms of hypertension, expressing wildly different views. In our discussion of the general subject of hypertension in the previous chapter we have seen that two main groups of cases may be recognized: (1) *Essential* or *primary hypertension*, which is the most common lethal disease of adult life, but the primary cause of which, we must confess, is still unknown. For this reason it is no exaggeration to say that the problem of essential hypertension is comparable to that of neoplasia in magnitude. (2) *Renal hypertension*, best exemplified by the Goldblatt experimental ischemic kidney, as well as by the ischemia produced by surrounding the kidney with cellophane, which induces a peripheral fibrosis with compression, but also by human chronic pyelonephritis, chronic glomerulonephritis, and nephrosclerosis. (3) *Radiation nephritis* which we have already discussed (p. 567) may be followed by hypertension both in man and the experimental animal. It is not known how the irradiation produces the hypertension, for in the animal (rat) the rise in blood pressure may occur before any structural damage is apparent in the kidney. In addition there are rare *extrarenal causes* such as *pheochromocytoma* and *primary aldosteronism*. The two problems which demand solution are: (1) What is the mechanism by which the blood pressure is raised and kept raised in renal hypertension? (2) What, if any, is the relation of the kidney to essential hypertension? To the latter question some workers, notably Goldblatt, answer categorically that so-called essential hypertension is of renal origin.

As regards the mechanism involved in the production of renal hypertension, attention is focussed on the polypeptide *hypertensin*, a powerful pressor substance which has been demonstrated in the circulating blood of dogs in experimental renal hypertension, as well as in the blood of the human subject with essential hypertension, being most abundant in the malignant form. The precursor of hypertensin is *renin*, a proteolytic enzyme contained principally in the granular cells of the juxtaglomerular apparatus, although possibly also in the cells of the proximal convoluted tubules. Renin acts on the renin substrate, *hypertensinogen*, continually produced by the liver, with the formation of the pressor substance hypertensin, also known as angiotonin, and *angiotensin*. Two different forms of hypertensin have been differentiated (Skeggs and Kahn). The first, hypertensin I, a decaptide, is a product of the action of renin on its substrate. This is changed to a vasoconstrictor octapeptide, hypertensin II, by an enzyme in the plasma. Knowledge of such chemical minutiæ may some day provide us with a key with which to control hypertension. The pressor mechanism seems to become active when the renal circulation is impaired, as in chronic glomerulonephritis, pyelonephritis, nephrosclerosis, and the Goldblatt kidney. Perhaps the strongest argument that an overproduction of renin is responsible for the hypertension of the Goldblatt kidney is the fact that this protein can be used to prepare a highly specific antibody, and that in animals with renal hypertension the active or passive immunity conferred by this antirenin is accompanied by marked lowering of the blood pressure (Wakerlin).

All the evidence outlined above seems to point to a humoral mechanism as the basis of experimental hypertension, a mechanism activated by acute renal ischemia. The blood pressure of a dog kept hypertensive for months or years owing to constriction of the main renal arteries can be returned to normal by the repeated subcutaneous injection of renin, which results in the development of antirenin in the blood. Renin is derived from the ischemic kidney. It does not follow, however, that other pressor enzymes and polypeptides may not be of non-renal origin, arising, although more slowly from other sites. Grollman and his associates have kept dogs with bilateral nephrectomy alive for 10 weeks by means of the artificial kidney or peritoneal lavage, and after an interval of a few days they have developed the clinical picture of hypertensive cardiovascular disease and the arterial lesions of malignant hypertension. Any theory relating to the pathogenesis of hypertension must take into account the fact that hypertension and arteriolar sclerosis may occur experimentally in the absence of renal tissue; indeed the presence of healthy renal tissue seems to act as a protection. The chief protective function of the kidney seems to be prompt removal of renin. It may be that the maintenance of normal blood pressure depends on a correct balance between the production of a pressor material by the

adrenal cortex and its elimination by the kidney, so that hypertension might be the result either of adrenal overactivity, which we know can happen, or of renal failure (Friedman and Friedman).

While the acute phase of experimental hypertension is due to sudden humoral action, in the chronic phase the pressor substances circulate in lesser amount, but at the same time there is a progressively reduced ability of the contralateral kidney to remove pressor polypeptides or their formative enzymes. When the ischemic kidney is unclamped the blood pressure falls, because the pressors can now be eliminated by the previously ischemic kidney.

Turning for a moment to *essential hypertension in man*, a subject discussed more fully in the preceding chapter, we have to face the fact that a person may have benign hypertension without vascular renal lesions other than those incidental to anyone of the same age. Even if specific vascular lesions are present, there may be little or no vascular occlusion with consequent renal damage. In view of the vast bulk of normal kidney tissue remaining, it does not seem likely that any minimal lesions which may be present could produce so striking a change in the blood pressure. It seems improbable that primary renal vascular disease is a common cause of hypertension in man, at any rate the so-called essential variety of hypertension. *The kidney is the victim rather than the culprit.* It appears more probable that essential hypertension is due to an unknown extrarenal factor, possibly adrenal in origin, but that in the later stages a renal component (ischemia) plays a part as the vicious circle develops. It is possible that studies on the juxtaglomerular apparatus may throw further light on the problem, for these cells seem to be related to the functional activity of the adrenal cortex (Hartroft and Hartroft).

The distinction between the renal hypertension of glomerulonephritis and primary (essential) hypertension may be easy for the clinician if the patient has been under observation for a considerable period. In the primary form high blood pressure develops early, whilst renal insufficiency is a late manifestation. Papilledema (in the malignant form), cerebral hemorrhage, coronary heart disease, and congestive heart failure are common features. In glomerulonephritis hypertension develops gradually *pari passu* with renal insufficiency, and marked secondary anemia is an early feature. If the patient is seen only after uremia has developed it may be very difficult to make the distinction.

The pathological distinction may be easy or difficult. In nephrosclerosis the lesions are much more patchy than in glomerulonephritis, and the remaining glomeruli are unaffected. Epithelial crescents, which may be fibrosed, indicate glomerulonephritis. The arterial lesions of nephrosclerosis, both benign and malignant, are characteristic. A serious difficulty is presented by the fact that hypertension in the uremic stage of glomerulonephritis may cause vascular lesions identical with those of malignant nephrosclerosis. In both diseases a vicious circle may be established. Hypertension leads to arteriolosclerosis, this produces ischemic lesions, and these in turn may intensify the hypertension. This is true also of chronic pyelonephritis.

Infarction.—The kidneys are one of the commonest sites of infarcts by reason of the enormous flow of blood which passes through them, and because of the "end-organ" type of circulation. The emboli responsible for the infarction come from three sites in the heart: (1) the left atrial appendage in mitral stenosis, (2) mural thrombi from the left ventricle in myocardial infarction, (3) the vegetations of bacterial endocarditis. Infarcts may be caused by emboli from an aortic aneurysm, and still more rarely by thrombosis in renal arteries or veins. Embolization by atheromatous material from aortic plaques may cause infarction, and this is particularly liable to happen as the result of the surgical treatment for aneurysm of the abdominal aorta and for aortic atherosclerosis with thrombotic occlusion. In such cases the infarcts produced by the emboli may be so numerous as to cause death from uremia. The infarct shows the usual characters which are described in Chapter 6. The necrotic area is surrounded by a zone of congestion, which in the earlier stages of the process may show much hemorrhage. For this reason there may be red cells in the urine at this stage. On the other hand, the urine is often normal. A renal infarct is usually without symptoms, there may be pain and tenderness over the kidney, and in exceptional cases the condition may simulate perforation of a viscus.

Bilateral Cortical Necrosis.—This rare condition, rare at least in the classic and fatal form in which it is recognized, and characterized by anuria at the outset, is also known as *symmetrical necrosis of the renal cortex*. For much of our knowledge of this fascinating subject we are indebted to the work of Sheehan and his associates. The cortical necrosis is ischemic in origin. The ischemia used to be attributed to thrombi which occlude the small arteries, but it appears probable that vascular spasm is the primary event, and that the thrombosis is a later complication. The vasospasm seems to be in the nature of an allergic reaction in the arterial wall, a view which would explain the suddenness of the onset (Duff and More). The walls of the small arteries and arterioles are necrotic at autopsy, and similar lesions may be present in the adrenals, pituitary, spleen and bowel. Cortical necrosis may be associated with a number of clinical conditions, but it is most frequently seen in the obstetrical catastrophe known as concealed accidental hemorrhage or uteroplacental apoplexy, the renal condition apparently starting at the same time as the development of the abdominal pain and shock. That vasospasm usually related to the later stages of pregnancy and therefore presumably on a hormonal basis is a prime factor in pathogenesis is suggested by the observation that in rats previously treated with ovarian hormones the injection of a large dose of oxytocin, the pituitary hormone which normally acts on plain uterine muscle at the end of pregnancy, produces vasoconstriction of the renal vessels with intense renal ischemia leading to massive cortical necrosis (Byrom and Pratt). The condition is twice as common in the late stage of pregnancy as in the non-pregnant state, but it may occur in both sexes and at any age. The *gross appearance* at autopsy is so characteristic that it can be recognized at a glance. Almost the entire cortex of both kidneys with the exception of a very thin

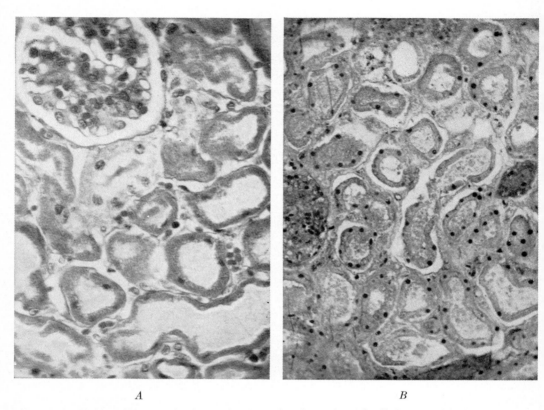

A   B

FIG. 344.—*A*, Necrosis of proximal convoluted tubules of a patient who died twenty-four hours after the onset of uteroplacental apoplexy (Hematoxylin and eosin stain. × 440.) The dead tubules have already lost their nuclei. *B*, Center of dead area in a case of gross cortical necrosis of six days duration. × 240. Hemotoxylin and eosin stain. Although the tubules have been dead for so many days, they retain their nuclei owing to the absence of any reflow. Compare with *A*. (Case Records of the Massachusetts General Hospital, N. Engl. J. Med.)

surface layer supplied by the capsular arteries, is a bright yellow outlined with red.

If death should occur early in the development of the condition, as from pulmonary embolism or cerebral hemorrhage, it is possible to trace the early steps of the process (Davis). These can be confirmed in the experimental animal. There is first the formation of numerous casts in the collecting tubules and lower nephrons, the result of albuminuria. This is followed by necrosis of the proximal convoluted tubules, then minor focal cortical necrosis, and finally gross cortical necrosis. The minor grades are probably reversible.

If the spasm of the intrarenal arteries lasts only one or two hours the proximal tubules, which are the most sensitive structures, develop coagulative necrosis as the result of the ischemia, the nuclei of their cells are lost, and the tubules are reduced to granular masses of débris. The picture is similar to that seen in mercuric chloride poisoning, although in that instance the process is toxic rather than ischemic in origin. Curiously enough these changes are due to reestablishment of the blood flow when the temporary ischemia passes off, for the fresh blood carries aerobic enzymes which reduce the dead tubules to granular débris lacking in nuclei. The patient becomes anuric, and remains so for a week or 10 days. With the stimulus of the new flow of blood the necrotic tubules become lined with low epithelium, the kidney begins to excrete a urine of low specific gravity as the tubules have not yet gained the power of reabsorption, and the prognosis is good provided treatment is directed to preventing the accumulation of water and potassium in the initial anuric phase, and their depletion in the subsequent phase of polyuria.

When the vasospasm is more severe and prolonged the blood flow is not reestablished, and a condition of permanent ischemia develops. As the dead tubules are not surrounded by fresh blood, the ordinary nuclear changes which depend on aerobic enzymes cannot take place, and the lining cells retain their morphology, including nuclei, for many days (Fig. 344). Moreover, the blood trapped in the ischemic area at the moment the circulation fails undergoes hemolysis, so that the infarct is deep red for the first few days, then pink, and finally a dull opaque yellow white. As regeneration of the tubules cannot occur, the patient dies of uremia. Thrombi are found in the later but not in the early stage, so it is evident that anticoagulant therapy is not indicated. Illustrations of the various lesions outlined above will be found in the discussion by Davis, from which much of the foregoing information is taken.

RENAL FAILURE

Renal failure is, of course, failure of function. The principal functions of the kidney are: (1) elimination of water not needed by body fluids, the amount depending on the balance between glomerular filtration rate and the degree of tubular reabsorption; (2) the excretion of certain substances normally present in the plasma when their concentration rises above a certain level (high threshold substances); (3) the selective reabsorption of substances such as glucose which are of value to the body; (4) the excretion of useless substances; and (5) the regulation of the acid-base balance. Disturbance of one or more of these functions is likely to manifest itself by the symptoms of disease. They are indications of renal failure.

Decrease in the glomerular filtration rate may be of extrarenal or of renal origin. *Extrarenal* causes are circulatory failure, severe hemorrhage, shock, *etc.*; *renal* causes are thickening of the glomerular tufts, arteriolar occlusion, or increased intrarenal pressure due to edema or obstruction.

Reduction in tubular capacity due to many causes results in decreased power to reabsorb solutes against pressure gradients (proximal tubules) or to excrete solutes at a normal rate (distal tubules). *Failure in tubular reabsorption* is due to interference with the necessary enzymes, with loss of solutes and water from the extracellular fluid. The enzyme loss is usually the result of destruction of a number of tubular units. We shall consider some instances in connection with electrolyte disturbances. *Failure in tubular excretion* on the part of the distal tubule is best illustrated by a failure to excrete ammonia. This is really a failure of metabolism, for the enzymes necessary for the synthesis of ammonia have ceased to function, and it is no longer available as a substitute for alkali cations, with acidosis as the result.

Renal failure may be acute or chronic. In actual practice this distinction may not be as simple as it sounds, but it is useful for the purpose of discussion.

Acute Renal Failure.—We may summarize the causes of acute renal failure by saying that they may be pre-renal, renal, and post-renal. Some of the principal of these causes are given in the table on page 606.

Chronic Renal Failure.—We have seen in our studies that the functions of the kidney may be interfered with by disease of the glomeruli, tubules, interstitial tissue or arteries. In the last analysis, it is the functions of the nephrons which matter. Two views are held as to the relation between the structural damage to the nephrons and the physiological disturbance observed by the clinician. (1) Structural damage to the vast majority of the nephrons allows these structures still to function, but interferes with important factors to a marked degree. This is the orthodox view. (2) Function is carried on by the surviving intact nephrons, but to a minimal degree by the affected ones. The reduced nephron population functions normally, but it is exposed to a relative increase in both solute and water load. Thus if 2,000,000 nephrons normally attend to the excretion of potassium, reduction of that number to 200,000 will mean that 10 times

PRINCIPAL CAUSES OF ACUTE RENAL FAILURE

Pre-Renal	Renal	Post-Renal

1. Circulatory failure:
  (1) cardiac;
  (2) peripheral;
  (3) occlusion of renal vessels.
2. Severe fluid and electrolyte depletion or imbalance.
3. Allergies and overwhelming toxemias
4. Addisonian crises
	1. Acute glomerulonephritis
	2. Anoxic (tubular) nephrosis
	3. Toxic (tubular) nephrosis
	4. Acute pyelonephritis
	5. Pyemic kidney
	6. Papillitis necroticans
	7. Bilateral cortical necrosis
	8. Eclampsia
	9. Malignant nephrosclerosis
	10. Radiation nephritis
		Obstruction in ureters, bladder or urethra.

the load will be placed on the remaining ones. The second theory is now increasing in popularity. As a matter of fact it was shown more than seventy years ago in the experimental animal that massive surgical reduction in the amount of functional renal tissue led to failure of the remaining nephrons. There is evidence to support both major theories in various types of renal disease, but certain it is that the overall flexibility of the diseased kidney decreases as the number of nephrons is decreased.

Uremia.—Uremia is a term used to describe a clinical and biochemical picture which is the result of renal failure due to renal rather than extrarenal causes. The three most important of these in order of frequency are *chronic pyelonephritis, benign nephrosclerosis* and *chronic glomerulonephritis,* but almost any of the conditions described in the foregoing pages may eventually terminate in uremia. The clinical picture is one of chronic renal failure. In acute failure the patient has a quiet end, without the convulsions and other distressing features which characterize the uremic state. It was Bright himself who first gave the name of uremia to the group of symptoms which constitute the clinical picture, because of the increase in the blood urea which he observed to be present. This observation, made well over one hundred years ago, is rather startling to us who regard blood chemistry as the latest child of modern medicine. A figure of over 50 mg. per ml. may be regarded as abnormal. Bright regarded urea as a highly toxic substance, but in this we now know that he was mis-

taken. Bright's original description of the clinical picture of uremia has never been equalled, ("the skin is dry, headaches occur with unusual frequency, or the calls to micturition disturb the night's repose"), and it should be consulted by the student with an ambition to write with clearness and vigor.

Uremia is a symptom complex in the make-up of which there are two principal factors: (1) *excess* of certain substances such as nitrogen-containing components of the urine, phosphates, potassium and acidic ions due to failure of excretion by the kidney; (2) *deficiency* of water and electrolytes, more particularly bicarbonate, leading to reduction of the alkali reserve as shown by decrease in the CO_2 content of the blood. This is due to excretion of fixed base in the urine consequent to the lack of ammonia formation, and is aggravated by the loss of water, sodium and chloride due to the vomiting which accompanies the condition.

The symptom complex of uremia is too varied in its manifestations to be considered here in detail. (1) The symptoms may be *cerebral,* with excitement, apathy, muscular twitchings, convulsions, and coma; (2) they may be *gastrointestinal,* with vomiting and diarrhea; or (3) they may be *pulmonary,* with the dyspnea of acidosis. Although always associated with the retention of urea in the blood, it is not caused by the urea. It is probable that different toxic products of metabolism may be at work in different cases. Uremia is the final manifestation of renal failure. Occasionally it is a cause of death in acute nephritis. It constitutes the

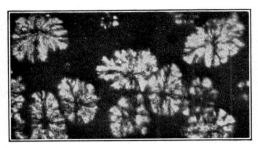

FIG. 345.—Xanthydrol urea crystals
(dark field). × 300.

usual termination of the chronic stage. Tiredness, both physical and mental, is a characteristic feature of chronic uremia. When tissues from a case of uremia are fixed in a solution of xanthydrol in glacial acetic acid, masses of crystals of xanthydrol urea are found in the cerebral cortex and other organs (*xanthydrol reaction*) (Fig. 345). The reaction is of value in determining whether or not a pericarditis or enteritis found at autopsy in a case of uremia should be considered uremic in nature. The *brain* in uremia usually shows marked edema (wet brain). *Uremic enteritis* and *pericarditis* may be found at autopsy. The entire *alimentary canal* may be affected (dry and glazed tongue, foul mouth, uremic breath, stomatitis, enteritis). Necrotizing and *ulcerative lesions* are commonest in the *lower part of the small intestine and the colon.* Some workers believe that the lesions are due to urea retention; others say that they are unrelated to urea retention and caused by infection of mucosal hemorrhages. The lungs may present a characteristic picture in the *x*-ray film, the so-called *butterfly shadow*, with one wing of the butterfly in the region of the hilus on each side. Microscopically the alveoli in the affected area are filled with a heavy protein exudate into which fibroblasts penetrate with eventual fibrosis.

Myocardial dysfunction may be due to retention of potassium and loss of calcium and sodium, so that an imbalance is established which may result in disorders of rhythm and electrocardiographic changes. The *skin*, particularly that of the face and hands, may present a characteristic "*café au lait*" discoloration, due to the oxidation of urochromogen to urochrome, the yellow pigment of the urine, in parts exposed to the light. The skin may also show flaky white deposits of urea known as urea frost in extreme cases. A good illustrtaion of this "frost" will be found in Allen's book. *Anemia,* is one of the most characteristic features, and is evidenced by the increasing pallor of the patient. The degree of the anemia is relative to the azotemia, so that it is a good indication of the progress of the case. It may be due to interference with the building up of hemoglobin in the liver or to toxic arrest of the maturation of red blood cells. It is difficult to overemphasize the importance of anemia in assessing the progress of a case of uremia. Estimation of the hemoglobin level is an economic and convenient substitute for periodic determination of the non-protein nitrogen in chronic cases.

THE KIDNEY AND ELECTROLYTE DISORDERS

In the discussion of renal function at the beginning of this chapter we have seen that the kidney is not merely an organ designed for the excretion of waste products. Of equal importance is the part it plays in the preservation of the internal environment by tubular reabsorption of water and electrolytes. Moreover, there is a two-way relationship of cause and effect between electrolytes and renal failure, for just as renal (tubular) failure may be responsible for a negative balance of sodium, potassium or calcium owing to excessive loss of these in the urine, so also a negative balance of sodium or potassium or an excessive urinary excretion of calcium may cause renal failure. The renal tubules represent the end-organ to some of the endocrine glands, and when they and their enzymes fail to respond to the hormones which these glands secrete, more particularly the antidiuretic hormone of the pituitary, aldosterone, and parathyroid hormone, water or electrolytes are lost to the body with consequences which may be serious or fatal (Platt). It is evident that a loss of electrolytes or water may be due to (1) failure of the tubular enzymes, or (2) overproduction of the corresponding hormone. We have already discussed the protein-losing kidney. We shall now consider briefly the water-losing, the salt-losing, the potassium-losing, and the phosphate-losing kidney.

The Water-losing Kidney.—This is failure of the lower distal tubule to respond to the antidiuretic hormone of the posterior pituitary. The failure may be acquired or congenital. The acquired form is called *water-losing nephritis*, and the congenital form *nephrogenic diabetes insipidus*. The symptoms are those of diabetes insipidus, namely intense thirst, marked polyuria, and an inability to concentrate the urine, but, unlike the symptoms of true diabetes insipidus, they do not respond to pitressin, because the defect lies in the tubules, not in the pituitary. The congenital cases of nephrogenic diabetes insipidus provide an interesting instance of an isolated breakdown of a renal mechanism, in this case an enzyme in the distal tubule, with preservation of all the other functions of the kidney. The symptoms develop in infants and children, who are known in their family as "water drinkers." Antidiuretic hormone alters the permeability of the distal and collecting tubules to water; when it is lacking these tubules become impermeable to water, and the fluid within them remains hypotonic. This change in permeability seems to be due to a change in the cement substance between the cells of the collecting tubules, a change caused by the secretion of hyaluronidase by the renal cells under the influence of antidiuretic hormone (Ginetzinsky). Congenital nephrogenic diabetes insipidus appears to behave as a sex-linked recessive on the x chromosome, affecting only the boys of the family, but being carried down through the female line. In this respect, of course, it resembles hemophilia.

The Salt-losing Kidney.—Some of the most serious and important symptoms of Addison's disease of the adrenals are due to absence of cortical aldosterone, the salt-saving hormone. Similar symptoms may be produced by a failure of the renal tubules to respond to aldosterone, although produced in normal amount, and so may lead to a mistaken diagnosis of Addison's disease. Some patients with chronic renal disease tend to lose salt, but the extreme cases of salt-losing nephritis are usually due to chronic pyelonephritis, often with little or no proteinuria and no hypertension, so that the renal basis of the clinical picture may easily be overlooked. In salt-losing renal disease there is usually marked hypertrophy of the adrenals in an effort to compensate for the defect in the tubules.

The Potassium-losing Kidney.—Potassium loss is much more important than potassium retention, although both may occur. The loss of potassium may be nonrenal or renal in origin. *Extrarenal causes* are primary aldosteronism, chronic ulcerative colitis of long duration and the sprue syndrome with steatorrhea, and the treatment of chronic congestive heart failure through the repeated use of mercurial diuretics. *Primary aldosteronism* or *Conn's syndrome* (first described by Conn in 1955) is characterized by increased excretion of potassium and retention of sodium with resulting hypopotassemia and hypernitremia. The clinical picture is one of intermittent tetany, paresthesias, periodic severe muscular weakness, and arterial hypertension. The cause of all this is an excessive secretion of aldosterone, the sodium-retaining adrenal corticoid produced by an adenoma of the adrenal cortex.

The *renal form* of potassium deficiency is seen when the tubules are extensively damaged, as in the so-called *renal tubular acidosis*. The kidney has two main methods of disposing of an excess of hydrogen ions. (1) It can produce a highly acid urine by the excretion of these ions as acid phosphate. (2) It can excrete ammonium salts, the ammonium being formed in the renal tubule by the combination of hydrogen ions with ammonia under enzyme influence. In ordinary chronic renal failure the first method is employed, so that the urine is highly acid, but in renal tubular acidosis the second mechanism comes into play. There seems to be an exchange of hydrogen ions from the renal cells for sodium, and as the sodium is reabsorbed the kidney may lose potassium instead.

Both in the renal and the commoner extrarenal forms of potassium deficiency there is a characteristic lesion known as

A

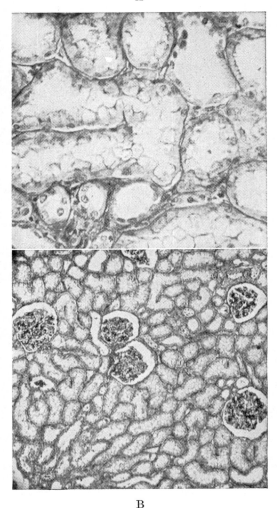

B

Fig. 346.—Biopsy of the kidney in a case of potassium deficiency at the height of the depletion—high power (A) and the low-power magnification (B) of the cortex. There is marked swelling of proximal tubular epithelium, with diffuse "foamy" degeneration of cytoplasm. The glomeruli are normal. (Relman and Schwartz, courtesy of N. Eng. J. Med.)

vacuolar nephropathy (Kulka *et al.*), a peculiar and distinctive vacuolation of the tubular epithelium, most marked in the proximal tubule, to a lesser degree in the distal tubule, and not at all in the loop of Henle (Fig. 346). The lesion, which has been called "clear cell nephrosis," must not be mistaken for the much finer vacuolated appearance produced

in the tubules by the parenteral administration of hypertonic sucrose solution. The most important clinical features are periodic paralysis and other puzzling forms of muscular paralysis due to the potassium deficiency, osteomalacia, and renal calcification.

Potassium retention with hyperpotassemia may be the precipitating cause of death in some cases of uremia. In the anuric patient tissue catabolism releases potassium from the cells, where the concentration is 30 times greater than that of the plasma, and sequestration of the electrolyte in the tissues may reach lethal levels. The clinical features are mainly cardiac, namely bradycardia, arrhythmia, characteristic changes in the electrocardiogram, and finally heart block.

The Phosphate-losing Kidney.—It is well known that in chronic renal disease there may be hypertrophy of the parathyroid glands, sometimes up to 100 times their normal size. This appears to be a work hypertrophy, due to failure of the kidney to respond to the parathyroid hormones. The most easily demonstrated action of the hormone on renal function is an increase in phosphate clearance due to a decrease of tubular reabsorption of phosphate. The hyperparathyroidism may be primary hyperaldosteronism. When secondary to renal failure the cause seems to be the stimulus to the parathyroids provided by a raised serum phosphate level due to the greatly lowered glomerular filtration rate. Here, as Platt points out, "we have another example of the kidney failing in its function as an end-organ of the endocrine system, but in this case it fails to excrete, whereas in the case of sodium and the adrenal it fails to conserve."

The Phosphate-retaining Kidney.—Retention of phosphate may occur under two very different conditions, the one known as renal osteodystrophy, the other the Fanconi syndrome. The latter is described on page 611 in connection with inborn defects of tubular function.

Renal Osteodystrophy.—This is also known by such descriptive names as *renal rickets*, renal osteitis fibrosa, renal dwarfism, and renal infantilism. Any chronic lesion of the urinary system, renal or extrarenal, congenital or acquired, may lead to osteodystrophy. The basic disturbance seems to be

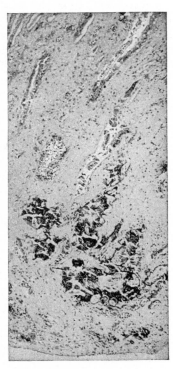

Fig. 347.—Randall's patch, showing deposit of calcium in renal papilla. × 50. (Boyd, *Pathology for the Surgeon*, courtesy of W. B. Saunders Co.)

an unexplained ability of the kidney to excrete phosphorus, with retention of that element in the blood. There is generally osteoporosis, more rarely osteosclerosis, together with secondary hyperplasia of the parathyroids. The chief *symptoms* are a failure to grow (dwarfism), infantilism if the patient reaches the age of puberty, bone deformities, polyuria and finally uremia. The urine always has a low specific gravity. The disease generally makes its appearance between the ages of seven and nine years, but it may be present from early infancy.

Calcium and Nephrocalcinosis.—It is convenient to refer to calcium in passing in this discussion of electrolytes and renal function. In contrast to the other electrolytes, however, we are more concerned with what calcium does to the kidney than what the kidney does to calcium. It is in the formation of urinary calculi that calcium is of particular importance, and the subject of stones will be taken up in relation to the

lower urinary tract (Chapter 31). In this place, however, we are interested in hypercalcemia with the resulting renal damage which may develop. This may occur in hyperparathyroidism, sarcoidosis, excessive vitamin D ingestion, idiopathic hypercalcemia of infants, and Burnett's milk-alkali syndrome, as well as metastatic carcinomatosis of bone and other conditions which will not be considered here. The nephrocalcinosis of hyperparathyroidism is discussed in the chapter on the parathyroid glands. Nephrocalcinosis as opposed to calculus or stone formation, is marked by deposits of calcium or calcium phosphate in the form of amorphous granular deposits in the tubules or the interstitial tissue, followed later by disintegration of the tubules and a granulomatous reaction in the surrounding stroma, with eventual fibrosis. The deposits are often most marked in the pyramids and papillæ (Fig. 347).

Sarcoidosis is associated with hypercalcemia and renal insufficiency in 20 to 45 per cent of cases. This is attributed to the production of a substance similar in action to vitamin D, which itself has an action like that of parathyroid hormone. The hypercalcemia leads in time to nephrocalcinosis and eventually to renal insufficiency.

Hypervitaminosis D can be studied in the experimental animal, and in the occasional patient who has continued on his own initiative to take the vitamin in large amounts for a prolonged period. The early symptoms of hypercalcemia are nausea, headache, diarrhea, lassitude and nocturia, followed later by evidence of renal insufficiency from calcinosis.

Idiopathic Hypercalcemia of Infants is a relatively common form of hypercalcemia in Great Britain, although virtually unknown in North America (Rhaney and Mitchell). In severe cases there may be physical and mental retardation, osteosclerosis, and finally renal failure with hypertension. The disorder, which is the cause of much ill health and interference with growth, would appear to be due to overaction of vitamin D in babies receiving more than they require or to intolerance to the vitamin.

The Milk-Alkali Syndrome or *Burnett's Syndrome* is a variety of hypercalcemia met with in patients with peptic ulcer who have received prolonged and excessive intake of milk (calcium) and absorbable alkali (Burnett *et al.*). The hypercalcemia is easily mistaken for that of primary hyperparathyroidism, obviously a serious error. Marked clinical and biochemical improvement follows withdrawal of the excessive amounts of calcium and absorbable alkali being administered therapeutically. The *lesions* are extensive and there is widespread calcification of the soft tissues and the arteries. The high calcium content in the milk damages the kidney with marked calcinosis and even stone formation. Fortunately only a very small percentage of patients ingesting large amounts of milk develop hypercalcemia. Preexisting renal disease appears to act as a predisposing cause.

Innate Functional Tubular Defects.—The concept of inborn defects of function in the renal tubules is a valuable and justifiable one, being first suggested by Fanconi to explain the baffling group of symptoms now known as the Fanconi syndrome. The defects are those of tubular reabsorption, probably depending on the absence of one or more enzymes in the cells lining the tubules. The resulting clinical conditions have been classed as unifactorial or multifactorial (Jackson and Linder). *Unifactorial* defects include water (renal diabetes insipidus), glucose (renal glycosuria), and bicarbonate (hyperchloremic nephrocalcinosis). *Multifactorial* defects include inability to reabsorb phosphate and sugar (glycosuric rickets or osteomalacia), and phosphate, sugar and amino acids (Fanconi syndrome). All these are inherited abnormalities, usually carried by a single recessive gene. There may, however, be other associated genetic anomalies, such as deaf-mutism and pigmentary retinal degeneration.

Fanconi Syndrome.—In this rare condition a profound disturbance of renal function may give rise to rickets and dwarfism in children, osteomalacia in adults. It is esentially a disease of childhood. There is a strong hereditary tendency, and it may be the tubular defect presently to be described which is inherited. The essence of the syndrome is a great diminution of tubular reabsorption, more particularly with regard to phosphate, glucose and amino acids, with in consequence a heavy phosphaturia, renal glycosuria despite a normal blood glucose level, and a striking amino-aciduria. The serum phosphate is low. In the classic Fanconi syndrome the urine never becomes acid. Polyuria and thirst are prominent clinical features, and there may be deposits of cystine in the cornea causing a ground-glass opacity. It may be mentioned that *cystinosis* can occur in two forms: (1) widespread deposition of cystine, including the cornea; (2) deposits in the form of renal calculi translucent to *x*-rays.

The *renal lesion* responsible for the condition seems to be a congenital and hereditary structural anomaly of the proximal convoluted tubule. By microdissection it is possible to demonstrate a narrow elongated swan-like neck of the beginning of the tubule, which itself is short and wide, together with a truncation of the remainder of the segment to a quarter or half of the normal length (Fig. 348). There is absence of phosphatase in the proximal tubules. Deficient phosphorylation in these abnormal tubules may account for the abnormal excretion of phosphates, amino acids and glucose.

Renal Tubular Acidosis.—This condition, known also as *renal hyperchloremic acidosis*, is a rare syndrome developing usually in infants and young children, and apparently due to a functional tubular defect. There is a curious association of chronic acidosis with secretion of a urine which is either alkaline or only weakly acid. The serum chloride is high and the bicarbonate is low. Nephrocalcinosis may also be present. In the presence of an acidosis the normal kidney increases the acidity of the urine and its ammonia content. This compensatory mechanism is impaired in renal tubular acidosis, perhaps as the result of an inborn defect in the enzyme carbonic anhydrase. The excretion of an acid urine is dependent on the ability of the tubular cells to excrete hydrogen ions, which are exchanged for ions of base that are reabsorbed by the tubular cells. Thus acidification of urine and conservation of base go hand in hand. It would appear that in tubular (hyperchloremic) acidosis the reabsorption of bicarbonate by

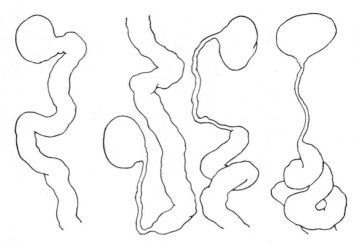

Fig. 348.—Outline drawing of the first part of three nephrons, showing that in the Fanconi syndrome the glomeruli are attached by a narrow elongated neck to the proximal convoluted tubule. A normal nephron is seen on the left. (Clay, Darmady and Hawkins, courtesy of Jour. Path. and Bact., Oliver and Boyd, Ltd.)

the proximal tubule is impaired as the result of some inborn and inherited defect.

Diuretics.—Whilst diuretics increase the flow of urine, the object of their use is to relieve the accumulation of water in the interstitial tissue, whether the accumulation is due to renal disease, cardiac disease, or from some other cause.

Organic Mercurials.—The administration of derivatives of mercury results in the rapid excretion of water by the renal tubules. Their presence in the cells lining the tubules inhibits the tubular reabsorption of chloride ions, and this automatically increases the urinary excretion of an equivalent quantity of cations. The result is an increased output of total solutes, so that the resulting osmotic diuresis removes the surplus of edema fluid.

Chlorothiazide.—This is an orally effective sulfonamide which promotes the renal excretion of chloride, sodium, and potassium. Chlorothiazide (Diuril) appears to differ from other diuretic agents in its mode of action on the renal tubule. The urine flow and the solute output are increased, but the *free* water clearance does not increase (Heinemann *et al.*). The addition of a mercurial diuretic such as meralluride induces a similar increase in flow of urine, but an increased excretion of free water, *i.e.* osmotically non-obligated water. Solute reab-

sorption is isomotic in the proximal tubule, but it may or may not be isomotic in the distal tubule. It would appear that the mercurial diuretic acts only in the proximal tubule, whereas chlorothiazide affects solute (sodium and chloride) reabsorption both in the proximal and the distal segments of the nephron.

Chlorothiazide, and to a much greater degree hydrochlorothiazide, is a mild *hypotensive* agent. Potent diuretics may lower the blood pressure by virtue of the diuresis reducing the plasma volume. They may also have a distinct and specific antihypertensive action. Such would seem to be the case with hydrochlorothiazide.

TUMORS OF THE KIDNEY

Tumors of the kidney may be divided into tumors of the kidney proper and tumors of the renal pelvis. Those of the kidney proper can be subdivided into tumors of the renal tubules and embryonal tumors. Tumors arising from renal tubules may be benign (adenoma), or malignant (carcinoma).

Adenoma.—Cortical adenomas are of common occurrence. They are small yellow nodules, frequently multiple, usually 1 cm. or less in diameter but occasionally large, circumscribed but often not encapsulated.

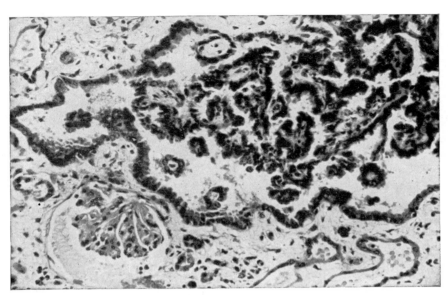

Fig. 349.—Adenoma of kidney with papillary cystadenomatous appearance.   × 200.
(Boyd, *Pathology for the Surgeon*, courtesy of W. B. Saunders Co.)

As is mentioned below, it is often not possible to draw a clear line between cortical adenoma and carcinoma. As a general rule tumors over 3 cm. in diameter prove to be malignant, but to this there are many exceptions. The lesions, indeed, seem at first to be focal compensatory hyperplasias in a damaged kidney, similar to what is seen in the liver and the thyroid (Fig. 349). They arise in areas damaged by vascular occlusion, so that they are met with in persons over middle age. In the ischemic nephron the glomerulus and most of the tubule goes, but if part remains it may form a cyst, the lining of which when supplied with new vessels develops papillary epithelial buds. The *microscopic picture* is curiously varied for a benign neoplasm. There is a general re-producing of renal tubules, but these may be irregular or dilated, papillary processes may project into them, so that the picture is that of a papillary cystadenoma, while in other places the cells form solid acini. Some of the cells are small, dark and compact, but others may be large clear cells, so as to resemble those of the clear cell carcinoma. There is either no strict delimitation from the surrounding tissue, or if a capsule is present it may be penetrated by the tumor

cells. The particular interest of the cortical adenoma is its possible relationship to car-cinoma. One grades into the other, and no sharp line can be drawn between the two. The characteristic clear cells are seen in both, and the only certain way to distin-guish the one tumor from the other is to look for the occurrence of metastases. As Willis puts it: "There are no structural criteria which will permit clear-cut separa-tion of the 'black sheep' from other members of the family."

Carcinoma ("Hypernephroma").—It is not necessary to fight once more the old battle about the origin of this tumor. It arises from the epithelium of the renal tubules, not as originally suggested by Grawitz from adrenal or hypernephroid tis-sue, so that it has no right to be called a hypernephroma. To call it a Grawitz tumor is to perpetuate still farther an erroneous theory suggested in 1883 and disproved a few years later. Unlike adrenal cortical tumors, it never produces an endocrine secretion nor the symptoms that go with hyperadrenalism. Many of these tumors must arise from the adenomas which they so closely resemble. It is perhaps significant that very small carcinomas are almost never

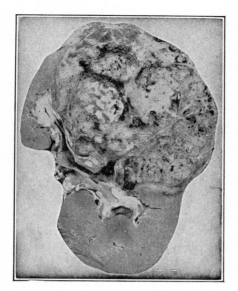

FIG. 350.—Renal carcinoma. The cut surface
has a variegated appearance

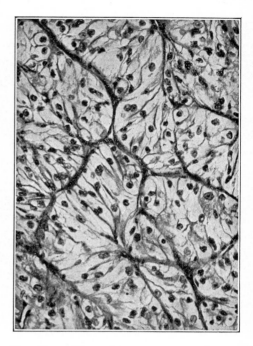

FIG. 351.—Microscopic appearance of a renal
carcinoma. The clear cells show a very marked
alveolar arrangement. × 200.

encountered, small tumors being classed as
adenomas.

The *gross appearance* is so characteristic
that it can usually be recognized at a glance
(Fig. 350). The tumor forms a rounded
mass usually in the upper or lower pole,
which may attain a large size. At first it
appears encapsulated, but later is invasive.
The great characteristic of the cut surface is
its variegated appearance. Yellow is the
chief color (due to lipid), but there are also
red hemorrhagic areas and cysts of varying
size, while only a small piece of normal
kidney tissue may be left. Some of the
cysts contain serous or mucinous fluid, but
others represent areas of necrosis into which
hemorrhage has occurred. There may be a
fibrous core in the center of the tumor.

The *microscopic picture* may be as varied
as the gross appearance. The tumor cells
are usually very characteristic, being large
and rounded with a peculiarly clear or
vacuolated cytoplasm (Fig. 351). This is
known as the *clear cell type*. The clearness
or vacuolation is due to the presence of a
large amount of lipid (mostly cholesterol
ester), and in part to the presence of glycogen, shown by Best's carmine stain after
alcohol fixation. Occasionally the tumor is

composed of dark granular cells; this *granular cell form* is much more malignant. The
arrangement of the cells is also variable.
There are three possibilities, which in their
order of frequency are: (1) a *cystic papillary
formation*, in which papillary processes project into indefinite cystic spaces, but with no
real tubular formation; (2) an *alveolar arrangement of solid cords*, divided into masses
by thin septa; (3) occasionally a definitely
tubular arrangement which irresistibly suggests that the tumor is of renal origin. The
stroma is scanty, but the blood vessels form
a striking feature of the picture; they are
usually numerous and very large, and the
vessel wall often seems to be formed of
tumor cells, thus accounting for the frequent
hemorrhage into the tumor and the tendency
to metastasize by the blood stream.

Spread.—The tumor may remain silent
for a long time, and metastases are often
the first evidence of a renal tumor. At first
the tumor is sharply separated from the
kidney by a fibrous capsule, but sooner or
later the malignant character becomes ob-

vious with *local invasion* and penetration of
the capsule. *Lymph spread* to the lumbar
nodes is found in about 50 per cent of cases
at autopsy. *Blood spread* is by far the most
important, owing to a special tendency to
invasion of veins, and the tumor may grow
into the renal vein and even into the inferior
vena cava, with widespread metastases as
the result. The *lungs* and *bones* are involved
most often, but the brain and the liver often
show metastases. In the lungs the metastases have a curiously clear-cut outline in
the roentgen-ray picture known as the
"cannon-ball" appearance. Renal carcinoma is one of the most important causes of
secondary tumors of bone, and the first manifestation that there is anything wrong with
the patient may be the occurrence of a
spontaneous fracture. A curious feature is
that in 60 per cent of the cases there is a
solitary bone metastasis, so that the possibility of removing the primary tumor and
the solitary metastasis may be entertained.
The order of frequency of involvement is in
upper end of humerus, spine, femur, pelvis,
and ribs.

Relation of Symptoms to Lesions.—Of the
symptoms *painless hematuria* is by far the
most important, and it occurs fairly early
in over 50 per cent of the cases. It is
accounted for by the numerous large thin-
walled blood spaces, which readily rupture
into the renal tubules. Pain is uncommon,
and a tumor can be felt only late in the
disease. The tumor causes *deformity of one
or more of the calyces of the renal pelvis*
at an early stage, and this may be detected
in a pyelogram. *Long-continued fever* is a
remarkable feature of some cases; it is
probably a protein fever due to breaking-
down of tissue. A pyelogram (roentgen-ray
of pelvis) shows the following: (1) spider
distortion due to stretching of the calyces,
(2) filling defects in the pelvis, and (3) displacement of the ureter outwards. In embryoma, on the other hand, the pyelogram
shadow is displaced by the tumor but not
otherwise altered until late, when the renal
pelvis is invaded. The symptoms which
bring the patient to the doctor may be due
to metastases in the bones or in the brain.
The *prognosis* is bad owing to the tendency

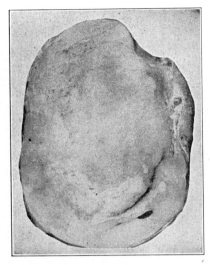

Fig. 352.—Embryoma. The homogeneous appearance of the cut surface is in striking contrast to
the variegated surface of hypernephroma. The
kidney is at the right of the tumor.

to blood spread, but early removal may be
followed by cure.

Embryoma, Wilms' Tumor.—This is the
*commonest abdominal malignant tumor of
early childhood.* It usually occurs during
the first three years of life and after the age
of five years it is infrequent, but it may very
rarely occur in adults. It may attain an
enormous size, nearly filling the abdomen.
Quite frequently it is bilateral. The diagnosis
cannot be made until a tumor appears, for
there is no hematuria and no pain, because
the renal pelvis is not invaded. Intravenous
urography may show a complete absence of
the normal roentgenogram shadow or distortion of the calyces. Fever occurs in 50
per cent of the cases. There is a marked
response in the size of the tumor to radiation,
a useful diagnostic point.

The tumor, which commences in the
cortex, is gray, soft, and has the homogeneous character of a sarcoma (Fig. 352),
but necrosis and hemorrhage may alter this
appearance. It tends to destroy the whole
kidney, and may spread to neighboring
organs, but distant metastases by the blood
stream are not frequent. In this respect it
differs completely from renal carcinoma.
The *microscopic appearance* varies in different parts of the same tumor. The general

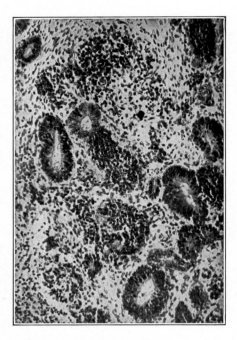

Fig. 353.—Wilms' tumor, showing a combined carcinomatous and sarcomatous appearance. × 150.

character is sarcomatous, and in the past the Wilms' tumor has been classed as "sarcoma of the kidney in children." The cells may be round or fusiform. Glandular (tubular) elements are often present, and such tumors have often been called *adenosarcoma* (Fig. 353). Smooth muscle and striated muscle are not uncommon, and in rare cases there may be cartilage and bone. The tumor is markedly radiosensitive.

The Wilms' tumor is a developmental tumor, and is best called an embryoma, a nephroblastoma, or an embryonal mixed tumor. It may seem strange that an epithelial organ such as the kidney should give rise to a developmental tumor with connective-tissue (sarcomatous) characteristics. This is readily explained by recalling that the epithelium of the urinary tract is derived from mesoderm (intermediate cell mass); the convoluted tubules develop from undifferentiated mesenchyma which has the appearance of cellular connective tissue in which glandular structures are formed. This is exactly the appearance presented by the usual form of Wilms' tumor. The occasional

formation of muscle and cartilage is a perversion of growth on the part of the embryonic mesenchymal cells.

It may not be out of place to point out that the name of the man who gave an early description of this tumor was Wilms, not Wilm. We can thus avoid the remarkably common mistake of writing the name of the lesion as "Wilm's tumor."

Other Tumors.—*Fibroma* occurs fairly often as a small circumscribed nodule in a pyramid or papilla. Narrow tubules are usually scattered throughout the fibrous tissue, so that the lesion should be regarded rather as a *hamartoma* than a true tumor, *i.e.*, a developmental defect in tissue combination (*hamartia*, defect) with a limited capacity for aberrant growth. *Lipoma* and *sarcoma* are rare tumors; most sarcomas develop from the capsule and invade the cortex secondarily. *Tumors of the renal pelvis* really belong to the lower urinary tract rather than to the kidney, so that they are considered in Chapter 31.

CYSTS OF THE KIDNEY

Polycystic Kidney.—Congenital Cystic Kidney.—This condition is found once in every 500 autopsies (Bell). It is nearly always bilateral, but in about 5 per cent of cases may be unilateral. There are two periods of life at which it is found. About 30 per cent occur in infants, the majority stillborn. The remaining cases present symptoms in early adult and middle life. The progressive atrophy of the parenchyma caused by continuous dilatation of the cysts is balanced during youth by compensatory hypertrophy, but by the third decade this compensatory power is lost. The kidneys may be enormously enlarged or only slightly so. They are converted into a series of cysts, which may occasionally communicate with one another but never with the renal pelvis (Fig. 354). The surface is grossly nodular owing to the large cysts. The contents may be thin or thick and viscid, clear amber or dark brown from hemorrhage, and sometimes contain urea. Hardly any renal tissue may be left, so that the occurrence of hypertension, renal insufficiency, and uremia is easily understood. Infection of the

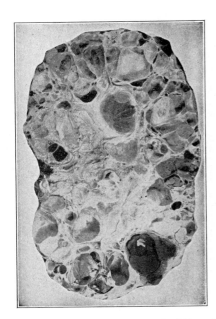

FIG. 354.—Polycystic kidney. The kidney is enlarged and converted into a series of cysts containing thick material which has been coagulated by the fixative.

cysts is not uncommon. *Microscopically* the cysts are lined by cubical epithelium, but in the large cysts it may be flattened. The remaining kidney tissue shows marked evidence of nephrosclerosis, with fibrosis of the glomeruli and disappearance of the tubules. The gross study of injected kidneys shows that the interlobar and interlobular arteries lie mainly in the cyst walls, often just under the lining epithelium. These vessels are easily ruptured as the result of hypertension or slight trauma, so that the cysts frequently contain fresh or old blood, and the patient suffers from attacks of lumbar pain. If the hemorrhage into a cyst should cause rupture into one of the calyces there will be hematuria—a not uncommon symptom. When the kidney is injected with an opaque substance and roentgen-rayed, there is found to be a great disappearance of vessels and occlusion of the arterial tree.

The congenital nature of the condition is suggested by the occasional occurrence of other congenital anomalies. Small cysts are sometimes present in the liver (due to malformation of the bile ducts), and more rarely

in the pancreas. There is, moreover, a strong hereditary tendency. It used to be supposed that the cysts were due to failure of the convoluted tubules to fuse with the collecting ones, but it is more probable that the cystic condition is merely a persistence of one stage of renal development. In the early embryo the convoluted tubules which first develop in connection with the collecting tubules are not permanent, but become detached and persist for a time as cystic structures. Normally these fetal cysts atrophy. If they persist they form a cystic kidney. *Clinically* it is justifiable to speak of a surgical and a medical type (but not with respect to treatment). In the *surgical type* the symptoms such as pain, tumor, and hematuria, are referable to one kidney. In the *medical type* there are symptoms of acute or chronic renal insufficiency, with arterial hypertension in over 50 per cent of the cases.

Solitary Cyst.—Sometimes a large single cyst is found projecting from one pole of the kidney, which may cause a degree of enlargement that can be detected clinically (Fig. 355). Some of these cysts may attain a very large size. There may be more than one of these "solitary" cysts. Often the cyst is quite small. The contents are serous and rarely contain urea. Hemorrhage may occur into the cyst. These cysts are rarely found in infants and children, a fact suggesting that they are acquired rather than congenital.

Obstruction and Calculus Formation.—Urinary obstruction and the formation of stones involve the bladder, ureters and renal pelvis. Although the first two, together with the urethra, constitute the lower urinary tract, while the renal pelvis is included with the kidney to form the upper urinary tract, the pelvis is merely the expanded funnel-shaped upper end of the ureter. It has everything in common in structure and in function, in health and in disease, with the lower part of the tract, and therefore will be considered together with it. For this reason the study of obstruction and calculus formation will be deferred until diseases of the lower urinary tract are discussed in Chapter 31.

The Myeloma Kidney.—Multiple mye-

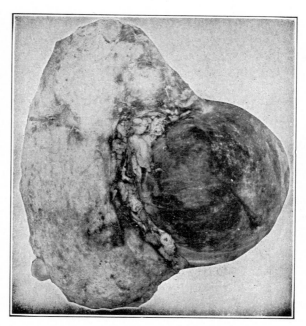

FIG. 355.—Large solitary cyst of the kidney.

loma is a widespread disease of bone in which the patient may develop anuria and die of uremia. At autopsy the renal glomeruli are normal, but the tubules are either atrophied or filled with peculiarly dense firm casts, which may excite a foreign body giant cell reaction (Fig. 356). In this disease the urine may contain a peculiar form of protein known as Bence-Jones protein, and it is this which forms the casts. The tubular atrophy is caused by obstruction. Apparently the uremia has an obstructive basis.

CONGENITAL ANOMALIES.—*Fetal lobulation* is the most common anomaly. The furrows which separate the original lobules fail to disappear, so that the surface remains lobulated (Fig. 356). *Horse-shoe kidney* is also common. The kidneys are fused together, usually by their lower poles. The ureters pass down in front of the connecting bridge of tissue. *Agenesia* or absence of one kidney is usually associated with absence of the ureter. The other kidney is double the normal weight (compensatory hypertrophy). There is no increase in the number of glomeruli and tubules, but they become larger. *Aplasia* or marked *hypoplasia* is not very rare. The kidney may be a mere structure-

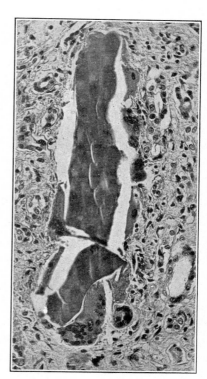

FIG. 356.—Kidney in multiple myeloma; cast with giant cells. × 150.

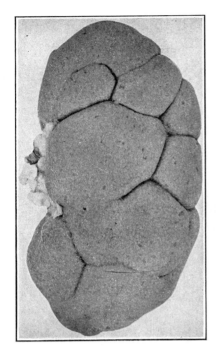

Fig. 357.—Fetal lobulation of the kidney.

less rudiment, or may appear to be a normal small kidney. The other kidney is correspondingly large. *Dystopia* means displacement of the kidney, but the displacement is not active; the kidney has failed to migrate upward to its normal position, and remains in its primitive position, usually at the pelvic brim or the bifurcation of the aorta. The ureter is naturally short, for it has never been of normal length, and as vascularization of the kidney does not occur until the final resting place is reached, the vessels will usually come off the lower end of the aorta. *Congenital cystic disease*, the most important of all the congenital anomalies of the kidney, has already been described.

HEMATURIA.—This subject may be considered in connection with circulatory disturbances, although it is usually due to quite different causes. Blood in the urine may come from the *urethra bladder*, *ureter* or *kidney*. Only the *renal causes* are considered here. In some cases the blood can be seen with the naked eye; in others it can only be seen with the microscope. In the latter group it is better to speak of red cells rather than blood in the urine. (1) The hematuria may be due to *circulatory disturbances, e.g.,* chronic venous congestion, infarction. (2) *Inflammatory* and *necrotic conditions, e.g.,* acute glomerulonephritis, embolic glomerulonephritis, focal nephritis, malignant nephrosclerosis. (3) *Tuberculosis* of the kidney. (4) *Tumors.* The common cause is renal carcinoma (hypernephroma), but papilloma or carcinoma of the renal pelvis may occasionally cause bleeding. (5) *Renal calculus*, the stone either remaining in the pelvis or passing down along the ureter. (6) *Essential hematuria* is a condition in which there is hemorrhage, sometimes severe, from one kidney, but when the condition is removed no cause is found. In most cases there is probably a focal nephritis which has been overlooked, or a varicosity in one of the renal papillæ.

ORTHOSTATIC ALBUMINURIA.—What has been called benign albuminuria is of common occurrence in children and young adults, and is due, certainly in many cases, to a circulatory disturbance of the kidney. The distinguishing feature of the albuminuria is that it is absent when the person is lying down and appears when he assumes the erect posture. For this reason it is called orthostatic or postural albuminuria. The albumin is most marked in a specimen passed after the person has been up for some little time in the morning. It is commonly associated with marked lordosis of the lumbar spine. When this lordosis is corrected, as by the child putting his foot on a stool, the albuminuria disappears even though the erect position is maintained. The vena cava lies to the right of the mid-line, so that the left renal vein has to cross the vertebral column, and is liable to be compressed if lordosis is at all marked. When catheters are placed in the ureters of a person who suffers from this condition, it will be found that when he assumes the erect (and lordotic) position the urine coming from the left ureter will contain albumin, while that coming from the right is normal. There may be anuria for one-half hour on the part of the ischemic left kidney, while the right kidney continues to secrete normal urine. The condition is an anomaly, but can hardly be called pathological. It tends to disappear as the person grows up and the lordosis lessens. The prognosis is excellent.

REFERENCES

ALLEN, A. C.: *The Kidney: Medical and Surgical Diseases*, New York, 1951. Arch. Path., 1941, *32*, 33. (Efferent arteriolar lesions in diabetes.) Am. J. Med., 1955, *18*, 277. (Nephrotic syndrome.)

BADENOCH, A. W. and DARMADY, E. M.: J. Path. and Bact., 1947, *59*, 79. (Acute tubular nephrosis.)

BAND, D.: Edin. Med. J., 1935, *42*, 162. (Tuberculosis of kidney.)

BARRIE, H. J., ASKANASZY, C. L. and SMITH, G. W.: Can. Med. Ass. J., 1952, *66*, 428. (Glomerular lesions in diabetes.)

BECKER, D. and MILLER, M.: New Eng. J. Med., 1960, *263*, 367. (Diabetic glomerulosclerosis in hemochromatosis.)

BELL, E. T.: *Renal Disease*, 2nd ed., Philadelphia, 1950.

————: Am. J. Path., 1935, *11*, 373. (Polycystic kidney.)

BELL, E. T. and CLAWSON, B. J.: Arch. Path., 1928, *5*, 939. (Arteriolosclerosis and hypertension.)

BERGSTRAND, A. and BUCHT, H.: Lab. Invest., 1957, *6*, 293. J. Path. and Bact., 1959, *77*, 231. (Electron microscopy of diabetic glomerulosclerosis.)

BROD, JAN.: Lancet, 1956, *1*, 973. (Chronic pyelonephritis.)

BURNETT, C. H. *et al.*: New Eng. J. Med., 1949, *240*, 787. (Milk-alkali syndrome.)

BYROM, F. B. and PRATT, O. E.: Lancet, 1959, *1*, 753. (Oxytocin and renal cortical necrosis.)

BYWATERS, E. G. L. and DIBLE, J. H.: J. Path. and Bact., 1942, *54*, 111. (Crush syndrome.)

CHURG, J. and GRISHMAN, E.: Am. J. Path., 1959, *35*, 25. (Membranous transformation in subacute glomerulonephritis.)

CLAY, R. D., DARMADY, E. M. and HAWKINS, M.: J. Path. and Bact., 1953, *65*, 551. (Nature of the renal lesion in the Fanconi syndrome.)

COGAN, S. R. and RITTER, I. I.: Am. J. Med., 1958, *24*, 530. (Radiation nephritis.)

COONS, A. H. and KAPLAN, M. H.: J. Exper. Med., 1950, *91*, 1. (Localization of antigen in tissue cells by microfluorescence.)

CROWSON, C. N. and MORE, R. H.: Arch. Path., 1955, *60*, 73. (Hepato-renal syndrome.)

DAVIS, J. C.: New Eng. J. Med., 1958, *258*, 1219. (Bilateral cortical necrosis.)

DEMOPOULOS, H., KALEY, G. and ZWEIFACH, B. W.: Am. J. Path., 1960, *37*, 443. (Distribution of renin in kidney.)

DE WARDENER, H. E.: *The Kidney: An Outline of Normal and Abnormal Structure and Function*, London, 1958.

DUFF, G. L. and MORE, R. H.: Am. J. Med. Sci., 1941, *201*, 428. (Bilateral cortical necrosis.)

DUNIHUE, F. W.: Anat. Rec., 1949, *103*, 442. (Juxtaglomerular cells.)

ELLIS, A.: Lancet, 1942, *1*, 34, 72. (Natural history of glomerulonephritis.)

FARQUHAR, M. G., HOPPER, J. JR. and MOON, H. D.: Am. J. Path., 1959, *35*, 721. (Diabetic glomerulosclerosis.)

FARQUHAR, M. G., VERNIER, R. L. and GOOD, R. A.: Am. J. Path., 1957, *33*, 791. (Glomerular changes in nephrosis.)

FRIEDMAN, M. and KAPLAN, A.: J. Exper. Med., 1943, *77*, 65. (Renal hypertension.)

FRIEDMAN, S. M. and FRIEDMAN, C. L.: Can. Med. Assn. J., 1949, *61*, 596. (Renal hypertension.)

GARCÍA-CÁCERES, U.: Am. J. Path., 1959, *35*, 755. (Proliferation of tubular epithelium in subacute glomerulonephritis.)

GINETZINSKY, A. G.: Nature, 1958, *182*, 1218. (Hyaluronidase in the reabsorption of water in the renal tubules.)

GOLDBLATT, H.: Am. J. Clin. Path., 1940, *10*, 40. (The kidney and hypertension.)

GOVAN, A. D. T.: J. Path. and Bact., 1954, *67*, 311. (Renal changes in eclampsia.)

GROLLMAN, A.: Arch. Int. Med., 1951, *87*, 379. (Renal hypertension.)

HALL, G. F. M.: J. Path. and Bact., 1952, *64*, 103. (Renal atheroma in diabetes.)

HAMILTON, J. D. and FREMES, N. E.: Am. J. Path., 1954, *30*, 127. (Natural history of experimental glomerulonephritis.)

HARDWICKE, J.: Proc. Roy. Soc. Med., 1954, *47*, 832. (Electrophoretic pattern of blood in nephrosis.)

HARRISON, C. V., MILNE, M. D. and STEINER, R. E.: Quart. J. Med., 1956, *15*, 285. (Renal vein thrombosis.)

HARTROFT, P. M.: J. Exper. Med., 1957, *105*, 501, and also to be published. (Juxtaglomerular cells and renin.)

HARTROFT, W. S.: Am. J. Path., 1953, *29*, 576. (Glomerular fat emboli in diabetes.)

HARTROFT, P. M. and HARTROFT, W. S.: J. Exper. Med., 1955, *102*, 205. (Juxtaglomerular cells.)

HEINEMANN, H. O., DEMARTINI, F. E. and LARAGH, J. H.: Am. J. Med., 1959, *26*, 853. (Effect of chlorothiazide on renal excretion of electrolytes and free water.)

JACKSON, W. P. U. and LINDER, G. C.: Quart. J. Med., 1953, *22*, 133. (Innate functional defects of renal tubules.)

JONES, D. B.: Am. J. Path., 1957, *33*, 313. (Nephrotic glomerulonephritis.)

KARK, R. M. *et al.*: Ann. Int. Med., 1958, *49*, 751. (The nephrotic syndrome in adults.)

KIMMELSTIEL, P.: Am. J. Path., 1938, *14*, 737. (Acute interstitial nephritis.)

————: South. Med. J., 1953, *46*, 175. (Classification of nephroses.)

KIMMELSTIEL, P. and WILSON, C.: Am. J. Path., 1936, *12*, 83. (Intercapillary glomerulosclerosis.)

KLEEMAN, C. R., HEWITT, W. L., and GUZE, L. B.: Medicine, 1960, *39*, 3. (Pyelonephritis.)

KRAKOWER, C. A. and GREENSPON, S. A.: Arch. Path., 1951, *51*, 629; 1958, *66*, 364. (Localization of nephrotonic antigens in extraglomerular tissues.)

KULKA, J. P., PEARSON, C. M. and ROBBINS, S. L.: Am. J. Path., 1950, *26*, 349. (Vacuolar nephropathy.)

KURTZ, S. M. and McMANUS, J. F. A.: Am. Heart J., 1959, *58*, 357. (Structure of glomerulus.)

LINDVALL, N.: Acta. Radiol., Stockholm, 1960, suppl. 192. (Papillary necrosis.)

LUCKÉ, B.: Mil. Surgeon, 1946, *99*, 371. (Lower nephron nephrosis.)

LUETSCHER, J. A. JR. and JOHNSON, B. B.: J. Clin. Investig., 1954, *33*, 276. (Sodium retention in nephrosis.)

Luxton, R. W.: Quart. J. Med., 1953, 22, 215. (Radiation nephritis.)

Maegraith, B. G., Havard, R. E. and Parsons, D. S.: Lancet, 1945, 2, 293. (Renal anoxia.)

Mallory, G. K., Crane, A. R. and Edwards, J. D.: Arch. Path., 1940, 30, 330. (Obstruction in pyelonephritis.)

Mallory, T. B.: Am. J. Clin. Path., 1947, 17, 427. (Acute tubular nephrosis.)

Masugi, M.: Beitr. Path. Anat., 1933, 91, 82. (Production of glomerulonephritis with heterologous antiserum.)

McManus, J. F. A.: Quart. J. Micro. Sc., 1947, 88, 39. (Glomerular root of vertebrate kidney.)

————: Proc. Am. Diabetes Assn., 1949, 9, 301. (Intercapillary glomerulosclerosis.)

————: Medical Diseases of the Kidney, Philadelphia, 1950.

————: South. Med. J., 1952, 45, 24. (Glomerular disappearance.)

McManus, J. F. A. and Mowry, R. W.: Bull. Int. Ass. Med. Museums, 1948, 28, 80. (Alkaline phosphatase.)

McManus, J. F. A. and Lupton, C. H. Jr.: Lab. Invest., 1953, 2, 76. (5-Nucleotidase); 1960, 9, 413. (Ischemic glomerular obsolescence.)

Mellors, R. C.: Am. J. Path., 1955, 31, 687. J. Histochem. and Cytochem., 1955, 3, 284. (Antigen-antibody reaction in glomerulonephritis.)

Mellors, R. C. and Ortega, L. G.: Am. J. Path., 1956, 32, 455. (Localizing gamma globulins in glomerulonephritis.)

Movat, H. Z.: Am. J. Path., 1959, 35, 708. (The glomerulus in renal amyloidosis.) Am. J. Path., 1959, 35, 670. (Fine structure of the glomerulus in nephrosis.)

Movat, H. Z. and MacGregor, D. D.: Am. J, Path., 1959, 35, 670. Am. J. Clin. Path., 1959. 32, 109. (Fine structure of the glomerulus in lipoid nephrosis.)

Muehrcke, R. C., Kark, R. M. and Pirani, C. L.: New Eng. J. Med., 1955, 253, 537. (Needle biopsy of kidney.)

Muirhead, E. E. et al.: J.A.M.A., 1950, 142, 627. (Papillitis necroticans.)

Nicholson, T. F.: Can. J. Biochem., 1957, 35, 419, 641. (Site of acidification in the dog's kidney.)

Oliver, J.: The Architecture of the Kidney in Chronic Bright's Disease, New York, 1939. Am. J. Med., 1950, 9, 88. (Dynamic morphology of the nephron.)

Ortega, L. G. and Mellors, R. C.: J. Exper. Med., 1956, 104, 151. (Fluorescent antibodies in nephrotoxic nephritis.)

Pitcock, J. A. and Hartroft, Phyllis, M.: Am. J. Path., 1958, 34, 863. (Juxtaglomerular cells.)

Platt, R.: Lancet, 1959, 1, 160. (The kidney and electrolyte loss.)

Pollak, V. E., Kark, R. M. et al.: Am. J. Med., 1956, 21, 496. (Renal vein thrombosis and the nephrotic kidney.)

Raphael, S. S. and Lynch, M. J. G.: Arch. Path., 1958, 65, 420. (Kimmelstiel-Wilson glomerulonephropathy.)

Relman, A. S. and Schwartz, W. B.: New Eng. J. Med., 1956, 255, 195. (Neuropathy of potassium depletion.)

Rich, A. R.: Bull. Johns Hopkins Hosp., 1942, 71, 123, 375. (Sulphonamide nephritis.)

Rhaney, K. and Mitchell, R. G.: Lancet, 1956, 1, 1028. (Idiopathic hypercalcemia of infants.)

Rosenheim, M. L.: Ann. Roy. Coll. Surg., 1951, 9, 102. (Uremia.)

Schreiner, G. E.: Arch. Int. Med., 1958, 102, 32. (Pyelonephritis.)

Sevitt, S.: Lancet, 1959, 2, 135. (Pathogenesis of traumatic uremia.)

Sheehan, H. L. and Moore, H. C.: Renal Cortical Necrosis and the Kidney of Concealed Accidental Haemorrhage, Oxford, 1952.

Skeggs, L. T. Jr. and Kahn, J. R.: Circulation, 1958, 17, 658. (Renal pressor system in hypertension.)

Smith, Homer W.: The Kidney: Structure and Function in Health and Disease, New York, 1951.

Spiro, D.: Am. J. Path., 1959, 35, 47. (Structural basis of proteinuria.)

Talbot, H. S.: J.A.M.A., 1958, 168, 1595. (The role of the ureter in ascending pyelonephritis.)

Thal, A.: Am. J. Path., 1955, 31, 233. (Bilateral cortical necrosis.)

Trueta, J., et al.: Lancet, 1946, 2, 237. (Renal anoxia.)

Volhard, F. and Fahr, K. T.: Die Brightsche Nierenkrankheit, Berlin, 1914.

Wachstein, M.: J. Histochem. and Cytochem., 1955, 3, 246. (Tubular enzymes.)

Wakerlin, G. C.: Circulation, 1958, 17, 653.

Weiss, S. and Parker, F. Jr.: Medicine, 1939, 18, 221. (Pyelonephritis.)

Willis, R. A.: Pathology of Tumors, London, 1953. (Adenoma of kidney.)

Wilson, G. and Byrom, F. B.: Quart. J. Med., 1941, 10, 65. (The vicious circle in chronic Bright's disease.)

Wilson, C., Ledingham, J. M. and Cohen, M.: Lancet, 1958, 1, 9. (Hypertension following irradiation of the kidneys.)

Chapter 24

The Respiratory System

THE NOSE
The Common Cold
Granulomata
    MALIGNANT GRANULOMA
Tumors

THE LARYNX
Laryngitis
    EDEMA OF THE GLOTTIS
Tumors
    PAPILLOMA
    CARCINOMA

THE BRONCHI
Bronchitis
    ACUTE TRACHEOBRONCHITIS
    CHRONIC BRONCHITIS
    FIBRINOUS BRONCHITIS
    BRONCHIOLITIS FIBROSA
      OBLITERANS
Bronchial Asthma
Bronchiectasis
    MIDDLE LOBE SYNDROME

THE LUNGS
General Considerations
    STRUCTURE
      Bronchopulmonary Segments
      Musculature
      Alveolar Membranes
    FUNCTION
      Ventilation
      Gaseous Interchange
The Bacterial Pneumonias
    LOBAR (PNEUMOCOCCAL)
      PNEUMONIA
    BRONCHOPNEUMONIA
      Streptococcal Pneumonia
      Staphylococcal Pneumonia
      Friedländer's Bacillus
      Pneumonia
The Viral Pneumonias
    INFLUENZAL PNEUMONIA
    PRIMARY ATYPICAL PNEUMONIA
    PSITTACOSIS
    Q FEVER
    GIANT CELL PNEUMONIA
    INCLUSION-DISEASE PNEU-
      MONITIS
Non-Bacterial Inflammations
    LIPOID PNEUMONIA
    LÖFFLER'S PNEUMONIA
    IRRADIATION PNEUMONITIS
    HAMMAN-RICH SYNDROME

CHOLESTEROL PNEUMONITIS
UREMIC PNEUMONITIS
PULMONARY MICROLITHIASIS
The Occupational Pneumoconioses
    SILICOSIS
    ANTHRACOSIS
      Rheumatoid Pneumoconiosis
    ASBESTOSIS
    ASPERGILLOSIS
    BERYLLIUM PNEUMONITIS
    BAUXITE FIBROSIS
    GRAPHITE FIBROSIS
    BYSSINOSIS
    SILO-FILLER'S DISEASE
    FARMER'S LUNG
Abscess and Gangrene
Tuberculosis
    PRIMARY INFECTION
    HEALING WITH FIBROSIS
    CHRONIC FIBROCASEOUS
      TUBERCULOSIS
    ACUTE TUBERCULOUS CASEOUS
      PNEUMONIA
    ACUTE MILIARY TUBERCULOSIS
    TUBERCULOUS LESIONS AFTER
      CHEMOTHERAPY
      Chromogenic Acid-fast
      Bacillary Infections
Syphilis
Mycotic and Other Granulomas
    BLASTOMYCOSIS
    ACTINOMYCOSIS
    STREPTOTHRICOSIS
    ASPERGILLOSIS
    COCCIDIOIDOMYCOSIS
    HISTOPLASMOSIS
    CRYPTOCOCCOSIS (TORULOSIS)
    PNEUMOCYSTIS PNEUMONIA
    OTHER MYCOTIC GRANULOMAS
    PULMONARY ALVEOLAR
      PROTEINOSIS
    PULMONARY SARCOIDOSIS
Circulatory Disturbances
    ACUTE CONGESTION
    PASSIVE CONGESTION
      Brown Induration
      Hypostatic Congestion
      Idiopathic Pulmonary Hemo-
      siderosis
    PULMONARY EDEMA
      Inflammatory Edema
      Mechanical Edema
    HYALINE MEMBRANE DISEASE

EMBOLISM AND INFARCTION
    Fat Embolism
PULMONARY HYPERTENSION
    AND ARTERIOSCLEROSIS
ARTERIOVENOUS ANEURYSM
    Digital Clubbing
Atelectasis
    CONGENITAL
    COMPRESSION
    OBSTRUCTIVE
    ACUTE MASSIVE COLLAPSE
Emphysema
    OBSTRUCTIVE
    COMPENSATORY
    ATROPHIC OR SENILE
    INTERSTITIAL
Tumors of the Lung
    BRONCHOGENIC CARCINOMA
      Incidence
      Etiology
    ALVEOLAR CELL CARCINOMA
    ADENOMA OF BRONCHUS
      Hamartoma
      Pancoast's Syndrome
    SECONDARY TUMORS
Congenital Anomalies
    CONGENITAL CYSTIC LUNG
    INTRALOBAR SEQUESTRATION

THE PLEURA
Pleurisy
    FIBRINOUS
    PLEURISY WITH EFFUSION
    EMPYEMA
Hydrothorax
    MEIGS' SYNDROME
Hemothorax
    CHYLOTHORAX
Pneumothorax
Tumors of the Pleura
    PRIMARY TUMORS
      Localized
      Diffuse: Mesothelioma
    SECONDARY CARCINOMA

THE MEDIASTINUM
Mediastinal Tumors and Cysts
    NEUROGENIC TUMORS
    TERATOID TUMORS
    MEDIASTINAL CYSTS
      Bronchial Cyst
      Other Cysts
    LYMPH NODE TUMORS

THE NOSE

THE COMMON COLD

THE common cold is an acute rhinitis or inflammation of the nasal cavities, with extension to the nasopharynx and it may be the nasal sinuses. This acute epidemic respiratory disease is characterized by rhinorrhea, nasal obstruction and sneezing. Nasal discharge is abundant, thin and watery for two or three days, then it becomes thick and purulent. The characteristic features of the secretion of the early stage are the great numbers of ciliated epithelial cells and the striking absence of bacteria. When the discharge becomes thick and purulent it is likely to contain pneumococci, staphylococci or streptococci. The disease may abort after twenty-four or forty-eight hours. Only too often, however, secondary invaders convert the acute into a chronic disease which may drag on for many weary weeks.

The etiological agent is a virus, which has already been discussed on page 342. The virus is spread with extreme readiness from one person to another, and, unlike most viruses, it fails to confer any immunity upon the infected person, so that he may suffer from several attacks in the course of a winter. *Contributing factors*, as is well known, play an important part. Of these the most important is chilling of the body as the result of sitting in a draught, wet feet, etc. In the absence of the virus no amount of chilling can cause a cold, as is shown by the immunity of travellers in the Arctic and of men compelled to spend many weeks at sea on rafts or in open boats.

The mucous membranes of the respiratory passages are acutely inflamed, with involvement first of the throat, then the nose, and later, if secondary infection is marked, the trachea, bronchi, and nasal sinuses. In the early acute stage the nasal mucosa is red from hyperemia and swollen from edema. *Microscopically*, there are small numbers of neutrophils, lymphocytes, plasma cells, and sometimes large numbers of eosinophils, but the striking feature is edema. As is but natural, in the later stages when secondary invaders assume command large numbers of neutrophils make their appearance.

GRANULOMATA

Many granulomatous infections may involve the nose. They all show a formation of new tissue, followed by necrosis, ulceration, and destruction of the septum.

SYPHILIS.—Syphilis of the nose used to be common. It may be congenital or acquired. The *congenital* form may cause an atrophic rhinitis with foul-smelling discharge. Or it may destroy the septum, cartilage, and bone so that the bridge falls in, giving the *saddle nose* so characteristic of congenital syphilis.

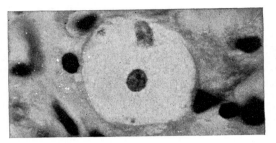

FIG. 358.—Mikulicz cell in rhinoscleroma. × 1000.

The *acquired* tertiary lesion is a gumma which perforates the septum and may destroy the bridge of the nose so as to give the more uncommon "saddle nose" of acquired syphilis.

TUBERCULOSIS.—Tuberculosis of the nose is rare, and is usually a complication of pulmonary tuberculosis. It is likely to produce an ulcerative lesion of the cartilaginous part of the septum.

LEPROSY.—Leprosy starts as a nodule which enlarges, undergoes ulceration, and may cause perforation of the septum.

RHINOSCLEROMA.—Rhinoscleroma is a disease of inhabitants of Eastern Europe. As the name implies, the lesion of the nose is peculiarly hard (*rhin*, nose; *sclera*, hard). The condition commences in the nose, but tends to spread to the pharynx. It is at first proliferative and then destructive. The microscopic diagnosis is made from the presence of peculiar large, round clear cells filled with a gelatinous material which may give the cytoplasm a foamy or reticulated appearance, and displace the nucleus to one side. These are known as Mikulicz cells. They are often filled with bacilli resembling Friedländer's pneumobacillus. This bacillus has been called Bacillus rhinoscleromatis, but it is by no means certain that the disease is caused by this organism.

GLANDERS.—Glanders is a very rare infection of the nose in man, although common in the horse. As usual, there is proliferation followed by destruction. The glanders bacilli are present in the secretion. The bacteriology and pathological lesions are given on page 280.

MALIGNANT GRANULOMA.—This rare, terrible and little understood disease may occur at any age. Following a prolonged prodromal period characterized by stuffiness of the nose, an ulcer develops on the nostril or nasal septum which slowly increases in size until the bones of the face and the palate are destroyed and death ensues from meningitis or bronchopneumonia. The final picture is one of hideous disfigurement of the face and erosion of the skull and large arteries.

The microscopic lesions are granulomatous in type with epithelioid cells, giant cells and lymphocytes, but the most striking feature is intense necrosis resembling that of an infarct and possibly due to a marked degree of obliterating arteritis which accompanies the condition. In spite of its name, which it owes to its relentless progress, there is no microscopic evidence of malignant neoplasia. The cause is unknown, possibly a virus or a local tissue hypersensitivity. A more detailed discussion of the nature of this baffling disease will be found in a well illustrated paper by Robertson and Milliken.

TUMORS

Tumors of the nasal cavity are usually polypoid in type. The commonest form of nasal polyp is not really a tumor, but an edematous mass of inflamed and hypertrophied mucous membrane. It is usually attached to the lateral wall near the opening of the antrum of Highmore, and hangs down as a soft mucoid globular mass with a well-defined pedicle. Sometimes a proliferation of mucous glands may suggest an adenoma. Carcinoma is uncommon and sarcoma still more rare.

THE LARYNX

LARYNGITIS

Infections of the nasopharynx will readily spread down and infections of the bronchi spread up to the larynx. We may recognize the following forms of laryngitis: simple, diphtheritic, tuberculous, and syphilitic.

Simple Laryngitis.—The inflammation is usually *acute*. It may form part of a common cold or may occur in the course of one of the infectious fevers, especially measles and scarlet fever. Pneumococci, streptococci, and Micrococcus catarrhalis are the commonest organisms. Non-bacterial irritants such as steam and chlorine gas may cause violent inflammation. The lesions are those of acute inflammation of any mucous membrane. The membrane is swollen and congested and is covered by mucus poured out by the glands. Microscopically it is infiltrated with inflammatory cells.

Chronic laryngitis may be caused by excessive smoking, chronic alcoholism, or undue use of the vocal cords. The surface of the mucous membrane is dry and covered by small papillary projections. The epithelium is thickened and opaque (pachydermia). The submucosa is infiltrated with chronic inflammatory cells. In typhoid fever there may be swelling of the lymphoid tissue of the larynx, and in rare cases ulceration of the cartilage.

DIPHTHERITIC LARYNGITIS. — Diphtheria is primarily a disease of the pharynx, but the infection frequently spreads to the larynx. A "false membrane" consisting of fibrin, leukocytes, and necrotic epithelial cells is formed on the surface, but is firmly attached to the underlying tissue. A membranous type of laryngitis may also occur in streptococcal and other severe infections.

TUBERCULOUS LARYNGITIS.—This is practically always secondary to pulmonary tuberculosis. It is fortunately not nearly as common as might be expected. Tubercles are formed in the subepithelial tissue. These undergo necrosis, and shallow lenticular ulcers are formed on the surface. The disease begins in the arytenoid region or the vocal cords, and may spread extensively so as to involve all other parts of the larynx. Eventually there may be widespread destruction of the cartilages and the epiglottis, a peculiarly distressing condition because food tends to pass down into the trachea and lungs.

SYPHILITIC LARYNGITIS.—In the secondary stage there may be catarrh or mucous patches. In the tertiary stage there is destruction followed by healing and scar formation. Papillary masses of new tissue may be formed. The scarring leads to distortion of the larynx, stenosis of the glottis, and a characteristic hoarseness of the voice.

Edema of the Glottis.—Edema of the glottis occurs in the course of an acute inflammation such as diphtheria or that caused by the inhalation of steam, irritating gases, etc. It may be part of an angioneurotic edema, but seldom forms part of a general cardiac or renal edema. There is great swelling of the loose tissue in the posterior wall of the pharynx, the false vocal cords, etc. The parts are very swollen and boggy. The edema may develop acutely and may cause death from suffocation.

TUMORS

Papilloma.—This is the commonest tumor of the larynx. It is a small warty growth composed of loose connective tissue, and usually arises from the vocal cords or the anterior commissure. It is common in singers and others who have to use the voice much. The tumor behaves differently in adults and children. In the adult it shows a strong tendency to recur after removal, and occasionally, though rarely, becomes malignant. In the child there is also a strong tendency to recur, no matter how radical the removal, but the new tumors are often at other sites in the larynx, and in time there is most likely to be spontaneous cure. In children, therefore, multiple recurrent papilloma is a benign self-limited disease.

Nodular Fibroma.—This is not uncommon in children. It is a small sessile growth composed of vascular connective tissue.

Carcinoma.—Cancer of the larynx is essentially a male disease, and often shows a definite relation to chronic irritation, such as overuse of the voice or abuse of tobacco and alcohol. Two forms may be recognized, intrinsic and extrinsic. The *intrinsic* form constitutes 80 per cent of the cases, and arises from the vocal cords, usually the anterior third. The tumor, originating from fully differentiated stratified squamous epithelium, often remains confined to the larynx for a considerable time, and offers a good chance of recovery after operative removal as well as being quite radiosensitive. The *extrinsic* form arises in the pyriform fossa, the aryepiglottic folds, or on the epiglottis itself. It involves the hypopharynx, invades the surrounding tissue, and gives rise to early lymph node metastases. This is one form of hypopharyngeal carcinoma. Carcinoma of the larynx begins as a small indurated patch or as a papillary tumor. In the later stages there is extensive destruction, ulceration, and sepsis with the danger of lung abscess or inhalation pneumonia. The intrinsic form is epidermoid, the extrinsic form usually transitional in type.

Sarcoma.—A rare tumor.

THE BRONCHI

BRONCHITIS

Acute Tracheobronchitis.—Acute inflammation of the bronchi affects either the large bronchi and trachea or the small bronchioles. The latter condition is associated with pneumonia, while the former occurs in a pure form which may be called tracheobronchitis.

Etiology.—The irritant may be bacterial, mechanical, or toxic. The bacteriology of acute bronchitis is by no means certain, but it is probable that the pneumococcus, micrococcus catarrhalis, streptococcus, staphylococcus, and influenza bacillus may at different times be responsible. Their presence in the sputum does not prove that they have caused the inflammation in the bronchial wall. Acute bronchitis may complicate any of the infectious fevers, especially the early stages of typhoid. Dust, steam, poisonous gases, and ether may all produce acute tracheobronchitis.

Lesions.—The mucous membrane of the trachea and large bronchi is red, swollen, and covered with a tenacious exudate which may be mucoid or purulent. Microscopically the mucosa is greatly congested and infiltrated with leukocytes. It is remarkable how often the latter are of mononuclear rather than polymorphonuclear type. The ciliated epithelium may be desquamated and the mucous glands are distended with mucus and show marked catarrhal change. The lumen of the bronchus is filled with pus.

Chronic Bronchitis.—Acute bronchitis is a relatively simple condition, which presents no particular problem. The reverse is true of chronic bronchitis. When I was a medical student in Edinburgh chronic bronchitis was one of the commonest diseases in the hospital, but when I came to Canada as a pathologist I seldom heard of the condition. The mortality from chronic bronchitis is said to be 45 times greater in England and Wales than it is in the United States (Flick and Paton). This suggests environmental factors such as climate, social and economic conditions, etc. Another and more potent reason is the fact that the connotation of the term is different in the two countries. In North America, the severe and serious chronic bronchitis of Britain is labelled asthma, emphysema, or bronchiectasis. This makes a satisfactory discussion of the subject singularly difficult.

It might be thought that chronic bronchitis was the result of repeated attacks of acute bronchitis. Such is not the case, for the acute attacks, which are frequent, are rather a result than a cause, and consequent on primary changes in the bronchial wall, more especially the mucous membrane, the normal folds of which become erased, with loss of power of arresting bacteria (Engel). The condition appears to begin with a slight dilatation of the bronchi (bronchiectasis), that leads to structural and functional disorder of the mucosa, which paves the way for further acute attacks, increasing the damage to the mucous membrane and the dilatation of the bronchi. In this way a vicious circle develops, with irreparable damage to the bronchial tree, secondary changes in the lungs, and eventually cor pulmonale.

The occurrence of chronic bronchitis, and more especially bronchiolitis, does not depend so much on the primary etiological agent, be it viral, bacterial or chemical, as on such factors as occlusion of the bronchial lumen by plugs of mucus with consequent retention of bacteria. Secondary bacterial infection is a major factor in the production of permanent damage. Moreover, evidence of old bacterial inflammatory damage of the bronchioles, including complete obliteration, is much more common than was previously believed (McLean).

It will be evident that chronic bronchitis is not, as the name might suggest, a matter of bacteria establishing themselves in the bronchial walls and keeping up the inflammation year after year. It is seldom or never a primary entity, being rather a complication of some preexisting pathological condition which may lie in the heart, the nasal sinuses, or the bronchi themselves. Combined with any of these may be added prolonged and excessive smoking of cigarettes.

Chronic heart disease, valvular or myocardial, is perhaps the most common cause, on account of the continued congestion of the bronchial tree which weakens its resistance to bacterial infection from the nose and throat. So long as the congestion remains, so long will the bronchitis persist.

Infection in the nasal sinuses is another common cause. An antrum or a sinus may be a regular cesspool of infection from which the bronchi are continually being reinfected. The same is true of septic conditions in the oral cavity. It has been well said that in suppurative conditions of the lungs and bronchi it is always well to look for the causes above the clavicle.

Dilatation of the bronchi, i.e., bronchiectasis, is now known to be at the bottom of many cases of chronic bronchitis, thanks to the diagnositic use of bronchography. With dilatation of the lumen a state of affairs is established in which conditions are ideal for a continuance of the infection, for efficient drainage becomes difficult or impossible. The subject of bronchiectasis is discussed later (page 629).

Cigarette smoking, when prolonged and persistent, can be shown statistically to be related to chronic bronchitis. It interferes gravely with the beating of the respiratory cilia whose constant motion night and day keeps the bronchial tubes clean of mucus.

Clinical Picture.—This will depend on the stage of the disease, and what is included in the term chronic bronchitis. The milder cases, which may be called simple chronic bronchitis, are characterized by a persistent cough with viscid mucus, especially in the morning, but no outstanding degree of dyspnea. The advanced cases of what in Britain is called chronic bronchitis and in North America bronchiectasis with emphysema were painted in vivid colors by Fothergill many years ago. "In the out-patient department of a chest hospital the old bronchitic people are still to be seen, a considerable proportion of the whole. With labored respiration and tardy step they enter, puffing and panting, scant of breath, which makes the speech difficult; while a significant shake of the head often tells more eloquently than words of the inward discomfort and that the breathing is embarrassed."

Lesions.—The mucous membrane may be swollen and hypertrophic, and bathed with mucus or pus. In old cases it may become atrophic, so that the wall has a reticulated appearance owing to strands of fibrous tissue which remain. Microscopically all the coats are infiltrated with round cells, but a replacement fibrosis which takes the place of the glands, muscle, and cartilage may be the chief feature. The epithelium is low and cubical, sometimes even flattened.

FIBRINOUS BRONCHITIS.—This is a rare and obscure condition in which the patient coughs up bronchial casts at periodic intervals. The casts are composed of mucin and epithelium rather than true fibrin. In diphtheria and pneumonia bronchial casts composed largely of fibrin may be formed.

Bronchiolitis Fibrosa Obliterans.—Obliterating bronchiolitis is often the result of inhalation of irritating gases, although it may also occur in the course of the infective fevers. Of the irritating gases nitrogen dioxide is the most important. This is formed as the result of the explosion of fuming nitric acid which is now of frequent use in certain industries, particularly in the oxidation of rocket fuel. The wall of the bronchiole may be extensively damaged, a fibrinous exudate forms in the necrotic wall and in the lumen; this becomes organized by fibroblasts and capillaries, so that first granulation tissue and later dense connective tissue replace the bronchiole and its lumen. The organizing exudate often assumes a striking polypoid appearance, projecting into the lumen from the wall of the bronchiole. Beautiful illustrations of the histological lesions will be found in McAdams' paper. The alveoli are collapsed and may be involved in the fibrosis. The gross appearance of obliterating bronchiolitis is that of numerous miliary nodules scattered through the lung. These resemble miliary tubercles, but a slit-like space representing all that remains of the lumen can often be distinguished in the center. In the roentgenogram the appearance may also suggest miliary tuberculosis. The *clinical picture* is what might be expected: an acute phase with marked unremitting dyspnea and cyanosis; a short intermission; a final return of the dyspnea and cyanosis in either an acute or a more slowly progressing form.

BRONCHOLITHIASIS.—Known also as bronchial calculus and lung stone, this term signifies the presence of calculi in a bronchus. The usual origin is a caseous tuberculous focus in the lung or lymph nodes or the inspissated pus of an old lung abscess. The calculus erodes through the bronchial wall, or it may be formed within the lumen of the bronchus. The calculi, which are often multiple, are hard and irregular. They may be expectorated or may remain within the bronchial lumen and cause obstruction. The *early symptoms* are hemoptysis and harassing cough. Later evidence of emphysema and bronchiectasis may develop.

BRONCHIAL ASTHMA

This difficult and distressing disease is well named, for it is derived from the Greek word meaning panting. Other forms of asthma are recognized, such as cardiac asthma in which shortness of breath is a striking feature, but we shall confine our attention to the classical variety of asthma which is *allergic* in origin. The hypersensitivity may be due to a variety of agents, in particular pollens, dusts, foods, drugs and bacteria. It may develop at any age, and it will be appreciated what a tragedy the disease may be when it manifests itself in childhood. We shall return to this subject and to the mode of production of the symptoms after the morbid anatomy has been described. A second etiologic factor is *heredity*. There may be a family history of asthma, and in over half the cases there is evidence of some form of allergy in the family. Finally a *psychosomatic factor* may be evident, the asthmatic attack being precipitated by some form of emotional stress, probably operating through the pituitary-adrenal axis.

Lesions.—In cases where the patient has died during an asthmatic attack the lungs are voluminous and emphysematous, filling the entire pleural cavities. Areas of emphysema alternate with areas of atelectasis or collapse. The meaning of emphysema and atelectasis are discussed later in this chapter.

In asthma, however, there may be no emphysema. A patient may have recurrent attacks of uncomplicated asthma for fifty years without the development of emphysema and the same is true of persons with severe asthma dying in status asthmaticus. On the other hand, patients with chronic bronchitis who die from cor pulmonale or respiratory failure are generally found to have well developed destructive emphysema. If the asthma is caused by or complicated by bronchitis, emphysema may be expected.

The smaller and medium-sized bronchi are occluded with thick, tough and tenacious mucus, which is responsible for the atelectasis (Fig. 358). *Microscopically*, the mucosa is thickened and markedly edematous, and it is infiltrated with cells which are mainly eosinophils, with which are mingled varying numbers of lymphocytes and plasma cells.

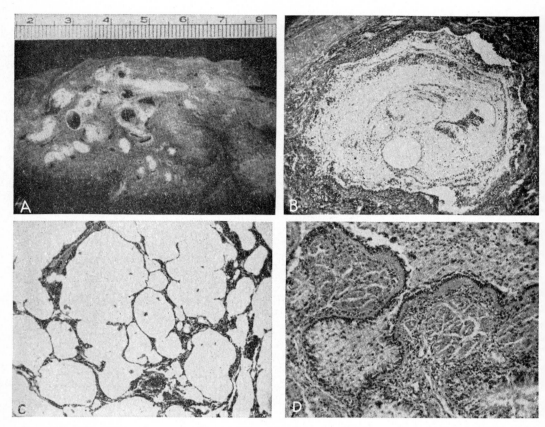

FIG. 359.—Bronchial asthma. *A*, Cross-section of the lung showing the medium sized and small bronchi filled with white mucous plugs, *B*, Low power of a bronchus filled with mucus. Basement membrane is thickened. × 30. *C*, Lung showing emphysema with rupture of alveolar walls. × 48. *D*, Section of bronchial wall showing the lumen filled with mucus, out-pouching, muscular hypertrophy and a thickened, hyalinized basement membrane. × 100. (Walton, Penner and Wilt, courtesy of Canad. Med. Assn. Jour.)

The basement membrane shows a characteristic hyalinized thickening. There may be well marked hypertrophy of the bronchial muscle. This may be regarded as primary, an essential part in the mechanism of the disease, or secondary to expel the air from the alveolar sacs. The submucosal glands are swollen and evidently very active. These various changes add up to a general thickening of the wall with partial or complete obliteration of the lumen by plugs of mucus. The distal pulmonary parenchyma shows emphysema alternating with areas of atelectasis.

Relation of Symptoms to Lesions.—The asthmatic suffers from recurring attacks of paroxysmal dyspnea, a wheezing cough, and a sense of constriction in the chest. Between the attacks he may feel well, but with the passage of time there is likely to be constant shortness of breath with characteristic expiratory wheezing. There can be no doubt that the attack is brought on by fresh or additional exposure to the allergen to which the patient is hypersensitive. The question is: What is the mechanism? The time-honored explanation is that the bronchial muscle undergoes spasmodic contraction, thus narrowing the lumen of the bronchioles with resulting dyspnea. The value of antispasmodics in relieving the attack would support this view. One cannot but be impressed, however, by the postmortem picture in those cases where death is evidently due to the acute asthmatic attack. Here the patient has evidently been choked by the amount of tenacious mucus poured out by the bronchial glands, and it is unnecessary to invoke any hypothetical contraction of plain muscle (Walton *et al.*). Although many asthmatics "pant on to a good old age," the disease is one of the occasional causes of sudden death, the patient dying of suffocation, often after the unwise use of sedatives. The beneficial effect of epinephrine may be explained by its action on the edematous mucosa rather than on the muscle, as is seen in the nose and elsewhere. Increased capillary permeability and edema are basic features of the allergic reaction, as is the presence of numerous eosinophils. These cells are present not only in the wall of the bronchus but also in the blood in greatly increased numbers (up to 30 per cent) and in the sputum. The combination of *blood*, *sputum*, and *tissue eosinophilia* is only found in this one disease. Spasmodic contraction of the bronchial musculature may well play a part in constricting the air passages, but we have already seen that the muscular hypertrophy may well be secondary rather than primary in character. Much of the respiratory disability in advanced chronic cases may be attributed to the emphysema and atelectasis caused by obstruction to the airways by mucous plugs. Auscultation in these cases reveals the sounds of inspiration to be brief and almost inaudible, compared with prolonged expiration which is accompanied by loud whistling, squeaking, groaning sounds that for some extraordinary reason are commonly described by the clinician as "musical" sounds. Curschmann spirals, often found in the sputum, consist of mucus poured out by the overactive glands. Charcot-Leyden crystals, also present, may be derived from the eosinophil cells.

The difficult prolongation of the expiratory phase of ventilation leads inevitably to a reduction of the vital capacity and diminution in the tidal air. There is therefore an increase in residual (stale) air and a corresponding reduction in the arterial oxygen saturation. The result of all this is retention of carbon dioxide with resulting fatigue of the respiratory center from overstrain so that it ceases to function normally. Respiration now becomes regulated by receptors in the carotid bodies and aorta, so that each breath is an effort stimulated by the insatiable demand for air.

BRONCHIECTASIS

A dilatation of the bronchi, either local or general is known as bronchiectasis. Stagnation of the bronchial contents follows the dilatation, with resulting infection and suppuration. Minor degrees of the condition are common, although often missed clinically unless bronchography is used.

Etiology.—The two main factors are infection and bronchial obstruction. The *infection* causes chronic inflammation of the bronchial walls with destruction of the musculo-elastic tissue resulting in dilatation of the part of the bronchial tree whose walls are damaged; the pathogenesis is the same as that of aortic aneurysm. The dilatation favors accumulation of secretion with added infection and further injury to the bronchial wall. There may be a physiological block due to paralysis of the cilia from infection or metaplasia of the columnar epithelium into a squamous type, thus interfering with the normal mechanism for the removal of secretion. A marked obliterating endarteritis may still further lower the resistance of the bronchial walls. In young children the process tends to be more acute, so that the first lesion is an ulcerative bronchitis with secondary destruction of the bronchial wall.

The acute infection, commonly occurring in childhood, may be measles or whooping cough, and occasionally influenza or pneumonia. The actual onset of symptoms is insidious, and is not ushered in by any acute illness. Neither gross upper respiratory tract infection nor chronic bronchitis is a common cause of bronchiectasis. Spirilla and fusiform bacilli are frequently found in the walls of the dilated bronchi, but it seems more probable that these are secondary invaders than primary etiological agents.

Obstruction of the bronchi leads to accumulation and stagnation of secretion, infection and weakening of the bronchial wall. The obstruction may be due to a tumor, a foreign body, or pressure from without by aneurysm, etc.

The pathogenesis of bronchiectasis is more involved, obscure and controversial than the

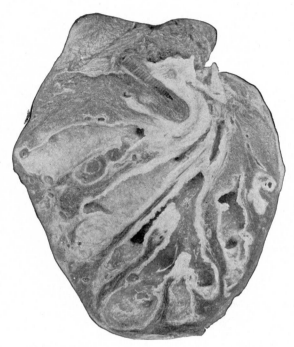

FIG. 360.—Bronchiectasis, showing widespread involvement of a lobe which has been removed surgically.

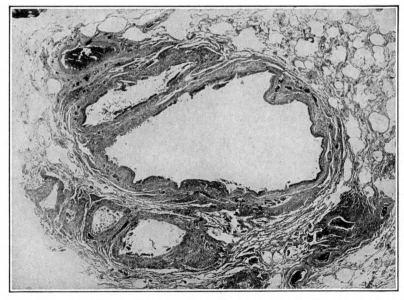

FIG. 361.—Bronchiectasis. Several small bronchi are dilated; their walls show fibrous thickening. × 12.

foregoing account would indicate. As Mallory points out, a single agent is seldom sufficient to produce the condition. In his opinion bronchial inflammation in combination with atelectasis or pneumonitis will account for most of the features of the disease.

Lesions.—Bronchiectasis may be diffuse (*cylindrical form*) or localized (*saccular form*). The former is the more common. It is usually bilateral, but it is rather remarkable that quite often it is unilateral. For some unknown reason the left lung is more often involved than the right, and the lower lobes more often than the upper owing to stasis. Only one lobe may be affected. The size of the cavity depends on the size of the bronchus. It is filled with pus which stagnates there owing to insufficient drainage, and still further weakens the wall of the bronchus. The mucosa is hypertrophic and may form tumor-like, highly vascular papillary masses. Later there may be atrophy. One of the most characteristic features is that the smaller bronchi and bronchioles are dilated to such a degree that they can be followed as far as the pleural surface. This is never the case in the normal lung. (Fig. 360). The *microscopic appearance* is similar to that of chronic abscess. The wall of the bronchus and the surrounding tissue is infiltrated with chronic inflammatory cells. The mucosa may be hypertrophic or atrophic, and in advanced cases the muscle, glands, elastic tissue, and even the cartilage may be replaced by fibrous tissue (Fig. 361). The most significant lesion is the destruction of the bronchial musculature and elastic tissue, for it is these which weaken the wall and allow the dilatation to occur. Septic thrombosis may occur with embolism and the formation of a secondary brain abscess.

Liebow and his associates have shown by preparing casts of the vessels by the vinylite corrosion technique that a remarkable enlargement of the bronchial arteries occurs and that a rich anastomosis with the pulmonary arteries develops. So great is this enlargement and anastomosis that they estimate that more than a liter of blood per minute flows through this collateral circulation, which may well have some physiological importance, for it tends to produce pulmonary hypertension.

Middle Lobe Syndrome.—This is a combination of atelectasis and bronchiectasis affecting the middle lobe of the right lung. It was first recognized in relation to tuberculosis, but it is now recognized that the same changes can develop in non-tuberculous cases. They are caused by compression of the bronchus to the middle lobe by enlarged firm mediastinal lymph nodes, which leave an indentation on the under surface of the bronchus (Graham *et al.*). In addition to atelectasis the bronchi are dilated and present the usual picture of bronchiectasis. The clinical picture is that of the latter disease.

Relation of Symptoms to Lesions.—The chief symptom is due to the chief lesion, the patient bringing up large quantities of *pus* at infrequent intervals, often when he changes position (*postural coughing* due to the pus coming in contact with a new and more sensitive part of the bronchial wall), or on awakening in the morning when the pools of stinking pus which have accumulated during the night are rapidly emptied. One of the biggest problems in *advanced* cases is the exceedingly foul breath which makes a social outcast of the unfortunate victim, so that he tends to live a life alone, apart, helpless and hopeless. The morbidity, indeed, is a greater problem than the mortality, and suicide may end the tragic history. *Hemorrhage* (*hemoptysis*) is common, occurring in 60 per cent of cases, and is due to the highly vascular papillary masses of mucosa which may line the walls, or to erosion of vessels passing through the cavity. *Clubbing of the fingers and toes* may develop in cases with marked ventilatory insufficiency, dyspnea and cyanosis. The intermingling of the pulmonary and systemic circulation demonstrated by Liebow's work may possibly be the cause of the clubbing, a matter which is discussed later on page 673. *Lipiodol* or other radioopaque material introduced into the bronchial tree outlines with beautiful distinctness the bronchial dilatations.

The development of knowledge of the *bronchopulmonary segments*, discussed in the next section, has greatly influenced the surgical approach to the disease, for these segments are not only anatomical units, but pathological units as well. The segment is a section of lung parenchyma more or less com-

pletely separated from neighboring segments by fibrous septa and supplied by a
bronchus of the second order of division.
The arteries follow the bronchi intraseg-
mentally, so that a segment rather than an
entire lobe can be removed. As bronchiectasis may be confined to one or more
segments, the practical importance of this
concept becomes apparent. The best illustration is provided by the lingula, the lowest
segment of the left upper lobe, corresponding
to the middle lobe of the right lung. The
lingula is involved in 80 per cent of left lower
lobe bronchiectasis, and can be dissected
free from the remainder of the left upper lobe.

THE LUNGS

GENERAL CONSIDERATIONS

The cardiovascular system, the kidneys,
and the lungs form an integrated mechanism
by means of which the constancy of the internal environment is maintained. We have
seen in the preceding chapter how the cardiovascular system and the kidneys work together to maintain electrolyte and acid-base
balance. Similarly the lungs and the heart
may be considered as a dual organ whose
function it is to supply the tissues with oxygen and to remove carbon dioxide. Two of
the most important symptoms of congestive
heart failure, namely dyspnea and cyanosis,
are pulmonary in origin, due to imbalance of
the two sides of the heart, increased output of
the right side or diminished output of the
left side resulting in congestion and dysfunction of the lungs. On the other side diffuse
pulmonary lesions may throw an intolerable
strain on the right heart.

Structure.—In this chapter we shall be
concerned with the structural changes in the
lung produced by various disease processes.
In addition it may be pointed out that the
lung differs from all other organs in being
able to hide nothing of its structure from the
roentgenologist, who regards it as a window
through which he may look into the body in
search of the disseminated disease. It is
indeed a delicate mirror in which is reflected
not only the evidence of pulmonary disease,
but lesions resulting from general or disseminated processes such as sarcoidosis and the
collagen diseases.

The *weight* of the right lung is 350 to 550
gm., that of the left lung 325 to 450 gm. The
texture is soft and pillowy. Owing to its *air
content* it crepitates when pressed between
the finger and thumb, and floats in water.
These properties are lost when the air has
been squeezed out of the lung by pressure
from without or has been replaced by inflammatory exudate or edema fluid. The
pleural lymphatics contain carbon, and thus
outline in black the polygonal lobules which
give the surface a mozaic appearance. In
actual practice it is rare to find a lung that is
perfectly normal throughout in color and
consistence, because during the last hours of
life blood tends to collect in the loose pulmonary tissue, and even after death blood
gravitates to the dependent part of the lung,
rendering it darker and firmer than normal.

The general structure of the lung is too
familiar to the reader to need recapitulation,
but reference may be made to the bronchopulmonary segments, the musculature, and
the alveolar membranes. For the comprehensive study of structural changes in the
lung, Gough's method of large sections of the
whole lung mounted on paper is unequalled.
These macrosections give an extremely informative morphologic map of the lung,
which is of particular value for the correlation of structure with function, and for comparison with radiograms taken during life
(Wyatt). We shall refer to this method
again in the discussion on emphysema
(page 675).

Bronchopulmonary Segments.—In the discussion on bronchiectasis we have seen that
the five lobes of the lungs are divided into
broncho-pulmonary segments, smaller and
more accurate units of localization which
correspond to smaller divisions of the bronchial vascular tree (Brock). Embryologically, each of the segments is represented by a
bronchial bud, so that many of the congenital
anomalies of the lung have a segmental basis.
Each segment is a complete anatomical unit,
having its own segmental bronchus of the
second order, pulmonary artery and vein,
and bronchial artery. It is an independent
unit, with little significant vascular and
bronchial communication with adjacent segments. Moreover it is also a pathological
unit, for aspirated material tends to be seg-

mental in distribution as we have seen in the case of bronchiectasis. Although the segments are more or less completely separated from the contiguous parenchyma by fibrous septa, they can hardly be recognized by the naked eye, but the surgeon is guided as to their location by the distribution of the bronchi and arteries, and by limiting his resection to the segments involved, he can conserve those unaffected. A discussion of the relation of gross congenital anomalies to the development of the bronchial segments as well as every other feature of segmental anatomy is contained in Boyden's great monograph on the subject.

Musculature.—In a very real sense the lungs are muscular organs, for in properly stained sections there is hardly an area without smooth muscle, and in many types of chronic pulmonary disease this muscle undergoes a remarkable degree of hypertrophy and hyperplasia (Liebow *et al.*). During inspiration the elastic recoil shortens the duct and contraction of the muscle narrows the lumen. As there is no elastic tissue in the walls of the alveoli they are not collapsed in expiration, so that the residual air which they contain can only escape by diffusion through the alveolar membrane. The part which spasm of the smooth muscle may play in asthma has already been mentioned.

Alveolar Membranes.—The respiratory parenchyma consists of thin partitions which separate the alveolar air-spaces. These partitions are perforated by the alveolar *pores of Kohn*, which provide a communication and therefore a means of collateral ventilation should the respiratory bronchiole become occluded. We shall return to the subject of a collateral ventilation in the discussion of emphysema. The alveolar walls, nourished by the bronchial arteries coming from the aorta, are composed of cells, capillaries of the pulmonary artery, and interstitial connective tissue. For one hundred years controversy has raged as to whether or not the alveolar walls are lined by epithelium, and as to the nature and function of the various cells present within the walls. Electron microscopy and histochemical methods have helped to answer these questions. (Bertalanffy and Leblond). The walls are now known to be lined by squamous epithelium, which in

electron micrographs are seen to be low flat cells with extremely attenuated nuclei. The periodic acid-Schiff stain reveals a definite basement membrane. The cells within the walls, which in the past have been known as septal cells, epicytes, dust cells, etc., are probably best named alveolar cells. They are connective tissue in nature, and are of two types, vacuolated and nonvacuolated. Both have the ability to ingest foreign particles and to progress by ameboid motion.

When the alveolar membranes become thickened as the result of disease the result is *alveolar-capillary block*. The block affects the passage of oxygen to a much greater degree than is the case with carbon dioxide, because the latter is much more diffusible. The result is arterial oxygen desaturation, but usually without a corresponding rise in CO_2. Alveolar-capillary block occurs in diffuse pulmonary fibrosis, in pulmonary edema, and in some of the dust diseases, berylliosis in particular.

Function.—Just as the kidney has two functions, namely excretion and the regulation of the internal environment, so the lungs have a double task, respiration and the maintenance of the acid-base balance. When the acid-base balance is temporarily upset it can be restored to normal much more quickly by blowing off CO_2 than by the excretion of acid by the kidneys. Normal pulmonary function depends on two entirely different processes: (1) ventilation, (2) gaseous interchange, which is the true respiratory and more important phase of pulmonary function. Needless to say, adequate pulmonary circulation is also essential, for without it respiration becomes meaningless.

Ventilation.—The term ventilation indicates the mechanical displacement of gases. This displacement, which represents the vital capacity, is effected by the muscles of the thoracic cage and the diaphragm, which have been compared to a pair of bellows. Ventilatory insufficiency resulting in dyspnea is far more common than inadequate gaseous interchange. It may be caused in two ways. (1) *By reduction in the vital capacity* either (a) by reason of weakening of the bellows from poliomyelitis or other causes, or (b) from displacement of the alveolar air by exudate or by collapse of the lung due to extrapulmonary pressure. (2) *By obstruction of the air passages* by mucus as in asthma, by a neoplasm, or by foreign bodies.

Pulmonary air volumes may be divided as follows. (1) *Tidal air* represents the amount of air breathed in and out during quiet respiration. It averages 500 cc. (2) *Vital capacity* signifies the maximum amount of air which can be expired after a maximum inspiration. It averages from 3500 to 5000 cc. In spite of its imposing name, which has at times misled surgeons into regarding it as a major criterion of operability, it is merely a measurement of air displacement and bears no relation to the absorption of oxygen from the air, which is what really matters. (3) *Residual air* is the amount left in the lungs after maximum expiration, amounting to 1800 to 2000 cc. It has the composition of alveolar air, namely oxygen 14 per cent and carbon dioxide 5 per cent. The residual air provides the homeostatic mechanism by which the normal ratio between H_2CO_3 and $BHCO_3$ is maintained. (4) *Dead space* is the term applied to the volume of the respiratory passages from the nose to the bronchioles. The air it contains takes no part in the exchange of gases.

Gaseous Interchange.—It is fundamental to realize that ventilation may be perfect in every respect, yet a person may die of dyspnea. Alveolar respiration is the exchange of oxygen and carbon dioxide across the alveolar membrane. This interchange is brought about by the difference in pressure gradients between the blood and the alveolar air. The two phases of alveolar respiration, absorption and O_2 and excretion of CO_2, may be dissociated. In emphysema for instance, sufficient O_2 may be absorbed, but retention of CO_2 may lead to severe acidosis and finally coma. On the other hand in diffuse pulmonary fibrosis the CO_2 diffusion rate is normal, but oxygen absorption may be poor. While CO_2 is absent from the atmosphere in any significant amount, it may be present if the inspired air is diluted with much residual air.

Interference with gaseous interchange is likely to be due to alveolar-capillary block or to bronchiolar obstruction. *Alveolar-capillary block* is a syndrome that includes a variety of pathological processes character-ized by changes in the alveolar wall and increased resistance to the diffusion of gases. Amongst these processes pulmonary scleroderma, beryllium granulomatosis, sarcoidosis, pulmonary fibrosis of unknown origin, and hyaline membrane disease of infants are specially worthy of mention.

It will be seen that profound biochemical disturbances may result from alveolar respiratory block. Primary excess of plasma CO_2 such as occurs in emphysema leads to depression of the respiratory center, while primary deficit of CO_2 may occur in the hyperventilation of psychoneurotics, in hyperthermia, and in those exposed to high altitudes.

THE BACTERIAL PNEUMONIAS

Pneumonia signifies an inflammatory consolidation of the lung, a consolidation which may be diffuse or patchy.

The lung is the one organ in the body which is in direct contact with the outside air. It is but natural, therefore, that bacterial infection is frequent. There might be cause for wonder, indeed, that it is not universal, and it might well be so were it not for the intricate series of defenses which the infecting agents have to circumvent. These include the sticky mucus of the bronchial mucosa which entraps the invaders, the cilia, whose ceaseless motion directs the flow upward, the cough reflex which serves to clear the lower segments of the bronchial tree, the lymphoid tissue of the bronchioles, and the mononuclear phagocytes lurking in the alveoli for any bacteria which may break through. The most important causes of acute bacterial pneumonias are Diplococcus pneumoniae, Streptococcus hemolyticus, Staphylococcus aureus, and Friedländer's bacillus. Pneumonia may be classified in a number of ways, more particularly with regard to (1) its distribution, whether diffuse (lobar) or patchy (lobular or bronchopneumonia), (2) the etiological agent concerned. Lobar pneumonia is nearly always caused by the pneumococcus, whilst bronchopneumonia is likely to be due to one of the other organisms just enumerated. These distinctions, while useful, are by no means absolute, as will at once become apparent in the discussion which follows.

Lobar (Pneumococcal) Pneumonia.—Lobar pneumonia is the ordinary result of pneumococcal infection, but it is not the invariable result. The lobar form is seen in the healthy adult, but in the very young and also in the old, in whom the disease so often blows out life's little candle, it appears as a bronchopneumonia. The disease, however, has changed its face and character as the result of the sulfonamides and antibiotics. To Osler it used to be "the Captain of the Men of Death" for those in the prime of life. Although displaced from that evil eminence it is still the terminal event in many elderly lives, because of the frequency of congestive heart failure in the old with its accumulation of fluid in the lung which provides a rich source of nourishment for stray bacteria and because of the damage to ciliary action resulting from repeated bronchial inflammation in these people (Sprunt).

Etiology.—With rare exceptions lobar pneumonia is caused by the pneumococcus, of which a large number of types are recognized. The type specificity depends on the capsular mucopolysaccharides, and it is the armor-plating of the capsule which protects the bacterium against phagocytes. Those strains which have no capsule (rough strains) are easily destroyed and are therefore nonvirulent. Species specificity depends on a carbohydrate known as the "C" substance (C for carbohydrate) present in the somatic portion of the micro-organism. This substance gives a precipitate with a protein in the blood in rheumatic fever and other acute infections, for which reason the protein is known as the *C-reactive protein*. Although the symptoms of pneumococcal infection are those of toxemia, the pneumococcus does not produce a toxin. The toxic picture seems to be due to the great invasiveness of the organism.

It is believed by many observers that *allergy* plays an important part in the pathogenesis of pneumonia. Certain it is that the age period at which the disease is most prevalent is that at which there is a high level of humoral immunity. Clinical observations also suggest that previous infections of the respiratory tract may sensitize the lungs so that pneumonia may be the result of a subsequent infection. An element of hypersensitivity would account in part for the sudden outpouring of edema fluid, with the cocci riding on the crest of the waves.

Predisposing factors lower the resistance of the patient and allow the organisms to pass from the upper to the lower respiratory tract. The best recognized of these are profound fatigue, chill, injury to the chest, severe fractures, debilitating diseases, and chronic alcoholism. Alcohol can be shown to inhibit the vascular inflammatory response in the experimental animal, and to prevent capillary dilatation and the emigration of leukocytes even in animals rendered highly immune by the intravenous injection of antipneumococcus serum, so that the bacteria can proliferate unchecked. Viral infections of the upper respiratory tract not only weaken the natural defences in the region, but are accompanied by an abundant production of mucin. The infected watery mucin can flow downward with little hindrance from ciliary action and thus gain entrance to the alveoli.

Pneumococci reach the pulmonary alveoli *via* the bronchial tree. The organisms pass in the inflammatory fluid from one alveolus to another through the interalveolar pores of Cohn. Thus the wave of infection sweeps throughout an entire lobe, but is often limited to that lobe. Spread of infection along the bronchial tree under the control of gravity is also of primary importance. Direction of spread depends on the bodily attitude of the sick person or animal. The capsular polysaccharide contains an edema-producing substance which can be extracted. It is natural, therefore, that the first feature of the exudate should be a marked inflammatory edema.

The mechanism by which the pneumococci are destroyed has been demonstrated in a remarkably beautiful series of experiments by Barry Wood and his associates. The all-important element is the leukocyte, mainly polymorphonuclear, but macrophage in the later stages. The organisms are carried outward by the advancing flood of edema fluid, pursued in turn by the leukocytes. If the tortoise is to catch up with the hare the pace of the latter must be slowed down. This may be effected by means of specific antibodies which cause agglutination of the pneumococci or by the bacteriostatic action of the sulfonamides and antibiotics. When the

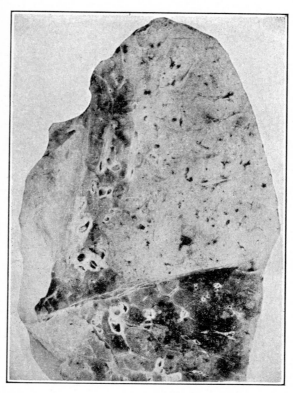

Fig. 362.—Lobar pneumonia. The upper lobe is completely consolidated, being in a state of gray
hepatization. The lower lobe, only part of which is shown, is not involved.

leukocytes have overtaken the pneumococci they pin them against the walls of the alveolar sacs, and only then are they able to engulf them.

Lesions.—The essential pathological feature is an out-pouring of an inflammatory exudate into the alveoli in response to the irritation produced by the pneumococci. The alveoli are filled by this exudate, the air is displaced, and the lung or part of it is converted into a solid and airless organ. This process is known as *consolidation* or *hepatization* because the lung becomes like the liver (hepar) in consistence. Four stages are recognized for descriptive purposes: congestion, red hepatization, gray hepatization and resolution, but these are really of very little importance. What is important is to realize that the process is a progressive one commencing at the hilus and sweeping out to the periphery, involving one or more lobes and sometimes both lungs. It follows that one part of the lung may be at one stage while another part is at another. The stage of the process can be determined by noting the freshness or the reverse of the exudate.

The *gross appearance* is very characteristic (Fig. 362). In the untreated case by the end of the second day the affected part of the lung is consolidated, red, and sinks in water. It is friable, and the cut surface is rough and granular like red granite. Later it is gray and moist. The pleural surface is covered with a fibrinous exudate and the bronchial nodes are enlarged.

The *microscopic picture* also depends much on the stage of the process. At the beginning the capillaries are congested, and the alveoli are filled with edema fluid containing great numbers of pneumococci (Fig. 363). Soon fibrin is formed and polymorphonuclears appear in great numbers, together with red cells and a few lymphocytes. All the elements are sharp and distinct (Fig. 364).

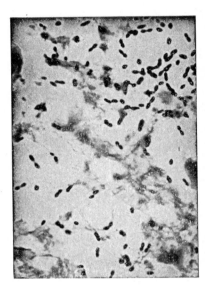

FIG. 363.—Lobar pneumonia, early stage. The alveoli, which are crowded with pneumococci, contain edema fluid but no leukocytes. × 1300.

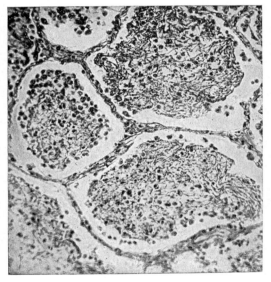

FIG. 364.—Lobar pneumonia. The alveoli are filled with an acute fibrinous exudate. × 100.

Later in the process (*gray hepatization*) this sharpness is blurred and lost owing to the action of proteolytic enzymes, the red cells are mere ghosts, the threads of fibrin become clumped, and the pneumococci disappear. The polymorphonuclears are replaced by macrophages which are now the active cells

(Robertson). These appear to be derived from the lymphocytes and monocytes of the alveolar exudate. In the final stage known as *resolution* the softened exudate is completely removed, partly by coughing, partly by transportation by phagocytes to lymph nodes, and partly by solution and absorption. By these means the consolidated lung is rapidly restored to normal.

Resolution is certainly the most remarkable phenomenon in the entire pathology of pneumonia. By means of this agency the huge mass of solidified exudate, consisting largely of fibrin, which has converted the airy lung into something resembling a lump of flesh, is completely removed, and the lung is restored, uninjured, to its former intact condition. This is so different from what occurs in the abdominal cavity, in the heart, in the brain, in the joints, etc., that it may well arouse surprise. One reason why so complete a return to the *status quo ante* is possible is that in lobar pneumonia there is no necrosis of the alveolar walls. The pneumococci pass so readily into the alveolar spaces, and there is so little real struggle in the interstitial tissue, that no destruction takes place. This offers a striking contrast to what occurs in staphylococcal and streptococcal pneumonia, as will be seen when these conditions are discussed. The solution of the fibrin must be brought about by proteolytic ferments, and these are most probably derived from the disintegrating leukocytes. It has long been known that purulent sputum has the power of dissolving fibrin, and that a portion of lung in a stage of gray hepatization will rapidly undergo autolysis, whereas this process is largely inhibited in a lung in a stage of red hepatization, but the exact chemical conditions necessary for the change are not yet thoroughly understood. Once the exudate is liquefied it becomes absorbed into the lymphatics and the blood vessels. Large numbers of macrophages are found in the bronchial lymph nodes, and occasionally one may be fortunate enough to catch them in their passage along the lymphatics. Little or none of the exudate seems to be got rid of by expectoration.

Complications.—Organization of the inflammatory exudate may occasionally occur. It becomes changed from fibrin into fibrous

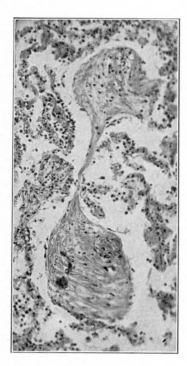

Fig. 365.—Organization of a pneumonic exudate. A strand of fibrous tissue passes through an opening in the alveolar wall.   × 150.

tissue. The strange thing is that this does not happen more frequently. Usually resolution occurs in time and the exudate melts away before fibroblasts have time to invade it. When organization occurs fibroblasts grow into the exudate from certain points of the alveolar wall, especially the angles, and these are soon followed by capillaries which later disappear. Long strands of fibrous tissue are formed which traverse the alveoli, often passing from one alveolus to another through what appear to be openings in the walls (Fig. 365). The end-result of these changes is to convert the lung into a dense elastic structure. As it is fleshy in consistence the process is known as *carnification*.

Pulmonary fibrosis secondary to pneumonia is seen more frequently than formerly. This may be attributed to two factors: the use of antibiotics and an increase in virus pneumonia. Both the clinical and the pathological picture of pneumonia are undergoing a change.

Suppuration and *abscess formation* are quite uncommon, and are due either to a very virulent infection or to poor resistance on the part of the patient. The alveolar walls are broken down and the exudate becomes purulent. It must be understood that although the exudate in lobar pneumonia may consist largely of polymorphonuclear leukocytes, this is not pus, and, as a rule, there is no suppuration, *i. e.*, breaking-down of tissue. Empyema may develop, but this is not common except in children, though a frequent complication of streptococcal penumonia. Spread of the infection may also cause pericarditis. As a result of pneumococcal septicemia there may be endocarditis, meningitis, and arthritis.

Relation of Symptoms to Lesions.—The clinical manifestations of lobar pneumonia are partly local, partly general. The *local* features are pain in the chest made worse by breathing, signs of consolidation of the lung (dullness on percussion, blowing breathing, increased vocal fremitus and resonance), moist rales during the period of resolution, and blood-stained sputum. The *general* symptoms are fever, dyspnea, evidence of severe toxemia, and a marked leukocytosis. In the untreated patient after a course of seven or eight days the illness suddenly terminates by crisis. Owing to the therapeutic revolution wrought by antibiotics it is seldom that the physician sees now the picture just described.

The *physical signs* are easily explained by the pathological findings. The dullness, blowing breathing, increased vocal fremitus and resonance are caused by a conversion of the lung into a solid organ which conducts sounds from the large bronchi to the chest with the greatest readiness. The moist râles heard during resolution are caused by the liquefied exudate in the bronchioles. The *pain* is due to pleurisy. It is an early symptom, because the pneumococci reach the surface long before consolidation has become complete. The *sputum* is rusty in color because it contains broken-down red cells. If there is much alveolar hemorrhage the sputum will contain bright blood. The sputum is very tenacious and stringy owing to its highly fibrinous character. The *blood* shows a high leukocytosis owing to the extensive character of the leukocytic exudate. Blood culture may be positive, but it is a sign of ill-omen except in the earliest stages. In cases which are going to recover the pneumococci usually soon disappear from the blood.

The *respiratory disturbances* (dyspnea, rapid shallow breathing, and in the more severe cases cyanosis) cannot be explained merely by the exudate in the lung, for they may be marked even though the pulmonary lesion is quite limited. They appear to be bound up with the condition of lowered oxygen saturation of the arterial blood known as *anoxemia*, the index of which is cyanosis. Anoxemia, which in some cases may be "the leak that sinks the ship," is difficult to explain. It has been attributed to the rapid very shallow respiration, which may ventilate only the dead space, so that the normal alveolar oxygen tension cannot be maintained, but the shallow respiration has then to be explained in a patient whom one would expect to be taking full deep breaths. Experimental work suggests that afferent impulses passing along the vagi from the inflamed lungs to the medulla may depress the respiratory center.

The *crisis* was the most dramatic clinical phenomenon seen in cases of lobar pneumonia before the days of antibiotics, for the patient passed in a few hours from a condition of grave peril to one of complete safety. The temperature would drop as much as 7° or 8° F. in the course of an hour, the dyspnea disappear, and the respirations return to normal, although the consolidation remained as before. In view of the fact that the crisis is never seen today on account of antibiotic therapy we do not need to concern ourselves with an explanation, which is fortunate, because no really satisfying explanation has been suggested.

Bronchopneumonia.—This condition, also called lobular pneumonia on account of its patchy character, is not a definite entity like lobar pneumonia. As a secondary condition complicating and often terminating other diseases it is extremely common. Indeed in hospital autopsies it is seldom that some degree of bronchopneumonia cannot be demonstrated. As a primary disease it occurs principally in childhood and old age. The susceptibility of the child may be due to poor expulsive power, to the delicate mucosa, or to the short wide bronchial tree. The pneumonias following *measles, whooping cough* and other *infectious fevers* are bronchopneumonic in type; so also are the *postoperative* and *terminal pneumonias*. It is usually due to streptococci, but pneumococci, staphylococci and influenza bacilli may be the predominant organisms.

Lesions.—As the name implies, this is a bronchial as well as a pulmonary infection and inflammation, the bronchi being the first to be involved. The infection begins in the upper respiratory passages, descends in droplets of secretion to the finer bronchioles which become inflamed, and finally invades the surrounding alveoli.

There is a patchy consolidation of both lungs, a lobular pneumonia which can often be felt better than seen. Sometimes the patches fuse together, giving a confluent bronchopneumonia which may simulate lobar pneumonia. Collapsed areas, dark purple in color and depressed below the surface, are seen on the outside of the lung especially in children. The collapse is caused by the bronchioles becoming filled with secretion, so that the air cannot enter the lobule; the imprisoned air in the alveoli is then absorbed and the lobule becomes collapsed. The collapsed areas are surrounded by emphysematous bullæ, a compensatory arrangement. A thin fibrinous exudate covers the surface. On the cut surface the patchy character of the lesions is very evident, areas of consolidation alternating with areas of collapse, of emphysema and of normal lung tissue. The patchiness can be seen even better with the naked eye in a stained section. The consolidated areas are then seen to be grouped around small bronchioles. The bronchial lymph nodes are enlarged and soft. It is interesting to note that the pleurisy, which is so common in pneumococcal pneumonia, is not a feature of bronchopneumonia.

Microscopically there is an intense inflammation of the bronchial wall, the lumen of which is filled with pus and desquamated epithelium. There is more of a bronchiolitis in streptococcal pneumonia than in the lobar form. The bronchiole is surrounded by a ring of alveoli filled with an inflammatory exudate consisting mainly of polymorpho-

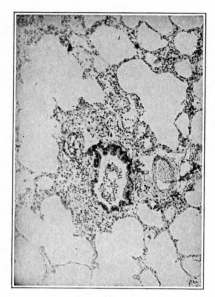

FIG. 366.—Streptococcal bronchopneumonia, showing patchy character of the exudate. × 60.

nuclear leukocytes with a moderate amount of fibrin (Fig. 366). Farther out the alveoli contain mononuclear cells and edematous fluid. The consolidated areas alternate with areas of congestion, collapse, and emphysema.

Recovery is often not complete. The walls of the bronchi are damaged, granulation tissue is formed followed by fibrosis, and permanent bronchiectasis may result. Moreover there is no distinct crisis, and absorption of the exudate tends to be delayed so that organization may occur. In these respects the disease differs from lobar pneumonia, which is a more satisfactory and honest type of infection and one easier to treat.

Streptococcal Pneumonia.—In the past the streptococcus has been the most important cause of bronchopneumonia, but at the moment it would appear as if its pride of place is being usurped by Staphylococcus aureus. In pneumonia in the young and in the aged the streptococcus is found fairly frequently, but the respiratory tract of the adult is able to withstand invasion unless resistance is weakened by infectious fevers such as measles, whooping cough and influenza, by chronic and debilitating illness (*terminal*

pneumonia), or by the inhalation of foreign material into the lung (*inhalation pneumonia*). Streptococcus hemolyticus attained a terrible prominence in the 1918–1919 epidemic of influenza, at which time hundreds of thousands of persons died of streptococcal pneumonia. But it was essentially as a secondary invader of weakened tissues, not as a primary agent, that it operated. In the case complicating influenza empyema was a very common and apparently lethal factor. The fluid was at first thin and watery though turbid, with innumerable streptococci, at a later period becoming frankly purulent.

Staphylococcal Pneumonia.—As has just been mentioned, at the present time Staphylococcus aureus, coagulase-positive, has taken the place of streptococci as dangerous secondary invaders in cases of Asian influenza. In one series this organism was responsible for 27 per cent of the deaths (Robertson *et al.*). In the staphylococcal cases the mortality was 47 per cent. The treatment of fulminating staphylococcal infections is very difficult, because it is necessary to treat not only the bacterial infection, which is often antibiotic-resistant, but also the attendant pulmonary edema and peripheral circulatory failure. Hemorrhage is the most characteristic feature, and abscess formation is likely to be marked in this form of bronchopenumonia.

Friedländer's Bacillus Pneumonia.—The causal bacillus (Klebsiella pneumoniae) is an encapsulated but, unlike the pneumococcus, a gram-negative organism, a very significant fact to the physician. Like the pneumococcus it also has a number of types. The disease, which is fortunately uncommon, used to have a mortality of 80 per cent, and even with modern treatment this has only been lowered to 20 per cent. The patches of consolidation, most frequent in the upper lobe, have a characteristic mucinous appearance, which corresponds to the sticky mucoid appearance of the colonies on culture. The patches tend to coalesce, undergo necrosis, and develop into abscesses. Death may take place in the course of a few days. When recovery takes place it is slow and protracted. During this period the condition is readily mistaken for tuberculosis both by the clinician and the radiologist, especially if it is confined to the upper lobes. As the organisms are gram-negative they are resistant to penicillin, but respond to a combination of streptomycin and the sulfonamides. The importance of using Gram's method of staining when examining the sputum in cases of pneumonia becomes self-evident.

THE VIRAL PNEUMONIAS

The concept of viral pneumonia, apart from the specific pneumonitis known to occur in influenza, vaccinia, measles and other diseases due to viruses, was first proposed in 1938 (Reimann). Viral pneumonias have become clinically delineated entities which now outnumber all other pneumonias, especially during epidemics. The non-committal and cumbersome term "primary atypical pneumonia of unknown etiology" may presently be abandoned, as it probably represents a group of conditions which are typical in their own right and atypical only if compared with lobar pneumonia. A stumbling block at present is the nomenclature, for the viruses are largely known by initials such as RI (respiratory infection), APC (adenoidal-pharyngeal-conjunctival), ARD (acute respiratory disease), and PAP (primary atypical pneumonia). It is to be hoped that in the course of time appropriate names may take the place of initials.

Influenzal Pneumonia.—Influenza is perhaps the most remarkable and challenging of all the infectious diseases. Usually it represents the mildest of endemic diseases affecting the upper respiratory tract, and referred to with a smile as "a touch of the flu." At intervals of a quarter of a century or more it suddenly assumes an epidemic or pandemic form and sweeps throughout the world. It is in the epidemic form that pneumonia constitutes the great threat. In the past century there have been three of these pandemics: in 1889–92, in 1918–19, the so-called Spanish influenza, and in 1957, the so-called Asian influenza, which spread from an initial focus in China. I know little or nothing about the first of these. The second, which I had the opportunity to study in Winnipeg, was marked by a very high mortality, mainly as the result of streptococcal pneumonia. In this pandemic there were

some 500,000,000 cases through the world, of whom 15,000,000 died. By comparison the pandemic of Asian influenza, caused by a variant of Type A influenza virus, was comparatively mild, most of the deaths being due to pneumonia caused by *Staphylococcus aureus*. Little can be said about the causal agent of the 1918–19 pandemic, because the virus of human influenza was not discovered until 1933. The virology of influenza has already been discussed in Chapter 14. The present account will be confined to *Asian influenza*.

The virus belongs to the group of influenza A virus, the other groups being B, C, and D. It is quite distinct immunologically from any of the types of influenza A virus isolated from earlier epidemics, so that no previous experience of influenza could be expected to provide immunity. The influenza virus consists of two parts, an outer protein shell and an inner core. The protein shell initiates the infection, and acts as an antigen which stimulates the formation of the antibodies responsible for immunity to influenza. The surface element remains constant during an epidemic, varies in a minor degree from one epidemic to another, but changes its pattern sharply every ten years or so. The central core carries an immunological character common to the group or species (A, B, etc.), thus allowing identification of the species to which the virus belongs, but it is not antigenic, and therefore plays no part in the production of immunity.

The infective period is from two days before symptoms develop to about nine days afterward. Infection incurred during the first three months of pregnancy may cause fetal abnormalities, in particular a failure of the brain to develop (Coffey and Jessop). This recalls the relation of another virus disease, German measles, during early pregnancy to imperfect cardiac development, with resulting congenital heart disease.

Lesions.—The infection begins in the upper respiratory tract, and the virus causes a widespread necrosis of the tracheal epithelium. The ulcerated surface of the mucosa is covered with a fibrin film. The resistance of the lung is depressed, and the way is opened to invasion by secondary bacterial infection. It is naturally very difficult to

41

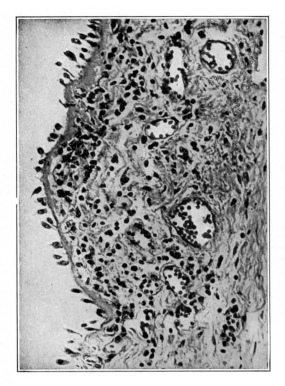

FIG. 367A.—Trachea in influenza. Desquamation of epithelium, congestion of mucosa, and infiltration with inflammatory cells. × 300.

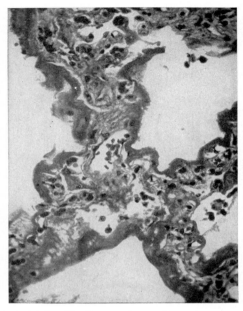

FIG. 367B.—Hyaline membrane disease in pregnant woman dying of influenza. (Boyd, *Pathology for the Physician*.)

distinguish between the lesions caused by the virus and those due to secondary infection. The trachea and bronchi are intensely congested, and the ciliated epithelium is desquamated (Fig. 367A). This in itself breaks down resistance to bacterial invasion. In pure viral infection, which is likely to be seen at the beginning of an epidemic, in addition to the bronchial lesions just mentioned there is a nodular peribronchial *interstitial pneumonitis* with widening of the interalveolar septa by cells of mononuclear type, edema of the alveoli, a hyaline membrane lining the alveoli (Fig. 367B), and a remarkable absence of inflammatory cells in the alveoli. The *hyaline membrane*, which is particularly characteristic, seems to represent fibrin derived from the albuminous fluid in the alveoli. The pure viral picture was seen much more frequently in the 1957 pandemic and many patients died of viral pneumonitis *per se*, the virus being isolated from pulmonary tissue, without bacterial infection.

The pneumonic lung varies in appearance, but the lesions are constantly bilateral. At the height of an epidemic, and sometimes in sporadic cases, the lungs are voluminous, covered by a thin fibrinous exudate, and of a vivid red color with splashes of a dusky purple. From the cut surface pours a bloody watery fluid due to a hemorrhagic edema which is the outstanding feature of the condition. In a marked case a correct diagnosis can be made at a glance. The lung is heavy, but without the firm consolidation of lobar pneumonia or the nodular consolidation of bronchopneumonia. The most marked feature of the microscopic picture is edema fluid filling the alveoli, with numerous red blood cells but few leukocytes and no fibrin. The other microscopic features already enumerated will also be evident. The tracheobronchial lymph nodes are enlarged, congested, succulent, and microscopically they show a sinusitis, with eventual necrosis of the follicles. Bacteria-free cases coming to autopsy have been not infrequent in the 1957 pandemic (Oseasohn *et al.*). Indeed, in one outbreak in the Netherlands there was a pure influenza-virus pneumonia in 20 per cent of the fatal cases (Hers *et al.*).

Relation of Symptoms to Lesions.—The most characteristic symptoms of influenza are profound prostration, a dry hacking cough, and leukopenia in place of the usual leukocytosis of acute infections. In addition, in the more severe cases with pulmonary complications there may be cyanosis, dyspnea, watery blood-stained sputum, pleurisy, and not infrequently empyema. The dry, hacking cough is due to the acute tracheitis and bronchitis. Cyanosis and dyspnea are probably due to interference with the exchange of gases in the alveoli, this in turn being caused by the copious outpouring of fluid. Death in the Asian influenza cases seemed to be mainly due to anoxemia resulting from a mechanical alveolar-capillary block due to interstitial inflammation and hyaline membrane formation (Soto *et al.*). The watery, frothy, hemorrhagic sputum merely represents an external appearance of the hemorrhagic edema of the lungs. The profound prostration, the most striking of all the symptoms of true influenza, is due to the general toxemia. So also is the Zenker degeneration of muscle and other changes of general character which are not discussed in this place.

During the pandemic of Asian influenza in many communities as many as one-quarter to one-third of the population was attacked. The case fatality rate was less than 1 per 1,000, apart from cases of mitral stenosis, chronic bronchitis, diabetes, and preexisting staphylococcal infections. Deaths were more common at the two extremes of life. The onset was often abrupt, and death might occur within a few hours or in two or three days. In young children influenzal pneumonia may be responsible for sudden and unexpected death. This may be due to a myocarditis, which is not infrequent, or to adrenal cortical insufficiency.

The *laboratory diagnosis* of Asian influenza is made by isolation of the virus from throat washings, which, after treatment with penicillin and streptomycin, are injected into the amniotic cavity of chick embryos. The amniotic fluid is then tested for its capacity to agglutinate red blood cells. The complement fixation test is of considerable value. Finally, the presence of degenerated and necrotic ciliated cells in nasal mucus stained with methylene blue indicates a similar condition in the ciliated epithelium of the trachea and bronchi.

Primary Atypical Pneumonia.—This relatively new arrival among the pneumonias is known under a variety of names such as virus pneumonia, virus pneumonitis and atypical pneumonia of unknown etiology. It seems probable that it constitutes a group rather than a specific entity, this group comprising pneumonic consolidations other than those caused by any known virus, rickettsia, bacterium or chemical agent. The various cases all seem to be caused by a *filterable virus*, which has been isolated from the sputum, and to which antibodies have been demonstrated in patients between the second and third week of the illness.

The distribution is widespread, and the disease may appear in small epidemics, usually in schools and army camps where young people are congregated, as a rule in the late fall and winter. The infection causes an acute inflammation of the mucous membranes of the upper respiratory tract, extending to the trachea and bronchi, and occasionally to the bronchi and lungs. The morbidity is high and the mortality low. The physical signs are largely negative, but there is roentgen-ray evidence of a patchy, ill-defined consolidation, seldom involving more than a part of a lobe. The course is usually mild, lasting two or three weeks, and a fatal outcome is rare. The chief feature of the fatal cases is a patchy, hemorrhagic, interstitial bronchopneumonia associated with acute bronchitis and bronchiolitis, in other words, the usual lesions of a virus pneumonitis.

Psittacosis.—This is a viral disease of South American parrots and parakeets (*psittakos*, parrot), which may be transmitted to man. The condition, which is of high mortality, has already been described on page 343. Viral disease of birds other than parrots is known as *ornithosis*.

Q Fever.—This disease, which derives its name from having been first described in Queensland, Australia, in 1937, is caused by a rickettsia, is carried by rodents, and is

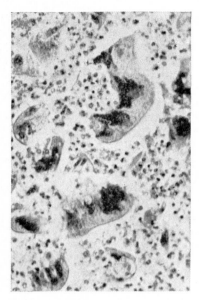

FIG. 368.—Giant-cell pneumonia. High magnification of the cells in the lumen of the bronchus. × 190. (Enders, McCarthy, Mitus and Cheathem, courtesy of New. Engl. J. Med.)

spread by ticks. The remarkable feature of the disease, which is widespread throughout the world, is the absence of any correlation between the pathological lesions in the lung and the clinical picture, which is that of a typhoid-like state. There is a definite pneumonitis, with soft patchy lesions in the x-ray film, but a complete absence of respiratory symptoms. Unlike psittacosis, the mortality is very low. The pathological *lesions* are similar to those of primary atypical pneumonia, namely mononuclear infiltration of the bronchial walls with edema and inflammatory cells in the lumen of the bronchi and alveoli.

Giant Cell Pneumonia.—This condition, first described by Hecht in 1910, is an *interstitial pneumonitis* of infants and young children characterized by the presence of large multinucleated giant cells derived from the lining of the alveoli and alveolar ducts. Large inclusions are present in the cytoplasm and smaller ones in the nuclei (Fig. 368). Similar lesions have been observed in the lungs in the early stage of fatal measles. We have already seen that giant cells are a hall mark of the measles virus in the tonsil and the appendix (page 340). It was natural,

therefore, that suspicion should be directed to the measles virus, but no direct evidence was available. It now becomes apparent that when young children are exposed to measles infection they may develop giant cell pneumonia, *but without a measles rash* (Enders *et al.*). A virus has been isolated from the lung which produces cytopathic changes in tissue culture indistinguishable from those induced by the measles virus. Monkeys inoculated intravenously with this virus develop antibodies against the measles virus. It would appear, therefore, that the virus of measles is the cause of some cases of giant cell pneumonia, although this may not be true of all cases.

Inclusion-disease Pneumonitis. — This condition known also as *cytomegalic inclusion disease* (Wyatt *et al.*) and generalized salivary gland virus infection has been described on page 348. It is a well-recognized disease of the newborn infants and young children. Occasional cases have been reported in adults suffering from some chronic debilitating condition (Fisher and Davis). The pulmonary lesion is a fibrosing interstitial pneumonitis, a fact which might suggest that other obscure forms of fibrosing pneumonitis, such as the Hamman-Rich syndrome to be described presently, may be of viral origin.

NON-BACTERIAL INFLAMMATIONS

Lipoid Pneumonia.—This term denotes an inflammatory condition of the lung caused by the presence in the alveoli of animal or mineral oil. It may develop when the throat has been repeatedly sprayed with mineral oils, liquid petrolatum, etc., especially in children. The habitual forced administration of cod-liver oil in children is another cause. It is important to realize that light oils can pass with ease from the upper respiratory passages to the lungs. The condition is much commoner than has been suspected, the incidence having increased greatly since the existence of the lesion was first demonstrated by Laughlen in 1925. This is due to the widespread habit of self-medication by the public who so frequently use oily sprays or drops for upper respiratory infections. Animal oils, particularly cod-liver oil, are highly irritating. Liquid petro-

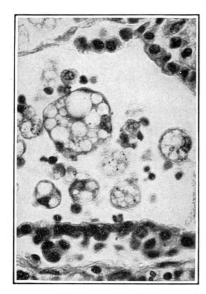

Fig. 369.—Oil pneumonia; phagocytes filled with globules. × 450.

latum, although less acutely damaging, produces severe chronic effects, as it leads to the formation of reticulum fibers, gaint cells, and finally extensive fibrosis. In the *gross* the affected areas are gray or yellow and moderately firm, projecting slightly above the pleural surface. The patches become firmer and grayish-white, and may be mistaken for tumor metastases. The alveoli are filled with large phagocytic cells (lipophages) distended with droplets of oil, giving a highly characteristic *microscopic* picture (Fig. 369). It must be pointed out that macrophages filled with lipid may be present in the alveoli apart from true lipoid pneumonia. They are seen in pulmonary tuberculosis, chronic suppuration, and in the vicinity of large infarcts. In such cases the lipid must be of endogenous rather than exogenous origin. It is possible that some of the fat has been transported from the liver, because much of the fat in a grossly fatty liver makes its way into the veins. Liquid petrolatum stains with scarlet red but does not reduce osmic acid, whereas cod-liver oil reduces osmic acid, and the same is true of vegetable oils. In the later stages fibrosis is marked, and giant cell formation is common. The disease occurs at the two ends of life, and the adult form is characterized by a dense fibrosis which is often so clearly localized that it may be mistaken for a neoplasm (paraffinoma of lung).

Löffler's Pneumonia.—The condition usually known as Löffler's syndrome, first described in 1932, is characterized by a mild clinical course, marked eosinophilia, and transitory pulmonary lesions which present a remarkable and alarming picture in the x-ray films. Little is known about the pathological lesions, because the patient seldom dies. In a careful study by Bayley, Lindberg and Baggenstoss, the following changes were observed. Scattered throughout the lungs were focal areas of consolidation. Some of these consisted of fibrous tissue with an intermingling of great numbers of eosinophilic leukocytes, so that the condition has been called *eosinophilic pneumonitis*, while others presented a granulomatous picture with epithelioid cells, numerous eosinophils, and fibrinoid degeneration of collagen. Widespread vascular lesions were present, in particular a necrotizing arteritis similar to that seen in periarteritis nodosa. In the bronchi there was marked hypertrophy of the muscle and extensive eosinophilic infiltration, lesions identical with those of bronchial asthma. The entire picture is strongly suggestive of an allergic reaction. The allergic agent may not be the same in every instance. In some cases the larvae of Ascaris lumbricoides which migrate through the lungs may be responsible, whilst in others the antigen responsible may be pollens or bacteria.

Irradiation Pneumonitis.—When the chest is exposed to repeated doses of therapeutic irradiation reactive changes may occur in the lungs. The alveolar lining cells enlarge, and some become very hypertrophic and bizarre like tumor giant cells. The bronchial epithelium shows similar but less extreme changes. The elastic tissue is ruptured and reduplicated. The alveoli may be lined by a hyaline membrane similar to that seen in epidemic influenza and in the newborn. The *triad* of *epithelial hyperplasia, changes in the elastic tissue,* and *hyaline membrane* lining the alveoli is pathognomonic. Injury to the tissues may lead to infection followed by fibrosis. It would appear that impaired

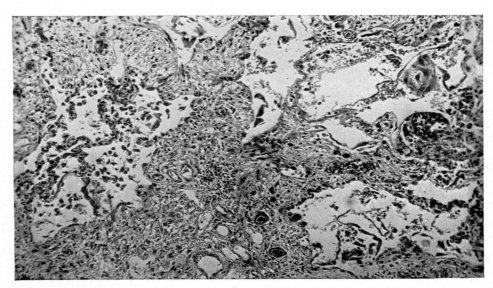

FIG. 370.—Hamman-Rich syndrome, showing diffuse interstitial fibrosis of the lung.
(Kindness of Dr. Ronald C. Sniffen.)

diffusion across the alveolar-capillary membrane plays an important part in the impairment of pulmonary function (Stone *et al.*). The *principal symptoms* are cough, sometimes severe and intractable, dyspnea, which is proportionate to the amount of fibrosis, and pain.

Hamman-Rich Syndrome.—As this condition of *diffuse interstitial fibrosis* appears to start as an inflammation rather than a fibrosis it will be considered here. The most striking symptom is shortness of breath, which is the earliest indication that anything is wrong, and which increases in severity until it reaches a fearful intensity. Cough, cyanosis, pain in the chest and clubbing of the fingers are accompanying features. The x-ray picture shows strand-like and patchy opacities throughout both lung fields. Death usually comes in a few months to release the sufferer, but sometimes not for several years.

It is now becoming evident that the Hamman-Rich syndrome is really a heterogeneous group of conditions characterized by diffuse fibrosis of unknown etiology. One member of the group constitutes a clinical and pathological entity seen in childhood, its chief features indicated by its name, *familial cystic fibrosis of the lung* (Donohue). It is a manifestation of a dominant gene of varying degrees of penetrance. Perhaps the basic genetic defect is failure of de-epithelialization of the alveoli, which are lined by metaplastic epithelium and develop into small emphysematous cysts.

At *autopsy* the lungs are heavy, firm and airless. At first the alveolar walls are infiltrated with lymphocytes, plasma cells and eosinophils, and there is formation of fibrin. Fibroblasts then lay down fibrous tissue which further thickens the walls and narrows the alveoli (Fig. 370). As the process is diffuse throughout both lungs giving widespread alveolar-capillary block, it is small wonder that the patient becomes increasingly dyspneic. The cells lining the alveoli may undergo hyperplasia to a degree that may suggest pulmonary adenomatosis. It is possible that the condition is the aftermath of previous viral infection. Another possibility, if not a probability, is that it is due to a tissue allergy (Read). Fibrosis may result from sensitivation to an external antigen such as arsenicals or it may represent a poststreptococcal allergic inflammation. Finally it may be that viral infection renders the alveolar lining cells antigenic.

Cholesterol Pneumonitis.—Another recent addition to the field of chronic interstitial pneumonitis is that described by Waddell,

Sniffen and Sweet, in which the characteristic features is an accumulation of *cholesterol-filled macrophages*, first in the alveoli and later in the alveolar walls. The cases are likely to be mistaken for bronchogenic carcinoma both by the clinican and the radiologist.

The affected portion of the lung is firm, bound to the chest wall by dense adhesions, and of an intense yellow color, due to the presence of innumerable minute yellow dots. Microscopically these prove to be due to flooding of the alveoli with macrophages filled with cholesterol and cholesterol ester. At a later stage the lung is gray and fibrosed, and this corresponds to a shifting of the macrophages from the lumen to the walls of the alveoli, and their subsequent replacement by dense fibrous tissue, which obliterates the alveolar lumen.

Neither the exact nature of the condition nor the origin of the cholesterol is known. Attention may be drawn, however, to two clues. (1) The lymphocytes and plasma cells in the interstitial tissue and the subsequent fibrosis, *i. e.*, chronic interstitial pneumonias, suggest a viral infection. (2) Accumulations of cholesterol-filled phagocytes are known to occur distal to stenosis of the large bronchi. It may be that the disease commences as an initial pneumonia, possibly viral in type, and that a viscid exudate obstructs the bronchioles, with resulting accumulation of cholesterol which is taken up by macrophages.

Uremic Pneumonitis.—Uremia may be complicated by a pneumonitis, which may develop within several days after the onset of the uremia or may de delayed as long as six months (Hopps and Wissler). The incidence is not high until the nonprotein nitrogen level has reached 100 mgm. per 100 cc. The cause of the pneumonitis is not clear.

The lungs are increased in weight and present a diffuse rubbery induration. Microscopically the alveoli are filled with a protein-rich edema, but the striking picture is an abundance of *fibrin* arranged as a fine network, but sometimes in dense hyaline masses or as hyaline asphyxial membrane. Polymorphonuclears are conspicuous by their absence, any cells present being mononuclear in type.

Pulmonary Microlithiasis.—This condition, which must not be confused with broncholithiasis to which it bears no relation, is a form of *diffuse pulmonary calcification* characterized by innumerable calcified intra-alveolar concretions (calcospherites) throughout the lung. The number of reported cases is few, but that may well be due to the fact that in the past the condition has not been recognized. There is little parenchymal involvement in the early stages, which corresponds with the remarkable absence of early symptoms. Interstitial fibrosis develops later, with corresponding interference with function.

At *autopsy* the lungs are large and remarkably heavy, weighing up to 5000 gm. They are said to feel like a sack of sand, and may have to be sawed open. The cut surface, from which minute concretions fall out, feels like sandpaper. Microscopically innumerable alveoli contain laminated concretions resembling corpora amylacea and consisting of calcium phosphate.

The most characteristic clinical feature is the x-ray appearance, from which the condition can be recognized on sight. It has aptly been compared to a snowstorm or more correctly a sandstorm. The other striking feature is the remarkable absence of symptoms.

The pathogenesis of the condition is quite obscure. There appears to be calcification of an unusual type of alveolar exudate which is not readily absorbed. There is a high familial incidence strongly suggesting a genetic factor (Sosman *et al.*).

THE OCCUPATIONAL PNEUMOCONIOSES

The inhalation of dust produced as the result of an industry over a long period of time gives rise to changes in the lung of a proliferative and fibrotic character. These dust diseases or pneumoconioses (*konis*, dust) differ in their course and prognosis, depending on the type of dust which is inhaled. The most important of these are silicosis, asbestosis and anthracosis, to which may be added hematite miner's lung, and bauxite and beryllium fibrosis. The pneumoconioses tend to progress to a fatal termination by way of tuberculosis or right-sided heart failure.

Silicosis.—Silicosis is the most widespread, the most serious, and the oldest of all occupational diseases. Silicon (Si) is the most widely distributed element in nature. The silicates merely give rise to a foreign body reaction, but silica (SiO_2), like asbestos, causes a progressive productive reaction ending in fibrosis and associated with marked impairment of pulmonary function. This condition, known as silicosis, is the most important of the dust diseases, and provides a serious hazard in the gold-mining industry in certain districts such as the South African Rand and northern Ontario. The worker is in great danger, but men mining any type of ore are liable to develop silicosis, provided the concentration of free silica in the aerial dust is great enough. If, in coal mining, hard rock has to be drilled through, coal miners may also suffer. Other occupations in which there is danger are tin-mining, stone-working, metal-grinding, sand-blasting, ceramic workers and makers of abrasive powders. In all of these cases dust containing fine particles of silica may be inhaled over long periods of time.

The particles of silica are taken up from the bronchioles, the epithelium of which is not ciliated, by phagocytes which carry them to the tiny lymphoid aggregations in the alveolar septa. The cell containing the silica undergoes changes similar to those seen in tuberculosis. The cytoplasm increases in amount and comes to contain lipid droplets, whilst the nucleus may divide repeatedly, so that a typical Langhans' giant cell may be formed. When silica is injected subcutaneously it produces necrosis, and the slow reaction in the lung results partly in necrosis but to a much greater degree in fibrosis. Both the rate and the extent of the fibrosis are in inverse proportion to the size of the silica particles. Previous disease processes, such as pneumonia, which may cause scarring of the delicate alveolar walls and lymphoid collections will facilitate the arrest of the particles and predispose to the production of silicosis. We have spoken as if the physical presence of the silica particles explained everything. A newer concept, the antigen theory, is coming into fashion. Silica, instead of having a simple toxic effect on the tissue, is now believed to combine with body protein to form an antigen, so that there may be some of the element of an antigen-antibody reaction. The fibrous tissue of the silicotic nodule is not merely collagen, but a mixture of collagen with α- and β-globulins having definite antigenic properties.

Lesions.—In this and in other fibroid conditions of the lung, the alveolar lining cells become cuboidal so that the alveoli assume a gland-like appearance like that of the early fetal lung, and the condition is, therefore, known as *fetalization of the alveolar lining* (Fig. 371A). This transformation is probably due to loss of respiratory function. The basic process is proliferation of reticular fibers, which later become transformed into collagen. The elastic fibers disappear completely. The *fibrosis* is at first patchy, corresponding to the deposits of silica in minute lymph follicles adjacent to the terminal bronchioles, and takes the form of "silicotic nodules" (Fig. 371B), composed of concentric layers of fibrous tissue and readily palpated in the lung. These nodules gradually coalesce, and the fibrosis becomes widespread. In extreme cases the lung becomes stony hard, and in one instance I had to saw the lung in two. When the lesions are produced by pure silica dust, as in gold miners and sand blasters, the nodules have the clean-cut laminated, onion-like character described above. When, however, as is frequently the case, the silica is mixed with other dusts, as in granite workers and anthracite coal miners, an interstitial fibrosis is added, and tongue-like projections extend from the nodules into the surrounding tissue. Moreover dust inclusions are commonly seen when the lesion is due to mixed dusts; these are seldom present in cases of pure silicosis. *Emphysema* is a common consequence of the extensive fibrosis, most marked, as a rule, at the base. The *lymph nodes* at the root of the lung are small, hard and fibrosed, with fibroblasts arranged in a characteristically whorled manner. The *pleura* is thickened and adhesions are common, due to deposits of silica in the subpleural lymphatics. The functional capacity of the lungs is greatly interfered with, and the chief symptom is marked *dyspnea*. The necrotizing action of the silica may lead to destruction and cavitation, but these changes

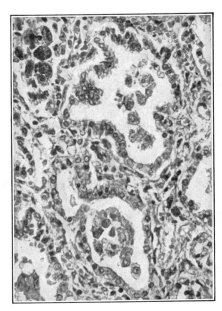

FIG. 371A.—Fetalization of alveolar lining in silicosis. × 160.

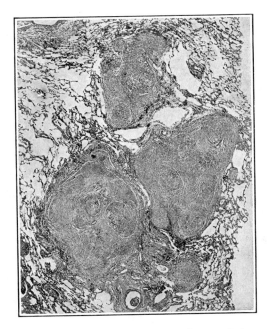

FIG. 371B.—Silicosis showing characteristic fibrous nodules. × 13.

are usually due to an accompanying tuberculosis.

Most silicotics die of tuberculosis because the presence of silica in the tissues favors the growth of tubercle bacilli to an astonishing degree. The lesions of silicosis and tuberculosis are at bottom essentially similar. As Gardner remarks, it is strange that a simple inorganic compound like silicon dioxide can give rise to the same cellular reactions as the tubercle bacillus with its proteins, carbohydrates and lipids.

The *radiological appearance* is of great importance, because it, together with a history of prolonged exposure to silica dust, forms the basis for the clinical diagnosis. The earliest change is an increase in the normal reticulation of the lung. The specific appearance, however, is that of clean-cut nodules scattered widely throughout both lungs, but in cases due to mixed dusts the outline of the nodules is much more hazy. When calcium is deposited in the nodules they stand out still more sharply. When tuberculous infection is added the nodules develop a fluffy outline, increase in size, and eventually coalesce to form large shadows;

this is in contrast to pure silicotic lesions which may remain discrete for years.

Silicotic lesions are not confined to the lung. Silica may occasionally be carried to the liver and spleen, where it causes necrosis and fibrosis.

Anthracosis.—A varying amount of coal dust is found in every lung at autopsy, and is usually of no significance. By itself coal dust appears to produce no harmful effect. In coal miners, however, it may give rise to the form of pneumoconiosis known as anthracosis. It does so because of the admixture of a certain amount of silica. In this mixed form the characteristic lesion is *dust-reticulation* (Belt), with corresponding fine net-like shadows (reticulation) in the roentgen-ray picture. Dust-reticulation is scattered diffusely throughout the lungs, forming a lace-like pattern along the lymphatic pathways and depots in which dust-laden macrophages are entrapped. The appearance of innumerable dust-ridden cobwebs is due to the formation of fine argentophil reticulum fibers; there is none of the collagen formation so characteristic of pure silicosis. The bronchial lymph nodes are masses of

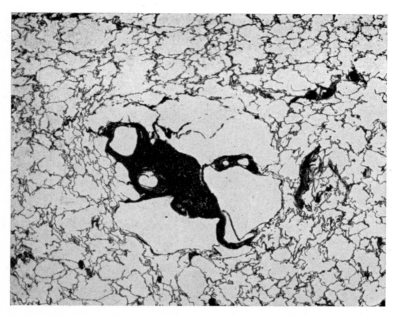

Fig. 372.—Centrally situated coal macule, with dust ensheathing and dilating several respiratory bronchioles of the third order (by serial section), creating morphological appearances of focal emphysema. No fibrosis associated with coal macule. Hematoxylin and eosin; × 120. (Wyatt, courtesy of Arch. Industrial Health.)

coal dust. In more advanced cases, which may be termed anthraco-silicosis, there may be *nodulation*, the formation of tiny nodules from 2 to 5 mm. in diameter. Finally there may be *confluent fibrosis*, a patchy confluence of the previous lesions. It is now believed that the massive fibrosis of coal-miner's pneumoconiosis is due to the admixture of coal dust with tubercle bacilli of low virulence. These lesions are really tuberculous scars, although the bacilli are hard to demonstrate. Emphysema may be marked, due perhaps to destruction of the elastic tissue. Belt remarks that the collier's lung is in a very real sense his occupational log book; it retains a qualitative and an indelible record of the mineral particles breathed during life.

It has now become apparent that under special conditions a distinctive form of pneumoconiosis may be caused by coal dust without the assistance of silica. This was first shown to be the case in South Wales coal miners (Heppleston), and the same condition has since been demonstrated in workers in the coal fields of Southern Illinois and other parts of the United States, particularly among men working at the coal face (Wyatt).

In these cases silica is minimal or absent as a cause of fibrosis. The basic lesion is a stellate nodule, (coal macule), heavily charged with coal, but free of the fibrosis which is the hall-mark of silicosis (Fig. 372). In spite of this the lesions are often associated with focal (centrilobular) emphysema. The coal is trapped in and around the respiratory bronchioles, causing stiffening of their walls, and apparently producing a terminal bronchiolectasia with increase in the residual lung volume. In Wyatt's cases, however, the emphysema extended far beyond the original central lobular site, perhaps owing to the rigid dilated bronchioles producing mechanical compression of the surrounding lung, thus interfering with the return air flow. One unfortunate feature is that there is poor correlation between the radiological picture and the degree of disability as assessed by clinical examination or physiological tests. This may become a serious matter as regards workmen's compensation.

Rheumatoid Pneumoconiosis.—In rheumatoid arthritis the characteristic rheumatoid nodules are rarely found in the connective tissue of the lung. Caplan has pointed out that in coal miners with pneumoconiosis who develop rheumatoid arthritis the x-ray picture is usually quite different from that of ordinary coal miner's pneumoconiosis. The shadows are multiple, round, well-defined, and distributed throughout both lungs. This condition has come to be known as *Caplan's syndrome*, and it must not be confused radiologically with multiple secondary carcinoma.

The *lesions* at autopsy are characteristic (Gough *et al.*). Discrete nodules are scattered throughout the lungs, but in the upper parts they may fuse to form large masses. Sometimes these masses contain cavities, apparently old, healed, tuberculous lesions. The nodules present a characteristic arrangement of lighter and darker layers. *Microscopically*, there is a central area of necrotic collagen, surrounded by a zone of active inflammation with macrophages and occasionally polymorphonuclears and giant cells. The picture may be mistaken for such fungal infections as histoplasmosis.

The condition is of interest in view of another possible immunological reaction, namely that in silicosis, to which reference has already been made.

Asbestosis.—This condition is due to the inhalation of asbestos dust which may contain over 50 per cent of silica. The disease is acquired either during the crushing of asbestos rock or in the process of carding the asbestos. The lung shows the airless and fibrosed condition found in silicosis, and on the cut surface there are areas of caseation with cavity formation. The characteristic microscopic feature, in addition to a large amount of silica dust, is the presence of large angular particles which are probably fragments of asbestos fibers, and curious golden-yellow bodies with a globular end and segmented body (Fig. 373). The latter structures, which may be called asbestos bodies, are pathognomonic of the condition. They appear to represent deposits around fragments of asbestos fiber.

There is a possible relationship between asbestosis and carcinoma of the lung, for the two conditions are not infrequently associated.

Beryllium Pneumonitis.—A modern industrial hazard is the pneumonitis produced by beryllium, used principally in the manu-

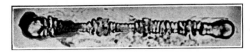

FIG. 373.—Asbestos body showing globular ends and segmented appearance. (Specimen of Dr. J. E. Pritchard.)

facture of fluorescent lamps and also in other industries. The illness may be acute, with recovery when the worker is removed from exposure to the irritant. More important is delayed beryllium poisoning, the symptoms appearing months or a year or two after exposure. The lesions take the form of *granulomatous nodules*, and resemble those of sarcoidosis. Conchoidal bodies similar to those seen in sarcoidosis are often present either in the giant cells or the granuloma. The hilar nodes are also involved. The end stage is *extensive fibrosis*, causing severe dyspnea and eventually right heart failure. The incidence among workers in a plant is low, the distribution spotty, and there is lack of relationship between the severity of the disease and the degree of exposure. Direct and obvious exposure is apparently not necessary, for persons living near a beryllium plant but not working in it have developed the chronic pulmonary form of the disease (Chesner).

Bauxite Fibrosis.—Quite different from the other pneumoconioses are the lesions produced by the dust of bauxite, from which alumina is extracted in the manufacture of carborundum abrasives. There is a diffuse reticulated fibrosis with none of the nodularity so characteristic of silicosis. Large emphysematous bullæ form a striking feature, and pneumothorax is a common consequence. Dyspnea is extreme, and the progress is rapid and fatal.

Graphite Fibrosis.—Graphite or plumbago is a crystalline form of carbon which is extensively used in the manufacture of lubricants, electric batteries, lead pencils, etc. Persons engaged in mining or grinding graphite appear to be exposed to the greatest dust hazard. The lung shows a granulomatous reaction, with areas of fibrosis, necrosis and caseation. Asteroid inclusions may be present in the numerous giant cells (Jaffe).

Byssinosis.—A very curious occupational

chronic respiratory disease due to the inhalation of dust has been observed in the textile workers of Lancashire for the past 200 years (Schilling). It has occasionally been reported in Europe and the United States. The disease is known as byssinosis, from the Greek word meaning linen or fine flax. The sufferers are cotton spinners and workers in the rooms where the bales of cotton are opened. The striking clinical feature is the occurrence of dyspnea and asthmatic symptoms on Mondays, so that it is known to the workers as *Monday Morning Fever*. As the disease progresses the disability is experienced throughout the week. Eventually it may prove fatal. There are no characteristic radiological changes, nor are any laboratory tests available, so that diagnosis has to depend on the patient's history. "It is therefore not surprising that it has been overlooked in this age of medicine in which doctors have so little time for history taking and hesitate to make a diagnosis without the aid of the laboratory and the radiologist" (Schilling). Few studies have been made on the *autopsy lesions*, and the findings fail to explain the clinical picture. The chief changes are chronic bronchitis with a moderate degree of emphysema. There is an absence of the distinctive fibrosis seen in silicosis and asbestosis. Black dust is present, although in small amount, but round or oval bodies comparable to the elongated bodies of asbestosis form a characteristic feature.

Silo-Filler's Disease.—The latest addition to the occupational respiratory disease is not one of the dust diseases, but it seems justifiable to include it in this place. Silo-filler's disease is due to the inhalation of irritating fumes in a freshly filled silo. These fumes are oxides of nitrogen, in particular nitrogen dioxide, similar to those given off in the famous Cleveland Clinic disaster of burning x-ray films. It has long been known that the inhalation of these gases can produce inflammatory changes in the lungs, and farmers have also been aware of the dangers of a freshly filled silo. These facts have now been brought together, with the recognition of a definite clear-cut, distinct clinical and pathological entity (Lowry and Schuman). The person becomes ill immediately with cough, dyspnea and a choking sensation.

This is followed by relative remission of symptoms for two or three weeks, at the end of which time a second phase of illness develops accompanied by fever, chills and increasing dyspnea and cyanosis, with death within six weeks of the initial exposure. The roentgenographic appearance may be indistinguishable from that of miliary tuberculosis.

The *lesions* at autopsy are highly characteristic. The lungs contain innumerable, uniformly distributed, firm nodules of miliary size. These nodules represent bronchioles filled with a fibrinous exudate, which becomes organized by the ingrowth of fibroblasts from the bronchial walls with occlusion of the lumen. The final result is a typical *bronchiolitis fibrosa obliterans*. If the exposure to the fumes in the silo has not been too severe, recovery may occur. The present trend in agriculture toward the greater use of commercial chemicals containing nitrogen may well intensify the danger of poisoning by nitrogen dioxide. Prevention consists of avoiding entrance to a freshly filled silo for a period of one week.

Farmer's Lung.—This disease with the non-committal name used to be confused with silo-filler's lung. The confusion was natural, because the condition is caused by breathing dust in the handling of hay or corn from moldy crops gathered when wet. A fungus is suspected as the causal agent, but hypersensitivity may play a part. The disease may be seen in an acute, subacute or chronic stage. In the acute stage dyspnea is the chief symptom, with varying degrees of fever, chills and weight loss. If the patient is removed from exposure to the dust, recovery takes place in one or two months. The chronic phase develops after exposure over a period of years. The patient is incapacitated with irreversible emphysema and pulmonary fibrosis. In the *x*-ray film the lungs present a nonspecific, sandstorm appearance with miliary nodules. Diagnosis is naturally difficult.

The lesions in the early phase, as seen in lung biopsy, are focal noncaseating granulomas surrounded by giant cells, with an interstitial infiltration of histiocytes and lymphocytes (Baldus and Peter). In the late stage fibrosis and emphysema dominate the picture.

ABSCESS AND GANGRENE

There is no sharp line to be drawn between abscess and gangrene of the lung. The former is a suppurative condition more or less circumscribed, while the latter is putrefactive and tends to be diffuse.

Etiology.—The cause may be divided into three groups: the inhalation, the embolic, and the pneumonic, depending on the method of causation.

1. The *inhalation group* is far the largest and most important. Abscess of the lung is a constant threat in operations on the mouth, nose, and throat. Tonsillectomy being the commonest operation is most often complicated by pulmonary sepsis, but this may happen with the removal of adenoids, operations on the nose, and the removal of teeth, and it may follow a local as well as a general anesthetic. The chief feature of the bacteriology of the inhalation group is its mixed character. This is in contrast to embolic abscesses or those due to staphylococcal pneumonia in which cases there is often only one infecting organism. The abscess is commoner in the right lung, perhaps because this lung has a more vertical bronchus. Foreign bodies may pass down the bronchial tree and give rise to abscess formation, especially in children. Septic material from the nasal sinuses, food regurgitated during general anesthesia, etc., may pass down the bronchial tree and cause an abscess. These foreign body abscesses must be distinguished sharply from other forms, because if the foreign body can be removed by means of the bronchoscope the prognosis is remarkably favorable. A metallic foreign body tends to cause hyperplasia rather than liquefaction of tissue, and when it is removed a complete cure may result. 2. The *embolic group* is caused by particles of a septic thrombus being carried to the lungs. As these particles are numerous the abscesses are nearly always multiple. 3. The *pneumonic group* is usually streptococcal or staphylococcal. In the lobar (pneumococcal) pneumonia it is very rare for the consolidated area to develop into an abscess. There remains a miscellaneous group, including mycotic abscess due to a variety of fungi, and spread of infection from a neighboring organ, *e. g.*, the esophagus, the vertebral column, or from below the diaphragm, as in amebic abscess. Bronchiectatic abscesses form a group which will be considered separately.

A particularly distressing form of inhalation accident is aspiration of stomach contents into the lungs during obstetrical anesthesia (Mendelson). In the production of this condition, sometimes referred to as *Mendelson's syndrome*, two factors play a part: gastric retention and laryngeal paralysis, both being related to the anesthetic used. The pylorus fails to relax, and if food has been taken just before or during labor, the stomach becomes distended with solid and liquid material. This material, more often liquid than solid, may be aspirated into the lungs as a result of the laryngeal reflexes being abolished during general anesthesia. If the material is solid there is bronchial obstruction with collapse of the lung. If it is liquid, as is usually the case, the irritating gastric hydrochloric acid produces bronchiolar spasm, and a peribronchiolar exudative and congestive reaction. The lungs are overdistended with air, and the blood in the lung is very dark, due to the chemical change produced by the acid. The condition is of particular importance to the anesthetist because a healthy young woman may be dead from this accident within an hour or two of delivery. The advisability of having an empty stomach during delivery is obvious.

Lesions.—Abscess is commoner in the right lung, and is as frequent in the upper lobe as in the lower. The lesion is at first a solid mass of yellow inflammatory tissue, but as liquefaction occurs a cavity is formed filled with pus. This cavity may be of any size, from the smallest to the largest. The wall is ragged and necrotic, but in the more chronic forms a wall of fibrous tissue is built up and the lining becomes smooth. Owing to the close relationship in the pulmonary lobule between the bronchus and blood vessels thrombosis is frequent, and this leads to extensive necrosis. The abscess is usually single at first, but secondary abscesses may occur at any time due to aspiration of infected material into other segments. The inhalation abscess is likely to communicate with a bronchus, the embolic abscess is not. Because the abscess is in the periphery of the lung the communicating bronchus is always small, rarely exceeding 2 to 3 mm. in diameter. A chronic abscess may show epithelialization of its wall from the bronchus. The *microscopic appearance* is that of an acute abscess with dense infiltration of polymorphonuclear leukocytes and a varying number of mononuclear phagocytes. The alveolar walls are destroyed, whereas in pneumonia they are preserved. As the condition becomes chronic fibroblasts multiply, and a wall of fibrous tissue is built up around the abscess.

The *odor* of the contents depends largely on whether the lesion is a suppurative or a gangrenous one. In an abscess uncomplicated by gangrene the contents may be inoffensive, but when gangrene supervenes the smell is horrible. This is due to decomposition of the proteins by saprophytes, of which the most abuntant are *spirochetes* and *fusiform bacilli*, which are found in the contents of the cavity, in the sputum, and in sections of the lung. They are largely responsible for the necrosis. These organisms are secondary invaders from the mouth, where they occur in connection with carious teeth and periodontal infection.

Gangrene may be preceded by abscess formation or may be the primary condition owing to the aspiration of heavily infected material. In debilitated persons a pneumonia may become gangrenous. Soft green areas are formed, and these break down with the production of ragged cavities filled with foul-smelling stuff. Blood vessels traversing the cavity may be opened, sometimes with fatal hemorrhage. Gangrene of the lung is likely to be rapidly fatal.

Relation of Symptoms to Lesions.—The chief clinical manifestations of abscess of the lung are (1) *cough and copious expectoration of pus*, (2) *foul breath and sputum*, (3) *elastic tissue in the sputum*, (4) *dullness on percussion*. The signs of gangrene are the same as those of abscess, and often the two conditions are combined.

Pus may be expectorated in large amount, but this depends on whether the abscess communicates with a bronchus. Such a communication exists in bronchiectasis, in an inhalation abscess, and when an abscess bursts into a bronchus. If the abscess can be drained by means of the bronchoscope or even by effective coughing and postural drainage combined with the control of inspection by an appropriate antibiotic, it may become healed. In an embolic abscess there is no communication with a bronchus, so that no pus is expectorated. The *sputum* may be very characteristic, thick, purulent, yellowish-green in color, and often very abundant. *Elastic tissue* in the sputum indicates destruction of the lung. *Pleurisy* is common, because the abscess is often subpleural in position. *Empyema* may be caused by rupture of the abscess into the pleural cavity. *Brain abscess* is an uncommon complication due to septic embolism. Two curious points should be noted: (1) that the cerebral abscess is often single, and (2) the nearly invariable absence of abscesses in the other organs. It is probable that the route of infection is by the vertebral series of veins described by Batson and others.

TUBERCULOSIS

The general problem of tuberculosis has already been discussed in Chapter 11, and in order to avoid needless repetition the reader is referred to that account for a consideration of such questions as the method of infection, primary and secondary infection, the relation of the type of lesion to the age of the patient, etc. Some of the conclusions will be briefly summarized here.

Tuberculosis of the lungs is the commonest of all forms of tuberculosis, partly because by whatever route the bacilli enter the body they pass *via* the lymphatics to the venous blood stream and thus reach the lungs, partly because the lungs are especially exposed to direct infection. In the adult the infection is acquired by inhalation. The inhaled material may be infected dust or infected droplets of sputum. Children may place infected material in the mouth and this may be inhaled into the bronchioles and alveoli. The disease is now being seen more often in old people than formerly.

The *incubation period* in so chronic a disease as pulmonary tuberculosis is difficult to

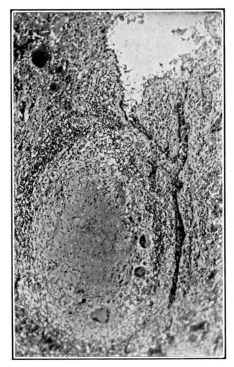

FIG. 374.—Tubercle rupturing into a bronchus. × 65.

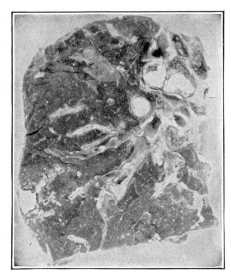

FIG. 375.—Active Ghon lesion. There is a subpleural caseous lesion in the lower lobe. The lymph nodes at the hilus are enlarged and caseous. Miliary tubercles are scattered through the lung, especially in the lower lobe. Some of the upper lobe has been removed. Death was due to general miliary tuberculosis.

determine, but it may be much shorter than anticipated as the following case in my own experience illustrates. A young man's tuberculin test was negative on June 25th. On July 12th he commenced animal experiments involving the use of living tubercle bacilli. On August 8th he developed general symptoms suggestive of infection and slight pain in the chest on breathing. On August 24th the tuberculin test was positive, on September 4th the roentgen-ray film was positive, and on October 17th the sputum contained tubercle bacilli.

Infection may *spread* throughout the lung from the original focus by the lymphatics, air passages, and blood stream.

1. *Lymphatics spread* is of special importance in the primary form. The lymphatics are perivascular and peribronchial and so are the lesions, which form a staphyloid group of tubercles around a central artery or bronchus. Such groups are often seen in the neighborhood of a caseous area. One of the tubercles may break through the wall of the bronchus or artery and rupture into its lumen causing a bronchial or blood spread of the infection.

2. *Bronchial spread* may occur when a focus opens into a bronchus (Fig. 374), and during the later stages infected material must be continually inhaled from one part of the lung to another, setting up fresh areas of bronchopneumonia. The massive forms of tuberculosis such as tuberculous caseous pneumonia are mainly due to this bronchogenic spread.

3. *Hematogenous spread* is caused by rupture of a focus into a blood vessel, usually a vein. This may cause miliary tuberculosis of the lungs as well as throughout the rest of the body.

Primary Infection.—The important distinction between primary infection and reinfection has already been discussed on page 288. Primary infection used to be synonymous with childhood infection, but as the result of public health measures infection is often not acquired for the first time until adult life. The primary or *Ghon lesion* is a small caseous focus, seldom more than 1 cm.

in diameter, usually though not always single, and situated in any part of the lung. In this it contrasts sharply with the secondary lesion which nearly always makes its first appearance at the apex. The primary lesion may be in the lower lobe and is often at the periphery of the lung (Fig. 375). The caseous center becomes surrounded with a fibrous capsule. Calcification and sometimes ossification occur, and the healed lesion is represented by a small scar or calcified nodule. Foci in the regional lymph nodes also become encapsulated and calcified, but some caseous material usually persists and may harbor viable tubercle bacilli for many years. Spread occurs primarily along the lymphatics, so that the regional lymph nodes are enlarged and caseous, again in contrast to what is found in secondary lesions. A chain of tubercles can be traced from the primary lesion to the infected lymph nodes. One of the caseous nodes may open into a blood vessel and cause general miliary tuberculosis.

The patient with primary infection either recovers or dies; the disease does not become chronic, nor is there any cavity formation. If recovery takes place there is healing of the pulmonary and the glandular lesions by encapsulation with subsequent calcification. These healed primary lesions are most readily detected at autopsy by taking roentgen-ray pictures of the lungs, but calcified subpleural nodules may also be felt. Sometimes actual bone is formed in the primary lesion. The results of healing are: (1) calcified parenchymal and lymph node foci; (2) a state of allergy shown by the tuberculin test. About one-half of the population of the United States is tuberculin-positive. If healing fails to occur there may be general blood infection (miliary tuberculosis) or invasion of a bronchus with rapidly fatal bronchopneumonia. The course of the disease depends on such factors as size of dose and protection against frequent reinfection.

Epituberculosis is a clinical term applied to certain tuberculin-positive children who develop a characteristic wedge-shaped x-ray shadow with the base at the pleura and the apex at the hilus that appears suddenly or slowly and then gradually disappears. Although the lesion may be extensive, the symptoms are remarkably mild, and the child may feel perfectly well. The condition is therefore usually discovered accidentally. It appears to be a form of absorption collapse due to bronchial obstruction caused by pressure upon the wall by enlarged tuberculous lymph nodes. These may merely constrict the lumen or may rupture into the interior with the formation of tuberculous granulations (Hutchison).

Reinfection or *secondary infection* is usually an infection from without (exogenous), but it is probable that endogenous infection may occur from a primary lesion which has failed to heal. There is a curious immunity between the ages of five and fifteen, and death from pulmonary tuberculosis during these years is extremely rare. The reaction of the now allergic tissues is quite different from that of the primary infection. The right lung is attacked much more often than the left, and the lesion is nearly always just below the apex.

This remarkable apical localization is characteristic of secondary as opposed to primary infection. All sorts of fanciful explanations have been offered, but the most satisfying and that which agrees best with observed facts is the one offered by Dock, which is based on the low pulmonary arterial pressure at the apex owing to the height of the column of blood from the right ventricle to the apex when the patient is erect. It is now known that the pressure at the apex is practically nil when an adult is in the erect posture. In tall, long-chested persons, notoriously susceptible to tuberculosis, the mean pressure will be negative. As a consequence there will be no production of tissue fluid or lymph in the erect posture, immune bodies will not reach the part, removal of oxygen from the alveoli will be minimal, and tubercle bacilli reaching the part will find optimum conditions for growth. Patients with mitral stenosis are almost immune from apical tuberculosis, and in them the pulmonary arterial pressure is sufficiently high to supply the needs of the part. On the other hand the disease is remarkably common in congenital stenosis of the pulmonary valve, a condition which produces the lowest known pulmonary arterial pressure. The higher incidence of right-sided apical lesions can be explained by the fact that the right pulmonary artery is longer and narrower than the left, winds around the aorta, and breaks into lobar branches at some distance before reaching the hilum of the lung. These considerations explain and emphasize the importance of rest in the recumbent posture in the treatment of pulmonary tuberculosis. As Dock puts it, "it is the erect posture, maintained for many consecutive hours, which has given man an 'Achilles heel' through which the acid-fast arrow may pass."

The *result* will depend on the size of dose and the degree of resistance. If the dose is small and the resistance high there will be complete healing or a quiet fibrocaseous lesion at the apex. If resistance is not so good there may be rapid excavation, and as the result of cavity formation bronchogenic spread may readily occur. At this stage spread by the lymph stream and blood is comparatively rare, so that lesions in lymph nodes are insignificant. If the dose is large and resistance low there will be a widespread tuberculous caseous pneumonia with fatal termination. If a massive dose is discharged from a caseous gland into the blood stream there will be a general miliary tuberculosis.

The principal features of *primary infection* are: (1) the lack of any constant site of the initial lesion, (2) caseous involvement of the lymph nodes, and (3) the absence of liquefaction and cavity formation. In *secondary infection* there may be: (1) healing with fibrosis, (2) chronic fibrocaseous tuberculosis, (3) acute tuberculous caseous pneumonia, and (4) acute miliary tuberculosis. We shall now consider these four very different tissue reactions in the previously infected person.

1. HEALING WITH FIBROSIS.—This is by far the commonest course for the infection to run. The lesion is usually at or just below the apex and takes the form of a small depressed pigmented scar which can often be better felt than seen, and is frequently adherent to the chest wall. The black pigment consists of carbon particles contained within phagocytes which have been arrested because of the blockage of the lymphatics by fibrosis (Fig. 376). Lime salts are usually present, and are seen in the x-ray film.

42

2. CHRONIC FIBROCASEOUS TUBERCULOSIS. —The characteristic reaction of a body already infected with tuberculosis to an additional heavy dose is breaking-down of the caseous tissue and the formation of a cavity. This is evidence of an allergic condition of the tissues, and is in no way connected with immunity. The softened tissue is discharged into a bronchus and coughed up in the sputum. When the disease has reached this stage it is called "open tuberculosis," and tubercle bacilli are found in the sputum. The bronchial wall is involved in the softening and undergoes dilatation, so that the cavity is formed partly as the result of caseation and softening, partly as the result of bronchiectasis. The first cavities are formed at the apex, and these are always the largest, but as the disease progresses other cavities may be formed in the lower lobe. The formation of a cavity is due to the elastic outward pull on an area of softening; this explains its regular outline in the roentgenogram and its comparatively sudden development. The wall of the cavity is smooth, quite unlike the ragged lining of an acute cavity. It may be traversed by bronchi and blood vessels, and erosion of the latter may lead to serious or even fatal hemorrhage (hemoptysis). In addition to the main areas of caseation and cavitation there are small acinar lesions on the outskirts, composed of yellow caseous acini surrounding a terminal bronchiole. The older these are the more are they fused together into larger masses, the younger and more distant they are the smaller are they likely to be. They are formed by invasion of the terminal bronchioles by tuberculous granulation tissue so that the corresponding acini collapse and become filled with an exudate which in turn becomes caseous. Just as the acinus is the fundamental unit of lung structure, so the acinar lesions form the fundamental units of the pathology of pulmonary tuberculosis.

So far we have spoken as if the disease were a steadily progressive one, but such is by no means the case. There is fibrosis as well as caseation, and this fibrosis is seen as a thickening of the bronchi, blood vessels, and pleura, and as numerous white strands on the cut surface. Chronic cavities have a thick and fairly smooth wall (Fig. 377).

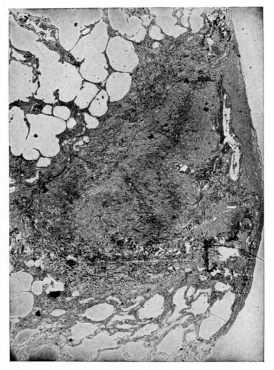

Fig. 376.—A healed tuberculous nodule in the lung.

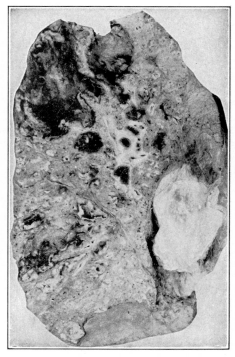

Fig. 377.—Pulmonary tuberculosis showing cavity formation and fibrosis.

Healing of a cavity may occur; this may take place either by scarring or by the cavity becoming filled with caseous material. A cavity of large size, as seen by x-ray, may entirely disappear. Sometimes a cavity may undergo healing in the clinical sense, *i. e.*, it no longer produces sputum filled with tubercle bacilli, and yet remains open, communicating with a bronchus. The caseous lining is shed, the tuberculous granulation tissue becomes fibrosed, and the inner surface of the wall may become epithelialized. A cavity may heal in the pathological sense as the result of occlusion of the draining bronchus, either by obstructive caseous bronchitis, or by the formation of a caseous plug.

When the lungs are freed from the normal pull of the chest by artificial pneumothorax they retract owing to their elasticity, and the cavity shares in this process and tends to collapse and become obliterated. The usual result is a solid nodule due to the retention, inspissation and calcification of the contents of the cavity. Pleural adhesions are very common, especially at the apex, and there

may be patches of recent pleurisy. All of this indicates a good defense, and the disease may either remain stationary or may retrogress to a marked degree if the patient receives the best treatment. This is the form of tuberculosis which can be treated with such encouraging results, especially in the early stages. The bronchial lymph nodes are either not involved or only to a slight degree. The five chief characteristics of this type of pulmonary tuberculosis are: (1) consolidation and caseation, (2) cavity formation, (3) acinar lesions, (4) fibrosis, (5) relative escape of the tracheobronchial lymph nodes, which contain very few bacilli.

The term *tuberculoma* is applied, more particularly by surgeons, to a circumscribed mass of encapsulated tuberculous tissue over 2 cm. in diameter. It is comparable to the tuberculoma of the brain. The lesion represents encapsulation of either an unusually large primary focus or a regressing secondary one. A tuberculous cavity blocked with dried necrotic material will give a similar picture. The lesion is likely first to attract attention during a routine x-ray examination of the lungs, for it does not give rise to symptoms.

The *microscopic picture* varies in different places. The basic lesion is the tubercle, consisting of epithelioid cells and lymphocytes with the usual addition of caseation and giant cells. As the tubercles fuse to form larger masses caseation becomes marked. Much of the elastic tissue remains intact and holds the caseous material together, but when secondary pyogenic infection occurs this tissue is destroyed so that softening soon develops. If the section is stained to show reticulum fibers, an abundance will be seen between the cells of the inflammatory exudate, in sharp contrast to what is found in the next form. Proliferation of fibroblasts and fibrosis are very marked, especially in those cases where resistance is good. The arteries may show an endarteritis obliterans which narrows or even closes the lumen, and this prevents hemorrhage if the wall of the vessel should become ulcerated. The surrounding alveoli may contain a cellular exudate, and in the more fibroid forms the alveolar epithelium may become cuboidal and gland-like (Fig. 371*A*, p. 649).

3. ACUTE TUBERCULOUS CASEOUS PNEUMONIA.—This is an acute form of the disease in which infection overwhelms resistance and sweeps through the lung, so that it gives rise to the clinical picture of "galloping consumption" or acute phthisis (wasting). The lesions ulcerate through the walls of the bronchi in many places and the infection is widely spread throughout the lung by inhalation. The lesions no longer remain discrete as they tend to do in the previous form, but fuse together to form large caseous areas which may involve the whole of a lobe or even the entire lung and give a pneumonic appearance like that of gray hepatization, so that the condition is called caseous pneumonia (Fig. 378). Acute cavities may form in the consolidated tissue, but these are seldom very large, and have the ragged lining characteristic of such cavities with none of the fibrous capsule which shuts off a chronic cavity from the surrounding lung. Pleurisy and bronchitis are present. The tracheobronchial lymph nodes are enlarged and caseous, for the lung is unable to hold back the bacilli which reach the nodes in great numbers.

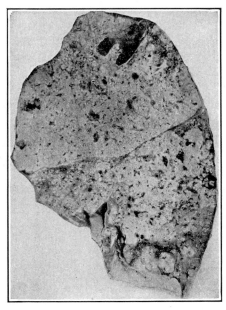

FIG. 378.—Pulmonary tuberculosis. Consolidation of the entire lung from caseous pneumonia with acute cavity formation in a boy, aged fifteen years.

The *microscopic picture* is one of rapid caseation and destruction with no evidence of resistance on the part of the tissues. The alveoli are filled with an acute cellular exudate, mainly mononuclear in type, which rapidly becomes caseous so that all detail is lost. Elastic tissue is destroyed, and no reticulum fibers are formed between the cells in the alveoli. Neither giant cells nor fibrosis are in evidence. Smears of the exudate and sections of the lung show enormous numbers of tubercle bacilli, far in excess of what is seen in any other form of pulmonary tuberculosis.

4. ACUTE MILIARY TUBERCULOSIS.—If a caseous tuberculous focus discharges its contents into a blood vessel the body is flooded with tubercle bacilli. A caseous bronchial lymph node may become adherent to a branch of the pulmonary artery and open into that vessel, in which case only the affected lung may show the tubercles. More often the vessel is a vein, and then tubercles are found in all the organs as well as in the lungs, the patient often dying of tuberculous meningitis.

The lungs are intensely congested and studded with minute tubercles, many of

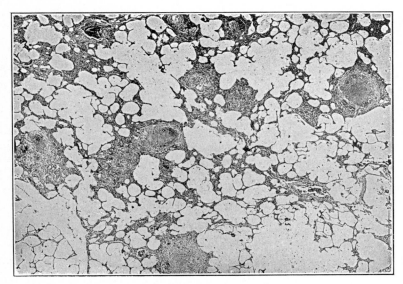

Fig. 379.—Acute miliary tuberculosis of the lung. Between the tubercles the lung tissue is practically normal. × 18.

which can only be seen with the aid of a magnifying glass. At first the lesions are pale and translucent but as caseation develops they become yellow and opaque. *Microscopically* the tubercles are seen to be everywhere in the fibrous framework of the lung, but the intervening alveoli are either empty or contain catarrhal cells (Fig. 379). The tubercles present the usual caseous center, epitheloid cells, lymphocytes, and giant cells.

A distinction must be drawn between tuberculous bacillemia and general miliary tuberculosis. A varying degree of bacillemia occurs in every case of tuberculosis; it is by this means that discrete foci in bone, kidney, etc., are set up. But it is only when resistance is overwhelmed that the condition becomes miliary tuberculosis, and it is overwhelmed because of the massive size of the dose, especially if this dose be continually repeated. Miliary tuberculosis may occasionally be *chronic* and the lesions may undergo healing by fibrosis.

Tuberculous Lesions After Chemotherapy. —The picture of tuberculosis which we have painted in the preceding pages is that of a disease taking its natural course. Modern chemotherapy has resulted in changes in the lesions observed by the pathologist. The effect will naturally be more marked in recent than in chronic lesions, and they are more striking after the use of isoniazid than after streptomycin, the two agents which have proved most useful (Dick). When observations are made from the second to the eighth week of treatment with isoniazid, recent lesions are found to disappear completely in a way never before believed possible in man. First there is increased vascularity with the formation of new capillaries, the epithelioid cells revert to macrophages which gradually disappear, and the tuberculous granulation tissue becomes converted into healing true granulation tissue. Only the giant cells tend to persist. At the same time there is vigorous regeneration of the specialized tissue. In recent lesions there is a complete absence of the dense fibrosis which follows streptomycin therapy. If the lesion is small it is completely absorbed, if somewhat larger it persists as loose granulation tissue, if still larger there will be extensive areas of open fibrous tissue which contract later to small scars.

"Cyst" formation after chemotherapy may result in thin-walled cyst-like structures detected in the lung by the radiologist, mostly in cases of recent consolidation receiving isoniazid therapy. As the development of

cysts is most apparent in recent cases which have responded particularly well to therapy, it is natural that pathological studies have been limited. Only one or two large cysts may develop, or the multiple cysts may suggest the presence of diffuse cystic disease. When the cysts are few in number they may attain 10 cm. in diameter. The cysts may be lined by bronchiolar epithelium, but usually the lining is composed of compressed alveolar walls or a thin layer of connective tissue (Berthrong). Some of the cysts will disappear, but others may persist as space-occupying lesions which require surgical treatment.

Relation of Symptoms to Lesions.—The *general symptoms* (fever, loss of weight, asthenia, etc.) are due to the absorption of toxins. They become more marked when secondary infection is added to the pure tuberculous infection. *Cough* is a bronchial symptom due to inflammation of the larger bronchi, the walls of which are much more sensitive than those of the bronchioles. *Pain* in the side is due to a tuberculous pleurisy. The character of the *sputum* depends entirely on the form which the lesions take. In miliary tuberculosis there may be no sputum. As long as the lesion remains closed the sputum remains scanty and contains no tubercle bacilli. When cavities form, the sputum becomes abundant and purulent and contains numbers of bacilli. It should be remembered that unless the bacilli number 100,000 per cc. of sputum, they will probably not be seen with the ordinary Ziehl-Neelsen method. Guinea pig inoculation is a thousand times more sensitive. The appearance of elastic tissue fibers in the sputum indicates lung destruction. *Hemoptysis* marks the end of the beginning or the beginning of the end. In the early stages there may be erosion of a small vessel in the process of softening. In the late stages a large artery crossing a chronic cavity may give way causing a severe and possibly a fatal hemorrhage.

The *physical signs* depend on the character of the lesions. The consolidation and cavitation of the fibrocaseous form are indicated by *dulness on percussion, increased tactile fremitus,* and *blowing breathing* which may become amphoric over a large cavity. All these signs are diminished if the pleura is much thickened. There is not the wooden dulness of lobar pneumonia except in the caseous pneumonic form. Moist râles intensified by coughing (post-tussic) indicate breaking down of caseous material; they become coarser as the cavities enlarge. Small calcified lesions, Ghon lesions, miliary tubercles, and, of course, more extensive consolidation and cavity formation are clearly shown by the roentgen ray films.

Chromogenic Acid-fast Bacillary Infections.—Acid-fast bacilli capable of producing infections used to be limited to those associated with tuberculosis and leprosy. It is now known that acid-fast bacilli which are not tubercle bacilli are occasionally found in lesions which resemble or are identical with those of tuberculosis (Weed). They have been named "anonymous mycobacteria," and they produce lung infections which masquerade as tuberculosis and may be called "pseudotuberculosis" (Lewis). The relationship of this new group to the lesions in which they are found is open to debate, but there can be no doubt of their importance as a possible source of serious errors in diagnosis.

The bacilli in question are indistinguishable morphologically from tubercle bacilli, but they *differ* from them in three important characteristics: (1) they grow on ordinary culture media, albeit slowly; (2) they are non-pathogenic to the guinea pig; (3) they are chromogenic, *i.e.* they produce pigment, so that the colonies are yellow, orange, or even red. The pigment is produced either in the light (photochromogens) or in the dark (non-photochromogens). It is the bacilli that produce yellow pigment, known for this reason by the somewhat confusing name of *yellow acid-fast bacilli,* which seem to be most intimately connected with the production of lesions similar to those of tuberculosis, although the pathogenicity of the atypical acid-fast organisms is still a highly controversial subject. The clinical condition with which they are associated in man is similar to tuberculosis; so are the x-ray findings and the gross and microscopic appearance. It is possible that the organisms are what may be termed *opportunist saprophytes.* They live mainly outside the body, but they can act as pathogens, producing lesions only rarely because most of the population is immune. The two important facts to bear in mind are: (1) that the presence of acid-fast bacilli in lesions with the microscopic picture of tuberculosis does not establish a diagnosis of tuberculosis, and (2) that *the chromogenic acid-fast bacilli are resistant to the chemotherapeutic agents effective against tuberculosis.*

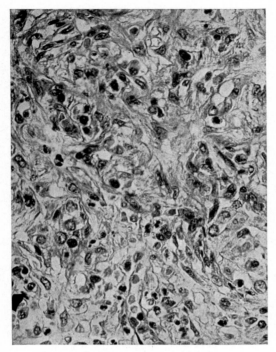

FIG. 380.—Congenital syphilis of the lung. × 300.

SYPHILIS OF THE LUNG

Syphilis of the lung may be congenital or acquired. The former is much commoner and much more characteristic than the latter.

The *congenital form* is seen in syphilitic infants. The child is either born dead or dies in a few days. The lung or part of it is consolidated so that it sinks in water, and is of a pale gray color. For this reason the condition is called *pneumonia alba*. It is an interstitial pneumonia caused by enormous number of spirochetes scattered through the lung, with the formation of a large amount of cellular fibrous tissue (Fig. 380). The alveoli are small, separated by the fibrous tissue, and lined by cubical epithelium so as to have a gland-like appearance. The picture is one of arrested development rather than active inflammation. I have seen nodular lesions, like gummata in the gross.

The *acquired* form is now so rare that it need only be mentioned. The usual lesion is ulceration of a bronchus with subsequent scarring and bronchial obstruction. Gummata are a remote possibility.

MYCOTIC AND OTHER GRANULOMAS

Perhaps as a result of the greatly increased (excessive ?) use of antibiotics mycotic infections of the lung due to the higher fungi are assuming greater importance, particularly in the Southern United States. Indeed these fungi seem to have usurped the place formerly occupied by bacterial invaders causing "terminal pneumonia." As will be seen, many of the fungi produce lesions which mimic tuberculosis. Even at autopsy the correct diagnosis may be overlooked, for in all the mycotic diseases there is caseation and cavity formation, so that they all resemble tuberculosis. A pulmonary granuloma, often giving the picture of a coin lesion in the x-ray film, should not be called a tuberculoma without bacteriological proof. For this purpose the periodic acid-Schiff (PAS) method of McManus is much superior to hematoxylin and eosin for the demonstration of fungi in the tissues. The organisms, which stain red against a greenish-blue background, are readily seen. Even better for demonstrating the remains of fungi which cannot be grown is Gomori's methenamine-silver nitrate stain. The cause of the majority of surgically excised pulmonary granulomas has not been determined, even with extensive bacteriological studies, but with this stain in one series of 138 cases it was possible to identify structures resembling Histoplasma capsulatum or Coccidioides immitis in 60 per cent (Segal *et al.*).

Blastomycosis.—This is probably the commonest of the pulmonary mycoses. The spores may be inhaled directly, or infection may spread by the blood stream from skin lesions to the lung. The lesions (consolidation and cavitation) are very much like those of tuberculosis, but there is more suppuration and giant cell formation. The blastomycetes are seen in the microscopic sections in large numbers and also in the sputum and pus. The prognosis is far worse than in tuberculosis.

Actinomycosis.—The actinomyces are inhaled into the lung or spread from the mouth. They never spread by the blood stream. The lesions are like those of fibrocaseous tuberculosis, but instead of cavitation there is abscess formation. Moreover the lower lobe is most often involved. As usual the disease spreads by contiguity, not by the lymph or blood stream, so that it extends to the chest wall, spine, and through the diaphragm, forming numerous sinuses, but not involving

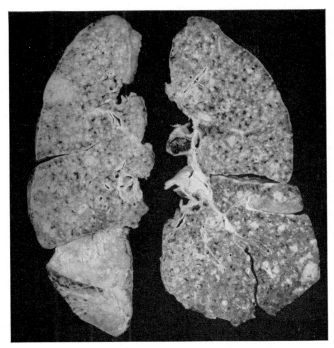

Fig. 381.—Pulmonary nocardiosis. The parenchyma of the lung is studded with
granular areas varying greatly in size.

the bronchial lymph nodes or distant organs. The fungus is found in the "sulfur granules" in the pus and sputum. The disease is usually fatal in from six months to a year.

Nocardiosis.—Nocardia asteroides belongs to the same family as Actinomyces bovis, but it differs sharply from that organism in being aerobic. Unlike actinomycosis, the main lesions are in the lung. Moreover nocardia is acid-fast, although weakly so, and this property leads to it being confused with the tubercle bacillus. The pulmonary lesions may resemble those of tuberculosis, but suppuration and abscess formation in the lung and the chest wall are frequent, and the draining sinuses may be mistaken for those of actinomycosis. The widespread character of the pulmonary involvement is evident in Fig. 381. In the past nocardiosis has generally been misdiagnosed for actinomycosis or tuberculosis. The distinction between the two fungus diseases is all-important, because Actinomyces bovis is extremely sensitive to penicillin, whereas Nocardia asteroides is relatively resistant, although it responds readily to sulfonamide therapy. "If you treat with penicillin all diseases caused by branching, fragmenting, filamentous fungi, then most patients with actinomycosis will recover, while almost all patients with nocardiosis will die" (Peabody and Seabury).

Streptothricosis.—A rare infection by a branching fungus, possibly a variant of actinomyces. The pulmonary lesions are of the septic type—abscess, gangrene and bronchiectasis. The infection may spread by the blood stream to the brain and elsewhere.

Coccidioidomycosis.—The characteristics of the fungus coccidioides are described in Chapter 13. The infection is widespread throughout Southern California, West Texas, and the regions of the United States bordering on Mexico. The spores of the fungus are inhaled from the soil, causing an acute pneumonia. While this usually clears up completely, many cases have incomplete resolution with residual infiltrations, of which nodular densities and cavities are the most characteristic x-ray feature. These may persist for many years unchanged. The residual pulmonary lesions, especially the cavities, may strongly suggest tuberculosis, but the patient presents no symptoms and feels quite well. The microscopic appearance resembles that of tuberculosis, but the pathognomonic feature is the presence of the double-contoured highly refractile coccidioides filled with spores (Fig. 180, page 323). Infection does not spread to other parts of the lung nor to distant organs. The fatal disseminated form of coccidioidal infection is a very different story.

Aspergillosis.—This is caused by Aspergillus fumigatus, a filamentous fungus with a basal stem and a stalk supporting a spore-bearing head. The disease occurs amongst bird fanciers, pigeon stuffers, and other grain handlers. The lesions are similar to those of tuberculosis, with necrosis and cavitation. Mats of mycelial threads may be seen in some areas. The x-ray picture may strongly suggest miliary tuberculosis or silicosis. Fatalities are now being reported, expecially in patients treated with antibiotics.

Histoplasmosis.—Like coccidiomycosis, histoplasmosis used to be regarded as a fatal systemic fungous disease. It is now known that a mild form exists. The geographic distribution is marked, namely the Mississippi valley and the Eastern Central states of North America. It is essentially a soil fungus. There is an unusually high incidence of pulmonary calcification with a negative tuberculin but a positive histoplasmin reaction in these areas, and there can be no doubt that this calcification indicates healed lesions in a benign form of pulmonary histoplasmosis. The yeast-like bodies which pack the reticuloendothelial cells in enormous numbers are so small that originally they were thought to be protozoa (Fig. 197, page 360).

The *primary localized* lesion resembles the Ghon lesion of childhood tuberculosis. A limited area of consolidation slowly resolves and becomes calcified. Strangely enough generalized lesions follow a similar pattern. It is natural that at this stage the disease is likely to be subclinical. If *reinfection* occurs, fibrocaseous lesions develop which may undergo cavitation and closely resemble chronic pulmonary tuberculosis. Were it not that the sputum and skin tests for tuberculosis are negative, while Histoplasma capsulatum is present in the sputum and the histoplasmin skin test is positive, it might be impossible to distinguish between the two conditions.

Cryptococcosis (Torulosis).—This also is an infection caused by a soil fungus, Cryptococcus neoformans (Torula histolytica) which enters the respiratory system but whose real threat is to the central nervous system. Massive inflammatory lesions like those of pneumonia may be seen in the x-ray film, yet with little or no clinical disturbance. In other cases there are rounded granulomatous masses. The most common pathological lesion is a subpleural nodule less than 1.5 cm. in diameter, but larger nodules with a tendency to necrosis and cavitation may be encountered. The histological diagnosis is made by recognizing the thick-walled yeast-like infecting cells in the sputum or the tissue. If infection reaches the brain, as it may well do, the result is a chronic but fatal meningitis, the true nature of which is indicated by finding cryptococci in the spinal fluid.

Pneumocystis Pneumonia.—This condition, caused by an *animal parasite* rather than a fungus, might better be called a pneumonitis than a pneumonia. It has a peculiarly well defined distribution, being relatively common in Europe but little known in North America (Hamperl). It is essentially a disease of infants, being hardly ever met with before the sixth week of life or after the sixth month. The incubation period is about six weeks. The mortality is from 30 to 40 per cent. At autopsy all lobes of both lungs show an extensive gray-white consolidation. *Microscopically* the alveoli are filled with an apparently fluid or foamy material. In addition there is an *interstitial plasma cell pneumonitis* (Fig. 383). The foamy material consists of myriads of tiny bodies in finely reticulated, honey-combed material which represents *cysts* and *spores* of the *parasite Pneumocystis Carinii*, named after Carini who first described it. As they contain mucopolysaccharides they are well shown by the PAS stain. Rodents, dogs and sheep are also infected.

Other Mycotic Granulomas.—It would be tedious to enumerate all the fungi which may

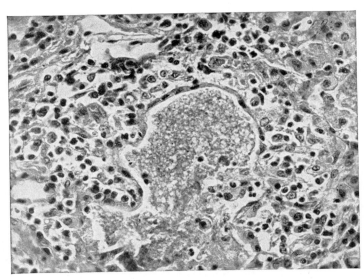

FIG. 382.—Pneumocystis carinii, showing foamy contents of alveolar sacs and plasma cell interstitial pneumonitis. (Kindness of Dr. F. Kuzma, Marquette University, Milwaukee.)

cause granulomatous reactions in the lung. The following, however, deserve brief mention. *Nocardiosis* is caused by infection with Nocardia asteroides. As this fungus is acid-fast, and as its filaments may become fragmented into bacillus-like rods, it is evident that mistakes may be made in the bacteriological examination of the sputum. Moreover, the pulmonary lesions may resemble those of tuberculosis, but suppuration and abscess formation in the lung and the chest wall are frequent, so that the condition may be mistaken for actinomycosis. *Moniliasis* is caused by the fungus, Monilia. The pulmonary lesions again resemble those of tuberculosis, taking the form of small yellow nodules, which fuse together, break down, and form cavities identical with those of tuberculosis. *Mucormycosis* is a newcomer to the field of pulmonary fungous infections (Baker), although the older German literature contains report of this condition, dating back to 1876. Its increasing incidence may be due to the use of antibiotics, which suppress the growth of bacteria, and thereby permit invasion of fungi. Inhalation of *Phycomycetes* as common contaminants is most likely to occur in the Southern United States. The fungus invades blood vessels, giving rise to thrombosis and infarction.

There is also involvement of the bronchi and alveoli. The lesions therefore present a characteristic combination of mild acute pneumonia and infarction. Some of the differential features of the important fungi are summarized in a table on page 329.

Pulmonary Alveolar Proteinosis.—The advisability of including in the present section this newcomer to the field of pulmonary pathology may well be questioned, for it is neither a known fungous disease nor is it a granuloma. It was in 1958 that Rosen, Castleman and Liebow described a new clinical entity which they called pulmonary alveolar proteinosis, because it was marked by filling of the alveoli with a proteinaceous material, strongly positive with the periodic acid-Schiff stain, and rich in lipid. This material appears to be produced by the lining "septal" cells, which slough into the lumen, ultimately becoming necrotic and adding granules and variable laminated bodies to the alveolar content. The condition bears some resemblance to pneumocystis infection of the lung. Indeed some of the 27 cases collected by Rosen and his associates had been reported as pneumocystis infection. This is the excuse for including proteinosis in this place. In truth, I did not know where else to put it.

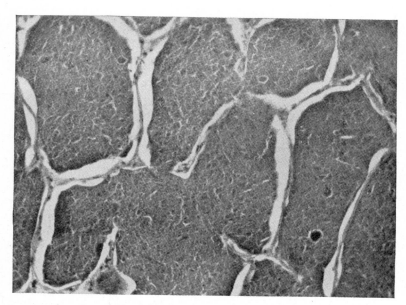

Fig. 383.—PAS-positive material. (Note thin alveolar walls, acicular spaces and rounded masses representing remnants of cells. (Rosen, Castleman and Liebow, courtesy of New Eng. J. Med.)

Clinically, the disease may or may not be ushered in by a febrile illness suggesting pneumonia. The most common and prominent complaint is *dyspnea*, usually accompanied by cough, sometimes with yellow sputum. Chest pain, fatiguability and slight loss of weight are less frequent symptoms. Cyanosis is associated with more severe involvement. Physical signs on percussion and auscultation are few or absent. Indeed *a clue to the diagnosis is offered by the disproportion between these symptoms and signs and the roentgenographic evidence of extensive pulmonary involvement simulating severe bilateral pulmonary edema.* The clinical course is variable, some cases showing definite improvement, others remaining unchanged, while still others progress to a fatal conclusion.

The *lesions* are remarkably constant and similar from one case to another. At autopsy large portions of the lung are consolidated. In earlier biopsy material multiple yellow-gray nodules are seen under the pleura. A fluid, either milky or like yellow pus, may ooze from the cut surface on gentle pressure. The weight of the lungs, which sink in water, is remarkable, many weighing from 3,000 to 4,000 gm.

The *microscopic appearance* has already been mentioned. The proteinaceous material which fills the alveolar spaces may be mistaken for edema, but with the PAS stain it has a characteristic granular appearance (Fig. 383). There is a striking absence of the interstitial plasma cell pneumonitis which is so constant a feature of pneumocystis pneumonia. The lesions must not be confused with those of cholesterol pneumonitis, in which a large portion of a lobe contains enormous numbers of phagocytes filled with fat, including cholesterol.

Both the *nature* and *cause* of the disease are unknown. The suggested relationship to pneumocystis infection in a modified form has already been mentioned, but no parasites have been demonstrated, and pneumocystis infection is mainly a disease of premature infants who usually die in the second or third month of life, whereas most of the patients with proteinosis are between twenty and fifty years of age. It may well be that this new disease is caused by some recently introduced inhalant, possibly commercial or industrial in character, and that the disease is "a penalty for the convenience of modern living."

Pulmonary Sarcoidosis.—The cause of

sarcoidosis is unknown. Indeed the disease itself is an enigma wrapped in a mystery. It is a disease mainly of lymphoid organs, so that it is discussed in Chapter 41. The reason why it is considered here is that the principal or the only lesions may be confined to the lung and that these lesions are granulomas.

The condition is discovered by the radiologist, often on a routine examination. One of the most suggestive features is the striking lack of symptoms, although the radiological findings may suggest such alarming possibilities as primary or secondary carcinoma or tuberculosis. There may be either no symptoms or merely a sense of tiredness, a little cough, low fever and mild dyspnea. In advanced cases extensive fibrosis with secondary emphysema may result in disabling dyspnea (McClement *et al.*). Frequently or as a rule, however, the lesions clear up and resolve spontaneously.

The *lesions* are those of sarcoidosis elsewhere. The basic lesion is the sarcoid, a tubercle-like, sharply circumscribed structure composed mainly of epithelioid and giant cells (Fig. 161, page 293), but with a notable *absence of caseation*. The lesions may be miliary in size or they may fuse to form large masses, and as the disease progresses fibrosis becomes more and more a prominent feature. If all other methods fail a lung biopsy or examination of a scalene lymph node may be necessary. From what has been said in this general section it will be evident that the responsible task of the pathologist may be none too easy, and that bacteriological and other methods may be needed in order to exclude granulomas caused by fungi and other agents.

CIRCULATORY DISTURBANCES

Active Congestion.—This is rather an ill-defined condition which may be the result of irritating gases or the initial stage of an acute inflammation. The vessels in the alveolar walls are distended with blood.

Passive Congestion.—In passive congestion the dilatation of the vessels is a passive affair due to mechanical causes. Two forms are recognized: (1) brown induration, a

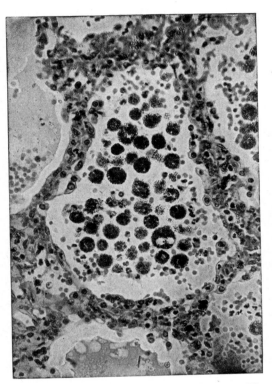

Fig. 384.—Heart failure cells in the lung. The alveolar walls are greatly thickened. × 250.

chronic process, (2) hypostatic congestion, usually a terminal one.

Brown Induration.—Brown induration of the lung is always associated with hypertension in the pulmonary circuit. This is most often due to mitral stenosis, but it may be caused by emphysema, extensive pleural adhesions, marked diminution in the lung volume, silicosis, or communication between the two sides of the heart due to a congenital defect. The lungs are voluminous, russet-brown in color, tough, and indurated (brown induration). *Microscopically* the lung is filled with blood, the alveolar vessels being widely distended, and the alveoli containing many red blood cells. The characteristic feature is the presence of great numbers of large phagocytic cells filled with yellow pigment. These cells are known as *heart failure cells* even when they occur in other than cardiac conditions, and may be derived from residual epithelial cells in the alveolar walls known as septal cells or epicytes (Macklin) or from histiocytes (reticuloendothelial cells) (Fig. 384). The pigment is hemosiderin, derived from the red blood cells in the alveoli, and gives the Prussian blue reaction for iron. There is also a marked increase in the connective tissue of the lung, which is partly responsible for the toughness and induration. This is probably caused by the pigment, which is carried by phagocytes into the lymphatics and distributed throughout the framework of the lung, where it excites fibrosis. The alveolar walls are thickened, so that the vascular endothelium is separated from the air in the alveoli. This interferes with oxygenation of the blood, and is responsible for some of the *dyspnea* of mitral stenosis. *Hemoptysis* is a common symptom of mitral stenosis, and is due to the hemorrhage into the alveoli. The blood in the alveoli is partly converted into bilirubin, and the bilirubin content of the plasma may be above normal, so that mitral stenosis is one of the conditions which may give rise to a latent jaundice.

Hypostatic Congestion.—An accumulation of blood in the lower and posterior part of the lung is found at every autopsy, and is due to relaxation of the vessels after death plus the force of gravity. A much more advanced condition is found in patients with some debilitating illness and weak heart action who have been kept on their back. The dependent part of the lung may appear to be consolidated, so that without the microscope it may be impossible to tell if the condition is hypostatic congestion or hypostatic pneumonia. The air in the alveoli is replaced by plasma and red blood cells, but a pneumonic process may be added as the result of terminal infection.

Idiopathic Pulmonary Hemosiderosis.—This rare condition, also known as essential brown induration of the lungs, is a disease of children. The lungs show an extreme degree of brown induration, but no cardiac or other lesions can be found to account for this. There are periodic attacks of severe anoxic anoxemia associated with massive intra-alveolar diapedesis of red cells. At autopsy the alveolar walls are thickened, the capillaries greatly dilated, and the alveolar spaces filled with red cells and macrophages containing hemosiderin. The cause is unknown.

Pulmonary Edema.—A slight degree of pulmonary edema is almost as common as congestion and may be seen at the base of the lung in nearly every autopsy. It is due to failure of the heart as the patient is dying. Pronounced edema may take two main forms, inflammatory and mechanical.

Inflammatory Edema.—This forms a part of any inflammatory exudate, the plasma readily passing from the vessels into the lumen of the alveoli. The amount varies depending on the irritant. It is very abundant in influenzal pneumonia, where the lung becomes water-logged. A varying amount of the plasma is converted into fibrin, the proportion being extremely large in pneumococcal pneumonia. The increased capillary permeability characteristic of shock results in edema. Many cases of so-called terminal edema are of this nature.

Mechanical Edema.—This variety is due to chronic heart failure. The edema is due to a disproportion between the working power of the two ventricles. If the left ventricle fails more rapidly than the right, the pulmonary vessels become distended and plasma leaks through the capillary walls into the alveoli. If we ask *why* the fluid leaks through, we find ourselves confronted with the difficult problem of edema which has already been discussed in Chapter 7.

Pulmonary edema of the mechanical type is naturally a chronic condition. An *acute pulmonary edema* may occasionally develop, for which no adequate cause can be found at autopsy. The patient usually has chronic nephritis or high blood pressure, and it appears as if some sudden strain had been thrown on the left side of the heart. An acute and fatal pulmonary edema may follow a surgical operation. I have seen this accident occur in a simple appendectomy. In rare cases acute edema of the lung may come on after removal of a pleural effusion. Here the lung which has been compressed for a long time suddenly expands, and for some reason fluid pours from the vessels into the alveoli.

As in other forms of edema, the great factor in the pathogenesis of pulmonary edema is increased capillary permeability. This may be due to increased intravascular pressure, to anoxia as in cerebral trauma, to poisonous gases such as chlorine, to severe smog, where the irritant is sulfur dioxide, and of course to bacterial toxins and viruses, as in influenza.

The *gross appearance* of the lung is characteristic. It is voluminous, heavy, firm, or doughy, and shows marked pitting on pressure. In the mechanical variety the edema is most marked in the dependent parts of the lung (base and posterior border). The consolidation may be so marked as to simulate pneumonia, but steady pressure will force the fluid out and leave the lung soft. When the lung is cut and squeezed, water pours from the cut surface and from the bronchi. If the condition is very marked as in influenzal pneumonia or acute edema of the lung the fluid pours out of the water-logged organ without any pressure being used. The color of the fluid depends on the presence or absence of congestion. If this is marked the fluid is bloody, if absent the fluid is clear and watery.

The *microscopic picture* is that of alveoli filled with fluid coagulated by the fixative (Fig. 385). The more albuminous the fluid, the more intensely does it stain with eosin. If the fluid has a very low protein content (mechanical edema), it may tend to be washed out by the fixative. In such cases the edema is best demonstrated by fixing the tissue for a few moments in boiling formalin which coagulates the fluid *in situ*. The material which fills the alveoli appears as a hyaline sheet, but sometimes it is granular. In inflammatory edema there may be a varying amount of fibrin formation. Before the alveolar edema which is so evident develops, there is first an interstitial edema because of the low pulmonary tissue pressure. It is only when the pulmonary lymphatics are no longer able to deal with the increased load that fluid passes from the interstitial spaces into the alveoli, and abnormal breath sounds are heard.

The *clinical picture* may be imagined from this description of the lesions. Severe and acute pulmonary edema presents the physician with a dramatic and alarming situation, with a profoundly anxious and cyanotic patient sitting bolt upright, gasping for air with wheezing respiration, his mouth and nose flecked with pink, frothy sputum. In more chronic edema the weakened patient

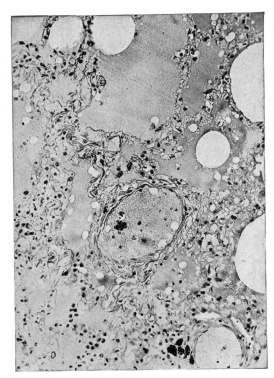

Fig. 385.—Edema of pulmonary alveoli filled with coagulated plasma. Dilated vessel in center of section. × 150.

is unable to expectorate the large volumes of fluid sputum produced, and he may actually drown in his own secretions. The breathing is difficult, with loud bubbling rhonchi, the face is cyanotic, and often there is visible engorgement of the superficial veins of the upper part of the body due to the increased venous pressure.

Hyaline Membrane Disease.—In a number of entirely unrelated disorders a striking feature of the pulmonary pathology is the presence of an eosinophilic hyaline membrane lining the inner wall of the alveoli and constituting in greater or less degree an alveolar-capillary block. We have already seen an example of it in influenzal pneumonia. It occurs in the reaction to the fumes of various metals such as cadmium, mercury and beryllium, as well as to certain viruses other than the virus of influenza, and to unknown causes, as in the Hamman-Rich syndrome.

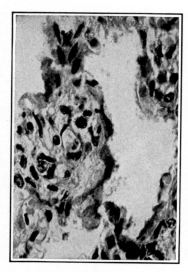

FIG. 386.—Hyaline membrane in pneumonia of
the newborn. × 500.

The one state, however, which is dignified
by the name hyaline membrane disease is
that which is observed in *infants*. This is a
serious respiratory condition which may not
be present at birth but becomes very evident
soon afterwards. The baby is born well,
but within a few hours he becomes acutely
dyspneic. If he dies, the terminal bronchioles and alveoli are filled with the fluid
which forms the hyaline-membrane-like layer
with which they are lined (Fig. 386).
The membrane does not stain with the
ordinary stains for fibrin. It is strongly
PAS-positive. Nevertheless it is believed
to be fibrin, perhaps modified, because
it gives a positive reaction with fluorescein-
labelled antibodies to blood proteins. Studies
with the electron microscope also point to
fibrin as a major component of the membrane. It used to be thought that aspiration
of amniotic sac contents may play a part
in some cases, but in view of the fact that
the hyaline membrane is commonly associated with pulmonary edema, severe pulmonary congestion, and intra-alveolar hemorrhage it seems best to regard the condition as a primary disorder in the pulmonary circulation. The easiest way to produce distinct hyaline membrane in the
animal lung is by oxygen poisoning. It
would seem that these small infants find the

sudden change from an intrauterine environment too much for their pulmonary circulation, so that plasma proteins are extravasated into the alveoli and pressed into a
membrane on the alveolar walls by the inhaled air. They may obstruct the alveolar
ducts, causing resorption atelectasis. Another suggestion is that hyaline membranes
represent a concentrated secretion from the
epithelial cells of the terminal bronchioles
and alveolar ducts. This is based on the
observation that special techniques show
this epithelium to contain a concentration
of granules with similar staining reactions
to those of the membranes (Lynch and
Mellor).

The condition occurs in those situations
where the mother could be expected to have
circulating hormones which might induce a
temporary increased permeability of the pulmonary capillaries of the child (Chapple).
Most of the cases occur in infants born: (1)
prematurely, (2) by cesarean section, and
(3) of diabetic mothers. Estrogen is known
to tighten cells and their membranes and
make them less permeable, whereas progesterone increases the permeability. In the
case of prematurity and cesarean section the
normal fall in the progesterone level which
marks the approach of normal delivery does
not occur so that the level in mother and
child remains high, whilst in diabetic mothers
the levels are frequently abnormal. It would
appear, therefore, as if hyaline membrane
formation in the newborn is due to an increased permeability of membranes, itself
conditioned by an abnormal hormonal situation.

Another concept which has been suggested
is that a predisposing factor in hyaline membrane formation in the newborn is the absence of plasminogen-activator activity in
the lung (Lieberman), an absence which may
have a genetic basis. The fibrinolytic
enzymes in man constitute a complex system
consisting of a circulating active enzyme
(fibrinolysin or plasmin), its inactive precursor (profibrinolysin or plasminogen), and
several blood and tissue activators. If the
activator is deficient the fibrinolysin which
dissolves unnecessary or harmful fibrin that
may be formed is not produced. The tissue
activator of plasminogen is found in the lung

as early as the third month of gestation, but in infants with hyaline membrane formation it is absent.

Perhaps an undue amount of space has been devoted to this discussion, but it seems probable that investigations of the type outlined above may lead to a solution of the problem, and open a way to the successful treatment of this dangerous and often fatal threat to the newborn or premature infant.

Embolism and Infarction. — This subject is fully discussed in connection with the general question of embolism in Chapter 6. The venous thrombosis which precedes the embolism is often postoperative, especially after operations on the female pelvis, but the condition is even more frequent in purely medical (chiefly cardiac) cases. The first embolus may prove fatal. As a rule, however, a fatal embolus is preceded by a number of smaller emboli which can be detected clinically and recognized as danger signals. In this case the use of anti-coagulents such as heparin and dicumarol can arrest the formation of thrombi in the veins and thus protect the patient against fatal embolism. In practice this procedure has proved of value. Ligation of the veins in the leg has a similar effect. If the embolus is large and blocks a main artery death may occur in the course of a few minutes from shock (Fig. 387). In this case there is no time for an infarct to be produced. *Death is believed to be due to the release of serotonin from platelets at the site of embolism.* Serotonin produced by carcinoid tumors is known to cause vasoconstrictor symptoms similar to those of pulmonary embolism. When the embolus is smaller a red infarct is formed with hemorrhage into the alveoli, hemoptysis, and pain in the side due to a patch of pleurisy over the infarct. When the infarct is larger there may be a hemorrhagic pleural effusion. As recovery takes place the infarct is partly replaced by a scar which can seldom be detected if the patient dies later. If, however, formalin is instilled into the trachea and the lungs are then inflated to their original size, healed infarcts can often be demonstrated. Chronic pleuritis and puckering are easily mistaken for healed tuberculosis. Persistence of elastic tissue and the demonstration of an organized embolus help to distinguish a

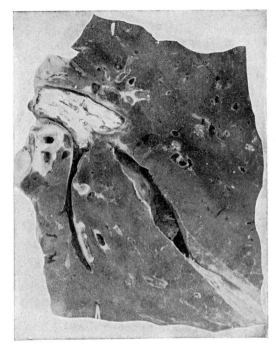

Fig. 387.—Large embolus astride the bifurcation of the pulmonary artery. (Boyd, *Pathology for the Physician.*)

healed infarct from tuberculosis. Further details will be found in Chaper 6.

Fat Embolism. — As a result of fracture, crushing injuries, and traumatic lesions of fat, globules of fat may enter the torn veins and be carried to the lungs. Here they seldom do much damage, but if present in very large amount there may be dyspnea and prostration. The gross appearance of the lung is normal, but in frozen sections stained for fat, globules and cylinders are seen in the capillaries. If the fat passes through the lungs it may reach the kidneys and be excreted, or it may lodge in the brain with fatal results.

Pulmonary Hypertension and Pulmonary Arteriolosclerosis. — Hypertension and associated changes in the arterioles of the lesser circulation present some of the problems which we have already encountered in the systematic circulation. Again there is a primary and a secondary type. Here, however, the situation is reversed, for the *primary* or idiopathic type of hypertension, in which there is no apparent cause, is very much more rare than the secondary form.

The *secondary* type is due to some pathological condition in the vascular arrangement. (1) *Heart disease*, either acquired or congenital, must be considered first. In the *acquired group* mitral stenosis produces the worst effect, followed by aortic stenosis. The *congenital group* consists of left-to-right shunts, more particularly patency of the interatrial or interventricular septum, or a patent ductus arteriosus. (2) *Pulmonary disease*, more especially diffuse fibrosis and the more extreme forms of emphysema, will cause great narrowing of the pulmonary arterioles. Multiple pulmonary emboli, referred to below, must also be considered. (3) *Kyphoscoliosis*, a backward curvature of the spine, decreases the volume of the thoracic cage to a marked degree, with resulting compression of the vascular bed.

The *vascular lesions* are very much those which we have already studied in connection with hypertension of the systemic system, so they need merely be mentioned. The *larger arteries* show atherosclerotic plaques, the *arterioles* are the site of hyperplastic arteriolosclerosis and elastosis, and the *capillaries* may be dilated or obliterated, depending on the causal factors responsible for the hypertension. Mitral stenosis naturally leads to back pressure in the pulmonary veins, with the result that the alveolar capillaries become intensely dilated and tortuous. On the other hand, in emphysema and diffuse pulmonary fibrosis the result is obliteration of the capillaries with secondary changes in the arterioles and small arteries. In congenital left to right shunts the brunt is borne by the large arteries, with the dreaded development of cor pulmonale with extreme hypertrophy of the right ventricle.

The relation of pulmonary arteriosclerosis to pulmonary hypertension and cor pulmonale is of particular interest. It is evident that widespread sclerosis of the pulmonary arterioles will result in elevation of the blood pressure in the pulmonary system. This is the condition which has been known in the past as *Ayerza's disease*, (black cardiacs), a vague entity in which the arteriosclerosis seemed to be primary. On the other hand the hypertension might be responsible for the arteriosclerosis, an everyday occurrence in the systemic circulation. Much has been written about Ayerza's disease, but it has been much ado about nothing. It now appears from animal autopsy and clinical evidence that the vascular sclerosis and hypertension may be the result of lodgment of multiple emboli in the arterioles. Repeated showers of small emboli may give rise to emboli numbered in the millions. The condition can be reproduced in rabbits by the intravenous injection of blood clots (Harrison). The emboli rapidly become organized and incorporated with the intima, so that the healed lesions are indistinguishable from those of a spontaneous arteriosclerosis.

That the hypertension is not responsible for the vascular sclerosis in the experimental animal is suggested by the fact that repeated injections of nonthrombotic material such as plastic beads results in pulmonary hypertension but not in pulmonary arteriosclerosis (Thomas *et al.*). In the human subject careful histories may reveal episodes suggestive of embolization. A number of these have dated from pregnancy. The interval between the production of vascular obstruction and clinical evidence or cor pulmonale may be measured in years rather than in weeks.

Glomoid hyperplasia of the pulmonary vessels is a curious lesion which may be associated with severe degrees of hypertension in the lesser circulation (Wagenvoort). It is seen in communications between the systemic and pulmonary circulation and occasionally in primary hypertension, but not in the pulmonary hypertension of mitral stenosis. In this condition tangled, hypercellular masses of small vessels or capillaries resembling renal glomeruli are observed within the lumen of the small arteries or veins, and occasionally in the alveolar walls. The glomus-like structure originates abruptly from a small artery and terminates equally abruptly in a small vein. The lesion, if so it can be called, is believed to be the result of necrosis of the arterioles caused by spasm, as in malignant systemic hypertension, the necrosis being followed by repair, or it may represent some form of hyperplastic arteriovenous shunt.

Arteriovenous Aneurysm.—When a young man suffering from dyspnea on effort but with no evidence of heart disease presents a picture of cyanosis, clubbing of the fingers, a secondary polycythemia, and a discrete density in the lung, a pulmonary arteriovenous aneurysm should be suspected. In this rare anomaly of the pulmonary circulation a large vascular cavity is in direct communication with one or more pulmonary arteries and veins, so that the venous blood in the pulmonary artery passes through the aneurysmal sac to the systemic circulation with consequent anoxia. For this reason cerebral symptoms are common, such as dizzy spells, brief periods of inability to speak, or even convulsions. Other vascular developmental defects such as telangiectases of the skin or the mucous membrane of the mouth and nose are often present.

Digital Clubbing.—This may be as convenient a place as any to consider clubbing of the fingers and toes, also known by the more formidable title of *hypertrophic pulmonary osteoarthropathy.* The condition is associated with (? caused by) a variety of intrathoracic lesions, more particularly congenital heart disease with cyanosis, and pulmonary lesions which interfere with the circulation through the lung and favor the development of arteriovenous anastomoses. Under such conditions clubbing is likely to develop. In rare cases of congenital anomalies of the great vessels mixed venous blood goes to the left arm and both legs, all of which show clubbing, whereas the right arm which receives normal arterial blood which has passed through the lung shows none.

The terminal phalanges are enlarged, their interstitial tissue is edematous, and there is dilatation of the arterioles and venules, but the capillaries are of normal size. The increased blood flow is believed to pass through dilated arteriovenous anastomoses, which causes congestion of the venules of the part with oxygenated blood under relatively high pressure, and therefore local tissue hypertrophy. The restriction of the hypertrophic changes to the fingers, toes, and occasionally the nose, is explained by the fact that these are the regions most richly endowed with arteriovenous anastomoses. It would seem as if the lungs had lost the ability to remove from mixed venous blood some substance

which is capable of dilating arteriovenous anastomoses, and so stimulating the developing of clubbing. The substance which seems to fit this description best is reduced ferritin, which is capable of inhibiting the vasoconstrictive action of circulating epinephrine. It has been suggested that if reduced ferritin in venous blood should escape oxidation in the lung and enter the systemic circulation in vasoactive form, it will dilate the arteriovenous anastomoses and produce the changes of digital clubbing (Hall). Experimental observations on patients with clubbed fingers tend to confirm this view. We need not suppose that there is only one cause of clubbing, but it seems probable that the clubbing associated with intrathoracic disease is produced by the shunting of a vasoactive substance past the lung, where it is normally destroyed, and that this substance may possibly be reduced ferritin.

It is interesting to know that pulmonary hypertrophic osteoarthopathy is common in the dog, the osseous lesions being associated with a major visceral disorder, usually intrathoracic in character. A comparable disease has been reported in horses, cattle and a lion, but much less commonly than in the dog.

ATELECTASIS

Atelectasis literally means incomplete expansion (*ateles,* incomplete + *ektasis,* expansion), but it is now synonymous with collapse of the lung. This may be: (1) congenital, (2) compression, or (3) obstruction.

Congenital Atelectasis.—This is the only form of collapse which deserves to be called atelectasis, for the alveoli have failed to expand. It is seen in the stillborn child who has never breathed, and in children who live only a few days and never breathe well, the lung shows many areas of atelectasis. The lung is dark, firm, and airless. If only a part is collapsed, that area is depressed below the surrounding surface. The collapsed lung sinks in water, a convenient practical test to determine if the child has breathed. The lung may have to be cut into separate pieces, for a small part may have become expanded. It is commonly stated that the alveolar epithelium of the full term fetus is cuboidal

43

in form, giving the alveoli a gland-like appearance. This is not correct. It is true for the earlier stages of development, but after the fifth month the cuboidal epithelium begins to disappear and the alveoli to be opened up. The difference between the lung which has inhaled air and the one which has not is quantitative rather than qualitative. As the result of extrauterine respiration the alveoli are more fully distended and their walls are thinner than if the child has never breathed. If the body has been kept for some time in a warm room the lung may float due to the production of gas by putrefying bacteria. In such cases bubble-like areas are seen microscopically in the septa and alveoli; these are easily distinguished from alveoli partially distended as the result of intrauterine respiration.

Resorption atelectasis is found in infants who have breathed well so that the lungs have been fully expanded. Then, owing to some interference with respiration, the air is slowly absorbed from many of the alveoli. This is seen to advantage in *hyaline membrane disease* of the newborn in which the alveolar ducts are blocked with protein-rich fluid and the alveolar walls are lined with hyaline material. The condition can be recognized by the fact that the flattened cells lining the alveoli do not return to their original cuboidal form.

Compression Atelectasis.—Pressure on the lung drives out the air and produces collapse. This may be *complete* when the pressure is great and uniform as in massive pleural effusion, empyema and pneumothorax, but only *partial* when the pressure is more local as in pressure by a tumor, an enlarged heart, or an elevated diaphragm. When the pressure is removed the lung will expand again, but a thick cortex of fibrous tissue (removal by decortication) may be formed (as in empyema) which may prevent re-expansion.

Obstructive Atelectasis.—In this form two factors are nearly always at work, *obstruction of a bronchus* and *weakening of the respiratory movements* (chest or diaphragm). If obstruction is due to a foreign body in a bronchus the second factor will not be present, but usually it is caused by an accumulation of mucus in the bronchioles

associated with poor respiratory movements. If deep breathing and coughing were possible the obstruction in the bronchioles would be cleared away. This type of atelectasis is commonest in debilitated children suffering from bronchitis, bronchopneumonia, etc. Indeed in such children even the normal amount of mucus in the bronchioles may lead to partial collapse. The two factors are present after an abdominal operation, for the anesthetic will stimulate the bronchial secretion, and the abdominal section will prevent the patient from breathing deeply. Tumors of the bronchus, enlarged lymph nodes, and tuberculous stenosis are frequent causes of obstructive atelectasis. In all of these instances the air in the affected part of the lung is absorbed into the blood, no more air can enter on account of the obstruction, and that part of the lung collapses.

Acute Massive Collapse.—This peculiar and rare complication is a special example of obstructive atelectasis caused by the two factors, bronchial obstruction and respiratory weakness. The clinical picture is a striking one. From a few hours to a few days after an operation, usually abdominal, the patient suddenly develops the symptoms of an acute thoracic catastrophe, *i.e.*, extreme dyspnea, marked cyanosis, and collapse. There is no respiratory movement on the affected side, the heart is displaced to that side, there are physical signs of consolidation of the lung, and the roentgen-ray films show a peculiarly dense shadow and the dome of the diaphragm high and immobile on the side of the collapse.

Although great difference of opinion exists regarding the mechanism by which acute massive collapse is produced, we are probably safe in saying that it is due to the two great factors, bronchial obstruction and weakness of the respiratory movements. The symptoms and the roentgen-ray picture of massive collapse are duplicated in cases of foreign body in the bronchi; indeed the roentgen-ray picture of collapse is one of the diagnostic features in favor of the presence of a foreign body. Removal of the body is followed by a rapid disappearance of the symptoms and the roentgen-ray shadow. Interference with the respiratory movements of the chest or diaphragm leads to the forma-

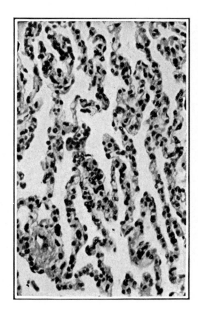

FIG. 388.—Atelectasis. × 225.

tion of plugs of mucus in the bronchi, and great debility, postoperative abdominal pain, etc., may prevent the patient from expelling them. The cough reflex is the watch-dog of the lungs, and when that reflex fails the lumen becomes completely obstructed. It is interesting to go back to 1853 and find Gairdner giving, as the three chief causes of pulmonary collapse in infancy, mucus in the bronchi, weakness of the respiratory power and inability to cough and thus remove the mucus.

Morbid Anatomy.—The condition of the lung is similar in all forms of atelectasis, whether congenital, acquired, or massive. In the massive form and in compression due to pleural effusion or pneumothorax the entire lung may be so collapsed that it no longer fills the cavity but lies against the posterior chest wall and vertebral column like a squeezed sponge. If only some parts are affected, these are firm, inelastic, airless, and sunk below the surrounding surface. These areas are steel-blue or slate-gray due to stasis of the circulation.

Microscopically, the alveolar walls are pressed together so that the lumen is nearly obliterated (Fig. 388). In the congenital form the fetal structure is still evident. If

the collapse is of long duration fibrosis may occur which will prevent full expansion.

EMPHYSEMA

Emphysema is one of the most important of pulmonary diseases. It is not only by far the commonest chronic disease of the lungs, but the most crippling over a long period and therefore the most to be feared, for the patient does not die quickly, but drags out a miserable existence for years, a trial and tribulation to himself, his family, and his doctor. He suffers with every breath he takes, and he must breathe some 20,000 times in the 24 hours. Fothergill's description of the chronic bronchitic (page 626) is really a description of the patient with obstructive emphysema.

It is unfortunate that the name emphysema is applied to four conditions which are entirely unrelated. These are: (1) chronic obstructive hypertrophic emphysema, a descriptive but somewhat cumbersome term for a condition often better referred to as bullous emphysema; (2) compensatory emphysema; (3) senile, atrophic or small-lung emphysema; and (4) interstitial emphysema. The first is a common and serious condition, the second and third are common but of no clinical importance, and the fourth is uncommon and does not really merit the name emphysema. When the physician thinks and speaks of emphysema he means the obstructive variety.

Obstructive Emphysema.—It is customary to start with the pathogenesis of a disease, then pass to the morbid anatomy, and finally the clinical results. In the present instance, for reasons which will become apparent, we shall reverse this order. In the investigation of the pathological anatomy of emphysema Gough's technique of whole lung sections of the organ distended with formalin, infiltrated with gelatin, frozen, cut at 200 to 300 microns, and mounted on translucent sheets of paper, has proved itself invaluable.

Lesions.—Emphysema is an increase in the size of the air spaces distal to the terminal bronchioles. This may be due to dilatation of the spaces or destruction of their

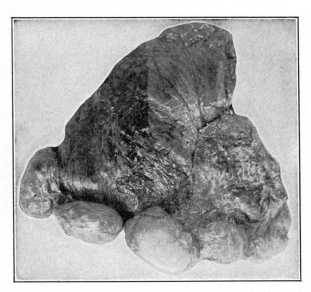

FIG. 389.—Pulmonary emphysema. Large bullous swellings at the base of the lung.
(Boyd, *Pathology for the Physician.*)

walls. To show the increase in size the lungs should be distended and fixed before being cut. Loss of elastic tissue is the prominent feature. The elastic tissue, however, is not in the alveolar walls, but in the bronchi, bronchioles, and alveolar ducts. *Obstructive emphysema* may be (1) *generalized* or (2) *localized*, the generalized being (a) *focal* or *centrilobular*, and (b) *diffuse* with no lobular pattern. Far the commonest is the centrilobular generalized form. The terms local and generalized apply to the distribution of the lesions in the lung as a whole, whereas focal or centrilobular and diffuse apply to the degree of involvement of the lobules (see below). *Panlobular emphysema* is a term applied to a uniform and diffuse change throughout the secondary lobules with over-distension and air sac rupture (Wyatt). It may be confined to a segment or a lobe, or may be widely diffused (generalized). This condition is more marked in the lower lobe, whereas generalized centrilibular emphysema is observed in the upper part of the lung. There is a limited degree of carbon pigmentation, in comparison with the concentration of pigment around the damaged bronchioles in the centrilobular form. Panlobular emphysema is associated with primary kyphotic

chest deformities, hilar sclerosis, and neoplasia of the airways.

The lungs are very voluminous, very pale due to ischemia, and quite dry. They may completely cover the heart, so that there is no cardiac dulness on percussion. Large blebs or bullae project on the surface in the more poorly supported regions (apex, anterior margin, base) (Fig. 389). Rupture of one of these bullae is the commonest cause of spontaneous pneumothorax. The lung has a peculiarly soft, dry, feathery feel. There is marked pitting on pressure due, not to edema, but to destruction of the elastic tissue.

The *microscopic appearance* is best studied in the large lung or whole lung section. In such a section one can readily distinguish the secondary lobules of Miller, which provide the keystone to the understanding of the anatomy of emphysema (Wyatt). The secondary lobules are made up of 6 to 12 primary lobules held together by connective tissue septa which radiate out from the root of the lung. The finer bronchiolar ramifications are accompanied by arterioles and occupy the central portions of the secondary lobule, the peripheral portions being composed of air ducts, saccules and terminal air

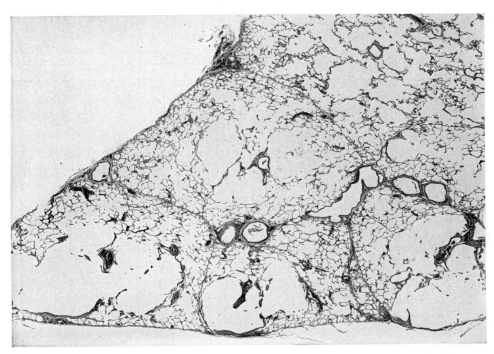

Fig. 390.—Centrilibular emphysema. (Gough in Harrison's *Recent Advances in Pathology*, courtesy of J. A. Churchill, Ltd.)

sacs. The emphysematous process begins as a distention and dissolution of the centrally situated terminal respiratory bronchioles, so that this form is called *centri-lobular emphysema* (Fig. 390). The surrounding air sacs are first distended and later disintegrate, the entire group forming a confluent pool of air, but air which is valueless because it does no work. Centrilobular emphysema may be localized to a segment of the lung or a lobe, or it may be generalized throughout the entire lung. In *diffuse emphysema* there is a diffuse distention of air ducts, saccules, atria and alveolar sacs throughout the secondary lobule, but without dissolution of the respiratory bronchioles.

In either form of generalized emphysema the lung presents a delicate lace-like structure. The air vesicles are few in number and of great size, and there is atrophy of the alveolar walls. Normally the alveoli present for the most part a closed appearance, because the lung is collapsed and random sections do not pass through the alveolar mouths as often as in expanded lungs. When the normal lung is fixed in a distended condition the alveoli open into the alveolar ducts, so that the walls may appear to be ruptured. In advanced cases the septa between the alveoli do become ruptured, and this is responsible for the formation of the large bullae on the surface. The three criteria which Hartroft suggests as pathognomonic of the emphysematous lung are: (1) marked decrease in the average alveolar depth, (2) a corresponding increase in the average alveolar diameter, and (3) flattening of the alveolar bases with loss of the zig-zag lines which form so striking a feature of the normal lung fixed in an expanded condition (Fig. 390). As a result of these changes there is a great diminution in the volume of the capillary bed. It is this avascularity which is responsible for the pallor of the lung, for the dryness of the cut surface, and for the obstruction to the pulmonary circulation.

In emphysema, and to a lesser extent in other chronic diseases of the lung, the broncho-pulmonary veins which drain the

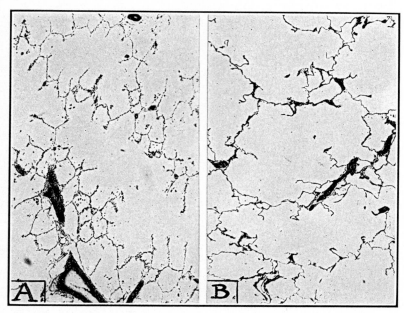

Fig. 391.—Emphysema. A, Normal lung. × 36. B, Emphysematous lung, showing increase in alveolar diameter, flattening of alveolar bases and loss of zig-zag lines. × 36. (Boyd, *Pathology for the Physician.*)

bronchi, bronchioles and pulmonary interstitial tissue are greatly enlarged (Liebow). These veins, which were first demonstrated by Zuckerkandl by means of injection in 1882, communicate both with the pulmonary and the azygos veins. They, therefore, act as a bypass when the pulmonary veins are occluded, and constitute a shunt between the right and left auricles. The flow at first is from left to right, but in advanced emphysema the valves between the broncho-pulmonary-azygos junctions become incompetent, and the flow may then be reversed. The expansion of the bronchopulmonary venous circulation may be compared with the expansion of the arterial collateral circulation which has been demonstrated so beautifully by Liebow in bronchiectasis, but the two do not necessarily go hand in hand.

Clinical Effects.—The effects of emphysema are far-reaching and serious. The chest has a barrel-shaped appearance, the ribs being raised and the sternum pushed forward, so that the antero-posterior equals the transverse diameter. The lungs are hyperresonant, and the area of superficial cardiac dullness obliterated. Respiratory movements are diminished, and expiration is difficult and prolonged. Owing to the vascular occlusion there is marked obstruction in the pulmonary circulation, so that there is great hypertrophy and dilatation of the right ventricle and general venous congestion throughout the body. This is the condition of cor pulmonale. The pulmonary artery may show arteriosclerosis, just as it does in the obstruction due to mitral stenosis. Dyspnea and cyanosis develop, with a compensatory increase in the number and size of the red blood corpuscles. One of the emphysematous bullae may rupture into the pleural cavity, giving rise to spontaneous pneumothorax.

The above-mentioned changes are merely mechanical effects. Far more significant to the patient are those involving the physiology of respiration with the attendant symptoms to which they give rise. The characteristic feature is hyperinflation of the lung after expiration due to obstruction caused either by bronchospasm or permanent narrowing of the bronchioles. The natural result is increase of the residual lung volume, that is to say the amount of air left after the maximum expiratory effort. The increased time and effort needed for exhalation is very characteristic. The large amount of stale air (residual volume) is reflected in the increased CO_2 content of the arterial blood. In consequence the respiratory center may become refractory. The patient is now dependent on hypoxemia for stimulation of respiration through chemoreceptors in the carotid bodies and the aorta which are sufficient to maintain life. If this mechanism is mistakenly depressed by opiates or the inhalation of oxygen, the result will be high CO_2 arterial blood content, with coma and finally death due to relative acidosis with lowering of the blood pH, an acidosis which the kidneys are unable to compensate when the terminal phase is reached.

The symptom which overshadows all others is *dyspnea*. "Perhaps the most compelling of all human appetites is the need for air and probably no distress is so agonizing as that which results from the inability to breathe adequately. The emotional component of dyspnea is invariably strong and must be given consideration by the sympathetic physician. The person who has never experienced true dyspnea has some difficulty in understanding the plight of one who has lost the ability to pump air in and out of the lungs without conscious effort." (Hinshaw and Garland.)

Pathogenesis.—What explanation can we find for these remarkable lesions and this distressing clinical picture? That the answer to this question is by no means easy can be seen from the number and variety of the theories which have been advanced. The dilatation of the alveoli and the atrophy or disruption of their walls recall the production of an arterial aneurysm, and suggest the operation of two factors: (1) increased intraluminal pressure, and (2) degeneration of the walls of the alveoli. Both of these may operate, or only one may be sufficient.

Increased intra-alveolar pressure is the most obvious factor, but the mechanism responsible for this increase is by no means self-evident. When I was a student I was taught that the playing of wind instruments was a causal factor, but this proved to be a myth, as will other "facts" which the student is taught at the present day. A patient with emphysema who performs in a band is as likely to play the big drum as the trombone.

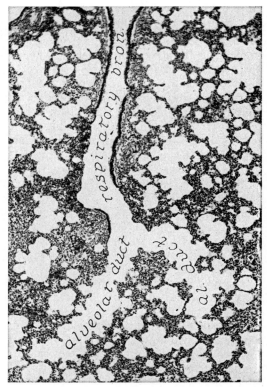

Fig. 392.—Very low-power photomicrograph of a section of the lung of a very young child. A respiratory bronchiole is cut longitudinally and may be seen to be opening into two alveolar ducts. (Ham, *Histology*, courtesy of J. B. Lippincot Company.)

It is "trapped air" in the alveoli which seems to constitute the great danger. It is generally believed that the mechanism responsible for the trapping is obstruction of the smaller bronchi and bronchioles by plugs of mucus. The obstruction is of the check-valve type, which allows air to be drawn in during inspiration, but prevents it passing out during expiration. This is in contrast to ball-valve obstruction, which blocks inspiration but allows air to pass out during expiration, thus leading to collapse rather than to emphysema. Obstruction may be spasmodic or permanent. Spasmodic obstruction is exemplified by paroxysmal bronchial asthma, in which the development of emphysema is a constant threat.

The great majority of cases of emphysema, however, are slow and insidious in onset. It is hard to visualize a plug of mucus remaining unaltered in a small bronchus and acting as a check-valve over a long period. It appears much more probable that the basic lesion is an obliteration of the bronchioles from bronchiolitis, and that the air enters and leaves the alveoli by the back-door route of the pores of Kohn, by which entry of air from neighboring lobules occurs more readily than does exit (McLean). This is a *collateral ventilation* corresponding to the collateral circulation which develops when an artery is occluded. If such a patient is subject to chronic coughing, the inevitable result must be distension of the alveoli with destruction of their walls.

The obstruction of the finer airways frequently seems to be due to a bronchiolitis. A brief study of Figure 392 will convince the reader of the ease with which the respiratory bronchioles can become occluded either by inflammatory swelling or by plugging, and the consequences that this will have for the alveolar ducts and then the alveoli. It is perhaps surprising that this is not more common. When mucus is aspirated into and beyond the respiratory bronchioles it will produce temporary plugging. Under normal conditions aeration of the affected area is maintained by collateral ventilation, and vigorous coughing will dislodge the plug. If, however, the plug remains static, bacterial growth will rapidly occur and set up an acute bronchiolitis, and if this is repeated a number of times, permanent occlusion will be the probable outcome. Any disturbance of what McLean terms the *homeostatic mechanism* of the bronchial passages will favor this result. The three elements of the mechanism are ciliary action, cough, and an effective collateral ventilation. The health of the cilia may be interfered with by viral infections such as influenza, bacterial infections, especially tuberculosis, and chemical agents such as toxic gases. The alveolar pores are the first to suffer as the result of damage to the walls by distension. In elderly, chronically ill patients the breathing is shallow, with reduced collateral ventilation and weakened coughing, so that plugs are not dislodged.

Perhaps the changes in the medium-sized and larger bronchi have not been sufficiently emphasized (Wright). These airways depend on the cartilaginous rings and plates for their rigidity and on their dense fibrous tissue content for support. When these are gone they collapse and obstruct the lumen, particularly as a result of chronic coughing. In obstructive emphysema the medium and large bronchi are collapsed and thin-walled with marked reduction in their cartilage and connective tissue content.

Atrophy of the alveolar walls and the elastic framework is the other etiological possibility to be considered. It is naturally difficult if not impossible to be certain if such an occurrence is primary in nature or merely secondary to alveolar distension. Many workers attach great weight to the primary aspect of this change. Impaired nutrition of the alveolar walls will impair their elasticity, and, as elsewhere in the body, this impairment may well be due to ischemia. Here again we are faced with the difficulty of deciding if the ischemia is primary, the result of sclerosis of the bronchial arterioles, or if it is caused by distension of the alveoli with disruption of their walls. My own feeling is that structural changes in the walls of the bronchioles are far more important than changes in the alveolar walls.

Compensatory Emphysema.—This form of emphysema is of interest to the pathologist rather than to the clinician. A portion of the lung becomes expanded in order to fill a space formerly occupied by pulmonary tissue. This occurs in atelectasis due to complete bronchial obstruction, in fibrosing conditions when these are localized, and after removal of segments of lung.

Atrophic or Senile Emphysema.—This condition is seen in old age (senile emphysema) and in wasting diseases. It is not a true emphysema, for there is no distention of the alveoli, no enlargement of the lungs, no bullae on the surface. The only resemblance lies in the microscopic picture, where there is atrophy and disappearance of the walls of the alveoli so that large spaces are formed. The condition is an atrophy from defective nutrition, and does not deserve to be called emphysema.

Interstitial Emphysema.—This also is not a true emphysema. The air escapes from the alveoli and makes its way into the interstitial tissue of the lung, particularly along the perivascular sheaths, as a result of which

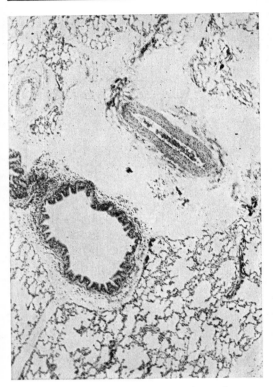

FIG. 393.—Pulmonary interstitial emphysema. Sheath of air around branch of pulmonary artery. × 58. (Boyd, *Pathology for the Physician.*)

there may be serious pressure on the vessels. (Fig. 393).

This is usually due to tearing of the lung by a fractured rib, wound, etc., but in children it is sometimes caused by overdistention and rupture of the alveoli during the violent paroxysms of whooping cough. Violent artificial respiration may produce the same result. The air collects in the lymphatics in the form of tiny beads, which are best seen under the pleura. It may then pass to the mediastinum and from there to the neck and down over the chest wall. The lung and the subcutaneous tissues have a peculiar and quite characteristic crackling feel.

The result of pulmonary interstitial emphysema and pneumomediastinum may be described as *airblock*, which is the combined effect on the circulation of the blood and the respiratory movements of the lung. Airblock is due both to impingement of bubbles of air on the pulmonary vessels,

heart and great vessels in the mediastinum, and to splinting or immobilization of large areas of the lung by air bubbles locked in the pulmonary connective tissue. Spontaneous recovery is the rule, but death may occur from interference with circulation, or a pneumothorax may supervene.

Hamman has described a *spontaneous mediastinal emphysema*, characterized by the sudden onset of severe pain in the chest radiating in a manner suggestive of coronary disease, and by an extraordinary crackling or crunching sound sometimes audible to the unaided ear at a distance of a foot or more. The pain is due to distention of the mediastinal tissues with air, and the crackling noise to vibrating pericardiac air bubbles. It is evident that the air must escape from ruptured pulmonary alveoli into the interstitial tissue of the lung and thence into the mediastinum. This condition is now known as *Hamman's syndrome*.

TUMORS OF THE LUNG

Primary tumors of the lung, with a few rare exceptions to be considered presently, are epithelial tumors of the bronchi, not of lung itself. This is but natural, as epithelium is only visible in the bronchial passages. There are three main types of bronchial neoplasm: (1) bronchogenic carcinoma, (2) bronchiolar carcinoma, more commonly known as alveolar cell carcinoma or alveolar cell tumor, and (3) adenoma of bronchus. Of these by far the most common and important is bronchogenic carcinoma. One of the commonest of secondary tumors is also carcinoma which has metastasized to the lung.

Bronchogenic Carcinoma.—At the present time carcinoma of the lung arising from a bronchus is perhaps the most interesting and challenging of all malignant tumors. It is interesting because of the problems it presents with respect to increased incidence, predilection for the male, and possible relation to external carcinogens. It is challenging because of the fact that it is the most readily seen of all malignant tumors of internal organs, and yet the prognosis is among the worst.

Incidence.—The tumor used to be regarded as a rarity, but during the past quarter of a century it has become one of the commonest, if not the commonest, of the killing cancers, especially in men. Indeed it has been said that it is important to think of a pulmonary neoplasm when a patient in the cancer age, showing no symptoms of cardiac, renal or arterial disease, begins to cough and is short winded. This tumor now causes over 24,000 deaths a year in the United States, which puts it in the category of epidemic diseases.

There has been much discussion as to whether this increase is real or only apparent, and if real, what has caused it. The answer is that we do not know for certain, because there are no figures on which the death rate from intrathoracic cancer of half a century ago can be compared with that of today. One can read papers proving that the increase in one country, such as Great Britain, is real or that it is only apparent. It was not until the beginning of the present century that coronary thrombosis and myocardial infarction were recognized, but no one suggests that the disease started then. There can be no doubt that the disease is recognized much more frequently nowadays by the internist, the radiologist, the bronchoscopist, the pathologist and the thoracic surgeon. Goethe once remarked "Was man weiss, sieht man," and we recognize what we know to be common and what we have been taught is common. When I was a student in Edinburgh we never heard of bronchogenic carcinoma, but we were continually shown both at the bedside and in the autopsy room examples of "mediastinal lymph node sarcoma" invading the lung, a tumor composed of round or oval cells. Indeed in the latest edition (1922) as well as many previous editions of Bland Sutton's *Tumors, Innocent and Malignant*, the standart text on the subject for very many years, there is a picture of a "mediastinal lymphosarcoma invading a bronchus," a picture which every medical student at the present day recognizes as an illustration of bronchogenic carcinoma invading a lymph node. This illustration must have been engraved on the memory of countless students, who when they became doctors would not dream of making a diagnosis of bronchogenic carcinoma.

It is also possible, indeed most probable, that there has been a true increase. Ochsner points out that from 1938 to 1948 the fatal cases of bronchogenic carcinoma increased 144 per cent, whilst the total cancer deaths increased only 31 per cent. In 1920 this tumor constituted only 1 per cent of cancers: in 1948 the figure was 8.3 per cent. The Canadian figures are almost identical. There has been a tremendous increase in the incidence in Britain in the last twenty-five years, as much as 15 fold according to Doll and Hill. The corresponding figure in the United States for a similar period is about half that amount. One point which deserves special mention is that the increase, whether real or apparent, is confined to men and to epidermoid carcinoma, not to adenocarcinoma or undifferentiated carcinoma. The mortality from cancer of the stomach has been stationary. On the other hand Steiner, in an analysis of the material examined in the Department of Pathology of the University of Chicago during the forty-year period between 1902 and 1941 came to the conclusion that there was no real increase in the frequency of bronchogenic carcinoma.

One of the best examples of the truth that what we know we see is afforded by the pulmonary disease endemic amongst the miners of Schneeberg and Joachimsthal in East Germany. Since 1500 A.D it has been known that a disease of the chest was endemic amongst these miners, but it was diagnosed as silicosis, tuberculosis, and other conditions until 1922. In that year a commission with Schmorl as chairman determined that the mysterious disease was, and presumably always had been, bronchogenic carcinoma. After that year there was naturally a sudden and dramatic change in the incidence of the disease amongst these men, as if a new and potent carcinogen had been introduced into the mines.

It is not my intention to suggest that the vastly increased incidence of carcinoma of the lung is to be explained merely by a truer appreciation and recognition of what has always been there. I have seized this as a pretext to point out that what on the surface is apparently true does not necessarily represent the whole truth. An excellent critical analysis of this contentious subject will be found in Willis' *Pathology of Tumors*,

1953, from which I take these words: "Is the increase real or only apparent?... Having read many of the contributions to the controversy, and having surveyed my own experience of the diagnostic errors made in this disease, my opinion is that it is still not possible either to affirm or to deny that there has been a real increase." Those wishing to pursue this intriguing and vitally important subject still farther will find it discussed in the monographs on cancer of the lung by Moyer and Maier and by Rosenblatt and Lisa, both published in 1956.

Etiology.—If there are differences of opinion as to the question of an increased incidence of bronchogenic carcinoma, these differences are multiplied many times when we come to the matter of etiology. The interdependence of these two problems will soon become apparent. In introduction, the obvious fact should be emphasized that as the neoplasm originates in the epithelium of one of the main or smaller bronchi it is reasonable to presume that the etiological agent is an external carcinogen or carcinogens which are inhaled. It is true that the very strong male sex incidence, as much as 9 to 1 in some figures, must be taken into consideration. This may or may not be related to carcinogens more likely to be inhaled by the male than the female. The carcinogen, whether inhaled in cigarette smoke or otherwise, is probably taken up by the mucus in the finer air passages, and moved upward in a progressively narrowing mucus sheet or raft, becoming greatly concentrated in the main bronchi in the region of the hilus. Finally we must not forget that it is a great mistake to think that one and only one carcinogen is responsible for producing cancer in any particular tissue. No better example of this truth could be afforded than cancer of the skin. Moreover it is reasonable to presume that the agent must operate for a period of years, probably twenty or more.

The fact that the disease is commoner in urban than in rural communities indicates the possibility that carcinogens are being produced in the city. Kotin and his associates have demonstrated the presence of carcinogenic hydrocarbons in the atmosphere of Los Angeles, and have produced epidermoid carcinoma of the skin of mice with this material. Kotin analyzed the exhaust gases and soot from automobiles, and found that gases were most dangerous during idling, accelerating and decelerating phases which are so common in the city. A somewhat unduly high incidence of the disease has been reported in workers in chromate plants, stokers inhaling hot tar fumes in generator plants, and asbestos workers. The disease among the general population, however, cannot be regarded as an occupational hazard, with the exception of Schneeberg and Joachimsthal, where the exact carcinogen is still uncertain, but is believed to be radioactive gases. The trouble is that we seem to swim throughout life in a sea of carcinogens that we continually inhale, amongst which may be mentioned smog rich in industrial carcinogens, tobacco smoke, the radioactive dust of certain mines, and now the fallout from thermonuclear explosions, so that the task of tracking down any particular one is difficult in the extreme. On the experimental side bronchial carcinoma has been induced in mice by means of a continuous emitter of gamma radiation, namely cobalt-60, introduced into the lung (Gates and Warren).

Cigarette smoking and lung cancer is the aspect of etiology which has aroused the keenest interest and the most heated debate. Three types of evidence may be considered: statistical, experimental and pathological. The *statistical evidence* at first sight is formidable. Wynder and Graham found that of 605 patients with cancer of the lung 51 per cent smoked more than 20 cigarettes a day, usually over a period of many years, while only 1.3 per cent were non-smokers. Hammond and Horn in the United States, Doll and Hill in Great Britain, and Kreyberg in Norway came to very similar statistical conclusions. As Kreyberg points out, it would appear that the epidermoid group of neoplasms, which with its subdivision, the anaplastic group, constitutes over 90 per cent of the cases and is essentially a male disease, is due to an external carcinogen, whereas in adenocarcinoma, a disease of women, an endogenous factor may play a part, whilst alveolar cell carcinoma may be due to a virus. Although there is still no *proof* in the usual sense of the word that cigarette smoking is a cause of lung cancer, statistics show that cigarette smokers have a greater risk of dying of lung cancer than have non-smokers, and the risk increases with the amount smoked. It is unfortunate for the statisticians that in the past fifty years there has been a far greater increase in cigarette smoking amongst women than amongst men, yet the increased incidence of cancer of the lung has been confined to men.

As I have had no training in the analysis of statistics and their pitfalls, it would be foolish for me to express an opinion on this matter. It should be mentioned, however, that other statistical authorities both in Britain (Sir Ronald Fisher) and the United States (Berkson) are of the opinion that the evidence as yet is far from conclusive, and there is much question about the *interpretation* of the accumulated statistical data. Indeed the leading authority on industrial cancer in the United States, Hueper of Washington, says: "It may be concluded that the existing evidence neither proves nor strongly indicates that tobacco smoking, and especially cigarette smoking, represents a major or even predominating causal factor in the production of cancers of the respiratory tract and is the main reason for the phenomenal increase of pulmonary tumors during recent decades."

The *experimental evidence* on this important problem has been disappointingly indefinite. No one has ever succeeded in producing carcinoma of the bronchial tree of a laboratory animal by the use of cigarette smoke. But the fact that in the past no one had ever succeeded in reproducing leprosy in any laboratory animal by inoculation with the leprosy bacillus was not taken as proof that organism was not the cause of leprosy. A cigarette tar concentrate obtained by means of a smoking machine produced cancer of the skin of mice when applied for over a year (Wynder *et al.*), but we have already seen that the same can be done with the atmosphere of large cities.

The *morbid anatomist* has been able to throw light on this contentious problem where the experimentalist has failed and the statistician has left us in doubt. It can be shown from autopsy material that changes in the bronchial mucosa vary proportionately with the smoking habits of the individual

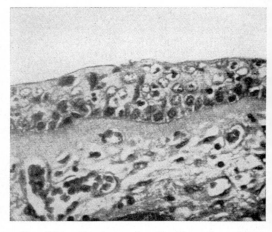

FIG. 394.—Carcinoma *in situ* of bronchus. Note the rather pronounced cellular pleomorphism, mitotic figures and scattered atypical hyperchromatic nuclei. × 480. (From a case of carcinoma of the opposite lung). (Hamilton, Sepps, Brown and MacDonald, courtesy of Can. Med. Assn. Jour.)

(Hamilton *et al.*). Such changes as basal cell hyperplasia, squamous metaplasia, and carcinoma-in-situ are observed diffusely distributed throughout the epithelium of the bronchial tree of both lungs in heavy smokers without carcinoma as well as in cases of carcinoma (Fig. 394). In non-smokers the changes are minimal or absent. Similar results have been obtained by other workers (Knudtson). This is the type of evidence which appeals to a pathologist.

It is of course possible to carry to a paralyzing extreme the demand for complete experimental evidence and absolute scientific proof, if indeed anything in the world can be proved completely and absolutely, above all with regard to the causation of cancer. It has been said that in order to obtain such proof in the present instance it would be necessary to paint the bronchial mucosa of human volunteers with an extract of cigarette smoke for twenty to twenty-five years, during which time the subject would have to reside in air-conditioned quarters lest he be exposed to atmospheric contamination. At the end of this period the lung would need to be removed, so that the bronchial tree would receive an adequate examination!

Reference has just been made to the long interval needed for the production of carcinoma in man. It should be pointed out that

PLATE IX

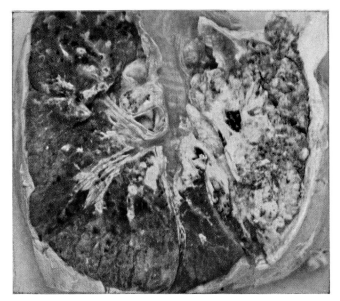

Bronchogenic Carcinoma

The carcinoma is arising from and occluding a bronchus to the lower lobe. The corresponding part of the lung and the pleura are infiltrated with tumor.

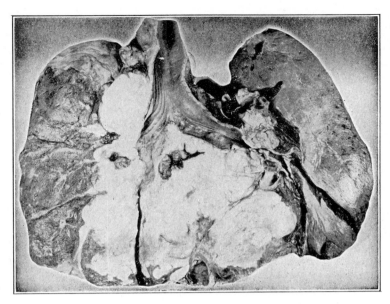

FIG. 395.—Primary carcinoma of the lung. Part of the new growth is the lung tumor, but part is the greatly enlarged bronchial lymph nodes.

the statistics regarding cigarette smoking and lung cancer, quoted so often and with such telling effect, are synchronized, thus disregarding the presumed latent period of twenty to forty years. The cancer cases observed in 1950 have no relation to the cigarettes smoked at that time, but rather to the consumption of tobacco from 1920 to 1935. The rise in the incidence of cancer of the lung began at the turn of the century, and preceded by two decades the widespread cigarette habit. To add still farther to our difficulties, if indeed that were possible, it is obvious that any discussion of the relationship between an increase of lung cancer and an increase in cigarette smoking would have to take into consideration the question as to whether the increase in the cancer was real or only apparent.

Further information on the cause or causes of lung cancer with a general discussion of possible etiological factors will be found in Weller's thoughtful monograph on the subject.

Lesions.—It is something of a relief to turn now to the more solid ground of morbid anatomy. Carcinoma of the lung is essentially bronchogenic in origin (Fig. 395). The *gross* appearance varies to an extraordinary degree, which is one of the reasons why in the past the correct diagnosis has been so often missed in the autopsy room. The most common finding is a firm grayish-white tumor arising from a bronchus to a lobe rather than from a main stem bronchus. It may project into the lumen as a papillary mass which may block the bronchus and cause atelectasis (Plate IX). The nature of such a lesion is self-evident. But it may merely cause a white fibrous thickening of the bronchial wall with narrowing of the lumen and only a suggestion of roughening of the mucosa. If one is not familiar with the existence of this type of lesion the diagnosis will probably be missed. Not rarely a microscopic examination of the suspected lesion is necessary before a definite report can be given. The size of the tumor varies greatly. It may be 1 to 2 cm. in diameter and yet may have caused large and multiple metastases responsible for the death of the patient. Usually, however, it extends outward for a considerable distance into the surrounding lung, and may fuse with the enlarged bronchial lymph nodes (Fig. 394). In a relatively small number of cases the tumor arises in the peripheral part of the lung from a small bronchus; such tumors tend to be more circumscribed, and are those best suited for surgical removal. Unfortunately this advantage is offset by the fact that for a long time these peripheral tumors give rise to no symptoms, so that the ultimate prognosis is no better than in the central form. In exceptional cases the tumor may arise in an old healed tuberculous scar at the apex.

Secondary changes may greatly alter the gross appearance. These changes are atelectasis, bronchiectasis and abscess formation. If a main bronchus is blocked a lobe or the entire lung may be completely collapsed. Massive pleural effusion, often blood-stained, may add to the collapse. A lobe or a lung may be riddled with bronchiectatic cavities, which may develop into abscesses. Sometimes the tumor itself is so completely destroyed by the abscess that microscopic examination is necessary to detect its presence.

The *microscopic appearance* is most varied. There is perhaps no tumor which is so pleomorphic as cancer of the lung, and this explains why in the past it has been so frequently mistaken for other tumors. The cells vary from the most undifferentiated or anaplastic to the most fully differentiated. Three main types can be distinguished, the epidermoid, the anaplastic and the adenocarcinomatous. As the anaplastic may be regarded as an undifferentiated variety of the epidermoid, it may be better to speak of two forms, epidermoid and adenocarcinoma. There is a striking sex difference between the two. Thus in Evarts Graham's experience 94 per cent of the male cases were epidermoid or anaplastic, whilst 35 per cent of the females were adenocarcinoma. The relationship to excessive and prolonged cigarette smoking is believed by many to be well marked in the epidermoid group, but is nonexistent in the adenocarcinomas. This suggests the possibility that the two are different diseases due to different carcinogens. In the epidermoid type differentiation is seldom marked, so that the line between this and the anaplastic type may be indefinite, but sometimes fully formed epithelial pearls are present (Fig. 396*A*). The development of the tumor may be preceded by metaplasia of the cylindrical bronchial epithelium into a squamous form, but this is not necessary nor indeed usual. In the *anaplastic* variety (Fig. 396*B*) the cells are spheroidal or oval (oat-cell type) or even spindle-shaped. Some workers recognize two groups of anaplastic tumors, small-cell and large-cell. These are the tumors which used to be regarded as mediastinal sarcoma, a very frequent diagnosis at the beginning of the century, when bronchogenic carcinoma was regarded as a rarity. Anaplastic is the popular American term, oat-cell the favorite British one. As a matter of fact the anaplasia is not necessarily as marked as the name suggests, for there may be evidence of differentiation into a histological pattern, such as streams of clumps of cells, ribbons, rosettes, and tubules containing PAS-positive mucin (Azzopardi). The *adenocarcinoma* is much the rarest. The cells, which may produce an abundance of mucin, are arranged around gland spaces (Fig. 396*C*), into which papillary processes may project. The stroma varies greatly in amount and density. *Epidermoid* carcinoma arises more insidiously, is of slower growth, and spreads electively to the lymph nodes, whereas the anaplastic form, being undifferentiated, behaves in more explosive fashion, invades the vessels and spreads by the blood stream. These statements of course are merely generalizations to which there are many exceptions.

The *prognosis* is best in epidermoid carcinoma, which tends to be circumscribed and slowly growing, so that surgical removal is possible, it is worst in the anaplastic type, especially the small cell variety which is likely to kill the patient in the course of six months, and intermediate in adenocarcinoma, which is often peripheral.

Spread.—The tumor tends to spread far and wide and the secondary growths may be the first announcement that there is anything wrong with the patient. Spread is threefold: (1) through the lung, (2) to the lymph nodes, and (3) to distant organs. *Spread through the lung* is mainly by way of the perivascular and peribronchial lymphatics with the formation of new nodules at a distance from the primary tumor (Fig. 397). The tumor cells may also creep along the bronchioles and

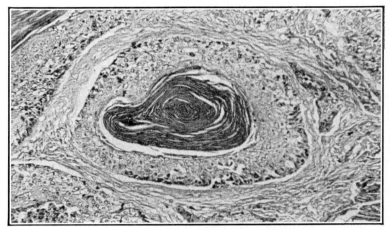

A, Epidermoid. $\times$ 150.

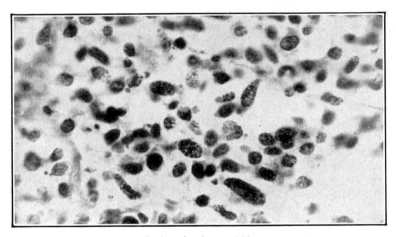

B, Anaplastic. $\times$ 700.

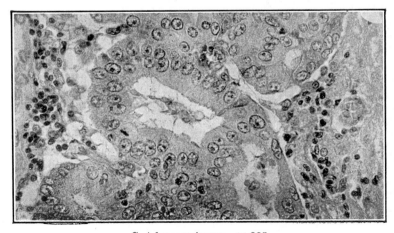

C, Adenocarcinoma. $\times$ 325.

Fig. 396.—Bronchogenic carcinoma.

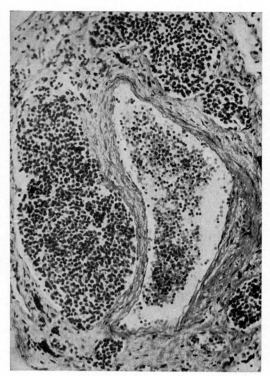

Fig. 397.—Dilated perivascular lymphatics filled with tumor cells. The lumen of the vessel contains red cells. × 175.

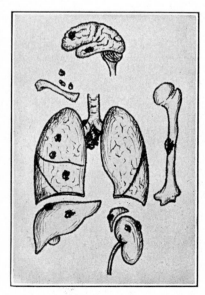

Fig. 398.—Diagram to illustrate sites of metastases in bronchogenic carcinoma.

form a new lining for the alveoli. There may be extension to neighboring structures (pericardium, parietal pleura, heart, etc.).

Spread to the lymph nodes is constant; first the regional nodes (tracheobronchial and mediastinal), but later more distant glands (supraclavicular, cervical, and retroperitoneal) may be involved. The mediastinal mass may be larger than that in the lung, and in the past a diagnosis has often been made of mediastinal sarcoma with secondary growth in the lung.

Spread to distant organs is very common. The order of frequency is as follows: (1) liver, (2) brain and bone, (3) kidney and adrenal (Fig. 398). Less commonly the pancreas, thyroid, etc., may be involved. The combination of metastases in brain and adrenal is remarkably common. In my material half the cases of all secondary tumors of the adrenal were due to bronchogenic carcinoma. The route of spread from lung to adrenals is probably mainly lymphatic *via* the abdominal lymph nodes, which receive efferents from both adrenals. The adrenals have direct lymphatic connection with the diaphragm and posterior mediastinum. In one case direct extension could be traced from a tumor in the hilum down through the mediastinum to the left adrenal. The brain metastasis is often mistaken clinically for a primary cerebral tumor, because the cerebral symptoms may precede the pulmonary ones. In one-third of Halpert's cases the central nervous system symptoms constituted the first complaint, but in one-third of the cases with cerebral metastases there were no symptoms suggesting such involvement.

The presence or absence of blood vessel invasion as seen microscopically in a surgical specimen bears a close relationship to the five-year survival period, and is therefore of value in determining the prognosis in a particular case (Collier *et al.*). In 100 cases of pulmonary resection the survival was 6 per cent with blood vessel invasion and 75 per cent without such invasion. Lymph node involvement proved to be of no significance for survival in the presence of invasion of blood vessels.

I may complete this discussion by quoting the opening words of Willis in his *Pathology of Tumors* when dealing with this subject, with every one of which I am in complete agreement: "With no other neoplasm is a knowledge of metastasis more important to the clinician than with pulmonary carcinoma. This tumor metastasizes with great frequency, often widely, and often at an early stage while the primary growth is still small and symptomless. More diagnostic mistakes due to metastases are made in this disease than in any other."

Relation of Symptoms to Lesions.—The patient is often remarkably well nourished in spite of his cancer, the symptoms being mainly those of pressure and obstruction. The chief symptoms are cough, blood-stained sputum, dyspnea, and pain in the chest. Although the patient is usually in the cancer age, I have seen a number of cases under twenty-five years of age. The x-ray film often fails to show any tumor, merely indicating such effects of the tumor as atelectasis, pleural effusion, enlarged mediastinal glands, paralysis of the diaphragm, etc. In secondary carcinoma, on the other hand, the tumor itself can be readily seen.

The persistent *cough* is due to irritation of a bronchus by the growth. *Bloody sputum* or actual hemorrhage is caused by ulceration of the bronchial mucosa. Occlusion of the bronchus leads to *atelectasis* with displacement of the heart and limitation of movement on the affected side. *Dyspnea* is a common and marked symptom and is probably due to *partial* blocking of a main bronchus, thus interfering with the ventilation (aeration) of a lobe or an entire lung. If the obstruction is complete and the other bronchi are patent there is no dyspnea because the lobe or lung is completely collapsed; there is no partial circulation through it, so that the aerated blood is not polluted by impure blood from the obstructed portions. This is also true of *cyanosis*, although not to the same extent. *Clubbing of the fingers* may be due to shunting of blood from the pulmonary to the systemic circulation.

Pain in the chest or back may be due to pleurisy, pressure on nerves, or metastases in the vertebral column. *Pleural effusion* is present in about 50 per cent of cases, and is due to carcinomatous involvement of the pleura. *The fluid is often blood-stained*, reaccumulates rapidly after removal, and

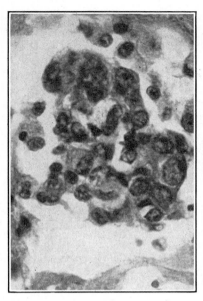

Fig. 399.—Carcinoma cells in sputum. × 630.

may contain clumps of tumor cells. There may be *pressure* on the esophagus, trachea, and recurrent laryngeal nerve with corresponding symptoms. *Fever* and *leukocytosis* may be due to occlusion of a bronchus and the accumulation of purulent material in the resulting abscess or bronchiectatic cavity.

Bronchoscopic examination is of great value. It may show a definite tumor, mucosal roughening, stenosis, or merely interference with the normal movements. Even though the bronchi do not seem correspondingly narrowed, there may be a remarkable absence of breath sounds over the affected area. It is usually possible to obtain a fragment of tumor for biopsy through the bronchoscope.

Exfoliative cytology has developed into a diagnostic method of great value, although the danger of false positives, even in the hands of experts, must always be kept in mind. The material may be obtained from the involved bronchus by means of the bronchoscope or smears of the sputum may be made (Fig. 399). The advantage of the latter method is that a series of specimens can be examined on successive days. False negatives may be due to blockings of the affected bronchus. The method is parti-

44

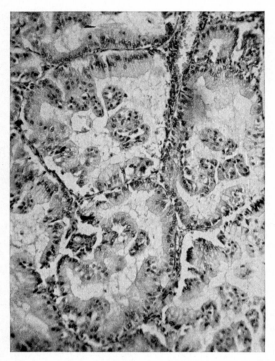

FIG. 400.—Pulmonary adenomatosis showing papillary processes and mucin in alveoli.

cularly valuable when the tumor is in a position in which bronchoscopic bite biopsy is impossible, and in tumors at the periphery of the lung which cannot be seen at all.

It not infrequently happens that the principal symptoms are due to metastases in other organs. Thus the patient may present a picture of cerebral tumor, cancer of the liver, or replacement of the bone marrow rather than carcinoma of the lung. If such cases do not come to autopsy the correct diagnosis may never be made. The higher the autopsy rate in a hospital, the higher will be the incidence of the disease.

Alveolar Cell Carcinoma.—This tumor is also known as *bronchiolar carcinoma*, in the belief that its origin is bronchiolar epithelium, and *pulmonary adenomatosis*, indicating that it may be a benign lesion and possibly not a true neoplasm. Perhaps no tumor has been given more names, and around none has raged so much controversy as to its nature and origin. Considering how the cellular lining of the alveoli, when it is evident under conditions of disease, blends with that

of the finer bronchioles, the matter seems rather immaterial. We have used the terms alveolar cell tumor or carcinoma because they are in such common use, and are so descriptive of the histological picture.

The tumor constitutes 3 or 4 per cent of pulmonary neoplasms, and it is equally common in both sexes. In my own experience it seems to be becoming more frequent, which means, of course, that it is being recognized more often by the clinician and the pathologist. It differs from bronchogenic carcinoma in almost every respect, in gross and microscopic appearance, in natural history, and in the symptoms which it produces. This form of lung cancer is probably the most suitable for surgical treatment by reason of its peripheral position and the absence of distant metastases.

Lesions.—The tumor may be of multiple nodular form or rarely diffuse. The nodular form is apt to be mistaken at autopsy for secondary carcinoma or miliary tuberculosis, whilst the diffuse form resembles the gray hepatization of lobar pneumonia. The cut surface has a glairy mucoid appearance owing to the mucin which can be squeezed out. The microscopic appearance has already been indicated. Papillary processes are common and the alveoli are filled with mucin (Fig. 400). Dense pleural adhesions are common. In about 25 per cent of cases there are metastases in the regional lymph nodes and there may be extension to distant organs. These are examples of malignant adenomatosis or alveolar cell carcinoma. Even in the cases which do not metastasize the condition may prove fatal because of the widespread replacement of alveoli with loss of their functional capacity. An infectious pneumonia of sheep known as *jaagsiekte*, possibly due to a virus, presents a similar microscopic picture.

Relation of Symptoms to Lesions.—As the large bronchi are not involved, the cough and hemoptysis so characteristic of bronchogenic carcinoma are usually absent. Their place is taken by a distressing *dyspnea*, often associated with *cyanosis*, both caused by the increasing involvement of pulmonary tissue. Atelectasis, bronchiectasis and other evidence of bronchial obstruction is absent. The sputum is mucoid or watery, and may be extremely copious. A complaint of increasing quantities of unusually thick sputum is always suggestive of this condition. *The finding of polypoid processes of mucin-filled cells in the sputum is pathognomonic.*

Adenoma of Bronchus.—This tumor, which is said to constitute from 6 to 10 per cent of primary lung tumors (Liebow), is remarkable for its long duration punctuated by repeated hemorrhages. Thus in a case of mine there were hemorrhages, sometimes copious, over a period of twenty-five years. The tumor is usually an adenomatous polyp growing in a main bronchus and causing obstruction of the lumen as well as hemorrhage. It may project on the surface, producing bronchial obstruction and forming a striking picture when seen with the bronchoscope. In other cases there is little to be seen on the surface, but there may be a large tumor growing into the lobe, a fact which emphasizes the necessity of lobectomy. *Microscopically* it consists of epithelial cells strikingly uniform in type, and usually forming solid masses reminiscent of a *carcinoid* tumor, so that the tumor is regarded by some as an argentaffinoma (Fig. 401). The cells may occasionally be arranged in *cylindrical* form around spaces in glandular formation. The origin of the tumor is a matter of dispute. It may arise from basal cells in the bronchial mucosa or even from epithelialized alveoli, which would explain the fact that there is often a distinct space between the tumor and the bronchial epithelium. Although the tumor is called an adenoma there is distinct invasion of the surrounding parenchyma and sometimes of the lymphatics. An adenoma may become carcinomatous, so that lobectomy is preferable to removal through the bronchoscope.

Like alveolar cell carcinoma (adenomatosis) but sharply differing from bronchogenic carcinoma, adenoma of the bronchus is as common in the female as in the male. There is no suggestion of the action of an external carcinogen. Mention has already been made of the resemblance of the neoplasm to the carcinoid tumor. It is therefore of interest to learn that in occasional cases the patient presents the clinical picture of the carcinoid syndrome, with periodic flushing of the face and the excretion of large amount of sero-

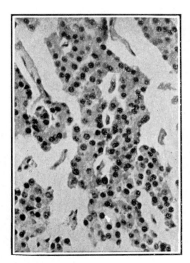

FIG. 401.—Adenoma of bronchus. $\times$ 275.

tonin (5-hydroxytryptamine) in the urine (Williams and Azzopardi) (Schneckloth *et al.*). In such cases autopsy will show multiple metastases in the liver and elsewhere.

HAMARTOMA.—This is a small benign lesion of the lung commonly situated at the periphery, usually symptomless and picked up in a routine radiological examination when it may arouse a suspicion of a more serious condition. A hamartoma (*hamartion*, a bodily defect), seen also in the kidney, is a developmental anomaly, well circumscribed, and consisting of the normal constituents of the part arranged in a jumbled and confused manner. Here it is composed principally of cartilage, often calcified, sometimes ossified, together with fat, fibrous tissue, muscle and glandlike structures. It may be presumed to originate as a faulty development of a bronchial anlage.

PANCOAST'S SYNDROME.—This is a clinical syndrome characterized by pain about the shoulder and down the arm, Horner's syndrome, local destruction of the first two or three ribs, atrophy of the hand, and a roentgen-ray shadow at the extreme apex. Pancoast suggested the name of *superior pulmonary sulcus tumor,* but it is better called Pancoast's syndrome. Most of these cases are examples of apical bronchogenic carcinoma pressing on the brachial plexus and the sympathetic cervical chain, but without symptoms or signs of pulmonary disease. In a few instances the lesion may be an epidermal carcinoma arising from embryonal remains rather than any adjacent normal structure.

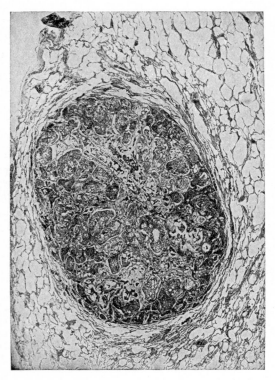

Fig. 402.—Secondary carcinoma of lung lying just under the pleura. × 12.

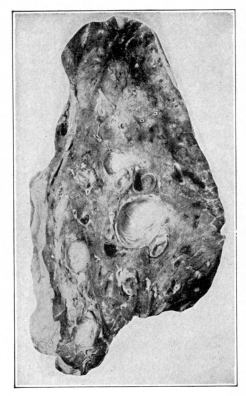

Fig. 403.—Congenital cystic lung. No communication could be demonstrated between the smooth-walled cysts and the bronchial tree. (Boyd, *Pathology for the Physician.*)

Secondary Tumors.—Secondary tumors of the lung are very common. Carcinoma may reach the lung by the blood stream or *via* the lymphatics (cancer of the breast). Many nodules are scattered through one or both lungs, and sometimes these nodules may be miliary in type. Microscopic clumps of tumor cells may be found where no gross tumor can be detected. In some cases the nodules are entirely subpleural, none being found in the substance of the lung (Fig. 402). Sarcoma of bone has a special tendency to metastasize to the lungs. Chorionepithelioma has the intensely hemorrhagic character of the primary tumor in the uterus.

CONGENITAL ANOMALIES

Congenital Cystic Lung.—Congenital cysts of the lung may be of bronchogenic type or of alveolar type. It seems probable that the type depends on the stage of development at which cyst formation occurs.

They are usually found in children and young adults, but they may occur at any age. They may be single, but as a rule are multiple, and they may be scattered or confluent. They are generally confined to one lobe or even a single segment, but they may involve the entire lung.

The *bronchogenic* cysts are lined by a bronchial mucosa, the ciliated cells of which may be columnar or cuboidal. They may communicate with bronchi, and when seen in childhood the condition is likely to be classified as congenital bronchiectasis. The cysts may contain fluid or pus, depending on whether the lesions communicate with the bronchial tree.

The *alveolar type cysts* are lined by the flattened cells characteristic of the air sacs, and they always communicate with bronchi. The cysts are filled with air. If the communication with the bronchus becomes closed, the air is absorbed, and the cyst may be obliterated. The large solitary so-called balloon cyst or pneumatocele appears to belong to this group. Although commoner in infants and children, the solitary cysts are also encountered in adults.

Pathogenesis.—"Congenital cystic disease of the lung results from an anonymous development of the lung anlage, and the characteristic cellular component of the malformation will be determined by the age of the individual at the time that the malformation occurs" (Cooke and Blades). The canalization of the mesodermal buds from which the bronchi develop seems to fail to progress at one point. A zone of atresia of varying length is produced, distal to which the smaller bronchi persist and develop. Such a condition results in the formation of multiple cysts of very varying size (Fig. 403).

The *clinical picture* may be one of two types. In the one the outstanding feature is attacks of dyspnea and cyanosis in early life. This is due to rupture of one of the cysts with the production of pneumothorax. The attacks may be recurrent and one of them may prove fatal. The other is characterized by cough, fever, purulent expectoration, and signs of pneumonitis. These are due to infection of the cysts from communications with the bronchi. There may be marked pulmonary hypertension as the result of vascular occlusion. In one of my cases the pulmonary artery was enormously dilated, measuring 12 cm. in diameter, whereas the aorta at the same level measured only 7 cm.

Intralobar Sequestration.—This may be regarded as a special variety of congenital cystic disease of the lung. It has two components: (1) a maldevelopment of part of the bronchial tree to a lower lobe giving a sequestrated or dislocated mass of lung; (2) distribution of arterial blood to the affected portion of lung by way of an anomalous artery arising from the aorta, just above or below the diaphragm, with corresponding failure of development of branches of the pulmonary artery to the affected part (Pryce). The anomalous vessel has the elastic structure of the pulmonary artery, not the muscular character of a bronchial artery. It appears to empty into the pulmonary vein, thus constituting an unusal type of vascular shunt which imposes added work upon the left ventricle and may be of some significance in older patients (Kergin). The vascular anomaly is probably primary, with resulting maldevelopment of the corresponding portion of the bronchial tree. At operation the lesion presents a characteristic picture of a rubbery mass of yellowish-pink, non-pigmented lung containing one or more cysts. The symptoms and radiological findings are those of cystic lung with superadded infection, namely chronic cough with purulent sputum and it may be hemoptysis.

Other congenital anomalies such as hamartoma and arteriovenous fistula or aneurysm have already been considered.

THE PLEURA

PLEURISY

Inflammation of the pleura, pleuritis, or pleurisy, is one of the commonest of autopsy findings, especially in its chronic form, as indicated by fibrous adhesions. Clinically, however, the condition is much less frequently encountered. The slighter degrees of pleurisy, therefore, may give rise to no clinical manifestations. In the great majority of cases the infection extends from the lung to the pleura. Occasionally, especially in the case of tuberculosis, it appears to originate in the pleura. In a third group the infection may spread from some neighboring part such as the chest wall.

Most cases of pleurisy are caused by one of three organisms, pneumococcus, streptococcus and tubercle bacillus. The usual classification employed, however, is not a bacteriological one, but depends on the type of the exudate.

This may be fibrinous, in which case we have a dry pleurisy, it may be serofibrinous, in which case we have a pleurisy with effusion, or it may be purulent, in which case we have an empyema. As with most pathological processes, however, the dividing line is not quite so sharp in practice as it is in theory. Dry pleurisy is usually associated with a slight increase in the amount of fluid normally found in the pleural sac, while the

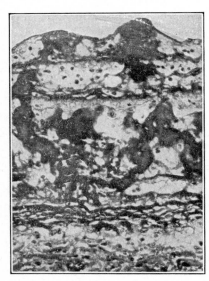

FIG. 404.—Pleursy showing fibrinous exudate. × 130

fluid in the serofibrinous form may contain considerable numbers of pus cells.

Fibrinous Pleurisy.—This form is characterized by the formation of an exudate consisting mainly of fibrin. Although a small amount of fluid is usually found in cases which come to autopsy, this is not present in sufficient quantity to be detected by clinical means. Fibrinous pleurisy may be *secondary* to such pulmonary conditions as pneumonia, tuberculosis, carcinoma, and infarct, or to a neighborhood infection such as pericarditis, periostitis of the rib, or peritonitis. In such cases it is likely to be of the dry variety. Or it may appear to be a *primary* pleural condition, either dry or with effusion. These cases are usually tuberculous in nature. The infection is not strictly primary, but probably begins in a subpleural focus in the lung from which it spreads to the pleura, both lesions subsequently becoming healed.

Epidemic pleurodynia is an uncommon condition which, as its name implies, may appear in mild epidemic form, and is characterized by severe pleural pain in the lower chest. It is believed to be caused by Coxsackie B$_5$ virus, which is also responsible for viral pericarditis.

LESIONS.—The fibrinous exudate may be so thin as merely to dull the luster of the membrane or so thick that it can be peeled

off in layers (Fig. 404). Both parietal and visceral layers are involved, and stringy fibrinous adhesions pass between the two layers and also between the lobes. Later these may become converted into permanent fibrous adhesions, and in extreme cases the entire cavity may be obliterated.

Pleurisy with Effusion.—This is also known as *serofibrinous pleurisy*, the serous part of the exudate being greatly in excess of the fibrinous part. The etiology is similar to that of dry pleurisy. Where the condition is apparently primary in the pleura with no clinically obvious lesion in the lung it should be regarded as tuberculous, although direct microscopic examination of the fluid for tubercle bacilli is seldom successful owing to their small numbers. Animal inoculation gives a positive result in about 50 per cent of cases, and the subsequent history shows only too frequently the tuberculous character of the infection. By far the most valuable method of determining the nature of a pleural effusion is by punch *needle biopsy of the pleura*, which was successful in establishing the correct diagnosis in 80 per cent of tuberculous and 60 per cent of malignant effusions (Mestitz *et al.*). Staining for acid-fast organisms was almost never successful, but the histological picture of tuberculosis or carcinoma was convincing and conclusive. A man would present a clinical picture confidently diagnosed as bronchogenic carcinoma, but pleural biopsy showed tubercles, and specific chemotherapy was accompanied by an uninterrupted recovery.

The *fluid* is clear or opalescent, depending on the number of cells it contains. The cells themselves vary with the infection, being mainly polymorphonuclears in infections by pyogenic bacteria, small lymphocytes (80 to 100 per cent) in tuberculous effusions. When the fluid is withdrawn a jelly-like clot forms, owing to the high fibrinogen content. Hemorrhagic effusion indicates malignancy. A fully fledged serofibrinous pleurisy very seldom turns into an empyema, unless infection is introduced from without. When the effusion is abundant the lung is collapsed, the heart pushed over to the other side, the diaphragm pushed down, and the intercostal spaces widened.

Empyema.—When this book was first written empyema or purulent pleurisy was

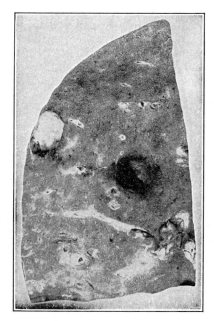

Fig. 405.—Subpleural abscess about to rupture. Rupture of such an abscess is certain to be followed by empyema.

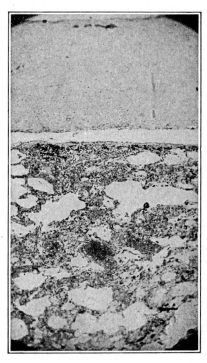

Fig. 406.—Empyema, showing greatly thickened pleura. × 40.

a common and dangerous complication of intrathoracic and sometimes extrathoracic disease. Now it has become uncommon and even rare, because most of the infections responsible for this complication can now be controlled by the sulfonamides and antibiotics. It is usually secondary to infection in the lung, sometimes to spread of infection from other organs—such as the pericardium, chest wall, or peritoneum. Pneumococcal empyema complicates lobar pneumonia in a small proportion of cases (2 to 5 per cent). Streptococcal empyemas are often due to rupture of a small subpleural abscess which floods the pleural cavity with the massive dose of organisms needed to produce suppuration (Fig. 405). In military surgery infection is introduced from without as a result of penetrating wounds. The three *common organisms* are pneumococcus, streptococcus and staphylococcus in that order of frequency although not of importance. Pneumococcal and streptococcal infections no longer present a real problem, because they can be so well controlled, but the staphylococcal empyemas due to antibiotic-resistant strains are a very different matter.

Lesions.—Here we have to consider the pleura, the lung, and the pus. The *pleura* is covered by a layer of inflammatory exudate, which is much thicker than in the other two forms of pleurisy. This thick layer covers the parietal as well as the visceral layer, so that an exploring needle may have to be pushed in a long way before it encounters pus. In course of time the exudate becomes converted into fibrous tissue (Fig. 406) and the lung may be bound down to such an extent that it fails to expand when the pus is evacuated. Very dense adhesions are likely to be formed.

The *lung* is collapsed to a degree depending on the amount of the fluid. In extreme cases it is flattened against the mediastinum and the posterior chest wall. Pressure of the pus may lead to necrosis and destruction of the lung at the seat of pressure. In longstanding cases there may be a diffuse fibrosis of the lung which combines with the adhesions and the pleural exudate to prevent expansion.

The *pus* varies in amount and in location. It is the exception rather than the rule for the entire pleural cavity to be involved; the the empyema may be either diffuse or encapsulated. Adhesions soon form which limit the pus to one region. The adhesions may pass from the common surface of the lung to the chest wall, or between the opposing surfaces of two lobes, or between the lung and the mediastinum. The pus is limited by these adhesions, so that an empyema is often not a pleural cavity filled with pus, but rather a pocket of pus tucked away in some obscure corner and very difficult of access by the exploring needle. In pneumococcal and staphylococcal cases the pus is yellowish-green in color, thick and creamy in consistence. In the streptococcal empyema of the great pandemic of influenza the fluid was often serous rather thean purulent, although swarming with hemolytic streptococci. In tuberculous empyema the pus tends to be thin and watery with masses of caseous material.

Relation of Symptoms to Lesions.—The symptoms of the various forms of pleurisy are very similar. *Pain* in the side made worse by breathing is the most characteristic symptom. It is not caused by friction of the inflamed and roughened surfaces as I was taught, for the friction rub may still be heard after the pain has ceased, and pleural pain may come on after pneumothorax. Like so many other pains it is due to tension, the inflamed and acutely sensitive parietal pleura being stretched every time the patient takes a deep breath. The visceral pleura is insensitive and so can take no part in producing the pain. Strapping of the chest relieves the pain by preventing the stretching of the parietal pleura; it does not prevent the friction. The pain disappears with the onset of effusion, because the fluid serves as a splint to immobilize the lower ribs. The *friction rub* is heard as long as the roughened surfaces are rubbing against one another; it disappears when the surfaces are separated by effusion.

HYDROTHORAX

Hydrothorax is a fluid transudate, as opposed to an inflammatory exudate, in the pleural cavity. The watery fluid has a specific gravity below 1.018 and protein content below 4 per cent. It is a part of cardiac or renal edema. For some reason hydrothorax due to cardiac disease is usually right-sided. This may possibly be due to pressure of the dilated right auricular appendix on the pulmonary veins on that side, but it must be admitted that that explanation sounds rather far-fetched. In renal edema the pleural effusion is usually bilateral, and if it happens to be unilateral it is as common on the left as on the right.

MEIGS' SYNDROME.—In 1937 Meigs and Cass reported a case of fluid in the pleural cavity and ascites associated with fibroma of the ovary, and more recently Meigs has reviewed a number of cases in the literature both before and after that date. The nature of this rare condition is completely obscure, although a number of ingenious suggestions have been made in an attempt to explain how a benign tumor of the ovary can cause pleural effusion. The fluid has nearly always been on the right side of the chest. After tapping, the fluid rapidly reaccumulates in the chest and abdomen. Removal of the tumor is followed by gradual disappearance of the pleural fluid and the ascites. The chief *symptoms* are difficulty in breathing and a sense of pressure and weight in the abdomen. The importance of the syndrome lies in the fact that it is apt to be mistaken for an inoperable malignant condition.

HEMOTHORAX

Blood in the pleural cavity is due to bleeding which may be traumatic or spontaneous. *Traumatic hemothorax* is due to penetrating wounds of the chest wall or lung. *Spontaneous hemothorax* may be the result of bleeding from a tuberculous lesion, a hemangioma of the lung, a ruptured pleural adhesion, and sometimes for no apparent reason. If the bleeding is slight the blood will be absorbed, but if massive it will become organized into a fibrous encasement of the atelectatic lung.

CHYLOTHORAX.—A milky fluid in the pleural cavity may be chyle, chyliform or pseudochylous. True *chyle* is due to rupture or obstruction of the thoracic duct by trauma, malignant disease, tuberculosis or filaria. *Chyliform* fluids, which closely resemble chylous fluid, are milky due to the presence of fine, fat droplets derived from fatty degeneration of cells in cancer of the lung or tuberculosis. A *pseudochylous* fluid does not contain fat, although it may have a milky appearance, which may be due to the presence of albuminous particles in fine subdivision.

PNEUMOTHORAX

Pneumothorax is air or gas in the pleural cavity. Sometimes this is accomplished by a serous or even purulent effusion. There is normally a negative pressure in the pleural cavity, and when the cavity communicates with the lung or the outside air rushes in, the negative pressure falls to zero, and as the opening is often valvular a positive pressure may take its place.

It used to be believed that pneumothorax was due to rupture of a subpleural tuberculous cavity, but it is now realized that this is a rare event. The condition is usually caused by rupture of an emphysematous bulla or subpleural bleb. Rarely it may be associated with carcinoma, abscess or bronchiectasis.

Lacerations of the pleura from without and tearing of the lung by a fractured rib are uncommon causes. Much more rare are perforation of the esophagus and rupture of an ulcer or cancer of of the stomach through the diaphragm. There remains a small group of cases of spontaneous pneumothorax, in which the condition suddenly develops without any obvious cause. Some of these may be due to rupture of an emphysematous vesicle.

LESIONS.—The air should be demonstrated before the chest is opened at autopsy. A needle may be pushed through the chest wall and the issuing gas may blow out a match. Or the skin may be reflected, and a small cup made in the intercostal muscles in which water is placed. When the pleura is punctured at this point bubbles of air appear in the water. When the chest is opened fluid will usually be found, which may be serous but is more often purulent (pyopneumothorax). The lung is collapsed, forming a small mass in the region of the hilus. The heart is pushed over to the opposite side and the diaphragm pushed down so that its under surface may become convex and the edge of the liver is far below the costal margin.

RELATION OF SYMPTOMS TO LESIONS.—The onset is often sudden with severe pain in the side and great dyspnea, or it may be quite gradual. The affected side is enlarged and immobile, with lack of vocal fremitus, hyper-resonance, absence of breath sounds, and the characteristically echoing coin sound. When the patient is shaken the Hippocratic succussion splash may be heard in some cases, but this is very rare. The abrupt onset is due to the air suddenly rushing into a cavity where there is a negative pressure. The pain is caused by stretching of the parietal pleura. The enlargement and immobility of the affected side, hyperresonance, and coin sound are due to the air which fills the pleural cavity. The dyspnea, lack of vocal fremitus, and absence of breath sounds are caused by collapse of the lung, and the succussion splash is caused by the movement of the fluid. The roentgen-ray picture is highly characteristic (air, fluid, and collapsed lung).

TUMORS OF THE PLEURA

Tumors of the pleura may be primary or secondary. Primary tumors are rare; secondary tumors (carcinoma) are fairly common.

Primary Tumors.—These may be divided into two groups, the localized and the diffuse. The *localized* tumors are of many histological types, but they have one characteristic in common; they arise from the tissues beneath the surface lining, whereas the diffuse tumors arise from this layer of cells. The localized tumors may grow from the parietal or visceral pleura. The most important member is the so-called *giant sarcoma* of the visceral pleura, which is of very slow growth and does not infiltrate nor metastasize, so that by the time it is discovered it may attain an enormous size and fill the entire pleural cavity. It has the microscopic structure of a fibrosarcoma, but does not behave like a malignant growth.

The *diffuse* tumor arises from the surface lining cells, and is commonly known as an endothelioma. It would be better called a *mesothelioma*, as the surface cells are mesothelial in character, the lining of the pleural cavity being derived from the coelomic epithelium, which in turn is developed by a splitting of the mesoderm. The tumor may present characteristics of either epithelial or connective tissue, due to the varied potentialities of the mesothelial cells. It causes a diffuse thickening of the pleura which may extend over a considerable area or even the entire lung and may be over 1 cm. in depth (Fig. 407). Both layers of the pleura may be involved. Pleural effusion is common, at first serous and later hemorrhagic. *Microscopically* the tumor consists of large spherical cells arranged in solid masses and columns, often within the lumen of lymphatics; they may have a definite glandular forma-

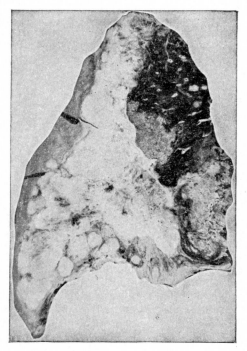

Fig. 407.—Mesothelioma of the pleura. The lung is enveloped by an enormously thickened pleura. (Boyd, *Pathology for the Physician*.)

tion as in an adenocarcinoma. The stroma is usually fibrous and abundant.

Secondary Carcinoma.—In secondary cancer of the lung the pleura may be involved, but not infrequently the pleura is studded with small tumors although none are to be seen in the lung. Sometimes a network of lymphatics is outlined as a series of white lines due to permeation by carcinoma cells. The primary tumor is usually in the breast.

THE MEDIASTINUM

MEDIASTINAL TUMORS AND CYSTS

The mediastinum is a complex structure containing a great variety of tissues. It is natural that an equal number of tumors have been reported. The primary tumors may be in the anterior or the posterior mediastinum. By and large, the anterior mediastinal tumors are teratomas; the posterior group are neurogenic tumors.

Neurogenic Tumors.—These tumors, which arise from the posterior roots of the spinal nerves, may be neurofibromas or ganglioneuromas. The great majority of the neurofibromas are benign and are picked up on routine mass x-ray examinations, but if they are left long enough they tend to become malignant. The *neurofibroma*, arising from the posterior nerve roots, grows forward pushing the parietal pleura in front of it, but it may grow backward through an intervertebral foramen and press on the spinal cord. This is the so-called dumb-bell tumor. The palisading of the nuclei or the whorled arrangement of the fusiform cells is characteristic of neurofibroma. When the tumor becomes malignant the growth is more disorderly and mitoses are frequent. The *ganglioneuroma*, more common in children, arises from sympathetic ganglia. It is a benign tumor composed of large adult ganglion cells with an admixture of small embryonal nerve cells. Neurogenic tumors are often symptomless, but they may give rise to root pain.

Teratoid Tumors.—Developmental tumors, solid or cystic, are confined to the anterior mediastinum. They are likely to be discovered in adolescence or early adult life. *The solid tumors are called teratomas, the cysts are dermoids*. The teratomas are composed of a variety of structures, whilst the dermoids are cysts with ectodermal and mesodermal tissues, *i.e.*, epithelium, glands, hair, cartilage, bone and teeth. No really satisfying explanation has ever been given for the occurrence of teratoid tumors and cysts in the mediastinum. The solid tumors may become malignant developing into an epidermoid carcinoma or adenocarcinoma. Cough is the most constant symptom, though there may be pain and dyspnea. The sputum may be blood-streaked. Expectoration of hair, known as *trichoptysis*, is the one pathognomonic symptom, although complaints by the patient of this occurrence have often been received with amused scepticism and incredulity. A circumscribed shadow is seen in the anterior mediastinum in the x-ray film, and the presence of teeth is pathognomonic.

Mediastinal Cysts.—Cysts, other than those of the teratoid group, never become malignant. They may be bronchial, esophageal, gastric, enteric, or pericardial in origin. They occur in the posterior mediastinum, with the exception of pericardial cysts, and are probably formed by a pinching off of a small bud of the bronchial tree.

The *bronchial* or *bronchiogenic cyst* is usually situated in the posterior part of the superior mediastinum at the bifurcation of the trachea or attached to a large bronchus. The wall consists of the normal constituents of the bronchial wall, and the cyst is lined by ciliated pseudostratified columnar epithelium. The esophageal cyst is lined by squamous stratified epithelium. *Gastric cysts* usually occur in young children; the wall is lined by gastric mucosa, and the contents are strongly acid. A peptic ulcer is liable to develop, which erodes the trachea and gives rise to hemoptysis. *Enteric cysts* are the rarest variety. They are lined by intestinal mucosa.

The *pericardial coelomic cyst* arises in the course of development of the pericardial cavity, and is situated in the anterior mediastinum, usually at the cardiophrenic angle. The lining is a single layer of flattened cells, and the contents are so clear and limpid that the lesion has been given the poetic name of "spring-water cyst." There are usually no symptoms.

Lymph Node Tumors.—These form the largest group of mediastinal tumors, and are situated in the anterior mediastinum. They may be primary or secondary. Tumors of the lumph nodes are discussed in Chapter 41, so that they will not be considered here.

REFERENCES

AZZOPARDI, J. G.: J. Path. and Bact., 1959, *78*, 513. (Oat-cell carcinoma of bronchus.)

BAKER, R. D.: Am. J. Path., 1956, *32*, 287 (Pulmonary mucormycosis.)

BALDUS, W. P. and PETER, J. B.: New Eng. J. Med., 1960, *262*, 700. (Farmer's lung.)

BAYLEY, E. C., LINDBERG, D. O. N. and BAGGENSTOSS, A. H.: Arch. Path., 1945, *40*, 376 (Löffler's syndrome.)

BELT, T. H.: Med. Res. Council, Spec. Rep. Series, No. 243, 1942. (Anthracosis.)

BERKSON, J.: Proc. Staff Meet. Mayo Clinic, 1955, *30*, 319; 1959, *34*, 206. (Statistical relationship of cigarette smoking to lung cancer.)

BERTALANFFY, F. D. and LEBLOND, C. P.: Lancet, 1955, *2*, 1365. (Structure of respiratory tissue.)

BERTHRONG, M.: Am. J. Clin. Path., 1956, *26*, 396. (Pulmonary cyst formation following chemotherapy.)

BOYDEN, E. A.: *Segmental Anatomy of the Lungs,* New York, 1955.

BROCK, R. C.: *The Anatomy of the Bronchial Tree,* London, 1946 (Bronchopulmonary segments).

CAPLAN, A.: Thorax, 1953, *8*, 29. (Rheumatoid pneumoconiosis.)

CHESNER, C.: Ann. Int. Med., 1950, *32*, 1029. (Beryllium pneumonitis.)

COFFEY, V. P. and JESSOP, W. J. E.: Lancet, 1959, *2*, 935. (Maternal influenza and congenital deformities.)

COLLIER, F. C. *et al.*: Ann. Surg., 1957, *146*, 417. (Blood vessel invasion in carcinoma of lung.)

COOKE, F. N. and BLADES, B. B.: J. Thoracic Surg., 1952, *23*, 546 (Congenital cystic lung).

DICK, J. C.: Lancet, 1955, *2*, 216. (Tuberculous lesions after chemotherapy.)

DOCK, W.: Am. Rev. Tuberc., 1947, *55*, 511. (Apical site of pulmonary tuberculosis.)

DOLL, R. and HILL, A. B.: Brit. Med. J., 1950, *2*, 739; 1956, *2*, 1071. (Incidence and relation of smoking to bronchogenic carcinoma.)

DONOHUE, W. L., *et al.*: Pediatrics, 1959, *24*, 786. (Familial cystic fibrosis of the lung.)

ENDERS, J. F., *et al*: New Eng. J. Med., 1959, *261*, 875. (Giant-cell pneumonia due to measles virus.)

ENGEL, S.: J. Clin. Path., 1958, *11*, 302. (Chronic bronchitis.)

FISHER, E. R. and DAVIS, E.: New Eng. J. Med., 1958, *258*, 1036. (Cytomegalic-inclusion disease in the adult.)

FISHER, SIR R.: *Smoking: The Cancer Controversy,* Edinburgh, 1959.

FLICK, A. L. and PATON, R. R.: Arch. Int. Med. 1959, *104*, 518. (Smoking and chronic bronchitis.)

GATES, O. and WARREN, S.: Am. J. Path., 1960, *36*, 653. (Bronchial carcinoma in mice produced by internal radiation.)

GOUGH, J.: In *Recent Advances in Pathology,* C. V. Harrison, editor, London, 1960.

GOUGH, J., RIVERS, D. and SEAL, R. M.: Thorax, 1955, *10*, 9. (Caplan's syndrome.)

GRAHAM, E. A., BURFORD, T. H. and MAYER, J. H.: Postgraduate Med., 1948, *4*, 29. (Middle lobe syndrome.)

HALL, G. H.: Lancet, 1959, *1*, 750. (Digital clubbing.)

HALPERT, B., FIELDS, W. S. and DEBAKEY, M.: Surgery, 1954, *35*, 346. (Cerebral metastasis in bronchogenic carcinoma.)

HAMILTON, J. D., BROWN, T. C. and MacDONALD, F. W.: Can. M. A. J., 1957, *77*, 177. (Morphological changes in smokers' lungs.)

HAMMAN, L.: Bull. Johns Hopkins Hosp., 1939, *64*, 1. Pulmonary interstitial emphysema.)

HAMMOND, E. C. and HORN, D.: J.A.M.A., 1954, *155*, 1316. (Relation of smoking to cancer of lung.)

HAMPERYL, H.: Am. J. Path., 1956, *32*, 1. (Pneumocystis pneumonia.)

HARRISON, C. V.: J. Path. & Bact., 1948, *60*, 289. (Multiple emboli and pulmonary arteriosclerosis and hypertension.)

HARTROFT, W. S.: Am. J. Path., 1945, *21*, 889. (Emphysema.)

HEPPLESTON A. G.: J. Path and Bact. 1953, *66*, 235. (Pneumoconiosis in coal workers).

HERS, J. F. PH., MASUREL, N. and MULDER, J.: Lancet, 1958, *2*, 1141. (Fatal Asian influenza.)

HESS, R.: Am. J. Path. 1960, *37*, 583. (Histochemistry of renal oxidative enzyme systems.)

HINSHAW, H. C. and GARLAND, L. H.: *Diseases of the Chest*, Philadelphia, 1956.

HOPPS, H. C. and WISSLER, R. W.: Am. J. Path., 1955, *31*, 261. (Uremic pneumonitis.)

HUEPER, W. C.: Indust. Med. & Surg., 1954, *23*, 1. (Relation of smoking to cancer of lung.)

HUTCHISON, J. H.: Quart. J. Med., 1949, *18*, 21. (Epituberculosis.)

JAFFÉ, F. A.: Am. J. Path., 1951, *27*, 909. (Graphite pneumoconiosis.)

KERGIN, F. G.: J. Thoracic Surg., 1952, *23*, 55. (Intralobar sequestration.)

KOTIN, P. *et al.:* Arch. Indust. Hyg., 1954, *9*, 153, 164. (Carcinogenic hydrocarbons in the atmosphere.)

KNUDTSON, K. P.: Am. J. Clin. Path., 1960, *33*, 310. (Smoking effects on bronchial mucosa.)

KREYBERG, L.: Brit. J. Prev. & Social Med., 1956, *10*, 145. (Bronchogenic carcinoma and cigarettes.)

LIEBERMAN, J.: New Eng. J. Med., 1959, *260*, 619. (Hyaline membrane disease.)

LIEBOW, A. A.: *Tumors of Lower Respiratory Tract*, Atlas of Tumor Pathology, Armed Forces Institute of Pathology, Washington, D.C., 1952.

————: Am. J. Path., 1949, *25*, 211. (Bronchiectasis.)

————: Am. J. Path., 1953, *29*, 251. (Bronchopulmonary veins in emphysema.)

LOWRY, T. and SCHUMAN, L. M.: J.A.M.A., 1956, *162*, 153. (Silo-filler's disease.)

LYNCH, M. J. G. and MELLOR, L. D.: J. Pediat., 1955, *47*, 275. (Hyaline membrane disease of newborn.)

MACKLIN, C. C.: Med. Rec., 1939, *150*, 5. (Pulmonary interstitial emphysema.) Canad. M. A. J., 1955, *72*, 664. (Lung fluid.) J. Thor. Surg., 1956, *31*, 238. (Concentration of carcinogens in outdrifting mucus.)

MALLORY, T. B.: New Eng. J. Med., 1947, *237*, 795. (Bronchiectasis.)

MAYER, E. and MAIER, H. C.: *Pulmonary Carcinoma*, New York, 1956.

McADAMS, A. J., JR.: Am. J. Med., 1955, *19*, 314. (Bronchiolitis obliterans.)

McCLEMENT, J. H. *et al.:* Am. Rev. Tuberc., 1953, *67*, 154. (Pulmonary sarcoidosis.)

McLEAN, K. H.: Am. J. Med., 1958, *25*, 62. (Pathogenesis of emphysema.)

————: Austral. Ann. Med., 1957, *6*, 29. (Permanent effects of acute bronchiolitis.)

MEIGS, J. V. and CASS, J. W.: Am. J. Obst. & Gynec., 1937, *33*, 249. (Meigs' syndrome.)

MENDELSON, C. L.: Am. J. Obstet. and Gynec., 1946, *52*, 191. (Aspiration of stomach contents during obstetrical anesthesia.)

MESTITZ, P., PURVES, M. J. and POLLARD, A. C.: Lancet, 1958, *2*, 1349. (Pleural biopsy in pleural effusion.)

MILLER, W. S.: *The Lung*, 2nd Ed., Springfield, Ill., 1947.

OCHSNER, A. *et al.:* J.A.M.A., 1952, *148*, 691. (Incidence of bronchogenic carcinoma.)

OSEASOHN, R., ADELSON, L. and KAJI, M.: New Eng. J. Med., 1959, *260*, 509. (Fatal Asian influenza.)

PEABODY, J. W., JR. and SEABURY, J. H.: Am. J. Med., 1960, *28*, 99. (Pulmonary nocardiosis.)

PRYCE, D. M.: J. Path. & Bact., 1946, *58*, 457. (Intralobar sequestration.)

READ, J.: Am. Rev. Tuberc., 1958, *78*, 353. (Pathogenesis of the Hamman-Rich syndrome.)

REIMAN, H. A.: J.A.M.A., 1938, *111*, 2357; 1956, *161*, 1078. (Viral pneumonias.)

ROBERTSON, A. L., CALEY, J. P. and MOORE, J.: Lancet, 1958, *2*, 233. (Staphylococcal pneumonia complicating influenza.)

ROBERTSON, D. M. and MILLIKEN, J. A.: Canad. M. A. J., 1958, *79*, 745. (Malignant granuloma of nose.)

ROBERTSON, O. H.: J.A.M.A., 1938, *111*, 1432. (Pneumococcal pneumonia.)

ROBINSON, W. L.: Brit. J. Surg., 1933, *21*, 203. (Bronchiectasis.)

ROSEN, S. H., CASTLEMAN, B. and LIEBOW, A. A.: New Eng. J. Med., 1958, *258*, 1123. (Pulmonary alveolar proteinosis.)

ROSENBLATT, M. B. and LISA, J. R.: *Cancer of the Lung*, New York, 1956.

SCHILLING, R. S. F.: Lancet, 1956, *2*, 261. (Byssynosis.)

SCHNECKLOTH, R. E., McISAAC, W. M. and PAGE, I. H.: J.A.M.A., 1959, *170*, 1143. (Carcinoid syndrome with metastatic bronchial adenoma.)

SEGAL, E. L., STARR, G. F. and WEED, L. A.: J.A. M.A., 1959, *170*, 515. (Staining of surgically excised pulmonary granulomas.)

SOSMAN, M. C. *et al.:* Am. J. Roentgenol., 1957, *77*, 947. (Pulmonary alveolar microlithiasis.)

SOTO, P. J., JR., BROUN, G. O. and WYATT, J. P.: Am. J. Med., 1959, *27*, 18. (Asian influenzal pneumonitis.)

STEINER, P. E.: *Cancer: Race and Geography*, Baltimore, 1954. (Geographic distribution of bronchogenic carcinoma.) Arch. Path., 1944, *37*, 185. (Incidence of bronchogenic carcinoma.)

STONE, D. J., SCHWARTZ, M. J. and GREEN, R. A.: Am. J. Med., 1956, *21*, 211. (Pulmonary insufficiency due to irradiation.)

THOMAS, W. A., O'NEAL, R. M. and LEE, K. T.: Arch. Path., 1956, *62*, 56. (Multiple emboli and pulmonary hypertension.)

TOTTEN, R. S. *et al.:* Am. J. Med., 1958, *25*, 803. (Farmer's lung.)

WADDELL, W. R., SNIFFEN, R. C. and SWEET, R. H.: J. Thor. Surg., 1949, *18*, 707. (Cholesterol pneumonitis.)

WAGENVOORT, C. A.: J. Path. and Bact., 1959, *78*, 503. (Vascular lesions in pulmonary hypertension).

WALTON, C. H. A., PENNER, D. W., and WILT, J. C.: Canad. M. A. J., 1951, *64*, 95. (Sudden death from asthma.)

WEED, L. A.: Proc. Staff Meet. Mayo Clinic, 1956, *31*, 238. (Granulomatous lesions associated with saprophytic acid-fast bacilli.)

WELLER, C. V.: *Causal Factors in Cancer of the Lung*, Springfield, Ill., 1956.

WILLIAMS, E. D. and AZZOPARDI J. C.: Thorax, 1960, *15*, 30. (Carcinoid syndrome with metastatic bronchial adenoma.)

WOOD, W. B. *et al.:* J. Exper. Med., 1941, *73*, 201; 1946, *84*, 365. (Recovery in pneumococcal pneumonia.)

WYATT, J. P.: Am. Rev. Resp. Dis., 1959, *80*, 94. Also personal communication. (Emphysema.)

WYATT, J. P.: Arch. Indust. Health, 1960, *21*, 445. (Pneumoconiosis in soft coal miners.)

WYATT, J. P. and RIDDELL, A. C. P.: Am. J. Path., 1949, *25*, 447. (Bauxite fibrosis.)

WYATT, J. P. *et al.:* Am. J. Clin. Path., 1953, *23*, 353. (Cytomegalic inclusion pneumonitis.)

WYNDER, E. L. *et al.:* J.A.M.A., 1950, *143*, 329. Cancer Res., 1953, *13*, 855. (Relation of smoking to cancer of lung.)

Chapter 25

The Mouth, Neck and Esophagus

THE LIPS
Carcinoma
Syphilis
Angioma

THE MOUTH
Tonsillitis
Diphtheria
Vincent's Angina
Syphilis
Carcinoma

THE TONGUE
Inflammation
Syphilis
Carcinoma
Tuberculosis
Ulcers of the Tongue
Innocent Tumors

THE PHARYNX
Retropharyngeal Abscess
Tumors of the Pharynx
    EPIDERMOID CARCINOMA

TRANSITIONAL CELL CARCINOMA
AND LYMPHO-EPITHELIOMA
LYMPHOSARCOMA

THE NECK
Cysts
    THYROGLOSSAL CYST
    BRANCHIAL CYST
    CYSTIC LYMPHANGIOMA
Tumors
    LYMPHOBLASTOMA
    BRANCHIAL CLEFT CARCINOMA
    CAROTID BODY TUMOR
    TUMOR OF GLOMUS JUGULARIS
    SECONDARY CARCINOMA

THE SALIVARY GLANDS
Acute Inflammation
Tumors
    MIXED TUMORS
    CARCINOMA
    ADENOLYMPHOMA
    HEMANGIOMA
    Sjögren's Syndrome

Uveo-Parotid Fever
Salivary Calculi and Cysts

THE ESOPHAGUS
General Considerations
Inflammation
    ESOPHAGITIS
    PEPTIC ULCER
    SCLERODERMA
Cicatricial Stricture
Achalasia: Cardiospasm
Diverticula
Hiatus Hernia
Varices
Carcinoma
    OTHER TUMORS
Congenital Anomalies
    HETEROTOPIC GASTRIC MUCOS
Spontaneous Rupture
Relation of Symptoms to Lesions
    DYSPHAGIA
    HEMATEMESIS

THE LIPS

THE important lesions of the lips are cancer, primary syphilis, and angioma.

Carcinoma.—Cancer of the lip is one of the commonest forms of malignant disease. But it is only common in one sex (male) and in one lip (lower). It is quite rare in women and in the upper lip. The high incidence in the lower lip may be attributed to its being much more exposed to irritation (biting, action of actinic rays, etc.). The disease is commonly preceded by some lesion caused by chronic irritation such as fissures, abrasions due to jagged teeth, a patch of seborrhea or leukoplakia, etc. The prognosis is excellent, whether treated by surgical removal or radiotherapy.

The disease begins as a local thickening and induration. If growth is mainly toward the surface a warty nodule is formed which soon becomes ulcerated. If growth is deep the chief lesion is a deep-seated induration, and there may be no surface tumor or ulceration for a considerable time. When an ulcer does form it has the usual hard raised edge of a malignant sore.

Microscopically the tumor is an epidermoid carcinoma. Most of the cases belong to Grades 1 and 2, and a fair number to Grade 3, but I have never seen a case of Grade 4. It may be pointed out here that a convenient practical method of grouping the *tumors of the oral cavity* from the point of view of malignancy is as follows: (1) tumors from lips to teeth—mostly low grade; (2 tumors from teeth to back of tongue—increasing in malignancy as we pass back; (3 tumors of pharynx—high grade of malignancy.

SPREAD.—The spread, which is very slow in the lower grade tumors, is by lymphatics seldom by the blood stream. The malignant ulcer may destroy the lip, the skin of the chin, and finally involve the mandible. The submaxillary lymph nodes are involved from the lateral part of the lip, the submenta from the central part, but the corresponding salivary glands are seldom involved. The tumor cells may then spread to all the superior cervical lymph nodes, both superficial and deep, but as there is no direct connection between the lip and the inferior cervical and supraclavicular groups, these nodes are seldom involved until very late in the disease.

Syphilis.—A primary chancre of the lip may be on either lip, but is commonly on the upper. It is usually caused by kissing, but an infant may be infected through being suckled by a syphilitic wet-nurse. The lesion begins as a hard nodule which may ulcerate and develop into a typical chancre. There is the usual regional lymph node involvement, the submental and submaxillary nodes becoming enlarged and hard. When ulceration occurs spirochetes are readily demonstrated by the darkfield method.

Angioma.—These are not uncommon tumors in children and are probably congenital. Both hemangioma and lymphangioma occur and cause a characteristic diffuse enlargement of the lip. A hemangioma has a bluish color, but a lymphangioma is colorless.

THE MOUTH

Large monographs are devoted to the pathology of the mouth. These are intended for oral surgeons and dentists. The very brief consideration given to the subject here must not suggest that it is one of little importance. A short outline of dental pathology is given for the benefit of the *medical* student at the end of the book in Chapter 47.

Tonsillitis.—Acute tonsillitis may be follicular or parenchymatous. *Follicular* tonsillitis is so called because the inflammation is confined to the lymph follicles surrounding the crypts. The tonsils are large and red, and the surface is covered with yellow spots of pus which can be wiped away. The *parenchymatous* form or *quinsy* is a diffuse inflammation involving the whole tonsil and spreading to the surrounding tissues. Quinsy is characterized by suppuration, swelling of the peritonsillar tissue and deviation of the uvula to one side. The cervical lymph nodes are enlarged and tender, for they also are inflamed. The *microscopic* picture is one of diffuse suppuration.

Diphtheria.—The lesions of diphtheria are chiefly in the throat, on the tonsil, pharynx, and soft palate. The lesions are usually localized, taking the form of a gray patch of inflammatory exudate known as a false membrane, which is firmly adherent to the underlying tissue so that when it is removed it leaves a raw surface. *Microscopically* the gray patch is composed of fibrin threads and necrotic epithelium. The fibrin is interwoven with the necrotic cells, thus explaining the firmness with which the exudate is attached. Large numbers of diphtheria bacilli are present in the membrane.

Vincent's Angina.—This is a destructive lesion associated with the presence of two organisms, a long fusiform bacillus with pointed ends and a spirochete which stains faintly with ordinary aniline dyes. These Vincent organisms, as they may be called, are probably closely related. They are readily demonstrated in direct smears (not culture), where the spirochetes may form tangled masses. The lesion, which is usually on or near the tonsil, is at first necrotic, and when the slough has separated a large cavity may be left. Before adopting drastic local treatment of a necrotic gingivitis a leukocyte count should be done to exclude agranulocytic angina.

Syphilis.—*Secondary* lesions take the form of bilateral grayish-white patches (mucous patches) like the track of a snail, or superficial ulcers. These lesions may occur on the tonsils, soft palate, or buccal mucous membrane. *Tertiary* lesions are gummata which break down and leave deep, punched-out ulcers. This lesion is most often seen on the hard palate, where it causes perforation of the palate and regurgitation of food through the nose, but it may also occur on the tonsil and fauces.

Carcinoma.—Cancer of the mouth is similar to the much commoner cancer of the tongue and will be merely mentioned. It occurs in the lower rather than the upper oral cavity, chiefly on the floor of the mouth, the cheek and the mandible. The lesion is at first a localized thickening, but later becomes a deep excavated ulcer. *Leukoplakia* is a frequent precancerous lesion, often associated with a badly fitting dental plate. Also probably precancerous in character are degenerative mucous membrane changes found in the majority of mouth cancers.

These are usually the result of a combination of avitaminosis with various forms of chronic irritation, e. g., tobacco, syphilis, and sepsis. Lack of vitamin B is the most frequent deficiency, and probably the most important from the point of view of carcinogenesis. *Microscopically* oral cancer is an epidermoid carcinoma, but of high grade and much more serious than cancer of the lip.

THE TONGUE

Inflammation.—Glossitis or simple inflammation of the tongue may take the form of an acute diffuse inflammation or of ulcers. *Acute glossitis* is not a common condition. It may be caused by the sting of a bee, an infected wound, etc. There is rapid swelling of the tongue and suppuration, and the patient may be nearly choked before the pus is let out. *Simple ulcers* occur at the edge or tip of the tongue, and are often due to the irritation of a jagged tooth or badly-fitting plate. The ulcer is at first shallow and acute in type, but if the irritant is not removed it may become more chronic with indurated edges, and may eventually become malignant. Shallow painful ulcers, usually of short duration, often develop in the mouth and on the tongue as the result of constitutional disturbances. Some persons are particularly susceptible. The pathogenesis of these lesions is not clear; they are probably surface infections. The condition commonly called *chronic glossitis* is nearly always syphilitic, and will be described under that heading.

Syphilis.—A syphilitic lesion of the tongue may be primary, secondary or tertiary. A *primary chancre* presents the usual appearance of the hard sore. Spirochetes can be demonstrated by the dark-field. The induration of the lesion and the fact that lymph nodes in the floor of the mouth are enlarged and hard may easily lead to a mistaken diagnosis of carcinoma, a much commoner condition. The *secondary* lesions are mucous patches or shallow ulcers. They are swarming with spirochetes and are highly infectious. The *tertiary* lesions may take the form of an ulcer or a diffuse glossitis. A *syphilitic ulcer* is caused by the breaking down of a gumma and is usually situated on the dorsum of the tongue. It is liable to be mistaken for

carcinoma, but it seldom shows the same degree of induration and the regional lymph nodes are not enlarged. *Syphilitic glossitis* causes an epithelial proliferation with the formation of lozenge-shaped white patches (leukoplakia) often separated by painful cracks and fissures. As carcinoma is apt to develop in one of the deep cracks, the lesion can be regarded as a precancerous one. Sometimes there is diffuse fibrosis which causes great enlargement of the tongue (syphilitic macroglossia). The foregoing description applies to syphilis as it used to be seen when I was a student. Modern chemotherapy has abolished the more advanced of these lesions in a well treated case.

Carcinoma.—Cancer of the tongue shows the same strong sex incidence as cancer of the lip, being quite rare in women. It seldom develops in a healthy tongue, being preceded by such precancerous conditions as chronic ulceration and syphilitic glossitis (leukoplakia, cracks, etc.). When a patient with a chronic ulcer on the dorsum of the tongue is found to have a positive Wassermann reaction, the case should be regarded as malignant until proved otherwise by biopsy. The tongue is divided into two portions by the V-shaped line of circumvallate papillae, the anterior two-thirds and the posterior one-third. *Cancer of the anterior two-thirds* is epidermoid in type, usually of distinctly higher grade than cancer of the lip. The edge is the common site, but the tumors which develop on a syphilitic basis are often on the dorsum. Cancer of the posterior third is fortunately much rarer, for it is usually markedly malignant although at the same time markedly radiosensitive. It is likely to be a high-grade epidermoid or occasionally a transitional cell carcinoma. The *gross appearance* at first presents merely a local induration; this may develop into a warty mass with early ulceration, but often the tumor takes a form of a deep infiltration and ulceration may be late. The *malignant ulcer* is characteristically hard with raised, indurated, rounded edges. Extensive necrosis, sloughing, destruction, and secondary infection constitute the finish of the picture. The *microscopic appearance* has already been indicated, i.e., epidermoid or transitional cell (posterior third). *Spread* is rapid, so that it is of the first importance not to temporize with a suspicious ulcer or indurated patch on the tongue. Time should be measured here in days, whereas in a similar lesion of the lip it may be measured in weeks or even months. An immediate biopsy is imperative. The most important reasons for the rapid spread are: (1) the extremely rich lymphatic drainage of the tongue, (2) the constant muscular movements, and (3) the high grade of the tumor. Lymph spread takes place into the submental and submaxillary lymph nodes, into the superior and inferior deep cervical nodes, and even into the supraclavicular nodes. In tumors of the posterior third the upper deep cervical group on both sides of the neck may be involved. Blood spread to distant organs is comparatively rare.

TUBERCULOSIS.—For practical purposes tuberculosis of the tongue may be taken to be secondary to pulmonary tuberculosis. It is remarkable how uncommon a complication it is. The squamous epithelium evidently acts as an efficient protection against the countless tubercle bacilli which must pass over it in a case of active phthisis. The lesion usually commences as an ulcer near the tip of the tongue with sinuous undermined edges, pale watery-looking granulations, and an absence of the induration characteristic of malignant disease. Nevertheless the condition is frequently mistaken for carcinoma. Sometimes it begins as a nodule which ulcerates later (Fig. 408).

Ulcers of the Tongue.—It is evident that an ulcer of the tongue may be inflammatory (simple), malignant, syphilitic, or tuberculous. A *simple* ulcer occurs on the edge or tip, is shallow and inflamed, and is often associated with a sharp tooth or jagged plate. A *malignant* ulcer occurs on the edge or center, is peculiarly hard with raised edges, and may be associated with syphilitic glossitis and enlargement of the regional lymph nodes. A *syphilitic* ulcer occurs on the dorsum, is serpiginous in outline, and is usually a tertiary lesion. A *tuberculous* ulcer occurs at the tip, has undermined edges without induration, and is secondary to pulmonary tuberculosis.

Innocent Tumors.—*Angioma* forms a soft bluish mass in the tongue, and is usually congenital. *Lymphangioma* causes a diffuse congenital enlargement (macroglossia). *Dermoid cysts* may occur under the tongue. A

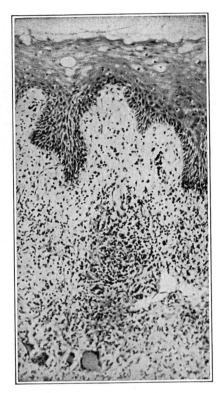

FIG. 408.—Tuberculosis of tongue not yet ulcerated. × 90.

thyroglossal cyst at the upper end of the thyroglossal duct may form a swelling at the base of the tongue.

THE PHARYNX

Many of the lesions of the pharynx have already been discussed in connection with the mouth, but one or two remain to be considered.

Retropharyngeal Abscess.—Pus may be formed as the result of suppuration in the loose tissue between the posterior wall of the pharynx and the vertebral column. It usually occurs in children suffering from some debilitating illness, and comes on acutely with rigidity of the neck, pain on swallowing, loss of voice, and a tense bulging on the posterior wall of the pharynx indicating the presence of pus. In tuberculosis of the cervical spine a chronic (cold) abscess may form in the same situation. *Ludwig's* *angina* is an acute diffuse streptococcal cellulitis involving the neck and tongue as well as the structures at the back of the throat. It usually occurs as a complication of the streptococcal fevers such as scarlet fever or erysipelas. There is a brawny induration of the neck with pressure on the trachea and edema of the glottis. The condition usually proves fatal in the course of a few days.

Tumors of the Pharynx.—A malignant tumor of the pharynx is likely to be an epidermoid carcinoma, transitional cell carcinoma, lympho-epithelioma or lymphosarcoma.

Epidermoid Carcinoma.—This may commence in the pharyngeal wall, the tonsil, or the soft palate. It produces a characteristic induration and soon ulcerates, leading to great destruction of the deeper tissues with secondary infection and a very foul breath. The lymph nodes at the angle of the jaw become enlarged and hard. Invasion of the jugular vein is a fairly common occurrence in epidermoid carcinoma of the head and neck with visceral metastases, especially in the liver. Nasopharyngeal carcinoma is the second commonest cancer in South-East Asia, especially amongst the Chinese. *Cancer of the hypopharynx* (postcricoid carcinoma) is confined almost exclusively to women. *This is the only malignant tumor of the alimentary canal which has this sex incidence.* It is often preceded over a number of years by a combination of dysphagia, dry atrophy of the pharyngeal mucosa, and hypochromic anemia (*Plummer-Vinson syndrome*). Both the anemia and the mucosal change have a dietetic iron-deficiency basis. The mucosal atrophy seems to act as a precancerous lesion. Adequate treatment of the anemia with iron may therefore prevent the onset of the cancer.

Transitional cell Carcinoma and Lympho-epithelioma.—There is difference of opinion as to whether these tumors are separate entities or are variants of the same lesion. The *gross character* and the *method of spread* is similar, so that they may be considered together. The tumor arises from epithelium covering lymphoid tissue, and originates in the nasopharynx, oropharynx and laryngopharynx (sinus pyriformis). Its *chief characteristic* is that the primary tumor, while still small and undetected, may give rise to *large secondary growths in the cervical lymph nodes on both sides.* The growth is centrifugal rather than centripetal. There is often invasion of the base of the skull with involvement of the cranial nerves, particularly the fifth and sixth. The growth may penetrate the cranial cavity. Secondary growths may occur in the lungs and liver at a later date. The tumor is markedly radiosensitive, and the mass in the neck may melt away for a time. *Microscopically* the transitional cell carcinoma is highly anaplastic, consisting of sheets of large pale cells showing numerous mitotic figures with no attempt at cornification. The lympho-epithelioma presents a similar picture, but in addition groups of lymphocytes are mingled with the epithelial cells, or they may be scattered more diffusely among these cells.

Lymphosarcoma.—This may arise in the tonsil or in the lymphoid tissue of the nasopharynx. The tonsillar cases are at first unilateral. The cervical and axillary lymph nodes are involved, and later the lymphoid tissue in the rest of the body. *Microscopically* the tumor may be of the lymphocytic or the reticuloendothelial type.

THE NECK

The neck is the most difficult region of the body about which to write in an orderly and organized manner. No classification of lesions can possibly give general satisfaction, and this is true not only for the reader but for the writer. It is, moreover, one of the most complex regions in the body. The esophagus, trachea, great veins and nerve trunks pass down it, the carotid arteries pass up it, while situated in it are the larynx, the thyroid and parathyroid glands, salivary glands and lymph nodes, in addition to such structures as the carotid body, sympathetic ganglia, etc.

The *severe inflammations* of the neck (Ludwig's angina and retropharyngeal abscess) have already been considered. Boils and carbuncles are common on the back of the neck owing to the friction of the collar.

Cysts.—A cyst of the neck may be mesial or lateral. The former is a thyroglossal cyst, the latter may be a branchial cyst or a cystic lymphangioma.

Thyroglossal Cyst.—The thyroglossal duct is a vestigial structure which passes from the foramen cecum at the base of the tongue to the isthmus of the thyroid gland. If a portion of the duct remains unclosed a cyst is formed lined by columnar epithelium. Such a cyst must always be in the middle line. It is usually below the hyoid bone, but occasionally is at the base of the tongue.

Branchial Cyst.—This is formed from an unclosed portion of a branchial cleft, usually the third, and is therefore at the level of the hyoid bone. If it arises from the second cleft it lies just below the mastoid process and projects into the mouth. The cyst is usually lined by columnar ciliated epithelium, but when quite superficial it is lined by stratified epithelium. The wall contains much lymphoid tissue. If the outer end of the cleft remains open the condition is a *branchial fistula*, which opens on the neck at the level of the angle of the jaw.

Cystic Lymphangioma.—The vessels of a lymphangioma may undergo marked dilatation so as to form a soft cystic swelling, usually in the anterior triangle of the neck, but sometimes in the axilla or on the chest wall. It is a congenital condition and is usually seen in children, tending to undergo spontaneous cure before adult life is reached. It is subject to recurring attacks of inflammation which probably play a part in the cure by closing the vessels. It is known clinically as *cystic hygroma* (fluid tumor), and may attain a very large size.

Tumors.—Tumors of the neck may be primary or secondary. Primary tumors may be accessory thyroid tissue (considered in connection with the thyroid gland), lymphoblastoma, branchial cleft carcinoma and carotid body tumor. Secondary tumors are examples of carcinoma. Salivary gland tumors are considered separately (see below).

Lymphoblastoma.—Enlargement of the cervical lymph nodes may be due to any member of the lymphoblastoma group, *i.e.*, lymphosarcoma, Hodgkin's disease, and lymphatic leukemia. The disease often commences in the cervical group involving first one and then both sides. Later the lymph nodes throughout the body become enlarged.

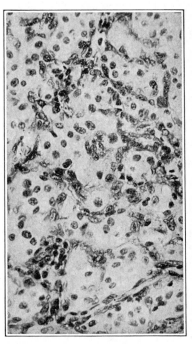

Fig. 409.—Carotid body tumor. × 275.

In leukemia the blood shows the characteristic leukemic change.

BRANCHIAL CLEFT CARCINOMA.—This rare tumor arises from remnants of branchial cleft epithelium. It is very much commoner in males than females. The tumor forms a very hard mass which starts deep in the neck near the bifurcation of the common carotid artery and infiltrates the surrounding tissue. The growth is a squamous cell carcinoma, but with little tendency to cornification or cell-nest formation.

CAROTID BODY TUMOR.—This is a firm, round, slowly-growing tumor in the bifurcation of the common carotid artery. Its firm and circumscribed character has earned for it the name of potato tumor. The tumor may grow around the artery, so that the vessel becomes embedded in the tumor. It may appear to be malignant, but the tumor does not infiltrate, and operation is inadvisable as the risk is so great. The cells, which are arranged in groups or sheets, are large, granular, and polyhedral, and may contain chromaffin substance (Fig. 409). The tumor is not a chromaffinoma as used to be thought, for the carotid body is not part of the chromaffin system.

TUMOR OF GLOMUS JUGULARIS.—Although this tumor arises in the vicinity of the middle ear rather than in the neck, it may be considered here because of its similarity to the carotid body tumor. The glomus jugularis or tympanic gland is a tiny structure analogous to the carotid body which lies along the tympanic branch of the glossopharyngeal nerve in its course either in the superior bulb of the jugular vein or in the bone canals of the middle ear. It resembles a ball of winding capillaries separated by a delicate stroma containing numerous epithelioid cells rich in cytoplasm. The tumor, which closely resembles the carotid body tumor, consists of these cells in alveolar arrangement with numerous sinusoidal vessels. It shows a strong tendency to recur on removal, but does not set up metastases. There is often a long history of throbbing and buzzing in the ear with slight loss of hearing.

Secondary Carcinoma.—Epidermoid carcinoma of the lip, tongue, mouth, larynx, and esophagus may metastasize to the cervical lymph nodes. The transitional cell type of carcinoma with a small often undiscovered primary growth in the pharynx or nasopharynx and large secondary tumors in the neck has already been described. Finally there may be lymphatic spread of carcinoma from more distant organs. Owing to the fact that the thoracic duct receives efferents from the supraclavicular and lower deep cervical nodes on the left side before it opens into the innominate vein, these nodes are often involved in abdominal and thoracic cancer. Gastric and bronchogenic carcinoma are the most frequent primary tumors responsible, but even the most distant tumors (ovarian, uterine, testicular) may metastasize to the neck by this route. Malignant supraclavicular nodes on the right side suggest cancer of the right lung (right lymphatic duct).

THE SALIVARY GLANDS

The salivary glands are divided into two groups, major and minor. The *major group* comprises the parotid, submaxillary and sublingual glands. Salivary gland tissue is also present in a number of other sites, such as the lips (usually the upper), gum, floor or mouth, hard and soft palate, tonsillar region, tongue and lacrimal gland. To this miscellaneous collection the term *minor salivary glands* is applied. The same lesions, inflammatory and neoplastic, which affect the major glands may also develop in the minor ones. These are rare, and the following discussion applies to the major glands and more particularly to the parotid.

The most important pathological conditions affecting the salivary glands are acute inflammation and tumors. The parotid is the common site of these disturbances, but the submaxillary and sublingual glands may on occasion be involved also.

Acute Inflammation.—This may be suppurative or non-suppurative. In *suppuration* the infection may be hematogenous as in acute fevers and pyemia. This is rare. Infection from the mouth by way of Stenson's duct is more common. The pus is prevented from reaching the surface by the dense fascia which covers the gland. It may form a retropharyngeal abscess.

The *non-suppurative* form is *mumps*, one of the commonest diseases of childhood. The gland on both sides is acutely inflamed, swollen, painful, and tender. There is little to be seen in the gland apart from a serous exudate. As there is no suppuration or necrosis, healing is by resolution and the gland is uninjured. A similar lesion is produced in monkeys by a filterable virus from the saliva of cases of mumps. Orchitis (inflammation of the testicle) is a common complication in the adult, but here recovery may not be complete and the testicle may undergo atrophy.

Tumors.—Tumors of the salivary glands form a large and confused subject because of the great histological diversification which they present. In many cases it is difficult to draw a line between the benign and malignant from the microscopic picture, so that no classification will be made on that basis. For further information on this difficult subject the reader has an abundance of articles to consult. Among the most noteworthy of these are those by Foote and Frazell, analyzing nearly 900 cases from the Memorial Hospital, New York, and Kirklin and his associates with an analysis of 717 cases from the Mayo Clinic. The three principal groups are: (1) so-called mixed tumors, (2) carcinoma with its various subgroups, and (3) adenolymphoma.

MIXED TUMORS.—This is the condition commonly called *parotid gland tumor* but,

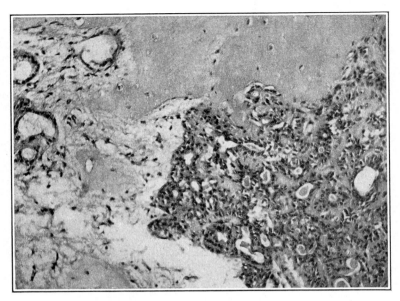

Fig. 410.—Mixed tumor of the parotid. Cartilage above, glandular tissue
to the right, mucoid tissue to the left. × 160.

as it may occasionally occur in any of the salivary glands, in the mucous membrane of the mouth, and in the palate, this name is undesirable and misleading. It is a fairly common slowly-growing tumor of early adult and middle life which begins either in the substance or the surface of the salivary gland and may continue to increase in size for many years, but at any time growth may stop. It is inherently benign, but after the usual operative procedure (enucleation of the tumor) there is recurrence in from 20 to 45 per cent of cases, the tumor then becoming locally destructive and invasive. Total excision of the gland with removal of the capsule gives infinitely better results. Sometimes after growing slowly for many years it may take on rapid growth and invade the surrounding tissue. The lymph nodes are rarely involved unless the tumor has been interfered with. It is usually encapsulated, but may not be.

The *microscopic appearance* is varied and perplexing, for the tumor appears to consist of both ectodermal and mesodermal elements. It is for this reason that it is called a mixed tumor. The following elements are commonly present in one or other part of the tumor, although it is very difficult to find them all combined in a single microscopic field (Fig. 410): (1) masses of epithelial cells often showing a glandular arrangement, (2) mucoid connective tissue with evidence of production of mucin, (3) cartilage, and (4) lymphoid tissue. The cartilage has been the chief stumbling block, as it seemed to be mesodermal in origin, while the epithelium was of ectodermal origin.

The *nature of the tumor* has long been a subject for discussion. It is possible that some of the tumors may arise as the result of the accidental sequestration of embryonal cells during the early and complicated development of the face; such tumors would be true "mixed tumors." It appears probable, however, that *the great majority are not really mixed tumors*, but are benign epithelial growths of the salivary glands in which there is an exaggerated latent potentiality of differentiation. In other words, they are *pleomorphic adenomas*. The difficulty presented by the cartilage is removed by the discovery that this material is not true cartilage. The tumor epithelial cells produce mucin, and this constitutes the origin of the mucinous "connective tissue." This myxomatous material, which stains well with muci-carmine, is homogenous like cartilage, and the cells which it contains may lie free in small spaces around which there may be a fibrillar condensation, so that a pseudo-cartilage may be produced. By means of histochemical methods and observing the action of hyaluronidase on the metachromasia of the mucin, it is possible to distinguish between two groups of mucins: (1) normal-appearing mucin (epithelial) with metachromasia unaltered by hyaluronidase, and (2) myxo-chondroid material similar to connective tissue mucin, markedly reduced by hyaluronidase (Azzopardi and Smith). It has been suggested that epithelial cells produce the ordinary mucin, whereas myo-epithelial cells produce the mucin of the myxochondroid areas (Lennox et al.). The latter mucins are of connective tissue type, being rich in acid mucopolysaccharides. Proliferating cells seem to be capable of inducing changes in adjacent tissues, so that metaplasia of the stroma of these tumors may give rise to true cartilage, bone, fat and lymphoid tissue. In studying these tumors one must separate sharply the neoplastic components which comprise the parenchyma from the metaplastic ones which are derived from the stroma (Morehead and Klein). Simard has reported a sweat gland adenoma of the palm with a structure identical with that of mixed tumor of the parotid. In this case the mucous secretion of the epithelial cells had undergone metaplasia into cartilage. Hellwig suggests that the tumor may be derived from misplaced elements of the notochord which resemble it in structure. The notochord comes into intimate relationship with the developing parotid and submaxillary glands and the palate, the three common sites of mixed tumors. One explanation may not fit all the cases.

CARCINOMA.—Carcinoma of the salivary glands varies greatly in its appearance and prognosis. In the previous edition of this book it was stated that this tumor "grows rapidly, infiltrates the whole gland, involves the regional lymph nodes, and sets up distant metastases." It may do so, but often it does not. An adenocarcinoma was removed from my own parotid gland in 1947, and then treated with implantation of radium, with highly satisfactory results so far.

Adenoid cystic carcinoma is a circumscribed

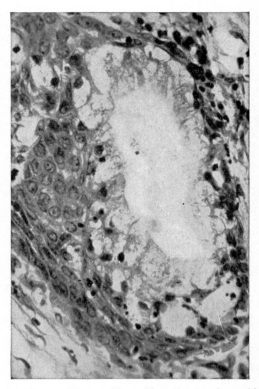

FIG. 411.—Muco-epidermoid carcinoma of parotid gland. × 375. (Boyd, *Pathology for the Surgeon*, courtesy of W. B. Saunders Co.)

but poorly encapsulated infiltrating tumor. It consists of anastomosing cords of small dark cells which are arranged around tubules or in a "Swiss cheese" pattern of rounded holes which is highly characteristic of the condition. These spaces may be empty or may be filled with mucin. Between the cords there may be similar acellular areas which may contain mucin. The tumor is believed to arise from the ducts, and is unique in being as common in the submaxillary as in the parotid gland. It is of slow growth and masquerades for a time as a mixed tumor. The growth, however, is relentless as well as slow, and local recurrence or lymph node involvement may occur over a period of many years.

Muco-epidermoid tumors constitute quite a large group, but they are usually unrecognized, although they were described by Masson and Berger in 1924 as tumors with "double metaplasia." Stewart, Foote and

Becker, who drew attention to the lesion (1945), originally described two groups, the one benign and the other malignant. They now consider them all to be malignant, one group of low, the other of high malignancy, the two groups being of equal size. In the gross the low group are poorly encapsulated and are often partly or mainly cystic, while the high are infiltrating. *Microscopically* the tumors consist of mucus-secreting cells with an admixture of cells of epidermoid character, together with some cells described as being intermediate in character (Fig. 411). In the low-grade tumors the mucoid and epidermoid cells are prominent, so that the lesion is taken for a mixed tumor. In the high-grade tumors the mucus-secreting cells are replaced by the epidermoid and intermediate types, and lymph node metastases are common. The prognosis is excellent in the low grade group, but poor in the high grade. I must have been fortunate in having a tumor of low grade.

Undifferentiated carcinoma need not be described in detail. The histological structure and the biological behavior are both implicit in the word "undifferentiated."

ADENOLYMPHOMA.—This uncommon tumor of the salivary glands occurs only in the parotid, usually in the fifth and sixth decades. It is benign, slowly growing, well encapsulated, and much commoner in males than females. The microscopic picture is characteristic: tubular alveoli lined by tall columnar epithelium supported by an abundant lymphoid stroma with active germ centers. (Fig. 412). There may be cystic spaces with papillary projections. The papillary projections may be so pronounced as to justify the high-sounding name of papillary cystadenoma lymphomatosum originally given to the lesion by Warthin. A characteristic feature is the *eosinophilic staining of the epithelium* which may be very marked. The tumor has been called an *onkocytoma,* because of the suggestion that it may arise from a special type of cell found in the parotid with advancing years characterized by its size (*onkos,* bulk), and known as an onkocyte. These cells are merely acidophilic granular cells which arise from the ducts and acini (Meza-Chávez), so that the term onkocytoma has become meaningless and should be dropped.

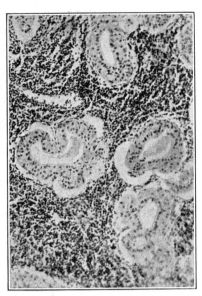

FIG. 412.—Adenolymphoma of parotid gland. × 100.

The *histogenesis* of adenolymphoma, with its curious combination of lymphoid and glandular tissue has long been a puzzle. It would now appear that it is derived from salivary tissue inclusions in lymph nodes, which themselves are often found in the parotid but not the submaxillary gland, *i.e.,* the distribution of the adenolymphoma. (Thompson and Bryant). It is of interest to note that these inclusions, which are in the nature of hamartomas, were reported by Neisse in 1898 as occurring in the parotid of the newborn. In spite of this suggested origin, the tumors are rare in childhood, the usual period being the fifth and sixth decades.

HEMANGIOMA.—This is a lesion of infancy. At least 90 per cent of parotid tumors before the age of one year are hemangiomas, either capillary or cavernous. These tumors are always benign.

SJÖGREN'S SYNDROME.—This rare condition is characterized by widespread degenerative and atrophic changes in the conjunctival, lacrymal and salivary glands, as well as in the submucous glands of the respiratory and upper alimentary tract, together with secondary changes in the associated mucosae. Rheumatoid arthritis is present in about two-thirds of the cases. It is in essence a *female disease,* from 85 to 95 per cent of the cases being in women. From the organs involved it will be realized that the serious and distressing symptoms are excessive dryness of the eyes with conjunctivitis, and of the mouth, nose and throat, with intermittent swelling of the salivary and lacrymal glands. *Microscopically* there is degeneration and atrophy of the parenchyma of the glands involved, together with a heavy cellular infiltration of lymphocytes, as well as some plasma cells and occasional eosinophils (Cardell and Gurling). The nature and cause of the condition is an enigma, but the fact that the lesions recall the early stage of Hashimoto's disease of the thyroid, the frequent association with rheumatoid arthritis, and the occurrence of polyarteritis nodosa in 2 of the 10 reported autopsies suggest the strong possibility of an auto-immune mechanism. It must be understood that only a few of the numerous lesions mentioned above may be present in a given case.

Mikulicz's disease is also marked by enlargement of one or more salivary and lacrymal glands. Often only one salivary and no lacrymal glands are involved. As Morgan and Castleman point out, the normal parenchyma of the glands is replaced not only by lymphoid tissue but also by the intraductal proliferation of cells with the formation of islands in which both epithelial and more peripheral myoepithelial elements can be distinguished. Mikulicz's disease is believed not to be a distinct entity, but merely one manifestation of the more generalized symptom-complex of Sjögren's syndrome (Morgan and Castleman). The salivary and lacrymal glands may also be enlarged in the course of leukemia or lymphosarcoma, a condition to which the rather misleading name of *Mikulicz's syndrome* is applied. In such a case the microscopic picture will be one of lymphosarcoma.

Uveo-parotid Fever.—This is a clinical syndrome characterized by chronic inflammation of the uveal tract (iris, ciliary body, choroid) and both parotids. The parotids are swollen, and the occasional enlargement of both lacrymal glands may lead to a mistaken diagnosis of Mikulicz's disease. Irido-cyclitis and facial paralysis are common. The course is generally febrile, but there is a marked tendency to spontaneous recovery. The condition used to be regarded as a low grade form of tuberculosis, but it is now believed to be a variety of sarcoidosis.

Salivary Calculi and Cysts.—A *salivary calculus* usually forms in Stenson's duct, and the saliva collects above the obstruction during a meal, causing a cystic swelling of the parotid which gradually subsides after the meal. A *ranula* is a cyst of the sublingual gland, and is therefore situated in the floor of the mouth under the tongue, where it forms a bluish nodule. Occasionally the submaxillary gland is involved.

THE ESOPHAGUS

General Considerations.—"When one considers how important eating is, one wonders why so little attention has been paid to the organ by which food is conveyed to the stomach. Even if we don't live to eat, as many people seem to, we must eat to live; hence the great importance of the esophagus." This is the opening statement of the monograph of Benedict and Nardi on the esophagus. It may be added that dysphagia or discomfort on swallowing, which is the commonest symptom of esophageal disease, interferes with the enjoyment of life more than is commonly realized. The importance of the subject has been greatly increased by the more widespread use of endoscopy, by means of which lesions can be visualized.

The esophagus is a soft muscular tube, about 10 inches in length, which extends from the lower border of the cricoid cartilage to the hiatus in the diaphragm. The muscle of the upper third is striated, the lower two-thirds are non-striated. The tube is narrowed at three points: (1) its origin, (2) the level of the aortic arch, (3) the point at which it passes through the diaphragm. The importance of these constrictions is that these are the places liable to perforation by foreign bodies. The esophagus lacks a serous coat, a fact which probably facilitates the spread of infection. The mucosa consists of a thick layer of stratified squamous epithelium, so that the carcinoma which so often arises from it is epidermoid in type, but the submucosa contains many mucous glands from which adenocarcinoma may develop. The venous drainage demands mention because of the importance of esophageal varices. The veins from the upper third of the esophagus drain into the subclavian veins, those from the middle third into the azygous veins, but those from the lower third by way of the coronary, left gastric and splenic veins into the portal vein. A communication is thus established between the portal and systemic circulations, so that in portal hypertension the lower esophageal veins tend to develop varices.

The only function of the esophagus is swallowing. From the physiological point of view the esophagus is a muscular tube closed at both ends by sphincters, the tube and its sphincters operating as one functional unit. Radiographic studies show that a pressure "barrier" exists between the stomach and the upper esophagus. This barrier, which plays the part of functional if not anatomical sphincter, ceases to exist in cases of esophageal reflux which have a neurogenic basis. Many persons have mucosal folds which, when drawn together, act as a cork to close the top of the stomach (Botha). These folds are not valvular, but are thrown up longitudinally by contractions of the muscularis mucosae. Swallowing is a function which in the beginning is voluntary, and then involuntary. It is dependent on peristalsis, but not in the case of fluids and semisolids. The average time occupied is five seconds, when the cardiac sphincter relaxes, allowing passage of food into the stomach. Then the sphincter quickly closes and prevents regurgitation. Reverse peristalsis results in belching, regurgitation and vomiting. In nervous persons there may be air-swallowing (*aerophagia*). Sometimes the air is stored in the esophagus between the closed pharyngeal and cardiac sphincters, with marked dilatation of the lumen.

Inflammation.—When we consider the number of irritants, both fluid and solid, both very hot and very cold, which we pour down the esophagus, it is remarkable that inflammation is not more frequent and more serious. The resulting lesions may be (1) diffuse in distribution and nonspecific in type, the condition known as esophagitis; (2) limited, sharply defined ulcers; (3) part of the systemic collagen disease, scleroderma.

ESOPHAGITIS.—As might be expected, a large variety of irritants may cause a nonspecific esophagitis. Of these the most important are: (1) corrosive fluids swallowed with suicidal intent by adults or accidentally by children; and (2) regurgitation of acid gastric juice in cases of persistent vomiting, especially after surgical operations. Excessive ingestion of alcohol or very hot foods may break down the resistance of the esophageal stratified squamous epithelium.

Other causes which will occur to the reader are general bacterial infections, spread of inflammation from the mediastinum, etc.

Routine microscopic examination of the esophagus at postmortem in a series of cases reveals the surprising fact that inflammatory lesions of the esophagus are much commoner in hospital patients than has been suspected, being present in 36 per cent of one series (Lodge). This may be attributed to long confinement to bed with the gravitational effects of recumbency. Even more surprising was the evidence of inflammation in 8 per cent of 100 cases of sudden death.

The *lesions* may be mild or severe, acute or chronic. The mucosa is red from congestion and swollen from edema. In the severe cases there may be areas of necrosis and ulcer formation. The acute lesions may become chronic when the irritation is frequently repeated. The result most to be feared is fibrosis with stenosis, which may become so extreme that food can no longer be swallowed. This complication is most to be feared in the cases of severe inflammation caused by the ingestion of corrosive poisons.

In milder and more chronic cases the common symptom is a sensation of burning substernal pain or heartburn. This is likely to develop as the result of repeated regurgitation of acid gastric juice into the lower end of the esophagus. Postoperative hematemesis may be attributed to inflammatory lesions produced in this manner.

PEPTIC ULCER.—A chronic solitary ulcer in the lower third of the esophagus may be regarded as similar in nature to the very much more common ulcers of the stomach and duodenum which are classed as peptic ulcers, being produced by digestion. Occasionally the ulcer occurs in the middle or upper third. For some reason it is 5 times more common in men than in women.

The most likely *cause* appears to be regurgitation of acid peptic secretions into the lower part of the esophagus. The ulcer may be related to heterotopic islands of gastric mucosa. In these cases the ulcer may be due to digestion of the surface produced by acid juice from the heterotopic gastric mucosa. This is particularly true of ulcers in the middle and upper thirds. The ulcer occurs not in the acid-producing island, but in the adjoining mucosa. The same is true, of gastric ulcer, as we shall see in the next chapter.

The ulcer is sharply circumscribed and similar in character to gastric and duodenal ulcers. Occasionally it may perforate the wall. If it opens into a blood vessel there will be severe bleeding. Long-continued ulceration may result in fibrosis and stenosis.

From what has been said about the lesions it is natural that the main *symptoms* are substernal pain and heartburn, difficulty in swallowing (dysphagia), vomiting, and occasionally hematemesis.

SCLERODERMA.—Scleroderma is a member of the group of so-called diffuse collagen diseases, which have been touched on in Chapter 4. The most striking feature of scleroderma, as its name implies, is a diffuse induration of the skin due to sclerosis of the connective tissue, so that it is considered in detail in connection with diseases of the skin. It is, however, a diffuse disease, and if a patient with the cutaneous manifestations of scleroderma develops dysphagia and substernal pain it is safe to conclude that the esophagus has become involved, and the prognosis is correspondingly more grave.

The *lesions* involve the submucosa and later the muscular coat, with secondary atrophy of the mucosa. The submucosa is indurated, thickened, and markedly fibrosed, and the muscularis is also fibrosed with atrophy of the muscle fibers. The end result is extreme rigidity and narrowing of the esophagus. There is loss of tone of the gastro-esophageal sphincter, allowing regurgitation of gastric contents, and also loss of contractile power in the lower two-thirds of the esophagus, which becomes unable to expell the foreign contents. Little wonder that the unfortunate sufferer is afflicted with dysphagia, heartburn and retrosternal pain, as well as induration and stiffening of the skin.

Cicatricial Stricture.—Organic stenosis is caused by scar formation due to the swallowing of corrosive or boiling fluids, and more rarely to laceration produced by impacted foreign bodies. Fibrous tissue is produced as the result of the injury usually at the upper or lower ends, and this becomes dense scar tissue which encircles the esophagus and causes an extreme degree of stenosis, which it may be very difficult to dilate. Cortisone and prednisone seem to be effective in preventing the stenosis caused by swallowing lye. The esophagus may be narrowed owing to pressure from without by an aneurysm of the aorta, a tumor of the lung, or a mass of enlarged lymph nodes.

Achalasia: Cardiospasm.—This can be regarded as a functional as opposed to an organic obstruction to the passage of food from the esophagus into the stomach. The term cardiospasm suggests a tonic contraction of the esophagus at its junction with the cardiac end of the stomach. Achalasia, on the other hand, indicates an inability of the sphincter to relax which is a truer concept.

Achalasia ranks next to carcinoma in being the commonest cause of esophageal obstruction. It may occur at any age, but it is commonest in the middle years, although it may develop for the first time in old age. It is in essence a disorder of the neuromuscular mechanism of the esophageal wall associated with degeneration or absence of the ganglionic cells of Auerbach's plexus. The patient is unable to initiate the peristaltic wave which is the key that opens the door to the stomach, *i. e.* the cardia. The patient can swallow, but the food is unable to enter the stomach. He can empty the esophagus by regurgitation, and "nocturnal overflowing" is a troublesome feature.

In distinction to what is found in organic stricture, there is a remarkable dilatation of the esophagus above the site of the obstruction (esophagectasia) with hypertrophy of the circular coat of muscle (Fig. 413). The esophagus may be lengthened as well as greatly dilated. The stretched mucous membrane may show secondary inflammatory changes. In the x-ray picture the lower end of the esophagus (filled with barium) has a characteristic conical or pointed appearance, quite different from what is seen in organic stricture.

The exact *nature of the condition* is still a matter of uncertainty. During life there appears to be distinct narrowing of the esophagus at the point where it passes through the diaphragm, but there is no thickening of the wall nor dilatation of the lumen at this point. The modern view is that the condition is due to some disturbance of the neuro-muscular mechanism of deglutition, an imbalance between the vagus (motor) and sympathetic (inhibitory) nerves. The name cardiospasm suggests that spasm due to overaction of the vagus is the essential factor, but it appears more probable the condition is an achalasia, an inability of the circular muscle to relax, due to preponderance of sympathetic control. Degenerative lesions in Auerbach's nerve plexus in the wall of the esophagus have been described. This finding is of interest in view of the fact that similar changes are present in the rectum in Hirschsprung's disease.

Other possible examples of achalasia are Hirschsprung's disease (inability of the rectal sphincter to relax), esophageal (pharyngeal) diverticulum, and the so-called *Plummer-Vinson syndrome*. In the latter condition there is *dysphagia with anemia* usually occurring in middle-aged women but sometimes in men. In this case there is failure of the cricopharyngeous sphincter between the pharynx and esophagus to relax during deglutition. The mucosa of the pharynx and tongue becomes very dry. The anemia may be due to the long-continued condition of semi-starvation. The great practical importance of the achalasias at either end of the esophagus is that they may be mistaken for malignant stricture.

Diverticula.—A diverticulum of the esophagus may be of the anterior or posterior variety. The *posterior* variety is much the commoner. It is really a pharyngeal rather than an esophageal diverticulum, occurring in the pharyngeal wall at its junction with the esophagus. It is usually found in men of middle age. The chief cause is probably prolonged intrapharyngeal pressure due to failure of what Chevalier Jackson calls the "cricopharyngeal pinchcock" to relax during swallowing. The mucous membrane of the lower part of the posterior wall of the pharynx becomes protruded between the oblique and transverse fibers of the cricopharyngeus muscle, so that a sac is formed behind the esophagus which pushes that structure forward. The condition tends to become steadily worse through the accumulation of food in the sac, and pressure on the eso-

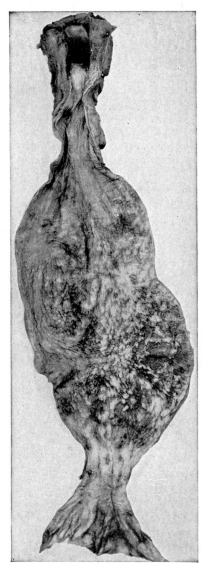

Fig. 413.—Dilatation of esophagus due to cardiospasm. (Boyd, *Pathology for the Surgeon*, courtesy of W. B. Saunders Co.)

phagus may cause difficulty in swallowing. The *anterior* variety occurs at the level of the bifurcation of the trachea, and is due to traction of tuberculous tracheobronchial lymph nodes which have become adherent to the esophagus. The posterior form is thus a pulsion diverticulum, the anterior form a traction diverticulum.

Hiatus Hernia.—This term signifies displacement of the cardiac end of the stomach and the distal portion of the esophagus, which is normally below the diaphragm, through the esophageal hiatus into the thorax. It is a common condition, and although it may be asymptomatic it is a frequent cause of discomfort and distress. It may occur at any age, but is most likely to be encountered in the fifth and sixth decades.

Three types of hiatus hernia must be distinguished, because they are quite distinct from one another. They are known as: (1) True hiatal or sliding, (2) parahiatal or rolling, and (3) short esophagus with thoracic stomach.

True hiatal or sliding hernia.—This is the common form and the one likely to need surgical treatment. The cardia of the stomach passes into the thorax through an enlarged esophageal hiatus. The esophagus may be of normal length, or it may be shortened owing to cicatricial contracture secondary to esophagitis with ulceration.

Parahiatal or rolling hernia is a condition in which the hiatus remains of normal size, the cardia remains in normal position, but a hernial opening develops at the site of the hiatus, and as this becomes larger a portion of the stomach rolls through it into the thorax and assumes an inverted position, the so-called "upsidedown stomach."

The short esophagus with thoracic stomach represents a secondary shortening due to esophagitis induced by reflux of gastric contents, so that the cardia is drawn through the hiatus into the thorax. In the occasional case the shortening appears to be congenital rather than acquired.

The *symptoms* depend on the type of the hernia rather than on its size. In the *sliding hernia* the symptoms are esophageal in origin. The upward displacement of the esophagogastric junction interferes with the valvular mechanism and allows regurgitation of gastric contents into the esophagus. This results in retrosternal pain and dysphagia. In *parahiatal hernia* there is no esophagitis, the symptoms being caused by the presence of the stomach in the hernial sac. Postprandial fullness, shortness of breath, and acute bouts of epigastric pain are the principal complaints. In *short eso-* *phagus with thoracic stomach* vomiting is frequent, and there may be symptoms of reflux esophagitis. Both in the hiatal and parahiatal forms there may be hematemesis and melena, due to bleeding from the esophagus or the inflamed and ulcerated segment of stomach trapped in the hernia. The bleeding may result in a marked degree of secondary anemia. There is a frequent curious association of hiatus hernia with cholecystitis and diverticulosis coli, a group known as *Saint's triad.*

Varices.—Esophageal varices are dilated tortuous veins in the wall of the esophagus. They constitute one of most important forms of esophageal lesion because of the danger of hemorrhage, frequently fatal. Apart from the bleeding they cause no symptoms, so that their presence may go unsuspected. They are invariably the result of portal hypertension, the blood flow through the coronary veins being reversed, with the portal blood draining through the esophageal veins into the systemic circulation. In the vast majority of cases the cause of the portal hypertension is cirrhosis of the liver, and the subject of esophageal varices is discussed in relation to that subject. These varices can be seen in the *x*-ray film in over 90 per cent of cases, although at autopsy they are much more difficult to visualize, because the varices collapse when the veins are divided. If adequate precautions are taken, however, they present a striking appearance (Fig. 414). Other rare causes are pressure on the portal vein by a malignant tumor, portal vein thrombosis, etc. The dilated and tortuous veins run in the mucosa in a longitudinal direction, and are most marked in the lower third of the esophagus.

As in the case of the similar varices of the hemorrhoidal veins of the rectum (hemorrhoids, piles), the great danger is rupture with massive hemorrhage, which may well prove fatal. This complication occurs in from 10 to 20 per cent of cases of cirrhosis of the liver.

Modern surgery has made such advances in the treatment of portal hypertension that it has become important to diagnose esophageal varices before they can present a threat to life. In cases of cirrhosis of the liver the two most valuable methods are

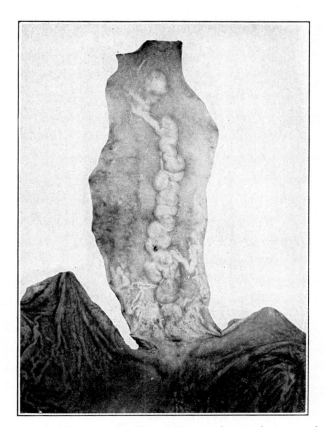

Fig. 414.—Esophageal varicosities which caused severe hematemesis.

roentgenography and esophagoscopy. Careful barium *x-ray studies* will usually show multiple filling defects produced by the varicosities (Fig. 415). During the phase of acute bleeding the veins collapse and may not be visible in the x-ray film, nor may they be seen in the early phase of portal hypertension. *Esophagoscopy* is of even greater value, especially in early cases. In a well-developed case the longitudinal bluish tortuous masses of veins may appear to fill the lumen and present a most striking and characteristic picture.

Carcinoma.—Carcinoma is naturally the most important and serious lesion of the esophagus. Unfortunately it is also a common one, ranking next in frequency to esophagitis and achalasia. Occasionally it apparently develops as a complication of a chronic lesion of many years duration. The tumor shows the usual sex incidence of alimentary canal neoplasms, over 80 per cent being in men. *Cancer of the hypopharynx (postcricoid cancer)* is sometimes included with cancer of the upper end of the esophagus; indeed it is often impossible to determine in which region the tumor originated. When this is done the sex incidence of upper end tumors is overwhelmingly female. The commonest site is the middle where the esophagus is crossed and constricted by the left bronchus, followed rather closely by the lower end. The middle, which is the narrowest part, and the lower end are the regions where irritants (food and drink) are delayed longest. The least common site is the upper end, but if cancer of the hypopharynx is included, the incidence practically equals that of the lower end. The tumor begins as a nodule in the mucous membrane, and sometimes grows into the lumen as a bulky mass, but usually takes the form of a diffuse in-

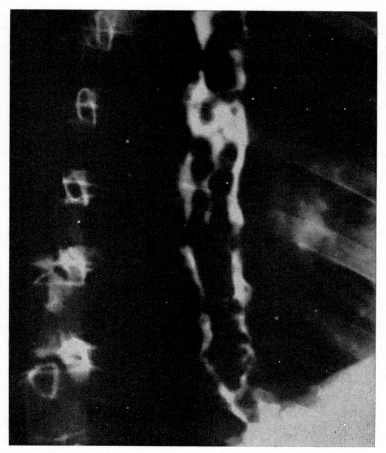

Fig. 415.—X-ray appearance of esophageal varices in a patient with cirrhosis of the liver who had severe rectal bleeding, with tarry stools and anemia. (Benedict, *The Esophagus*, courtesy of Little, Brown & Co.

filtration which showly encircles the esophagus and causes marked narrowing of the lumen with dilatation of the proximal part of the tube. (Fig. 416). Ulceration of the surface occurs sooner or later, and the growth may ulcerate into the trachea, into the aorta with fatal hemorrhage, or into the mediastinal tissues with gangrenous inflammation. The stenosis gives rise to marked difficulty in swallowing. The prognosis used to be hopeless, but modern surgery can remove the diseased esophagus and provide the patient with a new one. The earliest diagnosis can be made with the aid of the esophagoscope. *Microscopically* the tumor is an epidermoid carcinoma, but usually without epithelial pearls or much cornification. Occasionally it may be an adeno-

carcinoma, which probably arises from anomalous glands in the wall of the esophagus identical with the gastric glands.

Spread, as is usual in epidermoid carcinoma, is to the regional lymph nodes. These may be mediastinal, cervical, or abdominal. If the cancer is at the upper end of the esophagus, the cervical as well as the mediastinal glands will be involved; a tumor in the middle of the esophagus will spread to the mediastinal glands; with tumors of the lower end, metastases are formed below the diaphragm in the coelic chain of glands and in the liver.

The *symptoms* are due to stenosis. Unfortunately in the early stages the patient with cancer of the esophagus is completely free from symptoms, and even in the late

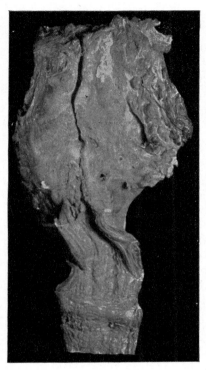

FIG. 416.—Carcinoma of esophagus with extreme stenosis. (Boyd, *Pathology for the Surgeon*, courtesy of W. B. Saunders Co.)

stages some 20 per cent of cases do not develop stenosis. The earliest and most frequent complaint is dysphagia. Other symptoms of stenosis are pain, regurgitation and vomiting, but 50 per cent of patients have no pain. Loss of weight is a common but not an early symptom.

OTHER TUMORS.—Both benign and malignant tumors are rare. The most frequent of the *benign tumors* is the *leiomyoma*, which forms a well-defined mass which encroaches on the lumen and may ulcerate the mucosa. In the lower third it may encircle and constrict the esophagus. Neurofibroma, fibroma and lipoma have been reported. The lipoma may hang by a pedicle in the lumen. *Malignant tumors*, apart from carcinoma, are rarities and need only be mentioned. Leiomyosarcoma rhabdomyosarcoma (in the upper part) and lymphosarcoma, may occur. For a beautifully illustrated account of tumors of the esophagus, both benign and malignant, the reader should consult the monograph on the subject by Stout and Lattes.

Congenital Anomalies.—Several congenital defects of the esophagus can now be treated by the surgeon. *Atresia with tracheo-esophageal fistula* is the commonest anomaly. It is easy to understand how the condition might occur. In the early stage of development there is no tubular communication between pharynx and the stomach. When the trachea and esophagus develop they have a common lumen at first, which later becomes divided by a septum. If part of the septum fails to develop, a fistulous communication between the two tubes will result. Part or the whole of the esophagus may be so narrowed that it is little more than a fibrous cord. Usually there is atresia with the fistula formation at the level of the bifurcation of the trachea. *Congenital shortness* of the esophagus is naturally accompanied by hiatus herniation of the stomach. Such persons are liable to suffer from esophagitis in the segment of esophagus just above the cardia due to regurgitation of hydrochloric acid. In this way a typical *peptic ulcer* will often develop in the lower third of the esophagus with eventual cicatrization and stenosis. *Webs* are thin membranes which project into the lumen, usually in the upper third. They may cause some difficulty in swallowing. Sometimes these webs are associated with the Plummer-Vinson syndrome, *i.e.* dysphagia with hypochromic anemia, to which reference has already been made (page 715).

HETEROTOPIC GASTRIC MUCOSA.—This might well be regarded as a congenital anomaly, and it also may occasionally be the cause of peptic ulceration. The heterotopic mucosa may occur anywhere in the esophagus, but is said to be most common in the postcricoid region (Rector). It is least frequent in the lower third, but it is in this region that peptic ulceration of the esophagus develops. The islands of mucosa are sharply delimited from the normal stratified epithelium.

Spontaneous Rupture.—Rupture of the esophagus may be traumatic as a result of the passage of a bougie or esophagoscope, or it may be spontaneous. Spontaneous rupture is a rare condition which occurs after prolonged vomiting, and is probably due to an acute esophagitis at the lower end of the tube produced by regurgitation of gastric juice. I have seen a case in which rupture occurred shortly after drinking home-made wine after a prolonged fast during a hunting trip. The pain is sudden and intense due to acute mediastinitis. The left pleural cavity is filled with dirty fluid, and the condition is rapidly fatal. In addition to complete rupture there may be lacerations of the mucosa associated with profuse bleeding and massive hematemesis (*Mallory-Weiss syndrome*). They take the form of longitudinal tears at the lower end of the esophagus, usually confined to the mucosa but occasionally penetrating more deeply. These lesions are most commonly found in chronic alcoholics who suffer severe bouts of vomiting which result in splitting of the mucosa. It is evident that the hematemesis may be confused with that caused by esophageal varices associated with alcoholic cirrhosis of the liver.

Relation of Symptoms to Lesions.—In the discussion of the various forms of esophageal disease two symptoms have received repeated mention, namely dysphagia and hematemesis. The significance of these to the clinician is rather different, for dysphagia points to the esophagus, whereas hematemesis is more likely to be due to a gastric lesion.

DYSPHAGIA.—Dysphagia, which means discomfort in swallowing, is due to esophageal obstruction. This may be organic or functional. In the *organic group* carcinoma should first be considered. Stenosis may be the result of cicatricial stricture caused by the healing of a benign ulcer or chronic esophagitis. In exceptional cases organic obstruction is due to pressure from without, as in bronchogenic carcinoma, aortic aneurysm, and enlarged mediastinal lymph nodes. In the *functional group* of dysphagias we must consider achalasia (cardiospasm) at the lower end of the esophagus and the Plummer-Vinson syndrome, the latter involving the pharynx rather than the esophagus. In the diagnosis of malignant lesions the clinician must depend on exfoliative cytology and biopsy in addition to roentgenology and esophagoscopy.

HEMATEMESIS.—In a case of hematemesis it is of prime importance to determine whether the blood is coming from the stomach as is usually the case, or from the esophagus. This may prove to be more difficult than it sounds. By far the most important esophageal lesion responsible for hematemesis is varices. At the same time mucosal lacerations should be considered. As both of these are usually associated with cirrhosis of the liver, clinical evidence of that condition will point to the esophagus rather than to the stomach as the source of the bleeding. Infrequent sources of massive bleeding are carcinoma, ulcer, and diverticula with erosion. Radiography and esophagoscopy are the diagnostic methods available. In the hands of the expert the esophagoscope is an invaluable instrument, as it allows direct inspection of the lesion, but the risk of rupturing large varices is self-evident.

REFERENCES

AZZOPARDI, J. G. and SMITH, O. D.: J. Path. and Bact., 1959, 77, 131. (Mucins of salivary gland tumors.)

BENEDICT, B. B. and NARDI, G. L.: *The Esophagus: Medical and Surgical Management*, Boston, 1958.

BOTHA, G. S. M.: Brit. J. Surg., 1958, 45, 569. (Mucosal folds at gastro-esophageal junction.)

CARDELL, B. S. and GURLING, K. J.: J. Path. and Bact., 1954, 68, 137. (Sjörgen's syndrome.)

FOOTE, F. W. and FRAZELL, E. L.: Cancer, 1953, 6, 1065. (Salivary gland tumors.)

HELLWIG, C. A.: Arch. Path., 1945, 40, 1. (Mixed salivary gland tumors.)

KIRKLIN, J. W., McDONALD, J. R., HARRINGTON, S. W. and NEW, G. B.: Surg., Gynec. and Obst. 1951, 92, 721. (Salivary gland tumors.)

LENNOX, B., PEARSE, A. G. E. and RICHARDS, H. G. H.: J. Path. and Bact., 1952, 64, 865. (Mucins of salivary gland tumors.)

LODGE, K. V.: J. Path. and Bact., 1955, 69, 17. (Non-specific esophagitis.)

MEZA-CHÁVEZ, L.: Am. J. Path., 1949, 25, 523. (Adenolymphoma of parotid.)

MOREHEAD, R. P. and KLEIN, R. E.: Am. J. Path., 1953, 29, 592. (Mixed salivary gland tumors.)

MORGAN, W. S. and CASTLEMAN, B.: Am. J. Path., 1953, 29, 471. (Mikulicz's disease.)

STOUT, A. P. and LATTES, R.: *Tumors of the Esophagus*, Washington, D.C., 1957.

THOMPSON, A. S. and BRYANT, H. C.: Am. J. Path., 1950, 26, 807. (Adenolymphoma of parotid.)

Chapter 26

The Stomach and Duodenum*

General Considerations
  STRUCTURE
  FUNCTION
    Uropepsinogen
    Nervous Control
    Hormonal Control
    Intrinsic Hematopoietic
      Factor
    Emptying
    Absorption
    Hunger and Appetite
Gastritis
  ACUTE GASTRITIS
  CHRONIC GASTRITIS

    Diffuse Giant Hypertrophic
      Gastritis
  GRANULOMAS
  EFFECTS OF GASTRITIS
Peptic Ulcer
  INCIDENCE
  ETIOLOGY
  HEALING
  MALIGNANT CHANGE
  JEJUNAL ULCER
Malignant Tumors
  CARCINOMA
    Exfoliative Cytology
  SARCOMA

Benign Tumors
  EPITHELIAL TUMORS
  MESENCHYMAL TUMORS
Miscellaneous Conditions
  CONGENITAL HYPERTROPHIC
    PYLORIC STENOSIS
    Primary Pyloric Hypertrophy
      in Adults
  ACUTE DILATATION OF THE
    STOMACH
  DUODENAL DIVERTICULA
  THE STOMACH IN PERNICIOUS
    ANEMIA
Summary of Gastric Disorders

GENERAL CONSIDERATIONS

THE stomach and the suprapapillary part of the duodenum have very much in common. Both are developed from the foregut and derive their blood supply from the celiac axis. The remainder of the duodenum is formed from the mid-gut and is supplied by the superior mesenteric artery. Most important of all, the first part of the duodenum, being above the entrance of the alkaline bile and pancreatic juice, is exposed like the stomach to the acid gastric juice. These factors have a bearing on the incidence of peptic ulcer. In other respects the stomach and the duodenum are very different. This is particularly true of the frequency of tumors, both benign and malignant. The two structures, therefore, will be considered both together and separately as the various lesions indicate.

Structure.—The stomach may be divided into two main portions, the *fundus*, which constitutes the great bulk of the organ, and the pyloric antrum, an area 1 or 2 inches in length proximal to the pylorus and extending to the angulation of the lesser curvature. The fundus is acid-producing, while the secretion of the antrum is alkaline. When the stomach is opened along the greater curvature a line can be drawn which separates the acid-producing fundus from the alkaline-producing antrum (Fig. 417). Peptic

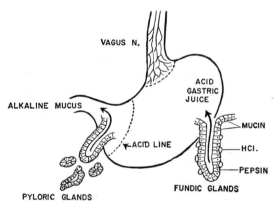

FIG. 417.—Diagram to show the gastric glands and the acid line. (Redrawn from Illingworth, *Peptic Ulcer*, in Boyd, *Pathology for the Surgeon*, courtesy of W. B. Saunders Co.)

ulcers occur most frequently in those portions where there are no acid-producing glands.

The glands of the fundus contain three types of cells. (1) *Parietal* or oxyntic cells (*oxys*, sour) which fringe the tubules and produce the hydrochloric acid, so that they have been called the fountainhead of the acid juice. As they stain red with eosin they are readily recognized. Their number varies

---

* The section on Structure and the opening paragraphs on Function are taken from the author's *Pathology for the Surgeon*, courtesy of W. B. Saunders Co.

enormously. The proportion of parietal cells which are engaged actively in secreting acid also varies greatly at different times, from a low of 20 or 30 per cent to a high of 70 per cent. Under the stimulus of histamine all of these cells may spring into activity. (2) *Chief* or central cells which form the bulk of the gland. They produce pepsin, and do not respond to histamine. (3) *Mucin-producing* cells which line the neck of the glands and cover the surface of the stomach. They pour out a protective film of mucin. The racemose glands of the pyloric antrum are deeper and may reach into the submucosa like Brunner's glands in the duodenum. They produce mucin, the proenzyme for pepsin, but not the anti-pernicious anemia factor. These histological features are worthy of note in relation to what is removed or left in operations on the stomach.

Function.—The function of the stomach is to initiate the process of digestion, to prepare the food mechanically and chemically so that it can be received into the small intestine for more complete digestion, and to eject the prepared material slowly and in small quantities into the duodenum. When one considers this physiological mechanism, it is hardly a matter for surprise that removal of the greater part of the stomach may sometimes be attended by digestive disturbances.

Uropepsinogen is the name applied to the precursor of pepsin which is excreted in the urine. The gastric glands have both exocrine and endocrine functions as regards pepsinogen, 99 per cent being secreted into the stomach, whilst 1 per cent is secreted into the blood and excreted in the urine uropepsinogen. Its estimation in the urine used to be cumbersome and difficult, but with simplified methods uropepsinogen values may offer a better index of gastric peptic activity than gastric intubation. It has proven useful in the diagnosis of peptic ulcer, carcinoma, macrocytic anemia associated with achlorhydria not altered by stimulation with histamine, and in massive hematemesis (Peak *et al.*). It is true that the normal range of values may overlap the range in duodenal ulcer in occasional instances, but over 90 per cent of cases of ulcer have a range higher than normal, generally three times as great. The fact that vagotomy

does not reduce the uropepsinogen may merely mean that it affects the exocrine but not the endocrine function. The values are lower in gastric carcinoma than in benign gastric ulcer, and they may be zero in linitis plastica.

The quantity and quality of the gastric secretion varies both in health and in disease. This variation may involve the hydrochloric acid, pepsin and mucin produced by the three types of cells. The production of hydrochloric acid is regulated by both nervous and chemical (hormonal) control.

NERVOUS CONTROL.—The stomach is supplied by the autonomic nervous system. Stimulation of the vagus increases the production of acid, while vagotomy decreases this action, at least for the time being. The transmission of nervous impulses to the parietal cells is through the agency of acetylcholine which results in the production of histamine. This stimulates the parietal cells to secrete acid. The stimulus to the nerves originates in the parasympathetic center in the hypothalamus, which in turn is played on by a variety of psychic stimuli. Nervous stimuli to the oxyntic cells may be interfered with either by secton of the vagus or by the use of ganglion-blocking agents such as hexamethonium and banthine. These agents have a chemical structure resembling acetylcholine, so that they compete with that substance and exclude it from the synapses.

The profound influence which psychic stimuli and stress may exert on the human stomach was first demonstrated by a series of direct observatons over a period of years made by William Beaumont on the Canadian voyageur, Alexis St. Martin, the interior of whose stomach was laid bare as the result of an accidental gunshot wound, the first of the observations being published in 1833. The conclusions drawn by Beaumont were fully confirmed 110 years later by Wolf and Wolff. Their subject, "Tom", the interior of whose stomach was also exposed, under varying emotional conditions would produce (1) a large volume of gastric juice of high acidity associated with great engorgement of the mucosa but no vigorous contractions, (2) a small volume of juice of high acidity associated with engorgement and vigorous contractions, or (3) a low volume of low acidity with a pale mucosa and almost no contractions. It will be evident that the emotions control the acidity, the motility and the mucosal blood supply. The same was true, in Tom's case, of varying situations involving stress and strain. Fear and sadness produced blanching and inhibition of secretion and motility in his stomach, while anxiety, hostility and resentment produced the opposite effect, with the later development of erosions and ultimately even of ulcers. Reference will be made presently to the relation of these observations to the production and also the healing or lack of healing of peptic ulcer.

HORMONAL CONTROL.—Emotional and systemic stress can act on the stomach by a hormonal as well as a nervous pathway, *viz.*: hypothalamus-anterior pituitary-ACTH-adrenals-cortisone-gastric glands. (Fig. 418) It is known that ACTH and cortisone may exacerbate the symptoms of peptic ulcer and even lead to perforation after resection of the antrum and division of the vagi. This would suggest that the hormones may act directly on the gastric glands without intervention of the nervous system. On the other hand, the secretion of gastric juice which follows stimulation of the anterior hypothalamus in the monkey is prevented by vagotomy (Porter *et al.*). Although these results are confusing they do serve to indicate that there are two great regulators of gastric secretion, the one nervous and the other hormonal. *Curling's ulcer* of the duodenum after extensive burns and other examples of what has been termed "stress ulcer" may be mediated through the hypothalamus-pituitary-adrenal axis, although in the Curling ulcer the marked increase of gastric secretion may be due to the presence in the blood of histamine or a histamine-like substance. The stomach, then, is a veritable sounding board of the emotions, and when one considers the bombardment it suffers from neurogenic, secretory and hormonal stimuli, not to mention exogenous irritants of every sort and description, the wonder is that anyone has a healthy digestion.

INTRINSIC HEMATOPOIETIC FACTOR. Apart from the production of pepsin, hydrochloric-

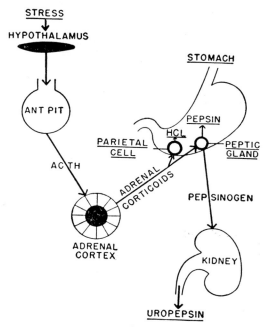

FIG. 418.—Hormonal pathway by which stress may be mediated to the stomach by way of the hypothalamus and the pituitary and adrenal glands, resulting in an increase of gastric acid and pepsin and an increased excretion of urinary uropepsin. (Gray in Harrison's *Principles of Internal Medicine*, courtesy of Blakiston Div. of McGraw-Hill.)

acid and mucus, the gastric mucosa exclusive of the antrum elaborates the intrinsic factor of Castle, which prevents pernicious anemia by facilitating the absorption and assimilation of viamin B_{12} from the intestine with consequent maturation of the erythrocytes. Removal of the body and fundus with anastomosis between the esophagus and the antrum results in pernicious anemia (MacLean). Such patients behave exactly as do those with pernicious anemia or total gastrectomy with regard to the absorption of radioactive B_{12}.

EMPTYING.—We have already seen that gastric motility is profoundly affected by emotional and other nervous stimuli. Gastric retention, often attributed to pylorospasm, is much more frequently of duodenal origin. The presence in the duodenum of such substances as fat, acid and hypertonic fluids acts not by causing contraction of the pyloric sphincter, but by inhibiting gastric motility with relaxation of the sphincter. Gastric retention is seldom due to pylorospasm. Duodenal inhibition of gastric motility acts through a dual mechanism. (1) Reflex action over the vagi (enterogastric) reflex; acid, peptone and hypertonic solutions act through this reflex. (2) A hormone (enterogastrone) which is liberated from the duodenal mucosa, especially by the presence of fat and carbohydrate.

ABSORPTION.—The stomach is not an organ designed for the absorption of food, but rather for the preparation of food for absorption by the small intestine. Some substances, however, are readily absorbed. This is particularly true of salicylate compounds and alcohol. Alcohol is quickly absorbed, especially when taken with carbonated beverages such as soda water. The intoxicating effect can be reduced (if that is desired) by substituting plain water, or by stirring the carbonated water until most of the carbon dioxide has been given off. Alcohol, like histamine, produces a maximum secretion of acid with very little pepsin, as is but natural.

HUNGER AND APPETITE.—In health our weight is maintained with remarkable constancy over long periods unless disease intervenes. This is accomplished by regulating the food intake so that it is sufficient for energy requirement, with the result that the body stores of fat vary only slightly. The taking of food is really a homeostatic mechanism, stimulated by appetite with the object of satisfying hunger, but the mechanism itself is complex and subtle, and there is much disagreement as to its components. Hunger is a physiological state characterized by an unpleasant sensation of abdominal emptiness or pangs of dull pain due to intermittent contractions of the empty stomach. Appetite, on the other hand, is a pleasant sensation conditioned by previous agreeable experiences with food. Hunger has to be converted into appetite, but it is difficult to say exactly how this is done. In many diseased states, as we all know, loss of appetite may be a dominant clinical feature. This may be due to local gastric lesions, such as gastritis, ulcer or cancer, or to a central mechanism located in the hypothalamus. Indeed there is said to be an "appetite center" in the lateral part of the hypothalamus and a "satiety center" in the central area. Gastric distention is telephoned to the satiety center via vagal afferent fibers arising from gastric stretch receptors.

This type of mechanism is designed for short-term regulation. Long-term regulation must be governed by biochemical factors, the information being transmitted from the food depots to the hypothalamus by the blood stream. Thus marked hypoglycemia is associated with hunger sensations and an increased food intake, and many other factors must play a part.

The water content of the body is governed not only by outflow of the excess through the kidneys, but also by adjustment of intake through the medium of *thirst*. This adjustment seems to be depend on two factors: (1) cellular dehydration, (2) contraction of the extracellular fluid volume, which in turn acts through a hypothalamic mechanism. Deficits in water are accompanied by reduction in the flow of saliva, and the resulting dry mouth acts as a powerful stimulus to water intake.

The *anorexia* or loss of appetite which accompanies generalized infections and other extra-gastric forms of disease must be central in origin. Two of the most striking examples are afforded by the virus diseases, influenza and hepatitis. It can be shown experimentally that many infections are accompanied by inhibition of gastric contractions. *Polyphagia* or the excessive ingestion of food without sensations of satiety, which may occur in conditions of augmented or impaired metabolism or in brain lesions, is often accompanied by exaggerated gastric hunger contractions.

GASTRITIS

When we consider the extraordinary assortment of substances, both fluid and solid, hot and cold, sour and sweet, alcoholic and aerated, to which the gastric mucosa is exposed, and also recall the striking changes which violent emotion and stress can produce as shown in the observations on Alexis St. Martin and on "Tom", it is a matter of wonder that we do not all have inflamed stomachs.

Opinions on the relation of gastritis to

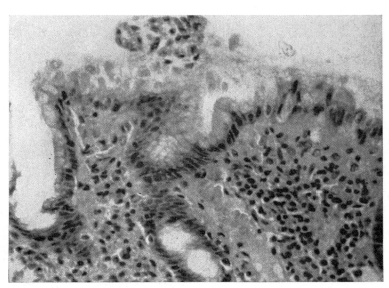

FIG. 419.—Acute gastritis. Gastric biopsy from a male patient aged 57 years, 3 days after a severe alcoholic bout followed by hematemesis. Necrotic superficial epithelial cells are visible in the surface mucus. They are irregular in height and show poor cell outlines. The lamina propria is edematous and infiltrated with plasma cells, lymphocytes and polymorphs (eosin and hematoxylin. × 600) (Wood and Taft, *Diffuse Lesions of the Stomach*, courtesy of Edward Arnold, Ltd.)

dyspepsia have undergone cyclic changes over the years. For a very long time it was believed that the two were almost synonymous. Then it was recognized that some of the most striking changes seen at autopsy were due to postmortem digestion. Surgical operations provided the pathologist with fresh material, but this suffered change from the manipulations of the surgeon. A most important advance was the contribution of Faber, who prevented postmortem digestion by injecting formalin immediately after death. Even in this fresh postmortem material there was the possibility of changes developing during the terminal illness. The final advance has been the inspection of the lining of the stomach with the gastroscope, and more particularly the obtaining of fresh tissue by means of the flexible gastric biopsy tube (Wood and Taft).

The inflammation of gastritis may be acute or chronic. In chronic gastritis the signs of inflammation may have faded into the past, leaving an atrophic mucosa.

Acute Gastritis.—Acute inflammation may be caused by powerful *surface irritants*. The commonest of such irritants, of course, is alcohol. Acute gastritis must be present to some extent after every severe alcoholic bout, and this is largely responsible for the too familiar "morning after" feeling. Mention must also be made of chemical poisons (lye, mercuric chloride) swallowed accidentally by children or with suicidal intent by adults, dietary irritants such as pepper and curry in excess, and very hot fluids. *Bacterial and viral infections*, especially in children, are often accompanied by acute gastritis with dyspepsia. *Emotional disturbances* have already been discussed.

LESIONS.—The mucosa is diffusely hyperemic and swollen by edema, with petechial hemorrhages and mucopurulent exudate. When damage is severe there may be erosions and even ulceration. The *microscopic changes* are best seen in gastric biopsy material (Fig. 419). In addition to necrosis of the superficial epithelium, the edematous lamina propria is infiltrated with polymorphonuclear leukocytes, and the normal number of plasma cells and lymphocytes is greatly increased. When the damage has been only superficial it is probable that regeneration is always complete, but when the deep glands are involved they may be replaced by mucus-secreting epithelium, while the deeper structures may be converted into granulation tissue. The acute gastritis of an alcoholic bout undergoes complete restitution, but if the bouts are severe and often repeated, the acute lesions will change to those of chronic gastritis and eventually gastric atrophy. *Membranous gastritis* and *phlegmonous gastritis* are terms applied to rare conditions in which there is extensive invasion of the stomach wall by bacteria, usually streptococci or staphylococci, with violent inflammation and necrosis over a wide area and to a great depth, with a fatal outcome.

Chronic Gastritis.—Chronic gastritis may be the end result of acute inflammation, or it may be chronic from the beginning. It is convenient to distinguish three main types of chronic gastritis: (1) superficial gastritis, (2) atrophic gastritis and (3) gastric atrophy (Wood and Taft).

In superficial gastritis there is a chronic inflammation of the surface of the mucosa without atrophy of the glands, so that complete restitution is possible, but the lesions may progress to those of the next variety. In *atrophic gastritis* the inflammation extends more deeply into the wall of the stomach, and the glands begin to disintegrate and disappear. In *gastric atrophy* we may be dealing with a secondary result of severe atrophic gastritis, or with what is believed to be a primary atrophy as seen in pernicious anemia. Finally there is the very rare diffuse giant hypertrophic gastritis, which will be considered later.

LESIONS.—The gross appearance, whether at autopsy or seen during life through the gastroscope, is apt to be misleading, for there may be little change from the normal. What used to be called hypertrophic gastritis, believed to be a common condition, is merely a marked rugosity of the mucosa due to contracture after death, or even seen during life in the undistended stomach.

The *microscopic appearance* will depend on the grade of the gastritis. In *superficial gastritis* the picture is similar to that of acute gastritis, although in more muted form. There is the same cellular infiltration of the lamina propria, although poly-

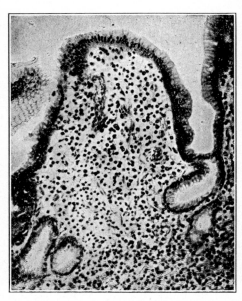

FIG. 420.—Chronic gastritis, showing highly cellular and vascular mucosa. × 140. (Boyd, *Pathology for the Physician.*)

morphonuclears are less in evidence than in the acute form. Regeneration of epithelium, both surface and glandular, may be apparent. In *atrophic gastritis* the inflammatory changes now extend to involve the whole thickness of the mucosa, but the characteristic feature is a varying degree of atrophy of the glandular elements (Fig. 420). Metaplasia of the epithelium to an intestinal type of gland with goblet cells and argentaffin cells is of common occurrence (Fig. 421). In *gastric atrophy*, whether secondary or primary, the glandular atrophy is much more prominent than the inflammatory element.

Diffuse giant hypertrophic gastritis is an exceedingly rare condition, perhaps rather more neoplastic than inflammatory in nature. The lesion may involve the entire mucosa or be quite limited. The prominent mucosal folds present a mammillary or cobblestone pattern. *Microscopically* the basic change is a benign hyperplasia of the surface epithelium and of the mucosal glands. It is evident that the lesion is more adenomatous than inflammatory in nature.

Etiology of Chronic Atrophic Gastritis.—From what has been said it will be apparent

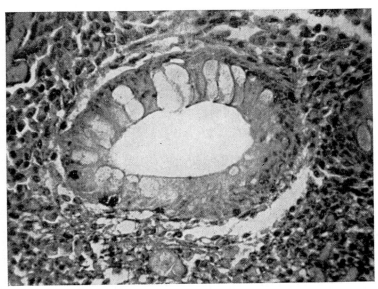

Fig. 421.—Chronic atrophic gastritis. Intestinal metaplasia. Argentaffin cells are visible at the base of the columnar cells, wedged in between them (Masson's silver impregnation, × 600). (Wood and Taft, *Diffuse Lesions of the Stomach*, courtesy of Edward Arnold, Ltd.)

that it is impossible to give a clear account of the etiology. Any of the causes of acute gastritis if repeated at intervals may set up chronic inflammation. In this respect *alcohol* demands special consideration. Although some persons seem to have stomachs which are immune to the poison, in the majority of cases chronic gastritis will be the penalty paid for continued heavy drinking or for repeated acute bouts. This has been denied on the basis of gastroscopic inspection, which may show little or no change even in the confirmed drunkard, but gastric biopsy tells another story. It is only fair to say, however, that some observers consider that chronic gastritis is rarely if ever a direct result of chronic alcohol (Palmer). Atrophy of the mucosa may be due in part to protein and vitamin group B deficiency, often present in chronic alcoholism. Similar atrophic changes are seen in the tongue. Other causal factors which deserve mention are *sex* (higher frequency in the female compared with the much commoner occurrence of diffuse hypertrophic gastritis in the male), *prolonged psychic stress*, and finally *irradiation* of the stomach, either in the treatment of abdominal malignancy or with the object of producing achlorhydria in duodenal ulcer.

Granulomas.—The stomach is an organ which does not lend itself to the development of the granulomas which are so common elsewhere. *Tuberculosis* is a great rarity. The lesions take the usual form, and may give rise to single or multiple ulcers. *Sarcoidosis* has been reported in rare cases. *Eosinophilic granuloma* is a peculiar and unusual condition characterized by granulomatous infiltrations of the stomach and occasionally the jejunum and ileum (Booker and Grant). The patient usually has a specific intolerance for certain foods and may show a constant eosinophilia suggesting an allergic basis. Barrie and Anderson report a case marked by massive eosinophilic infiltration of the submucosa of the pyloric antrum, duodenum and the first two feet of the jejunum with great thickening of the wall. Moran and Sherman suggest that at least some granulomatous lesions of the stomach are *foreign body granulomas* caused by the entry of gastric contents or gastric juice into the stomach wall through preexisting acute or chronic ulcers. In some of the lesions food particles can be identified.

Effects of Gastritis.—Chronic gastritis in the pyloric region may give rise to the classical symptoms of gastric ulcer, i. e., hunger pains, hypersecretion, and delayed emptying and stasis, but when gastrectomy is done no ulcer is found. European investigators find that gastric ulcer and chronic gastritis are frequently associated, and believe that the gastritis precedes the ulcer. In surgical material it is certainly the case that some degree of gastritis is almost always present in gastric and duodenal ulcer. When the gastritis is at all diffuse there is likely to be *achylia gastrica*. This is a very common consequence of chronic alcoholism, especially in elderly persons. Achylia may be due to hematogenous infection in the infective fevers such as influenza and typhoid, and may persist for years afterward. It occurs in over 30 per cent of cases of pulmonary tuberculosis, and in many cases of the toxemia of pregnancy. Complete achylia is always present in pernicious anemia and usually in cancer of the stomach.

PEPTIC ULCER

The stomach and the first part of the duodenum are both derived from the foregut, are both supplied with blood from the coeliac axis, and are both bathed by acid gastric juice, as the alkaline bile and pancreatic secretion flow into the second part of the duodenum. Ulcer of the duodenum is for practical purposes ulcer of the first part, and as gastric and duodenal ulcers are essentially the same in their pathology and are dependent for their production on the peptic juice, they may be considered together under the heading of peptic ulcer. Peptic ulcers also occur at the lower end of the esophagus, on the jejunal side of a gastro-enterostomy, and in Meckel's diverticulum.

Incidence.—Chronic peptic ulcers have a characteristic incidence in regard to site (stomach and duodenum), sex, and age, but this incidence has shown a curious and unexplained change during the past century. If we understood the change we might gain some insight into the difficult problem of pathogenesis. Illingworth, who devotes an entire chapter of his monograph on peptic ulcer to this subject, summarizes the matter as follows: "Peptic ulcer was once rare and is now common. Then gastric ulcer predominated, now duodenal. Then women were affected more often, now men. Then it was mainly a disease of early adult life, now it occurs at later ages too." To this may be added an increased tendency to perforation.

It is not easy to determine the true *relative frequency* of chronic gastric ulcer as compared with duodenal ulcer. Surgical statistics show that chronic ulcer is much commoner in the duodenum. In the Toronto General Hospital out of 875 cases of chronic ulcer coming to operation 70 per cent were in the duodenum and 30 per cent in the stomach. It must be remembered, however, that the surgeon sees a special class of cases, those in which symptoms of obstruction form a prominent feature. In the autopsy material of the same hospital gastric ulcers were nearly twice as common as duodenal. On the other hand Hurst and Stewart found duodenal ulcers somewhat more frequent in their autopsy material. The two are not infrequently combined. It is fairly common for gastric ulcer to be preceded by duodenal ulcer, but the reverse hardly ever occurs.

The *sex incidence* of peptic ulcer has also shown a curious change during the past seventy-five years. In the earlier part of this period Alsted found that in Denmark the incidence of males to females was 1 to 5; by the beginning of the century it was 1 to 1; in the decade from 1920 to 1930 it had risen to 3 to 1. Elsewhere in the world there has been a similar change in sex incidence. No doubt the increased frequency of duodenal ulcer, which is commoner in the male, is a factor of importance.

Blood groups also bear a relationship to the incidence of peptic ulcer, group O persons being more liable to ulcer than those in groups A and B (Aird *et al.*). The blood-group substances are mucopolysaccharides, and persons in group O have a mucopolysaccharide in larger amount than those in other groups. The mucopolysaccharides are present in much larger amounts in gastric and salivary secretions than in the red blood cells, where they are antigens responsible for group reactions. They are particularly abundant in the mucosal cells of the pyloric and prepyloric regions, as well as in the duodenum. Persons in group A are more prone to cancer of the stomach than members of the other groups. It may be that the mucopolysaccharides influence resistance to an exogenous ulcerogenic or carcinogenic factor, with blood group A protecting against ulcerogenic factors, and group O protecting against carcinogenic factors. We must remember defence as well as attack in the genesis of peptic ulcer.

Etiology.—It might be supposed that it would be an easy matter to determine the cause of a single simple ulcer of the stomach or the first part of the duodenum, just as it is in other parts of the body. In point of fact the reverse is the case. The pathogenesis of peptic ulcer has long been a matter of investigation and debate, nor has any agreement yet been reached. Perhaps the mistake has been to look for one instead of a number of etiological agents.

The current views may be summarized by saying (1) that the digestive power of the gastric juice may be so increased that it corrodes the normal healthy mucosa, or (2) that the damaged mucosa cannot resist the action of the normal hydrochloric acid and pepsin. Again we are faced with the problems of attack and defense. It can be said here that high acidity for long periods, especially at night when the stomach has emptied its contents into the duodenum, may possibly explain duodenal but not gastric ulcer. A biopsy taken through the gastroscope heals as quickly when the acidity is high and continuous as in cases of achlorhydria. The ulcer is produced by the action of the gastric juice, but no one has explained how it is that the stomach does not digest itself. Living healthy tissue evidently resists digestion, for when kidney or spleen with circulation intact are introduced into the stomach they are not digested, even when the cut surface is exposed to the gastric juice for weeks or months. *Pure* gastric juice, however, as secreted by the glands of the fundus and obtained from accessory stomach pouches in dogs has the capacity to digest and destroy all living tissue. A peptic ulcer, and in particular a chronic ulcer, is the result of the continued action of the gastric juice on an area of mucous membrane which is presumably of lowered resistance. The real

difficulty is to decide the cause of the lowered resistance. There are three principal views: the infective, the chemical and the neurogenic.

A plausible theory is that *hematogenous infection* with organisms of low grade virulence may cause inflammatory foci in the stomach wall leading to necrosis with subsequent digestion and ulcer formation. In one large series of cases an atrophic gastritis (gastritis leading to atrophy) affecting the antrum was an invariable accompainment of gastric and duodenal ulcer (Hebbel). It seems reasonable to suppose that the gastritis precedes and is the anatomical basis for the development of ulcer, and that chronic ulcer does not develop in a healthy mucosa. Gastritis is not nearly so frequent an accompaniment of gastric carcinoma, nor is it confined to the antrum.

Cushing revived the *neurogenic theory* that abnormal vagal impulses from the hypothalamic region of the diencephalon are responsible for vascular spasm and ischemia which cause the initial area of necrosis. Ulcer may complicate tumors and inflammation of this region. It is undoubtedly more common in the nervous high strung patient, in whom worry and strain may precipitate an attack. The neurogenic factor is the most important single etiologic agent in many cases of ulcer. Indeed the experimental and clinical observations of Dragstedt suggests *intimate connection between the neurogenic and chemical theories*, for the hypersecretion of gastric juice in ulcer patients appears to be due to a continuous hypertonus of the gastric secretory fibers in the vagus nerves. The paramount importance of this factor is emphasized by the spectacular therapeutic results which may follow bilateral division of the vagus nerves (vagotomy), the gastric secretion being greatly reduced and the ulcers tending to heal.

According to the *chemical theory* the essential factor is the action of excess acid. Hyperacidity is a constant accompaniment of peptic ulcer in the early stages, although it may disappear in old chronic ulcers. The fact that the ulcer occurs in non-acid-producing mucosa although in immediate juxtaposition to acid-producing mucosa must be significant. Of even greater significance is the fact that peptic ulcer occurs in a Meckel's diverticulum containing acid-producing gastric mucosa. Food, which is the normal stimulus for the formation of gastric juice, is the chief agent which protects the tissues against its corrosive activities. Also protecting the stomach and duodenum are the pancreatic juice, gastric mucus, duodenal juice and bile. It is important to remember that the gastric juice is secreted continuously even during prolonged fasting. It is during the night when the protective factors are absent that the worst damage may be expected. This damage may be better visualized when it is recalled that between 2,000 and 3,000 cc. of gastric juice are secreted in the space of twenty-four hours. The night secretion is reduced by vagotomy to the extent of 50 per cent. Worry and nervous strain are associated with hyperacidity, perhaps explaining the prevalence of ulcer amongst surgeons and its absence in pathologists. It has already been pointed out that the ulcer patient is frequently nervous and high strung. Food which causes hypersecretion may lead to the formation of ulcer. Thus in Abyssinia, where peptic ulcer was extraordinarily common, a favorite and universal sauce contained 50 per cent cayenne pepper (Bergsma). The experimental injection of histamine, which stimulates gastric acidity, results in the production of ulcers, especially when the histamine is implanted in beeswax to prolong its action. In severe burns histaminoid substances are produced, and it has long been known that such burns may be accompanied by the formation of acute ulcer in the stomach and particularly in the first part of the duodenum, a condition known as *Curling's ulcer*. This type of ulcer was found in 12 per cent of dogs in which large burns were produced. The subcutaneous injection of posterior pituitary extract produces acute hemorrhagic lesions, whilst repeated injections produce chronic ulcers of the peptic ulcer type (Dodds). If the stomach contents are rendered alkaline, injection of pituitary extract fails to produce ulcers. The most effective method of inducing an ulcer to heal, provided it is not too chronic, is by neutralizing the gastric acidity, especially by means of the continuous drip method. All of these facts point to

the paramount importance of gastric acidity in the production and maintenance of peptic ulcer, although they do not prove that some additional factor may not also be operative.

The *size of the stomach*, as indicated by the area of gastric mucosa varies markedly in different persons, and appears to bear a definite relationship to peptic ulcer (Cox). A large stomach containing great numbers of parietal cells, pours out an excess of acid gastric juice, and is associated with chronic duodenal ulcer. Persons with chronic gastric ulcer have a smaller average size of stomach.

In the case of *duodenal ulcer* the cause of the hypersecretion of gastric juice is of vagus or neural origin, so that excision of the pyloric antrum does not prevent the formation of new ulcers in the exposed gastrojejunal mucosa. When the vagus nerves to the stomach are completely divided in patients with duodenal ulcer, the output of acid in the fasting nocturnal gastric secretion falls below the level found in normal people (Dragstedt). Overstimulation of the vagus as occurs under stress and strain leads not only to the overproduction of gastric HCl, but to increased gastric peristalsis with the dumping of acid gastric juice into the duodenum.

A *gastric ulcer* is more likely to be hormonal in origin. Food in the pyloric antrum stimulates gastric secretion by causing the manufacture and release of a hormone, *gastrin*, from the antrum which passes into the circulation and stimulates the secretory activity of the parietal cells. Further gastric secretion results from the entry of neutral food into the duodenum, with the release of a gastrin-like hormone from the duodenal mucosa. This is the so-called intestinal phase of gastric secretion. It is evident that when the antrum is resected in patients with gastric ulcer, the cause of the hypersecretion of gastric juice is removed, and with it the threat of a secondary gastrojejunal ulcer.

Mention of gastrin brings up the question of *hormones* in the pathogenesis of ulcer and its attendant hyperacidity. It is generally believed that *hyperparathyroidism* and peptic ulcer are definitely linked, ulcer formation being fairly common in parathyroid hyperfunction. *Adrenocortical hypersecretion* may be the basis of the "stress ulcer" (the wound-stripe of civilization), and Curling's ulcer, the fulminating, acute, bleeding ulcer which may follow extensive burns. The long-continued use of cortisone and other adrenocortical steroids in the treatment of such conditions as rheumatoid arthritis may be accompanied by the development of acute peptic ulcers. These ulcers are usually atypical in site, being often situated on the greater curvature, show little or no inflammation nor tendency to healing, are often painless and therefore unsuspected, and yet may give rise to a fatal hemorrhage.

The *Zollinger-Ellison syndrome* provides the most dramatic example of the relation between peptic ulcer and endocrine activity. In 1955 Zollinger and Ellison described 2 cases of progressive peptic ulceration associated with a noninsulin-producing islet cell tumor of the pancreas. The hormone involved is uncertain, but it may well be glucagon. The syndrome appears to be a definite clinical entity consisting of (1) extreme gastric hypersecretion and hyperacidity; (2) severe recurrent peptic ulceration; (3) the presence of noninsulin-producing islet cell tumors of the pancreas (Ellison), or in some cases diffuse hyperplasia of the islet cells. The peptic ulcers are particularly frequent in the jejunum, but they may occur in the second and third part of the duodenum, as well as in the two usual sites, and even the lower end of the esophagus. Steatorrhea and intractable diarrhea are not infrequent. The steatorrhea is probably due to depression of the pancreatic lipase activity by the excess of HCl, with undigested fat in the stools, while the diarrhea has been attributed to the enormous quantities of acid gastric juice passing into the duodenum. The massive loss of electrolytes, potassium in particular, in the feces may prove fatal. In other cases the same type of adenoma causes no symptoms. The whole subject is well reviewed by Donaldson and his associates and by Rawson *et al.*, and is discussed again in connection with islet cell tumors.

That food deficiency may play a part in the pathogenesis of peptic ulcer in some regions is suggested by the extreme frequency of duodenal ulcer in Southern India, particularly Travancore. In this district food consists of rice and curry, poor in all the vitamins, particularly A and B_2. In some parts of Pakistan, such as the Punjab, where the diet is rich and well-balanced, peptic ulcer is singularly rare.

In spite of all the theories peptic ulcer still remains a mystery. We cannot explain the site, nor the sex incidence, nor why there has been an apparent shift from the stomach to the duodenum, from women to men, and from youth to middle age.

MORBID ANATOMY.—*Acute* ulcers may occur in any part of the stomach. They are usually shallow, more of the nature of erosions, but occasionally they may perforate the whole thickness of the wall. The *chronic* peptic ulcer is much more localized. Duodenal ulcers are practically always limited to the first part of the duodenum, usually on the anterior wall so that perforation is relatively common, as the ulcer in this position cannot become adherent to the abdominal wall. The vast majority of ulcers occur along the line of the lesser curvature or in close proximity to it. It is rare in the region of the cardia, in the fundus and on the greater curvature, and is uncommon in the pyloric canal (about 1 inch in length). The site of election is between 2 and 4 inches from the pylorus, whereas cancer is commonest in the juxtapyloric portion. Sometimes the ulcer is placed astride the lesser curvature (*saddle-shaped ulcer*). When such an ulcer heals the stomach will be divided into two parts, a condition known as *hour-glass stomach*. The fundus glands produce acid, whereas the glands in the pyloric (large) and cardiac (small) zones do not. The line between the acid and non-acid-producing areas is known as the *acid line* (Fig. 417, page 721). The zone of pyloric glands, and therefore the acid line, reaches much higher on the lesser than on the greater curvature. The line varies considerably in position in different stomachs, and can readily be determined by opening the stomach along the greater curvature and taking blocks of tissue along the lesser curvature.

Peptic ulcers do not arise in the area of acid production. They are formed immediately on the pyloric side of the varying acid line. It is of particular interest to note that peptic ulcers in Meckel's diverticulum are situated in the intestinal type of mucosa, not the heterotopic acid-producing mucosa.

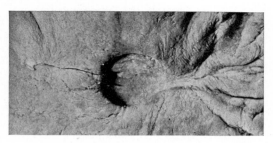

Fig. 422.—Peptic ulcer. This is a characteristic example of an innocent ulcer of the stomach.

The *gastric ulcer* is usually single but may be multiple (5 to 10 per cent). It is shaped like a funnel, penetrating the muscular coat sometimes as far as the peritoneal surface. Small ulcers tend to be circular and larger ones oval. The sides are generally sloping but may be steep; the cardiac side of the ulcer is steeper than the pyloric (Fig. 422). The edge is raised, often overhanging, and the floor is hard and indurated. The larger the ulcer, the more likely is it to be malignant. Most simple ulcers are less than 1 inch in diameter, but some may attain a much larger size. On the peritoneal surface the presence of the ulcer is indicated by pallor and well-marked induration, so that it can be felt better than seen.

A *duodenal ulcer* situated usually on the anterior wall of the first part of the duodenum, or more specifically the duodenal bulb (pyloric cap), is usually small and associated with marked cicatricial contraction, so that small diverticula are often formed between the ulcer and the pylorus. In very chronic and especially in healed ulcers cicatricial contraction may shorten the distance between the pylorus and the papilla from the normal 8 to 6.5 cm. or less.

Microscopically in well-fixed surgical material four zones can be distinguished in the floor of the ulcer (Fig. 423): (1) an inflammatory zone consisting of fibrin and polymorphonuclear leukocytes; (2) a zone of necrotic granulation tissue; (3) a zone of living granulation tissue; (4) a zone of dense scar tissue which forms one of the most important features of the ulcer. It extends in the submucosa for some distance under the intact mucous membrane, and materially interferes with healing in preventing the ap-

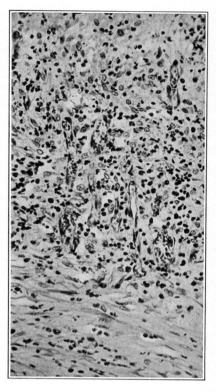

Fig. 423.—Peptic ulcer showing zones of necrosis, granulation tissue, and fibrosis. × 200.

proximation of the edges (Fig. 424). When a chronic peptic ulcer reaches a certain stage it simply cannot heal. There is nearly always greater destruction of the muscular coat than of the mucosa. Evidence of active inflammation in the shape of dilated vessels and foci of chronic inflammatory cells can be seen even in the most quiescent scar tissue, showing that irritation is still going on. The vessels are often narrowed by very marked endarteritis obliterans. At the *margin* of the ulcer there may be evidence of epithelial proliferation in the form of downgrowths, and glandular tissue may be found beneath the muscularis mucosæ. *These changes are apt to be wrongly interpreted as indicating carcinoma.*

Healing.—Acute ulcers and erosions heal rapidly and easily. Chronic ulcers may also heal though with difficulty. It appears likely that an ulcer may heal, recur, break down, and heal again, with each recurrence becoming deeper and more fibrotic. *Healing*

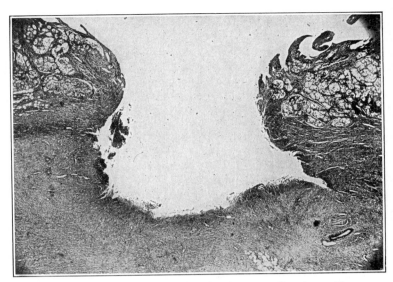

Fig. 424.—Chronic peptic ulcer showing great fibrosis. × 18.

is interfered with by (1) the acid gastric juice, (2) the necrotic layer on the base which covers the granulation tissue and provides no footing for the ingrowing epithelium, and (3) the dense scar tissue which prevents approximation of the edges. *Microscopically* the leukocytes and necrotic tissue disappear, the ulcer becomes filled with healthy granulation tissue, over which the mucosa grows as a single layer of flat cells which later become typically columnar and form tubular glands. The young mucosal cells are at first very fragile and easily destroyed by the passage of gastric contents over the ulcer.

Malignant Change in Peptic Ulcer.—On this important question much difference of opinion has existed. The matter is important because the outlook on treatment (medical or surgical) is so much influenced by the answer to the question. There is no doubt that a chronic ulcer *may* become carcinomatous, just as an ulcer in any part of the body may undergo malignant change. The important question is, *how often* does this occur? The difference of opinion depends largely on different interpretations of the microscopic appearance. To one pathologist the presence of isolated abnormal epithelial cells and aberrant tubules in the neighborhood of a tumor spells carcinoma, while to another they are the result of dis-

tortion produced by the contracting fibrous tissue or merely part of the regenerative process. In examining a malignant ulcer the following points would be in favor of it representing a malignant change in a peptic ulcer: (1) the edge is carcinomatous but not the base, for the latter is densely fibrous and resists invasion by carcinoma cells; (2) complete destruction of the muscular coat and its replacement by fibrous tissue; (3) fusion of the muscularis mucosae and the muscular coat at the margin of the ulcer due to healing.

The site of election of the lesion suggests that malignant change is not of common occurrence. The majority of cancers are situated at the pylorus, whereas the majority of ulcers are from 2 to 4 inches from the pylorus.

The *clinical evidence* is as important as the pathological. The true ulcer cases have a history of many years' duration whereas in cancer there is usually a history of only a few months' gastric disturbance, the patient often remarking that previously he was "able to digest nails." If cancer were often preceded by ulcer the reverse would be the case. Finally, ulcer of the duodenum is very common and cancer of the duodenum is extremely rare. Occasionally the symptoms of ulcer may change into those of cancer, the pain becoming continuous and losing its relation to food. Commonly accepted figures appear to be as follows: about 5 per cent of chronic gastric ulcers become malignant, while about 20 per cent of gastric cancers arise from a preëxisting ulcer. In some centers the figure is less. Thus at the Cleveland Clinic from 1945 to 1951 only 1.1 per cent of benign ulcers developed into cancer (Brown *et al.*).

Robbins at the Mallory Institute, Boston City Hospital, places the figure at under 1 per cent, and adds that "the possibility that a benign peptic ulcer may become malignant has been overemphasized." A carcinoma may undergo peptic digestion and thus simulate a benign ulcer which has become malignant. It is at best difficult to determine whether a cancer of the stomach may have arisen from a preexisting peptic ulcer, and often it is impossible. Moreover, the idea that an ulcer over 4 cm. in diameter is malignant and one under 4 cm. is benign is a gross oversimplification. It is all too easy to forget that a large ulcer may be benign, while a small one may be malignant. From what has been said previously, it is apparent that an ulcer in a patient of blood group A is more liable to become malignant than one in a patient of group O.

Relation of Symptoms to Lesions.—The great symptom is *pain*, relieved by the taking of food and alkalis. It is when the stomach is empty that the pain is most severe, so that the patient may have to get up in the middle of the night to eat a biscuit or drink a glass of milk. There are two possible explanations of the pain, both of which have warm supporters. (1) It may be due to the acid gastric juice acting on the raw surface of the ulcer. As the acidity is neutralized by food or alkalis the pain becomes relieved. When the ulcer becomes perforating the pain is no longer relieved by alkalis. (2) The pain may be muscular in nature and unconnected with the action of the acid juice on the ulcer. The inflammatory foci in the muscularis give rise to contractions in the neighborhood of the ulcer and especially at the pylorus. These increase the intragastric pressure and the tension of the muscle fibers, and this increase is reflected in the sensation of pain. In some cases the pain may be caused merely by the increased tension which accompanies the hyperemia and edema of inflammation.

It should be remembered that, unlike the somatic sensory nerves, the visceral afferents are relatively insensitive to such stimuli as cutting or burning. The effective stimulus for gastric pain is tension on the nerve endings produced by strong muscular contraction, distention, or inflammation. In addition to the discomfort felt in the viscus, there is generally pain "referred" to somatic structures, more especially the abdominal wall. The pain impulses pass to the dorsal root ganglia, and are then transferred to the neurones of somatic sensory nerves.

The pain in *gastric* ulcer tends to occur relatively soon after eating, as the acid gastric content is in immediate contact with the lesion. The pain in *duodenal* ulcer, usually described as a gnawing or an intense hunger sensation, comes on from one to two hours after a meal. This is probably the time when the acid secreted in response to a meal has reached a sufficient concentration and has acted at the ulcer site for a sufficient period to stimulate the visceral pain nerves, both by direct contact of the acid and by protective muscle spasm incited by the irritation.

A patient may present a typical history of peptic ulcer, yet operation may reveal no lesion in the stomach or duodenum. These organs receive the same double nerve supply (sympathetic and parasympathetic) as the other abdominal organs, and the possibility of reflected painful sensations must be borne in mind. The stomach is like a sensitive receiving set which tunes in to distant stations; at the same time it is an amplifier and loud speaker which magnifies any notes of distress it may receive. It cannot refrain from weeping when its neighbors are in trouble, and its voice may be so loud as to drown that of the others. Not only may all the symptoms of ulcer be present without an ulcer, but a well-developed ulcer may be present without symptoms. These facts do not make the task of explaining the clinical picture any easier.

Complications.—The other symptoms are rather in the nature of complications. *Hemorrhage* is very common. It is due to erosion of a vessel in the floor of the ulcer.

If the hemorrhage is severe the blood will be vomited; when the blood has been retained in the stomach and altered by digestion the vomitus will have a brown (coffee-ground) appearance. If the hemorrhage is slight it may only be detected in the form of occult blood in the stools. Minute erosions may cause oozing of blood from the mucosa (gastrostaxis). *Perforation* is more likely to occur in acute ulcers with a very short history in which there is rapid penetration of the muscular wall. In chronic ulcers of long standing there are likely to be adhesions between the ulcer on the posterior wall of the stomach and such organs as the liver and pancreas. Ulcers with continuous symptoms are more dangerous than those with intermissions, for in the former there is no healing and little fibrosis. The long-continued administration of cortisone has increased the danger of perforation. As duodenal ulcer is commoner on the anterior than the posterior wall, perforation is more likely to occur in this form of peptic ulcer. *Cicatricial contraction* at the pylorus will cause pyloric stenosis and great dilatation of the stomach. If the ulcer is on the lesser curvature the scar tissue may pull upon the greater curvature causing the constriction characteristic of *hour-glass stomach*.

Jejunal Ulcer.—After the operation of gastroenterostomy for peptic ulcer a secondary ulcer, also known as a *stomal ulcer*, may develop at the gastrojejunal junction or in the efferent loop of the jejunum within a few inches of the opening. This has all the characteristics of a peptic ulcer. It is caused by the unaccustomed action of the acid gastric juice on the mucosa of the jejunum, together with some accessory factor such as local injury of the mucosa due to the presence of an unabsorbable suture.

MALIGNANT TUMORS

Tumors of the stomach may be benign or malignant, and both may arise from the epithelium, muscle, nerves and lymphoid tissue of the stomach wall. Carcinoma of the stomach so transcends the others in frequency and importance that it will be considered first and in some detail.

Carcinoma.—Carcinoma of the stomach is one of the commonest forms of malignant disease affecting the internal organs. In the United States 40,000 persons die every year of the disease. In Great Britain it is nearly three times as common as cancer of the uterus and twice as common as cancer of the breast. Moreover, on account of its remarkable silence the cure-rate is the worst in malignant disease. About one-half of human cancers occur in the alimentary canal. Such cancers are very rare in all other series of animals. Thus in 142,000 mice only 15 had cancer of the stomach at autopsy (Wells). In the past it has not been possible to produce this very common form in the experimental animal, but squamous cell carcinoma of the forestomach of mice has been caused by the administration of carcinogenic hydrocarbons dissolved in olive oil (Stewart and Lorenz). The disease is much more frequent in the poorer classes than among the well-to-do. Thus in England it is three times commoner amongst the poor.

The *geographic incidence* is also of interest. In Britain the incidence is 22 per cent of all cancers in men, in America 42 per cent, in Holland 55 per cent, in Czechoslovakia 66 per cent. These differences are probably due to different habits in eating, drinking and chewing tobacco, possibly also to dental hygiene. All of these may lead to chronic gastritis, which is probably a precancerous condition of importance. It may be noted that the incidence is high among stokers and barmen, but low among clergymen. There is a peculiarly high incidence in North Wales, which has been attributed to "something in the soil," possibly in the nature of an enzyme.

Perhaps the most remarkable fact in the geographic pathology of gastric carcinoma is the almost complete absence of the disease amongst the Malays of Java and Sumatra, whereas primary cancer of the liver heads the list of malignant disease amongst these people (Bonne). Gastric ulcer is equally rare. On the other hand amongst the Chinese of these islands both gastric cancer and gastric ulcer are common, although surpassed in this respect by cancer of the liver. Pernicious anemia seems to be a predisposing cause, now that patients no longer die of that disease. The usual age period is about sixty, but it may occur much earlier. The

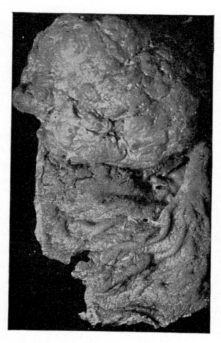

Fig. 425.—Polypoid form of carcinoma of stomach. (Boyd's *Pathology for the Surgeon*, courtesy of W. B. Saunders Co.)

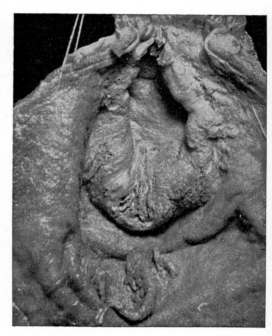

Fig. 426.—Excavating carcinoma of stomach. (Boyd's *Pathology for the Surgeon*, courtesy of W. B. Saunders Co.)

question of the relation of carcinoma to simple ulcer has already been discussed. About 5 per cent of chronic gastric ulcers may develop into carcinoma.

Blood groups seem to bear some relationship to the frequency and site of gastric cancer. In Great Britain patients belonging to blood group A are more liable to develop gastric cancer, just as we have already seen that those in group O are more liable to peptic (duodenal) ulcer (Aird *et al.*). Billington has carried the matter a step farther. He finds that in Sydney, Australia, patients with prepyloric ulcer and cancer at the cardia tend to belong to group A, whereas those with ulcer or cancer of the fundus tend to belong to group O. England seems to have a higher incidence of blood group gene A and also a higher incidence of prepyloric and cardiac cancer than does Sydney.

Morbid Anatomy.—The common *site* is the pyloric region, usually within 1 inch of, but not including, the pylorus. At least 70 per cent of cancers occur in this region. As benign ulcers are comparatively infrequent

in this region, an ulcer in this area should be regarded as malignant until proved not to be. About 25 per cent of the remaining tumors occur on the lesser curvature, and 5 per cent in the fundus.

The *gross appearance* varies greatly. (1) The tumor may form a large, soft, fungating mass which projects into the lumen of the stomach like a mushroom. Ulceration of the surface gives rise to infection and hemorrhage. This may be called the *polypoid form* (Fig. 425). (2) More often the tumor is only slightly elevated and early becomes ulcerated. The edges of the ulcer are raised and rounded, and its diameter may be much greater (above 2.5 cm.) than that of the usual peptic ulcer, although there are exceptions to this rule. This variety is the *excavating form* (Fig. 426). A simple ulcer which becomes malignant belongs to this group. The cut surface shows marked thickening of the wall with yellow flecks of necrosis, and sometimes nodules on the serous surface. (3) The *diffuse infiltrating form*, in which no real tumor is seen but a

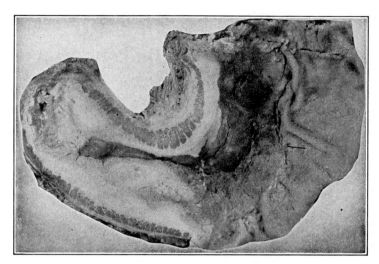

Fig. 427.—Carcinoma of the stomach. This is an example of the local pyloric form of the infiltrating variety.

great thickening of the stomach wall. This may be local or diffuse. The *local* form occurs at the pylorus, where there is a dense ring of sclerotic tissue which causes great pyloric stenosis and marked dilatation of the stomach (Fig. 427). The cut surface is greatly thickened and densely hard. The *diffuse* variety is known as *linitis plastica*, cirrhosis of the stomach, and leather-bottle stomach. The entire stomach is involved; it is very small and very thick walled. The normal stomach is about 12 inches long and contains 40 ounces; the leather-bottle stomach may only measure 4 inches and contain only 4 ounces. The wall may be an inch thick. The walls of the stomach are peculiarly stiff and rigid. There is no ulceration of the surface, but the mucosa is firmly tacked down to the underlying muscular coat. The stomach is involved from the cardia to the fundus; the thickening stops abruptly at the pyloric ring and does not invade the duodenum. On the other hand it may invade far into the esophagus. In the diffuse form it may be very difficult to demonstrate any cancer cells, most of which seem to die out, so that the condition is of low malignancy.

The *microscopic appearance* varies considerably. Although the stomach is a glandular organ, cancer frequently fails to form even rudimentary glands. The cells are usually arranged in cords or masses, or seen as isolated cells. This is in marked contrast to cancer of the bowel, in which an adenomatous arrangement is nearly always well marked. The *polypoid* (less malignant) form is likely to show the best examples of glandular arrangement (Fig. 428). The normal mucosa is replaced by atypical glandular tubules which penetrate the muscularis mucosae, spread widely in the submucous coat, and may finally appear on the serous surface. The glands are lined by one or several layers of cells with large hyperchromatic nuclei so that the tubules appear much darker than the surrounding normal ones. In other cases the tumor is more *anaplastic*, glandular acini are poorly formed or completely absent, and the cancer cells are arranged in masses or in single columns separated by a dense stroma of the scirrhous type. Such a picture is more likely to be seen in ulcerocarcinoma. The most extreme anaplasia is met with in the diffuse infiltrating variety, but in spite of the anaplasia this tumor is not of a high grade of malignancy. Here there is no attempt at gland formation, and the individual cells or clumps of cells are lost in a scar-like stroma so dense that it appears to be strangling them. Many of the cancer cells contain

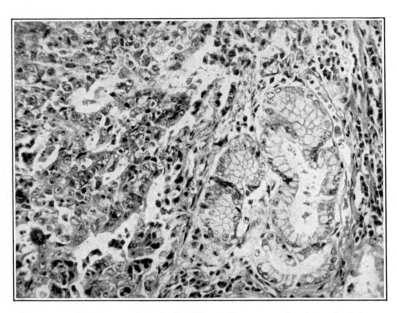

Fig. 428.—Carcinoma of stomach. The rudimentary glands to the left are highly malignant in type. × 300.

droplets of mucin which can best be demonstrated with the periodic acid-Schiff stain for acid mucopolysaccharides with alcian blue, a valuable method of identifying malignant cells embedded in dense fibrous tissue. When the mucin production is excessive the tumor is converted into a soft gelatinous mass; this variety is called *mucoid carcinoma,* formerly known as colloid cancer, and forms about 5 per cent of gastric carcinomas. The cells are distended and finally destroyed by clear mucinous material, but clumps of recognizable carcinoma cells are found here and there. The change does not affect the prognosis.

Gastritis and carcinoma are frequently associated. The mucous membrane not only in the immediate neighborhood of the tumor but also at a distance may show chronic gastritis, either atrophic or hyperplastic, with atrophy of the peptic cells and tubules, and a *transformation of the gastric into the intestinal type* of cells with many goblet cells. Although this metaplasia occurs in the normal stomach and is more frequent in peptic ulcer, it is most common in cancer, and it has been said that many cancers of the stomach arise from intestinal metaplasia. A high activity of the enzyme aminopeptidase can be demonstrated to be present in the cytoplasm of the cancer cells and of the metaplastic epithelium, but not in the normal gastric mucosa (Planteydt and Willighagen).

Spread.—Cancer of the stomach spreads locally, to the lymph nodes, and to distant organs. (1) *Local spread* occurs both in the stomach wall and to neighboring organs. Spread in the stomach wall takes place mainly in the loose submucous coat. In the diffuse infiltrating form the entire submucosa is first infiltrated and then becomes fibrosed. The tumor may penetrate the entire thickness of the wall and appear on the serous surface, from which the tumor cells may be spread by implantation over the abdomen (peritoneum, omentum, ovaries). The duodenum is never invaded, the tumor stopping short at the pylorus. Spread to neighboring organs usually involves the liver or the pancreas when the cancer is on the posterior wall of the stomach. (2) *Spread to the lymph nodes* is extremely common. At first the regional nodes draining the stomach are affected, but there may be distant spread along the thoracic duct, and the supraclavicular and cervical glands may be enlarged, especially on the left side. (3) *Spread to distant organs* is by the blood stream. The liver is involved first and most frequently *via* the portal vein. It may be enormously enlarged though the gastric tumor may be too small to be detected clinically. There may be blood spread to the lungs, central nervous system, kidneys and bones. The abdominal organs, especially the ovaries, may be the site of metastases, either by implantation or by lymphatic spread.

The Relation of Symptoms to Lesions.— When symptoms do make their appearance they are apt to be most indefinite. A "decline in health" often sums up the early picture. *Loss of appetite* is one of the earliest manifestations. This is probably due to the slow infiltration of the muscular wall of the stomach by tumor cells, thus interfering with the healthy tone on which the sense of appetite depends. (Fig. 429). The tolerance for food is upset, and there is a sense of fullness after meals, probably due again to the loss of tone. During this period the patient is likely to treat himself with antacids from the corner drug store in North America, from the chemist's shop in Great Britain, whilst every day the cancer is spreading.

Pain as an early symptom is unfortunately *absent in about one-half the cases* of cancer of the stomach, for it depends on destruction and irritation of the muscular coat; quiet infiltration by tumor cells may cause little irritation. Pain is likely to be present in ulcerocarcinoma, and when the tumor is at the pylorus where it excites spasm. If the pain of chronic peptic ulcer in a man in the cancer age changes its character, becomes continuous, and loses its relation to food, the possibility of a malignant change should be considered. *Absence of free hydrochloric acid* in the stomach contents is due partly to the destruction of the mucous membrane by the tumor, partly to secondary changes which develop in the rest of the mucosa leading to atrophy of the oxyntic cells. The suppression of hydrochloric acid is not so constant or complete as in pernicious anemia. In early carcinoma free hydrochloric acid is often present, and it can be demonstrated by the fractional method in about one-half the operable cases. *Lactic acid* appears as the

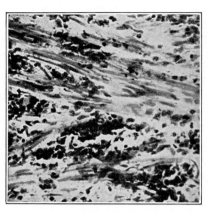

Fig. 429.—Carcinomatous invasion of the muscular wall of the stomach. It is this infiltration which destroys the muscle tone and is responsible for the loss of appetite. × 175.

result of pyloric obstruction and the decomposition of retained food. *Blood in the stool* (*occult blood*) is a most important and constant sign; it is due to ulceration and will therefore be absent in the diffuse infiltrating form. It can also be found in the stomach contents. *Anemia* is very common. It is usually of the so-called secondary type, but is occasionally indistinguishable from pernicious anemia. The anemia may be due partly to continued loss of blood, partly to ulceration and sepsis, but the more primary form may well be due to that loss of the power of the stomach to produce the hematopoietic principle (stored later in the liver) which is responsible for pernicious anemia.

Exfoliative cytology is the newest arrival in the diagnostic field. At first the results were disappointing, because the limitations of the method were not recognized, nor the fact that adequate preparation of the patient was as important as skilled examination of the smear. Gastric secretion rapidly digests any exfoliated cancer cells, so that they soon become unrecognizable and steps must be taken to prevent retention of food and secretions. This is done by means of a preliminary light diet, overnight fasting, and lavage if obstruction is present. The minimum delay in examination of the aspirated material (special technician and laboratory facilities) is also of great importance. The use of an abrasive balloon which is inflated at the fundus, carried by gastric motility to the pylorus, pulled back gently several times, and then deflated and withdrawn, has greatly incresed the number of positive results in some hands (Cooper and Papanicolaou). Peptic digestion will disfigure or destroy the cells on the necrotic surface of a large fungating tumor, whereas the smallest (earliest) tumor, by virtue of the loss of cohesion which is a characteristic of cancer cells, will exfoliate elements which can be collected by the abrasive balloon and recognized under the microscope. With this technique Cooper found that the only lesions giving negative findings were large fungating growths with a necrotic surface, the over-all results being 97 per cent correct in proved cases of carcinoma. This would appear, therefore, to be the most reliable diagnostic method at present available in cancer of the stomach.

The task of differentiating a benign from a malignant ulcer of the stomach may be far from easy. Every generalization has many exceptions, but some of the features given in the accompanying table may help the student in his thinking.

CANCER OF THE DUODENUM.—Although simple ulcer is so common, carcinoma is rare in the duodenum, but in my experience not so rare as in commonly stated. The usual site is the second part, not the first part as in ulcer. The tumor causes obstruction of the biliary and pancreatic ducts. It is easy to mistake cancer of the head of the pancreas for cancer of the second part of the duodenum.

Sarcoma.—Sarcoma of the stomach differs from carcinoma in a number of ways. It is as rare as carcinoma is common, and it tends to take one of two forms: (1) a large bulky mass within the wall which eventually fungates and ulcerates into the lumen, (2) a marked thickening and prominence of the rugae which gives a highly characteristic appearance. When seen in the operating room the tumor is likely to be large (unless of the rugose form), gray and soft. The microscopic appearance will depend on the cell of the origin, for the tumor may be a fibrosarcoma, leiomyosarcoma or lymphosarcoma. *Lymphosarcoma* is not merely a

BENIGN AND MALIGNANT GASTRIC ULCER

	Benign Ulcer	*Malignant Ulcer*
Age of Patient	Usually at younger age.	Usually in older persons.
Common location	Lessor curvature 2 to 4 inches proximal to pylorus.	Greater curvature in juxta-pyloric portion.
Size	Usually under 2 cm. in diameter.	Usually over 4 cm. in diameter
Symptoms	Often marked pain for years.	Often not apparent until late.
Gastric acidity	Generally hyper-acidity.	Often hypo-acidity.
Blood group	Group O more probable.	Group A more probable.
Microscopic appearance	1. Inflammatory zone. 2. Necrotic and living granulation tissue zone. 3. Dense scar zone.	Adenocarcinoma or varying grades of ana-plasia.
Cytology	No cancer cells.	Cancer cells present.

local manifestation of a generalized lymphosarcoma, but a lymphomatous neoplasm confined to the stomach and often responding well to surgical removal. In addition of course, the lesion in the stomach may be a part of a generalized malignant lymphomatosis. In such a case the lesion will be multiple, discrete, and, particularly in the reticulum cell variety, with a tendency to ulcerate into the lumen.

BENIGN TUMORS

Benign tumors of the stomach may be epithelian or mesenchymal.

Epithelial Tumors.—These may be *papilloma* or *adenoma*. They are really variations of the same tumor, and are of little clinical significance, except that the papilloma is said, on very insecure grounds, to have a tendency to become malignant.

Diffuse gastric polyposis is a condition in which soft nodules are scattered either over the entire mucosal surface or localized to one area. The *x*-ray picture is characteristic. Two of the most constant clinical features are severe anemia and achylia gastrica, both of which are easily understandable.

Mesenchymal Tumors. — These lesions although rare, are of clinical importance because they tend to ulcerate and cause hemorrhage, to obstruct the pylorus, to interfere with gastric motility and thus cause dyspepsia, and above all because of the diagnostic problems which they may present. The principal members of the group are *leiomyoma and neurilemmoma* (neurinoma, schwannoma). Although usually remaining small, they may attain a large size, forming a bulky mass which either projects into the lumen or grows outward. The mucosa over the tumor may become ulcerated, and the ulcer may be deep, with resulting hemorrhage. The usual *symptoms* in order of frequency are hematemesis, melena, indigestion and epigastric pain, symptoms which naturally suggest an ulcer. Most of these tumors are asymptomatic, even though they are quite large, provided they do not undergo ulceration or produce pyloric obstruction.

MISCELLANEOUS CONDITIONS

Congenital Hypertrophic Pyloric Stenosis. —This is a condition of congenital hypertrophy of the pylorus usually occurring in male breast-fed infants. The pylorus is greatly thickened so that it projects into the duodenum. The thickening extends for a few centimeters along the pyloric canal, then gradually disappears. The pyloric opening is greatly narrowed and is filled with closely-packed folds of mucous membrane. The thickening is caused by an enormous hypertrophy of the circular layer of muscle fibers. An element of spasm seems to be added to the hypertrophy, because the persistent vomiting which is the principal symptom of the stenosis does not begin for a week or two. The thickened pylorus can often be felt as a round firm mass. Surgery offers no more dramatic result than in the case of the Fredet-Rammstedt operation, which consists in dividing the hypertrophied muscle down to the mucosa; the vomiting stops as if by magic, and the starved child at once begins to put on weight.

PYLORIC HYPERTROPHY IN ADULTS.—Concentric hypertrophy of the pyloric muscle is a fairly common finding in autopsies on adults. This type is believed to develop late in life and is not a persistence of the congenital hypertrophy. It may be symptomless or associated with pain and vomiting and is recognizable in the *x*-ray film by the presence of a long, thin, pyloric canal. It is to be distinguished from the eccentric hypertrophy which so often develops just caudal to a healed ulcer of the duodenum or pyloric canal.

Acute Dilatation of the Stomach. —After an abdominal operation under general anesthesia the stomach may occasionally become very rapidly distended until it reaches an enormous size. The condition is likely to be fatal unless treated promptly. At autopsy the stomach may fill the greater part of the abdomen, its wall is very thin, and it contains a very large amount of fluid, although in the early stages the contents are entirely gaseous. The dilatation may stop at the pylorus or may extend as far as the point where the third part of the duodenum is crossed by the superior mesenteric vessels. It is probable that there are two etiological factors: (1) reflex atony of the stomach wall produced by trauma to the abdominal organs similar to the paralysis of the bladder which may follow operation on the perineum; (2) swallowing of air while the patient is under the anesthetic. In the later stages there is a great outpouring of watery fluid known as *gastric succorrhea*. The use of the stomach tube in the early stage soon relieves the condition.

Duodenal Diverticula.—Roentgen-ray studies have shown that diverticula of the duodenum are much commoner than used to be thought. Two types may be recognized, primary and secondary. A *primary* diverticulum usually arises from the second part of the duodenum, sometimes from the first part, rarely from the third part. It springs from the inner and posterior aspect of the bowel along the line of entrance of the vessels which weaken the wall. There is a herniation of the mucosa through the muscular coat, and the sac thus formed may be as small as a pea or as large as a plum. It may be single or multiple. It occurs in middle and late life. Often discovered accidentally, it may give rise to no symptoms, but when large it may cause dyspepsia, probably from pressure. *Secondary* diverticula are secondary to a duodenal ulcer, so that they occur in the first part of the duodenum. There may be bulging of one or both sides of a healed scar due to traction. The condition is of no clinical significance.

The Stomach in Pernicious Anemia.—In pernicious anemia the stomach presents a picture which is not seen in any other disease process, and which is the fundamental lesion of this blood dyscrasia. There is gross atrophy of the mucosa of the body and fundus, stopping abruptly at the junction of the body with the pyloric mucosa. Microscopically there is severe atrophy of all coats, only the surface epithelium and a few mucous glands remaining in the mucosa, with complete disappearance of the specialized oxyntic and peptic cells. To demonstrate this change the stomach must be fixed with formalin soon after death (Magnus and Ungley; Cox). It may be noted that the incidence of blood group A is unduly high in patients with pernicious anemia.

It must be realized that the gastric lesions outlined above are those seen at postmortem in cases of pernicious anemia. Biopsies of the gastric mucosa by means of the flexible gastric biopsy tube give a different picture. Thus in 100 patients with pernicious anemia only 40 showed the classical atrophic lesion; the remaining 60 showed atrophy combined with an inflammatory lesion characterized by widespread cellular infiltration of the mucosa (Joske *et al.*). We shall return to this matter again in the discussion on pernicious anemia in Chapter 39, and we may find that we have to modify our ideas about the relation of atrophy of the gastric mucosa to pernicious anemia.

SUMMARY OF GASTRIC DISORDERS

When we come to disorders of the intestine in the next chapter we shall encounter a bewildering array of possible pathological lesions. In the stomach, on the other hand, the physician has to consider only three main probabilities, namely gastritis, either acute or chronic, peptic ulcer, and carcinoma. Unfortunately the clinical manifestations of these three conditions may be confusingly

similar, the patient complaining of disturbance of digestion as manifested by loss of appetite, a sense of fullness in the epigastrium, nausea, perhaps vomiting and epigastric pain, and sometimes hematemesis. In many cases a consideration of the clinical facts such as age, sex, duration of the symptoms, and response to therapy may give a sufficient lead to a solution of the problem.

In other cases the assistance of the laboratory must be sought. The first of these of course is x-ray examination. Gastroscopy, and more particularly that uniquely useful instrument, the flexible gastric biopsy tube, may serve to solve the problem. Gastric chemical analysis in peptic ulcer, and cytological examination of the aspirated gastric contents in cases of carcinoma may be decisive. Even when all these aids have been utilized, the physician may still be in doubt, and surgical exploration aided by biopsy may be required.

Of the three main types of disorder gastritis is fortunately the most common. The acuteness of onset, the usually temporary character of the symptoms, and the response to antacid and antispasmodic therapy usually point to a correct diagnosis. Ulcer is the next most common lesion. When radiography shows an ulcer in the duodenum, the diagnosis is clear. In the stomach there is the possibility of a benign or malignant ulcer. Chemical analysis and cytological examination may serve to settle the question. Hematemesis points to peptic ulcer, then to cancer, and in occasional cases to esophageal varices.

REFERENCES

Aird, I. *et al.*: Brit. Med. Jour., 1954, *2*, 315. (Blood groups in peptic ulcer). Ibid., 1953, *1*, 799. (Blood group and gastric cancer.)

Alsted, G.: *Studies on the Changing Incidence of Peptic Ulcer of the Stomach and Duodenum*, London, 1939.

Barrie, H. J. and Anderson, J. C.: Lancet, 1948, *2*, 1007. (Eosinophilic granuloma.)

Billington, B. P.: Lancet, 1956, *2*, 859. (Gastric cancer and blood groups.)

Booker, R. J. and Grant, R. V.: Surgery, 1951, *30*, 388. (Eosinophilic granuloma.)

Brown, C. H., Fisher, E. R. and Hazard, J. B.: Gastroenterology, 1952, *22*, 103. (Malignant change in gastric ulcer.)

COOPER, W. A. and PAPANICOLAOU, G. N.: J.A.M.A., 1953, *151*, 10. (Exfoliative cytology in cancer of stomach.)

COX, A. J., JR.: Am. J. Path., 1943, *19*, 491. (The stomach in pernicious anemia.) Arch. Path., 1952, *54*, 407. (Stomach size in relation to chronic peptic ulcer.)

CUSHING, H.: Surg. Gyn. and Obstet., 1932, *55*, 1. (Neurogenic causation of peptic ulcer.)

DONALDSON, R. M., VON EIGEN, P. R. and DWIGHT, R. W.: New Eng. J. Med., 1957, *257*, 965. (Zollinger-Ellison syndrome.)

DORAN, F. S. A.: Lancet, 1951, *1*, 199. (Etiology of chronic gastric ulcer.)

DRAGSTEDT, L. R.: J.A.M.A., 1959, *169*, 83. (Cause of peptic ulcer.)

ELLISON, E. H.: Surgery, 1956, *40*, 147. (Ulcerogenic tumor of pancreas.)

FABER, K.: *Gastritis and Its Consequences*, London 1935.

GRAY, S. and SCHINDLER, R.: J.A.M.A., 1941, *117*, 1005. (Chronic gastritis.)

HEBBEL, R.: Am. J. Path., 1943, *19*, 43. (Peptic ulcer and gastritis.)

HURST, H. F. and STEWART, M. J.: *Gastric and Duodenal Ulcer*, London, 1929.

ILLINGWORTH, C. F. W.: *Peptic Ulcer*, Edinburgh, 1953.

JOSKE, R. A., FINCKH, E. S. and WOOD, I. J.: Quart. J. Med., 1955, *24*, 269. (The stomach in pernicious anemia.)

MACLEAN, L. D.: Gastroenterology, 1955, *29*, 653. (Intrinsic anti-pernicious anemia factor.)

MAGNUS, H. A. and UNGLEY, C. C.: Lancet, 1938, *1*, 420. (The stomach in pernicious anemia.)

MORAN, T. J. and SHERMAN, F. E.: Am. J. Clin. Path., 1954, *24*, 422. (Granulomas of stomach.)

PALMER, E. D.: Medicine, 1954, *33*, 199. (Gastritis.)

PEAK, W. P. *et al.*: J.A.M.A., 1956, *162*, 1441. (Uropepsinogen.)

PLANTEYDT, H. T. and WILLIGHAGEN, R. G. J.: J. Path. and Bact., 1960, *80*, 317. (Enzyme histochemistry of intestinal metaplasia in gastric cancer.)

PORTER, R. W., MOVIUS, H. J. and FRENCH, J. D.: Surgery, 1953, *33*, 875. (Hormonal control of gastric secretion.)

RAWSON, A. B. *et al.*: Lancet, 1960, *2*, 131. (Zollinger-Ellison syndrome.)

ROBBINS, S. L.: J.A.M.A., 1959, *171*, 2053. (Benign versus malignant peptic ulcers.)

WELLS, H. G. *et al.*: Am. J. Cancer, 1938, *33*, 223. (Cancer of stomach in mice.)

WOLF, S. and WOLFF, H. G.: *Human Gastric Function: An Experimental Study of a Man and His Stomach.* New York, 1943.

WOOD, I. J. and TAFT, L. I.: *Diffuse Lesions of the Stomach*, London, 1958.

ZOLLINGER, R. M. and ELLISON, E. H.: Ann. Surg., 1955, *142*, 709. (Jejunal ulcers and pancreatic islet-cell tumors.)

Chapter 27

The Intestine

General Considerations
  STRUCTURE
    Mucosal Biopsy
  FUNCTION
    Digestion
    Absorption
    Motility
Enteritis
  CATARRHAL ENTERITIS
  PSEUDOMEMBRANOUS AND
    STAPHYLOCOCCAL ENTERO-
    COLITIS
Chronic Ulcerative Colitis
  UREMIC ENTERITIS
Regional Enteritis
Bacillary Dysentery
Amebic Dysentery
Typhoid Fever
Cholera
Tuberculosis
Actinomycosis
Acute Appendicitis
  CHRONIC APPEDICITIS

THE OBLITERATED APPENDIX
Miscellaneous Lesions of the
  Appendix
  MUCOCELE
  MEASLES
  FOREIGN BODIES
  TUMORS
Intestinal Diverticula
  DIVERTICULITIS
  MECKEL'S DIVERTICULUM
    Enterogenous Cysts
Malabsorption Syndromes
  SPRUE
    Tropical
    Non-tropical
  CELIAC DISEASE
  INTESTINAL LIPODYSTROPHY
Tumors
  BENIGN TUMORS
    Villous Papilloma
    Polypoid Adenoma
    Multiple Polyposis
    Peutz-Jeghers Syndrome

  Benign Mesenchymal Tumors
  MALIGNANT TUMORS
    Carcinoma
    Carcinoid
    Serotonin
    The Carcinoid Syndrome
Intussusception
Volvulus
Hernia
Intestinal Obstruction
  ACUTE
    Pathological Physiology
  CHRONIC
  MECONIUM ILEUS
Hirschsprung's Disease
Mesenteric Vascular Occlusion
  Complete
  Partial
Miscellaneous Lesions
  HEMORRHOIDS
  MELANOSIS COLI
  INTESTINAL PNEUMATOSIS
  DEVELOPMENTAL DEFECTS

GENERAL CONSIDERATIONS

Structure.—Mention will be made of only a few points of structure which have a bearing on function, and which serve to differentiate the small from the large intestine. The function of the small intestine is to continue the digestion begun in the stomach, to absorb the products of digestion, and to move the contents onward. The fore-gut (jejunum), supplied by the coeliac axis, is concerned with *digestion*, the mid-gut (ileum, cecum and right colon), supplied by the superior mesenteric artery, with *absorption*, and the hind-gut (left colon, sigmoid and rectum), supplied by the inferior mesenteric artery, with *excretion*. The characteristic transverse folds of mucosa (folds of Kerckring), which serve as landmarks in a radiological barium meal study, increase the mucosal surfaces of the small bowel, but become less evident as we approach the lower end of the ileum. The myriads of villi in the small bowel are ideally designed for absorption. The mucous membrane of the bowel consists of three layers: surface epithelium,

lamina propria and muscularis mucosae. The lamina propria consists of areolar and lymphoid tissue and contains the tubular glands. The only submucosal glands are the Brunner's glands in the duodenum. The meaning of the very abundant lymphoid tissue is not clear. Possibly it acts as a filter against the bacteria which must continually penetrate the thin surface epithelium. Certain it is that enormous numbers of lymphocytes constantly move through the epithelium into the lumen of the bowel. The argentaffin or enterochromaffin system of cells, which are most numerous in the small bowel and produce 5-hydroxytryptamine or serotonin will be discussed in connection with carcinoid tumors of the bowel.

Small bowel mucosal biopsy by means of a peroral capsule triggered by suction promises to be a technique of value in investigating pathological changes in the small intestine (Smith *et al.*). The specimen removed consists of a small disc of mucosa measuring 7 mm. in diameter. Since 10 to 100 villi cover 1 square mm. of small intestine, several hundred such villi are available for study.

The finest details of the mucosa are visible in the microscopic sections.

Function.—We have already seen that the functions of the small intestine are digestion, absorption and motility, just as those of the large intestine are storage and movement of contents. As interference with any of these functions may result in disease, they will be briefly outlined.

DIGESTION.—The secretions by which digestion is carried on in the small intestine are the duodenal juice and the intestinal juice or succus entericus.

The *duodenal juice* is secreted by Brunner's glands which are the distinctive feature of the duodenal mucosa. It is alkaline in reaction and rich in mucus, resembling in these respects the secretion of the pyloric glands. It is increased by vagal stimulation, by the injection of secretin (which can be extracted from the mucosa), and by perfusing the lumen with dilute HCl. The response to food is partly nervous, partly under hormonal control, in these respects resembling gastric secretion.

The *intestinal juice* is alkaline, and contains mucus and two enzymes: (1) enterokinase, which activates pancreatic trypsinogen, and (2) amylase. The lining cells of the intestine also contain the enzymes erepsin, which converts peptones or polypeptides into amino acids, invertase which acts on cane sugar, maltase on maltose, and lactase on lactose. Mechanical stimuli, including colicky contractions, increase both the volume of the juice and the enzyme output.

ABSORPTION.—Digested food is absorbed in the small intestine. In the proximal half of the large bowel water and salts are absorbed, so that the contents are reduced in size, dried and converted into a formed fecal mass. The carbohydrates are absorbed mainly as monosaccharides, glucose or fructose, the proteins as amino acids, while 80 per cent of the fat is carried in the lymph to the thoracic duct and thence to the blood, the remainder passing to the liver by the portal vein.

Impaired absorption of fat is much more important than defective absorption of carbohydrates and protein. About 90 per cent of the daily intake of fat should be absorbed. When it is not absorbed in proper amount it is discharged in the stools, a condition known as *steatorrhea*, in which the feces are pale and very soft. The condition may be caused in a variety of ways which we shall have to study in this and other chapters. Thus there may be (1) a deficiency in bile salts or in pancreatic lipase owing to obstruction of the bile and pancreatic ducts or to disease of the pancreas; (2) structural defects in the mucosal cells, as in regional ileitis; (3) hyperperistalsis may move the contents along too quickly for absorption; (4) obstruction to the thoracic duct by tumors; (5) special conditions such as Whipple's lipodystrophy, celiac disease and sprue, which will be considered in their appropriate place.

As regards *reduced absorption in general*, this may be due to: (1) insufficient intake, (2) inadequate digestion from lack of pancreatic and other juices, (3) lack of materials necessary to promote absorption, *e.g.* bile salts, (4) disease of the bowel wall, and (5) extensive resection, short-circuiting operations, or gastro-colic fistula.

MOTILITY.—The dominant characteristic of the muscle of the *small intestine* is its rhythmicity, with alternating contractions and relaxations of surprisingly constant frequency. By contrast, peristaltic movements occur at irregular intervals, being initiated by stimuli provided by the intestinal contents. In the fasting animal the villi are inactive, lying flat on the surface of the mucosa. When in contact with fluids or in the fed animal they become highly active, showing both a lashing movement and a rhythmical shortening and lengthening.

Mass movements of the *colon* occur two or three times in twenty-four hours, the contents of the proximal part being transferred to the distal half. The time taken for the intestinal contents to pass along the bowel under normal conditions may be divided roughly into three periods: (1) from pylorus to cecum, six hours; (2) from cecum to sigmoid, twelve hours; (3) storage in sigmoid, six hours. The cecum and ascending colon are filled by the activity of the ileum. After each meal a gastro-colic reflex is set up, resulting in powerful massive peristalsis in the colon, the feces reaching the pelvic colon and accumulating there, but not passing into the rectum. When the correct stimulus together with the appropriate time and place are all together, a wave of peristalsis reaches the distal part of the bowel. The feces are forced into the rectum, and defecation occurs.

It is curious that the large intestine, apparently so passive, is more involved in emotional disturbances than any other part of the gastrointestinal tract, so that pale fear may loosen the bowels, as every medical student knows when he goes up for an examination insufficiently prepared. Similarly constipation may be due to psychic as well as organic factors. We shall encounter a number of instances of the latter in the pages which follow.

Constipation is likely to be associated with straining during defecation, which may be accompanied by notable changes in both arterial and venous blood pressures, especially with powerful straining efforts which initiate the Valsalva maneuver (trying to exhale against the closed glottis). The sudden change in pressure may have serious or even fatal consequences in such conditions as aneurysm, esophageal varices and cerebral vascular disease. It may also mobilize postoperative venous trombi with resulting pulmonary embolism. It is obvious that under these conditions the motility of the bowel must be kept in mind by the physician.

ENTERITIS

It is difficult to classify enteritis or inflammation of the bowel, for the causes are many. Some of these produce specific lesions, such as typhoid, dysentery and tuberculosis, but the majority do not. It is customary to group these nonspecific forms into catarrhal and membranous enteritis. In the former the lesions may be mild or severe, but no layer of inflammatory material is formed on the mucosal surface. The latter is characterized by a so-called pseudo-diphtheritic membrane.

Catarrhal Enteritis.—As we have already seen in the case of acute gastritis, it is small wonder that the bowel, particularly the small bowel, may become inflamed by reason of the many irritants which may reach it. *Acute enteritis* may be produced by: (1)

indigestible and irritating foods, (2) *food poisoning*, (3) *chemical poisons*, and (4) *food deficiencies*. So-called food poisoning is really due to the action of pathogenic bacteria contained in the decomposing food, the most important being *Bacillus enteritidis* (Gärtner) and the paratyphoid group. Many chemical poisons may irritate the intestine. Arsenic and mercury cause inflammation of the lower part of the ileum and most of the large bowel, apparently being excreted lower down after having been absorbed. In infective fevers, septicemia, and uremia enteritis may be present.

LESIONS.—The mucous membrane is swollen, edematous, covered with a slimy exudate, and flecked with red spots. It is seldom red throughout except in the severe inflammation produced by chemical poisons. The lymphoid follicles, particularly in children, are often swollen and the overlying mucosa may be shed off so as to form little, clear-cut shallow ulcers (follicular ulcers). *Microscopically* the change is confined to the mucosa and submucosa which are infiltrated with round cells and show marked edema. Polymorphonuclears are present in the more acute stages. The surface epithelium is degenerated, but in the intestine as in the stomach it is always difficult to separate antemortem from postmortem degenerative changes.

Pseudomembranous and Staphylococcal Enterocolitis.—The terminology here is complex, confusing, but at the same time important. Such names as pseudomembranous or membranous (diphtheritic) enteritis, staphylococcal enteritis and antibiotic enteritis are encountered in the literature. These names indicate that the small intestine is the site of election, that the characteristic lesion is the formation of a "false" membrane consisting of necrotic cells and fibrin resembling the lesion of diphtheria, that staphylococci may be concerned with the process, and that antibiotics, particularly those with a wide spectrum of action, have been incriminated. The condition has been long known under the name of diphtheritic or membranous enteritis or colitis. In 1893 Finney published a case of diphtheritic colitis ending in death fifteen days after a gastroenterostomy. Staphylococcal enteritis, on the other hand, what Finland has called staphylococcal dysentery, is a new arrival, although these cases also have been called pseudomembranous enteritis. A perusal of the literature is apt to leave the reader in a mental fog.

Perhaps the wise course at the present time is to assume that we are dealing with two distinct entities: (1) *pseudomembranous enterocolitis*, which usually but not necessarily follows abdominal operations or is associated with a state of shock; (2) *staphylococcal enteritis*, which is characterized by a similar pathological picture.

As a result of indiscriminate antibiotic therapy, especially the use of broad spectrum antibiotics such as chloromycetin, aureomycin and terramycin, resistant strains of staphylococci may invade the bowel from the nose and throat and multiply rapidly. These organisms are rarely found in the stools of normal persons, and never in large numbers. Unfortunately the incidence of resistant strains of staphylococci in the bowel is increasing as the result of broad spectrum antibiotics which displace the normal gram-negative inhabitants of the bowel. This increase is only observed in large institutions such as hospitals, where the mass effect of the newer therapy has room to operate, and where the personnel become carriers of the resistant stains.

This change in the intestinal bacterial flora is accompanied by an illness which may end fatally and which is marked by severe diarrhea together with excessive fatigue and exhaustion like that which accompanies influenza. There is an acute desquamative and membranous enterocolitis with enormous masses of hemolytic staphylococci in the exudate and membrane (Terplan). Large numbers of staphylococci are present in the stools.

There remains the group in which staphylococci do not appear to play a part. Infection is not a necessary agent for the production of the lesions, as is shown by the similarity of the histological picture in uremic and mercuric chloride enteritis. Some workers consider that the prime factor is the disturbance of the vasomotor mechanism which accompanies the state of shock (Penner and Bernheim). The dilatation of vessels in the submucosa and later the mucosa, the sub-mucosal edema and hemorrhage, may result in focal necrosis of the tips of the mucosal folds, with consequent infection and inflammation. The great difficulty is to explain the fulminating character of the clinical picture. Pettet and her associates believe that no one factor is sufficient to explain all the cases of postoperative pseudomembranous enteritis. More than one-half of their cases received no chemotherapeutic or antibiotic agents, because they occurred before the advent of these drugs. One set of factors may have been operative in the pre-antibiotic period and another set now. Baggenstoss, a member of the group, sums the matter up well in a personal communication as follows: "My own impression is that the manner in which the intestinal mucosa can react to injury is limited, and that the formation of a pseudomembrane probably represents a response to a wide variety of toxic and infectious agents."

Morbid Anatomy.—The picture at autopsy in a well-developed case is dramatic in the extreme. In large stretches of the small and often the large bowel the mucosa is covered or replaced by a yellow, gray or brown wrinkled membrane, which in the early stage is attached loosely, in the later stage more firmly, to the underlying eroded surface (Fig. 430). The segment of bowel involved is congested, atonic, and a little dilated. The *microscopic picture* corresponds to the gross appearance. The striking changes are in the mucosa and submucosa. In early cases the tips of the villi and the summits of the mucosal ridges are either necrotic or have disappeared as if they had been brushed or cut away. The mucosa in the crypts is generally not involved. In mild forms there may only be overproduction of a tenacious mucus. The mucosa is denuded in places, but is overlain by a thick layer (pseudomembrane) consisting of fibrin, necrotic cellular débris, and leukocytes. Masses of staphylococci may or may not be a feature (Fig. 431). The submucosa shows an intense hyperemia initially, followed by the development of edema and leukocytic infiltration.

The *clinical picture* is equally striking. In the postoperative cases in the course of a few days the patient rapidly develops symptoms

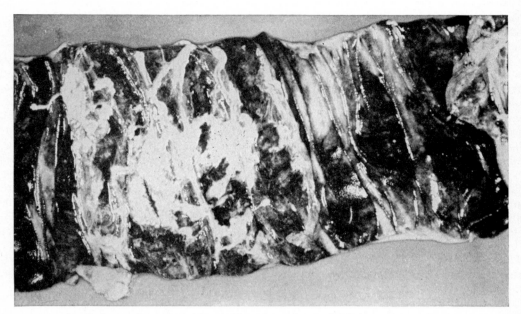

FIG. 430.—Staphylococcal enteritis. The patches of membrane (white) stand out against an intensely congested background (dark, but red in the original color). The condition developed after two and one-half days preoperative therapy with neomycin. (Boyd, *Pathology for the Physician.*)

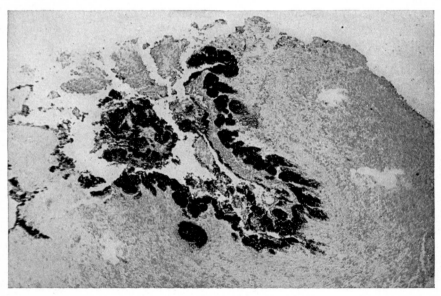

FIG. 431.—Staphylococcal enteritis. Masses of gram-positive cocci in exudate and necrotic mucosa. × 60. (Kindness of Dr. Kornel Terplan *in* Boyd, *Pathology for the Surgeon,* courtesy of W. B. Saunders Co.)

of acute circulatory collapse and irreversible shock, with death in a few hours or days; a similar picture to that of Asiatic cholera. Watery diarrhea is common, but I have seen cases where it was absent.

CHRONIC ULCERATIVE COLITIS

This chronic, distressing and intractable condition, characterized by alternating periods of exacerbations and remissions, shares with regional ileitis the distinction of being one of the most perplexing examples of an inflammatory lesion of the intestine. It is equally common in both sexes, and usually begins between twenty and forty years of age.

Etiology.—"Few diseases have been the subject of so many theories of causation and of so much research in an effort to establish the essential etiologic factor as ulcerative colitis. Despite the time and effort expended in searching for an answer to the perplexing problem, at the present writing the etiology remains competely obscure." This opening statement in the discussion on etiology in Bacon's monograph shows why the disease is often called idiopathic ulcerative colitis. The cause may be negative rather than positive in character, something lacking in the patient or the patient's bowel, possibly a food deficiency. In many cases there seems to be a strong psychogenic factor. It has been said that the sorrow which has no vent in tears may make other organs weep. Unexpressed anger and resentment may be reflected in the colon by hyperemia and hypermotility. The sufferer frequently presents an illusion of serenity: "he is actually hostile but appears sweet, anxious but calm, timid but rebellious" (Zetzel). The personality is likely to be marked by indecision, immaturity, and undue dependence on others, particularly the mother, who is apt to be dominating, if not overwhelming. It is of course possible to carry this line of thinking too far, but it is certainly safe to say that psychic trauma is often observed to precede recurrence of the signs and symptoms, and that emotional stimuli from the hypothalamic area influence the course of the disease. Treatment has to be directed to the mind as well as to the colon.

Under the best hygienic conditions the patient may recover for a time and remain well, but when he is subjected to strain, overwork and worry, the symptoms and lesions return once more. The disease is essentially chronic, continuing for years although marked by remissions and exacerbations, but occasionally it may run an acute course. In one of my cases the entire illness was of five weeks' duration, yet at autopsy the lesions were unbelievably extensive.

The *lysozyme theory* has attracted much attention. The earliest changes are in the rectum and sigmoid, spreading upward to the splenic flexure. These are the parts of the bowel supplied by the sacropelvic portion of the parasympathetic system, the remainder of the bowel being supplied by the vagus. The mucolytic enzyme, lysozyme, appears to be under nervous control and is greatly increased in amount as the result of emotional stimuli. This enzyme liquefies the mucus which normally protects the intestinal mucosa, so that excessive destruction of this protective layer will expose the mucosa to the action of bacteria and of pancreatic tryptic enzyme. In ulcerative colitis the lysozyme is enormously increased. It has been suggested that emotional stimuli from the hypothalamic area to the rectum and sigmoid cause overproduction of lysozyme with breakdown of defense and exposure of the mucosa to tryptic enzymal digestion (Portis). There is a sharp rise in the lysozyme titer in the stools during exacerbations, especially those induced by stress, resentment, etc. The trouble is that there is no proof that the increased lysozyme production has any *causal* relationship to the disease. It may just as well be an effect, a concomitant rather than a cause, reflecting the ulcerating process and serving as an index of its activity.

Morbid Anatomy.—The ulcers which form the principal lesion are usually confined to the colon and rectum. In fatal cases the entire large bowel may be covered with ulcers which vary from tiny erosions to ulcers several inches in diameter. Sometimes they are arranged along the line of the taenia coli. The ulcers are usually quite superficial, involving only the mucosa, but the muscular coat may also become necrotic, so

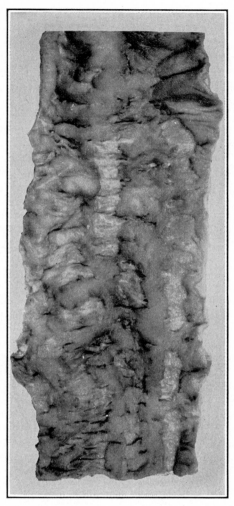

Fig. 432.—Ulcerative colitis. Ulcers are most marked along the line of the taenia coli. Pseudo-polyposis is apparent.

severe cases which have continued for several years. In one series the average duration of symptoms before the onset of cancer was 15 years. In another series carcinoma was found to be 30 times commoner than in the general population. It can be said, therefore that cancer is a very definite risk. The figures obviously have a bearing on the question of surgical treatment.

The *microscopic appearance* resembles that of chronic bacillary dysentery. At the site of the ulcer the mucosa has disappeared, but the submucosa is much thickened and infiltrated with round cells and leukocytes. The muscular coat is sometimes involved, and the peritoneum over the deep ulcers is thickened. The mucosa between the ulcers is thick, congested, and edematous. *Healing* occurs with very little scarring, so that there is no danger of stricture of the bowel.

Lesions of other organs are often found at autopsy. In some 40 per cent of cases necrotic and degenerative lesions are present in the *liver* (Kimmelstiel). These are probably metabolic in origin due to the diarrhea. In the *kidney* there may be glomerular and tubular changes (Jensen *et al.*). Glomerular endothelial proliferation is frequent and may cause obstruction to blood flow through the capillaries. Large vacuoles of undetermined nature are sometimes present in the tubular endothelium. In the *pancreas* there may be chronic interstitial inflammation, fibrosis and dilation of acini, the latter perhaps related to the marked protein deficiency (Ball *et al.*).

Relation of Symptoms to Lesions.—It takes only a cursory glance at the intestinal lesions at autopsy or seen through the sigmoidoscope to explain the distressing symptoms.

The dominant, consistant, and distressing symptom is *diarrhea*, with *blood, pus,* and *mucus in the stools,* which vary from 4 or 5 up to 30 a day. *Loss of weight* is common, and *secondary anemia* is always present. The anemia is attributed to chronic blood loss and diminished erythropoiesis secondary to chronic infection, but an auto-immune hemolytic component may sometimes be present. Secondary anemia and loss of weight are common. The roentgen rays show a hyperactive colon with loss of the normal haustrations (pipe-stem colon). With

that occasionally the base may come to be formed by the peritoneum with great danger of perforation. The intervening mucosa is often swollen and edematous so that polypoid masses project from the surface (colitis polyposa). One of these polypi may become malignant. The wall of the bowel may be very friable, so that the sigmoidoscope has to be used with care. The mesenteric lymph nodes are sometimes enlarged and inflamed. It is not possible to give exact figures as to the *risk of malignancy,* but the risk is very real. Cancer is most likely to be found in the sigmoidoscope ulcers are seen scattered over the reddened mucous membrane of the sigmoid and rectum. The ulcers are covered with mucus and bleed at the slightest touch, so that it is no wonder that blood in the stools is common. A dozen color photographs showing the varying appearance seen with the sigmoidoscope will be found in Jackman's *Lesions of the Lower Bowel.*

Exudative enteropathy may constitute a serious feature of ulcerative colitis. This is a *protein-losing gastroenteropathy* in which serum albumin is lost continuously in greater amount than it can be formed. The protein may be lost into the stomach in hypertrophic gastritis or into the large or small bowel in ulcerative colitis and regional enteritis, just as it is lost in the urine in the nephrotic syndrome. When the loss is severe the result is hypoproteinemia, it may be with generalized edema. We now have a method of determining the presence of abnormal permeability of the gastrointestinal tract to macromolecules by labelling an artificial plasma substitute, polyvinylpyrrolidone (P.V.P.) with I^{131}, and following its passage from the blood into the intestine (Gordon).

Uremic Enteritis.—In uremia there may be severe diarrhea, with purulent or bloody stools. The lesions are ulcerative and necrotizing. There are numerous ulcers in the large bowel and the lower part of the small bowel, particularly in the lymphoid tissue. The enteritis is associated in some way with urea retention, for similar lesions can be produced in dogs by the intravenous injection of urea.

REGIONAL ENTERITIS

In 1932 a nonspecific chronic inflammatory condition of the small bowel was described by Crohn and his associates under the name of regional enteritis. The site of election is the final 12 or 18 inches of the ileum, ending abruptly at the ileocecal valve (Fig. 433), so that it has been called terminal ileitis, but other segments of the small and even the large intestine may be involved. It may indeed be limited to the rectum. For this reason the term *Crohn's disease* is in some ways to be preferred. This name "avoids confusion, makes no pretence of pathological

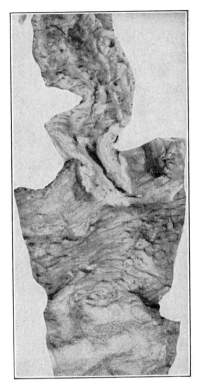

Fig. 433.—Regional enteritis ending abruptly at the ileocecal opening.

exactitude, conveys an exact meaning, is easily remembered by students, and pays a well-deserved tribute" (Armitage and Wilson). It is difficult to understand how so comparatively common a condition could have been overlooked before 1932, unless it is an example of the fact that what we don't know we don't see. Of equal importance is the fact that lesions change their names (see below).

Etiology.—Crohn's disease is as much of an etiological enigma as chronic ulcerative colitis. Almost every variety of etiological agent has been suggested, but their enumeration would be tedious as well as useless. The fact that elimination of certain foods from the diet has brought remissions may appear to support the idea of an intestinal allergy, as does an abundance of eosinophils about the lesions. Mesenteric lymphatic obstruction may play a part, with a bacterial or other agent entering the intestinal lymphat-

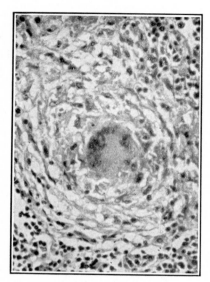

FIG. 434.—Tuberculoid lesion in Crohn's
disease.   × 192.

ics at the ileocecal angle, causing on the one hand a mesenteric lymphangitis and on the other edema and granulomatous lesions in the wall of the bowel. It has been suggested that regional enteritis, originally called terminal ileitis, and chronic ulcerative colitis are different manifestations of the same pathological process. Commenting on this idea Warren and Sommers in their valuable survey of 120 cases with 206 references to the literature remark that the two diseases are as different morphologically as are syphilis and gonorrhea. That does not rule out some element in the pathogenesis which is common to both. This element may be a psychogenic background, which is frequent in both diseases. Some writers, indeed, regard the condition as essentially a psychosomatic disorder. The patient is often frustrated for one reason or another. Emotional storms and upheavals may precede the onset of the disease and the occurrence of relapses. The patient as a rule is less dependent and more mentally mature than the victim of chronic ulcerative colitis. The histopathological changes, as we shall see, are suggestive of a reaction to irritative lipid substances, and the possibility should be borne in mind of a byproduct of some biochemical abnormality of lipid absorption.

Morbid Anatomy.—In 85 per cent of cases

the lesions are limited to the small intestine, usually the terminal ileum, where it begins abruptly at the ileocecal opening (Fig. 433). The lesions may be continuous, but often they are disconnected, although sharply delimited. The term "skip areas" signifies the alteration of areas of normal and diseased bowel. The affected part is thick and rigid like a hose-pipe, so that a correct diagnosis can often be made when the loop of bowel is taken in the hand. The mucosa presents a lumpy thickening known as the *cobblestone appearance*. The surface is usually ulcerated, and the hypertrophied mucosa between the ulcers projects in a polypoid manner, much as was seen in ulcerative colitis. The great thickening of the wall results in marked narrowing in the lumen and chronic obstruction, giving the characteristic *"string appearance"* of the terminal ileum in the x-ray film. The proximal segment of bowel is dilated. The mesentery is stiff and greatly thickened, and adhesion of the bowel to neighboring structures (bowel and abdominal wall) is followed by slow perforation and fistula formation. When I was a student I was told that this picture represented hyperplastic tuberculosis of the ileocecal region!

The *microscopic picture* is usually singularly nonspecific, consisting of marked edema of the submucosa and to a lesser degree of the other coats, together with lymphocytic infiltration and a varying degree of ulceration. The late stage of the disease at which the pathologist is likely to receive the specimen from the surgeon is probably the reason for the nonspecific character of the lesions. An early change, as Hadfield points out, is the formation of non-caseating granulomatous foci of large mononuclear phagocytes with foreign body giant cells resembling the lesions of sarcoidosis (Fig. 434). In the later stages ulceration may obscure and obliterate the primary lesion in the lamina propria or submucosa, but the giant cell systems may still be found in the regional lymph nodes. One of the most remarkable features is the patchiness of the lesions. As the disease progresses fibrosis and cicatrization dominate the picture. A curious finding is the occurrence of Brunner type glands, which probably represent a metaplasia rather than a true hyperplasia.

From what has been said it will be evident

that the over-all picture of Crohn's disease is very different from that of ulcerative colitis, although there are occasional cases in which the pathologist may be hard pressed in making the distinction. In *Crohn's disease* we appear to be dealing with a progressive sclerosing granulomatous lymphangitis, with an edematous, elephantiasis-like cicatrization of the entire thickness of the bowel wall, the mesentery and the regional lymph nodes. In *ulcerative colitis*, on the other hand, we have an exudative inflammatory condition mainly restricted in the colon to the mucosa and submucosa. It appears to be a disease of the body as a whole, with special emphasis on the colon, whereas in Crohn's disease the lesions are confined to the bowel.

Relation of Symptoms to Lesions.—The outstanding clinical features are a mass in the right iliac region, diarrhea and fever. The disease may begin with an attack like appendicitis, resembling actinomycosis of the cecum in this respect. Melena, due to bleeding from the intensely congested mucosa, is a suggestive symptom in a case of supposed appendicitis. The subacute and chronic forms are marked by recurring attacks of diarrhea with mucus in the stools, episodes of abdominal pain, and there may be vomiting. These symptoms are readily explained by the ulceration of the mucosa and the cicatrization leading to chronic obstruction. Loss of weight and of fat is marked. This becomes even more pronounced with the development of abscesses and fistulae, which must not be mistaken for those of actinomycosis of the ileocecal region. A particularly puzzling feature of the disease is the recurring nature of the attacks, with intervals of freedom. In this respect it resembles chronic ulcerative colitis. Sometimes symptoms reappear years after resection; in such a case it seems probable that the patient has suffered from a new attack of the disease rather than a recurrence from a skip area which has escaped the notice of the surgeon.

BACILLARY DYSENTERY

Dysentery, which means bowel trouble, was described by Hippocrates as a diarrhea characterized by the presence of blood and pus and accompanied by straining and tenesmus. This clinical definition by the father of medicine cannot be bettered at the present day. The laboratory, however, has shown that there are two forms of dysentery which constitute two entirely different diseases; these are bacillary dysentery and amebic dysentery. So different and distinct are these conditions that the only justification for grouping them under the heading of "dysentery" is historical usage. Bacillary dysentery has already been considered in relation to other bacillary infections in Chapter 11, page 276, so that it will not be discussed here.

AMEBIC DYSENTERY

Amebic dysentery is caused by the protozoal animal parasite, Entamoeba histolytica. The features of this ameba are considered in connection with the other parasites in Chapter 14, page 355. The lesions and clinical features will be described here.

The disease is gradual in onset and more protracted in its course than the bacillary form, sometimes lasting for months or years. The incubation period varies from ten to ninety days. Although primarily a disease of the tropics there is a growing incidence of infestation with the parasite in temperate regions, and serious localized epidemics are becoming more common. These can usually be traced to cooks and other handlers of food (in hotels, etc.) who are either *carriers* of the ameba or suffer from the disease in a mild form. An infected water supply is another source of danger. The parasite may be present in two forms, one active or ameboid (trophozoite), the other encysted. The latter is developed when conditions for growth are not favorable, and is the only infective form, for the active form is destroyed by the HCl as it passes through the stomach.

LESIONS.—When a cyst is swallowed in food or water it breaks up in the lower part of the small bowel and liberates a single ameba with 4 nuclei. These divide into 8, and 8 small amebae are formed. When they reach the large bowel they penetrate the lumen of the glands and, destroying the epithelium with which they come in contact by proteolytic enzymes, they penetrate the deeper tissues. No lesion is produced in the bowel unless the amebae colonize actively; they merely enter the portal venules and to a lesser extent the lymphatics. If they colonize in the submucosa, the result is dysentery. The parasites spread out in this coat and set up a colliquative necrosis by virtue of the proteolytic ferment which they produce. All this is quite different from bacillary dysentery where the organisms remain on the surface and by means of their diffusible toxins excite a suppurative inflammation instead of a quiet necrosis in the underlying tissue. The mucosa overlying the necrotic areas also dies and is cast off as a slough, so that ragged ulcers are formed. These ulcers have deeply undermined edges, because the submucosa is more extensively involved than the mucosa. The mucosa between the ulcers appear remarkably healthy because no diffusible toxin is at work. The ulcers are deeper than in the bacillary form, and the floor is often formed by the thickened peritoneum.

In a carrier the parasite is present in the active, not the encysted form. As the amebae in the stools contain intracellular red blood cells, it would appear that they have caused lesions in the carrier, although these have given rise to no symptoms. The state of equilibrium of the carrier may be disturbed at any time by factors which are largely unknown, but which apparently are more prevalent in tropical and subtropical areas than in temperate zones. Such disturbance of the state of equilibrium results in a pathological process which adversely affects the host and incidentally the parasite as well.

The *microscopic picture* is one of quiet necrosis with little or no inflammation. Large numbers of amebæ can be seen in the wall of the bowel. They digest the surrounding tissue by means of their proteolytic ferment, so that they frequently lie in small spaces, but they appear to excite comparatively little reaction. Any inflammatory cells in the floor of the ulcer are mononuclear in type. At a later date secondary infection may occur and this may cause some suppuration. The amebae penetrate the portal venules and can be seen within the lumen, so that they readily pass to the liver.

Liver abscess is thus a common complication of amebic dysentery. Although the lesion is commonly known as solitary abscess, it is multiple in over 50 per cent of the cases, being more frequent in the right lobe. There may be a few large or numerous small abscesses. The lesions are really not true abscesses, but are formed by the liquefaction necrosis of the liver cells produced by the digestive ferment of the amebae. The abscess may rupture into the abdominal cavity, or through the diaphragm into the lung, the patient expectorating a brown "anchovy sauce" material containing many amebae.

BACILLARY AND AMEBIC DYSENTERY COMPARED.—The chief symptom of dysentery—diarrhea with blood, mucus and pus in the stools—is the same in both forms. Bacteriological and immunological tests are of value in differentiating the two forms, but a rapid and useful method is the cytological examination of the stools, the type of cell depending on the histological reaction in the lesions. It will be remembered that there are three types of necrosis: lysis, pyknosis, and karyorrhexis. In *bacillary* infections cellular lysis is marked, the result being "ghost cells" from the macrophages and "ring nuclei" from the polymorphonuclear leukocytes. About 90 per cent of the cells are polymorphonuclears, but this loses its value from the fact that when amebic lesions become secondarily infected the exudates may be purulent. The most important cells are the macrophages and their ghost forms. Unfortunately these may bear a striking resemblance to amebae, and be a cause of mistaken diagnosis except in the hands of an expert, as happened in the epidemics both at Gallipoli and on Corregidor. In pure amebic infections the cells are few in number and are mainly mononuclears. They present either a "mouse-eaten" appearance due to the action of the digestive enzyme on parts of the cytoplasm or "pyknotic bodies" from the nuclear fragments. Large numbers of red blood cells are always present in addition to the amebae. Charcot-Leyden crystals are characteristic of amebic dysentery, and are not found in the bacillary form.

Some of the principal points in which bacillary differs from amebic dysentery are summarized as follows:

with Bacillus typhosus has been considered in Chapter 11 on bacillary infections, page 272.

	Bacillary dysentery	*Amebic dysentery*
1. Type of lesion	Suppurative	Necrotic
2. Depth of ulcer	Generally shallow	Generally deep
3. Edge of ulcer	Sharp	Undermined
4. Intervening mucosa	Inflamed	Normal
5. Organisms in lesions	Bacillus dysenteriæ	Entamœba histolytica
6. Cytology of stools	Polymorphonuclears	Mononuclears
7. Liver abscess	Rare	Common

TYPHOID FEVER

Typhoid or enteric fever is considered in this place for purposes of convenience. But, unlike both forms of dysentery, it is in no sense a disease of the intestine. It is true that intestinal ulcers are the rule, and that mishaps connected with these ulcers are a frequent cause of death. But for all that these lesions are merely incidental; the true basis of the disease lies elsewhere.

Little need be said regarding the clinical side of the disease. "Any fever lasting over a period of days, accompanied by malaise, headache, insomnia and diarrhea, ushered in by chill and nose-bleed, particularly when unaccompanied by definitely localizing symptoms, except possibly pain on epigastric pressure or sore throat, may be suspected of being typhoid fever. If the fever is at first marked by afternoon exacerbations with gradual rise, and is followed in a few days by a more continuous fever, with persistent abdominal symptoms and a stuporous condition, if the spleen becomes palpable and rose spots appear, the diagnosis becomes more assured" (Gay). Acute and subacute endocarditis and general miliary tuberculosis may closely simulate the disease and must always be kept in mind. Any or all of the usual symptoms may be absent. Indeed, a person may suffer from typhoid infection and yet manifest no symptoms of the disease. Such a person may become a carrier, though quite unaware that he has suffered from this infection.

For these reasons the subject of infection

CHOLERA

At the present day cholera is almost entirely a disease of tropical countries. It is caused by the spirillum of Koch, which is transmitted by water or by food. Although it is essentially an acute inflammation of the intestinal canal, it has no relation to the other forms of enteritis and colitis described in this place. For this reason it has been discussed in Chapter 11 on bacterial infections, page 278.

TUBERCULOSIS

The infection is usually secondary to pulmonary tuberculosis. Before the days of pasteurization of milk primary infection due to drinking tuberculous milk from infected cows was very common, particularly in children. The secondary type of lesion is due to massive infection from sputum which has been swallowed. A few bacilli do not seem to produce a recognizable lesion. For this reason the condition is usually associated with the presence of large cavities. Ulceration of the bowel is the commonest complication of pulmonary tuberculosis, and is found in from 50 to 80 per cent of the cases which come to autopsy; but it is by no means only a terminal occurrence.

The method of infection appears to be as follows: a massive dose of bacilli is swallowed and the organisms pass into the tubular glands of the intestinal mucosa, where an inflammatory exudate is produced in the depths of the gland. The bacilli are then

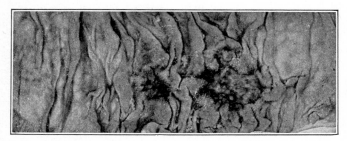

Fig. 435.—Tuberculosis of the bowel. There are two shallow tuberculous ulcers.

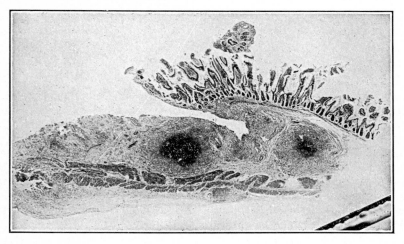

Fig. 436.—Tuberculous ulcer of bowel showing undermined edge and areas of
necrosis in the base.   × 15.

carried through the epithelial lining by phagocytic cells, and thus reach the submucosa where they give rise to the usual tuberculous lesions. The overlying mucosa may now be cast off with the formation of an ulcer, or it may remain intact so that the bowel may be tuberculous though not an ulcer can be seen. The bacilli may be carried from the submucosal lesion to the mesenteric lymph nodes which drain that segment of the bowel, and there produce caseous lesions. Mesenteric lymph node tuberculosis indicates intestinal tuberculosis but not necessarily intestinal ulceration.

Morbid Anatomy.—The first lesions appear in the ileocecal region, although at autopsy they may be scattered over a wide area. From this site of election the disease spreads up and down. As is usual with tuberculosis, the earliest lesions are in the lymphoid tissue and appear as small gray tubercles in the Peyer's patches and solitary follicles, which become yellow from caseation, soften, and break down (Fig. 435). The overlying mucosa undergoes necrosis and is cast off, the underlying caseous tissue is discharged, and an *ulcer* with ragged undermined edges is formed (Fig. 436). In the small bowel the ulcer may extend as far as the peritoneum, but in the large bowel it is shallower and seldom penetrates the muscularis. Small tubercles can be seen on the serous coat, or they may be covered up by a plastic exudate. The overlying peritoneum is usually thickened so that perforation is uncommon. The ulcer is supposed to spread transversely across the bowel (girdle ulcer), but quite often it lies in the long axis, especially when it is confined to a Peyer's patch. The *mesenteric lymph nodes* are enlarged and may be caseous. Extension of the inflammation outside the bowel leads to *adhesions*, and these by contracting produce acute *kinks* of the bowel which are a common cause of intestinal obstruction. The *microscopic picture* is one of tuberculous foci with epithelioid cells and lymphocytes, giant cells, and caseation (Fig. 437). Endarteritis obliterans is common, and this usually prevents a large hemorrhage from occurring.

Healing is common, especially with modern methods of treatment. The mucosa may be completely restored when the ulcer is shallow, and even deep ulcers become filled with granulation tissue and covered by a simple epithelium. But when destruction of tissue is extensive, cicatrization is correspondingly great, and if the ulcer is of the girdle type stenosis may result. These strictures are often multiple. Serious obstruction is much more likely to be due to kinks of the bowel produced by adhesions than to cicatrical stenosis, but in the primary lesions seen in children the cicatrices may lead to a marked degree of obstruction.

Perforation of a tuberculous ulcer may be complete or incomplete. *Complete* perforation in the general peritoneal cavity occurs in the small intestine where the ulcers are deeper, but it is not common owing to the thickening of the peritoneum. *Incomplete* perforation, which is much commoner, is seen in the large bowel, especially in the right iliac fossa, where it gives rise to a fecal abscess walled off by dense adhesions.

Relation of Symptoms to Lesions.—The symptoms are general and local. The general symptoms are those of pulmonary tuberculosis, *i.e.*, loss of weight, asthenia, etc. Every case of pulmonary tuberculosis which does poorly but with no increase in the physical signs should suggest intestinal ulceration. The *local symptoms* are abdominal pain, diarrhea, and the presence of pus and blood in the stools.

The *general symptoms* bear no relation to the lesions. The *pain* is not caused by the ulcers, for these are insensitive. It is due to spasm of the bowel, involvement of the peritoneum, or tuberculous lymphadenitis. The *diarrhea* is related to the hypermotility of the bowel which forms a striking feature of the roentgen-ray picture rather than to the ulceration. The hypermotility seems to depend in turn on inflammatory and de-

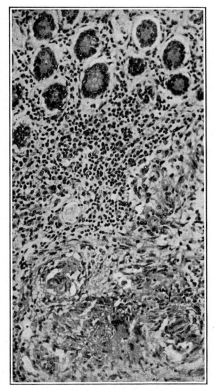

FIG. 437.—Tuberculosis of bowel. × 100.

generative lesions of the myenteric plexus of Auerbach. The site of the disease is also related to the diarrhea; lesions of the small bowel are generally associated with constipation, those of the large bowel and especially the descending colon with diarrhea. *Occult blood* in the stools and *pus* in small amount are due to the intestinal ulceration.

ACTINOMYCOSIS

Actinomycosis of the bowel usually occurs in the cecum or appendix, but occasionally in the pelvic colon. A mass of granulation tissue is formed in the submucosa, followed by ulceration of the mucous membrane. Suppuration occurs and the mass is converted into a nest of abscesses. The disease may spread to the abdominal wall with the formation of a sinus from which pus is discharged containing the characteristic sulfur granules in which the ray fungus is readily

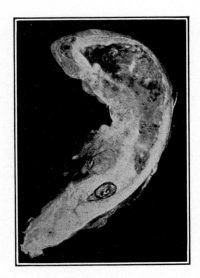

Fig. 438.—The obstructive element in acute appendicitis. Fibrous stenosis of proximal end, dilatation and thinning of distal half, and occlusion of lumen by fecalith.

demonstrated. The liver may become involved by way of the portal vein, and is eventually riddled with abscesses. Actinomycosis of the cecum is apt to be mistaken clinically for carcinoma.

ACUTE APPENDICITIS

The vermiform or worm-like appendix acts as a second stomach in some herbivora, but it has no known function in man and must therefore be regarded as a vestigial organ, albeit a very troublesome one. The mucosa and submucosa contain a remarkable abundance of lymphoid tissue, especially in the young in whom definite germinal follicles can be seen. With advancing years this lymphoid tissue undergoes atrophy and finally vanishes. The appendix may be enveloped in congenital fibrous bands, which may produce torsion or kinking of the organ. These structural features are mentioned because the symptoms of what the clinician vaguely refers to as "chronic appendicitis" may be caused by swelling of the lymphoid tissue or by distension of the lumen of the kinked appendix by feces or gas without any accompanying inflammation.

Etiology.—The etiological factors are exciting and predisposing. The two great *exciting* factors are obstruction and infection. It is becoming more and more apparent that the former is the dominant factor.

There is a sphincter-like mechanism at the base of the appendix which makes it a potential closed loop, and is probably responsible for the formation of concretions. Obstruction, then, may be caused not only by the easily recognized concretion (Fig. 438), but by contraction of the sphincter, as well as by swelling of the abundant lymphoid tissue in the wall, previous fibrosis of the proximal end, acute kinking by a band of old adhesions or by a congenital fold. Wangensteen and Bowers found obstruction in 72 per cent of cases of acute suppurative appendicitis and in 100 per cent of gangrenous appendicitis (80 per cent concretions). In most cases, then, obstruction seems to be a much more important initial factor than infection. The acute attack has been likened to a knock at the door saying, "Let me out." As the result of obstruction the lumen becomes distended, the intraluminal pressure increased and the venous return interfered with, so that the vessels rupture, hemorrhage occurs, the wall is poorly oxygenated and invaded by bacteria, the swelling increases, and perforation is the end-result. There is no doubt that a blow on the abdominal wall may occasionally precipitate an acute attack of appendicitis. As might be expected, mild cases are much more likely to have had multiple attacks, because the obstruction is slight and is overcome spontaneously, so that the patient can go on to another attack. The severe (gangrenous) cases have few previous attacks, because the obstruction can only be overcome by perforation of the appendix; it is natural that fecaliths causing complete obstruction should be common in these cases.

The infecting organisms appear to invade the mucosa from the lumen. They are probably the normal inhabitants of the appendix. Streptococci and E. coli are most commonly found, often in combination. The streptococcus is probably the chief infective agent, for the inflammation tends to spread throughout the organ in the same manner as streptococcal infections elsewhere. It is

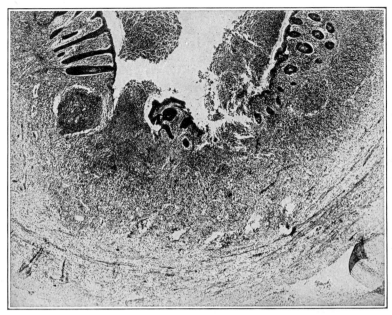

Fɪɢ. 439.—Acute appendicitis.   Small mucosal abscess rupturing into the lumen.   × 26.

probable that in exceptional cases infection may be by the blood stream, as when acute appendicitis occurs in the course of acute tonsillitis or septic sore throat.

The *predisposing causes* are indefinite. The disease is commonest in the second and third decades; it is rare in infancy and old age. Previous damage to the appendix with fibrosis predisposes to future attacks. The disease is common in highly civilized countries and urban communities, but rare in remote rural districts and among primitive peoples. Natives who live on a diet abundant in cellulose are immune from the disease, but when they adopt the diet of civilization they lose that immunity. The urgent gangrenous type of appendicitis is confined to meat-eating peoples.

Morbid Anatomy.—Acute inflammation of the appendix may take a variety of forms. It may be mild with correspondingly mild symptoms, a condition to which the clinician is fond of applying the quite unjustifiable term *catarrhal appendicitis*. A patient may suffer from a succession of mild attacks, and it is to these recurring attacks that the clinician applies his favorite name of *chronic appendicitis*. In other cases the inflammation is severe and purulent. These may be called *acute suppurative appendicitis*. Gangrene may be present, particularly when there is an element of obstruction; these are cases of *gangrenous appendicitis*.

In *acute suppurative appendicitis* the infection seems to begin at the bottom of one of the crypts, where a small focus of suppuration is formed in the mucosa (Fig. 439). The organisms apparently do not readily spread through the mucosa, because that coat may be apparently normal apart from one or two points of abscess formation although the rest of the appendix is acutely inflamed. The spread takes place in the loose submucosa, and from there through the muscularis along the line of the penetrating vessels to the subserous coat, where it again becomes diffuse. In looking for evidence of inflammation, therefore, attention should be directed to the submucous and subserous layers. By the time the appendix is removed the muscularis and peritoneal surface are usually also inflamed.

The appendix is swollen and elongated, bright red in color, with dilated subperitoneal vessels and a fibrinous or purulent exudate (sometimes very slight) on the surface.

There may be yellow spots on the surface indicating the beginning of an abscess. The tip is usually swollen, and the whole process is likely to be more marked in the distal than the proximal part. When the appendix is opened the mucosa is seen to be swollen and very congested. The surface is granular or warty. Superficial erosions are common, but there may also be ulcers which penetrate to the submucous coat and sometimes to the peritoneum. The lumen may be narrowed owing to swelling of the mucosa, but if that layer is destroyed it may be dilated and filled with pus.

Microscopically all the coats are congested, edematous, and infiltrated with polymorphonuclear leukocytes, but the mucous membrane may show little or no infiltration. The normal cellularity of this membrane makes it difficult to be certain of slight changes in the number and kind of cells. Eosinophils may be very abundant, especially when the acuteness of the inflammation is passing off. Necrosis of the mucosa is common, and masses of dead membrane may be cast off, thus forming ulcers especially at the points where the lymph follicles approach the surface. There may be hemorrhages in the mucosa which often leave a permanent pigmentation. The mesentery of the appendix shares in the inflammation, being thickened, edematous, and infiltrated with polymorphonuclear leukocytes. Thrombosis of the vessels may occasionally give rise to abscess formation in the liver (portal pyemia).

Gangrenous appendicitis is one variety of acute suppurative appendicitis. There is death and putrefaction of the tissues of the appendix due to interference with the blood supply. The gangrene is often local, appearing as a green or black patch at the distal end, often at the tip. A concretion which is sometimes quite hard is often found at the site of gangrene, and has no doubt played an etiological part by pressing on the stretched and inflamed wall.

Perforation may occur at any stage of acute appendicitis, but is commonly associated with gangrene. The ulceration of the mucosa already described may penetrate the muscular and serous coats causing perforation. A fecal concretion is often present at the site of the perforation, and evidently plays a part in its production. It may escape into the abdominal cavity. If the perforation occurs into the open peritoneal cavity *general peritonitis* will at once be caused by the flooding of the membrane with septic material. Often, however, the inflamed part of the appendix is surrounded by a layer of omentum which becomes adherent to it before perforation has time to occur. In this case a *local appendicular abscess* will be formed, and there may be no infection of the general peritoneal cavity. The abscess may involve the anterior abdominal wall, and when it is opened a *fecal fistula* may result, through which fecal matter is discharged from the appendix on to the abdominal wall. If the appendix hangs down into the pelvis the result will be an acute *pelvic appendicitis*. In the occasional case the distal end of the inflamed appendix becomes adherent to the bladder wall, with abscess formation, rupture into the bladder, and the production of an *appendiceal-vesical fistula*, with the passage of gas and feces in the urine.

Healing occurs as the acute process subsides. The tissue which has been destroyed will be replaced by fibrous tissue. In this way the entire mucosa may become converted into a fibrous mass with obliteration of the lumen. The submucosa and to a lesser extent the muscularis may also be fibrosed. In addition to the fibrosis, vascular dilatation and collections of inflammatory cells may be observed for a period varying from a few weeks to two or three months. These merely represent the aftermath of acute inflammation, and must not be taken as an indication of chronic inflammation.

Relation of Symptoms to Lesions.—Apart from fever and leukocytosis which are due to the infection, the chief symptoms are nausea, vomiting, and local pain and tenderness. In acute appendicitis the hyperemia and inflammatory exudate cause distention of the organ with stretching of the sympathetic plexus which lies in the outer part of the wall. The stimuli pass to the semilunar ganglia and give rise to nausea, vomiting, and general abdominal pain. The inflammation soon reaches the serous coat, and the inflammation of the

PLATE X

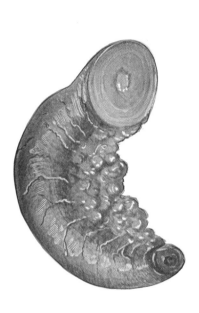 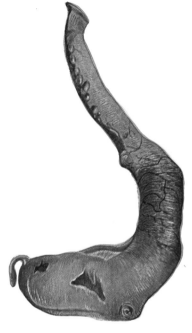

FIG. 1   FIG. 2

Fig. 1.—Carcinoid Tumor of Appendix Showing the Characteristic Yellow Ring.

Fig. 2.—Gangrenous Appendicitis. The Distal Third is Gangrenous, and is About to Perforate at the Lower Border.

(Boyd's Surgical Pathology, courtesy of W. B. Saunders Company.)

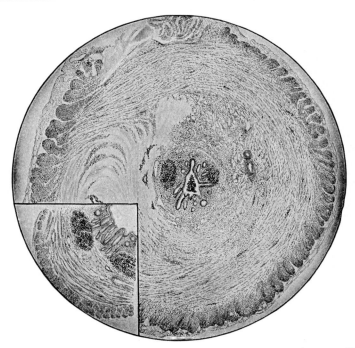

FIG. 440.—Fibroses of appendix; inset shows normal thickness of coats. (Boyd, *Pathology for the Surgeon*, courtesy of W. B. Saunders Co.)

parietal peritoneum is the cause of the local pain and rigidity. The local symptoms are more severe and more sudden in onset when acute obstruction is a marked feature, because the distention of the appendix is much greater. In the most severe and fulminating cases the local symptoms may be slight except at the very beginning, because the rapidly developing gangrene soon destroys the sympathetic nerve endings. The relation of the symptoms to the lesions in such complications as fecal fistula and appendiceal-vesical fistula is self-evident.

Chronic Appendicitis.—Chronic inflammation of the appendix is rare, despite the fact that it used to be a favorite surgical diagnosis, and indeed still is with some surgeons. It is not easy for the pathologist to recognize chronic inflammation. The appendix is thickened and fibrosed, and the wall infiltrated with mononuclear cells, particularly in the subserosa, and often associated with large lymphoid follicles. The great majority of the appendices labelled as showing chronic appendices are really examples of healing after a mild acute attack. In fact to many

it is doubtful if there is such an entity as chronic appendicitis in the sense of a slowly progressive inflammation without acute exacerbations.

No pathologist is in a position to answer with certainty the question often asked of him by the surgeon as to whether certain fibrotic changes could account for the symptoms complained of by the patient. He may well feel that the fibrotic and other changes are wholly inadequate to explain the symptoms ascribed to them. Removal of the appendix affords relief for a few weeks, largely because the patient is kept in bed, but when he returns home the abdominal discomfort soon returns and the operation is as unsatisfactory to the surgeon as to the patient.

The Obliterated Appendix.—Obliteration of the lumen of the appendix may be the result of: (1) former attacks of acute inflammation, (2) a physiological atrophy involving primarily the lymph follicles (appendicitis obliterans), and (3) hyperplasia of neuromuscular tissue in the wall.

Healing or subsiding appendicitis has al-

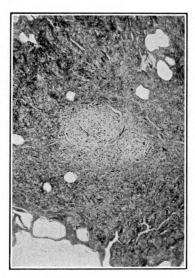

FIG. 441.—Neurinoma in fibrosed appendix.
(Masson's trichrome stain.)   × 50.

ready been discussed. When the appendix has been the scene of one or more acute attacks of inflammation there is a varying degree of replacement of the parenchyma by fibrous tissue, most marked in the submucous and subserous coats, leading to extreme narrowing or even complete obliteration of the lumen (Fig. 440).

Physiological atrophy is the condition which is wrongly named *appendicitis obliterans*. It is certainly not due to inflammation, being merely a premature abiotrophy similar to that which affects all structures of lymphoid character at succeeding stages in the journey through life, or the graying of the hair which may occur at an early age. The withered appendix, which is very firm, is atrophic and shrunken, sometimes to the dimensions of a piece of stout string. On section the appendix is seen to consist of two layers, an outer muscular layer, and an inner fibrous mass which includes what was once mucosa, submucosa and lumen. Perhaps this early senescence should not surprise us in an organ which we have already seen to be vestigial.

Neuromuscular hyperplasia involves the neuromuscular complex of Masson. In the infant plain muscle bundles accompanied by the nerves of Meissner's plexus can be seen to pass inward from the circular muscle coat and outward from the muscularis mucosae to anastomose in the submucosa and form a "neuromuscular complex." In the adult the presence of lymph follicles makes this arrangement less easily detected. Sometimes the submucosa shows a remarkable hypertrophy of the neuromuscular complex. The mucosa may also be thickened, and may contain numbers of small circumscribed neuromas (neurinomas). These are much more frequent than neuromuscular hyperplasia (Fig. 441). It has been claimed that these changes give rise to what has been termed "neurogenic appendicitis", but up to the present the evidence has not been convincing.

MISCELLANEOUS LESIONS OF APPENDIX

Before leaving the appendix one or two lesions of minor importance may be considered briefly.

Mucocele.—Mucocele of the appendix is a condition in which stenosis of the proximal part results in distention of the distal part with clear mucinous fluid to form a cyst. In rare cases the mucocele may be the starting point of *pseudomyxoma peritonei*, rupture of the cyst being followed by implantation of epithelial cells on the peritoneal surface, and the formation of large mucoid masses like frog's spawn.

Measles.—If the appendix happens to be removed in the prodromal stage of measles peculiar giant cells may be found in the germ centers of the lymphoid tissue of the appendix, and in the regional lymph nodes (Fig. 189, page 340). These cells may be 100 microns in diameter, and contain from 50 to 100 nuclei. They are similar to the cells first described by Warthin in the tonsil in the prodromal stage of measles, and are therefore known as Warthin cells. They represent a reaction to the measles virus, for monkeys injected with blood from measles patients show giant cells in the lymph nodes (Gordon and Knighton). Should the pathologist once in a lifetime (or less often) have the good fortune to encounter this lesion, he can surprise the surgeon by informing him that the patient is about to develop a measles rash.

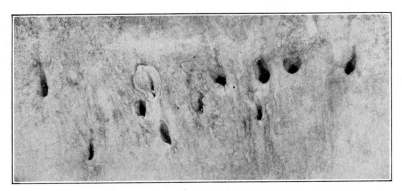

Fig. 442.—Intestinal diverticulosis, showing the openings of the diverticula on the mucosal surface.

Foreign Bodies.—In the diseased appendix it is common to find foreign bodies, which may simulate all kinds of familiar objects such as grape seeds, cherry stones, etc. It used to be commonly supposed that the stones of various fruits found frequent lodgment in the appendix, where they acted as the exciting cause of atttacks of acute inflammation. It is now known that these are of the rarest occurrence, although it is true that many curious objects may find their way into the appendix. Pins, bristles, grains of corn, even small shot have been found in the appendix, but in many cases the appendix may be quite normal. *Oxyuris vermicularis* is a common finding in children, but these worms seldom excite a pathological reaction. The common foreign bodies are fecal concretions. Some of these are as hard as stone, and it is they which were formerly mistaken for the stones of fruit. The formation of a concretion is favored by stenosis of the proximal end of the tube. The prominent part which an impacted concretion may play in the production of an acute attack of appendicitis has already been emphasized.

Tumors.—Tumors of the appendix, both benign and malignant, are remarkably rare. To this statement there is one notable exception, namely *carcinoid tumor*. Although this tumor is relatively frequent in the appendix, it is of low malignancy and importance in comparison with the less frequent carcinoid of the intestine. It will therefore be considered in connection with intestinal neoplasms.

INTESTINAL DIVERTICULA

Diverticula of the intestine usually occur in the duodenum and the lower part of the colon, but they may be met with in any part of the intestinal canal. Duodenal diverticula have already been described. The usual age period is in middle and late life. They are rare before the age of thirty years. In the small intestine they lie in the concavity of the bowel along the line of the mesenteric attachment, as the entering vessels serve to weaken the muscular wall. In the colon they are situated on the convexity, usually in two rows between the taenia coli. The commonest site is the sigmoid, but they usually stop abruptly at the commencement of the rectum, because here the taenia coli separate out into a broad muscular sheet. Occasionally diverticula occur in the rectum.

The diverticulum is a protrusion or herniation of the mucosa and submucosa through the muscular coat at some point of weakness. Diverticula may be present in great numbers, a condition of *diverticulosis*. The usual size is that of a large pea. The opening into the lumen of the bowel may be very small or wide and gaping (Fig. 442). In the small intestine the contents are fluid, but in the colon they are fecal and sometimes in the form of concretions.

The *cause* of the condition is uncertain. As in the case of aneurysm, there is probably a combination of weakness of the wall and increased pressure from within. The weakness seems to be due to the loss of tone and

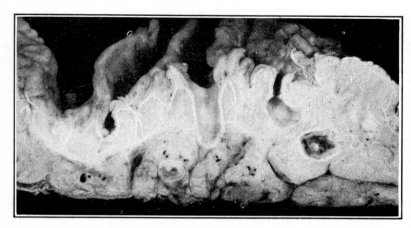

FIG. 443.—Multiple diverticula of bowel with peridiverticular fibrosis.

elasticity of muscle which is characteristic of the degenerative period of life.

Diverticulitis.—The condition of diverticulosis is unattended by symptoms, and is often discovered accidentally by the radiologist. But if inflammation occurs in the diverticula, symptoms will be produced. This is very rare in the small intestine where the contents are fluid and readily pass out of the diverticula, but it is fairly common in the colon. Fraser remarks that "in the Century and Oxford dictionaries a diverticulum is described as a 'way-side shelter or lodging,' with, from the context, the underlying meaning that they are houses of ill repute where trouble is apt to brew. In the large intestine they live up to their bad reputation, and as a temporary lodging for bowel contents can give rise to endless trouble." *Acute inflammation* often associated with the presence of a hard concretion in the diverticulum is similar to appendicitis, except that the symptoms are usually on the left side. Perforation may occur, with local abscess formation or general peritonitis.

Chronic inflammation is much commoner, and is accompanied by a *peridiverticulitis.* Toxins apparently leak through the mucosa and set up a chronic extramucosal inflammation, as a result of which a large amount of chronic inflammatory tissue is formed on the outside of the bowel (Fig. 443). This consists of granulation tissue which becomes converted into dense fibrous tissue. A large

mass is formed which may constrict the bowel and cause stenosis, so that it is readily mistaken for carcinoma even when the abdomen is opened. The diverticula may be completely covered up by the inflammatory mass. When the excised bowel is opened it may be impossible to detect the inner openings of the diverticula, as they may be hidden by the swollen mucosa. If thin slices are cut tangential to the outer surface of the mass the blind ends of the diverticula are exposed, and a probe can readily be passed through into the lumen of the bowel. On examining the gross specimen it may be difficult to decide if the condition is diverticulitis or carcinoma. A point of value is that in the former the mucosa is practically never ulcerated, while in cancer ulceration is almost always present.

Meckel's Diverticulum.—In about 3 per cent of cases the vitelline duct passing from the intestine to the umbilicus fails to become obliterated. If both ends are closed but not the middle portion, the result is a cyst. As a rule only the proximal part remains open and forms a pouch-like projection from the lower part of the ileum, usually within 2 feet of the ileocecal junction. This is known as Meckel's diverticulum. It may be a mere dimple, or may constitute a fistula which opens on the umbilicus. The proximal part may remain open and be continued to the umbilicus as a fibrous cord. A loop of bowel may be forced around this cord and becomes strangulated. Sometimes the diverticulum becomes acutely inflamed, with symptoms identical with those of appendicitis. It is a common cause of intussusception in children, the diverticulum becoming turned inside out. In a certain proportion of cases (12 to 44 per cent according to different authors) islands of gastric mucosa are found in the diverticulum. These produce gastric juice, as a result of which *peptic ulcer* may occur. This may cause *severe hemorrhage* from the bowel (especially in male children) or perforation. The dangers inherent in a Meckel's diverticulum are, therefore, three-fold, namely hemorrhage, inflammation and obstruction. Occasionally the diverticulum may contain pancreatic tissue.

ENTEROGENOUS CYSTS.—These are derived from diverticula of the intestine in which the communication with the bowel has been pinched off.

Intestinal structures, both epithelial and muscular, can often be demonstrated in the wall of the cyst.

MALABSORPTION SYNDROMES

The assimilation of foodstuffs into the body fluid takes place in two stages, namely digestion and absorption. *Digestion* depends on the presence of enzymes and other substances necessary for converting larger molecules into simpler material which can be readily absorbed by the small intestine. This depends on the normal and integrated function of the stomach, hepato-biliary system, pancreas and small intestine. Gross disease of any of these structures will cause a *secondary malabsorption syndrome*, the chief defect being in the absorption of fat. We shall encounter an example of secondary malabsorption in the case of partial occlusion of the superior mesenteric artery. The first step in the digestion of fat depends on the emulsifying action of bile, so that obstruction of the bile ducts is likely to lead to *steatorrhea*, the passage of fat in the stools. The next step is the addition of pancreatic lipase to the emulsified mixture, so that obstruction of the pancratic duct by stone or tumor may cause steatorrhea, and so may chronic pancreatitis. Malabsorption of fat may also be due to decreased absorption surface of the small bowel from extensive surgical resec-

tion, short circuiting operations, etc., inflammatory or neoplastic lesions of the small bowel as in regional ileitis and malignant lymphoma, or to abnormal bacterial flora causing increased mucus and decreased motility.

Absorption depends on (1) an adequate surface of intestinal mucosa available for absorption, (2) normally functioning mucosal cells, and (3) sufficient transit time through the small bowel to allow the absorption of nutriment to take place. In the absence of gross disease of the stomach, liver, bile ducts, pancreas or small intestine a defect in absorption gives rise to a *primary maladsorption syndrome*. The *chief defect* is in the *absorption of fat*, so that the outstanding symptom is steatorrhea, the stools being frequent, unformed, bulky, pale and greasy so that they float, and give off an unforgettable stench. The character of the stool is summed up vividly by the remark of the patient who said that his bowels moved once a day "but when they move it fills a bucket and drives everyone out of the house." The chief examples of primary malabsorption syndromes are (1) sprue, (2) idiopathic steatorrhea or celiac disease, and (3) intestinal lipodystrophy or Whipple's disease.

In the *primary malabsorption syndromes* the defect appears to be in the mucosal cells of the small intestine. Autopsy studies of the bowel are of little use, but the modern technique of jejunal biopsy shows blunting and atrophy of the intestinal villi to be a constant feature of idiopathic steatorrhea, although the cause of this change remains obscure. The condition may represent a genetically transmitted metabolic disorder. Celiac disease is often familial, and steatorrhea developing in adult life, as a tropical sprue, may represent a latent tendency to malabsorption which becomes overt owing to nutritional or environmental factors. It is now possible to follow the absorption of neutral fat by tagging it with radioactive iodine.

Sprue.—This was the first of the malabsorption syndromes to be described. It is sometimes called primary or idiopathic sprue in order to distinguish it from a secondary steatorrhea due to one of the causes outlined above. The word itself means thrush, and was applied in the 17th century because of the mouth lesions. The disease was first recognized in a severe tropical form, a less severe non-tropical variety being described later.

Tropical sprue is seen in the Orient, in the tropics, and to a minor degree in the southern United States, regions where the diet of the poor tends to be uniform and monotonous, restricted in amount, and low in protein. The disease is of insidious onset, with at first abdominal distention, flatulence, and epigastric pain, all made worse by eating, whilst later developments are glossitis and aphthous stomatitis (thrush), together with watery, frothy, foul-smelling and imperative steatorrhea, a condition readily mistaken for ulcerative colitis. The normal daily volume of feces is 100 to 200 ml., but in steatorrhea it may increase to 500 or 1000 ml. or even more. The increasing soreness of the mouth results in a very poor food intake, and this contributes to the progressive cachexia. The impairment of fat absorption is accompanied by defective absorption of the fat-soluble vitamins, A, K and D. A profound anemia may develop, and this may be due to impaired absorption of the hematopoietic vitamin, B_{12}. The administration of this vitamin not only produces a dramatic improvement in the blood, but seems to ameliorate the defective absorption of fat in the intestine. Carbohydrates are poorly absorbed, and the frothy character of the stool is due to fermentation of unabsorbed carbohydrate. It takes only a little sugar to make a lot of gas.

Non-tropical sprue is a less severe form of the disease, which appears to represent a disturbance in the dynamics of the intestinal mucosa, perhaps a primary defect in the phosphorylation of fats and sugars. The antianemia principle improves the anemia, but without any effect on the steatorrhea. This suggests a difference in the pathogenesis of tropical and non-tropical sprue.

Morbid Anatomy.—The *gross lesions* found at autopsy both in tropical and nontropical sprue are disappointing in comparison with the severity of the clinical picture. At most there are varying degrees of atrophy and thinning of the intestinal wall. The normal slightly velvety mucosal surface, however,

may be smooth and grayish-tan. *Microscopically* a jejunal biopsy shows widening and blunting of the villi, which must markedly diminish the absorptive area of the mucosa (Butterworth and Perez-Santingo). The finger-like villi which are normally in continual movement during digestion and separated by the small crypts of Lieberkuhn, are now swollen, fused and shortened to such a degree that they can no longer be distinguished. (Fig. 444). The crypts are deeper than normal, due apparently to hyperplasia and lack of maturation of the epithelial cells which line them. The absorptive surface is now greatly reduced, and the lamina propria may show a chronic inflammatory exudate.

Celiac Disease.—This disease of young children characterized by an inability to absorb fats from the intestine, is essentially a juvenile non-tropical sprue. It is also known as *idiopathic steatorrhea, Gee's disease,* and *intestinal infantilism* (marked impairment of development). It may be regarded as the infantile analogue of tropical sprue, a deficiency disease characterized by great wasting of fat, fatty stools, disturbance of calcium metabolism, and severe anemia. Owing to loss of subcutaneous fat and muscle the abdominal wall becomes very thin, so that the distention with gas and undigested food becomes intensified, giving a highly characteristic appearance, which is reflected in the name, meaning relating to the abdominal cavity (*koilia,* belly). The stools which are very bulky, are loaded with fat, and are white, soft, frothy and foul-smelling due to excessive fermentation. There is a high fecal output of calcium and in consequence osteoporosis and rickets are common, together with low blood calcium and tetany. Anemia is a marked feature; it is usually of the hypochromic type, but occasionally becomes hyperchromic and macrocytic late in the disease.

It is of interest to read the account of the disease by Aretaeus the Cappadocian in the second century A.D.: "Wherefore they have flatulence of the stomach, continued eructations, or a bad smell; but if these pass downwards the bowels rumble, evacuations are flatulent, thick, fluid or clayey, along with the phantasy, as if a fluid were passing

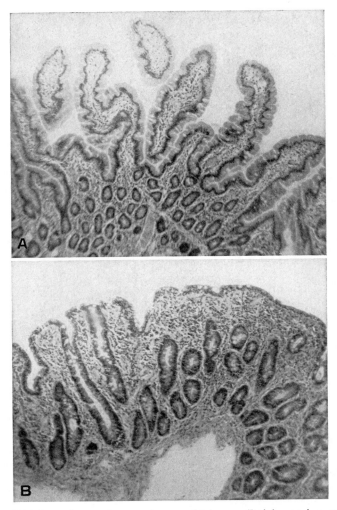

Fig. 444.—Malabsorption syndrome. A, normal jejunum. B, jejunum is a case of
idiopathic steatorrhea. (Kindness of Dr. A. J. Blanchard.)

through them"; and that of Samuel Gee in 1888: "Signs of the disease are yielded by the faeces, being loose, not formed, but not watery; more bulky than the food eaten would seem to account for; pale in colour as if devoid of bile; yeasty, frothy, an appearance due to fermentation; stinking, stench, often very great."

Whipple's Disease.—This very rare condition was first described by Whipple in 1907, and considered by him to be a malabsorption of fat, so that it was called *intestinal lipodystrophy*. The essential lesion was regarded as a deposit of lipids, for the most part neutral fat, in the mucosa of the small intestine and the mesenteric lymph nodes. Grossly the mucosa is flecked with minute yellowish deposits, whilst microscopically the fat is contained in dilated lymph spaces of the enlarged villi and submucosa, in mononuclear phagocytes, and in occasional multinucleated giant cells. Foam cells are present in the dilated sinusoids of the mucosa and of the greatly enlarged mesenteric and retroperitoneal nodes (Fig. 445). It is now realized that the great numbers of foamy histiocytes which form so prominent a feature in the lamina propria and the

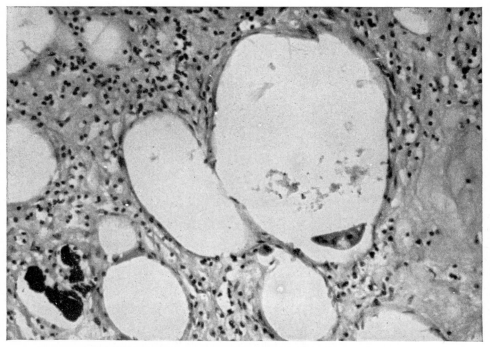

Fig. 445.—Whipple's disease, showing collection of fat in a mesenteric lymph node. (Kindness of Dr. G. B. Casselman.)　× 128.

lymph spaces are filled, not with lipid, but with a material which is periodic acid-Schiff-positive, *i.e.* a mucopolysaccharide (Casselman *et al.*). Some histiocytes, particularly in the lymph nodes, contain sudanophilic material, *i.e.* lipid. Clemmson noted pericardial fibrosis in 10 out of 16 cases reviewed; this was present in Whipple's first case.

The condition may be genetically determined, although remaining clinically silent until adult life. Cases of this rare disease have been reported in siblings, and the mucosa of the colon in young children with no symptoms of Whipple's disease has been found to be crowded with foamy histiocytes with histochemical features similar to those of classical Whipple's disease (Rowlands and Landing). There is much difference of opinion as to the mechanism of the condition. The mystery which shrouds it is as dense as when Whipple published his paper, and it combines with idiopathic sprue, Crohn's disease and ulcerative colitis to make a quartet with enigma variations. There

seems to be obstruction in the lymphatic drainage of the small bowel as well as interference with the absorption of fats, possibly due to faulty bile salt metabolism. In many of the reported cases systemic manifestations of disease outside the gastrointestinal tract antedated the local abdominal symptoms. These systemic symptoms resemble those of rheumatoid arthritis and disseminated lupus, and such lesions as arthritis, vegetative endocarditis and serositis are common. For this reason it has been suggested that Whipple's disease may be related to the rheumatic state (Peterson and Kampmeier). The chief *clinical features* are asthenia, anemia, arthritis, steatorrhea and abdominal distention in a middle-aged or elderly person. The disease usually proves fatal.

The *clinical effects of the malabsorption syndromes in general* constitute too large a subject to be entered into here. A dozen of these are enumerated in Volweiler's review. The most serious single feature of the malabsorption syndromes is the simple loss of calories. Metabolic bone disorders may be the result of: (1) defective formation of bone matrix from protein depletion (osteoporosis), and (2) dimeneralization from the long-standing negative calcium balance (osteomalacia). The hematological defects are protean, as iron, folic acid and vitamin B_{12} are all poorly absorbed.

TUMORS

Benign Tumors.—These may be epithelial or mesenchymal. Epithelial tumors are either villous papillomas or polypoid adenomas. The terms are confusingly alike, but have a different significance. *Villous papilloma* is a proliferation of surface epithelium on a connective tissue and vascular stalk from which hemorrhage occurs with great readiness. It is an uncommon tumor, occurring principally in the rectum, and, although covered with long villous-like processes giving it a velvety surface, it is not pedunculated. Evidence of adenocarcinoma has been found in 35 per cent of villous papillomas. (Fig. 446).

Polypoid adenoma is a pedunculated tumor composed of new glands. It may be single or multiple. Whilst adenomatous polyps may occur in the small intestine, they are much commoner in the large bowel. Their distribution in the rectum and sigmoid (75 per cent) closely parallels that of carcinoma, an indication of the relationship between these two forms of tumor. The malignant change may develop in the tip of the adenoma, in the center or at the base of the stalk. The change from adenoma into adenocarcinoma is often dramatically sharp. (Fig. 447).

Multiple Polyposis.—This condition, known also as *diffuse familial polyposis*, is a disease of the large bowel involving principally the descending and pelvic colon, but the rectum and cecum may also be affected. The younger the patient, the more widespread is the involvement. The patient is likely to be seen for the first time around the age of twenty, suffering from nausea and vomiting and a varying degree of abdominal pain. Blood in the stools and looseness and diarrhea are likely to develop in 95 per cent of cases either together or alone. The three most striking characteristics are (1) the

49

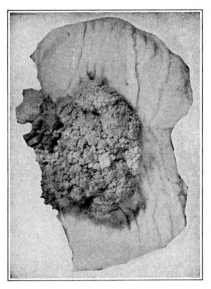

Fig. 446.—Malignant papilloma of rectum.

multiplicity of the lesions, (2) the hereditary character of the disease, and (3) the extreme tendency to malignant change. The polypi may number several thousand. The tendency to polyposis is inherited as a medelian characteristic and many members of a family may be affected, each in turn as they reach the critical age. In a case which came under my own observation 5 members out of a family of 7 were affected, and in 2 of the 5 carcinoma had developed. In the course of time, if nothing is done, this fate is likely to befall all sufferers from the disease.

Peutz-Jeghers Syndrome.—This rare form of polyposis is also hereditary and familial, but it primarily involves the *small intestine*, although the stomach, colon and rectum may also be affected, and *pigmented spots of melanin* occur on the mucous membrane of the mouth and lips (Jeghers *et al.*). Microscopically the lesions may show invasion, but no case of malignancy proved by metastases has been reported in this condition in the small intestine, although polyps in the stomach and colon may become malignant. There is something very curious about the resistance of the human small intestine to malignancy, lying as it does between two such cancer centers as the pylorus and the colon. For further information on this fascinating problem the student should consult the account by Dormandy based on 21 cases in members of 5 families, including illus-

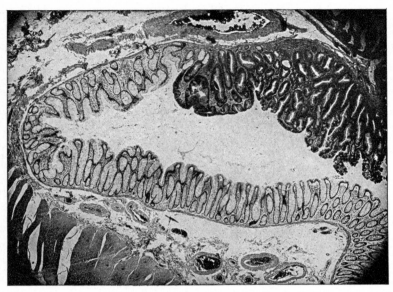

Fig. 447.—Transition from adenoma to carcinoma. × 20. (Boyd, *Pathology for the Surgeon*, courtesy of W. B. Saunders Co.)

trations of the characteristic pigmentation of the face and the misleading invasive appearance of the mucosa of the small bowel.

Benign Mesenchymal Tumors.—These tumors, which are more likely to occur in the small than the large intestine, are of little importance, were it not for the fact that they are uncommon causes of intestinal hemorrhage from an ulcerated surface, and of intussusception owing to their becoming pedunculated. Any of the structures forming the wall of the bowel may be the starting point of a tumor, which in order of frequency may be *leiomyoma*, *fibroma*, *neurinoma* and *lipoma*. The leiomyoma is the usual bleeding tumor in the small bowel.

Malignant Tumors.—The three principal groups of malignant tumors of the intestine are carcinoma, carcinoid, and lymphosarcoma. Carcinoma is very much commoner in the large bowel, carcinoid in the appendix and small bowel, and lymphosarcoma in the small bowel.

Carcinoma.—The *distribution of carcinoma* of the gastrointestinal canal is most peculiar and puzzling. One of the commonest sites of carcinoma in the body, particularly in the male, is the stomach. This is followed closely if not equally by carcinoma of the large bowel. Yet the disease is a rarity in the 20 feet or more of small intestine. This astonishing difference is seen in the very short distance which separates the prepyloric region of the stomach and the first part of the duodenum, and again in passing from the ileum to the beginning of the cecum. What does this mean? A possible carcinogen would be in contact with the gastric and colonic mucosa for many hours, but the rectum, in which carcinoma is more common than in all the rest of the bowel, is empty except during defecation. The usual sites of cancer are the rectum, cecum, and pelvic colon. Over 60 per cent of cancers of the bowel occur in the rectum. Precancerous lesions which may be followed later by carcinoma are papilloma, adenoma, and the papillary formation occurring in chronic ulcerative colitis. By far the greatest danger is familial multiple papillomata. Precancerous lesions in the rectum are of special significance. The site of cancer of the large bowel affects its behavior and characteristics to a marked degree. Thus cancer of the colon is more common in women, cancer of the rectum more common in men. The average duration of life without treatment is twice as long in cancer of the rectum as in cancer of the colon. Intestinal obstruction is much commoner in cancer of the descending colon and rectum than in cancer of the cecum, due to the fluid contents of the latter.

Morbid Anatomy.—The tumor may (1) grow into the lumen of the bowel in the form of a large fungating cauliflower-like mass which soon becomes ulcerated, or (2) it may infiltrate the wall and surround the bowel as an annular growth which may cause an extreme degree of stenosis (Fig. 448). The bowel above the stenosis is dilated and hypertrophied, that below the stenosis is collapsed. Hard fecal masses may be formed on the proximal side of the stricture and these may give rise to superficial erosions of the mucosa (*stercoral ulcers*). The fibrous stroma of the second form of tumor contracts, and from the outside it may look as if a tight string had been tied around the bowel (purse-string type). In this form ulceration occurs late. Mucoid degeneration may occur in the massive variety, and the large bowel is one of the common sites of *mucoid carcinoma*.

The *microscopic appearance* is that of adenocarcinoma. The fungating type is more likely to be well differentiated than the infiltrating form, which may develop a dense stroma. The prognosis depends largely on the degree of differentiation, *i. e.*, the grade to which the tumor belongs. In mucoid carcinoma the cells may be so distended with mucin that they disintegrate and disappear, so that in some areas not a cancer cell may be seen, yet the prognosis in this form is worse than in any of the others. There is an intriguing difference in the *reactive pattern of oxidative enzymes*, in particular of diaphorases and succinic dehydrogenases, of the epithelial cells of carcinoma of the large bowel in contrast to normal, hyperplastic and benign neoplastic cells of this region (Wattenberg). A marked decrease in staining for succinic dehydrogenase and a high degree of activity by the diaphorases is evident, particularly at the invading margin of the tumor. The method of exfoliative cytology is particularly useful and reliable in the preoperative diagnosis of cancer of the colon.

Spread.—This is comparatively slow, especially in cancer of the rectum, so that the

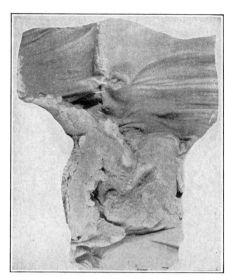

FIG. 448.—Carcinoma of the large bowel. There is almost complete obstruction, and above the obstruction the bowel is greatly dilated.

prognosis is correspondingly good. In a case of cancer of the rectum the tumor protruded from the anus, and was partially removed from time to time for seventeen years after the condition had been called inoperable, yet at autopsy there was no evidence of metastases. Spread is by the three usual methods: local extension, lymph spread and blood spread. Growth takes place easily towards the lumen and also in the long axis of the bowel; infiltration of the muscular coat is much slower. After penetration of the muscular coat there is again spread in the long axis in the subserous tissue; the lymphatics may be distended with cancer cells and appear as opaque white beaded lines which may be mistaken at operation for tubercles. The cancer cells may penetrate the serous coat and give rise to implantation growths on the peritoneum and the surface of the pelvic organs.

Lymph spread is the most important method for the surgeon who has to plan a possible resection, but the student should consult a book on surgical pathology for the details of this complex subject. *Blood spread* to the liver via the portal vein is fortunately usually a late occurrence, particularly in cancer of the rectum, but small lesions may

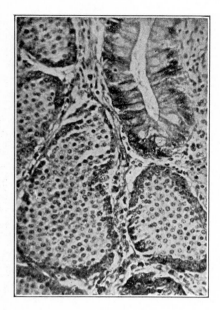

Fig. 449.—Carcinoid of appendix. There are masses of tumor cells in the mucosa and submucosa. × 150.

metastasize early, whereas large lesions may remain local. One of the largest livers I ever saw was the seat of carcinoma secondary to a growth so small that it was nearly overlooked at the autopsy. Nearly 50 per cent of the patients whose growths have been removed surgically with a hope of cure have recurrence in the liver owing to spread by the portal vein.

Carcinoid Tumors.—The story of carcinoid tumors and of serotonin, the hormone which they may produce, is one of the most remarkable in the history of medicine. The history of serotonin actually antedated and later paralleled that of carcinoid tumors without the two becoming fused until the work of Lembeck in 1953. It was in 1884 that a vasoconstrictor substance was first recognized to be present in clotted blood, whilst the tumor now known as carcinoid was described four years later. It was not christened carcinoid until 1907, the awkward name signifying a tumor which suggested carcinoma histologically and might be locally invasive, but which did not metastasize and could therefore be regarded as benign. The demonstration by Pierre Masson by means

of silver impregnation that the tumors arose from the argentaffin Kultschitsky cells of the gastrointestinal tract was a major advance. For this reason the tumors are called argentaffinomas.

A fundamental distinction must be drawn between carcinoids of the appendix, which are symptomless unless they cause obstruction at the proximal end, and carcinoids of the intestine, which may set up secondary growths in the liver that produce serotonin and the carcinoid syndrome. The figures usually given are appendicular carcinoids 90 per cent and intestinal carcinoids 10 per cent, but in MacDonald's series of 356 cases the figures were 58 and 42 per cent.

The *appendicular carcinoid* presents a very characteristic appearance. Usually at the tip of the appendix a firm nodule can be felt, which on cross-section appears as a yellow ring encircling the appendix and situated in the thickened submucous coat. *Microscopically* the tumor consists of masses of spheroidal or polyhedral cells with granular or finely vacuolated cytoplasm. These cells are rich in lipid, and it is to this that the yellow color of the tumor is due. The tumor cells are usually confined to the mucous and submucous coats, (Fig. 449), but they may reach the serous coat.

These tumors are *chromaffinomas* or tumors of the endocrine system, arising from the Kultschitsky cells of the intestinal mucosa which are found between the columnar cells of the crypts of Lieberkühn and belong to the chromaffin system. Both the Kultschitsky cells and the tumor cells are stained intensely by silver impregnation, so that the tumor is also called an *argentaffinoma* (Masson). The ferric ferricyanide reaction is simpler and more reliable. The azo coupling reaction is probably the most specific, and is particularly good in carcinoids of the stomach and rectum, where the silver reaction is usually negative (Lillie and Glenner).

The *intestinal carcinoid* is primarily a tumor of the ileum, but it may occur anywhere from the stomach to the rectum. It forms a yellow mass partly encircling the bowel and projecting into the lumen. Obstructive symptoms may develop quite early, but these seem to be due to peristaltic contractions caused by the secretion of the tumor rather than to mechanical obstruction.

Serotonin is a vasoconstrictor substance which was obtained from clotted blood in 1884, but not until 1948 was it crystallized and shown to be *5-hydroxytryptamine (5-HT)*. It is converted by deamination into 5-hydroxyindoleacetic acid, which is readily detected in the urine by Ehrlich's aldehyde reagent in the presence of a functioning carcinoid tumor. When serotonin is liberated into the blood it is taken up by the platelets which form a veritable storehouse from which it is set free according to the requirements of the organism. Its most constant biological activity is the stimulation of smooth muscle. In spite of its name it may have a depressor as well as a pressor effect. Unless this is borne in mind, such symptoms of excess serotonin production as flushing of the skin are apt to be confusing. It must be confessed that the primary physiological function of 5-HT is still unknown.

The *Carcinoid Syndrome* is a condition marked by symptoms pointing to involvement of the vessels of the skin, the valves on the right side of the heart, the respiratory and gastrointestinal symptoms, with high 5-hydroxytryptamine in the serum and increased excretion of 5-hydroxyindoleacetic acid in the urine, together with carcinoid metastases in the liver and possibly elsewhere in the abdomen. The most characteristic feature is the occurrence of *transient flushing*, or occasionally a *permanent* flush of the skin, particularly the face and neck. This may be accompanied by a fall in the systolic and diastolic pressure accompanied by increase in the pulse rate. In the course of time small *telangiectases* may develop, especially in the face and legs.

Respiratory distress similar to that of asthma may be attributed to spasm of bronchiolar muscle induced by the serotonin. The *digestive system disturbances* may be either in the nature of temporary obstruction or loose and watery diarrhea without pus or blood, both of which have been attributed to disordered peristalsis resulting from excess of serotonin. An associated peptic ulcer, either gastric or duodenal, has been found in nearly 40 per cent of cases.

The *right-sided cardiac lesions* are amongst the most serious and also the most puzzling, being unlike that produced by any other disease. There is fibrous thickening of the cusps limited to the right side with tricuspid and pulmonary stenosis, a combination practically unknown except in the presence of a metastasizing carcinoid tumor (Horsley and Prec). The substance (? vacoconstrictor) responsible for the changes on the right side of the heart is probably destroyed in its passage through the lungs. In one case all four valves were involved, and in this patient there was a patent foramen ovale. It must be understood that in many cases of malignant carcinoid with liver metastases there are no cardiac lesions, nor indeed any vasomotor disturbances of the skin.

In experimental work on rats the identity of the lesions of the renal vascular system with those of focal ischemia and necrosis produced by epinephrine has been established (MacDonald). Mucosal gastric ulceration was also produced, but only with large nonphysiological doses.

Relation of Symptoms to Lesions in Intestinal Neoplasms.—The symptoms produced by a malignant neoplasm depend on the part of the bowel and on the gross characterisitics of the cancer. The chief function of the *proximal colon* is absorption of water and electrolytes. The lumen is spacious, the contents are a highly infective fluid mush, and the tumor is likely to be voluminous, vascular and friable. Infection, occult blood in the stools and anemia are therefore the principal features, whereas signs of obstruction are absent. The anemia, which may bring the patient to the doctor, is microcytic and hypochromic in type, but occasionally it may be macrocytic, giving a blood picture resembling pernicious anemia. The former type is due to hemorrhage, the latter possibly to deficient absorption. The *distal colon* is concerned with storage of feces and absorption of water, its lumen is comparatively small, the contents are formed and firm, and the cancer is usually of a stenosing type. For these reasons increasing constipation progressing to definite obstruction is the chief complaint. The *rectum* is the organ of defecation, so that disturbance of this function is an early symptom. Speaking in general terms it may be said that cancer of the large bowel may manifest itself by a change in the patient's usual bowel habit, pain related to defecation, bleeding from the rectum (visible or occult), anemia, loss of weight and strength, and attacks of partial obstruction. Diarrhea may alternate with constipation, due to colitis developing above the obstruction.

In the *small intestine* the tumor is more likely to be benign than malignant. These tumors are commonly pedunculated, and their importance lies in the fact that they may form the starting point of an intussusception or may be responsible for an intestinal hemorrhage. *Hemangioma* is particularly liable to cause *bleeding from the bowel*. A diffuse reticulum cell sarcoma may form the basis for a secondary malabsorption syndrome.

The strange course of events, including obstruction, which may attend carcinoid of the small intestine with metastases in the liver has already been considered.

INTUSSUSCEPTION

This is the invagination of one segment of the intestine inside another. The common site is the ileocecal junction. There is usually an exciting cause in the shape of a focus of local irritation, an adherent tuberculous or malignant gland, the presence of a polypoid tumor (adenoma, lipoma, myoma), or Meckel's diverticulum. As a result of the irritation irregular peristaltic contractions are set up, and these force the upper segment of bowel into the one below which forms a sheath. The invaginated part is forced along the bowel by peristaltic contractions and may traverse the whole length of the colon, forming a curved thick sausage-shaped mass. The contraction of the sheath prevents the escape of blood from the enclosed part, so that there is great swelling and congestion; there is hemorrhage into the bowel, and discharge of blood from the rectum is the most characteristic symptom. At first intussusception can readily be undone by traction, but the two layers become inflamed and adhere together at the point of entry. The increasing contraction and pressure are apt to cause necrosis and gangrene of the bowel with symptoms of acute strangulation. The

condition usually occurs in boys under the age of one year. It is uncommon in the adult.

Multiple *agonal intussusceptions* are often seen in the small intestine of children at autopsy. They are probably caused by irregular spasmodic contractions at the time of death. There is no inflammation nor adhesions, so that the intussusception is readily undone by traction.

VOLVULUS

Volvulus is torsion of an organ. It is commonest in an ovarian cyst with pedicle and in the pelvic colon, but may occur elsewhere in the intestine, in the gallbladder, spleen, testicle, and uterus with fibroids. The cause is obscure. There is probably some predisposing cause (congenital defect of attachment, etc.), and the actual twisting may be due to irregular spasmodic contraction. The vessels, first the veins and then the arteries, are occluded by the twisting of the mesentery, so that first there is intense congestion of the organ and then gangrene. In the case of the bowel there is acute intestinal obstruction.

ADHESIONS.—Peritoneal adhesions are a common result of abdominal inflammation and may cause intestinal obstruction. The adhesion stretches as a fibrous band from the wall of the bowel to some fixed point, and as it contracts it causes kinking and obstruction.

HERNIA

A hernia is a protrusion of a viscus outside the cavity in which it is contained. The usual hernia is abdominal (although we speak of cerebral and other hernias), a loop of bowel, sometimes a piece of omentum, being protruded into a pouch of peritoneum which projects outward. This is an *external hernia*, and the common types are inguinal, femoral and umbilical, depending on the site of the peritoneal pouch. An *inguinal* hernia passes down the inguinal canal into the scrotum. A *femoral* hernia passes along the femoral vessels under Poupart's ligament and forms a soft swelling in the groin; it usually occurs in the female. An *umbilical* hernia appears at the umbilicus. A hernia may occur at the site of an abdominal wound owing to the scar giving way. This is a form of *ventral hernia*. The rare forms need not be mentioned. The *causes* are probably twofold: (1) local weakness, usually congenital; (2) increased pressure due to sudden muscular effort, straining at stool, etc.

In an *internal hernia* the protrusion occurs into one of the intra-abdominal pouches of the peritoneum, of which the principal are the paraduodenal pouch on the left side of the second part of the duodenum, the pouch behind the superior mesenteric artery, and the fossae in the neighborhood of the ileocecal junction. In rare cases there may be a hernia into the foramen of Winslow and other unusual sites.

Strangulation of the hernia is due to an increase of pressure in the hernial sac. A fresh piece of bowel may be forced through the opening, or there may merely be an accumulation of gas and feces. The loop of bowel is forced against the sharp edge of the opening so that the venous return is interfered with. This causes further swelling of the loop, more interference with the circulation and finally complete stasis. Necrosis and gangrene rapidly develop, the wall is invaded by bacteria, and general peritonitis is the result. The clinical and pathological picture is now one of acute intestinal obstruction.

INTESTINAL OBSTRUCTION

Obstruction of the intestine or ileus may be caused in two very different ways. It may be organic (mechanical) or paralytic (functional). *Organic* or *mechanical obstruction* may be due to a block (1) within the lumen, (2) in the wall, and (3) from outside. *Intraluminal obstruction* is a rare occurrence. It may be caused by a large gall stone or in the newborn by inspissated meconium. It is most frequently met with in the large bowel, where it is usually the result of a fecalith impaction (a common occurrence in horses), a mass of ascaris worms after a vermifuge, or a polypoid tumor. *Obstruction in the wall* may be caused by a tumor, either projecting into or constricting the lumen, by regional ileitis or tuberculosis, or by scars. These are more likely to produce chronic obstruction first, which later may become acute in type. *Obstruction from without* is of particular importance in the small bowel. It is commonly due to a strangulated hernia, often to bands and adhesions which cause kinking of the bowel, occasionally to volvulus, intussusception, or pressure from a mass of enlarged glands or a tumor.

Paralytic or *functional obstruction*, usually called *paralytic ileus* because the common site is the ileum, is frequently due to inflammation of a segment of bowel as a result of which peristaltic movements cannot pass from the segment above to the segment below, the bowels are unable to move, and the practical result is obstruction. A common cause used to be the pelvic peritonitis of acute appendicitis, in which a loop of ileum hangs down into a pool of pus in the pelvis and becomes completely paralyzed. The acute obstruction which follows mesenteric thrombosis or embolism is a variant of this form.

Functional ileus may be metabolic rather than reflex. The best example of metabolic ileus is that which accompanies *hypopotassemia* which is a preoperative and postoperative complication of increasing importance to the surgeon (Culligan). Potassium deficiency in the surgical patient may be due to: (1) limitation of potassium intake, (2) prolonged use of parenteral solutions containing no potassium, (3) loss of large amounts of gastrointestinal secretions through vomiting, suction or fistula, and (4) increased renal excretion of potassium resulting from surgical trauma with its attendant alarm reaction. Abdominal distention and paralytic ileus may develop as an accompaniment of the resulting hypopotassemia. Experimental studies have shown that induced potassium deficiency may cause paralysis of the gastrointestinal musculature. The administration of potassium in sufficient quantity quickly leads to a restoration of normal emptying of the stomach and bowel and disappearance of the abdominal distention.

Intestinal obstruction may be acute or chronic. In the acute form the blood supply to the bowel is cut off so that gangrene quickly develops; in the chronic form it is not interfered with. This difference is fundamental. The two varieties are so different that they must be considered separately.

Acute Obstruction.—Sudden obstruction may be caused by strangulation of a loop of bowel by a fibrous band or adhesion (strangulated hernia), twisting (volvulus), intussusception or infarction (mesenteric thrombosis or embolism). The last-named belongs to the paralytic group. Chronic obstruction due to carcinoma may suddenly become acute. The bowel below the obstruction empties and remains pale and contracted. The part above the obstruction is greatly dilated with fluid and gas and intensely congested so that it becomes deep purple in color as the veins are obstructed by the distention before the arteries. The mucous membrane undergoes necrosis, numerous small ulcers are formed, and bacteria pass through the wall of the bowel and cause general peritonitis. As the blood supply is cut off and bacterial invasion is severe, gangrene quickly develops.

Pathological Physiology.—The immediate danger to the patient in acute intestinal obstruction lies not so much in the local lesion as in the systemic disturbance produced by altered physiology. As the result of a combination of circumstances the body rapidly loses an enormous amount of water and electrolytes, so that a shock-like condition is produced. This is most pronounced in *high intestinal obstruction*, for in this section of the bowel there is very little absorbing surface compared with the large area below the obstruction. The higher, the deadlier. The huge amount of fluid in the shape of secretions which in the course of twenty-four hours normally enters the upper part of the gastrointestinal tract and is absorbed in the lower part is not generally appreciated. It amounts to between 5 and 7 liters daily. This amount is still further increased by acute distension of the bowel, which can be shown experimentally to act as a powerful stimulant to secretion. This fluid with accompanying electrolytes can no longer be absorbed and is therefore lost to the tissues, whether or not it be lost to the body through vomiting. In strangulation even more lethal factors come into play, so that the patient may die before serious loss of water and salts has occurred. For this reason careful clinical observation of the sick person may give more reliable information than reports from the biochemi-

cal laboratory. Here, as in so many other fields, the laboratory is a good servant but a poor master.

The *blood changes* of significance are four in number. (1) *Concentration* due to reduction in volume from loss of plasma, indicated by an elevated hematocrit reading and relative increase in the red cell count and hemoglobin. Concentration of the blood is a reflection, although not necessarily an accurate one, of dehydration of the tissues. (2) *Decrease in electrolytes.* All of the gastric secretions are lost, with their high content of *sodium chloride.* More chloride than sodium is lost, and this favors the development of alkalosis. The blood chlorides may fall from a normal average of 500 mg. per cent to as low as 350 mg. per cent. At these low levels the chlorides disappear from the urine, a danger signal of grave significance. An electrolyte of equal importance is *potassium,* the intracellular ions of which are essential to the normal functioning of voluntary and cardiac muscle and to the neuromuscular transmission of nerve impulses. Deficiency in potassium, a common complication of prolonged vomiting or gastric suction, is indicated by muscular weakness and atonia and by electrocardiographic changes. When hypopotassemia is severe it may cause death from cardiac failure. (3) *Alkalosis* is the result of the great chloride loss through vomiting. Bicarbonates are retained to maintain the electrolyte concentration of the blood, and there is a marked increase in the alkali reserve as indicated by the carbon dioxide combining power. (4) *Rise in the non-protein nitrogen,* which often precedes other blood changes, may be attributed mainly to the increased protein catabolism which accompanies cellular dehydration.

In *strangulation* death is not due to dehydration and electrolyte loss. If the affected loop is large there is a great outpouring of blood from the engorged wall into the lumen, and death may be due to a combination of *primary and secondary shock,* as it would be in massive internal hemorrhage. When the loop involved is small, death is more likely to be due to toxemia. The gangrenous wall of the bowel is readily permeable to putrefactive anaerobic bacteria and tissue toxins, and the toxic products can

PLATE XI

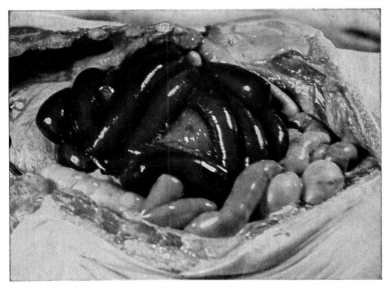

Acute Intestinal Obstruction Due to Volvulus

Body opened at autopsy showing gangrenous distended coils of small intestine.

be quickly absorbed from the peritoneal cavity. This exudate, which is toxic when injected into animals, contains small amounts of histamine and a substance which produces a toxic vasodepressor effect.

Chronic Obstruction.—Chronic obstruction is more likely to be encountered in the large intestine than in the small. In the *large bowel* the usual causes of obstruction are carcinoma, especially the infiltrating variety, cicatricial contraction of adhesions, and pressure from without. In the *small bowel* chronic obstruction is likely to be due to tuberculosis, regional enteritis and adhesions. Both the clinical and the pathological pictures are entirely different from those seen in the acute variety, nor does disordered physiology play a part of any significance.

Meconium Ileus.—A remarkable form of ileus certain to puzzle the uninitiated occurs in the new-born. There is no narrowing of the bowel but the lumen is blocked with thick meconium, and the wall may give way as the result of a "blowout" following on the first feeding. In one case reported from my laboratory the peritoneal cavity was filled with material so thick and tenacious as to suggest mucilage. In a number of cases there has been congenital stenosis of the opening of the pancreatic duct, with dilatation of the duct system and atrophy and fibrosis of the parenchyma (Kornblith and Otani). Farber (personal communication) observed this pancreatic lesion in twins, both of whom died of meconium ileus. The basis of the condition appears to be the mucosis or inspissated secretion which is the essential feature of fibrocystic disease of the pancreas (Farber).

HIRSCHSPRUNG'S DISEASE

This is a congenital idiopathic dilatation of the colon. For some reason the condition is much commoner in boys than in girls, 90 per cent of the cases being males. The pelvic colon and sometimes the entire large intestine are enormously dilated and hypertrophied. Indeed they may come to occupy the entire abdomen. The lower part of the rectum is rarely involved. The hypertrophy is due to great thickening of the circular muscular coat, but is probably not a primary condition. Chronic inflammatory changes in the mucosa and submucosa together with stercoral ulcers are due to the great accumu-

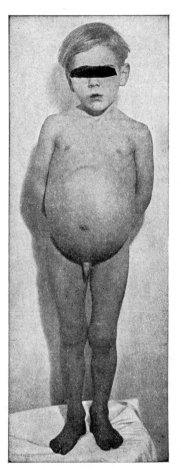

Fig. 450.—Hirschsprung's disease. (Boyd, *Pathology for the Surgeon*, courtesy of W. B. Saunders Co.)

lation of fecal matter in the sigmoid. The bowel is evacuated at long intervals of days or weeks, when a huge quantity is passed. The abdomen is greatly distended (Fig. 450). There are countless theories to account for this obscure condition, but it may be regarded as a form of *achalasia* or inability of the circular fibers at the junction of the sigmoid and rectum to relax. The basic lesion lies in a narrow spastic segment distal to the dilated hypertrophied colon. It is this segment which is responsible for the obstruction, and resection of this part has led to apparent cure of the condition. There is a complete absence of sympathetic ganglion cells in the affected part, together with the presence of abnormal nerve trunks at the sites of Auerbach's and Meissner's plexuses. In some cases the aganglionic segment has extended to the hepatic flexure. The physiological result is absence of peristalsis and increased tonus in the distal colonic segment.

MESENTERIC VASCULAR OCCLUSION

The occlusion may involve the superior mesenteric artery or the vein. Occlusion of the inferior mesenteric vessels is much less common and less serious, because they establish collateral communication with the superior mesenteric vessels above and the hemorrhoidal vessels below. It will not be considered here. *Arterial occlusion*, with which we are concerned, may be caused by thrombosis usually associated with atherosclerosis, and occasionally by embolism. *Venous occlusion* is naturally the result of thrombosis, the onset and course are slow, the result is often hemorrhagic gangrene, blood is always present in the stool, and spontaneous recovery is possible.

Occlusion of the superior mesenteric artery may be *complete* or *partial*. As in the case of other organs such as the heart, the distinction is fundamental, for the resulting clinical picture is entirely different in the two cases.

Complete Occlusion.—Complete obstruction is caused by thrombosis in an atherosclerotic vessel, and occasionally by embolism. The patient is usually over fifty years of age and presents evidence of cardiovascular disease, either as atherosclerosis or valvular heart disease. Auricular fibrillation is common. Sometimes the occlusion follows an abdominal operation. These points are mentioned because, as we shall soon see, an immediate diagnosis is essential if life is to be saved. The result of sudden complete obstruction is *infarction of the bowel*. The infarct is of the red or hemorrhagic variety, and usually occurs in the ileum or the lower part of the jejunum. The infarcted segment is sharply limited as a rule, thick, and darker red in color. Gangrene is likely to develop, resulting in perforation of the bowel.

The *symptoms* are extremely acute, for the onset is catastrophic. The first symptom is *sudden severe abdominal pain*, due to spasm of the bowel from sudden ischemia.

From the beginning, the patient is obviously and gravely ill. *Blood in the stools* is highly significant. There may be *immediate diarrhea*, but soon there is evidence of complete obstruction due to *paralytic ileus*. When gangrene of the bowel develops it leads to *perforation* or *general peritonitis*, which rapidly proves fatal. The leukocyte count and the temperature are both moderately elevated.

Until 1950 the only treatment was extensive resection of the infarcted segment of small bowel, an operation with a very high attendant mortality. In that year Klass in Winnipeg showed that if the artery is opened and the occluding element removed, be it a thrombus, an embolus, or an atherosclerotic plug, circulation would be reestablished in the ischemic segment if the diagnosis was made in time, for the wall of the bowel can tolerate total ischemia for twelve hours. Fortunately, the atherosclerotic process extends for only about 2 cm. down the mesenteric branches, leaving the terminal portions free of blockade.

Partial Occlusion.—Here, as in the coronary artery, there may be partial and gradual obstruction to the lumen of the artery, and here also the result may be the clinical state known as *intestinal angina*. It is in essence ischemia of the smooth muscle and the absorptive tissue of the bowel and it may manifest itself in three ways (Klass): (1) disturbance of muscular mobility, thereby producing *alterations in rhythm;* (2) disturbance of function resulting in one form of the *malabsorption syndrome;* (3) *effort pain,* the hallmark of muscular ischemia everywhere. Because of the disturbance in bowel rhythm, there are 4 or 5 bulky loose stools after a large meal. The disturbance of function with malabsorption leads to weakness, loss of weight, and an increased fat content of the stool. The effort pain occurs with maximal work, that is to say after the largest meal of the day, being felt mainly in the periumbilical area and sometimes radiating through to the back. This clinical picture is easily mistaken for occult gastrointestinal malignancy or chronic pancreatitis. Intestinal angina may be a prodromal symptom preceding acute mesenteric occlusion (Mikkelsen). It may be regarded as a protest reaction of ischemic muscle strained beyond endurance. Aortography provides a method of preoperative diagnosis, and thromboendarterectomy has proved of great value in both the anginal and the malabsorption cases (Shaw and Maynard).

MISCELLANEOUS LESIONS

HEMORRHOIDS.—Hemorrhoids or piles is a condition in which the poorly supported hemorrhoidal veins become dilated and varicose. *Internal* piles involve the superior hemorrhoidal veins and are covered by the mucous membrane of the rectum; *external* piles involve the inferior hemorrhoidal veins and are covered by skin. The causes are central and local. *Central causes* are cirrhosis of the liver (portal obstruction) and cardiac weakness. *Local causes* are constipation (causing straining at stool with dilatation of the veins), carcinoma of the rectum, and outside pressure from enlarged uterus, enlarged prostate, etc. *Every case of piles should first be examined for cancer of the rectum*, because cancer of the rectum can often be completely removed in the early stage. Some of the cases give a hereditary history.

The pile consists of a cluster of greatly dilated venules and may resemble a cavernous angioma. It is covered by mucous membrane or skin. Infection is frequent with accompanying phlebitis and thrombosis, known as an "attack of the piles." The thrombus may become fibrosed, a condition of spontaneous recovery. In rare cases the infected thrombus may become broken up and form septic emboli which are carried to the liver and there form abscesses. The tissue around the pile becomes fibrosed, and is often infiltrated with chronic inflammatory cells. Apart from the attacks of thrombophlebitis the principal symptom is repeated hemorrhage during defecation, which may lead to a marked secondary anemia.

MELANOSIS COLI.—This condition is described on page 404. Granules of melanin pigment are found in the large mononuclear cells in the mucosa, but not in the epithelium. The condition is often associated with chronic intestinal stasis, especially carcinoma of the bowel. The pigmentation is usually limited by the ileocecal valve,

but the appendix may be pigmented while the colon remains free. Marked pigmentation where the black color can be seen shining through the wall of the bowel is rare, but slight grades are common. The melanin is probably formed by the disintegration of proteins in intestinal stasis.

INTESTINAL PNEUMATOSIS.—This rare condition is characterized by the presence of gas in endothelial-lined spaces in the wall of the bowel and by a chronic productive inflammation. It may occur in infants or adults. In the former the cysts are mainly in the mucosa and submucosa, in the latter mainly in the serosa. Either the small or large intestine may be involved. It seems probable that the gas is derived from the intestinal lumen and enters the wall by a mechanical process through an ulceration in the mucosa. In many cases there is gross ulceration of the intestinal tract, and in others microscopic breaks in the mucosa are frequent.

DEVELOPMENTAL DEFECTS.—The commonest congenital anomaly is Meckel's diverticulum, which has already been described. Other diverticula (duodenal, intestinal) may possibly have a congenital basis, but this is doubtful as they are met with late in life. There may be *stenosis* or actual *atresia* of the bowel. The common site of atresia is the lower end of the rectum, where the the condition is known as *imperforate anus*. The anus is represented by a dimple of the skin, which is separated from the lower end of the rectum sometimes by a thin membrane, sometimes by a considerable interval filled with fibrous tissue. There may be congenital obliteration of the second part of the duodenum, and much more rarely at the lower end of the ileum.

Duplications of the Alimentary Tract.—In the development of the alimentary tract duplications may be formed. These are at first tubular structures with a wall of smooth muscle and a lining of mucous membrane which need not be of the same character as that normally present at that level. They are firmly attached to the alimentary tube. Owing to secretion of fluid by the lining epithelium they may become spherical and cystic, or they may remain tubular. These anomalies of development are encountered from the base of the tongue to the anus. The common sites are in relation to the esophagus and ileum, less commonly the cecum. The cysts contain clear mucoid fluid, which may occasionally be bloody. The lesions known as *enteric cysts* and gastric thoracic cysts belong to this category. They must not be confused with mesenteric cysts, which are lymphatic in origin, thin walled and readily peeled off from the surrounding structures.

The mode of production would seem to be a failure of the cystic spaces, which normally convert the solid stage of the canal into a tube, to join up with the main lumen. The condition manifests itself clinically by pain and signs of obstruction due to pressure. Sometimes there is hemorrhage from the bowel due to peptic erosion if the mucosa is gastric in type, just as occurs when heterotopic gastric mucosa is present in Meckel's diverticulum. These symptoms generally develop in the first year of life, and nearly always by the third year.

REFERENCES

ARMITAGE, G. and WILSON, M.: Brit. J. Surg., 1950, *38*, 182. (Regional enteritis.)

BACON, H. E.: *Ulcerative Colitis*, Philadelphia, 1958.

BALL, W. P., BAGGENSTOSS, A. H. and BARGEN, J.: Arch. Path., 1950, *50*, 347. (Pancreatic lesions in ulcerative colitis.)

BUTTERWORTH, C. E. and PEREZ-SANTIAGO, E.: Ann. Int. Med., 1958, *48*, 8. (Jejunal biopsies in sprue.)

CASSELMAN, W. G. B., MACRAE, A. I. and SIMMONS, E. H.: J. Path. and Bact., 1954, *68*, 67. (Histochemistry of Whipple's disease.)

CLEMMESON, J.: Acta. Med. Scandinav., 1945, *121*, 495. (Intestinal lipodystrophy.)

CROHN, B. B. and YARNIS, H.: *Regional Ileitis*, 2nd ed., New York, 1958.

CULLIGAN, L.: Minnesota Med., 1954, *17*, 198. (Intestinal obstruction and hypopotassemia.)

DORMANDY, T. L.: New Eng. J. Med., 1957, *256*, 1093, 1141, 1186. (Peutz-Jeghers syndrome.)

FARBER, S.: Arch. Path., 1944, *37*, 238. (Meconium ileus.)

GORDON, R. S.: Lancet, 1959, *1*, 325. (Exudative enteropathy.)

HORSLEY, D. B. and PREC, O.: Arch. Int. Med., 1956, *97*, 806. (Cardiac lesions in carcinoid tumors.)

JACKMAN, R. J.: *Lesions of the Lower Bowel*, Springfield, Ill., 1958.

JEGHERS, H., McKUSICK, V. A. and KATZ, K. H.: New Eng. J. Med., 1949, *241*, 993 and 1031. (Jeghers' syndrome.)

JENSEN, E. J., BAGGENSTOSS, A. H. and BARGEN, J.: Am. J. Med. Sci., 1950, *219*, 281. (Renal lesions in ulcerative colitis.)

KIMMELSTIEL, P., LARGE, H. L. JR. and VERNER, H. D.: Am. J. Path., 1952, *28*, 259. (Hepatic lesions in ulcerative colitis.)

KLASS, A. A.: Can. M. A. J., 1960, *82*, 620. (Intestinal angina and infarction.)

LILLIE, R. D. and GLENNER, G. G.: Am. J. Path., 1960, *36*, 623. (Histochemical reactions of carcinoid tumors.)

MacDONALD, R. A.: Am. J. Med., 1956, *21*, 867. (Carcinoids.)

————: Am. J. Path., 1959, *35*, 297. (Pathogenesis of lesions produced by serotonin.)

MASSON, P.: Am. J. Path., 1928, *4*, 181. (Carcinoid tumor.)

MIKKELSEN, W. P.: Am. J. Surg., 1957, *94*, 262. (Intestinal angina.)

PENNER, A. and BERNHEIM, A. J.: Arch. Path., 1939, *27*, 966. (Pseudomembranous enteritis.)

PETERSON, J. C. and KAMPMEIER, R. H.: Am. J. Med. Sci., 1951, *221*, 543. (Intestinal lipodystrophy.)

PETTET, J. D. *et al.:* Surg., Gynec. and Obst., 1954, *98*, 546. (Pseudomembranous enteritis.)

PORTIS, S. A.: J.A.M.A., 1949, *139*, 208. (Lysozyme in ulcerative colitis.)

ROWLANDS, D. T. JR. and LANDING, B. H.: Am. J. Path., 1960, *36*, 201. (Colonic histiocytosis in children.)

SHAW, R. S. and MAYNARD, E. P.: New Eng. J. Med., 1958, *258*, 874. (Mesenteric artery occlusion and malabsorption.)

SMITH, R. B. W. *et al.*: Am. J. Med., 1958, *25*, 391. (Peroral small bowel mucosal biopsy.)

TERPLAN, K.: Am. J. Path., 1953, *29*, 595. (Staphylococcal enteritis.)

WARREN, S. and SOMMERS, S. C.: Am. J. Path., 1948, *24*, 475. J.A.M.A., 1954, *154*, 189. (Regional enteritis.)

WATTENBERG, L. W.: Am. J. Path., 1959, *35*, 113. (Oxidative enzmyes in carcinoma of large bowel.)

WHIPPLE, G. H.: Bull. Johns Hopkins Hosp., 1907, *18*, 382. (Intestinal lipodystrophy.)

ZETZEL, L.: New Eng. J. Med., 1954, *251*, 610. (Pathogenesis of ulcerative colitis.)

Chapter 28

The Liver and Biliary Passages

THE LIVER
General Considerations
  STRUCTURE
    Hepatic Lobule
    Hepatic Circulation
  FUNCTION
    Liver Function Tests
    Needle Biopsy
Hepato-Cellular Failure
  JAUNDICE
  HEPATIC COMA
  ENDOCRINE IMBALANCE
  FETOR HEPATICUS
  ASCITES
Necrosis
Viral Hepatitis
  LUPOID HEPATITIS
Toxic Hepatitis
Deficiency Hepatitis
  KWASHIORKOR
  ALCOHOLISM
Cirrhosis
  PORTAL CIRRHOSIS
    Nutritional
    Post-hepatitic
    Post-necrotic
  BILIARY CIRRHOSIS
    Primary
    Secondary
  OTHER FORMS OF CIRRHOSIS
    Hemochromatosis

Hemosiderosis
Hepato-lenticular Degeneration
Schistosomal Cirrhosis
Sickle Cell Anemia Cirrhosis
Hereditary Disorders of
    Metabolism
Jaundice
  OBSTRUCTIVE
  HEMOLYTIC
  HEPATIC
    Familial Non-Hemolytic
      Gilbert's Disease
      Dubin-Johnson Disease
    Weil's Disease
      Canicola Fever
Circulatory Disturbances
  CHRONIC VENOUS CONGESTION
  INFARCTION
  THROMBOSIS OF HEPATIC VEIN:
    CHIARI SYNDROME
Infections
  ABSCESS
  AMEBIC ABSCESS
  ACTINOMYCOSIS
Granulomata
  SARCOIDOSIS
  SYPHILIS
  TUBERCULOSIS
Animal Parasites
  HYDATID DISEASE
  OTHER PARASITES

Tumors
  PRIMARY CARCINOMA
    Hepatoma
    Cholangioma
  SECONDARY CARCINOMA
  SARCOMA
  BENIGN TUMORS
Degenerations
  FATTY DEGENERATION
  AMYLOID DEGENERATION
  GLYCOGEN STORAGE: VON
    GIERKE'S DISEASE
  ATROPHY
  POSTMORTEM CHANGES
Developmental Defects
  POLYCYSTIC DISEASE

THE GALLBLADDER
General Considerations
Cholecystitis
  ACUTE CHOLECYSTITIS
  CHRONIC CHOLECYSTITIS
  CHOLESTEROLOSIS OF GALL-
    BLADDER
Gallstones
  PURE CHOLESTEROL STONE
  PURE PIGMENT STONE
  INFECTIVE OR MIXED STONES
Biliary Obstruction
  CARCINOMA OF THE GALL-
    BLADDER
    Carcinoma of the Bile Ducts

THE LIVER

GENERAL CONSIDERATIONS

THE liver is a singularly misleading organ. In structure it appears to be one of the simplest, but in function it proves to be one of the most complex. It is this combination of apparent simplicity with actual complexity which is the despair of all who attempt to correlate changes in structure with disorders of function. In the kidney a lesion of the glomerular basement membrane will produce one disturbance of function and a lesion of the distal convoluted tube will produce another of quite a different character. The liver cells, on the other hand, all look alike. Each can apparently do everything, being a jack-of-all trades. It can take in, build up, break down, and cast off. Moreover it has a unique power of repair like that of a primi-

tive animal, so that if a part is cut away, or destroyed, it can be replaced with matching parenchymatous tissue, not with the base substitute of fibrous tissue.

This apparent simplicity and similarity of cellular structure may be attributed to our relatively primitive histological technique. With the aid of biochemical cytology, that is to say the combination of electron microscopy, cytochemical staining of cells, and analysis of subcellular fractions isolated from tissue homogenates by differential centrifugation, we are beginning to gain a very different outlook, so that we can localize specific enzymes in different portions of the liver lobule. This will be elaborated in the next section. As a matter of fact the liver cell proves to be a mass of different enzymes, which are located in organelles such as the mitochondria and endoplasmic reticulum

(Novikoff and Essner). These can now be studied in living tissue by means of needle aspiration biopsy.

Structure—In order to appreciate the changes produced by disease we must recall some of the normal characters of the liver, including its size, shape, weight, color and consistence. The *size* is very constant in health, but as the result of disease it may be much increased (tumor, amyloid) or diminished (cirrhosis). The *shape* may be distorted by disease (syphilitic scars, etc.) or by Riedel's lobe, a tongue-like process occasionally extending downward from the lower margin of the liver external to the gallbladder. Grooves are not infrequently seen running across the upper surface of the right lobe in an antero-posterior direction; they are probably caused by folds in the diaphragm which occupy them. The *weight* is 1400 to 1600 grams in the male, 1200 to 1400 grams in the female. The *color* is a dark reddish-brown or chocolate, but the under surface is often of an indigo color due to the postmortem action of H_2S liberated from the large bowel on the iron pigment in the liver with the production of sulfide of iron; there may be greenish staining by bile from the gallbladder. The common pale and sometimes red patches under the capsule (pseudo-infarcts) must not be mistaken for true infarcts, which are extremely rare. The *consistence* is that of a soft solid, but the liver is friable and easily lacerated. When placed on a flat surface the dome-like curve of the upper surface becomes greatly flattened; any softening of the liver (fatty degeneration) will increase the flattening; any increase in consistence (amyloid) will prevent it.

The Hepatic Lobule.—For 150 years, indeed since Kiernan's paper in 1833, we have been educated to believe that the unit of hepatic structure is a hexagonal lobule composed of cords of identical cells centered around a terminal hepatic vein, known therefore as the central vein. The hexagonal pattern of the liver is the result of the tridimensional budding of the bile ducts by which the liver develops from its anlage. The picture on which the student of histology in the past has been brought up is that of the pig's liver. Indeed the pig may be regarded

as being responsible for the concept of the classic hexagonal lobule, for in that animal hexagonal areas are outlined by septa which are broad leaves of connective tissue carrying the portal canals, with the hepatic vein in the center. A lobule of a gland, the ultimate structural and functional unit, should be a group of secretory units that are grouped around a small afferent vessel and drain into a common duct. This is certainly not true of the Kiernan lobule, with its grouping around an efferent vessel. Moreover, septa outlining lobules are not present in the human liver.

That the hexagonal lobule does not represent the ultimate morphological or functional hepatic unit has been demonstrated by Rappaport and his associates. As the result of observations of the hepatic circulation *in vivo* Rappaport arrived at the conclusion that blood enters each unit of liver structure through a pair of terminal afferent portal and arterial twigs, and flows through the surrounding tissue which is not oriented around one of the central veins. The structural (and functional) unit of the liver, which Rappaport calls the *acinar unit*, a term previously used by Malpighi in 1666, proved to be a small berry-like or glomerular mass of parenchyma, irregular in size and shape situated around a trio of terminal branches of vein, artery and duct. Such pathological changes as ischemic necrosis, early fatty change and deficiency cirrhosis begin at the circulatory periphery of the acinar units, which thereby become outlined and conspicuous, especially when injected with India ink. The cells close to the axial afferent channels, being the first to be supplied with blood rich in oxygen and nutrients, remain for a time unaffected.

Perhaps it would be well to close this discussion on the structural relationship of cells to blood vessels by a quotation from Sheila Sherlock: "In our present state of knowledge, it would be a pity to dispense completely with the concept of lobular architecture. It has become firmly established as a convenient unit of reference."

We owe to Elias another fundamental change in our concept of liver structure. For one hundred years we have been taught to believe that the liver is made up of cords

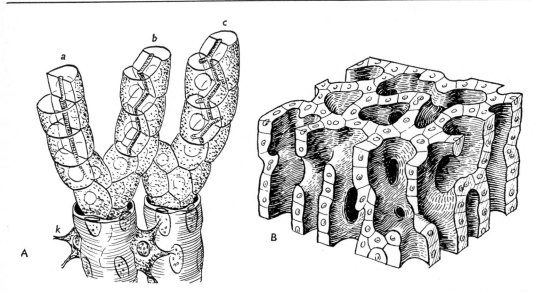

FIG. 451.—Stereograms of various concepts of mammation liver structure. *A*, liver cell cord, two cells thick, connected with each other, wrapped in endothelial sheaths in which spider-like phagocytes of Kupffer are incorporated; (*a*) cells arranged opposite each other, bile canaliculus straight (concept of Stohr); (*b*) cells arranged at alternate levels, bile canaliculus zigzag (concept of Braus); (*c*) cells arranged alternately, blind side branches projecting between liver cells (concept of McIndoe). *B*, Liver muralium, consisting of one-cell-thick plates, laminæ hepatis, a continuous mass of cells tunnelled by the lacunæ hepates which together form the labryinthus hepatis. (From original of Fig. 1, Elias, courtesy of Am J. Anat.).

of cells, each cord being two cells in thickness enclosing a bile canaliculus, wrapped in an endothelial sheet and bathed in blood. As a result of reconstructions from serial sections in a wide variety of animals Elias came to the conclusion that in place of cords of cells the mammalian liver, with the exception of the pig and a few other species, consists of a continuous system of plates or walls all connected with one another, the wallwork or muralium being tunnelled by a labyrinth of lacunæ in which the network of sinusoids is suspended (Fig. 451). Meshes of bile capillaries or canaliculi surround each individual liver cell, lying in grooves between the cells, and communicating with one another to form a chicken-wire meshwork which opens into the ductules. With such an arrangement it is little wonder that swelling of the cells in hepatitis may result in obstruction to the canaliculi.

The *hepatic cells* which constitute the lobules may appear identical in histological sections, and yet they may be very different in functional activity (Novikoff). On one side of each hepatic cell is the sinusoid, concerned with absorption, on the other side is the bile canaliculus concerned with secretion. The lining of the sinusoid, formed of the reticuloendothelial Kupffer cells, is separated from the hepatic cell by a potential space, the space of Disse, into which project innumerable *microvilli* which enormously increase the absorptive surface of the cell. Similar microvilli are present on the canalicular side. Both sets of microvilli contain phosphatases, but these are not the same in the two sets. On the canalicular surface there are adenosine triphosphatase and 5-nucleotidase, but on the sinusoidal surface there is only 5-nucleotidase. This enzymatic differentiation of the secretory and absorptive surfaces of the cell probably has important physiological significance (Novikoff). On either side of the bile canaliculus the cytoplasm is rich in acid phosphatase and Golgi apparatus.

The cells in the different parts of the lobule may look alike, but as regards enzymatic activity as revealed by the technique of biochemical cytology the lobule is heterogeneous rather than homogeneous. It is not what the cell looks like but what it does which matters. Thus there is more adenosine triphosphatase and alkaline phosphatase activity in the bile canaliculi of the peripheral zone than in those of the centrolobular zone, but higher 5-nucleotidase activity in the canaliculi of the centrolobular cells. Succinic dehydrogenase activity is high in the peripheral cells of the lobule, but very low in the cells adjacent to the central vein. Other examples of differing distribution of enzyme will be found in Novikoff's paper. Of special interest to the student of pathology is the concept that heterogeneity of enzyme distribution may be the basis of the selective localization in the hepatic lobule of lesions due to poisons, to toxins, and to infective agents.

Hepatic Circulation.—The liver is unique in that 80 per cent of the blood it receives is venous in character. As a natural result, the hepatic cells are peculiarly liable to necrosis from anoxia and from toxic agents. They live dangerously. The hepatic artery, however, is life-saving, for it maintains an oxygen tension incompatible with proliferation of the anaerobic bacteria from the bowel which would otherwise prove fatal. Two points of interest deserve mention. The first refers to the *activity of sphincters* which regulate the amount of blood passing from the distributing terminal branches of the portal vein into the sinusoids. Similar sphincteric activity also controls blood flow in the arteriovenous anastomoses between the hepatic artery and the portal vein and also in the termination of the sinusoids. As a result of this activity there are great variations in the total flow of blood through different lobules at different times. These variations may play a part in the otherwise puzzling pathological picture produced by hepatic poisons. The liver certainly does not work at full capacity and it has great reserve power.

The second point deals with the general distribution of the portal blood throughout the liver in the laboratory animal. By the injection of trypan blue it can be shown that *stream lines* exist in the blood of the portal vein, and that these correspond to the organs from which the blood is collected. Thus the blood from the stomach and spleen passes to the left lobe of the liver, whilst that from the duodenum, head of the pancreas and jejunum passes to the right lobe, with little or no intermingling of their streams. The blood from the colon passes to both lobes. Whether this stream-like phenomenon holds true for man is not certain. Liver metastases from carcinoma of the stomach are not confined to the left lobe, nor those of carcinoma of the cecum to the right lobe. On the other hand the distribution of abscesses secondary to abdominal infection seems to support the idea.

Function.—The liver plays a major role in the nutrition and maintenance of the body, for it dominates intermediary metabolism by which the food stuffs conveyed from the bowel are prepared for use by the tissues. It is indeed the master cook who makes the food digestible. From its anatomical position it is a receiving depot, as well as a storehouse and a chemical factory. It is both an exocrine and endocrine gland, the latter term being applicable to any organ which secretes substances into the blood, whether or not these are hormones. How grotesque, then, to speak of "liver pills" or "pills to improve the function of the liver", as do the advertisements for patent medicines!

Although any real discussion of the manifold functions of the liver would be out of place (as well as beyond the power of the author), an enumeration of the principal functions, as given by Wakim, may be of some little value in relation to the disturbances produced by the pathological processes to be considered in the course of this chapter. Without a knowledge of normal function, the student is unable to appreciate the results of disturbance of function, disturbance which is reflected in what we call the symptoms of disease.

1. *The Manufacture and Elimination of Bile.*—The parenchyma of the liver represents a barrier of cells separating the vascular bed from the biliary system, with an interchange of metabolites between these compartments. Bile consists of two very different and unrelated constituents: (*a*) bilirubin and (*b*) bile salts and acids.

Bilirubin is merely a waste product, an iron-free pigment derived from hemoglobin by the activity not of the liver but of the cells of the reticuloendothelial system. Its excretion depends on the action of enzymes in the liver cells, an action which may be stopped by death of the cells or depression by anoxia, poisons, viruses or chronic malnutrition. Elevation of pressure in the biliary system may stop the excretion. In all of these instances bilirubin will accumulate in the blood with resulting jaundice, a subject to be discussed on a later page.

Bile salts and acids are produced by the liver cells. They are in no sense a waste product, but are of physiological importance. Most of the salts which pass into the bowel are reabsorbed and returned to the liver, an enterohepatic circulation. In the gastrointestinal tract they aid in the emulsification, digestion and absorption of fats by lowering the surface tension of the fat globules. They perform a similar office for the cholesterol and for the fat-soluble vitamins, A, D, E and K. As vitamin D is antirachitic and as vitamin K is necessary for the manufacture of prothrombin, the importance of the bile salts is self-evident.

Cholesterol, whose name is derived from the Greek words meaning "solid bile," is an essential constituent of all cells and body fluids (as well as of gallstones), although little is known as to its function.

2. *Maintenance of the Blood Sugar Level.*— This subject will have to be discussed in relation to diabetes. Suffice it to say here that the hepatic cell is concerned with (*a*) glycogenesis or the formation of glycogen from glucose and its storage in the liver; (*b*) glycogenolysis or the breakdown of glycogen into glucose and its release into the sinusoids; and (*c*) gluconeogenesis or the formation of glucose from proteins and fats when the diet is deficient in carbohydrate. Sugar is as necessary for life as oxygen, and it is consumed continuously. The presence of large amounts of sugar in the blood is also harmful. It is the liver which provides the regulatory mechanism that maintains a constant level of blood sugar in spite of the ingestion of large amounts of sugar during meals. It first stores the sugar as glycogen and then releases it as glucose in response to the requirements of tissues.

3. *Regulation of Protein Metabolism.*—Deamination of amino acids and the synthesis

of urea are particularly involved in this regulation.

4. *Regulation of Fat Metabolism.*—Here may be mentioned the elaboration of unsaturated fatty acids and the phosphorylation of fats.

5. *Formation of Ketone Bodies.*—These are formed from fats, proteins and pyruvate.

6. *Formation of Plasma Proteins.*—The synthesis of serum albumin, prothrombin and fibrinogen occurs solely in the liver parenchyma. In hepatic insufficiency it is natural, therefore, that the serum albumin should be low, and that defective blood coagulation with a tendency to hemorrhage should be an ever-present threat. Gamma globulin, on the other hand, tends to rise in the presence of inflammatory processes involving the liver, whether primary or secondary to necrosis. This is because gamma globulin is not formed by the hepatic cells but by those of the reticuloendothelial system, which is particularly abundant in the human liver. A large increase in the gamma globulin fraction with a decrease in the albumin is the clearest abnormality of serum proteins in liver disease.

7. *Detoxication.*—This may be accomplished either by destruction of the poisonous substance, as in the case of strychnine, nicotine and drugs, or by excretion into the bile. The male and female sex hormones and the adrenal corticoids are excreted into the bile and then reabsorbed. It is evident that any breakdown of this mechanism may result in endocrine imbalance. This may account for the atrophy of the testes, gynecomastia, and the vascular spiders of the skin, the latter being attributed to concentration of circulating estrogens or related steroids. One cause of precocious puberty is the presence of a hepatoma.

8. *Erythropoiesis.*—In embryonic life the liver is the most important hemopoietic organ. This function can be resumed in severe anemia. Storage of the antianemic principle may be mentioned in this connection.

9. *Blood Coagulation.*—As has already been pointed out, the liver is the chief or only source of fibrinogen. Moreover the absorption of vitamin K from the intestine is dependent on the presence of bile salts.

Liver Function Tests.—When we remember

50

the multiplicity and complexity of liver functions it is obvious that no one test can tell us a great deal about disturbance of function. Perhaps for this reason the tests are continually changing in number and variety. Himsworth in his monograph on *The Liver and its Diseases* goes so far as to say: "There is yet no test which approaches in value a careful clinical examination of the patient." This is a remark which the student would do well to bear in mind, although it is undoubtedly easier to order a laboratory test than to make "a careful clinical examination" oneself. In spite of the limitations and lack of specificity of the tests, they can be of great value when selected with discrimination in relation to specific clinical problems, particularly the differential diagnosis of jaundice or hepatomegaly, and the confirmation of suspected liver damage together with a quantitative assessment of its degree.

In broad terms it may be said that tests for liver function fall into three general fields. (1) The *differential diagnosis of the various types of jaundice*, including that due to excessive hemolysis. This matter will be referred to when we come to the subject of jaundice. (2) The *estimation of liver damage in the absence of jaundice*. This is likely to include cases of suspected cirrhosis or non-icteric hepatitis. For this purpose the most sensitive are the excretory tests such as serum bilirubin and the tests for bile pigments in the urine, together with bromsulphthalein, which is the best test for estimating the total functioning mass of hepatic tissue in the nonjaundiced patient. (3) In addition the *flocculation or turbidity tests*, particularly zinc sulfate and thymol turbidity, may throw valuable light on liver function. It is a curious fact that many of this group of tests were the result of some chance observation and are therefore empirical in origin, but in this respect of course they are not alone in the multiplicity of useful techniques employed by the physician. The mechanism involved has been clarified by the introduction of electrophoresis, which has served to demonstrate that the gamma globulin is the protein fraction of the serum chiefly responsible for the precipitation. Moreover normal albumin acts as an inhibitor of the reaction. We have already seen that in liver disease

the gamma globulin tends to be increased and the albumin diminished, so that under these conditions positive flocculation tests are to be expected in hepatocellular disease. On the other hand it must be recognized that hyperglobulinemia does not necessarily go hand in hand with a positive flocculation test, for such a test is seldom positive in multiple myeloma.

In addition to the conventional liver function tests, observations on the behavior of liver enzymes in the blood have provided information of marked value. The two most important of these enzymes in indicating some functional change in the hepatic cells are glutamic oxaloacetic transaminase and alkaline phosphatase.

Serum glutamic oxaloacetic transaminase level is a highly specific index of hepatocellular injury. It is a much more sensitive indicator of minimal to moderate damage to the liver than are the other hepatic function tests. Transaminases are enzymes which transfer amino (NH_2) groups from one amino acid to another. The transaminase in question is so-called because glutamic acid and oxaloacetic acid are formed as the result of its activity. The catalyst is concentrated particularly in the heart, skeletal muscle, liver and brain. The transaminase activity parallels the degree of liver cell injury, and the blood level serves as a guide to recovery after acute injury. In this respect it is more sensitive than either alkaline phosphatase or serum cholinesterase (Molander *et al.*). The extent of the rise in infectious hepatitis is greater than in myocardial infarction and the increased activity is present for a longer period. The normal level is from 4 to 40 units, but in viral hepatitis it may be increased 100 times, and in carbon tetrachloride poisoning the level may go up to 27,000 units. The test is very useful in the differential diagnosis of jaundice, the serum level being much higher in jaundice due to hepatocellular disease than in that caused by extrahepatic obstruction. This is the reverse of what is seen when the serum alkaline phosphatase level is tested. The changing levels of serum transaminase may be due to an alteration of the state of the semipermeable membrane of the hepatic cell, allowing the passage of a large amount of enzyme into the blood.

Serum alkaline phosphatase estimation is a valuable indicator of liver disease, although, like the flocculation tests, it is not truly a liver function test seeing that it does not test any known liver function. Phosphatase, an enzyme produced by osteoblasts, is carried by the blood to the liver and excreted into the bile. High values are therefore found in the blood in obstructive jaundice. The test is often positive in the early stages of hepatitis when the liver is enlarged and tender, due perhaps to pressure on the smaller bile ducts. The raised values are not necessarily always due to simple retention, because there may be high values in the absence of jaundice, due perhaps to the deranged liver cells secreting the enzyme directly into the circulation rather than into the bile.

Needle Biopsy.—Transthoracic aspiration biopsy of the liver is proving itself as useful in its own way as many of the functional tests. Its potential value, indeed, seems to be unlimited. There are three fields in which it can be of great assistance to the physician: (1) it can give him insight into the metabolic activities of the liver, (2) it can throw light on the progress of the disease, and (3) it can indicate the effect of therapy. By means of this technique an estimate can be made of enzymatic activity, of lipid utilization, of vitamin A content, *etc*. With advances in histochemical methods fresh fields will continually be opened up.

The small size of the specimen removed is not as great a drawback as might be supposed, for so many of the puzzling disease conditions of the liver are characterized by diffuse lesions, and even localized lesions such as sarcoidosis are picked up in a surprising number of cases. The specimen received by the pathologist is one in depth, much preferable to the subcapsular tissue removed by surgical exploration, which is likely to be complicated by the acute inflammatory reactions which attend surgical intervention.

It must be realized that the microscopic picture of normal living liver tissue differs in several respects from that to which we are accustomed in autopsy material. The cells

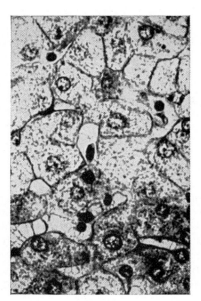

Fig. 452.—Glycogen in liver cells (pale and vacuolated). × 500.

are sharply outlined, there is a lack of the smudgy opacity which has been regarded as normal, and, in particular, there is an abundant glycogen content giving to the cytoplasm a ground-glass clarity which may be mistaken for vacuolation. (Fig. 452). Popper has emphasized the part which agonal changes and postmortem autolysis play in producing the picture seen in autopsy specimens and which may be mistaken for the effects of disease. In the moribund patient the hepatic circulation may fail, much as it does in shock, with resulting centrolobular necrosis. The glycogen disappears from the cells. The permeability of the sinusoidal wall for protein is increased, with resulting separation of the endothelial lining from the wall of liver cells, (space of Disse), an appearance which has been taken for serous hepatitis. Dissociation of the liver cells is also an agonal phenomenon observed in autopsy material.

HEPATO-CELLULAR FAILURE

In our study of disease of the kidney we have seen that in the majority of cases we could attribute the symptoms of renal failure to lesions of the glomeruli, the proximal or distal convoluted tubules, or the arterioles. This is much more difficult or impossible in the case of the liver, by reason of the uniform character of the cytological architecture. A person dead of hepatic coma, which corresponds to uremia in renal disease, may present a liver which gives no suggestion of a fatal outcome. Moreover, a bewildering variety of etiological agents may be responsible for the failure of hepatic function. This may be due to toxins, viruses, bacteria, anoxia, deficiency of essential food elements, or an overload with iron or copper. *The extent or diffuseness of the lesion seems to be more important than the histological appearance.* The outstanding manifestations of hepatocellular failure are: (1) jaundice, (2) hepatic coma, (3) endocrine imbalance, (testicular atrophy, gynecomastia, loss of body hair, arterial spiders, palmar erythema), (4) fetor hepaticus, and (5) ascites.

Jaundice.—There is no clinical manifestation which points more directly to the liver than jaundice, and yet, as in hemolytic jaundice, the liver may be completely innocent. The jaundice may be hepatogenous, due to sickness of liver cells and loss of their power to excrete bilirubin, or it may be extrahepatic and obstructive in origin. The general subject of jaundice is taken up on page 807, so that no more need be said in this place.

Hepatic Coma.—The manifestations of hepatic coma may be cerebral or psychiatric in character, the latter lasting for months or even for years. Hepatolenticular degeneration or Wilson's disease is considered in Chapter 42 in connection with diseases of the central nervous system.

Lesions.—The *hepatic lesions* responsible for coma are those which produce liver insufficiency, most often viral hepatitis, cirrhosis, or portocaval shunts. The catastrophe may follow the surgical production of an Eck fistula for the relief of portal hypertension when the liver is seriously damaged.

The *cerebral lesions* are marked by their widespread distribution. The outstanding histological change is a very great increase in the number of protoplasmic astrocytes, so that they may be twice as numerous as normal, together with an increase in the size of these cells. This diffuse hyperplasia of

protoplasmic astrocytes is found in the cerebral cortex, lenticular nucleus, thalamus, substantia nigra and the pontine nuclei. There is little or no change in the parenchyma. I do not know the relationship of the astrocytosis to the clinical picture, nor the mechanism by which it is produced.

Clinical Picture.—The cerebral condition may develop insidiously with personality changes and defects in judgment, and it has been remarked that these "jaundiced, pot-bellied, cirrhotic patients are usually the jovial clowns of the ward" (Murphy *et al.*). In other cases there is the sudden development of stupor deepening into coma. This is likely to be a complication of fulminating hepatitis with acute yellow atrophy. Motor disturbances pointing to lesions of the pyramidal tract may be a striking feature. These may take the form of grimacing and blinking, and a highly characteristic flapping tremor like the beating of a bird's wings, best seen when the arms are held out and the fingers extended. This *liver flap* or *asterixis* (Gr. *sterigma*, to support) is a series of rapid flexion-extension movements representing sudden loss of sustained dorsiflexion, and coming on within a minute of the arms being extended. Although characteristically seen in hepatic coma, asterixis is a non-specific phenomenon associated with a variety of conditions, such as pulmonary insufficiency, characterized by impaired cerebral metabolism. The electroencephalogram shows bilaterally synchronous slow waves in the delta range, which are also seen in the experimental dogs referred to above. The *classic triad of impending coma is mental confusion, a characteristic tremor, and specific encephalographic changes.*

Etiology.—It would appear that hepatic coma is due to cerebral intoxication by intestinal contents which have not been metabolized by the liver (Sherlock). We shall see that diffuse hepatic lesions are accompanied by the establishment of communications between the portal and caval systems, so that toxic nitrogenous material from the bowel either by-passes the liver or fails to be changed by the damaged liver cells or both. The shunt may be through the liver itself, or the portal blood may by-pass the liver through large natural collaterals, or an Eck fistula in a dog or a porta-caval anastomosis in man done to relieve portal hypertension may produce the same result. *Gastroentestinal hemorrhage* from esophageal varices is a precipitating factor of importance, especially if a shunt operation has been done for previous esophageal hemorrhage, thus increasing the nitrogen content of the bowel, and impairing liver function still further by virtue of hypotension and anemia. The particular culprit is believed to be *ammonia* produced from proteins in the bowel by the action of urea-splitting intestinal bacteria. The condition is ameliorated to a marked degree by the oral administration of broad-spectrum antibiotics which destroy the intestinal bacteria that convert nitrogenous substances into ammonia.

The *ammonia content* of the portal vein is three times that of the hepatic vein, the liver being the chief site of ammonia removal largely by the formation of urea. The increasing frequency of porta-caval shunt operations in man has brought the question of ammonia intoxication into prominence, especially with regard to the danger of a high protein diet in such cases. Ammonia is probably toxic to brain cells through inhibition of the aerobic metabolism of glucose by interfering with the citric acid cycle, together with a fall in glutamic acid and a rise in glutamine, a derivative of ammonia, in the nerve cells.

Endocrine Imbalance.—Certain clinical manifestations of liver disease may be the result of disturbed intrahepatic metabolism of steroid hormones, in particular estrogens and androgens. Simultaneous examination of the estrogen blood level in the hepatic vein and the femoral artery shows that a marked degree of inactivation has occurred in the liver, but this becomes very slight when the patient is severely undernourished.

Arterial spiders, so called because they consist of a central arteriole with radiating smaller vessels, are a feature of hepatic insufficiency (Bean). They have a curious and unexplained distribution, being rarely found below a line joining the nipples. These telangiectases quickly fade after death, so that it is not known if they involve internal organs. They are also observed in preg-

nancy, but only between the second and fifth months.

The following features indicate endocrine imbalance in liver disease. *Testicular atrophy* with accompanying loss of libido and potency is a common feature of cirrhosis of the liver. *Gynecomastia* or enlargement of the male breasts due to increased estrogen in the blood is seen in 40 per cent of men with portal cirrhosis. *Loss of body hair* may be marked on the chest and abdomen. *Arterial spiders* and *palmar erythema* (liver palms) are features of hepatic insufficiency with lack of estrogen inactivation. Diminished urinary excretion of 17-ketosteroids is the one constant biochemical finding in severe liver disease.

Fetor Hepaticus.—This common accompaniment of hepatic failure, which tells its tale to the educated nose, is sweetish, mousy, and slightly fecal in character, and the smell has been compared to that of a freshly opened corpse. It is probably due to the presence of an aromatic amine, which may also be present in the urine. The odor of the breath points to severe hepato-cellular damage, with failure to deaminate amino-acids from the intestine, and it often precedes the onset of hepatic coma, but it may also be due to the establishment of portal-systemic venous anastomoses, as a result of which the hepatic cells are by-passed.

Ascites.—The ascites of liver disease used to be attributed to back pressure in the portal vein the result of cirrhosis. But cirrhosis of the liver may not be associated with ascites even though evidence of portal hypertension is present, and the same is true of occlusion of the portal vein by thrombosis or experimental ligation in the dog. Ascites appears to depend on a multiplicity of factors, and it seems fair to consider the condition as evidence, either direct or indirect, of hepato-cellular failure. The following factors may play a part in different cases: (1) reduction in the serum colloid osmotic pressure, (2) retention of electrolytes owing to hormonal imbalance of debatable origin, and (3) back pressure in the portal venous system.

Lowered serum colloid osmotic pressure results from reduction of the serum albumin, which in turn is due to destruction of the albumin factory, the liver cells. By Starling's long-established principles the intra-vascular hydrostatic pressure tends to force fluid out of the vessels whilst the colloidal osmotic force of the plasma holds it back. Hepatic cell failure is inevitably accompanied by lowering of the plasma albumin manufactured by these cells, so that fluid may be expected to leave the vessels. This of course does not solve the problem of ascites, because it does not explain why fluid pours only into the peritoneal cavity and not into other serous sacs and subcutaneous tissue, nor does it account for the fact that a person may have hepato-cellular failure and cirrhosis for months or years, yet never develop ascites.

Salt retention with accompanying retention of water may be a factor of significance from the standpoint of therapy. This has probably a hormonal basis, although which hormone or hormones are involved is a matter on which opinions differ. Patients with cirrhosis but without ascites excrete sodium in a normal manner, but those with ascites show marked retention of sodium, sometimes only 1 mEq. of urinary sodium a day being eliminated. The excess sodium passes into the ascitic fluid. It is evident that repeated paracentesis may aggravate both the protein and electrolyte depletion, and thus do more harm than good. It seems probable that the salt-retaining adrenal cortical hormone is involved. Here there are two possibilities. The hormone may no longer be inactivated by the damaged liver. Or there may be adrenal cortical hyperfunction due to stimulation by the decreased sodium content of the extracellular fluid, itself caused by the passage of sodium into the ascitic fluid. Renal tubular resorption is the main custodian of the sodium ion. The electrolytic shifts seen in cirrhosis seem to be governed largely by the adrenal mineralocorticoids (DCA) and possibly by aldosterone.

Portal back pressure is an obvious factor which may explain the limitation of the fluid to the abdominal cavity, but we have already seen that portal hypertension alone is not a sufficient explanation of ascites. There may be ascites without hypertension and hypertension without ascites. Patients with Laennec's cirrhosis on whom a porta-

caval shunt has been performed, and who may therefore be presumed to have no portal hypertension, may still have ascites. There can be no doubt, however, that increased pressure in the portal system in conjunction with lowered colloid osmotic pressure form a powerful combination.

NECROSIS OF THE LIVER

In the liver the ordinary pathological conditions such as inflammation, tuberculosis and syphilis are of little importance. Necrosis of liver cells, on the other hand, is of the greatest significance. The necrosis may be divided into: (1) *diffuse necrosis*, in which all the cells in groups of lobules are affected, as in acute yellow atrophy; (2) *zonal necrosis* in which only the cells of a certain area in each lobule are affected; and (3) *focal necrosis* in which small areas of no uniform distribution are affected, as in severe bacterial infections such as streptococcal and typhoid. Zonal necrosis may be (a) *central*, this being the commonest type; (b) *mid-zone*, well seen in yellow fever; and (c) *peripheral*, as in eclampsia. From the clinical standpoint by far the most important variety is diffuse necrosis.

The characteristic reaction of liver cells to an injurious agent is necrosis. This may be called with equal truth either hepatic necrosis or hepatitis. The liver cells in comparison with other cells in the body are always living on the dangerous edge of things, for they exist in a condition of partial anoxia owing to the fact that their main source of blood is venous in origin. When the injury is slight and transient the dead cells are quickly removed and replaced by new liver cells, because no organ has greater power of reproduction. But when the injury is severe or prolonged there is likely to be a proliferation of fibroblasts resulting in fibrosis, which in the liver is known as cirrhosis. These two processes are as closely interwoven as inflammation and repair. The term hepatitis is often used for convenience to describe all stages of the process from necrosis to healing by fibrosis.

The *causes* of hepatic necrosis are many and varied. Indeed this richness of etiology is one of the chief reasons for the complexity of the subject. Our knowledge is dependent on observations on man and the experimental animal. Needless to say, we know much less about the former than the latter. At the same time it is well to remember that it is not wise to apply without reservation animal experimental observations to the human subject. On an etiological basis we can distinguish viral, toxic and deficiency hepatitis or necrosis.

VIRAL HEPATITIS

This is an acute diffuse hepatic necrosis which occurs in sporadic and epidemic form. The *sporadic form* is usually very mild, and has been called in the past *catarrhal jaundice*. The *epidemic form* was extremely common among the troops of all armies in World War II. The virus is excreted in the stools. A similar form of hepatitis associated with jaundice may follow the administration of pooled supposedly normal human serum, of mumps convalescent serum, of yellow fever vaccine, and of arsphenamine (syringe contaminated by an icterogenic agent from blood of other patients), as well as by dental injections with needles carrying a trace of the virus. Viral hepatitis has now become the third commonest reportable disease in the United States.

There are two hepatotropic viruses, which appear to be distinct from one another (Havens). These, for want of better names, are known as the virus of *infectious hepatitis* (IH) or *virus A* and the virus of *serum hepatitis* (SH) or *virus B*. Investigation has been hampered by the fact that no susceptible animals are known, and that all the work has had to be done on human volunteers. Moreover, the clinical picture in the two forms may be almost identical. *Virus IH* comes from the stools of a patient or carrier, and the route of infection is oral. Sporadic cases are due to person to person contact. As the virus is also present in the blood, the infection may be transmitted by blood transfusion. Explosive epidemics may be expected to occur under the insanitary conditions of wartime, as the result of contamination of a water supply from the flooding of rivers, *etc. Homologous serum* or *syringe hepatitis* (SH) is caused by a virus which is transmitted parenterally either by homologous human

serum or by a syringe or needle which has become infected by such serum or by use on a carrier. The common source of infection is pooled plasma or blood used for transfusion. In summary it may be said that there are only two known possible sources of infection, human feces in the case of spontaneous infective hepatitis and human blood in the case of serum or syringe hepatitis. It will be evident that in the SH form the stools are not infective, a point of importance in the nursing care. One attack usually conveys immunity against the specific virus responsible.

Lesions.—Viral hepatitis has a very broad spectrum as regards severity of lesions. In the most severe and fulminating cases, which used to be known as *acute yellow atrophy*, the lesions are mainly in the liver, but the kidneys are nearly always and the brain sometimes involved. The *liver*, in the fulminating cases, may lose 600 grams in weight in the course of a week. It is extremely soft, the capsule is wrinkled because of the rapid shrinkage, and the cut surface, which may resemble the spleen, presents bright yellow and darker red areas. The yellow color is due to remaining necrotic cells being stained with bile, the red represents areas in which the cells have vanished, leaving nothing but sinusoids distended with blood. *Microscopically* the astonishing feature is the complete disappearance of liver cells over wide areas. The virus seems to blow up the cells so that both cytoplasm and nucleus vanish without trace. The remaining cells are necrotic and disintegrating (Fig. 453). Inflammatory cells, often polymorphonuclears, are seen in the portal areas, and there may be endophlebitis of the portal veins. There is an inflammatory portal "triaditis," combined with a more central necrosis. An important feature is preservation of the reticulin outlining the columns of liver cells (Fig. 454). In those cases which recover (the vast majority) repeated aspiration biopsies show regenerating liver cells growing along this framework to form new columns. If no regeneration occurs the sinusoids collapse, the reticular fibers become fused together to form collagen, and cirrhosis may result.

Subacute necrosis with nodular hyperplasia is the name applied to those cases of massive

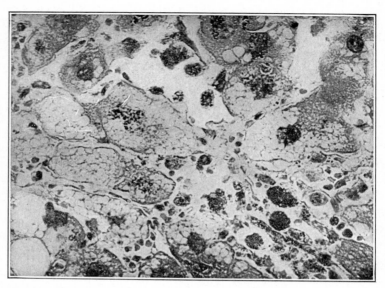

FIG. 453.—Acute diffuse hepatitis. There is an extreme degree of destruction of the liver cells. × 350.

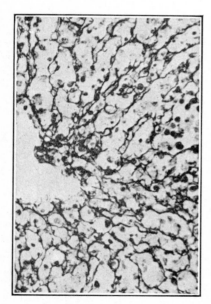

FIG. 454.—Preservation of reticulum around central vein in the necrosis of viral hepatitis.

necrosis which recover from one or more attacks. The patient frequently has had a number of recurring attacks of jaundice, epigastric pain, vomiting and fever. The liver is coarsely nodular and scarred, the nodules of regenerated liver tissue being often quite large. This is *healed yellow atrophy* or *post-necrotic cirrhosis*.

In the *kidneys* acute tubular degeneration (nephrosis) is the rule. Whether this is a primary effect or is secondary to liver damage is not certain. The presence of leucine and tyrosine in the urine, protein cleavage products of necrotic liver cells, is in favor of the second view. In the *brain* there was acute degeneration of the ganglion cells in 15 per cent of Lucké's 125 fatal cases, giving a clinical picture of encephalitis. This is a typical viral type of lesion, suggesting that it is probably not secondary to liver damage.

Relation of Symptoms to Lesions.—We have already seen that the lesions vary greatly in severity, and the same is true of the symptoms. In the most severe cases (acute yellow atrophy) the onset is sudden and the course very acute, with vomiting, profound jaundice, bile in the urine, diminution of liver dulness, delirium, coma and death. In civilian practice the fulminating cases are commoner in women in the later months of pregnancy, when there may be an element of dietary deficiency due to diversion of protein to the fetus. A low nutrition level greatly aggravates the condition and there are probably other accessory factors.

In the ordinary well-developed case the appearance of jaundice is preceded by loss of appetite. Indeed the earliest symptom is often *anorexia* so marked that the sight or even the thought of food is revolting, particularly so in the case of greasy foods. The same is true of alcohol and of smoking. This is accompanied by malaise and a general feeling of wretchedness, perhaps expressed in the old phrase "to feel liverish." *Fever* is present in about half the cases. The *liver* is somewhat *enlarged* and *tender*, and there is a dull ache under the right costal margin. The development of evident *jaundice* may be preceded by darkening of the urine and pallor of the stools. This is accompanied by loss of weight. A week or ten days after the onset of the jaundice it is likely to clear up, the stools to regain color, and the appetite to become voracious. The patient is out of the woods in from two to six weeks depending on the severity of the attack, but lassitude and fatigue may persist much longer. Complete clinical and biochemical recovery may be expected within four months.

Urobilinogen excretion in the urine is first increased owing to failure of the liver to excrete again that which has been absorbed from the bowel. At the peak of the jaundice urobilinogen disappears from the urine because so little bilirubin passes into the bowel. Reappearance of urobilinogen in the urine is a good indication of commencing recovery of liver function. Other functional tests give variable results and are unreliable. In difficult cases where it may be important to distinguish the jaundice from that of the obstructive variety, needle biopsy can be of great value.

The *prognosis* is usually favorable. Although the morbidity is high, the mortality is very low, generally 0.1 to 0.2 per cent; in other words 99.8 to 99.9 per cent of cases recover. Occasionally an SH epidemic will be more virulent, and a mortality as high as 20 per cent has been recorded. The fatal case is likely to be fulminant in type, death occurring within ten days of the onset of symptoms, but sometimes the course is subacute, lasting from three to eight weeks. In cases which have been followed by aspiration needle biopsy it is seen that the inflammatory lesions may be diffuse *or* zonal. The diffuse lesions generally heal rapidly and completely, but when the disease runs a longer course there may be residual fibrosis in the portal zones after apparent clinical recovery. The result in the occasional fulminating cases which recover will be postnecrotic cirrhosis, but in the milder cases it will be of the post-hepatitic type. There is no convincing evidence to show that viral hepatitis may produce Laennec's finely nodular cirrhosis.

Lupoid Hepatitis. — This term is applied to an active chronic hepatitis with a positive lupus erythematosus (L.E.) cell test (Mackay *et al.*). The lupoid hepatitis cases often show some manifestations of disseminated lupus erythematosus, but the two diseases appear to be separate entities, although with a similar pathogenesis, possibly mediated by way of an abnormal immunological responsiveness with autodestruction of the host's tissues. This is suggested by dense plasma cell and lymphocytic foci prominent in the portal tracts, a picture always suggestive of an immune body reaction. The liver disease is the initial and dominant lesion which determines the poor prognosis with death in liver failure.

TOXIC HEPATITIS

Necrosis of the liver may be caused by drugs (arsphenamine, chloroform, cincophen), by poisons used for suicidal or homicidal purposes (phosphorus, mercury), and by substances used in technical and manufacturing processes (carbon tetrachloride, tetrachlorethane and trinitrotoluene). The use of tranquilizing drugs such as chlorpromazine may occasionally be followed in the course of two or three weeks by the onset of jaundice and fever, with, in rare cases, a fatal termination, needle biopsy showing numerous "bile thrombi" in the bile canaliculi and minute foci of necrosis. The action of these substances can be observed both in man and in experimental animals. The effect depends both on the size of dose and on the length of the time that the poison acts. When rats are given a single dose, illness develops in a few hours, reaches its height in twenty-four hours, and is followed by complete recovery by the end of two weeks. The

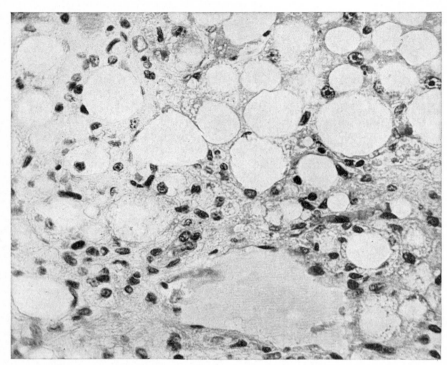

Fig. 455.—Fat cysts of liver in choline-deficiency rats. (Kindness of Dr. W. Stanley Hartroft.)

necrosis is zonal in type, central or peripheral depending on the poison, with restoration to normal in the course of a fortnight. When large doses are given at short intervals the necrosis is more massive and may be followed by cirrhosis.

DEFICIENCY HEPATITIS

Knowledge of this form of liver disease is due to feeding experiments on laboratory animals. Relatively little is known about the condition in man. *Lack of lipotropic factors* in the diet, especially choline and the sulfur-containing amino acids, methionine and cystine, results in an extreme degree of fatty infiltration of the liver followed by necrosis. Prolonged administration of a *low-protein diet* deficient in these essential amino acids also results in necrosis. These varied substances together with the B vitamins serve to protect the liver against the poisons mentioned above and also against virus infection. This is the basis of the high protein-low fat diet reinforced with B vitamins and

sulfur-containing amino acids in infectious and toxic hepatitis. In chronic alcoholism the diet is nearly always grossly deficient in the protective food substances. This is also true of races, such as the African Bantu, in whom cirrhosis (and carcinoma) of the liver is particularly prevalent. It is possible that in man toxic or viral attacks and deficiency in protective elements may be combined, particularly in the severe cases.

The beautiful experimental observations of Hartroft on the changes produced by a choline-deficient diet on the liver of the rat are highly suggestive in relation to human cirrhosis. The first change was an accumulation of fat in the cells farthest from the portal canals. The size of these fat spaces became ever larger, until they measured up to 100 microns in diameter, or 7 times the normal (Fig. 455). No single cell could be distended to this extent. It was found that these fat spaces represented many cells which had become fused owing to rupture of their over-stretched walls. In some cases as many as 80 nuclei could be seen in serial sections, so that the structure represented that number of liver cells. This fat unit Hartroft has named *fat cyst*. In the course of time the fat disappears, leaving the liver via the hepatic veins and bile ducts, the fat cysts atrophy, and at the same time become surrounded by fine fibrils of connective tissue which can be traced to the adventitial sheaths of nearby central veins. Identification of central and hepatic veins was facilitated by the injection of India ink into the respective veins. Cysts which have ruptured into bile canaliculi take on the appearance of atypical bile ducts lined by dedifferentiated hepatic cells, but their true nature at once becomes apparent in frozen sections stained for fat. This is the explanation of the apparent proliferation of bile ducts which is a striking feature of human cirrhosis. The fibrous tissue in the trabeculae represents consolidated, not proliferated, reticular stroma. Only a relatively small fraction of the components of "fibrous" trabeculae gives the characteristic reaction for collagen with connective tissue stains. The bulk of the trabeculae consists of remnants of fat cysts, interlacing channels lined by simple epithelium ("new bile ducts"), and aggregates of ceroid in atrophic cysts. It is small wonder that the fibrosis may appear extreme when it is recalled that a single fat cyst may represent as many as eighty hepatic cells which ultimately disappear. An abnormal accumulation of fat in the liver cells is therefore the basic lesion responsible for the cirrhosis in these animals. The fibrous trabeculæ around the central veins spread along the pathway to neighboring central veins, a pathway which runs midway between the nearest portal areas. Liver lobules are often arranged in petal form around main branches of the portal vein. Thus centrilobular areas lie close to the main portal canals at many points. The mimicry of bile ducts by the atrophic fat spaces in paraffin sections adds to the illusion of a portal distribution. The resulting cirrhosis, while not central in the sense of the centrilobular fibrosis of cardiac cirrhosis, is at least non-portal.

An additional feature of great interest observed by Hartroft in his experimental animals was the presence of fat emboli in the lung, kidney, and heart. The fat entered the pulmonary alveoli and was taken up by phagocytes. Hartroft found fat cysts to be an invariable accompaniment of alcoholic cirrhosis in man, and these cysts were larger than those of the rat. It seems reasonable to suggest that this fatty disintegration of liver cells is an important factor in the pathogenesis of many cases of human cirrhosis. The possibility that fat may be transported from the liver to other organs causing embolism with corresponding after-effects certainly provides food for thought.

It is one thing to observe clear-cut distinctions between deficiency and toxic necrosis in the experimental animal where conditions can be strictly regulated, but it is quite another matter to draw conclusions from observations on hepatic necrosis and cirrhosis in man. Cases of occupational toxic necrosis are fairly easy to recognize, but it is seldom indeed that unequivocal evidence of dietary deficiency can be demonstrated in human liver disease. "To the clinician, endeavouring to interpret these experimental results for a better understanding of the clinical issues at stake, the dangers of a naive overinterpretation are no less grave than a blind dismissal of animal results performed under circumstances which bear little relation to human conditions" (Sherlock).

When we turn to nutritional liver disease in man we are on much less certain ground, for in western countries it is difficult to recognize clear-cut examples of deficiency hepatitis. Two examples are of sufficient importance to demand brief consideration. These are kwashiorkor and alcoholism.

Kwashiorkor.—This is an African term meaning red boy. It is a widespread nutritional liver disease occurring particularly in East and Central Africa, the West Indies, and some parts of South America, regions where undernourishment is prevalent, particularly with regard to protein (Brock). It may be noted that in these areas cirrhosis and primary carcinoma of the liver have a high incidence. In Johannesburg, indeed, liver carcinoma is said to account for 52 per cent of all neoplastic diseases. The disease is prevalent in children as well as adults, and liver carcinoma is frequently seen in young adults from twenty to forty years of age. The striking lesion in the liver is an extreme degree of fatty infiltration with ensuing cirrhosis, a picture closely resembling that of alcoholic cirrhosis in man. The hair and skin shows a red pigmentation, particularly in children. The diet is very low in protein and high in carbohydrates, but the precise factor or factors responsible for the condition are not known. None of the recognized lipotropic agents are of any benefit.

Lesions of the liver in the Bantu fall into three main groups: (1) Fatty liver in infancy due mainly to kwashiorkor, rarely followed by necrosis and fibrosis. In children there is a characteristic zonal localization of fat in the liver lobule, commencing in the periportal area and spreading to the center. A similar lesion has been produced in the rhesus monkey by a protein-deficient diet, thus strongly supporting the theory of a deficiency disease (Deo and Ramalingaswami). (2) A fine symptomless portal fibrosis, generally apparent in the second half of life, and associated with heavy deposits of hemosiderin. (3) Severe cirrhosis, generally post-necrotic in type, with no special age incidence; more than half of these cases develop carcinoma. A factor of possible importance in producing liver damage is the wide variety of native medicines of unknown nature consumed by the adult Bantu.

Alcoholism.—Alcohol has been known for very many years to be associated with liver disease, particularly *cirrhosis*. It is possible that the alcohol has some direct hepatotoxic action. Much more important is the nutritional deficiency which is a constant accompaniment of chronic alcholism. The appetite of the chronic alcoholic is impaired by gastritis as well as by the high caloric value of the alcohol which takes the place of food. As Sherlock remarks, "the diet is particularly poor in protein, for protein-containing foods are expensive and little money is left after the preferred purchases of the equally expensive alcohol." Alcohol supplies calories which supplant the food. The truth is that a "gin-drinker's liver" depends not so much on gin *before* dinner as on gin *instead of* dinner. After a bout the alcoholic is more likely to seek relief from cups of coffee than from a beef steak. Everything, indeed, seems to rob the alcoholic of things his liver needs most. There is believed to be

choline deficiency in alcoholic cirrhosis. The liver is highly fatty in the earlier stages, but the fat may disappear when the fat depots have been exhausted. Acidophilic hyalinization of the cytoplasm with the formation of the so-called *alcoholic hyaline bodies* first described by Mallory, may be a striking feature, but these are also seen in viral hepatitis. A finely lobular cirrhosis of the Laennec type develops as the condition progresses.

Two types of alcoholism in relation to liver disease may be distinguished. In the *first type* the drinking is steady and continuous, but the signs of nutritional deficiency are not marked. The patient is likely to present himself with portal hypertension and ascites, but jaundice and evidence of hepatic failure are not necessarily present. Liver biopsy shows more or less advanced cirrhosis with little or no fatty change. In the *second type* the alcoholic is of the "skid row" variety. He has been drinking heavily and eating little for weeks or months, so that there is evidence of nutritional deficiency such as beriberi, Wernicke's encephalopathy, or severe macrocytic anemia. The liver is greatly enlarged and completely fatty, and death may occur in a week or two from hepatic failure with deep jaundice.

CIRRHOSIS OF THE LIVER

Cirrhosis of the liver is a progressive chronic destruction, diffuse in extent, accompanied by fibrosis, retrogressive changes in the parenchymal cells and proliferation of remaining cells in the direction of regeneration. The word is derived from the Greek *kirros*, meaning tawny, and was used by Laennec to describe the color of the liver. The connotation of the word has now completely changed. The essence of cirrhosis is a disturbance of lobular architecture with the formation of regenerative nodules and connective tissue septa.

A completely satisfactory *classification of cirrhosis* is not possible at the present time, by reason of formidable gaps in our knowledge of pathogenesis. These gaps are now becoming filled, and it is time that some of the older terms were discarded. It is natural that different systems of classification are used by different writers. We shall recognize two main groups: (1) *portal cirrhosis*, which used to be and still is known as Laennec's cirrhosis, and (2) *biliary cirrhosis*. In addition there is a *miscellaneous group* including pigmentary cirrhosis, cardiac cirrhosis, and cirrhosis due to infections with animal parasites such as schistosomiasis. Portal cirrhosis can be subdivided into: (1) *nutritional* (alcoholic) *cirrhosis*, (2) *post-hepatitic cirrhosis*, and (3) *post-necrotic cirrhosis* (Gall), while *biliary cirrhosis* is subdivided into (1) *primary* or *intrahepatic* and (2) *secondary* or *extrahepatic* cirrhosis. To add to the confusion some writers confine the terms portal and Laennec's cirrhosis to the finely nodular nutritional form.

Nutritional (Alcoholic) Cirrhosis.—This is usually regarded as the common type of what used to be known as portal or Laennec's cirrhosis. Of 755 examples of cirrhosis examined by Gall at the Cincinnati General Hospital, 65 per cent were placed in the nutritional and post-hepatitic groups.

Pathogenesis.—The first step in the development of nutritional cirrhosis is massive fatty infiltration or metamorphosis of the hepatic cells. The overstuffed cells become disrupted and lipid accumulates between the cells. There is a gradual nibbling away of liver cells and their replacement by fibrous tissue. When there is interference with tissue respiration and anoxia of the hepatic cells, efficient carbohydrate metabolism cannot take place, and the cells become infiltrated with fat which replaces the normal glycogen. There can be no doubt that chronic alcoholism is the principal although by no means the only cause of the condition. The pathologist must not be misled by a negative history of alcoholism in these cases, for chronic alcoholics are notorious liars in respect to their drinking habits. When the consumption of alcohol in a community is curtailed by reason of war or prohibition, the incidence of deaths from cirrhosis declines. When these phases of human behavior cease, the death rate from cirrhosis rises sharply. It must be remembered that nutritional cirrhosis may occur in children and in teetotalers.

It used to be thought that the alcohol poisoned the liver cells directly. We now know that it is deficiency of lipotropic substances such as choline and methionine in the diet which is responsible. This is indeed a nutritional cirrhosis. The subject of the relation of alcohol to the liver has already been discussed on page 796. There we saw that in the habitual addict alcohol takes the place of food. Moreover, if the addict cannot afford to buy both food and alcohol, he or she prefers alcohol to food.

The type of alcohol consumed does not appear to be related to the incidence of the disease, although opinions differ on this matter. Certainly the term gin-drinker's liver, synonymous with hobnail liver or finely nodular cirrhosis, is an unjust aspersion on a relatively pure form of alcohol unless, as already suggested, it takes the place of food. In beer-drinking countries a large fatty liver rather than a cirrhotic one is the rule. It may be pointed out that in Scotland, where the consumption of spirits is very high, the incidence of cirrhosis is low. This may be attributed to the good eating habits of the people or to the excellent quality of the whiskey.

It is difficult to make a statement of any value as to the incidence of cirrhosis in chronic alcoholics for the obvious reason that accurate data are not obtainable. It is apparently quite low, the figures quoted varying from 1 to 30 per cent. The average duration of the period of heavy drinking before the onset of symptoms is given as fifteen years.

Perhaps undue stress has been laid in this discussion on the subject of alcohol. This form of cirrhosis used to be called alcoholic. This is an inaccurate term, for other agents may interfere with hepatic cell respiration, long-continued severe malnutrition may result in this type of necrosis, and we have already seen that it may develop in those who have never touched alcohol.

Lesions.—The *liver* is atrophic in the later stages, but in the earlier stages it may be much larger than normal. This is especially the case when the fatty changes due to chronic alcoholism are marked. In extreme cases it is only one-half the normal weight. The consistence is very firm owing to the large amount of fibrous tissue and it is usually difficult to cut. The surface of the liver has a characteristic finely nodular appearance,

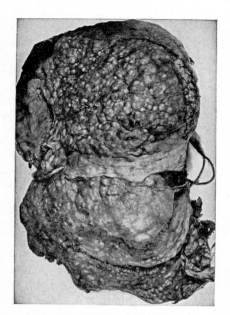

FIG. 456.—Nutritional cirrhosis of the liver. The external surface has a coarsely granular hob-nail appearance.

and the cut surface is correspondingly nodular and greasy (Fig. 456). The nodules are uniform in size. Large nodules over 2 cm. in diameter suggest the post-necrotic type cirrhosis, and these may be so large as to produce distortion of the liver. In nutritional cirrhosis the nodules are small (hobnail liver), averaging 2 to 3 mm. in diameter, and the surface may be merely granular. The color varies. The islands of liver tissue may show no change from the normal, but they are usually golden yellow from fatty changes. There is often a general brownish or tawny coloration, to which the name of cirrhosis was originally due, caused by the deposition of iron pigment.

Microscopically the earliest change is a proliferation of the connective tissue in the portal space. Normally there is sharp delineation of this space, but in cirrhosis the boundary is broken by proliferation of fibroblasts between the degenerated peripheral cells. In the early stages the tell-tale fatty infiltration of the parenchymal cells may be

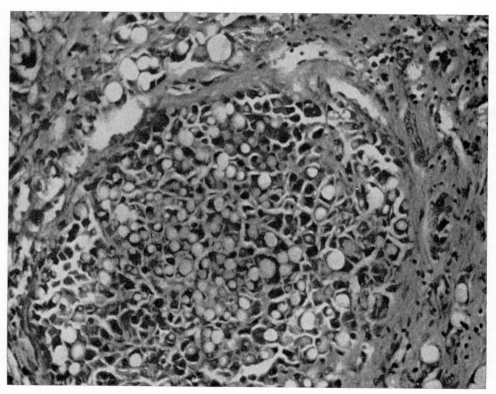

FIG. 457.—A pseudolobule in nutritional cirrhosis. Spherical nodule of fat-filled parenchyma is lacking in radial pattern or lobular landmarks. Nodule is outlined by a delicate frond of connective tissue. × 500. (Gall, courtesy of Am. J. Path.).

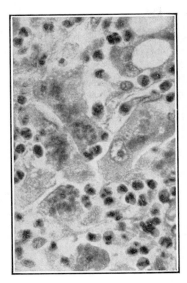

Fig. 458.—"Alcoholic hyaline" in
degenerating liver cells. × 450.

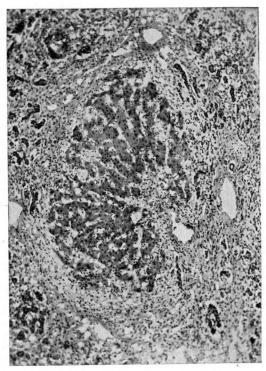

Fig. 459.—Nutritional cirrhosis of liver. Great
replacement of liver cells by fibrous tissue, with
formation of new bile ducts. × 50.

a marked feature, but later this ceases to be
evident. As the disease advances groups
of liver cells of very varying size are
separated by broad strands of fibrous tissue.
The islands of liver cells may resemble
lobules, but this appearance is fictitious;
there is no true lobular arrangement, for
there is no central vein in the center of the
islands, which for the most part represent
new formations due to regenerative hyperplasia (Fig. 457). The portal vein does not
drain into the new nodules, which get their
blood supply from the hepatic artery. The
salient feature is thus loss of hepatic architecture. The nodules are composed largely of
new cells which show irregularity of size and
arrangement. Between the nodules the liver
cells have disappeared. The most characteristic cytological feature is the presence of
hyaline droplets (*Mallory bodies*) in the
cytoplasm representing an acidophilic degeneration of that substance (Fig. 458).
Although it has been referred to as *alcoholic
hyalin*, it is now known that it may be
present in lesser degree in other liver lesions
such as viral hepatitis. The connective
tissue forms broad bands between the islands
of liver cells, and may be young and cellular
or old and fibrous (Fig. 459). Inflammatory
cells are present, but the chief feature is the

greatly increased number of bile ducts.
Cords of young liver cells may simulate new
bile ducts. There is evidently a proliferation
of biliary epithelium which establishes connection with the new groups of liver cells.
Jaundice only appears late in the disease;
even then it is seldom marked.

Testicular atrophy is a common finding in
hepatic cirrhosis. It is much more frequent
in those below the age of fifty years than in
those above that age. It has been suggested
from experimental evidence that there is
failure of normal inactivation of estrogens
by the liver, and that this results in atrophy
of the testes. The urine from patients with
cirrhosis of the liver contains increased
amounts of free estrogens, and it is well
known that administration of estrogens leads
to testicular atrophy. Hyperplasia of the
breasts in the male (*gynecomastia*) and metaplasia of the epithelium of the glands and
ducts of the prostate also occurs, though less
frequently (Bennett *et al.*).

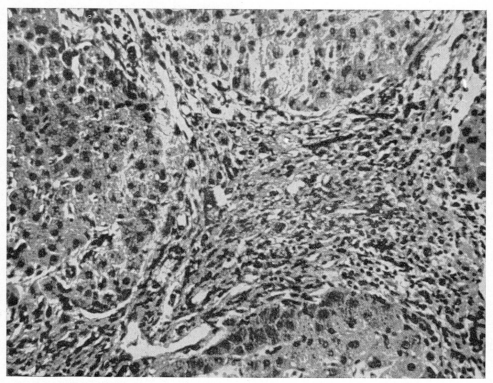

FIG. 460.—Post-hepatitic cirrhosis. From a stellate portal area, the seat of chronic inflammation, narrow fibrous trabeculæ extend to adjacent portal areas (not in photograph). (Gall, courtesy of Am. J. Path.)

Post-hepatitic Cirrhosis.—This form of cirrhosis appears to be the result of an underlying smoldering inflammation. It seems probable that this is viral in origin, but at the present time it is not possible to be more definite. We know that may persons are carriers of the virus of infectious hepatitis. It is they who are the source of infection in the homologous serum jaundice following blood transfusion. The hallmark of this subclinical infection is said to be the presence of lymphocytic exudates in every portal area. Post-hepatitic cirrhosis is believed to arise on the basis of such a condition (Gall).

Lesions.—In this variety of portal cirrhosis the liver is of normal color and normal or reduced size. The surface is uniformly nodular, but the nodules are larger than those of nutritional cirrhosis, averaging 0.5 to 1.5 cm. in diameter. On the cut surface a fine trabecular tracery can be made out. There is no suggestion of the characteristic greasy texture of nutritional cirrhosis nor the coarse scarring of post-necrotic cirrhosis.

Microscopically, narrow bands of fibrous tissue enclose group of lobules or single lobules (Fig. 460). The general architecture is preserved. There is none of the great accumulation of lipid within the liver cells which is so characteristic a feature of nutritional cirrhosis.

At the present time it is difficult to state the relative frequency of post-hepatitic cirrhosis. In Gall's material it slightly exceeded that of nutritional cirrhosis.

Post-necrotic Cirrhosis.—This is the condition known also as healed yellow atrophy, multiple nodular hyperplasia, coarsely nodular cirrhosis and toxic cirrhosis. It is much less common than the other two varieties of portal cirrhosis. In typical cases it is readily distinguished from nutritional and post-hepatitic cirrhosis, but not infrequently it is difficult to make this distinction.

Lesions.—The post-necrotic type of cirrhosis may be due to agents known to cause diffuse necrosis (cincophen, arsphenamine, trinitrotoluene) or there may be no obvious cause. There may be repeated attacks of jaundice with epigastric pain, vomiting and fever. At each attack large groups of liver cells are destroyed. If the patient survives, these areas are replaced by fibrous tissue, while the remaining cells undergo compensatory nodular hyperplasia. As the result of the hyperplasia quite large nodules of new liver tissue may be formed. These nodules are separated by depressed areas of fibrous tissue, the result being complete distortion and loss of the normal architecture. The lumina of central veins can be recognized, together with groups of complete portal triads, which are never seen in classical portal cirrhosis, although with the passage of time these become harder to recognize (Fig. 461). It is the resulting collapse, not the original necrosis, which is so self-evident (Steiner).

The regenerated nodules may cause distortion of the vascular arrangements as well as of the architecture, thus leading to necrosis of the newly formed tissue. "Cirrhosis, once established, sets in motion a series of events which are the sequelæ of disturbed architecture of the liver, and which may be quite distinct from the damage produced by the original agent" (Smetana). Thus a vicious circle is established which results in a never-ending cycle of degeneration and regeneration. Portal hypertension is not due to fibrous constriction of the vessels, but to the regenerative nodules that constitute the bulk of the hepatic tissue in the cirrhotic liver, nodules which compress and distort the portal and hepatic veins and sinusoids (Baggenstoss). Portal hypertension, with accompanying splenomegaly and bleeding varices, is much commoner in the nutritional type of cirrhosis, where the nodules are smaller, more numerous, and cause more vascular distortion.

Biliary Cirrhosis.—This term indicates that the cause of the cirrhosis is to be found in obstruction in the biliary system. The obstruction is usually extrahepatic, and is then known as secondary. When the lesion is intrahepatic the condition is called pri-

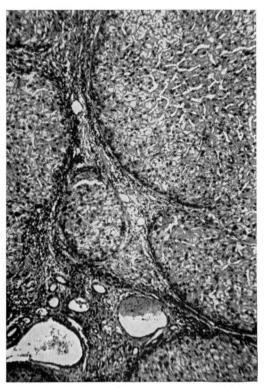

Fig. 461.—Post-necrotic cirrhosis. Moderately severe cirrhosis, showing in the left lower corner an area of old collapse believed to contain 3 portal tracts. The hepatic parenchyma all appears to be of the regenerated type. × 75. (Steiner, courtesy of Am. J. Path.).

mary. Biliary cirrhosis is much less common than portal cirrhosis.

Primary Intrahepatic Biliary Cirrhosis.—This rare condition was described by Hanot in 1876, and for long was called *Hanot's hypertrophic cirrhosis.* The term primary indicates that there is no obvious extrahepatic biliary obstruction. Unfortunately in the majority of cases there is no obvious etiological factor of any kind. It seems probable that a variety of agents may be responsible. The most important of these is drug sensitivity, in particular to chlorpromazine and methyl testosterone. There is ground to believe, for reasons discussed below, that these agents act by stimulating the development of auto-antibodies, and that an autoimmune reaction is responsible for the tissue injury (Hamilton).

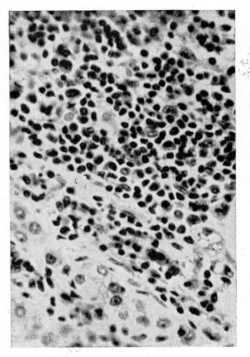

FIG. 462.—Primary biliary cirrhosis. Intense leukocytic infiltration, principally mononuclear, in the portal area. Duration of jaundice, 3 months. (Hamilton, courtesy of Laboratory Invest.)

The *lesions* are confined to the liver which is much enlarged, smooth, and dark green on account of staining with bile, so that it presents a very different picture from that of portal cirrhosis. *Microscopically* the most striking feature is the loss of the finest radicles of the bile ducts, with bile thrombi in the canaliculi. The primary injury results in degeneration and lysis of the cholangioles and neighboring liver cells, accompanied by an intense cellular infiltration, especially of plasma cells, in the portal connective tissue (Fig. 462). Hepatocellular degeneration is isolated, not diffuse or involving wide segments as in portal cirrhosis. As the disease progresses granulation tissue replaces the original infiltrate, and eventually this becomes fibrous tissue (MacMahon and Thannhauser). The fibrous tissue may encircle single lobules (monolobular cirrhosis), or many lobules. In the latter case it will be obvious that it may be very difficult to differentiate the lesions from those of portal cirrhosis.

The *pathogenesis* of the lesions is certainly obscure. Hamilton points out that the primary injury must be distinguished from the subsequent reaction. The primary injury may depend on an autoimmune mechanism, as suggested by the large numbers of plasma cells in the exudate, as well as lymphocytes and histiocytes. The plasma cell reaction is not nearly so marked in secondary biliary cirrhosis. At the same time there is lysis of the lining of the cholangioles and disruption of the limiting plate of liver cells. This allows the aberrant escape of bile into the space of Disse, the portal connective tissue, and even the regional lymph nodes, which are often enlarged. This aberrant bile may well be responsible for the later destruction and cirrhosis.

Complement-fixing antibodies to human tissue can be demonstrated in the blood. There may be circulating antibodies to more than one tissue (liver, kidney, thyroglobulin) in a single case, with dense lymphocytic and plasma cell infiltration in biopsy specimens of the liver, kidney and stomach (Mackay). This suggests the possibility that primary biliary cirrhosis may belong to the group of tissue-destroying immunopathies related to Hashimoto's disease and visceral lupus erythematosus.

Intrahepatic cholestasis is a term which indicates interference with flow in the biliary passages not due to obvious obstruction by stone, tumor or stricture (Popper and Schaffner). In the early stages induced by agents mentioned above (drugs, viruses), there may be no cholangitis. When this develops later it may be a result of the cholestasis rather than a cause. This is also true of the minor change referred to as *feathery degeneration* of the hepatic cells. That there is no impairment of hepatic cell function nor of glucuronide conjugation, is shown by the fact that the bile is of the direct-acting type in the van den Bergh test. The bile seems to be inspissated or altered in its constitution, as shown by the frequent presence of biliary concrements in the extrabiliary ducts. This again may be the result of an increase in permeability of the hepatic cell membrane lining the ductules, possibly affecting the microvilli (Watson and Hoffbauer). The increased permeability may lead: (1) to the regurgitation of bile from the ductules into the sinusoids, with a relatively greater backflow of fluid rather than solids, with a corresponding inspissation of the bile and the development of bile plugs; (2) to increased oozing of protoplasm from the hepatic cells into the bile (albumocholemia), with again an increase in the viscosity and inspissation of the bile. Some of the mechanisms which may cause this change are shown in Figure 463.

The *clinical picture* of primary nonobstructive cholangitis and intrahepatic cholestasis is characteristic, although often not to be distinguished from that of secondary obstructive biliary cirrhosis. *Pruritus* is generally the first symptom, which may antedate the others for a long period. The deepening *jaundice* is paralleled by a *rising serum bilirubin,* and accompanied by *elevated serum lipids* and *alkaline phosphatase.* Later there is a fall in the total serum lipids with a continued rise in serum bilirubin. *Steatorrhea* is common, due to the presence of soaps and increased free fatty acids, and this may eventually give rise to pathological fractures, owing to the development of osteomalacia, itself due to deficient absorption of vitamin D and also of calcium because of the formation of insoluble calcium soaps. *Xanthomatosis* in the form of flat yellowish deposits especially in the eyelids at the inner canthus, on the palms, and at pressure points is fairly common and is related to the high blood lipids. This condition has been called *biliary xanthomatosis* or *xanthomatous biliary cirrhosis* (MacMahon). The distinction between the clinical picture of biliary and portal cirrhosis is graphically drawn in the following passage: "In general, the patients are found to be fairly robust, active, jaundiced, itching, melanotic middle-aged women who differ strikingly from the typical cachectic, pale, pot-bellied males with portal cirrhosis. Jaundice, skin changes involving hyperpigmentation and xanthomatosis, and a markedly enlarged liver and spleen represent the characteristic physical signs" (Kunkel).

Secondary Extrahepatic Biliary Cirrhosis.— The *chief causes* of secondary biliary obstruction are *cancer of the head of the pancreas, stone in the common bile duct,* and

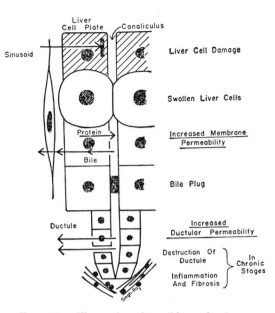

Fig. 463.—Illustration of possible mechanisms responsible for intrahepatic cholestasis (Popper and Schaffner, courtesy of Jour. Am. Med. Assn.)

benign stricture of the duct. Cancer of the head of the pancreas is likely to cause rapid dilatation of the hepatic ducts rather than cirrhosis, which is a slow process. Congenital obstruction of the bile passages in children leads to the obstructive type of cirrhosis.

The *liver* is usually of normal size, but it may be enlarged. The surface is smooth or very finely granular and the whole liver may be stained an intense green. The bile ducts are dilated and tortuous and new ducts appear to be formed. The connective tissue in the portal areas is increased and infiltrated with chronic inflammatory cells. Although sometimes the connective tissue encircles individual lobules (Fig. 464), in most cases the distribution cannot be distinguished from that of portal cirrhosis. The bile canaliculi in the interior of the liver cells are distended with thick bile to such an extent that the liver cells may be disintegrated (Fig. 465); they seem to burst, the canaliculi are ruptured, and the inspissated bile is seen between the liver cells and the walls of the sinusoids. There is marked jaundice but no ascites. The spleen may be enlarged.

For a masterly review of the histological variations and different types which may be

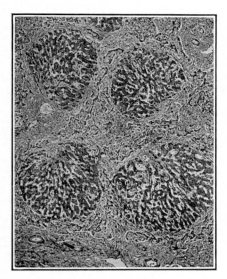

FIG. 464.—Biliary cirrhosis. The cirrhosis is monolobular in type. Numerous bile ducts in connective tissue. × 50.

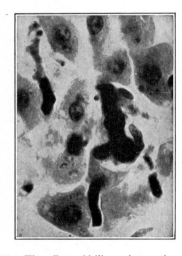

FIG. 465.—The effect of biliary obstruction. The bile canaliculi are distended with bile and the liver cells are disintegrating. × 600.

met with in biliary cirrhosis, MacMahon's paper on the subject should be consulted.

Relation of Symptoms to Lesions. — Although the cirrhotic liver may show marked disorganization and actual destruction of the parenchyma of the organ, there is a remarkable freedom from symptoms of hepatic insufficiency, owing to the great margin of safety which the liver possesses.

The symptoms are mainly those of obstruction, both portal and biliary.

Portal Hypertension.—The cause of portal hypertension may be intrahepatic or extrahepatic.

Intrahepatic portal hypertension is commonly caused by portal cirrhosis. The three factors responsible for the production of hypertension in cirrhosis are: (1) destruction and distortion of the portal vascular bed, well demonstrated by celloidin casts of injected specimens, (2) pressure of regenerating nodules on portal venous radicles with compression or obliteration, and (3) the development of direct hepatic artery-portal vein anastomoses, as a result of which the higher arterial pressure is transferred to the venous system. The resulting internal Eck fistula by-passes the sinusoids, with the regenerating nodules being supplied by the hepatic artery (Fig. 466).

Extrahepatic portal hypertension is caused by chronic thrombosis of the portal and splenic veins, which is said to occur in 10 per cent of cases of portal cirrhosis. It has been attributed to slowing the blood flow and the phlebosclerosis of the portal vein which accompanies cirrhosis. It may be due to malignant invasion of the vein wall, and in rare cases it is associated with polycythemia vera.

Portal hypertension is the chief effect of portal cirrhosis. There is congestion of the entire portal circulation with digestive disturbances, anorexia, etc. *Ascites* develops owing to transudation through the walls of the mesenteric veins. The *spleen* is enlarged. It differs from the cardiac spleen of heart disease in being much larger but not nearly so hard. In the cardiac spleen the sinusoids are distended with blood, while in the cirrhotic spleen there is a cellular increase of the pulp and marked deposits of hemosiderin. The splenic enlargement of cirrhosis is not always due to portal congestion, for it may be present in biliary cirrhosis. It is probable that the infective or toxic agent which acts on the liver acts also on the spleen. This is apparently the case in Banti's disease.

A *collateral circulation* is established with the systemic circulation, but this seldom proves sufficient. Moreover *varicose dilatations* are apt to develop at the points where

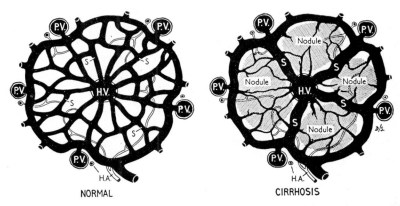

FIG. 466.—Cirrhosis of the liver. The formation of portal venous (P.V.) hepatic venous (H.V.) anastomosis of internal Eck fistulæ at the site of preexisting sinuoids (S.). Note that the regenerating nodules are supplied by the hepatic artery (H.A.). (Elias in Sherlock, *Diseases of the Liver and Biliary System*, courtesy of Charles C Thomas).

the two circulations communicate. Three of these are of clinical importance. (1) At the lower end of the esophagus and the cardiac end of the stomach the varicosities may give way, causing severe or fatal hemorrhage (hematemesis). The injudicious use of the stomach tube may cause rupture of these veins. They are easily overlooked at autopsy because the veins collapse when the liver is removed, so that the esophagus should be examined first in a case of cirrhosis. (2) Less frequently varicosities (hemorrhoids) are formed at the junction of the inferior mesenteric and hemorrhoidal veins. (3) The epigastric veins of the abdominal wall which communicate with the veins at the hilus of the liver by way of the round ligament become dilated, and there may be a ring of varicosities around the umbilicus known as the *caput medusæ*. Injection methods show that innumerable anastomoses develop between the portal and hepatic veins (Fig. 466).

Injection-corrosion studies show that the initial obstruction involves the small hepatic veins rather than the portal veins (Hales *et al.*). This is largely due to distortion and flattening of the hepatic veins by the large pseudolobules. The hepatic vascular bed is also reduced by the fibrosis. The hepatic veins appear to be more susceptible to pressure than the portal system, possibly because the latter is protected by the periportal connective tissue sheath. It will be evident that the major blood supply to the cirrhotic liver

is from the hepatic arteries, so that it has become a purely arterial organ.

There may be marked *hypoproteinemia* in portal cirrhosis. This causes a low serum colloid osmotic pressure, which probably accounts for the edema which may develop, and partly at least for the ascites.

Biliary Obstruction.—*Jaundice* is the great symptom of obstructive biliary cirrhosis, the bile being unable to escape from the bile ducts and accumulating in the blood. Cases of portal cirrhosis often develop jaundice in the terminal stages, but it is seldom severe. It may be explained by the extreme disorganization and distortion of the normal architecture of the liver. Indeed it is to be wondered at that jaundice is not a more marked feature of portal cirrhosis.

Other Forms of Cirrhosis.—In addition to the three main forms of cirrhosis, namely portal, post-necrotic and biliary, there is a miscellaneous group of conditions in which fibrosis may be associated with disturbance of liver architecture. Brief consideration will be given to the following conditions: (1) hemochromatosis and hemosiderosis, (2) hepatolenticular degeneration, (3) schistosomal cirrhosis, (4) sickle cell anemia cirrhosis, and (6) the cirrhosis of hereditary disorders of metabolism.

Hemochromatosis.—This rare condition, known also as bronzed diabetes, has already been considered on page 395 in connection with disturbances of pigments. It is not really a disease of the liver but a disturbance of iron metabolism. It is probably an *inborn error of metabolism*, and its genetic basis may account for the fact that it is practically confined to the male. The condition does not really merit its name, for the iron comes not from the blood but from the food, owing to a defect in the normal duodenal mucosal block.

Siderosis of the liver is very common amongst the South African Bantu suffering from pellagra, repeated needle biopsies showing a series of changes in the liver cells beginning with fatty degeneration and ending with massive accumulations of iron (Gillman and Gillman). The excess of iron appears to come from the diet. Natives who are heavy drinkers of Kaffir beer have a heavy incidence of siderosis as shown by needle biopsy. Kaffir beer contains 4 mg. of iron per 100 ml., and as it is not uncommon for an African to drink a gallon of Kaffir beer at one session (about 160 mg. of iron), this may well be the source of the iron enrichment of the diet (Lamont and Hathorn). The uptake of iron from iron-enriched diets is much greater in rats fed a "bad" (maize-meal) diet than in those fed a "good" (stock) diet (Gillman *et al.*). Moreover, the same choline-deficient diet which causes cirrhosis in rats may also lead to excess iron absorption from the diet. Relatively minor changes in the diet determine whether the end picture will be one of iron deposits in many organs with pigment cirrhosis (hemochromatosis) or without pigment cirrhosis (hemosiderosis) (MacDonald). The underlying lesion seems to be related to the intracellular iron-containing enzymes located on the mitochondria. Intracellular hypoxia, perhaps induced by malnutrition (the "bad" diet in the case of the rat), increases the speed and degree of iron uptake, suggesting that iron overload alone is not sufficient to produce dietary siderosis.

The liver in hemochromatosis contains enormous quantities of iron in the form of hemosiderin. The pigment is present in the liver cells, Kupffer cells and connective tissue. Owing to the continued irritation of the pigment the liver cells become necrosed and disappear, and there is a marked proliferation of connective tissue with a resulting

pigment cirrhosis, the microscopic appearance of which is identical with portal cirrhosis. The liver is usually enlarged and of a characteristic brown color. Carcinoma of the liver is a complication in about one-fifth of the cases. Liver biopsy is far better than skin biopsy for the purpose of diagnosis, as the color of the skin is due to melanin rather than to iron.

Exogenous hemochromatosis is a condition in which large deposits of iron are formed in the liver with subsequent cirrhosis, not on account of an inborn error of metabolism but by reason of an excessive exogenous supply of iron, usually as the result of repeated blood transfusions. It is a *hemosiderosis*. Although the iron is deposited first in the reticuloendothelial system, the parencyhmatous cells take up the excess when the depots are filled, with resulting degeneration and fibrosis, so that the morphological end result is similar to that of hemochromatosis. As a rule over 100 transfusions are required to produce this picture, although in some cases hemosiderosis has developed after only a dozen transfusions (Dubin).

Hepato-lenticular Degeneration (Wilson's Disease).—Although hemochromatosis and hepato-lenticular degeneration appear to be worlds apart, it is appropriate to consider them together, because both are fundamentally the result of an inborn defect in the nature of an enzyme deficiency in dealing with a metal, in the one case iron, in the other case copper. It is a rare disease of young people characterized by portal cirrhosis, degeneration of the lenticular nuclei in the basal ganglia, and pigmented rings in the periphery of the cornea. The defect is inherited as an Mendelian recessive, so that if it is to manifest itself it must be carried by both parents. The defect may be a deficiency in ceruloplasmin, a serum copper oxidase, a defect associated with the absorption of excessive amounts of copper, just as in hemochromatosis there is excessive absorption of iron. The clinical manifestations are neurological in character, and it is only late in the disease that hepatic insufficiency manifests itself, in spite of extensive destruction of the liver. The condition is therefore considered in more detail in connection with diseases of the nervous system.

In spite of what has just been said above it is now realized that Wilson's disease may manifest itself by symptoms of severe liver disease at a very early age long before the development of neurological symptoms (Chalmers *et al.*). Indeed the patient may die of hepatic failure before there is time for such development. Many cases of familial juvenile cirrhosis, some beginning before the age of one year, may really represent what has been called the abdominal form of Wilson's disease.

At autopsy the liver invariably shows a marked degree of cirrhosis, together with the presence of brown pigment in the hepatic cells. The type of cirrhosis varies much, in some cases being finely nodular, in others coarsely nodular as in the classic post-necrotic form.

In the main, however, it shows various stages of post-necrotic cirrhosis, but with the unusual addition of (1) fat-filled cells, suggesting a nutritional deficiency, (2) extremely large Kupffer cells, and (3) glycogen degeneration of the liver cell nuclei (Anderson and Popper).

Schistosomal Cirrhosis.—This condition, also called bilharzial cirrhosis, is a complication of schistosomiasis. It is a major form of cirrhosis in Egypt, Puerto Rico, and other centers of infestation by the parasite. The ova are deposited in the wall of the bowel or the bladder, depending on the species. Some of the ova are swept back into the liver, where they accumulate in the portal spaces, and set up a granulomatous reaction which gradually develops into a progressive fibrosis. The early *lesions* show pseudotubercles in the center of which ova may be detected. At this stage the correct diagnosis can be easily made by means of needle biopsy. As the fibrosis progresses there develops either (1) a coarse nodular or a diffuse cirrhosis, or (2) localized lesions peculiar to this condition to which the name of pipestem cirrhosis (white clay pipe) has been given. The granulomatous change may involve the walls of the intrahepatic veins with obliteration of the lumen and the establishment of vascular shunts between portal and hepatic vessels. The result is portal hypertension, splenomegaly, and hemorrhage from esophageal varices which often proves fatal. Pipestem cirrhosis is really an extraparenchymal portal fibrosis, and the resulting portal hypertension is similar in genesis to that of extrahepatic portal vein ob-

struction rather than to the intrasinusoidal hypertension characteristic of true cirrhosis.

Sickle Cell Anemia Cirrhosis.—A rare form of cirrhosis seen in the negro, often quite early in life, is that produced by sickle cell anemia (Song). The liver is nodular and the spleen enlarged. The lesions vary from areas of fresh necrosis to old fibrosis resulting in the formation of pseudolobules. It would appear that the damage is the result of the formation of agglutinative thrombi of sickle cells in the hepatic capillaries with further obstruction of the sinusoids by Kupffer cells swollen with erythrocytes.

Hereditary Disorders of Metabolism.—Two inborn errors of metabolism in which cirrhosis of the liver plays an important part, namely hemochromatosis and hepato-lenticular degeneration, have already been described. A number of other rare examples will be merely mentioned here. Because of the absence or even the abnormality of a single gene there may be lack of a single essential enzyme in the hepatic cells, and this lack may wreck the metabolism of carbohydrates, lipids, or amino acids. Examples of *carbohydrate defects* are galactosemia, glycogen storage disease, and gargoylism; of *lipid defects* Gaucher's and Niemann-Pick's disease; of *amino acids* cystinosis (Lignac-Fanconi disease). The result, mostly in children, will be degeneration of liver cells with the possible development of cirrhosis. Details of these conditions will be found in the paper by Gall and Landing.

JAUNDICE

The liver has far more important functions than the excretion of bile, but at present the estimation of those functions is a matter of great difficulty, and the study of the behavior of the bile pigments affords one of the most convenient methods for determining the state of health or disease of the liver cells. For this reason the study of jaundice or icterus is of interest to the pathologist as well as to the clinician. Jaundice is a coloration of the skin and sclerotics by bile pigment in the blood. The color varies from pale yellow to deep orange or even green. The internal organs are pigmented with the exception of the central nervous system, which usually escapes. The pigment is bound to elastin, which explains why the cornea and nervous tissue are not colored.

The investigation of a case of jaundice, in particular the all-important question as to whether medical or surgical treatment is

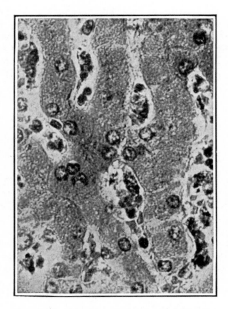

FIG. 467.—Swollen and detached Kupffer cells in liver sinusoids. × 525.

indicated, may be decided by clinical acumen or by laboratory tests. At the present day there is more likelihood of failure to depend on clinical acumen than failure to employ a formidable battery of laboratory tests. When an adequate history has been taken with attention to pertinent details it is remarkable how little place is often left for laboratory investigation except to provide confirmatory evidence. The age may give a clue; persons over the age of forty are more likely to have calculi (women) or carcinoma (men), whilst the younger they are the more chance there is of hepatitis. The occupation may provide an important lead. Bar tenders and brewery workers with jaundice are more likely than clergymen to have portal cirrhosis, cleaners are exposed to carbon tetrachloride vapor, workers in ammunition plants to trinitrotoluene, sewer workers, plumbers, garbage men and pig keepers to rats and Weil's disease, whilst laboratory workers handling human sera may develop virus hepatitis. A history of blood transfusions or even hypodermic and dental injections may point to viral hepatitis, whilst the use of arsenicals, sulfonamides, chlorpromazine or other occasionally hepatotoxic drugs may be significant.

Schiff, in his monograph on jaundice, emphasizes the value of simple observations on the color of the urine and stools. The appearance of dark urine is the best criterion of the onset of jaundice especially in colored patients, and may be detected several days before corresponding changes are apparent in the skin and scleræ. In infectious hepatitis the stools are likely to be clay-colored for about a week and then to acquire a normal color again. In obstruction of the common duct by calculus the stools may be alternately acholic and cholic for obvious reasons, whereas when the obstruction is due to carcinoma they will naturally remain acholic.

Bilirubin is formed from the hemoglobin of broken-down erythrocytes by the cells of the reticuloendothelial system, principally those of the bone marrow and spleen. If hemolysis is increased, the amount of bilirubin formed will be correspondingly increased. The bile acids are synthesized only by the liver. Jaundice may be the result either of excessive production or inadequate removal of the pigment.

When the bilirubin is formed it is carried to the liver for excretion. There are three elements in a liver lobule: (1) the hepatic cell; (2) the bile canaliculus, which we may call the bile duct; and (3) the sinusoid, which connects the portal with the hepatic vein and is lined intermittently by Kupffer cells (Fig. 467). The hepatic cell is flanked on one side by the vessel, on the other side by the bile duct. The bilirubin is carried to the lobule by the blood, passes through the wall of the vessel, is excreted by the hepatic cell into the bile duct, and escapes into the intestine. In the large bowel it is reduced by bacterial action to urobilinogen which is colorless. The greater part of the urobilinogen is excreted in the feces, but part is absorbed into the portal circulation and passes to the liver. Part of this fraction is again excreted by the hepatic cells, but part passes on into the general circulation and is excreted in the urine. In health a very small but fairly constant amount of urobilinogen is present in the urine. When bilirubin has passed through the hepatic cells as we shall see presently, it is conjugated with glucuronic acid, and in consequence becomes highly soluble in water, a fact of great significance.

If the altered bilirubin is then reabsorbed into the blood, as in obstructive jaundice, it is able to pass the barrier of the renal filter and appears in the urine. If it has not passed through the hepatic cells it is held up by the renal barrier and does not enter the urine, even though the amount in the blood is sufficient to produce jaundice; this is known as *acholuric jaundice*.

The bilirubin in the liver sinusoids is different from the bilirubin in the bile canaliculi. This was shown by van den Bergh in 1918 by means of Ehrlich's well-known diazo reagent (diazotized sulfanilic acid), which gives an immediate red color with bile or with the icteric serum of obstructive jaundice; this is known as the *direct van den Bergh reaction*. When the serum of a patient with hemolytic jaundice is added to the diazotized sulfanilic acid reagent an immediate reaction is obtained only on the addition of alcohol; this is therefore called the *indirect van den Bergh reaction*. The two types of bilirubin are known as direct reaction bilirubin, which has passed through the liver cells, and indirect reaction bilirubin which has not, or, more conveniently, as *cholebilirubin* and *hemobilirubin* (Harrison), although the latter terms are not yet of general acceptance. In hemolytic jaundice a positive reaction is obtained even without the use of alcohol after a delay of ten minutes; this is the *delayed direct* reaction. If the color develops at once in the absence of alcohol but deepens on standing, we have a combination of the two types, known as a *biphasic* reaction, which indicates the presence both of hemobilirubin and of cholebilirubin. Bilirubin is conjugated with glucuronic acid in its passage through the liver cells, and the resulting glucuronide is far more soluble in water than is unconjugated bilirubin. This is the explanation of the fact that conjugated bilirubin readily passes the renal filter, whereas pure bilirubin is held back. The glomeruli, indeed, are as efficient at distinguishing between the two types of bilirubin as is the van den Bergh qualitative reaction. *Direct-acting bilirubin is bilirubin glucuronide, whereas indirect-acting bilirubin is simply pure unconjugated bilirubin.*

We may summarize the principal features of the two pigments by saying that hemobilirubin gives an indirect van den Bergh reaction, is not present in bile nor in the urine of jaundice, has an affinity for brain tissue being lipophilic in nature, but does not stain the other tissues, and is raised in the blood in hemolytic jaundice. Conjugated bilirubin (cholebilirubin) offers a striking contrast, for it gives a direct van den Bergh reaction, it is present in the bile and in the urine of jaundice, it has no affinity for brain tissue, but, being water-soluble, it does stain the other tissues, and it is raised in the blood in obstructive jaundice (Billing and Lathe).

Before birth the placenta, not the liver, is responsible for removing bilirubin from the fetal blood, so that there is no jaundice at birth. Jaundice only develops if the enzyme glycuronyl transferase system in the hepatic cells responsible for bilirubin conjugation is not fully developed. This naturally is more likely to be the case in premature infants. A deficiency in the transferase enzyme is also present in Gilbert's disease, familial nonhemolytic jaundice (page 810).

The most rational classification of jaundice is based on the relation of the bilirubin to the liver cell. The lesion responsible for the jaundice may be *before, in* or *after* the bilirubin has passed through the liver cell, the result being respectively hemolytic, hepatic, or obstructive jaundice. The first two may be grouped together as retention jaundice, the liver being unable to excrete all the bilirubin, which therefore accumulates in the blood. This inability may be due to too much bilirubin being produced (hemolytic jaundice), or to sickness of the liver cells preventing them from excreting the normal amount of bilirubin (hepatic jaundice).

Of the great numbers of liver function tests, two are of special value in the study of a case of jaundice. A *negative cephalin-cholesterol flocculation test* shows that there is no primary disease of liver cells, and that the jaundice is not due to a hepatitis. A *high alkaline phosphatase* reading indicates obstruction either in the large bile ducts or hepato-cellular in character.

1. **Obstructive (Posthepatic) Jaundice.**—

The purest examples of obstructive jaundice are cases of obstruction of the common bile duct by cancer of the head of the pancreas, stone in the duct, or stricture of the duct. The pigment passes through the liver cells, but as it cannot escape, it is reabsorbed into the blood, produces clinical jaundice, and flows over into the urine. The *congenital jaundice* of children (not icterus neonatorum) due to atresia of the biliary passages belongs to this group. When the obstruction is severe little or no bile passes into the intestine, and the *stools* are *clay-colored*, because the fats remain undigested in the absence of bile. Owing to this absence no urobilinogen is formed, and as none is absorbed the urobilinogen normally present in the urine disappears completely. When obstructive jaundice is suspected, the clinician can resort to the technique of liver needle biopsy. We should bear in mind the fact that it is sometimes better to open the door and look by means of laparotomy than to peep through the key hole.

2. Hemolytic (Prehepatic) Jaundice.—

When there is excessive hemolysis the bilirubin carried to the liver cannot be all excreted so that some remains in the blood. This type of bilirubin cannot pass the kidney filter, so that the jaundice is of the acholuric type although there is a great increase of urobilinogen in the urine. The jaundice is never so intense as it may become in the obstructive form. This form of jaundice is best seen in the disease known as hemolytic jaundice (also called acholuric jaundice), in which there is overactivity of the reticuloendothelial system and increased fragility of the red blood cells, as a result of which the amount of hemolysis is considerably above normal. As might be expected, the amount of urobilinogen excreted in the feces is greatly increased.

Less degrees of jaundice may occur whenever there is marked hemolysis, *e.g.*, as the result of snake-bite, intraperitoneal hemorrhage, large pulmonary infarcts, ruptured tubal pregnancy, and blood infection with hemolytic streptococci. Sometimes, as in pernicious anemia, the blood bilirubin may be above normal but below the amount necessary to produce clinical jaundice. This is known as latent jaundice.

3. Hepatic (Hepatocellular) Jaundice.—

This form, also called toxic jaundice, is the jaundice of infectious (viral) hepatitis, or, more accurately, of liver necrosis. Hepatocellular jaundice is perhaps the most descriptive term for the condition. The first effect of disease of the hepatic cells is an inability to excrete all the bilirubin, some of which therefore accumulates in the blood. An even earlier result is a retention in the blood of the urobilinogen brought from the bowel, and a corresponding increase of the urobilinogen in the urine. With continued action of the virus the hepatic cells become more and more swollen so as to cause obstruction of the tiny bile canaliculi whose walls they form. Some of the bilirubin still passes through the sick cells, but as it cannot escape on account of the blockage of the canaliculi it is reabsorbed. If the chief effect of the lesion is retention, the bilirubin will not appear in the urine. If there is much obstruction of the canaliculi this reabsorbed bilirubin will accumulate in the blood and flow over into the urine. The milder forms constitute the common variety formerly known as catarrhal jaundice. In the most extreme forms little or no bile may enter the intestine. In this case the stools will be clay-colored, and the urobilinogen in the urine will first diminish and finally disappear altogether.

Some of the laboratory features which serve to distinguish the three main types of jaundice are summarized for convenience in the accompanying table. *In actual practice the results of the tests will not be as clear as indicated, depending on the phase of the disease and the presence of complications.*

Familial Non-Hemolytic Jaundice.—A rare form of constitutional jaundice, non-hemolytic, non-obstructive, and acholuric in type, was described by Gilbert and his associates in France in 1901 under the heading simple familial cholemia. *Gilbert's disease*, as it is now known, has been called constitutional hepatic dysfunction, and it is discussed here in connection with hepatocellular jaundice, although there is no evidence of structural damage to the liver cells, because there is no suggestion of hemolysis nor obstruction. It is probably best regarded as an *inborn error of hepatic function* resulting in a high excretory threshold for bilirubin. The genetic

SOME LABORATORY FEATURES OF THE PRINCIPAL TYPES OF JAUNDICE

Laboratory Studies	Hemolytic (Pre-Hepatic)	Obstructive (Post-Hepatic)	Hepatocellular (Retention)
Serum bilirubin	Indirect	Direct	Biphasic
Urine bilirubin	Negative	Positive	Positive
Urine urobilinogen	Increased	Low or absent	High
Stools	Dark	Clay-colored	Pale
Flocculation and turbidity tests	Negative	Negative (early)	Positive
Serum alkaline phosphatase	Normal	Increased	Normal
Total serum cholesterol	Normal	Increased	Decreased

defect is a deficiency in the transferase enzyme responsible for the conjugation of bilirubin with glucuronide into direct-acting bilirubin, soluble and therefore readily excreted by the kidneys. The jaundice, which is seldom intense and may only affect the scleræ, begins in youth and may last for many years. The patient is more icteric than sick, but he may complain of lassitude, fatigue and dyspepsia, and the jaundice itself is intermittent with exacerbations. The condition is familial, but, unlike familial hemolytic jaundice, there is no anemia, spherocytosis, or increased fragility of red cells. Liver function tests are normal, but urobilinogen is absent from the feces, and the elimination of injected bilirubin from the serum is delayed, as might be expected. Liver biopsy specimens show no microscopic evidence of disease, and the same is true of the very few autopsy cases on record.

Dubin-Johnson disease, (also called *Dubin-Sprinz disease*), is a variant of Gilbert's disease first described in 1954. The feature which sharply characterizes this variety of familial non-hemolytic jaundice is the presence in the parenchymatous cells, and occasionally in the Kupffer cells, of very large amounts of coarsely-granular, golden-brown pigment, which is not bile, iron nor ceroid (Fig. 468). The accumulation of pigment within liver cells probably represents a bloc due to an enzyme deficiency. The jaundice can be regarded as of the retention type. The distinction between this condition and Gilbert's disease seems to be that in Dubin-Johnson disease the metabolic disturbance is widespread, whereas in Gilbert's disease it is confined to the excretion of bilirubin. The diagnosis of these syndromes is important because of the risk such patients run of being labelled as cases of liver disease or being subjected to unnecessary surgical exploration.

Symptoms of Jaundice.—The principal symptoms are due to a retention of bile salts

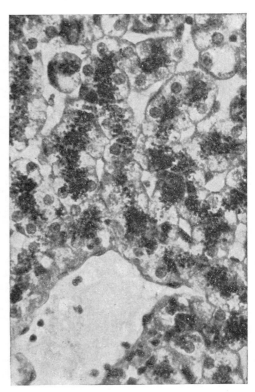

FIG. 468.—Dubin-Sprinz disease. Massive accumulation of coarse granular pigment within liver cells surrounding a central vein. Periodic acid-Schiff reaction. × 420. (Brown and Shnitaka, courtesy of Amer. Jour. Med.)

rather than to the bile pigment. In the disease known as hemolytic jaundice where the liver cells are normal there is no retention of bile salts, so that there are none of the characteristic symptoms. Such a dissociation between bile salts and bile pigment is spoken of as dissociated jaundice. In obstructive jaundice the salts as well as the pigment are retained, and the patient suffers from severe and sometimes uncontrollable itching, bradycardia (slow pulse), hemorrhage due to injury of the capillary endothelium by the bile salts, and various nervous symptoms. The blood cholesterol, which should normally escape in the bile, is increased, and there may be deposits of cholesterol in the skin which form small yellow nodules known as xanthomata. *Bleeding* is an important feature of jaundice, and postoperative bleeding may prove fatal. It is due to a marked fall in the plasma prothrombin, associated with prolonged clotting time. The low prothrombin level is due to: (1) failure of absorption of vitamin K from the intestine owing to absence of bile; (2) damage to the liver, in which organ prothrombin is formed from vitamin K. Administration of synthetic vitamin K before operation will bring the prothrombin level back to normal and prevent hemorrhage. In catarrhal jaundice there is a characteristic *leukopenia* or diminution in the white cells of the blood, which often fall to 4000 per c.mm. and sometimes even to 2000. The chief decrease is in the polymorphonuclears.

ICTERUS NEONATORUM.—Some degree of jaundice is very common in the newly-born. This is merely an exaggeration of a physiological condition present in all infants after birth. The jaundice is therefore hemolytic in type, and may remain latent or become visible. The reason for the hemolysis is that the child at birth has a polycythemia, an excessive number of red blood cells, because *in utero* it has been living in a condition of anoxemia or constant lack of oxygen. After birth the need for the polycythemia ceases, the excess red cells are destroyed by hemolysis, an increased amount of bilirubin is produced, and there is jaundice either latent or clinical.

WEIL'S DISEASE. SPIROCHÆTOSIS ICTEROHÆMORRHAGICA.—Weil's disease is a very acute epidemic infection, characterized by marked jaundice, hemorrhages from the mucous membranes, fever, enlargement of the spleen and nephritis. There is marked evidence of blood destruction, and blood and bile appear in the urine. The disease is caused by a specific spirochete (Spirochæta

icterohæmorrhagiæ). It occurs in troops on active service, and workers in mines, sewers and abattoirs. The factors common to these occupations are dampness of the soil and close association with rats.

The rat seems to act as a reservoir of infection, excreting great numbers of spirochetes in the urine. The spirochetes may penetrate the skin directly. Fleas may act as an intermediate host. A few cases have been caused by rat bites. The disease usually lasts about three weeks. During the first week the spirochetes are present in the blood. In the second week they disappear from the blood, but appear in the urine.

In addition to cloudy swelling the liver may show small areas of focal necrosis, in which mitoses or amitotic division can be seen. Even more striking than mitoses is the presence of binucleated liver cells, as if amitotic division of the nucleus had occurred. In some cases there is a striking *dissociation of liver cells*, the columns being broken up and the cells separated from one another (Fig. 469*A*). The renal tubules show degeneration or actual necrosis. There are degenerative changes in the muscle fibers, especially in the legs, and focal ischemic necrosis in the brain. The spirochetes, which often present a terminal hook like a shepherd's crook (Fig. 469*B*), lack the sharp spirals of the spirochete of syphilis. They are present in large numbers in the liver, kidney and adrenal, and in smaller numbers in other organs. If a guinea pig is inoculated with blood during the first week or with urine during the second week it will develop the disease and will show hemorrhages in the lungs and enormous numbers of spirochetes in the liver and kidney. Some strains, however, are not pathogenic for guinea pigs. The patient's urine may also be examined directly for spirochetes by the dark-field method. Immune bodies are developed in the blood, so that an agglutination test is of value for diagnosis.

CANICOLA FEVER.—This rare condition may be considered here because of the relation of the infecting spirochete to that of Weil's disease, but there is neither jaundice nor involvement of the liver. The organism is *Leptospira canicola*, so-called because the carrier host is canine, not rodent. The

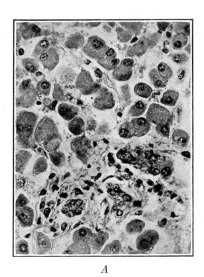

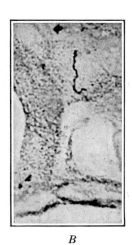

A   B

FIG. 469.—*A*, Dissociation of liver cells in Weil's disease. × 300.
B, Spirochete in kidney in Weil's disease. × 1350.

symptoms suggest involvement of the central nervous system, and the cases may be mistaken for meningitis or poliomyelitis. Both the protein and cell count of the cerebrospinal fluid are increased. Some degree of nephritis is almost always present, and the urine may contain albumen, casts, and red blood cells. Fever continues for about a week. The prognosis is good.

CIRCULATORY DISTURBANCES

Chronic Venous Congestion.—No organ shows chronic congestion so often as the liver, because when there is any back pressure on the venous circulation it is the hepatic vein which feels it first, as it practically opens into the right auricle. The common cause is valvular disease of the heart or myocardial failure. Emphysema which narrows or obliterates the pulmonary capillaries causes distention of the right side of the heart, and this is followed by congestion of the liver.

The liver is enlarged so that it can be felt below the costal margin, firm, and as the capsule is tightly stretched it may be painful and tender. In the later stages it may become smaller owing to atrophy of the parenchyma. The cut surface shows the characteristic appearance known as *nutmeg liver,*

characterized by undue distinctness of the lobules and a mottling with dark and light areas. The central vein and the surrounding sinusoids are filled with blood so that the center of the lobules is dark red; the periphery is pale because the cells are fatty and swollen, and the congestion of the sinusoids is much less there. *Microscopically* the central vein and the sinusoids of the central area of each lobule are so distended with blood that the liver cells may have largely disappeared owing to pressure atrophy. At the periphery of the lobule the congestion is usually much less marked, and the liver cells are fairly intact, but they show a considerable degree of fatty degeneration owing to the poor oxygenation. As the condition progresses the connective tissue stroma proliferates, giving *cardiac cirrhosis*.

Infarction.—An infarct of the liver may be produced as the result of embolism either of the hepatic artery or the portal vein. As a matter of fact, an aseptic infarct of the liver is very seldom seen in the autopsy room, owing probably to the abundant anastomosis which takes place between the two sets of vessels within the liver. On this account also the infarcted area is likely to be red, just as a pulmonary infarct is red. Occasionally a traumatic infarct may occur, produced by injury to the vessels going to the area. As this injury is likely to be of some extent, the anastomosis will be interfered with and the infarct will be pale. If septic emboli are carried to the liver by the portal vein there will be a suppurative phlebitis and the formation of multiple abscesses.

Thrombosis of the Heptic Vein.—Chiari Syndrome.—This very rare condition was described by Chiari in 1899, but previously by Budd in 1857, so that it is also known as the *Budd-Chiari syndrome*. The thrombosis may be due to malignant invasion of the vein wall, to thrombophlebitis migrans, or to polycythemia vera. The usual site of the thrombosis is the junction of the hepatic vein with the vena cava. The liver is large, tender, smooth, and purple in color. The cut surface gives the picture of the "nutmeg" liver. The microscopic appearance is that of chronic passive congestion. The onset is acute, with the rapid development of ascites, thus distinguishing the condition from portal vein thrombosis. Signs of portal hypertension soon appear, accompanied by those of hepatocellular failure.

INFECTIONS

Abscess.—An abscess may be caused by infection reaching the liver by way of (1) the hepatic artery, (2) the portal vein or (3) the bile duct.

(1) *Hepatic artery infection* is a manifestation of pyemia. Large numbers of small, even microscopic, abscesses are scattered through the liver. The condition is a terminal one, and death occurs before the abscesses have time to attain any size.

(2) *Portal vein infection* is usually due to septic embolism from a focus of suppuration in the appendix, or sometimes in the stomach or intestine. It is a portal pyemia, so that the abscesses are multiple, being most numerous in the right lobe. Occasionally there is direct extension of the inflammation from the septic focus in the gastrointestinal tract along the portal vein to the liver, a condition of *suppurative pylephlebitis* (*pyle*, a gate). The portal vein is filled with a soft infected thrombus, and when it is slit open it can be followed down to the original source of the infection.

(3) *Bile-duct infection* causes cholangitic abscesses. They are associated with calculus obstruction in the ducts or suppuration of the gallbladder. The abscesses are multiple, and the bile ducts are filled with pus.

Amebic Abscess.—Amebic abscess or tropical abscess is a special example of portal vein infection. It is a common complication of amebic dysentery, the amebæ being carried from the intestine to the liver by the portal circulation. The abscess may be single or multiple. The common site of the solitary abscess, which may attain a great size, is the upper part of the right lobe causing upward displacement of the right dome of the diaphragm. The contents are viscid and chocolate-colored, but are necrotic rather than purulent unless secondary infection occurs. The amebæ, however, are believed often to carry pyogenic bacteria with them on their way from the colon to the liver. The amebæ may die, leaving only sterile pus. It is hardly an exaggeration to say that all liver abscesses other than the small ones found in suppurative cholangitis and suppurative pylephlebitis are of amebic origin no matter whether amebæ or microorganisms are or are not found in the abscess. It may rupture into the peritoneum or lung. The condition is often a very chronic one.

Actinomycosis.—The fungus infection usually spreads from a primary focus in the cecum or appendix. Secondary abscesses are formed in the liver. These at first are arranged in small groups so that the affected area has a loculated or honeycomb appearance which is very characteristic. In some cases it resembles a sponge full of pus. Later large abscesses are formed containing the familiar sulfur granules in which the mycelia can be demonstrated.

GRANULOMATA

A variety of granulomatous lesions may occur in the liver. The interest of hepatic granulomas lies not in the damage which they do to the liver, which is minimal, but to the fact that they may offer a means of diagnosing the general condition by the use of needle biopsy.

Sarcoidosis.—The general condition of sarcoidosis is discussed in relation to the lymphatic system. The diagnosis can usually be made from biopsy of a superficial lymph node or skin. Occasionally these are not available, and in such cases needle biopsy of the liver may serve to clinch the diagnosis. It is remarkable how often the relatively small and scattered lesions can be picked up by the liver. Before giving a negative report the pathologist should make serial sections of the small block of tissue removed. The hepatic lesions do not in themselves give rise to any clinical disturbance. They may heal with scarring, but the fibrosis is always focal, never diffuse, so that there is not true cirrhosis.

Other granulomata may give a histological picture similar to that of sarcoidosis, e.g. brucellosis and beryllium poisoning, as well as fungous infections such as histoplasmosis, coccidioidomycosis, etc., but again the lesions are too minute to interfere with liver function.

SYPHILIS.—Syphilis of the liver used to be a subject of importance. Now it has sunken to the obscurity of small type. It may occur in two forms, congenital and acquired. The congenital lesions are usually diffuse, the acquired are localized.

CONGENITAL.—This form occurs in a child the subject of congenital syphilis. In the early stages the liver is enlarged; later it may be contracted. In Levaditi preparations the liver is found to be swarming with spirochetes, which are distributed diffusely through the entire organ. This serves to explain the lesion which is known as syphilitic cirrhosis, and takes the form of a fine diffuse fibrosis which penetrates the lobules and may separate the liver cells.

ACQUIRED.—The lesion of the acquired form is the tertiary gumma of which there may be several. They may be of considerable size. The left lobe tends to be more involved than the right. There may be tumor-like masses on the surface. As the gummata heal abundant scar tissue is formed, and when this contracts deep fissures are produced. These fissures divide the liver into irregular lobes, so that sometimes a remarkable degree of deformity is produced which is absolutely characteristic of the condition. Such a deformed and scarred liver is called hepar lobatum (Fig. 470). It must be added that gummata of the liver are hardly ever seen nowadays.

TUBERCULOSIS.—This may take two forms. (1) Miliary tubercles are scattered through the liver in general miliary tuberculosis. They are usually found in the region of the portal tract. (2) The solitary tubercle or tuberculoma is a rare condition in which a large caseous mass is formed

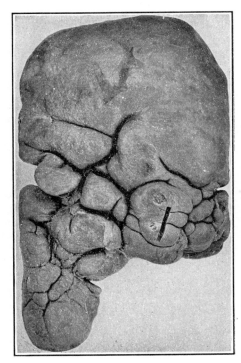

FIG. 470.—Hepar lobatum.

which is easily mistaken for a gumma. Indeed the differentiation may not be possible unless the tissue is stained for tubercle bacilli.

ANIMAL PARASITES

Hydatid Disease.—The presence of hydatid cysts in the liver causes a tumor-like enlargement. It is a comparatively rare disease except in those sheep-raising countries where men come into intimate contact with dogs, e.g., Australia, South America, etc. In these countries it is very common. The life cycle of *Tænia echinococcus*, of which the cystic stage is the hydatid, has already been traced in Chapter 14. The ingested embryos bore their way through the wall of the bowel, and are carried to the liver by the portal vein. Here they develop into the larval or cysticercus stage. The cyst wall is composed of a laminated membrane rather like the white of an egg, lined by a germinal layer from the cells of which daughter cysts grow. Scolices or heads of new individuals are formed within the cysts, and these are

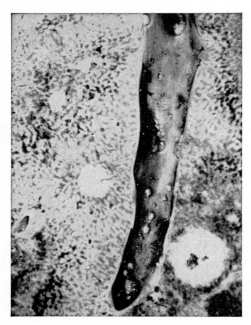

FIG. 471.—Invasion of portal vein by carcinoma of liver. (Boyd, *Pathology for the Surgeon*, courtesy of W. B. Saunders Co.)

Clonorchis sinensis, invades the bile ducts in large numbers and may cause jaundice. We have already seen that it may act as a carcinogen.

TUMORS

Although the liver has such remarkable powers of hyperplasia, primary tumors both innocent and malignant are quite rare. Secondary tumors are very common, because all the blood from the gastrointestinal canal and pancreas passes through the liver, and it is supplied in addition by the hepatic artery.

Primary Carcinoma.—Primary cancer is as rare as secondary cancer is common, with the exception of patients with cirrhosis of the liver, and certain peoples, such as the African Bantu, and in some parts of China. Before diagnosing a tumor as primary carcinoma, every other possible source of growth must be excluded. There are two forms of primary carcinoma of the liver: (1) *hepatoma* or liver cell carcinoma; (2) *cholangioma* or bile-duct carcinoma. Hepatoma is perhaps very much commoner than cholangioma. In typical cases the differentiation is very easy, but in atypical cases it is very difficult.

Hepatoma.—A more appropriate name for this neoplasm is *hepatocellular carcinoma.* There may be one large tumor with a few small outlying nodules, or more rarely multiple small nodules are scattered throughout the liver without any large primary growth. The massive tumors are soft, necrotic, and often show hemorrhage. When the growths are multiple there has usually been spread through the liver by the portal vein, for invasion of the vein is common (Fig.471). In some cases it appears probable that the tumors are of multicentric origin. This is especially so with the small multiple type of growth. The intervening portions of the liver may be very firm owing to portal cirrhosis which is commonly associated with primary carcinoma, and may give the liver a finely nodular appearance. *Microscopically* the tumor consists of liver cells very irregular in size and arrangement. They are arranged in interlacing strands, but sometimes show an attempted alveolar or even adenomatous formation which is easily confused with that of

armed with a row of small hooklets. The nature of the cyst can be recognized from the microscopic appearance of the laminated membrane, or the presence of the tiny hooklets in the watery fluid.

The liver may be greatly enlarged, and the mass caused by the large cysts is easily mistaken clinically for a tumor. The larvæ die out after some years, and the cyst may be converted into a putty-like mass with calcification of the capsule. Rupture may occur into the abdominal or pleural cavity, and the fluid may produce toxic effects. The fluid may be used as an antigen in a complement-fixation test or a precipitin test for the disease.

Other Parasites.—In *schistosomiasis* the ova may be carried by the portal blood stream to the liver, where they may set up a rather characteristic form of cirrhosis with areas of dense white connective tissue around the portal tracts. This is particularly liable to happen with *S. mansoni* and *S. japonicum* infections, as these flukes inhabit the mesenteric veins. The cirrhosis may be associated with carcinoma of the liver. The liver fluke, bile-duct carcinoma. Multinucleated giant cells may form a striking feature; indeed some of the largest carcinomatous cells occur in this tumor. The relation of carcinoma to cirrhosis is an intriguing one. It is probable that the cirrhosis is primary, and that the tumor arises from the associated hyperplastic nodules. In 682 cases of cirrhosis over a period of thirty-eight years hepatic neoplasia was present in 8.5 per cent of cases (Gall). The tumor, a hepatocellular carcinoma, showed a special predilection for posthepatitic and postnecrotic but not for nutritional cirrhosis. Carcinoma occurs as a complication of hemochromatosis in some 20 per cent of cases of that disease.

A point to be taken into consideration in cancer of the liver in the Chinese is the very common infestation with *Clonorchis sinensis* due to the ingestion of raw fish. The smallest bile ducts are not wide enough to accommodate the Clonorchis, the continual movements of the worms cause mechanical irritation and epithelial hyperplasia, with resulting multifocal adenocarcinoma of the bile ducts. This explanation may, of course, be quite wrong.

Cholangioma.—Bile-duct carcinoma is less common than hepatoma and less often associated with cirrhosis. The tumors are multiple, and the liver is enlarged and stained with bile. The *microscopic appearance* is that of an adenocarcinoma in typical cases, the lining cells resembling those of the bile ducts (Fig. 472). Giant cells are seldom seen. In the more atypical forms the structure resembles that of a hepatoma.

There seems to be general agreement that carcinoma of the liver is becoming more frequent. Thus at the Boston City Hospital the autopsy incidence of the disease in the period 1917-1946 was 0.34 per cent compared with 0.72 per cent during the period 1947-1954 (MacDonald). This was associated with an increased incidence of healed acute yellow atrophy and of fatty nutritional cirrhosis, but there was also a lesser increase in patients without cirrhosis. The increased longevity in recent years is of course a factor to be taken into account.

Symptoms.—The symptoms of primary carcinoma of the liver are often due as much to the cirrhosis as to the tumor. Jaundice

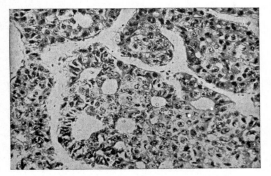

Fig. 472.—Cholangioma. The tumor cells in places are arranged around ducts.

and ascites are common. A very rapidly recurring ascites suggests malignant invasion of the portal vein. Fever is present in over 10 per cent of cases. It may be compared with the fever of gumma of the liver, and in both cases seems to depend on a mass of necrotic material in the liver.

Secondary Carcinoma.—Secondary carcinoma of the liver is very common. The spread may be: (1) from the gastrointestinal tract by way of the portal vein, (2) by the systemic circulation (hepatic artery), (3) by the lymphatics, (4) by direct spread from the gallbladder, stomach, or pancreas. Cancer of the stomach is the most common primary site, but cancer of the breast and the lung deserve special mention. Other sites are the kidney, adrenal, uterus, and eye (malignant melanoma.)

The liver may be enormously enlarged or of normal size. The tumors are multiple and are more on the surface than central in position. They vary greatly in size, are soft and necrotic, and may be yellow from necrosis, green from bile-staining, or red from hemorrhage. The superficial tumors show a falling-in of the center due to necrosis, which from the outside gives an appearance of dimpling known as *umbilication*. There is no cirrhosis.

Invasion of the larger portal tributaries in the liver by tumor growth is responsible for the multiplicity of nodules. There may be only one metastasis in the first place, but this mechanism, which can be demonstrated by cutting the liver into thin slices, is responsible for the multiplicity. Invasion of efferent veins is an important factor in further dissemination to the lungs.

SARCOMA.—Primary sarcoma is extremely rare. Secondary sarcoma is not common.

BENIGN TUMORS.—An *adenoma* is very rare. It usually remains small and is composed of irregular columns of liver cells; the normal architecture of the lobule is lost. The nodules in a cirrhotic liver when large may be mistaken for adenomata. A *solitary hyperplastic nodule* in an apparently normal liver may be several inches in diameter and press on the surrounding organs. It is not encapsulated like a true adenoma, but can be removed surgically. *Cavernous hemangioma* is fairly common. It is found by accident at autopsy and causes no symptoms. It forms a small red or purple area always situated on the surface and apt to be mistaken for an infarct. It consists of cavernous blood-filled spaces.

DEGENERATIONS

Fatty Degeneration.—So-called fatty degeneration of the liver has already been considered in Chapter 1. It is really an infiltration, fat being carried from the fat depots to the liver where it fails to be metabolized for various reasons. Accumulation of fat in the liver is one of the most delicate indicators of interference with the health of the organ. It is marked in diabetes, pernicious anemia, chronic alcoholism, etc. Starvation induces the condition, thus explaining in part the frequency with which it is found in hospital autopsy material. The part played by lipotropic factors in the experimental production of accumulation of fat in the liver has already been discussed on page 794. Extensive replacement of liver cells by fat in heavy drinkers may be the cause of entirely unexpected and abrupt death (Le Count, Singer, and Graham). In such cases the liver is huge, and the liver cells are represented by large fat globules. Replacement of glycogen is the probable cause of death. The fatty liver is yellow in color and greasy to the touch. The fat is either in the form of one large globule which pushes the nucleus to one side, or of many tiny droplets scattered through the cytoplasm. The latter probably indicates a greater disturbance in the health of the cell. Hartroft has shown that the huge globules really represent fat cysts formed by the fusion of many fat-filled cells to form one large globule of fat (see Fig. 455, page 794).

Amyloid Degeneration.—Amyloid disease

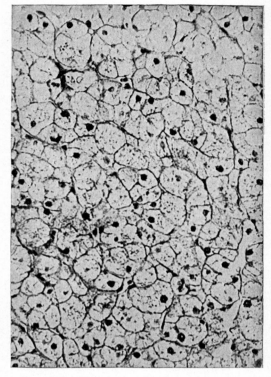

FIG. 473.—Liver in Von Gierke's glycogen storage disease. × 200. (Boyd, *Pathology for the Physician.*)

is described in Chapter 4. The spleen and the kidney are involved as well as the liver. The liver is much enlarged, smooth, and very firm and elastic in consistence. The cut surface has a characteristic translucent (waxy) look, with brown amyloid patches when treated with iodine. The essential change is an extreme hyaline (amyloid) swelling of the connective tissue, as a result of which the liver cells undergo a pressure atrophy and largely disappear. The veins and sinusoids are also compressed, yet ascites is a rare occurrence though sometimes it does develop. There is no jaundice. In advanced cases the microscopic changes are so extreme and the replacement of liver cells so great that it is remarkable that there is so little disturbance of liver function.

Glycogen Storage: Von Gierke's Disease.—The general features of von Gierke's disease has already been discussed on page 23, so that they do not need to be described here. The liver is greatly enlarged and this cause of hepatomegaly in a child must always be considered, for the disease, at any rate in its less severe forms, is probably less rare than has been supposed. The individual liver cells are enormously swollen and clear, and present an appearance liable to be mistaken for hydropic degeneration (Fig. 473). Glycogen in the normal liver is very difficult to demonstrate unless the tissue is examined immediately after death and fixed in absolute alcohol, for the glycogen is rapidly converted into glucose by the glycogenolytic ferment, and the glucose, being soluble in water, is readily dissolved out by a watery fixative such as 10 per cent formalin, which of course is 90 per cent water. In von Gierke's disease the glycogen can be demonstrated and stained by Best's carmine at least twenty-four hours after death, owing to the absence of the normal ferment, and even a watery fixative does not remove all of it. There is indeed very little decrease in the glycogen content even after the tissue has been kept under refrigeration for a week.

ATROPHY.—This is most marked in inanition, and in chronic starvation the liver may be quite shrunken and of a uniform brown color with loss of lobulation. In old age some atrophy is common. Pressure of a tumor, of amyloid deposits, etc., may produce local atrophy. Tight lacing (in the past) or continual stooping (occupational) may lead to the formation of grooves on its upper and anterior surface. There may be deep sagittal furrows corresponding to bulgings of the diaphragm.

POSTMORTEM CHANGES. — The commonest change is a bluish or greenish *discoloration* of the surface, due to the action of hydrogen sulfide liberated from the intestine and similar to the postmortem discoloration of the abdominal wall. It is seen first in those parts of the liver in contact with coils of intestine. *Foamy liver* is a condition in which the organ is filled with bubbles of gas, which are produced after death by gas-forming bacilli. It may resemble a sponge. The condition is most likely to occur in wound infections with the anaerobic gas-producing bacteria.

DEVELOPMENTAL DEFECTS

In rare cases one lobe of the liver may be absent or the left lobe may be very small. *Riedel's lobe* is a downward prolongation of the right lobe which may be mistaken for an abdominal tumor.

Polycystic Disease.—This condition, sometimes known as *cystic liver*, is a congenital and developmental defect, although it is usually seen in the adult. It is associated with the much commoner congenital cystic kidney, but the latter usually occurs without any cysts in the liver. Sometimes there are cysts in the pancreas. The cysts in the liver may be few and small, or the whole liver may be studded with large and small cysts so that the organ is greatly enlarged. In this case there will be great pressure atrophy of the liver parenchyma. As in the case of the cystic kidney the cysts tend to enlarge gradually. They contain a clear albuminous fluid and are lined by cubical epithelium. The condition is supposed to be due to some malformation of the smaller bile ducts, which fail to become connected with the main biliary tree and undergo cystic dilatation. Occasionally other congenital abnormalities such as hydrocephalus, spina bifida, and talipes may be present.

THE GALLBLADDER

GENERAL CONSIDERATIONS

The normal gallbladder is 3 to 4 inches long, and its capacity is about 45 cc. The liver produces nearly a liter of bile a day, but only some of this reaches the duodenum. The rest is absorbed, or rather the watery part is absorbed, by the wall of the gallbladder, so that the bile is greatly concentrated. The Graham visualization test depends on the concentrating power of the gallbladder. When this is lost the dye excreted by the liver is no longer sufficiently concentrated to be visible in the roentgen-ray picture. Loss of concentrating power is apparently an early result of gallbladder disease. The radiopaque contrast medium which used to be taken by mouth is now given intravenously. The inner surface of the gallbladder appears to be designed for absorption. The entire surface is divided into a series of polygonal spaces by delicate walls of mucous membrane, which are best appreciated if the gallbladder is examined under water by means of a magnifying glass or a binocular dissecting microscope. When this is done the transparent mucous folds,

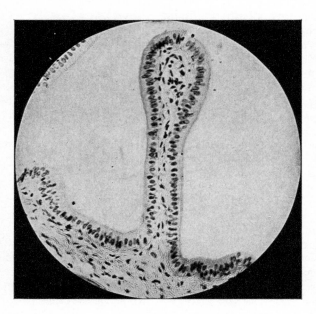

Fig. 474.—Normal gallbladder showing fold covered by tall columnar epithelium.   × 500.
(Boyd, *Pathology for the Surgeon*, courtesy of W. B. Saunders Co.)

gossamer-like in delicacy, are seen to float up like leaves of a water plant in a clear pool. In microscopic sections the membranes, cut transversely, appear as delicate villi. (Fig. 474). This is in striking contrast to the appearance in chronic cholecystitis.

A peculiar feature of the gallbladder is that polymorphonuclear leukocytes are frequently present in one or more layers of the organ without any other evidence of inflammation. These cells are also present in the dog's gallbladder. They do not indicate inflammation, and appear to be metabolic in function.

The muscle coat ceases abruptly at the neck of the gallbladder, and the bile ducts (cystic and common) are fibro-elastic tubes with only a few isolated muscle fibers. There is an abundance of nerve fibers in the outer part of the wall of the ducts. From these facts it is evident that biliary colic is due to distention of the duct and not to muscular spasm.

CHOLECYSTITIS

Cholecystitis may be acute or chronic. An acute attack may develop on top of the chronic form, or it may be followed by that form. Either may be associated with calculi. In the appendix acute inflammatory lesions completely outweigh chronic ones as a cause of symptoms. The opposite is the case in the gallbladder.

Acute Cholecystitis. — *Etiology.* — The causation of acute inflammation of the gallbladder is much more obscure than in the case of the appendix and is but dimly understood. A distinction must be drawn between acute inflammation of a previously normal gallbladder and that superimposed on chronic cholecystitis (Halpert). In the former stones are rarely present, whereas they are nearly always found in the latter. Two factors must be considered: (1) bacterial infection and (2) chemical irritation, but unfortunately it is often difficult or impossible to separate these. The infecting bacteria, such as Escherichia coli, non-hemolytic streptococci and Cl. welchii, are normal inhabitants of the bowel. They are carried to and excreted by the liver, and reach the gallbladder by way of an obstructed cystic duct, or they may spread directly from the liver to the gallbladder wall via the lymphatics. Hematogenous infection may also presumably occur. In the days when typhoid fever was common, acute cholecystitis could often be traced to this infection, but whether the bacilli came from the blood or from the gallbladder where they flourish who can tell? When present, organisms are found only in small numbers of the wall, and not in the lumen. This is in striking contrast to acute suppurative appendicitis, where bacteria are present in enormous numbers. The obstructed appendix has a high bacterial content, but the obstructed gallbladder has a high content of chemical irritants, the bile salts and acids. It is possible that chemical irritation may play a major role in acute inflammation of the gallbladder, and bacterial infection in most cases a relatively minor one.

Occlusion of the cystic duct is probably the most important single factor in the production of acute cholecystitis (Andrews). The lumen of the duct is small, and its wall is thick and deeply pocketed with sinuses, so that a slight degree of inflammation will cause narrowing or closure of the duct. Calculi causing obstruction may be associated either with acute or chronic inflammation. The intensity of the ensuing inflammation depends on the composition of the imprisoned bile (Womack and Bricker). When the cystic duct is tied after the gallbladder has been emptied and washed with saline, no inflammation develops. When the gallbladder contains bile there is edema, round cell infiltration and fibrosis. When the bile is replaced by a solution of dried bile double the concentration of that of normal bile, the wall undergoes complete necrosis, although when the cystic duct is open the changes are slight and transient. It is reasonable to suggest that in chronic as well as in acute cholecystitis the chemical factor is of great importance. This would serve to explain the extreme diffuseness of the lesions, so different from the patchy focal lesions of chronic inflammation in other organs, and also the association of cholecystitis with gallstones which are an important cause of biliary obstruction.

Morbid Anatomy.—The wall of the gallbladder is thickened, the serous surface is congested and covered by a fibrinous exudate, and the mucosa is bright red or purple. When obstruction of the cystic duct is com-

plete the lumen is distended with what appears to be purulent fluid, so that the condition is known as *empyema of the gallbladder*. This is often not a true empyema, for the "purulent" fluid is frequently found to consist of an emulsion of cholesterol crystals. *Microscopically* the most striking picture is a marked inflammatory edema, which is responsible for most of the thickening. Polymorphonuclears are relatively few in number in striking contrast to the abundant purulent exudate in acute appendicitis, suggesting a non-bacterial inflammation. Reference has already been made to the presence of polymorphonuclear leukocytes in the uninflamed gallbladder. In some cases the picture is that of an ordinary purulent inflammation, and in these the bacterial count in the bile is enormously increased.

Chronic Cholecystitis.—Chronic cholecystitis may be the result of an acute attack, but usually it is chronic from the outset and the symptoms develop gradually and insidiously. There is a low-grade inflammatory reaction commencing in the outer part of the wall and gradually spreading throughout the gallbladder. The gross appearance varies considerably. The bluish color of the thinwalled normal gallbladder is lost, and the surface may be opaque; it is sometimes yellow owing to an accumulation of subserous fat. The wall is thickened and fibrosed (Fig. 475), and the cavity may be of normal size, dilated or contracted. If there has been no obstruction at the neck of the gallbladder, the cavity is likely to be small from contraction of the new fibrous tissue. Sometimes the gallbladder is contracted upon one or two large stones, so that no room is left for any bile. Should obstruction be present owing to inflammatory swelling, cicatricial contraction, or the impaction of a stone at the neck of the bladder, there will be dilatation of the cavity as well as thickening of the wall. If obstruction becomes marked before the inflammatory changes have had time to cause thickening, the wall of the greatly dilated bladder may be quite thin. The cavity is filled with clear, colorless, watery fluid secreted by the lining epithelial cells, a condition known as *hydrops* of the gallbladder. The bile pigment is absorbed, and

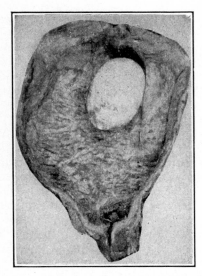

Fig. 475.—Chronic cholecystitis. The gallbladder is dilated, its wall moderately thickened, the fundus contains a large calculus, and the lining shows reticulation.

no more can enter owing to the obstruction. The condition of the gallbladder depends on the balance between inflammation and obstruction. In the milder cases the surgeon may have great difficulty in deciding at operation whether or not the gallbladder is diseased and should be removed. The cystic gland at the neck of the gallbladder is usually enlarged.

When the gallbladder is opened the appearance again varies. The color is usually not much changed, but it may be a deep red. With a hand lens or the dissecting microscope the thin folds of the normal mucosa are seen to be thick and swollen, but when the organ is markedly distended as in hydrops they may disappear completely. It is evident that the absorbing and concentrating power of the gallbladder will be greatly impaired or lost, so that no shadow is seen with Graham's visualization test. As a result of contraction of the fibrous tissue the surface may become reticulated and scarred, so as to present an interlacing network of fine bands which show through the atrophic mucosa with great distinctness.

The *microscopic appearance* is one of chronic inflammation usually involving the entire organ. There are definite groups of

lymphocytes, and occasionally large numbers of plasma cells and eosinophils, as well as a more diffuse infiltration. Single sections are of doubtful value, for serial sections show a high degree of patchiness of infiltration, which is often more marked on the hepatic then on the peritoneal surface. The folds of mucosa are thickened owing to edema. It must be remembered that the normal mucosa contains large numbers of round cells; these must not be mistaken for an inflammatory infiltration. The epithelium is usually intact in well-fixed tissue. Postmortem material is useless as, immediately after death, the bile digests away the epithelial lining in both the normal and pathological gallbladder. The same is true, though in a lesser degree, of gallbladders removed at operation unless they are at once opened and placed in formalin. The very best results are obtained by distending with formalin the freshly removed and emptied gallbladder. The mucosal folds are greatly widened by edema, and inspection of such folds do not remotely suggest an abortive organ (Fig. 476). To realize the full truth of this statement the student should compare figure 476 with figure 474. In the later stages there is an abundant formation of granulation tissue which causes great thickening of the wall (Fig. 477), and is ultimately replaced by fibrous tissue, so that the gallbladder is converted into an inert bag incapable of contraction. There may be a marked increase in the amount of elastic tissue, which normally is quite scanty (Riopelle). The elastic tissue increases both with age and with the duration of the disease. The increase seems to be dependent on intermittent dilatation of the viscus, and ceases after complete obstruction develops. It is comparable to the elastosis of benign hypertension. The *relation of the symptoms of acute and chronic cholecystitis to the lesions* is discussed together with the symptomatology of biliary calculi on page 826.

Cholesterolosis of the Gallbladder.—This is also known as the *lipid gallbladder* and the *strawberry gallbladder*. The wall is usually a little thickened, but the most striking change is in the mucosa, over the surface of which are scattered little yellow flecks like the seeds of a strawberry. The condition is best seen with the hand lens or under the dissecting

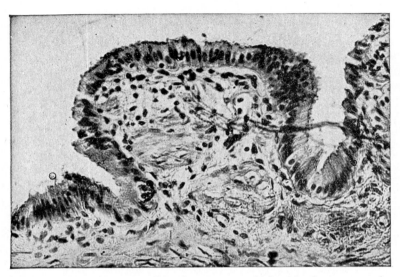

FIG. 476.—Chronic cholecystitis. The folds of mucosa are thickened, edematous, and contain dilated lymphatics. The epithelium is quite intact. × 300. (Boyd, *Pathology for the Surgeon*, courtesy of W. B. Saunders Co.)

microscope, which gives a much better idea of the lesion than a microscopic section (Fig. 478*A*). The normal delicate mucosal folds are seen to be loaded down by opaque yellow masses which first appear on the summit of the ridges. These are deposits of cholesterol ester which can be studied in frozen sections stained with a fat stain (Scharlach, osmic acid), or under crossed Nicol's prisms where their anisotrophic character is revealed. The lipid is found at the base of the epithelial cells of the mucosa and in phagocytic histiocytes in the deeper part of the wall (Fig. 478*B*). A mass of lipid in the mucosa may become pedunculated and is then readily detached, when it may act as the nucleus around which a gallstone may be formed (Fig. 479).

The explanation of the condition is not easy. Cholesterol seems to be absorbed by the gallbladder mucosa, although Elman and Graham believe that it is excreted, and that the excretion is increased by inflammation. In the condition of cholesterolosis there is storage of cholesterol under the mucosa. Two possible etiological factors may be at work. The first and most important is a disturbance of cholesterol metabolism, as a result of which the amount of cholesterol in

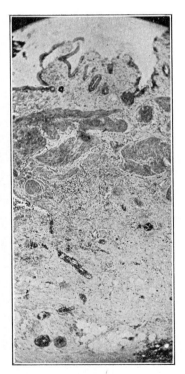

FIG. 477.—Chronic cholecystitis. The wall is greatly thickened and groups of inflammatory cells are scattered through it. The muscle is largely replaced by fibrous tissue. × 40.

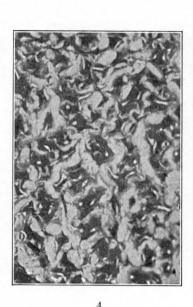
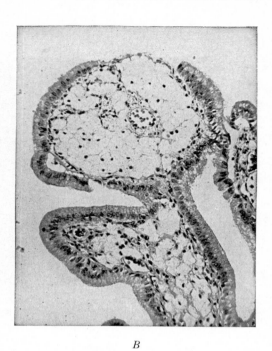

A *B*

Fig. 478.—*A*, Cholesterolosis of the gallbladder under the dissecting microscope. The ridges of mucosa are loaded with lipid.

B, Colesterolosis of the gallbladder. A villus is distended with large lipid-filled macrophages. The gap in the epithelium is an artefact. (Boyd, *Pathology for the Surgeon*, courtesy of W. B. Saunders Co.)

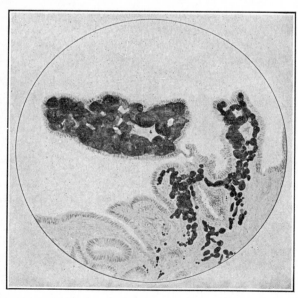

Fig. 479.—Cholesterolosis of the gallbladder. There are large masses of cholesterol in the mucosa and also in the deeper parts of the wall. A pedunculated mass is almost separated from its attachment. (Boyd, *Pathology for the Surgeon*, courtesy of W. B. Saunders Co.)

he blood and bile is increased. The second
s a mild degree of chronic inflammation. It
s probable that the condition of cholesterolosis is not necessarily a permanent one, and
that most if not all the cholesterol may
finally disappear. There is no convincing
evidence that these deposits can cause symptoms or that they are of any clinical significance.

CHOLECYSTITIS GLANDULARIS.—Sometimes, apparently as the result of chronic irritation, the
epithelium lining the gallbladder commences to
proliferate and form gland-like spaces. This proliferation may take the form of a papillary projection, commonly called papilloma of the gallbladder. In other cases the growth is into the
depth of the wall and new glands are formed
which may penetrate the entire thickness of the
wall and form a mass on the serous surface (Fig.
480). An apparent diverticulum or pocket may
thus be formed, and its communication with the
lumen of the gallbladder may or may not be apparent. These various appearances are merely
an exaggeration of the structures known variously
as *Luschka's crypts* and *Rokitansky-Aschoff sinuses*, which are merely diverticula of the gallbladder, similar to the diverticula occurring in the
colon and urinary bladder. They are protrusions
of the mucosa through the muscular coat, invaginations which are found in about half of all gallbladders removed in persons over thirty years of
age.

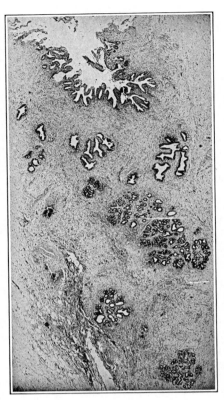

FIG. 480.—Formation of new glands in
whole thickness of gallbladder wall.

GALLSTONES

That profitable quarry, the gallbladder, is
a great former of stones or calculi. These
usually develop in the gallbladder itself, but
they may be formed in the bile passages,
especially those within the liver. They may
be single or multiple; sometimes there are
several hundred small stones. There are
three constituents: cholesterol, bilirubin,
and calcium. As the proportion of these
varies, so do the calculi vary in their gross
appearance. Three main varieties may be
recognized: (1) the pure cholesterol stone,
(2) the pure pigment stone, and (3) the common infective or mixed stone.

Etiology.—The etiology of gallstones is
still unsettled. We are certainly powerless
to prevent their formation. Three factors
may play a part: infection, stasis, and high
bile cholesterol. It does not follow that all
three need be present in any given case.

(1) *Infection.* This is the principal factor.
All the infective or mixed stones are associated with cholecystitis. The cholecystitis
causes the calculi, not *vice versa*. Cholesterol
is held in solution in the bile in a series of
loose chemical complexes with bile salts.
These may easily be broken up, *e.g.*, by
dialysis. When the bile salts are removed
the cholesterol is precipitated. There is no
differential absorption of cholesterol and bile
salts by the normal gallbladder. The infected gallbladder, on the other hand, absorbs bile salts rapidly but cholesterol very
slowly, so that the latter tends to be precipitated. When a nucleus of cholesterol is
established bilirubin is laid down around it
to form a mixed stone. (2) *Stasis* probably
plays a part. In pregnancy the gallbladder
does not empty in response to a fat meal.
Gallstones are much commoner in women (3
or 4 to 1), especially in those who have borne
children. Patients with gallstones are often

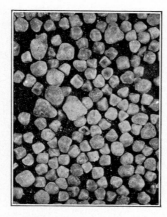

FIG. 481.—Infective gallstones. The facetted
stones are very uniform in size.

"fat, female, and forty." (3) *High bile cholesterol*, associated in turn with high blood
cholesterol, is a possible factor, although the
hypercholesterolemia may have disappeared
by the time symptoms have begun to manifest themselves. Deposits of cholesterol in
the mucosa may be come pedunculated, detached, and form the starting-point of calculi.

Pure Cholesterol Stone.—This is also
called the *metabolic stone*, because it is essentially due to a disturbance of cholesterol
metabolism. It is large, oval, white, usually
single, of light weight, and the cut surface
shows a characteristic radiate structure and
glistening crystals of cholesterol. The factors
which favor its formation are high bile cholesterol and stasis in the gallbladder. It is
a silent stone and usually causes no symptoms. There is no change in the gross
appearance of the gallbladder. The stone
may become impacted in the neck of the
gallbladder and lead to a condition of hydrops. Sometimes the impaction is followed
by infection. Should the stone now roll back
into the gallbladder and allow bile to enter,
bilirubin calcium is deposited on the surface
and a *combination stone* is formed.

Pure Pigment Stone.—These stones are
multiple, very small, black in color, friable,
and consist of bilirubin. They contain no
cholesterol. They are often present in
hemolytic jaundice, but are not confined to
that condition. Like the previous stone
they appear to be metabolic in origin. When

very small and numerous they constitut
biliary gravel.

Infective or Mixed Stones.—This is th
common variety, composed of cholestero
bilirubin, and calcium. It comprises abou
80 per cent of biliary calculi. The pigmen
and cholesterol are laid down in alternat
layers, so that the cut surface presents ;
concentric arrangement of laminæ. Th
general color is yellow or brown, and th
stones are facetted and polished unless ther
is only one (Fig. 481). There may be two o
three families of stones, all the members o
each family being about the same size and
probably starting life at the same time. I
the center there is usually a nucleus of mucu;
and cellular débris.

The *effect on the gallbladder* varies with th
kind of stone, for the changes are due to
inflammation. The metabolic stones (cholesterol and pigment) are likely to be associated with a gallbladder which appears
normal unless the stone causes obstruction.
The infective stone is associated with cholecystitis, so that the wall will be thickened
and the lumen usually contracted, but dilated
if impaction has occurred early (Fig. 482).
Stone in the common duct is seldom associated with dilatation (see below). The pressure of a stone may produce ulceration so
that a deep pocket is formed. This may perforate the wall, and the stone escapes into
the peritoneal cavity or into a cavity walled
off by adhesions. If the gallbladder becomes
adherent to the bowel the stone may perforate into the transverse colon or into the
ileum. If perforation is into the ileum the
stone may become impacted above the ileocecal valve, causing acute intestinal obstruction.

Relation of Symptoms to Lesions.—
Cholecystitis and calculi will be considered
together. In *acute cholecystitis* the severe
pain and tenderness over the gallbladder are
explained by the acute inflammatory swelling and tension of the wall. The picture is
that of an acute abdominal emergency, with
fever, nausea, vomiting, leukocytosis, abdominal rigidity, and a palpable gallbladder.
Particularly to be feared are such complications as perforation, liver abscesses due to an
ascending cholangitis, and subdiaphragmatic
abscess. There may be some jaundice owing

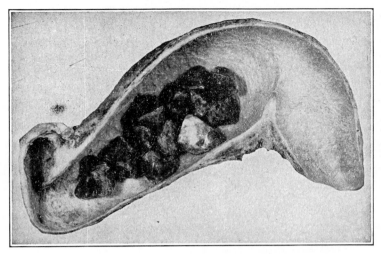

Fig. 482.—Facetted calculi in gallbladder with moderately thickened wall.

to spread of the inflammation to the common bile duct with obstruction. *Biliary colic* is due to the passage of a small stone along the cystic and common bile ducts, causing distention of these passages. It is true of the gallbladder as of the kidney that little stones like little dogs make the most noise. There is probably no spasm owing to the absence of muscle fibers. Colic is not a certain proof of a stone, for the passage of masses of pus or mucus may also produce colic. The mere presence of stones in the gallbladder may or may not be associated with symptoms. Stones are often found at postmortem examination when the patient had no symptoms to suggest gallbladder disease. When symptoms do occur, they are due to the associated cholecystitis. The metabolic pure cholesterol stone is silent.

The symptoms of *chronic cholecystitis* are for the most part referable to the stomach, *i.e.*, dyspepsia, nausea, belching of gas, and a feeling of fulness and bloating. These symptoms are aggravated by fatty foods. Food containing much fat causes the gallbladder to contract and empty itself, and if the wall is inflamed this may cause discomfort. The stomach suffers because it has the same double nerve supply (vagus and sympathetic from the ninth dorsal segment) as the gallbladder, and appears to be a specially sensitive and, as it were, sympathizing organ.

The most satisfactory results of surgical removal are obtained when stones as well as chronic inflammation are present. When there are no stones, the results of cholecystectomy may be as disappointing to the surgeon as to the patient.

It seems improbable that *cholesterolosis* of the gallbladder can of itself give rise to symptoms. The condition is not infrequently found at autopsy in persons who have never had any symptoms of gallbladder disease.

OBSTRUCTION OF THE BILIARY PASSAGES

The biliary passages may be obstructed in different ways and at different levels. The effect varies with these differences. *Courvoisier's law*, over a hundred years old, states that in jaundice due to pressure on the common bile duct from without, as by cancer of the head of the pancreas, the gallbladder is greatly distended, while in jaundice due to impaction of a stone in the common duct the gallbladder is not distended to such an extent that it can be detected clinically. This is a useful working rule which still holds good. The reason is that in obstruction due to stone there is already a cholecystitis, the wall of the gallbladder is thickened, so that it cannot be greatly distended; indeed it may be con-

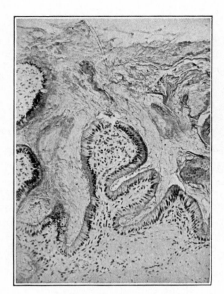

FIG. 483.—Thick secretion of mucus in gallbladder with obstructed cystic duct. × 85.

siderably contracted. It is important to remember that many stones may be lodged in the common duct; I have seen as many as 25 in one case, the gallbladder containing 23 more.

The site of the obstruction has an influence on the contents of the dilated ducts. (1) If the obstruction is in the common duct (the usual site) the biliary passages are still in free communication with the gallbladder, which concentrates the bile retained in the passages so that it becomes thick and dark. (2) If the obstruction is above the entrance of the cystic duct this concentrating mechanism can no longer operate, the bilirubin is absorbed, and the epithelial cells lining the hepatic ducts secrete a clear watery fluid, the so-called *white bile*, which fills and distends the biliary passages. It is evident that this fluid is not bile at all. If the wall of the gallbladder is degraded by disease so that it loses its concentrating power, an obstruction in the common duct will produce the same effect as if it was above the entrance of the cystic duct, and the entire biliary tract, including the gallbladder, will become filled with "white bile." (3) If the cystic duct is blocked by an impacted calculus or a tumor, the bile in the isolated gallbladder is first

absorbed, and is then replaced by clear fluid secreted by the lining epithelium. This fluid is much more mucoid than that secreted by the lining of the hepatic ducts, and the condition is called *mucocele* or *hydrops* of the gallbladder (Fig. 483).

Carcinoma of the Gallbladder.—Cancer of the gallbladder is a relatively common condition. This is not surprising when it is recalled that derivatives of cholic acid are amongst the most powerful of the chemical carcinogens. It bears a close relationship to the presence of gallstones, seldom occurring apart from calculi, so that the disease is four or five times commoner in women than in men. It thus offers a striking exception to the general rule that cancer of the digestive tract is much more common in the male sex.

The usual sites are the fundus and the neck of the gallbladder. It takes an *infiltrating form*, causing great thickening of the wall, but sometimes there is a large soft *papillomatous* mass which projects into the cavity of the organ (Fig. 484). *Microscopically* the structure is that of an adenocarcinoma, but in rare cases it may be that of an epidermoid carcinoma, owing to metaplasia of the columnar into squamous cell epithelium from the chronic irritation which precedes the development of the tumor. The clinical course is very insidious and there may be no symptoms for a long time. Jaundice does not develop until the bile ducts are invaded, the symptoms suggesting chronic cholecystitis. Early diagnosis is very difficult, and the prognosis is correspondingly bad.

Carcinoma of the Bile Ducts.—This usually grows at the lower end of the common bile duct, where it forms a small, hard, white mass readily mistaken for an impacted calculus. The tumor, which is less common than cancer of the gallbladder, has none of the remarkable female sex incidence so characteristic of that condition, and calculi are only present in one-third of the cases. When it is situated in the duodenal portion of the duct it is known as *carcinoma of the ampulla of Vater*. As the tumor gives rise to obstructive symptoms early, it is very small when diagnosed, and only a few metastases are present in the regional lymph nodes. The

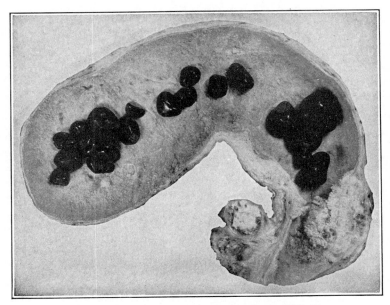

Fig. 484.—Papillary carcinoma at neck of gallbladder.

lesion usually appears as a scirrhous thickening of the wall of the duct with narrowing of the lumen, but occasionally it may be papillary or fungating. Microscopically it is an adenocarcinoma.

Owing to their rarity no mention has been made of *benign tumors of the gallbladder and bile ducts*. These may of course be epithelial (papilloma, adenoma), or arise from fibrous tissue, muscle, nerve, etc.

REFERENCES

Anderson, P. J. and Popper, H.: Am. J. Path., 1960, *36*, 483. (Hepatic lesions in Wilson's disease).

Andrews, E.: Arch. Surg., 1935, *31*, 767. (Acute cholecystitis.)

Baggenstoss, A. H.: Am. J. Clin. Path., 1955, *25*, 936. (Nodular hyperplasia in cirrhosis.)

Bean, W. B.: *Vascular Spiders and Related Lesions of the Skin*, Springfield, Ill., 1958.

Beeson, P. B., Brannon, E. S. and Warren, J. V.: J. Exper. Med., 1945, *81*, 9. (Removal of bacteria from blood in bacterial endocarditis.)

Billing, Barbara H. and Lathe, G. H.: Am. J. Med., 1958, *24*, 111. (Bilirubin metabolism in jaundice.)

Boyd, W.: Brit. J. Surg., 1923, *10*, 337. (Cholesterolosis of gallbladder.)

Brock, J. P.: Lancet, 1959, *2*, 859, 923. (Kwashiorkor).

Brown, N. L. and Shnitka, T. K.: Am. J. Med., 1956, *20*, 292. (Familial non-hemolytic jaundice.)

Chalmers, T. C., Iber, F. L. and Uzman, L. L.: New Eng. J. Med., 1957, *256*, 235. (Hepatolenticular degeneration.)

Connor, C. L.: Am. J. Path., 1938, *14*, 347. (Alcoholic cirrhosis.)

Deo, M. G. and Ramalingaswami, V.: Lab. Invest., 1960, *9*, 319. (Kwashiorkor.)

Dubin, I. N.: Am. J. Clin. Path., 1955, *25*, 514. (Transfusional hemosiderosis.)

Elias, H.: Biolog. Rev., 1955, *30*, 263; Am. J. Anat., 1949, *84*, 311; *85*, 379. (Structure of the liver.)

Elman, R. and Graham, E. A.: Arch. Surg., 1932, *24*, 14. (Cholesterolosis of gallbladder.)

Franz, Virginia K.: *Tumors of the Pancreas*, Atlas of Tumors Pathology, Section VIII, Fascides 27 and 28, 1959, Washington, D. C.

Gall, E. A.: Am. J. Path., 1960, *36*, 241. (Posthepatic, postnecrotic, and nutritional cirrhosis.)

————: Arch. Path., 1960, *70*, 226. (Relation of primary carcinoma to cirrhosis of liver.)

Gall, E. A. and Landing, B. H.: Am. J. Clin. Path., 1956, *26*, 1398. (Cirrhosis and hereditary disorders of metabolism.)

Gillman, J. and Gillman, T.: Arch. Path., 1945, *40*, 239. (Nutritional hemochromatosis.)

Gillman, T., Hathorn, M. and Canham, P. A. S.: Am. J. Path., 1959, *35*, 349. (Experimental dietary siderosis.)

Goldberg, L. and Smith, J. P.: Am. J. Path., 1960, *36*, 125. (Iron overloading and hepatic vulnerability.)

Graham, R. L.: Bull. Johns Hopkins Hosp., 1944, *74*, 16. (Sudden death in fatty liver.)

HALES, M. R., ALLAN, J. S. and HALL, E. M.: Am. J. Path., 1959, *35*, 909. (Injection-corrosion studies in cirrhosis.)

HALPERT, B.: Surgery, 1953, *33*, 444. (Acute cholecystitis.)

HAMILTON, J. D.: Lab. Invest., 1959, *8*, 701. (Primary biliary cirrhosis.)

HARRISON, G. A.: *Chemical Methods in Clinical Medicine*, London, 1947.

HIMSWORTH, H. P.: *Lectures on the Liver and its Diseases*, Cambridge, 1947.

KUNKEL, H. G. in SCHIFF, L.: *Diseases of the Liver*, Philadelphia, 1956.

LAMONT, N. M. and HATHORN, M.: (Personal communication.) (Liver siderosis in the Bantu.)

LE COUNT, E. R. and SINGER, H. A.: Arch. Path. and Lab. Med., 1926, *1*, 84. (Sudden death in fatty liver.)

LICHTENBERG, F.: Am. J. Path., 1955, *31*, 757. (Schistosomal cirrhosis.)

LUCKÉ, B.: Am. J. Path., 1944, *20*, 471. (Fatal epidemic hepatitis.)

MACDONALD, R. A.: New Eng. J. Med., 1956, *255*, 1179. (Increased incidence of liver carcinoma.)

MACKAY, J. R.: Lancet, 1960, *2*, 521. (Circulating antibodies in primary biliary cirrhosis.)

MACKAY, I. R., TAFT, L. I. and COWLING, D. C.: Lancet., 1959, *1*, 65. (Lupoid hepatitis.)

MACMAHON, H. E.: Am. J. Path., 1948, *24*, 527. (Xanthomatous biliary cirrhosis.)

————: Lab. Invest., 1956, *4*, 243. (Biliary cirrhosis.)

MOLANDER, D. W., WROBLEWSKI, F. and LA DUE, J. S.: J. Lab. and Clin. Med., 1955, *46*, 831, (Transaminase test for liver function.)

MURPHY, T. L. *et al.:* New Eng. J. Med., 1948, *239*, 605. (Hepatic coma.)

NOVIKOFF, A. B.: Bull. New York Acad. Med., 1959, *35*, 67. (Biochemical cytology of liver.)

NOVIKOFF, A. B. and ESSNER, E.: Am. J. Med., 1960, *29*, 102. (The liver cell.)

POPPER, H.: Arch. Path., 1948, *46*, 123. (Agonal changes.)

POPPER, H. and SCHAFFNER, F.: *Liver: Structure and Function*, New York, 1957.

————: J.A.M.A., 1959, *169*, 1447. (Intrahepatic cholestasis.)

RAPPAPORT, A. M. *et al.:* Anat. Rec., 1954, *119*, 11; 1958, *130*, 673. (The hepatic lobule.)

RIOPELLE, J. L.: Arch. Path., 1949, *48*, 55. (Elastosis of gallbladder.)

SHERLOCK, S.: *Diseases of the Liver and Biliary System*, 2nd. ed., London, 1958; Am. J. Med., 1958, *24*, 805, (Hepatic coma.)

SMETANA, H. F.: Lab. Invest., 1956, *5*, 175. (Histogenesis of coarse nodular cirrhosis.)

SONG, Y. S.: Arch. Path., 1955, *50*, 235. (Sickle cell anemia cirrhosis.)

STEINER, P. E.: Am. J. Path., 1960, *37*, 21. (Classification of cirrhosis of liver.)

WATSON, C. J. and HOFFBAUER, F. W.: Ann. Int. Med., 1946, *25*, 195. (Cell permeability in intrahepatic cholestasis.)

WOMACK, N. A. and BRICKER, E. M.: Arch. Surg., 1942, *44*, 658. (Occlusion of cystic duct in pathogenesis of cholecystitis.)

Chapter 29

The Pancreas

General Considerations
  STRUCTURE
  FUNCTION
    Exocrine Function
      Pancreatic Juice
      Pancreatic Function Tests
    Endocrine Function
      Insulin
      Glucagon
Pancreatitis
  ACUTE HEMORRHAGIC
  CHRONIC RELAPSING
Diabetes Mellitus
  THE NATURE OF DIABETES
  ETIOLOGY
    Heredity

Obesity
Pancreas
Pituitary
Adrenal
MORBID ANATOMY
  Pancreatic Lesions
  Renal Lesions
  Retinal Lesions
  Arterial Lesions
  Lipoid Lesions
Fibrocystic Disease: Muco-
  viscidosis
MORBID ANATOMY
  Pancreatic Lesions
  Pulmonary Lesions
  Hepatic Lesions

Tumors of the Pancreas
  CARCINOMA
    Primary
    Secondary
  ISLET CELL TUMORS
    Beta Cell Tumor: Hyper-
      insulinism
    Alpha Cell Tumor: Zollinger-
      Ellison Syndrome
Miscellaneous Conditions
  OBSTRUCTION OF PANCREATIC
    DUCT
  HEMOCHROMATOSIS
  CONGENITAL ANOMALIES

GENERAL CONSIDERATIONS

Structure.—The pancreas is in reality a double organ. It is an acinar digestive gland secreting the most powerful of all the digestive juices. For this reason postmortem changes occur very quickly, and the finer forms of investigation, such as an examination of the islet tissue for the specific A and B granules, should be carried out as soon after death as possible. It is also one of the endocrine glands, for the islets of Langerhans form one of the chief regulators of carbohydrate metabolism. The pathology of the pancreas therefore assumes a twofold aspect.

The pancreas arises as a bud from the intestinal canal in much the same way as the liver is developed. Its duct enters the duodenum at the same point as the common bile duct. This propinquity may be significant in the production of disease. The relationship of the two ducts varies a good deal, but they enter the duodenum through a single opening in about 85 per cent of cases, thus constituting a *common channel*, the opening being surrounded by the sphincter of Oddi. It is only if the septum separating the two ducts is short enough, *i.e.* sufficiently proximal to the sphincter, that closure of the common sphincter will allow mixing of bile

and pancreatic juice to occur. This is said to occur in 60 per cent of normal persons, but the published figures vary widely. The matter is not one merely of academic importance, to use a poor and deliberately slighting term. When we come shortly to the very difficult subject of the pathogenesis of acute pancreatitis, we shall see that it is of great practical importance.

It may be noted at this point that morphine increases the tonicity of the sphincter of Oddi, thus causing temporary obstruction not only of the common bile duct but of the common channel, if such exists, whereas the relaxing drugs, such as the nitrites, decrease the tonus of the sphincter, allowing the "common channel" to empty into the duodenum.

The pancreas consists of a large amount of acinar tissue, the cells of which are rich in zymogen granules and empty into ducts. Scattered throughout the gland, in greater numbers in the tail than elsewhere, are the islets first described by Langerhans in 1869. These represent the endocrine element of the gland. The specific granules in the so-called A and B or alpha and beta cells can be stained differentially. From 60 to 90 per cent of the cells are beta cells which manufacture insulin. The alpha cells produce glucagon, the other internal secretion.

(831)

As the pancreas is a dual organ, from the point of view of function we have to consider the pancreatic juice formed by the alveolar tissue and the insulin and glucagon produced by the islands of Langerhans.

Exocrine Function.—The pancreatic juice is a colorless, viscous fluid, alkaline in reaction owing to the presence of $NaHCO_3$. From 500 to 1200 cc. are secreted in the course of twenty-four hours. It contains three powerful digestive enzymes: trypsin, amylase and lipase. The secretion of the juice is regulated partly by nervous, partly by chemical stimuli.

Trypsin is not present as such in the pancreas, but is formed in the duodenum as the result of the activation of trypsinogen from the pancreas by enterokinase of the succus entericus. The resulting trypsin breaks down proteins into polypeptides, and it may eventually liberate such amino acids as leucine and tyrosine.

Amylase converts a variety of starches into maltase.

Lipase splits neutral fats into glycerol and free fatty acids, a reaction which is greatly increased by the presence of bile. The pancreatic enzymes do not merely split the lipids in the lumen of the bowel. They also combine them with the esterification of cholesterol within the intestinal mucosa. When lipase gains entry to the interstitial tissue of the pancreas and surrounding structures it produces the lesions of fat necrosis which are so characteristic of acute pancreatitis.

Pancreatic function tests.—These depend on an estimation of one or more of the three main digestive enzymes. The pancreatic juice obtained by duodenal intubation may be examined, but an analysis of the blood is much more widely used. The lipase and amylase levels in the serum give invaluable information. *Lipase estimation* occupies about 24 hours, but *serum amylase* can be measured within an hour, so that it is the method of choice in acute pancreatitis, which may constitute an acute abdominal emergency that has to be differentiated from acute appendicitis, perforated peptic ulcer, and biliary colic. Although amylase and lipase estimations are of the greatest use in acute inflammation, they are of little help in chronic pancreatitis. It is here that tests for *serum trypsin* levels may point to correct diagnosis. Very high levels are often present in chronic pancreatitis and carcinoma due to obstruction of the duct combined with continued secretion of the enzyme. Tests for endocrine dysfunction will be considered in connection with diabetes.

Endocrine Function.—We have seen that the alpha and beta cells of the islets of Langerhans are distinguished by the specific granules which they contain and that these granules are responsible for the endocrine secretions of the pancreas, insulin (*insula*, an island) being the secretion of the very numerous beta cells and glucagon of the alpha cells.

Insulin.—The power of the pancreas to produce insulin, the beta cells hormone, is related to the degree of granulation of these cells. Degranulation of the cells is related to diabetes mellitus of the growth-onset type (the type in which the diagnosis becomes apparent before skeletal growth is completed), but not necessarily in maturity-onset diabetes, which develops after the completion of skeletal growth. Both the level of the blood insulin and the level of the blood sugar influence the activity of the beta cells. Degranulation of the cells occurs under the administration of insulin, and if the insulin is given long enough a temporary diabetic state develops, with a return to normal when the insulin is stopped. The insulin content of the pancreas and the histology of the beta cells run parallel not only in diabetes of the growth-onset type in man, but also in the spontaneous diabetes of mature dogs and in the experimental diabetes of dogs produced either by partial pancreatectomy or by the administration of anterior pituitary extract. In all of these instances there is a progressive and profound loss of beta cells and of extractable insulin associated with a relatively acute onset of diabetes. This is in sharp contrast to the majority of cases of human diabetes of maturity-onset type, where the pancreatic insulin and the beta cell granulation are much more abundant, and show little change with the duration of the diabetes. In these patients the average insulin content is more than 20 times as high as the average in growth-onset diabetes of more than one year's duration, and about half as much as that of the controls (Wrenshall *et al.*). The beta cells are destroyed by alloxan, with resulting *alloxan diabetes*.

Three explanations have been given for the mode of action of insulin on carbohydrate metabolism. These may be called the permeability, the hexokinase and the oxidation phosphorylation hypotheses (Stadie).

The *permeability* concept is the most basic, because it involves the passage of glucose into the cells. It appears that the entrance of sugar into tissues is governed by a transfer system which is adapted to chemical structure. It is therefore possible to divide sugars into insulin-responsive and insulin-unresponsive.

The *hexokinase* hypothesis deals with the stage of activation once the glucose has penetrated to the interior of the cell. The activation of glucose is brought about by the formation of hexose-6-phosphates by reaction with adenosine triphosphate catalyzed by gluco-hexokinase.

Oxidation phosphorylation is involved in energy production. The oxidations of the Krebs citric acid cycle are concerned with the formation of high-energy phosphate bonds which are stored as adenosine triphosphate and creatine phosphate. These are needed for the initial phosphorylation of glucose and possibly its transfer across cell membranes. This oxidation phosphorylation is markedly increased by insulin.

Glucagon.—This is the alpha cell or hyperglycemic factor. It may be regarded as an opposite twin of insulin. It was first found in impure preparations of insulin from the pancreas. Glucagon is released into the portal blood when the blood sugar concentration is subnormal, just as insulin is released when it is above normal. The pituitary growth hormone increases this release into the blood. The liver is the chief organ directly affected by the glucagon released under physiological conditions, and in the liver it brings about the breakdown of liver glycogen to dextrose by activation of phosphorylase in the liver cells. Glucagon is therefore known as the glycogenolytic as well as the hyperglycemic factor of the pancreas. There is a prompt rise in the sugar content of the blood leaving

the liver. The action of glucagon may explain the difference between alloxan diabetes, in which glucagon is naturally present, and the diabetes of pancreatectomy in which it is of course absent. In pancreatectomy where 90 per cent of the gland is removed, the animal requires much more insulin for control of the glycosuria than does the animal in whom the entire pancreas has been removed, possibly because of the presence of alpha cells in the former case. Just as the beta cells are destroyed by alloxan, so can the alpha cells be destroyed by cobaltous chloride, although this effect is not complete and permanent.

Atrophy of endocrine gland cells is caused by the long-continued administration of the hormone which they produce. We have already seen that this is true with regard to insulin and beta cells. It is also true with regard to glucagon and alpha cells. The specific alpha granules are readily visualized as a silvery-white granulation in frozen sections of fresh unfixed material examined under dark-field illumination (Logothetopoulos and Salter.). In the course of three weeks the administration of glucogon produced nuclear and cytoplasmic shrinkage of the alpha cells, whereas prolonged treatment with insulin and multiple infusions of glucosa had no effect on these cells.

PANCREATITIS

There are four major diseases of the pancreas: (1) acute pancreatitis, (2) diabetes mellitus, (3) cystic fibrosis and (4) carcinoma. The first three of these have in common a cloak of mystery, as will soon become evident.

Acute Hemorrhagic Pancreatitis.—It has been customary in the past to draw a sharp line of distinction between acute and chronic pancreatitis, a line so sharp, indeed, as to justify the recognition of two separate diseases. With increasing knowledge it now becomes apparent that this is probably a mistake, that pancreatitis is a wide spectrum condition, both clinically and pathologically, and that relapsing pancreatitis may be regarded as a chronic malady with acute exacerbations separated by remissions. The incidence of acute pancreatitis has increased

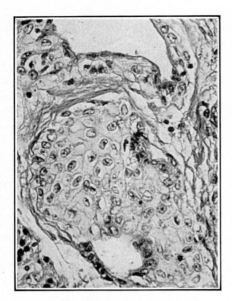

FIG. 485—Squamous metaplasia in
pancreatic duct. × 240.

very considerably in recent years. This may
be attributed to a greater awareness of the
condition and to the more frequent use of
serum pancreatic enzyme determinations
(Bockus *et al.*).

Acute hemorrhagic pancreatitis is really a
chemical autolytic pancreatic necrosis to
which hemorrhage may or may not be added.
A preferable name would therefore be *acute
pancreatic necrosis*. It constitutes one of the
acute abdominal catastrophies.

Pathogenesis.—The cause of the condition
is a matter of perennial dispute. The acute
necrosis is due to the action of the pancreatic
enzymes liberated from the ducts. The
problem is to explain how they escape. The
usual view is that it is due to the passage of
infected bile along the pancreatic duct; this
activates the trypsinogen in the pancreas
and converts it into trypsin, which proceeds
to digest the pancreas. This is the *common
channel theory*. More than one-half the
cases are associated with cholecystitis or
calculi. Opie originally pointed out that if
the common bile duct and pancreatic duct
open into a common chamber (as occurs in
70 per cent of persons), impaction of a
calculus at the ampulla of Vater will cause
the bile to flow into the pancreas. This is

a possible but very uncommon cause, yet
Opie's common-channel theory has dominated medical thought for half a century.
In the cat spasm of the muscle of Oddi at the
ampulla of Vater is followed by a flow of bile
into the pancreas, and such spasm may be
produced by pressure on the gallbladder or
by painting the ampulla with weak hydrochloric acid. This is a probable cause in
many cases.

Rich and Duff have suggested a different
explanation. They found that in both
human and experimental hemorrhagic pancreatitis the constant and specific lesion was
rapid necrosis of the walls of the arteries and
veins, hemorrhage being due to rupture of
the necrotic walls. Moreover, they found
that the pancreatic juice was able to produce
necrosis without activation of the trypsinogen by intestinal contents or bile. They
believe that the mechanism involved is
rupture of dilated thinned-out acini behind
an obstructed duct, this rupture being liable
to occur from increased pressure in the ducts
due to marked secretion after a large meal.
The main duct may be obstructed by a gall-
stone at the ampulla, but they found that
the obstruction was usually in one of the
smaller branches, being caused by squamous
metaplasia and piling up of the lining epithelium (Fig. 485). This lesion was present
in over half the cases of hemorrhagic pancreatitis. On the other hand Baggenstoss
found only one example of squamous metaplasia of the ducts in 29 cases of chronic
relapsing pancreatitis considered to be due
to repeated attacks of acute pancreatitis.

In dogs there seems to be a pathway between the pancreatic duct and the interstitial tissue of the pancreas (Stein *et al.*).
This means that following pancreatic duct
obstruction there is an increase in the level
of enzymes in the interstitial tissue without
the necessity of rupture of the pancreatic
ductules.

It seems probable that the basic factor in
the pathogenesis of acute pancreatitis is obstruction to the pancreatic duct, but this
obstruction may be caused in various ways
such as spasm of the sphincter of Oddi, impaction of a calculus (5 per cent), squamous
metaplasia of the lining of the small ducts,
duodenitis, even the presence of an ascaris,

Whatever be the mechanism by which the enzyme escapes from the ducts, the walls of the vessels are digested and undergo necrosis, and this is responsible for the hemorrhage. Yet in the last analysis it is perhaps wisest to keep an open mind and look for multiplicity of etiological factors rather than for a single one.

Cases of pancreatitis may be divided into two groups: (1) those with *stones in the gallbladder or common duct*, and (2) those without demonstrable biliary tract disease. In the latter group *alcoholism* plays a prominent part. As long ago as 1878 Friedreich spoke of drunkard's pancreatitis. In a series of reports the proportion of alcoholism varied from 20 up to 66 per cent (Richman). Many patients dying of acute alcoholism are found at autopsy to have acute pancreatitis. The exact mechanism involved is still unknown. The alcoholic cases are more severe, are more liable to complications, and are more likely to have frequent recurrences than the non-alcholic group (Bockus *et al.*). Acute pancreatitis is one of the important causes of unexplained abdominal pain in alcoholic patients, a cause which is often overlooked.

Morbid Anatomy.—In the severe and fulminating type of case the pancreas is swollen, soft, and dark in color. It may be red from hemorrhage or black and gangrenous. Hemorrhage is an accidental occurrence, which may or may not be present. Sometimes it dominates the picture. A pancreas may appear normal to the naked eye and yet may show the characteristic necrosis microscopically. The marked swelling is probably responsible for much of the intense pain, and also in part for the necrosis and hemorrhage due to the resulting infarction. Small necrotic areas may be replaced by fibrous tissue. Larger areas may be infected and form abscesses. The greater part of the pancreas may be destroyed. The peritoneal cavity contains a characteristic fluid, dirty, fatty, and beef-juice in character. The *microscopic appearance* is one of great necrosis of the acinar tissue, so that in the advanced cases no structure can be made out. A varying degree of hemorrhage takes place into this necrotic tissue.

Fat necrosis is often seen in acute pancreatitis and is pathognomonic of that con-

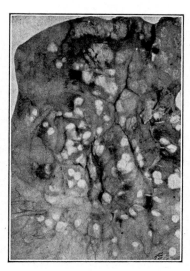

FIG. 486.—Fat necrosis of pancreas.

dition when encountered at operation. Small, dull, opaque white areas are scattered over the surface of the pancreas and the surrounding omentum and mesentery (Fig. 486). These represent areas of fat which have been broken down by the lipase in the liberated pancreatic juice. Areas of fat necrosis may be found at some distance from the pancreas and even in the thorax, owing to distribution of the lipase by the lymphatics. Glycerol and fatty acids are formed; the glycerol is absorbed, and the fatty acids are deposited in the cell as acicular crystals. The areas tend to be absorbed in the course of a few weeks, but the fatty acids may unite with calcium, so that some of the patches may become calcified. *Microscopically* the necrosed cells have an opaque appearance, in comparison with the clear cells of normal fat which is all dissolved out by the chloroform or xylol used for clearing the tissue. One part of a fat globule may show this opaque appearance while the rest of it is clear (Fig. 14, page 28). The necrotic area is usually surrounded by a zone of leukocytes. Associated with acute pancreatitis at autopsy there may be myocardial infarction or profound fatty change in the liver due to chronic alcoholism. Whether this association is by chance or has a basis in causality it is not possible to say.

Relation of Symptoms to Lesions.—There

is a definite relationship between the severity of the process and the intensity of the symptoms. In the milder forms there is merely digestive distress associated with some pain and nausea, the true nature of the condition being indicated by the elevated pancreatic enzymes. In the severe cases the picture, first drawn by Reginald Fitz of Boston in 1889, is an unforgettable one. The suddenness in onset, the illimitable agony which accompanies it, and the attendant mortality, all render it the most formidable of catastrophies. The pain, more terrible even than that of perforation of a gastric or duodenal ulcer, is noteworthy in that it so often follows a hearty meal or a drinking bout. The patient with biliary or renal colic changes his position every minute, seeking the relief which does not come. The patient with acute hemorrhagic pancreatitis, like the one with a perforated ulcer, remains motionless, although he may find that the pain is relieved by bending forward. The onset of shock, which may indeed be of a degree seen in no other condition, is always ominous. The face sometimes presents a peculiar cyanosis which is never seen in other acute abdominal conditions, and there may be patches of a slate-blue color on the surface of the abdomen. The cyanosis is often associated with dyspnea. It is important to realize that the classical picture is not always present. As a sobering illustration of this fact it may be mentioned that in one series of 21 patients who died of acute pancreatitis the usual symptoms were so notably absent that a correct diagnosis was made in only 3 cases (Donhauser and Bigelow). In some of these patients even acute epigastric pain, which is so characteristic a feature, was not noted.

Serum enzyme estimations are of great value, for the differential diagnosis may be very difficult, and the life of the patient may depend on a correct answer. We have already seen that acute pancreatic necrosis may mimic a number of abdominal emergencies which demand immediate surgical intervention, more particularly perforated peptic ulcer and acute appendicitis, as well as biliary and renal colic, and even myocardial infarction.

The most valuable single laboratory test is the demonstration of a *raised serum amylase*, the enzyme passing into the veins after injury to the pancreas. It is important to realize that the rise is usually transient, returning to normal in the course of two or three days. Moreover there is no relation between the level of the serum amylase and the severity of the disease. Indeed in very severe cases with early death the amylase may be subnormal owing to widespread destruction of the pancreas. The serum lipase is also of value, more particularly because the level may be elevated after that of the amylase has fallen. Glycosuria is present in about 10 per cent of cases. Glycosuria with hyperglycemia is diagnostically significant, but even more significant is the presence of hyperglycemia without glycosuria. Leukocytosis is a constant finding, but this is usually of little or no help.

The *cause of death* is probably the poisonous split-protein products formed as the result of partial digestion of the pancreatic tissue. These products are absorbed very quickly, and this, together with the profound degree of shock, perhaps accounts for the extraordinarily rapid termination of many of the cases.

Chronic Relapsing Pancreatitis.—If it is difficult to write a clear account of acute pancreatitis, it is infinitely more difficult to do so in the case of chronic pancreatitis. As seen in the experimental animal, such as the dog, chronic sclerosing pancreatitis can be shown to be the healed or healing stage of induced acute hemorrhagic pancreatitis. Whether this holds true of the human subject it is obviously extremely difficult to say. The present day view is that chronic pancreatitis represents a progressive destruction of the pancreas from repeated episodes of pancreatic edema or necrosis (Gross and Comfort). Each of the earlier attacks is of so slight a character that it is unlikely to give rise to a recognizable disturbance of function. It is only later that the destruction of structure is sufficiently extensive to produce permanent changes in function.

Pathogenesis.—The same factors which have been discussed in relation to acute pancreatitis may be involved in the chronic variety. Perhaps the most important of these is *chronic alcoholism*, with its stimulation of secretion of gastric hydrochloric acid, which in turn results in vigorous pancreatic stimulation. If this is accompanied by spasm of the sphincter of Oddi, the result may be recurring damage to the pancreas. *Disease of the biliary tract* is frequently present, but it is by no means certain which is cause and which is effect.

Morbid Anatomy.—Much will depend on the stage at which the pancreas is examined, whether by the pathologist or by the surgeon at exploratory operation. During an acute exacerbation the entire pancreas or only a part of it may be enlarged by diffuse edema, with areas of necrosis and infiltration by inflammatory cells. In the intervals the gland is firm, hard or nodular. These nodular areas of induration may present a very difficult problem to the surgeon, for they may closely simulate carcinoma. There may be pseudocysts of varying size containing clear or blood-stained fluid. In the final stage the pancreas is small, hard and calcareous. Such a gland consists largely of connective tissue which has replaced both acini and islets of Langerhans. The entire process may well be compared with what we have already studied in cirrhosis of the liver. In spite of what has just been said it must be admitted that in many cases where this type of pancreas is found at autopsy, no evidence of multiple subacute attacks is apparent in the history of the patient.

The *clinical picture* is naturally confused. At first the serum lipase may be elevated, but this is rarely true of serum amylase. As pancreatic destruction progresses not enough acinar tissue may remain to produce elevated enzyme levels, but there is likely to be steatorrhea, with bulky and fatty stools, and eventually frank diabetes.

DIABETES MELLITUS

The Nature of Diabetes.—Although considered in this chapter, diabetes mellitus is not fundamentally a disease of the pancreas, nor is its essence the presence of sugar in the urine. It is rather a syndrome which is characterized by *persistent hyperglycemia* with or without glycosuria, and which results from a derangement in the mechanism of blood sugar homeostasis (Lazarus and Volk). It is a carbohydrate metabolic block. It is indeed an inborn error of carbohydrate metabolism which manifests itself as an enzymatic defect that limits the production of insulin in the beta cells of certain individuals. As a result of this defect one link is missing in the complex mechanism which converts the sugar of the food into energy and heat. The various sugars of the diet are converted into glucose in the intestine, which is carried by the portal vein to the liver, where it is changed into glycogen and stored until reconverted into glucose in response to the demands of the body. The glucose is carried principally to the muscles, where it is changed back again into glycogen and oxidized with the liberation of energy or heat. Glucose is the form in which carbohydrate is transported, but glycogen is the active form in which it passes through the processes of metabolism.

In diabetes something goes wrong with the smooth working of the metabolic machine. As a result of this defect not only does carbohydrate metabolism no longer take place normally, but there is a disturbance in the metabolism of fats which is apt to prove of greater danger than the original disorder. That the missing link was connected with the pancreas was demonstrated as long ago as 1889 when Von Mering and Minkowski showed that removal of the entire pancreas in animals was followed by a fatal diabetes. We had to wait till 1922 for the demonstration in Toronto by Banting, Best and Collip that an extract of the islets would control the diabetes produced by pancreatectomy.

Insulin appears to produce three main effects: (1) It makes the storage of sugar as glycogen possible, especially by the liver and muscles; (2) it enables the tissues to burn sugar; (3) it prevents the formation of sugar from protein in the liver. *Perhaps the most fundamental of all the disturbances in diabetes is the inability to store sugar as glycogen.* As the sugar is not stored it accumulates in the blood, and appears in the glomerular filtrate in quantities too great to be absorbed by the renal tubules.

The importance of the disease is evident from the fact that there are some 3,000,000 diabetics in the United States at the present time, and the number is increasing, because the diabetic no longer dies early from the disease. We must also realize that the cause of death in diabetes has changed most dramatically in the past half century. Fifty years ago 50 per cent of the deaths were due to tuberculosis, now the figure is 0.2; for diabetic coma the figure was 64 per cent, now it is 1; at the present day 75 per cent of deaths are due to vascular disease of the heart, brain, or kidneys. The change is due, of course, to the discovery of insulin in 1922, and the resulting increased span of life.

Etiology.—The disease usually begins after middle life, but is more severe in the young. The essence of the condition appears to be a disturbance of the normal balance of the factors regulating carbohydrate metabolism. In this regulation the liver plays the most important part, but the hormonal output of the pancreas, pituitary and adrenals is also essential. In all cases of diabetes there is an insufficiency of insulin in relation to the needs of the organism, but the actual secretion may be normal or increased. In other words, it is not necessarily a disease of the pancreas. Indeed pancreatectomy may actually relieve diabetes, and persons with total pancreatectomy may require less insulin than do many diabetics. The pituitary, thyroid and adrenals have an action antagonistic to that of the pancreas. We shall consider the following possible factors: (1) heredity, (2) obesity, (3) pancreas, (4) pituitary, and (5) adrenals.

Heredity.—"Heredity is the basis of diabetes." This is the opening sentence of the chapter on etiology in Joslin's classic volume, *The Treatment of Diabetes Mellitus.* Certain persons are born with a diabetic tendency, a genetic defect. Such persons may develop the disease in childhood, or in later life, or not at all, depending on the severity of the defect and on the presence or absence of accessory factors. The last-named group serve as diabetic "carriers." The inheritance follows a recessive Mendelian pattern.

It is probable that there is a specific gene for every specific enzyme within a cell. When that gene is lost or altered the corresponding enzyme is also lost or altered. Hormones are believed to control the rate of reaction of enzyme systems. The gene in the nucleus will therefore determine whether a certain enzyme is present in the cell, whilst hormones (insulin, glucagon) will accelerate or inhibit the enzyme reaction. Both factors are needed for normal function.

It would appear, then, that diabetes is present from birth in the form of an inherently defective carbohydrate mechanism which can be triggered in a variety of ways. The defect may remain in a latent form for many years, but it may be brought to light by the stress of pregnancy, corticotrophin therapy, Cushing's syndrome or acromegaly, staphylococcal infections, or even overeating. If this view is accepted, the importance of unmasking potential diabetics who may show normal carbohydrate tolerance by present methods becomes apparent. For this purpose special tests can be used, which do not concern us here.

The hereditary aspect of diabetes is well summarized in the following statement by Warren and Le Compte: "When both parents have diabetes, all the children may be expected to develop the disease, if they live long enough; when one parent has diabetes and the other is a diabetic carrier, 40 per cent of their children may develop the disease; whereas if a diabetic or a carrier marries an individual who neither has diabetes nor is a diabetic carrier none of the children will have diabetes." The implications of the last statement for the elimination of the disease in the superstate of the future are obvious.

It has long been known that diabetic women give birth to large babies, which are often still-born. The newborn infant may present a picture of Cushing's disease, with macrosomia and a "tomato face" (ballooned cheeks and red skin). What is of equal or even greater significance is the fact that prediabetic mothers, women who may develop clinical diabetes many years later, show the same tendency. The still-born babies are red, flabby and edematous, with hepatomegaly, cardiac hypertrophy, and hyperplasia of the islets of Langerhans. Islet hyperplasia is seen in the still-born infant not only of the diabetic but also of the prediabetic mother, so that diabetes can sometimes be predicted 20 years before it becomes manifest merely by looking at the cells of another individual (Jackson).

Obesity.—Of the precipitating factors which help to bring out the inherited predisposition obesity is by far the most important, which is fortunate seeing that it is preventable. Abnormal food intake subjects the islets to constant strain, which results in degeneration of the islet cells. The glycosuria of middle-aged persons will often disappear when weight is reduced to a sufficient degree. The importance of obesity in diabetes is fully confirmed by insurance records.

Pancreas.—The most obvious immediate cause of diabetes is *insulin deficiency*, although it will be realized that the deficiency may be *actual* through lessened production or *relative* through increased demand on the part of the tissues. The difficulty is to determine the cause of the deficiency.

It has been suggested that an increased ratio of alpha to beta cells is responsible for the diabetic state, but the failure in many laboratories to produce permanent diabetes by the long-continued administration of glucagon has been used against the concept that glucagon is an "insulin-antagonist" and an important etiological factor in the pathogenesis of human diabetes. It will certainly produce an intense temporary diabetes both in the rat and in man. It has been shown in Best's laboratory that when immature rabbits (three days old) are given glucagon for a number of months a permanent diabetes results (Logothetopoulos *et al.*). This "meta-glucagon diabetes," as it has been called, is associated with extensive atrophy of the alpha cells and massive glycogen infiltration of the beta cells.

Selective necrosis of the islets can be produced by the intravenous injection of *alloxan*, one of the components of uric acid (Dunn *et al.*). Alloxan destroys all the beta cells in a dog in the course of two days. They simply vanish. Their place is taken by alpha cells which become greatly enlarged, so that in a hematoxylin and eosin section the islet may appear normal. Special granule stains such as that of Gomori tell the true story. The *alloxan diabetes* which results is characterized by a marked and fatal hypoglycemia, which is preceded by a puzzling transient hyperglycemia. There are three ways of producing

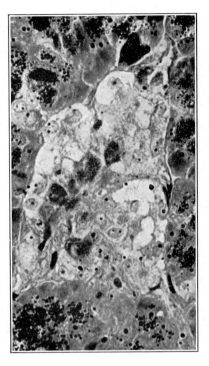

FIG. 487.—Islet of Langerhans in experimental diabetes showing extreme hydropic degeneration (glycogen infiltration) of the beta cells. × 500. (From a preparation by Dr. D. J. Bowie.)

diabetes experimentally: (1) by pancreatectomy, (2) by injection of anterior pituitary extract, (3) by injection of alloxan.

In man, as well as in the experimental animal, prolonged overactivity of the islets, as in continued hyperglycemia from any cause, may lead to "work exhaustion" of the beta cells and permanent diabetes. Corresponding lesions are seen in experimental diabetes produced by excision of nine-tenths of the pancreas followed by a carbohydrate diet. In the remaining portion of the pancreas the exhausted beta cells show loss of the specific granules and marked hydropic degeneration (glycogen accumulation) (Fig. 487); finally they rupture or degenerate and disappear.

Finally there remains the small but baffling group of cases in which the pathologist is unable to demonstrate any pancreatic lesions. This may be due to the inadequacy of our histological technique. The alpha cells may be at fault and responsible for the hyperglycemia. Or there may be an excessive demand for insulin which the islets are unable to meet. Or insulin which is released may be inactivated or antagonized.

Extrapancreatic Factors.—The question of factors other than pancreatic which may influence carbohydrate metabolism has already been alluded to. There is evidence suggesting that carbohydrate metabolism is disturbed at the level of the Krebs cycle. The basic action in the cycle, namely oxidative phosphorylation, seems to take place in the mitochondria of the *liver cells.* The question which has not yet been answered is whether it is insulin alone which is concerned with this mechanism, or whether other factors may play a part.

Pituitary.—There can be no question that pituitary hormones can influence the course of diabetes mellitus (Houssay). The growth hormone of the pituitary appears to have diabetogenic power. This is true both of the experimental animal and of man. Administration of the hormone leads to hydropic changes in the beta cells associated with an early reversible phase of diabetes, followed later by an irreversible phase with complete destruction of the beta cells. Diabetes may be associated with acromegaly. Hypophysectomy will arrest the course of diabetes in the experimental animal, and the operation has even been performed in malignant forms of human diabetes with the object of preventing blindness and irreparable renal damage. The result in the experimental animal is known as the *Houssay phenomenon.* In the human subject marked clinical improvement, reduction of insulin requirements, and the development of insulin sensitivity have resulted from hypopituitarism due to infarction of the anterior pituitary or for other reasons. The explanation still eludes us.

Adrenal.—Here again there is convincing evidence that adrenal cortical hormones may affect both the experimental and the human disease. Adrenalectomy will arrest or modify the progress of experimental diabetes. The onset of Addison's disease has an ameliorating effect on the human variety. Conversely, adrenal hyperplasia or tumors may be associated with diabetes, and the occasional case has been cured by the removal of such hyperplastic adrenals or

tumor. The administration of hydrocortisone causes diabetes with marked hyperglycemia in rabbits. The effect is intensified when adrenal hormone is combined with pituitary growth hormone (Volk and Lazarus).

Morbid Anatomy.—"The changes that may be found at autopsy on a diabetic patient are so varied, heterogeneous, and apparently unrelated that it is difficult to discuss them in a coherent manner." This arresting statement is the opening sentence of the chapter on the pathology of diabetes by Warren and LeCompte in Joslin's textbook. Some of these lesions may be regarded as primary, others secondary to the disturbances of carbohydrate and fat metabolism, although it is by no means always easy to be sure of these relationships nor, with the exception of intercapillary glomerulosclerosis and diabetic retinopathy, are they found only in diabetes. For the purpose of description it is convenient to recognize pancreatic, renal and retinal lesions, as well as lesions associated with abnormal carbohydrate and fat metabolism (Hamilton).

Pancreatic Lesions.—Although the patient may have died of diabetes, the pancreas generally appears normal to the naked eye, because the acinar tissue is unaffected. With hematoxylin and eosin staining the microscopic picture may also be disappointing. The islets may be greatly diminished in number, but they may be normally abundant and even hypertrophied. When granule stains are used, of which the best is that of Gomori, it is seen that the basic lesion is the disappearance of the granules in the beta cells (Fig. 488A). If these cells are replaced by hypertrophied alpha cells, the islets may seem to be normal.

Hyalinization of the islets was described by Opie in 1900 (Fig. 488B). Ever since that time controversy has raged as to its significance in relation to diabetes, for it is a common finding in nondiabetics as well as in diabetics with advancing years. Bell, whose views on the subject merit the most serious consideration, has analyzed the material in several thousand nondiabetics as well as diabetics. In his opinion the preponderance in diabetes is so marked that "no one can doubt that they are related in

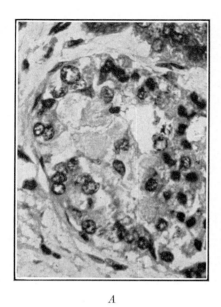

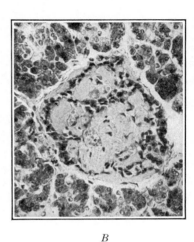

A   B

FIG. 488.—*A,* Loss of beta granules in diabetes. × 470.   *B,* Pancreas in diabetes. The islet of Langerhans shows an extreme degree of hyaline degeneration. × 325.

some way to the diabetic state." They are evidently not the cause of diabetes, as they are absent in nearly all young diabetics, and in one-half of older diabetics. They are much more frequent in nondiabetic males than in the corresponding group of females. The only evident relationship is to age. In 1901 Opie noted the resemblance of hyalinization of the islets to amyloidosis. More refined methods of staining than were at that time available have shown that the material really is amyloid (Ehrlick and Ratner). It has also been suggested that hyalinization of the islets may be an expression of unrecognized or potential diabetes. The fact that clinical diabetes is about twice as common in females as in males justifies the view that potential diabetes is about as frequent as overt diabetes in males, thus accounting for the higher incidence of hyaline islets in nondiabetic males.

Hydropic degeneration is an ancient term applied by Weichselbaum in 1901 to changes observed in the pancreas of diabetics dying in coma. The characteristic change is vacuolation of the cytoplasm of the islets, which was regarded as hydropic in character due to absorption of fluid from the surrounding tissues. (Fig. 486.) It now appears that this long-cherished idea is quite wrong, and that the vacuolar appearance is due to the artefactual removal of glycogen which has been deposited in the islets. The essence of the condition appears to be *glycogen infiltration* of the islets (Toreson). The glycogen can be best demonstrated by the periodic acid-Schiff (PAS) method, although this stains a number of other substances. Final proof is afforded by removal of the stainable substance by the enzyme, diastase. The presence of glycogen is positive evidence of diabetes.

Many diabetics do not die directly of diabetes but of such complications as arteriosclerosis, renal failure and gangrene. In such persons under insulin therapy the islets are no longer under strain and may have undergone regeneration. Finally it must be remembered that diabetes is the result of a disturbance of the normal balance of the factors regulating carbohydrate metabolism, and that in some cases the pancreas may not be the chief offender.

The diabetic under modern treatment is not likely to die of diabetic coma. He lives for many years and then dies from what are

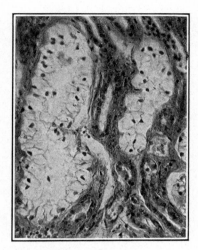

FIG. 489.—The kidney in diabetes. The clear cells of the loop of Henle are filled with glycogen. × 200.

called complications, but are really late manifestations of the upset in metabolism which is the essence of the disease. The late lesions are renal, retinal, arterial and lipoid.

Renal Lesions.—The renal lesions are of great importance, for the danger of death from diabetic coma has been replaced by the danger of death from renal failure. The younger the age of onset of the diabetes the shorter is the duration needed for the development of renal lesions. There are five principal lesions: (1) glycogen in the renal tubules, (2) arteriosclerosis, (3) the Kimmelstiel-Wilson lesion, (4) pyelonephritis, and (5) papillitis necroticans. The most charac-

teristic renal lesion used to be an accumulation of *glycogen in the tubules*, giving the cells a clear, transparent appearance (Fig. 489), a condition known as the *Armanni-Ebstein lesion*. The chief deposits are in the loop of Henle. Glycogen is seldom seen now owing to adequate treatment with insulin. *Renal arteriosclerosis* is common and severe in juvenile diabetics who have had the disease for fifteen years or more, particularly in females. It is likely to cause death from renal failure. The *Kimmelstiel-Wilson lesion* or intercapillary glomerulosclerosis when present in typical form is pathognomonic of diabetes. It is described on page 573. When present in marked degree it is pathognomonic of diabetes, but it is often absent, being seen in only 12 per cent of males and 19 per cent of females in one series (Bell). The material in the nodular deposits in the glomeruli stains brightly with PAS and is probably a mucopolysaccharide, possibly deposited from the blood (McManus). *Pyelonephritis* is again commoner in the female in the proportion of 2 to 1. In my own autopsy material more patients appeared to die from pyelonephritis than from any other renal lesion. *Papillitis necroticans* is the rarest of the lesions in my experience. It occurs in association with acute pyelonephritis, and pursues a fast and fatal course. The necrosis of one or more of the renal papillae seems to be due to vascular occlusion. The lesion is described on page 589. The renal lesions are summarized in the accompanying table.

THE RENAL LESIONS IN DIABETES

Lesions	Principal Features
Glycogen in the tubules (Armanni-Ebstein lesion)	Transparent cells in the loops of Henle of patients on improper insulin regimen.
Renal arteriosclerosis.	Especially severe in female juvenile diabetics.
Kimmelsteil-Wilson lesion (Intercapillary glomerulosclerosis).	PAS positive nodular deposits in the glomeruli of 12-20% of diabetics.
Pyelonephritis.	Accentuated lesions (female:male 2:1).
Papillitis necroticans.	A rare, rapid, and usual complication of acute pyelonephritis.

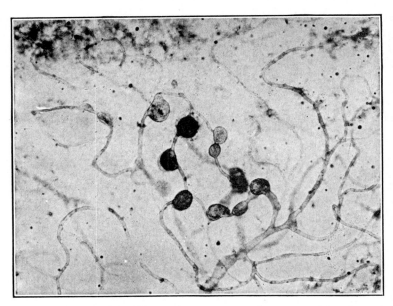

Fig. 490.—Diabetic retinopathy. Capillary micro-aneurysms demonstrated by the periodic acid-Schiff reagent method applied to whole mount of retina. (Dr. Jonas Friedenwald, courtesy of Amer. J. Ophth.)

Retinal Lesions.—Diabetic retinopathy develops especially in juvenile diabetics who have had the disease for upward of fifteen years. In those who have had the disease for twenty years it is present in 90 per cent of cases. The red spots seen with the ophthalmoscope, which used to be taken for punctate hemorrhages, are now known to be globular micro-aneurysms of capillaries in the inner molecular layer of the retina (Friedenwald). They are present in great numbers, and they may be the source of hemorrhage and thrombosis. To the physician who sees them they are an ominous sign. The lesions are best demonstrated when whole mounts of the retina are mounted flat without sectioning and stained with the periodic acid-Schiff method, which gives beautiful delineation of the capillary network and micro-aneurysms (Fig. 490).

The retinal lesions have been attributed to disturbed mucopolysaccharide metabolism with consequent weakening of the capillary wall. This might agree with their frequent association with the Kimmelstiel-Wilson lesions of the glomerular capillaries. All patients with Kimmelstiel-Wilson lesions have retinal micro-aneurysms, but less than 60 per cent of those with micro-aneurysms have Kimmelstiel-Wilson lesions. It has also been suggested on histochemical evidence that the micro-aneurysms are due to the accumulation of fat in the capillary wall with subsequent stretching, so that it herniates through the supporting reticulum network. A minute aneurysm then develops at this point of herniation (Pope). In addition to the micro-aneurysms there may be hard yellowish exudates, which are very different from the cotton-wool exudates of malignant hypertension.

These theories do not explain the fact that the aneurysms in diabetes are confined to the retina. This objection has been met by the suggestion that the micro-aneurysms are the result of capillary obstruction caused by swelling of the surrounding cells deep in the retina (Ashton). These cells depend largely on glucose for their energy, and the interruption of their normal metabolism in diabetes may well lead to the imbibition of water with swelling as a consequence.

Arterial Lesions.—Vascular lesions are of all varieties of arteriosclerosis. They result in gangrene, coronary artery disease and apoplexy. Hypertension is a good deal commoner in diabetics than in non-diabetics, bringing its own vascular troubles. The elderly diabetic is threatened with gangrene, coronary disease and cerebral hemorrhage. Indeed the diabetic is so susceptible to vascular disease that this has become a main problem in the care of the patient.

Some of the extrapancreatic lesions which have just been described may be regarded as complications of the disturbance in carbohydrate metabolism. In the case of others, more particularly the capillary lesions of intercapillary glomerulosclerosis and of retinal micro-aneurysms, there must be some other explanation. Lonergan and Robbins point out that hemochromatosis offers an interesting illustration of this fact. Hemochromatosis, which used to be called bronzed diabetes, is characterized by hemosiderosis of the islets on the one hand and hyperglycemia and glycosuria on the other. In 21 cases of diabetes due to hemochromatosis in which there was an interval of five to nineteen years between the onset of the diabetes and death, there was not a single instance of Kimmelstiel-Wilson lesions, and it may be assumed that there were no retinal capillary lesions. It is evident that diabetes associated with hemochromatosis differs from diabetes mellitus in not predisposing the patient to renal vascular disease. This would suggest that there are two separate and distinct features of diabetes mellitus, the one an anomaly of carbohydrate metabolism, the other a tendency to vascular disease.

Lipoid Lesions.—A variety of lesions occur as the result of abnormal fat metabolism. Lipemia may be marked. When the blood fat is high the plasma may be milky. In exceptional cases there is a remarkable *lipid storage* in the cells of the reticuloendothelial system. The cells become swollen with lipid which may take the form of globules. These large "foam cells" are seen in the spleen and liver (Kupffer cells). The lipid is usually cholesterol ester. There may be yellow patches in the aorta and yellow nodules in the skin (*xanthoma diabeticum*), which are deposits of the same material. The yellow color of the skin (xanthosis) sometimes seen in diabetics is not due to lipemia but to carotin, a pigment contained in carrots and other vegetables. There is a carotinemia, and the serum is bright yellow. The coloration of the skin is best seen in the nasolabial folds and on the palms of the hands and soles of the feet.

Relation of Symptoms to Lesions.— Glycosuria is the chief symptom of diabetes (*mellitus*, sweetened with honey), associated with polyuria (*diabetes*, a syphon or running through), excessive thirst and hunger, and marked loss of weight. Another group of symptoms due to incomplete combustion of fats are manifestations of acidosis, *e.g.*, air hunger, coma, ketone bodies in the urine, and lipemia. Pruritus, carotinemia, gallstones, arteriosclerosis, and gangrene of the extremities may occur. Neuritis is an unexplained accompaniment of many cases of diabetes. It bears some relation to the level of the blood sugar.

From what has already been said it will be evident that most of these symptoms are not related to any morphological lesion, but rather to a biochemical one.

All of the symptoms are in the last analysis due to the failure of the islets. The sugar absorbed from the bowel is not utilized; it accumulates in the blood, and when the renal threshold is exceeded it is lost in the urine, where it is followed by water so that very marked polyuria is the result. The large amount of sugar in the blood causes withdrawal of fluid from the tissues by reason of osmosis, so that there is great thirst. As the sugar is not utilized to satisfy the needs of the body, there is hunger, weakness and loss of weight, for the patient is being starved of carbohydrates. Much of the general weakness is due to the lack of insulin which is necessary for the regulation of the oxidative reaction in the Krebs tricarboxylic acid cycle, with resulting loss of energy production. Two other factors contribute to the loss of weight. When the sugar in the diet is cut down the tissue proteins become converted into sugar to satisfy the needs of the body. The fats also are used up to supply energy, although they are not properly oxidized because of the defective carbohydrate metabolism. Pruritus may be a prominent symptom and is apparently due to the accumulation of unused sugar in the tissues.

The most serious symptoms are due to disturbance in the metabolism of fats, not of carbohydrates, but these also are due, though indirectly, to the lesions of the islets. Fat metabolism cannot be completed unless carbohydrate oxidation is proceeding normally, and intermediate acid products, the ketone bodies, appear in the blood and give rise to acidosis, characterized by the violent deep respirations of air hunger (Kussmaul breathing), and it may be the onset of coma. The lips are cherry-red. The first of the ketone bodies to be formed is diacetic acid. Some of this is oxidized to acetone, some is reduced to β-hydroxybutric acid. The metabolic fire may be said to smoke with these poisonous products of incomplete fat combustion. The final coma is the result of acidosis and dehydration.

The relation of what may be called secondary lesions to symptoms is not difficult to understand. Thus renal failure may well result from the various lesions of the kidney, failure of vision from the retinal lesions, gangrene or myocardial infarction from arteriosclerosis. Infection both with bacteria and fungi are a constant threat in diabetes. The bacterial infections have long been familiar, but fungus infection is assuming increasing importance, especially in the Southern United States. Perhaps candidiasis (moniliasis) is the chief of these fungi, but mucormycosis can produce a rapid and fatal disease in the diabetic with cerebral and pulmonary manifestations. The condition is recognized by the striking appearance of the lesions in the nose and orbit (Baker).

Before leaving the subject of the relation of symptoms to lesions we may recall that diabetic patients can be divided into two groups, insulin-sensitive and insulin-resistant. In the former (growth-onset) group the diabetes is due to lack of insulin, whereas in the latter there is diminished responsiveness to insulin. The *insulin-sensitive group* are under thirty years of age, thin, and liable to develop ketosis. The islets may be reduced in number, and degranulation of the beta cells is marked. In the *insulin-resistant group* (maturity-onset) the diabetes develops after the age of forty years, the patients are obese, when insulin treatment is stopped there is no immediate threat of ketosis, and there appears to be an excessive demand for insulin secondary to an increased conversion of glucose to fat as part of the obesity. In these cases there are no significant abnormalities of the islet cells.

FIBROCYSTIC DISEASE: MUCOVISCIDOSIS

The story of the development of our knowledge of this disease is not only interesting but almost unbelievable. Twenty years ago the condition was virtually unheard of, although isolated cases had been reported. In 1938 Dorothy Anderson described a familial and fatal disease of young children with a basic pancreatic dysfunction, which is believed to affect 1 in 1000 live births. The genetic basis, reminiscent of diabetes mellitus, is transmitted as a simple *autosomal recessive gene*. Farber has shown that the basic defect is not confined to the pancreas, but is a generalized abnormality of mucous glandular secretion involving perhaps all the glands of the body. The condition appears to be a *mucoviscidosis*, an increased viscidity of mucous secretions. Finally Di Sant'Agnese *et al.* demonstrated an increased sodium chloride content of the sweat electrolytes.

In the course of a little over twenty years the disease has passed from the unknown to the commonplace. During the last ten years almost 3 per cent of autopsies at the Hospital for Sick Children, Toronto, have been on cases of fibrocystic disease, death being due to meconium ileus in 20 per cent of these, and to respiratory disease in 75 per cent. In six or seven years after the onset of the first symptoms 99 per cent of the children will be dead, although the very occasional patient may reach the age of twenty. It is evident that to make a diagnosis of fibrocystic disease or mucoviscidosis is virtually to give a death sentence.

Morbid Anatomy.—The main organs to be involved in gross lesions are the pancreas, the lungs and the liver. Not all of these need to be affected, but the pancreatic lesions always precede the others. From the functional standpoint there is also involvement of the sweat and salivary glands.

The *pancreatic lesions* are the most striking. Usually the pancreas is firmer and thinner than normal, but it may show no gross change or it may be nodular. The small and large ducts are dilated, converted into small cysts, and filled with homogeneous

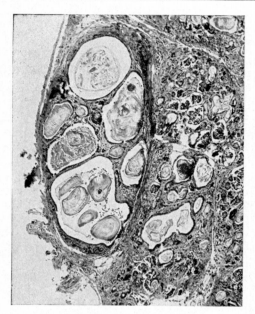

FIG. 491.—Fibrocystic disease of the pancreas.

eosinophilic material like inspissated secretion, and the acini may contain similar material (Fig. 491), with partial replacement by fibrous tissue. There may also be atresia of the interlobular and intralobular ducts. In the course of time the acinar tissue becomes atrophied and replaced by fibrous tissue, the fibrosis probably representing a reactive phenomenon. The Brünner's glands, which are mucus-secreting glands in the first part of the duodenum, are also distended and filled with inspissated material.

The *pulmonary lesions* may be just as important as those in the pancreas as a cause of clinical disturbance, but they may not be evident in infants dying in the neonatal period from meconium ileus. The two major elements in the pulmonary pathology are *obstruction* and *infection*. The mucous glands of the trachea and bronchi are filled with inspissated material which blocks the bronchi and bronchioles causing atelectasis and emphysema. The initial bacterial infection is nearly always due to coagulase-positive staphylococci. Almost all fibrocystics are persistent carriers of coagulase-positive staphylococci in the nasopharynx. It would appear that there is some lack of secretion in the respiratory track of these patients which enhances the growth of staphylococci.

It is perhaps significant to note that staphylococci are tolerant of a high concentration of sodium chloride, whereas most bacteria are not, and that 20 per cent of the parents and siblings of these children have raised sweat electrolytes and suffer to an unusual degree from respiratory disturbances. The inflammatory reaction is at first confined to the bronchi, but later the process may become purulent and destructive, leading to bronchiectasis and bronchopneumonia.

Lesions of the *liver* are characterized by hyperplasia of the ductules, together with dilatation with granular, brownish material. At an early stage of the disease there may be a focal *biliary fibrosis* (Bodian). If the child lives a sufficient number of years a true hepatic cirrhosis may develop with *portal hypertension*. In one case which I studied, a boy seventeen years of age with respiratory distress of long-standing, there was an extreme degree of coarsely nodular cirrhosis.

Occasionally the salivary glands and mucous glands of the cervix or prostate may show cystic and fibrotic changes similar to those encountered in the pancreas.

Relation of Symptoms to Lesions.—The symptoms are due to obstruction of the ducts of the pancreas, of the bronchioles, and if the child does not die, of the smaller bile ducts. The obstruction is due to mucoviscidosis, in which the mucous secretions are scanty and excessively viscid. The mucoviscidosis seems to be an expression of a genetic defect which causes the fully manifest disease in homozygotes and incomplete or no expression in heterozygotes.

Meconium ileus may be the first sign of the disease in the newborn infant. The obstruction is due to mucoprotein which is undigested because of pancreatic stoppage, a condition which will prove fatal without surgical intervention. If ileus does not occur, the child develops a remarkably healthy appetite, but fails to gain in weight by reason of lack of pancreatic digestive enzymes. The stools are frequent, large, pale and foul-smelling, with abdominal distention. This condition must not be confused with celiac disease, which develops later with impairment of appetite and severe hypochromic anemia.

The *respiratory symptoms* usually develop

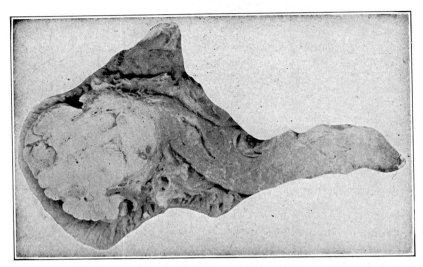

FIG. 492.—Carcinoma of the head of the pancreas causing marked displacement
of the second part of the duodenum.

by the age of six years, and often much earlier. The most prominent feature is persistent cough, which may go on to wheezing, hoarseness and recurring respiratory infections including bronchopneumonia. As the condition progresses there will be evidence of bronchial obstruction such as emphysema and segmental or even lobar atelectasis.

Involvement of the *sweat glands* will result in hyperhidrosis with loss of sodium, potassium and chloride. The continued loss of electrolytes renders the patients unduly susceptible to heat exhaustion during hot weather, and this condition may prove fatal. A simple and reliable diagnostic method depends on the presence of excessive chloride on the skin. The finger or palm of the hand is applied to a medium composed of silver nitrate and potassium chromate suspended in an agar base. If considerable chloride is present, an intense whitish-yellow discoloration of the medium occurs immediately.

It is now becoming evident that although full blown mucoviscidosis is a disease of childhood, minor manifestations and *formes frustes* are not uncommon in the adult. If close relatives of patients with the disease are screened by means of the finger-print test, many cases will be found with a raised sweat electrolyte level, pulmonary emphy-

sema, recurring duodenal ulcers, and unequal depression of the various pancreatic enzymes.

TUMORS OF THE PANCREAS

Carcinoma.—This is the common tumor of the pancreas. Like other cancers of the digestive tract, it is much commoner in men than in women. At least 70 per cent of the cases occur in the head of the pancreas (Fig. 492). This part of the gland is enlarged and remarkably hard. The hardness may simulate chronic pancreatitis, and the surgeon may find it difficult or even impossible to distinguish between the two conditions at an exploratory laparotomy. *Microscopically* the tumor may arise from the ducts or the acini. The duct tumor, which is far the commoner, is an adenocarcinoma; the columnar cells have clearly defined margins, a vesicular nucleus and a distinct nucleolus. In the acinar cell type there are lobular masses of polyhedral or rounded cells, with poorly defined cell margins, large hyperchromatic nuclei, and no visible nucleoli. Secondary growths occur in the regional lymph nodes and liver. The symptoms depend on the location of the tumor. In cancer of the head of the pancreas the chief symptom is persistant and increasing jaundice, due to pressure on the opening of the common bile duct. The bladder is dilated and thin-walled in accordance with Courvoisier's law. In cancer of the body and tail spread is a more striking feature, and this influences the symptoms (Duff). Deep-seated gnawing pain is due to spread along the perineural lymphatics, ascites is caused by implantation growths on the peritoneum or involvement of the portal vein, and distant metastases are more common than in cancer of the head.

One of the peculiar features of cancer of the body and tail of the pancreas is the frequency with which it is associated with multiple venous thromboses, the condition known as *migrating thrombophlebitis*. The great Trousseau observed and recorded the condition in himself when he was dying of carcinoma of the pancreas, so that the term *Trousseau's syndrome* has been fittingly applied to this association. It may be due to release of trypsin, which has a thromboplastic action, from the disrupted glandular tissue of the tumor bed (Gore). The only objection to this idea is that widely scattered venous thrombosis may complicate other cases of intra-abdominal malignancy. Thrombosis, more particularly in the femoral and iliac veins, has been observed in 22 per cent of cases of carcinoma of the pancreas (Smith and Albright). The occurrence of such thrombosis should therefore strongly suggest the possibility of pancreatic cancer.

Secondary Tumors.—Tumors secondary in the pancreas from a malignant growth elsewhere are uncommon. There may naturally be invasion from the stomach, gallbladder or bile duct. In rare instances metastases may occur from hypernephroma and other tumors. It is interesting and perhaps surprising to know that multiple venous thrombosis may be associated with secondary carcinoma of the pancreas, just as it may in the primary form of the disease.

Islet Cell Tumors.—These tumors form an uncommon but remarkably interesting group and the interest continues to grow at the present time. This interest is partly academic and partly clinical. The academic interest will soon become apparent. The clinical importance lies in the fact that here we have an example of a benign adenoma which may be no more than 1 cm. in diameter and yet may

result in the death of the patient unless a correct diagnosis is made. The tumor is usually benign but may be malignant. This seems to make little difference to its endocrine capability. There may be remarkably little difference between the histological appearance of the benign adenoma and the carcinoma which has metastasized to lymph nodes and liver.

The historical aspect of the subject is also not without interest. The first islet cell adenoma, an incidental finding at autopsy was described by Nicholls at McGill University in 1902. In 1922 Banting and Best discovered insulin in Toronto. In 1924, following a visit to Banting, Seale Harris of Birmingham, Alabama, postulated the possibility of a syndrome comprising hyperinsulinism with hypoglycemia and an islet cell tumor. In 1927 Wilder at the Mayo Clinic reported such a case (in this instance a carcinoma). In 1929 the first islet cell adenoma was removed by Roscoe Graham at the Toronto General Hospital with complete relief of the symptoms and the hypoglycemia. It was known that only 60 to 70 per cent of the tumors were associated with symptoms. The remainder were presumed to be "symptomless" or "non-functioning," which indeed they were with respect to the secretion of insulin. Then in 1955, Zollinger and Ellison of Ohio State University reported 2 cases of an association of recurring peptic ulcers, excessive gastric hyperacidity and hypersecretion, and a non-insulin producing islet cell tumor. This association has become known as the *Zollinger-Ellison syndrome*, but it would be better named the *Zollinger-Ellison triad*, because the concept of the syndrome has widened considerably.

Beta Cell Tumor.—The syndrome (happily unnamed) of hyperinsulinism, hypoglycemia and beta cell tumor may be caused by (1) islet cell adenoma, (2) adenomatosis of the islets, and (3) carcinoma of the islets with metastases. Some of the tumors may appear to be malignant histologically, but their behavior is benign. Finally there is hypoglycemia due to diffuse hyperplasia of the islets in infants born of diabetic mothers, a form of work hypertrophy.

The *gross lesion* is usually an adenoma no larger than 1 or 2 cm. in diameter and more

Recovery is complete, without memory of the accident. The attack is at once aborted by the administration of sugar. The so-called *Whipple triad* consists of: (1) attacks of hypoglycemia, (2) central nervous system symptoms, and (3) prompt relief of the attacks by the feeding or intravenous administration of glucose. One surgeon used to suffer from these attacks after an early breakfast and a long morning in the operating room. The occupational hazard for airplane pilots, engine and taxi drivers, house builders, window cleaners, *etc.* is all too obvious, and the beneficial result of enucleation of the adenoma is almost unbelievable to the despairing patient.

Alpha Cell Tumor.—We have already seen that until 1955 a considerable proportion of islet cell tumors, possibly 25 to 30 per cent, were considered to be symptomless and non-functioning. In that year Zollinger and Ellison showed that some of these tumors may be associated with a syndrome quite different from hyperinsulinism. What has come to be known as the *Zollinger-Ellison syndrome* or *triad* consists of (1) *recurring peptic ulcers*, often distal to the first part of the duodenum; (2) *marked gastric hypersecretion* and hyperacidity; and (3) an *alpha cell tumor* of islet tissue. It is now known that the clinical concept must be widened to include intractable watery diarrhea of long duration with accompanying dehydration, and serious or eventually fatal hypokalemia due to the continued loss of potassium and also sodium in the stools (Charles and Cochrane). It is of considerable interest to note that in Ellison's first case, diarrhea of eight years' duration preceded the development of two successive jejunal ulcers and two stomal ulcers, the lesion in the pancreas responsible for this prolonged and eventually fatal illness being a benign nodule only 1 cm. in diameter. Peptic ulcer is therefore not essential to the syndrome, although the feature most often recognized. In chronic refractory diarrhea associated with severe dehydration and profound potassium loss with accompanying fatigue and prostation, where no adequate cause can be found after careful investigation, an alpha cell tumor of islet tissue should be considered.

The *lesion* is similar in form to that of the

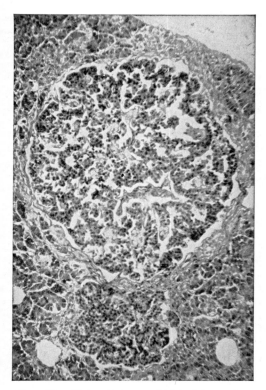

Fig. 493.—Beta cell tumor of islet of Langerhans. × 80. (Boyd, *Pathology for the Surgeon,* courtesy of W. B. Saunders Co.)

readily felt than seen by the surgeon. It is sharply circumscribed and easily enucleated. The carcinoma is infiltrating and more massive. *Microscopically* the adenoma usually duplicates the pattern of normal islets. It is indeed a gigantic islet, in which at times the cells may be arranged in ribbons (Fig. 493).

The *symptoms* are those of hyperinsulinism or insulin shock with marked hypoglycemia due to overactivity of the islet tissue. There may be attacks of faintness and unconsciousness when the interval after a meal is too long, and these can be averted by taking sugar. The condition is therefore the reverse of diabetes. A sense of weakness and extreme fatigue develops after a short fast. This may be followed by an overwhelming nervousness, often associated with mental confusion, finally developing into unconsciousness. The stupor may last for many hours, or it may be followed by convulsions.

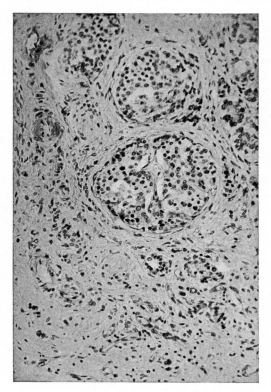

FIG. 494.—Almost complete disappearance of acini due to obstruction of the pancreatic duct. The islets remain intact. × 150.

beta cell tumor. It may be benign (adenoma) or malignant. One case of recurring perforating jejunal ulcers was relieved by resection of a carcinoma, but the diarrhea persisted until 3 metastases in the liver were also removed, when the diarrhea ceased and the patient was restored to health (MacKenzie *et al.*). The cytoplasm contains granules of the alpha cell type (page 831). The histology of the tumor resembles that of carcinoid tumor, with its well known secretion of serotonin. In the kidney the cells of the proximal convoluted tubules show the vacuolar change characteristic of marked potassium deficiency.

The *relation between the islet alpha cell tumor and the clinical picture* is at present quite obscure, being very different in this respect from the hyperinsulinism of the beta cell tumor. Excess of glucagon production naturally comes to mind, but it is more than difficult to explain all the clinical features on that basis. The extreme gastric hyper-

chlorhydria is probably responsible for the jejunal and other peptic ulcers. Different mechanisms may be involved in the gastric oversecretion and the watery diarrhea, for if the former causes the latter it is strange that a number of years may separate the onset of diarrhea and the development of peptic ulcers. Tumors of more than one endocrine gland have been reported in some cases, and yet we are faced with the fact that removal of the pancreatic tumor has cured both the ulcerogenic tendency and the persistent diarrhea.

MISCELLANEOUS CONDITIONS

Obstruction of the Pancreatic Duct.—Obstruction may be caused by cancer of the head of the pancreas, a gallstone impacted at the ampulla of Vater, a pancreatic calculus, or cicatricial contraction. The ducts become irregularly dilated, the acini atrophy and disappear and are replaced by fibrous tissue. The islets of Langerhans are unaffected, and as the pancreas shrinks in bulk, these structures appear to be more numerous and stand out with great distinctness. It was by producing experimental obstruction of the pancreatic duct by means of ligature that Banting and Best first succeeded in freeing the islet tissue from the trypsinogen-producing acini and were thus enabled to extract insulin. Carcinoma of the head of the pancreas may occasionally produce exactly the same effect (Fig. 494).

Hemochromatosis.—This rare condition has already been considered on page 395. It is a congenital inborn error of pigment metabolism in middle-aged males characterized by the most extreme hemosiderosis. The pancreas is of a rich brown color. Both the acinar tissue and the islet are loaded with granules of hemosiderin, so that they give an intense Prussian blue reaction. A slow process of necrosis occurs in the damaged cells, and gradually they atrophy, disappear, and are replaced by fibrous tissue. As the islets are destroyed as well as the acinar tissue, diabetes develops so that the condition used to be called bronzed diabetes, as it was thought that diabetes was an essential feature.

CONGENITAL ANOMALIES.—Malformations of various kinds may occur. The best defined of these is the condition known as *annular* or *ring pancreas*, in which the head of the pancreas surrounds the second part of the duodenum and may cause some constriction. Of more importance is *heterotopia of the pancreas*, a condition in which accessory pancreatic tissue is found in the pyloric end of the stomach, the duodenum, and more rarely in the ileum and even the mesentery.

REFERENCES

ANDERSON, D. H.: Am. J. Dis. Child., 1938, *56*, 344. (Fibrocystic disease.)

ASHTON, N.: Lancet, 1959, *2*, 625. (Diabetic retinopathy.)

BAGGENSTOSS, A. H.: Proc. Staff Meetings, Mayo Clinic, 1947, *22*, 542. (Chronic relapsing pancreatitis.)

————: Minn. Med., 1958, *41*, 599. (Pathogenesis of acute pancreatitis.)

BAKER, R. D.: Personal communication. (Mucormycosis infection in diabetes.

BELL, E. T.: Am. J. Clin. Path., 1955, *25*, 299. (Pathological diagnosis of diabetes.)

————: Am. J. Path., 1959, *35*, 801. (Hyalinization of islets in nondiabetics.)

BOCKUS, H. L. *et al.:* Arch. Int. Med., 1955, *96*, 308. (Acute pancreatitis.)

BODIAN, M.: *Fibro-cystic Disease of the Pancreas*, London, 1953.

CHARLES, B. and COCHRANE, W. A.: Can. M. A. J., 1960, *82*, 579. (Alpha cell tumor with chronic diarrhea and hypokalemia.)

DI SANT' AGNESE, P. A. *et al.:* Am. J. Med., 1953, *15*, 777. (Sweat electrolytes in fibrocystic disease.)

DONHAUSER, J. L. and BIGELOW, N. H.: Am. J. Surg., 1958, *96*, 61. (Acute pancreatitis.)

DUFF, G. L.: Bull. Johns Hopkins Hosp., 1939, *65*, 69. (Carcinoma of body of pancreas.)

————: Am. J. Med. Sci., 1942, *203*, 437. (Islet cell tumors.)

DUNN, J. S., SHEEHAN, H. L. and McLETCHIE, N. G. B.: J. Path. and Bact., 1943, *55*, 245. (Alloxan diabetes.)

EHRLICH, J. C. and RATNER, I. M.: Am. J. Path., 1961, *38*, 49. (Amyloidosis of islets of Langerhans.)

FARBER, S.: Arch. Path., 1944, *37*, 238. (Fibrocystic disease.)

FRANTZ, VIRGINIA K.: *Tumors of the Pancreas.* Atlas of Tumor Pathology, Section VII, Fascicles 27 and 28, Washington, D. C.

GORE, I.: Am. J. Path., 1953, *29*, 613. (Venous thrombosis in cancer of pancreas.)

GROSS, J. B. and COMFORT, M. W.: Am. J. Med., 1956, *21*, 596. (Chronic relapsing pancreatitis.)

HAMILTON, J. D.: Diabetes, 1953, *2*, 180. (Pathology of diabetes.)

HOUSSAY, B. A.: Am. J. Med. Sci., 1950, *219*, 353. (Diabetes and the anterior pituitary.)

JACKSON, W. P. U.: Brit. Med. J., 1952, *2*, 690. Lancet, 1955, *2*, 625. (The prediabetic state.)

JOSLIN, E. P., ROOT, H. F., WHITE, P. and MARBLE, A.: *The Treatment of Diabetes Mellitus*, 10th ed., Philadelphia, 1959.

LAZARUS, S. S. and VOLK, B. W.: Arch. Path., 1959, *67*, 456. (Pancreatic adaptation to diabetogenic hormones.)

LOGOTHETOPOULOS, J. *et al.:* New Eng. J. Med., 1959, *261*, 423. (Metaglucagon diabetes.)

LOGOTHETOPOULOS, J. and SALTER, J. M.: Diabetes, 1960, *9*, 31. (Alpha cells and glucagon.)

LONERGAN, P. and ROBBINS, S. L.: New Eng. J. Med., 1959, *260*, 367. (Absence of Kimmelstiel-Wilson lesions in diabetes due to hemochromatosis.)

MACKENZIE, W. C. *et al.:* Can. J. Surg., 1958, *2*, 6. (Alpha cell tumor with diarrhea and jejunal ulcers.)

McMANUS, J. F. A.: Proc. Am. Diabetes Assn., 1949, *9*, 303. (Nature of Kimmelstiel-Wilson lesion.)

POPE, C. H. JR.: Diabetes, 1960, *9*, 9. (Retinal capillary micro-aneurysms.)

RICH, A. R. and DUFF, G. L.: Bull. Johns Hopkins Hosp., 1936, *58*, 212. (Acute hemorrhagic pancreatitis.)

RICHMAN, A.: Am. J. Med., 1956, *21*, 246. (Acute pancreatitis.)

SMITH, B. K. and ALBRIGHT, E. C.: Ann. Surg., 1952, *36*, 90. (Carcinoma of body of pancreas.)

STADIE, W. C.: Am. J. Med. Sci., 1955, *229*, 233. (Action of insulin.)

STEIN, A. A., POWERS, JR. S. R. and BROWNE, H. H.: Ann. Surg., 1956, *143*, 508. (Experimental hemorrhagic pancreatitis.)

TORESON, W. E.: Am. J. Path., 1951, *27*, 327. (Glycogen infiltration of islets of Langerhans.)

VOLK, B. W. and LAZARUS, S. S.: Am. J. Path., 1958, *34*, 121. (Diabetogenic hormones.)

WARREN, S. and LE COMPTE, P. M.: *The Pathology of Diabetes Mellitus*, 3rd ed., Philadelphia, 1952.

WRENSHALL, G. A., HARTROFT, W. S. and BEST, C. H.: Diabetes, 1954, *3*, 444. (Extractable insulin and islet cell histology.)

ZOLLINGER, R. M. and ELLISON, E. H.: Ann. Surg., 1955, *142*, 709. (Clinical syndrome of alpha cell tumors.)

Chapter 30

The Peritoneum and Abdominal Wall

General Considerations
Acute Peritonitis
  PNEUMOCOCCAL PERITONITIS
  GONOCOCCAL PERITONITIS
  BILE PERITONITIS
  LOCALIZED PERITONITIS
  Subphrenic Abscess
Tuberculous Peritonitis

TALC AND LYCOPODIUM
  GRANULOMA
Tumors of the Peritoneum
  PRIMARY TUMORS
  SECONDARY CARCINOMA
Retroperitoneal Tumors
  LIPOMA

SARCOMA
Mesenteric Cysts
Ascites
  Pick's Disease
The Abdominal Wall
  TUMORS
  LESIONS OF UMBILICUS

GENERAL CONSIDERATIONS

THE peritoneum consists of a layer of flattened mesothelial cells supported by a small amount of connective tissue. As a result of irritation the lining cells may become cuboidal, proliferate, and enclose spaces to form tiny cysts. The normal peritoneal fluid contains about 2300 cells per cmm. The majority of these are mononuclear histiocytes, with many lymphocytes and a few polymorphonuclears and eosinophils.

Absorption of fluid can take place in great amount and at great speed from the vast surface of the peritoneum. The fluid passes by dialysis directly into the blood stream. In acute peritonitis the rapid absorption of bacterial toxins and toxic products constitutes one of the gravest dangers of the disease. The *semipermeable* character of the peritoneum and its vast extent have been utilized in the treatment of reversible renal injuries. It has a surface area of 22,000 square centimeters as compared with 15,000 in the glomeruli, and it can be made to play the part of a dialyzing membrane similar to the cellophane in the artificial kidney. Patients have been maintained in good condition by peritoneal lavage for as long as twenty-five days after the onset of uremia (Kelly and Vest).

Although there is no direct communication between the peritoneal and pleural cavities, yet septic and other material may pass indirectly from one to the other. The peritoneal surface of the diaphragm is studded with minute pits into which the membrane dips, and which come into close relationship with the *lymphatic plexus* of the diaphragm. Occasionally, though by no means frequently, bacteria may succeed in entering these lymphatics, whence they are carried to the mediastinal glands, and in this way the pleura may be secondarily infected.

The *omentum* is a specialized portion of the peritoneum which deserves special mention. It has marked absorptive powers, and plays an important part in the removal of bacterial and foreign substances. Indeed it has been shown that when bacteria are injected intraperitoneally in not too large quantities, none may be found in the peritoneal fluid at the time of death, and yet abundant cultures can be obtained from the omentum. This explains in part the frequent sterility of a peritoneal exudate, even when the condition proves to be fatal. The omentum plays the part of an abdominal policeman, hastening to the scene of trouble, localizing an infection, and even preventing a perforation. But the omentum plays a much more subtle role than that of a policeman, unless we remember that the most important function of a good policeman is the prevention of trouble. In response to intraperitoneal infection the omentum reacts actively by producing specific antibodies, and in this respect it far outstrips the peritoneum, the spleen or the liver (Walker *et al.*). The reactive omentum after the injection of an antigen becomes thickly populated with plasma cells, which can be shown to be the site of antibody formation by the use of fluorescence studies in which antibody is conjugated with fluorochrome.

ACUTE PERITONITIS

Etiology.—Acute inflammation of the peritoneum is the result of bacterial infection, although a local reaction may be caused by such aseptic irritants as a strip of gauze or a drainage tube, and a more general reaction by hemorrhage or the escape of fluid from a cyst. The common bacteria found are E. coli and streptococci; less frequent are staphylococcus, pneumococcus, gonococcus, Bacillus pyocyaneus, Bacillus typhosus, and certain anaerobic bacilli. The most acute and diffuse cases are those due to streptococci.

The infection may reach the peritoneum in three ways: (1) *From an abdominal organ.* This is much the commonest way, and the usual source is the gastrointestinal canal. Appendicitis easily heads the list, followed by gastric, typhoid, and dysentery ulcers, ulcerating carcinoma, etc. When the bowel becomes strangulated (hernia, etc.) or when it is gangrenous from infarction, peritonitis quickly develops. When the infection comes from the hollow viscera there may either be perforation with an outpouring of intestinal contents (ruptured appendix, perforated gastric ulcer), or the bacteria may pass through the intact but inflamed wall of the bowel. It is evident that in the former case the resulting peritonitis is more likely to be widespread and overwhelming. The female pelvic organs form a second important group, of which the principal members are puerperal sepsis, which is nearly always streptococcal, and gonococcal infection of the Fallopian tubes, which usually causes a local inflammation limited by adhesions. Other occasional sources of infection are acute cholecystitis, hemorrhagic pancreatitis, abscess of the liver, etc. (2) *From the exterior.* This may be due to an accident, or may occur in the course of a surgical operation. (3) *Hematogenous* infection is very rare; it is seen in the secondary form of pneumococcal peritonitis.

General peritonitis used to be a much dreaded and commonly fatal condition. The introduction of chemotherapy has profoundly changed the outlook.

Morbid Anatomy.—Peritonitis is at first a local condition. It may remain local or may become diffuse. At first the membrane merely appears pink and infected. Then the normal sheen is lost and replaced by a frosted appearance, due to the formation of a layer of fibrin on the surface. Finally the coils of bowel are glued together by a sticky exudate. Meanwhile a fluid exudate is being formed, and collects especially between the adherent coils of bowel. At first it is serous, but soon it becomes purulent. A thick creamy exudate is a better sign than a thin seropurulent one, which always suggests severe streptococcal infection with low resistance and a bad prognosis. Hemorrhagic fluid is seen in infarction of the bowel, strangulations, etc. The *microscopic appearance* is that of an inflamed serous membrane. The chief element of the exudate in the early stages is fibrin, but if the condition becomes purulent there may be a thick layer of polymorphonuclear leukocytes together with a variable number of red blood cells. The surface endothelium may be desquamated, but even in severe cases it sometimes remains intact under the exudate.

Spread may occur over the surface or *via* the lymphatics. *Surface spread* tends to be limited by protective adhesions, and by the action of the great omentum, which plays the part of the abdominal policeman, spreading itself over the inflamed area, sealing up a threatened perforation, and generally acting the part of guardian to the hollow viscera. It effectively prevents many a case of local peritonitis from becoming general. When the omentum is found in an abnormal position and adhering to a viscus, it is safe to assume that trouble is brewing. *Lymph spread* takes place with great rapidity in the subserous lymphatics in streptococcal infections, much as the infection spreads in erysipelas.

The *end-results* are complete recovery, the formation of fibrous adhesions, or death. The question of adhesions is considered later. They are not always permanent and may sometimes disappear.

Pneumococcal Peritonitis.—This variety is in a class by itself and should be separated in the mind from the other forms of acute peritonitis. It may be *secondary* to a primary focus elsewhere, usually in the lung or middle ear. The mode of infection is either by the blood stream or through the diaphragm.

This *primary form* usually occurs in girls under the age of ten years, for the most part in underprivileged classes living under unhygienic conditions. The vaginal secretion is still alkaline at this age, and pneumococci can reach the peritoneal cavity *via* the vaginal canal and Fallopian tubes. The disease commences as a pelvic peritonitis which spreads upwards. The gross appearance is so characteristic that it can often be recognized with the naked eye, the exudate being massive, sticky or stringy owing to the abundant fibrin formation, greenish in color, and without smell.

Gonococcal Peritonitis.—Gonococcal peritonitis is a disease of the female, the infection passing along the Fallopian tube. In rare cases it may follow infection of the seminal vesicles in the male. The peritonitis usually remains confined to the pelvis, and after a short acute phase soon becomes chronic, but occasionally the inflammation may be general. Its chief characteristic is the formation of very dense fibrous adhesions in the pelvis.

Bile Peritonitis.—The presence of bile in the peritoneal cavity is frequently associated with peritonitis. If the bile is sterile the peritonitis is bland in type, the local and constitutional symptoms are mild, and the pool of bile becomes walled off. If the bile is infected the course is stormy and often rapidly fatal, and the peritonitis is widespread. In laboratory animals the experimental introduction of sterile bile into the peritoneal cavity is followed by a fulminating peritonitis, with anaerobic bacilli of the Welch type swarming in the fluid. This does not occur in man.

Localized Peritonitis.—It is not usual for inflammation of the peritoneum to become generalized. Unless the infection is overwhelming, as in perforation of a hollow viscus or gangrene of the bowel which allows ready passage of enormous numbers of bacteria, there is a tendency for the process to be localized. Two things may happen. (1)

The inflammation may pass off and the membrane return to a normal state, or there may be thickening and adhesions. (2) Pus may be formed, which is limited by adhesions to form an abscess such as the periappendicular abscess which follows acute appendicitis. It is unusual for such an abscess to open into the peritoneal cavity; it is more likely to discharge onto the skin surface or into a hollow viscus. These localized peritoneal abscesses are often seen in the female pelvis. A special form is the subdiaphragmatic or subphrenic abscess.

Subphrenic Abscess.—A subphrenic abscess is a collection of pus between the diaphragm above, and the liver, stomach, or spleen below. In most of the cases the original inflammatory focus is in the upper part of the abdomen, especially gastric and duodenal ulcer and abscess of the liver, but the pus may trek up from below, *e.g.*, appendicular abscess, pelvic abscess. The site of the initial focus of infection determines whether the abscess be under the right dome of the diaphragm or the left. The abscess is shut off from the general abdominal cavity by adhesions. Usually the pus is intraperitoneal, but when the primary lesion is in the appendix, liver, or kidney, the pus is retroperitoneal. The diaphragm is pushed up on the affected side as shown by the roentgenray films and the liver is pushed down. The condition is progressive, and the abscess may burst into the peritoneal, pleural, or pericardial cavities.

TUBERCULOUS PERITONITIS

The peritoneum is infected with tuberculosis either from an abdominal organ or from outside the abdomen. There are three chief intra-abdominal sources: (1) tuberculosis of the bowel, (2) tuberculous mesenteric glands, and (3) tuberculosis of the Fallopian tube. In the first and third of these the infection may be limited to a few tubercles on the outside of the intestinal ulcer or the infected tube. We are concerned here with general infection of the membrane. Repeated infection may occur through the ostium of the tube, so that no treatment is of avail until the tube is removed, but usually the ostium is sealed up by adhesion of the fimbriae.

The extra-abdominal sources are the lungs and pleura (probably lymph spread through the diaphragm), and a distant focus in bones, joints, or bronchial lymph nodes (blood spread). The disease is commoner in children and young adults, and occurs in two main forms, the moist and the dry.

In the *moist form* the chief feature is the great distention of the abdomen, with its tight shiny dome overtopping the wasted body of the patient. The distention is caused by a great accumulation of thin, watery, pale yellow fluid which shows the characteristics of an exudate, *i.e.*, a specific gravity above 1018 and an albumin content about 4 per cent. It contains many lymphocytes and may be blood-stained. Blood in the abdominal fluid suggests tuberculosis or malignancy of the peritoneum. When the fluid is removed the surface of the peritoneum is seen to be studded with miliary tubercles. Sometimes the tubercles excite the formation of a plastic exudate which covers up and hides the tubercles. There may be larger caseous masses, and the mesenteric lymph nodes are usually large and caseous. The omentum may be thick and contracted, but this is more characteristic of the dry form. Occasionally the fluid may be encysted by adhesions, so as to simulate an abdominal cyst. Opening of the abdomen and drainage of the fluid is often followed by remarkable improvement which is difficult to explain, but unless the primary focus (Fallopian tube, etc.) is removed a permanent cure cannot be expected.

In the *dry form* there is little or no fluid, but a dense plastic exudate is produced which glues the intestines together and is followed by the formation of very firm adhesions. When the abdomen is opened the coils of intestine are matted together and cannot be separated, so that a detailed examination of the bowel for tuberculous ulcers may be a matter of great difficulty. The surface may be studded with tubercles, but often these are completely covered by the inflammatory exudate. The omentum is thickened and contracted so that it forms a flat mass like a pancake, or a rounded one like a sausage which can be felt through the abdominal wall. When the coils of bowel are partially separated collections of fluid may be found

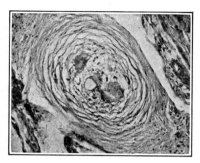

Fig. 495.—Lycopodium granuloma showing spores, giant cells and fibrosis. × 75.

between them. A fecal fistula may be formed owing to a loop of diseased bowel becoming adherent to the abdominal wall, followed by caseation of the wall and ulceration of the skin surface. The fistula may open at the umbilicus.

Talc and Lycopodium Granuloma.—Lycopodium spores which used to be a constituent of the dusting powder of surgical gloves may cause a localized peritonitis with the formation of adhesions or large numbers of small surface nodules which may be mistaken for tubercles or carcinomatosis. The surface of the spore (the edge as seen in a section) is furnished with firm spicules which cause it to adhere to any surface with which it comes in contact, and to be forced beneath that surface by any manipulation. The lesions consist of lymphocytes, plasma cells and foreign body giant cells which may contain the acid-fast spores. The whole forms a *lycopodium granuloma* (Fig. 495). Similar lesions are more commonly produced at the present day by talc powder (*talc granuloma*), which consists of crystals of magnesium silicate. It is in reality a silicious granuloma (Roberts). A table illustrating the various forms of granuloma will be found on page 63.

TUMORS OF THE PERITONEUM

Primary Tumors.—These are among the rarest of tumors. It would appear, however, that they actually do exist (Ackerman). The neoplasm is best called a *mesothelioma*. It usually takes the form of a spreading mass that consists of epithelial-like cells which may form acini and papillary processes, so that it is readily confused with secondary carcinoma.

Secondary Carcinoma.—The peritoneum may be infected from carcinoma of any intra-abdominal organ. There may be one or two masses in the mesentery and omentum, or a condition of diffuse carcinomatosis. The primary tumor is usually in the stomach, large bowel, or ovary (malignant papillary cystadenoma). The infection is caused by the tumor perforating the serous coat and scattering cells over the serous surface. The connection between the tumor on the inside and the tumor on the outside may be very evident to the naked eye, or the process of serous invasion may be seen only with the microscope. Tumor cells from a cancer of the stomach may drop down through the peritoneal cavity, forming little implantations on the serous surface to mark their track, and becoming seeded on the pelvic organs where they may form secondary growths. The ovaries form particularly favorable soil, and may present large tumors before a cancer of the stomach is suspected. Lymphatic spread may result in wide-spread dissemination. In such cases the wall of the bowel may be covered with a fine network of white lines representing lymph vessels distended by tumor cells. The irritation of the peritoneum causes ascites to develop, and *carcinoma cells may be found in the fluid. Unless the cells are in clumps or there are numerous undoubted individual malignant cells, it is very unsafe to diagnose them at indicating malignancy* (Saphir). The fluid is often hemorrhagic.

If the primary tumor is a colloid type of carcinoma, the secondary growths form large soft jelly-like masses. The curious condition of *pseudomyxoma peritonei* may be caused by rupture of a pseudomucinous cyst of the ovary and more rarely of a mucocele of the appendix. This condition, which is not really malignant, is considered in connection with ovarian cysts.

RETROPERITONEAL TUMORS

It is difficult to decide which tumors should be included in this group. Of the true retroperitoneal tumors by far the most numerous are the malignant lymphomas and metastatic carcinoma of the lymph nodes. The most frequent tumors growing from retroperitoneal tissue (exclusive of lymphoid tissue) are lipoma or liposarcoma and fibrosarcoma. Most of the other rare tumors arise from nervous structures, both nerve fibers and ganglia. The prognosis is extremely bad, in part because of the late date at which the correct diagnosis is made.

RETROPERITONEAL LIPOMA. — Retroperitoneal lipoma is really a mixed tumor, although consisting largely of fat. Some parts are myxomatous and some sarcomatous. It commences at one side of the vertebral column, usually at the level of the kidney, grows very slowly, and may reach an enormous size, filling the greater part of the abdominal cavity. It may creep through the intervertebral foramina and compress the cord. The tumor is more nearly related to the teratomata than to an innocent lipoma, and may occur in early childhood, although usually in middle age.

RETROPERITONEAL SARCOMA.—Retroperitoneal sarcoma is a fibrosarcoma which grows from the fascia of the posterior abdominal wall. It shows the usual gross and microscopic characters of a fibrosarcoma.

RETROPERITONEAL FIBROSIS.—This rare and very puzzling condition was first described in 1945. Although it is not a neoplasm, it is included here for convenience on account of its retroperitoneal character. A mat of dense fibrous tissue develops across the lower part of the vertebral column, usually between the fourth lumbar vertebra and the promontory of the sacrum, extending laterally to include the ureters and great vessels, any of which may be compressed with serious results (Stueber). In the only case with which I am familiar the mat of new tissue was 1 cm. thick. *Microscopically*, the most prominent feature is dense collagen, with varying numbers of fibroblasts and occasional collections of small round cells. The nature and cause of the condition is a complete mystery. It is usually described as being inflammatory, but there is no real support for this concept. Many reports are beginning to appear in the literature, which raises the question as to whether some new agent is at work. A similar fibrosis may occur in the mediastinum which may occasionally be associated with retroperitoneal fibrosis.

RETROPERITONEAL LYMPHOSARCOMA.—This is the commonest of the group of retroperitoneal tumors. The usual variety is a reticulum cell sarcoma. The characteristics of this and other lymphosarcomas are discussed in connection with diseases of lymphoid tissue.

MESENTERIC CYSTS

Cysts of the mesentery and omentum are rare. *Enterogenous cysts* are derived from diverticula or congenital reduplications of the intestine in which the communication with the bowel has been pinched off. Intestinal structures can often be demonstrated in the wall of the cyst.

Lymphatic cysts of the mesentery are probably lymphagiomata of congenital origin. They occur in childhood and early adult life. They are usually single and about the size of a hen's egg, but may attain a great size. The lining is a flat endothelium, and the contents are watery or milky. *Gas cysts* of the mesentery are very rare in humans, though common in the pig. They are quite small and are usually grouped in one segment of the bowel. Their nature is uncertain; the gas may be formed by bacteria, or may be produced by cells. *Hydatid cysts* are fairly common in the mesentery, where they form multiple masses which may reach a large size.

ASCITES

Ascites is an accumulation of serous fluid in the peritoneal cavity, so that the abdomen becomes converted into a bag of fluid (*askos*, a bag). The fluid may be dropsical in origin, *i.e.*, a transudate, or inflammatory, *i.e.*, an exudate. *Dropsical ascites* may be part of a general dropsy (*hydrops*, water), due to cardiac or renal disease, or it may be due to obstruction of the portal vein. Portal obstruction is usually caused by portal cirrhosis of the liver, but may be due to pressure on the vein by a tumor, enlarged glands, etc. The *exudative form* of ascites is caused by irritation of the peritoneum by tuberculosis or carcinomatosis, and the fluid may contain blood. Ascites in a woman with normal heart and kidneys should suggest carcinoma of the ovaries. The inflammatory fluid has a higher specific gravity (above 1018) and protein content (above 3 per cent) than the dropsical fluid.

PICK'S DISEASE.—This condition has already been discussed under the heading of chronic constrictive pericarditis, but it is mentioned here because the most striking features may be great thickening of the peritoneum and recurring ascites. In one case which I examined when the abdomen was opened it looked as if the viscera had been removed, so marked were the pressure effects of the ascites and so great was the peritoneal thickening. There is often a polyserositis, affecting peritoneum, pericardium, and pleura.

The accompanying table summarizes some of the major disorders producing ascites.

THE ABDOMINAL WALL

The abdominal wall suffers from the same pathological conditions as the rest of the surface of the body, but a few lesions deserve separate mention.

Tumors.—*Lipoma.*—A lipoma of the subcutaneous tissue is not uncommon. It must be differentiated from small extrusions of

COMMON DISORDERS PRODUCING ASCITES

Condition	SPECIAL FEATURES		
	Fluid	Abdominal Viscera	Miscellaneous
Right heart failure	Moderate, clear	Hepatomegaly	Dependent edema
Nephrotic syndrome	Moderate, clear	Severe renal disease	Edema and albuminuria
Portal cirrhosis	Abundant, clear	Small, hard, nodular liver; (large and fatty earlier).	Liver dysfunction and portal hypertension
Acute peritonitis	Moderate, turbid	Source—ruptured viscus, abscess, etc.	Local and systemic signs
Diffuse peritoneal carcinomatosis	Frequently abundant; contains tumor cells	Diffuse "seeding" of tumor over peritoneal surfaces	Evidence of tumor elsewhere

extraperitoneal fat in the middle line of the epigastric region.

Desmoid Tumor.—This perplexing neoplasm is a proliferation of fibrous tissue which seems to lie halfway between a benign fibroma and a malignant fibrosarcoma. The tumor grows from the sheath of the rectus and tends to infiltrate the muscle. It is densely hard, and interlacing bands of fibrous tissue are seen on the cut surface (*desmos*, a band). About 90 per cent of the cases occur in women who have borne children. In the remaining cases there is usually a history of injury to the abdominal wall. The enclosed muscle fibers may become converted into multinucleated plasmodial masses like giant cells. Some of these tumors show a tendency toward malignancy, for sometimes they recur after removal.

LESIONS OF UMBILICUS.—The umbilicus, though a small structure, suffers from many diseases, as may be seen in Cullen's monograph of 650 pages. The most important lesions are congenital anomalies, fistulae and tumors.

Patent Vitelline Duct.—The vitelline or omphalo-mesenteric duct, the original communication between the intestine and the yolk sac which normally becomes closed at the end of the second month of intra-uterine life, passes from the ileum a short distance above the ileocecal valve to the umbilicus. When the intestinal end remains open it is called *Meckel's diverticulum*; this is a common condition. Rarely the entire tract remains open, so that the intestine communicates with the surface; this is known as a patent Meckel's diverticulum. The distal end only may remain open while the intra-abdominal part is obliterated; the mucous membrane is prolapsed on the surface to form a raspberry-like tumor. If both ends are closed but the intervening portion remains open, a cyst is formed.

Patent Urachus.—The urachus is the communication between the urinary bladder and the allantois *via* the umbilicus. If it does not become obliterated, there is a fistulous opening at the umbilicus through which urine is discharged. A urachal cyst is formed if both ends of the duct are closed but the intervening part remains patent.

Fistulæ.—Examples of fistulæ of *congenital* origin have already been described. An abdominal *abscess* may point and rupture at the umbilicus. A *fecal fistula* is most often due to tuberculous peritonitis, a loop of diseased bowel becoming adherent to the umbilicus; caseation and breaking down then give rise to a fistula between the bowel and the skin.

Tumors.—Tumors of the umbilicus are usually *secondary carcinomas.* The primary growth is likely to be in the stomach, large bowel, gallbladder or ovary, and is usually an adenocarcinoma. It feels like a hard button. The tumor cells may reach the umbilicus *via* the round ligament. Secondary cancer of the umbilicus is a late manifestation, and indicates that the case is inoperable.

Primary carcinoma is very rare, although I happen to have seen 3 cases. It is usually an epidermoid carcinoma, but may be an adenocarcinoma. It is probable that most of the latter cases reported in the literature are really secondary. *Endometrioma* is an interesting tumor, in the form of a small red nodule from which blood may be discharged at the menstrual period. It consists of endometrial tissue (see discussion on Endometriosis). It is also known as an adenomyoma, because it may contain both glandular and muscular tissue.

REFERENCES

ACKERMAN, L. V.: *Tumors of the Peritoneum and Retroperitoneum,* Atlas of Tumor Pathology, Fascicles 23 and 24, Armed Forces Institute of Pathology, Washington, D.C., 1954.

KELLY, R. A. and VEST, S. A.: J. Urol., 1952, *68,* 539. (Peritoneal lavage in uremia.)

ROBERTS, G. B. S.: Brit. J. Surg., 1947, *34,* 417. (Talc granuloma.)

SAPHIR, O.: Am. J. Clin. Path., 1949, *19,* 309. (Cancer cells in peritoneal fluid.)

STUEBER, P. J.: J. Urol. 1959, *82,* 41. (Retroperitoneal fibrosis).

WALKER, F. C., THOMSON, J. D. and GRAY, J. C.: Brit. J. Surg., 1960, *48,* 89. (Antibody formation by the greater omentum.)

Chapter 31

The Lower Urinary Tract

RENAL PELVIS, URETER AND
  BLADDER
General Considerations
Effects of Obstruction
  HYDRONEPHROSIS
Inflammation
  CYSTITIS
    Cystitis Cystica
    Interstitial Cystitis (Hunner's
      Ulcer)
    Leukoplakia
  PARASITIC INFECTION

Tuberculosis
Calculi
  STONE IN THE KIDNEY
  STONE IN THE BLADDER
  STONE IN THE URETER
Epithelial Tumors
  TUMORS OF THE BLADDER
  TUMORS OF RENAL PELVIS
Other Tumors
Miscellaneous Conditions
  MALAKOPLAKIA

DIVERTICULUM
  Bone Formation
HEMATURIA

THE URETHRA
Gonorrheal Urethritis
  STRICTURE OF URETHRA
    Calculus of Urethra
Reiter's Syndrome
Congenital Anomalies of Lower
  Urinary Tract

THE upper urinary tract, *i.e.* the kidney with its one million nephrons, has already been considered in connection with those organs whose function it is to maintain the constancy of the internal environment. The term cardiovasculorenal disease indicates that this connection involves the pathological as well as the physiological. The lower urinary tract, namely the renal pelvis, ureter, bladder and urethra, plays no part in this regulating mechanism. It merely functions as a passive carrier of urine. At the same time it bears a close anatomical relationship to the male genital tract. For these reasons it seems preferable to consider the two parts of the urinary tract separately in a book which seeks to approach the study of disease from a physiological as well as from a structural point of view.

RENAL PELVIS AND BLADDER

GENERAL CONSIDERATIONS

The pelvis of the kidney, the ureter, and the bladder are so closely related embryologically, functionally, and structurally that it is natural that the pathological conditions from which they suffer should be very similar. All are lined by transitional epithelium, for the function of all three is either conduction or storage of urine, not secretion or absorption. The fact that a common epithelium lines the renal pelvis, ureter and bladder accounts for the similarity of the types of tumor which affect these structures. The incidence of these tumors is of course quite different in the three locations. It is commonest where the urine lingers longest and rarest where the urine flows most quickly.

The epithelial cells covering the pyramids contain cytoplasmic inclusions, which are seen in sections stained with histochemical technique for carbohydrates, such as the periodic acid-Schiff and the alcian blue methods. These inclusions are confined to the pyramids, and stop abruptly at the reflection of epithelium from the pyramid to the calyx. A particularly interesting point is the occurrence of similar inclusions not only in a primary carcinoma of the renal pelvis, but also in the metastases (Tucker *et al.*).

In the *development* of the epithelium of the urogenital system both entoderm and mesoderm participate. The bladder has a dual origin, in part from entoderm, in part from mesoderm. The mucosa of the trigone, which intervenes between the openings of the ureters and those of the ejaculatory ducts, is of mesodermal origin. So also is the floor of the internal urethra and the prostate which arises from the mesodermal floor. The remainder of the bladder (the dome) was originally part of the cloaca. As the digestive tract is formed from entoderm, it follows that the mucosa of the dome as well as that part of the urethra other than the

(859)

floor is of entodermal origin. These facts explain how it is that the lesions of cystitis glandularis in the dome resemble in structure the epithelium of the large intestine, whereas those in the trigone resemble the prostate. Adenocarcinoma of the dome resembles and may be mistaken for the same tumor in the large bowel, whilst adenocarcinoma of the trigone may be confused with cancer of the prostate (Pund *et al.*). The same is true for corresponding lesions in the internal urethra.

The *circulation* in the bladder depends on the degree of distention. When the bladder of the rat is examined by transillumination with the mercury vapor lamp it is seen that urethral obstruction soon leads to slowing of the blood flow, stasis, and hemorrhage into the wall and lumen (Mehrotra). The vessels are dilated and obstructed by clumps of red blood cells, and, if the urethral obstruction is complete, the blood comes to a standstill in forty-eight hours. By this time the epithelium is becoming lost, and acute inflammation may develop.

The bladder plays the part of a half way house between the upper and lower urinary tracts. It therefore runs a double risk of infection. As an offset to this it must be noted that the healthy bladder is peculiarly resistant to infections. Indeed it may safely be said that, with the exception of tumors, if a pathological condition be found in the bladder, the strong probability is that it is not primary in that organ. This is true for cystitis, for tuberculosis, and for calculi with the exception of those which occur in old men with prostatic retention. Finally, the bladder resembles the stomach in that it makes its voice heard above that of its neighbors, although usually it is they who are really suffering. Pus in the urine, painful micturition, and frequent micturition are apt to suggest bladder disease. They should not do so, but should rather be taken as an indication of renal disease.

EFFECTS OF OBSTRUCTION

Obstruction to the outflow of urine may cause dilatation of the bladder, ureter, or pelvis of the kidney, *i.e.*, *hydronephrosis*, depending on the site of the obstruction. The obstruction may be in the urethra, bladder or ureter. In the male urethra obstruction is due to *urethral stricture*, nearly always gonorrheal in origin. In the bladder the common cause is *enlargement of the prostate* but a *tumor of the bladder* may obstruct the opening of one, sometimes both ureters, producing hydronephrosis. A *calculus* may block the renal pelvis, ureter, or urethral opening in the bladder. *Stricture of the ureter* may be due to scarring following injury caused by the passage of a calculus, or, as shown by Hunner, there may be local inflammation of the wall of the ureter due to hematogenous infection with the formation of one or more strictures (*Hunner stricture of ureter*). Stenosis of the lower end of the ureter for no apparent reason is probably congenital. A rare cause of obstruction of the ureters is *retro-peritoneal fibrosis*, also called *periureteral fibrosis*, a mysterious condition which has already been discussed on page 856. Although it was only described for the first time by Ormond in 1945, many reports are now appearing in the literature. The condition must be considered in the differential diagnosis of renal failure due to ureteral obstruction, especially when associated with lower abdominal pain. *Moveable kidney*, a condition in which the normal supports of the kidney are relaxed, allowing the organ to slip downward, may lead to kinking of the ureter and intermittent hydronephrosis. An *aberrant renal artery* passing across the ureter to the lower pole of the kidney may in exceptional cases cause sufficient pressure on the ureter to produce hydronephrosis. It is evident that if the obstruction is in the urethra or bladder the hydronephrosis will be bilateral, whereas if it is in the ureter or the ureteric opening in the bladder, the hydronephrosis will be unilateral.

Obstruction in the urethra (male) leads to dilatation and hypertrophy of the bladder. The proportion varies, just as it does in the gallbladder and other hollow viscera when they are obstructed. The natural tendency is to dilatation, but there is a compensatory muscular hypertrophy, although this may be largely absent in old men. The hypertrophy leads to marked thickening of the wall of the bladder, and bands of muscle which normally have a reticulated arrangement under the mucosa become very prominent and stand out as trabeculae. The trabeculae are separated by depressions, and one or more of these may become enlarged so as to form a diverticulum. The dilatation of the urinary tract extends to the ureters and to the pelvis of the kidney. Infection is a common complication owing to the accumulation of stagnant urine, and the bladder, wall of the ureter and pelvis of the kidney show an inflammatory thickening in addition to the dilatation. The real danger of obstruction is its effect on the kidney, and this will now be considered.

Hydronephrosis.—This is a dilatation of the renal pelvis and calyces with destruction of the kidney substance (Fig. 496). Hydronephrosis is caused by obstruction to the outflow of urine. The obstruction may be *intrinsic* or *extrinsic* in relation to the lower urinary tract. Any extrinsic lesion pressing on the tract will naturally cause hydronephrosis. It is only the intrinsic causes of obstruction which will be considered here. These may be congenital or acquired.

Congenital obstruction takes the form of valve-like folds of the mucosa which are present in the fetus and sometimes at birth, or definite constrictions. These lesions, which are readily overlooked by the pathologist unless searched for with particular care, are commonest at the pelvi-ureteric junction, but also occur at the pelvic brim and in the intravesical portion of the ureter. The most extreme examples of hydronephrosis belong to this group, because the condition is symptomless until it becomes far advanced.

Acquired obstruction may take the form of: (1) obstruction in the *urethra* from stricture and enlargement of the prostate; (2) obstruction in the *bladder* due to a calculus or to the internal sphincter being unable to open owing to neuromuscular dysfunction (tabes, injury to cord, etc.); (3) obstruction in the *ureter* due to a stone at the upper or lower end, stricture of the ureter, pressure of an aberrant branch of the renal artery, or kinking of the ureter. The most extreme forms of dilatation are caused by gradual partial obstruction, but sudden complete obstruction, as from ligation of the ureter, may lead to a moderate degree of

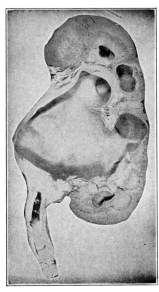

Fig. 496.—Hydronephrosis. The renal pelvis and calyces are dilated. The ureter is blocked by a calculus.

dilatation followed by hydronephrotic atrophy. If renal ischemia is added to urinary obstruction, the destruction of tissue is much more rapid. Experimental ligation of the posterior branch of the renal artery causes infarction of from one-third to one-half of the kidney; when this is combined with total ureteral obstruction enormous sacculations of the infarcted area are produced in a remarkably short time (Hinman and Hepler).

Some degree of dilatation of the ureter with hydronephrosis is common in *pregnancy*. This is not due, as used to be believed, merely to pressure on the ureters by the enlarged uterus. The main factor is the hormone complex of pregnancy, which causes not only relaxation of the smooth muscle of the uterus and gallbladder, but also of the ureters. The effect is dependant on the presence of the placenta, and can be observed to develop in the monkey long after the fetus has been removed (van Wagenen and Jenkins). Mechanical pressure no doubt plays a secondary part.

Megaloureter and *megalobladder* are conditions in which the ureter and bladder are greatly enlarged. This is comparable to the megalocolon of Hirschsprung's disease caused by absence of the cells of Auerbach's plexus. In megalobladder there is a decrease in the number and variety of nerve cells and bundles of nerves in the bladder wall. The enlargement of the ureter seems to be secondary to this defect.

Morbid Anatomy.—In other glands of the body obstruction of the corresponding duct is followed by primary atrophy of the gland. This is not true of the kidney, where the result of obstruction is first hydronephrosis, followed later by secondary hydronephrotic atrophy. The reason for this is reabsorption of the fluid, which is discussed below. The pelvis and calyces are dilated, sometimes to an enormous extent. The normal pelvis has an average capacity of 7 to 10 cc., but it may be distended so as to contain several liters. The pyramids are first destroyed by the dilatation of the calyces, and the cortex follows, until finally the kidney is converted into a thin-walled lobulated bag of watery fluid, the greatly distended calyces being separated by incomplete septa. Ischemia produced by pressure of the retained fluid is probably a large factor in the atrophy and destruction of the renal parenchyma. If infection is superimposed the condition becomes an infected hydronephrosis. The wall of the sac will be thicker and the lining more rough as the result of infection.

Microscopically the first change is marked by atrophy of the tubules, while the gloeruli may appear fairly normal. This dissociation of lesions may be very striking, and is quite peculiar to hydronephrosis. In course of time the glomeruli become fibrosed, and the renal parenchyma is replaced by fibrous tissue. Even in the advanced stages small areas can be found in which the glomeruli and tubules are apparently normal, and are probably continuing to secrete urine.

One of the problems of hydronephrosis is how it is that the contents of the hydronephrotic sac are fresh and clear instead of stagnant and stinking. Moreover, normal secreting tissue can be found even in cases of complete obstruction. It is evident that *absorption* of the fluid must occur, thus allowing a continual circulation. There has been difference of opinion as to the route taken by the fluid, but it would now appear that it may be (1) pyelovenous backflow from the minor calyces into the straight veins at the base of the pyramids, (2) pyelotubular backflow, which seems to occur more easily as time increases the size of the hydronephrosis, and (3) possibly by lymphatic channels.

INFLAMMATION

Infection of the pelvi-vesical tract may occur from the urethra, kidney, or neighboring organs. The short female urethra accounts for the frequency of lower urinary tract infection in women and children. In the male, infection from below is due to retention (stricture of urethra, enlarged prostate), or the passage of an infected catheter. Infection of the bladder usually comes from the kidney, unless there is some predisposing cause in the bladder such as retention or stone. The healthy bladder is remarkably resistant to infection, and when pyogenic bacteria are introduced into its cavity they rapidly disappear. Occasionally infection may come from a neighboring organ, as in inflammation of the appendix or the female pelvic organs. The common infecting organism is *E. coli*, with an acid urine. The pyogenic cocci are next in frequency, and they turn the urine alkaline owing to the production of ammonia. Two of the most troublesome organisms are *Bacillus proteus* and *Bacillus pyocyaneous*, because, being gram negative, they are resistant to penicillin. Fortunately they respond to streptomycin. Urinary infections due to resistant "hospital strains" of *Aerobacter aerogenes* are becoming a serious problem. This trend has developed since the widespread use of antibiotic therapy, just as we have already seen to be the case in hospital staphylococcal infections. The higher incidence of *A. aerogenes* infection occurs in chronic rather than acute urinary infections (Lattimer *et al.*).

A peculiar and important feature of the bacteriology of cystitis is that the flora of the bladder may change with a changed reaction of the urine. Thus a colon infection may replace a staphylococcus, or again a proteus may replace a colon infection. During treatment, therefore, both the reaction and the bacteriology of the urine should be carefully may become pavement or even squamous. The latter varieties present a more formidable barrier to the gonococcus than does the columnar epithelium, and for this reason a second attack is not so intense as the first.

The only common and important pathological condition affecting the urethra is acute inflammation due to the gonococcus, together with the consequences which may result from such inflammation.

GONORRHEAL URETHRITIS

This is a very acute suppurative condition. By the end of the second day the crypts in the wall of the anterior urethra are filled with pus cells containing gonococci, and by the third day the mucosa is extensively infiltrated, for the columnar epithelium offers no resistance. An acute inflammatory exudate is formed in the mucosa, and an abundance of pus is poured from the surface. The infection spreads in the submucosa until the posterior urethra (membranous and prostatic parts) is involved. Here the infection may linger for a long time in the glands which open on to the surface. The acute inflammation may subside in the course of a few weeks, the desquamated epithelium being replaced by epithelium of squamous type. In other cases the infection becomes chronic, being fed from foci in the posterior urethra. The mucous and submucous coats are converted into granulation tissue, which later becomes fibrosed and scarred. The scar tissue may contract, producing a stricture of the urethra.

Stricture of the Urethra.—This is a narrowing of the channel of the urethra due to the formation of fibrous tissue in the wall with subsequent contraction. It may be inflammatory or traumatic in type.

Inflammatory stricture is usually gonorrheal in origin. It may be single or multiple. The usual site is in the bulb of the urethra, but it may be in any part of the anterior urethra. The gonorrheal inflammation leads to the formation of granulation tissue in the mucosa and submucosa; this is followed by fibrosis and contraction of the scar tissue; finally a very narrow passage may be left, which is readily occluded by transient acute inflammatory edema.

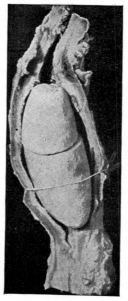

FIG. 502.—Urethral calculus which had been present in the penile urethra for thirty years. It consists of two parts. (Boyd, *Pathology for the Surgeon*, courtesy of W. B. Saunders Co.)

Traumatic stricture is nearly always in the membranous urethra. It is usually due to a fall on the perineum with rupture of the urethra, but sometimes to injury produced by the unskilled passage of an instrument. *Congenital stricture* is considered below.

The *effects* of a stricture are similar to those of prostatic obstruction. The bladder wall hypertrophies and later the cavity becomes dilated. There is bilateral hydronephrosis with dilatation of the ureters. The bladder is able to empty itself completely so that, unlike the condition in prostatic obstruction, there is no residual urine. For this reason secondary infection is less likely to occur in obstruction due to stricture. Nevertheless infection is almost certain to occur sooner or later, especially if a catheter has to be passed, and there is danger of an ascending pyelonephritis. Straining helps micturition in stricture, but not in prostatic obstruction.

Calculus of the urethra is a rare condition, usually due to the arrest of a renal or vesical calculus in its downward passage. I once performed an autopsy on a man who died at the age of seventy-eight, and who was aware of the

male has 44 autosomes and an XY-sex chromosome complex. It might be said that the essential difference between Romeo and Juliet was that Romeo had a Y chromosome determining genes on the single X chromosome, and the medulla of the indifferent gonads develops into testes while the cortex

functional relationship with the anterior
pituitary, the tubules and spermatogenesis
being stimulated by the gonadotrophic

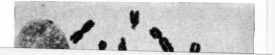

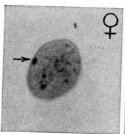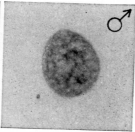

Fig. 505.—Nuclei in oral smear preparations from
human female and male. The sex chromatin is indicated by the arrow. Cresyl methyl violet stain.
× 1800. (Kindness of Dr. Murray L. Barr.)

regresses, but if it carries the XX-sex
chromosome complex, female-determiners on
the two X chromosomes outweigh male-
determiners on autosomes, so that the cortex
develops into ovaries and the medulla regresses. "Interference with this crucial step
of differentiation of bipotential gonads into
testes or ovaries at about the end of the
second month of embryonic development
appears to be the point of departure for most
sex anomalies in man." (Barr). It is of
interest to note in passing that the endocrine
component of the testis, namely the interstitial cells of Leydig, is well developed in
the embryonal testis and again after puberty,
but it is inconspicuous during the intervening period.

If the developing gonads are removed in
the experimental animal before differentiation of the rest of the reproductive system
has had time to occur, a contrast is apparent
in the two sexes. When the very early
ovaries in the rabbit embryo are removed,
there is still normal development of tubes,
uterus, vagina and external genitalia, but
when the testes are removed and the androgenic stimulus of the Leydig cells is lost, the
reproductive system again develops along
female lines, with the Wolffian ducts behaving as if they were Müllerian ducts. It
would appear that the neutral human form
is female and that the embryo has a normal
female tendency, which is perhaps a sobering
thought for the male.

Sex Chromatin.—Before considering the
difficult, confused and confusing subject of
sex reversal and intersex, reference must be
made to the relatively new and exciting topic
of sex chromatin. Thanks to the work of

Barr and his associates at the University of
Western Ontario we now know that the cells
of the body carry the finger prints of their
genetic sex, which may not correspond with
the *apparent* somatic sex of the person. Barr
has shown that a small mass of chromatin,
the sex chromatin, lies against the nuclear
membrane in about 85 per cent of cells of
normal females, but in less than 10 per cent
of cells in normal males (Fig. 505). This
chromatin mass is quite easy to see if you
know what you are looking for, but no one
before Barr realized its significance. The
female cells are said to be chromatin-positive,
the male cells chromatin-negative. The cells
can be obtained for examination from various
sources such as skin, blood (leukocytes),
etc., but the most convenient method is to
make a smear from the oral mucous membrane. The sex distinction in the leukocyte
depends on the presence of a small drum-
stick-like structure present in up to 6 per
cent of leukocytes of genetically female
persons but absent in genetic males. The
sex chromatin has been thought to be an
XX-sex chromosome marker, perhaps hetero-
pyknotic portions of the two X chromosomes
that adhere to each other, but it now appears
more probable that it is formed from one
X chromosome which has become condensed.
Nuclei with an XXY-sex chromosome complex would probably give a similar appearance, a point which will have to be referred
to presently. There is at present no explanation for the occurrence of sex chromatin
in a small proportion of male cells, unless
it is related to the XY-sex chromosome
complex.

Sex chromatin has been demonstrated in
a variety of *benign and malignant tumors*
from females, but it is often lying free in the
nucleoplasm instead of against the nuclear
membrane. (Myers). Identification in
more malignant tumors is often impossible.
In teratomas of the testes the nuclear sex is
as often female as male. There is at present
no adequate explanation of the presence of
chromatin masses identical with female sex
chromatin in teratomas from males.

Sex Anomalies.—Anomalies of sexual development are fortunately uncommon, but
are nevertheless important in medical practice. Even in the most normal person

neither sex represents a state of absolute unisexuality. Usually one sex predominates to such an extent that no doubt exists, but although the genitalia are an important criterion of sex, they are often unreliable indicators of chromosomal sex. Most of the anomalies are examples of *sex reversal*, a condition in which *chromosomal sex differs from anatomical sex. True hermaphroditism* (*Hermes,* messenger of the gods, and *Aphrodite* or Venus, goddess of love) in which both ovarian and testicular tissue are present with intersexual genitalia is very rare and need not detain us. In *pseudohermaphrodites* only testes or ovaries are present, yet there is an intersexual anatomy of the rest of the reproductive system; this is not uncommon. We shall consider four exmples of this intermingling: (1) Klinefelter's syndrome, (2) Turner's syndrome, (3) testicular feminization, and (4) the adrenogenital syndrome. The first three are examples of gonadal abnormality, but the fourth is due to an excessive production of androgens by the fetal adrenal cortex. Mention will also be made of mongolism, although it is not a sex anomaly.

Klinefelter's Syndrome.—This is the commonest of the sex anomalies, and it is said to occur about once in every 500 males. The testes are much smaller than normal, and testicular biopsy shows great changes in the seminiferous tubules, so that the condition is also known as *seminiferous tubule dysgenesis.* Some of the tubules are hyalinized, some closed by peritubular fibrosis, whilst in some cases they are lined by Sertoli cells in place of spermatogonia. The atrophic tubules are separated by large clumps of Leydig cells, which may actually resemble Leydig cell adenomata. There is thus a striking divorce between the tubular and the interstitial elements of the testis. In view of these findings it is natural that spermatogenesis is minimal and azoospermia is constant. The condition is therefore an important cause of male sterility. In some cases there is gynecomastia and eunuchoid traits (long limbs, scanty facial hair, etc.). The former probably reflects pituitary hypertrophy, the latter interstitial cell failure before puberty. The urinary gonadotrophins are usually elevated, as if the anterior pituitary was trying to flog a dying horse into action.

The sex-chromatin is positive (female) in about 75 per cent of the cases, but negative in the remainder. In patients with chromatin-positive nuclei the etiological factor apparently causes the gonads of the early embryo to develop into testes rather than ovaries as they would do normally. The chromatin-positive cases are known as *"true" Klinefelter's syndrome;* they are genetic females with atrophic tubules (ghost tubules) and hyperplasia of the interstitial cells which are collected in massive clumps. The chromatin-negative cases are known as *"false" Klinefelter's syndrome;* they are genetic males, with tubules of normal size lined by Sertoli cells, and the interstitial cells are normal in appearance and number but scattered diffusely (Figs. 506 and 507). The difference between the testicular biopsy picture in chromatin-positive (true) and chromatin-negative (false) cases is so striking that the nuclear sex can be determined by a glance at the microscopic section with a low-power lens (Ferguson-Smith *et al.*).

Mental deficiency is often a feature of the Klinefelter syndrome, as it is in other sex reversals. The syndrome was present in 1 per cent of male patients in a mental-deficiency hospital, and prepubertal testicular lesions were demonstrated in chromatin-positive mentally handicapped children (Ferguson-Smith). The psyche is masculine in the Klinefelter syndrome.

The *pathogenesis* of Klinefelter's syndrome is naturally obscure. The basic feature is the addition of a sex chromosome, so that the sex chromosome complex is XXY. Possibly the fault lies with the sex-determining genes in the zygote, a crossing over between an X-sex chromosome bearing female-determining genes and an autosome bearing male-determining genes. It is also known that when androgens are administered to female frogs (genetically female by nuclear sexing) at a critical stage of development, testes will develop instead of ovaries. Thus hormonal imbalance rather than an inborn genetic error may be responsible for a female-to-male sex reversal. The chromosomal sex of the human female infant is of course established at fertilization. During early gonadal dif-

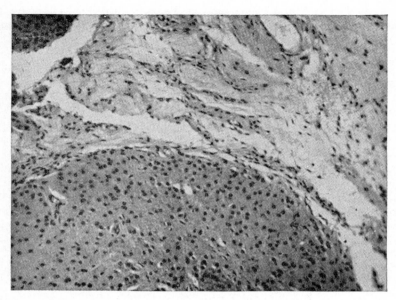

Fig. 506.—High-power view of testicular biopsy specimen from a thirty-seven year old man with chromatin-positive nuclei ("true" Klinefelter's syndrome). Note hyperplasia of interstitial cells (lower) and small atrophic hyalinized seminiferous tubules. Hematoxylin and eosin. × 240. (Augustine and Jaworski, courtesy of Arch. Path.)

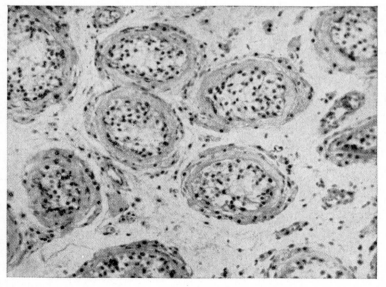

Fig. 507.—High-power view of testicular biopsy specimen from a twenty-seven-year-old man with chromatin-negative nuclei ("false" Klinefelter's syndrome). Note the normal size of the seminiferous tubules, thick basement membranes, and the absence of spermatogenesis. The interstitial cells are normal but scattered. (Augustine and Jaworksi, courtesy of Arch. Path.)

ferentiation, however, some unknown factor may cause the cortex of the indifferent gonads to degenerate, thus allowing testes to be differentiated from the medulla. The testes would then secrete androgens which would cause complete differentiation of the male accessory sex organs, with eventual descent of the testes into the scrotum. In this way the chromosomal female assumes the anatomical (somatic) appearance of the normal male (Moore).

Turner's Syndrome.—This forms an interesting contrast to the anomaly just described, for just as Klinefelter's syndrome may be regarded as the masculinization of the female with medullary dysgenesis of the gonads, so Turner's syndrome is a feminization of the male with cortical dysgenesis (ovarian agenesis) of the gonads. Persons with the syndrome are phenotypical females, but the nuclei lack sex chromatin in 80 per cent of cases. The chief defect is congenital absence of the gonads, the ovaries being represented by slender streaks of connective tissue. The nuclear sexing test shows that the majority of these "girls" are really males in whom the absence of testicular tissue with corresponding lack of androgens has permitted the maternal estrogens to promote the development of the Müllerian ducts and the female external genitalia with regression of the Wolffian system and the male external genitalia. Secondary sex characters naturally fail to develop at puberty, as does menstruation. Mental retardation may be present, but not so frequently as in the Klinefelter syndrome. Urinary gonadotrophins are elevated after the age of ten years, again an example of flogging the dead horse. The genetic defect is the presence of a single X-chromosome, unpaired with either an X- or a Y-chromosome. The psyche is feminine in Turner's syndrome.

Testicular Feminization.—Occasionally a woman with normal external genitalia seeks medical advice for amenorrhea, and is found to be suffering from an extreme form of *male pseudohermaphroditism*. Although the vulva and vagina are normal, the uterus and the tubes are missing, but testes are present either in the pelvis or in the inguinal region. The nuclei are always chromatin-negative in the oral smear, so that there is no doubt of the genetic sex. The interstitial cells of the testes in these patients can undoubtedly secrete considerable amounts of estrogen, for there is full development of female secondary sex characters at puberty, and removal of the testes brings on menopausal symptoms. One suggested explanation of the developmental anomaly is that the interstitial cells of the very early testes produce enough masculinizing hormone or evocator to suppress development of the Müllerian ducts but not enough to masculinize the external genitalia. The condition is hereditary, being transmitted by the normal mother, and the peculiar behavior of the interstitial cells is attributed to a mutant gene. The nuclei are chromatin-negative because they contain the XY-sex chromosome complex.

The Adrenogenital Syndrome.—This, the usual form of *female pseudohermaphroditism*, is quite unlike the other sex anomalies we have discussed, for the gonads and the rest of the reproductive system are normal with the exception of the external genitalia. These are partially masculinized in the female infant with hypertrophy of the clitoris and partial fusion of the labioscrotal folds. As the genetic and somatic sex are one and the same, the nuclei are always chromatin-positive, the sex chromosome complex being XX.

The *pathogenesis* seems to involve a recessive mutant gene which interferes with normal steroid metabolism in the adrenal cortex of the fetus and also postnatally. This is associated with hyperplasia of the cortex and the production of an excessive amount of androgens which are responsible for the masculinizing changes just described. Perhaps the greatest value of the nuclear sexing test is in the differential diagnosis of the adrenogenital syndrome from the various forms of male pseudo-hermaphroditism. A combination of chromatin-positive nuclei and raised urinary 17-ketosteroids points to the adrenogenital syndrome. Cortisone restrains the action of androgens and allows development to take place along feminine lines. For a good review of the important and rapidly expanding subject of nuclear sexing and its practical applications, consult the articles by Lennox (1956), Grumbach and Barr (1958), and Barr and Carr (1960).

The discussion of these rare sex anomalies seems justified because they serve to illustrate some general principles governing the male as well as the female reproductive system. We have seen that the influence of genetic, environmental or hormonal factors during the early stages of development may lead to a dichotomy between genetic and somatic sex, and that male secondary sex characteristics may develop irrespective of the fact that the genetic sex is female. To the doctor it will be apparent that the more appropriate sex from the clinical point of view will often be contrary to the chromosomal sex inferred from cytological tests in gonadal dysgenesis in which the somatic sex is female but the chromosomal sex is most often male.

About one-third of the patients with Klinefelter's syndrome have chromatin-negative nuclei, and about one-fifth of patients with Turner's syndrome have chromatin-positive nuclei. Such persons are not designated as intersexes, because there is no discrepancy between chromosomal and genital sex.

The following table serves to summarize some of the features of the sex anomalies which have been discussed.

Autosome Anomalies.—The new ability to examine and count the chromosomes during life has revealed the fact that just as sex chromosome disturbance may be responsible for anomalies in sex, so also aberrations of the somatic chromosomes (autosomes) may give rise to congenital disorders in infancy and childhood. The first example to be recognized was *mongolism*, that pathetic condition in which the newborn child has mongoloid (slanted) eyes, hyperextensibility of the finger joints, imbecile facies, and, as becomes apparent only too soon, an imbecile mind. The aberration responsible is an extra autosome in every cell, so that the chromosome count is 47 instead of 46. This is an acrocentric chromosome in the smallest size range, thus resembling the Y-sex chromosome. The condition appears to be an example of trisomy, *i.e.* the presence of a "mongol" autosome, No. 21, in triplicate, probably due to nondisjunction or failure of a pair of homologous chromosomes to segregate during miosis. Occasionally there are the normal number of 46 chromosomes, but one of the normal ones in group 13 to 15, the "wishbones," has been replaced by a much larger one, suggesting that a third No. 21 had been present and had fused with the missing "wishbone," thus producing the

DIFFERENTIAL CHARACTERISTICS OF THE MORE IMPORTANT SEX ANOMALIES

Disorder	*Characteristics*
Klinefelter's syndrome (masculinization of the female) (a) True: genetic females; atrophic tubules with Leydig cell aggregates. (b) False: genetic males; tubules normal in size but lined by Sertoli cells.	Males with atrophic testes. 47 chromosomes: 44 $+ \times \times$ Y. Chromatin positive.
Turner's syndrome (feminization of the male).	Female external genitalia in genetic males with absence of gonads. 45 chromosomes: 44 $+ \times$ O. Chromatin negative.
Male pseudohermaphroditism (testicular feminization).	Normal female external genitalia with pelvic or inguinal testes. Chromatin negative.
Adrenogenital syndrome (female pseudohermaphroditism).	Only external genitalia abnormal. Adrenal cortical hyperplasia. Chromatin positive.

larger chromosome, or that a *translocation* with exchange of material between two chromosomes had occurred rather than a true fusion. Thus we may speak of trisomy mongols and translocation mongols.

Other examples of trisomic syndromes are coming to light. Some are incompatible with life. It may be presumed that the larger the extra chromosome, the worse will be the disturbance. In one case the infant had a peculiar facies, webbing of the neck, congenital heart disease, and many minor abnormalities, chromosomal study at autopsy revealing an extra chromosome, apparently identical with the 17th pair (Edwards *et al.*). Mental deficiency is a frequent accompaniment. Mongolism and the Klinefelter syndrome may be combined in one patient, this being an example of two supernumerary chromosomes, one an additional sex chromosome, the other the small autosome characteristic of mongolism (Ford *et al.*).

INFLAMMATION

Inflammation is the commonest disease of the testicle, but it is common in the epididymis and not in the body of the testicle. The common form is inflammation of the epididymisis, is, or was, gonorrheal epididymitis. I am not sure of its frequency in this antibiotic age.

Gonorrheal Epididymitis. — Gonorrhea commences as an acute urethritis, with marked inflammatory change in the subepithelial connective tissue. The infection ascends the urethra and settles in the posterior urethra. The disease may clear up after an acute course of a few weeks, or the infection may linger in the posterior urethra and affect other parts of the genital tract. The epididymis is the chief sufferer, infection occurring usually in the second and third months. The first lesion is at the lower pole, the globus minor, but soon the whole organ is involved. It is seldom that the infection spreads to the testicle, although inflammation of the surrounding fibrous tissue may make that organ feel enlarged and hard. The epididymis is swollen and tender. Hydrocele is often present, and there may be some thickening of the spermatic cord. The type of inflammation is unusual. As the gonococcus is a pyogenic organism, there is suppuration with the formation of minute abscesses, yet there is no extensive abscess formation as might be expected, but rather a widespread inflammatory edema. The inflammation is acute and subsides quickly, but often leaves fibrous scars which obliterate the seminiferous tubules. Fortunately the epididymitis is usually unilateral. When it is bilateral, complete sterility may result.

Other gonorrheal lesions are prostatitis, stricture of the urethra, and blood infection of distant organs. The first two are considered below. Blood infection may give rise to inflammation of joints (gonorrheal arthritis) and of tendon sheaths (tenosynovitis).

Non-Gonorrheal Epididymitis.—Non-gonorrheal epididymitis is very much less common. It is usually caused by staphylococci, sometimes by streptococci or E. coli. The infection is secondary to stricture of the urethra, enlarged prostate, or inflammation of the seminal vesicles. There is abscess formation in the epididymis, marked hardness and thickening of the vas and seminal vesicle, and a tendency to chronicity and recurrences.

Spermatic Granulomas.—Many cases of granulomas of the epididymis caused by the liberation of spermatozoa in the interstitial tissue due to infection or trauma have been reported from the United States Armed Forces Institute of Pathology (Glassy and Mostofi). The onset is insidious, with pain and swelling in the majority of cases on the affected side. The average size of the lesion is 7 mm., usually in the superior pole of the epididymis. The early stage of the reaction is a neutrophilic response, followed later by a histiocytic and epithelioid reaction, and finally fibrosis.

Orchitis.—Inflammation of the testicle may be due to trauma or to acute infections. *Traumatic orchitis* is caused by a blow, which is followed by acute inflammatory edema of the organ. The condition is short and acute, but sometimes results in atrophy of the testicle. *Metastatic orchitis* is the term applied to infection from the blood stream which occurs in certain acute fevers. It is usually due to mumps, occasionally to typhoid fever and smallpox, and rarely to other febrile and septic conditions. Some-

56

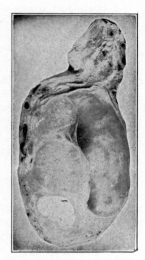

FIG. 508.—Tuberculosis of the epididymis. There is a caseous area in the lower pole and the spermatic cord is thickened.

times the *orchitis of mumps* has preceded the parotitis. It is usually unilateral, and is rarely seen before the age of puberty, being commonest in young men. The enlargement is not great owing to the firm fibrous tunica albuginea, but the tension is great and the pain correspondingly severe. The epididymis is rarely involved. The chief lesions are early edema, followed by diffuse lymphocytic infiltration of the interstitial tissue with focal hemorrhage, destruction of the germinal epithelium, and plugging of the tubules by epithelial débris and fibrin (Gall). The lesion is never suppurative, but may be followed by fibrosis and atrophy of the testicle. Infection by *extension* from the posterior urethra may occur. In severe gonorrheal epididymitis there may be slight involvement of the testicle. There may be colon bacillus infection from a cystitis. In these cases the lesions are suppurative.

TUBERCULOSIS OF THE GENITAL TRACT

As the entire genital tract, sometimes indeed the urogenital tract, may be involved by tuberculosis, it is convenient to consider all the organs together. The infection is usually blood-borne, and starts in the lower pole of the epididymis (Fig. 508), but occasionally in the seminal vesicle. In a small

proportion of cases the bacilli spread along the vas from the bladder, which itself is infected from a focus in the kidney. Nodules are formed throughout the epididymis, so that the organ is enlarged and hard. Caseation and liquefaction occur sooner or later, the skin of the scrotum is involved, and a tuberculous fistula is formed. By the time the patient is seen clinically the disease has usually spread throughout the genital tract, so that the vas, seminal vesicles, and prostate are all involved. The *testicle* is not involved early, but in time the disease spreads to it from the epididymis, invading first the body of Highmore. The *spermatic cord* is thickened and nodular. The *seminal vesicle* is involved early, and indeed the infection may commence there. The entire vesicle is usually destroyed. The *prostate* may be infected either from the genital tract or from the kidney. Caseous nodules are formed in the gland with destruction finally. The *tunica vaginalis* may be studded with tubercles, so that a hydrocele is a common accompaniment. The *other epididymis* is often involved at a later stage, probably by way of the lymphatics. The *bladder* shows tuberculous ulcers, especially in the trigone. The *kidneys* are occasionally involved by upward spread from the genital tract, but combined genito-urinary tuberculosis usually originates in the kidney, with secondary infection of the genital tract.

SYPHILIS OF THE TESTIS

Syphilis of the testicle has ceased to be a frequent lesion owing to modern chemotherapy. Unlike tuberculosis it affects the body, seldom the epididymis. It occurs in two forms which may be combined: (1) a diffuse interstitial inflammation, and (2) a gumma. (1) The *diffuse form* is the commoner, although usually overlooked because it gives rise to no symptoms. The testicle is not enlarged or tender, but it has a characteristic wooden hardness owing to diffuse fibrosis, and there is a loss of the normal testicular sensation when the organ is squeezed. The tunica albuginea is thickened, and the gland is pervaded with white bands of fibrous tissue, so that the cut surface remains flat instead of bulging forward in the normal manner. Microscopically there is at first a diffuse formation of cellular inflammatory tissue containing many spirochetes, followed later by fibrosis with atrophy and disappearance of the tubules. (2) A *gumma* causes enlargement of the testicle (Fig. 509). It is at first gray, but later becomes white and fibrous. Softening is uncommon, and the lesion tends to become scarred.

TUMORS OF THE TESTIS

It is doubtful if any branch of the subject of oncology is so confused as that of testicular tumors. This is due partly to the extremely varied histological features of the tumors, partly to the difficulty of determining the cell of origin. The tumors may be benign or malignant. Benign tumors are very uncommon. Of these adenoma and interstitial cell tumor will be described presently. If simplicity were everything it would be enough to say, as was done in previous editions of this book, that the remaining tumors of the testicle are malignant and of two types, seminoma and teratoma, the former arising from the cells of the seminiferous tubules and radiosensitive, the latter from primitive germ cells and radioresistant. The study by Friedman and Moore of 922 testicular tumors in men of the armed forces suggests that a further subdivision may be of value. At least 96 per cent of the tumors fall into the following groups (Friedman and Moore): (1) Seminoma (35 per cent); (2) embryonal carcinoma (19 per cent); (3) adult teratoma (7 per cent); and (4) teratocarcinoma (35 per cent). Choriocarcinoma forms a very small subgroup (1 per cent) which has been regarded, rightly or wrongly, as a variant of embryonal carcinoma.

Testicular tumors occur in early adult or middle life, the seminoma on the average ten years later than the other members of the group. The undescended testis is 30 times more liable to develop a tumor, either seminoma or teratoma, than is the organ in its normal position. Curiously enough, a person with a cryptorchid testis is liable to have a tumor in the opposite testicle.

Seminoma.—This is a solid tumor, sometimes of quick but often of comparatively slow growth, appearing in middle life. The cut surface is fleshy and homogeneous. The *microscopic picture* is generally as *uniform* as is the cut surface. The cells are polyhedral in form, with unusually distinct walls, unusually clear cytoplasm, and prominent

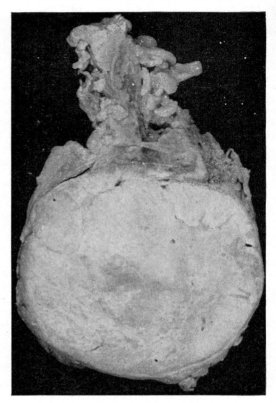

Fig. 509.—Gumma of testis.

nuclei and nucleoli (Fig. 510). The stroma may be infiltrated with large numbers of lymphocytes, occasionally with plasma cells and eosinophils. The tumor closely resembles the dysgerminoma of the ovary, which also has a stroma infiltrated with lymphocytes. It is believed that the lymphocytes represent an immunological or defense response to the tumor.

Embryonal Carcinoma.—This tumor is only half as common as the seminoma. There is *considerable variation* of cell type, but basically the cells are large with vacuolated or reticular basophilic cytoplasm and large nuclei. The pattern may be solid, glandular or papillary. Areas of hemorrhage and necrosis are common. There is early invasion and metastasis, and the prognosis is much worse than in seminoma. The question which naturally presents itself and which cannot be considered as settled is as to whether this tumor should be regarded as a separate entity or as a more malignant variant of the

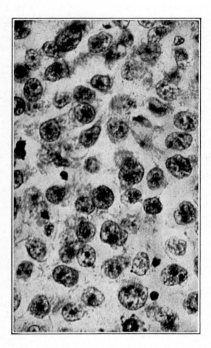

Fig. 510.—Seminoma. The cellular arrangement is anaplastic. The cytoplasm has for the most part disintegrated; only nuclei and nucleoli are seen. × 600.

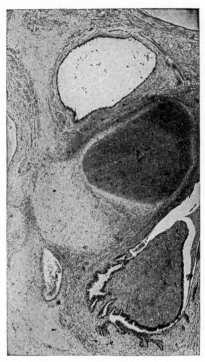

Fig. 511.—Embryoma of testicle. The structure is very varied showing tubular structures, cystic spaces, and cartilage in the center. × 30.

seminoma. It may be noted that Ewing's name for seminoma was embryonal carcinoma.

Teratoma.—This is a teratoid tumor which probably arises from a germinal blastomere or primitive germinal cell. As these cells are totipotent the tumor may contain structures derived from three embryonic layers. It is also called *embryoma*, mixed tumor of the testicle, and, in the older literature, fibrocystic disease. The tumor may attain a very great size. The cut surface usually presents a characteristic cystic appearance (hence the old name of fibrocystic disease), the cysts varying much in size in different specimens and sometimes being absent. The *microscopic appearance* is extremely varied, though in some cases the growth is almost confined to one type of tissue. From the *mesoderm* there may be cartilage, bone, plain and striated muscle, fat and lymphoid tissue; from the *entoderm* there may be tubular spaces lined by columnar cells, *i.e.*, abortive attempts at forming

an alimentary canal; from the *ectoderm* there may be stratified epithelium with typical cell nests. It is easy to understand how the tumor may be mistaken for a chondroma, myxosarcoma, adenocarcinoma, epidermoid carcinoma, lymphosarcoma, etc. A usual appearance is a mixture of lymphoid tissue, cartilage, and tubular spaces, many of which are dilated to form cysts of varying size (Fig. 511).

Teratocarcinoma.—This is a new term introduced by Friedman and Moore. It comprises a group characterized by a mixture of elements such as teratoma, embryonal carcinoma, seminoma and chorionephithelioma. It therefore forms a convenient group in which to place lesions which the pathologist is unable to classify in any of the preceding categories. Perhaps for this reason it forms one of the largest of the groups.

Chorionepithelioma.—This rare tumor is a special development of a teratoma in which fetal membranes have been formed, the chorionic epithelium giving rise to the chorionepithelioma. Other structures are also formed, but these tend to be destroyed by the malignant growth. In one case which I studied, typical choroid plexus was present. The tumor usually remains small, and its structure may be obscured by hemorrhage so that it is easily overlooked. The primary tumor may be only a few millimeters in size, but large secondary growths are formed in the lungs, liver, etc. The microscopic appearance is varied. In the so-called classical picture (which is seldom seen) there are two types: (1) trophoblastic cells resembling the Langhans cells of the similar tumor in the female, and (2) multinucleated syncytial structures. The Aschheim-Zondek test is positive. Gynecomastia (female type of breast development) is common.

TESTICULAR ADENOCARCINOMA OF INFANCY.—Testicular tumors are rare in childhood, but this group occurring in infancy is rather well defined (Magner et al.). The tumor is white or pale yellow, and often honey-combed by small cystic spaces, with the cut surface bathed with clear sticky fluid. The characteristic microscopic picture is one of heavily vacuolated tumor cells arranged in loosely woven masses, irregular tubular spaces and small cystic cavities. The tumor does not resemble any of the testicular neoplasms of adults described above. The origin of these tumors has not been determined with any certainty.

Spread of Malignant Tumors.—The great danger of testicular tumors is their tendency to metastasize, not their local destructiveness. Although some seminomas may remain localized for years, over 50 per cent of patients with testicular tumors have metastases when first seen by the doctor. In 95 per cent of cases the adult teratoma behaves as a benign tumor and remains localized.

All malignant types of testicular tumors are characterized by early metastases in the lymph nodes. The first to be involved are the upper lumbar glands; these may be greatly enlarged, while the primary growth in the testicle is still quite small. The inguinal nodes are not involved until the tumor invades the skin of the scrotum. The tumor reaches the epigastric group, passes along the prevertebral chain to the mediastinum and along the thoracic duct to the left supraclavicular fossa. Above the level of the epigastric nodes metastases from both testes follow the same route. Blood spread to the lungs is particularly characteristic of chorionepithelioma, but it may also occur in other malignant testicular tumors.

Benign Tumors.—All benign tumors of the testis are very rare. The only two which will be discussed are interstitial cell tumors and tubular adenoma.

Interstitial Cell Tumor.—This is a rare tumor which is met with both in man and the lower animals. It tends to be light brown in color. The cells of which it is composed are arranged in solid masses supported by a minimal amount of delicate connective tissue. They are polygonal, intensely acidophilic, and may present a foamy vacuolated appearance owing to the presence of fat. When the tumors develop before puberty there is evidence of sexual precocity, but when they occur at a later period there may be impotence, gynecomastia, and a positive Aschheim-Zondek reaction due to excess of estrogen. They are of slow growth, and are either benign or of a low grade of malignancy. Similar tumors can be induced in mice by the administration of estrogen.

Tubular Adenoma.—This benign tumor occurs in the undescended testis. As it apparently arises from Sertoli cells it might well be called *Sertoli cell tumor*. The majority of the cases in the literature are examples of Sertoli cell hyperplasia rather than true tumors.

Testicular Tumors and Sex Hormones.—It may be difficult to differentiate the smooth painless swelling of a tumor of the testicle from other lesions in this region. In such a case we may look for assistance to tests for abnormal hormones in the urine. In this connection two hormones must be considered: (1) the follicle-stimulating hormone of the pituitary (prolan A), and (2) the chorionic gonadotropic hormone (prolan B), produced by chorionic tissue and present in the urine of pregnant women as shown by the Aschheim-Zondek and Friedman tests. The pituitary hormone appears in the urine after castration and is an indication of decreased androgen activity, due to destruction of the interstitial cells of the testes. It may therefore be present as the result of any malignant

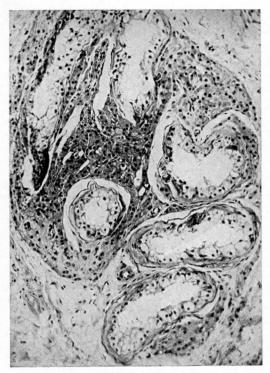

FIG. 512.—Hypertrophy of interstitial cells in undescended testicles. × 100.

some point in its descent. This may be in the neighborhood of the kidney, at the internal abdominal ring, in the inguinal canal, or at the external abdominal ring. The inguinal canal is much the commonest position. Here the testicle is exposed to trauma and therefore liable to attacks of orchitis. An undescended testicle is unusually prone to develop a malignant tumor. The gland is atrophic and the spermatogenic cells disappear, so that if the condition is bilateral the person is sterile. Virile power is retained, however, for the interstitial cells of Leydig do not share in the atrophy; indeed, they often appear to be more numerous than usual, and the best place to see these cells is in an undescended testicle (Fig. 512). Cryptorchism is now known to be due in some cases to lack of the gonadotropic hormone of the anterior pituitary which regulates the process. Administration of the hormone may be followed by descent of the testes. Curiously enough the gonadotropic hormone is present in the urine of these boys and disappears under treatment (Hess). It is known that when the testes have been removed (or are undescended) there is an excessive secretion of gonadotropic hormone.

testicular tumor. The chorionic gonadotropic hormone is naturally most abundant in chorionepithelioma, but it may occur in other tumors in which trophoblastic elements are present. On the whole the high expectations entertained for these hormonal tests as an aid in diagnosis and prognosis following treatment have not been fulfilled because of the inconstancy of the results and the number of false positives and negatives.

TORSION OF THE TESTIS

Torsion may occur either in the fully descended testicle or in the undescended testicle. The latter is the more frequent and the more severe. The usual exciting cause is some sudden muscular effort, but cases have been reported which have occurred during sleep. It is commonest in boys and young men.

UNDESCENDED TESTIS

Undescended testis or *cryptorchism* is a condition in which the testicle is arrested at

THE PROSTATE

GENERAL CONSIDERATIONS

The epithelial lining of the gland elements is tall columnar in type, and is much folded so that papillary processes may project into the lumen. This appearance must not be mistaken for evidence of hyperplasia or neoplasia. The stroma is a combination of fibrous tissue and plain muscle. Each gland element is surrounded normally by a sling of muscle. Venous thrombosis is frequent in the capsule in congestive failure, and forms a common source of emboli.

Effect of Age.—It has been said that it is possible to estimate the age of a man by the gross and microscopic examination of his prostate (Moore). By the end of the fourth decade changes can be detected. These may be divided into presenile and senile. In the *presenile* period, from the age of forty to sixty years, variations of the same nature can be detected in different parts. There is atrophy of the smooth muscle, relative increase of fibrous tissue which becomes more densely collagenous, while the papillae are less numerous and the epithelium lower. Individual acini may show hyperplastic papillae, but without involvement of the stroma in hyperplasia. There may be collections of lymphocytes in relation to the atrophic acini. The atrophy is irregular in distribution. In the *senile* period, over the age of sixty, most of the organ is diffusely involved in atrophy, and corpora amylacea, formed from retained and stagnating secretion, steadily increase in number. Similar changes are seen after castration.

Effect of Hormones.—The development and activity of the prostate are dependent on stimulation by testicular hormones. In the absence of testes the organ fails to develop. After castration it atrophies. The administration of estrogen leads to a change in the glandular epithelium from columnar to cuboidal type, squamous metaplasia may occur, and there is hypertrophy of the fibromuscular stroma. It is of interest to note that squamous metaplasia of epithelium is characteristically seen at the edge of an infarct, an area where the supply of androgen may be supposed to be greatly reduced. The posterior lobe of the prostate which lies behind the ejaculatory ducts, is purely male, while the middle and lateral lobes are ambisexual, being represented in both sexes. This difference is significant in relation to nodular hyperplasia.

Testicular Spermatogenic Cell Hypertrophy. —The spermatogenic cells of the tubules of the testis become hypertrophied as well as clear and hydropic as the result of excessive pituitary gonadotropic (follicle-stimulating hormone) or estrogenic stimulation, the latter coming in part at least from the adrenal cortex. This observation throws a suggestive side light on the pathology of the prostate, because it has been found that there are increased numbers of hypertrophied spermatogenic cells in 76 per cent of cases of prostatic hyperplasia, 63 per cent of cases of carcinoma, and only 23 per cent of normal prostates (Sommers). This suggests that estrogen secretion, probably partly of adrenal cortical origin following pituitary stimulation, is a significant factor in the

development both of prostatic hypertrophy and of cancer.

Phosphatase.—*Acid phosphatase* is an enzyme present only in the epithelial cells of the prostate of the sexually mature man and in prostatic carcinoma. It is called acid phosphatase because the activity of the enzyme is maximum at pH 5. Only a small amount is present in the serum because normally it enters the posterior urethra and the semen but not the blood. It owes its existence to the sustaining influence of the male sex hormone, and on that account has been called a chemical secondary sex characteristic (Nesbit and Baum). After castration the phosphatase promptly disappears from the epithelium and shrinkage of the gland occurs. *A sustained elevation of the level of acid phosphatase in the serum occurs only in metastatic carcinoma involving the bones or lymph nodes, and not in carcinoma confined to the prostate. It seems to be a question of absorption,* which is practically nil from the prostate but abundant from blood and lymph channels in the bone marrow and lymph nodes respectively.

Alkaline phosphatase is an enzyme produced by osteoblasts as an essential agent in the growth and repair of bone. Its maximum activity is at pH 9. Its level in the serum, in the absence of liver disease, reflects the degree of osteoblastic activity. Its elevation, therefore, is not pathognomonic of prostatic cancer, as is acid phosphatase, but is also present in metabolic bone disease and in disturbance of liver function. In known metastases from prostatic carcinoma the level of serum alkaline phosphatase is an indication of the osteoblastic reaction to the tumor, and a chemical index of the effectiveness of the treatment.

NODULAR HYPERPLASIA

This is the condition often called hypertrophy of the prostate, but nodular hyperplasia is a more accurate term suggested by Moore in his excellent review of the subject.

Enlargement of the prostate is very common in men over the age of sixty years, but only in a small number of cases (about 8 per cent) does it cause symptoms. It is essentially a disease of advancing years, and

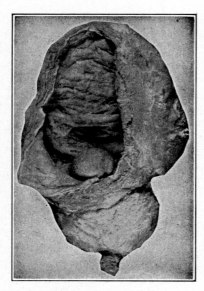

Fig. 513.—Hypertrophy of the prostate. The gland is considerably enlarged, and the middle lobe projects up into the bladder, the wall of which is hypertrophied.

is hardly ever seen in early life. The condition appears to be due to stimulation resulting from a disturbance in the ratio of androgens to estrogens which accompanies the decrease in testicular hormones that develops with advancing years. It is probably an expression of imbalance of the sex hormones in the male, analogous to cystic hyperplasia of the breast. When estrin is injected into castrated rats there is hyperplasia of epithelium, smooth muscle and connective tissue. These changes do not occur if testicular extract is injected at the same time, nor in normal rats which have not been castrated. This suggests that prostatic hyperplasia in elderly men is due to a disturbance in the balance between the production of testicular hormone and that of estrin (also produced by the testicle). It may be noted that the prostates of children at birth show similar changes, probably due to estrin from the placenta. The hope is that in the future it may be possible to control prostatic hypertrophy by means of hormone therapy. It is of interest to note that prostatic enlargement is common among domestic animals with the onset of old age. This is particularly well seen in the case of

the dog. Prostatic hyperplasia has a wide distribution throughout the animal kingdom.

Morbid Anatomy.—The condition of the prostate varies, depending on the proportion of glandular to fibrous tissue, so that it may be large and soft or relatively small and hard. Usually the enlargement is made up of a series of rather spongy nodules with clearly-defined margins; these nodules are clearly seen on the cut surface. Moore emphasizes the marked difference between the lobular architecture, both gross and microscopic, of the normal prostate and the nodular character of benign hyperplasia. The part of the gland containing the nodules enlarges so as to form a mass which compresses the surrounding tissue, and this in turn constitutes a false capsule which enables the nodular mass to be separated and shelled out with comparative ease. In other cases there is diffuse fibrosis rather than nodular hyperplasia, in which case no nodules can be seen and shelling out is impossible. The lateral lobes may be enlarged or a new *middle lobe* may be formed by hypertrophy of the group of glands which lies in the floor of the urethra. This middle lobe forms a conical mass which projects up from the floor of the bladder, carrying the urethral orifice with it (Fig. 513).

The *microscopic appearance* is one of glandular hyperplasia with overgrowth of fibrous tissue and muscle in varying degrees (Fig. 514). The picture may closely resemble that of lobular hyperplasia of the breast. The glandular tissue is increased, the acini are enlarged, and papillary processes of epithelium may project into the lumen. In other cases the glandular tissue is not hyperplastic, but there is a great increase of fibrous tissue and a good deal of plain muscle. Moore, whose studies of the structural variations of the normal prostate are so valuable, considers that the most striking feature of benign hyperplasia is the variation in appearance of the same structure in different parts of the prostate, compared with the uniform appearance of the normal prostate. As infection is a frequent complication, inflammatory foci may be scattered through the stoma.

Infarcts, either recent or healed, are frequently found. Although these are small

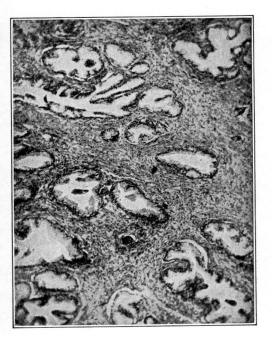

FIG. 514.—Hypertrophy of the prostate. There is marked epithelial proliferation in the acini and ducts. × 60.

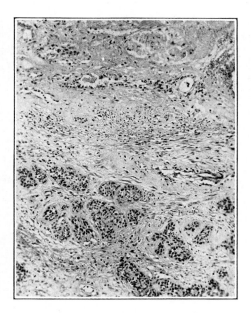

FIG. 515.—Infarct of prostate (above) with squamous metaplasia (below). × 110.

areas of coagulation necrosis similar to what is seen in infarcts elsewhere, there is no proof that they are due to vascular occlusion. At the margin of the healing infarcts can be seen solid masses of squamous epithelium (Fig. 515). This is a *squamous metaplasia* secondary to the necrosis, and must on no account be mistaken by the pathologist for epidermoid carcinoma, a tumor which is extremely rare in the prostate.

It may be noted in passing that the term prostatectomy to describe the operation for the removal of a hyperplastic (not a malignant) prostate is a misnomer, for the true prostate is left behind at operation. The hyperplastic nodules usually originate in the submucosal glands of the prostatic urethra. As the mass increases in size the normal prostatic tissue is compressed and displaced peripherally to form the so-called surgical capsule. At the usual operation it is this hyperplastic mass which is enucleated or resected, and the surgical capsule composed of the original normal prostatic tissue is left behind.

Effects.—Enlargement of the prostate is usually unaccompanied by symptoms. The symptoms when present are due entirely to the position of the gland at the urinary outlet. The effects are felt on the urethra, the bladder, and the kidneys. (1) The *prostatic urethra* may be elongated, compressed to a mere slit, and rendered tortuous. This is the most important cause of obstruction. (2) The *bladder* cannot be completely emptied, because the urinary outlet is lifted up above the surrounding floor and the enlarged middle lobe may exert a ball-valve action. Moreover the vesical sphincter is rendered incompetent through being stretched by the middle lobe which grows up from the floor of the urethra. There is therefore a constant dribbling of urine, and yet the bladder is never empty. The residual urine is readily infected and cystitis results. The bladder becomes hypertrophied in its efforts to overcome the obstruction, and the thick bands of muscle give the wall a ribbed appearance. Later there is dilatation, with pouching of the wall between the bands producing false diverticula. Owing to the cystitis and the stagnation of urine, phosphatic calculi are often formed in the bladder. (3) The *kidneys* suffer because of the obstruction and infection. The ureter and renal pelvis on both sides are dilated, so that hydronephrosis is produced. Infection ascends the dilated ureters, and causes pyelonephritis and pyonephrosis. Renal insufficiency now declares itself, non-protein nitrogen is retained in the blood, and the patient dies of uremia. The back-pressure of the kidney is associated with arterial hypertension, even though the kidney damage is only slight. When drainage of the bladder is established there is a marked fall in the systolic blood pressure within forty-eight hours.

Chapman sounds a word of warning which deserves repetition: "It is certainly unjustifiable to remove the prostate merely because it is enlarged and has been associated with some urinary symptoms. This fact should be made clear to the medical student. Prostatic enlargement should be regarded, like the arcus senilis of the cornea and the graying and thinning of the hair, as an anatomical feature of old age which occurs often enough to be regarded as a variety of the normal. Only when obstruction to the flow of urine is produced does it become a disease."

CARCINOMA

In 1900 Taylor, in a textbook devoted to genito-urinary diseases, makes the astonishing statement that "primary carcinoma and sarcoma of the prostate are extremely rare, but do occur." Now it is known to be one of the commonest forms of cancer in men, ranking third in frequency among the principal causes of death from cancer. It would serve no useful purpose to express this frequency in percentage figures because of the varied clinical manifestations of the lesion. The cancer may be (1) clinical, (2) occult and (3) latent. *Clinical carcinoma* manifests itself by producing symptoms of retention owing to invasion of the neck of the bladder. *Occult carcinoma* (hidden and active) causes no prostatic symptoms, but is recognized by the metastases to which it gives rise associated with an elevated serum acid phosphatase. *Latent carcinoma* (hidden and inactive) is detected at autopsy examination, and even then it is rarely recognized in the

gross. It is said to be present in a quarter of all persons over forty years of age (Moore). These latent tumors are small, slow-growing, and probably exist for many years without causing symptoms and with metastases. But they are real cancers, presenting a microscopic picture identical with that of metastasizing carcinomas, including invasion of perineural lymphatics. It would almost appear as if some hormonal stimulus were needed to release the trigger mechanism which causes the tumor to spring to activity. It should be pointed out that the figures quoted above are the result of examination of large numbers of blocks, because the minute lesions are so easily missed. The prostate happens to be of a convenient size for the thorough examination needed for the detection of latent cancer. It is possible that an unexpectedly large incidence might be found in other organs if they were submitted to a similar careful search.

Cancer of the prostate is often associated with nodular hyperplasia, but there is no proof that there is any etiological relationship between the two. The usual age incidence of cancer is about a decade beyond that of benign hyperplasia, although that, of course, is no argument against the existence of a relationship. Carcinoma arises in atrophic, not hypertrophic, areas, and in particular in a posterior lobe compressed by nodular hyperplasia. It is obvious that a prostatectomy, which leaves most of the posterior lobe intact, is no guarantee against the subsequent development of carcinoma in that lobe.

Morbid Anatomy.—The prostate may or may not be enlarged when the patient is first seen, but its chief characteristic is its hardness. It cuts with the gritty sensation of a scirrhous cancer of the breast. The cut surface is dry, does not bulge, is not nodular or lobulated, and shows little yellow islands of carcinoma cells like those seen in a scirrhous cancer of the breast. In all these respects it differs from nodular hyperplasia. At the same time it must be pointed out that in some cases the gross differentiation is impossible, and that microscopic examination of a number of blocks may be necessary before cancer can be excluded, as the malignant process may be confined to a

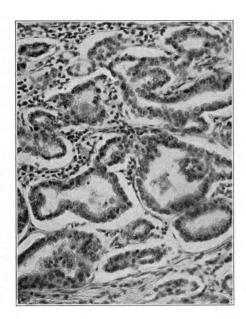

FIG. 516.—Carcinoma of the prostate. This glandular type may be mistaken in its early stages for simple hyperplasia. × 200.

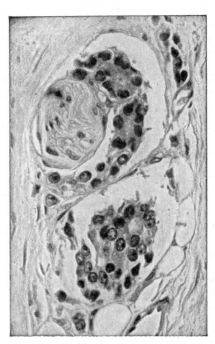

FIG. 517.—Perineural spread of carcinoma of prostate. × 400. Boyd, *Pathology for the Surgeon,* courtesy of W. B. Saunders Co.)

small part of the gland. Every prostate removed for hypertrophy should be cut up into a series of thin slices and examined for areas of malignancy indicated by increased hardness and lessened elasticity.

The *microscope picture* is adenocarcinoma of varying degree of differentiation. The acini may be so well formed that they are easily mistaken for normal acini (Fig. 516), but they lack the sling of muscle which surrounds each normal gland, so that nests of small acini seem to be invading the stroma which is frequently dense and scirrhous. The cells seldom show anaplasia, and mitotic figures are few or absent. The atypical pattern of the acini is more important than cellular abnormality.

Spread.—In the majority of cases when the patient is first seen by the doctor the condition has already become inoperable. This does not mean, however, that not a great deal can be done for the patient. The spread is both local and distant. The growth usually starts in the posterior part of the gland and spreads up along the line of ejaculatory ducts; it appears between the bladder and the seminal vesicles where it

can be felt on rectal examination. The floor of the bladder and the surrounding fibrous structures are invaded. An important method of spread is along the perineural lymphatics, which can often be seen distended with cancer cells. (Fig. 517). Perineural invasion of the capsule is one of the earliest changes, no matter how small the primary tumor may be. Bilateral sciatica in an elderly man is strongly suggestive of carcinoma of the prostate. The pelvic and lumbar lymph nodes are involved early, and there may be lymph spread to the thoracic and even the supraclavicular nodes. The inguinal nodes are involved in about 15 per cent of cases, probably due to lymphatic connection with the seminal vesicles and urethra and retrograde transport from these areas. It is evident that hardly a node in the body may escape.

Metastases are formed in the liver, lungs, etc., by systemic blood spread. But the commonest distant metastases are in the bones. In about 70 per cent of autopsies the skeleton is found to be involved. The pelvis and lumbar vertebrae are the commonest sites, followed by femur and ribs. These, of course, are the bones most readily examined at autopsy. Spread to the sacrum and lumbar vertebrae used to be thought to be by way of the perineural lymphatics, but, as Batson has pointed out, a far more frequent route is probably the vertebral system of veins. Some of the spread to bones is by the systemic circulation. When an elderly man is found to be suffering from a tumor of bone, the prostate should always be examined. Moreover the bone metastases in cancer of the prostate are different from those in other secondary carcinomas; the former are sclerosing in type, while the latter are rarefying, a distinction which can be readily recognized radiologically.

Phosphatase Activity.—The importance of the enzyme phosphatase in cancer of the prostate has already been indicated. *Acid phosphatase* can be demonstrated microscopically in the epithelium of both the normal and malignant gland by Gomori's method. There is, however, a striking difference in the histological pattern of acid phosphatase distribution in benign and malignant lesions (Mathes and Norman). In the normal gland and in benign nodular hyperplasia the pattern of enzyme activity is an arrangement of black material reproducing the glandular pattern of the prostate, whereas in carcinoma the pattern is completely lost in the area of malignant change. As the histological differentiation of benign and malignant disease of the prostate can be very difficult, especially in quick diagnosis on fresh frozen section, the value of this technique in selected cases is apparent.

The work of Huggins and his associates has shown that when the level of serum acid phosphatase exceeds 10 King-Armstrong units per 100 cc. disseminated prostatic cancer is present. But a patient with extensive metastases sometimes has normal phosphatase levels, while, on the other hand, one with no evident metastases may have a high level. Normal levels in the presence of metastases may be due to failure of the anaplastic tumor cells to produce phosphatase, while levels above normal in the apparent absence of metastases may be due to failure of bone changes which are recognizable on

the x-ray film to develop. On the other hand there may be no increase in the enzyme.

The level of the serum *alkaline phosphatase* is usually raised when skeletal metastases have occurred. This is an indication of osteoblastic activity, not of activity of prostatic epithelium. This agrees with the well known fact that the skeletal metastases are osteosclerotic rather than osteolytic in character.

Fibrinolysis in Cancer of Prostate.—Another enzyme activity of some importance in prostatic cancer is fibrinolysis. Widespread metastatic carcinoma of the prostate may be associated with hemorrhage from mucous surfaces such as the nose. This in turn is associated with increased fibrinolytic activity as shown by a blood test, deficiency of fibrinogen in the blood and a prolonged prothrombin time (Tagnon *et al.*). The normal prostate contains a proteolytic enzyme capable of digesting fibrinogen, and this activity is evidently increased in metastatic cancer.

Sex Hormones and Prostatic Carcinoma. —The development and activity of the prostate is dependent on stimuli from the testes. Castration before puberty prevents development of the prostate, and castration in adult life causes regression of the normal gland and decrease in size in cases of prostatic hypertrophy. Huggins and his associates have applied these facts to the problem of the control of cancer of the prostate with remarkable results. Orchidectomy is followed not only by an astonishing improvement in the subjective condition (bone pain, etc.), but also by such objective evidence as a great and permanent fall in the acid phosphatase in the blood and a shrinkage of the primary lesion. Injection of large amounts of estrogen has a similar effect on the acid phosphatase and to a lesser extent on the physical condition, owing apparently to neutralization of androgens which have an opposite effect. The estrogen has a marked effect on the cancer cells, which are either vacuolated due to accumulation of glycogen or may be actually necrotic.

Finally, there appears to be a relationship between the pituitary-adrenal axis and cancer of the prostate. Bilateral adrenalectomy in selected cases has resulted in remarkable improvement, particularly in relief of the distressing and intractable back pain.

Sarcoma.—Sarcoma of the prostate is very rare. It is probable that most of the tumors which in the past have been called sarcoma are examples of anaplastic, undifferentiated carcinomas.

Prostatic Calculi.—Prostatic calculi may form in the ducts of the gland. They are usually minute and give rise to no symptoms.

INFLAMMATION

Prostatitis may be acute or chronic. Both forms are usually due to gonococcal infection. The *acute* form is part of an acute posterior urethritis. It is usually mild in type, but some abscesses may be formed, and occasionally there is extensive suppuration. In *chronic* prostatitis foci of chronic inflammatory cells are scattered through the gland, with varying degrees of fibrosis. The prostate is hard, and may be larger or smaller than normal, depending on the amount of scarring which has taken place. In these chronic cases there is often a mixed infection with Bacillus coli, staphylococci, etc.

Granulomatous Prostatitis.—This uncommon condition, first described by Tanner and McDonald in 1943, is of importance because of the ease with which it is mistaken clinically for carcinoma and in other cases for nodular hyperplasia. Even on microscopic examination it may be confused with carcinoma and tuberculosis.

The prostate is always firm and may be stoney hard. Nodular hyperplasia is a constant accompaniment. *Microscopically* the acini and ducts are destroyed and replaced by an abundant exudate which varies in type. The principal cells are lymphocytes, but plasma cells and mononuclears may be abundant, and in some cases there have been great collections of eosinophils (Thompson and Albers). The ducts may contain polymorphonuclear leukocytes. Foreign body giant cells may be numerous, and pseudotubercles may form apparently around the ducts.

The nature of the condition is unknown, but the tuberculoid lesions recall in some respects those of plasma cell mastitis and chronic thyroiditis. In both of the latter

conditions it is believed that the chronic inflammation may represent a reaction to secretion which has escaped from the acini into the stroma, milk in the case of the breast, colloid in the case of the thyroid. Obstruction to the ducts might lead to a similar result in the case of the prostate.

PENIS AND SCROTUM

CARCINOMA

Cancer of the penis begins on the glans or prepuce. The tumor shows a striking geographical distribution, being rare in the America and Europe, but common among the Chinese, Malays, African Negroes, and in India. The disease is unknown in persons such as Jews who have been circumcised in infancy. It is rare in Mohammedans who are circumcised later (three to fourteen years). Circumcision in adolescence or adult life offers little protection, as the damage has apparently been done. In over 70 per cent of cases phimosis is or has been present, with retention of smegma which probably acts as a carcinogen. The lesion takes the form of a small wart at first, but a large fungating mass is formed later. The tumor is an epidermoid carcinoma. Secondary growths occur in the inguinal and later in the retroperitoneal lymph nodes. Blood spread is later still. *Cancer of the scrotum* used to occur in chimney sweeps and still does in workers handling coal tar and paraffin, owing to the long-continued action of these carcinogenic substances.

HYDROCELE

A hydrocele is a collection of fluid in the tunica vaginalis. It may be acute or chronic in type. The *acute* cases are due to spread of infection usually from the epididymis, occasionally from the body of the testicle, to the tunica vaginalis. The two infections commonly associated with acute hydrocele are gonorrhea and tuberculosis. The fluid, which is moderate in amount and somewhat turbid owing to the presence of pus cells, accumulates rapidly. The *chronic* variety is probably due to some low-grade infection, but this is not susceptible of proof. The fluid is clear and watery, rich in albumin,

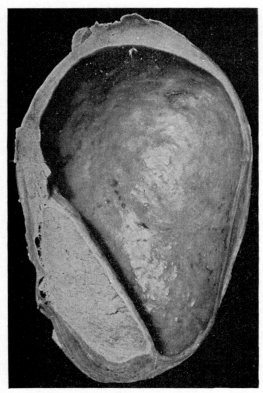

FIG. 518.—Large chronic hydrocele with thick-walled sac. The testicle shows the effects of compression. (Boyd, *Pathology for the Surgeon*, courtesy of W. B. Saunders Co.)

and may be so abundant as to cause great distention of the scrotum. It may contain shimmering cholesterol crystals, and in some cases fibrinous bodies may separate out. The sac tends to become greatly thickened, especially if there has been repeated tapping. In long-standing cases the pressure on the testicle may lead to atrophy. (Fig. 518).

Encysted hydrocele of the spermatic cord is a collection of fluid in an unobliterated portion of the processus vaginalis between the testicle and the internal abdominal ring. It does not communicate with the tunica vaginalis.

Hematocele.—Hematocele is the name given to a hemorrhage into a hydrocele. The hemorrhage is usually due to trauma of some kind. This may be a direct blow or kick, or it may be the result of tapping the hydrocele. In the latter case there is either injury to a vein by the needle, or the sudden reduction of pressure outside an unsupported vessel

may cause it to give way. Sometimes the hemorrhage may occur spontaneously. The cavity of the tunica vaginalis is occupied by breaking-down blood clot, and the walls are covered by ragged deposits of fibrin.

SPERMATOCELE

A spermatocele is a cystic dilatation of the spermatic ducts of the epididymis. The cyst is single or multilocular, and is situated at the upper end of the testicle. The fluid, which contains hardly any albumin, is of a peculiar milkiness owing to the presence of great numbers of spermatozoa.

VARICOCELE

This is a varicosity of the pampiniform plexus of veins in the spermatic cord. There is a primary and a secondary form. The *secondary* form is due to pressure on the spermatic vein, usually by a tumor of the kidney because of its proximity to the termination of that vein. It therefore is commoner over middle age. The *primary* form is very much more frequent. It is called primary because the cause is unknown. It is common in young unmarried men, and may be related to the congestion caused by unrelieved sexual stimulation. It is nearly always on the left side, so that a varicocele on the right side should suggest the presence of a tumor. The left spermatic vein enters the renal vein at right angles; the right spermatic vein enters the vena cava obliquely. There is therefore more resistance to the outflow of blood from the left vein. A loaded rectum may also press on the left vein. The veins of the plexus are elongated, tortuous, and feel like a bag of worms. They empty when the patient lies down. Thrombosis is rare.

CONGENITAL ANOMALIES

Undescended testis or *cryptorchism*, a condition in which the testis is arrested at some point in its descent so that the scrotum remains empty, has already been described on page 886. *Epispadias* is incomplete closure of the urethra on the dorsal aspect of the penis. *Hypospadias*, which is more common, is the same condition on the ventral aspect. *Hermaphroditism* is a blending of the male and female sexual organs. In very rare cases testicles and ovaries have been present together. The usual arrangement is for the gonads of one sex to be associated with the secondary sexual characters of the other. The commonest form is that in which the scrotum is split so as to resemble the labia majora, the penis is rudimentary, the testicles are undescended, and the secondary sex characters are of the female type.

MISCELLANEOUS LESIONS

PHIMOSIS.—Phimosis or narrowing of the prepuce is a congenital condition. In the more severe cases there may be marked urinary obstruction with hypertrophy of the bladder, dilatation of the ureters and hydronephrosis. The relation to carcinoma has already been mentioned.

CALCAREOUS DEPOSITS.—Calcareous deposits in the penis may occur in old people. They correspond to formations of bone in the lower animals.

SYPHILIS.—The primary chancre of the penis has already been described on page 301. A primary chancre sometimes occurs in the scrotum, but secondary lesions (condylomata) are much more frequent. The scrotum may be involved in a gumma of the testicle.

REFERENCES

BARR, M. L.: Science, 1959, *130*, 679. (Sex chromatin and sex anomalies.)

BARR, M. L. and BERTRAM, E. G.: Nature, 1949, *163*, 676. (Sex chromatin in nerve cells.)

BARR, M. L. and CARR, D. H.: Can. Med. Ass. J., 1960, *83*, 979. (Sex chromatin, sex chromosomes and sex anomalies).

CHAPMAN, T. L.: Lancet, 1949, *2*, 684. (Prostatic hypertrophy.)

EDWARDS, J. H. *et al.*: Lancet, 1960, *1*, 787. (Trisomic syndromes.)

FERGUSON-SMITH, M. A.: Lancet, 1959, *1*, 219. (Prepubertal testicular lesions in mentally handicapped children.)

FERGUSON-SMITH, M. A. *et al.*: Lancet, 1957, *2*, 167. (Testicular morphology in Klinefelter's syndrome.)

FORD, C. E.: Proc. Roy. Soc. Med., 1960, *53*, 491. (Technique of chromosome examination.)

FORD, C. E. *et al.*: Lancet, 1959, *1*, 709. (Mongolism and Klinefelter's syndrome.)

FRIEDMAN, N. B. and MOORE, R. A.: Mil. Surgeon, 1946, *99*, 573. (Tumors of testis.)

GALL, E. A.: Am. J. Path., 1947, *23*, 637. (Mumps orchitis.)

GLASSY, F. J. and MOSTOFI, F. K.: Am. J. Clin. Path., 1956, *26*, 1303. (Spermatic granulomas of epididymis.)

GRUMBACH, M. M. and BARR, M. L.: *Recent Progress in Hormone Research*, 1958, *14*, 255.

HUGGINS, C., STEVENS, R. E. JR. and HODGES, C. V.: Arch. Surg., 1941, *43*, 209. (Hormones and cancer of prostate.)

LENNOX, B.: Scot. Med. J., 1956, *1*, 97. (Nuclear sexing and its clinical applications.)

MAGNER, D., CAMPBELL, J. S. and WIGLESWORTH, F. W.: Cancer, 1956, *9*, 165. (Testicular adenocarcinoma in infancy.)

MATHES, G. L. and NORMAN, T. D.: Lab. Invest., 1956, *5*, 276. (Acid phosphatase pattern in benign and malignant lesions of prostate.)

MOORE, K. L.: Lancet, 1959, *1*, 217. (Sex reversal in newborn babies.)

MOORE, R. A.: J. Urol., 1935, *33*, 224. (Latent carcinoma of prostate.)

————: Am. J. Path., 1936, *12*, 599. (Evolution and involution of prostate.)

MYERS, L. M.: J. Path. & Bact., 1959, *78*, 29. (Sex chromatin in tumors.)

NESBIT, R. M. and BAUNN, W. C.: J.A.M.A., 1951, *145*, 1321. (Serum phosphatase and the prostate.)

SOMMERS, S. C.: Am. J. Path., 1956, *32*, 185. (Spermatogenic cell hypertrophy in prostatic hyperplasia and carcinoma.)

TAGNON, H. J. *et al.*: Cancer, 1953, *6*, 63. (Fibrinolysis in prostatic cancer.)

TANNER, F. H. and McDONALD, J. R.: Arch. Path., 1943, *36*, 358. (Granulomatous prostatitis.)

THOMPSON, G. J. and ALBERS, D. D.: J. Urol., 1953, *69*, 530. (Granulomatous prostatitis.)

Chapter 33

The Female Reproductive System

THE UTERUS
General Considerations
MENSTRUATION
   Ovarian Influence
   Pituitary Influence
   Placental Influence
   Endometrial Changes
Endometrial Hyperplasia and
Uterine Hemorrhage
Endometriosis
ENDOMETRIAL STROMATOSIS
Endometritis
PUERPERAL ENDOMETRITIS
PELVIC CELLULITIS (PARA-
   METRITIS)
ENDOCERVICITIS: "CERVICAL
   EROSION"
Syphilis
Tumors
LEIOMYOMA
   Cervical Fibroids
   Degenerations
ADENOMYOSIS
CARCINOMA OF CERVIX
   Carcinoma in Situ
   Exfoliative Cytology
CARCINOMA OF BODY
SARCOMA
   Endometrial Sarcoma
   Embryonal Tumors (Sarcoma
   Botryoides)
Pathology of the Placenta
HYDATIDIFORM MOLE
CHORIOEPITHELIOMA

TOXEMIAS OF PREGNANCY
RETAINED PLACENTA
UTERO-PLACENTAL APOPLEXY
PLACENTAL INFARCTS
ERYTHROBLASTOSIS FETALIS
SYPHILIS
TUBERCULOSIS

THE FALLOPIAN TUBES
Salpingitis
GONORRHEAL
TUBERCULOUS
Tubal Pregnancy
Cysts
Carcinoma

THE OVARY
General Considerations
STRUCTURE
HORMONE PRODUCTION
Inflammation
Ovarian Cysts
NON-NEOPLASTIC CYSTS
   Follicular Cysts
   Lutein Cysts: Corpus luteum,
   theca-lutein, hematoma
   Stein-Leventhal Syndrome
   Endometrial Cysts
Tumors of the Ovary
MUCINOUS CYSTADENOMA
SEROUS CYSTADENOMA
   Origin of Ovarian Cysts
PRIMARY SOLID CARCINOMA

   Secondary Carcinoma
    (*Krukenberg*)
DERMOID CYST
   Solid Ovarian Teratomas
   Fibroma
   Meigs' Syndrome
   Sarcoma
Special Ovarian Tumors
FEMINIZING TUMORS
   Granulosa Cell Tumor
    Theca Cell and Lutein Cell
    Tumor
MASCULINIZING TUMORS
   Arrhenoblastoma
   Hilus Cell Tumor
   Adrenal-like Tumor
   (Stein-Leventhal Syndrome)
DYSGERMINOMA
BRENNER TUMOR
Parovarian Cyst

THE VAGINA AND VULVA
Soft Chancre
Syphilis
Condyloma Acuminatum
Trichomonas Vaginalis Infection
Leukoplakia and Kraurosis
Tumors
Urethral Caruncle

CONGENITAL ANOMALIES
OF FEMALE GENTIAL TRACT
Uterus
Ovaries

THE UTERUS

GENERAL CONSIDERATIONS

WE have already seen in the previous chapter that during the first six weeks of development there is no apparent differentiation between the male and the female genital tracts. At first the gonad arising from the urogenital ridge is indifferent, consisting of an outer cortex and an inner medulla. The ovary develops from the medulla or the testis from the cortex. From there on, development proceeds smoothly in the vast majority of cases, but in the exceptional case, as we have also seen, something may go wrong, and there may be an intermingling of sexes.

Menstruation.—The basis for the study of gynecological pathology is an understanding of the changes which the endometrium undergoes during the menstrual cycle. Throughout the entire menstrual cycle of twenty-eight days the endometrium is responding to influences from the ovaries, so that the uterus may be said to be the mirror which reflects ovarian activity. If that activity becomes perverted, the changes in the endometrium will cross the boundary line between the physiological and the pathological.

Ovarian Influence.—The endometrium is continually played on by influences from the ovary, and the ovary is acted on in turn by the pituitary. The ovary produces two hormones, *estrogen* which is formed by the Graafian follicle, and *progesterone* which is formed by the corpus luteum. In the human subject ovulation occurs at the middle of the menstrual cycle, on the thirteenth or fourteenth day from the beginning of the last period. Immediately after ovulation the corpus luteum begins to be formed from the stratum granulosum of the ruptured follicle. As soon as the corpus luteum degenerates and becomes functionally impotent, which happens from twenty-four to thirty-six hours before menstruation, estrogen, the follicular principle, which has been present all the time though suppressed, reasserts itself and continues to do so until the development of the next corpus luteum. It is this resumption of follicular activity which is probably the direct cause of menstruation. If the ovum continues to live on account of being fertilized, the corpus luteum will persist and grow larger, and the amenorrhea (absence of menstruation) of pregnancy is established.

Pituitary Influence.—Just as the endometrium is under the influence of the ovary, so the ovary is under the influence of the anterior lobe of the pituitary. The periodicity of the ovary is not inherent in itself, but is dependent on the anterior pituitary which regulates it. Implants or extracts of the anterior lobe of the pituitary in an immature female animal rapidly bring on a state of maturity or premature puberty. As a result of rapid maturation of the follicles, estrogen is formed and this brings on all the phenomena of estrus. No changes are observed if the ovaries are first removed, for a castrated animal does not respond to anterior pituitary stimulation. The pituitary produces a follicle-stimulating hormone (F.S.H.) and a luteinizing hormone (L.H.). The former is related functionally to estrogen and the latter to progesterone.

Endometrial Changes.—The female sexual cycle can be divided into two phases: (1) an *estrogen* or *proliferative phase* from the close of menstruation to ovulation (from about the fifth to the twelfth day), and (2) a *progesterone* or *secretory phase* from ovulation to about twenty-four hours before the onset of menstruation. We shall find that these two phases are accurately reflected in the ovarian mirror—the endometrium (Figs. 519 and 520). In the proliferative phase there is repair of the tissues destroyed during menstruation; in the secretory phase the endo-

metrium is prepared for an approaching pregnancy (decidual reaction, pseudopregnancy), *i.e.* the implantation of a fertilized ovum. If the ovum remains unfertilized, all sign of these preparations is removed in the destructive and hemorrhagic process of menstruation.

The *proliferative phase* of the menstrual cycle is of about one week's duration, extending from the end of menstruation to ovulation. It provides the histological picture of what used to be considered the normal endometrium. During this period the endometrium is being acted on by the estrogen of the ripening follicle. It grows steadily in thickness, the low epithelium of the postmenstrual stage beomes tall and columnar, mitotic figures are numerous both in the glandular epithelium and the stroma, there may be a pseudostratification of the columnar epithelium which may be several layers thick in some of the glands, and the glands become more and more tortuous, particularly in the deeper part of the endometrium giving it a spongy appearance.

The *secretory* or *progesterone phase* begins after ovulation and formation of the corpus luteum, but the changes are only well developed about five days before menstruation. Soon after ovulation basic secretory vacuoles appear in the lining columnar epithelial cells, pushing the nuclei toward the lumen. A week later the mucinous vacuoles shift from the base of the cells toward the lumen, so that the nuclei are now at the base. This is the stage of glandular activity and secretion (not reproduction) and of decidual reaction. The secretory activity of the glands becomes more and more marked, the epithelium, which is at first distended with mucin, changes from high to low columnar and appears to melt into the mucin which passes into the lumen of the gland. As a result of this activity the glands develop a characteristic spirally twisted or corkscrew appearance, and in consequence buds project into the lumen like the teeth of a saw, giving a false suggestion of papillary formation (Fig. 520). It is this highly glandular but perfectly normal appearance which in the past was responsible for the very common diagnosis of "glandular endometritis." By this time the endometrium is divided into a superficial

57

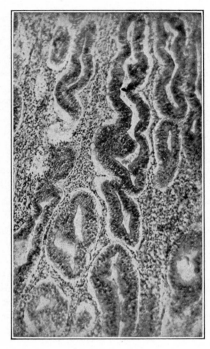

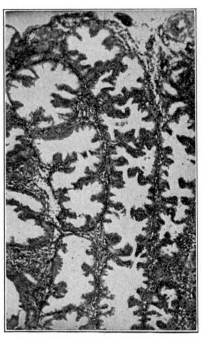

FIG. 519.—Estrogen phase.   FIG. 520.—Progesterone phase. × 45.

FIGS. 519 AND 520.—Endometrial phases.

compact layer and a deep spongy layer full of spiral glands. The stroma cells of the compact layer undergo the second change that is characteristic of the premenstrual or corpus luteum phase, the oval cells becoming enlarged, rounded, and epithelioid in type, and closely resembling the decidual cells of pregnancy. It is indeed a *decidual reaction*, for if pregnancy supervenes it is these cells which form the decidua of pregnancy. For this reason it is never safe in medico-legal work to make a diagnosis of pregnancy merely because decidual cells have been found in uterine scrapings. The decidual reaction has been called a pseudopregnancy. A day or two before menstruation the superficial layer is infiltrated with leukocytes. Widespread necrosis of the tissue on the surface now takes place, the compact layer is cast off, the walls of the capillaries are destroyed, and menstrual bleeding is the result. This necrosis and expulsion of tissue may be regarded as an expulsion or abortion of the pseudopregnancy. If impregnation has occurred and a

fertilized ovum reaches the uterus, menstruation does not occur, the decidua-like layer is retained, and developed into the decidua of pregnancy.

It is evident that these endometrial changes are the combined result of the follicular hormone and the lutein hormone. If ovulation fails to occur and no corpus luteum is formed, only the first set of changes will take place. We shall see that this is of profound importance, and that it is one of the principal causes of idiopathic uterine hemorrhage.

Brief reference must be made to changes in the *cervix* during the menstrual cycle. The cervical secretion is thick and impermeable to spermatozoa, but during the proliferative phase it becomes thin and serous allowing entrance of the sperms at the time of ovulation. Endocervicitis interferes with this adaptive mechanism and thus predisposes to sterility.

The *vagina* also is under the influence of estrogen stimulation. There is rapid proliferation and thickening of the lining epithelium, the cells of which become arranged in layers of three distinct types: basal, intermediate and superficial squamous. Recognition of these cells in vaginal Papanicolaou smears serves as a useful indicator of estrogenic functional activity.

When we come to the study of ovarian tumors we shall find that some of these are functioning tumors, producing estrogens, progesterone or even androgens, with corresponding clinical effects.

ENDOMETRIAL HYPERPLASIA AND UTERINE HEMORRHAGE

Just before or during the menopause a woman may begin to suffer from irregular uterine hemorrhage, which may take the form either of profuse periodic bleeding or of prolonged and continuous bleeding. This irregular hemorrhage may occur at earlier age periods, and sometimes in young women. When the uterus is curetted the endometrium is found to be thick; sometimes it forms papillary excrescences on the surface, and microscopically it presents a markedly glandular appearance. It is now known that the condition is due to ovarian dysfunction (pathological persistence of a ripening follicle), that there is no primary lesion in the uterus, and that the hemorrhage is really functional.

Menstruation is not necessarily dependent on ovulation. In the absence of ovulation there are no cyclic changes in the endometrium, no formation of a pseudopregnancy, but bleeding occurs just the same. This is known as *anovulatory menstruation*. In the condition under discussion the ovary shows two abnormalities. In addition to being somewhat atrophic, there is an entire absence of lutein tissue, but it does contain one or more ripening follicles. Apparently something prevents ovulation from occurring, and as no corpus luteum is formed the premenstrual changes in the endometrium do not occur. There is a continued overproduction of estrogen by the persistent ripening follicle, and the endometrium shows the effect of this overstimulation by manifesting in pathological form the first or hyperplastic phase of the menstrual cycle. It is the absence of the

normal secretory "topping-off" caused by progestin which is responsible for the type of endometrium seen in functional hemorrhage. Injection of estrogen into animals produces similar changes in the endometrium.

The *endometrium* is markedly thickened, and may measure 15 mm. Sometimes it shows polypoidal protrusions on the surface. *Microscopically* the endometrium presents a highly glandular appearance. The arrangement of the glands is disorderly as compared with the normal vertical extension from base to surface, they are increased in number, there is great variation in size and shape, and the epithelium may be several layers thick (pseudostratification). Some degree of *adenomyosis* is often present, *i.e.*, an invasion of the muscular wall by the glands of the endometrium; this is a minor form of true adenomyoma, which itself is a manifestation of endometriosis. Cystic dilatation of the glands in the deeper layers is common, so as to give what has come to be known as a "Swiss cheese appearance," and the condition has been called *Swiss cheese hyperplasia* (Fig. 521). The stroma cells show numerous mitoses, there is extremely marked vascular congestion and a good deal of edema. Decidual reaction is completely absent. If bleeding is going on when the curettage is done, two additional changes will be observed: (1) necrosis of the superficial layers and thrombosis of the small vessels; (2) extensive infiltration with polymorphonuclear leukocytes and mononuclears, but no plasma cells. The necrosis is patchy, not diffuse as in true menstruation. The two most characteristic features of the microscopic picture are the cystic glands and the patchy necrosis of the surface. The hemorrhage is due chiefly to the local necrosis, but the cause of the necrosis is uncertain. It may be due to cessation of corpus luteum influence as in normal menstruation, or more probably to overstimulation which may lead to thrombosis. From the physiological viewpoint it may be called "*hyperestrinism*," or from the morphological viewpoint "*cystic glandular hyperplasia of the endometrium*." Its great importance lies in the fact that it is the chief cause of functional uterine hemorrhage. The *ovaries* commonly present many small follicular cysts and a complete absence of lutein

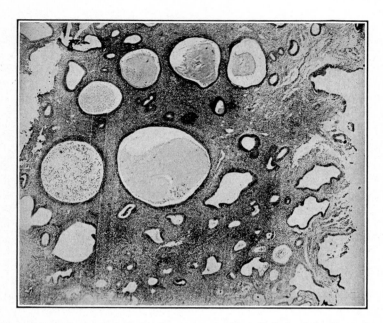

Fig. 521.—"Swiss cheese hyperplasia" of endometrium with marked glandular formation.   × 18.

tissue, this being the morphological basis of the hyperestrinism.

Corpus luteum overactivity is the converse of the condition just described. The endometrium shows excessive lutein phase changes, even a few days after the middle of the menstrual cycle, and the condition may resemble that of early pregnancy. In these cases the ovaries contain large corpora lutea or excess of lutein tissue.

ENDOMETRIOSIS

This conveniently noncommittal term is used to denote a condition characterized by the formation of endometrium-like masses in a variety of places in the female pelvis and abdominal cavity. As the masses may resemble tumors they are known as endometriomata. The origin of these lesions is a matter of dispute.

It was Sampson of Albany who in 1921 was the first to direct attention to that manifestation of endometriosis which he called endometrial implants. The occurrence of so-called chocolate-colored cysts of the ovary had long been recognized, and lesions of similar structure were found in the rectovaginal septum and other parts of the pelvis. Sampson suggested that these lesions were due to implantation of living endometrial cells on the surface of the ovary, peritoneum, etc. These cells were supposed to be cast into the cavity of the uterus during menstruation, pass along the tubes, and finally settle and grow at the site of the future lesion. The "implant" consists of gland-like spaces surrounded by columnar epithelium, and separated by the cellular stroma characteristic of the endometrium. Hemorrhage occurs at each menstrual period, so that the lesion contains either fresh blood or blood pigment. When the ovarian cyst ruptures the contents are scattered throughout the pelvis together with more desquamated endometrial cells which set up secondary endometrial implants.

Sampson's views have met both with support and opposition, the latter especially in Germany, where R. Mayer's theory of the serosal origin of the supposed implants is the popular one. The serosal theory, with which the writer is in agreement, is based on the fact that the entire epithelial apparatus of the female genital tract (endometrium, germinal epithelium of the surface of the ovary,

PLATE XII

FIG. 1

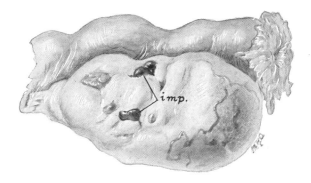

Endometriosis (Chocolate-colored Cysts) on Surface of Ovary.

(John A. Sampson, Surg., Gynec. and Obst., March, 1924.)

FIG. 2

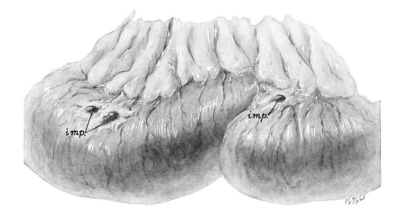

Endometriosis of Terminal Loop of Ileum.

(John A. Sampson, Surg., Gynec. and Obst., March, 1924.)

etc.) is derived originally from the primitive peritoneum which forms the epithelial lining of the celomic cavity. As the result of ovarian hormonal stimulus the serosa is believed to revert to its original function and form epithelium-lined cavities. Every pathologist is familiar with the fact that as the result of some stimulus such as chronic irritation the flattened serosal cells in either sex may become cuboidal, invade the underlying tissue, and surround gland-like spaces.

The question of ectopic decidual reaction is of interest in this connection (Weller). A nodular decidual reaction in the subserosa of the appendix is common during pregnancy. Similar lesions are found on the ovary, tube, broad ligament, rectal wall, etc., *i.e.*, a similar distribution to endometriosis. On the appendix the nodules are often mistaken by the surgeon for tubercles. It is evident that under appropriate hormonal stimulation decidual elements may develop from the connective tissue cells which lie under the serosal cells in the pelvis and lower abdomen. The mesothelial cells of the surface, especially when entrapped in adhesions, appear to form the epithelial elements of endometriosis. Excessive estrogen stimulation of the mesothelial and connective tissue is probably responsible for at least many cases of endometriosis, just as it is probably responsible for fibroadenoma of the breast, adenomyoma of the uterus, and possibly uterine fibroids. It may be noted that in all these conditions sterility and uterine hemorrhage are commonly associated features.

The older view that the chocolate-colored blood cysts of the ovary are follicular in origin has been revived by King. It has long been known that some cysts derived from the Graafian follicles, and especially from atretic follicles, may be lined by epithelium which cannot be distinguished from that of the endometrium. This is only natural, as the epithelium of both organs has a common developmental origin. Rupture of a chocolate-colored cyst may be followed by implants on the peritoneum. It is important to realize that the idea of normal adult tissues becoming implanted in other organs and growing there so as to produce irritation is quite without precedent in the science of pathology. Finally it must be recalled that

transplantation is not necessary to account for the presence of a tissue at a distance from the normal site of that tissue. Metaplasia will give the same result. It is possible that some of the lesions may be endometrial in origin, some serosal, and some ovarian.

The occurrence of the lesions is confined to the active reproductive period of the patient's life. Removal of the ovaries may be followed by atrophy and disappearance of the lesions. They are said occasionally to undergo malignant change, and Sampson believes that some of the malignant cystadenomas of the ovary arise in this way.

The majority of women suffering from endometriosis are sterile. The condition will regress spontaneously if pregnancy supervenes, so that it has been said that the best treatment is pregnancy, but it is evident that there are difficulties in the way.

The *lesions* are most often seen in the *ovary*, where they form one variety of ovarian hematoma, and are commonly known as *chocolate-colored cysts* (Plate XII, Fig. 1). The cysts, which are close to the surface, are quite small, are lined by columnar epithelium, and separated from one another by the highly cellular stroma so characteristic of the endometrium, in which are embedded many small glands like those of the uterus. There is no plain muscle in the ovary, but in the other lesions this is commonly present. The contents are hemorrhagic, and the blood is renewed at each menstrual period. Rupture of the cysts and liberation of the blood may be followed by the formation of peculiarly dense adhesions which in the past have been naturally thought to be inflammatory in nature.

Similar lesions may occur in the *rectovaginal septum*. The dense and hard adhesions may be mistaken for a malignant growth in this region. *Endometriomata* may occur in the Fallopian tubes, the broad and round ligaments, the appendix, the wall of the intestine (Plate XII, Fig. 2), the umbilicus, the groin and in abdominal scars after operations on the uterus. Blood may be discharged from an umbilical endometrioma at the menstrual period. Endometrioma of the groin is particularly puzzling. Here the mechanism cannot be that of endometrial implantation. Sampson has shown that endometrial tissue may be found within lymphatics and venous sinuses, and suggests that the cellular masses may spread in the same way as carcinoma, *i.e.*, by the lymph and blood stream as well as by the natural passages (tubes). An inguinal endometrioma may therefore be due to lymph spread. Or it may arise from the remains of an embryological peritoneal process in the inguinal canal, the processus vaginalis (serosal origin).

Endometrial Stromatosis.—In endometriosis the dominant element is epithelium. Occasionally the stromal cells of the endometrium assume invasive qualities under the influence, apparently, of hormonal stimulation. Under normal conditions root-like strands of these cells penetrate for a short distance into the muscularis. As the result of abnormal stimulation this invasion may become almost sarcomatoid in its character and form a tumor-like lesion. The stromal cell is in a constant state of flux during the sex life of the individual, and it has a high potentiality for differentiation, so that the mass may resemble a sarcoma (soft) or fibroma (hard) in both gross and microscopic appearance. Undoubtedly in the past this condition has frequently been diagnosed pathologically as sarcoma. A unique feature presented by some of these tumors is the presence on the cut surface of hundreds of *worm-like masses occupying the lymphatics* and occasionally the veins. In one case with which I am familiar the patient is alive and well four years after removal of the uterus, although long strings composed of masses of interstitial endometrial cells could be pulled out of the vessels of the uterine wall.

ENDOMETRITIS

Acute inflammation of the endometrium may affect the pregnant or non-pregnant uterus. The latter is relatively unimportant. It is commonly caused by the gonococcus, but gonorrhea is chiefly a disease of the cervix, and the infection may pass from there to the tubes producing very little change in the body of the uterus. In acute fevers there may occasionally be an acute endometritis (blood infection), and when the cervical canal is closed by carcinoma the body of the uterus may be distended with

pus, a condition of pyometra. Of far greater importance is puerperal endometritis, or acute inflammation of the pregnant uterus during the puerperium.

Puerperal Endometritis.—Puerperal sepsis used to be the greatest threat to the woman in childbirth. Now this river of death has shrunk to a mere trickle as the result of a combination of aseptic technique and antibiotic therapy. The invading organisms were aerobic hemolytic streptococci from the nose and throat of the attendants and the patient or anaerobic streptococci present in the vaginal canal of 40 per cent of women at birth.

The uterus is soft, flabby and enlarged because normal involution is prevented. The cavity is lined by dirty, breaking-down, necrotic material, under which there is a protective zone of leukocytes. When the infection is mild this zone is wide, and discharge of the infected material is followed by recovery, for blood invasion has not occurred. In the severe streptococcal infections, the leukocytic zone is thin, and the organisms are seen spreading into the deeper parts of the uterine wall. They may reach the serous coat and set up peritonitis, they may pass along the Fallopian tubes and flood the general peritoneal cavity, or they may spread throughout the body by the blood stream. The large venous sinuses are filled with septic thrombi, which break down and pass into the circulation as septic emboli, setting up pyemic abscesses in the lungs.

Pelvic Cellulitis (Parametritis).—This is a term commonly used by gynecologists. Cellulitis signifies an inflammation of connective tissue due to a wound infection. Pelvic cellulitis may result from infection of lacerations of cervix and vagina occurring during parturition or abortion, or from surgical operations on the cervix. It frequently occurs in conjunction with carcinoma of the cervix. Infection reaches the pelvic cellular tissue either by lymphatics or direct continuity of tissue. The common infecting organism is the streptococcus. Infection spreads in the retroperitoneal fascial planes and there may be abscess formation. While the condition may be a long drawn out one, resolution is usually complete and no impairment of reproductive function results.

Endocervicitis: "Cervical Erosion."—The endometrium of the body of the uterus does not provide a favorable nidus for chronic infection on account of its simple glandular structure and the fact that in large measure it is renewed every month. The reverse is true of the cervix. Here the complex racemose glands may harbor infecting microörganisms for long periods. Chronic inflammation of the cervix is accordingly the commonest of all gynecological lesions. By far the commonest cause is laceration of the cervix at childbirth, followed by pyogenic infection. The usual infecting organisms are staphylococci, streptococci, and E. coli. Gonorrheal infection of the cervix is the second common cause, but it is of minor importance compared with the first. The gonococcus may infect a laceration, or it may cause infection in a nullipara, as the gonococcus can readily penetrate intact columnar epithelium. The following description applies to the cases which follow laceration.

The infecting bacteria gain entrance to the racemose glands which arise from the columnar epithelium of the cervical canal and penetrate the depths of the muscle. These glands are not seen in the vaginal portion of the cervix which is covered by stratified squamous epithelium. The glands are irritated as the result of the infection, and pour out the thick, viscous, mucopurulent secretion which is characteristic of leukorrhea. It may be said that leukorrhea is almost always a sign of cervicitis. The stroma of the endometrium shows edema and an infiltration with lymphocytes and plasma cells, the latter being the most characteristic cells of chronic inflammation in the female genital tract. In time the inflammation extends to the fibromuscular layer, so that the condition becomes a true cervicitis and not merely an endocervicitis. The columnar epithelium of the surface is curiously resistant and is not desquamated.

Owing to the constant irritation of the infected leukorrheal discharge or for some other reasons at present unknown, a patch of squamous epithelium at the external os undergoes maceration and becomes separated, leaving a raw surface which partially or completely surrounds the os. The raw surface is quickly covered by an outgrowth of the columnar epithelium of the cervical canal. The covered patch remains red, however, for the underlying vascular tissue shines through the thin layer of epithelium. This is the condition which has been known in the past as *"cervical erosion,"* a mere clinical nickname for the raspberry red appearance of what used to be thought was a true granulating ulcerated surface. If the cervix has been badly lacerated the os may become everted and patulous. The new epithelium appears to be stimulated by the constant irritation, and give rise to new racemose glands in the portio vaginalis. In course of time the inflammation dies down, and as a sign of healing the squamous epithelium once more replaces the columnar type over the disputed patch, either by growing under it from the edge or by a conversion of the columnar into the squamous stratified type. The new epithelium tends to close the mouths of the ducts of the new glands, and these may undergo cystic dilatations so as to form the bluish swellings on the portio vaginalis known as *Nabothian follicles* (Fig. 522). In some cases the squamous epithelium may grow down into the ducts, forming epithelial plugs which may be mistaken for commencing carcinoma. In the deeper parts of the cervix there is fibrosis and scarring, so that the cervix becomes hard, and owing to contraction of the scar tissue there may be marked eversion of the os.

SYPHILIS

The cervix is the only part of the uterus affected by syphilis. The lesion may be primary, secondary or tertiary. The primary lesion is a *chancre*, which can only be diagnosed with certainty by finding the Treponema pallidum with the dark-field method. Many cervical chancres have been diagnosed clinically as carcinoma. The secondary lesion is a *mucous patch*. The tertiary lesion is a *gumma*, which may also be mistaken clinically for carcinoma, but can easily be distinguished from it in microscopic sections. All of these conditions are uncommon.

TUMORS OF THE UTERUS

Leiomyoma.—The tumor known as myoma, fibromyoma and fibroid tumor of the

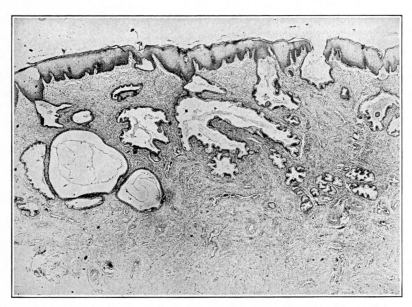

Fig. 522.—Endocervicitis with marked glandular proliferation and Nabothian follicles.   × 16.

uterus is the commonest of all neoplasms. It is even more frequent in colored than in white women. Although not strictly accurate the condition is commonly called a *fibroid*. The tumors are confined to the reproductive period of life. This suggests that they may bear some relation to ovarian activity. The ovaries are often enlarged, and contain cysts and large unruptured follicles. In the breast the common fibroadenoma, which is often more of a fibroma, is most probably due to abnormal ovarian stimulation. The same may be true of the fibromyomas of the uterus. They never appear after the menopause, and usually tend to retrogress in that period. When estrogenic hormone is introduced under the skin of a guinea pig in tablet form, uterine fibromyomata are produced; these cease to grow and retrogress when the hormone ceases to act. The tumors occur chiefly in the body of the uterus. Cervical tumors are relatively uncommon.

Morbid Anatomy.—In its *gross appearance* the fibroid tumor varies considerably. There may be a single tumor or large numbers: they may be very small or very large, and their consistence may be much changed by degeneration. As a rule, the tumor is hard, circumscribed, and the cut surface presents a whorled appearance, due to interlacing bundles being cut in different planes. The more fibrous tissue it contains, the harder and whiter it is, contrasting with the relatively soft and brownish-red surrounding muscle (Fig. 523). As it grows expansively it compresses the muscle and thus forms for itself a capsule from which it can often be shelled out. According to its site the tumor is divided into interstitial, submucous, and subperitoneal varieties. The *interstitial* is the common form, for every leiomyoma commences in the substance of the muscle. It is well supplied with blood from the surrounding muscle, so that degeneration is not very common in this form. The *submucous* fibroid is formed by the centripetal growth of an interstitial tumor. It projects into the uterine cavity, and, owing to the uterine contractions it may become more and more polypoid, until finally it may appear in the vagina. Even when quite small it may cause marked uterine hemorrhage owing to the irritation of the endometrium which it produces. The overlying endometrium may be remarkably thickened. A large tumor may distend the uterine cavity, giving an appearance which may so closely simulate

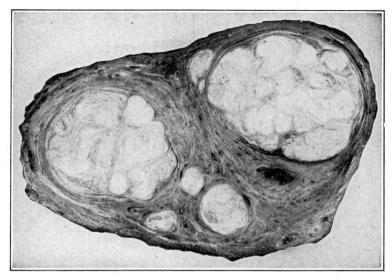

Fig. 523.—Leiomyomata of uterus. The white color is due to the large amount of fibrous tissue.

pregnancy that a correct diagnosis may be impossible even when the abdomen has been opened. In rare cases the cavity of the uterus may be covered with small tumors. The *subperitoneal* fibroid is centrifugal in growth, so that it becomes subserous and may be pedunculated. *Twisting of the pedicle* may interfere with the blood supply, so that degenerations are most common in this form. In rare cases the tumor may become adherent to the omentum and derive its chief blood from that source (parasitic fibroid). The subperitoneal tumors are usually multiple and may attain an enormous size. It is common to find two or all three varieties present in the same uterus.

The *microscopic appearance* is a mixture of plain muscle and fibrous tissue in varying proportions. The muscle fibers run in interlacing bundles, some of which are cut longitudinally, some transversely (Fig. 524). The small tumors consist mostly of muscle, but as they grow in size the proportion of fibrous tissue becomes greater, and tumors of long standing may be almost entirely fibrous. The nuclei of the muscle fibers are short, plump, and fusiform, while those of the fibroblasts are longer, slender and curved.

Cervical Fibroids.—Fibroid tumors of the cervix, *i.e.*, tumors originating in the cervix, are not common, although fibroids of the body may invade the cervix. A true cervical fibroid is single. As it grows in size the uterus becomes perched on the summit of the tumor, and if the patient becomes pregnant normal delivery is impossible.

Degenerations.—The blood supply of a fibroid is easily interfered with, so that degenerations are common. The subperitoneal form is nourished solely through its pedicle, and it is in this variety that degeneration is most frequent. *Atrophy* may occur after the menopause, due probably to loss of the ovarian stimulus, and a similar result may follow removal of the ovaries. *Hyaline degeneration* is the commonest change, and is due to an insufficient blood supply. The fibrous tissue becomes hyaline, and the muscle fibers tend to disappear. *Cystic degeneration* may follow the hyaline change. The hyaline material becomes liquefied, and cyst-like spaces are formed, but they have no epithelial lining. *Fatty degeneration* is seen in old fibroids. The cut surface is yellow and homogeneous, and the muscle fibers contain fat droplets which can be demonstrated by means of the special stains for fat. *Calcification* may be a sequel to fatty degeneration, and is seen in the subserous fibroids of elderly women. The entire tumor may become converted into a mass of stone, which forms a striking feature in the roent-

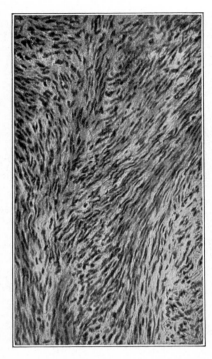

Fig. 524.—Leiomyoma of uterus. The fibers run in interlacing bundles. × 225.

gen-ray picture, but gives rise to no special symptoms. *Red degeneration* is a peculiar change which is commonly regarded as being much commoner in pregnancy. This has not been the case in my own experience. In 38 examples of this condition operated on at the Toronto General Hospital over a period of eight years, 11 (29 per cent) were associated with pregnancy whilst 27 (71 per cent) bore no such relationship. The change is marked by sudden pain and tenderness in the tumor. The latter becomes quite soft and of a bright red color like that of raw beef. The red color is due to a collection of blood in the tissue which becomes hemolyzed and causes diffuse staining of the entire tumor. The condition is probably the result of thrombosis of the veins, so that it may be regarded as a red infarct. The venous obstruction may be attributed to pressure, contractions of the uterus, or torsion of the tumor. The change is commonest in the interstitial variety. *Sarcomatous degeneration* of a myoma is discussed in connnection with Sarcoma of the Uterus.

Adenomyosis.—In this condition there is an intermingling of glandular and muscular elements. It is not a true tumor, so that the term adenomyoma, formerly applied to it, is a misnomer. Areas of decidua have been found in the lesion shortly after labor, and even in cases of tubal pregnancy. Although the lesion is sometimes spoken of as a variety of endometriosis, it will be apparent that the relation of the two conditions is merely casual and in no way intimate. Adenomyosis consists of and is derived from endometrium, but in endometriosis the new tissue is more probably of serosal origin.

The *gross appearance* is usually characteristic. The lesion may be limited to the anterior or posterior wall or may form a mantle just outside the mucosa. Although the uterus may be enlarged to two or three times its normal size, and the affected part may be markedly thickened, the normal outline of the organ is usually retained. When the uterus is opened the diagnosis can often be made from the gross appearance. The anterior or posterior wall is diffusely thickened, with a complete absence of the sharp demarcation so characteristic of the ordinary fibroid. The thickened portion of muscle is coarsely striated, and homogeneous translucent areas resembling mucous membrane may be scattered through it. These areas often present a brownish discoloration due to the presence of extravasated menstrual blood. Small cystic spaces filled with chocolate-colored contents may be scattered throughout these mucosal areas. The line of demarcation between the lesion and the normal mucous membrane is always sharp; it extends to, but never into, the endometrium.

Microscopically, the growth is made up of fibromyomatous tissue, only differing from that of an ordinary fibroid in that it is not encapsulated, together with glandular structures. The latter resemble the normal endometrium, although not so regular in appearance (Fig. 525). "The uterine mucosa is often of normal thickness and looks perfectly normal, but as we approach the underlying diffuse myomatous tissue the mucosa is seen to penetrate it in all directions, sometimes as an individual gland, but often large areas of mucosa are seen extending into the depth. In favorable sections one can follow a prolongation of the mucosa half way through the uterus" (Cullen).

Carcinoma of the Cervix.—Cancer of the uterus is one of the commonest forms of cancer in women, and carcinoma of the cervix is 3 or 4 times commoner than carcinoma of the body of the uterus (endometrial carcinoma) and much more fatal. Unfortunately the disease commences in a very insidious fashion, and is often well advanced before a correct diagnosis is made, in spite of the fact that we are dealing with a neoplasm arising from superficial tissue. Small wonder, then, that great stress is laid at the present time on early diagnosis.

Etiology.—Two etiological factors are worthy of consideration. I used to be taught that laceration of the cervix was all-important, because over 90 per cent of the cases occur in women who have born children, and the fecundity of these patients is above the average. But carcinoma of the cervix can develop in women who have been delivered by cesarean section, and in whom there can be no question of cervical laceration. In one case with which I am familiar carcinoma developed ten years after delivery by section. It is much more probable that *hormonal stimulation* is the connecting link between fecundity and cancer of the cervix. The prolonged administration of estrogen produces cancer of the cervix in the mouse, an animal in which this form of cancer is unknown as a spontaneous disease (Gardner *et al.*). The highest incidence of female genital cancer occurs at or after the menopause when ovulation has stopped. There is therefore no progesterone from the corpus luteum, but the output of estrogen may continue, especially if the ovaries are cystic. It is evident that hormonal imbalance is a possible or probable factor.

A second factor may be *smegma*, which is believed to act as a carcinogen in cancer of the penis. The rate of cancer of the cervix is only one-quarter as high in Jewish as in non-Jewish white women both in Israel and in New York City (Casper). The incidence is also much lower in Moslems, a group in which circumcision is practiced. It may be noted that the rate for negro women in New York is more than 11 times and for Puerto Rican women in New York 23 times that

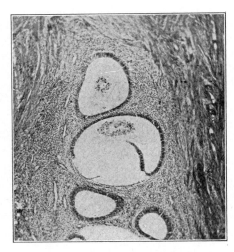

Fig. 525.—Adenomyosis of the uterus. Deep in the wall of the uterus there are dilated endometrial glands surrounded by the cellular stroma of the endometrium.

for Jewish women in New York and Israel. A puzzling feature is the incidence of the disease among the Indian population of Canada. The incidence of cancer among Canadian Indians is less than among the white population, but the incidence of cancer of the cervix is much greater, and it tends to occur earlier in life (Warwick and Phillips).

Morbid Anatomy.—The *gross appearance* may take a papillary form or an infiltrating form. (1) The *papillary variety* forms a large fungating mass, projecting into the cavity of the vagina, and appearing to arise from the lip of the external os. There is little tendency to invasion of the deeper tissues, and as hemorrhage, especially after coitus, is an early symptom, diagnosis may be made fairly early, so that the prognosis is less unfavorable. (2) The *infiltrating variety* (Fig. 526), which is the common one, may give little sign of a tumor on the surface, but extends deeply in the direction of the internal os, causing enlargement and hardening of the cervix, but unaccompanied by symptoms for a considerable time. In the course of time there is extensive necrosis and sloughing, with destruction of the cervix and the formation of a ragged, badly infected cavity (Fig. 527). Sometimes the cervical canal becomes blocked by the tumor, so that drainage from

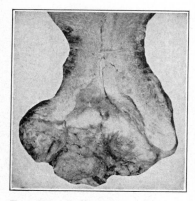

FIG. 526.—Infiltrating carcinoma of
the cervix uteri.

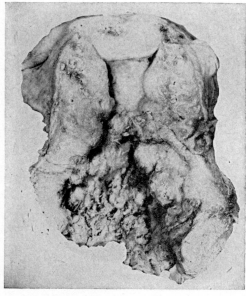

FIG. 527.—Carcinoma of cervix. The cervix is
converted into a ragged fungating mass.

the uterine cavity is impossible and pus
accumulates, often under very high pressure,
a condition known as pyometria. A similar
state of affairs may be produced by fibrosis
and cicatricial contraction of the canal
caused by treatment (often cure) of the
tumor by radium. When the cervix is
painted with Lugol's solution the normal
epithelium is colored a deep brown by the
iodine (glycogen reaction), while diseased
epithelium and cancer is unstained. This is
used as a guide for the site of biopsy in early

cancer (Schiller test), but unfortunately cervical erosion also remains unstained.

The *stage of the disease* is of obvious importance in statistical reports of the results
of treatment. The International Classification now generally adopted is as follows:

Stage O.—Carcinoma in situ.

Stage I.—Carcinoma confined to the cervix.

Stage II.—Carcinoma extending beyond
the cervix but not reaching the pelvic wall.

Stage III.—Carcinoma which has reached
the pelvic wall and the lower third of the
vagina.

Stage IV.—Carcinoma involving the bladder or rectum (widespread metastases).

The *microscopic appearance* has caused
most of the difficulties of classification. Two
types of epithelium are found in the cervix.
The vaginal portion (portio vaginalis or
simply portio) is covered by stratified squamous epithelium of the epidermal type, while
the cervical canal is lined by a single layer
of columnar epithelium. Corresponding to
these two types of epithelium we find two
types of tumor, a *common epidermoid carcinoma*, and a *rarer adenocarcinoma* which
forms less than 4 per cent of the total. But
it is not safe to conclude that the former must
arise from the portio and the latter from the
cervical canal, for squamous epithelium may
extend into the canal, and the racemose
glands of the portio may be the starting point
of an adenocarcinoma. It seems probable
that in the majority of cases the tumor originates at the external os which has been the
seat of a cervical erosion with change from a
squamous to a columnar type of epithelium
and reversion again to a squamous type with
gradual development of an epidermoid carcinoma (Fig. 528). Columns of cells grow
down into the deeper tissues, usually showing
numerous mitotic figures.

Gynecologists have made minute subdivisions according to the type of cell (spinous,
transitional, spindle, etc.) in the hope that
the radiosensitivity of the tumors might be
determined, seeing that radiation therapy
plays such an important part in the treatment of the condition. It seems better to
speak merely of the degree of differentiation
which the tumor exhibits. The cases of
epidermoid carcinoma may be divided into

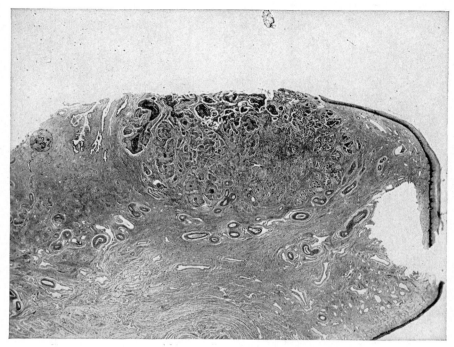

Fig. 528.—Very early carcinoma of the cervix showing origin at external os. × 8.
(Kindness of Dr. A. T. Hertig, A.F.I.P. acc. No. 520594.)

three groups according to their degree of radiosensitivity. Group 1 (20 per cent) is the *adult type*, made up of highly differentiated cells with a tendency to cornification and the formation of pearls. It is radioresistant. Group 2 (60 per cent) is the *plexiform type* in which the cells have lost most of their squamous character, show a plexiform arrangement, a tendency to infiltration, and a moderate degree of anaplasia (Fig. 529). The tumor is more radiosensitive. Group 3 (20 per cent) is the *anaplastic type* in which the cells have lost all squamous characters, are completely undifferentiated and diffusely invasive. They are highly radiosensitive. When the results of radiation therapy are analyzed the curious position is revealed that the best results (permanent cure) are obtained with the most malignant tumors, *i.e.*, those of Group 3. The reverse is the case when the growths are removed surgically. In about 5 per cent of cervical cancers the tumor is an *adenocarcinoma* arising from the cervical canal. The microscopic appearance is often deceiving,

for the lesion may look benign but behave in a malignant manner. On the whole, these tumors are more malignant than the epidermoid carcinomas. A peculiar feature is the occasional occurrence of adenocarcinoma in children.

Effects of Radiation.—The therapeutic application of radium produces both gross and microscopic changes in carcinoma of the cervix. The *gross changes* may be divided into the following 5 stages (Farrar). (1) Hyperemia within one week; (2) slough formation three weeks later; (3) separation of the slough at the end of the second month; (4) contraction of newly formed fibrous tissue at the end of the third month; (5) final sclerotic contraction at the end of the fourth month.

The *microscopic changes* consist in degenerative changes in the cytoplasm and nuclei of the cancer cells. The cytoplasm becomes vacuolated and the nuclei pyknotic and bizarre looking. Finally the radiated cells disappear. In the stroma there is a marked infiltration with chronic inflammatory cells,

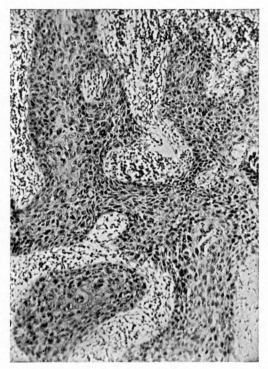

FIG. 529.—Carcinoma of cervix. The plexiform arrangement of the epidermoid cell is well shown. × 115.

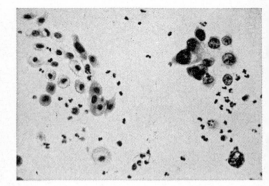

FIG. 530.—Group at right typical, unradiated, undifferentiated, malignant cells. Group at left shows pyknosis of basal cells. (Graham, courtesy of Surg. Gynec. and Obst.)

endarteritic occlusion of the vessels, and progressive scarring.

The *prognosis* of cases treated with radiation can be estimated by means of vaginal smears, this estimate being fairly accurate in 75 per cent of cases (Graham). Malignant cells disappear during treatment, but the epithelial cells of the vaginal smear show such radiation effects as vacuolization of the cytoplasm, increase in the size of both nucleus and cytoplasm, and various nuclear degenerations (Fig. 530). The percentage of cells showing these changes is an index of the degree of the radiation effect, which varies considerably in different people.

Carcinoma in Situ.—This condition is also known as intraepithelial carcinoma and pre-invasive carcinoma. The *entire thickness* of the squamous epithelium is replaced by cells identical in appearance with those seen in an invasive carcinoma, but the basement membrane is intact (Fig. 531). The *histological diagnosis* may be self-evident to the trained eye or it may be extremely difficult. The

picture is one of cellular unrest, and it is liable to cause similar unrest in the mind of the pathologist. The features which he has to weigh, as elsewhere in the body, are: (1) hyperchromatism of the nuclei; (2) variations in size and shape of nuclei; (3) abnormal mitoses, and (4) alteration in the polarity of the basal cells (cellular unrest). The last of these is the most important. These changes may extend down into the cervical glands. This must not be mistaken for malignancy. It may be noted that immediately deep to the carcinoma in situ there is often a heavy infiltration of plasma cells and lymphocytes. These are not due to infection, because in an invading and ulcerated lesion they are often absent. It is more likely that they represent some immunity defense mechanism against metabolites passing from the cancer cells into the underlying tissue. Another illustration of carcinoma in situ will be found on page 206.

Theoretically there are three *possible terminations* for such a lesion: (1) it may become invasive; (2) it may remain non-invasive for an indefinite period, and (3) it may possibly undergo regression, although this is by no means certain. It is impossible for the pathologist looking down the microscope to predict which course of the three the lesion will take. Nor is it possible to give statistics indicating the percentage of cases which will become invasive. So much depends on the connotation of the word invasion. One extreme is represented by the presence of

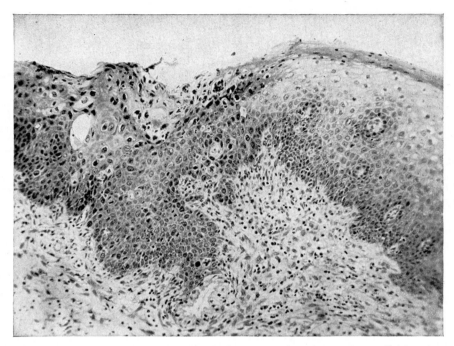

Fig. 531.—Carcinoma in situ. Junctional zone between preinvasive carcinoma (left) and normal cell epithelium (right). × 110. (Boyd, *Pathology for the Surgeon*, courtesy of W. B. Saunders Co.)

clumps of tumor cells in the lymphatics under the epithelium, the other extreme by a mere transgression of the basement membrane. The figures relating to invasion will differ widely (and wildly) depending on which criterion is adopted. In 419 cases of intraepithelial carcinoma of the cervix at the Vancouver General Hospital, 6 per cent were found to have microscopic foci of invasion, as distinguished from occult frank invasion (Fidler and Boyes).

Two facts *may* or *may not* be significant in this connection. (1) The average age at which carcinoma in situ is detected is about ten years earlier than that at which invasive carcinoma makes its appearance. (2) The preinvasive lesions are much more frequent than is the incidence of invasive carcinoma. This suggests that the terms preinvasive carcinoma and carcinoma in situ are not quite synonymous. The former implies that invasion may be expected to occur eventually, whereas the latter is non-committal. One undoubted fact must be emphasized. An increasing number of cases are being reported in which the preinvasive variety has been followed in the course of some years by the true invasive form.

Pregnancy is a complicating factor. A picture of *basal cell hyperplasia* strongly suggestive of carcinoma in situ may develop in the later months of pregnancy. Sometimes the two conditions are indistinguishable. The change is most marked between the twentieth and thirty-second week, it tends to regress as full term approaches, and it disappears a few weeks after delivery when the hormonal stimulus is withdrawn. A similar picture may develop as the result of the irritation of trichomonas infection.

Exfoliative Cytology.—Cancer cells are less cohesive than those of normal epithelium. They are thus liable to be exfoliated and desquamated. This is true both of preinvasive and invasive carcinoma. The examination of the cells of a vaginal smear, first suggested by Papanicolaou in 1928, has become a standard procedure which is fortunately of particular value in early cases. When necrosis and infection of the fungating

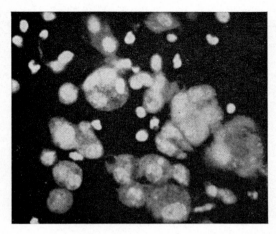

Fig. 532.—Smear from patient with carcinoma in situ of cervix, showing marked pleomorphism of cells. Fluorescence microscopy. × 280. In the original slide the cells were flaming red-orange in color. (Bertalanffy *et al.*, courtesy of Cancer.)

surface has occurred the desquamated cells naturally lose their characteristic features, but by that time the test has become unnecessary. Indeed the principal value of the method may be the detection of carcinoma in situ. The *cytological features* looked for are: (1) great variety in form and size of the cells; (2) atypical structure of their nuclei; and (3) vacuolization of the cytoplasm. *Fluorescent microscopy* may prove to be a more rapid method of identifying malignant cells in vaginal smears, and one not requiring the services of a highly trained observer. With the fluorescent dye acridine orange malignant cells show an intense red-orange fluorescence, whereas other cells fluoresce green to orange. The method is based on the differentiation of the two nucleic acids of the cell, DNA and RNA, by acridine orange. The DNA in the nucleus gives green fluorescence, but the RNA in the cytoplasm and nucleolus fluoresces in reddish to brilliant orange colors. (Bertalanffy *et al.*). Proliferating malignant cells have a high content of cytoplasmic RNA, which is readily seen under low magnification (Fig. 532). It must be strongly emphasized that a positive smear must be followed in every case by a biopsy, conization of the cervix offering the best opportunity of a thorough search for an early lesion. Finally, the changes which develop in the cervical epithelium during

pregnancy may be reflected in the vaginal smear, with the production of cells indistinguishable from those of carcinoma.

Spread.—The malignancy of cancer of the cervix is due to its invasive character, and we have already seen that this invasion may be most insidious, so that the disease may be far advanced before it is recognized. Spread may occur by permeation, by the lymph vessels, or by the blood stream. *Permeation* may carry the tumor cells outward to the parametrium, forward to the bladder, backward to the rectum, and downward to the vagina. It is very seldom that the tumor spreads so as to invade the body of the uterus, although the entire cervix may be involved. Obstruction of the ureters is common, causing an ascending infection which may prove fatal. *Lymphatic spread* leads to involvement of the iliac, hypogastric and sacral groups of lymph nodes. The tumor generally metastasizes late; only about 50 per cent of autopsy cases show gross metastases, and in radical hysterectomies lymph node involvement averages about 30 per cent. *Blood spread* is not common and is only found in advanced cases, in accordance with the rule that epidermoid carcinoma does not tend to invade the blood vessels.

Carcinoma of the Body.—Cancer of the body of the uterus (endometrial carcinoma) is much less common than cancer of the cervix, being outnumbered as 3 or 4 to 1. It occurs later in life, usually after the menopause, so that irregular bleeding is more likely to cause alarm. It is much less infiltrative than cervical carcinoma. For these reasons the prognosis is more favorable. Childbearing is not an etiological factor, for it is even more common in nulliparæ than multiparæ.

Morbid Anatomy.—The tumor usually begins in the endometrium of the fundus and spreads superficially so that a large surface may be involved (Fig. 533). It assumes the papillary rather than the infiltrating form, and may constitute a mass which occupies the greater part of the uterine cavity, and causes a moderate degree of enlargement of the organ. Involvement of the cervix is very rare. Invasion of the muscular wall occurs in time, so that care must be exercised in performing a diagnostic curettage to avoid

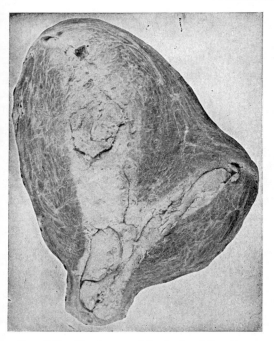

FIG. 533.—Carcinoma of the body of the uterus. The uterus is bicornuate, and the carcinoma fills the cavity of both horns.

carcinoma may be epidermoid in type. In rare cases the tumor may take the form of *adeno-acanthoma*, *i.e.*, a combination of glandular and epidermoid carcinoma.

Spread.—Spread takes place through the muscular wall, with eventual perforation. Fragments of tumor may be carried through the Fallopian tubes and infect the ovaries, so that the ovaries must always be removed together with the uterus. Lymph spread to the paravertebral glands and blood spread to lungs and liver occur in the later stages.

Sarcoma.—Sarcoma of the uterus is an uncommon tumor. It usually occurs as a *malignant change in a myoma*, so that it may be called a *myosarcoma* or malignant myoma. Occasionally it may arise from the normal uterine wall. The *gross appearance* is characteristic, for the whorled or striated appearance of the fibroid is lost, the cut surface is homogeneous and brain-like, and the tumor is soft and may be of a yellowish color. Cyst formation and hemorrhage are frequent. *Microscopically* the tumor is composed of large fusiform cells, in many of which the nuclei are remarkably large and may show numerous mitoses. It is almost impossible to be certain if these cells are derived from plain muscle or from fibroblasts.

Endometrial Sarcoma.—This neoplasm is usually circumscribed but may be diffuse. It originates in the fundus, and often forms a polypoid bulky mass in which necrosis may occur as well as cystic areas of hemorrhage. Microscopically it consists of a mixture of fusiform and large spherical cells. The degree of mitosis parallels the clinical malignancy of the tumor. Invasion of the uterine muscle occurs, and spreads to peritoneum, regional lymph nodes and distant organs.

Embryonal Tumors (Carcinosarcoma, Sarcoma Botryoides).—These are very rare tumors containing a variety of tissue of mesodermal origin, of which striated muscle is the chief. The general structure is sarcomatous and they are usually called sarcomas or rhabdomyomas. The best-defined variety is the so-called *grape-like sarcoma* or *sarcoma botryoides* (*botrys*, a cluster of grapes), of the cervix or vagina, which usually occurs in young children, and projects into the vagina in polypoid masses that may become so edematous as to resemble a bunch of grapes

perforating the uterus, but there is never the early involvement of the parametrium which is so characteristic of cancer of the cervix. Curettage gives definite chunks of cancer tissue; if the scrapings are scanty, soft and pink, they are almost certain not to be malignant.

Microscopically, the picture is usually that of a typical adenocarcinoma with irregular malignant tubules invading the underlying muscle. Sometimes the structure is more anaplastic with little glandular formation. Diagnosis from fragments of scrapings is not always easy unless some muscle is included, for the new-formed glands may resemble those of endometrial hyperplasia. Attention must be paid to irregularity of staining, mitosis and evidence of invasion. Generally speaking the cytological rather than the histological features are those which count. When the pathologist is in doubt, it is generally not cancer. Histological grading of biopsy material is singularly disappointing and of little prognostic value, as different blocks may show widely varying pictures (Cosbie and Henderson). Occasionally the

58

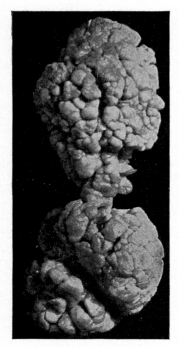

FIG. 534.—Sarcoma botryoides of cervix. This specimen was removed from a child one year of age. (Boyd, *Pathology for the Surgeon*, courtesy of W. B. Saunders Co.)

(Fig. 534). Most of the cells are round or fusiform, but striated muscle is usually present. Epithelial and glandular structures similar to those occurring normally in the female genital tract may be intermingled with the mesodermal structures. The tumor is very malignant, spreads both locally and by the blood stream, and kills the patient within a year.

PATHOLOGY OF THE PLACENTA

Hydatidiform Mole.—The word mole means mass. A hydatidiform mole is a not uncommon condition (1 in 2500 or 3000 cases) in which the placenta is converted into a mass of grape-like bodies resembling hydatid cysts (Fig. 535). The cysts, which may be as small as a pin's head or as large as a grape, represent *a cystic degeneration of the connective tissue of the chorionic villi*. Hydatidiform mole has been an enigma since the days of Virchow, and it still manages to retain its sphinx-like character. It presents *three basic changes*. These are: (1) hydropic degeneration of the stroma of the villi, which gives them their cystic appearance; (2) trophoblastic proliferation in which both

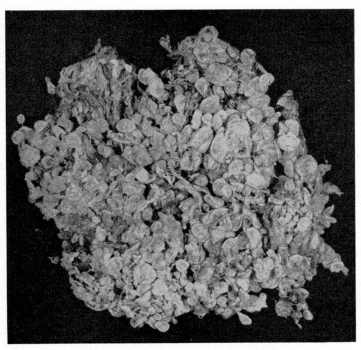

FIG. 535.—Hydatidiform mole. This mass was aborted in the third month of pregnancy.

Langhans' cells and syncytium take part, so that there are several layers of the former and the syncytial cells are unduly prominent; (3) scantiness of the blood vessels in the villi. Each of these has been stressed in turn and considered to be at the root of the trouble. In spontaneous abortion, where the ovum is said to be "blighted," the villi often show the same characteristic hyaline swelling and cystic degeneration. Indeed it may be that an early stage of hydatidiform mole is the explanation of many "spontaneous" abortions. The proliferation of the trophoblast is regarded by many as the essential feature, so that condition might be regarded as a benign epithelial tumor, of which the malignant variety is the chorionepithelioma. By still others stress is laid on the absence of blood vessels. The affected villi are totally or partially ischemic, and this absence of fetal circulation has been blamed for the accumulation of fluid that cannot be absorbed. It will be realized that we are faced with the old dilemma of determining when confronted with two associated events, which is cause and which is effect. It was in 1895 that Marchand stated that the most important factor was the trophoblastic proliferation, involving both sets of cells. But we are at once confronted with the awkward question as to why many of the sections show none of this hyperplasia.

When the change in the villi occurs early the fetus and placenta disappear, being replaced by a mass or mole composed of cyst-like bodies. When the change takes place later there may be a small atrophic fetus and remnants of placenta. Sometimes the changes may be microscopic; these cases are much commoner than the fully developed ones (Fig. 536). The formation of a mole leads to abortion and may cause severe hemorrhage. At least part of the hormone which appears in the urine during pregnancy and gives the Aschheim-Zondek test for that condition is produced by the placenta. With the termination of pregnancy and complete removal of the placenta the test at once becomes negative. If portions of the placenta are retained or if hydatidiform mole or chorionepithelioma develop, the hormone continues to be produced and the test remains positive. When an innocent mole is

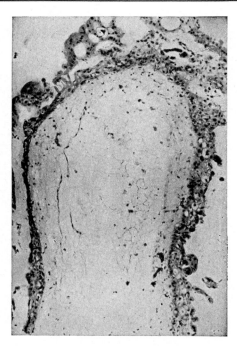

Fig. 536.—Hydatidiform degeneration of a chorionic villus. There is mucoid degeneration of the connective tissue and proliferation of the epithelium covering the villus. × 25.

removed the test becomes negative. If it remains positive it indicates that chorionepithelioma has developed. As long as active chorionic epithelium remains in the uterus, the test remains positive.

One of the most difficult tasks with which the pathologist can be confronted is to determine from an examination of the mole alone whether it is purely benign or whether it has developed into the malignant form, in which case a hysterectomy is indicated. The criteria of malignancy are never absolute, only relative (Hertig and Sheldon). The histological picture varies in different parts of the mole, and a number of blocks should be examined. The absolute indication is invasion, and this can only be determined when the uterus is examined. When the picture of malignancy is fully developed (see below) there need be no difficulty. It is the indeterminate picture which causes the headaches. False negative diagnoses are rare, but false positives are common. It is probably true to say that only about half the cases

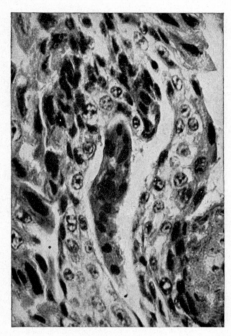

Fig. 537.—Chorionepithelioma consisting of clear Langhans' cells and dark syncytial masses. × 350.

in which the microscopic picture suggests malignancy prove to be malignant clinically.

Chorionepithelioma.—This remarkable tumor is unique in that it is derived not from the tissues of the patient but from those of another individual, for it arises from the epithelial cells covering the chorionic villi, from fetal and not from maternal tissue. It is therefore the highly malignant counterpart of the hydatidiform mole. It usually follows an abortion, sometimes is the result of a full-term pregnancy, and in rare cases has been found in the ovary and in the testicle. In about 50 per cent of the cases it is preceded by a hydatidiform mole, a benign epithelial tumor of the chorionic villi which will be described in connection with the pathology of the placenta. It is said that about 15 per cent of hydatidiform moles may show this malignant change, but it is impossible to get accurate figures, and this proportion is probably much too high. Both chorionepithelioma and hydatidiform mole are often associated with an unusually large corpus luteum or bilateral lutein cysts. The connection is not certain, but it is probable that they are a result rather than a cause of the uterine condition. The tumor may develop very soon after pregnancy, or there may be an interval of months or years. The *Aschheim-Zondek* test for pregnancy is markedly positive.

Morbid Anatomy.—The tumor commences at the placental site, usually in the fundus of the uterus. It forms a soft, red, highly hemorrhagic mass which projects into the cavity and at the same time invades the muscular wall. Secondary growths may be formed in the lower part of the uterus and in the vaginal wall; in the latter position the progress of the disease can be watched and the effect of treatment noted. Later the tumor appears on the outer surface of the uterus.

Microscopically the chorionepithelioma is an exaggeration of the condition normally found in pregnancy. The fetal part of the placenta consists of the chorionic villi, and the essential part of the villus is the trophoblast, the function of which is to invade the maternal blood sinuses. The trophoblast presents two types of epithelium, an inner layer of clear cubical cells with large pale nuclei known as *Langhans' cells*, and an outer layer of large dark multinucleated masses of cytoplasm known as the *syncytial cells*. The *chorionepithelioma consists mainly of clear Langhans' cells* with a varying proportion of dark syncytial masses lying in large pools of blood (Fig. 537). The normal relationship of the two types of cell is lost, for the exuberant Langhans' cells have burst through the outer syncytial layer. There is no stroma nor blood vessels, as the tumor is nourished by the blood in the vessels it invades.

Spread.—Spread is almost entirely by the *blood stream*, owing to the fundamental tendency of the trophoblastic cells to invade blood vessels. Distant metastases in the lungs, etc., may be set up at an extraordinarily early date after an abortion. The secondary tumors are as hemorrhagic as the primary growth and show the same microscopic structure. Secondary nodules may appear in the vaginal wall. These are not implantations, for the tumor cells lie within vessels.

Not all cases run the rapidly fatal course of the ordinary chorionepithelioma. Some cases make a complete recovery when the primary growth is removed, and spontaneous disappearance of the metastatic growths has even been reported after this operation; this disappearance may be watched in the case of secondary nodules in the vagina. There is one small group of tumors (about 5 per cent) in which the structure is comparatively benign with a corresponding absence of blood vessel invasion and formation of metastases. The growth consists of syncytial cells only, with no admixture of Langhans' cells. The tumor is therefore known as a *syncytioma*.

Perhaps a better term is *syncytial endometritis* suggested by Novak and Novak, who point out that the condition is a postpregnancy syncytial infiltration of the uterine wall together with marked inflammatory reaction and perhaps necrosis rather than a true neoplasm. A second subdivision is known as *chorioadenoma destruens* or *malignant hydatidiform mole*, characterized by a tendency to invade uterine and pelvic blood vessels, but without the formation of distant metastases except in rare instances. The third group is the *chorionepithelioma malignum* or *choriocarcinoma*, which we have already considered.

Owing to the large amount of gonadotropic hormone produced by the chorionic epithelium, the Aschheim-Zondek test in markedly positive. This test is of value for prognosis as well as diagnosis. It quickly becomes negative after complete removal of the tumor, but if metastasis has occurred it remains positive or again becomes positive after an interval sufficient for the development of the secondary tumors.

Toxemiasis of Pregnancy.—This serious complication of the last trimester of pregnancy is divided into *preeclampsia* and *eclampsia*. The former, which is much the commoner, consists of (1) edema and (2) albuminuria with (3) the significant addition of hypertension. *If convulsions develop the condition becomes eclampsia.* The toxemia of pregnancy is still the most common major obstetrical complication in young primigravidas.

The chief *lesions* are in the kidney, liver and placenta. Both kidneys are swollen, and the glomeruli present a solid ischemic appearance (Glomerulosclerosis) which has been described on page 577. Symmetrical necrosis of the renal cortex is a very rare complication (page 603). The liver lesions, take the form of characteristic patches of hemorrhagic necrosis. They are not nearly so constant nor fundamental as the renal lesions. In the placenta the characteristic change is a premature ageing as evidenced by syncytial degeneration, together with more numerous infarcts than are found in normal pregnancy. The convulsions appear to be due to hypertensive vasoconstriction of the cerebral arterioles, with resulting ischemia and edema.

Generalized edema of varying degree is found in over 60 per cent of normal pregnant women. An increase over the normal in the retention of water is the first warning of impending toxemia signalled by the patient to her doctor, it may be by tightening of the wedding ring. The hypertension of toxemia usually disappears after delivery. On the other hand mild toxemia may be followed by permanent hypertension in the female.

Eclampsia has been called "the disease of theories." Although pregnancy is a physiological state, the extensive changes in the maternal organism place gestation on the dim borderline between the normal and the pathological. Whether toxemia represents only an exaggeration of the normal changes incident to pregnancy such as fluid and electrolyte retention, or whether it is the result of entirely different pathological processes, is still an unresolved question. There is no doubt that *salt retention* plays a major role. In the Negroes of Tanganyika and Haiti, where almost no salt is consumed, eclampsia is unknown, whereas among American Negroes whose sodium intake is high, preeclamptic and eclamptic toxemias are frequent. The renal lesions reduce glomerular filtration, with resulting retention of sodium and water. The importance of a low-salt diet becomes obvious in the all-important matter of prognosis. Placental ischemia is said to counteract the normal control of the adrenocortical hyperactivity of pregnancy. Or the placenta may produce a *pressor substance* which acts directly on the arterioles. It has also been suggested that the disturbance leading to the pathological changes found at autopsy may be a sudden

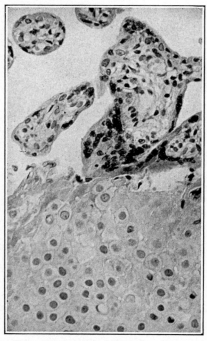

Fig. 538.—Placenta at full term. Above are vascularized villi with syncytial cells; below is decidua. × 225.

intravascular deposition of fibrin which is caused by a mechanism similar to the generalized Shwartzman phenomenon in experimental animals (McKay *et al.*). This process may be the result of the autoinjection of *thromboplastic material* derived from amniotic fluid, decidua or trophoblast in an individual "prepared" by pregnancy. This would bring the toxemias of pregnancy into the autoimmunity group of disturbances. A similar mechanism may be responsible in bilateral renal cortical necrosis.

One thing is certain and that is that vasoconstriction does occur, for it can be observed with the ophthalmoscope in the retinal arteries. *Generalized arteriolar vasoconstriction may, indeed, be regarded as the basic lesion of eclampsia*, being responsible for the cerebral changes leading to convulsions, as well as decreased blood flow to the uterus causing anoxia which may result in the death of the fetus. If the vasoconstriction and hypertension persist for more than a few weeks, permanent vascular changes may develop and the hypertension becomes irre-

versible. A full discussion of the problem will be found in the monograph by Dexter and Weiss.

Retained Placenta.—After an abortion or a full-term pregnancy portions of placenta may be retained in the uterus. The villi may remain alive for many months and may appear perfectly normal when removed by the curette. The pathologist must therefore be cautious about expressing an opinion as to how long a time may have elasped after the last pregnancy, especially in medico-legal cases. In the course of time the villi undergo hyaline degeneration. The stage to which pregnancy has advanced may be roughly estimated by remembering that before mid-term the villi are relatively avascular and the Langhans' cells are prominent, while after that time the villi become vascular and are covered only by syncytial cells, the Langhans' cells disappearing (Fig. 538).

Utero-placental Apoplexy.—This is a complication (possibly a cause) of premature separation of the normally implanted placenta. There may be most extensive hemorrhagic infiltration of the decidua and the uterine wall. In one case which I examined the muscle fibers in places seemed to be floating in pools of blood. In this case the decidual vessels showed acute inflammatory changes which may have been the primary cause both of the uterine apoplexy and the separation of the placenta.

Placental Infarcts.—These are localized areas in the placenta, which may be red when they consist chiefly of coagulated blood, or pale yellow when the blood is decolorized and there is much necrosis of tissue. They constitute one of the commonest abnormalities of the placenta. Minute infarcts are indeed present in every placenta. Sometimes large wedge-shaped segments are involved. The accepted basis for the condition is an endarteritis of the vessels in the chorionic villi causing necrosis of the villi followed by coagulation of the blood between the villi, and matting together of the latter by fibrin. In many cases, however, no endarteritis can be found, so that another explanation must be sought. After the seventh month the Langhans' cells disappear and the syncytium may also atrophy in patches, as a result of which fibrin becomes deposited on the rough surface. The layer of fibrin cuts off the villi from their blood supply in the maternal sinuses so that they undergo necrosis. In this case the process is an ischemic necrosis but not an infarction. *Calcification* is not uncommon in these necrotic areas.

Erythroblastosis Fetalis.—The placenta is very large and edematous, particularly in the

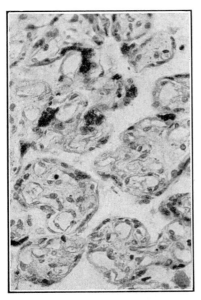

FIG. 539.—Normal placenta. × 280.

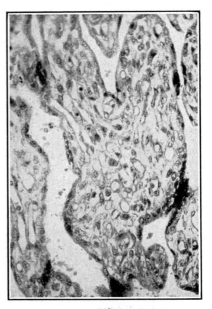

FIG. 540.—Placenta in erythroblastosis. × 280.

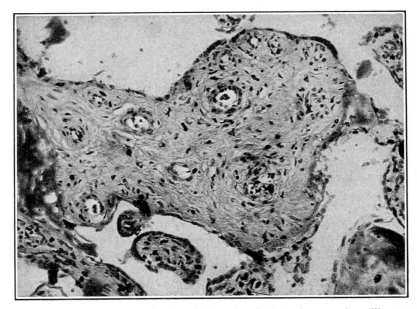

FIG. 541.—Syphilitic placenta showing thickened and relatively avascular villi. × 175.

hydropic form of the disease. *Microscopically* the villi are swollen, the Langhans' cells which normally disappear about the middle of pregnancy still persist, and the capillaries contain numerous erythroblasts. These changes make a diagnosis possible even when the fetus has become completely macerated (Figs. 539 and 540).

SYPHILIS.—When the fetus is syphilitic the placenta may be normal, but often it is thick and pale. The pallor is due to avascularity. The normal villi are very vascular, but in syphilis they may become markedly avascular owing to endarteritis, and considerably thickened (Fig. 541). In judging of avascularity it must be borne in mind that it is only in the second half of pregnancy that the villi are vascular for in the earlier months they contain very few vessels.

TUBERCULOSIS.—Tuberculosis is rare. Miliary tubercles may occur, or larger caseous masses.

THE FALLOPIAN TUBES

Although the only function of the Fallopian tubes is to carry the ovum from the ovary to the uterus, the mucous membrane shares in the general cyclic changes of menstruation. There are two types of epithelial cells, ciliated and non-ciliated. In the advanced secretory phase the ciliated cells become much lower, and the non-ciliated cells project between them, with bulbous herniation into the lumen of the tube. During menstruation both sets of cells become low. This lowness is greatly accentuated during pregnancy, when they become almost flat. After menstruation the cells regain their normal height in three or four days.

It would almost appear as if nature had designed the Fallopian tubes to become the seat of an infective process, and were this the case the attempt has certainly been a successful one, for few organs are more frequently affected by inflammation, both acute and chronic. Tumors and other lesions are of little importance. The tubes may be infected from either end as well as from the blood stream. The narrow uterine opening, which is so easily closed by swelling of the wall, and the very numerous folds of mucous membrane tend to make an infection of long duration. *Salpingitis* or inflammation of the tubes is due to infection with the gonococcus in about 80 per cent of cases. Pyogenic cocci, especially streptococci, are responsible in about 15 per cent, and the tubercle bacillus in the remaining 5 per cent. Streptococci can be grown from the tubes many months or years after the primary infection, but the gonococcus may die out in the course of a few months.

Gonorrhea of Female Genital Tract.— Before describing gonorrheal salpingitis it is convenient to make a brief survey of gonorrheal infection of the female genital tract. The primary infection is usually in the urethra, occasionally in the cervical mucosa. Both of these are lined by a layer of epithelium which is readily penetrated by the gonococcus. The cornified squamous epithelium of the vulva and vagina is seldom infected except in children, in which it is soft and delicate. It is evident that when smears are made they must *not* be taken from the vagina, but from the cervix and urethra. The infection in the urethra usually gives rise to little or no clinical disturbance, so that it is difficult to determine with accuracy the date of infection. *Bartholin's glands*, situated on either side of the posterior commissure of the vaginal entrance, may become infected from the urethra, with the formation of an acute abscess. Acute bartholinitis is almost always gonococcal in nature. The *cervix* is involved primarily or secondarily in most cases of gonorrhea, but as it is a very insensitive organ there are often no symptoms. It is in the mucous membrane of the cervical canal that the infection becomes chronic, for the branching racemose glands of the endocervix form an ideal lurking place for the gonococcus, from which it may issue periodically to infect other parts of the genital tract. Laceration after childbirth and gonorrhea account for nearly all cases of endocervicitis and cervicitis. The *endometrium of the body* of the uterus is seldom seriously infected. When first invaded by the gonococcus there are no doubt suppurative lesions of the superficial layers, but these are swept away at the next menstrual period, and it is seldom that chronic infection of a serious nature occurs. When the gonococcus reaches the *tubes* it finds as favorable a habitat as the endocervix, and the most serious results of gonorrhea in the female occur in the tubes. Before considering gonococcal salpingitis a few words may be devoted to gonorrhea in children.

Gonorrheal vulvovaginitis is practically confined to children, because in them the vaginal epithelium is not yet cornified and is readily penetrated by the gonococcus. The disease is extraordinarily contagious, and may sweep like a fire through a school or a children's hospital. The infection is spread by towels, sponges, etc., but often it is difficult to determine the exact means of spread. Once the infection is established it is very resistant to treatment. Anyone who has had practical experience with this disease in a hospital will be struck by the marked discrepancy between the laboratory findings and the clinical evidence of the disease. When routine vaginal smears are made in a hospital, gram-negative intracellular diplococci are not infrequently found in children who show no symptoms of any kind. It is possible that in many cases the organisms seen are not gonococci but Micrococcus catarrhalis, which is morphologically indistinguishable from the gonococcus and is known to be capable of causing vaginitis in children. The distinction can readily be made by culture.

Gonorrheal Salpingitis.—Infection of the tubes may occur early in the disease, but there is often a considerable interval. During this time the gonococcus is lurking in the racemose glands of the cervix, from which retreat it may invade the tubes at any time. The infection is practically always bilateral. The effect depends entirely on the intensity of the inflammation. In mild cases it has the character of a catarrh, while in more severe form it becomes purulent. There is a tendency for both ends of the tubes to become closed even though the inflammation be mild. The outer end may be closed by the inflamed fimbriæ becoming withdrawn into the ostium of the tube and adhering together, or by becoming adherent to the ovary. The inner end, which normally is less than 1 mm. in diameter, is easily closed by inflammatory swelling of the mucosa. The tube is now a closed cavity, and if a fluid exudate is poured out as the result of inflammation the tube will be distended. The distention is most marked at the distal end, and the tube becomes curved into a form like a retort. When the exudate is more or less serous (catarrhal salpingitis) the result is hydrosalpinx; when it is purulent a pyosalpinx is formed.

In *hydrosalpinx* the distention of the tube may be great, but the wall is thin and translucent, for there is no pronounced inflammatory thickening. The mucosa is atrophic, and the contents clear and watery, though rich in albumin. In *pyosalpinx* the wall is much thickened and the distended tube is filled with thick pus. The wall is infiltrated with inflammatory cells, polymorphonuclears in the early stages and lymphocytes and plasma cells later. In the tube as in the cervix the plasma cell is the characteristic cell of chronic inflammation. It is seldom that the gonococcus can be found in the pus except in recent cases, but secondary infection with Bacillus coli is rather frequent. If the inner end of the tube is not closed, there is no distention and the condition is called a *pus tube*. In *tubo-ovarian abscess* the inflamed fimbriæ adhere to the ovary, and infection of the ruptured Graafian follicle is a natural result. The gonococci flourish in the hemorrhagic tissue of the corpus luteum, and an abscess is formed which distends the ovary and communicates with the pyosalpinx by a narrow opening. The tube and ovary together form one large retort-shaped bag of pus. Very dense pelvic adhesions around the tubes and ovaries are a common result. *Salpingitis isthmica nodosa* is a peculiar condition in which nodules are formed at the inner end (isthmus) of the tube. As the result of persistent inflammation areas of mucosa are included in the deeper layers and may become separated from the lumen so as to give an adenomatous appearance. The condition is nearly always gonorrheal in origin, but is occasionally found in tuberculous salpingitis. It causes closure of the tube. From what has been said it is easy to see the relation which gonorrhea bears to sterility and chronic invalidism in women.

Tuberculous Salpingitis. — Tuberculous salpingitis resembles gonorrheal salpingitis in some respects, but differs from it in others. The mode of infection is quite different, being nearly always hematogenous from some distant focus, rarely from the peritoneal cavity in abdominal tuberculosis, and never from the lower genital tract. It is almost always bilateral, like the gonorrheal form, and is accompanied by adhesions which are even firmer and may make removal of the tubes quite impossible.

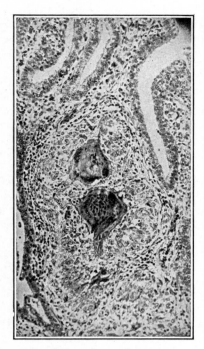

FIG. 542.—Tuberculous salpingitis. × 125.

The tubes are thickened, and there may be tubercles on the serous surface. The ostium usually remains open, in contrast to what occurs in gonorrheal salpingitis. Occasionally it may be closed, so that a *tuberculous pyosalpinx* develops, which may be indistinguishable from the gonorrheal form. The contents are characteristically thick and in old cases may become putty-like. Caseation, tubercle formation, epithelioid cells, and giant cells in the mucosa and other layers form a characteristic microscopic picture (Fig. 542).

Infection may spread from the tubes to the peritoneum. Persistently recurring tuberculous peritonitis in the female sometimes clears up only when the tubes are removed.

Tubal Pregnancy.—The ovum takes nearly a week to pass along the Fallopian tube from the ovary to the uterus, and it is during its passage down the tube that it becomes fertilized. If the impregnated ovum is arrested in the tube it may develop there and form a tubal pregnancy. The arrest is usually due to chronic salpingitis, as a result of which the folds of the tube are thickened

and deep glandular pockets are formed in which the ovum is entrapped. This explains the rarity of the condition in nulliparæ, and the fact that there is often a long interval of sterility between the last pregnancy and the occurrence of the tubal pregnancy.

A very different explanation of tubal pregnancy is offered by Asherman, who reports that in 325 patients who developed tubal pregnancy in Tel-Aviv, Israel, only one had had gonorrhea. He points out that full patency or lack of structural changes of the Fallopian tubes will not necessarily suffice to insure their normal functioning. Movements of the tubal muscles are as dependent on the hormonal as on the nervous system. Asherman considers that the predominant cause in his patients is functional disturbance of the autonomic nervous system resulting from emotional conflicts and causing *tubal dyskinesia*. This does not, of course, rule out the possibility or indeed the likelihood of organic obstruction of the tubes in other cases. The ovum is usually arrested in the outer end of the tube, the ostium becoming closed by the end of the second month. When development takes place in the inner part of the tube the ostium remains open.

There may be slight decidual formation in the tube, but it is never marked. The normal uterine decidua offers a good deal of resistance to invasion by the chorionic villi, and as this resistance is absent in the tube the villi are able to penetrate deeply into its wall. The ovum may burrow into the muscle, becoming separated from the lumen by the mucosa and some of the muscular layer. It now lies in a cavity in the wall of the tube, a cavity bounded on both sides by muscle and completely separated from the lumen which may be much narrowed (Fig. 543). A well-marked decidua is formed in the empty uterus, and this is sometimes expelled as a decidual cast. The uterus becomes enlarged owing to muscular hypertrophy caused by hormonal stimulation. Uterine scrapings show decidual cells but no chorionic villi, a dissociation only found in extra-uterine pregnancy.

The pregnancy is usually terminated before or at the end of the second month, although in rare cases it may go on much longer or even to full term. *Tubal abortion*

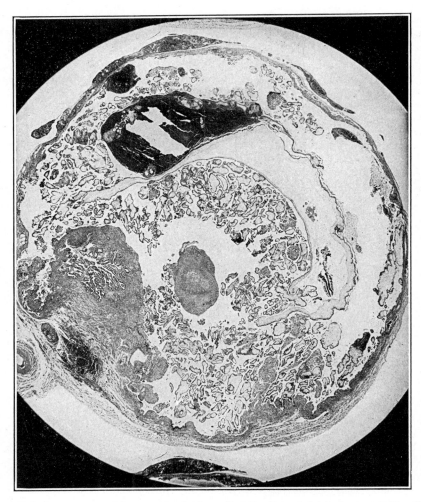

Fig. 543.—Tubal pregnancy. A large cavity in the wall of the distended tube is occupied by (1) chorionic villi; (2) dark blood clot; and (3) the gestation sac, which is the crescentic structure to the right with the body cavity in its lowest part. The lumen of the tube is seen to the left. × 7.

is the common method of termination. Hemorrhage occurs into the gestation sac, destroying the embryo, distending the tube with blood so that it forms a *hematosalpinx*, and converting the products of conception into a *tubal mole* (*mole*, mass). The mole consists of firm blood clot in which chorionic villi are found under the microscope, but no fetal parts. Blood escapes through the ostium if it is still open, the mole becomes detached, and may be extruded by the muscular contractions of the tube into the abdominal cavity. In very rare cases a mole

formed in the isthmus of the tube has escaped into the uterus. At the time of the abortion there is a flow of blood from the uterus. This really comes from the uterus, not from the tube, being due to breaking down and discharge of the decidua. *Tubal rupture* occurs in about 25 per cent of cases. The wall of the tube is perforated by the trophoblast of the chorionic villi, bleeding occurs into the abdominal cavity, and the patient may die of internal hemorrhage. In rare cases the fetus may be slowly extruded through the ostium without severe hemorrhage. It may then be converted into a *lithopedion*, a mummified mass in which calcium salts are deposited.

TUBAL CYSTS.—Small *subserous cysts* about the size of a pin's head are common and are readily mistaken for miliary tubercles. They are probably formed from the peritoneum as the result of mild inflammation. *Cysts of the hydatids of Morgagni* are also fairly common. The cyst is about the size of a pea, filled with clear fluid, and attached by a slender stalk to one of the fimbriæ of the tube.

CARCINOMA.—Carcinoma of the Fallopian tube is the rarest of the primary cancers of the female reproductive tract, but the most malignant. The lumen is distended by adenocarcinoma. The clinical features are vaginal bleeding, a pelvic mass, lower abdominal pain and masses of cancer cells in the vaginal smears.

THE OVARY

GENERAL CONSIDERATIONS

Structure.—It is important to realize the gross appearance of the ovary in health, otherwise the surgeon may remove a normal organ. Each ovary is an elongated flattened body, the surface of which presents bosses (follicles, corpora lutea) separated by fissures and scars. The length is 2.5 to 5 cm., the width 1.5 to 3 cm., and the thickness 0.5 to 1.5 cm. The weight is 5 to 7 grams. Most of the surface is covered by glistening peritoneal mesothelium, but this changes to a lusterless surface (germinal epithelium) along the *white line* which marks the hilum of the ovary, *i.e.*, the site of attachment of the mesovarium. The ovary presents a cortex and medulla, although not clearly demarcated. The *cortical zone* contains ripening Graafian follicles forming cysts of varying size, sometimes up to 1.5 cm. in diameter. Still larger, and often mistaken by the ignorant for a pathological lesion, is the corpus luteum. In some cases it may occupy one-third of the ovary. The center is filled with fresh blood, and the wall is of a characteristic bright yellow color and an equally characteristic wavy convoluted outline.

Apart from the Graafian follicles in various stages of development, the *cortex* consists of closely packed spindle cells resembling plump fibroblasts, an appearance which might be mistaken by the unwary for evidence of inflammation or neoplasia. The subserous zone, on the other hand, consists of a thin layer of acellular fibrous tissue, thickening of which may prevent rupture of the follicles and ovulation with corresponding functional disturbances (see Stein-Leventhal syndrome, page 926). The *medulla* consists of looser mesenchymal tissue. A few large epithelial-like cells occur in the so-called hilar region. These are derived from the primordial gonad, and correspond to the Leydig interstitial cells of the testis, so that they are called *hilar Leydig cells* or hilus cells. They may contain the same crystalloids of Reinke which have already been noted in the testis. *Hyperplasia or neoplasia of these cells may give rise to a picture of masculinization.*

At birth the germinal epithelium covers the surface of the organ, but during development all the Graafian follicles are derived from this tissue. During the course of the menstrual cycle a number of follicles approach maturity, the germinal epithelium proliferating to form several layers of *granulosa cells*. These follicles may develop along one of two lines. (1) The ripe follicle at mid-term of the cycle approaches the surface, discharges the ovum, and becomes converted into the *corpus luteum*, the granulosa cells proliferating and acquiring a high lipid content which gives the new structure its yellow or lutein color. The corpus luteum is an organ of internal secretion which acts on the endometrium and the other developing follicles, but after menstruation it undergoes rapid hyaline degeneration, and becomes changed into a structureless white mass, the *corpus albicans*. If pregnancy supervenes the corpus luteum does not degenerate, and continues to increase in size. (2) Under the influence of the lutein hormone the other maturing follicles undergo retrogression or *atresia*. It is from these atretic follicles, which may be regarded as examples of arrested development and are still lined by granulosa cells, that the majority of retention cysts probably arise. The stromal cells in contact with the developing follicle are known as *theca cells*. During atresia they become enlarged, acquire a lipid content, and assume an epithelioid character, being known as *theca-lutein cells*.

Hormone Production.—Just as we have

already seen in the case of the testis, so also in the ovary the cells may produce male as well as female hormones. There is, however, much difference of opinion as to which cells elaborate which hormone. *Estrogens* are believed to be produced by the theca and theca-lutein cells, as they behave in a positive manner with histochemical reactions found to be characteristic for ketosteroids, whereas granulosa cells react negatively. *Progesterone* seems to be produced by the corpus luteum, although the exact cell concerned is uncertain. *Androgens* are probably elaborated by the hilar Leydig cells, and perhaps by granulosa and theca cells, judging from what is observed in patients with tumors of these cells. Further information on the hormonal functions of the ovary and the endocrine effects which may accompany functioning tumors and other ovarian lesions will be found in Morris and Scully's *Endocrine Pathology of the Ovary*.

INFLAMMATION

Inflammation of the ovary is usually the result of infection of the ovary from the Fallopian tube in the course of puerperal sepsis or gonorrhea. It is occasionally infected from the blood stream in infectious fevers.

Acute diffuse inflammation (oöphoritis) is generally caused by puerperal sepsis. The ovary is covered by the tough fibrous tunica albuginea which lies under the germinal epithelium and forms a formidable barrier to invading microörganisms. In puerperal sepsis there is pelvic peritonitis, so that the ovary may be bathed in pus containing virulent streptococci which overcome the barrier of the tunica albuginea and may cause an acute inflammation. Both ovaries are enlarged, congested, and contain numerous small abscesses. In general septicemia acute oöphoritis is a rare complication due to blood infection. The inflammation which may accompany mumps is non-suppurative.

Ovarian abscess is usually due to invasion of the ruptured Graafian follicle by the gonococcus. This may be rendered easy by fusion of the fimbriæ of the tube with the ovary. It sometimes occurs in puerperal sepsis. The wall of the abscess is at first formed by the yellow wall of the corpus luteum, but in time the abscess involves the entire ovary which becomes converted into a bag of pus. This may fuse and communicate with the tubal abscess so as to form a tubo-ovarian abscess.

NON-NEOPLASTIC CYSTS

No organ in the body is so frequently the site of cyst formation as the ovary. These cysts vary greatly in nature. Some appear to be the result of inflammation, retention, or degeneration, while others are true tumors or cystadenomata. The latter will be considered in connection with ovarian tumors.

Ovarian cysts may therefore be classified into non-neoplastic and neoplastic groups as follows:

   I. Non-neoplastic.
      1. Follicular cysts.
      2. Lutein cysts.
         a. Corpus luteum cysts.
         b. Theca lutein cysts.
      3. Endometrial cysts.
  II. Neoplastic cysts.
      1. Cystadenoma.
         a. Mucinous.
         b. Serous.
      2. Dermoid cysts.

Follicular Cysts.—These very common lesions of the ovary are retention cysts of atretic follicles. The cysts are small, seldom more than 3 cm. in diameter, multiple, and sometimes are so numerous as to involve the entire ovary, producing some enlargement. The cyst is lined by epithelium which is cuboidal in the small cysts but flattened in the large ones. There is generally an associated fibrosis of the ovary, hence the old name of sclerocystic disease of the ovary. One cyst may grow at the expense of the others which it absorbs, and may reach the size of a plum or even a tangerine orange, the remaining cysts disappearing. The contents are clear and watery, and there is no trace of an epithelial lining in these larger cysts. In the ovaries of infants and even in the newborn there may be large numbers of small follicular cysts. These must be due to some abnormal hormonal stimuli (maternal); possibly some similar mechanism may be responsible for follicular cysts in the adult.

Lutein Cysts.—These cysts may represent degeneration of the corpus luteum formed after ovulation, or they may be *theca-lutein cysts* formed from atretic follicles lined by luteinized cells. The distinction between the two types is often difficult. Each cyst is lined by the characteristic wavy yellow lutein tissue, the cells of which are loaded with anisotropic lipid. Hemorrhage is frequent into both varieties. The hemorrhage may be severe, extend into the interstitial tissue, and form a *hematoma*. This may rupture into the abdominal cavity causing severe internal hemorrhage with symptoms simulating ruptured tubal pregnancy or some other abdominal catastrophe. The hemorrhage may prove fatal unless the ovary is at once removed.

Stein-Leventhal Syndrome.—In 1935 Stein and Leventhal described a syndrome consisting of menstrual irregularity or actual amenorrhea, sterility, obesity, uterine hypoplasia and underdeveloped breasts, with in some cases evidence of virilism such as hirsutism of masculine distribution and hypertrophy of the clitoris. In other cases reported arterial hypertension has been present. Both ovaries are enlarged, presenting an oyster-gray appearance with a firm smooth surface. The tunica is markedly thickened and fibrosed, and beneath it are many unruptured follicles in various stages of arrested maturation and atresia with varying numbers of follicular cysts. It is a condition of bilateral microcystic ovaries. There is a striking absence of corpora lutea, and it is evident that no ovulation is taking place. Marked hyperplasia of the theca interna cells lining the atretic follicles is common, and these may show a striking degree of luteinization. In one series of 45 cases endometrial carcinoma was present in 9 (Jackson and Dockerty).

No satisfactory explanation of the clinical picture is so far forthcoming, in particular as to whether the ovarian changes should be regarded as primary or secondary to some anterior pituitary dysfunction. It is of interest that wedge resection of the fibrotic cortex has produced marked clinical improvement in a number of cases. This has been explained on the basis of removing the barrier to ovulation, or by the reduction of the ovarian "target area," thus allowing a better pituitary-ovarian hormonal balance.

Endometrial (Chocolate-colored) Cysts.—These are examples of endometriosis, *i.e.*, ectopic development of endometrium-like tissue. They are small, often multiple, and of a dark reddish-brown color (chocolate) due to the presence of old blood. (Plate XII, page 900). They are situated on the surface of the ovary and may show evidence of previous perforation, with dense adhesions consisting of endometrial tissue. The cysts represent endometrial glands into which menstrual hemorrhage has occurred. The condition is probably an example of metaplasia due to hormonal stimulation of a tissue which is related developmentally to the endometrium rather than a result of endometrial implants. This matter has already been discussed fully in connection with endometriosis (page 900).

TUMORS OF THE OVARY

The classification of ovarian tumors is particularly difficult, because they consist of tissues which are different from those of the normal ovary, whereas in other organs the tumor is at least in some degree a duplication of that organ. The tumors may be *cystic* or *solid*. The former are very much more common, and are known as cystadenomas. They are for the most part innocent, though they may become malignant; the solid epithelial tumors, on the other hand, are practically all malignant. The cystadenomas may be divided into two main groups, the mucinous and the serous. These differ not only in their contents, but also in structure and behavior. There is a rare third group of tumors associated as a rule with sexual endocrine dysfunction for which there is no very appropriate name, but which may be called the *special group*.

Mucinous Cystadenoma.—This is a common tumor, usually unilateral, and may reach very large dimensions. It is always multilocular, owing to the formation of daughter cysts from projecting buds of the lining epithelium. The daughter cysts vary greatly in size, a few may grow to a large size at the expense of the others, the intervening walls becoming broken down. The

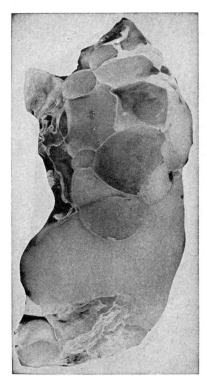

Fig. 544.—Mucinous cystadenoma of the ovary. The cysts are filled with thick mucinous material which has been coagulated by the fixative.

contents are very thick, mucoid, and stringy (Fig. 544). The fluid may be turbid and tinged with blood, or it may be shimmering with crystals of cholesterol. The cyst develops a well-marked pedicle, and this may become twisted, producing intense congestion of the wall, hemorrhage into the cavities, and a clinical picture of acute strangulation.

The *microscopic picture* is characteristic. The cysts are lined by a layer of very tall columnar epithelial cells with extremely clear cytoplasm (due to the mucinous content) and nuclei situated at the base of the cells (Fig. 545). The cells are not ciliated, in contrast to the cells of serous cystadenoma. There may be small papillary projections from the wall of the cyst, but these are seldom pronounced. In the exceptional cases where there is marked papillary formation there is danger of malignancy; such cases are often bilateral (Fig. 546).

There is a tendency to spontaneous perforation, but the mucin seems to do little harm in the peritoneal cavity. In exceptional cases the tumor cells may become implanted on the peritoneum and produce large jelly-like masses, a condition known as *pseudomyxoma peritonei*. The prognosis is then bad, for the irritation of the new material sets up a chronic peritonitis, and repeated removal may fail to cure the patient.

Serous Cystadenoma.—This form, which constitutes about one-third of the cystic tumors of the ovary, may show different degrees of development. Thus there is the simple serous cyst which it may be difficult to distinguish from a large follicular cyst, the multiloculated serous cyst without papillary processes, and the multiloculated papillary serous cyst. The cystadenoma, which is frequently bilateral, resembles externally the mucinous form, but it seldom has a well-developed pedicle. The *contents* of the cysts are clear and watery; they contain no mucin, but are highly albuminous. *Microscopically* the cysts are lined by an epithelium which is low compared with that of the mucinous variety, nor are the cells filled with mucin. The cells are usually ciliated (Fig. 547), thus differing from the epithelium of the mucinous cystadenoma.

The most characteristic feature of these tumors is the presence of papillary processes, although these are not always present, so that the name papillary cystadenoma cannot be applied to the whole group. The presence of papillomata indicates a greater proliferative activity on the part of the epithelium, and the papillomata may appear on the outer as well as the inner surface, owing to invasion of the wall by the tumor cells (Fig. 548). This penetration does not prove that the condition has become malignant, but it is always suggestive. The papillary cystadenomas have a marked tendency toward malignant change, which is indicated by the soft character of the papillomata and the irregular arrangement of the epithelium. More or less of the original cyst structure may remain, with the malignant tissue represented by firm knobby areas, or the tumor, if highly cellular, may be soft and friable. In other cases the original cyst has been almost entirely replaced by tumor, so that the mode of origin may be more than doubtful. The malignant change may only be

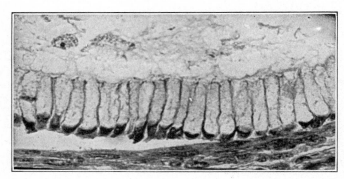

FIG. 545.—Mucinous cystadenoma of the ovary. The palisade cells, which are non-ciliated, are filled with pseudomucin and the nuclei are displaced to the base. × 500.

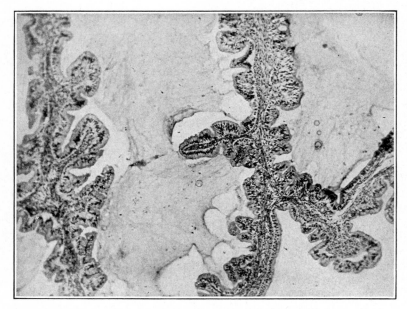

FIG. 546.—Mucinous cystadenoma with papillary formation. × 600.

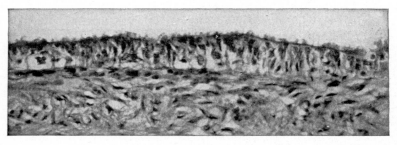

FIG. 547.—Ciliated epithelium in serous cystadenoma. × 240. (Boyd, *Pathology for the Surgeon*, courtesy of the W. B. Saunders Co.)

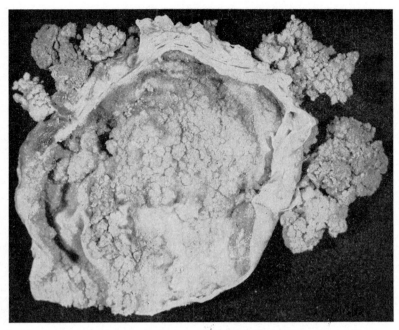

Fig. 548.—Papillary serous cystadenoma of ovary. The interior is filled with papillary processes, and many have penetrated to the serous surface.

recognized microscopically. Concentric rounded *psammoma bodies*, apparently a product of the interaction of pelvic peritoneum and underlying stroma, may be of value in identifying the germinal epithelial origin in poorly differentiated malignant examples, although they are most frequently seen in well-differentiated forms. The percentage of these tumors which become malignant varies in different statistics from 20 to 65. The mere fact that carcinoma is found in such a tumor does not mean that the prognosis is necessarily bad, for the malignancy is not high, the growth is often circumscribed, and removal may be followed by complete cure. Secondary papillomata may be scattered over the peritoneum producing an ascites which recurs repeatedly after tapping. The microscopic picture does not always correspond with the clinical course. There may be no microscopic evidence of malignancy, and yet the peritoneum may be covered with papillomata. On the other hand, cases of undoubted malignancy may run a very slow course and live as long as ten years. Calcification may sometimes occur; in one of my

cases this involved a large area; it may even affect the glandular metastases.

The important features of the two types of ovarian cystadenoma are shown in the table on page 930 from Ackerman's *Surgical Pathology*.

Origin of Ovarian Cysts.—The three main types of ovarian cysts, namely mucinous, serous and endometrial, may all be formed, as Hertig suggests, from infoldings of the pelvic Müllerian germinal epithelium from which the tubal mucosa, the endometrium and the endocervix are developed. If such an infolding gives rise to a cervical type of mucin-forming gland the result will be a *mucinous cystadenoma*, if to a fallopian tube type of ciliated epithelium the result will be a *serous cystadenoma*, and if to an endometrial type of epithelium the result will be the *cysts of endometriosis*. Another view as to the origin of the mucinous cystadenoma is that it represents a one-sided development of a teratoma in which the tall columnar intestinal type of epithelium has replaced the other elements of the growth, just as the cartilage of a testicular teratoma may pro-

CYSTADENOMAS OF THE OVARY

	Serous	*Mucinous*
Bilateral	50 per cent	5 per cent
Size	Moderate	Often huge
Malignant	High percentage	Low percentage
Lymph node metastases in malignant form.	High percentage	Low percentage
Implants	Frequent	Moderate
Microscopic type	Cuboidal	High columnar, basally situated nucleus.
Cilia	Often present	Never present
Psammoma bodies	Frequent in well-differentiated types.	Never present

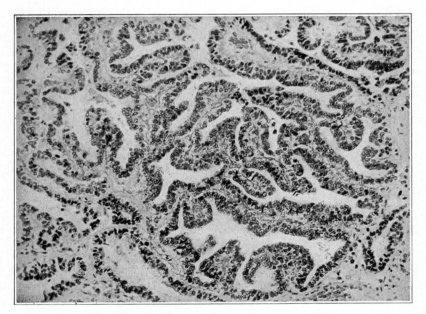

Fig. 549.—Papillary carcinoma of ovary. × 100.

liferate and give rise to a chondroma. It is probable that some mucinous cystadenomas may arise in this way, because in an ovarian teratoma one may find small cysts lined by typical mucinous epithelium. In support of the view that the epithelium is intestinal in nature Novak points out that in mucocele of the appendix, a lesion which may give rise to pseudomyxoma peritonei, the epithelium is of the same mucinous nature. A serious objection to the theory is that mucinous cystadenoma is very common and teratoma is equally rare.

Carcinoma.—Carcinoma originating in the ovary is uncommon in comparison with metastatic carcinoma. The tumor is usually bilateral, one ovary being infected from the other. The tumor is of moderate size, and is usually soft and friable, though it may be firm if the stroma is abundant. The great majority of cancers of the ovary are malignant papillary cystadenomas, although the papillæ may coalesce so as to give a solid appearance (Fig. 549). Thus a solid carcinoma may be a papillary cystadenoma which has become solid or it may be solid from the start. The latter may be of adenocarcinomatous or medullary type. The medullary form is usually composed of solid masses of carcinoma cells separated by a varying amount of stroma, but sometimes the cellular arrangement is diffuse and the structure highly anaplastic. Such tumors are easily mistaken for sarcoma, and their carcinomatous character is often not recognized.

Metastases are scattered over the surface of the peritoneum, and are responsible for the hemorrhagic ascites which is characteristic of the condition, and in a woman should always suggest the possibility of cancer of the ovary. There may be metastases in the uterus owing to infection by way of the Fallopian tube. In such cases it may be difficult or impossible to be certain if the cancer started in the endometrium or the ovary, for both are derived from a common type of epithelium.

Secondary Carcinoma (Krukenberg).— These growths, which are nearly always bilateral, are of fairly frequent occurrence. The common primary sites are the stomach, large bowel, and uterus. The so-called *Krukenberg tumor* is characterized by large, round, vesicular cells with the nucleus pressed to one side by mucoid material so as to present a signet-ring appearance (Fig. 550), and separated by connective tissue showing mucoid degeneration. As a rule the primary tumor in the stomach or large bowel is a mucoid carcinoma, but this is not always the case. Apparently cancer cells growing in the ovary may acquire an ability to produce mucin which they do not possess in the primary lesion. For this reason the tumor has been well named *carcinoma mucocellulare*. The route of infection probably varies. In some cases it is no doubt due to implantation of cancer cells on the surface of the ovary. On the other hand the tumors are usually in the interior rather than on the surface of the ovaries. Retrograde lymph spread to the lumbar nodes and thence to the ovaries is a reasonable explanation in most cases. Blood spread is an occasional possibility.

Dermoid Cyst.—This is a *teratoma*, and is one of the common tumors of the ovary. In about 10 per cent of cases it is bilateral. It is of slow growth, and is almost invariably innocent, but in rare cases one of the elements

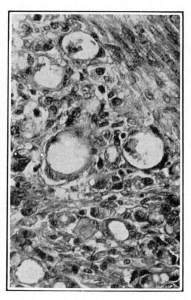

Fig. 550.—Krukenberg tumor showing signet-ring cells. × 275.

of which it is composed may undergo malignant change. Its appearance is very characteristic, for it is of a yellow color and of a doughy consistence when removed from the body, although at body temperature the contents are fluid. The *contents* consist of a yellow, greasy, buttery material containing a considerable amount of hair (Fig. 551). The wall, which is lined by cubical epithelium, gives rise at one place to a nipple-shaped process covered by stratified epithelium and known as the *dermoid process*. This is the real tumor, for the other solid elements are derived from it. The commonest of these are skin and hair (hence the name dermoid), but bone, teeth, cartilage, brain, intestine, striated muscle, thyroid, adrenal, etc., may occur. In exceptional cases the thyroid tissue may proliferate to such a degree that the tumor consists almost entirely of this tissue. Such a condition is known as *struma ovarii*. It will be seen that the tumor contains constituents derived from all three germinal layers, and is therefore a true teratoma. The oily material which distends the cyst is produced by the numerous sebaceous glands with which the skin of the dermoid process is studded (Fig. 552). A dermoid begins as a

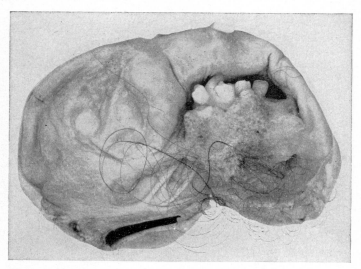

FIG. 551.—Dermoid cyst of ovary containing hair and teeth.

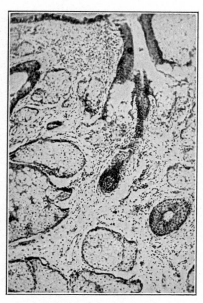

FIG. 552.—Dermoid cyst showing stratified epithelium and sebaceous glands. × 60.

solid tumor, and the cyst formation is secondary.

The dermoid cyst and the solid ovarian teratoma are commonly supposed to arise from one of the original blastomeres formed by the primary segmentation of the ovum, which has become separated and included in the ovary. It appears equally or even more probable that the tumor arises from one of the sex cells (ova) of the ovary, what has been called "the spontaneous growth of the unfertilized ovum."

Solid Ovarian Teratomas.—Solid ovarian teratomas are very rare tumors. They contain no fully formed structures such as skin and bone, but a variety of tissues usually in a rudimentary state, although well formed thyroid and other structures are sometimes present. They form soft solid masses which are highly malignant.

Fibroma.—Fibroma of the ovary is rare. Many of the lesions which used to be regarded as fibroma are now known to be examples of Brenner's tumor. It is a small, hard, white circumscribed tumor, and may arise in some cases from a corpus albicans.

Meigs' Syndrome.—This term denotes a strange association of ascites, hydrothorax (usually right-sided), and a tumor of the ovary, usually but by no means invariably fibroma. Ascites is said to develop in association with 40 to 70 per cent of ovarian fibromas. Many theories have been suggested to explain the ascites and the less common hydrothorax. Rubin and his associates, recalling an old observation of Geibel's that an ovarian fibroma weighing 3200 grams lost 1150 grams of water in twenty-four hours, adduce evidence in support of the view that the fluid comes from the numerous and large lymphatics at the hilum of the ovary. As ovarian tumors are covered by a single layer of low highly permeable epithelium, the fluid may readily escape. Transfer from the abdominal to the pleural cavity may be through the channels which connect the lymphatic networks on both sides of the diaphragm.

Sarcoma.—Sarcoma is very rare. Most of the tumors taken for sarcoma are probably anaplastic carcinomas. True sarcomas may occur as bilateral tumors in children, and present the usual soft homogeneous appearance of a sarcoma. They are composed of round undifferentiated cells.

SPECIAL OVARIAN TUMORS

I have found it singularly difficult to give an appropriate title to the next group of tumors. Obviously I have not succeeded. Indeed, the term is not my own. It is intended to indicate that the ovary may be the seat of a group of uncommon tumors which do not belong to the common run of the mill. They are all characterized by a probable common origin from embryonic remnants and in some instances marked by sex hormone disturbances. Three of these (granulosa cell tumor, arrhenoblastoma and dysgerminoma) have a common origin from the primitive mesenchyme of the ovary; the fourth (Brenner tumor) is unrelated. For the correlation of the lesions with clinical symptoms it will be convenient to recognize two groups of these tumors, namely functioning and nonfunctioning. The functioning neoplasms produce hormonal effects which may be either masculinizing or feminizing, the nonfunctioning naturally produce neither.

In the developing ovary the granulosa layer of the follicles is formed by differentiation of the mesenchymal core of the gonad, not from the surface epithelium as used to be thought. The primitive granulosa cells are therefore connective tissue in type; only later do they develop an epithelial form. It follows that unripe tumors arising from these cells resemble connective tissue and are called theca cell tumors, whilst ripe tumors resemble epithelium and are called granulosa cell tumors; sometimes there may be a mixture of types.

The primitive gonad is neither ovary nor testicle, but may develop into either, the direction of development perhaps depending on the sex of the germ cells which invade the gonad from the primordial gut. Three errors of development are possible. (1) Embryonic rests of undifferentiated mesenchyme may remain and develop years later into a *granulosa cell tumor*. Such a tumor will produce the female hormone with corresponding structural and functional disturbances. (2) In the primitive gonad male cells may be formed as a result of faulty development; these may remain as rests, and give rise in later life to an *arrhenoblastoma*, so-called because it produces a male hormone (*arrhen*, male) with corresponding functional disturbance. (3) Cells may be formed which do not develop along either a male or female line, and may be regarded as neuter. Years later these may give rise to tumors which naturally lack the power of producing hormones. In the ovary such a tumor is a *dysgerminoma;* in the testicle it is known as a seminoma. The *Brenner tumor* does not arise from the primitive mesenchyme of the ovary. Its origin is uncertain.

Feminizing Tumors.—The term "feminization" has its drawbacks when applied to a woman. It denotes a prolonged estrogen effect, which may better be termed *estrinism*. In infancy and early childhood it produces precocious puberty, with development of the breasts and genital tract, uterine bleeding, the appearance of pubic and axillary hair, and accelerated somatic growth. In postmenopausal women the major symptom is uterine bleeding. The principal neoplasm in this group is the granulosa cell tumor, to which may be added theca cell and lutein cell tumors.

Granulosa Cell Tumor.—This tumor is also called granulosa cell carcinoma, but in less than 30 per cent of cases has evidence of malignancy developed. The size varies greatly from 1 to 2 cm. in diameter to a mass the size of an infant's head. Usually unilateral, the outline is sharply defined, the outer surface smooth, and the cut surface has a characteristic yellow tinge but is sometimes gray. It may present cysts of varying size, although the smaller tumors as a rule are solid.

The *microscopic appearance* is confusingly varied, and as different parts of the tumor may differ in structure, it is important to cut a number of blocks. Three main types may be distinguished: the follicular, diffuse, and cylindrical. In the *follicular type*, which is perhaps the most common, the granulosa

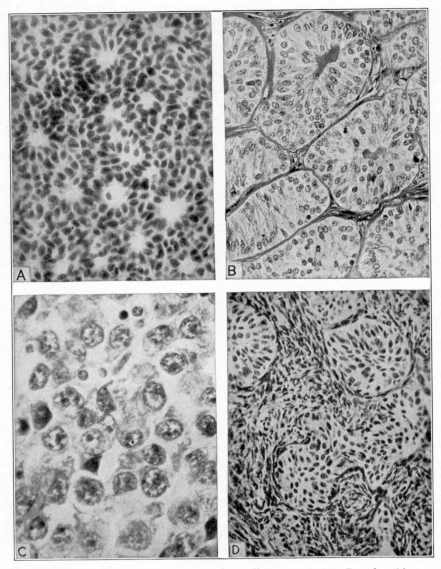

FIG. 553.—Special ovarian tumors: *A*, granulosa cell tumor. × 240; *B*, arrhenoblastoma. × 240; *C*, dysgerminoma. × 510; *D*, Brenner tumor. × 200.

cells are arranged in little clusters or rosettes around a central lumen (Fig. 553, *A*). To be distinguished from this lumen are the so-called *Call-Exner bodies*, which are spaces in larger masses of granulosa cells produced by liquefaction. These spaces may contain bodies resembling and formerly mistaken for ova, but in reality they are secretion or degeneration products. In the *diffuse type* the granulosa cells are arranged diffusely rather than in rosettes. In the *cylindroid* or cylindromatous form masses of epithelial cells are separated by invasion and overgrowth of connective-tissue elements so that the appearance is one of anastomosing cylinders. Luteinization may occur, *i.e.*, an accumulation of lipid in the tumor cells. This is readily demonstrated by fat stains. The more marked is this process, the more striking is the yellow color of the tumor.

When the process is widespread the tumor is spoken of as a luteoma.

The *malignancy* is variable. Most cases pursue a benign course, the tumor often being found incidentally. In other cases there may be peritoneal recurrence a few months after removal of the tumor. *The microscopic picture is of no value in determining the degree of malignancy.*

Occasional tumors of this series present a connective-tissue appearance and are known as *theca cell tumors*. The tumor, which is hard and fibrous, consists of interlacing bands of spindle cells rich in doubly refractive lipid and therefore giving the tumor a yellow color (*lutein cell tumors*).

The *genesis* of these tumors is usually considered to be granulosa cell rests which have not been used in the process of follicle formation. When one considers the intimate relationship which exists between the granulosa cell and theca cell tumors, it seems more probable that their origin may be traced to primitive mesenchyme which antedates the differentiation of granulosa and theca cells.

The *clinical effects* of what has been called the feminizing tumor depend on the period of life at which the tumor develops. The granulosa cells produce estrogenic hormone, so that there will be abnormal menstrual bleeding before puberty or after the menopause, but during the reproductive years the only effect is likely to be increase in the flow. In the child there will be precocious puberty, *i.e.*, early menstruation, development of the breasts and external genitalia, and hypertrophy of the uterus. In the adult endometrial hyperplasia may be a marked feature. Carcinoma of the endometrium has developed in a number of cases, a point of interest in connection with the relation of sex hormones to carcinogenesis. Removal of the tumor in the prepuberty and postmenopausal cases is followed by disappearance of the abnormal clinical features.

Masculinizing Tumors.—The two principal members of this group are the arrhenoblastoma (*arrhen*, male), and the lipoid cell tumors, which include the Leydig cell and the adrenal-like or hypernephroid tumors.

Arrhenoblastoma.—This masculinizing tumor is the rarest member of the special ovarian tumors. It arises from the cells of the primitive ovarian mesenchyme which have a male tendency, and it is often found in the region of the rete ovarii, which is the homologue of the male testis. The *gross* appearance is similar to that of the granulosa cell tumor. The *microscopic* picture varies even more widely than that of the latter tumor. In some cases, but these are the exception, there is perfect reproduction of the seminiferous tubules of the testis, a condition described long ago by Ludwig Pick as *testicular adenoma of the ovary* (Fig. 553 B). More usual is a very imperfect attempt at tubule formation, the cells being arranged for the most part in irregular columns. The lining cells are cuboidal or columnar with basal nuclei resembling the Sertoli cells of the seminiferous tubules. The nuclei often show a step-ladder arrangement which may suggest to the observer the true nature of the tumor (Fig. 554). At the far end of the scale the cells are completely undifferentiated, giving a picture of sarcoma. In such cases the pathologist is dependent on the characteristic clinical history. In spite of the sarcomatous appearance the tumor is either benign or of low malignancy. The stroma of the arrhenoblastoma often contains large, polyhedral, eosinophilic cells resembling Leydig cells, cells which are found at the hilus in 80 per cent of normal ovaries. Indeed *three types of arrhenoblastoma* have been recognized: (1) a *Sertoli cell type*, (2) a *Leydig cell type*, and (3) a *mixed type* (Langley). Further reference to Leydig cells will be found in relation to the hilus cell tumor.

The *clinical effects* are at first defeminizing, later masculinizing. Amenorrhea and extreme atrophy of the breasts are the early signs. These are followed later by hirsutism with masculine distribution of hair, roughening and deepening of the voice, and hypertrophy of the clitoris. The picture is similar to that of tumor of the adrenal cortex, a structure with which the ovary is closely related developmentally.

Hilus Cell Tumor.—This tumor arises from cells at the ovarian hilus which are androgenic in function and are analogous to the Leydig cells of the testis. Both sets of cells contain lipids, lipochrome pigment, and the peculiar and characteristic rod-like structures known as the *crystalloids of Reinke*. It

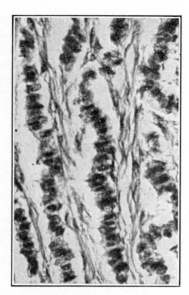

FIG. 554.—Arrhenoblastoma showing step-ladder arrangement of cells. × 220.

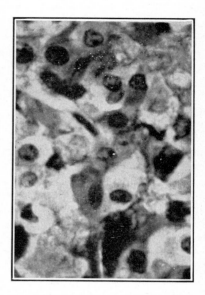

FIG. 555.—Reinke crystalloid in hilus cell tumor. × 670.

was Berger who in 1922 first recognized the significance of these hilar cells and their identity with the similar cells of the testis. He named them sympathicotropic cells because of their constant relationship to the nonmyelinated nerves of the hilus, the cells ensheathing the nerve fibers, and sometimes lying within a nerve trunk. Berger was also the first in 1942 to report a case of masculinization associated with a small tumor of ovarian hilus cells. The pathognomonic feature is the presence of intracellular Reinke crystalloids (Fig. 555). These tumors in the past have been mistaken for other masculinizing tumors of the ovary such as arrhenoblastoma and adrenal rest tumors.

Adrenal-like Tumors.—These lesions, like their name, constitute an indeterminate group of rare tumors which may be masculinizing. They originate in the hilar region, so whether or not they represent adrenal elements as has been suggested is a question which cannot be answered with certainty. Although usually only a few centimeters in diameter they may, especially when malignant, largely replace the ovary. The cytoplasm is clear owing to a high glycogen or lipid content, and the cellular arrangement may closely resemble that of the zona

glomerulosa and fasciculata of the adrenal cortex.

The *Stein-Leventhal syndrome* has already been described on page 926. This is an example of a defeminizing condition which may or may not be associated with definite masculinization, but in which the lesion in the ovaries is a non-neoplastic one, so that it does not really deserve to be mentioned here.

Dysgerminoma.—This tumor, the name of which is also spelt disgerminoma, arises from indifferent cells of the mesenchyme in the gonad which fail to develop in either a male or female direction. It may occur in the ovary or testis. In the ovary it is often bilateral, may grow to a considerable size, and shows a characteristic yellow staining of the cut surface due to lipoid degeneration.

Microscopically the tumor is simple in structure, and does not show the marked variation characteristic of the granulosa cell tumor and arrhenoblastoma. The cells are large and round with vesicular nuclei (Fig. 553, C), but they shrink to a marked degree when embedded in paraffin, and are best seen in frozen or celloidin sections. They are grouped in solid alveoli or in columns, separated by septa of fibrous tissue in which there may be large numbers of lymphocytes.

These tumors vary greatly in malignancy, nor does the microscopic picture help much in the prognosis, although the presence of numerous mitoses is of course a bad sign. The tumor is less malignant than the granulosa cell tumor but more malignant than the arrhenoblastoma. In about 25 per cent of cases there are extrapelvic metastases.

The *clinical effects* are in striking contrast to those of granulosa cell tumors and arrhenoblastoma, as might be expected from the fact that the tumor originates from indifferent sex cells. It usually arises in children and adolescents, but may occur in adults. As a rule the patient is normal sexually, but in a number of cases there has been pseudohermaphroditism, sexual hypoplasia or infantilism. This disturbance of development does not appear to be dependent on the presence of the tumor, because after surgical removal there has been no change in the clinical condition.

Brenner Tumor.—This lesion, described by Brenner in 1907, but clarified by Robert Meyer in 1932, differs sharply from the group of three "special" ovarian tumors already discussed. In the gross the tumor may take two forms, solid or cystic. The solid form, which is the usual type, tends to be small and resembles a fibroma, for which it is readily mistaken. When large, for reasons which soon will be apparent, it may take the form of mucinous cystadenoma with nodular masses of tumor persisting in the wall. There are wide variations in size; it may be minute or it may be enormous.

The *microscopic picture* has none of the extreme variability so characteristic of granulosa cell tumor and arrhenoblastoma. There are two essential elements: (1) nests of epithelial cells, and (2) fibromatous connective tissue separating these nests (Fig. 553, *D*). The epithelial cells are for the most part strikingly uniform in type, and recall the appearance of a carcinoid tumor of the appendix or bowel. There are no mitoses, nor any suggestion of malignancy. Cystic degeneration in the center of the nests is common, giving rise to an appearance which may be mistaken for follicles. One striking variation from the usual picture may occur, the cells becoming columnar and clear, secreting mucus, and lining spaces, a picture similar

to that of a mucinous cystadenoma. When this condition is widespread, the gross appearance may be identical with the ordinary cystadenoma, and the essential character of the original tumor may be overlooked. The connective-tissue elements vary, but may be so abundant that the lesion is mistaken for a fibroma.

The *origin* of the tumor has long been a matter of dispute. It used to be thought that the starting point was the so-called Walthard inclusions, which arise by metaplasia of serosal cells in the young child, but there are definite histochemical differences between the Brenner tumor cells and those of the Walthard nests. Serial sections of minute tumors show no connection with germinal epithelium, as has been suggested. It seems probable that the *origin is from follicular epithelium*, as in the case of the granulosa cell tumor (Teoh). The epithelium of the larger tumors is similar to that of granulosa cell tumors and follicular epithelium. It may be noted that there is a frequent association with mucinous cystadenoma.

For references to the group of special ovarian tumors the reader should consult the monograph of Morris and Scully and the textbook by Novak and Novak.

A summary of the special tumors and some of their principal characteristics are given in the following table.

PAROVARIAN CYST

The parovarium, which represents a remnant of the sexual part of the Wolffian body, is situated in the mesosalpinx between the ovary and the Fallopian tube. It consists of a horizontal tube, the duct of Gartner, homologous with the vas deferens, and a series of vertical tubes homologous to the vasa efferentia and epididymis. A parovarian cyst is situated between the layers of the broad ligament and may attain a great size. The wall is thick and lined by low, columnar, ciliated epithelium. Sometimes it shows warty papillary processes, but usually it is quite smooth. As the cyst occupies the broad ligament it may be mistaken for a serous cystadenoma of the ovary growing in that position. The intact ovary is attached to the side of the cyst, and the tube is stretched

vagina, so-called sarcoma of the vagina, is the same tumor as the *"grape-like sarcoma"* of the cervix. It is a malignant tumor of children, and is composed of mucoid tissue,

(Tubal pregnancy.)

COSBIE, W. G. and HENDERSON, D. N.: J. Obst. and Gyn. Brit. Empire, 1936, *43*, 655. (Carcinoma of body of uterus.)

Dexter, L. and Weiss, S.: *Preeclamptic and Eclamptic Toxemia of Pregnancy*, Boston, 1941.

Fidler, H. K. and Boyes, D. A.: Cancer, 1959, *12*, 673. (Patterns of early invasion from intra-epithelial carcinoma of cervix.)

Gardner, W. U. *et al.:* J.A.M.A., 1938, *110*, 1182. (Hormonal stimulation in carcinoma of cervix.)

Graham, R. M.: Surg., Gyn., and Obst., 1947, *84*, 153; 1951, *93*, 767. (Vaginal smears in radiation of cervical cancer.)

Hertig, A. T. and Sheldon, W. H.: Am. J. Obst. and Gyn., 1947, *53*, 1. (Hydatidiform mole.)

Jackson, R. L. and Dockerty, M. B.: Am. J. Obst. and Gynec., 1957, *73*, 161. (Stein-Leventhal syndrome.)

Langley, F. A.: J. Clin. Path., 1954, *7*, 10. (Sertoli and Leydig cells in ovarian tumors.)

McKay, D. G. *et al.:* Am. J. Obst. and Gynec., 1953, *66*, 507. (Pathological anatomy of eclampsia.)

Morris, J. M. and Scully, R. E.: *Endocrine Pathology of the Ovary*, St. Louis, 1958.

Novak, E. and Novak, E. R.: *Gynecologic and Obstetric Pathology*, Philadelphia, 1958.

Sampson, J. A.: Arch. Surg., 1921, *3*, 245. (Endometriosis.)

Stein, I. F. and Leventhal, M. L.: Am. J. Obst. and Gynec., 1935, *29*, 181. (Stein-Leventhal syndrome.)

Teoh, T. B.: J. Path. and Bact., 1959, *78*, 145. (Origin of Brenner tumor.)

Warwick, O. H. and Phillips, A. J.: Brit. J. Cancer, 1954, *8*, 223. (Cancer of cervix in Canadian Indians.)

Weller, C. V.: Am. J. Path., 1935, *11*, 287. (Endometriosis.)

Chapter 34

The Breast

General Considerations
  STRUCTURE
  DEVELOPMENT
  HORMONAL STIMULATION
    Gynecomastia
Cystic Hyperplasia
  RELATION TO CARCINOMA
Sclerosing Adenosis
Fibroepithelial Tumors
  FIBROADENOMA
    Intracanalicular
    Pericanalicular
    Giant Fibroadenoma (Cysto-
    sarcoma Phyllodes)
  DUCT PAPILLOMA
Carcinoma
  CAUSAL FACTORS

Hormonal Stimulation
The Milk Factor
Retention of Secretion
CLASSIFICATION
SCIRRHOUS CARCINOMA
MEDULLARY CARCINOMA
  Acute Carcinoma
ADENOCARCINOMA
PAPILLARY DUCT CARCINOMA
PAGET'S DISEASE
  Extramammary Paget's
  Disease
SPREAD
  Infiltration
  Lymph Spread
  Blood Spread

RELATION OF SYMPTOMS TO
  LESIONS
EFFECT OF RADIATION
PROGNOSIS
CARCINOMA OF THE MALE
  BREAST
BLEEDING FROM THE NIPPLE
SARCOMA
Cysts of the Breast
Acute Mastitis
Other Lesions of the Breast
  FAT NECROSIS
  PLASMA CELL MASTITIS
  TUBERCULOSIS
  ACTINOMYCOSIS
  HYPERTROPHY
  CONGENITAL ANOMALIES

GENERAL CONSIDERATIONS

Structure.—The breast is in essence a modified sweat gland. The normal virgin breast in the intermenstrual period consists of a small number of ducts with rudimentary acini. They are surrounded by a specialized loose connective tissue, the periductal tissue, which is under hormonal influence and is quite distinct from the general stroma of the breast. The combined glandular and specialized connective tissue form a series of islands known as lobules or gland fields (Fig. 556, p. 942).

The epithelium lining the commencement of the lactiferous duct is stratified as far as the ampulla, where it gives place to tall columnar epithelium. When the small ducts are reached the epithelium becomes cuboidal, and the terminal acini are lined with the same variety. Although at first sight it appears as if the ducts were lined by one layer of epithelial cells, there is in reality a second flattened layer outside, which may be described as a *reserve layer* for reproducing the lining cells, much as the basal layer of the epidermis replaces the cells lying superficial to it. Its cells proliferate and enlarge in pathological conditions, so that it is common to find the ducts and acini lined by a definite double layer of cells. A single layer can seldom be found in a fibro-adenoma, in cystic hyperplasia the cells are frequently several layers in depth, and in carcinoma they have begun to invade the connective tissue stroma.

In addition to the ordinary epithelial lining of the ducts *myo-epithelial cells* may be observed at short intervals lying beneath the low columnar epithelium and within the basement membrane. These cells have their long axis tangential to the circumference of the duct, intensely hyperchromatic nuclei, and cytoplasm which stains red with Masson's hematoxylin-erythrosin-saffron technique. It is of interest to note, in view of the fact that the breast is a modified sweat gland, that in the sweat glands of the skin spindle-shaped cells resembling smooth muscle cells are arranged longitudinally around the secretory portions of the tubules, their contractions possibly assisting in expelling the sweat. We shall encounter these myo-epithelial cells again in the discussion of gynecomastia and sclerosing adenosis.

The *lymphatics* of the breast are extremely numerous, unfortunately for the woman who develops carcinoma. They drain into two main basins, namely the axillary nodes and the nodes of the internal mammary chain. A rich plexus surrounds the lobules which communicates with the subareolar plexus and by large vessels with the deep fascial plexus underlying the pectoral fascia. Main trunks pass to the axillary and supraclavicular groups of nodes. On the medial side of the breast lymphatics follow the perforating branches of the internal mammary artery, draining into the nodes along that vessel and into the mediastinal nodes. There are also crossed anastomoses with the lymphatics in the opposite breast and also with the abdominal network. From this account it will be evident that removal of the axillary nodes is but a feeble attempt to arrest the outward march of carcinoma cells by the lymphatic route.

Development.—The development of the breasts is first indicated by an ectodermal thickening along a line running from the axilla to the groin on both sides; these are known as the *milk lines*. The epithelial cells along these lines have the potential ability to grow into the underlying mesenchyme and form mammary glands. In the human the breast only develops at one site, but in pigs and other animals with numerous offspring two rows of mammary glands develop in order to feed their large families. In the human female supernumerary nipples and even breasts may develop along this line, and require surgical removal. The enlargement of the breasts at puberty is due to an accumulation of fat in these modified sweat glands. These changes at puberty are due to the action of estrogen, so that they do not occur in the male. The development of true secretory units must await the complex stimulus of pregnancy.

Hormonal Stimulation.—Just as the endometrium is not a static structure but shows cyclic changes due to ovarian stimulation, so also does the breast. Indeed there is no organ which shows a wider range of structural variation in health. Up to the time of puberty the parenchyma consists only of ducts. At puberty under the influence of estrogen active budding of the ducts occurs, and from these buds the acini are formed later. It is during pregnancy and lactation that the changes are most marked. The breast in pregnancy consists of a mass of glandular tissue which entirely replaces the fat, and which has been likened to the pancreas in structure. When the placental stimulus is

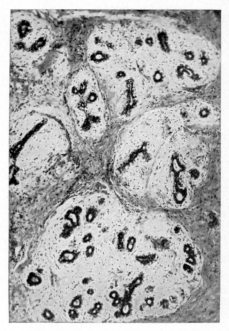

FIG. 556.—Gland fields of the breast. Six units are shown, each consisting of a group of ducts surrounded by specialized pale connective tissue. Changes in these units are the basis of cystic hyperplasia and fibroadenoma. × 75.

withdrawn lactation (secretion) begins, and this is accompanied by a marked invasion of lymphocytes. After lactation comes involution, but this is never complete and the glandular overgrowth does not entirely disappear. At the menopause the glandular tissue is replaced by connective tissue. This is complete involution.

During each menstrual cycle these structural changes are reproduced in miniature. The normal virgin breast in the intermenstrual period consists of a small number of ducts with rudimentary acini. These are surrounded by a specialized loose connective tissue, the *periductal tissue*, which is under hormonal influence and is quite distinct from the general stroma of the breast. The combined glandular and specialized connective tissue form a series of islands known as lobules or gland fields (Fig. 556). Only a certain proportion of the gland fields undergo menstrual changes. At the menses some of the epithelial cells are desquamated, the remainder atrophy and there is shrinkage of the ducts. A few days after the period the duct system begins to proliferate, the epithelial cells increase in size and number, and here is development of soft, pale, periductal connective tissue, mucoid in character and infiltrated with lymphocytes. Wide morphological variations may occur, which are beautifully illustrated in Helen Ingleby's paper.

Conflicting explanations which we cannot go into here are given for the changes which characterize the breast in pregnancy as the result of hormonal stimulation. It is obvious that *estrogen* from the placenta and *progesterone* at first from the corpus luteum and later from the placenta are all-important, but *anterior pituitary hormones* also play a part. In animals from whom the ovaries have been removed anterior pituitary extract causes enlargement of the breasts, and in the absence of the pituitary estrogen and progesterone are without effect. It would appear that growth of the breast is dependent on these three groups of hormones.

During pregnancy the breast secretes colostrum, a fluid rich in protein and poor in fat, but no milk, because the release of lactogenic hormone from the anterior pituitary is inhibited by the large amounts of estrogen from the placenta. It is only after delivery and removal of the placenta that the resulting decrease of estrogen allows full production of the *lactogenic hormone*, which ensures the prompt delivery of milk.

Gynecomastia.—Gynecomastia is a hypertrophy of the male breast, being commonest in adolescent boys, but also occurring later in life. It is the result of hormonal imbalance, due to a relative or absolute increase in estrogen (Karsner). It may occur as a complication of the rare *feminizing tumor of the adrenal*, of *pituitary* and *testicular tumors*, and of *diffuse liver disease* such as cirrhosis, because the liver is the chief organ responsible for inactivation of estrogenic hormones. One or both breasts are enlarged and tender. The periductal tissue is increased in amount compared with that of the normal male breast, loose and myxomatous in character, and rich in hyaluronic acid (Fisher and Creed). The same mucopolysaccharide is found in fibroadenoma in the female. Proliferation of myo-epithelium plays an important part in the ductal hyperplasia of

gynecomastia (Karnauchow). This may proliferate alone or with the ordinary ductal epithelium to form benign intraductal papillary growths, and may even extend into the periductal connective tissue, although still confined by the basement membrane. The condition has no relation to carcinoma.

The infinitely delicate balance between the ovarian hormonal stimuli is easily upset, and this upset is reflected in the mirror of the breast. The ducts become hypertrophied and dilated and the connective tissue is increased. These changes may be within physiological limits, (*mazoplasia*), or they may form the basis of *mammary dysplasia* (Ingleby and Gershon-Cohen) with such lesions as cystic hyperplasia, fibroadenoma and duct papilloma (Fig. 557).

CYSTIC HYPERPLASIA

In our study of most other organs we have seen that acute inflammation, granulomas, vascular disturbances, etc. were among the most common conditions to be considered. This is not true of the breast. In the breast the common presenting lesion is in the form of a lump or mass, and this mass usually represents one of three conditions, namely cystic hyperplasia, fibroadenoma and carcinoma. It is obvious that the last of these three, which is the commonest form of cancer in women, must first be excluded before the other two can be considered, and it is here that the work of the pathologist proves invaluable and often indispensable.

Nature of the Condition.—Cystic hyperplasia, the commonest structural lesion of the breast, is an exaggeration of the normal cyclic physiological changes outlined above. Countless names have been attached to the condition over the years. Until recently the common name was *chronic mastitis*, although this is in no sense an inflammation of the breast. One of the best terms is lobular hyperplasia with or without cyst formation (Smith). This was used in previous editions of this book, but it has never been generally accepted. Cystic hyperplasia is admittedly inadequate, as there may be no gross cysts but merely dilation of the ducts. It is, however, a convenient makeshift. The basis of the condition is *hormonal imbalance*, prob-

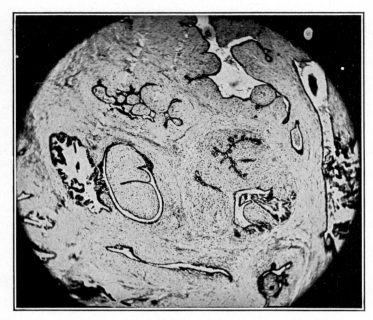

Fig. 557.—Section of breast showing a combination of cystic hyperplasia and fibroadenoma. × 40.

ably corpus luteum deficiency combined with an excess of estrogenic stimulation. It is, therefore, chiefly seen in the last decade of reproductive life when hormonal production becomes irregular but the main symptoms may not appear till after the menopause.

Morbid Anatomy.—The *gross appearance* is characteristic, and it is usually easy to make a naked-eye diagnosis when the specimen is removed in the operating room. As the involvement of the lobules is so variable the condition may be general or local, and each of these may be cystic or non-cystic, at least to the naked eye. The generalized cystic form is known as *Schimmelbusch's disease*, in which the breast may be riddled with large smooth-wall cysts. Sometimes there is a single large cyst tensely filled with fluid and known as the *blue-domed cyst.* Cysts of varying size and number are usually present (Fig. 558), but usually they are small. The cause of the cyst formation is obscure. The dilated ducts may be filled with putty-like material which can be squeezed out like worm casts. The lesion is characteristically tough and like rubber in consistence, but without the hardness of

carcinoma, nor has it the circumscribed character of a malignant mass, shading off into the surrounding tissue. The color is gray.

The varied *microscopic picture* presents one or more of the following features: (1) *Glandular hyperplasia* is usually marked as evidenced by the number and prominence of the gland fields. The acini are represented by solid buds of cells which stain darkly. This appearance is likely to be found in younger women. (2) *Cyst formation* is so common that it has been incorporated in such names as cystic mastitis (Fig. 559). The cysts are usually small, they may be microscopic in size, or they may be as large as a cherry. The cysts are formed from the ducts, not as the result of obstruction by fibrous tissue nor distention by secretion, but because the hyperplastic duct has not undergone complete involution to the normal size. When a cyst is once formed, secretion may add to its size. (3) *Papillary formation* may be very striking owing to the epithelial cells growing in bud-like formation into the cyst spaces. This intraductal epithelial proliferation may progress to such a degree that the entire lumen

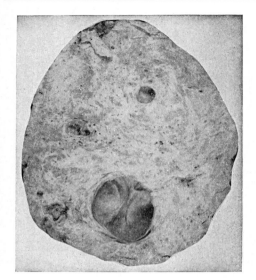

Fig. 558.—Cystic hyperplasia. All of the tissue shown is the seat of a diffuse induration. There are several cysts of varying size and many very minute cysts.

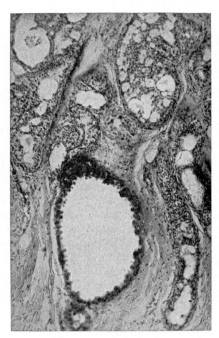

Fig. 559.—Cystic hyperplasia. Both epithelial proliferation and cyst formation are present. There is commencing papillary formation in the large cyst.

becomes packed with cells. It may be very difficult to distinguish this condition from carcinoma, and in some cases actual invasion of the surrounding tissue may occur. (4) *Acidophilic epithelial cells* may line the cyst or form the papillary processes (Fig. 560). Part of a cyst may be lined by normal cells, and part by the large cells, the cytoplasm of which stains pink with eosin. The change appears to be due to hyalinization of the epithelium. The cytoplasm of these cells when suitably stained is found to be filled with granules, and the appearance of these cells is identical with that of the cells of the specialized apocrine sweat glands in the axilla and elsewhere (Lendrum). Both mammary epithelium and the epithelium of apocrine glands arise from primitive sweat gland epithelium, and the mammary epithelium may become dedifferentiated to the primitive sweat gland type, and in the subsequent regeneration acquire the characteristics of apocrine sweat gland epithelium. Bunting, on the other hand, has shown that true apocrine sweat glands with eosinophilic epithelium are normal constituents of the breast, presenting the same patterns of lipid and iron which are characteristic of the apocrine glands in the axilla and elsewhere. (5) *Connective tissue hyperplasia* is an inte-

gral part of the process, but varies greatly in amount. It is the specialized connective tissue of the gland fields which is involved, not the stroma of the breast. The overgrowth may be so great that the condition is practically one of pericanalicular fibroma. (6) *Lymphocytic infiltration* is a very common feature, and is responsible for the misconception that the condition is a mastitis.

Relation of Symptoms to Lesions.—The patient is usually in the involutionary period of life, at a time when the ovarian function is irregular and declining. Another group is seen in young unmarried women who often present evidence of disturbance of ovarian function. They really suffer from hypoactivity of the ovaries (short and scanty menstruation) with overactive or persistent corpora lutea. The condition is commoner in multiparæ, whose breasts have repeatedly passed through the periodic hyperplasia and involution of pregnancy and lactation. The woman complains either of pain or a lump in the breast; the pain is usually worse at the menstrual period. There is tenderness as well as pain. Both breasts are often in-

60

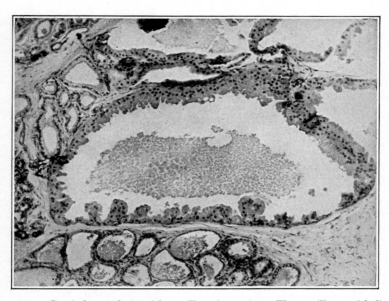

FIG. 560.—Cystic hyperplasia with papillary formation. The papillary epithelium
stained pink with eosin. × 90.

volved, and there may be several lumps in each breast, which always suggests an innocent condition. The breast may feel coarsely granular owing to the presence of small cysts; such cysts always feel as hard as a tumor, never soft and fluctuating. The axillary lymph nodes may be enlarged and tender for a reason which is not obvious. The natural history of the disease varies greatly. New cysts often continue to form over a period of years, but in some cases when a single cyst is removed no more develop. In the course of time the active phase ceases, the cysts become smaller, and by the time of the menopause with the cessation of hormonal stimulation the disease has usually run its course.

The Relation of Cystic Hyperplasia to Carcinoma.—The question of the relation of cystic hyperplasia to carcinoma is a very difficult one, regarding which there are great differences of opinion. The condition is commonly regarded as precancerous and a radical operation is often done lest a worse thing should befall the patient. This may be advisable in an elderly patient, but is certainly unjustifiable in a young woman. The writer feels that from the pathological point of view it is possible to trace a long series of progressive changes in the duct epithelium, until the ducts are filled with masses of cells which are indistinguishable histologically from cancer cells and which may finally break through the wall and invade the surrounding tissues (Fig. 561). Actively proliferating lesions such as intraduct papilloma and cysts with papillary epithelium are of graver import than large cysts with atrophic epithelium. Greene has observed a strain of rabbits many of whom developed cystic disease of the breast followed by carcinoma. The cystic disease phase was identical with Schimmelbusch's disease in women. Within the cysts there occurred first epithelial hyperplasia, then neoplasia, and finally invasion. These changes were watched by means of repeated biopsies. From the pathological standpoint, therefore, the condition may be regarded as precancerous. The final court of appeal should be studies on women who have had complete (but not radical) removal of the gross lesion. Unfortunately there is no unanimity on this point in the published reports. Clinicians of great experience conclude from such studies that there is no causal relationship between the two conditions, although cystic hyperplasia may be

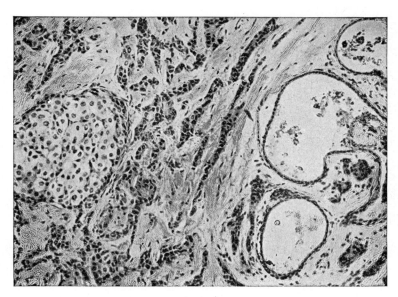

FIG. 561.—Carcinoma of the breast associated with cystic hyperplasia. (Boyd, *Pathology for the Surgeon*, courtesy of W. B. Saunders Co.)

combined with carcinoma in 75 to 80 per cent of cases. Such figures mean little or nothing. When two diseases are common in the same sex and in the same age period they must inevitably be associated very frequently. Shields Warren, as the result of careful histological and follow-up studies, believes that a woman who has had cystic hyperplasia is in far greater danger of developing cancer, even though all the apparently abnormal tissue has been removed, but once she has passed the menopause there is no greater danger than in any control group.

It is important to distinguish between possibility and probability, as in the case of gastric ulcer and carcinoma. No one would deny the *possibility* of certain forms of cystic hyperplasia passing into carcinoma, but the question is, how often? If it is frequent, mastectomy, often bilateral, must become a common prophylactic procedure; if but seldom, the risk of cancer developing may be too small to justify an operation entailing physical mutilation and psychic trauma. If the majority of surgeons were women rather than men the outlook on the best practical procedure might possibly be different!

SCLEROSING ADENOSIS

The importance of this condition, also known as *fibrosing adenosis*, is the ease with which it can be mistaken for carcinoma, especially in frozen sections. In 1000 female breasts removed surgically there were 12 cases in which sclerosing adenosis was the primary lesion and 73 in which it was an incidental finding (Sandison). The condition is commoner in young women. The breast contains a number of hard discrete nodules, the cut surface of which is uniform in contrast with that of carcinoma. *Microscopically* there is hyperplasia and distortion of the mammary lobules, with a disorderly arrangement of an abundant collagenous stroma which accentuates the irregular lobular arrangement. This can best be seen with the low power of the microscope (Fig. 562). It has been suggested that the new material is formed of myo-epithelial cells and that the condition should be called myoid sclerosis (Ingleby and Gershon-Cohen). The fibrosis gradually dominates the picture, finally leading to atrophy, with a tendency for the acini to break up into small groups and clumps of cells, a picture which may readily be mistaken for carcinoma in frozen

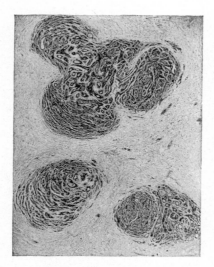

FIG. 562.—Fibrosing adenosis. × 22. (Boyd, *Pathology for the Surgeon,* courtesy of W. B. Saunders Co.)

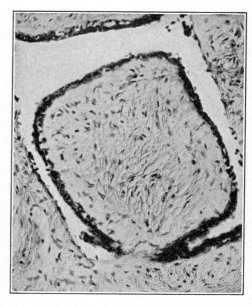

FIG. 563.—Intracanalicular fibroadenoma. The process of formation is shown here, but usually no connection can be seen between the mass within the duct and the surrounding wall. × 75.

sections. For excellent illustrations of this important lesion the papers by E.K. Dawson and by Urban and Adair should be consulted. The condition bears no relation to malignancy.

FIBROEPITHELIAL TUMORS

When the hyperplasia which is characteristic of aberrant breast physiology is localized, a nodular condition is produced which is commonly regarded as a tumor. The hyperplastic area may be semi-encapsulated, being sharply demarcated on one side but continuous with the breast tissue on the other. The hypertrophy may be great enough to push the fibrous tissue aside so that a complete capsule is formed. If the overgrowth chiefly affects the connective tissue we speak of a *fibroma.* As a rule both epithelial and fibrous tissues share in the overgrowth, giving a *fibroadenoma.* Localized epithelial overgrowth into a dilated duct forms a *duct papilloma.*

Fibroadenoma.—A fibroadenoma occurs chiefly in young women, originating perhaps at puberty and growing during the years of developing sexual activity. It is commoner in nulliparæ than in those who have borne children, differing in this respect from cystic hyperplasia. It is a slowly growing tumor, but growth may be more rapid during adolescence, in pregnancy and toward the menopause periods, when the concentration of estrogen is high.

It is customary to recognize two forms of tumor, the intracanalicular and the pericanalicular. The *intracanalicular fibroadenoma* is the common variety (Fig. 563). As the hyperplasia involves particularly the specialized connective tissue of the lobules, the tumor is more a fibroma than an adenoma. It is usually well encapsulated, has a soft consistency and a rather moist appearance, and the cut surface may show many narrow slits or splits (the ducts), so that the appearance may resemble the leaves of a book; sometimes little masses can be distinguished enclosed within small spaces. The encapsulation may be only partial, the tumor blending on one side with the surrounding breast tissue. *Microscopically* there is a great proliferation of loose connective tissue of open structure which invaginates the wall of the ducts, projecting into the lumen to form polypoid masses, and producing great dilatation, elongation, and distortion of the ducts (Fig. 564). The connection of these

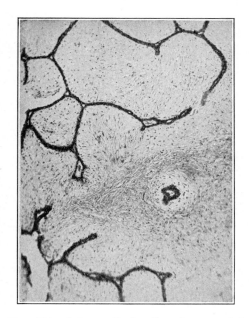

FIG. 564.—Intracanalicular fibroadenoma of the breast. The ducts are elongated and distorted by the new fibrous tissue. × 75.

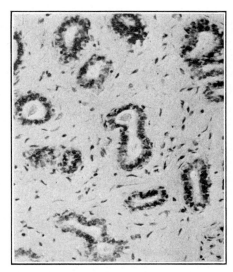

FIG. 565.—Pericanalicular fibroadenoma. The ducts are surrounded by the new fibrous tissue. × 200.

polypoid growths with the wall of the duct is often not seen in the section, so that fibrous masses covered by a layer of epithelium appear to be lying free in the lumen. The ordinary connective stroma of the breast takes no part in the overgrowth. The lobules of the surrounding tissue often show hyperplasia, and in those cases where the encapsulation is only partial the similarity of structure of the tumor and the adjacent tissue may be very striking.

The *pericanalicular fibroadenoma* is a much harder tumor, and seldom becomes as large as the preceding variety. It is well encapsulated, and when the sheath is incised it can usually be shelled out quite readily. It has a characteristic mobility when palpated. The cut surface is white, dry, and homogeneous. *Microscopically* there is a proliferation of glandular and fibrous tissue. The new connective tissue surrounds the ducts without invaginating them, hence the name pericanalicular (Fig. 565). The picture suggests less active growth than that of the preceding variety.

The distinction between the two forms, however, is not fundamental. Examine the intracanalicular type and many areas of pericanalicular formation will be found. Taking the broader view we may say that a fibroadenoma may be predominantly intracanalicular or pericanalicular in type. The recognition of the two forms is customary but somewhat unnecessary.

Cystosarcoma Phyllodes.—This is a very rare tumor for which Stewart lists 44 synonyms. Of these should be mentioned *giant fibroadenoma, giant intracanalicular myxoma* (Owens and Adams), and *adenosarcoma phyllodes,* for they all give some insight into the nature of the lesion. It is a giant variant of fibroadenoma, with an average weight of $7\frac{1}{2}$ lbs. (Lee and Pack) and one recorded example of 35 lbs. When the tumor starts to enlarge the connective tissue takes on a myxomatous character. The tumor was first described in 1838 by Johannes Müller, who gave it the name of cystosarcoma phyllodes, because it contained cysts, was fleshy, and presented clefts like the leaves of a book (*phyllon,* leaf). In those days the term sarcoma denoted flesh, not malignancy. Myxomatous processes which grow into the numerous cysts are crowded together to give a leaf-like appearance. The tumor usually remains benign, but occasionally may become truly sarcomatous and metastasize to the lungs or lymph nodes.

Duct Papilloma.—This condition is also known as adenocystoma, papillary cystoma,

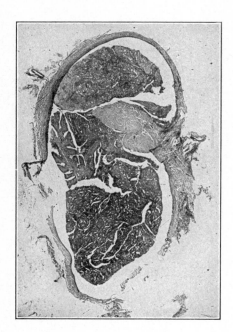

Fig. 566.—Duct papilloma of the breast. The duct is greatly distended by a raspberry-like mass. × 10.

intracystic papilloma, and many other names. The papilloma projects into a dilated duct, usually in the vicinity of the nipple. At first it is composed of a series of folds so that it resembles a small raspberry, but as it increases in size the folds or villi adhere together so that the surface becomes smoother. Finally it distends the ducts and becomes a solid compact mass. *Microscopically* the tumor consists at first of numerous delicate villi covered by epithelium, but as it increases in size and the processes are pressed together, adhere and interlace, gland-like spaces are formed so that the appearance becomes adenomatous (Fig. 566). This explains the use of such a term as adenocystoma. The blood vessels are numerous and thin-walled so that hemorrhage is common, and a blood-stained discharge from the nipple is one of the characteristic symptoms. In some cases a malignant change seems to develop and the condition becomes a duct carcinoma. Other observers consider that benign intraduct papilloma is a fairly common lesion, that papillary carcinoma is very rare and arises de novo, that there is no evi-

dence of a change of the benign into the malignant type even after many years, and that the papilloma does not recur if properly removed by local excision rather than by mastectomy (Haagensen and Stout).

CARCINOMA

Carcinoma of the breast is the commonest form of cancer in women. It is twice as common as cancer of the cervix, the next most common variety. The disease is said to occur in 5 per cent of the adult female population. Such a figure proves, were such proof needed, that every lump in the breast should be regarded as a possible carcinoma until proved otherwise. It usually occurs during the involution period, *i.e.*, in the years before the menopause, and it is rare before the age of thirty-five years. There is a higher incidence in nulliparæ, and the disease bears no relation to repeated suckling. Pregnancy, indeed, appears to have a protective influence.

Causal Factors.—We shall discuss possible causal factors rather than etiology, which suggests a single agent. As a matter of fact disease is seldom caused by a single factor. Certainly the presence in the body of the diphtheria bacillus or the tubercle bacillus is not enough to produce diphtheria or tuberculosis. Three types of agent have been incriminated in the pathogenesis of carcinoma of the breast: (1) hormonal stimulation; (2) the Bittner milk factor, a virus in the mother's milk; (3) retention of secretion. As in our previous studies of carcinogenesis we must try to distinguish between an inducing factor and a continuing one, although in the present instance such a distinction is difficult if not impossible.

1. *Hormonal Stimulation.*—In the section on General Considerations we have seen that the development and growth of the breast are under the influence of the ovary, the adrenal and the pituitary. This is true also of mammary carcinoma. Indeed no other tumor exhibits such a wide range of endocrine influences. Four hormones are principally involved: (1) estrogen, (2) progesterone, (3) pituitary lactogenic hormone, and (4) pituitary mammotrophic or mammogentic hormone (prolactin). The endocrine

organs involved in the production of this hormonal tetrad are of course the ovary, adrenal and anterior pituitary. Some idea of the amount of hormones being produced may be gained from a measurement of their excretion in the urine. It will be realized that when we say that mammary carcinoma is extremely susceptible to endocrine influence, we do not mean to imply that such influence is necessarily responsible for the original induction of the tumor. Moreover not all cancers of the breast are *hormone-dependent*. Only 50 per cent belong to this group (Hadfield), although some clinicians give a figure as high as 60 per cent, and only 40 per cent are markedly dependent. The remainder have the gloomy and mysterious attribute of "autonomy", so often regarded as the essential biological characteristic of all malignant tumors. Unfortunately the histology of the tumor gives no indication of its dependence or otherwise. It is now recognized, however, that the enzyme content of the cancer cells may give us some lead in this respect. A histochemical study of breast tumors showed abundant esterase, lipase and succinic dehydrogenase in well differentiated adenocarcinomas, less in scirrhous carcinomas, and none in medullary carcinomas (Melnick and Bullock). There is histochemical evidence that in estrogen-sensitive tissues estrogen acts as a co-factor for transhydrogenase, thus releasing more energy for metabolic activities.

Both clinical and experimental observations support the concept of endocrine influence on breast cancer. The highest *incidence of cancer* is between the ages of forty and fifty years, when the influence of estrogen is especially strong, women with a delayed menopause appear to be excessively prone to develop the disease, the incidence is low in women who have had an ovariectomy, and the tumor is 100 times commoner in the female breast than in the male. If the ovaries are removed in young mice with a high mammary cancer strain the danger of development of the tumor will be completely averted. The repeated injection of estrogen into mice will produce mammary cancer in a high percentage of cases, including males of a non-susceptible strain (Lacassagne). None of this, of course, is proof that human breast cancer is induced by hormonal stimulation, nor has cancer been produced in the higher mammals closely related to man by the use of estrogens.

It is of interest to note that in a series of 207 cases of cancer of the breast in all but a few instances there was hyperplasia of pituitary amphophils and basophils, adrenal cortex, and ovarian stroma, combined with thyroid atrophy, with evidence of continuous estrogen stimulation of the epithelium of the breast (Sommers). In these cases the breast and ovaries appeared to act as target organs.

Normal breast growth is controlled by the synergistic action of the pituitary hormone prolactin acting at a relatively high concentration with ovarian estrogen acting at a relatively low one. Growth of cancer is affected by these and the other hormones just mentioned. Combined oophorectomy and adrenalectomy deprive the breast cancer of estrogenic steroids, and growth regression follows if the tumor is hormone-dependent. This effect seems to be almost always temporary, although the remarkable relief to the symptoms caused by both the primary tumor and the metastases have been justifiable described as "a superb palliation." The effect is an all-or-nothing one; either all the tumors are affected or none of them are. Similarly none of the hormone-independent tumors, primary or secondary, are affected. When growth of the cancer is resumed it may again be arrested by hypophysectomy, a last resort for metastic breast cancer, but once more the effect is temporary. If the urine of a woman with breast cancer has no mammotrophic activity, it seems very probable that her cancer would not be hormone-dependent and that hypophysectomy would be of no benefit.

The concept of the endocrine relationships of breast cancer, although by no means new, has hit both the experimentalist and the clinician with explosive violence. Several symposia devoted to this subject have been published in book form, including one edited by Currie with 88 contributors. Unfortunately (or fortunately) what is true of this subject today is apt to be out of date tomorrow. Hormone therapy, both additive and subtractive, has given marked relief in many inoperable cases. Androgens may benefit one case and estrogens another. The possible value of oophorectomy, adrenalectomy and hypophysectomy has already been mentioned. We are still in the dark as to why the benefit of these procedures is only temporary; they never cure the patient, but that does not mean that they are of little value. It has been suggested that overgrowth of accessory adrenal tissue restores the original hormonal balance, but how do we account for the relapse after hypophysectomy? The explanation may be similar to that which we are accustomed to apply to the emergence of antibiotic-resistance in a bacterial population. When the sensitive bacteria are eliminated, the resistant ones take possession. In the same way destruction of hormone-dependent cancer cells may be followed by proliferation of hormone-resistant ones. We may close this discussion with the sobering thought that removal of a target organ such as the steroid-producing endocrines may increase and accelerate the production of the breast-stimulating hormones of the pituitary. Harm may be done as well as help given, and, as we have so often seen already in this book, what is powerful for good may become potent for evil. From this discussion the student will gather that the subject of the endocrinology of breast cancer is as important practically as it is fascinating intellectually.

2. *The Milk Factor.*—The importance of heredity in the etiology of cancer is well recognized, but Bittner has shown that in mouse mammary cancer some extrachromosomal influence may be transmitted in the mother's milk. If the young of a high breast tumor stock are suckled by mothers of a low breast tumor stock the incidence of breast cancer is greatly reduced. Bittner has succeeded in extracting the cancer-producing factor in the breast of animals with high spontaneous carcinoma of the breast. When this factor was given to animals with a normal incidence of this tumor the incidence rose from 1 per cent to 67 per cent. It seems certain that the carcinogenic factor is a filterable virus. It is rather startling to learn that the factor may be transmitted by the male mouse as well as by the female. Wood and Darling report a cancer family in which a number of instances of bilateral mammary carcinoma occurred in the course of four generations. In the third generation three sisters developed breast cancer. The cancer occurred only in those women who had been nursed by their mothers, a fact suggesting the operation of a factor similar to the "milk influence" demonstrated by Bittner in mice. It is obvious that it would be most desirable to learn to what extent Bittner's work on the mouse can be applied to the human female, but the difficulties in the way are also obvious. It is possible that a virus in the mother's milk may be the *fons et origo* of the entire complex process, the spark which kindles the neoplastic fire in later life when conditioning factors such as hormonal imbalance or irritation in the ducts prepare the stage for the final act.

3. *Retention of Secretion.*—Breast drainage may be interfered with as the result of anomalies of the duct, a plug of desquamated cells in the duct, etc. The breast of the typical spinster has an underdeveloped, small, hard, fibrosed nipple, and we have already seen that cancer is commoner in those who have never borne children. According to Adair only 8.5 per cent of patients with cancer of the breast give a normal nursing history. Bagg has shown that in a strain of mice with a low incidence of cancer of the breast, ligation of the ducts to the nipples on one side of the body half way through pregnancy frequently produced carcinoma. By means of very rapid breeding without accompanying suckling he also produced a high proportion of cancer. After all, the animal with the most over-worked mammary gland in the world, namely, the cow, never develops mammary cancer.

Infiltrating carcinoma may originate *de novo* from normal breast tissue. In many cases, however, there is a preliminary epithelial hyperplasia followed by neoplasia within the ducts before infiltration occurs. This may affect many groups of cells, so that the tumor may be of multicentric origin (Muir), an illustration of wide field of origin of carcinoma. Greene has observed a similar process in rabbits in whom, by means

PLATE XIII

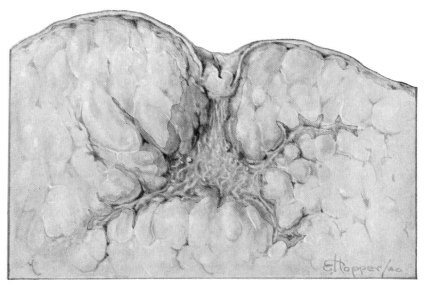

Carcinoma of Breast

The concave surface, the indrawn nipple, the infiltration, and the yellowish-grey
streaks are all shown.

of repeated biopsies, he was able to watch the gradual evolution of the tumor.

Trauma and external irritation bear no relation to cancer of the breast. If trauma were a factor, the disease would be more frequent among the laboring and agricultural classes. That a physical trauma should produce breast cancer is contrary to the dictum that the stimulus to cancer must be of the same type as that to which the particular tissue is biologically best adapted to respond with proliferation.

Classification.—A great variety of forms of breast carcinoma have been described. Some of the names apply to the gross appearance, some to the microscopic structure, and some to the clinical behavior. The great majority of cases can be placed in one of the following five groups: (1) scirrhous carcinoma, (2) medullary carcinoma, (3) adenocarcinoma, (4) duct carcinoma, and (5) Paget's disease. Rarely the tumor is so undifferentiated that it cannot be placed in any of these groups; this may be called the anaplastic form.

When the names of these five types are analysed it will be realized that scirrhous means hard, medullary means soft (like bone marrow), adenocarcinoma indicates the histological structure, duct carcinoma signifies cancer of a duct, whilst Paget's disease means nothing at all except that the condition was first described by Paget. This is hardly a classification of which to be proud, but it seems to work. For those desirous of a more scientific and comprehensive classification, that given by Foote and Stewart can be recommended. Their material is illustrated both in their paper and in Stewart's superb monograph and atlas on *Tumors of the Breast,* from which I quote this penetrating comment on classification: "Classification of tumor types is one of the bugbears of pathology. Not only are there many classifications, but there are many useless classifications. The same words do not signify the same things to different pathologists, and rarely do they mean anything at all to clinicians." It need hardly be mentioned that a pathologist is speaking. Finally it may be pointed out that cancer of the breast is probably not one neoplastic disease but a group of various cancers, which have dif-

ferent modes of origin and different natural histories, and which in many instances require different forms of therapy. The diversity of histological structure is well illustrated in the beautiful pictures in Lewison's monograph on breast cancer. The doctor who undertakes to treat this condition is not faced with a simple problem.

Scirrhous Carcinoma.—This is much the commonest form of cancer of the breast. It usually begins in the upper and outer quadrant of the breast, where it forms a hard nodule which can best be appreciated with the palm of the hand. It becomes fixed to the deep fascia and later to the skin, but if the growth occurs midway between fascia and skin the tumor may be freely movable for some time. There may be slight dimpling of the skin due to lymphatic edema. Fixation and retraction of the nipple is a late symptom, caused by involvement of the large milk ducts. The breast is small and flattened. It must be understood that in the *early* (operable) *stage* the only sign may be a hard nodule in the breast. Any such nodule in the breast of a woman in the cancer period may be carcinoma, and should at once be examined. Scirrhous carcinoma grows more slowly than the medullary form, but the ultimate prognosis is no better, because though local growth is slow, dissemination occurs early.

Morbid Anatomy.—The lesion is definitely circumscribed in comparison with cystic hyperplasia, although of course it is not encapsulated and sends processes into the surrounding tissue. It forms a definite *tumor;* an absolutely diffuse lesion is almost certain to be cystic hyperplasia, not carcinoma. It is peculiarly hard, a feature from which it derives its name (*skirros,* hard). It cuts with the grittiness of an unripe pear, so that a diagnosis can often be made the moment the knife enters the tumor. As Bichat put it long, long ago: "Il crie sous le scalpel." The cut surface is gray, and is seldom homogeneous, presenting yellow or gray streaks which represent clumps of necrotic fatty tumor cells (Plate XIII). The cut surface is concave, retracting below the general level (Fig. 567). Small cysts may be present. The gross appearance of a scirrhous cancer is usually quite characteristic. When

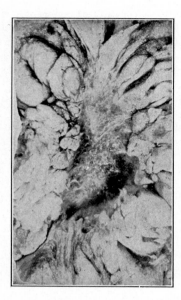

FIG. 567.—Scirrhous carcinoma of the breast. The tumor is in the center of the specimen. It is fairly well circumscribed and depressed below the surrounding tissue; the cut surface is marked by streaks.

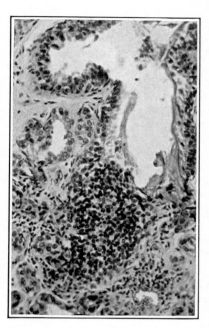

FIG. 568.—Carcinoma of breast arising from wall of duct. × 145.

the tumor is exposed it is incised. This is not attended by any danger of dissemination as used to be feared. If the tumor is found to be malignant, by frozen section if necessary, radical removal of the breast and the surrounding structures is done at once, whereas if it appears to be benign the entire lump is removed and the diagnosis verified by frozen section on the spot or later paraffin sections. Prior to operation no surgeon in the world can be certain that a localized lump in the breast is not a carcinoma, however innocent it may appear to be.

The *microscopic appearance* is also readily recognized. The tumor originates from the epithelium lining a duct (Fig. 568), so that in reality the tumor is a variant of adenocarcinoma, but soon the normal glandular structure becomes replaced by tumor growth, consisting of masses of epithelial cells separated by a dense and abundant fibrous stroma (Fig. 569). This may be so dense that the cancer cells are only present in single file, lying within lymph spaces, and in places they may have disappeared completely. The cells are polygonal and distorted by the dense fibrous tissue; they are small and stain

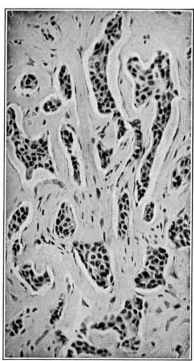

FIG. 569.—Scirrhous carcinoma of the breast. The compressed groups of tumor cells are separated by a dense stroma. × 175.

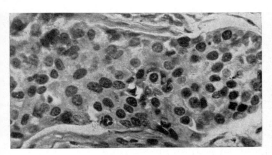

FIG. 570.—Medullary carcinoma of the breast. The cells are massed together with no stroma between them. × 250.

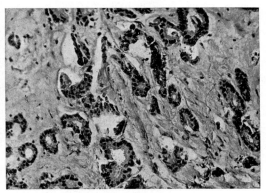

FIG. 571.—Adenocarcinoma of breast. × 125.

darkly, and mitotic figures are rare. Round-cell infiltration may be present in places.

Parenchymal ducts in apparently normal tissue in the immediate neighborhood of the tumor often show marked periductal lymphoid infiltration (Black and Speer). These infiltrates are distinct from and not necessarily accompanied by lymphoid infiltration within the invading tumor. It may well be that these periductal infiltrates may indicate a preinvasive stage in which epithelial cells antigenically foreign to their site of origin arouse an immunological response. The lymphoid infiltrate is not seen around invading cancer cells, possibly owing to complete loss of "identity proteins" of the cancer cell, so that heterotopic localization incites no reaction. In Chapter 8 on the general pathology of tumors we have already studied the concept of an antigenic change in the cell proteins as a result of which "tumor recognition" is lost.

Medullary Carcinoma.—This tumor presents a marked contrast to the preceding group which is probably 30 times more common. It is bulky, often measuring from 4 to 6 cm. in diameter when first seen, rounded, circumscribed, and of soft consistence. It is usually situated deep in the central part of the breast, and hemorrhage and cyst formation are frequent. The soft character of the lesion has earned it the name of *encephaloid carcinoma*. It is also known as bulky mammary carcinoma. The cells lack the invasive biological activity of the scirrhous type, so that the tumor is not adherent to the skin, although eventually it may fungate and axillary node involvement is late. *Microscopically* the cells, which are arranged in large masses, have abundant cytoplasm with large vesicular nuclei and many mitoses. Infiltration of the scanty stroma with small lymphocytes is a highly characteristic feature, in some cases these cells forming the bulk of the tumor. This may indicate a host reaction against the tumor, as is the case in carcinoma in situ in the skin and cervix. This is a threatening picture, but the threat is more a show than a reality. In Stewart's material at the Memorial Hospital only 11.5 per cent were dead of cancer at the end of five years compared with 56 per cent of scirrhous cancers, while 50 per cent were well at the end of five years compared with 27 per cent of the scirrhous form.

Acute Carcinoma.—This tumor is of the medullary type, although usually more diffuse. It generally develops during lactation, and there is rapid dissemination throughout the breast and skin. It is easily mistaken for the acute mastitis which may complicate lactation, for the breast is hot, swollen, painful, and tender, and there is often a well-marked leukocytosis. The course is very acute and seldom lasts more than a few months.

Adenocarcinoma.—This is a rare tumor of the breast in its fully differentiated form. It is of soft consistence and may become quite bulky, but it is of slow growth, of rather low malignancy and may remain localized for a long time. The *microscopic* appearance is that of gland spaces surrounded by columnar epithelium (Fig. 571).

Papillary Duct Carcinoma.—This tumor usually arises from one of the large ducts

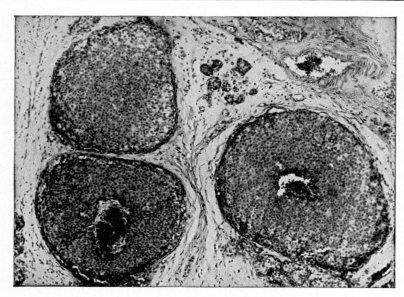

Fig. 572.—Intraduct carcinoma of the breast (comedo form). The tumor cells are confined within the ducts. × 85. (Boyd, *Pathology for the Surgeon*, courtesy of W. B. Saunders Co.)

near the nipple, and is commonly called *duct carcinoma*. The growth may originate from duct papilloma. Owing to fusion of the papillary processes a gland-like condition may be produced, so that the lesion has been called *cystadenocarcinoma*. The tumor is only slowly invasive. Bleeding from the nipple is a common symptom.

Intraduct carcinoma is a convenient term applied to those cases of cystic hyperplasia in which a malignant change is added to epithelial hyperplasia, but the tumor cells are still confined within the walls of the ducts (Fig. 572). Such a condition tends to be diffuse in contrast to papillary carcinoma of the main ducts which is a localized lesion. It may be very difficult for the pathologist to decide before invasion has occurred whether such a specimen is malignant or not. Destruction of the basement membrane and invasion by carcinoma may not be detectable in sections stained with hematoxylin and eosin, although quite evident with modification of the PAS method. The *"comedo carcinoma"* of Bloodgood (so called because worm-like casts can be expressed from the cut surface) belongs to this group.

Paget's Disease.—The condition described by Sir James Paget in 1874, and since known as Paget's disease of the nipple (to distinguish it from Paget's disease of bone), is a chronic eczema of the nipple with the development after some years (sometimes as long as ten years) of a cancer in the breast. In the past there has been much difference of opinion as to whether the skin condition or the cancer was the primary lesion. The skin lesion is malignant, but of very slow growth and without glandular involvement. The breast tumor may be of rapid growth. The eczematous area at the nipple is usually bright red and either moist and weeping or dry and scaly. *Microscopically* the skin in the affected area shows marked epidermal hypertrophy before ulceration takes place. The most characteristic feature is the presence of the peculiar structures known as *Paget's cells* (Fig. 573). These are large, clear, vacuolated cells with small pyknotic nuclei. They look like clear spaces punched out of the epidermis. They are most abundant in the basal layers, but may permeate the entire thickness of the epidermis. The underlying dermis shows infiltration with lymphocytes and plasma cells. In the later stages there is ulceration of the epidermis.

The *pathogenesis* of the condition is still a matter of dispute. Muir and others believe that it begins as an intraduct carcinoma, and that the cancer cells spread along the duct

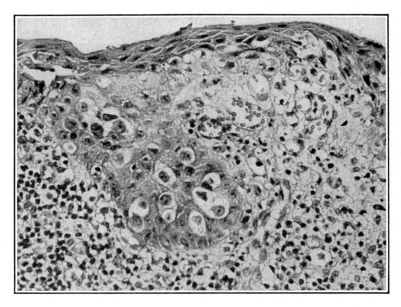

Fig. 573.—Paget's disease of the breast showing clear Paget's cells in the hypertrophic epidermis. × 325.

and penetrate between the cells of the epidermis (intraepithelial spread of carcinoma). Frequently the tumor appears to begin as a local lesion at or near the outlet of a lactiferous duct, whence it spreads centrifugally both in the duct epithelium and in the epidermis, but the continuity is broken when some parts die while others remain alive, so that there may be no connection between the epidermal lesion and the tumor in the breast (Inglis). Another suggestion is that the carcinogenic agent has acted both on the epidermis and on the breast tissue at a distance, a view with which the writer is in agreement. In support of this is the fact that a series of ducts may show neoplastic change.

Extramammary Paget's Disease.—In rare instances the lesion has occurred outside the breast. Paget himself described such a case. The tumor is usually in the region of the *anus* or *vulva.* There may or may not be an underlying carcinoma. All the acceptable reported cases have involved regions where apocrine sweat glands are known to occur and it has been suggested that the condition may represent an apocrine sweat gland carcinoma with extension into the overlying epidermis (Eisenberg and Theuerkauf).

Spread.—Cancer of the breast derives its evil power from its ability to invade lymphatics and spread even in its earliest stage. It is true that some of its forms such as the comedo and medullary varieties do not exhibit this tendency, but they are hopelessly outnumbered by the infiltrating scirrhous form. Spread may be by infiltration, by the lymphatics, and by the blood.

Infiltration.—This is the means by which the malignant cells spread throughout the breast. They infiltrate the tissue spaces between the fat cells and connective tissue bundles, as can be best seen in the scirrhous form of cancer. It is in this way that the deep fascia and skin are involved. Adenocarcinoma and duct carcinoma show a comparatively slight tendency to infiltration. Microscopic sections of the whole thickness of the breast show that the pectoral muscle is involved in over one-half the cases of scirrhous carcinoma at the time of operation, although no gross evidence of involvement may be apparent.

Lymph Spread.—Spread by the lymphatics carries the tumor cells to a distance. There are two ways in which this spread may occur. The cells may grow along the lymphatics by a process originally described by Sampson Handley and named by him lymphatic permeation. Or they may be carried by the lymph stream in the form of tumor emboli. It appears probable that embolism is a much more important method than permeation, although for a long time it was thought that permeation was the chief method of spread. The tumor cells reach the *axillary lymph nodes* early in the disease especially in the scirrhous form of carcinoma. These nodes show *microscopic* involvement in over 60 per cent of cases at the time of operation. The *mediastinal nodes* may occasionally be involved quite early, sometimes even before the axillary nodes. It is in these cases that surgery is so helpless. Adenocarcinoma and duct carcinoma rarely invade the nodes, but unfortunately these are uncommon forms of cancer of the breast. R. S. Handley points out that the *internal mammary lymphatic chain* may be involved without invasion of the axillary nodes. This may explain why early cases of carcinoma of the breast shows a recurrence of about 25 per cent within five years of radical mastectomy.

Enlargement of the regional lymph nodes may be due not to metastases but to *hyperplasia of histiocytes* which fill and distend the sinusoids, a sinus histiocytosis, which when present in high grade indicates a favorable prognosis, for it is an immunological reaction, a sign of host resistance (Black *et al.*). A similar change is seen in the follicles. A high grade of sinus histiocytosis, regardless of metastases to the nodes, is usually associated with a survival period of five years or more. Conversely, absence of histiocytosis, even though no cancer cells can be found in the nodes, is likely to be associated with recurrence within five years of operation.

The plexus of lymphatics which lies upon the deep fascia becomes filled with tumor cells, and it is along the planes of the deep fascia and the muscular aponeuroses that the principal spread takes place. The nodules which often appear in the skin after removal of the tumor owe their origin to this deep supply of tumor cells. Obliteration of the deep lymphatics may cause a lymphatic edema of the skin, and as the epidermis is anchored at many points by hair follicles, the intervening skin becomes swollen so as

to give a characteristic dimpled appearance known as *pig skin* or *peau d'orange*. The condition spoken of as *cancer en cuirasse* is due to lymphatic edema rather than to invasion of the skin by tumor cells. The pleural and peritoneal cavities may be invaded by lymphatic spread along the fascial and aponeurotic planes. The lung may be invaded from the bronchial lymph nodes, and the liver by way of the lymphatics in the falciform ligament.

Staging of cancer of the breast is dependent on lymph spread. It is customary to divide the disease into four stages. *Stage 1:* the growth is limited to the breast. *Stage 2:* the axillary nodes are involved in addition to the breast. *Stage 3:* the growth has spread to extramammary structures such as the pectoral fascia, the chest wall, and the skin beyond the breast. *Stage 4:* spread has occurred in distant parts such as the opposite breast, the cervical nodes, and the viscera, in particular the lung, liver and bones. This may be simplified by recognizing three stages. Stage I: the tumor is confined to the breast. Stage II. the tumor has not transgressed the limits of the standard radical mastectomy. Stage III: the tumor has extended beyond these limits.

Blood Spread.—When the blood stream is invaded, the tumor cells are carried far and wide. The organs most frequently the site of *metastases* are the lungs, liver, bones and brain in that order. Other organs, however, may be involved. In 43 cases of carcinoma of the breast coming to autopsy there were metastases to the spleen in 10, the adrenals in 19, and the ovaries in 7 (Saphir and Parker). In one of these cases, a girl twenty-two years of age, the patient died eight months after the removal of an anaplastic adenocarcinoma. At autopsy metastases were found in the lungs, liver, spleen, kidneys, adrenals, ovaries, sternum, ribs, spine, pelvis, femur, thyroid, myocardium, uterus, pleura, pericardium and skin. It would appear to be the small and clinically unnoticed carcinomas which give rise to the most widespread metastases. Involvement of the lungs and liver may also be by lymphatic spread. Skeletal metastases are usually confined to bones containing richly vascular red marrow such as the vertebral column, the skull, and the upper ends of the humerus and femur. Spread to the vertebrae and skull can also take place by Baston's vertebral system of veins.

Relation of Symptoms to Lesions.— Reference has already been made to the effect of lesions in producing various clinical manifestations in the discussion of the morbid anatomy of the various types of cancer, but a brief recapitulation may be useful. Careful and expert palpation of the breast will reveal a tumor when it measures only 4 or 5 mm. in diameter. The cardinal clinical triad is *increased consistency, lack of circumscription,* and *loss of mobility.* These are all dependent on fibrosis within the tumor and extension to the surrounding parts including the skin. But some at least of these may be misleading. A medullary carcinoma may be circumscribed, papillary and mucoid carcinomas may be soft, and a fibroadenoma and a blue-domed cyst may be hard. These facts emphasize the importance of the biopsy. *Dimpling of the skin* is due to contraction of the fibrous tissue with traction on the ligaments of Cooper. Such contraction may lead to shrinkage of the entire breast. The pull of scar tissue on the fascial septa may cause *deviation of the axis of the nipple,* and flattening or even retraction of the nipple. In scirrhous growths the skin over the tumor becomes tied down. *Edema of the skin* in the advanced stage is due to blockage of the dermal lymphatics, first by tumor embolism and later by permeation of the lymphatics. *Erosion of the nipple* in Paget's disease is due to involvement of the skin by tumor cells. The first clinical indications of a tumor may be those produced by metastases, such as pleural effusion, cerebral symptoms, etc., although this is not so likely to be the case as in carcinoma of the bronchus or prostate.

Effect of Radiation.—The radiosensitivity of cancer of the breast varies markedly with the type of growth. About 20 per cent of the cases are radiosensitive, 20 per cent are resistant, and 60 per cent are intermediate. Unfortunately radiosensitivity is no criterion of certain cure. The more sensitive the tumor, the more cellular it must be, and the more cellular the more dangerous on account of the earlier formation of metastases. Scirrhous carcinoma, as might be expected, is highly radioresistant. The medullary form, on the other hand, may be quite radiosensitive. Adenocarcinoma and duct carcinoma do not respond well to radiation. The rapidly growing anaplastic forms respond best, but have the worst prognosis.

Prognosis.—In estimating the prognosis in cancer of the breast clinical features are of greater value than the microscopic appearance. At the same time we must admit that the scirrhous and medullary types (the common varieties) have a worse prognosis than adenocarcinoma, duct carcinoma, and Paget's disease. The size of the tumor is not as important a factor as might be supposed, but rather its biological character. The smallest tumor may have invaded the lymphatics and blood stream by the time it is recognized, whereas a bulky one may remain circumscribed. It used to be thought that the younger the patient, the worse was the outlook, but this has now been challenged. Certainly rapidity of growth spells disaster. Lymph node involvement is the most important single factor, and the internal mammary chain has been called the principal highway of death. Reference has already been made to the relation which a histiocytic reaction in the nodes may have to the prognosis.

In determining the prognosis of a given case the question of treatment is obviously all-important. If the patient is not treated, she will die. But here we enter a region of great difficulty, perplexity and confusion. It was in 1856 that Velpeau wrote: "To destroy a cancerous tumor of the breast by surgical means is usually an easy matter and but little dangerous in itself, but the question arises whether such a proceeding affords a chance of radically curing the patient." This question still remains unanswered. Surgical removal of the tumor used to be followed by a very high percentage of recurrence at the site of operation or in the surrounding chest wall. This threat was met by Halstead at Johns Hopkins Hospital, when in 1894 he introduced the method of radical mastectomy with removal of the breast, the surrounding skin, the pectoralis major, and the axillary lymph nodes. In the sixty-five years which have elapsed since then there has been no major change in the surgical attack apart from extending its scope to include the internal mammary chain and even the supraclavicular nodes. Now radiation therapy, either preoperative or postoperative, has been added to the attack.

It is singularly difficult to determine the value of all this in terms of life expectancy. The individual patient can be cured in very many cases, using the term cure in the limited sense appropriate to a disease in which secondary growths may develop after long intervals of time. The difficulty becomes apparent when we come to large groups which can be dealt with statistically. These, of course, must be compared with control groups. When this is done it may be found that the average survival in the treated group is six years and in the control untreated group only three and one-half years. The five-year survival of a series of 742 cases treated at the Toronto General Hospital as measured from the onset of symptoms was 32.5 per cent (Janes), whilst the corresponding figure for a series of 100 untreated cases was 21 per cent (Daland). One very important point which is commonly overlooked in comparisons of series of treated and untreated cases is that the former are inevitably *selected* cases with exclusion of the hopeless cases, whereas in the untreated group all cases are included. The result of this omission will be evident to the reader. Adair sums up his own very extensive surgical experience in these somber words: "I doubt very much that the average patient with early breast cancer has any better opportunity for cure today than sixty years ago."

Since Halstead's pioneer work the patient is not likely to die of a fungating local lesion, but of the metastases in the lymph nodes and and viscera. (This in itself is a big step in advance from the point of view of the woman, if not of her surgeon.) It is the invasive character of the tumor rather than the treatment which determines the outcome. The tumor cells may be in the lymphatics and in the blood stream at a time when the mass can hardly be detected by the clinician. In 59 patients with cancer of the breast definite cancer cells were found in blood from a regional vein and from a peripheral vein in 36 cases and atypical cells in 5

cases (Moore *et al.*). It is true that these were advanced cases, but they were not terminal. Tumor cells are also often present in the bone marrow. These figures must not lead us to think that every cancer cell in the blood stream is going to set up a secondary growth, any more than bacteria circulating in the blood need necessarily cause a pyemia. The *resistance of the host* is even more important than the presence of the cancer cell, but unfortunately at present we have no means of measuring this resistance. With regard to lymph node metastases it is easy to see how clumsy manipulation of the primary lesion during removal of the breast may dislodge tumor cells in the lymphatics with involvement of the internal mammary chain of nodes.

Discouraged with the poor prospect of a five-year cure in the average case with radical mastectomy, McWhirter of Edinburgh has organized a program in which simple mastectomy is followed by intensive radiation to the axillary, supraclavicular and internal mammary areas. It is claimed that if the axillary nodes are not involved a radical operation is unnecessary, and if they are involved it is of no avail.

This healthy feeling of dissatisfaction with his results has caused the surgeon to turn to other therapeutic measures. Reference has already been made to the possibility of restraining tumor growth for considerable periods of time by giving or withholding hormones from the ovaries, adrenals and anterior pituitary through removal of the corresponding glands, and great activity is being shown in this field. An interesting example of the combination of endocrine with chemotherapy is the report of marked inhibition of growth in 30 out of 34 cases of advanced breast cancer by the use of "thiotepa," an alkylating antimitotic drug of the nitrogen mustard group together with testosterone, which holds in check proliferation of the hormone-dependent cells (Watson and Turner).

In concluding this discussion of prognosis in relation to therapy, we may reiterate what has been said before, namely that breast cancer may be several diseases rather than a single entity, and that it is the biological activity of the tumor cells which counts

Unfortunately the microscopist has no method of assessing this activity. As Greene remarks: "The conception of the divinity of morphology is not a product of the morphologist, but owes its origin to the naive faith of biologists, chemists, and surgeons who place the microscope on a pedestal." Be that as it may, it becomes more and more evident that to form a rational prognosis in carcinoma of the breast is a superhuman task. We can adopt the face-saving attitude that we can cure only those patients capable of being cured because of the inherent nature of their disease, and whether the patient will be cured depends not only on the kind of cancer but on the degree of immunity of the patient.

Carcinoma of the Male Breast.—This is rare and usually occurs at an older age than cancer of the female breast. The prognosis is much worse, owing to the ease with which the tumor involves the pectoral fascia and deeper structures on account of the small size of the breast. Fixation and ulceration of the skin are marked features.

BLEEDING FROM THE NIPPLE.—The two common causes of discharge of blood or bloodstained fluid from the nipple are *duct papilloma* and *duct carcinoma*. There is much difference of opinion as to whether or not the symptom usually indicates malignancy, but it seems probable that about 50 per cent of the cases are benign and 50 per cent are malignant. It is important to realize that the discharge may not contain blood although the patient says that it does, and in every case a microscopic examination should be made of a smear. Cystic hyperplasia may cause a discharge from the nipple which is chocolate, green, or yellow in color, but which contains no blood. A dark, stagnant, bloody discharge is practically pathognomonic of duct carcinoma. Transillumination of the breast is useful for localizing the lesion, for a collection of blood appears black with this method.

SARCOMA.—This is quite uncommon. It may attain a great size. The cut surface presents a characteristic homogeneous appearance like fish-flesh, and shows none of the yellow necrotic areas and striations characteristic of carcinoma. This, combined with its softness, usually allows a correct diagnosis of the tumor to be made with the naked eye. The sarcoma may develop from a fibroadenoma, in which case it is composed of spindle cells arranged around ducts. In the ordinary form which arises *de novo* it is made up entirely of spindle cells, many of which show mitotic figures. The lymph nodes are seldom involved, but there may be distant blood spread.

Other tumors which may rarely be found in the breast are *angioma, lipoma, myxoma, osteogenic sarcoma,* and *chondroma.*

CYSTS OF THE BREAST

The common cysts of the breast are those of cystic disease. These are not retention cysts due to obstruction of the ducts, but are first produced by dilatation from epithelial hyperplasia, followed by incomplete involution which leaves the duct dilated. Obstruction may then be superadded, so that continued secretion may lead to a great increase in size. A feature of these cysts is that the clear fluid which they contain may be under marked tension, so that it spurts out violently when the cyst is incised. A *galactocele* is a very rare condition in which a large cyst containing milk is formed during lactation. Being a dilatation of one of the main milk ducts, it is situated close to the nipple. *Hydatid cysts* are extremely rare.

ACUTE MASTITIS

Acute inflammation of the breast is practically confined to the first few weeks of lactation. Physiological hyperplasia may occur immediately, after birth and at puberty, and when unduly marked this may cause symptoms which are described clinically as acute mastitis, but it is not a true inflammation. The common infecting organism is the Staphylococcus aureus, which produces a localized inflammation. More rarely a steptococcus may cause a diffuse inflammation. Infection takes place through the milk ducts or cracks in the nipple. Suppuration occurs and an *abscess* may be formed. This may be subcutaneous, intramammary, or retromammary. In the latter form the breast is pushed forward. Only one segment of the breast may be involved, or a number of abscesses may be formed in adjoining lobes so that multiple incisions are required. Acute mastitis may be closely simulated by acute carcinoma, a condition characterized by pain, swelling, heat, and fever.

OTHER LESIONS OF THE BREAST

FAT NECROSIS.—It has long been known that a quiet necrosis with saponification may occur in traumatized or ischemic fat in any part of the body, a process similar to pancreatic fat necrosis but of slower *tempo* due to absence of the active pancreatic lipase. Within recent years it has been recognized that such a process in the breast may give rise to a lesion which closely *simulates scirrhous carcinoma*. A history of trauma to the breast shortly before the appearance of the lesion is obtained in many cases, so that the condition is commonly called traumatic fat necrosis, but in about one-half the cases there is no such history. The patients are usually corpulent with large full breasts, and most cases occur in the fourth and fifth decades. A hard localized mass is formed, which is often adherent to the skin, so that the condition is readily mistaken for cancer.

The *gross appearance* of the lesion is characteristic, and should be recognized in the operating room. The affected area is of an opaque, white, chalky appearance, which is well shown in one of Hadfield's illustrations. This area is composed of necrotic fat. As saponification proceeds liquefaction takes place, and a cavity is formed containing a pool of yellow oily fluid. This pseudocyst is surrounded by dense tissue which represents a reaction to the fatty irritant. Lime salts combine with the liberated fatty acids, so that some degree of calcification is common. The cicatricial contraction, the concave surface, and the yellow streaks of scirrhous carcinoma are absent.

The *microsopic appearance* is similar to that of fat necrosis elsewhere in the body. The fat cells are broken into droplets which remain attached to the cell envelope and stain faintly with hematoxylin. Fatty acid crystals may be present. The surrounding tissue shows a chronic productive inflammation, and contains large numbers of phagocytic cells filled with lipoid material. Foreign body giant cells form a striking feature of the lesion. Lymphocytic infiltration and an obliterating endarteritis complete the picture.

PLASMA CELLS MASTITIS.—This rare condition is an acute or subacute inflammation which begins suddenly with pain, tenderness, diffuse swelling, and enlargement of the axillary lymph nodes. The acute symptoms soon subside, leaving the breast hard, the skin adherent, and the lymph nodes firm, so that to mistake it at this stage for carcinoma is almost inevitable. The *gross* appearance is that of a hard diffuse mass, so that again there is resemblance to carcinoma. The *microscopic* appearance is explained by the pathogenesis. The condition is an inflammation initiated by stasis and inspissation of secretions with rupture of the dilated mammary ducts, often associated with a history of difficult nursing. It is an *endogenous granuloma*, and has been called *split milk mastitis*. The lesion, which may resemble tuberculosis but without caseation, consists of large numbers of plasma cells, together with varying numbers of polymorphonuclears, epithelioid cells, foam cells and giant cells which may be clustered around fatty acid crystals. A developing fibrosis increases the induration.

TUBERCULOSIS.—Tuberculosis of the breast is uncommon but not rare. At first it takes the form of a hard mass, which is easily mistaken for carcinoma. Softening occurs, with the formation of large tuberculous cavities and sinuses opening on the surface. The microscopic picture is characteristic of tuberculosis.

ACTINOMYCOSIS.—This is one of the rarest of breast diseases. It may involve the breast by extension through the chest wall from the pleura.

HYPERTROPHY.—Hypertrophy of the breasts usually comes on soon after puberty, but may occur during pregnancy or lactation. It is probably of endocrine origin, due to some abnormal action of the ovarian hormone. The hypertrophy involves both glandular and connective tissue, but as a rule most of the enlargement is due to a great increase of the connective tissue, which is soft and of open structure.

CONGENITAL ANOMALIES.—*Amastia* or congenital absence of the breast is usually bilateral but may be unilateral. *Athelia* or absence of the nipple is rare. It may be associated with amastia, or the breast may be well developed. *Polymastia* or abnormal number of breasts is much more common than either of the preceding conditions. The "milk-line" extends from the axilla to the groin, and accessory or supernumerary breasts may occur anywhere along this line, the most common site being the axilla. The accessory mammary tissue may or may not be provided with a nipple. The mass enlarges during lactation and may secrete milk. *Polythelia* or accessory nipples are rare. They may occur on the breast or elsewhere along the milk-line. In the latter case they have underlying mammary tissue (polymastia).

REFERENCES

ADAIR, F. E.: New York State J. Med., 1934, *34*, 61. (Duct obstruction in pathogenesis of breast cancer.)

————: S. Clin. North America, 1953, April, 313. (Curability of breast cancer.)

BAGG, H. J.: J. Cancer Research, 1925, *9*, 498. (Obstruction of ducts in breast cancer.)

BITTNER, J. J.: Am. J. Cancer, 1937, *30*, 530; 1939, *35*, 90. (Milk factor in breast cancer.)

BLACK, M. M., KEYSE, S. and SPEER, F. D.: Am. J. Path., 1953, *29*, 505. (Histiocytosis in metastatic nodes.)

BLACK, M. M. and SPEER, F. D.: Arch. Path., 1955, *60*, 457. (Periductal lymphoid infiltration.)

BUNTING, H.: Bull. Internat. Assn. Med. Museums, 1948, *28*, 48. (Cystic hyperplasia.)

CURRIE, A. R.: Edit.: *Endocrine Aspects of Breast Cancer*, Edinburgh, 1958.

DALAND, E. M.: Surg., Gynec. and Obst., 1927, *44*, 264. (Prognosis of breast cancer.)

DAWSON, E. K.: Edin. Med. J., 1954, *61*, 391. (Sclerosing adenosis.)

EISENBERG, R. B. and THEUERKAUF, F. J.: Am. J. Clin. Path., 1955, *25*, 642. (Extramammary Paget's disease.)

FISHER, E. R. and CREED, D. L.: Lab. Invest., 1956, *5*, 267. (The periductal stroma in gynecomastia.)

GREENE, H. S. N.: J. Exper. Med., 1939, *70*, 147, 159 and 167. (Multicentric origin of cancer of breast.)

GREENE, H. S. N. and LUND, P. K.: Cancer Res., 1944, *4*, 352. (Curability of breast cancer.)

HAAGENSEN, C. D.: *Diseases of the Breast*, Philadelphia, 1956.

HADFIELD, G.: Brit. J. Surg., 1929, *17*, 673. (Fat necrosis.)

————: Brit. M. J., 1956, *1*, 1507. (Endocrine aspects of breast cancer.)

HANDLEY, R. S. and THACKRAY, A. C.: Brit. Med. J., 1954, *1*, 61. (Lymph node metastases.)

INGLEBY, H.: Arch. Path., 1942, *33*, 573. (Morphological variations.)

INGLEBY, H. and GERSHON-COHEN, J.: *Comparative Anatomy, Pathology and Roentgenology of the Breast*, Philadelphia, 1960. Surg., Gyn. and Obst., 1954, *99*, 199. (Myo-epithelium in sclerosing adenosis.)

INGLIS, K.: *Paget's Disease of the Nipple*, London, 1936. Am. J. Path., 1946, *22*, 1. (Paget's disease.)

JANES, R. M.: Can. J. Surg., 1959, *2*, 252. (Prognosis of breast cancer.)

KARNAUCHOW, P. N.: Am. J. Path., 1954, *30*, 1169. (Myo-epithelium in gynecomastia.)

KARSNER, H. T.: Am. J. Path., 1946, *22*, 235. (Gynecomastia.)

LACASSAGNE, A. and MYKA, W.: Compt., rend. Soc. de biol., 1934, *116*, 844. (Experimental production of breast cancer.)

LENDRUM, A. C.: J. Path. and Bact., 1945, *57*, 267. (Cystic hyperplasia.)

LEWISON, E. F.: *Breast Cancer and its Diagnosis and Treatment*, Baltimore, 1959.

McWHIRTER, R.: Brit. M. J., 1947, *2*, 542. (Treatment of breast cancer.)

MELNICK, P. J. and BULLOCK, W. K.: Am. J. Path., 1959, *35*, 706. (Histochemical study of breast neoplasms.)

MOORE, G. E., SANDBERG, A. and SCHUBORG, J. R.: Ann. Surg., 1957, *146*, 580. (Cancer cells in blood stream.)

MUIR, R.: J. Path. and Bact., 1927, *30*, 451. (Paget's disease.)

————: J. Path. and Bact., 1941, *52*, 155. (Multicentric origin of cancer of breast.)

SANDISON, A. T.: J. Clin. Path., 1958, *11*, 101. (Sclerosing adenosis.)

SAPHIR, O. and PARKER, M. L.: Arch. Surg., 1941, *42*, 1003. (Spread of breast cancer.)

SMITH, R. P.: Can. M.A.J., 1940, *43*, 70. (Cystic hyperplasia.)

SOMMERS, S. C.: Lab. Invest., 1955, *4*, 160. (Endocrine abnormalities in women with breast cancer.)

URBAN, J. A. and ADAIR, F. E.: Cancer, 1949, *2*, 625. (Sclerosing adenosis.)

WATSON, G. W. and TURNER, R. L.: Brit. M. J., 1959, *1*, 1315. (Thiotepa and testosterone therapy in breast cancer.)

Chapter 35

The Pituitary

General Considerations
  GENERAL ENDOCRINE
    INTEGRATION
    Fluid and Electrolyte
      Metabolism
    Endocrine Mediators of Injury
  STRUCTURE
    Adenohypophysis
    Neurohypophysis
  FUNCTIONS OF THE ADENO-
    HYPOPHYSIS
    Growth Hormone
    Thyrotrophic Hormone
    Adrenocorticotrophic Hormones
    Gonadotrophic Hormones

FUNCTIONS OF THE NEURO-
    HYPOPHYSIS
  Vasopressin (Antidiuretic
    Hormone)
  Oxytocin
Vascular Lesions
Inflammations
Tumors
  ADENOMA
    Chromophobe Adenoma
    Acidophil Adenoma
    Basophil Adenoma
    Neighborhood Symptoms
  CARCINOMA
  CRANIOPHARYNGIOMA

Congenital Anomalies
Hypopituitarism
  SIMMONDS' SYNDROME
  LORAIN-LEVI SYNDROME
  FRÖHLICH'S SYNDROME
    Laurence-Moon-Biedl
      Syndrome
  DIABETES INSIPIDUS
Hyperpituitarism
  GROWTH HORMONE
    Gigantism
    Acromegaly
  ADRENOCORTICOTROPHIC
    HORMONE
    Cushing's Syndrome
  THYROTROPHIC HORMONE

GENERAL CONSIDERATIONS

General Endocrine Integration.—Before taking up in detail the lesions and malfunction of the individual endocrine glands, and in this chapter those of the pituitary, it may be well to devote a few thoughts to the general *physiology and integration* of these remarkable structures. The ductless glands are members of the endocrine system, but they are also members one of another in the Biblical sense, for at least some of them exert an important influence on other members of the series. What used to be the uncharted sea of the endocrines strewn with the wrecks of shattered hypotheses has now become as well surveyed a group of waterways as the canals of Venice. No place for an interpolation of this discussion could be more appropriate than the present chapter, for the pituitary is not only the conductor of the endocrine orchestra, but it itself plays several important instruments in the ensemble, as well as acting as a link or mediator between soma and psyche.

The endocrine or ductless glands are the chemical regulators of the body by virtue of the hormones (*hormao*, to excite) which they produce. The hormones govern the processes concerned with growth, metabolism, and reproduction. Of special importance in pathol-

ogy is the fact that some of the hormones control the metabolism of certain inorganic elements, and that upset of this control may have serious effects. Thus the adrenal cortex controls sodium metabolism, the thyroid iodine metabolism, and the parathyroids the metabolism of calcium and phosphorus. No reference need be made to the relation of the islets of Langerhans to carbohydrate metabolism and diabetes, a subject which has already been considered in Chapter 29.

The endocrine system shares with the nervous system the function of *biological integration*, the channels in the one case being the blood vessels, in the other case the nerves. Not only do the endocrine integrators produce a train of chemical reactions; there are also negative feed-back regulators which tend to prevent excessive overaction, thus playing the part of a safety valve or rather a governor. As one of the chief objects of hormonal activity is to supply energy, it is obvious that this action would be harmful if overdone.

Many of the hormones, particularly those of the pituitary, are trophic in character. They act not directly on the body cells, but on another endocrine organ, which may be called the target gland, for example the thyroid, the adrenal and gonads. The target gland in turn produces its own hormone

(964)

which acts on the cells of the tissues, and which may at the same time lay a restraining hand on the original source of the stimuli. The brain may play an essential part in this complex mechanism, again best seen in the case of the pituitary. This neuro-endocrine-somatic relationship is thus brain $\rightarrow$ pituitary $\rightarrow$ target gland $\rightarrow$ body cells. The mechanism by which a trophic hormone releases the specific hormone of the target gland is uncertain, possibly by increasing the permeability of the cell membrane. The afferent impulses of what may be termed neuroendocrine reflexes may reach the brain through nerve pathways, or through the circulation. Finally it may be psychogenic in origin. Thus fear stimulates the secretion of epinephrine, which in turn increases the function of the pituitary, thyroid, adrenal cortex and pancreas. The efferent nervous signals to the pituitary are carried mainly through the hypophysial stalk. The antidiuretic hormone of the neurohypophysis no longer operates when the hypophysial stalk is divided.

(It may be remarked here that the hormones have the suffix *trophin* attached to them, derived from the Greek *trophe*, meaning nourishment. It has become fashionable to change trophic to tropic, but I prefer to remain old-fashioned in this respect. The student will understand that both spellings are correct and he may well prefer to use the newer one).

The trophic hormones may be decreased or increased in amount, with corresponding changes in the hormones of the target glands. Most endocrine disease is due to too much or too little hormone. *Hypotrophism* is followed by atrophy of the target gland, though the concentration of hormone in the gland remains constant; less is made, but less is released into the circulation. *Hypertrophism* results in hyperplasia of the target gland, with increased production and discharge of the hormone, but decreased concentration in the gland. Administration of the target gland hormone inhibits the production of the corresponding trophic hormone, an illustration of the feed-back mechanism.

The sensitivity of the end organs (cells) differs with different hormones. Thus the thyroid hormone and the growth hormone of the pituitary stimulate metabolism in all the cells of the body, but estrogens act only on the female genital structures, breasts and hips, whilst androgens stimulate growth of hair in the axilla and pubis.

The *mechanism of action* of hormones is to intensify existing biochemical reactions, not to start new ones. They seem to act as catalysts, greatly augmenting enzymatic reactions. Under normal conditions there may be no apparent clinical insufficiency, even though 70 per cent of the gland is destroyed. If, however, great demands are made on the hormone, a relative insufficiency may develop, even though the gland is working overtime. Thus a patient with severe thyrotoxicosis may develop relative adrenal insufficiency, and the administration of dessicated thyroid to a patient with Addison's disease may greatly intensify the symptoms.

The signal for more or less hormone is generally given by the concentration in the blood of some special substance, but this may start a more complex train of events. Thus hypocalcemia stimulates the parathyroids and increases parathormone production with consequent excessive renal excretion of phosphorus, which in turn upsets the calcium-phosphorus balance in the body with resulting osteolysis and an increase of serum calcium. A rise in the serum osmolarity of the blood stimulates the hypothalamic nuclei, and this tends to stimulation of the neurohypophysis with an increased production of antidiuretic hormone and increased reabsorption of water from the renal tubules.

As regards *chemical structure*, hormones may be proteins, steroids, or small molecular weight amines. *Protein hormones* are secreted by endocrines which originate from the alimentary tract; such are the anterior pituitary, thyroid, parathyroids and pancreas. *Steroid hormones* are produced by glands derived from the celomic mesothelium, *e.g.* testis, ovary and adrenal cortex, the chief variations being in the attachments to the 3, 11 and 17 carbon atoms. The *small molecular weight amines* are secreted by cells of nervous origin, such as the neurohypophysis and the adrenal medulla. Hormone synthesis takes place within the cells of the gland, and the hormone remains in the cell until discharged into the circulation. In the case of the thyroid and ovary, however, it is stored in special receptacles.

Antibodies to hormones can be produced in the experimental animal. When such an antibody is injected into a second animal, there is complete protection against that particular hormone.

A practical illustration of the value of a working knowledge of endocrine integration to the practitioner of medicine is afforded by (1) the influence of endocrines on fluid and electrolyte metabolism, and (2) the endocrine mediators of injury.

Fluid and Electrolyte Metabolism.—A posterior pituitary hormone, the *antidiuretic hormone* or *vasopressin*, acts directly on the renal tubules to promote the reabsorption of water, and in this way it regulates the volume of water in the body. The effect on electrolytes is negligible. The stimulus for the production of this hormone is an increase in the effective osmotic pressure of the serum and extracellular fluid, which itself is brought about primarily by an increase in serum sodium.

The *adrenal cortical hormone* of importance in this respect is *aldosterone*. This has the same action as desoxycorticosterone, that is to say retention of sodium by increasing its reabsorption through the tubules, and in consequence retention of water and potassium diuresis.

These two hormones, the one from the posterior pituitary, the other from the adrenal cortex, thus provide an automatic and simultaneous regulation of the volume and the effective osmotic pressure of the extracellular fluid. A reasonable concept as to the sequence of events is that aldosterone increases the tubular reabsorption of sodium; this increases the effective osmotic pressure of the serum, which then stimulates the supra-optic-hypophyseal system to produce antidiuretic hormone, with resulting water reabsorption and lowering of the serum osmotic pressure, thus inhibiting the further production of antidiuretic hormone. Naturally the extracellular fluid volume participates in these changes.

Endocrine mediators of injury.—Here the doctor is interested in the problem of post-traumatic metabolism which may follow surgical injury (Moore). This subject has already been discussed in relation to the healing of wounds (page 68). The four endocrine mediators which bring to the tissues remote from the injury a call for help from the site of the injury are as follows. (1) The *hypothalamic-pituitary-hydroxycorticosteroid system*. ACTH and hydrocorticosteroids are at once produced in increased amounts after the injury. Patients who have no adrenals on account of disease or adrenalectomy do not tolerate trauma unless given replacement therapy. (2) The *aldosterone-renal tubular system*. In the posttraumatic patient sodium excretion is diminished. There is a lowered sodium-potassium ratio in the urine, together with an increased tubular resorption of sodium. (3) The *antidiuretic hormone* of the posterior pituitary may produce marked water retention after the most trivial form of trauma or even emotional excitement. (4) *Epinephrine and nor-epinephrine* is increased after injury, fright, and psychic stimuli, with effects on carbohydrate metabolism and blood flow. The importance of a knowledge of these facts to a surgeon treating an injured patient are self-evident.

Further information on the general subject of endocrine physiology and its relation to disease will be found in such monographs as those of Soffer, of Williams, and of Simpson, which contain striking illustrations of the various clinical disturbances that may result from such disease.

Structure.—"Here in this well-concealed spot, almost to be covered by a thumb-nail, lies the very mainspring of primitive existence, vegetative, emotional, reproductive." In these striking words Harvey Cushing describes the pituitary body, one of the smallest of the endocrines, but the master gland of the body. The pituitary consists of an anterior lobe or adenohypophysis and a posterior lobe or neurohypophysis. The adult pituitary gland only weighs from 0.4 to 0.6 Gm., and up to 0.8 Gm. in women who have been pregnant. Of the total weight 75 to 80 per cent is anterior lobe tissue. The *anterior lobe* is epithelial in structure, and is derived from Rathke's pouch, an up-growth from the pharynx. The stalk connecting it

PLATE XIV

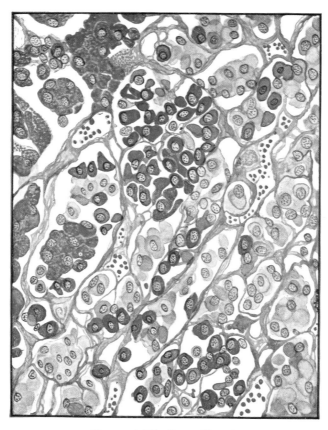

Normal Pituitary Gland.

The acidophil (eosinophil), basophil and chromophobe cells are present in normal
proportions.   (Acid fuchsin and methylene blue.)

with the pharynx disappears, but epithelial rests may remain from which tumors may arise known as Rathke pouch tumors or craniopharyngiomas. The posterior lobe, of nervous structure, is developed from the floor of the third ventricle, and remains attached to the hypothalamic region of the brain by a stalk or infundibulum, in which a very narrow channel of communication with the ventricle remains open. The *posterior lobe* consists of a pars nervosa and a pars intermedia. The *pars nervosa* consists of non-medullated nerve fibers, which connect the pituitary with the hypothalamus, and a varying amount of nerve cells and neuroglia. The *pars intermedia* is an epithelial investment of the pars nervosa, derived from Rathke's pouch. It is composed of basophil cells.

Anterior Lobe.— (Adenohypophysis).— In the days when hematoxylin-eosin was a satisfying stain the structure of the adeno-hypophysis was delightfully simple, for it consisted of three sets of cells: (1) *acidophils* or eosinophils, their cytoplasm filled with granules staining red with eosin; (2) *baso-phils*, and (3) *chromophobes*, with non-granular cytoplasm which stained faintly or not at all. The proportion of the various forms was roughly as follows: chromophobes, 50 per cent; acidophils, 40 per cent; basophils, 10 per cent (Plate XIV).

Those days are past, and newer staining methods have not only given us new pictures, but perplexing and ever-changing terminology. The introduction of the McManus periodic acid-Schiff (PAS) method of staining with orange G as a counterstain has provided a new histological picture more closely related to the biological and hormonal activity of the cells. The PAS method gives a bright red color with polysaccharides, and, using this technique, Pearse has been able to localize the pituitary mucoprotein hormones in the cells which produce them. With this method the following groups of cells can be recognized: (1) *chromophobes* which are non-granular and PAS-negative; (2) *acidophils* which are granular and PAS-negative, although staining with orange G; and (3) *PAS-positive basophils*. The basophils have been farther divided into two groups: (1) *normal basophils* with dense granules,

strongly PAS-positive, and (2) *amphophils*, sparsely granular and weakly PAS-positive, called amphophil because they stain variably with Mallory's aniline blue technique (*ampho*, both). A commonly employed classification at the present time is into: (1) *acidophils*, (2) *basophils*, (3) *amphophils*, and (4) *chromophobes*, with the addition of (5) *hypertrophic amphophils*, which resemble a giant chromophobe with a nucleus about twice the normal size, and which are seen in human adrenocortical hyperfunctional states such as Cushing's syndrome, adrenal virilism and the adrenogenital syndrome, as well as in invasive carcinoma.

Ezrin and his associates have introduced a further modification of technique, treating the section with dialyzed iron and potassium ferrocyanide before staining with PAS and orange G. Five types of cells can be distinguished with the iron-PAS technique: (1) *alpha cells* (acidophils), (2) *beta* and (3) *delta cells* (two types of basophils, the beta cell staining red and the delta cell blue-purple with PAS), (4) *gamma cells* (heterogeneous group of lightly PAS-positive cells), and (5) *chromophobes* (small nongranular cells). The alpha cells (acidophils) are increased in conditions of prolonged adrenal glucocorticoid excess, as in Cushing's syndrome; the beta cells are constantly reduced in Addison's disease; In Cushing's syndrome many of the beta cells show a striking hyaline degeneration; while the delta cells are present in abundance (about 8 per cent) in the normal pituitary of a healthy person who has died suddenly. If the illness last longer than twenty-four hours, the proportion of delta cells steadily decreases (Ezrin). The densely granulated basophils of the classification in the preceding paragraph now constitute the beta and delta cells, while the lightly granulated basophils, now called gamma cells, correspond to the amphophils.

It is, of course, the *function* of the various cells of the adenohypophysis in which we are interested, in other words, which hormones they may be expected to produce. The only answer to this question lies in a comparison of the histological picture with a variety of endocrine disturbances. As may well be imagined, there is no consensus of opinion on this thorny subject. Any conclusions

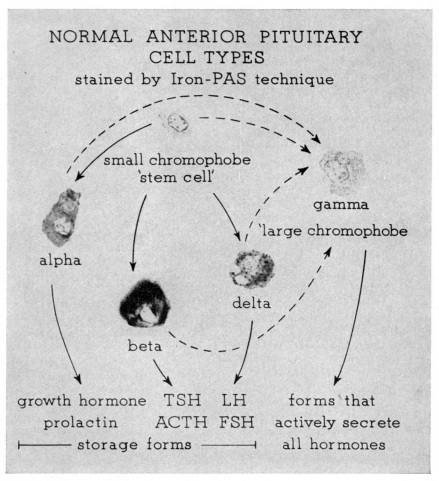

NORMAL ANTERIOR PITUITARY
CELL TYPES
stained by Iron-PAS technique

small chromophobe
'stem cell'

gamma
'large chromophobe

alpha

delta

beta

growth hormone TSH LH   forms that
prolactin   ACTH FSH   actively secrete
|——— storage forms ———| all hormones

Fig. 574.—Cell types of the anterior pituitary and the hormones they are believed to secrete. (From a colored drawing, kindness of Dr. Calvin Ezrin.)

which may be drawn are purely tentative. Russfield and her associates from an analysis of clinical and pathological material in man consider that the growth hormone, ACTH thyrothrophin, gonadotrophin and the lactogenic hormone are secreted by the amphophil cells, although not necessarily simultaneously. Sommers, from a consideration of a large amount of similar material, is of the opinion that growth hormone and prolactin are produced by the acidophils, gonadotrophin by the basophils, and thyrotrophin by the amphophils. The chromophobes appear to be functionally hypoactive. Ezrin believes that the delta cell makes one or more of the pituitary gonadotrophins because of the absence of these cells in children under ten years of age and their disappearance after the first trimester of pregnancy, in both of which periods the pituitary contains virtually no gonadotrophins. Some of the suggested relationships of staining properties of the cells to function are shown in Figure 574.

The cells have been usefully divided into actively secreting cells and storage cells (Golden). The actively secreting cells, both basophil and acidophil, are prominent during adolescence, and reflect increased pubertal gonadotrophic and growth-hormone secretion. These cells are larger, with prominent nuclei, and delicate cytoplasmic stippling. The storage cells are smaller and densely granulated. *It is now believed that all the cells of the adenohypophysis may be variants of a single cell type, their histological and histochemical changes merely indicating functional changes.*

Posterior Lobe.—(Neurohypophysis).—The posterior lobe has never suggested in its structure that it has an endocrine function, and yet it was from this part of the pituitary that the first hormones were isolated. The paradox is explained by the *neurosecretory concept* which we owe to the Sharrers and to Bargmann. The hormones, it now appears, are not made in the pars nervosa of the posterior lobe but in the supra-optic and paraventricular nuclei of the hypothalamus, passing down the corresponding axons in the hypothalamic-hypophyseal tract to the neurohypophysis, where they are absorbed into capillaries. If this tract is interrupted, the neurosecretion cannot reach the neurohypophysis to be absorbed and diabetes insipidus results. Colored illustrations of the neurosecretory material in its various stages of transit will be found in Ham's *Textbook of Histology*, 4th edition, 1961.

The neurosecretory material does not stain with the usual pituitary stains, but it can be demonstrated by means of Alcian blue or Gomori's chromealum-hematoxylin. The neurohypophysis seems to act as a storage and release center, a depot for these hormones, rather than as their factory, a depot from which they can be obtained in a hurry in certain emergencies such as dehydration and parturition. It may also act as the location of specialized osmoreceptors that serve to regulate the liberation of the antidiuretic hormone by detecting small changes in the osmotic pressure of the interstitial fluid bathing it. It is of interest to note that the neurohypophysis is one of the few portions of the central nervous system which is situated outside of the so-called "blood-brain barrier," so that it is in a specially favored position to influence and be influenced by changes in the humoral environment.

Neurosecretory cells must be of fundamental biological significance, for they are found in all vertebrates, as well as in worms, molluscs and insects, the material being particularly well shown in the cerebral ganglia of that primitive animal, the earthworm (Sharrer and Sharrer).

The *blood supply* of the pituitary is attracting wide attention, mainly with reference to the *hypophyseal portal system* of vessels. This system appears to act as a vascular link between the nervous system and the adenohypophysis, arising in one set of capillaries and ending in another, hence its claim to the name portal system. The veins of the system originate in the neurohypophysis, not the hypothalamus as was previously believed. It has been suggested that other hypothalamic hormones that are trophic for the anterior pituitary are transported as neurosecretory material to the portal capillaries in the neurohypophysis, and thence to the adenohypophysis where they regulate the release of adenohypophyseal hormones. Such material could therefore be regarded as trophic in character, bearing the same relation to the trophic hormones of the pituitary as the latter bear to the hormones of other endocrine glands, as exemplified by adrenocorticotrophic hormone and cortisone.

Cutting the stalk or infundibulum results in massive infarction of the greater part of the anterior lobe. It has therefore been suggested that in cases where hypophysectomy is considered desirable, as in carcinoma of the breast, this procedure might be preferable to the more serious and hazardous operation. Unfortunately mitotic figures indicating regeneration may be observed in the remaining fragments in the experimental animal.

Functions of the Anterior Lobe.—We have already seen that the pituitary has been called the conductor of the glandular orchestra, and with each advance in knowledge it becomes more and more apparent that the metaphor is an appropriate one. As the hormones of the endocrine glands affect the activities of every body cell and influence the metabolism of carbohydrates, fats, proteins, minerals and vitamins, the pituitary may well be regarded as the master gland of the body. All the different members report to it regularly about their activities, and by secreting trophic hormones it regulates their structure and function. The cells of the pars anterior behave as if they performed a chemical assay on the blood which flows around them

The Pituitary

in the sinusoids. The result of the assay determines whether more or less trophic hormone shall be despatched to each target gland.

The anterior pituitary secretes at least 6 distinct hormonal principles. These are (1) the growth hormone (GH) or somatotrophic hormone (STH); (2) the adrenocorticotrophic hormone (ACTH); (3) the thyrotrophic hormone (TSH); and three gonadotrophic hormones, namely (4) the follicle-stimulating hormone (FSH); (5) the luteinizing hormone (LH) or interstitial cell-stimulating hormone (ICSH), depending on the sex; (6) the lactogenic hormone. The follicle-stimulating hormone produces a ripening of the ovarian follicles in the female and stimulates the seminiferous tubules to form sperm in the male. The luteinizing hormone causes luteinization of the ripe follicle in the female and stimulates the Leydig cells of the testis to produce testosterone in the male. There is evidence to suggest that LH or ICSH may stimulate the zona reticularis of the adrenal cortex to produce 17-ketosteroids, which are excreted in the urine.

The problem of the individual secretory functions of the various types of cell is still unsolved. Pearse divides the six hormones into two groups on the basis of their carbohydrate content as shown by PAS staining, namely a *carbohydrate-containing group* (1) follicle-stimulating, (2) luteinizing and (3) thyrotrophic, and a *carbohydrate-free group* (4) growth, (5) lactogenic and (6) adrenocorticotrophic. It would appear that the mucoid cells, *i.e.* the basophils and those chromophobes with mucoprotein granules or vesicles, the total exceeding in numbers the basophils shown by the older methods from 12 to 25 per cent, are responsible for the first group, as well as for ACTH, whilst the growth and lactogenic hormones are produced by the acidophils.

Growth Hormone.—This, the so-called somatotrophic hormone, does not operate through the mediation of any target gland. It is therefore not really entitled to the suffix trophic. Unlike the other pituitary hormones, the growth hormone is more of less species-specific. Thus bovine growth hormone has little effect on man, whereas human and monkey growth hormone exert striking anabolic effects in human subjects. This is a good example of how easy it is to make mistakes when transferring the result of animal observation to man. The hormone acts on all cell systems, whether epithelial, mesothelial or endothelial, and it influences the metabolism of protein, carbohydrate and fat (Weil). The rate of protein formation is increased, in part owing to an increased utilization of depot fat, thus sparing protein. The clinical effects of overproduction of the growth hormone are gigantism or acromegaly, depending on the age of the patient. The long-continued administration of the hormone leads to a decrease in the size and number of the acidophils in the experimental animal, and an increase in the basophils and chromophobes.

Thyrotrophic Hormone.—There is evidence to suggest that the thyroid-stimulating hormone is made up of 3 factors, one causing the thyroid to secrete an increased amount of hormone, a second inducing increased growth (hyperplasia) of the gland, and a third producing exophthalmos. The growth factor is apparently dependent upon direct continuity with the hypothalamus for its production, but the metabolic factor is independent. Thyroidectomy often aggravates the exophthalmos of Graves' disease, while the administration of thyroid hormone may relieve the condition to some extent through inhibition of the pituitary. A week or more after hypophysectomy the thyroid atrophies, and the production of thyroid hormone fall to 10 per cent or less of normal.

Adrenocorticotrophic Hormone.—The adrenotrophic hormone, corticotrophin, or ACTH, as its name indicates, stimulates the adrenal cortex but not the medulla. The adrenals of most patients are enlarged at the time of death in contrast with persons who are killed suddenly. This is because *nonspecific stress* of a wide variety of kinds may activate the pituitary-adrenal axis. Among the stimuli are trauma, hemorrhage, emotional stress, drugs, chemical or bacterial toxic agents, as well as such hormones as insulin, thyroxine, vasopressin and epinephrine. It is for this reason that the response to the most diverse forms of stress follows a relatively uniform physiological pattern.

The anatomical site from which the mechanism is triggered is the hypothalamus, a humoral agent of unknown nature passing to the adenohypophysis *via* the hypophyseal portal vessels. The stimulus which activates the mechanism may be either hormonal when the stress is not sudden or severe, or neurogenic when it is of this character. Hydrocortisone is a powerful inhibitor of ACTH production, so that it can be used when the physician wishes to depress adrenal cortical function in cases of adrenal hyperplasia.

In general terms it may be said that the ACTH-adrenal mechanism serves to regulate the mobilization of protein, the amount of liver glycogen and the blood glucose level, the depot fat in the liver, renal tubular reabsorption of water and electrolytes, the processes of inflammation and the immune response, the amount of lymphoid tissue, and the integrity of the connective tissue.

Gonadotrophic Hormones.—These are three in number: (1) follicle-stimulating hormone, (2) luteinizing, or, in the male, interstitial cell-stimulating hormone, and (3) lactogenic hormone. The action of these hormones and the effects produced by disturbance of their function have already been discussed in connection with diseases of the male and female reproductive systems.

Functions of the Neurohypophysis.—The neurohypophysis, to use a more accurate term than that of posterior lobe, produces at least two hormones, vasopressin and oxytocin. *Vasopressin* can produce a marked elevation in the blood pressure owing to peripheral vasoconstriction. It exerts a perhaps even more important *antidiuretic action* on the renal tubules, and some workers speak of three instead of two hormones. The *antidiuretic hormone* or ADH increases the rate of reabsorption of water and electrolytes by the tubular epithelium in the loop of Henle. It therefore reduces the output of urine, and thus performs the extremely important function of guarding the organism against excessive water loss. Lack of the hormone results in the development of diabetes insipidus, with its characteristic polydipsia and polyuria with urine of low specific gravity and low chloride content.

Oxytocin derives its name from its ability to cause contraction of smooth muscle, notably the uterus (*oxus*, swift; *tokos*, birth). The hormone is of value in inducing *uterine contractions* during labor. The effect can be inhibited by progesterone. Oxytocin also acts on the contractile cells of the mammary gland, thus stimulating a *flow of milk* in the lactating breast. Mechanical stimulation of the nipple in suckling and also in milking leads to an excitation which reaches the central nervous system by a neural path, and there causes release of oxytocin, which is carried by the blood to the breast.

This brings us to the question of the hypothalamic centers in the diencephalon, and the *hypothalamic-hypophyseal system.* Although we have spoken of the hormones of the neurohypophysis, we are faced with the fact that the posterior lobe of the pituitary contains no typical glandular cells such as we see in other endocrine glands. It does contain a very dense network of fine nerve fibers, which are extensions of neurones of the diencephalon, itself the most ancient part of the cerebrum, which has remained almost unchanged in the course of development, and governs the primitive functions such as sleep and water balance, and the primitive sensations such as hunger and thirst. The fibers of the neurohypophysis arise in two nuclei of the hypothalamus, the supraoptic and the paraventricular. The cells of these nuclei have long been known to contain granules and colloid droplets, so that they have been called "glandular nerve cells". A definite secretory pathway has now been traced between these cells and the network of nerves in the neurohypophysis, first by staining with chrome-hematoxylin and more recently by electron micrography. By these methods secretory material can be shown to fill the cells in the diencephalon and to pass along the fibers which traverse the infundibulum, ending in the terminal arborizations of the fibrils in the neurohypophysis which appear to act as a storage site (Bargmann). It is easy to understand now why cutting the stalk of the pituitary, the infundibulum, in the experimental animal is followed by a heavy flow of urine, and why in the human subject hypothalamic tumors and even tumors pressing on the hypothalamus may give rise to polyuria and diabetes insipidus, as well as to adiposity and pathological somnolence. Perhaps we should begin to speak of hypothalamic hormones rather than those of the posterior pituitary.

The variety of functions of the pituitary is fortunately not paralleled by a variety of lesions. Only three groups merit mention: (1) vascular lesions, (2) inflammations, and (3) tumors. The pituitary has a remarkable faculty of functional reserve, so that only very extensive lesions are likely to produce functional disorder and clinical symptoms.

VASCULAR LESIONS

It is not unusual to find microscopic areas of necrosis in the anterior lobe at autopsy. In the absence of inflammation, these may be presumed to be arteriolosclerotic or vascular in origin. They are without clinical significance.

Sheehan made a notable contribution to the subject when he associated pituitary necrosis occurring after delivery with shock and hemorrhage. During pregnancy the pituitary enlarges and its circulation increases. If acute blood loss or shock occurs at the time of delivery, the enlarged pituitary becomes ischemic, and thrombi form with infarction and necrosis of the gland. The endocrinological result of the destruction to the pituitary has come, justifiably, to be known as *Sheehan's syndrome*, the clinical features of which we shall consider presently. It is now recognized that this syndrome may be produced by a variety of pathological processes which destroy at least two-thirds of the gland in man as well as women. The pituitary is soft and pale due to the ischemia, unless hemorrhage has occurred. With the passage of time the dead tissue is replaced by fibrous tissue, with subsequent shrinkage and atrophy, so that the gland may be reduced to a mere nubbin. The results may not become apparent for many months or even years. The same is true also of the only other lesion which frequently leads to profound destruction of the anterior pituitary, namely the chromophobe adenoma.

INFLAMMATIONS

Inflammatory lesions, which are so important in other organs, are of negligible importance in the pituitary, for they rarely cause functional disturbance. This is indeed true of the other endocrine glands. The granulomas, more especially tuberculosis and sarcoidosis, are not infrequent, but they are seldom of sufficient size to disturb function.

TUMORS

Adenoma.—In our study of the various organs of the body we have encountered no instance in which benign tumors are more important than malignant ones, but this is true in the case of the pituitary. It is the adenoma which produces the symptoms, which may be those of hyperactivity or underactivity of the gland. It is easy to understand how symptoms of hyperpituitarism should result from proliferation of a gland secreting hormones. Hypopituitarism may be the result of the anatomical site of the pituitary within the sella turcica, the pressure of the rigid walls on the expanding mass causing loss of function if not actual necrosis.

We speak of acidophil (eosinophil), basophil and chromophobe adenomas, as if each tumor was composed of a different type of cell. With our increasing insight into the meaning of the staining reactions of the cells, this concept is gradually being discarded. One or other type of cell may dominate, but these cells represent a storage, not a production, of hormone. Although acromegaly is supposed to be associated with an acidophil adenoma, the tumor found at operation is more often a chromophobe than an acidophil one. Both the lesions conventionally called chromophobe and acidophil adenomas may really be cells with sparse PAS-positive granules. These cells should rather be regarded as amphophils, which produce trophic hormones acting on various target organs. Possibly deficiency in the target organ may induce hyperplasia in the pituitary (Russfield *et al.*). This can be shown by removal of the adrenals or gonads in the experimental animal. With these previsos we shall still use the time-honoured classification of chromophobe, acidophil and basophil adenomas.

Chromophobe Adenoma.—This is much the commonest form of pituitary tumor. The chromophobe cells are non-granular, so that the cells of the tumor appear clear, but with special stains many of them prove to be sparsely granular. Most of these tumors show a very characteristic alveolar grouping, with fibrous septa between the groups, but in some the cells are arranged diffusely. The tumors about to be described are those which produce symptoms either local or general. Much more common are collections of cells which have been called subclinical adenomas, usually miliary or microscopic in size and producing no symptoms. The cell pattern differs from the normal and may be that of a convoluted papilloma or a compound tubular gland. These cell collections are not encapsulated. When symptoms are present they are those of *pituitary insufficiency*, similar to the changes produced in an animal when the anterior lobe is removed. The negative symptoms of insufficiency are the result of compression of the functioning eosinophil and basophilic cells. The adenoma often remains confined to the sella, causing interference with skeletal and sexual development. If it breaks through the membranous roof and presses on the tuber cinereum, hypothalamic adiposity will be superadded.

Acidophil Adenoma.—The eosinophil adenoma is a good deal less common. It is composed of cells filled with red-staining granules, the cells are large and often multinucleated, and they are arranged diffusely, with complete absence of the alveolar grouping so characteristic of the chromophobe adenoma. The eosinophil cells are concerned with skeletal growth, so that the tumor is associated with the syndrome of overgrowth, *i.e.*, *gigantism* or *acromegaly*. The acidophil adenoma may give rise to the nearest approach to pure hyperpituitarism (skeletal overgrowth, connective tissue hyperplasia, hypertrichosis, glycosuria, increased metabolic rate), but later in the disease insufficiency symptoms may become apparent. The tumor found at autopsy is often a chromophobe adenoma, although with one of the special strains such as PAS-orange G the cells are seen to be sparsely granulated, but it is probable that it was acidophilic in type in the earlier phase of the disease.

Basophil Adenoma.—This is by far the rarest form of adenoma associated with symptoms, although minute examples are not an uncommon incidental finding at autopsy. Cushing thought that the syndrome which goes by his name was caused by this tumor, but it is now evident that the lesion is only secondary, an effect rather than a cause. The constant pituitary lesion in *Cushing's syndrome* is *hyalinization of the basophil* cells with disappearance of their granules first described by Crooke. Hyalinization is an indication of inactivity of the basophils, and the occurrence of small basophil adenomas may indicate merely an attempt to compensate for the depressed basophil function.

Heinbecker, in an excellent review of the subject, points out that at least three primary lesions may be precursors of the all-important hyalinization of the basophil cells; these are (1) a tumor of the adrenal cortex, (2) a tumor of the thymus, and (3) atrophy of the nuclei of the hypothalamus. Experimental lesions of the hypothalamus in the dog are followed by marked loss of basophil cells, with degenerative changes in the remaining basophils. The most frequent primary lesion is a tumor (usually a benign adenoma) or hyperplasia of the adrenal cortex. Every case of Cushing's syndrome should therefore be explored for adrenal tumor.

Neighborhood Syndrome.—The effects of a pituitary tumor may be divided into general tumor symptoms, endocrine symptoms, and neighborhood symptoms. The first group comprises the symptoms of cerebral tumor in general, particularly increased intracranial pressure. If the tumor is small and confined to the sella these symptoms will be absent. The endocrine symptoms are about to be discussed. The neighborhood symptoms are caused by pressure on neighboring structures. Pressure on the optic nerve causes optic atrophy of the primary type. The most characteristic pressure symptom is bitemporal hemianopsia due to compression of the inner fibers of the optic chiasma. There may be pressure on the hypothalamus with production of the hypothalamic syndrome (adiposity, polyuria). This is more likely to be caused by a chromophobe than a chromophil adenoma, as the latter remains confined to the sella long after the development of symptoms of hyperpituitarism. The sella is always expanded by the tumor, and may be markedly ballooned, with absorption of the clinoid processes.

Carcinoma. (Malignant Adenoma).—This is a rare condition. In Cushing's series there were only 3 malignant tumors compared with 159 innocent ones. The tumor destroys the base of the skull, bursts through the roof of the sella, and invades the floor of the third ventricle. I have seen it cause cerebrospinal rhinorrhea or discharge of cerebrospinal fluid from the nose. The cells, which are of the *chromophobe type*, are grouped in irregular masses.

Craniopharyngioma.—Tumors of Rathke's pharyngeal pouch or the hypophyseal duct, conveniently called craniopharyngeal tumors, arise from vestigial remnants of the epithelial tract from which the anterior lobe of the pituitary is originally formed. They are usually suprasellar tumors, but may originate and be confined within the sella. They may be quite minute, about the size of a pea, or may form huge calcareous masses as large as a tennis ball. *The tumor usually appears under the age of fifteen years, and attains a much larger size than the average pituitary adenoma. Cystic degeneration* and *calcification* of the wall of the cyst are common, and suprasellar calcification (*x*-ray) is a clinical sign of great value. The tumor may compress the pituitary, causing retardation of growth, but the most marked symptom may be adiposity due to pressure on the hypothalamus. *Microscopically* the tumor is usually an epidermoid carcinoma, but it may be a basal cell cancer of the adamantinoma type. Cystic degeneration is common, and the entire tumor may be converted into a cyst.

The *symptoms* are a combination of hypopituitarism and the hypothalamic syndrome owing to the pressure of the tumor both upward and downward. Among these symptoms are amenorrhea, failing libido, low basal metabolic rate, loss of hair, stunting of growth, obesity in young adults, sleepiness and polyuria, the last-named differentiating it from adenoma of the pituitary. *Suprasellar calcification* is a sign of the greatest value.

CONGENITAL ANOMALIES

The anterior lobe of the pituitary is formed from a diverticulum from the roof of the buccopharyn-geal junction. A remnant of this process is practically constant under the pharyngeal mucosa, where it is known as the *pharyngeal hypophysis*. Other remnants may be left along the course of the craniopharyngeal canal where they may give rise to the craniopharyngiomas. Congenital hypoplasia of the gland is found in various types of dwarf. *Dermoid tumors* are of rare occurrence in this region. They are due to invagination of the cranial epidermis during closure of the neural canal.

HYPOPITUITARISM

Three main types of hypopituitarism are recognized: (1) the *Simmonds' syndrome*, occurring in adult life, marked by profound cachexia and premature senility, and usually caused by Sheehan's postpartum pituitary necrosis; (2) the *Lorain-Levi syndrome*, occurring in childhood, characterized by dwarfism, and in most cases due to destruction of the pituitary by a craniopharyngioma; and (3) the *Fröhlich syndrome*, most frequent at the time of puberty, a combination of genital atrophy and adiposity, and associated either with a chromophobe adenoma or craniopharyngioma.

This is undoubtedly an oversimplification of a very complex problem. Thus *Sheehan's syndrome* has been separated from Simmonds' syndrome, being distinguished by such features as (1) gonadal atrophy with its secondary consequences; (2) absence of normal pigmentation; and (3) thyroid atrophy with resulting increased sensitivity to cold, a flabby facies with thinning of the eyebrows, mental torpor, a low basal metabolic rate, and a very low urinary excretion of 17-keto-steroids. Such a woman has a characteristic facial appearance, but it is often diagnosed as myxedema. She does indeed have myxedema, but it is a secondary or pituitary myxedema. It is evident that if the destruction of the anterior pituitary is complete and the hypopituitarism also complete, all the other target glands will suffer in unison, so that the clinical picture may become all-embracing.

Lesions.—The lesions in hypopituitarism are varied. The usual organic cause is *craniopharyngioma.* Such tumors press upon the hypothalamus as well as upon the pituitary, and as they are congenital in origin and usually develop early in life, they cause some of the most extreme forms of adiposogenital dystrophy in children. *Chromophobe adenoma* of the pituitary may sometimes be responsible. This seldom develops before the age of twenty years, and therefore fails to explain the cases occurring in childhood. As the adenoma is often confined to the sella and therefore may not press on the hypothalamus, adiposity may be slight or absent. A much rarer group is that of *pituitary necrosis* (Simmonds). Many of these cases of pituitary old age have been attributed to puerperal sepsis. In other cases nothing is found beyond a hypoplasia of the pituitary, which is indicated clinically by the very small size of the sella turcica. In addition to these gross organic causes there can be little doubt that in the majority of cases there is no tumor or necrosis, but merely a hypofunction of the gland, often temporary in character, as a result of which there may be some retardation of growth, lack of sexual development, or undue adiposity, all of which may be remedied in the course of a few years.

Simmonds' Syndrome.—The Simmonds' syndrome may develop in adult life or in childhood. Both are examples of premature senility or *progeria*. When the disease appears in childhood the patient remains a dwarf. A person suffering from pituitary old age presents a remarkable clinical picture, for a child often may have the aspect of a decrepit old man (Fig. 575). Many years ago Jonathan Hutchinson of London reported the case of a patient who when only fifteen years of age had the aspect of a decrepit old man, 3 feet 5 inches in height and weighing only 38 pounds. He died two years later of apparent senility. There is a general *microsplanchnia*, all the organs being small and underweight in contrast to the large heavy organs of acromegaly. The atrophy may affect the thyroid causing thyroid insufficiency (myxedema), or the adrenals causing adrenal insufficiency. The structure of the anterior pituitary is wiped out. Simmonds attributed this to embolism, but the blood reaches the anterior lobe by many channels, and there was no good evidence of the presence of emboli in his cases. Sheehan pointed out that extensive necrosis of the anterior pituitary is not uncommon in women during delivery, and this he attributed to thrombosis of the pituitary

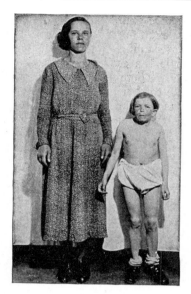

Fig. 575.—Simmonds' disease. The patient on the right is twenty-seven years old but looks much older. Her sister (left) is twenty-three years old. (Boyd, *Pathology for the Physician*.)

vessels caused by collapse after severe hemorrhage. It is possible that the necrosis, at least in some cases, may be anoxic rather than ischemic, owing partly to the high metabolic rate which is known to exist at least in the rat's pituitary during parturition, and partly to pressure of the sella on the enlarged pituitary of pregnancy.

Lorain-Levi Syndrome.—This is a rare prepubertal association of infantilism and even dwarfism with destructive lesions of the pituitary. Destruction of the sella turcica is often evident in the x-ray film, being caused by a suprasellar cyst or craniopharyngioma. There is a retention of infantile proportions, lack of sexual development, and bright mentality. The patient remains a graceful and attractive child, a Peter Pan who refuses to grow up. In such a case it is evident that the growth and gonadotrophic hormones are deficient, whilst the thyrotrophic hormone and ACTH are unimpaired. In other cases there may be an appearance of premature senility due to a dry, yellowish, wrinkled condition of the skin. If the hypothalamus is involved, obesity may change the picture.

Fröhlich's Syndrome.—This is a *dystro-*

phia adiposo-genitalis that commonly develops about the time of puberty, but may appear later in life. Depression of the sexual function is the earliest and most constant symptom. There is amenorrhea in the female, due to absence of the hormone which stimulates ovarian function, and loss of libido in the male. The sexual organs remain undeveloped or atrophy. Of equal importance is atrophy of the skin and hair, in striking contrast to what is found in acromegaly. The skin is thin, delicate, smooth like a child's and dry. This is due to atrophy of the dermal connective tissue. The hair of the head is normal in amount but soft and fine; the facial, axillary and pubic hair is scanty; the skin of the trunk and legs is hairless. After the age of thirty-five years the soft skin becomes finely wrinkled owing to the lack of fibrous tissue in the dermis. Adiposity may be very marked or may be absent. When the condition develops in an adult male, deposits of fat in the breasts, hip, buttocks, and lower abdomen give the figure a distinctly feminine cast. Sudden fluctuations of weight are characteristic. The basal metabolic rate is usually low. Mental dullness of varying degree is common. Sugar tolerance is not really high as is commonly supposed, for after the administration of glucose the blood-sugar curve takes an unusually long time to return to normal owing to the general slowing up of metabolic processes, but glycosuria never occurs, so that in that sense the patient has a good sugar tolerance. A variation of this syndrome is the adipose type, illustrated to perfection by the Fat Boy in Pickwick. His face is round and chubby, his mind is slow, and he is ready to drop asleep at a moment's notice.

It is singularly difficult to give a satisfying pathological (morbid anatomical) explanation of this striking clinical picture. It may well be that this is more an example of hypothalamo-hypophysial dystrophy than of pure hypopituitarism. The dysfunction is due to pressure on the hypothalamic centers from without such as a craniopharingiona or chromophobe adenoma rather than a lesion of the centers themselves. Experimental destruction of the hypothalamus in dogs produces a much more severe and rapid obesity than does hypophysectomy. This is prob-

ably due to a disorder of fat metabolism, a metabolism which is regulated by the hypothalamic nuclei, together with an increased appetite. It is interesting to note that in 1904 Erdheim suggested that the obesity in Fröhlich's was due to involvement of the hypothalamic region. Genital atrophy may also be due to hypothalamic damage. The unsolved problem is how it is that in the majority of cases no lesion can be found. To this there is no answer.

A rare apparent variation of the Fröhlich type is the *Laurence-Moon-Biedl syndrome.* I say apparent, because it seems to be a *genotypic inherited* character defect rather than one of pituitary origin. The condition is characterized by a strong familial tendency, adiposity, genital dystrophy, mental deficiency, retinitis pigmentosa, and polydactylism. A patient with adiposity, partial blindness, and six fingers or six toes is easily recognized as belonging to this group, especially when it is found that other members of the family present the same condition. It has been suggested that the adiposity and genital atrophy are caused by a congenital malformation in the hypothalamic region.

Diabetes Insipidus.—This is another result of failure of the hypothalamic-hypophysial system which produces the antidiuretic hormone. The condition is marked by the passage of large quantities of urine of a very low specific gravity, so that the essential defect is the renal loss of water. The polyuria often amounts to 8 to 12 liters a day, in exceptional cases even 25 liters! The specific gravity may be as low as 0.001. The total excretion of chloride is reduced. There is a lowered water content in the vascular, interstitial and intracellular compartments, and this gives rise to thirst so intense that the patient has been known to drink his own urine.

The polyuria is due to decreased secretion of the antidiuretic hormone, which controls resorption of water from the loop of Henle and the distal convoluted tubule. It is fortunate that 80 per cent of the glomerular filtrate is absorbed by the proximal tubules, otherwise the hard-pressed patient might have total loss of the concentrating power of his kidneys.

The hormone is secreted by the pars

nervosa of the pituitary, but the secretion is under the control of stimuli from the hypothalamic nuclei. It is evident, therefore, that a variety of lesions in different sites such as the hypothalamic nuclei, the connecting nerve tracts, the pituitary stalk or the neurohypophysis may be responsible for the hormonal failure. The lesion may be large, such as a pituitary tumor or one pressing on the hypothalamus, trauma, as in fracture of the base of the skull, and meningitis. In other cases it is microscopic, as in encephalitis.

HYPERPITUITARISM

In the discussion of hypopituitarism it was pointed out that the clinical manifestations were those of a general inadequacy of pituitary hormones rather than of any one in particular. This is not the case in hyperpituitarism, where the effect may be due to overaction of the growth hormone, of the adrenocorticotrophic hormone, or possibly of the thyrotrophic hormone. It must be borne in mind that the cause of the disturbance of function is often a tumor, an adenoma, and that this tumor in addition to elaborating an excess of the hormone normally produced by its cells of origin will usually destroy the other types of cell. Even in the purest forms of hyperpituitarism we shall not expect to find an exaggeration of all the normal functions of the gland. There will nearly always be some insufficiency to mar the perfect picture. The main effect of hyperpituitarism is excessive growth of the connective tissues and especially of the bones.

Growth Hormone.—Here the clinical result will depend on the age of the patient at which the hormonal hyperfunction becomes apparent. If in early years the result will be gigantism, if at a later date it will be acromegaly, depending on whether or not ossification has been completed.

Gigantism.—This is always due to pituitary hyperplasia. A definite tumor is usually present with enlargement of the sella turcica, but in the milder forms there may merely be hyperplasia of the anterior lobe. The acceleration of growth may be extraordinary, as in the case of the boy who weighed 9 pounds at birth, 62 pounds at one and

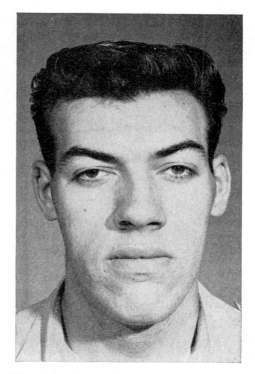

Fig. 576.—Acromegaly. Note the large face, heavy features, prognathous jaw, and coarse and thick hair.

one-half years, and at nine years he was 6 feet, 1 inch in height, weighed 178 pounds, and was able to pick up his father and carry him about (Behrens and Barr).

Associated with the skeletal overgrowth there may be a later development of symptoms of pituitary insufficiency, especially impotence in men and amenorrhea in women. The skeletal overgrowth is caused by hyperplasia of the eosinophil cells of the anterior lobe, while the subsequent sexual insufficiency is due to pressure on the cells of that lobe which are concerned with sexual stimulation. The pituitary activity may inhibit the action of insulin so that glycosuria develops, and it is common for giants to die with symptoms of diabetes. Later in the disease the tumor may be converted into a cyst so that the pituitary is greatly shrunken, but the skeletal changes are permanent, and the expanded sella bears witness to the former size of the gland.

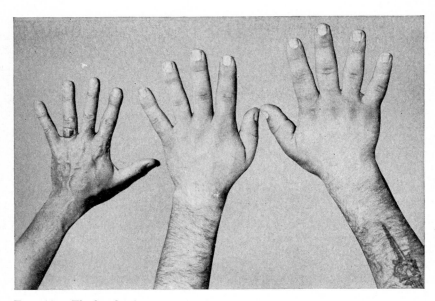

Fig. 577.—The hands of acromegaly compared with a normal hand. Same patient
as shown in Figure 576.

Acromegaly.—Acromegaly is the result of hyperpituitarism after ossification is completed. The chief changes are enlargement of the bones, hypertrophy of the connective tissue, and changes in the skin and hair, to which may be added later in the disease symptoms suggestive of hypopituitarism such as depression of the sexual function. The tumor found at operation or autopsy is more often a chromophobe than an acidophil adenoma, but it is probable that the cells were acidophil in the early phase of the disease. It was Pierre Marie who, in 1886, recognized the pituitary origin of the disease and named it from the great enlargement of the hands and feet (*akros*, extremity; *megale*, large). The face is large, the frontal sinuses prominent, the eyes deeply set, the lower jaw is heavily undershot and prognathous (Fig. 576), so that the lower teeth project beyond the upper ones, the teeth themselves are widely separated, the hands and feet are huge and clumsy (Fig. 577), with exostoses on the phalanges and a characteristic tufting of the terminal phalanx seen in the roentgen-ray picture. Kyphosis may be marked, and the patient with his bent back, huge hands reaching to the knees and protruding lower jaw presents a gorilla-like picture. In addition to the osseous changes there is marked connective tissue hyperplasia which produces enlargement of the lips, tongue, nose, hands, and feet. Owing to this fibrosis the skin becomes thick, coarse, and furrowed, a change that is most strikingly evident in the scalp which is deeply corrugated like that of a bulldog. There is marked increase in the hair, which is thick and coarse, and profuse sweating is common. In the active stage of the disease there may be increased sexual excitement. Lactation after pregnancy may continue for a number of years. Changes in the basal metabolic rate are not constant, but during the active stage it may be increased and the appetite is sometimes voracious. Glycosuria occurs in about 20 per cent of the cases, but it is curiously inconstant in the same patient. The disease is self-limited, and the signs of overactivity become replaced by those of hypopituitarism, *i.e.*, adiposity, somnolence, and sexual impotence. The structural changes (bone and connective tissue) are of course permanent.

There is a general overgrowth of the viscera, a *macrosplanchnia*, which may be compared with the microsplanchnia in Simmonds'

PLATE XV

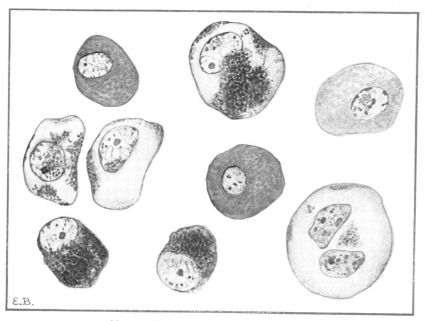

Hyaline Changes in Pituitary Basophils.

Crooke's hyaline change in the basophil cells of the pituitary in Cushing's syndrome. Two normal basophils are seen in the lower left corner. A normal chromophobe and two normal acidophils are also included.

disease. Hyperplasia of the adrenals is particularly marked.

Adrenocorticotrophic Hormone. — Cushing's Syndrome. — When Harvey Cushing first described the condition now known as Cushing's syndrome he naturally attributed the remarkable clinical picture to the basophil adenoma which was present in a number of his cases, although he was aware of the presence of adrenal cortical hyperplasia or adenoma. These lesions are now believed to be responsible for the symptoms in 90 per cent of the cases. In the remaining 10 per cent, however, no lesions of the adrenals can be demonstrated, and in such cases a small *basophil adenoma* of the pituitary is often found. In these instances it may well be that an excessive secretion of ACTH is responsible for adrenal cortical hyperfunction, which may be followed later by cortical hyperplasia. Cushing's disease may be regarded as the result of an *altered pituitary-adrenocortical balance*, the primary upset being usually adrenal but occasionally pituitary in origin. Cases have been reported recently where bilateral adrenalectomy for hyperadrenocorticism has been followed in the course of two or three years by the development of a chromophobe tumor of the pituitary secreting large quantities of ACTH. A more detailed discussion of the Cushing syndrome will be found in the chapter on the adrenals, page 991.

A constant lesion which points to a disturbance of the normal pituitary-adrenocortical relationship is the *hyalinization* of the *pituitary basophil cells* first described by Crooke in 1935 (Plate XV). Instead of the condition being a manifestation of overactivity of the basophil cells, so-called basophilism, it appears rather to be a result of inactivity of these cells (Heinbecker). Loss of the basophil cell function leads to regressive changes in the thyroid, gonads and islets of Langerhans, which are probably responsible for some of the protean manifestations.

Thyrotrophic Hormone. — The thyroid is under the direct control of the pituitary thyroid-stimulating hormone, which in turn is increased by stimuli arising in the hypothalamus. This might be connected with the well known occurrence of symptoms of thyrotoxicosis following severe emotional and psychic stress. Hyperthyroidism may also be associated with acromegaly. Such facts offer the tempting idea that the hyperplasia and hyperfunctioning of the thyroid in Graves' disease are due to an increase of TSH secretion, but the evidence at present available is hardly sufficient to justify its acceptance.

REFERENCES

BARGMANN, W.: Endeavour, 1960, 125. (The neurosecretory system of the diencephalon). *Das Zwischenhirn-Hypophysensystem*, Berlin, 1954.

BEHRENS, L. H. and BARR, D. P.: Endocrinology, 1932, *16*, 120. (Gigantism.)

EZRIN, C. *et al.*: J. Clin. Endocrinol. and Metab., 1958, *18*, 917 (delta cell in acute and chronic illness); 1959, *19*, 621 (beta and delta cells in adrenocortical disorders); 1959, *19*, 958 (pituitary cells in thyroid disorders.)

GOLDEN, A.: Lab. Invest., 1959, *8*, 925. (Actively-secreting and storage cells of anterior pituitary.)

MOORE, F. D.: Can. M.A.J., 1958, *78*, 85. (Endocrine mediators of surgical injury.)

PEARSE, A. G. E.: J. Path. and Bact., 1949, *61*, 195; 1952, *64*, 791; 1953, *65*, 355. (Cytochemistry of anterior pituitary.)

RUSSFIELD, A. B., REINER, L. and KLAUS, H.: Am. J. Path., 1956, 32, 1055. (Endocrine significance of pituitary tumors.)

SHARRER, E. and SHARRER, B.: Recent Progress in Hormone Research, 1954, Vol. 10, New York. (Hormones produced by neurosecretory cells.)

SHEEHAN, H. L. and SUMMERS, V. K.: Quart. J. Med., 1949, *18*, 319. (Syndrome of hypopituitarism.)

SIMPSON, S. L.: *Major Endocrine Disorders*, 3rd ed., London, 1959.

SLOPER, J. C. and ADAMS, C. W. M.: J. Path. and Bact., 1956, *72*, 587. (Hypothalamic elaboration of posterior pituitary principles in man.)

SOFFER, L. J.: *Diseases of the Endocrine Glands*, 2nd ed., Philadelphia, 1956.

SOMMERS, S. C.: Lab. Invest., 1959, *8*, 588. (Cell types in relation to function.)

WEIL, R.: Arch. Int. Med., 1955, *95*, 739. (Growth hormone.)

WILLIAMS, R. H.: *Textbook of Endocrinology*, 2nd ed., Philadelphia, 1955.

WOLMAN, L.: J. Path. and Bact., 1956, *72*, 575. (Pituitary necrosis in raised intracranial pressure.)

Chapter 36

The Adrenals

General Considerations
  STRUCTURE AND DEVELOPMENT
  CORTICAL PHYSIOLOGY
    Mineralocorticoids:
      Aldosterone
    Glucocorticoids: Hydrocortisone
    Sex or Nitrogen Hormones:
      17-Ketosteroids
    Pituitary-Adrenal Relation-
      ship
  MEDULLARY PHYSIOLOGY
    Noradrenalin
  STRESS
Hypoadrenalism

ACUTE ADRENAL INSUFFICIENCY
CHRONIC ADRENAL INSUFFI-
    CIENCY. ADDISON'S
    DISEASE
  Relation of Symptoms to
    Lesions
Hyperadrenalism
  CUSHING'S SYNDROME
  ADRENOGENITAL SYNDROME
  PRIMARY ALDOSTERONISM:
    CONN'S SYNDROME
    Secondary Aldosteronism
  NORADRENALISM
Tumors

CORTICAL TUMORS
  Adenoma
  Carcinoma
MEDULLARY TUMORS
  Neuroblastoma
  Pheochromocytoma
  Ganglioneuroma
SECONDARY TUMORS
Miscellaneous Lesions
  POSTMORTEM CHANGES
  NECROSIS
  MASSIVE HEMORRHAGE
  AMYLOIDOSIS
  MYELOLIPOMA

GENERAL CONSIDERATIONS

Structure and Development.—The human adrenal is an organ of dual character. It consists of a cortex and a medulla which are perfectly distinct in development, in structure, and in function. The cortex is developed from the mesoderm of the Wolffian ridge in conjunction with the sex glands. The medulla is ectodermal in origin and arises from the neural crest together with the anlage of the sympathetic nerve cells. These embryological relationships are of the greatest importance in connection with adrenal physiology and pathology.

In the adult the adrenals have a combined weight of 12 to 15 gm., but this figure can vary widely. The *cortex*, which is yellow in color on account of its high lipid content, consists of 3 zones: an outer *zona glomerulosa*, so called because the cells are arranged in clusters bearing a feeble resemblance to glomeruli, a very wide middle *zona fasciculata* with parallel cords of cells at right angles to the capsule, and a *zona reticularis* made up of interlacing strands of cells. The three zones produce different kinds of hormones, a matter which is discussed in the section on cortical physiology. The zona reticularis is dark brown and often shows softening or cavitation at autopsy. It is easy to mistake this inner layer for the medulla, especially when there happens to be no medulla in the

slice inspected. The cortical cells in all three zones are rich in lipids of three types: (1) cholesterol, (2) neutral fats, and (3) functionally active steroids. These vary with different disease states, but it must be remembered that ordinary histological technique with its use of fat solvents for paraffin sections completely removes all three sets of lipids.

The *medulla* belongs to the chromaffin system, that is to say, it stains brown with chrome salts such as potassium bichromate. The abdominal sympathetic, the carotid body, and the organ of Zuckerkandl found in children at the bifurcation of the aorta, belong to the same system. Destruction of the medulla is, therefore, more readily compensated than destruction of the cortex.

The *development* of the adrenals presents some curious features. In fetal life the adrenal is almost all cortex, and at the third month it is actually larger than the kidney. Unlike the cortex after birth the fetal cortex contains no lipids. The rate of weight compared with that of the kidney is 1 to 3.5, whereas in the adult it is only 1 to 30. Immediately after birth a strange change takes place. The entire fetal cortex rapidly degenerates and is slowly replaced by adult cortex and medulla, but it is not until the twelfth year that the original size of the adrenal at birth is regained. Massive hemorrhage may occur into the degenerating cortex at birth, and as the hemorrhage is often bilateral it may prove fatal to the child. In the *anencephalic fetus* the cortex is absent, so that the adrenals are very atrophic. This maldevelopment of the adrenals is probably the result of interference with the development of the pituitary, for the posterior lobe of the pituitary is often missing (Angevine). Accessory cortical tissue is common at birth, but it soon atrophies and disappears. Occasionally it persists into adult life as small bright yellow nodules which are found under the capsule of the liver and in the line of descent of the gonads, *i.e.*, in the kidney, along the spermatic vein, in the broad ligament, testicle and ovary.

Cortical Physiology.—It is just over 100 years since Addison opened the door and allowed us our first peep into the working of the adrenals, at the same time laying the foundation stone of the temple of endocrinology. He observed that patients with adrenal insufficiency often died from minor infections and stresses. We now know that it is the adrenal which enables the body to withstand the large variety of environmental stresses and strains to which it is subjected. The adrenal plays perhaps the largest single role in determining whether any person is sick or well, and, more particularly, if he *feels* sick or well. Removal or destruction of the cortex of both adrenals is invariably followed by death in the absence of replacement therapy. The adrenals are more essential to life than is the pituitary. The result of removal of the adrenals is increase in the urinary excretion of sodium, accompanied by marked loss of water, reduction in the circulating plasma volume, and eventually dehydration and shock. There is a corresponding though less marked increase in the excretion of chloride, but a decreased excretion of potassium which accordingly accumulates in the serum. These changes seem to be due to loss of control of the permeability of membranes. Renal failure may develop as the result of the dehydration and shock caused by the loss of salt and water. A similar clinical picture develops as the result of chronic adrenal insufficiency in Addison's disease. Hypoglycemia may also occur. In both the experimental animal and in the patient the entire picture can be reversed by the administration of adrenal cortical hormone.

The three zones of the cortex have differing physiological significance. The *zona glomerulosa* is particularly rich in lipids, especially cholesterol, the raw sterol material from which the corticoids are formed. This zone is the source of aldosterone with its desoxycorticosterone-like property of retaining salt and water and increasing the loss of potassium. It appears to function autonomously, whereas the other two zones are thought to be under the control of ACTH, the adrenocorticotrophic hormone (corticotrophin) of the anterior pituitary. It is felt that the *zona fasciculata* is the probable source of the 17-hydroxycorticosteroids, whilst the *zona reticularis* supplies the 17-ketosteroids or androgen-like hormones. Under ACTH stimulation in the experimental animal the cells of the zona reticularis spread toward the zona fasciculata which shrinks almost to nothingness in the course of a few days. *The zona fasciculata may be considered to be the storehouse of the precursors of both corticoids and androgens, while the zona reticularis is the site of biosynthesis*, the factory in which the end products are produced.

The steroid nucleus of all the adrenocortical steroids has the same basic four-ring structure, differing only in the presence or absence of an O or OH group at carbon positions 11 or 17. Thus cortisone (Compound E) is the same as hydrocortisone (Compound F), except for the presence in the latter of an H atom at position 11, both having a hydroxyl group at position 17. This becomes more evident when the full chemical names are used, cortisone being 11-dehydro-17-hydroxycorticosterone whereas hydrocortisone is 17-hydroxycorticosterone, there already being an OH group at position 11.

Using a physiological or functional basis of classification we may recognize three groups of steroids. (1) Those concerned *mainly* with *the control of water and electrolyte metabolism*, and known therefore as *mineralocorticoids*, the naturally occurring hormone being aldosterone and the synthetic hormone desoxycorticosterone. (2) Those concerned *mainly* with *carbohydrate me-*

tabolism, (hence known as *glucocorticoids*), but also with the metabolism of protein and fat. Examples of this group are corticosterone, with an OH at position 11 and therefore more correctly termed hydroxycorticosterone, cortisone, with an O at position 11 and an OH at position 17 (11-dehydro-17-hydroxycorticosterone) and Compound F, with an OH at both the 11 and 17 positions. Neither of these groups is mutually exclusive, for the mineralocorticoids influence general metabolism to some degree, and the glucocorticoids influence electrolytes and water. (3) The *sex hormones* or *androgens* (androsterone), containing only 19 carbon atoms. They have an O atom at the 17 position, and 17-ketosteroids are normally excreted in the urine. A small amount of estrogen may be produced in addition to the androgen, so that a tumor of the adrenal cortex may on rare occasions be associated with feminizing rather than masculinizing effects. *The mineralocorticoids come from the zone glomerulosa, the glucocorticoids from the zona fasciculata, and the androgens from the zona reticularis.* This grouping of the internal secretions of the adrenal cortex, which is the golden thread to guide the hapless wayfarer through the labyrinth, may be referred to colloquially, though not academically, as the salt, sugar and sex hormones.

1. *Mineralocorticoids. Salt and Water Metabolism. Aldosterone,* produced by the zona glomerulosa, and the synthetic *desoxycorticosterone* represent the mineralocorticoids. As in the case of desoxycorticosterone, aldosterone promotes to a marked degree the reabsorption of sodium and water by the renal proximal convoluted tubules with corresponding loss of potassium. This retention of sodium and excretion of potassium leads to an exchange in these electrolytes, first in the extracellular and then in the intracellular fluid. The retention of sodium leads to an increased osmotic pressure of the serum, which stimulates the supraoptic-hypophyseal system to produce more antidiuretic hormone. This in turn leads to water reabsorption, which lowers the serum solute concentration, thus inhibiting the further output of ADH. At the same time it results in an increase in the volume of the extracellular fluid (ECF). As the final

regulator of aldosterone production in this dual feed-back mechanism is the volume of ECF, it is evident that no more aldosterone will be secreted. Aldosterone, then, provides the mechanism by which sodium, potassium and the extracellular fluid are maintained in normal balance (Bartter *et al.*). It is probable that some control of aldosterone production comes from the cells of the juxtaglomerular apparatus of the kidney. A correlation can be shown between the degree of granulation of the juxtaglomerular cells, the level of serum sodium, and the width of the zona glomerulosa (Pitcock and Hartroft). This matter has been discussed in detail on page 553.

The adrenal regulation of sodium metabolism appears to be independent of anterior pituitary control. Aldosterone is detectable in the urine even after hypophysectomy, whilst stimulation with ACTH, which greatly increases the urinary output of 17-hydroxycorticoids in healthy people, has only a small and transient effect on aldosterone output. *It is the zona fasciculata producing the glucocorticoids, not the zona glomerulosa producing aldosterone, which is involved in the pituitary-adrenal axis.* There does appear to be a hormone in the posterior portion of the diencephalon, more particularly the pineal gland, which stimulates aldosterone secretion. This diencephalic hormone can be demonstrated in the urine of adrenalectomized rats.

Hyperaldosteronism may occur: (1) in normal persons with low sodium intake, (2) in certain pathological states. In the former it may be regarded as an effect, in the latter it may possibly be a cause. The pathological group includes: (1) generalized edema, such as occurs in heart failure, nephrosis and cirrhosis of the liver; (2) in the persistent elevation of blood pressure which accompanies Cushing's disease, primary aldosteronism, the toxemias of pregnancy, and essential hypertension. It is evident that in secondary hypoadrenalism due to hypopituitarism it is not necessary to give mineralocorticoids, because aldosterone secretion is independent of ACTH control. The subject of primary aldosteronism is discussed in relation to hyperadrenalism on page 993.

2. *Glucocorticoids. Intermediate Carbo-*

hydrate Metabolism.—The principal members of this group produced by the zona fasciculata are hydrocortisone (17-hydroxycorticosterone, Compound F) and cortisone (17-hydroxy-11-dehydrocorticosterone, Compound E), which, as its chemical name indicates, differs from hydrocortisone only in lacking an H atom at the 11 carbon position of the steroid nucleus. Both are 11-oxygenated steroids. Hydrocortisone is more potent than cortisone in its carbohydrate-regulating capacity, and probably participates more actively than cortisone in physiological reactions under conditions of stress.

Hormones of this type are gluconeogenic, *i.e.*, they convert amino acids into sugar instead of into protein, increasing blood sugar and liver glycogen. In this sense they may be regarded as antianabolic. They cause *lysis of lymphocytes*, both those in the blood and those in the lymph nodes, and *circulating eosinophils* are *almost completely eliminated*. In excess they produce the picture of Cushing's disease, while deficiency is associated with the lesions seen in Selye's alarm reaction in experimental animals, and possibly with the collagen diseases.

Cortisone, in addition to influencing protein, carbohydrate and fat metabolism, seems to act on the intercellular substance and to *affect the permeability of cell membranes*. It also interferes with the antigen-antibody response, and it *inhibits the formation of antibodies* due probably to the rapid atrophy of lymphoid tissue which it induces. Cortisone *suppresses the inflammatory response* of the tissues to practically all forms of irritation, so that it eliminates the natural barriers to infection. This is spoken of as the anti-inflammatory or *antiphlogistic action* (*phlogistos*, burnt, and old term for inflammation). The hormone may act through suppressing the permeability of membranes lining the vessels, the joint, and the serous cavities. In this respect it is the antithesis of the mineralocorticoid, desoxycorticosterone, which increases permeability and is said to be *phlogistic*.

In experimental infections the microörganisms grow unrestrained, a fulminating bacteremia develops, and the animals remain active and happy until they die. In other words, cortisone relieves the symptoms of disease without influencing the cause. Although it may be dangerous in infections, its greatest use is in those non-bacterial inflammations which are grouped as the collagen diseases. If the inflammation is short-lived, as in rheumatic fever, cortisone may be of great value, but in long-continued inflammation such as periarteritis nodosa and disseminated lupus, when the hormone is withdrawn the inflammation starts up again. As Hench, the discoverer of the clinical use of cortisone, puts it in his Nobel prize lecture, the hormone acts as an asbestos suit behind which the patient protects his tissues from the fire. It does not put out the fire nor does it repair the fire damage. Indeed very large doses in certain species prevent the formation of granulation tissue and inhibit fibroblastic proliferation, but in clinical therapeutic doses it does not interfere with the healing of clean wounds. On the other hand perforation of a peptic ulcer is commoner in patients on prolonged cortisone therapy, and in some persons there is a tendency to develop an acute gastric ulcer, often on the greater curvature, with minimal inflammatory changes, but the danger of serious and sometimes fatal hemorrhage.

The glucocorticoids are effective in the treatment of such presumably allergic conditions as rheumatoid arthritis and the collagen diseases, the classic allergies such as asthma and drug hypersensitivity, skin inflammation (local application), eye inflammation (local application), metabolic diseases, *e.g.* gout, gastrointestinal lesions, *e.g.* ulcerative colitis and regional enteritis, and various granulomas. The combination of a steroid with the appropriate antibiotic will lessen inflammatory resistance to the infection, but at the same time provide an antidote to the infection.

One of the chief drawbacks of the earlier steroids of the glucocorticoid group such as cortisone and hydrocortisone is the fact that prolonged administration for a chronic inflammation such as rheumatoid arthritis is apt to lead to retention of salt and water with resulting edema, because of the mixed character of the steroid. Modification of the steroid nucleus as in the case of prednisone and prednisolone has resulted in a greatly intensified anti-inflammatory action with much less retention of sodium and water. Still further advances have been made by the introduction of a methyl group at the C-16 position with much greater biological activity. These developments represent chemical analogs, which are not so readily degraded by the enzymes of the liver.

3. *The Sex or Nitrogen Hormones.*—This group is called the nitrogen or N group, because the hormones are *anabolic as well as androgenic in function*. These hormones masculinize the body, and increase the synthesis of amino-acids and protein from nitrogen. As they are anabolic in effect they tend to counteract the action of the previous group. They favor retention of nitrogen, phosphorus, potassium, sodium, and chloride. These steroids when metabolized possess a ketone group on the 17th carbon atom. They are usually excreted in the urine, where they provide a valuable index of the activity of the adrenal cortex and the testes. The urinary excretion of 17-keto-steroids is greatly increased in tumors and hyperplasia of the cortex, in virilism, and in Cushing's syndrome. It is extremely low in Addison's disease and in Simmonds' disease, the latter caused by destruction of the anterior pituitary.

One more hormonal effect of the adrenal sex hormones may be alluded to, namely their influence on breast carcinoma. Bilateral adrenalectomy may result in a remarkable degree of palliation, with an astonishing regression of the primary and secondary growths. Similar results may follow hypophysectomy and castration, indicating the involvement of sex hormones.

Pituitary-Adrenal Relationship.—That the adrenal cortex is stimulated by the anterior pituitary has been known for many years. Hypophysectomy leads to atrophy of the adrenal cortex, whilst the administration of ACTH causes a marked increase in the size and activity of that structure. This relationship is a reciprocal one, for both atrophy and hypertrophy of the adrenal cortex lead to structural changes in the anterior pituitary. It is probable that ACTH is produced by the basophils of the pituitary. An intact adrenal cortex is necessary for an adequate response. *Prolonged administration of ACTH will lead to adrenal hyperplasia, whereas similar use of cortisone will result in atrophy both of the adrenal and the anterior pituitary.*

The hypothalamus is an essential link in pituitary-adrenal activation. Epinephrine and various forms of stress can stimulate hypothalamic centers to secrete a humoral substance that excites production of ACTH. Subcutaneous injection of epinephrine reduces the eosinophils 50 per cent or more. The pituitary is evidently under the influence of hormones not only of the adrenal cortex but also of the medulla.

Some of the relationships of the pituitary to the cortex and medulla of the adrenal are indicated in the accompanying diagram (Fig. 578).

Medullary Physiology.—The earliest work on adrenal hormones concerned the medulla, for it was from it that the first hormone, adrenalin (epinephrine), was isolated. Now another closely related medullary hormone has come to the fore. This is noradrenalin (norepinephrine), an amino-homologue or first cousin of adrenalin without its terminal CH_3 group. Both these amines are present in the adrenal medulla, but noradrenalin is also present in the adrenergic sympathetic nerves. The fresh human adrenal contains 80 per cent adrenalin and 20 per cent noradrenalin. In the fetus the adrenal contains no noradrenalin, but it is present in abundance in the chromaffin organ of Zuckerkandl.

Noradrenalin has displaced adrenalin as the predominant chemical transmitter of the effects of adrenergic nerve impulses, mainly in the postganglionic sympathetic fibers to the effector cells. It is present in all organs rich in adrenergic nerves, but it disappears after sympathetic denervation. In general terms, noradrenalin is always vasoconstrictor, whereas adrenalin is vasodilator in some regions, especially the coronary arteries. In pheochromocytoma of the adrenal medulla the urinary output of adrenalin is normal or on occasion somewhat increased, but that of noradrenalin is greatly increased. The urinary concentration of the two amines reflects that found in the tumor.

Stress.—The subject of stress in relation to adrenal and pituitary activation has attained much prominence through the animal experimental work of Selye, and

THE ADRENAL, ITS RELATIONSHIP TO THE PITUITARY AND ITS NORMAL FUNCTIONS

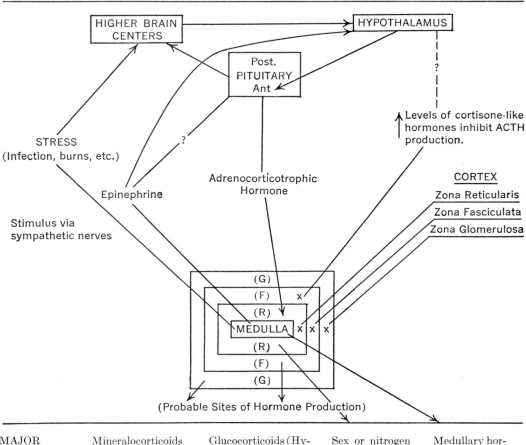

(Probable Sites of Hormone Production)

MAJOR PRODUCTS	Mineralocorticoids (Aldosterone, desoxycorticosterone).	Glucocorticoids (Hydrocortisone, cortisone).	Sex or nitrogen hormones (Adrenosterone)	Medullary hormones (Epinephrine, norepinephrine).
PRINCIPAL NORMAL FUNCTIONS	Maintenance of electrolyte balance (promote *retention* of Na and diuresis K^+; H_2O balance; blood pressure secondarily).	Gluconeogenesis and protein catabolism. Control of circulating eosinophils and and lymphocytes.	Masculinizing and anabolic.	Vasoconstriction. Adrenalin acts as a vasodilator in some areas (coronaries etc).
		(Urinary 11-oxysteroids and 17 hydroxycorticosteroids (Porter-Silver chromogens).	(Urinary 17-ketosteroids) (Zimmerman chromogens).	Stimulates general metabolism.

FIG. 578.

there is a widespread tendency to apply to human disease not only the experimental results but the hypothesis of the "general adaption syndrome" which has been erected on this work. It is important to keep in mind that effects observed in the rat are not necessarily duplicated in man, and that in the field of the adrenal hormones the response varies markedly in different species.

The idea of *specific* adaptation is, of course, an old one. Every physiological response to a stimulus or "stress" is such an adaptation. In the bacteriological field the production of a specific antibody to a given antigen is a classic example. The part played by the adrenal in the body's adaptation to stress was recognized in Cannon's emergency theory, in which epinephrine was produced by the adrenal medulla in times of anger, combat and flight when the immediate conversion of glycogen into fuel was urgently needed.

Selye's contribution is the idea that in addition to specific adaptation there is a *general* adaptation mechanism or syndrome which helps to raise resistance to stress (infections, trauma, nervous strain, heat, cold, muscular fatigue, and *x*-radiation) irrespective of the specific nature of the stimulus. In this mechanism the endocrine system, and in particular the pituitary-adrenal axis, plays an essential part. In the experimental animal the general adaptation syndrome is characterized by enlargement of the adrenal cortex with increased secretion of corticoids, involution of the thymus and lymphoid organs, gastrointestinal ulcers, and certain metabolic changes. If the stress continues, the general adaptation evolves in three stages. (1) The *alarm reaction* or "call to arms" is the result of sudden exposure to stimuli for which the individual is not prepared. Fear, anger, trauma, etc., act on the adrenal medulla by way of the para-sympathetic nerves with the production of epinephrine, and the resulting conversion of the glycogen reserve into glucose for the purpose of energy. This is Cannon's emergency mechanism. There then follows ACTH stimulation of the adrenal cortex with the production of corticoids. (2) The *stage of resistance*, that is to say optimal non-specific resistance to prolonged stimuli. (3)

The *stage of exhaustion*, in which the general adaptation fails. Examples of the three stages of alarm, resistance and exhaustion are the severely burned man who, after receiving treatment, returns to help put out the fire and dies a day or two later, and the wounded soldier who fights on, seems to do well for a while, and then succumbs to secondary shock.

Selye also suggests a new concept under the title of *diseases of adaptation*, or even better, maladaptation. Some of the most common diseases of man have been included under this heading, *i.e.*, hypertension, nephritis, nephrosclerosis, the rheumatic and other collagen diseases, and ulcerative colitis. These are said to be due to a "derailment" of the defence mechanism. These derailment diseases are manifestations of hypercorticoidism, the particular target organ (joint, artery, bowel) being determined by such conditioning factors as constitution, diet, etc. The basis for this hypothesis is that the administration of mineralocorticoids (the salt or electrolyte group) such as desoxy-corticosterone produces in animals experimental replicas of the rheumatic and hypertensive diseases such as arthritis, polyarteritis nodosa, and hyaline necrosis of arterioles. These are relieved by the glucocorticoids (cortisone). The suggestion is that an imbalance between mineralocorticoids and glucocorticoids is the basis for this large group of diseases. In the final analysis the imbalance may be pituitary rather than adrenal, for whilst the output of glucocorticoids is dependent on ACTH, the output of mineralocorticoids seems to depend on STH, the somatotropic or growth hormone of the pituitary. This may be true in the rat but not in man.

Selye's experimental work and theoretical explanations are of great interest, and have served as a stimulus to much investigation and thinking. In essence the idea of the general adaptation syndrome (which is not a syndrome in the proper use of the word but a mechanism) is that the body reacts to all varieties of stress by pituitary stimulation of the adrenal cortex. Sometimes, for some unknown reason, the cortex reacts by producing an excess or imbalance of mineralocorticoids. This results in a host of ills which have been collected under the umbrella term diseases of adaptation. Now, there is a world of difference between a hypothesis and a principle. As Sir George Pickering remarks in this connection: "The history of medicine shows how great is the tendency for a tentative hypothesis to assume the guise of a so-called fundamental principle." The suggestion of excess production of mineralocorticoids is a pure guess, a hypothesis which future work may prove or disprove. The introduction of a number of new names must not be confused with the discovery of new facts. There is a large group of diseases of unknown etiology. Many of these have been attributed in the past to focal infection and more recently to psychosomatic disorder. To now call them diseases of adaptation and attribute them to stress may be an important advance. It must be remembered, however, that in many examples of these diseases there is no evidence of stress, and there are many examples of stress without accompanying disease. It is difficult to understand how diseases having such different incidence, different lesions, and different course can arise from one and the same mechanism. ACTH works wonders in the collagen diseases, but there is no laboratory evidence of altered adrenal function in these diseases, nor proof of increased production of mineralocorticoids. It must not be forgotten, however, that, apart from the estimation of eosinophils in the blood and 17-ketosteroids in the urine, our tests for adrenal cortical function are still only the shadow of a shadow.

Finally it must be remembered that stress is not necessarily harmful. Without stress, as Arnold points out in a thoughtful and stimulating address to which I had the pleasure of listening in Honolulu, plants, animals, men and even civilizations tend to degenerate and wither away. Orchids need comparative drought to produce their best blooms, bones freed from the stress of weight-bearing undergo osteoporosis, a climate with marked variations in temperature is likely to produce a people physically and intellectually superior, and the great civilizations have developed in lands where conditions were hard and life was difficult.

HYPOADRENALISM

Acute Adrenal Insufficiency.—Hypoadrenalism used to be regarded as essentially chronic in character. This was the condition which Addison described. Acute insufficiency is now coming to assume a position of increasing importance, partly because of the development of adrenalectomy, partly on account of the great popularity of steroid therapy with its organic and functional effects on the adrenal cortex.

An *acute adrenal crisis* may be precipitated in three ways. 1. *Bilateral adrenalectomy* will obviously produce an acute insufficiency unless this threat is met by appropriate replacement (substitution) steroid therapy. At the present time the adrenals are removed for a number of reasons, amongst which may be mentioned carcinoma of the breast and progressive, intractable arterial hypertension. 2. *Massive adrenal hemorrhage* destroying the glands or widespread *thrombosis*. This may occur in the newborn, or at any age due to overwhelming infection, usually meningococcal. *Hemorrhage in the newborn* is not infrequent, and when bilateral and massive it may be a cause of death. The hemorrhage follows the necrosis of the inner layer of the cortex which always occurs at birth, possibly as the result of the sudden withdrawal of the maternal sex hormones. Massive hemorrhage is also apt to occur in overwhelming meningococcal and also in staphylococcal septicemia, this combination of infection and massive bilateral adrenal hemorrhage giving rise to the *Waterhouse-Friderichsen syndrome*, marked by acute and fatal peripheral circulatory collapse. It is in the meningococcemia of childhood, even without evidence of meningitis, that this catastrophic complication is most likely to occur, but even here it is fortunately rare. The subject is discussed more in detail on page 998. 3. *Sudden stress* (trauma, surgical operation, acute illness) superimposed on adrenals gravely damaged by chronic disease or atrophied as the result of prolonged administration of cortisone with consequent suppression of the normal ACTH response of the pituitary-adrenal axis to stress. The abrupt withdrawal of oral cortisone under these conditions will inevitably precipitate a crisis of insufficiency. Even without withdrawal the patient receiving long-term steroid therapy may not be able to stand the stress of infections, subsequent operations, etc.

The *clinical picture of acute crisis* will naturally vary markedly in intensity as well as in completeness. In its fully developed form the patient will suffer from pain in the abdomen or the costovertebral angle, headache and lassitude, which may be accompanied by nausea, vomiting and diarrhea. The temperature may shoot up to hyperpyrexic levels. Unless treatment is prompt the patient becomes confused and very restless, circulatory collapse develops, the final picture being one of coma terminating in death.

It is important to realize that the adrenal crisis represents a synthesis of two distinct syndromes: (1) sodium loss, and (2) deficiency of 17-hydroxycorticosteroids (Lipsett and Pearson). Originally all the stress was laid on sodium loss, and therapeutic effort was directed to replacing the sodium and the administration of desoxycorticosterone acetate (DOCA). When the sodium loss dominated the picture this therapy worked well, but it came to be realized that a patient could die while in sodium balance and with normal serum electrolytes, death being due to loss of the steroids by means of which the body withstands stress. This loss can be made good by the administration of the missing steroids, hydrocortisone in particular.

Chronic Adrenal Insufficiency.—Addison's Disease.—It was Thomas Addison's recognition of the fact that disease of the adrenals could give rise to a highly characteristic clinical picture which first directed attention to the endocrine system in general and the adrenal glands in particular. That was in 1855, and it is remarkable how little Addison left to be added to his clinical description of hypoadrenalism or his account of the lesions responsible.

The *clinical picture* has been painted for us by Addison in words so simple yet graphic that they must not be paraphrased. The principal features are "general languor and debility, remarkable feebleness of the heart's action, irritability of the stomach, and a peculiar change of color in the skin, occurring in connection with a diseased condition of the supra-renal capsules." The color of the skin presents "a dingy or smoky appearance, or various tints or shades of deep amber or chestnut brown, and in one instance the skin was so universally and so deeply darkened that but for the features the patient might have been mistaken for a mulatto." "This singular discoloration usually increases with the advance of the disease; the anemia, languor, failure of appetite and feebleness of the heart become aggravated; a darkish streak usually appears on the commissure of the lips; the body wastes, but without the emaciation and dry, harsh condition of the surface so commonly observed in ordinary malignant diseases; the pulse becomes smaller and weaker, and without any special complaint of pain or uneasiness the patient at length gradually sinks and expires." Addison did not have a blood pressure apparatus, but he noted that the pulse was always soft and compressible, thus indicating the characteristic hypotension.

Lesions.—The usual lesions of the adrenals (always bilateral) may be of three varieties: tuberculosis, atrophy, and secondary tumors. (1) *Tuberculosis* used to be the most common (Fig. 579). It is of the chronic fibrocaseous type. The patient seldom shows clinical evidence of tuberculosis, and it may be difficult to find the primary lesion which is the cause of the infection. Both cortex and medulla are destroyed, but a small portion of cortex always remains, otherwise life could not have been supported. Calcification of the adrenals may be seen in the x-ray film, a feature of diagnostic value. The disease is confined to the adrenals and the kidneys are not involved, nor does renal tuberculosis spread to the adrenals and cause Addison's disease. (2) *Simple atrophy* (so-called) is a *necrosis of the adrenals* rather than an atrophy, although all trace of the active process may have been lost. It is apparently very much commoner than it used to be. Duffin found necrosis to be the causal factor in 41 per cent of the cases studied in my department. Many of these patients (male) have scanty hair on the face and body, a feature which makes it possible to prophesy that necrotic atrophy will be found in such cases. The adrenal

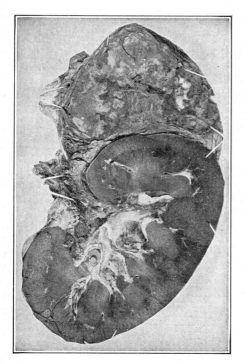

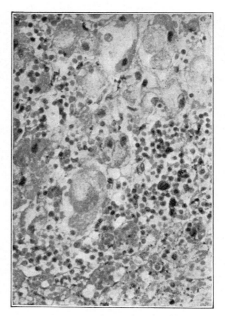

Fig. 580.—Idiopathic atrophy of adrenal cortex with lymphocytic infiltration. × 250.

Fig. 579.—Addison's disease. Enlargement of the adrenal the results of caseous tuberculosis.

glands are very small, and usually show marked lymphocytic infiltration (Fig. 580). The cause of the atrophy and the reason for its increased frequency are obscure. It is possible that the condition may be iatrogenic in origin, *i.e.*, caused by one of the countless new drugs poured into the bodies of patients, some of whom may have had an idiosyncrasy for it. More appealing is the idea that the lesion may be analgous to Hashimato's disease of the thyroid (page 1016), which is also characterized by atrophy of the parenchyma and a striking infiltration with lymphoid cells, and is believed to be due to autoimmunization to thyroglobulin with circulating thyroid autibodies in the serum. Anderson and his associates have now shown by means of the complement fixation test that antibodies to human adrenal are present in the blood of some cases of idiopathic Addison's disease, so that the progressive destruction of the adrenal cortex in simple atrophy may be the result of an autoimmune reaction. (3) *Bilateral tumor formation* is an uncommon cause. The tumor is usually a secondary bronchogenic carcinoma. In rare cases primary carcinoma of the cortex on both sides has given rise to the picture of Addison's disease. Bilateral *amyloid disease* and *histoplasmosis* are occasional causes. The possibility of histoplasmosis should be considered especially in persons who live or have lived in the Central Mississippi Valley where the disease is prevalent.

The *pituitary* shows changes which are presumably secondary in nature. The chromophobe cells are increased in number, with many exceptionally large examples, the acidophils are slightly reduced, and there is extreme reduction in the number of basophils, many of which are of abnormal type (Crooke and Russell). It has been suggested that the loss of basophils may be related to the low blood pressure and possibly the hypoglycemia. Hyperplasia of the *islets of Langerhans* is commonly present, which may be a compensatory reaction to the hypoglycemia.

Relation of Symptoms to Lesions.—The characteristic asthenia is gradual in onset, the heart's action is feeble, the blood pressure remarkably low. The gastrointestinal symptoms are nausea, vomiting, and attacks of diarrhea. The pigmentation, which ranges from light yellow to deep brown, is most marked on exposed parts and in regions where normal pigmentation is well marked (areola of nipples, genitals, etc.). The mucous membranes of the mouth and vagina are often pigmented. There is a loss of hair over the body and axilla. Although the downward course is generally gradual, there may be remissions and exacerbations. The latter are known as *crises*, and are marked by extreme arterial hypotension, decrease in the blood volume, gastrointestinal symptoms, and shock, sometimes terminating in sudden death. Hypoglycemia is apt to develop, and death may be due to hypoglycemic shock.

All of these changes are due in the final analysis to lesions of the adrenal cortex or secondary changes in the anterior pituitary. To pin-point the symptoms to any particular hormonal disturbance is a very different and far more difficult task. It is allowable, however, to recognize two main groups of disturbance; (1) cortical insufficiency resulting in ionic and fluid imbalance, and (2) cortical insufficiency causing changes in general metabolism.

Loss of salt and water balance includes depletion of sodium and chloride together with a rise in the plasma potassium. This involves a flow of water from the extracellular into the intracellular compartment, with an accompanying decrease in plasma volume. These changes in turn lead to circulatory failure with fall in blood pressure and decreased blood flow to the organs. In the kidneys the fall in blood flow is accompanied by a decreased glomerular filtration rate resulting in renal failure which, in conjunction with failure of the circulation, may finally prove fatal. It is easy to see how many of the symptoms such as weakness, hypotension, and gastrointestinal disturbance may be caused by interference with salt and water balance, which in turn may be traced to a lesion of the zona glomerulosa.

Changes in general metabolism affecting principally carbohydrates, but also protein and fat, are due to insufficiency of 17-hydroxycorticosteroids produced by the zona fasciculata. The hypoglycemia may be attributed to failure of gluconeogenesis owing to the proteins not being broken down in the liver to amino acids from which sugar can be formed. The muscular weakness and the hypotension may also be due in part to interference with protein metabolism. The loss of body and axillary hair as well as the loss in weight may be associated with lack of anabolic hormones from the zona reticularis.

Pigmentation is under *the influence of the pituitary, not of the adrenals*. The intermediate lobe of the pituitary secretes a *melanocyte-stimulating hormone*, MSH, which determines the color in Addison's disease, the melasma of pregnancy and the loss of pigment in panhypopituitarism (Lerner *et al.*). The pituitary control of pigment of the skin has been demonstrated experimentally in fish and frogs. MSH governs the condition necessary for tyrosinase-tyrosin reaction in the melanocyte with the production of melanin. In Addison's disease nevi darken, and new ones appear. The hormone is extremely potent. When large doses were given to one patient, an increase of pigmentation was observed in the course of a few hours. Hydrocortisone and cortisone appear to inhibit the release of MSH. In Addison's disease the output of MSH is increased because the hydrocortisone inhibition of the pituitary is decreased. If the adrenal medulla is also destroyed inhibition of MSH by adrenalin and noradrenalin is decreased still farther. In panhypopituitarism the output of MSH is decreased. An excellent illustration of the pigmentation in Addison's disease will be found in Thorn's monograph on adrenal insufficiency

HYPERADRENALISM

Hyperfunction of the adrenals may involve either the cortex or the medulla. Of these by far the more important is that involving the cortex. Theoretically any of the three layers of the cortex may be involved, although it is natural that absolutely pure forms are the exception rather than the rule. Over-function of the *zona glomerulosa* will involve the mineralocorticoids and lead to *aldosteronism*; over-function of the *zona fasciculata* will involve the glucocorticoids with the clinical picture of the *Cushing syndrome.* Over-function of the *zona reticularis* leads to undue production of sex hormones with resulting adrenal virilism, the *adreno-genital* syndrome. Over function of the *medulla* results in *noradrenalism.*

Cushing's Syndrome.—This is a strange clinical complex first described by Harvey Cushing in 1932 in association with small basophil tumors of the anterior pituitary. It is now recognized to result from an excess of circulating hydrocortisone.

Clinical Picture.—The syndrome is characterized by the following features: (1) painful adiposity which is confined to the face, neck and trunk but spares the limbs (buffalo type of obesity); (2) hirsutism in females and preadolescent males; (3) a dusky plethoric appearance; (4) peculiar striations of the skin of the abdominal wall giving an appearance of pregnancy; (5) sexual dystrophy (amenorrhea in females, impotence in males); (6) muscular weakness and atrophy; (7) kyphosis of the upper thoracic spine and generalized osteoporosis; (8) vascular hypertension; and (9) a tendency to diabetes. The most helpful diagnostic feature in Cushing's syndrome is the deep red, round, full-moon face. There is nothing else which simulates it closely except perhaps the red face of a burly brewer's drayman (Fig. 581).

The picture is antianabolic as evidenced by atrophy of such tissues as muscle, bone and skin, in marked contrast to the anabolic picture presented by the infant Hercules of the adrenogenital syndrome. *The glucocorticoids divert body tissue into the metabolic pool for the ultimate formation of carbohydrate and fat at the expense of muscle and bone matrix.* With this in mind many of the features of the complex clinical picture become intelligible and acquire a meaning, *e. g.*, the adiposity, muscular weakness, skin striations, kyphosis and hyperglycemia. Hormonal imbalance and interference with the other corticoids may account for other features such as the sexual dystrophy.

Estimation of corticosteroid excretion in the urine serves to distinguish between the Cushing and the adrenogenital syndromes. An elevated resting level of urinary 17-hydroxycorticoids in the absence of an increase in the 17-ketosteroids suggests pure

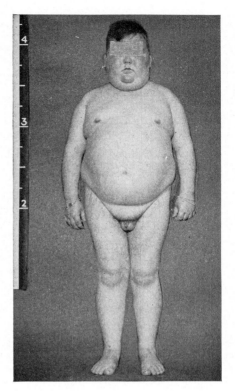

Fig. 581.—Cushing's syndrome. Age eleven years, height 52 inches, weight 119 lbs. urinary 17-ketosteroids 11.5 mg. per twenty-four hours. (Kindness of Dr. E. Perry McCullagh.)

Cushing's syndrome. The reverse is characteristic of pure adrenal virilism. An increased urinary level of both corresponds with a mixed type of clinical picture.

Lesions.—The lesion may be adenoma or carcinoma of the adrenal cortex, bilateral (rarely unilateral) cortical hyperplasia, basophil adenoma of the anterior pituitary as in Cushing's first cases, and even hypothalamic lesions. When the disease is congenital, the lesion is always bilateral hyperplasia. In the prepubertal period adrenal carcinoma is often responsible. In the adult about 60 per cent of cases are associated with bilateral cortical hyperplasia, mainly involving the zona fasciculata; in about 30 per cent there is a malignant or a benign tumor; in about 10 per cent of cases no change in the adrenal, gross or microscopic can be detected. The tumors will be described in their appropriate place. The appearance of the hyperplastic

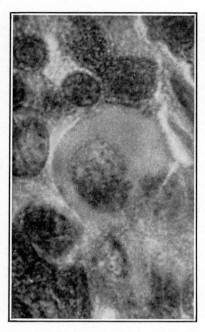

Fig. 582.—Crooke's hyaline change in basophil cells. × 1000. (Kindness of Dr. W. L. Donahue.)

cortex is characteristic. In the normal gland the cortex presents an outer bright-yellow zone 1 mm. thick and a very thin, scarcely visible inner zone of dark brown. In hyperplasia the outer yellow zone is thickened, and, more important, the inner brown zone is equally broad, the entire cortex measuring 2 mm. or more. In adrenals removed surgically from patients with Cushing's disease the zona glomerulosa has been found to be atrophic, and, in many areas, completely absent (Ashworth and Garvey). This was interpreted as compatible with a reduction in the normal inhibitory effect of adrenocortical hormone upon the pituitary, resulting, in turn, in an increased adrenocorticotrophic (ACTH) effect.

The most constant *pituitary lesion* is hyalinization of the basophil cells with disappearance of the basophil granules, a change first described by Crooke and known as *Crooke's hyaline change* (Fig. 582).

Hyalinization is an indication of inactivity of the basophils, such cells being no longer capable of producing hormones, as shown by investigation of the cells' chemistry

(Wilton *et al.*). It seems probable that the basophilic degeneration is a result rather than a cause of the hyperadrenalism, being caused by inhibition of ACTH secretion by an excess of circulating adrenal cortical hormones, as is well known to occur. It is still true, of course, that the long continued administration of ACTH may lead to the development of some of the features of Cushing's syndrome such as the adiposity, the round full-moon face and the hirsutism, just as is seen in the over-use of cortisone. It is difficult to associate hyalinization of the basophils with over production of ACTH, which these cells are believed to secrete. The unfortunate results of the misuse of steroid therapy have transformed Cushing's syndrome from a rare clinical curiosity to a condition of significance to every doctor using these hormones.

When we try to formulate a concept of the *pathogenesis* of the Cushing syndrome we are confronted with a problem which, to me at any rate, appears insoluble at the present time. In those cases in which an adenoma or carcinoma is present in the adrenal cortex it would seem reasonable to presume that these lesions are responsible for an over-production of cortical hormones. The real difficulty is presented by the 60 per cent of cases in which only cortical hyperplasia is present. It is well recognized that such hyperplasia is produced by continued stimulation by ACTH. This would suggest that, in these cases at any rate, the primary wrong-doer is the pituitary, if not the hypothalamus, with the adrenals playing a secondary role. This would seem not unreasonable in those exceptional cases where a basophil adenoma is present, but how are we to explain the cases where no such lesion is present, and in particular the usual occurrence of hyalinization of the basophils? Perhaps future work will provide us with an answer.

Apart from lesions in the endocrine glands, cardiovascular and renal changes are often important features of Cushing's syndrome (Scholz *et al.*). *Cardiac enlargement* is a very common and *arteriolosclerosis*, either hyaline or necrotizing in type, a frequent accompaniment and result of the constant hypertension. *Renal calculi* and *renal calcinosis* are not uncommon. They are probably connected with the generalized osteoporosis, which itself is a manifestation of the accelerated destruction of tissue which is an integral part of the disease.

The *results of treatment* depend on the cause of the condition. Removal of the adrenal tumor may be followed by an amazing clinical transformation, the hirsutism, adiposity, sex disturbance, etc., quickly disappearing and the patient returning to a normal condition. A primary adrenal cortical carcinoma is often operable, but the condition soon relapses owing to the growth of functioning secondary deposits. Removal of an adenoma results in a permanent cure, but it may take many months for the remaining adrenal to resume normal function. Adrenal cortical hyperplasia is best treated by total adrenalectomy, but large doses of intramuscular steroid must be given to cover the operation, and the patient has to have replacement therapy for the rest of his life.

Adrenogenital Syndrome: Adrenal Virilism.—In this condition the presence of an excess of masculinizing hormones (androgens) produces a striking variety of clinical changes, depending on age and sex. In girls if the abnormality is present in the first few weeks of intrauterine life the result is female pseudohermaphroditism; if late in intrauterine life or in boys the result is precocious puberty. In some cases the excess of androgen may be associated with a severe deficiency of hydrocortisone, due probably to an enzyme disorder blocking the normal pathways of steroid synthesis in the zona fasciculata and reticularis. This results in a marked loss of sodium, which may precipitate dangerous weakness and vomiting in infants that may resemble an Addisonian crisis.

The *clinical picture* is characterized by hirsutism, virilism, and great muscularity, so that a boy may present the picture graphically termed the infant Hercules with premature development of the sex organs although often associated with impotence. In girls there is a development of both primary and secondary male characters; the clitoris becomes enlarged, and hair develops on the face and body (hirsutism). In women the sex organs atrophy, amenorrhea and obesity develop, the voice is deep, and

hirsutism is marked both on the face and body. Adult males show no sexual change, except in rare cases where there is a feminizing effect. Urinary 17-ketosteroids are elevated, serum sodium and blood sugar levels are low, and serum potassium is high.

The *lesions* are similar to those found in Cushing's syndrome, namely bilateral cortical hyperplasia, adenoma or carcinoma, but involving the zona reticularis, the androgenic zone, rather than the zona fasciculata. If both zones should happen to be involved, the result will be a combination of the adrenogenital and Cushing syndromes.

Early recognition of the condition and adequate substitution therapy with cortisone may allow normal puberty to be attained through suppression of pituitary function. If a tumor is present it must be removed if possible.

Primary Aldosteronism.—Aldosterone is the astonishingly powerful mineralocorticoid produced by the most superficial layer of the cortex, the zona glomerulosa, which plays a major part in maintaining fluid and electrolyte homeostasis by regulating the excretion of electrolytes, causing retention of sodium and increased loss of potassium. It differs from the glucocorticoids and androgen of the zona fasciculata and zona reticularis in that ACTH influences its secretion by the adrenal only to a slight degree. Primary aldosteronism, more properly termed primary hyperaldosteronism, refers to the clinical condition caused by an overproduction of aldosterone by the adrenal.

The *clinical picture* is spoken of as *Conn's syndrome*, as the first case was described by J.W. Conn in 1954. It is characterized by *periodic* severe muscular weakness or paralysis; intermittent tetany and paresthesias; hypertension; renal dysfunction shown by polyuria, nocturia and albuminuria. The *laboratory findings* are a low potassium and a moderately raised sodium level in the blood, alkalosis shown by elevation of the pH and CO_2-combining power of the blood and inability of the kidney to secrete an acid urine after a loading dose of ammonium chloride. The urinary aldosterone level is extremely high, whilst the 17-hydroxycorticoids and the 17-ketosteroids are normal. There is evident imbalance between mineralocortocid and glucocorticoid activity, the biochemical lesion being confined to electrolyte metabolism, with organic metabolism remaining normal. A puzzling feature is the absence of edema. In the early stages the correct diagnosis may be suggested by a combination of hypertension and hypokalemia, which may be suspected from the electrocardiogram. The *serum potassium* may be extremely low, yet of this there may be little evidence apart from the periodic muscular weakness. Many cases in the past have undoubtedly been diagnosed as potassium-losing nephritis. Muscle biopsy reveals a great decrease of intracellular potassium and a corresponding increase of intracellular sodium. Renal biopsy shows a diffuse vacuolar nephropathy, the so-called "*clear cell nephrosis*," which is characteristic of chronic hypokalemia. This is the basis for the loss of power to excrete a concentrated urine. Renal arteriolosclerosis is a frequent finding at autopsy, possibly related to the hypertension.

The *adrenal lesions* are those with which we have become familiar in the Cushing and adrenogenital syndromes, namely adenoma, carcinoma and bilateral cortical hyperplasia, but in the present instance adenoma is very much more common than the other two.

The aldosterone content of the cortical tumor is 30 times greater than in tumors responsible for Cushing's syndrome. Following surgical removal of the tumor, (which has been called an *aldosteronoma*), there is a dramatic and complete disappearance of the clinical signs and symptoms, including the hypertension, together with the electrolyte disturbance, in the course of two weeks. As primary aldosteronism belongs to the small group of causes of hypertension where a permanent cure may be achieved by surgical intervention, and as the hypertension may be the only manifestation of the disease, the importance of a plasma potassium determination of serious cases of hypertension becomes evident. One man had had hypertension for twelve years with systolic pressures ranging from 236 to 160 mm. Hg., and diastolic pressures from 160 to 100 mm. Hg. His serum potassium level was found to be 2.5 MEV. per liter. The entire right adrenal and 90 per cent of the left adrenal

were removed, both being the seat of nodular hyperplasia. In four days the serum potassium levels had returned to normal, and in five weeks the blood pressure was 110/80 mm. Hg., at which level it has remained (Richardson).

The *problem of the control* of the all-important secretion of aldosterone is an intriguing and still a distinctly baffling one. We have already seen that ACTH only slightly influences the secretion of aldosterone. Observations on dogs suggest that secretion is stimulated by a neurohormone from the brain. Exactly where the neurohormone is produced is uncertain, although it may be in the region of the pineal and the subcommissural body. As regards the afferent pathway the studies of Bartter *et al.* have established that changes in intravascular volume influence aldosterone secretion. The increase in aldosterone secretion associated with salt restriction seems to be due to contraction of blood volume. Construction of the inferior vena cava in dogs increases aldosterone secretion (Davis), and it would seem that stimulation of the neurohormone mechanism is effected by volume receptors sensitive to changes in blood volume located along the arterial tree. It still remains to be seen whether the mechanism in the dog operates also in man. The relation of renin produced by the juxtaglomerular cells of the kidney to the secretion of aldosterone is discussed on page 553.

Secondary Aldosteronism.—Increased production and excretion of aldosterone may occur under such conditions as the nephrotic syndrome, hepatic cirrhosis with ascites, and congestive heart failure. It will be seen that in all of these there is loss of fluid into the tissues, the peritoneal cavity, etc. In all of these there is decrease of the intravascular volume, with resulting stimulation of aldosterone production through the mechanism outlined above.

Noradrenalism.—This term signifies hypersecretion of the hormones of the adrenal medulla, of which noradrenalin (norepinephrine) is infinitely more potent, although less abundant, than adrenalin. These pressor amines are produced in excess by the *pheochromocytoma*, a tumor of the adrenal *medulla* which is usually benign and unilateral, but may be malignant, bilateral, or familial. It secretes more of the potent noradrenalin than adrenalin.

The classical *clinical picture* is characterized by symptoms of hypertension, which may be paroxysmal or continuous. The episodes of hypertension are marked by headache, palpitation, dyspnea, weakness, chest or abdominal pain, nausea, vomiting, flushing, pallor, dizziness, tingling, or convulsive twitching in various combinations. The paroxysms may be precipitated by emotional disturbance, changes in position such as stooping, abdominal palpation, trauma, or histamine administered for gastric analysis.

The *laboratory tests* used in this differential diagnosis are useful, but by no means easy. They consist of the determination of an excess of pressor amines in the blood and urine, and "provocative" and "inhibitory" pharmacological tests which will not be discussed here.

TUMORS OF THE ADRENAL

Primary tumors of the adrenal are rare in comparison with the relatively common hypernephroma of the kidney. Although the cortex is of mesoblastic origin, its cells are epithelial in type, so that the cortical tumors are adenoma or carcinoma. The medulla is composed of nerve cells and belongs to the chromaffin system, so that a medullary tumor may be a neuroblastoma, ganglioneuroma, or chromaffinoma, (pheochromocytoma).

Tumors of the endocrine glands are peculiar in that the functional disturbances which they produce are of greater importance, variety and complexity than the neoplastic lesions themselves. These disturbances, for which both benign and malignant tumors may be responsible, have already been discussed in relation to hyperadrenalism involving the cortex and the medulla. The lesions themselves will be considered here, without reference to the symptoms which they may produce.

Cortical Tumors.—From our study of hyperadrenalism we have seen that it is the tumors of the cortex, either adenoma or carcinoma which produce the picture of Cushing's syndrome, the adrenogenital syndrome, and primary aldosteronism, although a more common cause of the first two is bilateral cortical hyperplasia.

Adenoma.—The cortical adenoma forms a yellow or brown circumscribed mass, which varies enormously in size. It may remain a nodule, but functioning tumors removed surgically are frequently 100 to 200 gm. in weight. The cells resemble those of the zona glomerulosa in appearance and arrangement, but the structure varies in different cases and even in different parts of the tumor. Atrophy of the cortex of the opposite adrenal and even of the uninvolved part of the gland containing the adenoma is constant, a point to be borne in mind as regards substitution therapy when removal of the adenoma is undertaken.

Carcinoma.—This rare tumor resembles hypernephroma of the kidney (renal carcinoma) in its gross appearance. It is yellow in color, often hemorrhagic, and may attain a large size (Fig. 583). Not infrequently it is bilateral. The *microscopic* picture varies in its degree of differentiation. Some cases are distinguished with difficulty from an adenoma, the acini and columns of the cortex being fairly well reproduced; although appearing rather benign, they may be quite malignant clinically. Others may be called malignant adenoma; a suggestion of acinar grouping still remains, and the cells are large and contain lipid, but the arrangement is quite atypical and the picture evidently carcinomatous. Giant cells may form a marked feature. In a third group the structure is anaplastic, consisting of solid cords of small dark cells. Sometimes sarcomatous characters are evident in adrenal carcinoma, the cells being fusiform and arranged diffusely. Such a picture recalls the fact that the cortex is mesoblastic in origin.

The tumor may *spread* widely. The adrenal disappears and the kidney may be involved, so that difficulty may arise in distinguishing the tumor from renal carcinoma. This can be done by remembering that in the latter condition the adrenal is usually intact. The adrenal and renal veins are invaded, and the tumor may grow along the renal vein into the vena cava. The opposite adrenal is often affected, and *metastases* are common in the retroperitoneal, mesenteric

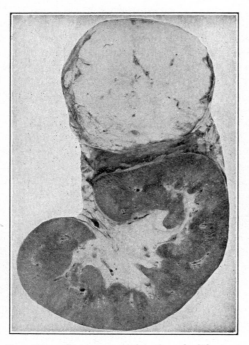

FIG. 583.—Carcinoma of the adrenal. The tumor is entirely confined to the adrenal, and has not invaded the kidney.

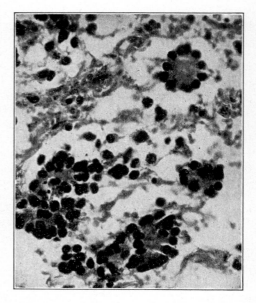

FIG. 584.—Neuroblastoma showing rosettes. × 300.

and mediastinal lymph nodes, and in the liver, lungs, brain, and other organs. The bones are seldom involved; in this respect the tumor differs markedly from renal carcinoma.

It must be noted that although the clinical picture caused by adrenal carcinoma may be dramatic, it is the exception rather than the rule for endocrine symptoms to develop. I have seen a tumor the size of a football which was a complete surprise at autopsy because of the total absence of endocrine symptoms.

Medullary Tumors.—The primitive sympathetic neuroblasts which form the anlage of the adrenal medulla develop either into nerve ganglion cells or into chromaffin cells (pheochromocytes). Three types of tumor may thus arise from the medulla: (1) the *neuroblastoma*, from the primitive neuroblasts; (2) the *ganglioneuroma*, from the mature ganglion cells; (3) the *chromaffinoma* or *pheochromocytoma* (*phaios*, dark), from the chromaffin cells. The first is much the commonest (although itself rare), and being

primitive in type is highly malignant. The other two arise from adult cells and are innocent.

Neuroblastoma.—The tumor is almost confined to children, usually under four years of age. I have seen a case in a stillborn infant. Very rarely it may occur in adults, and I have observed a case in a boy nine years of age. It is soft and may grow to a great size. Often it is bilateral. Occasionally it does not arise from the adrenal, but from sympathetic nerve tissue in the abdomen or thorax. The *microscopic picture* resembles that of a sarcoma, and formerly this tumor used to be called "adrenal sarcoma of children." Most of the so-called retroperitoneal round-cell sarcomas of infants are of this character, arising from the abdominal sympathetic ganglia. The tumor consists of undifferentiated small round cells (neuroblasts), a few imperfect ganglion cells, and fibrils. The fibrils form the distinctive feature, for they are nerve fibrils and are arranged either in longitudinal bundles or in little rounded masses around which the cells are grouped in a *"rosette"* form (Fig. 584). These rosettes are highly characteracteristic of the tumor, but sometimes they are found with difficulty. They are absent in un-differentiated forms.

Spread of the tumor often gives rise to the formation of remarkable *metastases in the skull, particularly in the orbit*, so that the first sign of the disease may be the appearance of a hemorrhagic area in the neighborhood of the eye, followed later by protrusion of the eyeball (proptosis). When proptosis develops in a young child it is well to examine the abdomen. Other bones besides the skull may also be involved. This picture is referred to as the *Hutchinson type*. It seems likely that spread to the skull takes place by the vertebral system of veins. In other cases there is a great and uniform enlargement of the liver due to diffuse infiltration with tumor cells. The mesenteric nodes are involved. This is spoken of as the *Pepper type*. It is natural that tumor cells should spread more readily to the liver from the right than from the left adrenal, possibly by the lymphatics but there is little justification for the statement that the Hutchinson type indicates a left adrenal tumor, the Pepper type a tumor in the right adrenal.

The skeletal metastases are associated with multiple tumors in the lungs. Cases of this type are likely to be met with over the age of six months. In the Pepper type with massive liver involvement the lungs are usually spared. These cases are usually infants under six months of age. In the older group spread takes place by the post-natal circulation, but in the young infant spread may have occurred before birth. In intra-uterine life most of the blood in the umbilical vein passes through the liver, whilst the lungs are by-passed by way of the foramen ovale and ductus arteriosus.

The *prognosis* was at one time regarded as invariably hopeless, but this view has had to be modified. The neuroblastoma, indeed, offers one of the best examples of that remarkable phenomenon which we have already discussed (page 199), the spontaneous regression of cancer (Boyd). Incredible though it may sound, complete recovery may take place spontaneously or after incomplete removal or inadequate radiation (Farber). In a case with which I am familiar at the Toronto Hospital for Sick Children, part of a neuroblastoma in a child aged 9

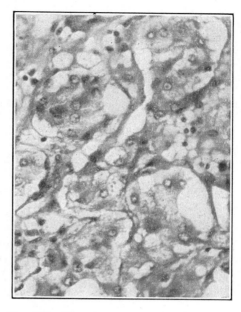

Fig. 585.—Pheochromocytoma. The large ragged cells resemble those of the adrenal medulla. × 320.

months was removed surgically, but the remainder had to be left in the abdomen, yet the girl made an uninterrupted recovery and is well sixteen years later. Usually the regression is due to necrosis of the tumor cells, but in rare cases the neuroblasts seem to become differentiated into ganglion cells.

Pheochromocytoma. (*Phaios*, dark).—This rare tumor is also known as *chromaffinoma* and *paraganglioma*. It is usually innocent, small, well encapsulated, and may be found by accident at autopsy in elderly persons. It may be familial, and is sometimes associated with von Recklinghausen's neurofibromatosis. Several cases which I have studied have presented a characteristic cystic degeneration. The tumor may be brown in color. About 20 per cent of the cases are said to be bilateral, and these are usually malignant. Occasionally it may attain a great size, as in one case reported by Soffer and his associates where the tumor weighed 2000 grams. The most interesting clinical feature is the frequent occurrence of *arterial hypertension, often paroxysmal* in type, for the tumor contains a large amount of *nor-*

adrenalin, often much more than the normal adrenal, and a pressor substance can be demonstrated in the blood. During the attacks the systolic blood pressure may rise to 250 or even 300 mm. of mercury, and an accompanying hypoglycemia may lead to shock. The attack may last for minutes or hours, and if prolonged it may prove fatal. The tumor may be demonstrated radiographically by perirenal insufflation or by depression of the renal pelvis in a pyelogram. These tumors are found in other parts of the *chromaffin system*, such as the carotid body, the abdominal paraganglia and the organ of Zuckerkandl at the bifurcation of the aorta. It is best to use the name chromaffinoma for the whole group, pheochromocytoma for the adrenal tumors, and paraganglioma for the extra-adrenal tumors. The tumor is composed of large epithelium-like cells (Fig. 585) which are often pigmented and may stain brown when fixed in chrome salts. In a number of cases there has been an associated neurofibromatosis.

Ganglioneuroma.—This rare form of innocent tumor occurs both in children and adults, and is found in the brain and abdominal sympathetic as well as in the adrenal medulla. It is composed of adult ganglion nerve cells, spherical or pyramidal, and nerve fibers which may be medullated or non-medullated, and it produces no hormonal secretion.

Secondary Tumors.—Metastatic tumors are remarkably common in the adrenals, considering the small size of the glands. In my experience the commonest type of primary tumor is *bronchogenic carcinoma*, but others give precedence to cancer of the *breast* and *stomach*. In bronchogenic carcinoma the only metastases may be in the adrenal. Secondary tumors develop first in the medulla, but they soon involve the entire organ, so that when bilateral they may cause Addison's disease, as Addison was the first to recognize.

MISCELLANEOUS LESIONS

Postmortem Change.—This is extremely common in the adrenal and must not be mistaken by the beginner for evidence of disease. The inner layer of the cortex softens and is converted into a brown mush, so that only a rind of cortex is left.

Necrosis.—Necrosis of individual cells is seen in various acute infections, and this may be associated with a striking transformation of the solid cords of the zona fasciculata into tubular structures resembling renal tubules and containing an acute inflammatory exudate (Rich). Such lesions may serve to explain the acute collapse of circulatory failure.

Massive Hemorrhage.—The adrenals are liable in an unusual degree to massive bilateral hemorrhage, with resulting adrenal insufficiency. By this we do not mean that the condition is common, for it is fortunately rare, but that this type of hemorrhage is not seen in other organs. It is seen in fulminating meningococcal septicemia and occasionally in other septicemias. Such a combination is likely to be associated with profound circulatory collapse.

The association of circulatory collapse with overwhelming septicemia is known as the *Waterhouse-Friderichsen syndrome*. The syndrome is not necessarily associated with massive hemorrhage, for it is seen in meningococcemia without hemorrhage. The condition is the cause of many unexplained sudden deaths in children and young adults. The incidence is from 2 to 4 per cent of meningococcal infections, and 90 per cent of the cases occur under the age of nine years (Nelson and Goldstein). The meningococcal cases are characterized by a hemorrhagic rash, circulatory collapse, cyanosis, hypotension, an almost death-like lividity, and it may kill in twenty-four hours. Signs of meningitis are often not pronounced and may be absent. The cyanosis is due to dilatation of capillaries, arterioles and venules, with swelling and breaking of the lining endothelium, large numbers of platelet thrombi, ischemic necrosis and hemorrhage into the perivascular spaces.

This brings up the matter of the adrenal hemorrhage. The massive hemorrhage is not due to an acute bacterial endocarditis. It seems more likely that the vascular lesion responsible for the hemorrhage is in the nature of an immunological reaction of the nature of a *Shwartzman phenomenon*. Meningococci are known to contain a necrotizing factor for blood vessels, which can produce the Shwartzman phenomenon (Black-Schaffer *et al.*). I have seen massive bilateral hemorrhage causing extreme enlargement of both adrenals, which together weighed 40 gm., in a case of abdominal suppuration due to a ruptured gastric ulcer. Some of the adrenal vessels showed definite fibrinoid necrosis. In those cases where massive hemorrhage has not wiped out evidence of cellular damage there may be degeneration of the cell cords which opens them to dissection by blood elements and conversion into tube-like structures (Rich). Such a change might be the first step toward a massive hemorrhage, to which the rich blood supply of the adrenal predisposes the organ. The rapid loss of lipid in response to the stress of severe infections may result in cytolysis, which might in turn lead to the tubular change of Rich. In rare instances spontaneous hemorrhage has been reported without infection. In such cases we may seek refuge in vague thoughts about an autoimmunization reaction. Reference has already been made to the special variety of massive and it may be fatal hemorrhage occurring in the developing adrenal in the new born.

Amyloidosis.—The *secondary* form of amyloid degeneration may involve the adrenals at the same time as the liver, spleen and kidney. The deposit begins in the connective tissue and the basement membrane of the cells of the zona glomerulosa, so that disturbance of salt and water metabolism may be prominent. In course of time the greater part of both glands is involved, so that amyloidosis is an occasional cause of Addison's disease.

MYELOLIPOMA.—This condition is also known incorrectly, as myeloid metaplasia, because of the presence of fat cells and varying numbers of hemic cells, so that the appearance may resemble that of bone marrow. The lesion is circumscribed, and grossly resembles a lipoma. It seems probable that it is the result of infection.

Lymphocytic infiltrations are often observed in the cortex associated with focal necrosis.

REFERENCES

ANDERSON, J. R. *et al.*: Lancet, 1957, *2*, 1123. (Autoantibodies in Addison's disease.)

ANGEVINE, D. M.: Arch. Path., 1938, *26*, 507. (The adrenals in anencephaly.)

ASHWORTH, C. T. and GARVEY, R. F.: Am. J. Path., 1958, *34*, 1161. (Diffuse adrenal lesion in Cushing's disease.)

BARTTER, F. C. *et al.*: *Aldosterone*, London, 1957.

BLACK-SCHAFFER, B., HIEBERT, T. G. and KERBY, G. P.: Arch. Path., 1947, 43, 28. (Waterhouse-Friderichsen syndrome.)

BOYD, W.: Can. J. Radiolog., 1957, *8*, 45, 63. (Spontaneous regression of neuroblastoma.)

CONN, J. W.: Arch. Int. Med., 1956, *97*, 135. (Aldosterone.)

CROOKE, A. C. and RUSSELL, D. S.: J. Path. and Bact., 1935, *40*, 255. (The pituitary in Addison's disease.)

DAVIS, J. O. *et al.*: J. Clin. Invest., 1957, *36*, 689. (Aldosterone secretion.)

FARBER, S.: Am. J. Dis. Child., 1940, *60*, 749. (Regression of neuroblastoma.)

HILL, S. R. *et al.*: Arch. Int. Med., 1959, *104*, 982. (Hypertension in primary hyperaldosteronism.)

LERNER, A. B., SHIZUME, K. and BUNDING, I.: J. Clin. Endocrinol. and Metab., 1954, *14*, 1463. (Endocrine control of melanin pigmentation.)

LIPSETT, M. B. and PEARSON, O. H.: New Eng. J. Med., 1956, *254*, 511. (Adrenal crisis.)

NELSON, J. and GOLDSTEIN, N.: J.A.M.A., 1951, *146*, 1193. (Waterhouse-Friderichsen syndrome.)

PICKERING, G. W.: Lancet, 1950, *1*, 81. (Stress.)

PITCOCK, J. A. and HARTROFT, P. M.: Am. J. Path., 1958, *34*, 863. (The juxtaglomerular cells and the zona glomerulosa.)

RICH, A. R.: Bull. Johns Hopkins Hosp., 1944, *74*, 1. (Adrenal lesion in acute infections.)

SCHOLZ, D. A., SPRAGUE, R. G. and KERNOHAN, J. W.: New Eng. J. Med., 1957, *256*, 833. (Cardiovascular and renal complications of Cushing's syndrome.)

SELYE, H.: *The Physiology and Pathology of Exposure to Stress*, Montreal, 1950.

THORN, G. W.: *Diagnosis and Treatment of Adrenal Insufficiency*, Springfield, Ill., 1951.

WILTON, A., TORELL, B. and SUNDWALL, W.: J. Path. and Bact., 1954, *67*, 65. (Pituitary changes in Cushing's syndrome.)

Chapter 37

The Thyroid

General Considerations
  Structure
  Function
    Iodine Metabolism
    Pituitary-Thyroid Axis
    Antithyroid Drugs
    Radioactive Iodine
  Hyperplasia-Involution
    Cycle
    Goiter
Diffuse Colloid Goiter
Nodular (Adenomatous) Goiter
  Relation to Carcinoma

Graves' Disease
  Relation of Symptoms to
    Lesions of Goiter
    Exophthalmos
    Pretibial myxedema
Cretinism and Myxedema
  Cretinism
  Myxedema
Thyroiditis
  Acute Infectious Thyroiditis
  Subacute Thyroiditis
  Chronic Thyroiditis
    Hashimoto's Disease
    Riedel's Struma

Autoimmunity in Thyroiditis
Tumors
  Adenoma
    Follicular
    Papillary
  Carcinoma
    Papillary
    Follicular
    Undifferentiated
  Secondary Tumors
Miscellaneous Lesions
  Infective Granulomas
  Congenital Anomalies

GENERAL CONSIDERATIONS

Structure.—The thyroid gland is one of the most labile organs in the body. It is continually being played upon by various influences (endocrine, etc.), and responding to the varying demands of thyroxin. On this account the structure is not fixed, any more than the structure of the breast or endometrium is fixed. Physiological variations as evidenced by a certain amount of hyperplasia and involution are common in autopsy specimens, although in some cases no doubt they are terminal. Such compensatory hyperplasia is not necessarily associated with any symptom of hyperthyroidism. The pathological thyroid gland differs from the normal in degree rather than in kind of change, and it is often extremely hard to draw a line between the two. It may well be that under normal conditions the acini of the thyroid are in various phases of function, which may be called the resting, secretory and resorptive phases (Halpert). In the *resting phase* the acini are large, lined by flattened cells, and filled with deeply stained homogeneous colloid. This is the picture in colloid goiter and in the gland of hyperthyroidism treated with a solution of iodine. In the *secretory phase* the acini are lined by cuboidal epithelium and the colloid is stained moderately darkly. This is the picture seen in the normal thyroid. In the *resorptive phase* the acini are lined by columnar epithelium, and contain lightly stained, vacuolated and scalloped colloid. This is the picture seen in hyperthyroidism and in patients treated with thiouracil. The normal thyroid gland in non-goitrous districts weighs from 25 to 35 grams, but it weighs more in women than in men, more in the summer than the winter, more during pregnancy and lactation, and more in goitrous districts even though it may appear to be quite normal.

Function.—The chief function of the thyroid gland is to maintain a higher rate of metabolism, as evidenced by heat production, than would otherwise be possible, and to regulate this rate according to the needs of the body. This is done by means of its iodine-containing hormone, thyroxin. The physiological effect of feeding thyroid gland is to raise the rate of metabolism. Removal of the thyroid gland is followed not only by a loss of heat production, but in the growing animal by poor physical, mental and sexual development. The thyroid gland has a remarkable affinity for iodine, and is the only organ in the body which has the power of storing that element. The iodine content of a dog's thyroid can be increased several hundred per cent in the space of five minutes by the intravenous injection of 50 mg. of potassium iodide. The rapidly stored iodine is at first inactive, but gradually becomes converted into an active form. Apparently the iodine is converted by the epithelium of the acini into thyroxin. Some of this passes into the circulation in response to the demand of the tissues. The rest is stored in the form of colloid within the acini, where it constitutes an emergency ration which can be used when the need arises. The normal iodine content of the gland is about 0.2 per cent. If it falls below 0.1 per cent morphological changes at once become apparent in the acinar epithelium, and the gland becomes enlarged in consequence. This fall may be due to an increased demand on the part of the tissues for thyroxin, or to an inadequate supply of iodine to the gland. The morphological changes are hypertrophy and hyperplasia of the acinar epithelium together with an increased vascularity. As a result of this cellular activity the emergency ration in the colloid is made use of and depleted, and the demand of the tissues for thyroxin is met. If this demand is moderate the hypertrophy may be regarded as physiological; when it is excessive or long-continued the response of the thyroid becomes pathological. When the iodine supply is insufficient the epithelial activity is an indication that the gland is engaged in the attempt to make bricks without sufficient straw, and if the strain is not too great the attempt may be successful. The administration of iodine, even in minute doses, soon relieves the strain, and the epithelial activity subsides, while the iodine-containing colloid collects once again within the acini. The process is known as involution.

In dogs and in other experimental animals the process of hyperplasia is diffuse, so that there is a uniform enlargement of the entire gland. In man, on the other hand, it tends to be patchy and localized, with the result that nodules tend to be formed. These are known as adenomas, although in the great majority of cases they are not true tumors, so that the name is misleading. Some of these nodules or adenomas respond to iodine treatment like the rest of the gland, but others may not.

Iodine Metabolism.—Iodine is one of the necessities of life, for without iodine the thyroid hormone cannot be built and with-out that hormone normal life is impossible, although one may still survive. Iodine, of course, does not exist in free form either in the blood or in the tissues. Iodine metabolism has been described as a grand cycle in which iodine in the form of iodide ions is extracted from the blood by the thyroid, converted into thyroxine and possibly other hormones, discharged as such into the blood, and carried to every cell in the body, where it exerts a profound effect on metabolic and enzymatic activities (Berson). Iodine comprises two-thirds by weight of the thyroid hormone which exercises this far-flung control.

The iodides consumed in food and water are absorbed and carried to the *iodide pool* in the extracellular fluid. Here they are competed for by two organs, the thyroid and the kidney. When more iodides are ingested than are needed, they are excreted in the urine. The thyroid takes from the blood whatever it requires for its uses, uses which are determined by the demands of the tissues. Five main events occur within the thyroid: (1) trapping of iodide, (2) oxidation of the iodide to organic iodine by a peroxidase enzyme system, (3) synthesis of the hormone, (4) storage of the hormone as thyroglobulin in the thyroid follicle, and (5) discharge of the hormone to the circulation. In addition there is the matter of transport to targets, action upon targets, and the final fate of the hormone (Means).

The thyroid has been called with justification an *iodide trap*, the only one in the body. It functions to the iodide in the blood flowing through its vessels as a flypaper does to the flies in its neighborhood. It is TSH, the thyroid-stimulating hormone from the anterior pituitary, which sets or springs the trap. The trapping mechanism can be blocked by thiocyanate and perchlorate compounds, just as the oxidation and synthesis mechanism can be blocked by thiouracil and sulfonamides. The trapping of iodine can be followed in radioiodine tracer studies both in health and under the disturbed conditions of disease.

Thyroxine is unique among hormones in being an amino acid. There are three iodine-bearing amino acids in the thyroid, thyroxine being tetraiodothyronine. A fourth

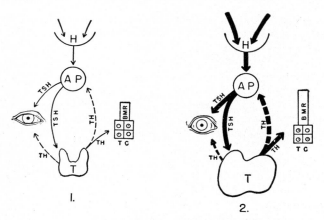

Fig. 586.—The pituitary thyroid axes, showing interrelationship of hypothalmus, anterior pituitary, thyroid, tissue cells and eye in normal person (1) and Graves' disease (2). (Means, courtesy of Ann. Int. Med.)

and very much more potent member of the series, *triiodothyronine*, is now known to be present in small amounts. This produces a much more rapid effect in the treatment of myxedema than does thyroxine, and it has been suggested that many of the clinical effects in Graves' disease are due to triiodothyronine. Iodine is found in the blood in two forms: (1) inorganic iodide, and (2) organic or *protein-bound iodine*. Both thyroxine and triiodothyronine are protein bound, but triiodothyronine is bound much more loosely than thyroxine, and therefore dissociates more quickly and diffuses much more freely into the body cells. *The level of organic (protein-bound) iodine is a reliable index of thyroid secretory activity.* The normal level is 4–8 μg. per cent, in myxedema it is 0.2–2.5 μg. per cent, whilst in hyperthyroidism it is usually around 15 μg., but may go up as high as 30 μg. per cent.

The *salivary glands* as well as the thyroid seem to be concerned with the iodine cycle. These glands concentrate iodide ions into the saliva, the concentration being 30 times that of the plasma. There seems to be some relation between thyroid and salivary gland function. By means of isotope studies a remarkable correlation between the radioiodine secreted by the salivary glands and thyroid activity can be demonstrated both in hyperthyroid and in hypothyroid states (Jaimet and Thode). The salivary glands are responsible, at least in part, for the degrading of thyroxine in the body and the recycling of the iodine to the thyroid as iodide ion. The *saliva test* for radioiodine secreted by the glands is of marked diagnostic value in thyroid disease.

Pituitary-Thyroid Axis.—An intimate relationship exists between the thyroid and the anterior pituitary, a mechanism which has been called the pituitary-thyroid axis. The thyrotrophic or thyroid-stimulating hormone (TSH) of the pituitary is the most powerful known stimulant of thyroid activity. In the experimental animal it causes extreme enlargement of the gland, great epithelial hyperplasia, and corresponding elevation of the basal metabolic rate. The pituitary itself is under the influence of nervous stimuli from the hypothalamus, the controlling center of emotional activity. It is evident that emotional disturbance may be expected to play a part in thyroid hyperactivity. The TSH probably acts mainly by increasing the collection or trapping of iodide, but it may also have some effect on hormone synthesis. The stimulating effect is only temporary; after a time a refractory stage is reached and hypothyroidism may develop. In man the TSH must be continually playing on the thyroid, but as the term axis suggests, there is a two-way activity, and the thyroid hormone in turn inhibits the production of TSH in the pituitary, so that a balance is maintained (Fig. 586). This balance may theoretically be upset at either end.

We have spoken as if the thyroid-stimulating hormone was the only pituitary hormone involved in thyroid disease. This is not necessarily true. For long it has been evident that Graves' disease is not merely an aggravated form of thyrotoxicosis, because no amount of thyroxin will give rise to exophthalmos when administered either to animals or man. It would now appear that another pituitary hormone, the *exophthalmos-producing substance* (EPS), which is separable from TSH in anterior pituitary extracts, is responsible for the lesions in the orbit, lesions which will be discussed in relation to Graves' disease.

Antithyroid Drugs.—Certain sulfur-containing substances interfere with the cycle of iodine metabolism in the thyroid at one or other point, causing a curious dissociation of the usually associated thyroid hyperplasia and increased basal metabolic rate, stimulating the former and depressing the latter. Chief among these are thiocyanate, the sulfonamide drugs, and sulfur-containing thiourea and its non-toxic derivative, thiouracil. These may block the trapping mechanism or they may block the synthesis process.

Block of trapping is produced by thiocyanate. This gives rise to the apparently contradictory combination of thyroid cellular hyperplasia and hypothyroidism. The contradiction vanishes when it is realized that these substances paralyze the iodide trap, so that thyroxine cannot be formed on account of lack of iodine, thus causing hypothyroidism. The normal inhibition of the pituitary by thyroxine is now missing, so that excess of TSH is produced with resulting thyroid hyperplasia. *Blocking of thyroxine synthesis* is simply the production of the same result at a different point in the assembly line. The sulfonamides and thiouracil prevent the synthesis of thyroxine at a normal rate. Iodine when given to control thyrotoxicosis appears to push the finished product into the warehouse (thyroid follicles) and thus prevent the distribution of thyroxine to the body.

Radioactive Iodine.—Much of our more accurate knowledge of disturbed thyroid physiology we owe to the introduction of I^{131} or radioactive iodine. The labelled iodine could now be followed from the source of the raw material to the factory, to the warehouse, and finally to the users. The radioiodine uptake by the thyroid and the level of protein-bound iodine in the blood can now be estimated and compared, as can the efficacy of the thyroid trap for iodine, the deposition and departure of labelled iodine being followed by means of a Geiger counter placed over the gland. The serum bound iodine (PBI), of which the normal level is 4 to 8 micrograms per 100 ml., gives a level of the circulating hormone, both thyroxine and triiodothyronine, and is the the most reliable single criterion for hyperthyroidism. The normal I^{131} uptake range is from 15 to 45 per cent, below 10 and above 50 being abnormal. An increased uptake is an index of increased thyroid function. For a full discussion of the newer views of thyroid function, the monograph edited by Werner should be consulted.

The Hyperplasia-Involution Cycle.—We have already seen under the heading of structure that the normal thyroid acini may be in various phases of activity designated as resting, secretory and resorptive. Under pathological conditions the gland may show the exaggerated phases of hyperplasia and involution. When three-quarters of the thyroid gland of a dog are removed the remainder soon begins to show changes which may be classed as hypertrophy and hyperplasia. The remnant becomes larger until the original size of the gland may be restored. At the same time there is a proliferation of the epithelial cells, a true hyperplasia. The histological changes are briefly as follows. The lining epithelium becomes tall and columnar, the cytoplasm stains feebly and contains presecretion products in the form of granules and globules, and there is a great increase of mitochondria. In order that the acinus may accommodate the increased number of cells the acinar space becomes enlarged, and soon the proliferating epithelium is seen to project into this space in the form of processes, until the acinus comes to assume an almost solid appearance. At the same time the colloid becomes thinned, vacuolated, and finally disappears. The store of iodine varies inversely with the hyperplasia, and becomes more and more depleted as the hyperplasia increases. There is an increase in the lympho-

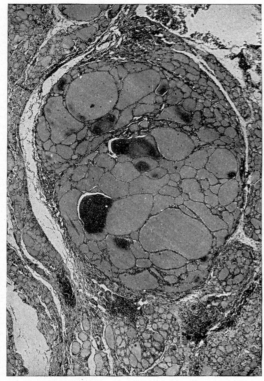

Fig. 587.—Colloid nodule developing in a diffuse colloid goiter. × 30. (Boyd, *Pathology for the Surgeon*, courtesy of W. B. Saunders Co.)

cytes of the stroma. This is an illustration of *compensatory or work hypertrophy* and hyperplasia, the remaining portion of the thyroid having to perform more work to supply more iodine to the body in the form of thyroxine. We shall encounter the same compensatory hyperplasia in relation to shortage in the supply of iodine.

Involution is the sequel of hyperplasia. It may be result of exhaustion or it can be induced by the administration of iodine to the animal. When the supply of this raw material falls below a certain level, only a feverish activity on the part of the gland will suffice for the normal metabolic processes. The epithelial proliferation disappears, the distended acini are lined by low cuboidal or flattened epithelium, and colloid once again accumulates. The fibrous stroma is increased, dividing the gland into areas of varying size, an appearance which is intensified by the patchy character of the hyper-

plasia-involution process. This gives the gland a nodular appearance (Fig. 587). These areas are so discrete that in the past they have been regarded as adenomas, but it will be obvious that they are in no sense neoplastic.

Goiter.—This is an indefinite term applied to enlargement of the thyroid. From what has been said it is evident that theoretically this enlargement might be evidence: (1) of a primary hyperplasia; (2) of a compensatory hyperplasia to meet increased demands of the tissues for hormone; and (3) of increased storage of colloid. There is no satisfactory *classification* of goiter. It is usual to recognize three main types: diffuse colloid goiter, exophthalmic goiter (Graves' disease), and nodular or adenomatous goiter. It will be noticed that the first type is named from a microscopic feature, the second from a leading symptom (which may be absent), and the third from the gross appearance.

The *geographic pathology* of goiter varies greatly (Hellwig). This serves to explain the conflicting accounts which are found in the writings of observers in different parts of the world. The goiter of North America, for instance, is very different from that of the Himalayas and the Alpine districts of Switzerland. In the former the common variety is the diffuse and nodular colloid goiter with large acini distended with colloid (macrofollicular type), whilst in the latter parenchymatous goiter is the usual form characterized by small follicles poor or lacking in colloid (microfollicular type). Thyrotoxic symptoms are commoner in North America than in any other country. Thus in Berne, Switzerland, 3 per cent of goiters are associated with thyrotoxicosis, whereas in Portland, Oregon, 67 per cent fall in the toxic group. In mountainous countries the microfollicular non-toxic type is prevalent; in level countries the macrofollicular, often associated with toxic symptoms, is common.

Perhaps not enough attention has been paid to the role of the microfollicle in goiter. The macrofollicles and the microfollicles, present in varying proportions in most goiters as indicated above, are believed by some to constitute two distinct morphological and functional units (Stein). In the ordinary mixed goiters the macrofollicles

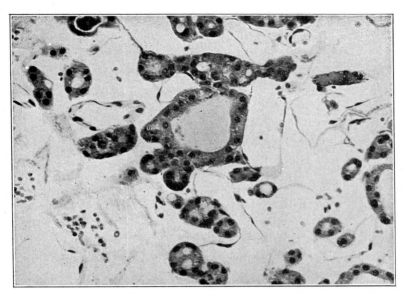

Fig. 588.—Adenoma of the thyroid. The acini are very small and are widely separated by a structureless material. The vessels are markedly dilated. There is microfollicular budding of the acinar epithelium, with formation of new acini. × 250.

respond to iodine therapy, indicating that they are related to iodine deficiency, but the microfollicles show no response. Microfollicular hyperplasia is accomplished by budding of the parent follicles (Fig. 588). It is in the Hashimoto struma (goiter) and in the so-called fetal adenoma that microfollicles are dominant.

DIFFUSE COLLOID GOITER

This type of goiter includes those varieties known as simple goiter, endemic goiter and adolescent goiter, although these various terms are by no means synonymous. It is the most physiological form of thyroid disease, for it commences as a compensatory or work hypertrophy, but physiological limits in the thyroid are easily transgressed, and when the gland has met the demand of the tissues it may be unable to return to its former size.

The main *causal factor* in endemic goiter is an insufficient supply of iodine to the thyroid, which in consequence develops a work hyperplasia followed later by involution. The soil of high countries is denuded of iodine, so that the drinking water is poor in that element. In the endemic region of North America, particularly the region of the Great Lakes and the valley of the St. Lawrence, the soil is iodine-poor, having been deposited from the melting of the ice of the last glacial epoch. Animals as well as men living in endemic regions suffer from simple goiter. This type of goiter is a deficiency disease due to lack of iodine.

Simple colloid goiter is much commoner in women than in men. It commonly appears in girls at the time of puberty or soon after. It tends to disappear after a few years, so that the usual age period is from fifteen to twenty-five years. In endemic regions the condition tends to appear earlier and last longer. It may be due to a relative rather than an absolute lack of iodine. There may be enough iodine in the food and water for ordinary purposes, but not for the in-increased demand for thyroxin at adolescence and puberty in the female. Similar enlargement may occur during pregnancy and lactation and for a similar reason. Such goiter responds remarkably to the administration of iodine when in the hyperplastic stage. "The normal physiological rhythm of colloid storage during rest and colloid

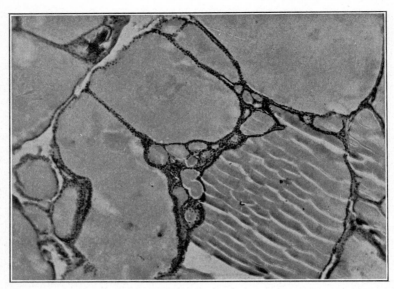

Fig. 589.—Colloid goiter. The acini vary much in size, some being widely dilated. The colloid is abundant and stains deeply. The epithelium is flattened. × 75.

release during activity is changed into a different gear by the demands of puberty, pregnancy and parturition. Undue stress and strain will eventually throw this finely equilibrated balance out of rhythm." (Levitt).

Lesions.—It is very seldom that one has the opportunity to study the goiter of adolescence during the hyperplastic stage, for it should never be removed surgically. When the gland is removed in the involutionary or colloid stage, as may have to be done on account of its increasing size, it is found to be uniformly and diffusely enlarged and of soft consistence. The cut surface is amber in color, and presents a finely honeycombed translucent appearance, owing to the distended acini being filled with colloid.

The *microscopic appearance* may resemble that of normal thyroid tissue, but there is greater irregularity. Many acini are greatly enlarged. Some are of normal size and some are smaller than normal. All are filled with densely stained colloid (Fig. 589). The epithelium is low, and in the larger acini it may be flattened. A few small islands of hyperplasia may still be present, and evidence of former hyperplasia is apparent in the form of withered spurs which still project here and there from the acinar walls.

NODULAR GOITER

As the years pass a goiter tends to become nodular. Some of these nodules may be new formations of tissue, so that they are called adenomas. Some may be associated with symptoms of thyrotoxicosis, so that they are referred to as *toxic adenomas.* There is no difference in structure between toxic and non-toxic adenomas. They merely cause pressure symptoms. The number increases with age. We have used the general term nodular rather than adenomatous goiter, although the latter is commonly employed by clinicians. From what has already been said it is obvious that the great majority of nodules in the thyroid are not true neoplasms, but merely discrete areas affected by the hyperplasia-involution process. Adenomas which appear to be true neoplasms are considered in the section on thyroid tumors.

Lesions.—Nodular goiter is the common type of goiter demanding surgical treatment in North America. The nodule may be single, but more often it is multiple (Fig. 590). The larger nodules are well encapsulated. Degenerative changes such as softening, cyst formation and hemorrhage are common. When a thyroid nodule suddenly enlarges it is probably due to hemorrhage into a cyst. Calcification is frequent. The *microscopic appearance* is the same as that of the surrounding gland. It may or may not show hyperplastic changes. These may be more marked than those of the surrounding gland. In young persons the lesion is often the so-called *fetal adenoma*, because of the resemblance to the fetal thyroid. The cut surface in such a case is dense, opaque and pale, and the nodule is composed of small acini with little or no colloid. This is the picture of the microfollicular parenchymatous goiter so common in the endemic regions of Europe, although that lesion is diffuse and not localized. Mucoid degeneration may cause the acini to be widely separated (Fig. 588).

In toxic nodular goiter *the uptake of* I^{131} *is a reliable index of the rate of secretory activity of the thyroid cells*. This can be determined by scanning the thyroid with a gamma-ray detector, by excision of a slice of thyroid tissue and making an autoradiogram, or by determining the proportion of the tracer substance excreted in the urine. In the examination of thyroid nodules by this technique a wide range will be encountered from tumors taking up I^{131} and therefore totally inactive, the so-called "cold nodule," to those taking up the tracer substance with great avidity, the "hot nodule," while the remainder of the thyroid takes up little or none. Contrary to what might be expected, hyperfunction of a nodule seems to be good insurance against the presence or subsequent development of malignancy. It is the cold nodule which is the threat. Hyperplasia and malignant neoplasia appear to be mutually exclusive. This, of course, has long been known in relation to Graves' disease.

The Relation of Nodular Goiter to Carcinoma.—This is one of the most contentious subjects in clinical medicine, and it is still far from settled. Some authorities consider that nearly all cancers develop in *normal* thyroids (Crile); others of equal distinction take the opposite view (Taylor). It has been said that 24 per cent of nontoxic nodular goiters are carcinomatous; it has also been said that carcinoma of the thyroid is a rare form of malignancy.

There are probably two main reasons for

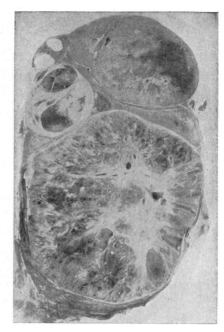

Fig. 590.—Nodular goiter. The large nodules are of the colloid type, while the small nodules at the top left-hand corner are of the so-called fetal type.

this violent difference of opinion. (1) It is often difficult and sometimes impossible for the pathologist to draw a sharp line of distinction between a benign nodule of the thyroid and a malignant adenoma or carcinoma. Different pathologists will disagree sharply over the same section. The tendency is to favor a diagnosis of malignancy so that the patient may have the benefit of an early operation. (2) The reports in the medical surgical literature naturally come from large thyroid clinics where the nodular goiters are highly, although unconsciously, selected. They do not represent nodular goiter in the general population. It has been estimated from painstaking surveys that among the total population of persons with nodular goiter the prevalance of cancer of the thyroid is less than 0.1 per cent, compared with about 8 per cent among persons with nodular goiter submitted to thyroidectomy in well known clinics (Sokal). As a matter of fact it may well be the patient who makes the selection, because she has probably noticed that her goiter had begun to change in character. Well over half of all thyroid glands when examined at autopsy are found to contain single or multiple nodules, and the occurrence of carcinoma in one of these nodules is a rarity (Hull). It is possible that both the surgeon and the patient are right, the surgeon in removing most of the nodular goiters sent to him, the patient in not getting alarmed about a nodular goiter which is showing no change.

EXOPHTHALMIC GOITER: GRAVES' DISEASE

It is difficult to give a satisfactory definition of Graves' disease. Clinically it is marked by the classic triad of: (1) *hyperthyroidism*, the picture produced by an excess of thyroxine, (2) *exophthalmos* or protrusion of the eyeballs, and (3) *goiter*. Unfortunately, one or other of these may be absent, at least for a time. That is why Graves' disease is a more satisfying name than exophthalmic goiter. Pathologically, the trade-mark of Graves' disease is *diffuse* hyperplastic enlargement of the thyroid, although, as we have just seen, the goiterous enlargement is sometimes not evident clinically. It is obvious that the lesion with which Graves' disease may be confused is nodular goiter with thyrotoxicosis. We shall return to this matter presently.

Etiology.—Graves' disease remains an enigma, for it provides an example of an entire organ starting and continuing to hyperfunction without any regard to the needs of the body. The etiology remains obscure. It bears no apparent relation to iodine deficiency. There is often a very definite history of nervous or psychic shock, not infrequently sexual in character. In some cases the onset of the disease has followed such a shock within a few days. The tendency at present is to look beyond the thyroid in seeking the essential cause of Graves' disease. The pituitary is a possibility, since the thyrotrophic hormone of that gland is the most powerful stimulator of thyroid hyperplasia. As there is excitement of the sympathetic system the adrenals may play a part. Most persons who develop Graves' disease belong to a certain type, the so-called *Graves' constitution*. They are of slender build, temperamental, easily over-stimulated, with rapid pulse and slight tremors, and especially sensitive to the administration of thyroid extract. It would appear that in such persons something serves to upset the normal balance which should exist between the ductless glands (pituitary, adrenals, thyroid), one result of which is overstimulation of the thyroid, and that this balance may never be permanently regained.

Lesions.—The thyroid gland is moderately or considerably enlarged, but the largest goiters do not occur in Graves' disease but in the nodular and colloid forms. It must be remembered that no enlargement may be detected clinically, as the hypertrophied lobes may be behind the trachea. The gland, over which greatly dilated veins may course is firm, pink in color owing to the increased vascularity, and of a dense meaty appearance which is in marked contrast to the translucency of the normal thyroid. If the patient has been given iodine (Lugol's solution) before the thyroid gland was removed, the characteristically dense appearance is lost owing to the temporary change from a hyperplastic to a colloid condition. The enlargement is diffuse, but the cut surface shows a fine lobulation which, together with the meaty appearance, suggests a resemblance to the cut surface of the pancreas.

The *microscopic picture* shows three characteristic changes: (1) epithelial hypertrophy and hyperplasia, (2) disappearance of colloid, and (3) lymphoid hyperplasia. The epithelium is tall and columnar, and mitotic figures may be numerous. The acini are greatly enlarged and very irregular, but this enlargement is not readily obvious unless a wax reconstruction is made, for they are filled with the papillary processes which form in order to accommodate the new formation of cells (Fig. 591). Sometimes there is no enlargement of acini with infolding of their walls, but a formation of great numbers of small rounded acini lined by columnar epithelium. In both forms the colloid is thin and scanty or has completely disappeared. The change in the colloid is most marked where it comes in contact with the lining epithelium, as if it is being absorbed by the acutely active cells. Scattered throughout the stroma are lymphoid follicles with definite germinal centers (Fig. 592), in

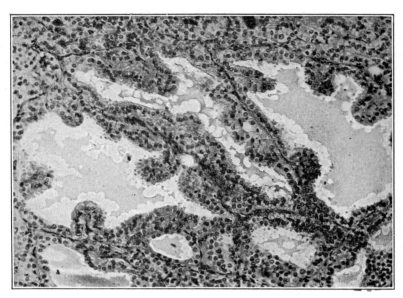

FIG. 591.—Thyroid of Graves' disease undergoing involution under iodine treatment. The papillary processes are being withdrawn from the enlarged acini, and the colloid is reappearing. Above and below there is still dense hyperplastic tissue. × 150.

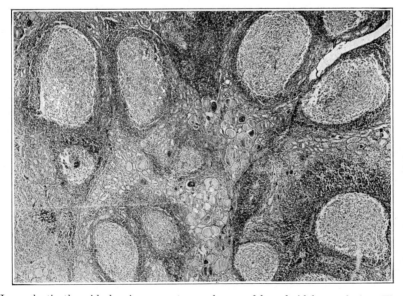

FIG. 592.—Hyperplastic thyroid showing an extreme degree of lymphoid hyperplasia. The patient had been treated with Lugol's solution. × 40.

addition to which there may be a more diffuse infiltration with lymphocytes. The lymph follicles become larger and more distinct after prolonged treatment with Lugol's solution. It is probable that they are a result of the hyperplasia and hypersecretion of the thyroid. There is a marked increase in the vascularity in keeping with the general increase in glandular activity.

Histochemical methods throw additional light on the histological picture (Haley *et al.*). Decreased intensity of staining with the periodic acid Schiff (PAS) reaction of McManus suggests enhanced peroxidase activity which transforms iodide into iodine and increased mucinase activity in the colloid prior to its resorption. The scalloping of the colloid reflects the increase in intra-follicular proteolysis characteristic of hyper-thyroidism. In nontoxic nodular goiter, on the other hand, there is an abnormally slow turnover as evidenced by strong staining with PAS.

When the patient has had a short pre-operative course of Lugol's solution the picture is markedly changed, corresponding with the great abatement in the symptoms of thyrotoxicosis. The epithelial hypertrophy and hyperplasia subside, colloid reappears, and the lymphoid tissue is less abundant. But when the administration of iodine is prolonged for weeks or months a different picture develops, which bears a spurious resemblance to the resting colloid gland. Epithelial hypertrophy is still absent and the atrophic looking follicles are lined by a low type of cell, but the colloid is thin and watery, lymphoid hyperplasia is very marked, the germinal centers of the follicles are remarkably large and pale, and there is proliferation of the stroma. The symptoms meanwhile may have returned in full force.

Thiouracil, a derivative of thiourea, produces a curiously contrasted effect. The clinical symptoms of hyperthyroidism are relieved and the basal metabolic rate lowered, but the resorptive phase of thyroid physiology appears to be intensified, for the colloid is diminished in quantity and density and may finally disappear, whilst the epithelium is tall and columnar. The picture resembles the histology of toxic goiter before the days of preoperative preparation with iodine

(Halpert). Thiouracil, as we have already seen, blocks the synthesis of thyroxine, so that the normal inhibition of the pituitary by thyroxine is now lacking, and an excess of TSH is produced with resulting thyroid hyperplasia.

It is interesting to consider the condition of the remaining thyroid tissue after the two major forms of treatment of Graves' disease, namely subtotal thyroidectomy and I^{131} radioactive iodine. Normal thyroid balance may be achieved by either method, but the end results differ in both the histological and the functional activity of the remaining thyroid tissue (Curran *et al.*). Some years after partial thyroidectomy there is decrease of cellular hyperplasia and increase of colloid storage; the longer the interval, the more marked becomes this change. In patients who die within two or three months of I^{131} therapy there is nuclear pyknosis, cellular necrosis, breakdown of follicles, thrombosis of capillaries and small blood vessels, with edema of the stroma. There is evidence of continuing hyperactivity of functioning tissue for many years after irradiation even in euthyroid patients. The protein-bound iodine remains at a high level for many years after irradiation, but after partial thyroidectomy this level gradually falls. This result indicates that after irradiation a small mass of highly active tissue remains, the reason being that the distribution of I^{131} in autoradiographs is seen to be patchy. Finally it may be mentioned that in no case was there any evidence of neoplasia as the result of irradiation.

Lesions in other organs deserve at least passing mention. The hyperplasia of the *thymus* and *lymphoid tissue* has already been mentioned. A persistent and enlarged thymus is found at autopsy in the majority of cases of typical exophthalmic goiter. The lymph nodes, tonsils, Peyer's patches, and lymphoid follicles in the spleen may all show hypertrophy similar to that of status lymphaticus. In some of my fatal cases there has been tremendous lymphoid hyperplasia of the appendix, the lymphocytes obliterating the mucosa and lumen and infiltrating the muscular wall. The *blood* shows a relative lymphocytosis. The heart is often enlarged, and may show myocardial degeneration and fibrosis, but there are no specific lesions. The *muscles* may show fatty degeneration. This can hardly account for the muscular weakness, which may manifest itself in the difficulty the patient has in lifting his foot to a height (quadriceps sign). Sometimes the muscular weakness is the most prominent clinical feature, a condition known as chronic thyrotoxic myopathy. The basis of this disorder may be a deficiency of steroid hormone, as indicated by low urinary excretion of 17-ketosteroids, testicular atrophy and degeneration of the adrenal cortex. In the *orbit* there is an increase of fat and water content, and the extraorbital muscles are greatly swollen, and firm and india-rubbery in consistence. The *adrenals* may be atrophic, but there are no specific lesions. The *liver* often shows passive congestion, and degenerative lesions are common. Fatty change is extremely frequent. There may be acute necrosis, both focal and central. Cirrhosis has been reported in from one-third to one-half of the cases. It is most marked in the subcapsular zone. Liver function tests often show a marked degree of impairment. It has been suggested that in thyrotoxicosis the over-stimulated metabolism results in combustion of the protective glycogen of the liver beyond the degree of safety. When that point is reached there develops sudden and extreme hyperpyrexia, an almost uncountable pulse, vomiting, diarrhea, and restlessness which may pass into delirium, coma and death. This picture is known as *thyroid crisis* or thyroid storm. The *bones* often show marked rarefaction and decalcification due to a lacunar absorption brought about by osteoclasts and associated with a great excretion of calcium.

Relation of Symptoms to the Lesions of Goiter.—*Diffuse colloid goiter* usually produces no symptoms, except possibly those of pressure. On the other hand there may be mild degrees of thyrotoxicosis or of hypothyroidism. Microscopic examination of the thyroid fails to give a satisfactory explanation of these differences. The parenchymatous, microfollicular, colloid-poor goiter so prevalent in the mountainous regions of Europe is hardly ever associated with toxic symptoms.

Nodular Goiter (adenomatous goiter) may exert local pressure on the trachea, which may cause marked narrowing of that structure with dyspnea. Hemorrhage into an adenomatous cyst may aggravate the condition in a sudden and alarming manner. A *retrosternal goiter*, usually due to the downward extension of an adenoma, is a cause of dyspnea which may escape detection for some time. *Thyrotoxicosis* may or may not be present; the adenoma is said by the clinician to be toxic or non-toxic. The validity of the concept of toxic adenoma has long been disputed, but the matter has been settled by the use of tracer doses of radioactive iodine. The uptake of labelled iodine is an index of the rate of secretory activity of the thyroid cells as shown by an externally applied Geiger counter or by autoradiograms with excised tissue. In toxic adenoma the tumor alone is actively secreting, whereas in Graves' disease the entire gland is active. In both the epithelium is taller than in the normal thyroid. The non-toxic adenoma may take up no labelled iodine. As shown by this test, malignant tumors secrete very slightly or not at all. It is extremely rare to find carcinoma in a thyrotoxic gland, whether adenomatous or diffusely hyperplastic. Indeed hyperplasia and malignancy are largely exclusive.

Graves' disease is much commoner in women than in men in the proportion of 5 to 1. It usually begins in early adult life and the onset is often sudden and acute. When it develops in later years the onset is more gradual. The symptoms of Graves' disease are due to excitation of the sympathetic system. The four *cardinal signs* are enlargement of the thyroid, exophthalmos, tachycardia, and tremors (Fig. 593). The skin is moist and liable to vasomotor disorders such as flushing; the patient is excitable; palpitation, diarrhea, and vomiting may occur; there is loss of weight and an enormously increased body metabolism as indicated by calorimetric observations. This seems to be caused by the direct action of thyrotoxine on the cells. It is as if some blast were blowing on the metabolic furnace of the body, fanning it into a state of furious activity. The course of the disease varies.

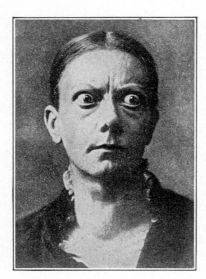

Fig. 593.—Graves' disease. (Byrom Bramwell's *Atlas of Clinical Medicine.*)

It may be acute and fulminating, the patient dying with all the classical symptoms of exophthalmic goiter; sometimes he dies in a so-called *thyroid storm* after thyroidectomy. In other cases the course is less violent, and is marked by a series of remissions and exacerbations. Gradually the fire burns itself out, the thyroid breaks down under the constant stimulation, and a condition of partial thyroid insufficiency (myxedema) may develop. There is profound disturbance in iodine metabolism, as indicated by raised blood iodine, increased excretion of iodine, and a negative iodine balance. This increased mobilization of iodine in hyperthyroidism resembles the disturbed calcium metabolism of hyperparathyroidism.

In Graves' disease the cardiovascular phenomena and the increased basal metabolic rate are manifestations of hyperthyroidism, which itself is presumably caused by epithelial hyperplasia. But there are difficulties. A patient may have well marked symptoms of hyperthyroidism without epithelial hyperplasia, especially when iodine treatment has been too prolonged. Goiter in adolescents in regions of severe goiter may show all the microscopic changes characteristic in Graves' disease, yet thyroid function may be normal. Here, of course

the hyperplasia is secondary or compensatory in character, whereas in Graves' disease it appears to be primary. The administration of thyroxine does not produce the exophthalmos and other neurological phenomena of Graves' disease. Thyroidectomy removes the inhibitory effect of the thyroid on the pituitary, thus explaining the occasional postoperative intensification of the exophthalmos. It has been suggested that in Graves' disease the thyroid allows thyroxine to leak from the gland (thyroid diarrhea), and that the hyperplasia is an attempt to compensate for the rapid loss of hormone, and therefore merely a secondary phenomenon. This sounds well, but it may have more sound than meaning.

Exophthalmos is one of the major problems of Graves' disease. It may be present in patients with little or no evidence of hyperthyroidism. Indeed the onset of hypothyroidism may aggravate the eye changes, although they are never present in primary myxedema. The ophthalmopathy consists of two elements: (1) *lid-lag*, the inability of the upper lid to follow the movement of the lid, together with retraction of the upper lid, giving the eyes a staring appearance; (2) *proptosis* or true exophthalmos. The first group may possibly be a manifestation of the tension of thyrotoxicosis. There is no close relationship between hyperthyroidism and exophthalmos. Exophthalmos may appear years before hyperthyroidism or years after its control and without its recurrence (McCullagh).

There is reason to believe that the exophthalmos is related to overactivity of the anterior pituitary, more particularly to EPS, the exophthalmos-producing substance. Exophthalmos is produced by injection of crude pituitary extracts into animals which have been thyroidectomized, in whom, therefore, there could be no thyrotrophic effect. Thyroidectomy may greatly aggravate the condition in the human subject, with the development of the so-called malignant exophthalmos in which the eyeball may be destroyed. The operation has removed the normal inhibitory effect of the thyroid on the pituitary. Thyroid feeding does not cause exophthalmos in man.

The eye displacement is due to edema of

the orbit, which may be so marked as to produce an extreme degree of proptosis. There is a deposition of mucopolysaccharides rich in hyaluronic acid in the fat tissue of the orbit, which is of the same nature as the material formed in the ground substance in collagen disease. At this stage the condition is still reversible. Later, when there is replacement by connective tissue, the condition becomes irreversible.

Pretibial myxedema is a thickening of the skin and the underlying connective tissue in the pretibial area and the dorsum of the foot. The lesions resemble those of myxedema in that they do not pit on pressure, but they do pit when injected with hyaluronidase, suggesting that the tissue is infiltrated with mucopolysaccharide containing hyaluronic acid. The lesions are almost invariably limited to patients with severe or malignant exophthalmos, in which mucopolysaccharide is also found in excess in the tissue.

In concluding this discussion of Graves' disease it may be interesting, although not enlightening, to compare the condition with toxic nodular goiter, what in this connection we may term hyperfunctioning adenoma. Both are characterized by thyrotoxicosis, but in the case of the adenoma we are dealing with a hypersecreting mass of endocrine tissue, whereas in Graves' disease the stimulus is unknown, nor can all its features be explained on the basis of an abnormal production of thyroxine. In Graves' disease there is a general emotional instability, exophthalmos, and a remarkable response to iodine therapy in the course of a few days. None of these features are observed in toxic adenoma. While, therefore, there is a similarity in the clinical response to the two lesions, there are fundamental differences which so far defy explanation.

CRETINISM AND MYXEDEMA

Deficiency of the thyroid secretion gives rise to very characteristic symptoms and may be caused in a variety of ways. The basis of the condition may be congenital or acquired. The former is known as cretinism, the latter as myxedema.

Cretinism.—If the thyroid does not develop properly during fetal life, or if it is acted on during that period by goitrogenous influences, the child is born a cretin. Cretinism may be endemic or sporadic. The *endemic* form is common in the great regions of endemic goiter, the Alps and the Himalayas. It has been said that goiter is the first step on the road to cretinism. The mother almost always suffers from simple (endemic) goiter. The child at birth does not have a goiter, but in a few years he usually develops one unless removed to a non-goitrous district. At first the thyroid may show a compensatory hyperplasia, but later there is exhaustion atrophy although the gland is still enlarged. Endemic cretinism can be prevented by giving the pregnant woman a sufficient amount of iodine. The *sporadic* form occurs in non-endemic regions. The cause is not known, but is apparently something that interferes with the development of the thyroid, which is represented by a fibrous remnant. Indeed it may be difficult to find any trace of thyroid tissue, so that goiter does not develop.

The cretin is a dwarf physically and mentally. The mind, the skeleton, and the sexual organs do not develop. Like Peter Pan, the cretin never grows up, but he has none of Peter's vivacity, for the vitalizing influence of the thyroid is lacking. He is a sad, old child. The stature is stunted, the head large, the face broad, the features coarse, the arms short and curved, the sexual organs undeveloped, and the mental powers little better than those of an imbecile. What was intended to be created in the image of God has become what has been called the pariah of Nature, and all for want of a little iodine.

Myxedema.—This is the condition of thyroid deficiency in the adult, which usually appears about the age of forty years. Like other diseases of the thyroid, it is commoner in women. It has no relation to goiter, and is not more frequent in the regions of endemic goiter.

The *etiology* of myxedema is in most cases obscure, or rather unknown. Two classes of case are easily accepted: (1) *Thyroid deficiency* due to thyroidectomy, neoplasms, chronic thyroiditis, or radioiodine therapy; (2) *pituitary deficiency* of the thyroid-stimulating hormone due to tumors or

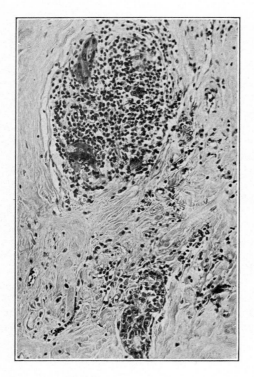

FIG. 594.—The thyroid in myxedema. The glandular tissue has been replaced by fibrous tissue; remnants of acinar epithelium remain surrounded by lymphocytes. × 125.

granulomas of the pituitary, to Simmonds' disease, or possibly failure to produce TSH. Such cases have been called *pituitary myxedema* (Means). The TSH test serves to differentiate between the thyroid and pituitary forms. Usually, however, there is no clinical evidence of pituitary disease in myxedema, nor any significant histological changes in the pituitary. Such cases are known as *primary myxedema*. These cases are associated with a high level of circulating thyroid antibodies in the blood, and it has been suggested that the destruction of thyroid tissue may be due to an auto-immune reaction similar to that of Hashimoto's disease, a condition which may terminate in myxedema. Doniach, indeed, says that primary myxedema is the end result of Hashimoto's thyroiditis without goiter, representing submerged non-goitrous examples of the same disease.

As regards *local lesions*, the thyroid gland

is atrophic, hard, and in the most severe cases is converted into a mass of fibrous tissue. As a rule areas of atrophic glandular tissue remain separated by an abundant fibrous stroma. Lymphoid collections are frequent, and they may form nodules strongly reminiscent of the similar condition in Hashimoto's disease (Fig. 594).

The *clinical picture* in an advanced case is so characteristic that the diagnosis can be made at a glance, but owing to the efficacy of treatment with thyroid extract such cases are seldom seen nowadays. The woman is heavy and intensely phlegmatic, the face broad and devoid of all expression, the skin rough, dry, and singularly sensitive to cold. Persons with hyperthyroidism have a moist skin and rarely feel the cold, those with hypothyroidism have a dry skin and continually feel cold because the metabolic fire is burning so low. The hair is dry and falls out, often beginning first in the outer third of the eyebrows. The basal metabolic rate is characteristically low. The serum cholesterol is invariably high in untreated cases and decreases on treatment.

Laboratory features of value are: (1) a low BMR (20 to 40 per cent below normal), (2) low serum protein-bound iodine indicating a deficiency of circulating thyroid hormone, (3) a very low radio-active iodine uptake by the thyroid, and (4) a high serum cholesterol level, which decreases on treatment. It must be remembered that cases encountered in practice are not likely to show the full-blown clinical picture and have to be recognized when the symptoms are much less marked. That is where the laboratory tests are of value. The transformation of a severe case of myxedema under adequate thyroid therapy is the most miraculous in the whole realm of clinical medicine, as can be seen in Figure 595 showing one of the original cases in which substitution therapy was used. Incidentally those wishing to see the variety of startling clinical appearances presented by the various forms of thyroid disease, together with pictures of lesions in color, may consult Levitt's *The Thyroid*.

The disease owes its name to a solid pseudo-edema of the skin and mucous membranes caused by infiltration with an acid mucopolysaccharide (hyaluronic acid) so that the

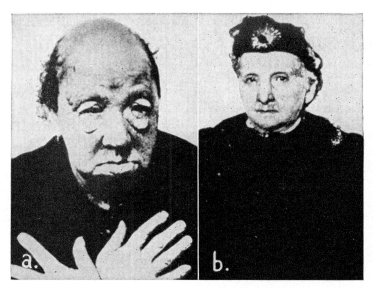

Fig. 595.—The result of thyroid therapy in myxedema. *A*, This is a photograph of the patient in 1893, when she was sixty-five years of age, bed-ridden and imbecile from myxedema of twenty years standing. *B*, This is a photograph of the same patient in 1923 when she was ninety-four years old, after thirty years of thyroid therapy. She was in normal health, happy and mentally active. The patient died in January 1924. (C. R. Harrington, courtesy of Brit. Med. Jour.)

tissue appears to be myxomatous. It is this infiltration which serves to iron out the expressive wrinkles and folds of the face, so that all the patients have a strong family resemblance to one another. The change is most marked in the face, neck, supraclavicular fossæ and the backs of the hands, which are fat and clumsy. The mucous membranes are also infiltrated, so that the tongue is thick, and there is swelling of the mucous membrane in the nose, mouth, larynx, bronchi, and alimentary canal. The heart may appear to be markedly enlarged on clinical and roentgenological examination (myxedema heart). This is in the main due to pericardial effusion, in part to myxomatous infiltration of the myocardium and dilatation of the chambers. The walls of the capillaries of the heart are thickened due to an infiltration with glycoprotein, with resulting increased permeability of the capillaries (Paker and Hamilton). The enlargement of the heart shadow rapidly returns to normal under thyroid therapy. Cardiac edema is not associated with increased capillary permeability. There is advanced atrophy of the interstitial cells of the testis,

accounting for such gonadal symptoms as impotency and loss of desire (Marine).

Cachexia strumipriva is postoperative myxedema caused by too radical removal of a goiter (struma). The condition, which is characterized by marked wasting as well as the ordinary symptoms of myxedema, was common in the early days of goiter surgery, but is very rarely seen at the present time.

THYROIDITIS

Although the thyroid is simple in structure and apparently simple in function, we have already seen that the pathological processes present many problems. In no field is there greater difficulty and confusion than in the inflammations of the gland. Hazard in his exhaustive review of the entire subject enumerates a large number of varieties. Two of the main groups are infectious thyroiditis and thyroiditis of unknown etiology. We shall divide the lesions into acute, subacute and chronic. We shall not consider the localized infective granulomas such as tuberculosis and syphilis, which are of little importance and are discussed on page 1024.

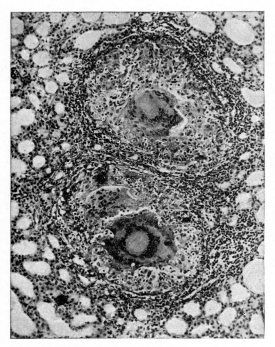

Fig. 596.—Subacute thyroiditis. The appearance is suggestive of tuberculosis. × 100.

Acute Infectious Thyroiditis.—This may be caused by infection with streptococcus hemolyticus, staphylococcus aureus, pneumococcus and other less common organisms. It may also complicate many specific fevers. The disease is of abrupt onset with fever, chills and local pain and tenderness. The condition may be suppurative with abscess formation or it may be nonsuppurative. It is obvious that this form of thyroiditis presents no problem.

Subacute Thyroiditis.—Other names for this condition are *granulomatous thyroiditis*, *pseudotuberculous thyroiditis*, *giant cell thyroiditis*, and *de Quervain's thyroiditis*. It pursues a chronic course, but is usually acute in onset.

The disease often begins abruptly, it is some 5 times commoner in women than in men, it subsides even without treatment after some weeks or months, and its etiology remains unknown, although a viral origin is suspected. In keeping with its acute onset, the thyroid is often exquisitely tender with accompanying pain on swallowing, whilst fever, constitutional disturbances, and an elevated sedimentation rate point to an infectious process. Thyroid function is not permanently damaged, and the BMR is unaffected. The response to radiation therapy is rapid and remarkable, and the patient may be well in two or three weeks. The entire gland is uniformly enlarged, so that it deserves the term goiter, which is never applied to it. *Microscopically* the striking feature is the presence of numerous *foreign body giant cells*, which may be surrounded by focal collections of chronic inflammatory cells, an appearance responsible for the name pseudotuberculous thyroiditis (Fig. 596). It has been suggested that the giant cells represent a reaction to colloid, some of which has been "spilled" from the follicles as a result of destruction of the basement membrane.

Chronic Thyroiditis.—The really puzzling group is that which includes the conditions known as Riedel's and Hashimoto's struma (an old name for goiter). Endless controversy has raged as to the relationship of these two forms of goiter, one group giving weighty evidence that they are distinct and separate entities, the other group producing equally weighty evidence that Riedel's struma is the end product of Hashimoto's disease. The reader seeking support for the idea that the conditions are unrelated should consult Crile's paper. If he wishes to believe that the different forms of thyroiditis are varying manifestations of one process, he will find the arguments ably marshalled by Levitt. My own feeling is that the Hashimoto does not progress to the Riedel lesion for reasons which will become apparent as we proceed, and more particularly because the histological appearance in repeated biopsies may remain unchanged, even up to twenty-three years (Crile and Hazard). It is of interest to note, as pointed out by Levitt, that Riedel in the years between 1896 and 1910 described only three cases, of which the first alone was a true fibrosis, the others belonging to the group of subacute thyroiditis described above, whilst Hashimoto described four cases, only two of which by his own admission were typical, the fourth being characteristic of the Riedel group.

Hashimoto's Disease.—This condition, also known as *lymphadenoid goiter* and *struma lymphomatosa*, is very much commoner in women, usually about the time of the menopause. Indeed some observers claim that it is practically confined to the female. This sex and age incidence must mean something, possibly endocrine in nature. The thyroid is uniformly enlarged, moderately firm, but not adherent to the surrounding structures. Hypothyroidism may be prominent, slight or absent.

Microscopically the striking feature is a change to an oxyphilic (eosinophilic) type of epithelium. The cells become larger than normal, the cytoplasm is abundant and and acidophilic, the nuclei are variable in size and shape to such a degree that the pathologist may suspect malignancy. These large oxyphilic cells have been called Hürthle cells, oncocytes, and still other names. Perhaps the best name is *Askanazy cells*, as they were originally described by Askanazy in 1898. Doniach considers that the Askanazy cell change is a metaplasia analogous to squamous metaplasia of the bronchial mucosa or intestinal metaplasia of the gastric mucosa. They are certainly not degenerated cells, for their cytoplasm is stuffed with mitochondria and rich in oxidative enzymes (Tremblay and Pearse). They may be arranged in small follicles, or in clusters without a follicular structure. The most arresting feature, which gives the condition its alternative name, is the abundance of lymphoid tissue, the cells of which may be collected into lymphoid follicles with germinal centers, or arranged diffusely (Fig. 597). There is reason to believe that this lesion is secondary, not primary, in character. There may be a varying degree of fibrosis which is naturally most marked in They may be arranged in small follicles, or in clusters without a follicular structure. The cases of long standing. This may progress to a condition of myxedema, and we have already seen that primary myxedema may well represent non-goitrous examples of Hashimoto's disease.

The *nature of the condition* is the real puzzle. Evidence is now forthcoming independently from both Buffalo and London that autoimmunization to thyroglobulin may be the answer. As this matter has wider implications than merely for Hashi-

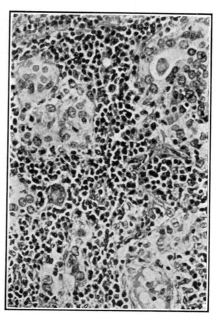

Fig. 597.—Hashimoto's struma, showing diffuse infiltration with lymphocytes and groups of Askanazy cells. × 250.

moto's disease, discussion of the question is deferred till later (Page 1018).

Riedel's Struma.—This used to be known as woody or iron-hard thyroiditis, graphic descriptive terms, although the consistence is rather that of leather than of wood or iron. It is considerably harder than the Hashimoto thyroid, it is adherent to surrounding tissue, it is more rare, it is not commoner in females, and it occurs at a younger age. There is often contraction rather than enlargement of the thyroid, and the involvement of the gland is less symmetrical than in the Hashimoto struma.

The *gross features* are marked by (1) extreme hardness so that the lesion may cut like cartilage, (2) dense fibrous adhesions to surrounding structures, and (3) asymmetrical involvement, the process usually involving only one lobe or even the isthmus. In all of these respects it differs from Hashimoto's disease. The gross character is really of greater diagnostic value than the microscopic, and is responsible for the pressure symptoms which are marked in over 50 per cent of the cases, including tracheal obstruc-

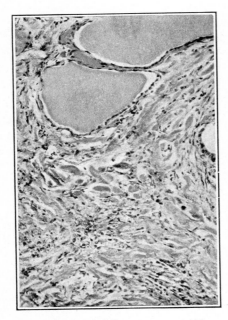

Fig. 598.—Riedel's struma. × 120.

tion which may be a distressing feature. It is natural that these symptoms, together with the hardness and asymmetry of the lesions and the adhesion to surrounding structures, should often suggest and be mistaken for carcinoma.

The *microscopic picture* will vary with the stage of the disease. In the early phase, which I have never seen, there is said to be lymphocytic infiltration, but later this is replaced by peculiarly dense fibrous tissue, which in turn replaces the parenchyma (Fig. 598). Fragments of colloid may be surrounded by clusters of epithelial cells, so as to give an appearance of foreign body giant cells with the formation of pseudo-tubercles, which may be responsible for a mistaken diagnosis of tuberculosis. Some of these cells may be macrophages which have ingested colloid (colloidophages).

The *nature of the disease* presents the usual thyroid problem to which we have become accustomed. The picture suggests chronic inflammation but no infective agent has been incriminated. It has been suggested that it is a later development of "subacute" thyroiditis, but the insidious onset, the absence of pain, and the fibroblastic invasion

of the capsule do not support this idea. The irritant in Riedel's struma may be a chemical one in the nature of what has been termed "colloid spillage," which may be compared with the "spilled milk" of plasma cell mastitis and with bile salt chronic cholecystitis. We are faced with the problem as to what causes the colloid to be spilled. It is obvious that the concept of a direct chemical irritant in Riedel's struma is quite different from that of an autoimmunization mechanism as in Hashimoto's disease.

It is possible that although each of the various forms of chronic thyroiditis may have its own etiological approach, involvement of the basement membrane of the follicles may be common to all. Diffuse degenerative changes and discontinuities in the follicular basement membrane can be demonstrated in the various members of the group by the McManus-Mowry (sulfuric acid-hematoxylin) stain (Sommers and Meissner). The membrane becomes smudgy, vacuolated and discontinuous. The basic lesion, particularly in Riedel's disease, may be one of the thyroid stromal matrix, followed by exposure and consequent degeneration of the parenchymal cells, colloidophagy, lymphocytic infiltration, and follicular breakdown and atrophy.

Autoimmunity in Thyroiditis.—We have already seen that in various forms of subacute and chronic thyroiditis we are confronted with the problem of an inflammatory reaction without a satisfactory cause. The work of Witebsky and his associates in Buffalo and of Roitt *et al.* in London suggests that an autoimmune reaction to thyroid antigens may be involved, more particularly in Hashimoto's disease and also in primary myxedema. In Hashimoto's disease the normal reaction to incipient hypothyroidism, namely the production of increased thyroid-stimulating hormone by the pituitary, results in goiter through hyperplasia of the remaining healthy thyroid tissue, whereas in primary myxedema not enough healthy thyroid tissue remains to respond to the stimulus.

When thyroglobulin is injected into laboratory animals it acts as an antigen which stimulates the formation of antibodies. It has been suggested that these react with the thyroid of the animal to produce lesions resembling those of Hashimoto's disease. Such lesions have been produced by the injection of antithyroid serum, and by the injection of rabbit thyroid extract into rabbits immunized against such extract (Rose and Witebsky; Terplan *et al.*). Circulating antibodies can be demonstrated not only in the inoculated animal but also in Hashimoto's disease (98 per cent), primary myxedema (83 per cent), and to a lesser degree in subacute thyroiditis and thyrotoxic goiter (Roitt and Doniach). Demonstration of the antibodies can be effected by the agglutination of tanned red blood cells coated with thyroglobulin, precipitation and complement fixation tests, and Coons' fluorescent antibody technique.

It would now seem that two antigens rather than one may be involved in these thyroid reactions: (1) thyroglobulin from within the acini, antibodies to which are best demonstrated by tanned red cells agglutination, and (2) an intracellular antigen localized predominantly in the microsome fraction of thyroid homogenates and responsible for complement-fixing antibodies. The initial event in Hashimoto's disease (thyroiditis) may be leakage of thyroglobulin out of the acini into the gland. Within the acinus the thyroglobulin leads a secluded life cut off from all contact with antibody-forming cells. The thyroglobin leak attracts lymphocytes and plasma cells, which themselves make antibodies locally. The thyroglobulin antibody in the circulation thus appears to be derived from reticuloendothelial elements within the thyroid itself. (It may be noted in passing that alternative names for the condition are lymphadenoid goiter and lymphoid thyroiditis. We have already seen that in Graves' disease and in myxedema collections of lymphocytes form a prominent feature). The resulting antigen-antibody reaction causes cellular destruction, which releases more antigen, thus setting up a self-perpetuating chain reaction. Some of the antigen may pass into the adjacent lymph nodes, where thyroglobulin can be demonstrated by means of antibody labelled with fluorescent technique. The last stage is that in which thyroglobulin escapes into the general circulation, so that antibodies

are produced by other tissues and intensify the reaction in the thyroid. It is interesting to know that intradermal skin tests, using extract of human thyroid as antigen, give a strongly positive Arthus type of reaction, for which precipitating antibody is essential, in Hashimoto's disease and myxedema (Buchanan *et al.*). There still remains the all-important question: Are the circulating antibodies the cause of the disease or only an effect?

Striking evidence of the presence of a cytotoxic agent in Hashimoto serum acting against human thyroid cells is provided by tissue culture technique (Pulvertaft *et al.*). Within thirty seconds of the addition of the serum to a young culture of thyroid cells cytotoxic changes can be observed. The pale, thin mitochondria become dark and thick, then dark solid spheres, and finally large hollow vesicles. This is followed by lysis of the cells, which are then phagocytosed by monocytes and polymorphonuclears.

Basement membranes changes may play an important part in thyroid disease (Sommers and Meissner). The normal basement membrane stains intensely, and completely seals off the contents of the follicles from the blood in the surrounding capillaries. Abnormal basement membrane changes are found in patients with high antibody titer as shown by the tanned red cell agglutination technique (Stuart and Allan). The damage is focal, consisting of fragmentation, beading and duplication (Fig. 599). The changes are more severe and diffuse in Hashimoto's disease than in subacute thyroiditis, but it cannot be said that a direct relationship between basement membrane change and antigen-antibody reaction has yet been established.

An intriguing extension of the concept of autoimmunity in thyroid disease involves the pathogenesis of at least some cases of *cretinism*. Antithyroid antibodies have been demonstrated in the serum of the mothers of cretins more frequently than in other groups, suggesting that cretinism is sometimes causally related to thyroid autoimmunization in the mother (Blizzard *et al.*). When antithyroid antibodies cross the placenta, which, being gamma globulins, they can

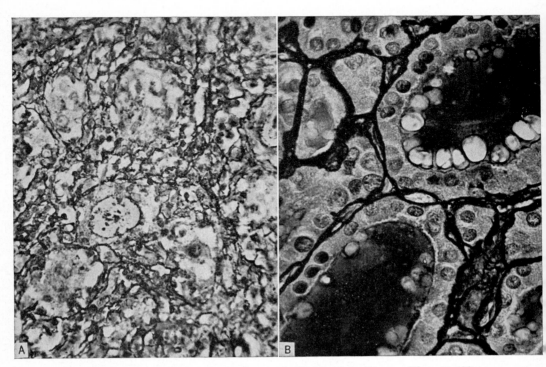

FIG. 599.—*A*, Severe basement membrane damage in Hashimoto's disease. Silver × 400.
  B, Normal appearance of basement membranes of thyroid follicles. Silver × 650. (Kindness of Dr. Angus E. Stuart, Edinburgh.)

readily do, either normal children or athyrotic cretins may be born. One woman with circulating antibodies gave birth to three infants who were hypothyroid and athyrotic at birth. It is also more than possible that myxedema, the hypothyroid state in the adult, may also have an autoimmunity basis. We have already discussed the probable relationship of primary myxedema to clinical and subclinical Hashimoto's thyroiditis.

From what has just been said it might be thought that the perplexing problem of chronic thyroiditis and its variants had been solved, and that the subject was closed. Such is very far from being the case. Although auto-antibodies found in the sera of patients with thyroid disease react *in vitro* with thyroglobulin, it is not yet certain whether these are auto-aggressive *in vivo* in the human subject. Moreover, while thyroglobulin antibodies were present in the sera of 59 per cent of patients with thyroid disease, they were also present, using the tanned-cell hemagglutination technique, in

18 per cent of 387 hospital patients in Adelaide, Australia, in whom there was no clinical evidence of disorder of the thyroid (Hackett *et al.*). This is disturbing to our concept of pathogenesis. But it has also been found that Hashimoto-like lesions, with clumps of Hürthle cells and collections of lymphocytes may be present at autopsy in 6 per cent of males and 30 per cent of females over forty years of age (Goudie *et al.*). In these patients there had been no clinical evidence of thyroid disease, but there was a positive thyroid antibody complement fixation test, which is more sensitive than the precipitin test. It may be, indeed, that a finding of thyroglobulin antibodies in a person without clinical thyroid disease indicates a condition of subacute subclinical thyroiditis with corresponding lesions, and it seems probable that attacks of subacute and even acute thyroiditis are frequently overlooked.

One final question remains unanswered: Why is it that abnormal serological findings with their characteristic lesions are so much more frequent in elderly females, especially those with disease of the liver? The answer may involve the interrelationship of hepatic, thyroid and ovarian function, for the normal liver is known to metabolize both thyroid and ovarian hormones.

TUMORS OF THE THYROID

The subject of thyroid neoplasms is perhaps the most confused and contentious branch of thyroid pathology. This is particularly true of classification of the incidence of tumors in the general population, of the relation of microscopic structure to prognosis, and of the development of carcinoma in benign lesions. Some of these problems have already been encountered earlier in this chapter. The confusion depends on a number of factors.

(1) The geographic variation of goiter, including the nodular and adenomatous forms, has already been referred to. Papers coming from different regions will vary in their statistical content. The material in a special thyroid clinic is not representative of the population in general. (2) The classification and subdivision of types has been carried to such an extreme that it is difficult to compare reports from one center or country with those from another. (3) The frequency of malignancy depends on the pathologist's report, and the criteria insisted on in one center may not be considered so important in another. This is illustrated by the question of venous invasion (p. 1023). (4) The difficulty of adequate follow-up studies. Thus a malignant papillary adenoma may not show its true character until long past the usual five or ten year follow-up period.

We shall avoid the complicated classifications which can be found in monographs dealing with the thyroid, and content ourselves with recognizing the adenoma and the carcinoma, both of which may be follicular or papillary. We have already considered the extreme difficulty there may be in distinguishing a regenerative nodule from a benign neoplasm.

Adenoma.—In general terms, the chief characteristics of a true adenoma are the

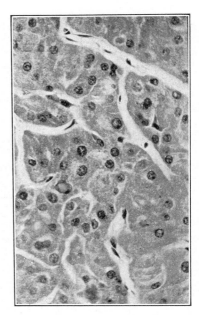

Fig. 600.—Hürthle-cell adenoma. × 240.

presence of a single nodule compared with the multiple nodules of nodular goiter, good encapsulation, a fairly uniform structure, a different growth pattern from that of the surrounding gland, and evidence of compression of the adjacent thyroid tissue by the nodule (Warren and Meissner).

Follicular Adenoma.—This is marked by the formation of new follicles and is the usual type. Degenerative changes are common, with cyst formation and hemorrhage. The histological picture varies considerably from case to case, and this variation has given rise to endless subdivisions which need not concern us here. Two names, however, deserve mention. *Fetal adenoma* consists of great numbers of small follicles (microfollicular), giving an appearance somewhat suggestive of a developing gland. The *Hürthle cell adenoma* is a rare tumor consisting of large, polygonal cells with abundant strongly acidophilic cytoplasm arranged in solid masses of columns, so that the picture bears a marked resemblance to that of the liver (Fig. 600). It is believed that the cytological change represents some form of degeneration. Occasionally the tumor becomes invasive, a condition to which the term Langhans' tumor has been applied by European writers.

Papillary Adenoma.—This is much less common than the follicular variety. The formation of papillary processes with delicate fronds of epithelium is the characteristic feature, frequently with the formation of true cysts, so that the lesion becomes a papillary cystadenoma. The pathologist may be hard put to it to distinguish a very active papillary adenoma from a papillary carcinoma.

Carcinoma.—"No other kind of carcinoma shows a wider range of rate of growth and metastatic behaviour than thyroid carcinoma. At one extreme there are the very indolent, highly differentiated cystic papillary growths which metastasize to the neighbouring cervical lymph glands and spread slowly from gland to gland over a long period of years; at the other extreme, there are the highly anaplastic sarcoma-like growths which grow quickly to a huge bulk or disseminate rapidly and widely by the blood-stream" (Willis).

In spite of the wide range of tumors so well described by Willis, it is possible to divide them into three main groups, which differ as much in their biological behavior as in their histological structure. These are (1) papillary carcinoma, (2) follicular carcinoma, and (3) undifferentiated carcinoma.

Cancers of the thyroid are not necessarily autonomous from the beginning, but, like tumors of other endocrine glands, they may for a time be under *endocrine control*. It is well known that tumors of various endocrine glands can be induced in the experimental animal by disturbing the balance of the endocrine system. Cancer of the thyroid in rats can be produced by feeding thiouracil (Purves *et al.*). First adenomas and then metastasizing carcinomas develop. At first these cancers are transplantable only in rats conditioned with thiouracil, but in the course of time they lose their endocrine dependency and become transplantable into rats which are not thyroxine conditioned. In passing, it is of interest to note that the transplanted tumors develop into a number of lines of widely differing histological appearance. The mechanism of tumor production and of continued growth is evidently a function of the pituitary-thyroid axis. When the production of thyroxine is depressed by thiouracil or other agents, the normal inhibition of the anterior pituitary by this hormone is removed, and TSH, the pituitary thyroid-stimulating hormone, now takes full control. The result may be the development first of an adenoma and then of carcinoma. Later the conditioned or dependent neoplasm changes into an autonomous one.

Realization of this truth is beginning to influence the therapeutic approach to the control of thyroid tumors. If the tumor is dependent, the aim will be to restore the disturbed endocrine balance; if it is autonomous, the aim must be to destroy the malignant cells. Remarkable results have already been achieved in the control or even the cure of metastasizing cancer by means of continued feeding with dessicated thyroid (Crile). This applies to the papillary and follicular forms, but not to undifferentiated cancers. This, of course, is what might be expected. In assessing the results of any form of treatment it must be remembered that some thyroid cancers grow very slowly, and may persist or recur over a period of ten or even twenty years. This is sometimes true even of undifferentiated carcinomas which to the pathologist may look most forbidding.

Papillary Carcinoma.—This can be regarded as the malignant variant of the benign papillary adenoma. It is the commonest form of thyroid cancer and the least malignant. Its three most striking characteristics are its occurrence in young women, particularly in the second and third decades, although it may develop at a later period, the prolonged character of its course, and its tendency to invade lymphatics but not blood vessels. There may be spread to the regional lymph nodes, even when the tumor is less than 1 cm. in diameter. This is the basis for the former erroneous concept of *lateral aberrant thyroid tumors* occurring in young adults in whom the primary tumor remained undetected. These lymph node metastases are equally sluggish in behavior. The tumors have low functional activity, a low radioactive iodine uptake, and they are insensitive to external radiation, which may

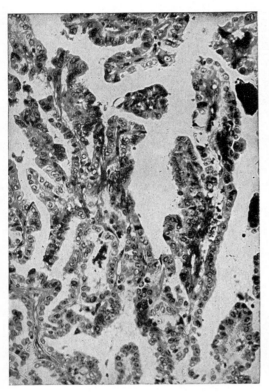

Fig. 601.—Papillary adenocarcinoma of thyroid. × 175. (Boyd, *Pathology for the Surgeon*, courtesy of W. B. Saunders Co.)

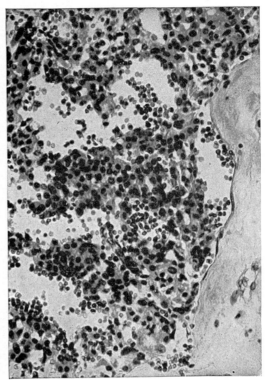

Fig. 602.—Carcinoma of thyroid with mass of tumor cells lying in lumen of vein. × 275. (Boyd, *Pathology for the Surgeon*, courtesy of W. B. Saunders Co.)

indeed be harmful inasmuch as it depresses the production of thyroxine and thus allows free play to the pituitary. It is in this variety of cancer that therapy with dessicated thyroid is particularly effective.

Microscopically the papillary processes have no longer the delicate appearance of the papillary adenoma, and they may present several layers of cells, together with the cytological changes of malignancy (Fig. 601). Curiously enough there seems to be no relation between the histological appearance and the biological behavior. No matter how wild the picture may be, growth is characteristically sluggish. Perhaps this is related to the hormone-dependent character of the tumor.

Follicular Carcinoma.—This type of tumor, formerly called adenocarcinoma, usually, but not necessarily, arises in a pre-existing follicular adenoma. Sometimes it represents a tiny microscopic lesion, but as a rule it takes

the form of a mass which may either remain encapsulated or may penetrate the capsule of the gland, invading the muscles, skin, trachea and recurrent laryngeal nerve, and causing dysphagia, hoarseness and cough. Its most striking characteristic, however, is a tendency to invade veins, so that metastases are set up in distant organs, especially the bones (Fig. 602). This is in marked contrast to the tendency of the papillary type to invade and spread by the lymphatics. The basal metabolic rate usually remains within normal limits, but some patients are hypothyroid and a few are hyperthyroid. In the latter group the lesions are well differentiated, and may show a vigorous uptake of radioactive iodine.

Microscopically the degree of differentiation may vary greatly. In some cases the acini are remarkably well formed and contain colloid. Under these circumstances the metastases may simulate and be mistaken

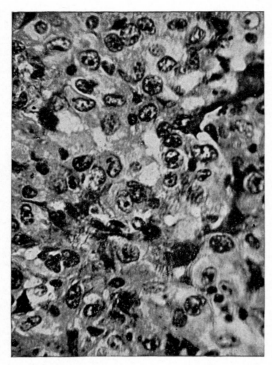

FIG. 603.—Undifferentiated carcinoma of the thyroid showing complete disorder of the normal cellular arrangement. × 500. (Boyd, *Pathology for the Surgeon*, courtesy of W. B. Saunders Co.)

for normal thyroid tissue. This is the basis of the former term *"benign metastasizing goiter."* In such cases the primary tumor has frequently remained small, encapsulated, and therefore undetected. In other cases the tumor is less well differentiated and deserves to be called an adenocarcinoma.

Undifferentiated Carcinoma.—This type follows the general pattern of cancer in other organs. It is a disease of middle and older age, the incidence increasing with the years. *Microscopically* the tumor may be completely undifferentiated (Fig. 603) or may show some recognizable features of adenocarcinoma. The undifferentiated cancers may be small cell or giant cell. The small cell carcinomas are easily mistaken for lymphosarcoma. The *giant cell tumors* are amongst the most malignant, the microscopic picture suggesting an anaplastic fibrosarcoma with numerous elongated tumor giant cells. Not only do different tumors differ from one another, but different parts

of the same tumor may show widely varying structure. Invasion of the surrounding tissue occurs early, together with spread by the lymphatics and by the blood stream to the lungs and bones, more particularly the cranium. Venous invasion may be very striking in the primary tumor. The tumor cells have no functional capacity as might be expected, so that as a rule there is little or no uptake of radioactive iodine. Although they are usually markedly sensitive to external radiation, the effect is transient, and few patients survive as long as two years after the diagnosis has been established.

Secondary Tumors.—Secondary tumors of the thyroid are rare, with the exception of malignant melanoma and bronchogenic carcinoma.

MISCELLANEOUS LESIONS

INFECTIVE GRANULOMAS.—*Tuberculosis* of the thyroid gland is rare, the gland showing a remarkable resistance to this infection. Miliary tubercles may occur, but must be distinguished from the pseudotubercles of Riedel's struma, and from similar structures which are very occasionally seen in diffuse and nodular goiters. Large areas of caseation may be formed, but this is extremely rare. *Syphilis* may not uncommonly cause enlargement of the thyroid in the secondary stage. Tertiary gummata are very rare.

CONGENITAL ANOMALIES.—The thyroid may be absent. Normally the gland is developed as a downgrowth from the anterior wall of the pharynx, the stalk connecting it with the pharynx forming the *thyroglossal duct*, which at birth is represented only by the dimple of the foramen cecum at the posterior part of the tongue. Portions may be displaced during the course of development. A nodule at the base of the tongue may form a *lingual thyroid*. There may be small masses in the neck known as *accessory thyroids*, and pieces may be found at some distance from the normal position. A portion of the duct may remain unobliterated and form a *thyroglossal cyst*, which is recognized by always being in the middle line of the neck. Pieces of parathyroid or thymus may be embedded in the thyroid.

REFERENCES

BAKER, S. M. and HAMILTON, J. D.: Lab. Invest., 1957, *6*, 218. (Capillary changes in myxedema.)
BERSON, S. A.: Am. J. Med., 1956, *20*, 653. (Pathways of iodine metabolism.)

BLIZZARD, R. M., *et al.*: New Eng. J. Med., 1960, *263*, 327. (Maternal autoimmunization in cretinism.)

BUCHANAN, W. W., *et al.*: Lancet, 1958, *2*, 928. (Skin test in thyroid disease.)

CRILE, G., JR.: Ann. Surg., 1948, *127*, 640. (Chronic thyroiditis.)

————.: Cancer, 1957, *10*, 1119. (Endocrine dependent cancers.)

CRILE, G., JR. and HAZARD, J. B.: J. Clin. Endocrinol., 1951, *11*, 1123. (Chronic thyroiditis.)

CURRAN, R. C., ECKERT, H. and WILSON, G. M.: J. Path. and Bact., 1958, *76*, 541. (Thyroid in Graves' disease after treatment of hyperthyroidism.)

DOBYNS, B. M.: Am. J. Med., 1956, *20*, 684. (Physiologic concepts in Graves' disease.)

DONIACH, J.: in *Recent Advances in Pathology*, edit. by Harrison, C. V., 7th ed., London, 1960. (Hashimoto's thyroiditis and myxedema.)

GOUDIE, R. B., ANDERSON, J. R. and GRAY, K. G.: J. Path. and Bact., 1959, *77*, 389. (Complement-fixing antithyroid antibodies and asymptomatic thyroid lesions.)

HACKETT, E., BEECH, M. and FORBES, I. J.: Lancet, 1960, *2*, 402. (Thyroglobulin antibodies without disease of thyroid.)

HALEY, H. L., DEWS, G. M., SOMMERS, S. C.: Arch. Path., 1955, *59*, 635. (Histochemistry of thyrotoxic goiter.)

HALPERT, B., CAVANAUGH, J. W. and KELTZ, B. F.: Arch. Path., 1946, *41*, 155. (Phases of thyroid activity.)

HELLWIG, C.: Surg., Gynec. and Obst., 1932, *55*, 35. (Geographic pathology of goiter.)

HULL, O. H.: Arch. Path., 1955, *59*, 291. (Incidence of thyroid nodules in autopsy material.)

JAIMET, C. H. and THODE, H. G.: Can. Med. Ass. J., 1956, *74*, 865. (Relation of thyroid and salivary gland function.)

LEVITT, T.: *The Thyroid, a Physiological, Pathological, Clinical and Surgical Study*, Edinburgh, 1954.

————.: Lancet, 1951, *2*, 957; Ann. Roy. Coll. Surg. Eng., 1952, *10*, 369. (Chronic thyroiditis.)

MEANS, J. H.: Trans. Ass. Am. Phys., 1940, *55*, 32. (Pituitary myxedema.)

PULVERTAFT, R. J. V., *et al.*: Lancet, 1959, *2*, 214. (Cytotoxic effects of Hashimoto's serum on thyroid tissue culture.)

PURVES, H. D., GRIESBACK, W. E. and KENNEDY, T. H.: Brit. J. Cancer, 1951, *5*, 301. (Endocrine dependent cancers.)

ROITT, I. M., *et al.*: Lancet, 1956, *2*, 820. (Auto-antibodies in Hashimoto's disease.)

ROITT, I. M. and DONIACH, D.: Lancet, 1958, *2*, 1027. (Immune bodies in various forms of goiter.)

ROSE, N. R. and WITEBSKY, E.: J. Immunol., 1956, *76*, 417. (Autoimmunity in thyroiditis.)

SOKAL, J. E.: J.A.M.A., 1959, *170*, 405. (Malignancy in nodular goiter.)

SOMMERS, S. C. and MEISSNER, W. A.: Am. J. Clin. Path., 1954, *24*, 434. (Basement membranes in chronic thyroiditis.)

STEIN, A.: Arch. Path., 1959, *67*, 168. (The microfollicle in goiter.)

STUART, A. E., and ALLAN, W. S. A.: Lancet, 1958, *2*, 1204. (Basement membrane changes.)

TERPLAN, K. L., *et al.*: Am. J. Path., 1960, *36*, 213. (Experimental thyroiditis.)

TREMBLAY, G. and PEARSE, A. G. E.: J. Path. and Bact., 1960, *80*, 353. (Oxidative enzymes in Askanazy cells.)

WERNER, S. C.: *The Thyroid*, New York, 1955.

WILLIS, R. A.: *Pathology of Tumors*, London, 2nd ed., 1949, page 609.

WITEBSKY, E., *et al.*: J.A.M.A., 1957, *164*, 1439; Lancet, 1958, *1*, 808. (Auto-antibodies in Hashimoto's disease.)

Chapter 38

The Parathyroids

General Considerations
   Structure
   Function
Hyperparathyroidism
   Bone Lesions
   Renal Lesions

Gastrointestinal Symptoms
Biochemical Changes
Hypoparathyroidism
Tumors
   Adenoma

Primary Hyperplasia
Secondary Hyperplasia
Carcinoma
Clinical Picture
Other Lesions

GENERAL CONSIDERATIONS

Structure.—The parathyroid glands are minute structures, not more than 5 mm. in diameter, four or more in number, and frequently difficult to demonstrate, especially as the inferior group may be embedded in the substance of the thyroid. The glands consist of sheets of epithelial cells arranged in groups separated by sinusoids. Three main types of cells may be encountered under different conditions. (1) *Chief cells*, which are the only cells until puberty, have scanty cytoplasm and a relatively large, deeply-stained nucleus. (2) *Oxyphil cells* appear after puberty and increase in number with age. As the name implies, they stain red with acid dyes, owing to the presence of acidophilic granules. They are rich in phospholipid. For some reason they are more numerous in women, and the few reported cases of oxyphil cell adenoma have nearly all been in women. They do not appear to elaborate the parathyroid hormone, and in one case a tumor of these cells weighed 52 gm. without causing evidence of hyperparathyroidism. (3) *Water-clear cells*, usually known for some strange reason by their German name, *wasserhelle* cells, appear in very small numbers after puberty, but they may be the principal constituent in hyperplasia and adenoma. The water-clear cells appear to be derived from the chief cells. They are rich in glycogen which is soluble in water, thus accounting for their water-clear character.

The parathyroids are the most difficult organs in the body to find at autopsy, partly on account of their small size, partly because of their resemblance to lobules of fat. Excellent instructions for their demonstration will be found in the appendix to Gilmour's paper.

Function.—The function of the parathyroids is to regulate the metabolism of calcium, phosphorus and bone. At a given pH there is a strong tendency for the solubility product of calcium and phosphorus to remain constant, the one rising as the other falls, and this constancy depends on the parathyroid hormone. With an increase in parathyroid activity there is an increase in serum calcium (average 10 mg. per 100 cc., normal range 9 to 11 mg.) and a fall in serum phosphorus (average 3 mg., normal range 2 to 4 mg. per 100 cc.), the reverse occurring in hypoparathyroidism. Normally the calcium and phosphate ions of the blood and calcium phosphate of the bones are in a state of equilibrium and are subject to the law of ionic dissociation, *i.e.*, concentration of the ions, if altered, must vary inversely with one another. This helps to maintain the acid-base equilibrium. Removal of the parathyroids results in hypocalcemia, and the level of serum calcium may drop to 6 mg. per 100 cc. The administration of parathyroid extract will send the calcium level up to 20 mg. per 100 cc., and the phosphate may fall to 1 mg. per 100 cc.; both are excreted in increased amounts in the urine.

Renal disease may cause retention of inorganic phosphorus; this tends to depress the calcium, and would do so were it not for increased function of the parathyroids and consequent hyperplasia. Just as renal lesions can influence the parathyroids, so

(1026)

also can parathyroid overactivity cause renal lesions. The pathological physiology of the gland may vary in the direction of hyperfunction or hypofunction. *Pure hyperparathyroidism gives rise to generalized osteitis fibrosa; pure hypoparathyroidism gives rise to tetany.*

The mode and site of action of the parathyroid hormone has long been a matter of dispute, Collip, who originally isolated the hormone, maintaining that the action was on bone, whereas Albright considered that the effects of the hormone could be explained by increased renal excretion of phosphorus, with resulting upset of the normal serum calcium-phosphorus ration and consequent withdrawal of calcium from the bones. It would now appear that both of these views are in part correct, for there is evidence to show that there are not one but two parathyroid hormones (Dent), which can be separated by dialysis from the crude extract, the one acting on bone, the other on the kidney. The equilibrium between the bone crystals, which are estimated to have a total surface of some 30 acres, and the tissue fluid must be the major factor in determining the serum calcium level, which is extremely constant at about 10 mg. per 100 cc. in normal indivduals. It is the parathyroid secretion which sets the level at which this homeostatic mechanism operates, and which must therefore regulate the living barrier between the bone salt and the tissue fluid. The bone is slow to respond, being relatively insensitive, but the reaction is unlimited. The second hormone appears to decrease the renal tubular reabsorption of phosphate, thus permitting phosphaturia to occur, with lowering of the serum phosphorus level and a compensatory increase in serum calcium. An elevated serum calcium may therefore be due to both actions. The kidney is very sensitive, so that the reaction is rapid, but it is quite limited.

It is evident that the functional activity of the parathyroids is regulated by changes in the serum level of ionized calcium. They differ diametrically from the thyroid and the adrenals in not being under the influence of the pituitary, nor does their secretion affect that gland.

HYPERPARATHYROIDISM

Hypersecretion of parahormone, the hormone of the parathyroids, may be primary or secondary. *Primary hyperparathyroidism* may be caused by adenoma, carcinoma, or diffuse hyperplasia of all four glands involving usually the water-clear cells, but occasionally the chief cells. These various lesions are described on page 1029. *Secondary hyperparathyroidism* is associated with secondary hyperplasia, which results from calcium deprivation, and in turn may produce an excess of hormone causing further decalcification (page 1029). In this discussion we shall confine our thinking to primary hyperparathyroidism such as is produced by adenoma of one of the parathyroids. The chief evidence of disturbance is seen in the skeleton, kidney, gastrointestinal tract, and blood chemistry. Diagnosis would be simple if all of these were combined in every case. Unfortunately there may be (1) renal signs only, (2) evidence of bone disease only, (3) evidence of both bone and renal disease, and (4) neither renal nor bone disease, but signs and symptoms of hypercalcemia pointing to the gastrointestinal canal. In addition the muscles are hypotonic, for the tissues are flooded with mobilized calcium, neuromuscular irritability is accordingly diminished, and there is great muscular weakness.

Bone Lesions.—The great effect of hyperparathyroidism is decalcification. There is first *halisteresis*, a removal of lime salts due to some change in the relationship between the plasma bathing the bone and the bone itself. This is followed by *osteoporosis*, a removal of the decalcified organic material by osteoclasts, the phagocytes of bone. Coincident with the removal of bone there is a formation of a fibrous material between the bony trabecula, and thin trabeculæ of new bone are formed in these fibrous foci. There is thus a continuous process of bone destruction and formation, but the former predominates, so that the bone becomes very pliable and marked deformities develop, the condition known as *von Recklinghausen's disease of bone* (Fig. 604). In extreme cases the degree of decalcification is unbelievable. Cysts may develop in the newly formed fibrous tissue often giving rise

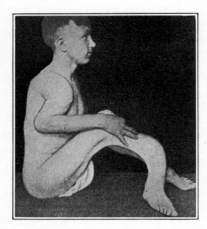

Fig. 604.—Osteitis fibrosa. The extremely marked bony deformities are the result of hyperparathyroidism.

to fractures, but these are not an invariable feature, so that it is better to name the bony lesions *osteitis fibrosa* rather than osteitis fibrosa cystica. The cysts are usually small, but may attain a considerable size, and may lead to pathological fracture. Brownish areas may be visible in the medullary cavity which represent *giant cell tumors* containing large numbers of osteoclasts and representing part of the reaction caused by the disturbance of calcium metabolism.

Renal Lesions.—Lesions of the kidney may be just as important as those in the skeleton. Indeed about 30 per cent of cases do not show changes in the bones, and when the disease proves fatal, death is due to renal failure. Renal insufficiency itself may give rise to secondary hyperparathyroidism, which in turn may be responsible for further renal damage. This is more likely to occur in children with a long history of renal insufficiency.

A fine deposit of calcium occurs in the renal tubules and the interstitial tissue of the pyramids. There may be calcification of the tubular epithelium and the tubular basement membrane. Renal calculi may develop with accompanying pyelonephritis and renal insufficiency. The frequency of this complication differs materially in the reports of different workers, varying from 1 to 8 per cent or higher. It may at least be said that in every case of renal calculi the possibility

of hyperparathyroidism should be considered, all the more so if the stones are bilateral and recurrent. It may not be possible to distinguish sharply between the renal lesion of primary and secondary hyperparathyroidism, as calcification of the tubules may occur in both forms (Morgan and Maclagan).

Gastrointestinal Symptoms.—Hyperparathyroidism has been called "a disease of stones and bones." It might be recognized more frequently if it were regarded as "a disease of stones, bones and abdominal groans" (St. Goar). Hyperkalemia is responsible for the principle abdominal symptoms, which are of special value in early diagnosis when the changes in bones and disturbance of renal function are still reversible by surgical intervention. It would appear that an increased calcium ion concentration in the sympathetic ganglia impedes the transmission of afferent stimuli and diminishes their efferent discharges. The frequent result is marked constipation, probably due to atony of the large intestine, and gastric atony, with dyspepsia, nausea and vomiting. Peptic ulcer, usually duodenal, develops in about 8 per cent of cases.

Biochemical Changes.—These are usually highly characteristic and it is from them that the final diagnosis has to be made. The *calcium* which is extracted from the bones appears in the blood in large amount, and the blood calcium may rise from the normal figure of 10 mg. per 100 cc. to 20 or more, although a more usual figure is 15 or 16. Should the excretion of calcium by the kidney keep pace with the increased mobilization from the bones, the blood calcium may be normal, a confusing point which must be borne in mind in making a diagnosis. The *blood phosphorus* is below normal and may be as low as 1.1 mg. (normal, 3 mg.), because the renal threshold for phosphorus is lowered by excess of parathyroid hormone. It must be remembered, however, that many of these patients have associated renal disease when first seen, and consequently phosphate retention, so that the serum phosphorus may be misleading. The *urinary excretion of calcium* is greatly increased, so that there is a negative calcium balance. In normal persons 70 to 90 per cent of the calcium output goes through the stools and only 10 to 30 per cent appears in the urine. In osteitis fibrosa this relation is reversed. There is also an increased phosphorus excretion. *Metastatic calcification* is a natural accompaniment of the extensive decalcification of the skeleton. The calcium is deposited particularly in the arteries, the renal pelvis (to form a calculus), and in the renal tubules.

HYPOPARATHYROIDISM

The clinical manifestation of this condition is *tetany*. Tetany may be produced in a variety of ways, all of which are connected directly or remotely with the low calcium in the tissues. Pure parathyroid tetany is best seen when the parathyroids have been removed intentionally in animals or unintentionally in man in the course of an operation for goiter. There is a marked drop in the blood calcium and a decreased excretion of calcium in the urine. The phosphorus of the blood is normal or raised. The tissues are depleted of calcium, and tetany develops owing to the increased neuromuscular irritability. This hyperexcitability is shown by twitching of the muscles and severe clonic carpopedal spasms and convulsions. When the nerves are stimulated electrically and even when pressed upon, the muscles may go into a persistent tetanic spasm. *The low calcium is the key to the clinical picture,* for it facilitates the transmission of nervous impulses across the myoneural junction, with, as a result, a great increase in neuromuscular excitability.

In idiopathic hypoparathyroidism due to hypoplasia of the glands the blood phosphorus is markedly raised and the calcium very low. Contrary to what might be expected, metastatic calcification may be encountered, more particularly in the walls of the vessels of the basal ganglia, which are thereby rendered visible in radiograms of the head.

TUMORS

The term tumor is used here in the clinical sense of an enlargement of one or more of the glands. This enlargement may be due to: (1) adenoma (much the commonest), (2) primary hyperplasia, (3) secondary hyperplasia, and (4) carcinoma (much the rarest). All may be associated with symptoms of hyperparathyroidism.

Adenoma.—These tumors vary from 1 to 7 cm. in diameter, but occasionally they may weigh as much as 50 or 60 gm. Fortunately only one gland, and at first only one part of that gland, is involved, but sometimes two glands may be the site of tumors. There is no relation between the size and functional activity of the adenoma. Even a large tumor may not be palpable, because it is tucked away behind the trachea or hidden in the mediastinum, a point the surgeon must keep in mind. It may be embedded in the thyroid, where it is apt to be mistaken for a thyroid adenoma. The tumor is grayish-white in color, usually nodular, and very often cystic. *Microscopically* all three types of cells, chief, water-clear and oxyphil are usually represented, but the chief or water-clear cells are the commonest (Fig. 605), and one or other of these may dominate the picture. The pleomorphism of cell type is in contrast to the uniformity of hyperplasia.

Primary Hyperplasia.—Hyperplasia rather than neoplasia may be the basis of hyperparathyroidism (Castleman and Mallory). All of the parathyroids are diffusely enlarged, in contrast to the limited and localized enlargement of adenomas. The hyperplastic glands present a singularly uniform appearance; the cells are large and extremely clear, so that the condition has been called parathyroid hypernephroma; the outlines are sharp, the nuclei are at the base of the cells, and there is a marked acinar arrangement. Oxyphil cells are not present. There appears to be a much rarer form consisting entirely of chief cells. The degree of hyperplasia is remarkable. They may be 100 times the weight of normal tissue, whereas in Graves' disease there is only a 5- or 10-fold hypertrophy of the thyroid. The diffuse character of the hyperplasia affecting all the glands suggests the action of an external continuous stimulus.

Secondary Hyperplasia.—Enlargement of the parathyroids may be a secondary rather than a primary phenomenon. Much confusion existed before this fact was recognized. Thus enlargement of the glands was noted in two such unrelated but apparently similar conditions as osteitis fibrosa (von Reckling-

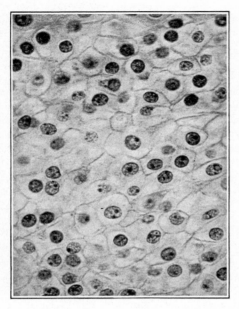

Fig. 605.—Parathyroid adenoma. The lesion is composed of water-clear cells. × 500.

hausen's disease) and osteomalacia, and this fact was used to link the two together. It is now known that in the former condition the hyperplasia is a cause, whereas in the latter it is an effect. The matter is not so simple, however, as this statement might suggest, because secondary hyperplasia may also be hyperfunctioning and may give rise to the same skeletal and other changes seen in primary hyperplasia, so that the differentiation may be very difficult. The bone lesions have been called renal hyperparathyroidism, renal rickets, *etc.*, but perhaps the most satisfactory term is *renal osteodystrophy* (Snapper).

The most important cause of secondary hyperplasia is *chronic renal insufficiency* in childhood, particularly pyelonephritis. Retention of phosphate due to renal tubular damage is accompanied by rise in serum phosphorus and a corresponding fall in serum calcium. This is compensated for by withdrawal of calcium from the skeleton, which is mediated by overactivity of the parathyroids with corresponding hyperplasia. Decalcifying diseases such as rickets, osteomalacia, multiple myeloma, and secondary carcinomatosis of bone may also be respon-

sible for secondary parathyroid hyperplasia. The histological picture differs from that of primary hyperplasia in that there is *variation rather than uniformity of cell type*, with the chief cells usually predominant.

Carcinoma.—This is fortunately by far the rarest cause of parathyroid enlargement. The tumor infiltrates the thyroid and surrounding tissues, and metastasizes to the regional lymph nodes, lungs and bones. Usually it produces no hormone, but in some cases it is responsible for hyperparathyroidism (Rapoport *et al.*). The microscopic distinction between parathyroid adenoma and carcinoma is often extremely difficult, although the presence of mitotic figures are strongly in favor of carcinoma.

Clinical Picture.—The symptoms of parathyroid tumor and hyperplasia are those of hyperparathyroidism. The main features of this condition evidenced by disturbances in the bones, kidneys, gastrointestinal tract and blood chemistry have already been outlined earlier in this chapter. The symptoms fall into three main groups: (1) those due to hyperkalemia, such as weakness, lassitude and hypotonia; (2) those due to renal changes associated with a greatly increased excretion of calcium with resulting polyuria, thirst, and calculi with their complications; (3) bone changes. In a full-blown classical case the picture is as follows: The patient, usually young, shows marked *skeletal deformities*, pain is a dominant feature in the early stage, muscular weakness and hypotonia may cause him to be bedridden, the electrical irritability of the muscles is diminished, there is generally decalcification of the skeleton and cyst formation in the long bones, giant cell tumors of bone may develop, the urine may contain blood and pus owing to calcium deposits in the renal pelvis, and the blood chemistry is characteristic of hyperparathyroidism. Even more frequently the primary manifestations are *renal* in character, such as colic, hematuria, and "passing sand." A very long drawn-out history is in favor of hyperparathyroidism. Sometimes the chief symptoms are *gastrointestinal*, including anorexia, nausea, vomiting, constipation and abdominal pain. These are probably related to the hypercalcemia.

The classical picture of osteitis fibrosa

is rare and easy to recognize. Other slighter and less typical manifestations of hyperparathyroidism are much more common. The condition should be suspected in every case of renal calculus. The calculus cases due to parathyroid tumor are more often not associated with bone disease than with it. The replacement of the marrow by fibrous tissue may lead to anemia and leukopenia. Bone pain and tenderness may be present for a long time before deformities appear. Multiple myeloma and metastatic carcinoma in the skeleton may give a similar picture of decalcification of bone with high blood calcium, but the blood phosphorus is also high, thus distinguishing the condition from hyperparathyroidism. In one of my cases of secondary carcinoma of bone the blood calcium was above 18 mg. per 100 cc. Senile osteoporosis is the most difficult condition to differentiate from mild hyperparathyroidism.

OTHER PARATHYROID LESIONS

Many other lesions of the parathyroid glands have been reported, but none of them appears to be of any importance. Hemorrhage may occur into the parathyroids of the child during labor, but enough tissue is left to perform the normal function of the glands. Even when all four parathyroids have been destroyed by secondary carcinoma, there have been no symptoms of tetany. Fibrosis and scarring is often found in elderly persons. Cysts are not uncommon. In none of these cases is there any evidence of functional disturbance.

REFERENCES

ALBRIGHT, F. and REIFENSTEIN, E. C., JR.: *Parathyroid Glands and Metabolic Bone Disease*, Baltimore, 1948.

CASTLEMAN, B.: *Tumors of the Parathyroid Glands*. Atlas of Tumor Pathology, Fascicle 15, Washington, D. C., 1952.

CASTLEMAN, B. and MALLORY, T. B.: Am. J. Path., 1935, *11*, 1. (Primary hyperplasia of parathyroids.)

DENT, C. E.: Proc. Roy. Soc. Med., 1953, *46*, 291. (Two parathyroid hormones.)

GILMOUR. J. R.: *The Parathyroid Glands and Skeleton in Renal Disease*, London, 1947. J. Path. and Bact., 1938, *46*, 133. (Gross anatomy of parathyroids.)

MORGAN, A. D. and MACLAGAN, N. F.: Am. J. Path., 1954, *30*, 1141. (Renal lesions in hyperparathyroidism.)

RAPOPORT, A., SEPP, A. H. and BROWN, W. HURST.: Am. J. Med., 1960, *29*, 443. (Carcinoma of the parathyroid.)

SNAPPER, I.: *Medical Clinics on Bone Diseases*, 2nd ed., New York, 1949.

ST. GOAR, W. T.: Ann. Int. Med., 1957, *46*, 102. (Gastrointestinal symptoms in hyperparathyroidism.)

Chapter 39

The Blood

General Considerations
  THE BONE MARROW
  THE ERYTHROCYTE
    Development
    Abnormal Forms
    Life Span
    Sedimentation Rate
    Abnormal Hemoglobins
      Heme Moiety
      Globin Moiety
  THE LEUKOCYTES
    Function
      Granulocytes
      Monocytes
      Lymphocytes
    Biochemistry
  THE BLOOD PLATELETS
    Function
  BLOOD GROUPS
    Rh Blood Groups
      Blocking Antibodies
      Coombs' Test
  TRANSFUSION REACTIONS
  ABNORMAL GLOBULINS
    Cryoglobulinemia
    Macroglobulinemia
    Agammaglobulinemia
      Congenital
      Acquired
      Transient in infancy
      Secondary
The Anemias
  CLASSIFICATION
Macrocytic Anemias
  PERNICIOUS ANEMIA
    Sprue
    Dibothriocephalus Latus
    Pregnancy
    Gastrectomy
    Hepatic Cirrhosis

Iron Deficiency Anemia
  MICROCYTIC HYPOCHROMIC
    ANEMIA
    Chlorosis
    Pyridoxine Deficiency Anemia
**Hereditary (Intracorpuscular)
  Hemolytic Anemias**
  CONGENITAL SPHEROCYTIC
    ANEMIA
    Hypersplenism
  DRUG-INDUCED HEMOLYTIC
    ANEMIA
  HEREDITARY HEMOGLOBIN-
    OPATHIES
    Sickle cell Anemia
    Thalassemia
    Other Hemoglobinopathies
    *Paroxysmal Nocturnal Hemo-
      globinuria*
**Acquired (Extracorpuscular)
  Hemolytic Anemias**
  EXTRANEOUS AGENTS
  AUTO-IMMUNE ANTIBODIES
    *Paroxysmal Cold Hemo-
      globinuria*
  ISO-IMMUNE ANTIBODIES
    *Hemolytic Disease of the
      Newborn*
      Rh factor in blood trans-
        fusion
      Rh factor in pregnancy
Bone Marrow Hypofunction
  APLASTIC ANEMIA
  MYELOPHTHISIC ANEMIA
Secondary Anemia
  ANEMIA OF INFECTION, CHRONIC
    RENAL DISEASE, PREGNANCY
    AND MALIGNANCY
  LEAD POISONING

Polycythemia
  POLYCYTHEMIA VERA:
    ERYTHREMIA
  ERYTHROCYTOSIS
    Relative Polycythemia
The Purpuras
  IDIOPATHIC THROMBOCYTO-
    PENIC PURPURA
    *Neonatal Thrombocytopenic
      Purpura*
  THROMBOTIC THROMBOCYTO-
    PENIC PURPURA
  SECONDARY PURPURA
  VASCULAR PURPURA
    Purpura Simplex
    Henoch's Purpura
    Schönlein's Purpura
The Bleeding Diseases
  HEMOPHILIA (fibrinogen)
  CHRISTMAS DISEASE (thrombo-
    plastin)
  HEMORRHAGIC DISEASE OF
    NEWBORN (prothrombin)
    Afibrinogenemia
The Leukemias
  CHRONIC MYELOGENOUS
    LEUKEMIA
  LYMPHATIC LEUKEMIA
  ACUTE LEUKEMIA
    Monocytic Leukemia
    Plasma Cell Leukemia
  MYELOPROLIFERATIVE DISEASE
    Chloroma
Agranulocytosis
  PRIMARY SPLENIC NEUTRO-
    PENIA
Infectious Mononucleosis
**Blood Diseases and Auto-
  Immunity**

GENERAL CONSIDERATIONS

THE blood is the most precious fluid in the body, a fact expressed in such common terms as "the life blood." It is surprising, therefore, that from very early times we find references to the value of *"blood letting"* by means of venesection, perhaps with the idea of letting loose some evil spirit or matter imprisoned in the body. The best time for drawing the blood was ascertained by study of the moon or the conjunction of the planets. Blood letting, indeed, represents one of the oldest human efforts at therapy.

This procedure was carried to its most absurd extreme in the 18th century, "the age of reason," when a doctor who was at a loss as to what to do for his patient would drain off as much blood as possible. It was at least calculated to take the patient's mind off his ills, and make him feel that something was being done for him. It is hard to believe but true that for centuries normal people were bled periodically to insure a continued state of health, just as today healthy people take vitamins in order to remain well. In the 18th century one celebrated French physician had himself bled 7 times for a simple cold in the

(1032)

head. Even in the time of Laennec at the beginning of the 19th century it was necessary to import 42 million leeches into France in one year for the purpose of blood letting, but no one paused to inquire whether it was good for the patient to be deprived of so much blood. Finally light began to break through the darkness, and the lancet was denounced as "a minute instrument of mighty mischief." Now, as so often happens, the pendulum has swung violently in the opposite direction, and blood is poured into the patient's veins at the least excuse, often with disastrous results, either immediate or remote, a subject to which we shall return later.

THE BONE MARROW

The factory for the cells of the blood is the bone marrow. But this is only true of extra-uterine life and of a state of health. In the second month of intrauterine the liver begins to form primitive blood cells. In the fifth month the spleen commences to share in this activity, and now for the first time the marrow becomes a hematopoietic structure. By the time of birth the spleen has lost its blood-forming capacity, the liver still shows a few islands of hematopoiesis, and the bone marrow has now taken over all the work.

The cells of the blood in extrauterine life are formed in the bone marrow. It is only the red marrow which is blood-forming, the yellow marrow consisting of nothing but fat. In the adult the red marrow is confined to the flat bones, i.e., vertebræ, sternum, ribs, skull, and pelvic bones. In the child, on the other hand, all the bones are filled with red marrow. About the seventh year microscopic evidence can be detected of a change from the red to the yellow marrow, the change being evident to the naked eye at the fourteenth year, and by the twenty-first year all the red marrow of the long bones has become replaced by fat and is therefore of the yellow type. The change first appears in the distal bones and is always most complete in them. A little red marrow is left in the proximal bones, and at the proximal end of these bones, i.e., at the upper end of the femur and humerus. When functional hyperplasia of the marrow occurs, it first becomes apparent in the proximal bones and only later involves the distal bones. The marrow of the femur is often red when that of the tibia is still yellow. Red marrow is much more vascular than yellow marrow. It is natural, therefore that secondary carcinoma should be more common in the humerus and femur than in the bones of the forearm or the tibia. Marrow occurs only in bone. This is true even for such heterotopic bone as may be formed in a tuberculous scar in the lung or in the media of an artery. The explanation of this constant association appears to lie in the fact that marrow can be observed to arise from the endosteum of bone in the experimental animal (Steinberg and Hufford). The technique employed was complete extirpation of the marrow of the tibia, with subsequent regeneration. The presence of fat spaces is a prerequisite to the formation of myeloid elements.

It is in the bone marrow that the three types of blood cells are formed, the erythrocyte, the leukocyte, and the thrombocyte. It seems probable, although not certain, that all three cells are derived from a primitive mesenchymal stem cell, the *hemocytoblast*, which is large, with a finely granular basophilic cytoplasm, a very large nucleus, and several prominent nucleoli.

The bone marrow readily undergoes *functional hyperplasia*, as a result of which a very extensive actively functioning tissue is formed. The chief evidence of hyperplastic activity is the conversion of the yellow marrow into the red variety. The bony trabeculæ of the yellow marrow become absorbed, and if the hyperplasia is marked there may be absorption of the compact bone so that the medullary canal is widened. First the proximal and then the distal bones become filled with red marrow. If the marrow of the femur is examined routinely at autopsy the observer will be surprised to find how often it is red instead of yellow owing to the presence of terminal infections, etc. The two *chief causes* of functional hyperplasia are anemia and infection; in the first the response is mainly erythroblastic, in the second it is mainly leukoblastic, but pure forms of the reaction are seldom seen. In the leukoblastic reaction the new cells are mainly myelocytes. In the erythroblastic reaction they may be either normoblasts or megaloblasts.

THE ERYTHROCYTE

The red blood cell is a unique and extraordinary structure. It is the only cell in the body without a nucleus or cytoplasmic particles such as microsomes and mitochondria. In consequence its life span is limited to about one-hundred-twenty days. We have grown so accustomed to the fact that the erythrocyte has no nucleus that we have ceased to wonder. But in all animals except mammals these cells are nucleated, and even in mammals, including man, they have a nucleus before they enter the circulation. Why do they lose it?

The cytoplasm has a stroma and a membrane envelope. The *stroma* consists of protein and lipids, with a very little carbohydrate. The lipids lie mostly at the surface to which they impart an intensely negative charge. As all the cells are charged alike they repel one another, and probably never touch during their millions of collisions. When hemolysis does occur it is a dissolution of the bond between stroma and hemoglobin rather than a puncturing of a balloon (Crosby). The shape is that of a biconcave disc, because this gives the largest interface between each erythrocyte and plasma, thus insuring not only efficient absorption and release of gases, but ready penetration of gases from the surface to the center of the cell. Under disease conditions the biconcave shape may be lost (spherocytosis) with unfortunate results.

The red cell is not the inert blob of hemoglobin which its microscopic appearance might suggest, but rather a hive of activity depending on numerous *enyzme systems* (Altman). There are indeed dozens of enzymes, but we know next to nothing of their function. One function is undoubtedly the maintenance of the unnatural shape of the cell. Hemoglobin is constantly shifting back and forth from the functional reduced state to oxidized ferric hemoglobin. The reducing system capable of reconverting methemoglobin glycolysis. Most of the needed energy for enzyme action comes from the anaerobic glycolysis of glucose into lactic acid by glucose-6-phosphate dehydrogenase, the energy being transmitted to the enzyme systems by adenosine triphosphate. The erythrocyte has indeed become adapted to a cellular metabolism dependent almost entirely on *anaerobic glycolysis*. Glucose penetrates the cell membrane not by diffusion but as the result of transfer by enzymes present in the membrane. We shall see presently in relation to acquired hemolytic anemias that a coating of the surface of the erythrocyte with iso-immune antibodies may alter the environment so as to bring about inactivation of the critical enzymes at an abnormally rapid rate, with early disintegration of the cell.

Development.—The adult erythrocyte is purely and simply a carrier of oxygen by reason of the hemoglobin of which it is composed. Some 900 billion are produced daily. The total surface area of the circulating erythrocytes is about 3800 square meters, being 2000 times greater than the total body surface. The active marrow, occupying only one-half of the total marrow cavity, comprises an organ the size of the liver; with capacity to enlarge greatly under the appropriate stimulus.

Erythropoiesis is controlled not by the level of the red cells but by the level of circulating hemoglobin. The stimulus comes from a lowering of the oxygen content of the arterial blood (anoxia), whether due to loss or destruction of erythrocytes, to high altitude, or to disease of the heart or lung. Regulation of erythropoiesis seems to be under the influence of a hormone, *erythropoietin* (hemopoietin), which is present in small amount in normal blood and in increased amount in conditions of anoxia. In the laboratory animal the hormone appears to be formed in the kidney, an origin which may explain the anemia of renal disease and the polycythemia sometimes seen in renal carcinoma. When the size of the red cell mass shrinks, information is fed back to the bone marrow, and red cells are released until the mass is again normal.

Development takes place from the nucleated erythroblast, through the normoblast, to the adult erythrocyte. The cytoplasm of the precursors is basophilic owing to the presence of ribonucleic acid, but as hemoglobin gradually begins to make its appearance the cytoplasm no longer stains a pure blue, but presents a slaty color, a mixture of red and blue, the condition known as *polychromatophilia*. When a wet film is stained with brilliant cresyl blue the basophilic substance appears in the form of a fine reticulum with no diffuse staining. Young erythrocytes which stain in this manner are known as *reticulocytes*. As a result of pathological processes the basophilic substance may become aggregated into granules in the fixed film, the condition known as *basophilic stippling* or *punctate basophilia* of the red cells. This may be observed in many forms of anemia, but is seen to best advantage in cases of lead poisoning. It is thus evident that polychromatophilia, reticulation of the red cells and punctate basophilia are merely variations of the same condition.

Erythropoiesis is extravascular, and red blood cells must lose their nuclei in maturing before entering the marrow capillaries. First, however, they must spend some two days in the *reticulocyte pool*, from which reticulocytes can be drawn immediately on sudden demand.

Abnormal Forms of the Erythrocyte.—The normal red blood cell is a circular biconcave disc without a nucleus, the average diameter being 7.5 μ. In pernicious anemia the diameter varies from 4 to 12 μ. with a mean of 7.5 to 8.5 μ., an obvious macrocytic anemia. By reason of the biconcave character of the disc, the center of the cell is paler than the periphery. Should the cell become spherical instead of biconcave (spherocyte) this central pallor will disappear. The erythrocyte possesses a stromal framework revealed by the electron microscope, which supports the hemoglobin and prevents it from being spilled when the cell is fragmented.

The erythrocytes of the peripheral blood may be abnormal either by reason of immaturity or because of senescence, which may be normal or pathological. Prematurity may be evidenced by the presence of nuclei. Nucleated cells may be *normoblasts* or, if still more immature, *megaloblasts*. The gateway from the bone marrow has been opened too wide or too early, or the press of immature cells in the marrow has been too great. *Reticulocytes* are juvenile erythrocytes containing remnants of basophilic material of the cytoplasm of the erythrocyte precursors. These are seen particularly in the hemolytic anemias where the demand for new cells is excessive, and in myelophthisic anemia, where the erythroid tissue is replaced by tumor or fibrous tissue before it has time to mature. It indicates the response of pernicious anemia to treatment, falling to normal when the therapy is adequate. It may also be present in spite of the presence of hemopoietic agents when hemorrhage is acute, but not in chronic loss of blood. *Anisocytosis* or variation in size, *poikilocytosis* or variation in shape, and *basophilic stippling* are indications of erythrocyte immaturity. Anisocytosis is seen very early in pernicious anemia, poikilocytosis and basophilic stippling at a later stage. Poikilocytosis is very marked in sickle cell anemia, basophilic stippling in myelophthisic anemia.

It is more difficult to designate the signs of senescence of the erythrocyte. The *spherocyte* is a cell on its way to destruction; its life span is short. *Increased osmotic fragility* is almost diagnostic of hemolytic anemia, although it does not determine its type.

Life Span.—The red blood cell lacks a nucleus, so that it has no power of repair and reproduction. Its days are strictly numbered, the average life of the erythrocyte being about 120 days. This figure is arrived at either by injecting cells of a different but compatible blood group, or by withdrawing blood, tagging the erythrocytes with an isotope such as radiochromium, and then reinjecting them. With either method samples of blood are taken from time to time, and the period required for disappearance of the injected cells is noted. It has been calculated that each erythrocyte travels some 175 miles in the course of its comparatively short life.

Every anemia is due either to faulty production of erythrocytes or to a shortening of the life-span, although the bone marrow may compensate for a time by increasing the output. In chronic hemolytic anemia where the marrow is not hampered by disease the output of erythrocytes may be 8 times the normal. The life span seems to be predetermined by limitation of the metabolic system of these cells. When the erythrocyte loses its nucleus and mitochondria it loses much of its capacity for respiration, and when it passes the reticulocyte stage more and more of the enzymes which govern its metabolic activities wear out. The end comes, not as the result of hemolysis, as might be expected, but by fragmentation of the cell.

When the red cell is destroyed its iron and protein is used again, but the porphyrin is excreted as bile pigment. The pigment is transported in the plasma as bilirubin bound to albumin. In this form it is insoluble in water, and therefore will not react in chemical tests until dissolved in alcohol; this is so-called *indirect-reacting bilirubin.* The liver clears it from the plasma, and converts it into water-soluble *direct-reacting bilirubin,* which is excreted into the blood.

Sedimentation Rate.—The sedimentation rate is an indication of the suspension stability of the red cells, and may be taken as an non-specific index of the presence and intensity of organic disease, being comparable in this respect to fever and leukocytosis. When blood is drawn and prevented from coagulating, the red cells slowly settle to the bottom of the tube. The rate of sedimentation is expressed as the distance in millimeters which the cells fall in one hour. The rate depends on the type of tube in which the test is carried out. With the Wintrobe tube the average rate for men is about 3.5 and for women 9.5. With the Westergren tube the figures are somewhat higher. There is, however, a wide normal variation. An increase of rate indicates an active disease process, just as does a rise of temperature. In chronic disorders, however, and in local infections the temperature and white cell count may be normal, yet the sedimentation rate may be increased. The test is particularly valuable as an index of activity of pre-existing pulmonary tuberculosis and rheumatic fever.

Abnormal Hemoglobins.—In considering the subject of the erythrocyte we must not forget its all-important component, hemoglobin. Hemoglobin consists of a protein, globin, united with a pigment, heme. Heme is an iron-containing porphyrin, the nucleus consisting of 4 pyrrol rings. Abnormalities of hemoglobin may involve either the heme moiety or the globin moiety of the hemoglobin molecule.

Heme Moiety.—A change in the nature of the heme moiety is likely to be reflected in a change in the color of the patient. This is best seen in methemoglobinemia and sulfhemoglobinemia.

Methemoglobinemia may be *acquired* as the result of exposure to industrial substances or therapeutic agents or it may be congenital. Among the commoner toxic agents are anilin, phenacetin, the sulfonamides, and various nitrites and nitrates. Even the wearing of freshly dyed ladies' shoes may be responsible. The principal symptoms are a blue cyanosis involving the entire body, headache, confusion, and drowsiness. A *congenital* form is a rare hereditary disorder, most commonly seen in Greeks. Sulfhemoglobinemia is a similar condition due to the reaction of hemoglobin with inorganic sulfides. The most common cause is the habitual use of acetanilid, often in the form of Bromo-seltzer. The continued use of phenacetin is frequently responsible. Porphyria is an uncommon disorder of pyrrol metabolism. It belongs to the group of inborn errors of metabolism, and it has already been considered on page 398.

Globin Moiety.—*Hemoglobin variants* are dependent on changes in the globin moiety of the hemoglobin molecule. It has long been known that in hemoglobins of different species the globin moiety varies whereas the heme structure does not change. It has also been known that fetal (F) hemoglobin differs from adult (A) hemoglobin in a number of respects, such as crystalline form, solubility, electrophoretic mobility, and amino acid composition. The difference lies in the globin component, which in the earlier months of fetal life is made in the liver, not in the bone marrow. At twenty weeks of pregnancy 94 per cent of the hemoglobin is still fetal in type, at birth from 55 to 85 per cent. The F variant disappears in early infancy. In certain congenital blood disorders, more particularly sickle cell anemia and thalassemia, there seems to be a renewal or persistence of production of fetal hemoglobin. The occurrence of F hemoglobin, however, appears to be of no pathological significance.

In addition to the normal A and F hemoglobins a number of *abnormal variants* with a difference in isoelectric points have been discovered by electrophoretic analysis. They have the same heme moiety, but they differ in the nature of their globins. Like A, all the other known variants are inherited on simple Mendelian principles, one gene coming from each parent. Various combinations are therefore possible, and clinical disturbance in the form of an increased rate of red cell destruction may be in evidence when the inherited trait is homozygous. Sickle cell anemia is now known to be due to the presence of an abnormal hemoglobin (S) which, when deoxygenated, is able to form long rods that twist the erythrocytes out of shape. It was in 1949 that Pauling and his associates described sickle cell hemoglobin and thus introduced into medicine the new concept of *molecule diseases*, a concept that implies that certain diseases are caused by genetically determined abnormalities of protein synthesis on a molecular level (Chernoff).

Normal A hemoglobin may be inherited from one parent, while an abnormal hemoglobin is inherited from another, so that a heterozygote results. This individual will be a carrier of the abnormal trait, but the presence of the normal A gene prevents the development of serious anemia. If both A genes are replaced by a variant, anemia will usually result. Thus the genetic constitution SS will develop sickle cell anemia. Abnormal hemoglobins other than S are designated C, D, E, G, H and I. The only variants of clinical importance are S (sickle cell), C, and D (Rh factor). The clinical results of hemoglobin abnormalities will be discussed in relation to the hemolytic anemias.

The accuracy with which the experts have succeeded in pin-pointing the site of the various defects in the hemoglobin molecule arouses the wonder and admiration of the amateur. The globin part of the molecule contains some 600 amino acids of 19 different kinds arranged in two chains, each with 300. Trypsin hydrolyses an amino acid chain only at points where lysine or arginine occurs, resulting in fragments, each a peptide, containing about one dozen amino acids. By means of electrophoresis and chromatography these peptides can be separated and identified. They have been called *hemoglobin fingerprints*. The difference between hemoglobin A, S and C consists of one particular peptide containing nine amino acids, but one of the nine is different in each case. glutamic acid in hemoglobin A, valine in hemoglobin S, and lysine in hemoglobin C. The formation of hemoglobin S instead of normal adult hemoglobin A, with resulting sickle cell anemia, is apparently the result of the action of a gene which affects the synthesis of hemoglobin so delicately that all but one of the 300 amino acids in the chain in the molecule are in their normal positions (Ingram).

The *geographic* and *racial distribution* of the abnormal hemoglobins is being worked out. Sickle cell anemia and the sickle cell trait is prevalent all over tropical Africa, more especially in Eastern and Central Africa. It was first described in the American Negro. Thalassemia, named from *thalassa*, the Greek word for sea and applied to the Mediterranean, is naturally found along the shores of the Mediterranean, but not in tropical Africa. Hemoglobin C is mainly restricted to West Africa, but has been encountered in American Negros originating in that area. Other variants have still other distribution (Lehmann).

THE LEUKOCYTES

The so-called white cells of the blood (which of course are not white but colorless) form three groups: granulocytes, monocytes and lymphocytes. The granulocytes may be neutrophil, eosinophil or basophil, depending on the staining character of the granules in their cytoplasm. The neutrophils are usually called polymorphonuclears (a term which may be abreviated considerably) because of the variable form of their nucleus. It appears probable that the granulocytes and the monocytes are formed in the marrow and that the lymphocytes are formed in the lymphoid tissue. The earliest granulocyte is the myeloblast, although at first it is not a granular cell at all. As the cytoplasm becomes less basophilic, the specific granules appear, and these are well marked in the next stage, the myelocyte. As this cell develops it becomes smaller, its large indented nucleus becomes lobed, and the fully-formed ameboid polymorphonuclear leukocyte passes through the wall of the vessel and enters the circulation. As the lymphocytes are produced in enormous numbers in the lymphoid tissue throughout the body, the spleen and lymph nodes in particular, they are considered in the two succeeding chapters.

It is of prime importance to be able to distinguish between immature and adult cells in the peripheral blood smear. Generally speaking the larger the cell, the more immature it is. The immature cell has a larger nucleus in relation to the size of the cell and one with lightly staining chromatin. The clearer the nucleoli, the greater the immaturity. The great exception to these general principles is the lymphocyte, with its high nuclear-cytoplasmic ratio and its spherical nucleus. Increase of lobulation or irregularity in the shape of the nucleus indicates maturity of the cell and the length of time it has been in circulation. In the granular leukocytes, the poorer the definition of the granules in their cytoplasm, the greater is the immaturity. Basophilia of the cytoplasm is characteristic of the primitive and blast forms. As the granules develop, the diffuse basophilic staining is lost.

Function.—The function of the leukocytes is quite different in the different forms. The *polymorphonuclear* is the great phagocytic cell for bacteria, and shows its highest activity in acute inflammatory lesions. When the call for help is heard the bone marrow pours these cells in huge numbers into the circulating blood, and when they reach the scene of action they leave the blood and migrate into the tissues.

The *eosinophils* present a very much more difficult problem. The normal number of 250 c. mm. may be increased (eosinophilia) in a wide variety of disorders. *Eosinophilia* is encountered in allergic disorders, many skin diseases, animal parasite infestation of tissue, Loeffler's syndrome and tropical eosinophilia (bronchial symptoms and mottling of the lungs in the x-ray film), Hodgkin's disease, and periarteritis nodosa. What are we to make of this confusing collection? Nothing definite, except that allergic inflammation seems to be a recurring theme running through at least some of these variations, often a reaction to animal parasites. Even if we do not know what the eosinophils are doing, their presence in the blood film in excess numbers often provides a valuable diagnostic clue. *Eosinopenia* also presents a puzzle, for it is under endocrine control, being caused by release of adrenocortical hormones through stimulation of the anterior pituitary. Within a few hours of injury or burning, the number of eosinophils in the peripheral blood begins to drop, soon reaching low or even zero values. The degree of eosinopenia may be taken as an indication of the severity of the stress.

The *basophils*, which represent only about 1 per cent of the leukocytes in circulating blood, are also a mystery. They are believed to contain heparin and possibly histamine, which are released when the cells disintegrate. The *mast cell* of the tissue is also intensely basophilic. It is believed to arise from mesenchymal tissue cells, but it does not have the multilobed nucleus of the basophilic leukocyte, and it is believed to arise from mesenchymal tissue cells rather than from cells of the marrow.

The *monocytes* are *par excellence* scavengers for a wide variety of particulate matter as well as as for bacteria. As befits scavengers, they come along to clean up after the shock troops in the inflammatory struggle, the polymorphonuclears, have begun to disintegrate. Their power of phagocytosis is greatly argumented by the motility of their cytoplasm, a matter which has already been discussed on page 47 in connection with the inflammatory process. These macrophages are rich in lipases that can digest the lipoid capsule of tubercle and leprosy bacilli, thus allowing the monocyte to ingest these bacteria, which in the case of leprosy can be seen within the cytoplasm in enormous numbers.

The *lymphocytes*, not being of myeloid origin, need not be considered here. This is perhaps fortunate, because with none of the cells of the blood does greater uncertainty exist as regards function. The matter is discussed in the chapter on the Lymph Nodes (page 1104).

Biochemistry.—The biochemistry of the leukocytes is a wide and complex field in which active and expanding studies are in progress. Only one or two highlights can be mentioned. Glycogen is stored in the white cells, which utilize glucose with consumption of oxygen and the production of lactic acid. This glycogen activity is limited to the granulocytes, the myelocytes in particular. It is substantially higher in normal leukocytes than in those of myelogenous leukemia. The white cells contain a bewildering variety of enzymes, of which acid and alkaline phosphatase, nucleotidase and transaminase may be mentioned. Both the phosphatases are present in abundance. Alkaline phosphatase activity is diminished in myelogenous leukemia, but increased in the leukocytosis of infection and in situations of stress such as myocardial infarction, diabetic acidosis and trauma, being also increased by the administration of ACTH in normal persons but not in patients with Addison's disease. Histamine is largely confined to the granulocytes, particularly the basophils. Radioactive phosphorus can be incorporated in the DNA of the leukocyte nucleus to show that the *average life span* of the granulocyte is 9 days, that of the lymphocyte from 3 to 30 days.

THE BLOOD PLATELETS

The third formed element of the blood, the platelet, the last to have its function recognized, is in a very different category from the erythrocyte and the leukocyte. For one thing the platelets are unique in that they *seem* only to function when they disintegrate. They are capable of great good, but they may also do great harm.

The *number* may be taken as from 250,000 to 300,000 per c. mm., but the very multiplicity of the counting methods suggested is an indication that none are satisfactory in every respect. This is in the main due to the extreme tendency to *agglutination* which is their most striking characteristic. They are small irregularly-rounded, oval or rod-shaped bodies, from 2 to 4 μ in diameter, but becoming much larger in active blood regeneration. They consist largely of ribonucleoprotein, and have a variety of enzymatic activities. Many fine fibrils project from the surface, appearing after any change in environment and sometimes existing even in normal venous circulation. The fibrils are related to carbon dioxide and oxygen tension, thus explaining the phlebothrombosis which occurs in venous blood and especially that following

the anoxemia of surgery and shock. Observations with the electron microscope suggest that the platelets function as intact units in the coagulation of blood, and that disintegration is not necessary (Hutter). The form previously described as "lysed" seems to be derived from a transitional form in which there is accentuation of side branches with a great degree of arborization.

The *origin* of the platelets is from pseudopodia of the megakaryocytes of the bone marrow, which become pinched off and enter the circulation. Eventually the cytoplasm of the megakaryocyte becomes completely broken away. The entire number of platelets in the circulation can be replaced in 3 or 4 days, the *average life span* being about 5 days. Trauma results in a marked increase in the number. This is particularly pronounced after a major surgical operation, the greatest rise occurring after one or two weeks, a fact with an obvious bearing on postoperative thrombosis. Splenectomy causes the greatest rise.

Function.—The function of the platelets is hemostasis, the arrest of hemorrhage. This is brought about partly by their extreme tendency to agglutination when they encounter any roughness, the process of thrombosis, partly by their role in coagulation, a very different and much more innocuous process. Closure of a ruptured vessel is also aided by vasoconstriction, which is mediated by the liberation of serotonin and possibly noradrenalin, which may be stored rather than produced by the disintegrating platelets.

BLOOD GROUPS

The fact that the red blood cells of one individual may become clumped when mixed with the blood of many others, with fatal results if transfusion is done, is old knowledge. The modern era was inaugurated in 1900 by Karl Landsteiner when he showed that all persons can be divided into four groups as regards the reaction of the serum of one on the red cells of another. This original method of grouping is Landsteiner's classic ABO system. This comprises 4 groups: A, B, AB and O. The red cells of A contain one agglutinogen, B another, AB both, and O neither. Group A was then found to consist of two subgroups, A_1 and A_2, so that the number of groups in the ABO system was increased from 4 to 6, namely A_1, A_2, B, A_1B, A_2B, and O. Since the original work on the ABO system at least 8 other systems have been discovered, of which the most important are the Rh system, disclosed again by Landsteiner in 1940, and the M-N system. These three main systems represent groups of "factors" present in human red blood corpuscles, (and indeed in the cells of all tissues except epithelium, nerve tissue, skin appendages, bone and cartilage), which enable individuals to be differentiated from one another. The results have proved of profound importance from the clinical, the medico-legal (determination of identity and of paternity), and the genetic standpoints.

The group reaction is due to the presence of group specific *antigenic substances*, polysaccharide in character, in the erythrocytes. These are agglutinogens, so that the red cells containing them will be agglutinated if injected into a blood stream containing the corresponding agglutinin antibody. In transfusions we are concerned with the effect of serum agglutinins of the recipient on the cells (agglutinogens) of the donor. It is evident that if an agglutinogen is present in the red blood cells of a person, the corresponding agglutinin must be absent from the plasma. Were it not so and both were present in the same blood, agglutination of the red cells would speedily make circulation impossible. In the case of the ABO system the converse is also true; absence of the agglutinogen means that the corresponding agglutinin must be present. This does not apply to the Rh and M-N systems, in both of which the absence of agglutinogen is not accompanied by the normal presence of corresponding agglutinin.

The AB group, having no agglutinins in the serum, is a universal recipient, whilst group O, having no agglutinogens in the red cells, used to be regarded as a universal donor. The term "universal" unfortunately ignores the Rh factor, so that safety in blood transfusion demands cross matching of the serum of the recipient against the red cells of the donor. This serves to safeguard against the Rh factor as well as possible ABO incompatibility.

Reference has already been made on page 736 to the puzzling *relationship* between the *ABO blood groups* and *lesions of the stomach*. Patients with carcinoma of the stomach are more likely to belong to group A than are controls, whilst those with peptic ulcer are more likely to belong to group O. The incidence of duodenal ulcer in group O is particularly high. Further discussion of this intriguing matter will be found in the section on peptic ulcer. We must be careful not to draw too sweeping conclusions on this subject, because the material on which opinions are based is almost entirely statistical, and in this field there are many fallacies and pitfalls, especially in the selection of control material.

Further discussion of blood groups, of their relation to disease, of their distribution in human tissues, and other allied subjects, will be found in the British Medical Bulletin, May, 1959, which is devoted entirely to this subject.

Rh Blood Groups.—When Landsteiner found, forty years after his epoch-making discovery of the classical ABO blood groups, that injection of red cells of the rhesus monkey into rabbits evoked the production of an agglutinin to these cells which would also agglutinate human erythrocytes in 85 per cent of white persons, the idea of a new Rh (rhesus) agglutinogen in human red cells was born. These people are said to be Rh positive because their red cells contain Rh agglutinogen, and their serum naturally contains no corresponding agglutinin. The remaining 15 per cent are Rh negative, and their serum also contains no agglutinin antibodies, unless (1) they are transfused with Rh positive blood, or (2) an Rh negative woman has had one or more pregnancies with an Rh positive fetus, in which case the Rh factor, derived from an Rh positive father, can pass in the red cells from the fetus to the mother in whom antibodies are formed. These then return to the fetus by the placental circulation and there give rise to hemolytic disease of the new born. The Rh factor is considered again in connection with the latter disease on page 1064.

Blocking Antibodies.—These, also called

incomplete antibodies, owe their name to the fact that they do not cause agglutination of red blood cells suspended in saline, yet the cells so exposed can no longer be agglutinated by ordinary antibodies, whose action is "blocked" by the presence of the first antibody contained in globulin on the surface of the red cells. Blocking antibodies, however, do cause agglutination of red cells suspended in a protein medium. In Rh blood testing it is the serum of the recipient that is tested for the presence of antibody against the red cells of the donor. Although there may be no iso-agglutination of donor's red cells suspended in saline (the standard technique), yet a violent hemolytic reaction may occur as the result of transfusion owing to the presence of the globulin of the plasma.

The *Coombs test* has proved invaluable for detecting dangerous blocking antibodies contained in globulin attached to the surface of the erythrocytes. An antiglobulin testing serum is prepared by injecting rabbits with human globulin. This serum will reveal the presence of blocking antibodies, because, being an antiglobulin, it reacts with the globulin part of the antibody attached to the surface of sensitized red cells. The reaction is not connected with the *specificity* of the antibody, nor is the Coombs test specific for Rh immunization. The actual presence of a coating of globulin on the surface of the erythrocytes when the Coombs test is positive can be seen in electron microphotographs.

TRANSFUSION REACTIONS

Blood transfusion is one of the most valuable therapeutic measures, but, like other good things, it is open to abuse. It is ordered by the clinician, who unfortunately has nothing to do with the procedure which determines whether a given donor is the right one. The collection of the blood and the performance of the tests is done by highly trained technicians (sometimes not so highly), but we must not forget that to err is human, and even a wrong donor's name may be attached to a flask of blood. The mistake may cost the patient his life. Enough has been said to indicate that *blood transfusion should only be ordered when it is deemed essential*. Whole blood transfusion is indicated: (1) to *restore blood volume* after acute hemorrhage or shock; (2) to *maintain the concentration of circulating hemoglobin* in those anemias who do not respond to other therapeutic measures.

The bad effects of transfusion are due to incompatibility of the blood of the donor with that of the recipient. In 95 per cent of the transfusion reactions groups A or B or the Rh factor (also known as group D) are involved. The chief cause of these reactions is ABO incompatibility due to human errors in typing, *intragroup reactions* being usually due to Rh sensitivity. A reaction to the first transfusion will occur in the case of A and B, because anti-A and anti-B agglutinins occur normally. In the case of the Rh factor the first transfusion to an Rh-negative man has no harmful effect, because, as we have seen, his blood contains no natural antibodies. A second transfusion finds him sensitized, and the usual ill effects will follow. The special case of the Rh-negative pregnant woman with an Rh-positive fetus is considered in connection with hemolytic disease of the newborn or erythroblastosis fetalis on page 1065.

The *result of transfusion with mismatched or incompatible blood* is first *agglutination* of red cells followed by *hemolysis*. There are three different types of clinical disturbance, differing in degree rather than in kind. (1) Simple febrile reactions, occurring in from 1 to 15 per cent of cases in different reports. There may be an inapparent degree of hemolysis, the blood returning to normal in the course of a week. The reaction is often due to technical errors connected with tubing, saline, *etc.* (2) A mild degree of hemolytic jaundice due to an excessive formation of bilirubin. (3) A severe reaction with hemoglobinuria and renal failure. *Symptoms* often develop quickly before much blood has been given. These have been attributed to clumps of agglutinated red cells blocking the capillaries before hemolysis has time to develop. Restlessness, anxiety, and precordial oppression are followed by nausea and vomiting, terminating in shock and coma. These features are accompanied by the development of hemoglobinuria, jaundice, oliguria and finally anuria and uremia. At any stage, assisted by therapeutic measures, diuresis and recovery may set in. The renal failure is caused by disruption of renal tubules owing to cortical ischemia. This disruption may occur in any part of the nephron, either upper or lower. It is not due to so-called hemoglobinemic nephrosis, the precipitation of hemoglobin in the tubules being secondary to a functional change in the nephrons associated with circulatory failure rather than primary and causal in character. In addition to the hemolytic phenomena there may be circulatory failure due to an overloading of the cardiovascular system caused by the administration of too large a volume of blood. To these purely transfusional complications must be added the occasional transmission of hepatitis and other viral or bacterial infections.

The possible hazards of blood transfusion need continued emphasis. As many as 3,500,000 transfusions are administered yearly in the United States, and fatalities due to transfusion reactions have been estimated at one death in 1,000 to 3,000 transfusions. Transfusion should only be ordered when it is really necessary. Blood from a husband should never, except as a last desperate resort, be used to transfuse a wife, for reasons which will be obvious from the preceding discussion and from that which is to follow. Hemolytic reactions due to specific antibodies can occur in patients with a history of previous pregnancies or transfusions even when no incompatibility can be demonstrated by the most sensitive methods now available.

It is not only the acute complications which are to be feared. Repeated transfusions may sustain life in protracted cases of refractory, hemolytic or aplastic anemia, but they carry with them the danger of *hemosiderosis*. Every pint of blood transfused carries some 250 mg. of iron into the body, and this iron is unable to escape. After a period that differs in different persons it is inevitable that hemosiderosis of the liver, spleen and pancreas should occur, which with the accompanying fibrosis will interfere with their function. The bone marrow, myocardium, kidneys and adrenals in time will be involved. As with antibiotics, anesthetics and tranquilizers, blood trans-fusion is a priceless gift, but it is well to remember that what is potent for good can also be powerful for evil.

ABNORMAL GLOBULINS

The general subject of normal and abnormal serum globulins has already been discussed in Chapter 5 in relation to immunity and resistance. Some aspects of the subject of more particular interest in connection with diseases of the blood will be reviewed briefly in this place.

Cryoglobulinemia.—As the name implies, this condition is characterized by the presence in the circulating blood of an abnormal globulin which is precipitated on exposure to cold (Volpé *et al.*). It has a low cold solubility, but it must not be confused with cold agglutinins, with which it has no relation. It is present in small amounts in a confusing variety of disease states, including multiple myeloma, disseminated lupus, periarteritis nodosa, rheumatoid arthritis, lymphosarcoma, leukemia and polycythemia vera. In most cases it is present only in small amount and does not give rise to symptoms. In rare cases the amount is so large that symptoms result. This is most often seen in multiple myeloma, where the huge numbers of plasma cells may be responsible for the production of the abnormal globulin. It is generally related to hypergammaglobulinemia, but cold insolubility may also affect the alpha and beta fractions. Very exceptionally the condition appears to be primary rather than secondary to some other disease. In these "essential" cases there is often a long history of abnormal sensitivity to cold.

The *symptoms* are due to precipitation of the abnormal protein in the capillaries and veins or in the arteries. In the case of the *capillaries* there may be tender, ulcerating skin lesions which heal slowly, hemorrhagic stomatitis, epistaxis, retinal hemorrhages, cerebral purpura, intestinal petechiæ, *etc.* Involvement of the larger *veins* will lead to thrombosis and pulmonary embolism. Precipitation in the *arteries* is associated with gangrene of the digits and visceral infarctions, followed by organization and recanalization. The condition, which usually affects men in the sixth and seventh decades, may be marked by sensitivity to cold and Raynaud's phenomenon.

Macroglobulinemia.—This is a very uncommon condition characterized by the presence of macroglobulins in the blood similar to those found in multiple myeloma, bleeding from mucous membranes and into the retina, marked fatigue, and frequently lymphadenopathy. The condition must be distinguished from *purpura hyperglobulinemia of Waldenström* in which purpura, mostly on the legs and provoked by prolonged standing or walking is associated with increased gamma globulin. It is doubtful if this constitutes a true entity, for purpura and hyperglobulinemia are associated in a number of syndromes.

Agammaglobulinemia.—This condition is of interest to us in relation to decreased resistance to infection. The gamma globulins may be increased in chronic infection due to repeated antigenic stimulation, but they may also be decreased, with a consequent deficiency of specific antibodies, because of impaired protein synthesis (Gitlin *et al.*). As a matter of fact the term agammaglobulinemia is usually a misnomer, because only in a minority of patients with this disorder are the gamma globulins completely absent. It is rather a *hypogammaglobulinemia*. The normal serum gamma globulin level is from 15 to 20 per cent of the total protein, but in agammaglobulinemia it is usually around 0.4 per cent as shown by electrophoresis or chemoimmunological methods. The critical level of serum gamma globulin concentration seems to be about 100 mg. per cent. Below this level, susceptibility to infection increases. Active synthesis of gamma globulin does not begin until the infant is about six weeks old, but it does begin to appear at the end of the second or third week. The condition may be (1) congenital, (2) acquired, (3) transient, or (4) secondary.

Congenital agammaglobulinemia manifests itself in infancy or early childhood by repeated bacterial infections, the organisms being usually of the pyogenic coccal group, including meningococcus. Otitis media and sinusitis are particularly common in these children with lowered resistance unable to produce antibodies to meet the infective

agents. Curiously enough there is no decreased resistance to viral infection. In this type there is a complete failure to synthesize gamma globulins and antibodies. The deficiency is inherited as a *sex-linked recessive* trait in males. The protein deficiency is associated with a corresponding cellular deficiency, for there is an absence of plasma cells which are believed to produce antibodies, and a general deficiency of lymphoid elements in the lymph nodes, spleen, thymus, gastrointestinal tract, and even the bone marrow. Neutropenia also occurs frequently, particularly with severe infections in infancy.

Acquired agammaglobulinemia is very uncommon. Its name might suggest that we know the cause of its development. Nothing could be farther from the truth. It merely signifies that the condition develops in adults of either sex and that there is no suggestion of a genetic element. Again there is the familiar liability to recurring infections, with a corresponding relative paucity of plasma cells. Pneumonia is the most frequent infection. The serum gamma globulin concentration is higher than in the congenital variety, usually between 25 and 75 mg. per 100 ml.

Transient hypogammaglobulinemia of infancy depends on delay on the part of the infant to synthesize gamma globulins to replace those passively transferred from the maternal circulation and lost in the course of a few weeks. It takes at least four weeks for the gamma globulins to fall below 300 mg. per 100 ml. Again there is the lowered resistance to bacterial infection. It has been suggested that the tragic cases of sudden unexpected death in infants, usually between two and six months of age, often attributed to suffocation in bed and now known to be due to overwhelming infection, may have a basis of hypogammaglobulinemia.

Secondary hypogammaglobulinemia may occur as the result of some other disease, more particularly the nephrotic syndrome, and neoplasms of lymphoid tissues. In the *nephrotic syndrome* of children the agammaglobulinemia may be due to: (1) loss of gamma globulins in the urine (proteinuria); (2) increased catabolism, the half-life of gamma globulins in the full blown disease being only one-third or one-quarter the normal. These two mechanisms are frequently combined. The average concentration of gamma globulins in children suffering from the nephrotic syndrome is about 200 mg. per 100 ml. In the *adult*, proteinuria is the only important cause of loss of gamma globulins. It will be noticed that in this variety of the secondary form of hypogammaglobulinemia there is no question of failure to synthesize gamma globulins.

Some neoplasms of the lymphocytic and plasmacytic cells may be associated with hypogammaglobulinemia. This is particularly true of lymphosarcoma, lymphatic leukemia and multiple myeloma, but not myelogenous leukemia. It is true that the myeloma is composed of plasma cells, but in some individuals neoplasia seems to interfere with their ability to synthesize gamma globulin.

The only advantage which agammaglobulinemia confers on the individual is that it makes homologous skin grafting and perhaps even organ transplantation possible, because of the absence of an antigen-antibody reaction.

THE ANEMIAS

The term anemia signifies a reduction in the amount of oxygen-carrying hemoglobin in a given volume of blood. This reduction involves the number of red cells, the quantity of hemoglobin, and the volume of packed red cells in a given unit of blood. The decrease may be more marked in the number of red cells or in the amount of hemoglobin they contain.

There is however, just one thing which really defines anemia, and that is a concentration of hemoglobin which is less than normal. The presence of anemia is detected by estimation of the amount of hemoglobin or measurement of the packed red cell volume in the hematocrit (Wintrobe), not by counting the number of red cells, for in some hypochromic anemias the red cell count may be normal or even above normal.

Classification.—There are endless classifications of the anemias but none is ideal, that is to say ideal for everyone. It is common to base the classification on the morphology of the red blood cells as seen in a smear, a system which naturally appeals to the hematologist and which I have used else-

where. The red cells may be normal in size, or larger or smaller than normal. Similarly their hemoglobin content may be normal, or greater or less than normal. On this basis we may recognize four main types of anemia from an examination of the blood smear. These are: (1) *macrocytic anemia, e.g.* pernicious and related forms of anemia; (2) *hypochromic microcytic anemia, e.g.* the iron deficiency anemias; (3) *simple microcytic anemia, e.g.* impaired blood production, as in the anemia of chronic inflammation; (4) *normocytic anemia, e.g.* the anemia of sudden blood loss, the hemolytic anemias, the anemias due to abnormal hemoglobins, etc.

For the student beginning the study of the anemias who has to think his way through this complex subject it seems preferable to use a classification based on etiology or pathogenesis, keeping in mind the fact that an anemia is not necessarily the result of a single causal agent. The quantity of red cells carrying hemoglobin in circulation represents a balance between production and destruction. The turnover rate in the average man is about 9 billion per hour, so that a fine balance must be maintained between the two forces.

It is obvious that there are two main ways in which anemia may develop: (1) *too much blood may be lost*, and (2) *too little blood may be formed*. This is shown in the following table.

CLASSIFICATION OF ANEMIAS

I. *Increased loss of red cells, due to*
   A. Hemolysis (destruction within the body).
   B. Acute hemorrhage (loss outside the body.)

II. *Diminished production of red cells, due to*
   A. Deficiency of
     1. Iron
     2. Vitamin B_{12} and folic acid, etc.
   B. Bone marrow hypofunction.

(Watson and Lichtman, Med., Clinics N. Amer., 1955, *39*, 735.)

These general groups may be subdivided to one's heart's content. Thus the anemia may be due to: (1) *loss of blood* outside the body, which in the male is likely to be due to peptic ulcer or carcinoma of the colon, in the female to excessive loss of menstrual blood; (2) *hemolysis*, or destruction of red cells within the body, which may be (a) intracorpuscular (hereditary hemolytic anemia, or (b)) extracorpuscular (acquired hemolytic anemia); (3) *impaired blood production*, as in iron deficiency and the vitamin B deficiency anemias; and (4) *faulty construction of red cells*, which may be hereditary, as in sickle cell anemia and thalassemia, or *acquired*, as in the anemia of infection, renal failure, irradiation, etc. When the student has considered the details of the various anemias he will be better qualified to pass judgment on this brief summary. Moreover, he may feel qualified to challenge some of the statements in the summary, especially in view of his knowledge of the various hemoglobinopathies or defects in the formation of hemoglobin.

MACROCYTIC ANEMIAS

Pernicious Anemia.—The form of anemia commonly called pernicious was first described by Addison, so that it is sometimes known as Addison's anemia, a more appropriate term than pernicious anemia, as the disease is no longer "pernicious" since the introduction of liver therapy. But old names in medicine are hard to displace.

Pathogenesis.—Like the iron deficiency hypochromic microcytic anemias, pernicious anemia is also a deficiency anemia, but hyperchromic and macrocytic in type. Nor is the deficiency one of supply, but rather one involving the mechanism of absorption. The normal development of red blood cells in the bone marrow depends on a *maturation principle*. In pernicious anemia the marrow is packed with immature cells which are unable to enter the blood stream in any numbers. To borrow a catchword from the political economist, there is poverty in the midst of plenty. The maturation principle has been believed to be formed, as originally suggested in the brilliant hypothesis of Castle, by the interaction of an extrinsic factor in the diet, now known to be vitamin B_{12}, and an intrinsic factor in the stomach, produced by the cells of the gastric glands in the upper two-thirds of the stomach, but not by the pyloric glands of the distal or pyloric region.

It has been said that the underlying defect in pernicious anemia is vitamin B_{12} deficiency, but it is more correct to regard it as the result of a lack of the intrinsic factor in the stomach which is necessary for absorption of the vitamin in the small intestine. Moreover, the original idea of the intrinsic and extrinsic factors uniting to form a maturation or antianemic principle which was stored in the liver has been replaced by the belief that the intrinsic factor merely permits the passage of the very large molecules of the essential vitamin B_{12} across the intestinal mucosa, the vitamin being then stored in the liver and used as required. The intrinsic factor deficiency is undoubtedly related to the atrophic lesion in the gastric mucosa presently to be described, but the natural idea that this relationship was a simple one of cause and effect has been called in question. This doubt has been expressed by Magnus as follows: "The changes in the gastric mucosa may well be endogenous in origin and due to the fact that the intrinsic factor or its percursors are necessary for the maintenance of its normal structure and function. The basic lesion would appear to be an inherited chemical defect, perhaps expressed by the inability of certain cells of the gastric mucosa to manufacture an essential enzyme."

The relation of the intrinsic to the extrinsic factor can be demonstrated by feeding radioactive B_{12} to pernicious anemia patients. Little is absorbed, the great bulk being recovered from the stool. Healthy persons, on the other hand, absorb nearly all the tagged vitamin. In patients with pernicious anemia absorption of the radioactive vitamin can be rendered normal if it is first mixed with normal gastric juice containing the intrinsic factor. This technique enables us to make an exact diagnosis of intrinsic factor deficiency. The intrinsic factor is believed to be an enzyme, it has been named *hemopoietin*, but so far it has not been isolated. The absence of this factor, which is the basis of this form of macrocytic anemia, is associated with achylia and achlorhydria. There may be no free acid in the gastric juice for many years before the development of the anemia. Other members of the family may show achylia without anemia, and the disease often has a hereditary basis, pointing strongly to a genetic defect.

Another member of the vitamin B group,

pteroylglutamic acid, commonly known as *folic acid,* is also a growth factor which provides a powerful stimulus for maturation and has been used in the treatment of pernicious anemia. Vitamin B_{12} has the great advantage of preventing the development of central nervous system lesions and of clearing them up when they have developed, whereas folic acid has no such effect, and in some instances may even accentuate them. On the other hand the macrocytic anemia of pregnancy as well as other macrocytic anemias respond well to folic acid, but poorly to B_{12}, so that they may be regarded as due to folic acid deficiency. Deficiency in folic acid can be induced in the experimental animal by means of succinyl-sulfathiazole, which inhibits the bacterial synthesis of folic acid in the intestine and leads to macrocytic anemia and severe granulocytopenia (Endicott *et al.*).

*The Clinical Picture.—*The following description is that of the untreated disease seldom seen nowadays, but the classical picture when I was an undergraduate.

The disease is usually one of middle age, affecting the two sexes equally, although occurring at an earlier age in women. The symptoms are those of a gradually progressive anemia. As Addison remarked in his original contribution: "It makes its approach in so slow and insidious a manner that the patient can hardly fix a date of his earliest feeling of the languor which is shortly to become so extreme." There may be very remarkable intermissions during which the symptoms clear up and the blood returns toward the normal. In exceptional cases the red cell count may rise from 1,000,000 to 3,000,000 in the course of two or three weeks without any treatment whatever. Before the introduction of liver therapy the course was progressive and uniformly ended fatally, but varied extremely in its degree of acuteness. Now that patients no longer die, they show a tendency to develop cancer of the stomach. The symptoms are those of any severe anemia, *i.e.,* pallor, shortness of breath, palpitatiom, edema. But there are two features which are characteristic of the pernicious form of anemia; these are achlorhydria and spinal cord symptoms.

The *achlorhydria* is often spoken of as *achylia gastrica.* The two terms are not synonymous, for the latter indicates suppression of all the elements of the gastric juice—pepsin and rennin as well as hydrochloric acid. This suppression often occurs in pernicious anemia, but it is not so constant as achlorhydria. It is a complete achlorhydria, whereas that of carcinoma of the stomach is never constantly complete. It is probable that the achlorhydria antedates the development of the anemia by a considerable period. It is often associated with loss of appetite (anorexia), which may cause a wrong diagnosis of cancer of the stomach. *Spinal cord symptoms* appear in about 5 per cent of the cases, and take the form of ataxia, sensory disturbances, spasticity, and loss of vibration sense in the bones of the leg. The symptoms bear no relation to the severity of the blood changes nor even to their presence, for they may develop before the appearance of any alteration in the blood. In addition to spinal cord symptoms minor nervous symptoms are very common, occurring in about 80 per cent of the cases. They take the form of numbness, tingling, and paresthesias in the arms and legs. These common symptoms are not related to cord lesions, being due to a mild peripheral neuritis.

*The Blood Picture.*The blood picture varies greatly with the stage of the disease, being very abnormal during an exacerbation but often showing little change during an intermission. The changes described below are those of a severe relapse. All the formed elements of the blood are diminished in number, the red cells, the leukocytes, and the platelets. It is the qualitative rather than the quantitative change however, which is significant, the picture being that of a *hyperchromic macrocytic anemia.* In severe cases the *red cells* may only number 1,000,000 or less. Any anemia in which the red cell count is below 2,000,000 is probably, but not necessarily, pernicious in type. In remissions the count may be as high as 4,000,000. The hemoglobin is also diminished but not in proportion, so that the *color index* (ratio of hemoglobin percentage to percentage of red cells) is high and may be above 1, even as high as 1.5. The red cells, at least many of them, are well colored; they are hyperchromic, in striking contrast to the condition

PLATE XVI

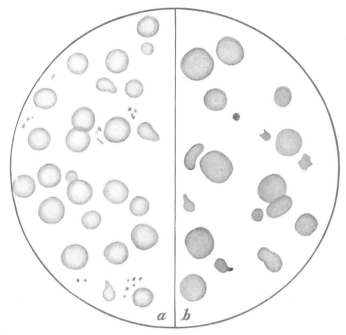

a. Hypochromic Anemia

The cells are pale and none are larger than normal.   Platelets are present.

b. Hyperchromic Anemia

Film of pernicious anemia showing macrocytosis as well as poikilocytosis, anisocytosis
and hyperchromia.   There are no platelets.

in the hypochromic or achromic forms of anemia (Plate XV, *b*). More important than the number of red cells is the presence of qualitative changes. Just as the characteristic lesion of pernicious anemia is a megaloblastic reaction in the bone marrow, so the characteristic change in the blood is a megalocytic or macrocytic anemia. The large *macrocytes* can be seen readily in a stained film, but more important than the presence of occasional large cells is the fact that the *average* size of the red cells is above normal. The average diameter of normal red cells is 7.5 microns, while the average in pernicious anemia may be as high as 8.5 microns. The variation in size, which normally is from 6 to 9 microns, in pernicious anemia may be from 4 to 12 microns. Many of the red cells are therefore smaller than normal. These are called *microcytes*, and the variation is known as *anisocytosis*. The large cells are hyperchromic, but the microcytes are hypochromic. The average size of the cells is estimated by the measurement of *mean corpuscular volume*. This can be done simply by dividing the red cell count into the the volume of packed red cells as determined in the hematocrit. Poikilocytosis (*poikilos*, manifold) may be marked, the cells varying greatly in shape, many being tailed or shaped like a cocked hat. At this point it may be remarked that in pernicious anemia, as in other blood diseases including leukemia, examination of a *properly made* and properly stained film provides for more valuable and reliable information than a red cell count or hemoglobin estimation, in which there is great room for inaccuracies.

The tendency in pernicious anemia is for the red cells to revert to a more primitive or embryonic type, for the essence of the disease is a failure on the part of the red cells of the marrow to mature sufficiently quickly. The megaloblastic reaction of the marrow and the macrocytic type of anemia are evidence of this tendency. Many of the cells show *polychromatophilia*, the cytoplasm being of a slaty color owing to having taken up both the red and blue stain. This is most marked in the megaloblasts. The cytoplasm of the original red cell is entirely basophilic. It becomes partly acidophilic as hemoglobin begins to appear, and at this stage shows

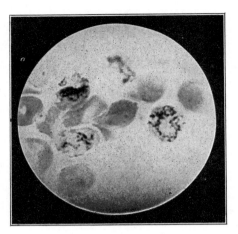

FIG. 606.—Increase of reticulocytes in pernicious anemia. Four of the red cells show reticulation. × 1400.

polychromatophilia. It is only when the cell is mature that it becomes completely acidophilic. *Basophilic stippling* (granular degeneration) may be present; it is merely another manifestation of the same basophilic substance, which in this instance takes the form of fine granules staining blue. The presence of *reticulocytes* is an indication of immaturity, for the reticulum is another form of the same basophilic material. In health reticulated red cells form 1 per cent of the total count, but in pernicious anemia they usually form 5 per cent (Fig. 606). The best indication of successful activity on the part of the marrow is an increase in the reticulocyte count. There is a marked rise in a remission, and a specially great increase when liver therapy is commenced. In aplastic anemia, where the bone marrow shows no activity, there is a complete absence of reticulocytes. The reticulation is not shown in an ordinary film; vital staining has to be used.

Nucleated red cells provide another indication of immaturity. They may be normoblasts or megaloblasts. The latter are commoner and much more characteristic, as normoblasts may occur in any severe anemia, but megaloblasts are seldom found except in pernicious anemia. The megaloblast is much larger than a normoblast, its nucleus is larger and more open, and the cytoplasm is polychromatophilic or even basophilic.

The nucleus may show mitosis. They can always be found if the count is below 2,000-000, but when it is above 2,500,000 it may be difficult to find a single megaloblast. Owing to the immaturity of the red cells in pernicious anemia, their fragility is diminished rather than increased, for it is the older cells which become more fragile when tested with hypotonic salt solution.

A word may be devoted here to what is known in hematology as the "megaloblast problem." The term megaloblast has been used in two different senses. Ehrlich applied the word originally to an essentially abnormal cell which is only present in pernicious anemia, and this practice has been followed by European hematologists. Florence Sabin, on the other hand, in her studies on the development of the blood cells used the term to denote the earliest identifiable member of the maturing normal red cell series. It would appear that red cells can develop along two different but parallel routes, one normal and the other abnormal (pernicious anemia). It is possible to distinguish the Ehrlich megaloblast (abnormal) from the Sabin megaloblast (normal) in stained marrow films. The *abnormal megaloblast* is larger, has a finer reticular nuclear chromatin, and more or less hemoglobin content than the corresponding cell of the normal series. The end result is a macrocyte, whereas the end result of the normal series is an erythrocyte.

The *leukocytes* diminish in number, so that there is a *leukopenia*. This affects chiefly the polymorphonuclears, so that there is a relative lymphocytosis. The polymorphonuclears are much more lobed in pernicious than in other forms of anemia. This is a useful practical point. Indeed it has been said that in studying the anemias more may be learned from looking at the white cells than at the erythrocytes. There is no leukocytosis even in acute infections. The fault lies in the marrow. This is filled with myelocytes, but they fail to mature, so that there is a decrease in the polymorphonuclears. Myelocytes are not infrequently found in the blood. The *platelets* are much diminished in number (thrombocytopenia), and they may disappear altogether. The *plasma* shows a characteristic yellow tinge due to an increased bilirubin content, the result of increased blood destruction, and there is a positive indirect van den Bergh reaction, with an increase of urobilinogen in the urine. These serological findings are of great value in those difficult cases where the cytological picture is so indeterminate that no definite diagnosis can be made.

Morbid Anatomy.—The following account of the lesions seen at autopsy applies only to cases which have not received specific therapy and in which the patient really did die of his disease.

The lesions of pernicious anemia are partly primary in character, but mostly secondary either to the anemia or to increased blood destruction. The two most constant pathological findings are a *megaloblastic type of bone marrow* and marked *siderosis*. The intensity of these lesions will depend on the stage of the disease at the time of death. If the patient dies during an acute exacerbation, the megaloblastic reaction, the siderosis, and all the secondary lesions will be marked, whereas they may be trivial if the patient dies of some intercurrent disease during a remission. This is not true of lesions of the spinal cord and possibly those of the alimentary tract. It will be seen from the following description that the *lesions* may be divided into five groups: (1) *Those due to the anemia* (fatty degeneration, hemorrhages); (2) *bone marrow changes;* (3) siderosis, increased phagocytosis by the reticuloendothelial cells, and other *evidences of blood destruction;* (4) *lesions of the alimentary tract;* (5) *lesions of the nervous system.*

The *skin* is of a lemon-yellow color, and has not the pure pallor of secondary anemia. There is a remarkable absence of wasting, and the abundant fat is also lemon-yellow. The *muscles* are normal or deep red in color. Petechial *hemorrhages* are common in the serous membranes and can be seen during life in the retina. These changes are due to fatty degeneration of the walls of the small vessels. The fatty degeneration is caused by the anemia. The fatty change is best seen in the *heart*, which is pale, very flabby, so that it collapses when held up by the apex, and the wall of the left ventricle and the papillary muscles show a yellow speckling known as the "thrush breast" or "faded leaf" appearance (Fig. 261, page 490). This is marked when the anemia is severe, but may be slight or absent if death occurs during a remission. The *liver* shows two changes: fatty degeneration and siderosis. The fatty change may be extreme. The yellow granules of hemosiderin, which give the Prussian blue reaction for iron, are mainly deposited in the liver cells, especially in the outer two-thirds of the lobule. They are present, but to a lesser degree, in the Kupffer cells. Hepatocellular siderosis in pernicious anemia is usually attributed to hemolysis, but it seems probable that at least some if not most of the iron is derived from the disruption of intracellular iron-containing enzymes and not from hemoglobin (Gillman). Myeloid areas may be present; these are discussed below. The *spleen* is usually slightly enlarged; during a relapse it may be red and markedly swollen. The chief microscopic change is evidence of marked phagocytic activity on the part of the reticuloendothelial cells, which contain pigment and fragments of red blood cells. These changes are most pronounced during a relapse. There are also deposits of iron pigment, but the siderosis is not nearly so marked as in the liver. It is evident that though the spleen may play a part in destroying the red cells, it is the liver which stores the blood pigment. Small islands of myelocytes and nucleated red cells are occasionally present. The *lymph nodes* show no special change. In the *kidneys*, as in the liver, there is a combination of fatty degeneration and hemosiderosis. This combination may be seen in lesser degree in many of the other organs.

The *bone marrow* changes are by far the most important. There is a very marked erythroblastic reaction, as a result of which the yellow marrow becomes red and resembles red currant jelly. This change is patchy, so that examination of a small piece of marrow may be quite misleading. The marrow of one long bone may be red, while in another it is quite yellow, or the change may only affect part of the marrow of a bone. The hyperplasia always involves the femur before the tibia. During a remission the marrow of the tibia may be normal, while that of the femur shows marked hyperplasia. The earliest change is seen in the upper end of the femur and humerus, regions in which nor-

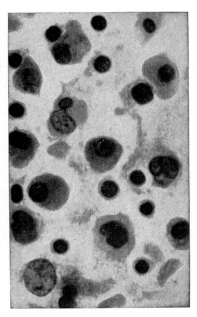

Fig. 607.—Megaloblastic reaction of the bone marrow in pernicious anemia. All of the cells are either megaloblasts or normoblasts. × 1000.

mally there is a certain amount of red marrow. As a result of the hyperplasia the trabeculæ of the medullary cavity are absorbed and the cavity may be enlarged at the expense of the shaft.

The *microscopic picture* is quite different from that of the functional hyperplasia which follows hemorrhage. The latter is a normoblastic reaction, whereas the reaction in pernicious anemia is of the megaloblastic (Ehrlich) type (Fig. 607). The *megaloblast* changes directly into a macrocyte, with loss of the normal multiplication which should occur at the normoblastic level. Megaloblasts have no place in the development of normal red blood cells in extrauterine life, but only when the normal activity of the hemopoietic principle of the liver is lacking. This explains the drop in the red cell count and the relatively few normoblasts in the circulatory blood. This reaction is the one and only pathognomonic finding in the disease. During a remission there is a return to the normoblastic type of reaction. It must not be thought that the megaloblasts are the only abnormal cells of the hyperplastic marrow. Primitive white cells (*myelo-*

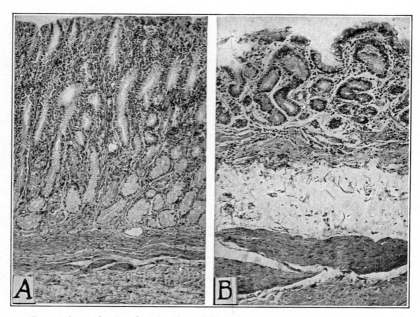

FIG. 608.—Comparison of normal stomach wall (*A*) with that of pernicious anemia (*B*). × 65.

cytes and *myeloblasts*) are always numerous, and at first sight it is remarkable that such numbers of primitive leukocytes in the marrow can be associated with a marked leukopenia. The answer to the riddle is that the white cells, like the red cells, fail to mature, and until they mature they are unable to enter the circulation. It looks as if some factor (possibly a liver factor) which is normally responsible for the maturation of myelocytes into polymorphonuclears is lacking in pernicious anemia. Adult polymorphonuclears are much less numerous in the marrow of pernicious anemia than in the normal marrow. The *megakaryocytes* are reduced in number, and those which are present are small and degenerated; this explains the *thrombocytopenia*. Phagocytic cells containing hemosiderin or erythrocytes are prominent during a relapse.

Extramedullary blood formation may occur, but it is difficult to know to what extent. Before the fifth month of fetal life the blood is formed by the liver and spleen. When there is great demand for more blood in pernicious anemia small islands of myeloid tissue may develop in the liver and possibly in the spleen. It is doubtful if these extramedullary foci play a part of any importance,

for even in severe exacerbations it will seldom be found that all the bone marrow of the body is hyperplastic.

The lesions of the *alimentary tract* affect chiefly the tongue and stomach. Soreness of the *tongue* is a frequent feature of the early stage of the disease. At the time of death there may be a severe glossitis, the tongue being fiery red and resembling a beefsteak. In more chronic cases the tongue is atrophic and smooth as if it had been ironed, with disappearance of the papillæ and atrophy of mucous membrane and muscle. Scrapings from the surface of the tongue and smears of saliva show epithelial cells with a cytoplasmic diameter smaller than normal but a larger nucleus. These changes are also observed in other macrocytic anemias and even in iron deficiency anemias, but they are most frequent in pernicious anemia. They may be related to the gastric lesions about to be described. Vitamin B_{12} seems to be necessary for the maturation of many cells besides red and white cells, and it may be an essential factor for normal nuclear metabolism in the buccal, gastric, nasal and vaginal epithelium.

The *stomach* shows severe atrophy in its proximal two-thirds. In some cases the wall may be not thicker than parchment, so that the diagnosis may be made with the naked eye. The atrophy involves all of the coats (Fig. 608), and in the mucosa the specialized oxyntic and peptic cells have disappeared. At the junction of fundus with pyloric mucosa there is an abrupt change to normal thickness. This characteristic atrophy of the proximal part of the gastric mucosa was regarded not only as pathognomonic of pernicious anemia, but as constituting the basic lesion responsible for the absence of the intrinsic factor. In support of this idea it was pointed out that lifelong therapy with vitamin B_{12} is required, since the gastric lesion responsible for the deficit of the intrinsic factor cannot be repaired. This concept is now challenged in two respects. (1) The introduction of the flexible gastric biopsy tube by Wood and his associates in Melbourne has shown that the picture of gastric atrophy merely represents an end stage seen at autopsy (Joske *et al.*). When biopsies are taken at an earlier stage and at repeated intervals it is found that in only about 40 per cent of cases of pernicious anemia is the so-called typical atrophic lesion found, the remainder showing varying degrees of atrophic gastritis, with widespread cellular infiltrate in the substantia propria and atrophy of the tubules. (2) The second challenge to the concept is the suggestion that the gastric lesion may be the result rather than the cause of the fundamental defect, due to an endogenous lack in the intrinsic factor, a defect which may be genetic in origin. This idea has already been discussed on page 1045.

Spinal cord lesions occur in about 5 per cent of the cases. It is a *subacute combined degeneration*, affecting both posterior and lateral columns, more especially the former. The cord is swollen, and shows translucent patches first in the posterior columns, then the lateral columns, and finally the anterior columns. *Microscopically* there is breaking up and degeneration of the medullary sheaths, followed later by disappearance of the axis cylinders. The lesions are shown by means of the Weigert myelin sheath stain (Fig. 675, page 1190). These changes are responsible for the ataxia and spasticity already described. The cord lesions bear no

relation to the severity of the anemia, and may appear before any anemia can be detected. Nor are they responsible for the numbness, tingling, and paresthesias which are so common an accompaniment of the anemia. It seems probable that the condition is caused by deficiency either of vitamin B_{12} or of some other extrinsic factor, for the symptoms and possibly also the lesions are greatly benefitted by administration of the vitamin.

A number of macrocytic anemias must be mentioned in addition to Addisonian pernicious anemia. Of these the most important are the anemia of sprue, of Dibothriocephalus latus, and of pregnancy. In these, and in other examples of less importance, the blood picture may be that of pernicious anemia, but lack of the gastric intrinsic factor plays no part in the pathogenesis. Moreover, in some the extrinsic factor that is lacking appears to be folic (pteroylglutamic) acid rather than vitamin B_{12}.

Sprue.—This is a tropical intestinal infection characterized by abdominal distention, the passage of large pale bulky stools with a high fat content, atrophy of the tongue and the intestinal mucous membrane, gastric anacidity in about one-half the cases, and the development of a blood picture which may be indistinguishable from that of pernicious anemia. The *anemia is macrocytic* and the reaction of the marrow is megaloblastic in type. It seems probable that the *intestinal lesions* (thinning and atrophy of the mucosa, disappearance of the epithelium) may so *interfere with absorption* that a condition of chronic deficiency develops, with the same effect on the marrow as in pernicious anemia. Other tropical macrocytic anemias are due to lack of the extrinsic factor in the food of poorly nourished natives.

Dibothriocephalus Latus.—The fish tapeworm is a common parasite among fish-eating peoples. A very small percentage of such infected persons develop a macrocytic anemia identical with pernicious anemia. Achlorhydria is present in over 80 per cent of these patients. If the worm is expelled, the patient is cured, but the blood can be brought back to normal by means of liver treatment, even though the worm is still present in the bowel. Some additional factor besides the worm must be necessary to produce the anemia, possibly absence of something akin to the pernicious anemia-preventing principle. Fish tapeworm infestation is very common in Japan but is never associated with anemia, and pernicious anemia is also unknown in that country. Most of the cases of Dibothriocephalus anemia occur in Finland, suggesting that there may be some racial factor.

Pregnancy.—A small number of women develop an anemia identical with pernicious anemia during the later months of pregnancy and in the early puerperium (this must not be confused with the common hypochromic anemia of pregnancy). It responds in the usual way to liver treatment, and the prognosis is much better than in pernicious anemia. *Gastrectomy* may be followed by macrocytic anemia if the acid-bearing part of the stomach has been removed. Only a few cases of gastrectomy develop the anemia, and a long interval elapses between the gastrectomy and the change in the blood picture. Diffuse disease of the liver such as *cirrhosis* may interfere so much with storage of the hemopoietic principle that the same type of anemia may sometimes develop.

IRON DEFICIENCY ANEMIAS

Any anemia which responds to adequate doses of iron may be classed as an iron-deficiency anemia. The total amount of hemoglobin is low, but the red blood cells are not diminished in equal proportion, so that the color-index is low and the anemia is *hypochromic*. The red cells may be smaller than normal (*microcytic anemia*) or of normal size. There are two supplies of iron for the manufacture of hemoglobin: (1) the food, and (2) the iron stores in the liver, spleen and bone marrow. Examination of the marrow for stainable iron is the best clinical method for differentiating iron deficiency from other forms of anemia. The iron is stained a brilliant blue with potassium ferrocyanide and hydrochloric acid (Prussian blue method). In health only minute quantities of iron are absorbed, but in experimental iron-deficiency large amounts are absorbed. The course of the iron can be followed by rendering it radioactive and thus labelling

it. Absorption occurs mainly from the duodenum, and as this is dependent on gastric acidity it is evident that achlorhydria will often be associated with hypochromic anemia.

Causes.—Iron-deficiency anemia may be caused: (1) by blood loss, (2) by deficient iron intake, (3) by a demand so great that absorption and the iron stores are unable to satisfy it, and (4) by defective use. *Blood-loss* factor needs continual emphasis. A man may slowly lose half his blood and make it up again, but in doing so he has exhausted his store of iron, and any further loss of blood will produce anemia. Gastric and uterine hemorrhage are common causes of continued blood loss. In the adult male and in the post-menopausal female iron deficiency anemia is a signal of chronic loss of blood, the cause of which must be searched for and found; it is not enough to treat the anemia. *Deficient intake* may be due to poverty, faulty dietary habits, or organic disease of the stomach and esophagus. *Excessive demand* is physiological and depends on age and sex. There is an increased demand for iron during the first two years of life, and on account of menstruation, pregnancy and lactation. For these reasons hypochromic anemia is common in infancy and in women during the reproductive period. Bottle-fed babies get an infinitesimal amount of iron, and prematurity may have prevented the accumulation of a sufficient store of iron.

The question of *defective use* of iron is a more difficult and contentious matter. It raises the problem of *intracellular iron-containing enzymes*, basic disorders of which may underlie some of these anemias (Gillman). The need for iron varies in different cells in health. Siderosis may be due to cellular metabolic change, not necessarily to iron overload. Thus in the experimental animal siderosis may be increased by exposure to simulated high altitudes. Certainly the iron uptake can be altered by anoxia. The body's capacity to use iron may be made to vary by bleeding and anoxia as well as by deficient diet. Finally, iron metabolism may be deranged in many cells of the body other than those concerned with hematopoiesis.

Microcytic Hypochromic Anemia.—Many names have been given to this condition, *e.g.*

idiopathic hypochromia, simple achlorhydric anemia, chronic chlorosis, etc. The condition is a disease of middle-aged women, among whom it is a more common cause of ill-health than pernicious anemia. It often follows pregnancy, or rather the anemia is a continuation of the anemia which normally occurs in the later months of pregnancy. Occasionally it may occur in men. It is remarkable for its chronicity, and average period being ten years. The patient presents a curious *combination of the clinical picture of pernicious anemia and the blood picture of hypochromic anemia.* Digestive symptoms are marked. There is evidence of gastritis— poor appetite, frequent absence of free hydrochloric acid in the stomach, and much mucus in the stomach contents so that the gastric juice is very viscid. Examination of the *gastric mucosa* by means of the flexible gastric biopsy tube shows histological changes in 75 per cent of cases, varying from superficial inflammation to extreme atrophy (Davidson and Markson). The *tongue* is bald and glazed even more commonly than in pernicious anemia; in the severe cases it is angry red. The *nails* often present a very characteristic appearance; they are dry and brittle, longitudinally striated, and turned up at the edges so that they become "*spoon-shaped*," a change never seen in pernicious anemia. *Paresthesias* such as numbness and tingling may be present in the arms and legs. The *spleen* is often palpable, but is never greatly enlarged. *The triad characteristic of the disease is anemia, atrophy of the mucous membrane of the tongue, and brittleness or spoon-shaped deformity of the nails.*

The *blood changes* are the reverse of those which we studied in pernicious anemia, for the red cells are hypochromic instead of hyperchromic and microcytic instead of macrocytic, while the bone marrow is normoblastic instead of megaloblastic in type.

The *red cells* are diminished in number, but the decrease in hemoglobin is still greater, so that the color index is low and hypochromia (achromia) is marked (Plate XV, *a*, and Fig. 610). The average diameter of the red cells is smaller than normal, while in pernicious anemia it is greater than normal (Fig. 609). It is therefore a *microcytic anemia.* Indeed it may be said that small pale

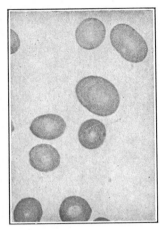

Fig. 609.—Hyperchromic anemia (pernicious anemia). The cells are macrocytic. × 1000.

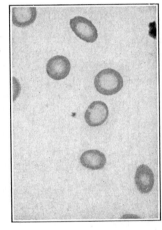

Fig. 610.—Hypochromic anemia. The cells are microcytic with a pale center. × 1000.

red cells are the hallmark of iron deficiency anemia, for in all other anemias the cells are either of normal size and color or are larger than normal. There is no evidence of the hemolysis characteristic of pernicious anemia. There is leukopenia, relative lymphocytosis and thrombocytopenia. The lack of iron seems to interfere with the normal maturation of the normoblasts, nor is the hemoglobin molecule properly built up in these cells. The result is a stuffing of the bone marrow with normoblasts and a deficiency of mature erythrocytes in the peripheral blood, those present being poorly supplied with hemoglobin.

The symptoms of iron deficiency may be due more to *depletion of iron enzymes* with resulting disturbance of tissue metabolism than to mere reduction in the circulating hemoglobin (Beutler). There is no correlation between the severity of symptoms and the degree of anemia. Iron-deficiency patients receiving iron therapy, particularly when given parenterally, may show marked symptomatic improvement before there is any rise in the hemoglobin. A general depletion of iron stores and enzymes precedes the development of frank anemia. Rats fed on an iron-deficient diet and then bled show a marked decrease in cytochrome content of the liver and kidneys, but a very slight reduction in hemoglobin concentration. Moreover the epithelial signs of iron deficiency such as the changes in the tongue, mouth and stomach cannot be explained on a basis of anemia alone, for they may occur without anemia. The gastric mucosal changes respond specifically to iron therapy in early cases. It is more than possible that the hypochlorhydria and achlorhydria may be the result and not the cause of iron deficiency. The precarious state of iron balance in menstruating women is well known. A high proportion of abnormally tired women have depleted bone marrow iron stores, although the circulating hemoglobin may be normal.

The so-called *Plummer-Vinson syndrome* is practically the same disease with the addition of dysphagia. It occurs in middle-aged women, although occasionally in men, and is characterized by hypochromic anemia, dysphagia, dryness and atrophy of the mucous membrane of the tongue, pharynx, and esophagus, painful cracks at the angles of the mouth, achlorhydria, brittleness of the nails, and enlargement of the spleen. There is a tendency for the condition to act as a predisposing cause of cancer of the hypopharynx in women. Owing to the dysphagia the patient will be found to have been living on slops for a prolonged period, and the anemia is doubtless due to the deficiency of iron in the diet. It responds remarkably to the administration of iron.

Chlorosis.—Chlorosis, the green sickness, is an example of an iron-deficiency anemia whose interest is mainly historical although it may still be seen at the present day. The disease is entirely confined to the female sex; if the condition is seen in the male it may be assumed that the diagnosis is incorrect. The age incidence is equally striking. Chlorosis usually appears at the time of puberty, but may develop at any time between the age of fifteen and twenty-five years. It was called by the ancients "the disease of virgins." The onset of the disease coincides, therefore, with a period in which a great strain is placed upon the blood-forming tissue, and in this connection it may be remarked that amenorrhea is one of the most constant symptoms.

The *blood* shows the picture of hypochromic microcytic anemia, the red cells having a pronounced central pallor. The blood platelets are greatly increased in number, an increase which is of interest in relation to the tendency to thrombosis which is often observed, usually in the veins of the leg, but occasionally in the cerebral sinuses. An important feature is a great increase in the plasma, so that the blood volume is above normal. Much of the anemia is therefore more apparent than real.

PYRIDOXINE DEFICIENCY ANEMIA.—An interesting link between the two principal forms of nutritional anemia in man, namely, pernicious anemia and iron-deficiency anemia, is provided by experimental pyridoxine deficiency anemia in swine (Wintrobe *et al.*). When the diet of the pig is lacking in pyridoxine but adequate in all the other elements of the vitamin B complex, the animal develops a severe anemia characterized by microcytosis, polychromatophilia, reticulocytes and nucleated red cells in the blood, a rise in the serum iron, hemosiderosis and bone marrow hyperplasia. The microcytic anemia resembles that due to iron deficiency, whilst the hemosiderosis and elevated serum iron suggest pernicious anemia. It is evident that in the pig pyridoxine plays some essential part in erythropoiesis and the synthesis of hemoglobin.

THE HEMOLYTIC ANEMIAS

The hemolytic anemias form a large and heterogeneous group, but the basis of each member of the group is a shortened life-span of the red blood cell, that is to say, premature destruction and death. This is accompanied by evidence of increased regeneration of red cells. The mechanism by which the life-span of the erythrocytes is shortened may be one of two profoundly different types. In the first the defect is *hereditary* (genetic), intrinsic, intracorpuscular, the defect residing within the cells, the resulting disease being congenital in type; in the second it is *acquired*, extrinsic, extracorpuscular. As Dameshek puts in, the red cell is either *born* vulnerable so that its normal life-span of four months is reduced and it can make fewer round trips through the capillaries before its defective enzyme systems are worn out, or it *becomes* so as the result of external factors, especially auto-immune bodies which are developed when the specific tissue cell concerned is sufficiently altered to become antigenic, the antibodies becoming adherent to the red cells and thus rendering them vulnerable to hemolysis acting in combination with complement. Some of the more common hemolytic disorders are now known to be the result of abnormalities in the synthesis of protein—hemoglobin protein and enzyme protein in the hereditary group, antibody protein in the acquired group. In the case of hemoglobin protein the defect may involve the heme fraction or the globin (Young).

The *hereditary* type is characterized by an intracorpuscular defect in the red cells which is transmitted by a gene. We have already seen that the red blood cell is not the inert bag of hemoglobin we are apt to picture it, but a highly complex and active structure. In addition to the structural proteins of which it is composed there are at least 40 related to glycolysis and respiration. A change in one enzyme or in a single amino acid of the 300 present in the hemoglobin molecule is enough to upset the delicate balance, the result being one of the hemolytic anemias. *Abnormal erythrocytes* due to an *enzyme deficiency* is the basis of hereditary spherocytic anemia, although a rather similar anemia is encountered in the acquired group. *Abnormal hemoglobin* due to a *defect in hemoglobin protein synthesis* is seen in the group known as the *hemoglobinopathies*, of which the more important members are sickle cell anemia, thalassemia or Mediterranean anemia, and the drug-induced hemolytic anemias, examples of which are given below.

The *acquired type*, which is the commoner of the two, comprises anemias that are related to extracorpuscular factors, so that the Coombs test is frequently positive. It includes cases which may be described as idiopathic with circulating antibodies and spherocytes (probably the commonest variety of hemolytic anemia), erythroblastosis fetalis, and the paroxysmal hemoglobinuria associated with exposure to cold. At least some of the anemia of neoplastic diseases such as the malignant lymphomas and leukemia may be of this type, as circulating hemolysins have been demonstrated in the blood in a number of cases, and the survival time of transfused red cells is markedly decreased. It is of interest that abundant *intracytoplasmic bodies* giving a strongly positive reaction with the periodic acid-Schiff method have been found in neoplastic lymphocytes in the lymphoid tissues in cases of lymphatic leukemia and lymphosarcoma (Rappaport). This raises the question as to whether the lymphocytes may not be connected in some way with the production of the auto-antibodies responsible for the Coombs reaction which is positive in these cases.

The *Coombs test* is designed to show the presence of *antibodies (agglutinins) adsorbed to the surface of the red cells in the acquired but not in the hereditary forms.* A rabbit is immunized with human serum globulin, a human globulin antiserum being produced in the rabbit. When the red cells of the patient are tested with this serum there is agglutination only in the acquired form.

Normal red cells can be tagged with an isotope such as radioactive iron. Their life varies from 100 to 120 days. When the red cells (spherocytes) of a patient with hereditary hemolytic anemia are injected into the circulation of a normal person they disappear completely within 14 to 19 days. On the other hand, normal red cells are rapidly destroyed by patients with acquired hemolytic anemia, whereas cells of acquired hemolytic anemia survive normally when transfused into normal persons. This indicates that in the hereditary form the fault lies in the red cells, whereas in the acquired form it lies in the environment. For this reason removal of the spleen, the graveyard of the red cells, is markedly beneficial in hereditary spherocytosis, whereas ACTH or cortisone, with their anti-hypersensitivity action, may be equally beneficial in the acquired forms.

Hemolytic disease may be compensated or uncompensated by bone marrow activity (Crosby). The result will naturally depend on the degree of destruction and of repair. *Hemolytic disease* occurs when, in the absence of a hemolytic factor, the average life span of the red blood cells is less than normal. *Hemolytic anemia* occurs when the marrow is unable to compensate for the shortened life span. In hemolytic anemia the destruction of hemoglobin may be 6 or 8 times the normal rate, the same being true of the production of bile pigment. The best single signpost of hemolytic anemia is a reticulocytosis of 5 per cent or over. Other evidence of bone marrow overactivity is leukocytosis, increased platelets, and the presence of nucleated red cells in the peripheral blood.

Having considered the general principles of hemolytic disease and the hemolytic anemias we may now turn our attention to some of the more important examples, first of the hereditary and then of the acquired group.

HEREDITARY (INTRACORPUSCULAR)

We have already seen that the hereditary defect may involve abnormal erythrocytes or abnormal hemoglobin, the latter group, being known as the hemoglobinopathies. The outstanding example of a defect in the make up of the erythrocyte is hereditary spherocytosis, which gives rise to congenital spherocytic anemia.

Congenital Sphercyotic Anemia.—The obvious blood anomaly in this condition is the spheroidal shape of the erythrocytes in place of the normal biconcave discs. The basic genetic defect, however, is one involving the metabolism of the cells. Metabolism in the mature red cell is predominantly glycolytic, the energy gained from the anerobic breakdown of glucose being stored in chemical form within the cell as adenosine triphosphate. As the red cell is the only cell entirely dependent upon glycolysis, it is particularly vulnerable to defects in the

enzyme involved which has to do with the maintenance of normal amounts of adenosine triphosphate in the cell. Such a basic intracellular defect in phosphorylation has been found in hereditary spherocytosis, but not in thalassemia or sickle cell anemia, with the exception of cells which have already become sickled. Such a basic defect could well be included in Garrod's original concept of "inborn errors of metabolism," even though in this case the defect is an intracellular one. "Accepting the evidence that the red cells in hereditary spherocytosis pass sluggishly through and stagnate in the splenic pulp, the hemoconcentration that ensues would create conditions in which the supply of glucose per cell is reduced, and the cells, being incapable of normal glycosis, can no longer maintain their normal chemical stores of energy, so that hemolysis ensues" (Prankerd).

It is the spheroidal shape of the erythrocytes which seems to be responsible for increased fragility of these cells, and the excessive blood destruction gives rise to a hemolytic jaundice, also known as *acholuric jaundice* because no bile appears in the urine. So striking is this feature that a common name for the condition is congenital hemolytic jaundice. The most precise name for the blood dyscrasia would be *hereditary spherocytosis*, because there may be spherocytosis without either anemia or jaundice. It must be noted that spherocytes are also found in acquired hemolytic anemias, but here they are not gene-induced.

Hereditary spherocytic anemia is familial and congenital, though it may not manifest itself until the second decade. One case is reported in which the disease remained latent until the age of seventy-five years, when treatment by splenectomy was successful (Mandelbaum). Some members of the family may have fragile red cells, but no anemia or jaundice. The *jaundice* persists throughout life, usually in mild form but with occasional exacerbations due to the characteristic "crises," in which there is increased blood destruction with attacks of pain in the region of the liver and spleen. This is in reality the result of an acute aplastic condition in the erythropoietic tissue with complete cessation of formation of red cells (Owren). As the average lifetime of the red cells in this disease is only 15 days (compared with the normal 120) it is evident that an acute crisis may be expected when the cells cease to be formed. The jaundice is due to increased production of bilirubin owing to excessive blood destruction. There is therefore an excess of bilirubin in the stools, increased production of urobilinogen, which is excreted in the urine, but bilirubin does not appear in the urine, hence the name acholuric jaundice. The blood gives an indirect van den Bergh reaction. *Gallstones* of the pure bilirubin type without any admixture of cholesterol are frequently present. The *spleen* is considerably enlarged. The *long bones* show longitudinal striation and a patchy moth-eaten appearance in the roentgen-ray picture, owing to osteoporosis produced by the hyperplastic marrow. *Intractable ulcers of the leg* not associated with varicose veins are a rather frequent complication. As a rule they heal quickly after splenectomy. Similar ulcers are not uncommon in sickle cell anemia. We may presume that the ulcers are caused by some interference with circulation to the leg, but the nature of that disturbance I do not know.

The *blood* shows an anemia, usually mild, but severe in the crises. The patient may have a count as low as 3,000,000, and yet be without symptoms and able to play his part in the world. If the anemia becomes severe it may closely resemble the pernicious anemia type. The two chief characteristics of the film are microspherulocytes and reticulocytes. A spherocyte is smaller and thicker than normal; it is spherical instead of biconcave. This characteristic can be recognized in wet preparations; in dry smears the cells merely appear as densely stained microcytes. As biconcave cells become globular when placed in hypotonic saline, it is evident that the more globular cells will rupture more readily. Reticulated red cells are more numerous than in any other disease. In place of the usual 1 per cent there may be 20 per cent; in the acquired form there may be 50 per cent or more. This is an indication of compensatory bone marrow activity. The white cells share in this activity, and the leukocyte count is generally from 12,000 to 15,000. In crises it may go up to 80,000. Normoblasts may be numerous, and these

may be mistaken for leukocytes in the counting chamber and cause error in the count. There is an increased fragility of the red cells, *i.e.*, they are hemolyzed by salt solution of a strength which leaves normal red cells untouched. It is only the small spherical cells which are abnormally fragile, and these are selectively removed by the spleen where they are found in large numbers.

Lesions.—The most striking change is in the *spleen*, which is markedly enlarged and weighs about 1000 grams. It is firm and of a bright red color like a beefsteak. It is stuffed with blood, so that after removal it loses considerably in bulk unless the vessels are clamped. The capsule is thickened. *Microscopically* the pulp is entirely occupied by red cells, thus presenting a very characteristic appearance. The sinuses are empty, and the lining cells may resemble glandular epithelium. The phagocytic cells contain a large amount of hemosiderin, especially during the hemolytic crises. The other reticuloendothelial organs (liver and bone marrow) also show *hemosiderosis*, as do the epithelial cells of the liver and kidney. Hemosiderosis may occur in any condition associated with long-continued hemolysis.

RELATION OF SYMPTOMS TO LESIONS. —The essential symptoms are anemia and jaundice; the essential lesions are splenomegaly and hemosiderosis. The connecting link between the two groups is the *increased fragility of the red cells, which itself is due to spherulocytosis.* Owing to this fragility the red cells are unduly exposed to the inimical influence of the reticuloendothelial cells, particularly those of the spleen, and are thereby broken down. The anemia and jaundice are relieved promptly, completely and permanently by splenectomy. It has been said that the hemolytic diseases are the children, and the spleen is their mother, whereas their father is unknown. It would appear that in the case of congenital spherocytic anemia we are justified in saying that the father is an inborn error of metabolism involving a glycolytic enzyme system in the erythrocytes with a resulting or accompanying change in shape which shortens the life span of the red cells, since they are unable to pass through the splenic pulp as readily as do the normal discoid erythrocytes, so that they are held up, filtered off and disintegrate, with accompanying splenomegaly. It has been calculated that every red cell spends two and a half days of its short life in the spleen. That is not a thing any red cell can do with complete impunity, and it is simply asking for trouble when the cell is a spherocyte.

Hypersplenism.—This is the term applied to a hypothesis designed to explain an association of splenic enlargement with marked diminution in the circulating blood of erythrocytes (congenital hemolytic icterus), platelets (thrombocytopenic purpura), granulocytes (splenic neutropneia), or all three (panhematopenia). As Wiseman and Doan put it: "The reticuloendothelial cells of the spleen when on a rampage of destruction may selectively choose as victim any *one* of the elements of marrow origin passing through this organ, but more often than not other innocent bystanding elements suffer likewise in some degree. Splenectomy always is followed by an increase in *all* circulating blood elements whenever applied in any one of these conditions." Two explanations have been offered for this association of splenomegaly with depression in the formed elements of the blood. The first, championed particularly by Dameshek, is that of *marrow inhibition*. The spleen is believed to depress marrow function by some influence, probably hormonal. The second view is that of *splenic hypersequestration.* The fact that splenectomy produces immediate improvement in the blood picture, and that marrow hyperplasia is a feature of the syndrome, appears to favor the second view. The unique anatomical arrangements of the spleen, with its combination of a smooth muscle capsule, pulp, and large fenestrated sinusoids, provide an ideal reservoir for blood storage. "The human spleen has a semi-open circulation controlled by a filter-mesh mechanism in the sinus wall which by heredity or under pathological conditions may become more or less permeable to blood" (Doan). There is abnormal stasis in the sinusoids or pulp and loss of plasma and erythrocyte potassium. This leads to increased fragility of the red cells, and exposes them to the phagocytic activity of the reticuloendothelial cells, an ideal environment

for cell destruction. The principal microscopic change is a prominent marginal zone of the Malpighian follicles (Leffler). The degree of sequestration and the possible need for splenectomy can be measured by comparison of splenic and hepatic radioactivity by surface counting (scanning) after injection of red cells tagged with P^{32}. Excessive trapping and destruction of erythrocytes by a large spleen may be due to abnormal red blood cells or to an abnormal spleen.

It must be emphasized that primary hypersplenism is still a hypothesis rather than a fact or an entity. The question which remains unanswered is: Does the splenomegaly represent a cause or an effect? The chief support for the concept comes from those cases in which splenectomy relieves or abolishes a pre-existing cytopenia.

In addition to the primary hypersplenism which has just been described there is a less common *secondary form*, which may give the same picture of specific splenic sequestration. This is seen in such conditions as *Banti's*, *Gaucher's*, and *Hodgkin's disease*, *sarcoidosis*, and *Felty's syndrome* in which splenomegaly and blood cytopenia are associated with rheumatoid arthritis.

Drug-Induced Hemolytic Anemia.—At first sight it might seem a mistake to include hemolytic anemias induced by drugs in the intrinsic rather than the extrinsic group. The reason will soon become apparent. It is well known that drugs which are harmless to most persons produce hemolytic reactions in a few sensitive persons. This is particularly true of the antimalarial drug, primaquine, and to a lesser degree of some aniline derivatives such as sulfanilamide, phenacetin, acetanilid, and others. Dark intracorpuscular bodies known as *Heinz bodies* are seen in wet unstained preparations, although not in fixed films stained with the ordinary dyes. They can be stained supravitally with brilliant cresyl blue. Their presence in a case of hemolytic anemia *suggests the action of some toxic drug to which the patient is sensitive.* The susceptible persons are mostly Negroes, whose red cells are deficient in the enzyme glucose-6-phosphate dehydrogenase. It is said that 10 per cent of American Negroes and a very small number of Caucasians suffer from drug sensitivity (Motulsky). The *dehydrogenase deficiency is genetically determined*, probably by a sex-linked gene in the X-chromosome. The enzyme catalyzes the first step in the oxidation of glucose by the red blood cell. Absence of the enzyme is associated with inability of the red cells to maintain the compound glutathione in a reduced state, and reduced glutathione seems to be the main defence of the red cell against injury by drugs and possibly other poisons. Its chemical activity is related to the sulfydryl (SH) group of cysteine, one of its three amino acids, so that glutathione is referred to as GSH. These facts form the basis of the *in vitro reduced glutathione (GSH) stability test* for drug sensitivity, with lowering of the level when the red cells are sensitive.

Favism or acute hemolysis following ingestion of Vicia fava beans, may have a similar basis. A deficiency of dehydrogenase activity has been demonstrated in the red cells of patients with favism, and glutathione stability tests on red cells from such cases are also normal. Favism is racial in distribution, and it is most common among Greeks, Sards, and other Mediterranean stocks. The hypersusceptibility seems to depend on an enzymatic deficiency of genetic origin.

It seems probable that damage by drugs to other cells (liver, etc.) may be determined by genetic enzymatic defects. This may explain qualitative differences between species, and also susceptibility or resistance to diseases other than drug idiosyncrasies.

Hereditary Hemoglobinopathies.—In the discussion of hemoglobin and its abnormalities under the heading of General Considerations we have seen that new techniques, paper chromatography in particular, have served to reveal new concepts relating to some of the hemolytic diseases. These can be included under the general heading of the hemoglobinopathies or molecular diseases. The more important of these will now be considered. For greater detail, monographs devoted to the subject must be consulted.

The majority of the hemolytic syndromes in childhood belong to this group (Smith). The racial incidence and geographic distribution of the different hemoglobins is becoming recognized. Thus hemoglobin S (sickle cell) and C is confined to Negroes, whether African or American, whereas hemoglobin E is encountered in the natives of Thailand. The highest proportion of fetal hemoglobin (F) is met with in thalassemia. Here again, as in hereditary spherocytosis, we must distinguish between compensated hemolytic disease and hemolytic anemia. Thus the output of hemoglobin is 3 times the normal in thalassemia, whereas it is 5 or 6 times the normal in sickle cell anemia, indicating the greater need of transfusion in the former. Here again we have an index of bone marrow activity in the reticulocyte count, nucleated red cells, bilirubinemia, and increased urobilinogen excretion in the stools. Complicating an already complex subject is the fact that more than one abnormal hemoglobin may be present. Thus sickle cell and thalassemia anemia may be combined, as may hemoglobin C and E.

The distinctive type of erythrocyte known as *target cell* or Mexican hat cell is commonly present in the hemoglobinopathies, although not confined to these conditions. The target cell has a central rounded area of pigment, surrounded by a clear zone, with further out a thick pigmented capsule. The envelope is thick in relation to the content of the cell, being the opposite to the spherocyte in this respect. Target cells up to 10 per cent are seen in thalassemia, they are more frequent in sickle cell anemia, and most numerous in sickle cell hemoglobin C disease where they may constitute from 40 to 90 per cent of all the red cells. They are also seen in hemoglobin E disease, but not in D, G, M, I or J hemoglobinopathies.

Sickle Cell Anemia.—Although this disease is dependent on an inherited anomaly in the formation of the hemoglobin molecule, it has much in common with spherocytosis in which there is an enzyme deficiency in the structure of the erythrocyte. Both are familial and hereditary, and both are characterized by a hemolytic type of anemia, acholuric jaundice, hemosiderosis, and the appearance of large numbers of reticulocytes. The genetic defect is largely confined to the Negro race, and the disease is very prevalent in the colored population of the United States, particularly in the deep South. It is estimated that about 30,000 United States Negroes suffer from the disease, and that

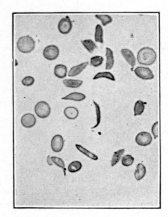

FIG. 611.—Sickle cell anemia. Many erythrocytes are sickle-shaped. × 500.

some 1,500,000 carry the sickle cell trait (see below).

The disease, which was first described by Herrick in 1910, offers many points of resemblance to hemolytic spherocytosis and to the hemolytic anemia of young children described in the next section. It is a congenital disease, being present at birth, is familial as well as hereditary, and is apparently confined to the Negro race.

Two different phases are described by those who have studied this disease, the latent and the active. It seems better, however, to regard the former as a tendency to sickle cell formation, a *sickle cell trait*, rather than a latent form of an anemia. It is this tendency which is inherited as a dominant Mendelian trait, and it has been observed in the white man as well as in the Negro. The active phase is the development of a hemolytic type of anemia. In the latent phase the patient presents few or no symptoms beyond the sickle cell trait. We may speak, then, of *sickle cell disease*, which includes the sickle cell trait and sickle cell anemia. In this case the term disease is used to indicate a defect in constitution, which may or may not be associated with symptoms. It would appear that *the sickle cell trait represents a heterozygous state, whilst sickle cell anemia is homozygous*, the defective gene being inherited from both parents. Moreover in the sickle cell trait both A (normal adult) and S (sickle cell) hemoglobins are present, whereas in sickle

cell anemia the hemoglobins are S and F (fetal), the bulk, from 60 to 98 per cent, being of the S type. Sickle cell hemoglobin is an abnormal hemoglobin electrophoretically different from normal hemoglobin, its formation being determined by a single abnormal gene. The sickle cell trait is an anomaly of the Negro race in Africa and of their descendants in North and South America, although it has occasionally been reported in white person for reasons which may readily be guessed. In Africa the incidence varies greatly from tribe to tribe, being over 45 per cent in one group in East Africa. Similarly the incidence varies in different parts of the Southern United States, although to a much lesser degree, with an average of from 8 to 10 per cent. In the American Negro about 1 in 40 with the sickle cell trait develop anemia.

It is in the examination of the blood that we find the chief difference between the two phases of this condition. In the *latent phase* there is no actual disease, so that no anemia is found. The blood appears normal. In the *active phase*, on the other hand, there is marked anemia and leukocytosis, the red cells averaging 2,000,000 and the leukocytes 20,000. The film shows an extraordinary change in the shape of the red cells, for large numbers of these are of crescentic, sickle or stellate form (Fig. 611). Many of the abnormal cells are being phagocytosed by macrophages. Reticulated red cells form a prominent feature. The serum is deep yellow due to the great increase of bilirubin. The sickling seems to be due to a greatly decreased solubility of reduced sickle cell hemoglobin, so that intracellular crystallization occurs in the absence of oxygen. After an initial period of cytoplasmic unrest the cells are gradually or at times suddenly changed into crescent or scimitar shaped bodies. We have already seen that hemoglobin S differs in its molecular structure from normal hemoglobin A, and this may account for its reduced solubility under anoxic conditions.

Although sickle cells are not found *in vivo* in the latent phase, they are readily demonstrated *in vitro*. A wet film is made and covered, and the preparation sealed so as to prevent evaporation and exclude air. In the course of eighteen or twenty-four hours large numbers of the red cells will be found to have assumed the sickle form. The factor which leads to the actual production of sickle cells *in vitro* appears to be a diminution in the oxygen tension. Sickling is probably due to a process of gelation. Hemoglobin S has a low solubility, so that it forms a gel more readily than other hemoglobins, and removal of its oxygen reduces its solubility still farther. The molecules become oriented in long axes, this stiffening and straightening overcomes the pliant fabric of the stroma, the cell suddenly opens like a switch knife, and is now rigid and sickled (Crosby). These rigid sickled cells are not only more easily destroyed, but also increase the viscosity of the blood, and are thus responsible for the infarctions which characterize the disease.

Persons with a *sickle cell trait* rarely suffer from any disability unless exposed to conditions involving some degree of anoxia. Those who inherit the defective gene from a single parent not only suffer no ill effect, but are actually benefitted through being resistant to malaria. On the other hand colored personnel flying at high altitude in unpressurized planes during the Second World War would develop splenic infarction. Such people were naturally found to have a sickle cell trait. Under physiological conditions most red cells are deoxygenated for only about ten seconds, but if anything holds up the flow of cells through the tissues, the proportion of sickled cells will rapidly rise. The sickled cells themselves tend to intensify the hold-up by sludging and blocking blood vessels. When we consider the slow passage of red cells as they wander through the pathless forest of the spleen, it is little wonder that they lose oxygen, undergo sickling, block vessels, and thus lead to infarction.

Clinical Picture.—The state of health of the patient will vary greatly. At times he feels well, at other times he presents the symptoms of a severe anemia in addition to the peculiar set of symptoms outlined below. The patient, although outwardly well, has to bear the burden of a blood dyscrasia whose outstanding feature is an abnormally high rate of destruction of red blood cells. At the same time he manages to live on good terms with his disease, and is able to adapt

himself to a remarkable degree to a state of chronic anemia and jaundice. He is apt, however, to break down under stress, and his normal life span, like that of his red blood cells, is considerably shortened.

Crises may occur periodically. These are not merely an exacerbation of pre-existing symptoms of anemia. There may be recurring attacks of pain in the joints and muscles, fever, leukocytosis, and general disability with protean manifestations which may be referred to almost any organ of the body. Particularly confusing are the acute attacks of abdominal pain in the epigastrium or right or left hypochondrium, associated with rigidity of the abdominal wall, prostration, fever and leukocytosis. It is evident that *before the abdomen of a colored patient is opened for an expected ruptured peptic ulcer, intestinal obstruction or acute appendicitis, it is advisable to look at a blood film.* The varied manifestations of the acute crises are best explained by sudden sickling and agglutination of the affected cells leading to localized areas of anoxia.

In addition to the usual symptoms of anemia there are numerous other features peculiar to the disease. The *physical appearance* may be characteristic in cases of long duration, the patient being under-weight, the trunk short, the limbs long and slender, and the skull high domed, the "tower skull." The *heart* is enlarged both to right and left, and a systolic murmur and thrill may be evident, which may readily be mistaken for evidence of mitral valvular or congenital heart disease. *Bone deformities* with corresponding x-ray changes may be seen in the spine and other bones. *Neurological manifestations* are common, and may suggest cerebral hemorrhage (hemiplegia, aphasia), meningitis (irritability, stiffness of the neck), or even poliomyelitis. *Chronic ulcers in the lower half of the leg* such as have already been described in connection with spherocytosis are of common occurrence. These varied symptoms are due to vascular obstruction caused by agglutination of the sickled red cells.

Lesions.—The *bone marrow* is soft, dark red, and intensely hyperplastic, as might be expected from the extent it can compensate for the short life span of the red blood cells.

The *spleen* is enlarged in the earlier years, but with advancing age it becomes much smaller, largely due to the multiple infarcts with which it becomes studded. Splenomegaly is present in one-third of the cases in the first decade, but in only 10 per cent in later life. The malpighian follicles are surrounded by pools of blood, and the sinusoids may be collapsed owing to the accumulation of blood between them. This is a pathognomonic appearance (Rich). It may be due to obstruction caused by clumps of sickled cells. In the later stages the lesions develop into siderotic nodules. The incredibly small size to which the spleen may shrink came as a shock and a surprise to me when I first encountered it in an autopsy room in the Southern United States, although it was quite familiar to the local pathologists. The *liver* showed evidence of hepatic cell damage in every one of 31 autopsies, and in 9 there was cirrhosis of the macronodular or postnecrotic type (Song). The lesions may be due to sinusoidal blocking similar to that which occurs in the spleen. *In all of the organs sickle cells may be seen in the capillaries.*

Thalassemia.—This variety of hemoglobinopathy is known by many names, such as *Cooley's anemia, erythroblastic anemia, leptocytosis* (see below), and Mediterranean anemia. It is due to a homozygous defect in hemoglobin formation, the gene responsible being distributed among the peoples of the eastern Mediterranean basin. For this reason it has long been known as Mediterranean fever or thalassemia from the Greek word, *thalasse*, meaning sea, for in olden times there only was one sea, the Mediterranean. The trait has now been carried far and wide throughout the world by the migration of peoples.

No specific *abnormal* hemoglobin seems to be responsible for the anemia, but fetal hemoglobin (F) is formed in place of the more difficult synthesis of adult hemoglobin (A). In severe forms of the disease there may be an extraordinary amount of fetal hemoglobin, from 40 up to 100 per cent. This results in a decreased life span of the circulating red cells. The resistance of the red cells to hypotonic saline is not decreased, but their mechanical fragility is said to be greater than normal.

Thalassemia is characterized by a constant familial and racial incidence, a typical facial appearance, distinctive changes in the bones, and enlargement of the spleen. It usually appears in the first two years of life and sometimes in the newborn. The familial (hereditary) incidence is marked; it has been reported in identical twins. Originally it was a disease of the Mediterranean races, most often in Greeks, but also in Italians and Armenians. The skin is yellow, the face mongoloid, the head enlarged, the abdomen prominent, the stature stunted. Owing to hyperplasia of the marrow the bones show medullary trabeculations in the roentgen-ray picture, and the skull is thickened by the thick diploë. There is a moderate or marked anemia, the platelets are increased, and there is a leukocytosis which may reach 50,000. The splenomegaly is due to foci of hemopoietic tissue and hyperplasia of reticuloendothelial cells.

The characteristic features of the blood film are the great numbers of erythroblasts and the presence of *leptocytes* or thin cells (*leptos*, thin), oval cells, and *target cells*, which have already been described (page 105). The leptocytes are comparable to the sickle cells, both representing a departure from the normal. Target cells are not confined to Mediterranean anemia. Indeed they are more likely to be seen in cases of cirrhosis of the liver and after splenectomy. The *pathognomonic* feature is the presence of great numbers of nucleated red cells, both normoblasts and megaloblasts. In one case in the newborn there were 90 per cent of erythroblasts. The immature red cells suffer at the hands of the reticuloendothelial cells, which accounts for the anemia and the deposits of hemosiderin in the spleen, liver, pancreas, and other viscera, almost like hemochromatosis. Excessive erythropoiesis is present in the marrow and in the spleen and liver. The course is usually chronic and may last a number of years.

Thalassemia minor is the heterozygous form of the dyscrasia. It is more of a carrier state than an actual disease, corresponding to the sickle cell trait, because usually there are no symptoms, and the condition is discovered by chance. There may or may not be anemia, but the red cells show hypochromia, microcytosis, stippling, target cells and oval cells. In spite of these rather startling changes the life span of the red cells does not appear to be shorter than normal.

Other Hemoglobinopathies.—Other rare forms of hemolytic anemia due to genetic defects in the synthesis of hemoglobin have been described, such as *hemoglobin C disease*, confined generally to the Negro, and *hemoglobin E disease*, occurring in the people of Thailand. For details of these rare forms special monographs may be consulted.

Paroxysmal Nocturnal Hemoglobinuria.— This condition, also known as the *Marchiafava-Micheli* syndrome, is a chronic hemoglobinuria which occurs only during sleep or is more marked at that time. The morning urine is deeply colored. The fundamental abnormality does not lie in the serum, as in the ordinary form, but in the erythrocytes, which are abnormally susceptible to hemolysis in plasma of *increased acidity* such as results from reduced pulmonary ventilation during sleep. The increased susceptibility of the erythrocytes, which is the essence of nocturnal hemoglobinuria, is an acquired condition which does not have a genetic basis. The blood often shows a well-marked anemia, usually macrocytic in type, with numerous reticulocytes. This is accompanied by jaundice and splenomegaly. There is marked hemosiderosis of the kidneys, which are enlarged and brown in color, but the liver, spleen and other usual sites of hemosiderosis are not involved.

March hemoglobinuria is a condition in which hemoglobin appears in the urine after prolonged walking, and is seen particularly in young soldiers on forced marches and in long-distance runners. There is no anemia, because the loss of hemoglobin is too transient.

ACQUIRED (EXTRACORPUSCULAR) HEMOLYTIC ANEMIAS

The hemolytic anemias which have so far been discussed have been of the hereditary type. There remains to be considered the rather miscellaneous group of the acquired hemolytic anemias. We have already seen that these may be (1) due to extraneous agents or (2) idiopathic in character, of a so-called auto-immune type. Hemolytic disease of the newborn can be regarded as one of the acquired group, but it is of so special a character that it seems better to consider it separately.

Extraneous Agents.—A number of these have been mentioned already. They fall into the following groups. (1) *Protozoan parasites*, such as those of malaria, which destroy the red blood cells. Anemia due to malaria is by far the commonest variety of hemolytic anemia in the world. (2) Viruses, more particularly that of primary atypical pneumonia, in which cold antibodies can usually be demonstrated, although hemolytic anemia is rare; when it does occur it develops suddenly toward the end of the second week. (3) *Bacterial infections*, such as those of hemolytic streptococci and B. Welchii, may cause hemolysis. (4) *Chemical agents*, particularly toxic substances used in industry, such as trinitrotoluene. The drug-induced hemolytic anemias have already been considered in connection with the hereditary group of erythrocyte abnormalities. (5) *Animal and vegetable poisons*, of which the most dramatic example is snake venom.

IMMUNE ANTIBODY ANEMIAS

The remaining members of the acquired group of hemolytic anemias represent the action of antibodies on erythrocytes. Here again the fault lies with the environment, not the enzyme structure of the red cells or the synthesis of hemoglobin. The antibodies may be *auto-immune*, as in paroxysmal cold hemoglobinuria, or *iso-immune*, as in hemolytic disease of the newborn, and they may be hot or cold. *Warm auto-antibodies* react well at 37° C. and are not potentiated at lower temperatures, whereas *cold antibodies* are markedly potentiated by reducing the temperature below 37° C. Spherocytosis frequently accompanies acquired hemolytic anemia. Both agglutinating and incomplete antibodies can provoke this change. When normal red cells are transfused into the patient they are rapidly eliminated, whereas normal cells transfused into patients with congenital hemolytic anemia survive for the normal span. The *Coombs test*, which detects auto-antibodies attached to the surface of the red cells, is naturally positive in the acquired and negative in the congenital form. In the treatment of the anemias which have an antibody basis cortisone or ACTH may be remarkably effective, relieving the anemia promptly and sometimes permanently.

Paroxysmal Cold Hemoglobinuria.—This rare condition is characterized by sudden attacks of fever and chills accompanied by the appearance of hemoglobin in the urine. There are two etiological factors, *syphilis* and *exposure to cold*. The exposure to cold may be very slight, such as washing the hands in cold water or even drinking cold water. Usually cold weather is needed, and the most bloody urine that I have seen was passed on a day of 60° of frost. Shortly after exposure to cold the patient develops pain in the muscles and abdomen, followed by severe chills and fever. The urine is full of hemoglobin and may be of a port-wine color. It contains no well formed red cells, but numerous ghosts of hemolyzed cells; the urine is therefore clear, not smoky or cloudy as when it contains ordinary blood. The spectroscope shows the absorption bands of oxyhemoglobin or methemoglobin. There may be transient jaundice, due to the formation of bilirubin from the liberated hemoglobin. The spleen may be temporarily enlarged. The blood shows a hemolytic anemia, followed by very rapid regeneration. There is a transient leukopenia due to the protein shock caused by the rapid liberation of hemoglobin.

The hemolysis is due to the presence of an autohemolysin which is present in the blood of some syphilitic patients. This unites with red blood cells in the presence of complement but, strange to say, only at a low temperature. When the two factors of syphilitic hemolysin and a low temperature are both present, a sudden reaction takes place with marked hemolysis and the liberation of large quantities of hemoglobin in the blood. This causes transient hemolytic jaundice and is excreted in the urine giving hemoglobinuria. Hemolysis with hemoglobinemia and hemoglobinuria may be caused by malaria, by drugs of the coal-tar series, or by blood transfusion, but in these cases the mechanism is quite different and bears no relation to cold.

Hemolytic Disease of the Newborn.—We now pass from auto-immune hemolytic reactions, where the patient's own blood is at fault, to *iso-immune* reactions, where the factor responsible for hemolysis comes from the blood of another individual. This may be due to a transfusion of incompatible blood, a subject which has already been considered, or to *incompatible iso-antibodies transferred across the placenta during pregnancy*, resulting in hemolytic disease of the newborn. It is obvious that the latter condition can occur only when there is a difference between the blood groups of a mother and her fetus. The difference lies mainly in the Rh blood group system or the ABO blood group system. Of these, Rh incompatibility is much the more severe, and it is to it that we shall direct our attention. It is an interaction of fetal antigens and maternal antibodies. This disease may take various forms, which are known by such names as *congenital hemolytic disease, erythroblastosis fetalis, icterus gravis,* and *hydrops fetalis*. The condition is essentially an Rh incompatibility, a term more descriptive than the common designation erythroblastosis fetalis, for erythroblasts may be present in excess in the fetal blood and tissues as the result of other causes.

The red blood cells of the majority of human beings contain the agglutinogen known as Rh antigen D, the Rh or rhesus factor. This has already been discussed on page 1040 in connection with the question of blood groups.

About 85 per cent of persons possess the Rh factor so that they are Rh-positive, whilst 15 per cent lack the factor and are Rh-negative. There is a racial distribution of the factor as indicated by the fact that 90 per cent of Negroes and 99 per cent of Chinese are Rh-positive. Anti-Rh agglutinins may be formed in Rh-negative persons following the transfusion of Rh-positive blood. An Rh-positive father can transmit the factor to the fetus as a simple Mendelian dominant. If the mother is Rh-negative, anti-Rh agglutinins may be formed in her blood as the result of immunization or sensitization by the Rh factor of the fetus (Fig. 612).

The stage is now set for disaster in two

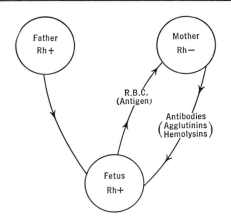

FIG. 612.—Diagram to illustrate Rh factor.
(Courtesy of Dr. I. Erb.)

possible forms. (1) If the mother is transfused with Rh-positive blood, even though belonging to the same general blood group, there may be an intra-group transfusion accident. (2) If the maternal anti-Rh agglutinins reach the fetal blood through the placenta, they will react with the agglutinogen in the fetal red cells, as a result of which there will be a slow continuous hemolysis of those cells, although in the test tube the reaction takes the form of agglutination.

Hemolytic disease of the newborn may also result from incompatibility in the ABO system, the agglutinins in this case being anti-A or anti-B. The exciting cause is blood transfusion. Thus hemolytic disease may occur even though the mother is not Rh negative. She is almost invariably group O. In these cases there may be no anemia and the antiglobulin test may be negative, but in some instances anemia may occur with marked jaundice and even with kernicterus. *Thus the pregnant woman may be sensitized either from the paternal Rh agglutinogen via the fetus or by blood transfusion.* Hemolytic disease of the newborn is not common, nor yet is it rare. It occurs once in every 200 pregnancies, and accounts for 2 to 3 per cent of all neonatal deaths. There is an unknown factor influencing susceptibility to the antigenic stimulation, for some women become sensitized during the second pregnancy, some after repeated pregnancies, and some never. In the homozygous Rh-positive both chromosomes will carry D (DD), so that all the

sex cells will contain D, and all children will inherit D and be Rh-positive. In the heterozygous Rh positive, one chromosome will carry D and the other d. Some of the children will therefore inherit D and others d.

The simplest and best means of detecting the passive transfer of maternal antibody to the infant's circulation is to determine whether the infant's erythrocytes have been coated with antibody. This is demonstrated by the direct anti-globulin (Coombs) test, which remains positive for up to two months in the absence of exchange transfusion.

In prenatal care the mother's blood must be tested for the Rh factor and the ABO blood group. If she proves to be Rh-negative then it becomes necessary to determine the Rh type and blood group of the father. A diagnosis of Rh type hemolytic disease can be made during pregnancy. This is not true of ABO hemolytic disease, but the clinical manifestations of the latter condition are usually mild.

The Rh Factor in Pregnancy.—In pregnancy the presence of the Rh factor in the red cells of the fetus carries a twofold threat, first to the mother and secondly to the child. The former, the danger of a transfusion reaction due to the presence of Rh antibodies in the woman's blood, has already been discussed. In the child the threat is the development of hemolytic disease of the fetus and the newborn. The chance of dangerous consequences is not as great as might be feared, as will be evident from the following figures. One out of 12 marriages involves an Rh-positive husband and an Rh-negative wife. The incidence of hemolytic disease of the infant is about 1 in 250 to 500 deliveries, that of the severe jaundiced form of erythroblastosis fetalis 1 in 1500 deliveries, and the fatal hydrops form 1 in 2000 deliveries. While the condition may arise in the first pregnancy, it may not develop until after the tenth normal child has been born. Not all mothers who are Rh-negative become sensitized by an Rh-positive fetus. The exact percentage who escape and the reason for this is unknown.

The child may be born dead, especially in the hydrops cases, it may live only a few days, or it may survive. About 7 per cent of those which survive are mental defectives.

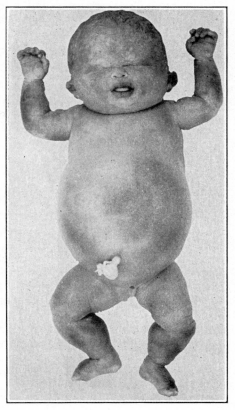

Fig. 613.—Hydrops fetalis in hemolytic disease of the newborn.

If jaundice develops it usually does not do so until some days after birth. This is apparently due to excretion of the excess of bilirubin through the placenta. In the most severe form of all, hydrops fetalis, jaundice is absent.

It sometimes happens that the titer of agglutinins in the maternal blood bears no relation to the severity of the hemolytic disease in the child. Indeed in the hydrops cases there may be an apparently complete absence of maternal agglutinins. This paradox is explained by the discovery in the maternal serum of what have been called *blocking antibodies* in addition to the usual agglutinating antibodies (page 1040). The blocking antibodies interfere with the union in the test tube between the antigens and the agglutinating antibodies, so that the presence of the latter is readily overlooked.

The *clinical picture* in the child is one of *congenital anemia* with *erythroblastosis fetalis*. *Jaundice* may or may not be present. Any baby who becomes jaundiced within the first day of life should be investigated for hemolytic disease. There are great numbers of nucleated red cells, a compensatory phenomenon, and active erythropoiesis in the liver and spleen, together with hemosiderosis in these and other organs. In a small number of cases there is necrosis of the liver, and still more rarely actual cirrhosis occurs. The child may die in the course of a few days of *malignant icterus neonatorum* or *icterus gravis*. In such a case the nuclear structures of the brain (caudate nucleus, optic thalamus) show intense staining with bile ("*Kernicterus*"). It is estimated that brain damage associated with kernicterus is present in some 15 per cent of cases. About 70 per cent of the babies with this lesion die within seven days of birth, and those which do not die are liable to have permanent neurologic sequelæ, such as cerebral palsy. The principal changes are degenerating neurones, petechial hemorrhages and crystals of bilirubin. The damage develops late in the second day, with opisthotonos as the characteristic symptom. It bears a close relation to the severity of the jaundice. Possibly the fact that the "blood-brain barrier" of the adult is not yet built up in the fetus and premature infant may play some part in allowing bilirubin to produce a toxic encephalopathy. If the serum bilirubin is kept below 20 mg. per 100 cc. by means of exchange transfusion, this serious complication can be almost completely prevented. Obviously the appropriate blood type must be used—Rh negative or the same ABO group as the mother.

In *congenital hydrops* the child is likely to be born dead with edema and marked ascites (Fig. 613). The cause of the edema appears to be an increased permeability of the capillary walls due to anoxemia. The hydrops variety is associated with a greatly enlarged and edematous placenta, the surface being made up of large, friable, pale cotyledons. Microscopically the villi show evidence of immaturity, such as large size (Fig. 614), the persistence of Langhan's cells which normally disappear about the middle of pregnancy, and the presence of numerous erythroblasts in the capillaries. In the jaundiced

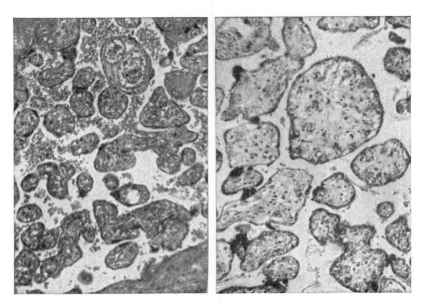

Fig. 614.—*A*, Normal placenta, 8 months. × 100. *B*, Placenta in erythroblastosis, 8 months, enlarged villi. × 100. (Boyd, *Pathology for the Physician*.)

form of erythroblastosis the changes in the placenta are similar but of much milder degree. If the fetus has died before the onset of labor and become macerated it may be very difficult to establish a diagnosis. Here again the presence of placental changes and of numerous erythroblasts in the pulmonary capillaries is of great value.

It may be helpful here to recall what we have already learned about the two types of bilirubin, namely pure bilirubin (hemobilirubin) and bilirubin conjugated with glucuronic acid, the latter being formed by the enzyme bilirubin glucuronyl transferase during passage through the liver cells (page 809). Bilirubin is the pigment of hemolytic jaundice, while conjugated bilirubin is the pigment of obstructive jaundice. Jaundice may develop in the newborn infant apart from hemolytic disease of the newborn. The absence of conjugated bilirubin in the plasma of these babies suggests a metabolic block in the excretory process at the stage at which bilirubin is converted to the conjugated pigment. The infant is not born jaundiced, because before birth the placenta, not the liver, is responsible for removal of bilirubin from the fetal blood. He only becomes

jaundiced if the enzyme system in the liver cells responsible for the conjugation and excretion of bilirubin has not been fully developed (Billing *et al.*). In small and premature babies with immature livers there is a natural tendency for the plasma bilirubin level to be elevated. By the end of a week the bilirubin transferase activity seems to have risen to the adult level, and any jaundice which may have been present disappears.

In hemolytic disease of the newborn there is a marked additional increase of pigment formation due to the blood destruction, an increase with which the underdeveloped liver is unable to cope, and the result is a much higher concentration of bilirubin in the blood than occurs in adults with either obstructive or hemolytic jaundice. The toxicity of bilirubin in cases of kernicterus seems to depend on the lipophylic nature of unconjugated bilirubin, and to be due to an inhibitory effect on the oxygen consumption of brain tissue mediated by an uncoupling action on the oxidative phosphorylation of brain mitochondria. (Claireause *et al.*). Conjugated bilirubin is non-toxic, and the water-souble bilirubin glucuronides do not stain the brain tissue. This serves to explain the absence of kernicterus in the adult with even intense degrees of obstructive jaundice. It may be noted that a rare familial congenital hyperbilirubinemia in both adults and children in whom the blood contains only traces of conjugated bilirubin is due to a deficiency in the transferase enzyme.

The historical and comparative aspects of the subject are not without interest (Roberts). It is rather sobering to learn that although our knowledge of the Rh factor dates only from 1940, hemolytic disease of the newborn with its accompanying jaundice has long been known to the veterinarian to occur in the horse and mule, and now the piglet is added to the list. Indeed the condition was described in the mule foal in 1774. In 1609 a midwife to the Court of France published her reminiscences, in which she mentioned delivering a pair of twins, one a stillborn girl with hydrops, the other a living boy with marked jaundice. In 1900, the year the human blood groups were first discovered by Landsteiner, it was suggested that an exchange of antibodies might occur between the mother and the fetus. It will be seen that although the discovery of the Rh factor has thrown a flood of fresh light on the pathogenesis, the general subject of this disorder has aroused the interest of the medical and veterinary professions for several hundred years.

The Rh Factor in Blood Transfusion.— Intra-group blood transfusion reactions are usually due to the Rh factor. The danger arises if an Rh-negative person is transfused with Rh-positive blood a number of times. (In rare instances a single transfusion is sufficient.) Once sensitization occurs it appears to be permanently imprinted on the individual's constitution, and a further transfusion years later may be followed by a severe reaction. In women an initial transfusion is not necessary, provided they have become sensitized by having had an Rh-positive child. Thus Rh-negative women who have borne children should be transfused only with Rh-negative blood.

BONE MARROW HYPOFUNCTION

We have considered the deficiency anemias (iron and maturation factor deficiency) and the hemolytic anemias, both hereditary and acquired. There remains a somewhat miscellaneous group in which the basic defect is hypofunction of the bone marrow. The cause of the hypofunction may be obvious, as when there are associated lesions of the marrow, or it may be quite obscure.

Aplastic Anemia.—Aplasia of the bone marrow and the anemia which accompanies it may be due to some obvious cause (secondary form), but occasionally there is no obvious cause (primary form). *Primary aplastic anemia* is fortunately a rare disease occurring in young people usually between the ages of fifteen and thirty years. It may be very acute and extremely fatal, killing the patient in a few weeks, or at the most some months. Fever is very common, due probably to interference with the heat regulating mechanism. The cause is unknown. Some agent depresses the activity of the bone marrow until no more blood is formed. The normal amount of blood destruction is going on, but there is nothing to take the place of the destroyed erythrocytes. The anemia becomes extreme, but the blood film remains strangely normal; there are none of the changes such as the presence of macrocytes, nucleated red cells, polychromatophilia, reticulocytes, etc., which indicate that the marrow is struggling to make good the wastage. The change is quantitative not qualitative. All the formed elements of the blood are diminished, the leukocytes and platelets as well as the red cells. On account of the extreme thrombocytopenia purpuric hemorrhages form an important feature of the clinical picture, and it may be very difficult to distinguish the condition from true purpura hæmorrhagica. The color index is below normal, but not extremely low. There is no evidence of hemolysis such as an increase of bilirubin in the blood or the appearance of urobilinogen in the urine. The red bone marrow is profoundly aplastic, consisting of little more than fat, and contains very few cells (Fig. 615), but some islands of hyperplasia may be found.

Secondary aplastic anemia is due to some external agent which interferes with the production of blood. *Industrial poisons* may cause a dangerous or fatal anemia. *Benzol* and its parent substance, crude benzene, are

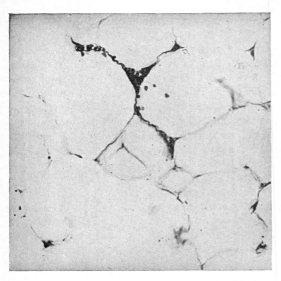

Fig. 615.—Bone marrow in aplastic anemia, showing complete absence of hyperplasia. × 275.

used as a solvent for rubber, gum and resins, as well as in dozens of industries where there may be danger of inhalation of the fumes. The blood picture is usually aplastic in type, with in severe cases the characteristic triad of extreme anemia, leukopenia and thrombocytopenia, but sometimes it may be hemolytic and regenerative in type so that the bone marrow is usually aplastic but occasionally hyperplastic. Symptoms of benzol poisoning may appear after a few weeks of exposure or not for many years, suggestive of an element of individual idiosyncrasy. *Drugs* may produce a refractory anemia in the susceptible person. Amongst these may be mentioned the organic arsenicals such as neoarsphenamine, chloramphenicol and gold compounds. *Ionizing radiation* has long been known to produce an aplastic anemia, and at the present time the subject is of course becoming of major importance. The radiation may come from a diagnostic x-ray machine, from radiation therapy or from an atomic explosion. In the near future we shall have to add atomic sources of industrial power. The hemopoietic tissues are the most sensitive in the body to radiation, taking precedence even of the epithelium of the testes and ovaries. All elements of the bone marrow are depressed, so that the resulting blood picture is anaplastic in character.

Myelophthisic Anemia.—This is a wasting (phthisis) or replacement of the marrow and a *leuko-erythroblastic anemia*, mild in degree and characterized by an increased number of primitive red and white cells. The commonest cause is replacement of the marrow by *carcinomatous metastases*, more particularly from the breast, prostate, lungs, adrenals and thyroid. Extensive replacement of the marrow in *multiple myeloma* may be associated with myelophthisic anemia in some 5 per cent of cases. An equally extreme replacement of marrow may be caused by the condition known as *myelofibrosis* or *myelosclerosis*, in which there is an irregular formation of fibrous and finally osseous tissue in the marrow, together with *splenomegaly* which may be extreme in degree due to *myeloid metaplasia*, with lesser involvement of the liver. This is the condition to which the unnecessarily esoteric designation of *agnogenic myeloid metaplasia* has been applied, agnogenic merely meaning idiopathic. In the rare condition known as osteosclerosis in which the bone is thickened and the marrow reduced an aplastic anemia (*osteosclerotic anemia*) may develop.

The *blood* in leuko-erythroblastic anemia shows an anemia with nucleated red cells out of proportion in number to the degree of the anemia, which may be quite slight. Most of these cells are erythroblasts, but there may be a few more primitive cells. The leukocytes are variable, in some cases being reduced, in others reaching the proportion of a mild leukemia, with myelocytes and even more primitive white cells. The diagnosis may be suspected in the presence of nucleated red cells or myelocytes with little anemia.

SECONDARY ANEMIA

This term, while somewhat old fashioned, is a convenient one, for it comprises a miscellaneous collection of anemias which form one feature of a group of diseases or states of health. Amongst these the more important are the anemias of infection, chronic renal disease, malignancy and pregnancy, to which may be added lead poisoning.

In general it may be said that the life-span of the erythrocytes is reduced, as shown by tagging these cells with radioactive chromium and following their subsequent life history. This is presumably due to some enhancement of blood destruction, although this fails to produce the usual concomitants of hemolysis such as jaundice and urobilinuria which could be compensated readily by a normal marrow.

Anemia of chronic infection is of common occurrence, a striking example being subacute bacterial endocarditis. It seems probable that the anemia is due to some abnormality of hemoglobin synthesis apparently dependent on the presence of infection. Such anemias are refractory to iron and liver therapy. Wintrobe and his associates have shown that in this condition the plasma iron is very much below normal, nor does the administration of iron raise the plasma iron as it does in the normal person. There appears to be a failure in the utilization of iron for hemoglobin regeneration during chronic infections due probably to some unknown "persistent and urgent demand for iron to fulfill some function in relation to infection which has a greater priority for iron than hemoglobin formation." There is reason to believe that iron accumulates in inflammatory tissue and in the reticulendothelial system in experimental infections. In chronic infection there is also a marked increase in copper in the plasma (Cartwright and Wintrobe), the meaning of which is still obscure.

Anemia of chronic renal disease is observed in many types of renal insufficiency, especially chronic nephritis, and it has been blamed on nitrogen retention. It now seems more probable that it is due to failure to elaborate erythropoietin, a marrow stimulating hormone believed from experimental evidence to be produced by the kidney.

Anemia of pregnancy is common, but is usually only moderate in degree. More than one factor may be involved. The condition is in part a pseudo-anemia, due to the progressive increase in plasma volume during pregnancy. In many cases there is some degree of iron-deficiency, leading to a hypochromic microcytic anemia. In exceptional cases (although common in India) a macrocytic anemia may develop similar to pernicious anemia.

Anemia of malignancy is of common occurrence. The cause may be obvious, such as chronic loss of blood from the gastrointestinal tract, interference with production of the intrinsic factor in carcinoma of the stomach, etc. By far the commonest form, however, is the simple chronic type of anemia with an apparently normal blood film. There is a reduced life span of the erythrocytes coupled with failure on the part of the bone marrow to meet the increased demand. In the case of the malignant *lymphomas* at least there is evidence to believe that autoimmune antibodies are produced which may coat the erythrocytes and thus interfere with their normal enzyme activity. In the *anemia of leukemia* as well as that of malignant lymphoma the most common erythroid defect is hemolysis, which is often associated with marrow insufficiency that may occur apart from infiltration of the marrow. Leukemia may occasionally first manifest itself clinically as acquired hemolytic anemia with a life span of the red cells of less than two weeks and a positive Coombs' test many months before leukemia could be recognized in blood smear or marrow biopsy (Desforges *et al.*).

Lead poisoning gives rise to a mild normocytic anemia. The characteristic feature is stippling or *punctate basophilia* of the red cells. This is believed to be due to the lead interfering with the synthesis of porphyrin and thus with the formation of hemoglobin. Stippling is more intense in early than in late cases of severe plumbism. It is of particular importance in the detection of industrial lead poisoning. The presence of *stippled cells* is no proof of *lead poisoning*, for they are seen in *pernicious anemia* and *leukemia*. It is probably safe to take anything over 200 stippled cells per 1,000,000 erythrocytes as positive evidence, especially if supported by a history of exposure to lead and not accompanied by other marked changes in the blood. A blue-black *lead line* along the gums serves to confirm a diagnosis of lead poisoning.

POLYCYTHEMIA

The term polycythemia means an increase in the number of the cells of the blood, but in practice this increase applies only to the red cells, so that a more accurate although less popular name is erythremia. The two terms are used interchangeably. The condition may be *primary, secondary* or *relative*.

Polycythemia Vera. Erythremia.—This is true primary erythremia, known also as *polycythemia rubra* and *Vaquez-Osler's disease*. In true erythremia there is an increase of the red cells irrespective of the needs of the body; they usually number from 7,000,-000 to 10,000,000 per c.mm. In addition there is an increase in the volume of the blood, a true plethora, so that the total increase of red cells is greater than is indicated by the hemocytometer count. The blood becomes more viscid owing to the great number of red cells. The hemoglobin is increased to 125 or 150 per cent, and the color index is about 1. There is a moderate leukocytosis with a polymorphonuclear count of over 80 per cent. Occasional primitive red and white cells (normoblasts and myelocytes) may be seen in the film. The bone marrow is markedly hyperplastic, the change being chiefly erythroblastic (normoblastic) in type, but with areas of myelocytic reaction. It also shows capillary thickening and marked subintimal and adventitial fibrosis of the arterioles. Splenomegaly is present, usually moderate, but sometimes marked. Absence of splenomegaly practically rules out primary polycythemia. The visceral vessels are greatly distended with blood.

Relation of Symptoms to Lesions.—The polycythemia appears to be due to a primary erythroblastic hyperplasia of the bone marrow which may be neoplastic in character. It has been classed with chronic myeloid leukemia and myelofibrosis as one of the "myeloproliferative" disorders (page 1085). A relationship to leukemia is suggested by the fact that occasional cases have changed from erythremia into leukemia of myelogenous type. A myeloblastosis in which the primary effect is on the erythroblastic tissue results in erythremia; when the primary effect is on leukoblastic tissue leukemia develops. The appearance of the patient is striking; the skin and mucous membrane of the mouth are red or bluish-red and the conjunctiva is blood-shot. The color is due to the increased number of red cells. For some unknown reason the disease is twice as common in males as in females. It is also relatively common in the Jew and uncommon in the Negro. In a number of cases it is associated with renal carcinoma. At postmortem the visceral vessels are greatly distended owing to the increased blood volume; this is best seen in the mesenteric veins and these vessels may be thrombosed. Vertigo and sensations of fullness in the head are common; they are due to the great distention of the cerebral vessels, so that when the patient stoops he feels as if there was a rush of blood to the head. Hemorrhage from the mucous membranes or into the retina may occur on account of this vascular fullness. Peptic ulcer (usually duodenal) is a not uncommon complication. Possibly this is due to thrombosis of small vessels. The enlargement of the spleen may be regarded as a compensatory arrangement to deal with the increased number of red cells. A helpful test is the estimation of arterial oxygen saturation, which distinguishes primary polycythemia from the secondary form due to hypoxia (Pike). A test for alkaline phosphatase activity in the polymorphonuclears gives a strongly positive result in primary polycythemia, a normal moderate result in secondary polycythemia, and a negative result in myelogenous leukemia (Leonard *et al.*).

Erythrocytosis.—This is secondary polycythemia, a compensating increase of red cells in conditions of *insufficient oxygenation* such as congenital heart disease, congestive heart failure, emphysema, pulmonary arteriosclerosis and residence at high altitudes. Erythrocytosis is a temporary condition, and corresponds to leukocytosis. There is no increase in leukocytes, a diagnositic point of great value in distinguishing the condition from polycythemia vera.

Relative Polycythemia.—This is merely an apparent increase in the number of blood cells, both red and white, owing to loss of plasma with resulting concentration of the circulating blood. The red cell mass is not increased. It may be caused by low fluid intake, marked loss of body fluids from persistent vomiting, severe diarrhea, etc., or a shift of fluid into tissue cells owing to loss of electrolyte from the extracellular compartment.

THE PURPURAS

The *hemorrhagic disorders* is a convenient term which covers a variety of conditions in which hemorrhage is a principal feature. A satisfactory classification and listing of the endless variations would be so extensive as to defeat the purpose of this book. For a more detailed study the reader is referred to the monograph by Stefanini and Dameshek. Suffice it to say that the hemorrhagic tendency may be due: (1) to a primary *defect in the vessel wall*, as in vascular purpuras; (2) to a much more serious *platelet deficiency*, either quantitative or qualitative, as in idiopathic thrombocytopenic purpura; or (3) to a *deficiency in the blood coagylation mechanism*, as in the so-called bleeding diseases.

Purpura is a condition characterized by a tendency to bleeding into the skin and from the mucous membranes. As a term it has less exact pathological significance than has anemia. There are endless ways of subdividing and classifying the purpuras, but for our purpose we may consider three main groups: (1) thrombocytopenic purpura hæmorrhagica, (2) thrombotic thromocytopenic purpura, and (3) allergic purpura. This omits the hundred and one miscellaneous conditions in which some degree of purpuric bleeding may occur in the skin and mucous membranes as a complication of other diseases.

Idiopathic Thrombocytopenic Purpura.— This condition, also called *Werlhof's disease*, and named idiopathic (I.T.P.) to distinguish it from thrombocytopenic purpura secondary to replacement of the bone marrow, was described by Werlhof in 1740, but it was not until 1910 that Duke demonstrated that the essential basis of the condition was a thrombocytopenia or decrease in the number of the blood platelets (thrombocytes).

SYMPTOMS.—The disease is commoner in young people of the female sex. The hemorrhages which form the chief clinical feature may be small petechiæ or large ecchymoses. There may be hemorrhages into the skin, hemorrhage from the mucous membrane of the nose, mouth, stomach, intestine, and uterus, and blood in the urine. The hemorrhage may be spontaneous or traumatic. Hemorrhage due to trauma may last for an hour or more; the bleeding-time is prolonged, but the clotting-time is normal. In hemophilia, on the other hand, the clotting-time is prolonged, but the bleeding-time is normal. A tourniquet applied to the arm so as to obstruct the venous but not the arterial flow causes petechiæ to appear below the tourniquet. The spleen may be moderately enlarged, and splenectomy may be attended by brilliant results. In this connection it must be recognized that the disease may follow an acute or a chronic course. The *acute* cases prove fatal in the course of a few weeks, and splenectomy is not of the slightest use. The *chronic* cases may go on for months or years, and for some unexplained reason there may be intermissions when the patient is free from all signs of the disease. It is in these cases that splenectomy gives the best results.

The most striking *change in the blood* is the thrombocytopenia. The normal number of platelets is 200,000 or 250,000 per c.mm. In purpura hæmorrhagica the number is usually below 60 000, and in severe cases they may entirely disappear. We can only guess at the cause of this remarkable disappearance. It seems probable that the platelets are defective in quality, just as are the red cells in hereditary hemolytic anemia and the hemoglobin in sickle cell anemia. They therefore fall an easy prey to the destructive and phagocytic powers of the reticuloendothelial cells in the spleen, liver, bone marrow, and lymph nodes. Splenectomy removes the largest collection of these cells, so that the fragile platelets are now able to hold their own. On the other hand a thrombocytopenic factor not of splenic origin has been demonstrated in the plasma of a number of these patients. When the plasma is injected into normal persons there is a prompt decrease in the number of platelets, often apparent within one hour and lasting nearly a week, due apparently to destruction of the platelets. The same result is obtained with the blood of patients from whom the spleen has been removed. The factor seems to be a constituent of the globulin fraction. It is possible to prepare an antiplatelet serum which when injected into an animal causes an extreme fall in the number of platelets with the appearance of purpuric symptoms. In some cases there may be no marked change in the platelet count, but in these there may be a qualitative change. In the general discussion of blood platelets we have seen that it is the small (young) platelets which are active in stopping bleeding, the larger ones being inactive. In purpura hæmorrhagica there may be many large and giant platelets, but although giants morphologically they are dwarfs functionally.

The blood shows other changes. There is an anemia of varying severity, depending on the degree of the hemorrhage. Leukocytosis is present after the hemorrhages. The clotting-time is normal and the bleeding-time greatly prolonged. A very characteristic feature due to the absence of platelets is loss of contraction power of the clot, so that it is unable to shrink from the side of the test tube in which the blood is collected.

Bone marrow changes are confined to the *megakaryocytes*, but these are of great significance. Although not reduced in number they show a variety of appearances which add up to arrest of maturation with failure to produce platelets in normal sensations of fullness in the head or a rush of blood to the head. Hemorrhages from mucous membranes or into the tissues (brain, retina *etc.*) are not uncommon. One of the most characteristic symptoms is great vascular engorgement with redness or cyanosis of the skin. The *spleen* is moderately enlarged and firm, and in some cases it may reach beyond the umbilicus. The *liver* is often slightly enlarged. A characteristic finding is the presence of megakaryocytes in the sinusoids of the spleen, the lining cells of which are swollen and resemble glandular epithelium.

Relation of Symptoms to Lesions.—The main symptom is the hemorrhage, the main lesion thrombocytopenia. In discussing the relation between these two it is fundamental to distinguish between spontaneous hemorrhage and the hemorrhage which follows trauma, both of which are present in purpura. The prolonged bleeding-time after an incision is due to the lack of platelets. Hemorrhage from a vessel is first arrested not by the production of fibrin but by the formation of a plug of platelets which adhere together and close the hole temporarily until a permanent clot is produced. In the absence of the platelets this all-important clot cannot be formed. The platelets also initiate the process of clotting, for when they disintegrate owing to injury they liberate the necessary thromboplastin. Only a small number of platelets are necessary for this purpose, and there are sufficient in most cases of purpura, so that the coagulation-time is normal. The excess of platelets causes retraction of the clot in some unknown way. In purpura there is no excess, so that the clot in the test tube fails to retract.

The cause of the spontaneous hemorrhage, which after all is much more common and important than hemorrhage due to trauma, remains a mystery. Presumably it bears some relation to the thrombocytopenia. It is as if the vascular pipes normally leaked, perhaps as the result of minimal trauma, but the leaks are continually plugged by the platelets. In thrombocytopenia such plugging is no longer possible. The long intermissions in the chronic cases are also difficult to explain. A final difficulty is the therapeutic effect of splenectomy. The theoretical basis for this form of treatment is the observation that removal of the spleen in a normal animal is followed by a marked rise in platelets. This occurs also in man, but in the course of a few weeks or months the platelets may fall again to their original level, and yet the patient may remain free from purpuric manifestations. There must be more in splenectomy than meets the eye. It is important to note that removal of the spleen may produce a temporary but not a permanent cure; the patient may remain well for a year or two, and then the purpuric manifestations may return. Cases should be followed for from three to five years before one can be certain that the condition is cured.

The possiblity or probability of some *immune anti-platelet (thrombocytopenic) factor* in the plasma which damages the megakaryocytes and destroys the platelets has come much to the fore. Platelet agglutinating antibodies, apparently a gamma globulin, have been demonstrated in the serum of some 70 patients. The transfusion of plasma from patients into normal persons may be followed by severe thrombocytopenic purpura and even changes in the megakaryocytes suggesting immaturity. The platelet-agglutinating factor is retained even after splenec-

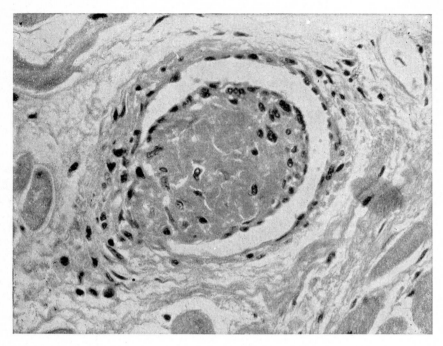

Fig. 616.—Thrombotic thrombocytopenic purpura. Polypoid occlusion in small vessels in myocardium. Crescentic-shaped lumen remains open. Segmental necrosis of vessel wall at point of attachment. × 320. (Kindness of Dr. John H. Fisher.)

tomy and when the platelet count has returned to normal. Nevertheless splenectomy may be invaluable in these patients. Normal platelets transfused into a patient with purpura survive only a few hours.

Neonatal thrombocytopenic purpura seems also to be due to the presence of circulating antiplatelet antibodies. These are maternal auto-agglutinins which are transmitted across the placenta to the fetus. Purpura due to antiplatelet antibodies both in the adult and in the child respond best to splenectomy or adrenocortical hormones.

Thrombotic Thrombocytopenic Purpura.— This uncommon disease is a real puzzle, if ever there was one. In spite of its name, sometimes abreviated for convenience of discussion to T.T.P., it bears no relation to purpura hæmorrhagica. The characteristic *clinical triad* is: (1) thrombocytopenic purpura, (2) severe hemolytic anemia, and (3) transitory neurological signs and symptoms such as mental confusion, stupor and convulsions, which wax and wane. The essence of the disease is the occurrence of myriads of tiny occlusions in the arterioles and larger capillaries (Fig. 616), but the nature of these occlusions is quite obscure. They would appear to be secondary to degenerative lesions of the vessels, which may be associated with microaneurysms (Meacham *et al.*). Others think that they represent masses of platelets, but investigation with fluorescent-antibody technique suggests that they are composed of fibrin. It would appear that a *serum platelet-destructive factor* is operative, with or without poor manufacture of platelets by the megakaryocytes. As the lesions are almost as widely distributed as those of polyarteritis nodosa, it is small wonder that the clinical picture may be varied. *Ischemic effects* are evident principally in the myocardium, adrenal and renal cortex, pancreas, and gray matter of the brain. The disease is usually acute and fatal in a few days or weeks, but in rare cases it is relapsing. The liver and spleen are generally enlarged. A hypersensitivity mechanism might account for the lesions, but there is no evidence of auto or isohemolysins or agglutinins.

Secondary Purpura.—So-called purpuric hemorrhages into the skin and mucous membranes may occur in a variety of pathological conditions. Toxic injury to the vessel walls may cause such hemorrhages in septicemia and in the infectious fevers, especially meningococcal meningitis, scarlet and typhus fevers, where they form a purpuric or hemorrhagic rash. Lesions of the bone marrow with reduction in the number of blood platelets may cause purpuric manifestations more nearly related to those of primary thrombocytopenic purpura, though the platelets seldom fall to so low a level. Widespread secondary carcinoma of the marrow, lymphatic leukemia, and pernicious anemia may produce secondary purpura of this type, but the most striking example is aplastic anemia with its great reduction in the number of megakaryocytes from which the platelets are formed.

Vascular Purpura.—In some persons there is an increased permeability of the small blood vessels, as a result of which both plasma and red cells can pass out into the tissues. The platelets are normal. The condition is not permanent, but comes on in attacks resembling anaphylaxis. These cases are calssed as *allergic purpura*, perhaps on insufficient grounds. At least it can be said that they are associated with one of several symptoms of allergy, such as erythema, urticaria, and effusions into serous cavities or loose connective tissue. The escape of red cells from the vessels causes purpuric lesions, but the escape of plasma may cause urticaria in the skin and even more important visceral lesions. The following forms of the *exudative diathesis* may be distinguished:

Purpura Simplex.—A mild condition of purpura occurring in children. The hemorrhages are confined to the skin and clear up in a week or two.

Henoch's Purpura.—In this form of the diathesis there are lesions in the skin, mucous membranes, and wall of the alimentary canal. Hemorrhage, urticaria, and erythema occur in the skin. There may be hemorrhage from the nose, stomach, bowel, and kidney. The most distinctive feature of this variety is the occurrence of *transudation of serum* into the wall of the stomach and intestine, thus causing pain, vomiting and diarrhea. Intus-

susception may occur. If the skin manifestations are absent or delayed, the patient is in danger of having his abdomen opened and his appendix removed. The occurrence of fever and leukocytosis makes this danger even greater. The renal lesions constitute the gravest complication, for in occasional cases they may lead to rapidly developing renal failure and death (Norkin and Wiener). The renal changes are identical with those of acute glomerulonephritis (type I nephritis of Ellis) with hypercellular glomerular tufts and even crescent formation.

Schönlein's Purpura.—This hardly deserves a special name. It is merely a form of the exudative diathesis in which the main manifestations are in the joints. The skin shows purpuric spots, urticaria, and erythema. There is a serous exudation into the joints causing an *acute arthritis* which is easily mistaken for rheumatic fever, especially as the temperature may be raised.

There seem to be grounds for believing that Schönlein-Henoch purpura is a generalized vascular disease of immunological origin (Kreidberg *et al.*). The clinical features and the histological lesions have been reproduced experimentally by the use of hetero-immune anti-blood vessel serums. The features of the disease have much in common with such a collagen disease as periarteritis nodosa, a condition generally considered to be of immunological origin. In some cases it is difficult to distinguish between acute vascular purpura and periarteritis nodosa. It would appear that an antigenic storm, with an antigen-antibody reaction at the end organ, in this case the small blood vessels, may determine the clinical and pathological picture.

THE BLEEDING DISEASES

The bleeding diseases are those in which the normal mechanism for the control of hemorrhage is deficient or deranged. The two most important tests in the study of these diseases are the *bleeding time* and the *coagulation time*. The former measures the vascular response and is independent of the coagulation mechanism, whereas the latter provides a criterion of the blood clotting mechanism. The two tests form a useful basis for the classification of the bleeding diseases into 3 main classes: (1) *bleeding and coagulation times normal;* (2) *bleeding time prolonged and coagulation time normal;* (3) *coagulation time prolonged and bleeding time normal.*

The infinitely complex subject of blood coagulation has already been considered in Chapter 6, page 126. With every year that passes the subject becomes more complicated. The essence of the problem, however, the bare skeleton on which the superstructure is built, remains more or less the same and may be compressed into one sentence: *In the process of coagulation thromboplastin acts on prothrombin in the presence of calcium to form thrombin, which in turn causes fibrinogen to change to fibrin.* The complications involve certain accessory factors which can accelerate the process, and unfortunately many of these factors parade under a variety of names. Hemophilia is dependent on an abnormality in fibrinogen, Christmas disease on thromboplastin production, and hemorrhagic disease of the newborn on deficiency of prothrombin.

Quick points out that the protection of the body against loss of blood depends on a series of integrated reactions. The three most important of these reactions are: (1) vascular, (2) platelet agglutination, and (3) coagulation of fibrinogen. Failure of any of these may result in hemorrhage. It has been well said that blood clotting studies "represent only one leg of a four-legged stool, of which the other legs are the vascular, the platelet and the fibrinolytic mechanism" (Stefanini and Dameshek.)

The *vascular reaction, i.e.* contraction of the injured vessel, is the first line of defense. In purpura hemorrhage occurs because the injured vessels fail to contract. The platelets and the coagulation time are normal. In hemophilia the vascular response is normal, so that bleeding stops promptly after a tooth extraction, but it may begin again in the course of a few hours when the vessel relaxes, because no permanent closure is possible.

Platelet agglutination may (or may not) succeed in arresting hemorrhage in the absence of a fibrin clot, as in afibrinogenemia. This mechanism is impaired in hemophilia, and here we may speculate on the possibility

of a thromboplastin deficiency due to the abnormal stability of the platelets.

Coagulation of fibrinogen is a slow process. Time is required for the thromboplastin liberated from the disintegrating platelets to accumulate. Clot formation is naturally imperfect in thrombocytopenic purpura.

After this brief review of the hemorrhagic diseases we may now proceed to a consideration of the condition which is par excellence "the bleeding disease," namely hemophilia.

Hemophilia.—Hemophilia, as everyone knows, is characterized by prolonged bleeding following a cut or trauma, but not by spontaneous hemorrhage. It is the most hereditary of all hereditary diseases, and repeats itself in generation after generation. Famous examples which occurred in the royal families of Europe are known to everyone, for the tragic gene weaved itself across the tapestry of modern Europe like a scarlet thread, probably originating as a mutation in one of the parents of Queen Victoria. It is almost invariably confined to males but transmitted by females of the family. It is, therefore, an example of sex-linked heredity. The hemorrhagic tendency appears in early childhood. A simple injury such as the extraction of a tooth or circumcision may give rise to a fatal hemorrhage. Hemorrhage into the large joints after slight trauma is common. The hemophilic joint, usually the knee or elbow, develops a condition like chronic arthritis; some of the blood is not absorbed, and this causes proliferation of the synovial membrane and erosion of the cartilage.

The striking *blood change* is the very *prolonged coagulation time,* sometimes several hours in length. The bleeding time, *i. e.,* the time blood continues to flow from a minute puncture of the skin, is normal in the majority of cases, as there is no thrombocytopenia; it is the platelets which plug such a puncture. When the clot does form it shows normal retraction. In these respects hemophilia differs from thrombocytopenic purpura hæmorrhagica, and also in the fact that spontaneous hemorrhage is the characteristic feature of the latter but not the former. The reason why blood continues to flow from a cut but not from the puncture made in estimating the bleeding-time is that hemorrhage from a cut is arrested primarily by the formation of a clot, whereas hemorrhage from a puncture is stopped by a plug of platelets.

The cause of this remarkable disease has long been a matter of dispute. In hemophilia the fibrinogen, prothrombin and calcium are present in normal amount. The thrombokinase liberated by the tissue cells is also normal, so that in testing the coagulation-time it is essential to collect the blood direct from a vein, and thus avoid the tissue juices. The essential deficiency is that of a plasma factor necessary for coagulation. This *anti-hemophilic factor* (AHF) is associated with the globulin or fibrinogen fractions of the plasma proteins, so that it is also known as anti-hemophilic globulin (AHG). The injection of normal blood freed from platelets markedly reduces the coagulation time of the hemophilic. Deficiency of another factor, the plasma thromboplastin component (PTC), is responsible for the variety of hemophilia known as Christmas disease. Still other factors have been described, for an account of which one of the several monographs devoted to hemophilia must be consulted.

It is now known that a bleeding disease identical with human hemophilia occurs in at least one strain of dogs. This provided us for the first time with an experimental animal in the study of hemophilia. By mating a hemophilic male with a carrier female it was possible to produce hemophilic female pups. This serves to confirm the occasional rare reported occurrence of hemophilia in the human female.

Christmas Disease.—It used to be thought that the bleeding disease was due to a specific defect in a single clotting factor, anti-hemophilic globulin (AHG). It is now known that any one of three different defects in the blood-clotting mechanism can cause the clotting characteristics and the clinical picture of hemophilia. The plasma components involved are: (1) *anti-hemophilic globulin* (AHG), deficiency for which is responsible for true hemophilia, (2) *plasma thromboplastin component* (PTC), lack of which will cause Christmas disease, and (3) *plasma thromboplastin antecedent* (PTA). The distinction between the three is more than academic, for the management and prognosis vary with each disease. Hemorrhage, joint involvement, and hematuria are most severe in AHG deficiency, of moderate severity in PTC deficiency, and mildest in PTA deficiency.

Christmas disease is due to *deficiency in the thromboplastin component* (PTC). Like hemophilia it is transmitted as a sex-linked recessive trait by the female to the male. The rather queer name is taken from the first English family in whom the trait was observed, and this was at Christmas. A more helpful name would be hemophilia B. The clinical picture may be distinguishable from that of true hemophilia, but the treatment is quite different. Hemophilia is at least 7 times as common as the Christmas variety.

Like the anti-hemophilic factor the plasma thromboplastin component takes part in the first stage of coagulation through the formation of thromboplastin, but it is not consumed in the process of clotting, so that it is present in good quantity in the serum, as opposed to plasma. In this respect the Christmas factor differs profoundly from the anti-hemophilic factor, which is used up in the process of clotting, and is therefore not present in serum. The Christmas factor is very stable on storage, so that it is not necessary to use fresh blood or plasma, in contrast to the case of the anti-hemophilic factor. The *thromboplastin generation test* is a simple method of detecting the deficiency in Christmas disease.

Hemorrhagic Disease of the Newborn.—This bleeding disorder is a self-limited condition confined to the first few days of life, but if severe it may prove fatal. It can be distinguished from neonatal thrombocytopenic purpura (page 1074) by the absence of any hereditary or familial factor, and by the presence of a normal level of blood platelets. The basis of the condition is an extremely *low plasma prothrombin*. As vitamin K is necessary for the formation of prothrombin, as there is no reservoir of vitamin K in the fetus, and as the infant's food contains very little of this vitamin during the first few days of life, it is but natural that the prothrombin level is distinctly low in the normal infant. Indeed it is curious that hemorrhage is not more frequent at this period. Severe bleeding may be expected when the plasma pro-thrombin is below 15 per cent of normal.

The most frequent loss of blood is from the gastrointestinal tract, followed by bleed-ing into the skin and subcutaneous tissue, the umbilical cord, and the viscera, including the adrenals. Visceral involvement may be accompanied by corresponding clinical man-ifestations but the hemorrhage is seldom massive. This disorder is responsible for the wise injunction in the Mosaic law which postponed circumcision until the eighth day after birth. Transfusion of whole blood and the administration of vitamin K will quickly restore the prothrombin level to normal

Afibrinogenemia.—This is a very rare bleeding disease due to a deficiency or rather absence of fibrinogen. The absence of the protein is de-tected by electrophoresis. The *clinical picture* is that of a hemorrhagic diathesis from birth. In contrast to hemophilia there is no sex incidence, and the blood is *incoagulable*, not merely delayed in clotting as in hemophilia. On the other hand all the other factors concerned with the arrest of hemorrhage such as vasoconstriction, forma ion of platelet thrombi, *etc.*, are normal, so that there is much less disability than in classical hemo-philia. The condition is recognized by observing that the plasma remains clear when heated to 60 °C; fibrinogen is coagulated at a temperature of 58 °C. It has been suggested that the defect is the result of an enzymatic destruction of fibrinogen. A particularly puzzling feature is the occurrence of a chronic arthritis, apparently of the rheumatoid type, in a considerable number of cases.

THE LEUKEMIAS

The essential feature of leukemia is a neoplastic proliferation of the leukoblastic tissues, as a result of which there is usually a great increase in the white cells of the blood. It is important to realize that, in spite of its name leukemia is essentially a disease of tissue, not of the blood. The increase may affect the myeloid cells (myelo-genous leukemia), the lymphoid cells (lymphoid leukemia), or the monocytes (monocytic leukemia). Occasionally there is proliferation of white cells in the tissues, but they fail to appear in the blood stream. Such a condition is called *aleukemic leukemia*, but it would be much better to speak of aleukemic myelosis, aleukemic lymphaden-osis, or aleukemic reticuloendotheliosis, de-pending on which of the leukoblastic tissues is affected. It is not a separate disease entity, but merely a phase of the leukemic state, for sooner or later the blood becomes flooded with white cells. Even before this happens abnormal types of leukocytes may be found in the blood, although the total count is not raised. The leukemia is usually of the lymphatic type. It is evident that it may be difficult or impossible to draw any sharp distinction between aleukemic lymph-adenosis and lymphosarcoma, for the latter condition may also terminate with a leu-kemic blood picture. There can be little doubt that from the pathological standpoint these conditions are closely related.

The disease is not peculiar to man. A leukemic condition characterized by the formation of tumor-like masses and a great increase in the white cells of the blood is found in the fowl, but as it differs in a num-ber of ways from the human disease it is better called leukosis. Conditions more closely resembling human leukemia are found in horses, dogs, mice and other animals Study of the leukoses, particularly in the fowl and the mouse, has yielded much valu-able information to which brief reference will be made presently.

The leukemias fall into three main groups *myelogenous*, *lymphatic*, and *monocytic leu-kemias*. To these may be added a fourth *acute leukemia*. Rare cases in which plasma cells are present in the blood and leukoblastic tissues in large numbers are known as *plasma cell leukemia*. The distinction between the fully developed and classical types is very easy. Sometimes the distinction is very difficult. The more acute the disease, the more difficult is it to be certain of the nature of the abnormal white cells, for it is the prim-itive blood cells which appear in the acute cases, and these lack distinguishing charac-teristics.

In all forms of leukemia there is a marked increase in the number of the white cells But such an increase is not of itself pathog-nomonic. Temporary counts as high as 100,000 may be met with in infective condi-tions, and as the result of treatment the white cell count may fall to normal in a

PLATE XVII

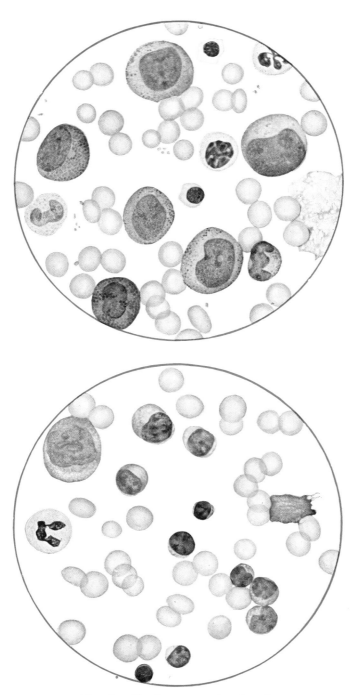

Fig. 1. Myelogenous Leukemia

Myelocytes in various stages of development, an eosinophilic myelocyte, an eosinophil
polymorphonuclears, normoblasts and platelets.

Fig. 2. Lymphatic Leukemia

Numerous small lymphocytes and one nuclear smudge, but no platelets.

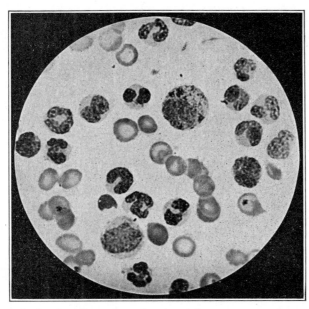

FIG. 617.—Myelogenous leukemia. Several myelocytes and very many polymorphonuclear leukocytes.
× 1000.

leukemia. Much more characteristic is the presence of immature white cells, but these also may occur in other conditions which throw a strain on the bone marrow, and a terminal leukemoid blood picture may closely simulate an acute terminal leukemia. At the same time it must be understood that in the great majority of cases the correct diagnosis can be made without the slightest difficulty merely by a glance at the stained blood film.

Myelogenous Leukemia.—The essential lesion in this disease is a hyperplasia of the myeloid tissue. The nature of this hyperplasia will be discussed later. Myeloid cells are found in abundance in the spleen, lymph nodes, liver, kidney, and other organs. This probably represents an infiltration by the cells of the blood, but in such organs as the liver and spleen it may well represent an extramedullary formation of new cells, a question discussed in connection with Myeloproliferative Disease (page 1085).

The Blood.—In myelogenous leukemia there is a great increase in the granular series of cells, both primitive (myelocytic) and adult (polymorphonuclear) in type (Fig. 617); the cells in either of these groups may

be neutrophil, eosinophil, or basophil. The myelocyte usually forms the prominent feature of the film (Plate XVI, Fig. 1). It is a large cell about double the size of the polymorphonuclear, with an indented or lobed nucleus and abundant cytoplasm containing granules which may be fine and neutrophil, or coarse and eosinophil, or basophil. Neutrophil granulocytes contain a highly labile alkaline phosphatase. This only makes its appearance about the myelocyte stage of development. In chronic myeloid leukemia the activity of this enzyme is greatly reduced. More primitive leukocytes are seen in the terminal stages or in the acute form of leukemia; these are myeloblasts with non-granular cytoplasm. The total leukocyte count averages 200,000, but it may go as high as 500,000 or even 1,000,000. As a result of radiation, benzol treatment or an acute infection such as pneumonia, there may be a great drop in the cell count, sometimes to normal. All the elements of myeloid tissue tend to take part in the abnormal activity; in other words, there may be a complete myelosis. Primitive red cells, therefore, appear in the blood, and normoblasts are more numerous than in any other disease—far more numerous than in pernicious anemia. Sometimes there are macrocytes and megaloblasts in considerable numbers. In spite of this activity in the bone marrow there is a marked and progressive anemia, owing to the erythroblastic tissue being crowded out by the myeloid cells. In extreme cases there may be equal numbers of red and white cells. The megakaryocytes also take part in the myelosis, and there is, therefore, a great increase of platelets in the blood, sometimes to 2,000,000. The megakaryocytes themselves may be found in the blood. If it is remembered that there may be 1,000,000 white cells, 1,000,000 red cells, and 1,000,000 platelets, some of the principal features of the blood picture may be recalled. As the lymphocytes are not formed in the marrow, the percentage count is greatly reduced.

The most important feature in any form of leukemia is the presence of *stem cells*. These show that the case is definitely one of leukemia; the adult forms indicate the type of leukemia. Stem cells are recognized by their deeply basophilic cytoplasm, relatively large nucleus, and the nature of their nuclear pattern, the latter serving to distinguish them from adult lymphocytes. In the lymphocytes the nuclear chromatin forms a coarse pattern in heavy blocks, but no nucleoli can be distinguished. In contrast to this the nuclear chromatin of the stem cell is arranged in very fine strands like a sieve, and one or more nucleoli can usually be seen.

Bone Marrow.—In *myelogenous leukemia*, as the name implies, the basis of the disease is a leukoblastic overactivity of the myeloid tissues. The red marrow becomes filled with immature white cells, and the fatty yellow marrow is converted into actively functioning tissue. Its gross appearance varies. It is firm, and may be gray, brown, or red; sometimes it is soft and purulent. The principal cell is the neutrophil myelocyte, but the microscopic picture is a complex one, for all varieties of leukocytes and of myelocytes are present. There are also groups of non-granular myeloblasts, and these cells may enter the blood in considerable numbers in the terminal stage of the disease. The megakaryocytes are increased in number, thus accounting for the rise in the platelet count. The erythroblastic tissue is largely replaced by leukoblastic elements.

Spleen.—In myelogenous leukemia the spleen is greatly enlarged and may fill the entire abdomen, sometimes weighing as much as 10,000 grams. It is dark in color, and infarcts are common, due probably to the formation of leukocytic thrombi in the small vessels. Microscopically the lymphoid tissue has disappeared, and the pulp has the same structure as the marrow, being crowded with myeloid cells of every description. It is probable that most of these cells have been arrested by the splenic filter, but there may possibly be some myeloid metaplasia, an assumption by the spleen of its primitive blood-forming function.

Liver.—The liver may be moderately or markedly enlarged, and small nodules may be seen on the cut surface. Microscopically the arrangement of the leukemic cells is often strikingly different in the myelogenous and lymphatic types. In myelogenous leukemia the myelocytes distend the sinusoids to a marked degree, whereas in the lymphatic form the leukemic cells are for the most part gathered in large collections in the portal areas, although many are also seen in the sinusoids. In typical cases the distinction can be made at a glance at the liver sections (Fig. 618), but unfortunately every case is not a typical one.

Other Organs.—The *lymph nodes* may be of normal size or slightly enlarged. Even when not enlarged they often present a microscopic appearance similar to that of the spleen, a crowding of the vessels and sinusoids with myeloid cells. The *kidneys* are slightly enlarged and show the usual myeloid engorgement. The heart, lungs and other organs show a similar condition.

In addition to these specific changes the effects of anemia may be observed, such as fatty degeneration of the heart. Cerebral hemorrhage is a not infrequent cause of death. Hemorrhage from the mucous membranes is characteristic of the acute rather than the chronic form of leukemia, but in any of the forms there may be hemorrhage into the retina or into the inner ear, resulting in impairment of vision and sudden deafness.

Lymphatic Leukemia.—In the lymphatic form of leukemia the lymphoid cells of the

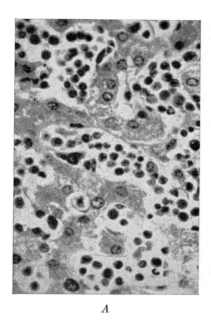 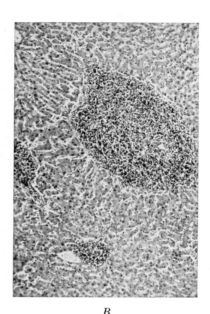

A   B

Fig. 618.—Liver in leukemia.   *A*, myelogenous, *B*, lymphatic.

blood are increased, the myeloid cells being unaffected. This does not mean that the bone marrow is uninvolved, for lesions are always found in that tissue. Indeed hyperplasia of the marrow may be so great as to cause bone pain, and the sternum may be tender on percussion. The chief *clinical feature* is an enlargement of the superficial lymph nodes all over the body. The spleen also is moderately enlarged, sometimes very markedly so. The clinical picture varies in different cases. For many months or even for a number of years the patient may remain in reasonably good health, while the lymph nodes and spleen slowly increase in size and the leukocyte count creeps upward without any change in the hemoglobin and platelets. Many of the older patients may die *with* rather than *from* the disease. Sooner or later evidence of bone marrow failure makes its appearance, the hemoglobin level falls, and death follows rapidly from anemia and exhaustion.

The Blood.—In lymphatic leukemia only the lymphoid cells are increased, and may form as much as 99 per cent of the total count, although 90 per cent is a commoner figure (Plate XVI, Fig. 2). The average count is 50,000 to 100,000, rather lower than in the myelogenous form. The lymphocytes contain less cytoplasm than the normal small lymphocytes, so that they may appear as naked nuclei, and the cytoplasm usually contains no azurophil granules. Many of the lymphocytes appear to be dead, so that in the slide they look like a smeared nucleus, the so-called smudge. Primitive myeloid cells may appear in the later stages, owing to irritation of the marrow produced by deposits of lymphoid cells. This appearance coincides in time with the development of points of tenderness in the bones. Secondary anemia becomes marked when the marrow replacement reaches a severe degree, but there is none of the erythroblastic activity characteristic of myelogenous leukemia, so that there are no normoblasts or only a very few. For the same reason blood platelets are much diminished in the later stages.

A consideration of the red cells and the platelets is of more use for differentiating myelogenous from lymphatic leukemia in difficult cases than is a study of the primitive white cells. Anemia is much more marked in the myelogenous than in the lymphatic form and megaloblasts are frequent. In lymphatic leukemia there is a great fall or complete disappearance of the platelets associated with bleeding, as indicated by petechiæ in the skin and occult blood in the stool and stomach contents, whereas in the myelogenous form the platelets are not greatly affected until the late stages of the disease.

Morbid Anatomy.—The lymph nodes are everywhere enlarged, the most extreme change being in the abdominal glands, which may be as large as walnuts. The normal structure is entirely replaced by lymphocytes, and the microscopic picture cannot be distinguished from that of lymphosarcoma. The intestinal and other lymphoid tissues show the same enlargement. In the *spleen* the hyperplasia of lymph follicles is so great that the pulp has completely disappeared. The organ is moderately enlarged, occasionally greatly so. The *liver* is slightly enlarged, and shows the characteristic large accumulations of lymphocytes in the portal tracts to which reference has already been made, and which serve to distinguish the microscopic picture from that of myelogenous leukemia (Fig. 618, p. 1081). The *skin* and *mucous membranes* may contain nodules of leukemic cells. It has been suggested that mycosis fungoides, a disease in which multiple nodules develop in the skin, is essentially akin to lymphatic leukemia. The *bone marrow* is similar in gross appearance to that of myelogenous leukemia. Microscopically in the late stages the myeloid tissue is largely replaced by lymphocytes.

Acute Leukemia.—The acute forms of leukemia offer a striking contrast to the chronic forms both clinically and pathologically. The disease may commence with startling suddenness, and its true character may not be suspected until near the end. In many cases the correct diagnosis is missed. Indeed, it is probable that acute leukemia is a good deal more common than either of the chronic forms. It is a disease of early life, being commonest in the first decade, and rarely seen over the age of twenty-five years. The diagnosis must be made with caution for two reasons. In the first place acute infections about the mouth and throat in children may be associated with a very high leukocyte count and swelling of the lymph glands. In the second place it must be remembered that a chronic myelogenous leukemia may terminate with an acute picture and a flooding of the blood by primitive cells (myeloblasts). Bleeding from the nose and gums, septic infections of the mouth and tonsils, sudden enlargement of the cervical glands, and a pronounced degree of fever are common and naturally misleading early symptoms. Purpuric hemorrhages in the skin are common. The disease runs a very acute and malignant course, usually terminating fatally in a few weeks or months.

The Blood.—The white cell count is seldom very high, and in the early stages it may be subleukemic (below 30,000) or aleukemic. At first sight nearly all the cells appear to be large lymphocytes (Plate XVII), and it used to be thought that most cases of acute leukemia were of the lymphatic type. It now appears probable that the acute cases are mostly myeloid in type and that the predominant cells are myeloid stem cells. It is often impossible to distinguish with certainty between a myeloblast and a lymphoblast, although the hematologists give a number of fine points of difference. The ordinary worker who is not a specialist in hematology will learn more by the indirect method of studying the more fully developed cells than by trying to stain stem cells by peroxidase or other special methods. If the primitive cells are myeloblasts, some myelocytes and a few polymorphonuclears will be noticed. If they are lymphoblasts the only differentiation is toward the lymphocyte. In such cases there may be very large lymphocytes with pale nuclei, the so-called *Rieder's cells.* When moving pictures of tissue cultures of stem cells are studied, striking differences at once become apparent, both in form and in method of locomotion (Rich, Wintrobe and Lewis). The myeloblasts become elongated and wriggle through the culture in a highly characteristic twisting, writhing, worm-like manner, whereas the lymphoblasts maintain a rather fixed shape like that of a hand mirror with a tail-like process, and move forward in a steady unperturbed manner, whilst monocytes continually throw out pseudopodia bordered by a broad, filmy, undulating, ruffle-like margin, and dart now in one direction, now in

PLATE XVIII

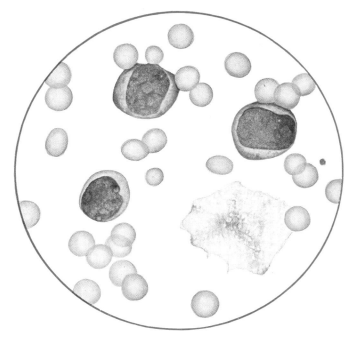

Acute Leukemia

Three blast cells and one nuclear smudge.

another. Roentgen-ray therapy causes an initial drop in the white cell count; when it again goes up, the cells will be much more mature and readily recognized. There is severe anemia and great diminution of the platelets. Megaloblasts may be numerous, so that in the early aleukemic stage the disease may be mistaken for pernicious anemia.

Morbid Anatomy.—The tonsils are often enlarged. The lymph glands are nearly always enlarged, but not invariably. The spleen is moderately enlarged, sometimes greatly so, but in the very acute cases it may be of almost normal size. Its sinuses are packed with myeloblasts, and the endothelial cells lining the sinuses may be very prominent. The heart muscle fibers may be separated by great numbers of myeloblasts. The bone marrow is red and is packed with myeloblasts, together with a few myelocytes and a very few red cells. The erythroblastic tissue of the marrow is so rapidly and completely replaced that a profound anemia may develop in the course of a week or two. In response to chemotherapeutic agents the marrow may return to an apparently normal state for a brief period. Such marrow has been obtained by multiple aspirations of the iliac bone, stored at $-70°C.$ and used as an infusion of autologous marrow during a relapse (McGovern *et al.*).

Monocytic Leukemia.—A rare form of so-called monocytic leukemia has been described, which presents the clinical picture of acute leukemia, and usually kills the patient in three or four months. It is probable that at least the majority of cases represent an atypical phase of myelogenous leukemia, because a large percentage have ended as the latter disease. The majority of the cells appear to be monocytes.

Plasma Cell Leukemia.—This is the condition commonly known as *multiple myeloma* or *plasma cell myeloma*, and since, as the name suggests, the most striking lesions are usually those of the bone marrow, it is customary to regard it as a bone disease, for which reason it is discussed in Chapter 43. On the other hand it can be regarded as a chronic form of leukemia involving plasma cells with the conspicuous lesions localized in the flat bones, but with minimal invasion of the blood stream (Dameshek and Gunz). From the hematological point of view the condition is aleukemic or subleukemic, there usually being only from 1 to 5 per cent of plasma cells in the peripheral blood. There is a general proliferation of plasmacytes throughout the marrow, as well as in other tissues. Neoplastic masses of these cells encroach on the cortex, causing osteolysis with danger of resulting fracture. The flat bones and skull are most involved, owing to their abundant content of red marrow. The plasma cell has a remarkable property of producing protein in large amount, more particularly globulin. There is accordingly a hyperglobulinemia, mostly gamma globulins, and this is responsible for such features as: (1) great elevation of the sedimentation rate, (2) red cell rouleaux formation in blood smears, (3) Bence-Jones' proteinuria, (4) interference with normal antibody production and therefore increased susceptibility to infection, (5) renal damage, and (6) amyloidosis. All of these will be discussed in connection with plasma cell myeloma (page 1262).

Relation of Symptoms to Lesions.—The clinical manifestations of the three main forms of leukemia naturally differ considerably. The *age incidence* of acute leukemia is in early life, being commonest in the first five years; myelogenous leukemia usually occurs between the ages of twenty-five and forty-five years, and lymphatic leukemia between the ages of forty-five and sixty years. The patient suffers from the usual weakness, dyspnea and palpitation of *severe anemia*, due to replacement of the erythroblastic tissue in the bone marrow. There may be a fullness and dragging sensation in the abdomen due to the great *splenic enlargement*. This enlargement may sometimes be as great in the lymphatic as in the myelogenous form. The condition of the superficial *lymph nodes* is not always a reliable indication as to the presence or absence of general lymphoid hyperplasia, for the deep nodes (abdominal and mediastinal) may be greatly enlarged though the superficial ones are barely palpable. *Pain and tenderness of the sternum* and more rarely of the long bones may be quite striking; this is caused by the hyperplastic-neoplastic process going on in the interior of the bone. *Hemorrhages* are common in all the varieties, particularly in the acute form, so that leukemia is classed as one of the "bleeding diseases." There may be hemorrhage from the nose, mouth, or bowel, or into the brain or retina. Bleeding gums and necrotic processes in the mouth, associated with fever and severe and progressive anemia are characteristic features of acute leukemia. The cause of the hemorrhage in leukemia is obscure. The coagulability of the blood is greatly decreased, but the reason for this is also unknown. *Priapism* may occur in the myelogenous form, due probably to engorgement of the penile cavernous tissue. *Ascites*, sometimes chylous, and chylous effusions in the chest may be due to pressure of enlarged glands on the thoracic duct. The *basal metabolic rate* is high owing probably to the increased metabolic activity of the great numbers of immature cells. The *fever*, which is most marked in acute leukemia, may be due to the same cause. A large amount of uric acid may appear in the urine owing to disintegration of nuclear material and liberation of nucleoproteins. The presence of Bence-Jones' protein in the urine is characteristic of bone marrow lesions, being also found in chloroma and more particularly in multiple myeloma.

The accompanying table summarizes some of the features of the various forms of leukemia, and may therefore be of use in reviewing the subject.

The Etiology of Leukemia.—The leukemic process is one of the most interesting in the whole realm of pathology, for it is not quite like anything else. It presents us with a double problem, for we are not certain as to its nature, and we know even less about its causation. In being a disorderly non_

THE PRINCIPAL TYPES OF LEUKEMIA AND THEIR IMPORTANT PATHOLOGICAL CHARACTERISTICS

Characteristics	Stem cell (Acute)	Chronic Granulocytic	Chronic Lymphocytic	Plasmacytic (Multiple Myeloma)
Anemia	Marked	Moderate	None to slight	Moderate
Fever	Marked	None to slight	Marked	Slight to moderate
Bone pain	Moderate	None to slight	None to slight	Marked
Lymph node enlargement	Slight to moderate	None to slight	Moderate to marked	Slight
Splenomegaly	Slight	Greatest enlargement, up to 10,000 grams	Moderate	Slight
Hepatomegaly	None to slight	Moderate to marked	None to slight	Normal to slight
Leukocyte count	3,000–200,000	200,000–1,000,000	50,000–100,000	10,000–40,000
Peripheral blood differential	Stem cells (blasts)	Myelocytes, segmented cells	Mature lymphocytes	Plasma cells Rouleaux formation
Platelet count	Very low	Increased initially; falls terminally	Very low to absent (late)	Normal early; low terminally
Bleeding tendency	Marked	Moderate terminally	Marked terminally	Slight
Predilection	Children	Young adults	Older adults	Males past middle age

altruistic proliferation of the cellular elements of the blood it certainly suggests neoplasia more than anything else.

There are two principal features of the process. The first is the hyperplasia of marrow or lymphoid tissue; the second what has been called the release mechanism, which regulates the escape of the proliferating cells into the circulation. When this mechanism shuts down, the proliferating cells remain at the site of production and the disease is in the aleukemic phase. We do, however, know something of two agents: ionizing radiation in human leukemia, viruses in animals.

Ionizing radiation is definitely leukemogenic. This is seen in the higher incidence of the disease in patients who have been exposed to therapeutic radiation, and even more in radiologists, amongst whom the disease is 8 to 10 times as common as in non-radiologists. It is also said that the incidence is twice as great in doctors as in the general population. The part which *atomic radiation* may play is of course illustrated by the numerous cases of leukemia which developed subsequent to the bomb explosions at Hiroshima and Nagasaki. More than half of these cases were acute, the remainder being of chronic myelogenous type.

Viruses can produce leukemic-like conditions in animals. *Fowl leukosis*, a very serious economic disease, is marked by greatly increased numbers of red cells, as well as myelocytes and lymphocytes, so that it is hardly comparable with human leukemia. The work of Ludwik Gross on *transmissable mouse leukemia* has aroused the greatest interest. Gross used an inbred strain of mice, Ak, 70 per cent of which develop lymphatic leukemia at middle age (seven to ten months) and a C3H strain in which the incidence of spontaneous leukemia is only 0.5 per cent. The carrier mice, earmarked to develop leukemia later on, remain in perfect health till the appointed time. When cell-free filtrates from the organs of leukemic Ak mice are inoculated into newborn C3H mice, less than 24 hours old, over 80 per cent develop leukemia when they reach middle age. As we have seen in the discussion of the etiology of cancer,

newborn mice are used because antibody development has not yet begun at that age. If the inoculated mice are more than 7 days old, no leukemia develops in later life. In support of the hypothesis that the leukemogenic agent or agents are viruses is the work of Stewart and her associates, who showed that these agents when grown in tissue culture would induce parotid tumors, although not leukemia. When leukemic extracts are examined with the electron microscope, large quantities of small particles become apparent. Inoculation of these particles into newborn mice is followed in some instances by the development of leukemia in the course of from 6 to 12 months.

The passage of the disease from one generation to another is explained by what Gross terms *"vertical transmission,"* the pathogenic agent being transmitted by germinal cells or occasionally, as in the mammary cancer of mice, through the mother's milk. The agent remains latent for a considerable period of the animal's life span, so that the host appears in perfect health, but can still transmit the seeds of the disease to its offspring. This still leaves room for the action of activating agents such as ionizing radiation and chemical poisons.

To what extent, if any, these results can be applied to leukemia in man is a moot point. We have no proof that mouse leukemia is identical with human leukemia. It may be noted that in the mouse there is nothing corresponding to the acute leukemia of childhood. Mouse leukemia seems to be due to an inter-relationship of a number of factors, including a genetic one. It may well be that the different forms of human leukemia have different causes, just as do the infective granulomata which may resemble one another so closely histologically, but which may be caused by such different agents. Indeed it is now believed that acute leukemia may differ from the chronic forms of leukemia in being the result of changes in the genetic material of the cell. In acute but not in chronic leukemia chromosome abnormalities have been reported with reduction in the chromosome count.

Myeloproliferative Disease.—This term has been suggested to describe a primarily proliferative disease in which the marrow as well as the extramedullary sites of prenatal erythropoiesis are involved (Vaughan and Harrison). It is a panmyelopathy in which, in response to some unknown stimulus, there is proliferation of red cells, leukocytes, monocytes, and megakaryocytes with their offspring, the platelets. It is therefore the reverse of a pancytopenia, and represents a proliferation of blood-forming cells *en masse* or as a unit rather than as single elements. Extramedullary myeloid proliferation is one of the basic features of the disease. This results in splenomegaly which may be extreme, and in lesser enlargement of the liver. The splenic lesions are described in connection with *myeloid metaplasia of the spleen* on page 1099. These extramedullary features may precede any marked changes in the blood by a considerable period. New myeloid tissue may also be formed in the kidneys, adrenals, pancreas and pituitary. This new tissue may be the site of hemorrhage or thrombosis.

One of the most puzzling features of the disease is the development of *myelofibrosis* in the later stages. This may be due to cells from which the hemopoietic cells originate, finally involving the fibroblasts and reticular cells, with a laying down of ground substance and eventually fibrosis and osteogenesis. Repeated marrow biopsies reveal this fibrosis to be progressive (Taylor and Simpson).

The blood picture will naturally vary greatly, depending on the stage of the disease. In the proliferative phase there may be (1) a normoblastosis and reticulocytosis; (2) neutrophilia with immature myeloid cells; and (3) thrombocytosis. Abnormal cells, including megakaryocytes, may appear in the peripheral blood in large numbers, where they may be mistaken for cancer cells if the patient has cancer. As myelofibrosis develops there will be a corresponding impoverishment in the blood elements with hypochromic anemia. Deep bone pain may be an early feature of the disease. Hemorrhages and thrombotic complications are frequent, and these may be responsible for the development of fresh clinical features such as sudden adrenal insufficiency. The disease tends to run a rather static course

for a number of years unless interrupted by some vascular complication.

CHLOROMA.—This very rare tumor is of theoretical interest, because it forms a link between leukemia and tumor growth; it is a malignant tumor with a leukemic blood picture. Green tumors (*kloros*, green) are formed in the flat bones of children and young adults, especially in the face and skull, where they may fill the orbit and push the eye forward. The sternum, spine, ribs and pelvic bones (red-marrow bones) are involved, and occasionally the long bones. There may be green tumors in the liver, kidneys, muscles and skin. The spleen and lymph nodes are often enlarged. The green color fades on exposure to air; the nature of the pigment is unknown. The bone marrow of the long bones is filled with green tumor tissue. The tumors which can be detected clinically are under the periosteum, but it is probable that the primary growth is in the marrow, and that the periosteal tumors are secondary. The lesions consist of large non-granular cells similar to those of acute leukemia; there may be numerous granular myelocytes. The tissues (frozen sections) give the oxidase reaction. The tumors are much more invasive than the cellular collections of leukemia. The *blood* shows a picture of acute leukemia, although the total white cell count is not always increased. It used to be thought that the abnormal cells belonged to the lymphoid series, but it is now believed that they are myeloblasts. The distribution of the lesions in chloroma resembles that of multiple myeloma, the chief distinction between the two being that in myeloma the tumor cells do not usually enter the blood stream. Both are invariably fatal.

AGRANULOCYTOSIS

This condition is characterized by a remarkable disappearance of the granulocyte series of leukocytes from the blood and an accompanying drop in the total white cell count. It may not be possible to distinguish some cases from acute leukemia in the aleukemic stage. A differential point of value is that the *platelet count* is high in agranulocytosis but low in aleukemic leukemia. Most of the patients have been middle-aged women, and when accompanied, as is commonly the case, by necrotizing gangrenous lesions of the mouth involving the tonsils, gums, and even the bone of the jaw, it has in the past been nearly invariably fatal. The striking characteristic of the necrotic lesions of agranulocytosis is the almost entire absence of polymorphonuclears. There may be multiple ulcers of the stomach and intestine, and sometimes of the vulva. The association of leukopenia and destructive lesions of the mouth is known as *agranulocytic angina*. The condition is not a disease *sui generis*, but rather a symptom complex, an indication of the action of some powerful leukocidal poison, some destroyer of the bone marrow, which may or may not be accompanied by severe infection of the mouth. Three groups of cases may be recognized: (1) A primary form with fever, ulcerative mouth lesions, and agranulocytosis, so that leukocytes are absent from the necrotic ulcers. No definite cause such as a constant and specific microörganism can be found. (2) Malignant leukopenia of bacterial origin, as in pneumonia, osteomyelitis, etc. (3) Malignant leukopenia of toxic origin; benzol, antisyphilitic arsenical preparations, and certain analgesic and antipyretic drugs such as amidopyrine and the barbiturate series, *i.e.*, chemicals containing the benzene ring, may so depress the bone marrow that leukopenia results and bacterial infection of the mouth may develop in consequence. Should the patient continue to take the drug, as all too often happens, a fatal termination can hardly be avoided. Many of the patients display a hypersensitiveness to drugs, and probably this is a factor of great importance.

The *pathogenesis* of the second and third groups is easy to understand. That of the first group is much more obscure. It is known that certain pyogenic bacteria are capable of producing a leukocidin, a toxin specifically lethal for the leukocytes, the granular series in particular. Staphylococcus aureus, Streptococcus hemolyticus, and Streptococcus viridans are the most powerful members of this group. Pyogenic bacteria can produce agranulocytosis only when prevented from active penetration of the tissues, otherwise they merely excite leukocytosis. This suggests that some circumscribed focus of infection is present in the primary cases.

The *bone marrow* in the acute cases shows lack of maturation in the granular series of cells which therefore largely disappear, together with hyperplasia of the stem cells. The essence of the disease seems to be a maturation arrest affecting the granular leukocytes, so that they are unable to enter the circulation (poverty in the midst of plenty), a situation strictly comparable to that of pernicious anemia. In the more prolonged cases there may be hypoplasia of the myeloid tissue which contains large numbers of plasma cells and lymphocytes. In recovery there is a rapid change of stem cells into myelocytes and polymorphonuclears. In the neutropenia of overwhelming sepsis and arsphenamine poisoning there is not the same disappearance of adult granular cells from the marrow, and segmented forms can be seen.

The prognosis in the past has been extremely grave. This, however, has been greatly altered for the better by the use of antibiotics to combat the infection, and of pyridoxin (vitamin B_6) and blood transfusions, empirical but occasionally beneficial forms of therapy.

Primary Splenic Neutropenia.—This condition, described by Wiseman and Doan in 1939, is characterized by marked neutropenia, splenomegaly and marrow hyperplasia. The white cell count may be extraordinarily low owing to disappearance of the neutrophils, in one case. falling to 150 per c.mm. In a few hours after splenectomy the count may be increased 20 times. The condition is apparently a *manifestation of hypersplenism*, there being an accelerated destruction of the granular leukocytes by the reticuloendothelial cells of the spleen. It is permanently cured by splenectomy. The spleen is rich in highly phagocytic cells containing polymorphonuclear leukocytes and erythrocytes. There is often a hemolytic anemia and a diminution of platelets. The condition may therefore be compared to congenital hemolytic anemia and thrombocytopenic purpura, to which it evidently is related as far as the spleen is concerned. "The reticuloendothelial cells of the spleen when on a rampage of destruction may selectively choose as victim any *one* of the elements of marrow origin passing through this organ, but more often than not other innocent bystanding elements suffer likewise in some degree. Splenectomy is always followed by an increase in all circulating blood elements whenever applied in any one of these conditions" (Wiseman and Doan).

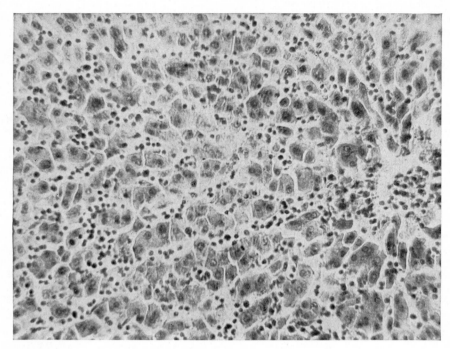

FIG. 619.—Liver in infectious mononucleosis. Central vein and sinusoids packed with "mononucleosis" cells. Note similarity to leukemia. × 230. (Kindness of Dr. John H. Fisher.)

INFECTIOUS MONONUCLEOSIS

The condition about to be discussed can hardly be described as essentially a blood disease, any more than can leukemia. Its older and alternative name is *glandular fever*, indicating the important part played by the lymph glands or nodes. It has indeed been classified as a leukemoid condition, and even as "an atypical form of acute leukemia with a self-limiting cou se and in which reversal to the previously no mal status always takes place" (Dameshek and Gunz).

The *lesions* are seldom seen, because recovery is the almost invariable rule unless one of the complications such as rupture of the spleen proves fatal. There is a widespread proliferation of a characteristic mononuclear cell in the lymphoid tissue throughout the body. This is most pronounced in the *spleen*, particularly in cases of spontaneous rupture, but leukemic-like infiltrations are also present in the lymph nodes, marrow and liver (Fig. 619). Two other sites deserve special mention by reason of their

relation to the clinical picture. These are: (1) the nasopharynx and gastrointestinal tract which are the site of lymphoid collections with ulceration of the overlying mucosa and resulting hemorrhage in these regions; (2) the nerve roots and meninges which are infiltrated with the characteristic cells, these lesions being reponsible for degeneration of the myelin sheaths and the development of a slowly ascending motor paralysis associated with severe root pains, the picture known as the *Guillain-Barré syndrome*.

Although sporadic cases occur, the disease is most readily recognized in epidemic form, the high degree of infectivity being indicated in the name. The *clinical features* are a mild degree of *fever* lasting for two or three weeks in young persons, nearly always under the age of thirty and frequently medical students or nurses, a very *sore throat*, enlarged and tender cervical *lymph nodes* and sometimes the axillary and inguinal groups, moderate enlargement of the *spleen*, and an increase of the mononuclear cells of the blood. In less than 1 per cent of cases there may be severe neurological disturbances including stiffness of the neck, convulsions, and other signs of acute meningitis or encephalitis suggestive of a viral infection as well as the symptoms of the Guillain-Barré syndrome already alluded to. The spleen is moderately enlarged in about 50 per cent of cases. The disease is not fatal apart from the *complications* already alluded to, namely (1) *spontaneous rupture of the enlarged spleen*, due apparently to the lesions responsible for the enlargement, or, more rarely, (2) *hemorrhage from the nasopharynx* or the *gastrointestinal tract*, and (3) the *Guillain-Barré syndrome.*

The *blood* shows a striking and constant increase in the mononuclear cells. This increase does not coincide with the onset of the illness, but only appears after some days have passed, a point to be remembered in the diagnosis of suspected cases during an epidemic. The total leukocyte count rarely exceeds 20,000, but the percentage of mononuclears may be from 50 to 95 per cent of the total count, so that at first a distinction from lymphatic leukemia may be impossible. There is, however, no anemia and the platelets are normal, features which serve to differentiate it from acute leukemia. Three varieties of mononuclears may be seen: (1) small lymphocytes similar to those of normal blood; (2) the large mononuclears of the normal blood; (3) mononuclears of an unusual type. These cells, which usually predominate, are larger than the small lympocyte, with more abundant cytoplasm, an indented nucleus, and a variable amount of azurophil granules. For want of a better name they are known as *infectious mononucleosis cells.* There is not the cell monotony that is characteristic of acute leukemia, but the relationship of the widespread lymphoid lesions to the blood picture is certainly suggestive of a temporary leukemic or at least leukemoid state.

The condition is apparently due to infection, most probably viral in nature, through the tonsils or the upper respiratory tract, as a result of which lymphoid tissue is unduly stimulated, many of the newly formed cells appearing in the blood stream. In this connection it is of interest to recall our discussion of the etiology of leukemia. The blood of patients with or recovering from

infectious mononucleosis contains heterophile antibodies, *i.e.* the serum will clump sheep's red cells even in high dilution. This is the *Paul-Bunnell test*, a useful test in doubtful cases, but by no means specific, for it may be negative in infectious mononucleosis and positive in virus pneumonia. The test is an indicator of an immunological process at work. Almost all cases give a positive cephalin flocculation test, indicating some degree of liver involvement, and they often show a false positive serological test for syphilis.

BLOOD DISEASES AND AUTO-IMMUNITY

In various forms of diseases of the blood we can discern, without straining the imagination too severely, some relationship, either obvious or vague, to immunological processes. Suggestive evidence in support of such an idea may be found in diseases involving red cells, white cells and blood platelets. This is particularly true of the auto-immune hemolytic anemias such as hemolytic disease of the newborn, of idiopathic thrombocytopenic purpura, and of the acute vascular purpuras. It must be admitted that in the vast majority of instances we are ignorant of the particular antigen responsible, but we have definite evidence of the action of antibodies, which are present in the blood as a gamma globulin type of protein. Normal platelets injected into the blood of a patient with idiopathic thrombocytopenic purpura are soon destroyed by an antibody in the serum. An adsorbed antibody can change a normal erythrocyte into a spherocyte. Henoch's purpura is essentially an immunological process involving small blood vessels and joints. Systemic lupus erythematosus, a disease with a sound immunological basis, is often intimately associated with idiopathic thrombocytopenic purpura. In some cases the antigenic agent appears to be a virus. I.T.P. may develop after chicken pox, measles, or vaccination against poliomyelitis and influenza.

We know that an auto-immune reaction, once begun, tends to be self-perpetuating. At the cellular level there may be an abnormal self-replicating proliferation of cells producing an abnormal harmful protein. In this respect leukemia naturally comes to mind (Dameshek and Schwartz). In leukemia in the experimental animal a recognizable external stimulus such as irradiation, carcinogenic chemicals, or a virus may initiate the mutation, so that a new race of cells arises. The same is true of irradiation in the human subject. About 20 per cent of cases of chronic lymphatic leukemia develop an auto-immune hemolytic anemia, which is not unnatural when we consider that lymphocytes belong to the antibody-producing group of cells. Infectious mononucleosis, a self-limited lymphoproliferative disorder probably caused by a virus, is associated with a peculiar heterophile antibody against sheep red blood cells, an antibody which must be produced by the abnormal lymphocytes.

We may close this discussion with a reference to two conditions which provide suggestive links between cellular proliferation and an auto-immune mechanism, namely multiple myeloma and macroglobulinemia. *Multiple myeloma* may be regarded as a leukemic type of disorder involving plasma cells and characterized by (1) a great proliferation of plasma cells, and (2) the production of large amounts of an abnormal protein of globulin type in the serum. It is surely significant that plasma cells are the great producers of antibody. *Macroglobulinemia* is also marked by (1) an increase in an abnormal heavy globulin, and (2) proliferation of a peculiar type of lymphocyte ("reticular lymphocytes") which are believed to produce the heavy globulin. Both of these may be regarded as "double diseases" in which there is also a proliferation of cells and the production of an abnormal protein.

Thought and work along these lines may in the future throw fresh light on some of the dark corners of the field of blood diseases, and more particularly on the nature and eventual control of the leukemias.

REFERENCES

ALTMAN, K. I.: Am. J. Med., 1959, *27*, 936. (Erythrocyte enzymes.)

BEUTLER, E.: Am. J. Med. Sci., 1957, *234*, 517. (Iron enzymes in iron deficiency.)

BILLING, BARBARA H., COLE, P. G. and LATHE, G. H.: Brit. Med. J., 1953, *2*, 1263. (Plasma bilirubin in the newborn infant.)

BILLING, BARBARA H. and LATHE, G. H.: Am. J. Med., 1958, *24*, 111. (Bilirubin metablism in jaundice.)

BODDINGTON, M. M.: J. Clin. Path., 1959, *12*, 222. (Changes in buccal cells in the anemias.)

CARTWRIGHT, G. E. and WINTROBE, M. M.: Advances in Internal Medicine, 1952, *5*, 165. (Anemia of infection: a review.)

CHERNOFF, A. I.: New Eng. J. Med., 1955, *253*, 322. (Human hemoglobins in health and disease.)

CLAIREAUX, A. E., COLE, P. G. and LATHE, G. H.: Lancet, 1953, 2, 1226. (Icterus of brain in newborn.)

CROSBY, W. H.: Am. J. Med., 1955, *18*, 112. (Metabolism of hemoglobin and bile pigments in hemolytic disease.) Ann. Rev. of Med., 1957, *8*, 151. (The red blood cells.)

DAMESHEK, W.: Am. J. Med., 1955, *18*, 315. (Hemolytic anemia.)

DAMESHEK, W. and SCHWARTZ, R. S.: Blood, 1959, *14*, 1151. (Leukemia and auto-immunity.)

DAMESHEK, W. and GUNZ, F.: *Leukemia*, New York, 1958.

DAVIDSON, W. M. B. and MARKSON, J. L.: Lancet, 1955, *2*, 639. (Gastric mucosa in iron deficiency anemia.)

DESFORGES, J. F., ROSS, J. D. and MOLONEY, W. C.: Am. J. Med., 1960, *29*, 69. (Anemia in leukemia and malignant lymphoma.)

DOAN, C. A.: Bull. New York Acad. Med., 1949, *25*, 625. (Hypersplenism.)

ENDICOTT, K. M., DAFT, F. S. and ORR, M.: Arch. Path., 1945, *40*, 364. (Experimental folic acid deficiency anemia.)

GILLMAN, T.: Nutrition Reviews, 1958, *16*, 353. (Cell enzymes and iron metabolism in anemia.)

GITLIN, D., GROSS, P. A. M. and JANEWAY, C. A.: New Eng. J. Med., 1959, *260*, 72. (Hypogammaglobulinemia.)

GROSS, L.: Blood, 1954, *9*, 557. Ann. N. Y. Acad. Sci., 1957, *68*, 501. (Vertical transmission of mouse leukemia.)

HUTTER, R. V. P.: Am. J. Clin. Path., 1957, *28* 447. (Blood platelets under electron microscope.)

INGRAM, V. M.: Nature, 1956, *178*, 792; 1957, *180*, 326. (Genes and hemoglobinopathies.)

JACOBS, A.: J. Clin. Path., 1960, *15*, 463. (Buccal mucosa in anemia.)

JOSKE, R. A., FINCKH, E. S. and WOOD, I. J.: Quart. J. Med., 1955, *24*, 269. (Gastric biopsy.)

KRIEDBERG, M. B., DAMESHEK, W. and LATTORACA, R.: New Eng. J. Med., 1955, *253*, 1014. (Schönlein-Henoch purpura.)

LEHMANN, H.: J. Clin. Path., 1955, *8*, 178. (Human hemoglobin variants.)

LEONARD, B. J., ISRAELS, M. C. G. and WILKINSON, J. F.: Lancet, 1958, *1*, 289. (Alkaline phosphatase test in polycythemia.)

MAGNUS, H. A.: J. Clin. Path., 1958, *11*, 289. (The relation of the gastric lesion to the intrinsic factor in pernicious anemia.)

MANDELBAUM, H.: Ann. Int. Med., 1939, *13*, 872. (Splenectomy in hereditary spherocytic anemia.)

McGOVERN, J. J., JR.: New Eng. J. Med., 1959, *260*, 675. (Stored autologous bone marrow in treatment of leukemia.)

MEACHAM, G. C., *et al.*: Blood, 1951, *6*, 706. (Thrombotic thrombocytopenic purpura.)

MOTULSKY, A. G.: J.A.M.A., 1957, *165*, 835. (Drug reactions, enzymes and biochemical genetics.)

NORKIN, S. and WIENER, J.: Am. J. Clin. Path., 1960, *33*, 55. (Pathology of Henoch-Schönlein syndrome.)

OWREN, P. A.: Blood, 1948, *3*, 231. (Hereditary spherocytic anemia.)

PAULING, L.: *The Harvey Lectures*, New York, 1955. (Abnormality of hemoglobin molecules in hereditary hemolytic anemias.)

PIKE, G. M.: New Eng. J. Med., 1958, *258*, 1250. (Arterial oxygen saturation test in polycythemia.)

PRANKERD, T. A. J.: Am. J. Med., 1957, *22*, 724. (Inborn errors of metabolism in red cells of hereditary hemolytic anemias.)

QUICK, A. J.: *The Hemorrhagic Diseases*, Philadelphia, 1957.

RAPPAPORT, H.: Am. J. Path., 1953, *29*, 590. (Hemolytic anemia in lymphoblastomas.)

RICH, A. R.: Bull. Johns Hopkins Hosp., 1928, *43*, 398. (Splenic lesions in sickle cell anemia.)

RICH, A. R., WINTROBE, M. M. and LEWIS, M. R.: Bull. Johns Hopkins Hosp., 1939, *65*, 291. (Locomotion of myeloblasts and lymphoblasts.)

ROBERTS, G. F.: *Comparative Aspects of Hemolytic Disease of the Newborn*, London, 1957.

SONG, Y. S.: Am. J. Path., 1957, *33*, 331. (Hepatic lesions in sickle cell anemia.)

STEFANINI, M. and DAMESHEK, W.: *The Hemorrhagic Disorders*, New York, 1955.

STEINBERG, B. and HUFFORD, B. V.: Arch. Path., 1947, *43*, 117. (Bone marrow development.)

STEWART, S. E., *et al.*: Virology, 1957, *3*, 380. (Virus etiology of mouse leukemia.)

TAYLOR, H. E. and SIMPSON, W. W.: Blood, 1950, *5*, 348. (Myelofibrosis in aleukemic myelosis.)

VAUGHAN, J. M. and HARRISON, C. V.: J. Path. and Bact., 1939, *48*, 339. (Myeloproliferative disease.)

VOLPÉ, R. and OGRYZLO, M. A.: Blood, 1955, *10*, 493. (Cryoglobulin inclusion cell.)

VOLPÉ, R., BRUCE-ROBERTSON, A., FLETCHER, A. A. and CHARLES, A. B.: Am. J. Med., 1956, *30*, 533. (Cell enzymes and iron metabolism in anemia.)

WATSON, R. J. and LICHTMAN, H. C.: Med. Clin. N. Amer., 1955, *39*, 735. (The anemias.)

WINTROBE, M. M.: *Clinical Hematology*, Philadelphia, 4th ed., 1956.

WISEMAN, B. K. and DOAN, C. A.: Ann. Int. Med., 1942, *16*, 1097. (Primary splenic neutropenia.)

YOUNG, L. E.: Ann. Int. Med., 1958, *49*, 1073. (The hemolytic anemias.)

Chapter 40

The Spleen

General Considerations
  STRUCTURE
  FUNCTION
    Blood Formation
    Blood Destruction
    Reservoir Function
    Defense Reactions
    Hypersplenism
    Splenic Puncture
Acute Splenitis
Chronic Splenomegaly
  CONGESTIVE SPLENOMEGALY:
    BANTI'S DISEASE
  PRIMARY RETICULOENDO-
    THELIAL GRANULOMAS
    Gaucher's Disease

Niemann-Pick Disease
Schüller-Christian Disease
Letterer-Siwe Disease
Hypercholesterolemic Spleno-
  megaly
BLOOD DYSCRASIAS
  Erythrocytes
  Leukocytes
  Platelets
  Hypersplenism
  Myeloid Metaplasia
Infections
  TYPHOID
  MALARIA
  TUBERCULOSIS
  SYPHILIS

KALA-AZAR
Tumors
  PRIMARY
  SECONDARY
Miscellaneous
  SARCOIDOSIS
  AMYLOIDOSIS
  INFARCTION
  RUPTURE
    Cysts
    Atrophy
    Perisplenitis
    Accessory Spleens
Review of Splenic Enlargements
  SPLENECTOMY

GENERAL CONSIDERATIONS

Structure.—The size of the spleen varies much within normal limits, depending on age, physiological state, etc. The average length is about 12 cm., the breadth 7 cm., and the thickness 3 cm. The weight is 150 to 200 gm. The color is a reddish-purple, indicating its great content of blood. In consistency it is rather soft and quite friable. Unlike the liver, the kidney and the pancreas it is a large abdominal organ without a duct. It may be regarded as a vast reticuloendothelial sponge with a supporting framework of trabeculae and reticulum, and a certain amount of lymphoid tissue superadded, an apparatus admirably designed to detain and alter the blood which is filtered through it.

The larger arteries are clothed with a sheath of lymphoid tissue, the Malpighian bodies. Each arteriole ends abruptly in a globular mass of cells known as an ellipsoid. The ellipsoid represents an elongated collection of reticuloendothelial cells. The capillary which leaves the ellipsoid is believed by some to open into the wide marsh of the splenic pulp before being gathered into the sinusoids, by others to pass directly to a sinusoid. With the light microscope the walls of the sinusoids present slit-like openings between the elongated endothelial cells, giving an appearance of a barrel with alter-

nate staves removed, an arrangement which allows the red cells wandering through the marsh to enter in the freest manner into the venous channels.

There is considerable difference of opinion as to whether the circulation through the spleen is really of this *open type*, or if it is not rather a *closed circulation*. With the electron microscope the cells lining the sinusoids do not present the barrel-stave appearance referred to above, for they fit together as the result of the pseudopodia of one cell being invaginated into the cytoplasm of its neighbors. This observation was made on the rat, and what is true for the rat is not necessarily true for man.

A rather different conception of splenic circulation is afforded by Knisely's direct microscopic observations of living trans-illuminated mammalian spleen. By this technique the sinusoids appear to be separated by partitions of pulp and lined by walls which are readily permeable to fluid and colloids but not to red blood cells. There seems to be a phase of storage of blood and a phase of flow, the flow being regulated by sphincters situated on the arterial and venous sides of the sinusoids. The cycle begins with closure of the sphincter on the venous side, as a result of which the sinus becomes distended with blood and fluid passes through the wall into the pulp.

(1092)

When the sinus is completely distended with red cells the sphincter on the arterial side shuts, and the corpuscles lie free from plasma for a varying period, sometimes up to ten hours. The sphincter on the venous side then opens, and a soft mass of red cells passes into the vein. During the phase of storage or separation the erythrocyte-plasma interface is profoundly changed, as a result of which the cells become spherical instead of biconcave and are therefore more readily hemolyzed.

In addition to the structures already mentioned the spleen contains a fibro-muscular framework and pulp, the latter composed of reticuloendothelial cells and constituting the bulk of the organ. As the spleen is part of the hematopoietic system it is a little hard to believe that the erythrocytes do not come into contact with this important mass of tissue.

Function.—For nearly 2000 years the spleen has been described as "an organ full of mystery." It cannot be said that it has even yet discarded its cloak, but experimental and clinical observations have served to lighten the darkness. The mystery remains how one of the largest of the organs can be removed without producing any noticeable change in the physiology of the body in health. Perhaps the abundance of reticuloendothelial and lymphoid tissue elsewhere enables the functions with which the spleen is concerned to be carried on without faltering after splenectomy. When other organs are removed, evidence of deficiency or impairment becomes apparent which indicates to the physiologist or the physician at least some aspect of normal function. It is the unconcern with which the body treats splenectomy which has been one of the chief stumbling blocks to an understanding of splenic function. The principal functions are. (1) blood formation, (2) blood destruction, (3) blood reservoir function, (4) hemolysin formation, (5) defence reactions. To these may be added the hypothetical function known as hypersplenism.

1. *Blood Formation.*—In the embryo at one stage all the blood elements are produced in the spleen. After birth this function is taken over by the bone marrow, but if the marrow is put out of action, the spleen may resume its hematopoietic role, undergoing the change known as *myeloid metaplasia*. It is believed by some workers that the spleen also exerts a subtle control over blood formation in the marrow, possibly by means of a hormone, regulating the maturation of all the blood elements and the rate at which they are allowed to escape into the peripheral blood. We shall return to this subject in the discussion of hypersplenism.

2. *Blood Destruction.*—The spleen removes from the peripheral blood those elements which are aged, damaged or deteriorated. This is particularly true of the red blood cells as they wander through the pathless forest of the pulp and are trapped by the reticuloendothelial cells. It may be argued whether the spleen is the graveyard or the slaughterhouse of the red cells (Dameshek and Welch). It is undoubtedly the decrepid and defunct cells which find their last resting place here, but it seems probable that the great reticuloendothelial mass of the pulp plays an active part in the final destruction. Abnormal cells such as the spherocytes of hereditary hemolytic anemia have little chance of making the passage successfully.

3. *Reservoir Function.*—The spleen has been likened to a reservoir or blood bank, which can empty itself of blood when there is a sudden demand as in violent exercise, asphyxia or hemorrhage. This is much more true of animals such as the cat and dog whose spleen has an abundance of plain muscle compared with that of man.

4. *Defense Reactions.*—Although a person can get along without a spleen, there seems to be little doubt that his immunological defense mechanism is impaired. One of the most striking demonstrations of the truth of this statement is the fact that rats and dogs from whom the spleen has been removed may develop serious bartonella infections, whereas the same animals with intact spleens, living under identical conditions, are able to control such infections without difficulty. The parasites of kala-azar are present in the splenic macrophages in enormous numbers, and the same cells quickly engulf bacteria injected intravenously. Lymphocytes when destroyed release gamma globulin. Histological evidence of such destruction can be seen in the germinal

centers of lymph nodes, and the same is probably true of the spleen.

Hypersplenism.—The contentious subject of primary hypersplenism has already been discussed in connection with diseases of the blood (page 1058).

The complete hypersplenic syndrome, if we may use the expression, consists of: (1) splenomegaly to such a degree that there may be an equivalent of 2, 3 or even more spleens; (2) a blood cytopenia which may be *selective* with anemia, neutropenia or thrombocytopenia, or *total* with a decrease in the number of red cells, leukocytes and platelets, *i.e.*, a pancytopenia; (3) a "full" marrow, hypercellular but free from proliferating cells, the condition reflecting either a maturation arrest or a blocked delivery; (4) relief of the cytopenias by splenectomy. The chief support for the concept of primary hypersplenism comes from those cases in which splenectomy relieves or abolishes a preexisting cytopenia.

In *secondary hypersplenism* the splenomegaly may be due to: (1) chronic infections such as subacute bacterial endocarditis; (2) portal hypertension; (3) lipid cellular disease such as Gaucher's disease; (4) primary lymphosarcoma of the spleen; (5) nonspecific splenomegalies. In all of these there may be a decrease in one or more formed elements of the blood. The question which still remains unanswered is: Does the splenomegaly represent a cause or an effect of the hematopoietic phenomena?

Splenic Puncture.—Puncture of the spleen, using a 20 gauge needle and syringe for aspiration, may provide material of value for diagnostic smears (Block and Jacobson.) This is particularly true in cases of splenomegaly with a normal blood picture and in "dry" bone marrow punctures where no material can be obtained from the sternum. This is likely to be due to myelosclerosis, and the reason for the splenomegaly is myeloid metaplasia. The method is of value in the diagnosis of neoplasms such as lymphosarcoma, and in atypical leukemias. The large lipid-filled cells of Gaucher's disease are readily recognized. Sheets or clumps of large mesothelial cells derived from the normal serosa must not be mistaken for pathological elements. Splenic puncture

is naturally contraindicated in any form of hemorrhagic disease.

ACUTE SPLENITIS

The spleen has a greater capacity for rapid change in size in acute infections than any other organ in the body. The normal spleen weighs about 150 grams, but in acute infections it soon becomes two or three times that size. It is not likely to be palpable until it is about three times the normal size, especially if it is soft. This acute enlargement is often called acute splenic swelling or acute splenic tumor. The most striking examples are shown by what may be termed the *septic spleen*, which is seen in pneumonia, septicemia, acute endocarditis, and other acute infections. It is enlarged, often very soft, and of a grayish-pink color. The pulp swells up in a pouting fashion on the cut surface, and is so soft that it can be wiped away with the knife. The softest spleens are seen in septicemia and pyemia. The swelling is due partly to enormous numbers of cells trapped in the pathless forest of the pulp, partly to local proliferation. Rich and his associates have shown by motion picture studies of tissue cultures that the large, basophilic, mononuclear cells which predominate have the same method of locomotion as lymphocytes, and are therefore probably lymphoid in character. In *typhoid fever* the spleen is enlarged so as usually to be palpable, soft, and deep red in color. The cut surface may resemble red jelly. The splenic pulp and sinuses are crowded with red blood corpuscles, together with large numbers of the macrophages characteristic of typhoid infection. Many of the macrophages contain erythrocytes which have been phagocytosed. In diphtheria and other acute infections of childhood there may be marked swelling of the lymph follicles so that they become visible to the naked eye.

CHRONIC SPLENOMEGALY

It is impossible to make any satisfactory classification of the chronic enlargements of the spleen, as so little is known regarding their real nature, but we may recognize disease conditions affecting the principal elements of which the organ is composed, *i.e.*, lesions of the *vascular structures*, the *reticulo-endothelial structures*, and the *lymphoid structures*. In the first group we have congestive splenomegaly, and infarction, the second group includes Gaucher's disease, Niemann-Pick disease, Schüller-Christian disease, Letterer-Siwe disease, hypercholesterolemic splenomegaly, and hemolytic jaundice, while in the third group there are the leukemias.

Congestive Splenomegaly : Banti's Disease. —*Banti's disease* is a name which has long been applied to those cases in which there is first enlargement of the spleen with anemia and leukopenia, followed later by cirrhosis of the liver with ascites and a tendency to gastric hemorrhage. This association is so variable and the clinical picture is so indefinite that little is to be gained by preserving the name. One may speak of the Banti syndrome, but it is certainly not a separate disease entity. The development of clinically evident cirrhosis of the liver in splenic anemia is an uncommon occurrence. Microscopic evidence of cirrhosis, however, can be found in 70 to 80 per cent of cases. The ordinary case displays a characteristic *triad of symptoms*, *i.e.*, splenomegaly, secondary anemia and leukopenia, and gastric hemorrhage.

The *nature of the condition* has long been a matter for discussion. Banti's view that the splenic condition was primary has become untenable, in spite of the fact that removal of the spleen may sometimes cure the condition. This is true of other diseases where the changes in the spleen cannot be regarded as fundamental (hemolytic jaundice, thrombocytopenic purpura). Evidence is accumulating that splenic anemia is a *vascular disturbance of the spleen due to high portal blood pressure*. There is a valvular mechanism in the splenic arterioles at the point where they end in the ellipsoids, so that the back-pressure is not transmitted to the splenic artery, but makes its effects felt on the splenic pulp. The question of how much the spleen will enlarge depends a good deal on the age of the patient, marked enlargement occurring more readily in young persons. Cirrhosis of the liver is a sufficient cause, but splenomegaly usually develops long before there is any indication of cir-

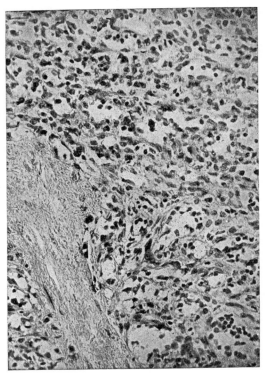

Fig. 620.—Banti's disease. General fibrous thickening of splenic reticulum and dilatation of the sinuses. × 250.

rhosis. Measurements of the diameter of the branches of the portal vein in the liver show that there may be considerable narrowing with little or no cirrhosis in the ordinary sense of the word. Other causes of portal back-pressure are thrombosis of the portal or splenic veins, and vasodilatation of the hepatic artery.

Lesions.—The spleen is much enlarged and very firm. The average weight is 800 to 900 grams. The capsule is thickened, and the cut surface, from which no blood escapes, has a fibrosed or beefy appearance. The *microscopic lesions* are similar to the changes found in portal cirrhosis. The chief features are dilatation of the sinuses and thickening of the fibrous framework of the organ (Fig. 620). The fibrosis is periarterial in origin, extending throughout the reticulum, and finally involving the main trabeculæ. The arteries usually show hyaline degeneration, but this change is of such common occurrence beyond the first decade that it has no

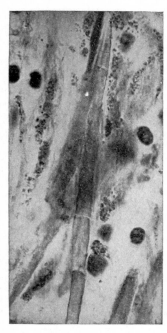

FIG. 621.—Siderotic nodule in spleen. The bamboo-shaped crystals are very characteristic. × 1000

special significance. Periarterial hemorrhages are frequent. A common finding is the presence of yellowish-brown flecks like flakes of tobacco leaf on the cut surface. Microscopically these may present a peculiar filamentous appearance, so that the lesions have been mistaken by some observers for the mycelia of fungi. The filaments are merely elastic fibers on which iron has been deposited, and the so-called fructification organs of the supposed fungi are pale green crystals jointed together like a bamboo cane. In addition to the filaments and crystals there are masses of hemosiderin, some of which is intracellular and some extracellular, together with giant cells and deposits of calcium. The whole mass gives an intense reaction for iron, and may be called a *siderotic nodule* (Fig. 621). These nodules are probably caused by hemorrhage at the point of termination of the arteriole in the ellipsoid where there is a valvular arrangement, so that raised portal blood pressure may cause rupture of the vessel at this point. The hemorrhage is followed by organization and fibrosis. Much of the iron-containing blood pigment is carried away by phagocytes, but

some may be taken up by fibroblasts. These cells proliferate and lay down collagen fibers, and in this way the splenic reticulum becomes more and more fibrosed. All cases of splenic anemia do not show siderotic nodules, nor are the nodules confined to this disease. Their great importance lies in the fact that they indicate an increase in the portal blood pressure, which is the chief cause of the hemorrhages. The nodules are also found in the intensely congested spleen of hemolytic jaundice, in which hemorrhage may readily occur.

Degenerative changes in the splenic vein and portal vein are of common occurrence, and there may be thrombosis. These lesions are probably secondary to heightened portal blood pressure. If they are sufficiently great they may produce some of the splenic changes. Thickening of the wall (phlebosclerosis), endophlebitis, atheromatous change, and calcification are the chief lesions. The vein may be greatly distended, and huge collateral channels may connect the spleen with the stomach and diaphragm. The liver may or may not show cirrhosis of the portal type, but even when there is no cirrhosis it is probable that there is narrowing of the terminal branches of the portal vein.

Relation of Symptoms to Lesions.—The enlargement of the spleen is probably the result of the increased portal pressure, which causes the dilatation of the sinuses, the hemorrhages, and indirectly the fibrosis. The gastric hemorrhage, one of the most constant and often one of the earliest of the symptoms, can best be explained by the same mechanism. These hemorrhages are analogous to the siderotic nodules in the spleen. In the former the blood escapes on a free surface, while in the latter it is imprisoned within a solid organ. The cause of the anemia may possibly be hypersplenism, if we admit the existence of such an entity. The anemia, usually associated with leukopenia, is not of the hemolytic type, for there is no evidence of undue hemolysis, and the fragility of the red cells is not increased. It may not develop until long after the splenomegaly has been detected, but it appears to be related to the lesions in the spleen, for splenectomy may cure the disease if it is not too far advanced. The gastric hemorrhages may contribute to the condition, but cannot account for all the cases. It must be remembered that in portal cirrhosis of the liver a progressive anemia is the rule. The three conditions which are most benefited by splenectomy are hemolytic jaundice, thrombocytopenic purpura, and splenic anemia.

Primary Reticuloendothelial Granulomas. —There exists a group of five rare diseases characterized by an accumulation of large pale reticuloendothelial cells. These cells contain lipids varying in amount with the members of the group. Two of these reticuloses, Gaucher's disease and Niemann-Pick disease, are lipid in character; there is a true disturbance of lipid metabolism associated with hyperlipemia. They are *lipid-storage diseases* or *lipidoses*. The other three, Schüller-Christian's disease, Letterer-Siwe disease and eosinophilic granuloma of bone, are non-lipid reticuloses. As suggested by Farber they appear to be variants of the same basic disease disorder of the reticuloendothelial system. Common to all three there are collections of large pale mononuclear cells, often phagocytic and containing lipid. Eosinophils are common to all three, but are most numerous in the earlier stage of eosinophilic granuloma, disappearing with the advancing age of the lesion and the conversion of the mononuclears into foam cells. The clinical variations seem to depend largely on the effect of age on the reactions (Dennis and Rosahn). The younger the age, the more acute and malignant the process. Lesions of the skin and the lymph nodes are common both to Letterer-Siwe disease and Schüller-Christian disease.

Gaucher's Disease.—This rare condition is a disorder of the reticuloendothelial system. It commences in early life and is sometimes familial. Very exceptionally it appears to develop in the adult, when it runs a mild and prolonged course. There is an extreme degree of splenomegaly, moderate enlargement of the liver, some secondary anemia and rather pronounced leukopenia, a brownish-yellow coloration of the skin, and yellow wedge-shaped patches in the conjunctiva on each side of the cornea. Splenic puncture shows the very characteristic large, pale Gaucher cells. Roentgen-ray examination shows rarefaction of the bones, flattening of

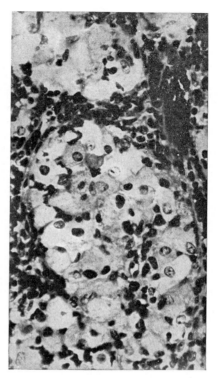

Fig. 622.—Gaucher's disease. × 315.

the head of the femur, and a fusiform expansion of the lower end of that bone. As the vertebræ are involved in the rarefaction, the stature may be stunted.

The spleen may be enormous, filling the greater part of the abdomen. White spots are scattered over the surface, and these consist of very large, peculiarly pale cells filled with lipid (Fig. 622). These are the Gaucher cells, and represent the reticuloendothelial cells of the organ filled with the cerebroside, kerasin. The cerebroside is in the form of a lipoprotein. It stains feebly with the ordinary fat stains, but intensely with McManus' periodic acid-Schiff reaction and with Weigert's method designed for the more complex lipids. It is the swelling of these cells which causes the great enlargement of the spleen. The lesions are not confined to the spleen, but are found also in the liver, lymph nodes, bone marrow, and other parts of the reticuloendothelial system. The anemia and leukopenia are caused by the bone marrow lesions. In one form of Gaucher's disease the lesions are mainly osseous. All the affected members of a family may suffer from this form. Pick mentions a family in which five brothers developed skeletal lesions. Scarcely a bone in the body may be spared. The disease is an example of lipid storage by the cells of the reticuloendothelial system. The basis of the condition is a disturbance of lipid metabolism, the nature of which is at present unknown.

Niemann-Pick Disease.—This is an even rarer condition than Gaucher's disease, of which it may be regarded as a variation. It is a familial condition, occurring nearly always in Jewish infants, and the child does not live beyond the second year. In addition to involvement of the spleen, liver, lymph nodes and bone marrow as in Gaucher's disease, the characteristic lipid-filled cells are found in the adrenal, pancreas, thymus, intestinal mucosa, lung, brain, and renal glomeruli. The affected cells are much more vacuolated than in Gaucher's disease. With the McManus stain the cells remain colorless, whereas Gaucher's disease cells stain rose-purple. The histiocytes as well as the endothelial and reticular cells are involved, so that it is a true lipid histiocytosis. Many epithelial cells may contain the lipid, *e.g.*, thyroid and kidney, and the monocytes of the blood may also be filled with this material. Widespread involvement of the ganglion cells of the brain and retina is the basis of amaurotic family idiocy. The lipid differs from that of Gaucher's disease in being a phospholipid, namely, sphingomyelin.

Schüller-Christian Disease.—This very rare condition is characterized by defects in the membranous bones, especially the skull, exophthalmos, and diabetes insipidus—at first sight a curious mixture. The lesions are the result of accumulations of reticuloendothelial cells which contain lipid (cholesterol) at some time in the disease. It seems to be a primary xanthomatosis often associated with giant cell formation. The bone defects are due to erosion caused by periosteal deposits of xanthoma cells, the exophthalmos to deposits in the orbit, and the diabetes insipidus to deposits around the pituitary. The pituitary lesion may also cause dwarfism. Almost any organ may be involved. Lesions in the lung may result in pulmonary fibrosis. The disease shows extreme variations in its course, the localization of the lesions and the clinical manifestations. It generally affects young adults, and may be very chronic in character, lasting for many years. In early childhood it is rapidly fatal.

Letterer-Siwe Disease.—This is a *nonlipid reticuloendotheliosis*, but with many features in common with the lipid reticuloendothelioses described above. It is a disease of infants and young children which runs a rapid and fatal course marked by a skin eruption, hepatomegaly, splenomegaly, lymphadenophathy and progressive anemia. There is universal proliferation of the reticuloendothelial cells, with an increase in size of those organs containing large numbers of these cells. Few organs escape. The cellular proliferation is both diffuse and focal with the formation of nodules.

Hypercholesterolemic Splenomegaly.—This is a rare example of lipid storage, the nature of which is indicated by the descriptive name. If the escape of bile is obstructed for a considerable period as by chronic pancreatitis, the blood cholesterol is raised, and there may be lipid storage in the reticuloendothelial system, especially the spleen, with a considerable degree of splenomegaly.

In summary, the various lipidoses may be classified according to the type of lipid principally involved (Thannhauser). *A, Cerebroside lipidosis:* Gaucher's disease. *B, Phosphatide lipidosis*: (1) Niemann-Pick disease; (2) amaurotic family idiocy. *C, Cholesterol lipidosis* (xanthomatosis): (1) idiopathic—various forms, of which the Schüller-Christian syndrome is the best known; (2) secondary to diabetes, jaundice, nephritis.

Hypercholesterolemia.—A word may be devoted here to the general subject of hypercholesterolemia. The blood lipids, cholesterol in particular, may be elevated in a number of unrelated conditions. *Primary hypercholesterolemia* is a rare familial condition with a genetic basis. *Secondary hypercholesterolemia*, in which other lipids may be involved, occurs in a variety of diseases. Of these atherosclerosis is the most important. It may also be marked in diabetes mellitus, hypothyroidism, lipoid nephrosis, and xanthomatous biliary cirrhosis. Soft yellow nodules known as *xanthomas* (*xanthos*, yellow) may be formed, more particularly in the

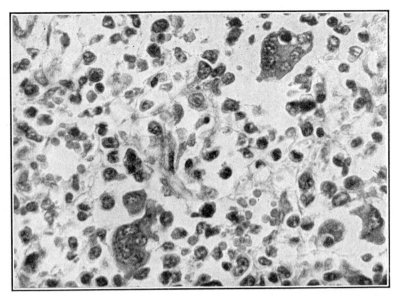

Fig. 623.—Myeloid metaplasia of spleen showing marrow-like picture and multinucleated giant cells. × 610. (Boyd, *Pathology for the Physician.*)

eyelids, but also in wrinkles (below the breasts, in the palms of the hands) or over pressure points (elbow, etc.). These consist of collections of macrophages filled with lipid in the subcutaneous tissue.

Blood Dyscrasias.—An important cause of chronic splenomegaly is one or other of the blood dyscrasias, so that the first thing to do when the spleen is found to be enlarged is to examine the blood. We have already considered these disorders of the blood in detail in the previous chapter, so that little more than mention will be made of them here. The disorders associated with splenomegaly may involve the red cells, the white cells or the platelets.

Erythrocytes.—Sickle cell anemia must always be considered as a possible cause of splenomegaly in the Negro, but this is true only of the *early stages* of the disease. The sinusoids are distended with sickle cells, and pools of blood are formed around the Malpighian corpuscles. Over the years a progressive fibrosis develops, and the spleen may shrink to an incredibly small size. In *congenital hemolytic jaundice (hereditary spherocytosis)* marked enlargement of the spleen is a feature of the disease, for it is in the spleen that the spherocytes are destroyed. The empty sinusoids are lined by hypertrophic endothelium, while the pulp is packed with erythrocytes being destroyed. In *polycythemia vera* the splenomegaly is rarely marked. Thromboses with resulting infarcts are characteristic of the condition. In *thalassemia (erythroblastic anemia)* the spleen is markedly enlarged and firm, infarcts are common, and there are foci of extramedullary hematopoiesis together with accumulations of peculiar foam cells.

Leukocytes.—In *chronic myelogenous leukemia* the spleen is massively involved, sometimes to such an extent as to fill the abdomen. Numerous small infarcts are practically constant. In the *chronic lymphatic form* the splenomegaly is much more moderate. In *acute leukemia* the spleen may or may not be enlarged, never to a marked degree.

Platelets.—In *thrombocytopenic purpura* the spleen may or may not be enlarged, and never to a marked degree. It is in the cases of long standing that splenomegaly is likely to be a feature.

Myeloid Metaplasia.—An uncommon cause of splenomegaly is the development of abundant active marrow tissue in the organ. Large multinucleated cells of megakaryocyte type form a prominent feature (Fig. 623). Similar changes but less marked in degree may be present in the liver and lymph nodes. Immature red and white cells are seen in the circulating blood. The condition may be *secondary* to fibrosis of the bone marrow or osteosclerosis, but in other cases the marrow is normal. The name *agnogenic* (idiopathic) *myeloid metaplasia* has been applied to this *primary* group (Jackson *et al.*). In their useful review of the subject in which they regard the condition as a specific entity Linman and Bethell mention 10 alternative names. An extreme degree of splenomegaly, often reaching 1500 gm. and accompanied by hepatomegaly, may occur when the marrow is still cellular, myelofibrosis occurring later (Taylor and Simpson). It would appear that in such cases the reticuloendothelial cells of the spleen have responded to a leukemic-like stimulus to a greater degree than those of the marrow, so that the condition may be regarded as an *aleukemic myelosis*. The blood is likely to present a leuko-erythroblastic picture, but it may simulate that of myeloid leukemia or, more rarely, acquired hemolytic anemia. It used to be thought that splenectomy was dangerous and indeed likely to be fatal owing to removal of a large area of essential blood-forming tissue. There appears to be no ground for this belief. The bad results of splenectomy in the past were due in large part to the surgical risks of a formidable procedure in patients who were seriously ill.

INFECTIONS

Typhoid.—The features of typhoid infection have been considered elsewhere (page 272). The spleen shows a moderate degree of enlargement, from 250 to 500 gm., the pulp being crowded with reticuloendothelial cells, many of which contain phagocytozed red blood cells. The condition can be regarded as an acute splenitis.

Malaria.—Enlargement of the spleen is one of the commonest lesions in malaria. In an acute attack the spleen is moderately enlarged and soft, but as a result of long-continued infection it becomes greatly enlarged and very hard (*ague-cake spleen*). In malarial districts the greater part of the population may have enlarged spleens, giving the children in particular a pot-bellied appearance.

Tuberculosis.—Tuberculosis of the spleen is of little importance. In general miliary tuberculosis the spleen is enlarged and may be studded with tubercles, which are easily mistaken for enlarged lymph follicles. Occasionally large caseous masses are scattered throughout the spleen causing marked enlargement of the organ. The primary lesion in the lung or lymph nodes may be so small and quiescent that it is readily overlooked, and the condition is described as primary tuberculosis of the spleen. A large solitary tubercle (tuberculoma) is of very rare occurrence. The lesions of sarcoidosis have been mistaken in the past for those of tuberculosis.

Syphilis.—In congenital syphilis the spleen is frequently enlarged and contains large numbers of spirochetes. The condition is often associated with marked anemia.

Kala-azar.—Kala-azar is a common cause of splenomegaly in the tropics. The spleen is very greatly enlarged, fibrosis is marked, and the pulp is filled with macrophages containing the Leishman-Donovan parasites which have already been described on page 359. The parasites are readily demonstrated by means of splenic puncture.

TUMORS

All tumors of the spleen are uncommon, perhaps we should say rare. They may be benign or malignant. *Benign tumors* are likely to be *lymphangioma* or *hemangioma*. *Primary malignant tumors* of the spleen are curiously rare. Most of the articles in the literature are reports of single cases. The tumors may arise from any of the three main types of splenic tissue. (1) From the capsule and trabecular framework there may be a *fibrosarcoma* and *spindle cell sarcoma*. (2) From the lymphoid tissue there may be *lymphosarcoma* and *reticulum cells sarcoma*. Some of these tumors may attain an enormous size, weighing as much as 5000 gm. and filling the abdomen. A lymphosarcoma arising elsewhere may of course involve the spleen, and the same is true of *Hodgkin's disease*. (3) From the sinus endothelium may arise an *angiosarcoma* as well as a *benign cavernous angioma*.

Secondary carcinoma might be expected to be of common occurrence. The tumor cells must reach the spleen, but apparently they do not find conditions favorable for growth. In this respect the spleen differs sharply from lymph nodes, an arresting and unexplained fact. The tumor cells can reach the spleen by the lymphatics which accompany the blood vessels as well as by the blood stream. The usual site of the primary tumor is the breast or lung.

MISCELLANEOUS

Sarcoidosis.—The spleen is often involved in general sarcoidosis, but occasionally splenomegaly is the most conspicuous feature, dwarfing all the others. In such cases the spleen is studded with large discrete granulomatous nodules composed mainly of epithelioid cells. In spite of the absence of caseation the histological picture has been mistaken in the past for that of tuberculosis, and there can be no doubt that most of the cases diagnosed formerly as primary tuberculosis of the spleen were really examples of sarcoidosis.

Amyloidosis.—The splenic lesions have already been described in connection with amyloid disease (page 90). The spleen is much enlarged, elastic, and very firm. The common lesions affect the arterioles of the lymph follicles, but the fibrous reticulum is sometimes involved. The disease is almost never confined to the spleen.

Infarction.—An infarct of the spleen may be caused in the usual way by embolic occlusion of the artery. If the embolus is infected an abscess will be formed in the spleen. Or it may develop as the result of vascular disturbances in the spleen (thrombosis of the splenic vein) in such conditions as splenic anemia and leukemia, and injury to the organ, especially rupture. It presents the usual characters of an ischemic infarct, but in addition siderotic nodules may be present. The infarct reaches the surface which it involves, in contrast to infarct of the kidney where a thin rim of uninvolved tissue separates the infarct from the capsule. This explains why pain is a symptom more characteristic of splenic infarct than of renal infarct.

Rupture.—The normal spleen may of course be ruptured by *severe injury* such as automobile accidents. An enlarged spleen (due to malaria, etc.) may be ruptured by a comparatively *minor injury*. In rare cases there is *spontaneous rupture* of an enlarged spleen, the best example being *infectious mononucleosis*. A correct diagnosis of rupture of an enlarged spleen, whether traumatic or spontaneous, is essential, because immediate splenectomy is necessary if the life of the patient is to be saved. The bleeding from the torn surface is usually very severe, which is not surprising when we consider that the spleen is primarily a vascular organ, and the patient may die in a few hours from internal hemorrhage. In other cases there may be a curious latent interval for several days after the injury, at the end of which time symptoms of severe hemorrhage suddenly manifest themselves. In these cases the splenic pulp is torn, but the capsule remains intact and prevents the excape of blood, only to give way later with resulting copious hemorrhage.

Cysts.—Cysts of the spleen are rare. Primary cysts of unknown origin may occur. Echinococcus cysts are less uncommon in countries where the disease prevails. Hemangioma and lymphangioma may cause cystic formation.

Atrophy.—The spleen becomes markedly atrophic in old age, and may be only one-third of the normal weight. Similar atrophy may occur in wasting diseases of long duration and also in sickle cell anemia. The capsule is thickened and wrinkled, and the cut surface has a markedly fibrosed appearance. The lymphoid tissue disappears, and the pulp is atrophic.

PERISPLENITIS.—Perisplenitis is a rather indefinite term which denotes fibrous thickening of the capsule, sometimes extreme in degree. It is seen in senile atrophy, and in some enlarged spleens the surface is covered with thick fibrous patches. The most extreme thickening is seen in Pick's disease.

Accessory Spleens.—Accessory spleens or spleniculi are common. Usually there is only one, sometimes two, but in rare cases several hundred have been present. This is a reversion to the primitive condition in which the splenic tissue is not collected into a definite organ, but is strewn throughout the subserous coat of the gastrointestinal tract. The importance of an accessory spleen lies in the fact that in conditions benefited by splenectomy recurrence of the symptoms may be due to hyperplasia of the accessary organ.

GENERAL REVIEW OF SPLENIC ENLARGEMENT

Enlargement of the spleen may be due to very different causes. The spleen is a contractile sponge, which may rapidly undergo marked variation in size. (1) In *acute splenic swellings* there is a great accumulation of inflammatory cells in the pulp, to which is probably added proliferation of the local endothelium. (2) The splenomegaly of *hereditary spherocytic anemia* is characterized by an enormous accumulation of red blood cells in the splenic pulp, but the condition must be regarded as a reticuloendothelial rather than a vascular disorder. (3) In *polycythemia vera* the spleen is moderately enlarged and firm owing to an accumulation of the excess red cells in the splenic reservoir. There may be cystic spaces filled with blood. (4) *Congestive splenomegaly* appears to be due to vascular disturbances in the spleen caused by back-pressure in the portal and splenic veins. (5) The splenic enlargement of *portal cirrhosis* and the much lesser enlargement in chronic valvular disease of the heart is due to a similar cause. The increase in the fibrous reticulum which occurs in these conditions may be responsible for some of the enlargement. (6) The enlargement of *amyloid disease* is due to the great swelling of the individual connective-tissue fibers. (7) In the *lymphoblastoma* group (Hodgkin's disease, lymphosarcoma and leukemia), there may be hyperplasia both of the lymphoid and the reticuloendothelial structures in the spleen. (8) The *lipid storage* diseases (Gaucher's disease, Niemann-Pick disease, and hypercholesterolemic splenomegaly) form a group in which distention of the reticuloendothelial cells with lipid is attended by great enlargement of the spleen. (9) The splenomegaly of *kala-azar* and possibly of *malaria* is due to a reticuloendothelial proliferation.

Splenectomy.—The question of which splenomegalies should be treated by surgical removal of the enlarged spleen has long been a subject of debate. In spite of our lack of precise knowledge of the functions of the spleen, splenectomy is an empirical form of treatment which may do great good in certain blood diseases. It is indicated particularly in: (1) rupture of the spleen from trauma or disease such as infectious mononucleosis; (2) hereditary spherocytic anemia in which the best results are obtained (75 per cent of cases), and in which the subsequent development of gallstones can be prevented; (3) In 6 out of 7 cases of idoipathic thrombocytopenic purpura splenectomy was followed by immediate cessation of bleeding, restoration of the bleeding time to normal, and rise in the platelet count (Nelson); (4) Cases of hypersplenism may be completely relieved by reason of removal of the supposed inhibitory influence of the spleen on the bone marrow. In considering the advisability of splenectomy in any given case we must remember that many, perhaps all, of the activities of the spleen seem to be shared by other tissues in the body.

REFERENCES

BLOCK, M. and JACOBSON, L. O.: J.A.M.A., 1950, *142*, 641. (Splenic puncture.)

DAMESHEK, W.: Bull. New York Acad. Med., 1955, *31*, 113. (Hypersplenism.)

DAMESHEK, W. and WELCH, C. S.: *Hypersplenism and Surgery of the Spleen*, New York, 1952.

DENNIS, J. W. and ROSAHN, P. D.: Am. J. Path., 1951, *27*, 627. (Primary reticuloendothelial granulomas.)

DOAN, C. A.: Bull. New York Acad. Med., 1949, *25*, 625. (Hypersplenism.)

FARBER, S.: Am. J. Path., 1941, *17*, 625. (Non-lipid reticuloses.)

PICK, L.: Am. J. Med. Sci., 1933, *185*, 453. (Gaucher's disease.)

RICH, A. R., LEWIS, M. R. and WINTROBE, M. M.: Bull. Johns Hopkins Hosp., 1939, *65*, 311. (Acute splenic swelling.)

THANNHAUSER, S. J.: *Lipidosis: Diseases of Cellular Lipid Metabolism*, 3rd ed., New York, 1958.

WISEMAN, B. K. and DOAN, C. A.: Ann. Int. Med., 1942, *16*, 1097. (Splenic neutropenia.)

Chapter 41

The Lymphatic System

General Considerations
STRUCTURE
FUNCTION
LYMPH NODE BIOPSY

THE LYMPH VESSELS
Lymphangitis
Tumors of the Lymphatics
LYMPHANGIOMA

THE LYMPH NODES
Lymphadenitis
ACUTE LYMPHADENITIS
CHRONIC LYMPHADENITIS

Mesenteric Lymphadenitis
Dermatopathic Lymphadenitis
Chronic Granulomas
TUBERCULOSIS
TULAREMIA
BRUCELLOSIS
TOXOPLASMOSIS
FUNGUS GRANULOMAS
CAT SCRATCH DISEASE
LYMPHOGRANULOMA VENEREUM
SYPHILIS
SARCOIDOSIS
Tumors of Lymphoid Tissue
LYMPHOSARCOMA

MACROFOLLICULAR LYMPHOMA
RETICULUM CELL SARCOMA
HODGKIN'S DISEASE
Reticular Lymphoma
BENIGN LYMPHOMA
LEUKEMIA
SECONDARY TUMORS
LYMPHADENOPATHY

THE THYMUS GLAND
Status Thymico-Lymphaticus
Tumors of the Thymus

GENERAL CONSIDERATIONS

Structure.—The lymphatic system forms one of the most all-pervasive, important and indispensable parts of our anatomy, although it is very little in evidence in a state of health. It consists of lymphatic vessels and lymphoid tissue, the latter forming three groups: (1) lymph nodes situated in the lymph stream, (2) lymphatic tissue in mucous membranes, and (3) lymphatic tissue situated in the blood stream. For convenience in this chapter we shall include the thymus, although it consists of epithelium as well as lymphoid tissue. The spleen has already been considered. Lymphatics appear first in the round worm, but they reach their highest development in amphibia, which have actually got lymph hearts. Lymph nodes are only well developed in mammals, in whom valves appear in the vessels. The valves and contractions of muscles take the place of the lymph heart.

The *lymphatics* commence as blind diverticula from which first a network and then a series of collecting vessels arise. They share with the capillaries the regulation of tissue fluid, especially the absorption from the tissue spaces of particles of high molecular weight, including extravascular protein, for their endothelium is much more permeable than that lining the blood vessels. The lymphatics therefore constitute a me-

chanism for cleansing the tissues of substances not readily removed by the blood stream, and for returning to the blood proteins which have leaked from the capillaries. It is the readiness with which particulate matter can enter the lymphatics which gives these vessels their great importance as a pathway for the spread of infection and of cancer. Fortunately the lymph nodes stand as sentinels along the course of this pathway, although, like human sentinels, they may be overwhelmed when the attack is too powerful. The lymph channels may therefore be likened to an absorbent sponge, but the nodes play the part of a filter. There is no need for lymphatics in the brain, as the production and absorption of cerebrospinal fluid is so rapid. Perhaps this is one reason why malignant tumors of the brain do not spread outside the cranial cavity.

A *lymph node* consists of a cortex containing a large number of spherical germinal centers and a medulla made up of medullary cords separated by lymphatic sinusoids. Lymphoid tissue, in the nodes and elsewhere, consists of (1) lymphocytes, which are free cells in a framework of (2) reticulum cells, which are part of the reticuloendothelial system and are both supporting and phagocytic. The reticulum cells are attached to a fine reticulum network, and are phagocytic both in situ and after becoming detached into the blood stream. The germinal centers have

(1103)

pale centers made up of larger more loosely packed cells showing mitotic figures, and which may be regarded as lymphoblasts.

All the lymph passes through one or more nodes. The lymph reaches the nodes by afferent lymphatics well supplied with valves, and first enters the peripheral subcapsular sinus known as the corridor. It is here that cancer cells are first arrested. When the rest of a suspected node appears to be clear of secondary involvement, special attention should be paid to this sinus. The structure of a lymph node is ideal for filtration. The pressure of the lymph falls when it enters the peripheral sinus and makes its leisurely way through the labyrinth of sinusoids, lined by endothelium and intersected by strands of reticulum, which still farther retard the flow and give time for the reticuloendothelial phagocytes to function. It is the reticuloendothelial apparatus which plays the part of a filter, holding up foreign particles, bacteria, etc., probably by the mechanism of adsorption, so that the nodes become in truth the dust bins of the body. The precise details of regional lymph node drainage have been determined by the use of radioactive tracers (isotopes) and by the injection of fluorescein.

Function.—The function of lymphoid tissue seems to be threefold: (1) filtration, (2) production of antibodies, (3) production of lymphocytes. The subject of *filtration* has already been discussed. *Antibody formation* is believed to be a function of lymphoid tissue, at least in the laboratory animal. It appears that the rate of liberation of antibody from lymphoid tissue is under the control of pituitary adrenal cortical secretion (Dougherty and White). Single injections of ACTH in mice, rats and rabbits produce an absolute lymphopenia, associated with degenerative changes in the lymphoid tissue and serum globulin release. Unfortunately similar changes have not been observed in man. It has been thought that the reticulum cell rather than the lymphocyte is the producer of antibodies. Recently, and especially in view of the deficiency of plasma cells in agammaglobulinemia, attention has been focussed on the plasma cell as the antibody factory. This leaves the *function of the lymphocyte*, perhaps the most ubiquitous

cell in the body and one which is involved in all sorts of pathological processes, rather up in the air. There can be no question that it is intimately involved in immunological processes, but at the present time its role seems to be that of a carrier rather than a manufacturer of antibodies. It is claimed that its chief function is to synthesize and store nucleoproteins for use by other cells. The *production of lymphocytes* goes on with remarkable abandon. In the dog lymphocytes labelled with P^{32} entered the thoracic duct at the rate of 430 million per hour, a sufficient number to replace the entire mass of circulating blood lymphocytes 7 times a day (Perry *et al.*). It would certainly appear that the lymphocyte has some task of importance to perform. The life span of these intriguing cells has not been firmly established, but it seems likely that it is only a few days.

Lymph Node Biopsy.—The student when he becomes a clinician will readily turn for help to the lymph node biopsy when confronted by an obscure clinical problem in which the nodes are enlarged. It is well for him to realize that the pathologist also has his difficulties. As Ackerman remarks in the opening sentence of the discussion of the subject in his *Surgical Pathology:* "The microscopic diagnosis of lymph node lesions is extremely difficult; probably more errors are made in this field than in any other organ. The more common error is in the incorrect diagnosis of a benign node as malignant lymphoma." The chief reason for the difficulty is the fact that the reticuloendothelial cells possess a remarkable power of reacting to an irritant by proliferation and hyperplasia, so that it may be almost impossible to tell whether we are dealing with an inflammatory condition or a true neoplasm. The histological picture of Hodgkin's disease illustrates this dilemma of the pathologist only too well. It is unfortunately true that various pathological processes give similar morphological patterns in the lymph nodes.

The clinician must bear the following points in mind. (1) At least one sentence of information should accompany the specimen, such as the site of the lymph node removed, the fact that the part had been recently scratched by a cat, that the skin drained by the node was the seat of a chronic dermatitis, etc. Too often the specimen is sent in without a word of history. This might be taken as a tribute to the pathologist's omniscience, but it is grossly unfair to the patient. (2) When there is a generalized enlargement of nodes the worst possible selection is one of the inguinal group, (although often chosen for the sake of convenience), because these nodes so frequently show evidence of previous infection (from legs and genitalia) in the shape of fibrosis and distortion which obscure the underlying pathological process. (3) When the possibility of a malignant lymphoma is suspected, a lymph node biopsy should never be done until after careful study of a blood film, a study which will often given information of greater value than histological examination of a node. (4) Bacteriological examination of a node may give more valuable information than the histological picture, because different microorganisms may stimulate tissue reactions which are identical histoligically, and a given species of organism may produce a wide variety of histological patterns. In these days of chemotherapy and antibiotics an exact bacteriological diagnosis has now become of pressing practical importance. If such a diagnosis is to be made it is obvious that the excised node must not be placed in a fixative which will kill any bacteria present. The ideal procedure is to divide the node into two pieces, putting one immediately into the fixative, whilst the other is placed in a sterile container and stored if necessary in the ice box.

THE LYMPH VESSELS

LYMPHANGITIS

Inflammation of the lymphatic vessels is due to the entrance of bacteria through a wound or abrasion of the skin which may be so minute as to escape detection. Some of the most serious forms of lymphangitis before the days of antibiotics were due to puncture of a finger at an operation or an autopsy on a septic case. The streptococcus is the usual offending organism.

The inflammation commences in the lymphatic network of the skin, and may spread throughout that network, a spread accompanied by the phenomena of *erysipelas,* or it may pass rapidly up the collecting vessels to the nearest lymph nodes, which become swollen, tender, and painful, and in some cases may suppurate. In a superficial infection the inflamed lymphatics are seen as wavy, red lines passing up the limb, but if infection is deep these lines need not be looked for, although the part will be swollen and will pit on pressure.

As a rule the inflammation ends in resolution, although *suppuration* at the site of infection is common. Occasionally a severe infection, arrested at the group of nodes into which the lymphatics empty, may set up *abscess* formation. Should the bacteria pass the line of defense furnished by the nodes a *general infection* will ensue, with pyrexia, chills, delirium and, it may be death.

If the inflammation is at all severe, the sequel may be connective tissue formation with lymphatic obstruction and the production of a brawny edema. If the obstruction is at all extensive, it may give rise to a condition of *lymphedema* in one of its various forms. As the pressure in the lymphatics raises the valves become competent, fluid rich in protein collects in the tissue spaces, and fibroblasts proliferate rapidly in this excellent tissue culture medium. The resulting fibrosis still further aggravates the stasis. Fluid medium is good not only for the growth of cells but also of bacteria, so that recurring attacks of acute inflammation are frequent. Eventually the limb may become swollen to such fantastic proportions as to justify the term *elephantiasis* given to the condition many centuries ago. The most severe forms of elephantiasis, in which the legs of the unhappy sufferer may really come to resemble those of a young elephant, are those due to obstruction of the lymphatics by Filaria bancrofti.

TUMORS OF THE LYMPHATICS

It is difficult and sometimes impossible to draw a dividing line between simple dilatation of the lymphatics or lymphangiectasis and true neoplasms or lymphangiomas. The neoplasms are more circumscribed, but they are not encapsulated and tend to extend into the surrounding tissue.

Lymphangioma.—A tumor composed of lymphatics is much less common than a hemangioma. It is usually localized but may be diffuse. The diffuse form may occur in the tongue giving rise to *macroglossia*, or in the lip giving *macrocheilia*. The localized form may be a capillary, but more usually a *cavernous lymphangioma*. It occurs most frequently in the skin and subcutaneous tissues, forming a doughy swelling which may be mistaken for a cold abscess. In the neck it may form a cystic mass, known clinically as a *cystic hygroma*. This and the other forms of lymphangioma are more common in children. *Microscopically* the picture is the same as a hemangioma, except that the endothelial-lined spaces are filled with clear lymph and a few lymphocytes instead of blood.

THE LYMPH NODES

Lymph nodes, like the spleen and thyroid gland, respond to disease by enlargement. There are therefore many causes of lymph node enlargement, but the more important of these may be divided into four main groups: (1) inflammation, (2) chronic granulomas, (3) lymphoblastomas or malignant lymphomas, and (4) secondary tumors.

LYMPHADENITIS

Reduced to the simplest terms, the two disease processes in which the lymph nodes may become involved are inflammation and neoplasia. As the nodes are situated on the course of the lymphatics which drain not only the skin but also internal mucosal surfaces, it is inevitable that they should be exposed to irritants of every description, bacterial, fungal, viral and inorganic. In consequence lymphadenitis, either acute or chronic, is of frequent occurrence.

Acute Lymphadenitis.—This is the result of virulent bacteria (staphylococcus, streptococcus) being arrested in the lymph node. The node is enlarged, painful, and tender, the cut surface varies from pink to gray, and a milky juice can be scraped from the surface. The *microscopic picture* varies with the severity of the inflammation. If this is extreme, the sinuses will be crowded with polymorphonuclear leukocytes, and patches of necrosis will be scattered through the gland which eventually is converted into an abscess. It is comparatively seldom that the inflammation proceeds to suppuration. Usually the lesion clears up by resolution, and in such cases there is no necrosis, but merely marked hyperplasia of lymphoid and reticuloendothelial tissue to which the enlargement of the gland is due.

It is the regional lymph nodes which drain an area of acute inflammation that develop acute adenitis. Some of the more important examples are the following: occipital and superficial cervical glands infected from pediculosis and wounds of scalp and ear, deep cervical glands from teeth and mouth, lateral pharyngeal glands from the pharynx with suppuration and the formation of a retropharyngeal abscess, axillary glands from the hands, inguinal glands from the genitals, leg, or foot. In all of these instances there may be a chronic lymphadenitis if the infection is less acute in type.

Chronic Lymphadenitis.—Chronic enlargement of a lymph node occurs when the node drains a focus of chronic inflammation. The gland is moderately enlarged, firm and homogenous. *Microscopically* the change is a proliferative rather than an exudative one. There is hyperplasia of the reticuloendothelial cells, large numbers of the endothelial cells becoming swollen, rounded and cast off into the greatly dilated lymph sinuses, an appearance to which the name of *sinus catarrh* is given (Fig. 624). It may be noted in passing that lymphoid structures and hematopoietic structures in general respond to irritation by hyperplasia, so that it may be very difficult to distinguish between inflammatory and neoplastic conditions. This is a matter of supreme importance in connection with the lymphoblastoma group. Chronic lymphadenitis is a very common condition. The cervical group is most often involved, due to infection from the mouth, tonsils, and teeth. Infection of the leg or the male genitalia will cause enlargement of the inguinal glands; infection in the lung, lesions in the bronchial glands, etc.

Mesenteric Lymphadenitis.—In children

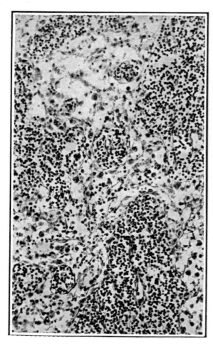

FIG. 624.—Chronic lymphadenitis. × 150.

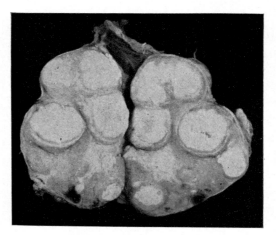

FIG. 625.—Tuberculosis of a lymph node showing several large caseous areas in the enlarged node.

and young adolescents there sometimes occurs an acute abdominal condition simulating appendicitis, diverticulitis, renal colic, etc., but in which the major finding at operation is inflammatory enlargement of the mesenteric lymph nodes in the ileocecal angle. In only a few cases can bacteria be demonstrated, and these are usually streptococci. Some of the cases are tuberculous. It is difficult to explain how the lesion in the lymph nodes gives rise to the clinical picture. Some of the symptoms may be due to spasm of the bowel.

Dermatopathic Lymphadenitis.—Chronic dermatitis associated with pruritus may cause a characteristic type of hyperplasia of lymph nodes (Laipply). The hyperplasia may be extensive enough to be mistaken for lymphoblastoma. It is the reticular cells of the pulp which undergo hyperplasia. They frequently contain lipid vacuoles, and melanin pigment is found in large mononuclear cells. On this account an alternative name is *lipomelanotic reticular hyperplasia.* The fat and melanin are released from the skin by scratching and carried to the nodes,

which they color yellow (fat) or brown (melanin).

CHRONIC GRANULOMAS

Tuberculosis.—Tuberculosis is one of the common causes of enlargement of lymph nodes. The three groups most commonly involved are the *cervical, bronchial,* and *mesenteric.* The first is infected from the mouth and throat, usually the tonsils, the second from the lung, the third from the bowel. Mesenteric lymph nodes tuberculosis is likely to be caused by drinking tuberculous milk or swallowing tuberculous sputum. Although theoretically it is possible for the bacilli to pass through the intact wall of the bowel, in practice the more careful the examination the more often will an intestinal lesion be found. When the ileocecal group is involved in children, as we have just seen, there may be symptoms like those of acute appendictis, *i.e.,* sudden onset of abdominal pain and rigidity, fever, vomiting, and a moderate leukocytosis. These symptoms are apparently due to spasm of the bowel.

The glands are at first discrete and firm, but when periadenitis occurs they become matted together. The cut surface shows tuberculous areas which are at first gray and translucent, but later become yellow, opaque and caseous (Fig. 625). The entire gland may eventually become caseous and break down, so that a mere shell is left. In this way a cold

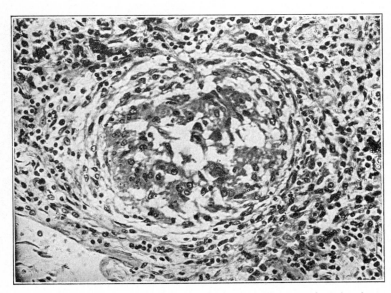

Fig. 626.—A tubercle. Epithelioid cells form the principal part of the tubercle. × 250.

abscess is formed which discharges on the surface (best seen in the neck), with the establishment of persistent sinuses which finally heal with deep scar formation. It must not be thought that this steady progression is the usual course. As a rule in response to appropriate treatment the condition clears up and does not go on to extensive caseation.

The *microscopic picture* shows the usual tuberculous follicles composed largely of epithelioid cells with a few giant cells (Fig. 626). In the caseous case much of the structure of the node has disappeared. There is no tissue in which it is so hard to find tubercle bacilli; when present they are never numerous; it seems as if they are destroyed in the gland in some way. As healing occurs fibroblasts proliferate and dense collagen fibers are laid down. Calcification is common in the caseous glands, particularly in the bronchial lymph nodes. However quiet the lesion may appear to be, there is always a danger that it may set up another focus elsewhere (bone, adrenal, etc.), by way of the blood stream. Sometimes the lesions are not discrete tubercles, but take the form of a *diffuse hyperplastic tuberculosis*, characterized by reticuloendothelial hyperplasia and sheets of epithelioid cells, but no caseation and no giant cell formation. It is more than probable in the light of recent knowledge that many, perhaps all, of these cases are really examples of sarcoidosis.

Tularemia.—The glandular lesions of tularemia may be indistinguishable from those of tuberculosis. There is the same caseation, necrosis, epithelioid cell proliferation and giant cell formation. In other cases the lesions are acute in nature, with focal necrosis and suppuration. The infection, which is due to a small plague-like bacillus, comes from a reservoir in rodents, particularly the ground squirrel and the jack-rabbit. It therefore occurs in farmers, hunters, butchers and housewives who may handle the contaminated skins or internal organs of infected rabbits. Infection may also be due to the bites of ticks or flies. The site of inoculation and the regional nodes draining it both develop lesions about the same time. The primary lesion may be insignificant. The *diagnosis* is made by agglutination of *Pasteurella tularensis* by the blood serum or by isolation of the organism from guinea pigs inoculated with material from the node.

Brucellosis.—In chronic cases of brucellosis the lymph nodes may be enlarged. Biopsy from such a node is easily mistaken either for tuberculosis or Hodgkin's disease, because large cells resembling Reed-Sternberg cells may suggest the latter condition.

Here again diagnosis is made by agglutination or culture of the tissue for brucella.

Toxoplasmosis.—Glandular toxoplasmosis caused by the intracellular protozoan parasite *Toxoplasma*, is said to give a histological picture similar to that of so-called benign Hodgkin paragranuloma (Saxen and Saxen). It is a medullary reticulosis characterized by clusters of large, pale, epithelioid-like cells, so that the histological picture may resemble that of sarcoidosis. The diagnosis usually depends on the demonstration of neutral antibodies in the serum.

Fungus Granulomas.—Rather similar reactions in the lymph nodes may be produced in *blastomycosis, histoplasmosis* and *coccidioidomycosis*. It is worthy of note that the nodes are not involved in actinomycosis. The histological diagnosis is most readily made by demonstration of the fungus in the tissue. Minute fungi such as *Histoplasma capsulatum* may not be distinguished in sections stained with hematoxylin and eosin, but they may be vividly shown by the periodic acid-Schiff stain.

Cat Scratch Disease.—As this condition has already been described on page 348 it will only be referred to here. It is probably caused by a virus, the infection coming from a cat, although not necessarily by way of a scratch or bite. The *microscopic picture* in the involved node is that of a granuloma with hyperplasia of the reticular cells and occasional giant cells.

Lymphogranuloma Venereum.—This condition, also called *lymphopathia venereum*, is caused by a filterable virus. The method of transmission is usually venereal, and the condition is commoner in the Negro. The inguinal nodes become enlarged, owing to an accumulation of large mononuclear cells which form small solid granulomas. Ischemic necrosis follows, the invasions by polymorphonuclear leukocytes and the formation of a characteristic *stellate abscess* (Smith and Custer). The clinical diagnosis is confirmed by the Frei allergic skin reaction.

Syphilis.—Syphilis used to be one of the first of the granulomata to be considered in the differential diagnosis of an enlarged lymph node. In the primary stage the regional nodes and in the secondary stage the nodes throughout the body were regularly involved. Those days are past, thanks to antibiotic therapy, but the possibility of syphilis must be kept in mind, as the occasional case may escape diagnosis and treatment. The *microscopic picture* is the usual indefinite one characteristic of syphilis: a proliferation of mononuclear cells, lymphocytes, and plasma cells. In the primary and to a lesser extent in the secondary stage the nodes are swarming with spirochetes.

Sarcoidosis.—Chronic lymphadenopathy is an important feature of sarcoidosis. The *microscopic picture* may so closely resemble that of tuberculosis that precise differentiation may be impossible without bacteriological examination. Sarcoidosis is still an enigma, its etiology and nature remaining obscure, so that it is not possible to say if it deserves to be included with the other granulomas. This matter is discussed in more detail on page 292, in connection with the granulomata. Several etiological agents are known to produce a similar histological picture, so that sarcoidosis remains "the disease of unknown etiology" after the others have been eliminated. It is known that the disease is endemic in regions of pine forests, such as the Scandinavian countries, and the South, North Central and New England states of the United States (Michael). Pine pollen has acid-fast staining characteristics similar to those of the tubercle bacillus, and is capable of evoking epithelioid cell granulomata in normal animals (Cummings and Hudgins). It is therefore possible that pine pollen may be at least one etiological agent which can excite the reaction characteristic of sarcoidosis.

TUMORS OF LYMPHOID TISSUE

These tumors, which may originate in the lymph nodes, the lymphoid tissue of the alimentary canal, or the spleen, are unique among neoplasms in several ways and constitute a most intriguing group. We have already seen that the tendency of lymphoid tissue to react to irritation by hyperplasia rather than by exudation is responsible for the frequent difficulty which the pathologist experiences in differentiating between a benign inflammatory and a neoplastic process. The tumors are peculiar in the following respects.

(1) They may arise from either of the two types of cell which constitute lymphoid tissue, namely the lymphocyte (including the lymphoblast) and the reticular cell. Our classification is based on the recognition of this fact. When, however, we follow the life history of one such tumor by means of repeated biopsies we may find evidence of permutation and transformation from one cell type into another. This can be explained by recalling that both lymphocytes and reticular cells have a common ancestor of mesenchymal origin, the reticuloendothelial cell. It may be remarked that in tissue culture lymphocytes may be seen to develop into epithelioid cells and giant cells.

(2) The tumor may apparently start in a single node, but in the course of time there may be involvement of other nodes in the group, then of other groups of nodes, and finally not only of nearly every node in the body, but also of the lymphoid tissue of the spleen and liver. Although we have specially mentioned the nodes as the starting point of these neoplasms, they may of course originate in the lymphoid tissue of the bowel, where they form one of the commonest malignant tumors of the small intestine. It is difficult (or impossible) to decide if this widespread involvement really signifies spread of the tumor or whether it may not represent multiple origin.

(3) Sooner or later the neoplastic cells may pour into the circulating blood, and the case then becomes one of lymphatic leukemia, chronic in type if the cells are lymphocytes, acute if they are lymphoblasts.

(4) There is an extreme variation in the malignancy of the lymphoblastomas. Some, such as the reticulum cell sarcoma may kill in one or two years, while others, such as the macrofollicular lymphoma, usually run a course of ten to fifteen years. Indeed the patient may die before the tumor has begun to show any signs of spread, and such cases are responsible for the difference of opinion as to whether or not we should recognize a benign as well as a malignant type of lymphoma.

The lymphoid tumors present many difficulties both to the clinician and to the pathologist, and one of the greatest of these is nomenclature, which in turn depends on classification. Each writer seems to have his own classification, and Willis, in his monograph on tumors, gives a list of 20 of the "more usual" names. Writers on this and allied subjects may be divided into "lumpers" and "splitters", the former taking delight in gathering everything together into one or two groups, the latter taking even greater delight in splitting up these groups into subdivisions. Speaking generally, the clinician tends to be a lumper and the pathologist a splitter. It may be observed in passing that a very good lumper's term (which we owe to the pathologists) is lymphoblastoma, but this does not signify a tumor of lymphoblasts, the precursors of lymphocytes, but a malignant tumor or blastoma of lymphoid tissue.

There are *four main subgroups* of the *malignant lymphomas* or *lymphoblastomas*, but these may be subdivided endlessly by the splitter. They are all more frequent in the male in the proportion of about 3 to 1. The subgroups are (1) *giant follicle lymphoma* or *follicular lymphoma*, in which the follicular architecture is preserved, at least for long periods; (2) *lymphosarcoma*, in which the stem cells have differentiated along the lymphocytic line; (3) *reticulum cell sarcoma*, in which they have differentiated along the reticular line; and (4) *Hodgkin's disease*, in which is manifested the full pluripotentiality of the reticular stem cells, and in which additional reactive inflammatory cells make their appearance in varying degree. Of these Hodgkin's disease is the commonest, while follicular lymphoma brings up the rear. Opinions differ regarding the relative frequency of the other two.

Lymphosarcoma.—The characteristic feature of this tumor is the fact that it arises in one group of lymph nodes or in one collection of lymphoid tissue and, after a varying interval, spreads to other groups of nodes apparently by way of the lymphatics. In addition to the nodes there may be widespread involvement of the lymphoid tissue in the pharynx (tonsils, etc.), gastrointestinal canal, spleen, bone marrow, liver and other organs. The spleen may be enlarged, although splenomegaly is not nearly so

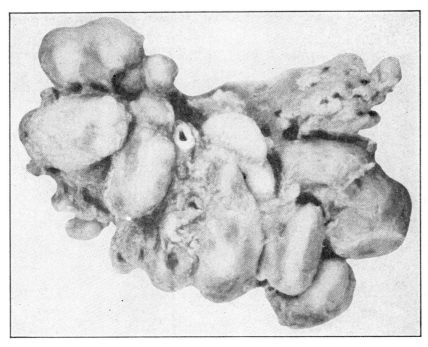

Fig. 627.—Lymphosarcoma. Mass of enlarged abdominal lymph nodes.

frequent as in Hodgkin's disease, fever is a common complication, and changes in the blood point to involvement of the bone marrow. The most constant of these changes is a progressive secondary anemia, but there may be a relative or absolute lymphocytosis. Many cases are undoubtedly examples of aleukemic leukemia which have been unrecognized. It is often not realized by the physician that *examination of a blood smear is more valuable than a biopsy*. Pure classical lymphosarcoma of the type described originally by Kundrat is not a common disease. Few tumors are more susceptible to the effect of radiation, and the growth may completely disappear under this treatment. The disappearance, however, may be followed by the death of the patient from asthenia.

The *gross appearance* of the lesions is very similar to that of Hodgkin's disease, but in lymphosarcoma there is a greater tendency to rupture of the capsule of the glands with invasion and destruction of the surrounding tissues. The *cervical* group of nodes is most often involved, first on one side and then on the other. Closely allied to this group is the *pharyngeal* form, in which the first lesions are in the tonsil, the laryngeal sinus or the nasopharynx. From these sites the cervical nodes become secondarily involved. The primary growth is often quite small, and is frequently overlooked. The *mediastinal form* is common and important. In it are seen some of the best examples of infiltration, for the lungs and bronchi are extensively invaded. When I was a student mediastinal lymphosarcoma was a common diagnosis, because anaplastic bronchogenic carcinoma spreading to the regional nodes was mistaken for lymphosarcoma of the nodes invading the bronchi. The lymphoid tissue of the *bowel* may be much swollen so as to form nodular masses on the inner surface. The abdominal and thoracic cavities may be filled with tumor masses of remarkable size considering the state of the superficial nodes (Fig. 627).

The *microscopic appearance* shows complete replacement of the mature lymphocytes by much larger hyperchromatic cells with a small amount of basophilic cytoplasm and a

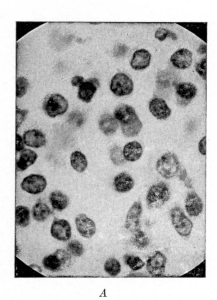

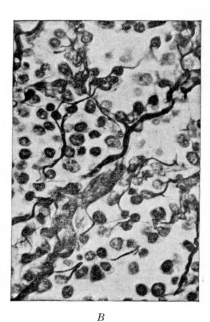

A   *B*

Fɪɢ. 628.—Lymphosarcoma. *A*, There is great uniformity of cell type. × 650. *B*, Reticulum stain. × 510.

round or oval nucleus with a fairly prominent nucleolus; mitoses may be present, but are not easy to recognize. These cells may be lymphocytes or lymphoblasts. The uniformity of cell type is an outstanding feature in comparison with the multiplicity of cell forms seen in Hodgkin's disease (Fig. 628*A*). There is no increase in reticulum as shown by silver stains. Those reticulum fibers which are present represent the original content of the node, and these are dispersed by the infiltration of neoplastic cells, so that in a given field they appear to be decreased in number (Fig. 628*B*).

In some cases there is a generalized lymph enlargement rather than a neoplasia commencing in one region and gradually extending and becoming disseminated. In these cases the normal architecture is replaced by mature lymphocytes, and the picture is indistinguishable from that of lymphatic leukemia; only a blood examination can differentiate the two lesions. Such a condition may be called *lymphocytoma;* it may terminate as a lymphatic leukemia.

Macrofollicular Lymphoma.—This condition is also known as *giant follicle lymphoma,* *follicular lymphoma,* follicular lymphoblastoma, and Brill-Symmers' disease. It is the most benign member of the group and one of the least common. It is a highly differentiated lymphosarcoma, so that it seems a pity to refer to it as a lymphoblastoma. It is slowly progressive, with 50 per cent of the cases surviving for more than five years, and about 15 per cent for ten years or more (Gall and Mallory). In spite of the good differentiation the lesion is extremely radiosensitive. The usual age of onset is around forty years. There may be a single enlarged node, usually in the neck, remaining localized for a number of years, and not recurring on removal, or there may be multiple nodes forming one or more groups, extending slowly, with the final development of lymphosarcoma, Hodgkin's disease, and even leukemia. The spleen is also usually enlarged, weighing often well over 1000 grams. From an analysis of 136 cases Wright came to the conclusion that, with a few possible exceptions, the condition is a malignant tumor from its outset. Perhaps it would be better to call it a potentially malignant lesion.

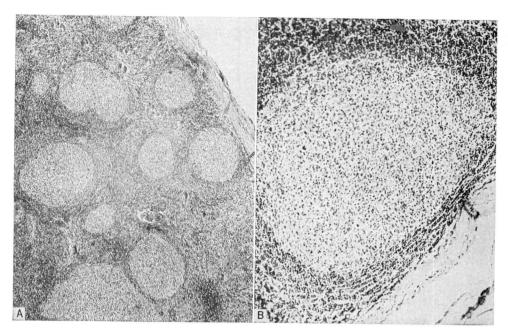

Fig. 629.—Follicular lymphoma. *A*, The varying size of the large follicles is evident. × 45. *B*, The same, more highly magnified. Note uniformity of the cells in the giant follicle. × 135. (Kindness of Dr. Desmond Magner, Ottawa.)

The nodes are not adherent to one another and are freely movable. On the cut surface the large follicles can be seen with the naked eye. *Microscopically* the follicular structure is preserved and the germinal centers are greatly enlarged (Fig. 629) consisting of closely packed, rather large lymphoblasts, with the surrounding lymphocytes compressed into concentric layers. The sinusoids are obliterated in contradistinction to the dilated sinusoids characteristic of chronic lymphadenitis, with which the lesion may be confused. Phagocytosis, so common in chronic inflammation, is absent. With the onset of actual malignancy there is a loss of follicular structure and destruction of the stromal framework as shown by one of the silver stains for reticulin fibers.

Reticulum Cell Sarcoma.—This tumor is commonly regarded as a form of lymphosarcoma under the name reticulum cell lymphosarcoma. This is permissible in regard to tumors of lymph nodes, where the tumor arises from the reticular cells of the node. It may occur, however, in many other situations, including bone, where it forms

one variety of bone sarcoma, so that it is better to speak of it as reticulum cell sarcoma. It is a highly malignant disease, the average duration being less than two years. Although behaving like lymphsarcoma, it may occasionally occur as an isolated lesion. radical removal of which may result in apparent cure. Reticulum cell sarcoma is a much commoner lesion of lymph nodes than pure lymphosarcoma.

The *microscopic appearance* is characteristic, but this is only true if the material is properly fixed, so as to prevent distortion by shrinkage, and suitably stained. The cytoplasm of the reticulum cell is usually abundant and faintly acidophilic (Fig. 630). The nucleus is double the size of that of a lymphocyte, and is commonly infolded, giving it a reniform appearance. Highly characteristic in well-fixed material is the presence of pseudopod-like processes of both cytoplasm and nucleus, indicating ameboid activity in the living cell. The tumor cells may often be seen infiltrating the vein walls and almost closing the lumen. The pathognomonic feature is the distribution of

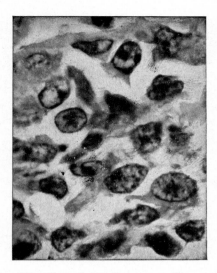

FIG. 630.—Reticulum cell sarcoma. Compare the size and form of the cells with those in Figure 627. × 650.

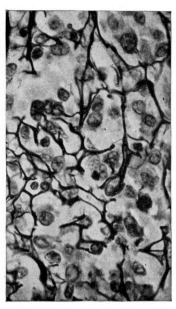

FIG. 631.—Reticulum cell sarcoma; reticulum stain. × 510.

reticulum in silver preparations. In addition to a general increase of reticulum the fibers show an intimate relationship to the tumor cells, encircling groups of cells and sending fibrils between and around individual cells (Fig. 631).

Hodgkin's Disease.—It is now nearly 130 years since the pathologist to Guy's Hospital in London described "some morbid appearances of the absorbent glands and spleen." Since that time endless controversy has raged as to the nature of the condition, whether inflammatory, neoplastic, or in the dim borderland between the two. Various bacteria have been incriminated, and of course viruses have been dragged in. The pleomorphism of the histological picture has suggested inflammation, while the malignant progress of the disease indicates a neoplasm. One of the major obstacles in the investigation has been the fact that no comparable disease in animals is known. The debate can now be regarded as closed. Hodgkin's disease is a *malignant neoplasm* involving both sets of the cells which constitute lymphoid tissue, namely lymphocytes and reticulum cells, although the basic element is the reticulum cell.

Lesions.—The affected *lymph nodes* are enlarged, usually in groups The greatest enlargement may be in the mediastinal, mesenteric, and retroperitoneal groups. The groups are not continuous with one another, thus differing from the usual picture of lymphosarcoma. For long the nodes may remain discrete, but eventually they may become fused as in tuberculosis. Sometimes there may be invasion of the surrounding tissue; thus invasion of the lung may take place from the mediastinal glands. The cut surface is pale gray, homogeneous, translucent, and moist, and has been likened, not inaptly, to fish flesh. Later it may become yellow owing to necrosis. The *spleen* is large and firm, but it often has not the homogeneous appearance of the lymph nodes, for scattered through it are numerous opaque patches, gray or yellow, like pieces of suet (Fig. 632). These represent areas of "Hodgkin tissue," the change having commenced in the lymphoid follicles. Later the process becomes more diffuse. Small gray areas may be seen on the enlarged *liver;* these are lesions confined to the portal tracts. The *bone marrow* may appear red and hyperplastic. Other organs may more rarely show lesions, *e.g.*, intestine, stomach, kidney, and wherever there happens to be lymphoid tissue.

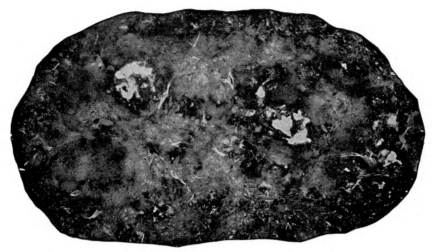

Fig. 632.—Enlarged spleen of Hodgkin's disease showing suet-like areas.
(Boyd, *Pathology for the Surgeon*, courtesy of W. B. Saunders Co.)

In exceptional cases the disease may be mainly or entirely confined to one organ, so that it is possible to have Hodgkin's disease of the lung, stomach, etc.

The capsule of the glands is usually intact, but in the later stages there may be invasion of the surrounding tissue. The vertebræ may be invaded with consequent pressure on the spinal cord. Other bones may also be involved. Craver and Copeland found that out of 172 cases 27 had bone lesions, generally of the spine and pelvis. Fracture is rare, but collapse of a vertebra is common. The discs are seldom involved. Osteoplastic and osteolytic changes are often combined. The invasive quality is best seen in the mediastinal form, but it is probable that many of these cases are in reality examples of thymoma, a true tumor arising in the thymus. Lesions are said to occur in the lung in 40 per cent of cases. In about 10 per cent of these cases the disease seems to have started in the lung (Moolten). Such cases may be called *Hodgkin's disease of the lung*. The main lesions are in the bronchi, and the spread is peribronchial in type. In one case which I studied the involvement was so diffuse as to present the gross appearance of lobar pneumonia.

The *microscopic appearance* is the same wherever the lesions occur, but in any one site it may be extremely varied in character.

Indeed its *pleomorphism* is its most characteristic feature. The lesion is mainly composed of large pale cells of "epithelioid" type. These large cells are probably derived from the reticuloendothelial cells of the node. Even more characteristic is the appearance of very large or giant cells, some of which are mononuclear but many are multinucleated; when the nucleus is single it may be convoluted or ring-shaped. These giant cells are the cells known as the *Dorothy Reed* or *Sternberg cells* (Fig. 633). The Reed-Sternberg cells, derived from the reticular cells, is the specific diagnostic feature. These cells were first described in 1878 by Greenfield, my own professor of pathology in Edinburgh. The multinucleated forms frequently have two nuclei, one of which is the mirror-image of the other, the so-called "mirror-image giant cell." Lymphocytes, plasma cells, polymorphonuclear leukocytes and eosinophils may all be present. Eosinophils are particularly characteristic, and help to settle the diagnosis when it is in doubt, but it must not be thought that they are invariably present. Necrosis may appear later, but this is best seen in the spleen. It must be noted that *necrosis* is not a feature in the other forms of lymphoblastoma. There is a marked and characteristic increase of reticulum shown by silver staining. In the later stages there is dense fibrosis. In the earlier

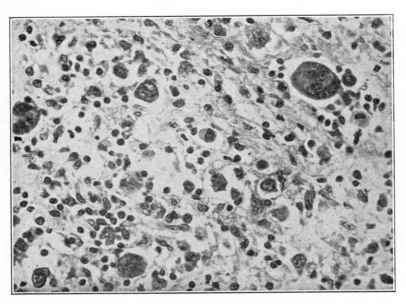

FIG. 633.—Hodgkin's disease. The cytological picture is characteristically pleomorphic. There are several large multinucleated cells in the Reed-Sternberg type. × 350.

cellular stage the lesion will respond for a time to radiation, but not in the late fibrotic stages.   Sometimes there is not the pleomorphism of inflammation but rather the uniform cellular picture of neoplasia.   The cells are large, of uniform size, with abundant cytoplasm and the large prominent nucleolus characteristic of malignancy.   Mitoses are common.   Reticulum formation is at a minimum.   The lesion is much more invasive than is the ordinary form.   Such cases have been called *Hodgkin's sarcoma*.

Jackson and Parker analyzed a large series of lymphadenopathies at the Boston City Hospital in which Reed-Sternberg cells were present and which may therefore be regarded as Hodgkin's disease.   They find that the cases fall into 3 groups, which they call *paragranuloma* (38 cases), *granuloma* (237 cases) and *sarcoma* (51 cases).   In the *paragranuloma* the disease is confined to the cervical lymph nodes although the spleen may also be involved, the capsule remains intact, the principal cell is the lymphocyte, and Reed-Sternberg cells are few and difficult to find; the lesion is easily mistaken for lymphadenitis.   The granuloma is the common phase of the disease.   Its characteristics

and those of the sarcomatous form have already been outlined.

Reticular lymphoma is the term suggested by Lumb in place of Hodgkin's paragranuloma.   The normal architecture of the node is replaced by a proliferation almost entirely composed of mature lymphocytes, among which are scattered occasional reticulum cells, which tend to remain isolated rather than to occur in clumps.   Robb-Smith's title lympho-reticular medullary reticulosis describes the cell types found in the tumor, but it must be admitted that it is rather forbidding.   There is no tendency for invasion of the capsule or necrosis,   Fibrous thickening of the capsule is frequent, with collagen strands passing through the node giving it an irregular lobulation which may be detected with the naked eye or hand lens (Harrison).   The lesion should be regarded as a potentially malignant one.

Relation of Symptoms to Lesions.—This discussion is concerned more particularly with Hodgkin's disease, but it will be obvious that many of the observations apply also in some degree to the other members of the lymphoblastoma group.   The disease may occur at any age, but is commonest in middle life, usually in men. It is nearly always fatal, but not invariably so. There are acute and chronic forms, just as there are in other types of cancer. The more acute cases have general involvement of the nodes from the beginning, and do not do well with any form of treatment. The chronic form, on the other hand may smoulder for years without seriously handicapping the patient's way of life (Warwick and Sellers). One-third of the Ontario cases reviewed by Warwick and Sellers died within a year of diagnosis, but those who survived to the five-year and especially the ten-year mark had an increasingly favorable prognosis. One medical student developed enlarged left cervical nodes and some time later right axillary nodes, both treated by radiation. After graduating he engaged in active medical practice, dying twenty-two years later of coronary thrombosis. Another patient presented himself in 1932 with a node in the left axilla the size of a large egg, nodes in the right axilla in 1935, a large mass in the abdomen in 1944, and evidence of mediastinal and left hilar node involvement in 1950. The various lesions disappeared after radiation, and the patient was well twenty-six years after the first evidence of the disease. Needless to say, the diagnosis in both these cases was confirmed by biopsy. I know of one case where a patient applied for life insurance sixteen years after a diagnosis of Hodgkin's disease had been made independently in two first class laboratories of surgical pathology.

The *prognosis* depends partly on the type of histological change, partly on the clinical behavior of the process. The "paragranuloma" or reticular lymphoma type generally carries a good prognosis, whereas the presence of many giant cells in mitosis and signs of much reticulum cell activity are correspondly grave. The survival period depends on the clinical class to which the case belongs (Warwick and Sellers). In *class I* the disease is limited to a single area without constitutional symptoms and signs; in *class II* two or more lymphatic areas are involved in a single anatomical region, (*a*) without and (*b*) with constitutional symptoms and signs; in *class III* several anatomical areas are involved and constitutional symptoms and signs are serious. Radiation therapy and chemotherapy with nitrogen mustard and other alklylating agents may be expected to benefit the first but not the third class.

In adults Hodgkin's disease is about twice as common as lymphosarcoma, but in children the incidence of the two diseases is about equal. The disease is usually first detected by an enlargement of the cervical glands, first on one side and then on the other, but deep glands (mediastinal, mesenteric) may have been enlarged long before the superficial ones become palpable. The spleen is enlarged to a considerable degree in 75 per cent of cases. The liver shows a slighter degree of enlargement in 50 per cent of the cases. A *progressive anemia* is constant, but the leukocytes show no uniform change. They may be increased or diminished in numbers, monocytes may be more numerous than normal, and occasionally there is a well-marked eosinophilia. Megakaryocytes have been found in the blood, and the blood platelets are often increased. *Fever* is common. Occasionally this assumes the so-called *Pel-Ebstein type*, characterized by spells of mild fever lasting for a few days and separated by intervals of a week or two of normal temperature. In other cases the fever is more continuous. Less common symptoms, but worthy of mention, are pruritus (itching), which may be present long before the glandular enlargement, pigmentation, and in rare instances infiltration of the skin. There may be dyspnea, cyanosis, paralysis, and other signs of pressure by the enlarged lymph nodes.

It is easy to correlate such symptoms as dyspnea and cyanosis with pressure of enlarged lymph glands in the neck or mediastinum. The glandular masses may press on the spinal nerves as they issue from the canal causing pain, paralysis, etc., or masses may be found lying within the spinal canal and pressing directly on the cord. The enlarged spleen will cause a sensation of abdominal fullness or heaviness. The anemia and the variations in the blood picture (eosinophilia, etc.) have been attributed to involvement of the bone marrow.

It is possible that the anemia, which is hemolytic in character, and the cachexia of the later stages, as well as other puzzling clinical features such as fever, may be due to an *auto-immune state* involving cells concerned with antibody formation (Kaplan and Smithers). If lymphoid tumor cells become differentiated from the cells of the host by the loss of antigen they retain the capacity to make antigens, and thus acquire the ability to react against and destroy the patient's normal lymphoid cells. Suggestive *clinical evidence* in support of this concept are: (1) the multiple infections and poor immune reactions which occur in patients with malignant lymphomas (Ewing used to say that tuberculosis follows Hodgkin's disease like a shadow, and a great variety of fungus infections, especially torulosis, may be found at autopsy); (2) the already mentioned hemolytic anemia, wasting, and lymphoid destruction seen in these diseases; (3) the presence of auto-immune antibodies in the blood in some patients with lymphomas; (4) the dramatic if temporary response to steroid therapy in some cases, particularly with regard to continued or intermittent fever, hemolytic anemia, and the cutaneous disturbances. It is possible, therefore, that some of the clinical and histological features of Hodgkin's disease which suggest inflammation rather than neoplasia may have a basis in auto-immunity, that convenient explanation which is invoked perhaps too readily nowadays to account for obscure phenomena.

BENIGN LYMPHOMA.—This is an innocent tumor of a lymph node or group of nodes. It is very *uncommon*, and it is never safe to make the diagnosis from the microscopic picture alone, since this may be identical with that of lymphosarcoma. Indeed in all of these conditions the pathologist should be supplied with all the information possible before making a diagnosis. But if an enlarged gland or cluster of glands in the neck or groin increases slowly in size or remains stationary for a number of years without evidence of involvement of the rest of the lymphatic system, and if this gland when removed shows a replacement of the normal structure by a diffuse arrangement of small round cells such as is seen in lymphosarcoma, the blood meanwhile remaining normal, then it seems justifiable to make a diagnosis of benign lymphoma.

Leukemia.—The morbid anatomy of leukemia as well as the blood changes has al-

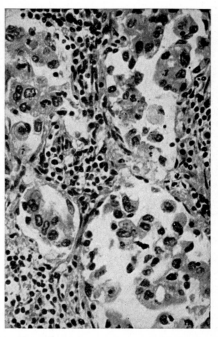

FIG. 634.—Secondary carcinoma of a lymph node. The lymph sinuses are distended by carcinoma cells.

ready been considered in Chapter 39, but it is convenient to mention the condition of the lymph nodes in this place. In the lymphatic form of leukemia there is a general enlargement of the lymph nodes. Sometimes this is almost confined to the deep nodes in the thorax and abdomen so that the superficial glands may show little change. The *microscopic picture* is the same as that of lymphosarcoma, for the nodes are so crowded with lymphocytes that all normal structure disappears. Lymph node enlargement does not form an essential part of the myelogenous form of leukemia, but it may occur, owing to the newly-formed primitive leukocytes (myelocytes) being detained in the sinuses of the nodes or possibly to a local formation by a process of myeloid metaplasia. The nodes are often enlarged in multiple myeloma (plasma cell leukemia).

Secondary Tumors.—A carcinoma tends to metastasize to the regional lymph nodes. The cancer cells are first found in the peripheral lymph sinus and then in the medullary sinuses (Fig. 634). As the tumor cells grow they destroy the lymphoid tissue, until finally the entire node is a mass of carcinoma.

The secondary growth may be more or less differentiated than the primary tumor. When the tumor cells break through the capsule the gland becomes firmly adherent to the surrounding tissues, being then inoperable. Malignant melanomas also metastasize to the lymph nodes, but sarcomas rarely do, spreading as a rule by the blood stream.

Lymphadenopathy.—In his clinical work the student will continually encounter examples of enlargement of the lymph nodes, a condition known by the rather inaccurate term of lymphadenopathy. It may assist him on occasion to consult the table of contents at the beginning of this chapter. There he will see a list of the three main groups of conditions which may cause either local or general enlargement of the nodes. These are: (1) *acute* and *chronic lymphadenitis;* (2) *chronic granulomas,* which may be of bacterial, fungal or unknown etiology; and (3) the *lymphoblastomas,* including the four main subtypes plus lymphatic leukemia and infectious mononucleosis. The task for the clinical observer is to endeavor to correlate what he sees in the patient with one of the conditions contained in the list of lesions. This may be a task of extreme difficulty, and frequently the assistance of the pathologist is required. We have already considered some of the pitfalls of the lymph node biopsy, in particular the need for: (1) Examination of a blood film before considering removal of a node when the enlargement is generalized, and (2) bacteriological examination of the node after removal.

THE THYMUS GLAND

The thymus is partly epithelial and partly lymphoid in structure. At first it is entirely epithelial, being derived from the third branchial cleft, but later in embryonic life it becomes invaded with lymphocytes. The epithelium persists as the Hassall's corpuscles and the cells of the reticulum. The cytoreticulum is derived from the endodermal third branchial pouch, the Hassall corpuscles from the ectodermal cervical sinus.

The size of the thymus is its most important feature. No idea of the size during life can be obtained unless the patient has died suddenly, for the gland undergoes a rapid and remarkable *shrinking* as the result of infection, starvation, and other hostile influences; this shrinkage takes place at the expense of the lymphocytes. In emaciated children the gland may weigh only 2 to 3 grams instead of the normal 15 or 20 grams. It follows that in cases of sudden death, whether in the child or adult, the thymus may appear to be abnormally large. The average weight at birth is 13 grams, and this gradually increases until at puberty it weighs 35 grams or more. After that period there is a gradual atrophy. The fall in weight after puberty suggests that the thymus exerts some influence on genital development, but the real *function* of the thymus is obscure, which is a nice way of saying that it is unknown.

Hyperplasia of the thymus is a constant feature of Graves' disease, where it forms part of a general thymico-lymphatic hyperplasia. There is said to be hyperplasia in Addison's disease, acromegaly, castration, myasthenia gravis, and after thyroid feeding.

STATUS THYMICO-LYMPHATICUS

In cases of sudden death from no obvious cause the thymus and the lymphoid tissue throughout the body may be found to be enlarged, and it is the custom to attribute death in these cases, especially when there is a coroner's inquest, to "status lymphaticus" or "enlarged thymus." There is a remarkable difference of opinion regarding the importance and even the existence of status lymphaticus. Marine, Warthin, and others described the condition as a constitutional defect associated with lowered resistance and characterized by hyperplasia of the thymus, lymph nodes and lymphoid tissue in general, together with underdevelopment of the adrenals, gonads, and cardiovascular system. Greenwood and Woods, on the other hand, after a most careful statistical investigation describe status thymico-lymphaticus as a good example of the growth of medical mythology, in which a nucleus of truth is buried beneath a pile of intellectual rubbish, conjecture, bad observations, and rash generalization, and that it is as accurate to attribute the cause of death to "an act of God" as to status lymphaticus.

The writer has not had sufficient experience with cases of sudden death to enable him to express an opinion on this difficult matter. Two facts, however, must be admitted. The first is that certain persons have an abnormally low resistance to drugs, anesthetics, vaccines, serums, and such poisons as arsphenamine and cocaine. In such persons death may follow the most trivial of causes, such as extraction of a tooth, tonsillectomy, a slight blow, or taking a cold bath. The second fact is that in some persons there is a remarkable lymphoid hyperplasia affecting the lymphoid tissue of the throat, nasopharynx, intestinal canal, lymph nodes, and frequently the thymus, associated with hypoplasia of the adrenals, heart, and great vessels. It has been shown experimentally that removal of the adrenals lowers the resistance of rats to morphine as much as 400 times. Modern knowledge regarding the relationship of the adrenal cortex to resistance to stress and lymphoid tissue development suggests that it is the small adrenal rather than the large thymus which is the source of danger. It seems to me that there can be no doubt that the *constitutional disturbance* known as status lymphaticus is a real entity and that its most striking clinical feature is a great lowering of resistance. It *may* explain some of the sudden and unexplained deaths in infants and young children, especially those cases in which an apparently healthy infant is found dead in its crib, although the more careful and searching the autopsy examination is on such cases, the more often will some more satisfying explanation be found such as a hidden and unsuspected infection.

TUMORS OF THE THYMUS

The only tumor which need be mentioned is the *malignant thymoma*. This constitutes one variety of mediastinal tumor and is commonly taken for a lymphosarcoma. It is highly malignant, compresses the trachea and other structures, invades the lungs, and metastasizes to bronchial, cervical and axillary glands, and sometimes to distant organs. The structure varies, and this is natural, be-

cause the thymus arises from two cell systems, the one lymphoid and the other epithelial. The usual type of picture is lymphosarcomatous, but occasionally it is frankly carcinomatous. It seems probable that these two types arise from one or other of the two cell systems. Finally the tumor may be of a composite nature consisting of the various cells which go to make up the normal thymus. It is to this group that the term thymoma should be applied. For illustrations of the various thymic tumors Castleman's Atlas should be consulted.

Different *microscopic* fields from the same tumor may show great variation in structure, depending on the degree of differentiation from the epithelial anlage. Of particular significance is the presence of "granulomatous" areas, where epithelial cells intermingle with lymphocytes and eosinophils, the areas being separated by dense collagen bands which are particularly characteristic of thymic tumors. The epithelial cells are large and pale, and giant cells are common. With such a histological picture it is easy to understand how confusion with Hodgkin's disease may occur, and why some workers believe that lesions of the thymus form an integral part of the latter disease.

Iverson at the Armed Forces Institute of Pathology in Washington has analyzed 50 cases diagnosed by the pathologist as thymoma, only 27 of which proved to be true tumors of the thymus.

Of particular interest is the division by Iverson of her cases into two groups. (1) Those without myasthenic symptoms; here there is lymphoid proliferation, spindle cell proliferation and stromal proliferation. (2) Those with evidence of myasthenia gravis; the lesions consist of large pale epithelial cells loosely mixed with lymphocytes and often arranged in cords or characteristic clusters around blood sinusoids, suggesting the possibility of an endocrine function. Of the 27 cases, 14 were not associated with myasthenia, the symptoms being those of a slowly growing mediastinal mass in a patient of an average age of fifty years. The remaining 13 cases were associated with myasthenia gravis, the average age being thirty-eight years. The difficult question of the relationship of the thymus and thymic tumors to myasthenia gravis will be discussed in connection with diseases of muscle. Suffice it to say here that: (1) 15 to 25 per cent of cases of myasthenia are associated with thymoma; (2) most thymic tumors are not associated with myasthenia gravis; and (3) contrary to what might be expected, the prognosis is better when a non-neoplastic thymus is removed than in the case of a thymoma (Keynes).

REFERENCES

CASTLEMAN, B.: *Tumors of the Thymus Gland*, Atlas of Tumor Pathology, Section V, Fascicle 19, Armed Forces Institute of Pathology, Washington, D. C., 1955.

CRAVER, L. E. and COPELAND, M. M.: Arch. Surg., 1934, *28*, 1062. (Bone Lesions in Hodgkin's disease.)

CUMMINGS, M. M. and HUDGKINS, P. C.: Am. J. Med. Sci., 1958, *236*, 311. (Pine pollen and sarcoidosis.)

DOUGHERTY, T. F. and WHITE, A.: Physiol. Rev., 1952, *32*, 379. (Influence of hormones on lymphoid tissue.)

GALL, E. A. and MALLORY, T. B.: Am. J. Path., 1942, *18*, 381. (Classification of lymphoblastomas.)

GREENWOOD, M. and WOODS, H. M.: J. Hyg., 1927, *26*, 205. (Status thymico-lymphaticus.)

HARRISON, C. V.: J. Path. and Bact., 1952, *64*, 513. (Benign Hodgkin's disease, Hodgkin's paragranuloma.)

IVERSON, L.: Am. J. Path., 1956, *32*, 695. (Thymomas.)

JACKSON, H., JR. and PARKER, F., JR.: *Hodgkin's Disease and Allied Disorders*, New York, 1947.

KAPLAN, H. S. and SMITHERS, D. W.: Lancet, 1959, *2*, 1. (Auto-immunity in malignant lymphomas.)

KEYNES, G.: Brit. J. Surg., 1955, *42*, 449. (Thymic tumors in relation to myasthenia gravis.)

LUMB, G.: *Tumours of Lymphoid Tissue*, Edinburgh, 1954.

MARINE, D.: Arch. Path., 1928, *5*, 661. (Status thymico-lymphaticus.)

MICHAEL, M., JR.: Ann. Int. Med., 1956, *45*, 151. (Pine forests and sarcoidosis.)

PERRY, S., *et al.*: Arch. Int. Med., 1959, *103*, 224. (Life span of the lymphocyte.)

SAXÉN, E. and SAXÉN, L.: Lab. Invest., 1959, *8*, 386. (Glandular toxoplasmosis.)

WARWICK, O. H. and SELLERS, A. H.: Can. Med. Ass. J., 1959, *80*, 423. (Life history of Hodgkin's disease.)

WEISS, S.: New Eng. J. Med., 1940, *223*, 793. (Sudden death.)

WRIGHT, C. J. E.: Am. J. Path., 1956, *32*, 201. (Macrofollicular lymphoma.)

Chapter 42

The Nervous System

General Considerations
THE NEURONE
   Neuronal Degeneration
THE NEUROGLIA
PATHS OF INFECTION
THE BLOOD-BRAIN BARRIER
PATHOLOGICAL PHYSIOLOGY
THE CEREBROSPINAL FLUID
HYDROCEPHALUS
INCREASED INTRACRANIAL
   PRESSURE
Cerebrovascular Disease
Strokes
   Thrombosis with Athero-
     sclerosis
   Cerebral Embolism
   Cerebral Hemorrhage
ANTERIOR SPINAL ARTERY
   OCCLUSION
COLLAGEN DISEASE LESIONS
Intracranial Aneurysms
CONGENITAL
MYCOTIC
ATHEROSCLEROTIC
Meningeal Hemorrhage
EXTRADURAL
SUBDURAL
SUBARACHNOID
Brain and Cord Injuries
LACERATION
CONCUSSION
TRAUMATIC EDEMA
METABOLIC EFFECTS OF BRAIN
   INJURY
EPILEPSY
SPINAL CORD INJURIES
Intracranial Suppuration
EXTRADURAL ABSCESS
ABSCESS OF THE BRAIN
SINUS THROMBOPHLEBITIS
Meningitis
MENINGOCOCCAL MENINGITIS
OTHER FORMS OF SUPPURATIVE
   MENINGITIS
TUBERCULOUS MENINGITIS
Virus Diseases
ENCEPHALITIS
   Type A (Lethargic)
   Type B (St. Louis)
   Equine Encephalitis
   Mumps Meningoencephalitis

ACUTE DISSEMINATED ENCEPH-
   ALOMYELITIS
   Post-vaccinal Encephalitis
ASEPTIC MENINGITIS
   Lymphocytic Choriomeningitis
   Coxsackie Group B Meningitis
   Echo Meningitis
ACUTE ANTERIOR POLIO-
   MYELITIS
COXSACKIE VIRUS INFECTIONS
HERPES
RABIES
Non-Viral Encephalitis
LEAD ENCEPHALITIS
DRUG ENCEPHALITIS
CEREBRAL TOXOPLASMOSIS
Myelitis
Syphilis of the Nervous System
GUMMA
MENINGOENCEPHALITIS
TABES DORSALIS
GENERAL PARESIS
Fungus Infections
CRYPTOCOCCOSIS
MUCORMYCOSIS
COCCIDIOIDOMYCOSIS
HISTOPLASMOSIS
Demyelinating Diseases
MULTIPLE SCLEROSIS
SCHILDER'S DISEASE
ACUTE DISSEMINATED EN-
   CEPHALOMYELITIS
ACUTE NECROTIZING HEMOR-
   RHAGIC ENCEPHALOMYELITIS
Metabolic Disorders
HEPÀTO-LENTICULAR DEGENER-
   ATION (WILSON'S DISEASE)
AMAUROTIC FAMILY IDIOCY
   (TAY-SACHS DISEASE)
Nutritional Deficiencies
SUBACUTE COMBINED DEGENER-
   ATION
WERNICKE'S ENCEPHALOPATHY
PELLAGRA
Idiopathic Degenerations
CHRONIC MOTOR NEURONE
   DEGENERATION
   Amyotrophic Lateral Sclerosis
   Progressive Muscular Atrophy
   Progressive Bulbar Palsy
   Cerebral Palsy

PARKINSON'S DISEASE
KURU
HUNTINGTON'S CHOREA
SYDENHAM'S CHOREA
FRIEDREICH'S ATAXIA
SYRINGOMYELIA
PICK'S CONVULUTIONAL
   ATROPHY
ALZHEIMER'S DISEASE
Intracranial Tumors
GLIOMA
   Glioblastoma Multiforme
   Astrocytoma
   Medulloblastoma
   Ependymoma
Sheath Tumors
   Meningioma
   Acoustic Nerve Tumor
Miscellaneous Tumors
   Pinealoma
   Ganglioneuroma
   Retinoblastoma
   Hemangioma
   Cholesteatoma
METASTATIC TUMORS
   Subacute Cerebellar Disease
     in Cancer
Spinal Cord Tumors
EXTRAMEDULLARY
   Extradural
   Intradural
INTRAMEDULLARY
The Nerves
INJURY AND REPAIR
NEURITIS
   Acute Primary Polyneuropathy
     Guillain-Barré syndrome
     Carcinomatous neuropathy.
     Brachial neuritis
   Secondary Neuritis
TUMORS
   Neurofibroma
   Neurofibromatosis
   Neurogenic Sarcoma
Defects of Development
BRAIN
   Miscellaneous Conditions
   Tuberous Sclerosis
   Arnold-Chiari Malformation
SPINAL CORD
   (Sacrococcygeal Pilonidal
     Sinus)

GENERAL CONSIDERATIONS

THE student approaching the pathology of the nervous system need not expect his task to be an easy one. The structure of liver, kidney, pancreas or lung seems childishly simple when compared with that of the brain, the spinal cord, the various ganglia, and the peripheral nerves. This complexity of structure is more than matched by complexity of function, as is evident from the infinitely varied clinical disturbances which may be

(1122)

encountered. Moreover specialized techniques have been developed over the past century designed to demonstrate some particular structure such as the Nissl granules in the nerve cells, the myelin sheaths of the fibers, and the various glial elements, techniques which may involve the use not only of different stains from those of general pathology, but different methods of fixation. The disadvantage of these special methods is that while they reveal particular structures, they may fail to demonstrate the relation of these structures to others which are not rendered visible. This difficulty has been overcome by the advent of the electron microscope, which not only shows *all* the structures present in a given area with a preciseness and minuteness hitherto unattainable, but without the confusing artefacts which were unavoidable with standard technique. Greenfield points out in his great book that not only does neuropathology demand a technique different from that of general pathology, but it also uses a different language, in so far as it deals with different tissues, so that we have Nissl's degeneration, demyelination, and a host of other terms that are new to us.

Other respects in which the central nervous system is unique will be referred to in the discussion which follows. Among these of particular importance are the blood-brain barrier, as a result of which the normal brain lives in a peculiar state of apparent isolation by comparison with other organs, the interneuronal system of glial cells which were once regarded as mere passive supporters (*glia*, glue), and the series of synapses by means of which the nerve impulse is transmitted from one unit to another and which may break down from various causes.

The respect in which disease of the brain differs most fundamentally from that of other organs is the distinction between "organic" and "functional" disease. In organic disorders some definite structural cause for the symptoms can be demonstrated, whereas in so-called functional disease no organic cause can be found to account for the disordered function, which is often described as "mental" in character. The nature of these disturbances, however, suggests impaired integration of neuronal activity which may be related to abnormal neurohumoral intersynaptic transmission (Fazakas). Indeed the whole subject of the biochemical basis of mental disorders promises to be a thrilling field for future investigation.

The *average weight of the brain* in the male is 1400 grams, in the female 1250 grams. There is a minimal amount of cerebrospinal fluid in the subarachnoid space, much more in the basal cisterns. The pia-arachnoid is glistening, translucent, and is stripped off readily without tearing the brain (decortication). The subarachnoid space may be distended with fluid in conditions of edema. The convolutions are rounded and the sulci of moderate size. In cerebral atrophy the convolutions become shrunken and the sulci wide and deep, whereas in increased intracranial pressure the convolutions are flattened and the sulci obliterated. Not only the size but also the lining of the ventricles must be noted; it becomes granular in general paresis. The substantia nigra is examined for loss of pigment in chronic encephalitis lethargica. The vessels at the base should be soft and free from atheroma.

When a stained section of any part of the brain is examined it is seen to consist of a medley of cells and fibers. These can be divided into two groups, the first composed of the neurones, the second of the interstitial tissue, the neuroglia. The typical large motor cells are easily recognized, but in a hematoxylin and eosin preparation it is not possible to distinguish with certainty between the smaller nerve cells and the cells of the neuroglia. When appropriate stains are employed these two groups can be readily differentiated.

The Neurone.—The neurone, the essential unit of the central nervous system, of which there are 10 billion, consists of a nerve cell and nerve fiber. The *nerve cell* has certain peculiarities which distinguish it from all other cells. Two of its most striking characteristics are its longevity and its great susceptibility to environmental and metabolic disturbances. It can live for 100 years (compare this with the short life of the lymphocyte), but it cannot be replaced if it is destroyed, nor does it undergo mitotic division. Small wonder that we so seldom encounter tumors of adult nerve cells. On the other hand the nerve cell has great metabolic activity, requiring a constant large supply of oxygen and glucose, so that the cells of the cerebral cortex cannot survive five minutes of anoxia due to complete arrest of the circulation at normal body temperature, and a fall in blood sugar level to 20 mg. per 100 ml. results in loss of consciousness. *Nissl granules* constitute the most characteristic feature in the cytoplasm of the healthy cell. With the electron microscope they appear as ergastoplasmic structures.

The *nerve fiber* is made up of 3 constituents: the axis cylinder or axon, the medullary or myelin sheath, and the neurolemma (neurilemma) or nucleated sheath of Schwann. Within the central nervous system the fibers consist only of the first two elements, the sheath of Schwann being added when the fiber becomes peripheral. After giving off one or more collateral fibers the larger axons may run for long distances in the central nervous system, as they do in the peripheral nerves, without branching. Near their termination they lose their myelin sheath and break up into a number of five terminal twigs, which either enter the peripheral end-organ or make synaptic connection with the cell bodies of other neurones by means of ring-like endings known as *boutons terminaux*, or with dendrites of these neurones.

The *myelin sheath* is one of the most characteristic features of the neurone. It is a lipid structure. The electron microscope has shown that myelin is laid down in concentric laminæ like the rings of a tree. In the peripheral nerves the laminæ are deposited spirally on the axon by successive rotations around it of the enclosing Schwann cells. In the central nervous system the oligodendroglia takes the place of the Schwann cells, but without this wrapping-around process. We used to regard myelin as a passive element which merely protected the axis cylinder, just as we used to regard neuroglia as a nerve glue. That view must be abandoned. From 50 to 60 per cent of the dry weight of the brain is made up of *lipid*. This consists largely of cholesterol, sphingomyelin and cerebroside, to which more recently has been added ganglioside, the last three being grouped as sphingolipids.

There is no esterified cholesterol. When a nerve such as the sciatic is cut the myelin components decrease, and there is a marked increase of water, but of particular significance is the appearance for the first time of esterified cholesterol. The demyelination in multiple sclerosis, that disease of mystery, follows a very similar pattern, more particularly in the active plaques (Cumings). Similar lipid findings are observed in Schilder's disease, the so-called sudanophilic type of diffuse sclerosis. The great increase of esterified cholesterol is absolutely characteristic of these two types of demyelination. It seems probable that this is due to a deficiency in an enzyme factor, very likely on a genetic basis. When we come later to the complex and obscure subject of the demyelinating diseases, we shall have to return to these theoretical matters. Moreover in the discussion of the neuroglia which follows we shall see that the oligodendroglia maintains an intimate relationship with the myelin sheath, being concerned with its preservation and possibly with its formation.

We are accustomed to think of the neurones of the brain and spinal cord as structural units consisting of cells and long fibers, with specific functions, either motor or sensory. To these we must add the *reticular formation* of the central core of the brain stem consisting of a multitude of small cells with fine, short fibers which have many synapses and therefore diffuse interconnections. This non-specific neural system can exert an influence at various levels either to diminish or raise the activity of other functions. The *ascending reticular system* seems to exert an influence on the cerebral hemispheres which initiates and maintains such states as wakefulness and attention (Magoun). Injury to this system results in partial or complete loss of consciousness. In addition the reticular system appears to influence neuroendocrine control of visceral function through the anterior pituitary secretion. Lesions in this region will cause corresponding disturbance of this control. Excitation of the reticular system by peripheral stimuli or cortical stress in the experimental animal can result in increased secretion of gastric hydrochloric acid and the production of peptic ulcer.

Neuronal Degeneration. — Degenerative changes affecting the various parts of the neurone are of the greatest importance in neuropathology. When any part of the neurone is injured the remainder of the neurone will show constant and characteristic changes. By the use of this method experimentally and in some cases in man it is possible to follow the course of a fiber arising from an injured nerve cell, and also to determine from which cell an injured fiber arises.

Wallerian degeneration is the term applied to the characteristic changes in the *distal part* of the nerve fiber when any level of the fiber is divided or when the cell from which it arises is killed. These changes were first observed and described by Waller in the experimental animal in 1850, a date which shows that neuropathology is not entirely modern. The axis cylinder becomes fibrillated and disintegrates, the medullary sheath breaks up into droplets of myelin which can be stained black by Marchi's method, (Fig. 635), and the cells of the sheath of Schwann are converted into phagocytes which remove the remnants of the medullary sheath and axis cylinder. These cells also play an essential part in regeneration, a process which will be studied when the healing of nerve is considered. As the sheath of Schwann is not present in the central nervous system it is evident that healing after injury cannot occur in the brain and spinal cord. The complete process of Wallerian degeneration is best studied in a peripheral nerve, but the axonal and medullary sheath changes take place in the central nervous system also and have proved of extreme value in the experimental study of the path of fibers and tracts owing to the ease with which the degenerating myelin can be stained. The *proximal part* of the divided fiber also shows changes. The medullary sheath degenerates up to the first node of Ranvier, and the nuclei of the sheath of Schwann multiply in this segment of the nerve, and help to bridge the gap between the two ends of the divided fiber in a way which will be described in connection with injuries to nerves. The nerve cell from which the fiber arises undergoes Nissl's degeneration (see below).

Wallerian degeneration readily occurs as

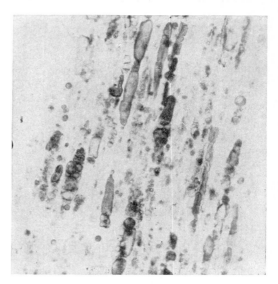

FIG. 635.—Wallerian degeneration. Early degeneration of myelin sheath thirteen days after section of a nerve. Weigert's stain. × 90. (Kindness of Dr. Mary Tom.)

the result of *avitaminosis*, for the health of the medullary sheath is dependent on vitamins, especially B_1. There is, however, no activity on the part of the Schwann cells. When vitamin B_{12} is withheld experimentally degeneration of the anterolateral and dorsal tracts of the cord occurs as well as myelin degeneration of the peripheral nerves.

Nissl's degeneration is the characteristic change which the nerve cell undergoes when the nerve fiber which arises from it is injured, or when the cell is acted on by chemical or bacterial toxins, or by viruses. The same secondary changes in the cell occur as the result of alcoholic and other forms of neuritis. The cell becomes swollen and rounded, the nucleus becomes eccentric in position and may be situated at the extreme margin, and the Nissl granules in the cytoplasm disintegrate and disappear (Fig. 636). It is this condition, known as *chromatolysis*, to which the degeneration owes its name. It is evident from what has been said that Nissl's degeneration is complementary to Wallerian degeneration. When degeneration is sufficiently far advanced the phenomenon of *neuronophagia* may be observed, the cell body being surrounded by phagocytes, known in this regard by the somewhat

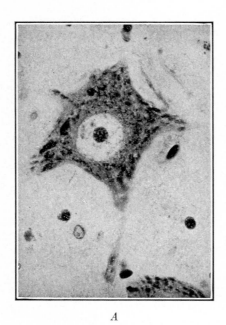

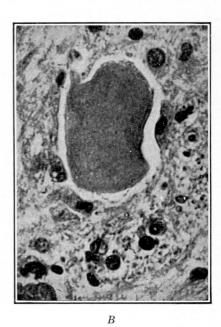

A   B

Fig. 636.—*A*, Normal nerve cell showing processes, concave borders, Nissl granules, nucleus and nucleolus. × 600. *B*, Degenerated nerve cell; borders convex, loss of processes, Nissl granules and nucleus. × 600.

sinister term of satellites, which assist in its disintegration. These cells are derived from two constituents of the interstitial tissues, the *microglia* and the *oligodendroglia*. About three weeks after the division of a nerve, regeneration begins, the granules reappear, and the cell body is restored to normal. These regenerative changes are not seen in the cells of the upper motor neurone, just as no regeneration occurs in the fibers of these neurones. They just die.

The *distinction between upper and lower motor neurone lesions* is one of the most fundamental in neuropathology. *Upper motor neurone lesions* affect any part of the pyramidal tract from the motor cells in the cortex to the termination of the fibers around the anterior horn cells of the cord or the motor nuclei of the cranial nerves. *Lower motor neurone lesions* involve the anterior horn cells and their fibers or the motor nuclei of the cranial nerves and their fibers. Lesions of either the upper or lower neurone cause paralysis of muscles, but they can usually be readily distinguished from one another. The characteristics of *upper neurone lesions* are spasticity (increased muscle tone), exagger-

ated deep reflexes, and Babinski's sign (dorsiflexion of great toe on stimulation of sole of foot). *Lower motor neurone lesions* are characterized by flaccidity of the paralyzed muscles, loss of the deep reflexes, muscular atrophy and severe trophic disturbances, fibrillary twitchings in the affected muscles, and the reaction of degeneration in these muscles. The commonest example of an upper motor neurone lesion is afforded by a hemorrhage into the internal capsule which destroys the pyramidal tract fibers. Examples of lower motor lesions are poliomyelitis (infantile paralysis), transverse myelitis, and the ordinary form of facial paralysis.

The Neuroglia.—The interstitial tissue of the central nervous system has long been known as the neuroglia. Glia means glue, and the neuroglia was regarded as a kind of putty which served the humble purpose of holding together the more noble neurones. In ordinary preparations the interstitial elements appear for the most part as naked nuclei. Gold and silver impregnation, however, gives an entirely different picture, and in place of naked nuclei we now see cells pro-

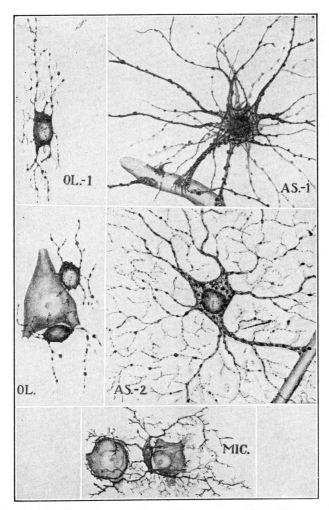

FIG. 637.—The interstitial cells of the central nervous system. AS.–1, Fibrous astrocyte with several perivascular feet on blood vessel. AS.–2, Protoplasmic astrocyte showing numerous processes but no fibrils. OL–1, Oligodendroglia. OL., Two oligodendroglia cells as perineuronal satellites around nerve cell in which nucleolus is distinctly shown. MIC., Microglia cells with numerous processes placed between and in contact with two nerve cells: in the latter the nucleolus can be distinguished. (Penfield, in Cowdry's *Special Cytology,* courtesy of P. B. Hoeber.)

vided with a forest of fibers. By the aid of these methods, it is possible to distinguish three elements in the interstitial tissue: these are the *astrocytes,* the *oligodendroglia,* and the *microglia.* The first two are ectodermal in origin, and together make up the neuroglia. The third is mesodermal in origin and is un-related to the neuroglia. The astrocytes and the microglia are the great indicators of dis-ease in the central nervous system. Stim-ulation of the brain in the experimental animal results in a marked increase in the content of enzyme proteins in the neurones, with a corresponding drop in that of the glial cells.

Astrocytes.—The astrocytes, the cells of the classical neuroglia, are of two types, protoplasmic and fibrous. The *protoplasmic astrocytes* are found almost entirely in the gray matter, particularly in the middle and deep layers of the cerebral cortex and in the molecular layer of the cerebellum. When

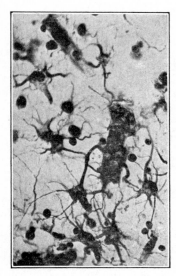

FIG. 638.—Astrocytes with sucker feet attached to vessels. Gliosis (gold sublimate.) × 315.

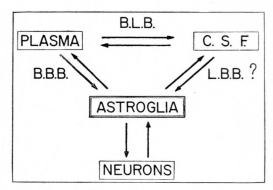

FIG. 639.—Diagrammatic representation of the hypothetic relationships between plasma and cerebrospinal fluid with the neuron through the astroglia. LBB, liquor-brain barrier, BLB, blood liquor barrier, BBB, blood-brain barrier. (Gerschenfeld, Wald, Zadunaisky and De Robertis, courtesy of Neurology.)

examined with the electron microscope the cells have an abundant but relatively empty ("watery") cytoplasm, with few mitochondria and only an occasional Golgi apparatus, the material being evidently in a highly soluble state. This appearance acquires significance when we turn to the subject of function. They have wavy branching cytoplasmic processes that extend out from all aspects of the cell body, so that they resemble bushy shrubs. The *fibrous astrocytes* are characterized by the presence of fine firm fibers running through the cytoplasm and processes, which are not seen in the protoplasmic type (Fig. 637). The fibrous type is found in the white matter, but it is also arranged in a dense layer in the most superficial zone of the cortex immediately under the pia mater to form a *superficial limiting membrane*. Both types of astrocyte are large cells with many processes, best demonstrated by Cajal's gold-sublimate method. At least one of these processes is attached by a pyramidal expansion called a vascular foot plate or sucker foot (Fig. 638). The extent to which a capillary may be enveloped by vascular feet must be seen to be realized. It seems probable that these structures form the most important element of the blood-brain barrier (page 1130). The sucker feet may also envelope nerve cells. Penfield describes in graphic yet concise manner the arrangement of the astroglia when he says that the octopus-like astrocytes hold the manifold structures of the nervous system within their tentacles, and are attached to the pia and the vascular tree by specialized expansions. In tissue culture the astrocytes form mucoprotein or mucopolysaccharide staining with PAS, which accounts in part for the watery appearance of the cytoplasm.

It will be evident that the *function of the astroglia* must be far more vital than that of a humble filler-in, as used to be supposed. Studies with the electron microscope suggest that the astroglia constitutes a water-ion compartment interposed between the capillaries and cerebrospinal fluid on one side and the cellular compartment proper on the other (Gerschenfeld *et al.*). It has, indeed, taken the place of the concepts of a perivascular space and of an intercellular ground substance which used to be generally accepted. The astroglia seems to be involved in the selection and transport of metabolites and fluid interchanges between the vascular spaces and the nerve cells (Fig. 639).

The astrocyte plays an active part *in disease*. Hortega and Penfield have shown that the repair of wounds in the brain is due entirely to the activity of the astrocytes, which enlarge, multiply, and fill in the gap, just as fibroblasts do in other parts of the body. The *gliosis* seen in general paresis and other chronic inflammations consists of astrocytes and their fibers. In experimental intoxications the perivascular astrocytes develop into ameboid cells, the processes and sucker feet being much swollen at first and later becoming absorbed into the body of the cell. Finally, the astrocyte is the cell from which the great majority of *gliomas* (astrocytomas, glioblastomas) arise. The oligodendroglia rarely and the microglia apparently never take on neoplastic growth.

Oligodendroglia.—This is the largest group of the interstitial cells, but the one about which the least is known. In ordinary sections they appear as naked nuclei arranged in rows between the nerve fibers in the white matter, and in the gray matter as satellites adhering to the nerve cells. When stained by Hortega's silver carbonate method the cells, which are much smaller than the astrocytes, are seen to possess a small number of fine processes (*oligos,* few) (Fig. 637). The *function* of these cells is obscure. They seem to bear the same relation to the myelin sheath of the nerve fibers in the central nervous system as the cells of the sheath of Schwann do in the peripheral nerves, so that they may have something to do with the preservation of the myelin. *In disease* they appear to play a part of no importance. They are evidently very sensitive to noxious agents, for they readily undergo acute swelling, becoming pale, vacuolated, and losing their processes. The cells are seldom seen in perfect form in human postmortem material, for they rapidly undergo autolysis after death.

Microglia.—The microglia differs fundamentally from the other two elements in being mesodermal in origin, while they originate from ectoderm. The cells are very small (hence the name), and are provided with numerous fine branching processes which are stained by the silver carbonate method. Some of them form satellites to the nerve cells (Fig. 637). The microglia is not present at birth, but invades the brain from the pia in the course of a few weeks. These cells may be regarded as forming part of the reticuloendothelial sys-

tem, for when studied in tissue cultures by vital staining they behave in exactly the same way.

The *function of the microglia* is phagocytic; the cells are indeed the phagocytes of the central nervous system. Under pathological conditions they develop into the rod cells of general paresis and the scavenger cells (also known as compound granular corpuscles, fat granule cells and Gitterzellen) seen in brain softening. The transformation of the quiescent microglial cell into the ameboid and phagocytic scavenger cell is a remarkable one. The cell body becomes swollen and rounded, the processes are thickened and then withdrawn into the cell, and the cytoplasm becomes filled with fat globules derived from the disintegrating myelin. The cells collect in enormous numbers at the site of injury, and then appear to carry the ingested myelin to the nearest vessels, into which they possibly discharge their content.

If the student would care to get a glimpse of the thrilling new world of the neuroglia as seen by the electron microscope, he could not do better than glance at *Biology of Neuroglia*, (1958), edited by W. F. Windle.

Corpora Amylacea.—These are small spherical hyaline bodies, sometimes displaying a concentric structure, which are seen in large numbers in the nervous system in old age, and may occur earlier as a result of degenerative diseases. It used to be thought that they arose from the medullary sheath of degenerating nerves or possibly from nerve cells, but it now appears more probable that they represent degenerated microglial cells, or in some cases they may be formed from the oligodendroglia.

Paths of Infection.—Infection may reach the central nervous system by way of the blood stream or the lymph stream, or it may pass along the axis cylinders of motor or sensory nerves.

Blood infection may be very obvious, as in the solitary abscess of the brain which may complicate bronchiectasis or endocarditis, and which is due to infected material carried by the arteries, or in the minute miliary abscesses of septicemia.

Perineural lymphatics may convey both bacteria and their toxins to the brain and cord. It can be shown in the experimental animal that the histological picture produced by the action of toxins on the central nervous system is that of cord degeneration with edema and hyaline thrombosis but no inflammation of the tissues if spread is by the blood vessels, while there is a primary inflammation of the fixed tissues if spread is by the lymphatics.

It is possible that in many cases this spread is *along the axis cylinders* rather than along the perineural lymphatics. Goodpasture's work on the virus of herpes simplex, described in a later section, is particularly suggestive in this regard. Some at least of the poison of tetanus passes by this route. This spread within the nerve itself appears to be of particular importance in virus diseases.

The methods of spread within the central nervous system itself need further investigation. When the virus of poliomyelitis or herpes is inoculated into the brain it is rapidly diffused through the whole brain and cord. Does the infection spread by the cerebrospinal fluid, or may the virus be passed up and down the cord by way of the axis cylinders? These are important questions which still await an answer.

The Blood-Brain Barrier.—For many years it has been known that the cerebral vessels differ from other blood vessels in their permeability. Thus when large molecule dyes are introduced into the circulation they appear in the histiocytes of the liver, spleen and lymph nodes, but not in the cerebral histiocytes, except where the brain is injured or inflamed. The intravenous injection of methylene blue results in a rapid and clear picture of the peripheral nervous system, but there is no immediate coloring of the nerve cells and fibers in the brain unless the capillary barrier has been broken down by cell poisons mixed with the methylene blue.

The foregoing statement regarding permeability of cerebral vessels is apt to be misleading. *The barrier is against large molecules, which include a wide variety of toxic substances, not against water and electrolytes.* It is obvious that the neurones with their high metabolic level need an abundance of water, oxygen and glucose. It is when radioactive isotopes of electrolytes are given

intravenously that the labelled ions are found to behave in a physiological manner, and to play a role in the normal metabolism of the central nervous system (Bakay). The clear glia cells seem to provide an intracellular transport system for nutrients and electrolytes, so that this system functions in the cerebrum as the extracellular space does in other organs. The application of cold to the exposed brain of the mouse results in a localized swelling, which is due to enlargement of the cytoplasmic volume of glia cells with clear cytoplasm and does not involve the intercellular space (Torack *et al.*). The blood-brain barrier is essentially a defence mechanism against noxious agents. Most bacteria and viruses can only penetrate the barrier with difficulty. At the same time the barrier prevents the brain and cord from being flooded with fluid in pathological states which result in marked edema of the other tissues of the body.

It is evident that the blood-brain barrier is related to the close application of the cytoplasmic foot processes of innumerable astrocytes to the endothelium of the capillaries. Certain toxic substances can break down the barrier and allow the passage of colloidal material injurious to the neurones.

Pathological Physiology.—The normal physiology of the brain may be changed into dysfunction involving the motor or sensory fields or those of intellect or behavior. It is customary to classify examples of cerebral dysfunction as either organic or functional. In *"organic" syndromes* gross or microscopic lesions can be demonstrated. These are associated with interference with the supply of carbohydrate or oxygen to the brain, or abnormalities of cerebral enzyme activity, or disordered energy utilization. In *"functional" syndromes* there are no demonstrable anatomical, biochemical or physiological abnormalities, but "their nature suggests impaired integration of neuronal activity, which may be related to abnormal neurohumoral intersynaptic transmission" (Fazekas). *What in the past we have called mental disease and stigmatized as insanity or madness is probably in most cases merely a biochemical disturbance of nerve cells which will be corrected in the future by biochemical means.* It seems likely that most of the popular neuropharmacological agents such as ataractics, "psychic energisers," etc. act upon neurohumoral mediators and thus change the utilization of cerebral energy.

The neuronal impulse is a form of energy derived from oxidative reactions mediated by enzymes acting on a carbohydrate substrate in the presence of oxygen. *Enzyme activity* is dependant on the action of a number of the B-complex vitamins which are constituents of co-enzymes necessary for the production of energy from carbohydrate degradation. Nutritional deficiencies involving these vitamins, more particularly thiamin, riboflavin and pyridoxine (necessary for the biosynthesis of serotonin), will impair enzymatic activity with results which will be encountered in the course of this chapter. Many drugs inhibit these enzyme systems, with consequent impairment of cerebral function. *Substrate insufficiency* may ruin enzyme activity, and a decrease in blood glucose concentration may prove disastrous. *Oxygen insufficiency* is equally harmful, for cerebral metabolism is almost completely aerobic. The brain, indeed, is responsible for one-fifth the oxygen consumption of the entire body, and total interference with the oxygen supply results in irreversible damage to the cerebral cortex in five to eight minutes. *Cerebral anoxia* is most often the result of surgical shock such as may follow an operation, but sometimes it may be due to severe respiratory disease. The result is a diffuse disorder of function which is reversible if the anoxia is not too severe and prolonged, together with signs of focal damage which are more apt to be persistent. A state of confusion is first induced, with the danger of a later development of mental impairment.

Serotonin.—The general subject of the pharmacological action of serotonin has already been discussed on page 773 in connection with carcinoid tumors of the intestine. Its original name, *enteramine*, is descriptive both of its origin and its chemical nature, for it is an indole-amine, 5-hydroxytryptamine (5-HT), obtained originally in tissue extract of intestinal mucosa and found to be active against blood vessels and smooth muscle. Serotonin is now known to be a normal constituent of the gray matter of the brain, the highest concentration being in the hypothalamus, midbrain, limbic lobe, and floor of the fourth ventricle. As it does not pass the blood-brain barrier it is formed locally from 5-hydroxytryptophan.

What serotonin does and should do in the brain is largely unknown country at the present time, although it has been shown to have an excitatory action on neural structures. A number of ingenious suggestions have been made, linking this substance to schizophrenia and other mental disorders through disturbed chemical regulation of cerebral synaptic transmission. Serotonin is known to powerfully depress such transmission, whereas tranquilizing drugs block this action and restore nervous and therefore mental equilibrium. Again, LSD (lysergic acid diethylamide), a substance which produces mental changes in man, is a potent antagonist of serotonin in its peripheral effects. At the present time it seems safe to say that 5-hydroxytryptamine is one of the most powerful metabolites known, and that this hormone is apparently of vital concern in the metabolism of the brain, and in maintaining normal mental processes.

Schizophrenia.—It would be obviously absurd even to think of considering the all-important subject of mental disease in this place. A word, however, may be devoted to schizophrenia in this discussion of pathological physiology, for it is the principal cause of chronic mental illness, and is said to affect in some degree nearly 1 per cent of the population, and to be responsible for more disability than any other illness in the whole of medicine. It manifests itself most often between the ages of fifteen and twenty-five years (hence the older name of dementia praecox), first by a gradual social withdrawal, followed by the development of all sorts of bizarre hallucinations. It involves a fragmentation, a breaking-up, of all the processes of thought and feeling which enable a healthy person to remain in touch with his world, and might be regarded as a cancer of the mind gnawing into the very soul of the patient. What interests us at this point is that similar hallucinations can be induced in a normal person by means of the so-called hallucinogenic drugs. The volunteer subject may experience distortions of reality, a feeling of fantastic bodily lightness, and the self seems to be dissociated from the body and to watch it from the outside. The significance of these observations is that they indicate that *a chemical abnormality in a brain that is structurally normal may result in a condition of insanity.* The mechanism may be an interference with cell enzymes by antimetabolites, but it seems possible that too great or too little a production of serotonin might result in a similar mental state through disturbance of the biochemistry of the synapses. Finally it must be added that a genetic factor seems to be involved, and as genes are believed to control enzymatic activity a mutation involving certain genes could lead to abnormal enzymatic reaction in the cerebral metabolism.

Phenylpyruvic Oligophrenia.—This is a condition in which there is a low level of 5-hydroxytryptamine in the serum, so that it may be mentioned here. It is an inborn error of metabolism resulting in a severe hereditary mental deficiency in children, oligophrenia coming from the Greek meaning feeblemindedness. There is defective hydroxylation of phenylalanine, an essential amino acid, so that phenylpyruvic acid is excreted in the urine, a condition known as *phenylketonuria.* In some cases there is generalized demyelination of the brain and spinal cord, but in other cases no lesions can be distinguished, even in the presence of severe mental deficiency.

The Cerebrospinal Fluid.—The cerebrospinal fluid, or spinal fluid as it is often called for convenience, is the sensitive mirror in which is reflected many a picture of disease of the central nervous system, although we shall find as we proceed that the picture is often blurred and indistinct. The fluid is *secreted* in the lateral ventricles and the third ventricle by the choroid plexus, passes along the aqueduct of Sylvius to the fourth ventricle, and escapes thence into the cerebral subarachnoid space through the small openings in the membranous roof of that ventricle, namely the median foramen of Magendie and the two lateral foramina of Luschka. The *subarachnoid space* is extremely narrow over the upper surface of the brain, but widens out into cavernous cisterns at the base. From here it passes

down to the third piece of the sacrum, and as the spinal cord ends at the lower border of the first lumbar vertebra, the fluid may safely be withdrawn by means of lumbar puncture from any part of the intervening space.

The brain and spinal cord are suspended floating in the cerebrospinal fluid, which provides these structures with the best mechanical protection. Absorption takes place in the great venous sinuses through the medium of the arachnoid villi, which are prolongations of the subarachnoid space projecting for the most part into the superior longitudinal sinus, and perhaps also directly from the subarachnoid space into the cerebral capillaries. The greater part of the absorption occurs above the level of the tentorium cerebelli, so that if some form of obstruction should prevent the flow of the fluid from the lower to the upper part of the cranial cavity, hydrocephalus will result even though the aqueduct of Sylvius and the foramen of Magendie are both open.

We have been accustomed to think of the cerebrospinal fluid bathing the neurones by virtue of the sleeve-like extension of the subarachnoid space supposed to be carried by the cerebral arteries into the brain substance. We now believe in a sheath of astroglia rather than a sleeve of subarachnoid space. There is, however, a *blood-fluid barrier* furnished by the choroidal epithelium which protects the brain by the selection and control of vital chemical compounds and blocks harmful materials.

The *normal pressure* varies from 80 to 190 mm. of water with the patient recumbent. The *total protein* is 20 to 30 or by some methods up to 45 or 50 mg. per 100 cc. The globulin content is nil, because of the larger size of its molecule compared with that of albumin. The *sugar content* is 45 to 75 mg. per 100 cc., being decreased by pyogenic infections. The *chloride content* is 720 to 750 mg. per 100 cc., being decreased in tuberculous meningitis, a feature which may be of the greatest diagnostic value. The *cells* (lymphocytes) are 3 to 5 per cmm. Reference to variations in the character of the spinal fluid under pathological conditions will be made in the appropriate place.

Enzymes may be found in the cerebrospinal fluid under conditions of disease. They are not likely to come from the blood on account of the blood-brain barrier. *Glutamic oxalacetic transaminase* (GOT), an enzyme which is increased in the blood in acute damage to the myocardium, liver and skeletal muscle, appears in quantity in the cerebrospinal fluid in experimental cerebral infarction in dogs, and a similar rise in transaminase level was found in 7 out of 11 patients suffering from this condition (Green *et al.*). *Nucleases* are of special significance in poliomyelitis and other virus infections (Kovacs). Neither ribonuclease nor desoxyribonuclease can be detected in the spinal fluid of healthy persons. With bacterial infections such as meningitis both of the nucleases are present in proportion to the acuteness of the infection. In poliomyelitis and other viral infections, on the other hand, there is intense ribonuclease activity but with no accompanying desoxyribonuclease activity.

Hydrocephalus.—Hydrocephalus or water on the brain is a condition in which the cerebrospinal fluid collects inside (and sometimes outside) the ventricles, so that these cavities become greatly dilated with an accompanying pressure atrophy of the cerebral tissue. We have already seen that the cerebrospinal fluid is secreted by the choroid plexus of the lateral and other ventricles, passes along the aqueduct of Sylvius to the fourth ventricle, and escapes through the foramina in the roof of that ventricle to enter the basal cisterns of the subarachnoid space. From there it flows upward through the narrows between the brain stem and the incisura in the tentorium, to expand again into the shallow lake of the cerebral portion of the subarachnoid space. It also passes down from the basal cisterns into the spinal canal. The fluid is absorbed into the large venous sinuses, especially the superior longitudinal sinus, by way of the arachnoid villi, which are diverticula of the subarachnoid space that project into the lumen of the sinuses. The Pacchionian bodies are hypertrophied villi which are only found in adult life. It is evident that if the fluid is unable to escape from the ventricles absorption is impossible, if it cannot pass from the basal cisterns to the cortical subarachnoid space

absorption will be impaired, and there may local interference with absorption if the arachnoid villi and Pacchionian bodies are blocked. The obstruction may occur at three points: (1) in the aqueduct, (2) in the roof of the fourth ventricle, and (3) around the mesencephalon where it passes through the narrow opening in the tentorium. The first two cause *internal hydrocephalus*, the third causes *communicating hydrocephalus*, the ventricles being in open communication with the basal cisterns and the spinal canal. All three are obstructing. Hydrocephalus has been divided into (1) congenital, (2) acquired, and (3) relative due to cerebral atrophy. It is often difficult if not impossible to distinguish between the congenital and the acquired forms, particularly in young children.

The ordinary hydrocephalus of children is due to obstruction either in the roof of the fourth ventricle or in the aqueduct. The exact *cause of the obstruction* is not certain. As Dorothy Russell remarks, quoting Spiller: "It is not necessary to study the different works on hydrocephalus very exhaustively to find that actually observed lesions are much rarer than theories explanatory of the causes of hydrocephalus." It is probable that adhesions due to a mild meningitis are the most frequent cause of obstruction in the roof of the ventricle. The aqueduct may be occluded by a delicate veil-like membrane which is probably the result of a developmental defect, but may in some cases be due to slight intra-uterine inflammation. Congenital hydrocephalus is due to obstruction of the aqueduct.

A rare cause is the so-called *Arnold-Chiari malformation*, a congenital deformity of the hind-brain in which the brain stem is displaced through the foramen magnum, plugging of which prevents the cerebrospinal fluid from passing upward to reach the cerebral subarachnoid space, there to be absorbed. It is possible, however, that the hydrocephalus may be the cause rather than the result of the displacement (see page 1217). Hydrocephalus may complicate meningitis or brain tumors. Tuberculous meningitis, the lesions of which are essentially basilar, is always accompanied by dilatation of the ventricles, due to the formation of a plastic

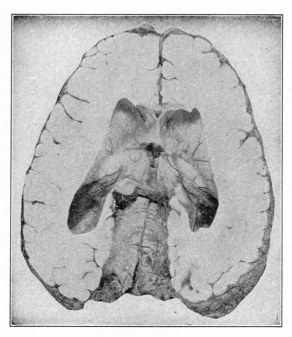

FIG. 640.—Hydrocephalus. The ventricles are moderately dilated.

exudate on the roof of the fourth ventricle with blockage of the foramina of Magendie and Luschka. Various lesions of the arachnoid villi and Pacchionian bodies may prevent absorption and cause the fluid to accumulate over the cortex in the subarachnoid space. Aplasia of the villi may cause congenital hydrocephalus. Blocking of the villi by exudate occurs in acute and tuberculous meningitis and as the result of hemorrhage into the subarachnoid space. It is therefore advisable to remove as much blood as possible by lumbar puncture. Hydrocephalus is a common accompaniment of brain tumors and is the chief cause of such classical symptoms as headache, vomiting, and optic neuritis. It may be produced in a variety of ways. (1) A glioma of the fourth ventricle or mid-brain may cause complete obstruction of the aqueduct. (2) A tumor above the tentorium may press the cerebrum down so as to wedge the brain stem into the opening in the tentorium, thus producing obstruction to the flow of fluid from the basal cisterns to the cortical subarachnoid space and so preventing absorption. (3) If the brain is pressed upward against the vault of the skull the subarachnoid space will be obliterated and again absorption will be interfered with. It is small-wonder, then, that hydrocephalus is a common accompaniment of brain tumor.

The greatest degree of hydrocephalus is seen in young children, in whom the head is still capable of enlargement. The enlargement may be enormous, with wide separation of the cranial bones, islands of bone in a sea of membrane. The little wizened face is surmounted by the huge dome-like cranium, which toward the end becomes little more than a bag of jelly. The degree of dilatation of the ventricles varies from the slightest to the most extreme (Fig. 640). In the latter the cerebral tissue is reduced to a mere shell from pressure atrophy, but the subtentorial structures remain wonderfully intact. This is one of the saddest features of the disease, for the mental deterioration may be complete, yet the intact vital centers in the medulla allow the child to continue its miserable and vegetative existence.

Hydrocephalus is unfortunately a more common condition than one might imagine. The incidence in infants is estimated at 1 in

500 to 1 in 1000, so that there may be as many as 6,000 cases of some degree of hydrocephalus a year among infants born in the United States. Encouraging results have been reported from the establishment of a ventriculo-venous shunt between the lateral ventricle and the internal jugular vein, with the aid of a valve placed in a subcutaneous pathway behind the ear (Carrington).

Increased Intracranial Pressure.—The brain is confined within a rigid bony box and contains the most sensitive cells in the body. An increase of pressure is therefore of great importance, and may give rise to the clinical picture known as *compression*. The four chief causes of compression are *hemorrhage*, *abscess*, *tumor*, and *edema*. Edema may complicate any of the other three, and is the cause of compression (in conjunction with hydrocephalus) in laceration of the brain and fracture of the skull. At the site of the pressure the vessels are emptied of blood, and it is the medullary ischemia thus produced which renders the condition so dangerous. The fluid is driven out of the cerebral subarachnoid space into the spinal canal, thus giving the brain a little more elbow-room, but the relief is only temporary. The dura is tense and the convolutions flattened so that the sulci can hardly be detected. In the traumatic cases where the brain is forced up against the skull, the subarachnoid space may be empty when the dura is incised. In general cerebral edema and in cases where the cerebrospinal fluid eliminating mechanism is blocked (arachnoid villi and Pacchionian bodies) there may be an abundance of fluid over the cortex.

When the cause of the increased pressure is supratentorial, the brain may be forced down so that herniations occur through the foramen magnum and the incisura tentorii. The latter is commoner and of more serious import. The medulla may be compressed between the herniated cerebellar tonsil and the rim of the foramen magnum, so that a groove is formed delimiting what is known as the pressure cone. Under these circumstances the withdrawal of even a few drops of cerebrospinal fluid by lumbar puncture may be attended by the risk of sudden death from cardiac or respiratory failure

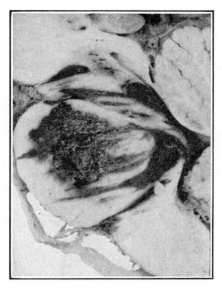

Fig. 641.—Splinter hemorrhages in pons and midbrain.

owing to increased pressure on the medulla. In massive cerebral hemorrhage the cause of death often seems to be the so-called *splinter* or *crow's feet hemorrhages in the pons*, which take the form of small linear streaks (Fig. 641). These are associated with herniation of the hippocampal uncus through the opening in the tentorium. As the venous drainage of the brain stem flows upward to join the vein of Galen or downward into the spinal venous plexuses, the pressure of the herniated uncus causes the veins to rupture, with fatal venous hemorrhage. In a study of 43 brains with morphological evidence of intracranial hypertension due to supratentorial space-occupying lesions, in 17 there was pontine or mid-brain hemorrhage (Fields and Halpert). Such hemorrhage occurred only in those patients in whom there was a sudden change in the intracranial hydrodynamics, as brought about by direct trauma, lumbar puncture, ventriculography or craniotomy, with accompanying herniation through the tentorial incisura. The third nerve may also be stretched by the herniated uncus, thus explaining the fixed dilated pupil often seen in fatal head injury.

Relation of Symptoms to Lesions.—The symptoms of compression are the same no matter what the original cause may be. The higher centers suffer first, so that the mind is dulled and the patient gradually sinks into coma. It must be said, however, that unconsciousness is not necessarily due to cortical injury or compression. It may rather be due to disturbance of the brain stem and hypothalamus, involving the ascending reticular system to which reference has already been made.

Pressure on the motor centers may first cause convulsive movements, followed later by paralysis. The vital centers in the medulla are first stimulated and then depressed, so that the pulse, respirations, and blood pressure are all affected. It is not too much to say that, with the exception of motor paralysis, nearly all the really important symptoms of intracranial lesions are due to increase of the intracranial pressure. This is particularly true of brain tumor. The classical symptoms of that condition—headache, vomiting, and optic neuritis—are late manifestations of increased pressure. Nearly all the surgeon's troubles in the operating room are due to this cause, and every effort must be made to combat the increase.

CEREBROVASCULAR DISEASE

The most frequent organic lesions of the brain are the result of vascular disturbances. Cerebrovascular disease is indeed the foremost crippler and the third ranking killer of all diseases in the United States. It has three main aspects which demand consideration. (1) *Changes in the vessel wall and lumen*, leading to either a narrowing with final closure of the lumen or a break in the wall, results which have been colloquially referred to as "plugs" and "leaks." (2) *Changes in the brain*, which may be (*a*) infarction from a plug or (*b*) hemorrhage from a leak. (3) *Neurological changes* resulting from the infarction or the hemorrhage. Infarction is caused by cerebral anoxia, which may be due either to thrombosis or embolism. The clinical condition which develops as the result of infarction or hemorrhage is best described by the old fashioned term, stroke. Apoplexy means to be struck down, but it has come to connote cerebral hemorrhage,

usually massive, whereas a stroke may be caused by thrombosis, embolism or hemorrhage.

A few words to refresh our memory of the *arterial supply* to the brain may not be out of order. This supply falls into two main divisions. (1) The *internal carotid artery* dividing into the anterior and middle cerebral, (2) the *basilar artery* formed by the junction of the two vertebrals, and itself dividing at the tentorial opening into the posterior cerebrals, which are connected by the posterior communicating arteries to form the posterior part of the circle of Willis, the anterior portion being formed by the anterior communicating connecting the two anterior cerebrals. The connecting vessels which have just been mentioned, together with other anastomotic channels of lesser caliber, are often sufficient to prevent serious damage from occlusion on one side, provided that the vessels of the other side are adequate. The *posterior cerebral artery* supplying the inferior surface of the temporal lobe and the entire occipital lobe, usually comes from the basilar, but in about 10 per cent of cases it may arise from the internal carotid. The circle of Willis serves to connect not only the two sides, but also the internal carotid and the basilar systems. Penetrating arteries run to the basal ganglia from the middle cerebral, to the thalamus from the basilar and posterior cerebrals, and to the pons and medulla from the basilar and vertebral. It should be noted that the brain stem and thalamus are not supplied by the middle cerebral but by the basilar system.

STROKES

We have already seen how sensitive the brain is to even temporary ischemia. If the anoxia is severe or complete the nerve cells may suffer irreparable damage in the course of a few minutes, the earliest damage being in the hippocampus and the Purkinje cells of the cerebellar cortex, followed by the cells in the deeper layer of the cerebral cortex. It is obvious that the amount of blood reaching the brain depends on two factors, namely the efficiency of the heart and the condition of the arteries carrying the blood to the cranium and within the brain substance. Cerebral symptoms may be cardiac or vascular in origin, and both factors may be combined. A simple fainting attack is a manifestation of temporary cerebral anoxia due to cardiac failure and so fleeting in character that no structural damage ensues. Sudden transient focal cerebral disturbances may occur marked by hemiplegia, monoplegia, hemianesthesia, aphasia, and visual disturbances. These attacks by reason of their transient character have long been a puzzle to the clinician and the pathologist. Cerebral angiospasm has been a popular explanation for many years, especially when the condition is associated with hypertension.

The concept of "little strokes" being caused by arteriolar spasm has lost much of its former appeal. There can be no doubt, however, that the larger cerebral arteries, which are well supplied with muscle and with nerves, are capable of contraction. This has been observed by neurosurgeons in the course of an operation, and after subarachnoid hemorrhage due to a ruptured berry aneurysm reversible narrowing of the cerebral arteries can be demonstrated by arteriography (Potter). Many of the *minor strokes* may be explained on a basis of cerebrovascular insufficiency (Rothenberg and Corday). This insufficiency will result from a combination of cerebrovascular narrowing and a hypotensive state, which may be induced by a variety of conditions such as myocardial infarction, cardiac arrythmias, the shock of hemorrhage, and carotid sinus hypersensitivity.

What has been called the *carotid sinus syndrome* is the occurrence of spontaneous symptoms precipitated by a hypersensitive carotid sinus reflex and mediated through the vagus nerve. External stimulation of the sinus reproduces the spontaneous symptoms. The first onset of symptoms is sudden and dramatic. The chief features are vertigo and syncope, focal motor or sensory disturbance in the limbs, and mental confusion (Hutchinson and Stock).

A great change has taken place in our thinking regarding *major strokes*. Not so long ago a stroke used to be synonymous with cerebral hemorrhage, which in turn used to be said to be caused by a strong heart breaking weak vessels. One disturb-

ing feature was our inability to demonstrate the broken vessel. Another was our total neglect of the main arteries carrying the blood to the cranial cavity, namely (1) the internal carotids in the neck and more particularly in the petrous, temporal, and cavernous sinuses, and (2) the vertebral arteries. Only the arteries removed with the brain at autopsy were examined with any thoroughness. Miller Fisher points out that the cervical portion of the internal carotid artery, the main vessel of supply of blood to the brain, lies in a no-man's land between general pathology and neuropathology, so that its examination at autopsy in the past was largely neglected. It is now realized that the local ischemia responsib'e for a stroke may be due to thrombosis, embolism or hemorrhage, and that the site of occlusion is more likely to be extracranial than intracranial. This changed concept has brought about a startling change in our outlook on the subject of strokes. It has also directed attention to the vital importance of focal diagnosis. Formerly it was sufficient for the physician to make a general diagnosis of a stroke, because there was nothing he could do to assist the patient. Revolutionary changes in the medical and surgical treatment of strokes demand accurate focal diagnosis by means of cerebral angiography.

The *clinical manifestations* of a stroke vary within the widest limits, as we shall see. It may take the form of a violent assault, in which the patient falls as if felled by an axe, deprived of sense and motion. This is the only variety which used to be recognized, and which earned the condition its title of stroke or apoplexy. Far the most frequent type is that in which there is only a slight defect of speech, thought, motion, sensation or vision; consciousness is not lost or even affected, and some degree of recovery is nearly invariable. It is obvious that the former type is likely to be caused by massive cerebral hemorrhage, the latter type by thrombosis. The neurological disturbances may be: (1) *focal*, as evidenced by hemiplegia, homonomous hemianopia, slurred speech, etc.; or (2) *diffuse disturbance of function*, with drowsiness, confusion and stupor, due to general cerebral shock, increased intracranial pressure, etc., a disturbance which is often transitory. Many strokes are preceded by transient warning episodes of weakness or numbness. Naturally such warnings will suggest a diagnosis of thrombosis rather than embolism or hemorrhage.

Thrombosis with Atherosclerosis.— *This is the most common cause of strokes,* comprising probably 50 per cent of all cases. The atherosclerosis is the primary lesion, the occluding thrombus being added at a late stage to produce an *ischemic* stroke. Arterial hypertension aggravates the process. The carotid and basilar systems are equally affected, the result depending largely on to the extent to which a collateral circulation has developed.

For many years thrombosis was overshadowed by hemorrhage and embolism as a cause of strokes, but now it is coming into its own. The main reason for this neglect may be attributed to the term cerebral thrombosis, which suggests that thrombi are to be found in the cerebral vessels, whereas *the main site of obstruction is the extracerebral arteries*, particularly the internal carotid, which have been neglected in the past in routine autopsies. Apart from the very occasional instances where thrombosis is due to the arteritis of tuberculous meningitis, polyarteritis nodosa, *etc.*, the vast majority of cases are associated with atherosclerosis, particularly at bifurcations, branchings and bends. Miller Fisher, to whose papers on strokes I am much indebted, gives the following order of frequency of involvement: the carotid sinus, the paraclinoid portion of the internal carotid artery, the bifurcation of the internal carotid into the anterior and middle cerebrals, the union of the vertebrals to form the basilar, and the bifurcation of the basilar. It will be recalled that the internal carotid begins at the bifurcation of the common carotid as a localized dilatation, the carotid sinus, and consists of four portions: a *cervical*, including the carotid sinus, 8 cm. long, a *petrous* in the carotid canal in the petrous temporal bone, 4.5 cm. long, a cavernous in the *cavernous* sinus, 4.5 cm. long, and a *cerebral*, only 1 cm. long. The atheromatous plaques do not ulcerate as they do in the aorta, but they slow down

the blood flow distal to the narrowing and thus predispose to thrombosis. After the internal carotid as a site of thrombotic occlusion come the vertebrals, the basilar and the posterior cerebral arteries. Thrombosis of the basilar is usually preceded by thrombosis of one or both vertebrals.

The *aortic arch syndrome* or *Takayashu's syndrome* is a very rare but remarkably interesting example of the association of extracranial thrombosis with cerebral softening. It is also known as the *pulseless disease*, owing to the frequent absence of the radial pulse, although this is not necessarily the case. Takayashu's syndrome, also known as "young female arteritis," is predominantly a disease of the female in the reproductive years. The lesions consist of a thickening of the wall of the arch of the aorta and of the origins of the main vessels which arise from it, together with an associated thrombosis. The result is malnutrition of the cranial half of the body, the development of collaterals from the caudal half, and, not infrequently, raised blood pressure in the legs, which in some cases is due to narrowing of the origin of the renal arteries. The combination of absent radial pulse and hypertension in the legs is indeed a dramatic clinical finding. *Microscopically* there is an arteritis suggestive of the lesion of temporal (giant cell) arteritis. The condition, which was originally reported from Japan, may be hyperergic in character, although of this there is no proof. The cerebral manifestations are identical with those of thrombosis of the internal carotid artery. Vertigo, especially on rising from the horizontal position, is the most common symptom, to which may be added very distressing headache, hemiplegia, and loss of consciousness (Ross and McKusick).

Trauma may play a major part in the causation of arterial thrombosis, and this may form an important or fatal feature of injuries to the head and neck, for the violence may be indirect as well as direct. There may be hemorrhage in the wall of the artery, but the most important lesion is rupture of the internal elastic lamina.

Lesions.—When an area of the brain is deprived of its blood supply it undergoes *infarction*. The infarct may be red or pale,

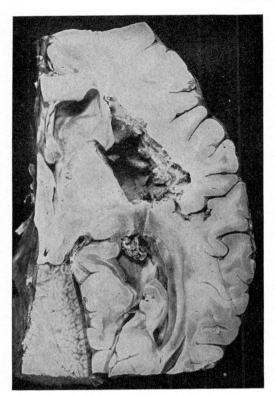

FIG. 642.—Large area of softening in the lenticular nucleus with cyst formation, due to vascular occlusion.

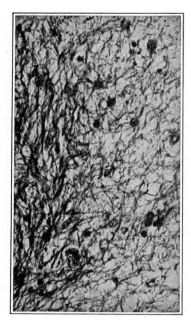

FIG. 643.—Gliosis at margin of softened area. × 300.

depending on the efficiency of the collateral circulation able to pour blood into the part, and on the tempo of the infarction. The necrotic material becomes liquefied and converted into a creamy material, the condition of *cerebral softening* or *encephalomalacia* (Fig. 642).

In cases of cerebral softening following upon complete occlusion of a cerebral artery the area of infarction is often less extensive than anticipated. The reason is the rich anastomotic network of perforating leptomeningeal vessels and the larger arteries supplying the area. This is not true of the deep penetrating arteries of the base of the brain which have no anastomoses, so that in the basal ganglia the softened area is always as extensive as the irrigation area of the occluded artery.

In the experimental animal temporary arrest of the circulation for five minutes causes necrosis and softening of the cerebral cortex; if the arrest is maintained for over seven minutes there is complete destruction and liquefaction of the brain substance (Weinberger *et al.*). The color is usually pale, but in the course of time becomes yellow owing to blood pigment and the lipid liberated from breaking down myelin. In exceptional cases it is red on account of marked congestion. The sequence of events is similar to that which occurs in hemorrhage. As liquefaction proceeds a cyst is formed with clear or milky contents and a yellow margin. The neuroglia proliferates and forms a limiting zone around the cavity. (Fig. 643). When the cortex is involved a cyst is formed beneath the meninges, or there may simply be atrophy of the convolutions with depression of the affected area.

The *microscopic changes* involve both the neurones and the interstitial tissue. A smear of the liquefied material shows at first granules and globules of lipid, the remains of cells and fibers, and large numbers of scavenger cells. In sections of the affected area there is complete necrosis and loss of all structure. Secondary (Wallerian) degeneration can be traced down the course of the motor fibers through pons, medulla, and

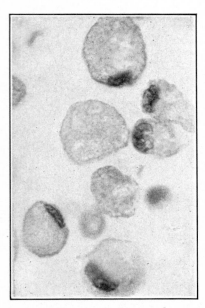

FIG. 644.—Scavenger cells of the brain (Hortega cells) filled with lipid. These cells are derived from the microglia. × 1000.

cord, the droplets of myelin being demonstrated by the Marchi method. At a later date Weigert's myelin sheath stain shows complete disappearance of the fibers, whose place is occupied by proliferated neuroglia. A zone of gliosis is seen around the wall of the cyst. But the most characteristic feature of a recent softening is the presence of enormous numbers of large pale scavenger cells derived from the microglia and filled with lipid globules taken up from the disintegrating myelin (Fig. 644). These cells are known by a variety of names such as compound granular corpuscles, fat granule cells, Gitterzellen (lattice cells), and Hortega cells on account of the demonstration by del Rio Hortega that they are *microglial in origin*. Frozen sections stained for fat with Scharlach show in a beautiful manner the lipid character of the cell contents. The walls of the vessels are infiltrated with these cells, which seem to be discharging their contents into the lumen.

Relation of Symptoms to Lesions.—The clinical evidence of thrombotic occlusion is that of a stroke, although when the occlusion is purely atherosclerotic the onset of symptoms may be so gradual as not to deserve the designation of strokes. When we consider the variety of vessels which may be involved it is natural that there may be a great variety of clinical syndromes, such as those of the middle cerebral, anterior cerebral, posterior cerebral, internal carotid, vertebral and basilar arteries. Even to mention the neurological manifestations of such syndromes would take us much too far afield. In the early stages of a stroke the nature of onset and the intimate details of the prodromal symptoms are of prime importance in making a diagnosis. In the present instance the most important single factor is the *history of prodromal transient episodes*. In no other form of stroke is this encountered with the exception of that due to a ruptured berry aneurysm.

The *neurological symptoms proper* may take several days to develop. Compare this with the stroke of a cerebral hemorrhage where the period if measured in minutes or at the most in hours, or cerebral embolism where the period is so short that it cannot be measured. Hemiplegia develops in fits and starts, in contrast to the smooth and gradual onset of hemiplegia due to a brain tumor, an abscess, or a subdural hematoma. There is a tendency for the stroke to develop while the patient is asleep, or within an hour of arising, or during a period of hypotension after hemorrhage or myocardial infarction. A stroke due to hemorrhage is likely to develop during waking hours, whilst that due to embolism may of course occur at any time. A finding of monocular blindness with contralateral hemiplegia is almost pathognomonic of carotid artery thrombosis. Palpation may reveal lack of pulsation in the neck, unless the occlusion happens to be in the intracranial course of the vessel. A carotid and cranial bruit can be heard in some 20 per cent of cases. Pressure in the central artery of the retina on the same side is decreased. Diagnosis of occlusion can be established with certainty by cerebral angiography. The clinical effects of occlusion will naturally depend on the collateral circulation, in particular the flow from the meningeal vessels. Excision of the occluded segment of the artery and anastomosis or insertion of an arterial or other graft may yield highly gratifying results in selected cases.

The *clinical picture* of cerebral infarction will naturally be influenced by the distribution of the occluded vessel. *Acute occlusion of the internal carotid artery*, as by an embolus, results in unconsciousness, complete loss of function of the opposite side, followed by death. In *chronic occlusion* there may be recurring episodes of transient loss of function involving the face, arm or leg, followed later by permanent paralysis. The *anterior cerebral artery* supplies the anterior part of the internal capsule, the orbital surface of the frontal lobe, and the mesial surface of the hemisphere with the exception of the occipital lobe. Infarction results in loss of consciousness, followed by mental symptoms and a hemiplegia involving the leg to a greater degree than the arm. The *middle cerebral* artery has, of course, a very wide distribution over the cerebral cortex, and in addition it sends penetrating branches to the internal capsule and the basal ganglia. Infarction due to occlusion of branches of this artery is the commonest cause of hemiplegia, and of aphasia when the left side is involved. Occlusion of the main artery produces very much the same picture as occlusion of the internal carotid from which it arises. The *posterior cerebral artery* supplies the midbrain, the posterior part of the internal capsule and thalamus including the lateral geniculate body, and the medial surface of the temporal and occipital lobes. Occlusion of branches to the thalamus and lateral geniculate body results in contralateral hemianopsia and hemianesthesia, while if the medial surface of the occipital lobe is involved there may again be hemianopsia.

Thrombosis of the posterior inferior cerebellar artery is of special interest to the pathologist as well as to the clinician, because it is possible to correlate the autopsy findings with the clinical symptoms with a singular degree of accuracy. The posterior inferior cerebellar artery is a branch of the vertebral which supplies the lateral surface of the medulla. The distribution of the artery is variable, and the lesions (and symptoms) vary accordingly. The commonest symptoms are hemianesthesia of the face on the side of the lesion and the body on the opposite side, laryngo-palatine palsy, and Horner's syndrome on the side of the lesion. In addition there may be cerebellar ataxia, Ménière's syndrome, paralysis of deglutition, and absence of sweating over one side of the face. The hemianesthesia of the body is due to destruction of the spinothalamic tract at the mid-olivary level of the medulla. The hemianesthesia of the face is due to involvement of the spinal nucleus of the fifth nerve in the medulla, the main sensory nucleus in the pons remaining unaffected. The paralysis of the larynx and palate is due to damage to the motor nuclei of the ninth and tenth nerves, particularly the nucleus ambiguus. The Horner's syndrome is due to destruction of the sympathetic fibers from the hypothalamus.

Venous Obstruction.—This is caused by thrombosis of the venous sinuses. Not infrequently the cerebral thrombosis is part of a general venous thrombosis. In other cases it is of local infective origin, as in sinus thrombophlebitis due to spread of infection from the middle ear, nose, etc. The superior longitudinal sinus is most often affected. In severe cases there may be a remarkable dilatation of the superficial veins which become completely thrombosed, so that the surface of the brain seems to be covered with dark worms.

Cerebral Embolism.—The second great cause of strokes is embolism of the cerebral vessels. The embolus most often originates in the *left side of the heart*, either as a vegetation on the mitral or aortic valve, as a clot in the appendix of the left atrium, or as a mural thrombus which has formed in the left ventricle as the result of myocardial infarction. The last named should always be considered in an apparent case of cerebral hemorrhage in persons under 40 years of age. A frequent source is a thrombus in the *carotid sinus*, a fact only recently recognized. A hazard of modern cardiac surgery is thrombosis with consequent cerebral embolism. The possibility of the embolus originating in a *pulmonary vein* may be borne in mind, it being well recognized that cerebral abscess is a not infrequent complication of suppuration in the lung. The embolus usually passes into the left carotid artery and is most likely to stick in the middle cerebral. If it blocks that artery before the branches to the basal ganglia are given off, the accompanying paralysis will be very extensive. A septic embolus will set up an inflammatory process in the vessel wall with resulting weakening, which may lead to the formation of a mycotic aneurysm or to rupture of the artery without aneurysm formation.

This *lesion* differs from that produced by thrombosis by reason of the suddeness of the arrest of circulation. There is no time for collateral blood flow to the part, and all the tissues supplied by the affected vessel become infarcted. In thrombosis there may be no visible infarct. The infarct may be pale or hemorrhagic, hemorrhage possibly being due to the embolus disintegrating and moving on. Red infarction is the hall mark of embolism, not of thrombosis.

The *clinical picture* is similar in a general way to the other varieties of strokes, being marked by hemiplegia, paresthesia, aphasia, *etc*. Its distinguishing features are: (1) the suddeness of the onset of symptoms, with complete development in from 10 to 30 seconds; (2) the absence of prodromal warnings; (3) evidence of a likely source of an embolus or of emboli elsewhere. If the collateral circulation is good the symtpoms may be very fleeting, in which case the condition is apt to be mistaken for vasospasm.

Cerebral Hemorrhage.—Massive as distinguished from petechial hemorrhage in the brain may be divided into two main groups: (1) primary or spontaneous hemorrhage, and (2) secondary hemorrhage due to aneurysm, hemangioma, embolism, trauma, tumor, or one of the bleeding diseases. Of the latter group special mention will be made of hemorrhage due to trauma. A stroke due to hemorrhage from a *ruptured berry aneurysm* is characterized by sudden loss of conciousness followed by severe headache but no paralysis, a combination which is quite specific, especially in a young person. This subject is discussed in connection with cerebral aneurysms (p. 1147).

Spontaneous Hemorrhage.—Nothing in life is ever spontaneous, for there is always a cause, although it may not be apparent. Massive hemorrhage constitutes what is commonly known as *apoplexy*, and represents about 25 per cent of the cases of stroke encountered at autopsy.

The hemorrhage usually occurs in middle-aged men with high blood pressure and arterial degeneration. Hemorrhage may occur in the absence of hypertension. The opinion is gaining ground that apoplectic hemorrhage is not merely a question of a blood vessel bursting. It takes place into soil which has been prepared by vascular thrombosis or occlusion. As a result of the ischemia a focal encephalomalacia is produced, and it would appear that such softening is an essential precursor to rupture of a vessel (Fig. 645). An infected embolus lodging in one of the cerebral vessels may give rise to a mycotic aneurysm, which on rupturing may cause a massive hemorrhage. An occasional cause of hemorrhage is rupture of a congenital aneurysm on the circle of Willis or one of its branches; this usually leads to subarachnoid hemorrhage, but the blood may make its way into the brain substance. Such an aneurysm should be looked for in cerebral hemorrhage in a younger person.

In *hypertensive encephalopathy* three types of lesion may be encountered: (1) edema, causing such symptoms of increased intracranial pressure as headache, nausea, vomiting, dulness, etc.; (2) multiple miliary destructive lesions (ischemic), causing a wide variety of symptoms such as vertigo, transient hemiplegias and aphasias, convulsions, etc.; and (3) massive hemorrhage into larger areas of softening.

Lesions.—The common site of massive hemorrhage is the *internal capsule and lenticular nucleus*. The small arteries to the basal ganglia come directly off the middle cerebral, so that the pressure is not "stepped down" by continuous branching as in the case of the cortical branches. The lenticulostriate artery was long ago called "the artery of cerebral hemorrhage." The next most common site is the *white matter of the frontal lobe*, the hemorrhage coming from the anterior cerebral artery. Next come the *pons and cerebellum*. Hemorrhage into the pons may be due to unilateral increase of intracranial pressure, such as may be caused by a large hemorrhage into a

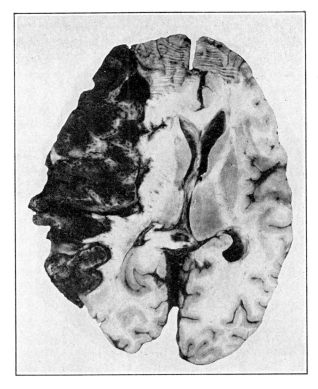

Fig. 645.—Hemorrhage in area of softening in distribution of middle cerebral artery.

hemisphere. The hippocampal uncus is herniated through the opening in the tentorium, and the resulting pressure leads to pontine hemorrhage which may be the direct cause of death. The hemorrhage takes the form of small linear streaks, often termed splinter or crow's feet hemorrhages (Fig. 641; page 1135). Spontaneous hemorrhage in the cerebral cortex is rare. Hemorrhage in the basal ganglia may extend inward, and more rarely outward. When it passes inward it may penetrate the caudate nucleus and *rupture into the lateral ventricle* (Fig. 646). About 40 per cent of fatal capsular hemorrhages rupture into the lateral ventricle before death. Pontine hemorrhages almost invariably rupture into the fourth ventricle. Spontaneous intracerebral hemorrhage only very rarely ruptures outward into the subarachnoid space. The blood passes through the aqueduct and fills the entire ventricular system, passing thence to the subarachnoid space *via* the foramina in the roof of the fourth ventricle and filling the cisterns at the base of the brain. The original hemorrhage may be into the ventricles, usually from the anterior cerebral artery which supplies the tip of the caudate nucleus.

A clot is formed at the site of the hemorrhage, and this may be surrounded by petechial hemorrhages, caused probably by the sudden disturbance of pressure. The mass of blood grows in volume as the bleeding proceeds, and may shift the midline structures to the opposite side. The brain tissue in which the hemorrhage has occurred is torn up and completely disintegrated. The clot becomes softened and the destroyed brain substance liquefied, so that if the patient lives the hemorrhage is replaced by a cyst containing yellow or milky fluid. The surrounding tissue is stained yellow, and this discoloration may persist for a long time.

Microscopically there is great destruction of neurones. The nerve cells are degenerated and the medullary sheaths are broken up into

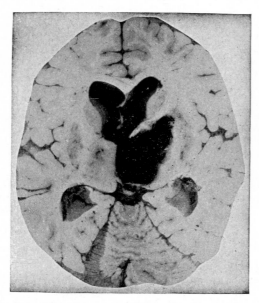

FIG. 646.—Intraventricular cerebral hemorrhage. The hemorrhage has started in the internal capsule, passed inward through the optic thalamus, and ruptured into the lateral ventricle.

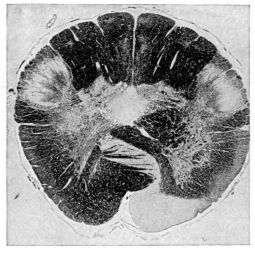

FIG. 647.—Section of medulla at level of decussation of the pyramids showing degenerated pyramidal tract (white) crossing to the opposite side. From a case of old left-sided cerebral hemorrhage. (Myelin sheath stain). × 6. (Boyd, *Pathology for the Physician*.)

droplets of myelin; presently the entire neurone disappears. In the case of the motor paths the degenerated fibers can be traced down through the brain stem (Fig. 647) into the cord. Two elements of the interstitial tissue, the astrocytes and the microglia, show marked activity. The *microglia* gives rise to large numbers of scavenger cells, which take up the myelin droplets and pigment granules, carrying them to the nearest vessels and perhaps discharging them into the lumen. The *astrocytes* proliferate and form abundant fibers, so that a small cyst may be obliterated, while a larger cyst is shut off from the surrounding tissue by a glial zone. Granules of blood pigment indicate for many years the hemorrhagic origin of the cyst.

Relation of Symptoms to Lesions.—Depending on the size of the hemorrhage, the patient with apoplexy either feels faint or loses consciousness. He may fall as though struck to the ground (*plexis*, to strike down), but sudden death is rarely due to cerebral hemorrhage unless it be into the ventricles or the pons or medulla. The immediate loss of consciousness is due to the sudden cerebral anoxia caused by compression of the capillaries by the hemorrhage, and the coma into which the patient may pass is to be attributed to the rapidly developing edema. It is the compression of the vital centers in the medulla by the edema which is the usual cause of death. The condition of the *cerebrospinal fluid* is of help in the diagnosis. In hemorrhage into the ventricles a large amount of blood is present in the fluid. When the hemorrhage does not communicate with the ventricles the fluid is at first normal, but in the course of three days it assumes a yellow tinge owing to blood pigment having seeped through into the ventricles, a condition known as *xanthochromia*. This is not found in any of the other comatose states which simulate cerebral hemorrhage.

Traumatic Hemorrhage.—Although this form of hemorrhage does not give rise to the clinical picture of stroke, it is convenient to consider it in this place. It is important to remember that a patient who has had a trauma to his head may nevertheless be suffering from a spontaneous hemorrhage. The hemorrhage may come first, causing him to fall, injure his head, even fracture his skull. This is particularly true when the hemorrhage is in the internal capsule.

Trauma may cause cerebral hemorrhage in two ways. (1) Hemorrhage is a more or less constant accompaniment of *laceration of the brain.* Fracture of the base or vault of the skull may be present, but it is important to realize that large cortical hemorrhage may occur without fracture. *Contrecoup* hemorrhage, which is situated on the side opposite the site of trauma, usually occurs without fracture; it is caused by the brain being thrown forcibly against the opposite side of the skull. A large hemorrhage due to trauma is very rarely (perhaps never) in the internal capsule, such hemorrhage being spontaneous. (2) *Multiple punctate hemorrhages* in the basal ganglia and elsewhere may be caused by trauma.

The condition known to prize-fighters as "punch-drunk" may be of this nature. Many old fighters develop corpus striatum symptoms (paralysis agitans, etc). The punctate hemorrhages used to be thought to be due to a wave of cerebrospinal which the blow on the head caused to pass from the subarachnoid space into the perivascular prolongations of that space. With our newer views on the relation of the astroglia to the small vessels, this explanation has lost its former appeal.

Fisher found complete or almost complete occlusion of one or both internal carotids in 8 per cent of routine autopsies, the incidence being greatest between sixty-five and eighty years of age. The occlusion was due to atherosclerosis, which is most marked in the *carotid sinus,* a site prone to atheroma second only to the abdominal aorta (Fig. 648). Thrombosis is naturally a frequent accompaniment, and the thrombus may give rise to otherwise unexplained emboli.

These vitally important facts are not new. In 1905 Chiari found thrombi on atheromatous plaques in the carotid sinus in seven cases in 400 consecutive autopsies, some of which were the source of cerebral emboli. Hultquist in 1942 studied the entire carotid system in 1400 autopsies and wrote a monograph on the subject. Carotid artery arteriography has shown many cases of occlusion in the living patient.

Fisher emphasizes the fact that internal carotid occlusion seems to be a frequent cause of single and double hemiplegia and

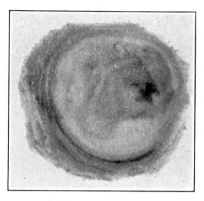

FIG. 648.—Occlusion of internal carotid artery at site of carotid sinus. (Kindness of Dr. C. Miller Fisher.)

may be associated with the picture of senile dementia. Moreover, hemiplegia occurring as a result of the shock of myocardial infarction, severe hemorrhage and major surgery may be determined by unsuspected carotid artery blockage. As in the case of the coronary arteries the occlusion may be silent owing to an adequate collateral circulation.

The plan of the circulation in the brain would seem to include the ability to counteract the effects of occlusion of any of the major arteries. In this plan *anastomoses between meningeal and cerebral arteries* play an important part. The reason for these arrangements is, of course, the fact that the effects of vascular occlusion are more far-reaching in the brain than in any of the other viscera with the single exception of the heart.

Developmental anomalies of the circle of Willis may impair the adequacy of the collateral circulation. Cerebral softening and hemorrhage may therefore occur in the absence of occlusive thrombotic lesions of the cerebral arteries, being caused by the coexistence of congenital vascular defects, heart failure, and cerebral arteriosclerosis.

Punctiform Hemorrhages.—Punctiform or petechial hemorrhages occur in a great variety of conditions, and they present a striking microscopic picture. They are seen in acute bacterial and viral infections, in chemical poisoning, more particularly that due to carbon monoxide, in bleeding diseases such as leukemia and hemorrhagic purpura, in systemic lupus erythematosus, and in the neighborhood of a massive cerebral hemorrhage. The hemorrhages surround small vessels, the bleeding apparently coming from the ring of capillaries around each cerebral arteriole.

The accompnaying tabular summary may be found useful for recalling to mind some of the clinical features of the cerebrovascular catastrophies just described.

fracture, aortic occlusion during operation, dissecting aneurysm of the aorta, and even severe physical work involving the shoulders and back. In many cases no satisfactory antecedent can be named. The anterior spinal artery is formed by the union of a branch from each vertebral artery to which branches from vessels adjoining the vertebral column contribute largely.

The anterior horn cells are extremely

IMPORTANT CLINICAL CHARACTERISTICS OF THE PRINCIPAL CEREBROVASCULAR DISORDERS

General Features of Intracerebral Hemorrhage	Primary Subarachnoid Hemorrhage	Hemorrhage of a Vascular Anomaly	Cerebral Thrombosis and Infarction	Cerebral Embolism
Hypertension.	Sudden onset of severe headache.	Young person without hypertension.	Prodromal episodes, (recurrent cerebral ischemic attacks).	Sudden onset of cerebrovascular symptoms.
Onset usually during physical activity.	Transitory disturbance of consciousness.	Antecedent symptoms (epilepsy, etc).	Presence of atherosclerosis and/or other associated disorders.	Consciousness usually partially maintained.
Headache (if conscious).	Kernig and Brudzinski signs.	Repeated subarachnoid hemorrhages.	Gradual onset and progression of symptoms.	Occasionally improvement apparent.
Rapidly developing hemiplegia.	No focal neurologic signs.	Cranial bruit.	Consciousness usually partially maintained.	Special arterial syndromes or focal signs.
Early progression to coma.	Preretinal hemorrhages.	Preretinal hemorrhage and retinal angiomas.	Frequently a grouping of symptoms as syndromes	Source of emboli often apparent.
Cerebrospinal fluid bloody.	Cerebrospinal fluid bloody.	Cerebrospinal fluid bloody.	Cerebrospinal fluid clear.	Cerebrospinal fluid clear.

(Adapted from "A Classification and Outline of Cerebrovascular Diseases," Neurology 1958, 8, 5.)

Anterior Spinal Artery Occlusion.—The syndrome of occlusion of the anterior spinal artery is of interest because of the striking clinical picture, which in the past has been mistaken for that of acute anterior poliomyelitis. This picture is the result of hypoxia, to which the anterior horn cells are extremely vulnerable. A variety of conditions can apparently be responsible for the hypoxia. Syphilitic vascular disease used to receive the most attention, but vascular occlusion may be associated with vertebral

vulnerable to hypoxia, and it is these which suffer, particularly in the lower cervical and lower thoracic region (Peterman et al.). The onset is usually abrupt, and the clinical picture is fully developed in the course of a few hours. In lower dorsal involvement there is sudden loss of power in the lower limbs, the bladder and bowels are paralyzed, and appreciation of pain and temperature is lost below the level of the lesion, but joint-position sense, touch, and vibration sensibility are spared, as the posterior columns are not involved. In cervical cases there may be severe permanent disability of the upper limbs, particularly the hands. The association of an anterior horn cell disorder at the level of the lesion with sparing of the posterior columns is strongly suggestive of occlusion of the anterior spinal artery.

Collagen Disease Lesions.—This may be as convenient a place as any to mention the occasional central nervous system lesions which may occur in some of the collagen diseases. These principally involve the small vessels, but secondary changes develop in the surrounding tissue as a result of the ischemia. *Systemic lupus erythematosus* may be accompanied by cerebral lesions in its acute stage. In one series of 6 fatal cases there was endarteritis of the cerebral small arteries and arterioles in no less than 3, with resulting focal or disseminated encephalomalacia principally involving the gray matter of the cerebral cortex (Glaser). Neurological signs and symptoms were absent in two of the cases despite extensive cerebral lesions, but in the third there were generalized seizures and coma. *Rheumatoid Arthritis* may also be associated with meningeal and cerebral vascular lesions (Steiner and Gelbloom). These take the form of early fibrinoid deposits and later rheumatoid nodules in the dura and subarachnoid space, together with secondary ischemic lesions both in the cortex and the white matter of the cerebrum.

INTRACRANIAL ANEURYSMS

These aneurysms are nearly always extracerebral, for they are situated on the circle of Willis or its main branches. Aneurysmal dilatations in the brain substance are seldom true aneurysms. There are three main types of intracranial aneurysms. In their order of frequency these are the *congenital*, the *mycotic*, and the *arteriosclerotic*. Aneurysms due to syphilis are practically non-existent.

1. Congenital Aneurysm.—These aneurysms, which may be multiple, form small swellings on the vessels of the circle of Willis, the middle cerebral, anterior cerebral, and anterior communicating arteries (Fig. 649). They are commonly known as *berry aneurysms*. Although often present in young

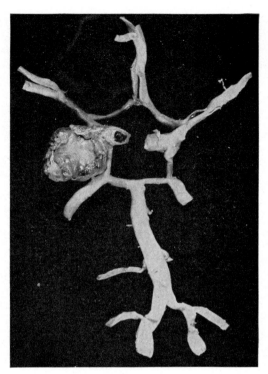

Fig. 649.—Aneurysm of circle of Willis. The aneurysm, which is of unusually large size and still unruptured, arises from the internal carotid artery. The location adjacent to a bifurcation is characteristic. (University of Alabama Medical School.)

persons, the usual age period is between forty and sixty years. The most striking peculiarity of the aneurysm is that in every case it is situated at the bifurcation of the vessel. At this point there is often an absence of the muscular tissue of the middle coat in normal persons, which may be looked on as a vascular malformation or defect. The same localized medial defect is found in the berry aneurysm, the wall of which is formed by greatly thickened intima, with complete absence of media and internal elastic lamina. It has been the fashion to regard these defects as congenital in nature and the cause of berry aneurysms. But the anatomical distribution of the defects is not the same as that of the aneurysms, they increase in frequency with age which is not in support of the view that they are congenital in character, and there is no evidence to suggest that they represent areas of weakness (Stehbens). Glynn finds such defects as common among controls as in cases of aneurysm (80 per cent in each group). He points out that in the vessels of the circle of Willis all the elastic fibers are concentrated in the internal elastic lamina, not distributed throughout the media and adventitia as in other arteries. For this reason a patch of atheroma may destroy all the elastic tissue and thus produce an aneurysm. Atheroma is almost constantly present in these aneurysms, but has been regarded as secondary rather than primary. If this interpretation is correct, berry aneurysms must be regarded as atheromatous, not congenital, in origin. Carmichael has suggested that in most cases of atheroma the commonly associated fibrohyaline thickening of the wall compensates for the destruction of the elastica. Whatever the truth may be it would seem that the term berry aneurysm is to be preferred to congenital aneurysm as a description of the arterial lesion. Rupture of the aneurysm leads to hemorrhage into the subarachnoid space which is usually fatal. If the aneurysm is on the anterior cerebral or the anterior communicating artery and therefore wedged in between the frontal lobes, it may rupture into the brain substance. The same is true of the middle cerebral. These cases are easily mistaken in the autopsy room for ordinary cerebral hemorrhage, the aneurysm being lost in the hemorrhage and readily overlooked.

2. **Mycotic Aneurysm.**—An infected embolus, usually from a vegetation on a heart valve, lodges in the middle or anterior cerebral artery and sets up an acute arteritis. This weakens the wall so much that a small mycotic aneurysm is formed, which is certain to rupture unless the patient dies before that happens.

3. **Atherosclerotic Aneurysm.**—These aneurysms may be fusiform, diffuse or globular, and they consist of enlargement of the entire circumference of the artery, thus differing from the saccular or berry aneurysm which is a thin-walled blister protruding from the artery. It is not certain if they are atherosclerotic in nature, for they may occur apart from that condition. They seldom rupture or give rise to clinical symptoms.

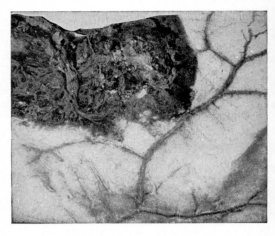

FIG. 650.—Extradural hemorrhage.

MENINGEAL HEMORRHAGE

Meningeal hemorrhage may be *extradural, subdural, or subarachnoid.*

1. EXTRADURAL HEMORRHAGE.—This is commonly called *middle meningeal hemorrhage*, being due to injury to the middle meningeal artery from fracture of the lower part of the parietal bone or the squamous portion of the temporal bone. It is caused by a direct blow; the elastic recoil of the skull separates the dura from the bone, and the spaces become filled with blood. A large clot is formed outside the dura over the vertex and this presses on the brain (Fig. 650). Prompt operation with ligation of the bleeding vessel is needed, otherwise the patient will die from compression of the brain. The *clinical picture* is highly characteristic. There may be brief loss of consciousness owing to the blow. This is followed by a *lucid interval* of some hours, at the end of which time symptoms of compression appear owing to the gradual accumulation of blood between the skull and the brain. There is no blood in the cerebrospinal fluid. A useful localizing sign is a fixed dilated pupil on the *same side* as the lesion, due probably to herniation of the hippocampal uncus with pressure on the third nerve as it crosses the greater wing of the sphenoid. There may also be conjugate deviation of the eyes to the opposite side due to irritation of the oculomotor center in the second frontal convulution.

PLATE XIX

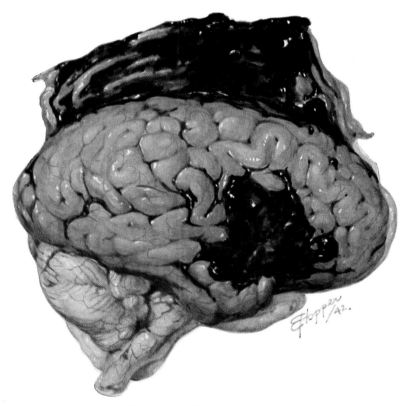

Subdural Hemorrhage

In addition to the blood clot on the brain and the inner surface of the dura there is diffuse staining of the cerebrum.

SUBDURAL HEMORRHAGE.—Subdural hemorrhage (Plate XIX) may be regarded as venous, just as extradural hemorrhage is arterial in origin. The condition, which is at least 4 times as common as extradural hemorrhage, is of great importance, because the life of the patient depends on a correct diagnosis and this is easily missed. It is customary to recognize a traumatic and a spontaneous form, but it is becoming doubtful if the latter is more than a myth, for the traumatic factor in the etiology is often slight and easily overlooked. The cause is a blow in the frontal or occipital region (*e.g.*, knocking the head against a shelf or door), which injures the cerebral veins passing into the sagittal sinus. As there are no septa to localize the extravasated blood, it may spread from the frontal to the occipital pole and from the sagittal sinus to the Sylvian fissure. The symptoms may not come on for weeks or even months after the injury. This is explained by the unique subsequent behavior of the clot. This is not absorbed as it would be in other serous sacs, for the subdural space is closed and without lymphatics. The clot becomes liquefied and surrounded by a mesothelial membrane, so that a cyst is formed which separates the dura from the brain. Into this cyst cerebrospinal fluid is drawn by the osmotic pressure of the blood, so that the tension in the cyst continually increases, with corresponding pressure on the brain. At the site of a subdural hematoma, therefore, the dura is lined by a dirty-green, gelatinous membrane which is easily detached, and the cyst contains dark green, thin fluid under pressure. *Pachymeningitis hæmorrhagica interna* is a term which was long applied to the supposedly spontaneous form in which a membrane containing great numbers of large blood spaces is found on the inner surface of the dura. Hemorrhage is supposed to occur at intervals from these giant capillaries, but they are also present in traumatic cases.

Intracranial Hemorrhage of the Newborn.—This is a variety of subdural hemorrhage. It is a common cause of death in the newborn. The child is cyanosed, the respirations difficult, the pulse slow, the fontanelle bulging, and there may be twitching movements. Death may occur in a few hours or in the course of a day or two. If the child survives, paralytic and mental symptoms may develop later. The hemorrhage is due to tears in the tentorium cerebelli or the falx cerebri or to injury to the cerebral veins passing from the cortex across the subdural space into the superior longitudinal sinus. These injuries are produced by the severe molding of the head which occurs at birth, and not necessarily by the use of instruments. The hemorrhage is largely supratentorial and often bilateral. It is commoner in the premature than in the full-term infant owing to immaturity of the fibers of the dural septa. The arachnoid is often torn, so that blood is found in the cerebrospinal fluid. Lumbar puncture is of great use in doubtful cases. The gravity of the condition depends not merely on the extent of the lesion, but on whether the child suffers from a hemorrhagic diathesis which interferes with the clotting of the blood. This is due to a low prothrombin content of the blood, and the condition can be treated by injections of vitamin K, or prevented by giving the vitamin to the mother before delivery.

Among the more immediate *symptoms* are a tendency to asphyxia, slow pulse, irregular respiration and a bulging of the fontanelle. Paralytic symptoms appear later, notably spastic paraplegia or hemiplegia. In place of motor symptoms there may be serious mental defects, epilepsy, and other disastrous sequelæ.

3. SUBARACHNOID HEMORRHAGE. — Hemorrhage into the subarachnoid space may be spontaneous or traumatic. The distinction between these two is fundamental, and the resulting clinical picture is very different.

(1) *Spontaneous Subarachnoid Hemorrhage.*—This intracranial catastrope, which may resemble a stroke in the suddenness of its onset, results in more than 80 per cent of cases from the rupture of a "congenital" aneurysm of the circle of Willis or of the vessels in the immediate vicinity (Richardson and Hyland) (Fig. 648). These so-called *berry aneurysms*, which when minute may hang like berries on the arterial stalk, have already been described on page 1147. The little aneurysm is covered with blood clot, so that it is easily missed at autopsy

unless specially looked for. Bleeding from an *angiomatous malformation* accounts for another 10 per cent of cases. The lesions occur in adolescents or young adults, and the clinical picture develops more slowly and in less dramatic fashion. The remaining cases are due to bleeding from a brain tumor, inflammatory lesion, or to a blood dyscrasia. We shall confine our attention to rupture of a congenital aneurysm.

It must not be thought that the lesion is confined to the presence of blood in the subarachnoid space. In perhaps half the cases the hemorrhage encroaches on the cerebral substance, and bleeding occurs into the subdural space in up to 5 per cent of cases. Moreover *cerebral infarction* is a common and important complication, a fact which has been overlooked in the past. In one series of 32 consecutive fatal cases massive infarction was present in 46 per cent (Tomlinson). Of particular importance is the high incidence of focal infarction found on microscopic examination of tissue appearing normal in the gross (Birse and Tom). Infarction, rather than intracerebral hemorrhage, may be the main cause of residual disability in patients who survive. Blood tends to collect between the frontal lobes, in the Sylvian fissure, and in the depths of sulci exerting pressure on the parent vessel. In addition there may be tearing of perforating branches at the time of the hemorrhage, or arterial spasm following trauma to the cerebral vessels.

Perhaps some of the damage should be attributed to the localized arterial spasm which can be shown by cerebral angiography to accompany subarachnoid hemorrhage. This may lead to a reduction in blood flow varying from 25-fold to 400-fold (Potter). The basilar artery is required to transmit an enormous excess of blood if it is to compensate for deficiency of the carotids resulting from spasm. The blood appears to be carried from the basilar to the fringes of the carotid territory by small peripheral anastomotic cerebral and more particularly leptomeningeal arteries.

Relation of Symptoms to Lesions.—The sudden onset of severe headache, cranial nerve paralysis, signs of meningeal irritation such as extreme stiffness of the neck, and the appearance of blood in the cerebrospinal fluid in the previously healthy person, often although not necessarily young, constitutes a clinical picture easily recognized. With the first attack of bleeding there is an immediate mortality of 20 to 35 per cent. The initial bleeding may subside spontaneously, but 20 per cent of the survivors will have a second and even more violent attack in the course of a few days or weeks. It is in these recurrent cases that modern methods of localization and treatment are so important. Cerebral angiography serves not only to determine the origin of the hemorrhage, but also to indicate the presence of a hematoma which will require evacuation, to evaluate the status of the collateral circulation through the circle of Willis, and to demonstrate whether or not there are multiple aneurysms. Vertebral arteriography may indicate the presence of an aneurysm in the basilar rather than the carotid system. Operation is performed shortly after the initial episode and before the period of high recurrence, which is usually the second to the fourth week.

Because the majority of aneurysms are situated along the branches of the internal carotid artery or on the circle of Willis, the second to the sixth cranial nerves are most often involved by compression. The optic nerve is also involved, with disturbance of function, in 10 to 20 per cent of cases. Almost half the cases give evidence of paresis of the third nerve before or after rupture of the aneurysm, with ptosis of the lid, dilatation of the pupil, and external deviation of the eye. Intermittent headache is quite frequent before rupture of the aneurysm, and if this is associated with third nerve palsy, the possibility of a congenital aneurysm should be investigated at a time when successful surgical treatment is still possible.

The most significant evidence of subarachnoid hemorrhage is of course the presence of blood in the cerebrospinal fluid. This can be distinguished from accidental blood due to the lumbar puncture by the fact that there is some hemolysis with *xanthochromia* or yellow coloration of the fluid after the red blood cells have been removed by centrifugation. It is obvious that, because of the intracranial bleeding and increase in pressure, a minimum of fluid must be withdrawn very slowly to prevent any possibility of herniation through the foramen magnum, otherwise the result of the lumbar puncture may be fatal.

(2) *Traumatic Subarachnoid Hemorrhage.* —Traumatic hemorrhage is likely to occur in all lacerations of the brain, so that blood will appear in the spinal fluid. The presence of blood in the subarachnoid space may irritate the cells of the arachnoid and cause blockage of the arachnoid villi through which the cerebrospinal fluid is absorbed into the venous blood sinuses. As the fluid cannot escape in the normal way it may collect in pools and cause pressure atrophy of the underlying cortex. It is possible that this may partly explain the puzzling post-traumatic neuroses and psychoses. The presence of pressure atrophy can be demonstrated in the living patient by means of encephalography or injection of air into the subarachnoid space.

The reader desirous of more detailed information on the subject of cerebrovascular diseases could not do better than consult the report on the subject in *Neurology*, 1958, *8*, 395.

INJURIES OF THE BRAIN AND SPINAL CORD

Laceration.—Most head injuries are acceleration injuries especially in this age of automobile accidents; the moving head hits an immobile object, or the stationary head is struck by a moving object. Varying degrees of laceration are common results of head injury. This may occur with or without fracture of the skull. Fracture, indeed, seems to act as a safety valve for the brain, as in a case which I observed of a child who fell on his head from a height of two stories and sustained a fracture of the skull which extended from the base over the vertex to the base on the other side, but suffered no permanent ill effects. Often the laceration is most marked on the side opposite to that on which the blow is struck, the condition known as *contrecoup*. Contrecoup injury, which is commonly seen on the under surface of the frontal lobes and the temporal

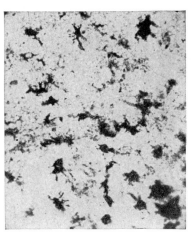

Fig. 651.—Mobilization of microglia with indrawing of the processes 3 days after wounding of the brain. Silver impregnation. × 200. (Kindness of Dr. Mary Tom.

and occipital poles, may be more or less severe than the lesion at the site of the original injury. Occasionally the only hemorrhage found is in the pons or mid-brain due to impact of the brain stem against the basiocciput. When the patient dies months or years later, cortical defects may be seen at the summits of the convolutions. The end result is a worm-eaten scarred area of cortex to which are attached the overlying arachnoid and dura. There is demyelination and neuroglial scarring of the underlying white matter (Fig. 651). These lesions, often small and easily overlooked, may be yellowish-brown in color due to the presence of old blood pigment. The acutely injured brain is swollen, a swelling usually attributed to edema, although some workers question this explanation. Petechial hemorrhages are common. Under the microscope they take the form of so-called ring hemorrhages, a ring of red blood cells around a central necrotic area. The lesions are really in the nature of hemorrhagic infarcts rather than true hemorrhages; blockage of a small vessel leads to necrosis, with diapedesis of red cells into the necrotic zone.

Concussion.—This is a transient state following head injury, of instantaneous onset, with purely paralytic symptoms, no sign of cerebral damage, and always followed by amnesia for the actual moment of the accident. As the result of a blow on the head, which as a rule does not produce a fracture, the patient instantaneously loses consciousness, and at the same time passes into a condition of profound shock. The face is pale and the body covered with a cold sweat, the temperature is subnormal, the pulse imperceptible, and the respiration almost suspended. The patient soon recovers consciousness, and as reaction sets in the temperature rises and the pulse becomes bounding. In some cases an unpleasant sequel is a marked degree of irritability, a condition of "cerebral irritation" which may last for a long time.

If a patient suffering from concussion should die, the autopsy findings are inconclusive. There may be laceration of the brain especially on the under surface of the frontal and temporal lobes, with hemorrhage into the subarachnoid space. These lesions can have nothing to do with the sudden loss of consciousness and development of shock. Petechial hemorrhages may be scattered through the brain. Unconsciousness in head injury is not necessarily due to cortical injury or compression, but to disturbances of the brain stem and thalamus and the ascending reticular activating system which contains the waking center or arousal mechanism. The most important sign to be watched for after head injury is a deterioration in the level of consciousness, although the orginal blackout may be followed by a so-called "lucid interval." Coma and death are likely to be due to compression of the midbrain by herniation of the hippocampal uncus at the hiatus tentorii.

Traumatic Edema.—The edema which follows trauma is of extreme practical importance on account of the disturbance which it causes in the circulation of the cerebrospinal fluid. The best example of this type of edema is seen in fracture of the skull. It is not the injury to the bone which is of importance but the laceration of the brain, as a result of which local edema and swelling rapidly develop. If the swelling is marked and persistent the brain tends to be pushed up or down, depending on the site of the hemorrhage. If it is pushed up against the skull, the subarachnoid space over the vertex is obliterated so that no absorption of fluid

can occur. If it is pushed down, the opening in the tentorium is plugged so that the fluid cannot pass from the basal cisterns to the upper subarachnoid space. In both cases the result is the same—a great accumulation of fluid at the base of the brain with increasing pressure on the vital centers in the medulla, as indicated by slowing of the pulse and respiration. This clinical picture of compression is usually attributed to "medullary edema," but it is evident that the effects are not due to a local edema of the medulla but to disturbance of the cerebrospinal fluid circulation.

Metabolic Effects of Brain Injury.—Since the days of the great Magendie we have known that damage to the floor of the fourth ventricle in the experimental animal results in hyperglycemia and glycosuria, and that a unilateral lesion in this area causes diuresis without hyperglycemia, accompanied by an increased excretion of chloride ions. This probably results from damage to or irritation of descending fibers which ultimately impinge on the sympathetic outflow from the spinal cord. We are now aware of the fact that the hypothalamus is particularly concerned with water, electrolyte and carbohydrate metabolism, and that experimental lesions in this region may cause hyperglycemia with glycosuria, hypoglycemia, diabetes insipidus, hyperchloremia with hypochloruria, and disturbances of corticotrophin. It is not surprising then to learn that in man injury to the brain may cause many disturbances in metabolism, more particularly (1) diabetes insipidus, (2) hypothalamic obesity, (3) hyperglycemia and glycosuria, and (4) respiratory alkalosis due to overstimulation of the respiratory centers by irritative lesions in the brain stem causing hyperventilation with excessive loss of carbon dioxide. In addition there may be hypernatremia and hyperchloremia with hyponatruria and hypochloruria, due apparently to excessive tubular reabsorption of sodium and chloride.

Epilepsy.—There is no ideal spot in a textbook of pathology in which to discuss epilepsy, but as many cases may be attributed to some type of brain injury, using that term in its wider sense, we may be allowed to consider it here.

Epilepsy may be either idiopathic or secondary to some cause, obvious or doubtful as the case may be. In the so-called *idiopathic* category one of the largest groups is that characterized by temporal lobe seizures (dreamy states, feeling of unreality, unpleasant odors). Penfield and his associates have drawn attention to the presence of *temporal lobe lesions* in these cases, ischemic in nature and apparently due to pressure on vessels at the time of birth. In 157 cases of temporal lobe seizures this type of lesion was present in 100, the remaining 57 cases showing evidence of post-natal injury, intracranial infection or neoplasm in the temporal region (Earle, Baldwin and Penfield). The seizures may begin in childhood or may be delayed to the second or third decade. In one-quarter of the cases there was a history of difficult birth. The gross lesions are sclerotic areas involving a single gyrus or it may be the entire lobe. These areas are tough, yellow, avascular and shrunken. *Microscopically* there is a striking increase in the astrocytes, sometimes giving the appearance of an astrocytoma. There may or may not be a focal loss of nerve cells and fibers. The hippocampus and uncus are supplied principally by the anterior choroidal artery, which at birth is as large as the middle cerebral. This and other vessels have to cross the sharp edge of the tentorium against which they may be compressed. It is common knowledge that in the adult increased intracranial pressure can cause hippocampal and uncal herniation through the incisuria tentorii. Penfield has shown that the same can happen in the newborn if labor is prolonged, with resulting ischemia and eventual sclerosis, a condition to which he has given the name of *incisural sclerosis*.

The *secondary* cases are due to such gross lesions of the brain as tumor, abscess, etc. In post-traumatic *epilepsy* the pia-arachnoid is thickened, and localized collections of fluid with atrophy of the corresponding convolutions can be seen on the operating table, although not in the postmortem room. It is possible that the initial lesion is an arachnoiditis, the effect of which is to block the villi and to divide the subarachnoid space into areas in which the excess of fluid is confined.

73

INTRACRANIAL SUPPURATION

Suppuration within the cranial cavity may take the form of *extradural abscess*, *abscess of the brain*, and *sinus thrombophlebitis*. Acute meningitis is also a suppurative condition, but is more conveniently considered under a separate heading.

The following account applies to cases which have not received the benefit of antibiotic therapy.

Extradural Abscess.—The infection spreads from the skull as the result of osteomyelitis of the cranium, a compound fracture, middle-ear disease, or frontal sinus infection. A collection of pus is formed external to the dura, and as that membrane offers a stout barrier to the spread of infection, the abscess may remain localized for a considerable time. The scalp over the inflamed area of bone becomes swollen and edematous, forming what is known as *Pott's puffy tumor*, a condition described by Percival Pott in 1760.

Abscess of the Brain.—The infection may spread from a local focus or may be carried from a distance by the blood stream. The common *local focus* is middle-ear suppuration. It may also result from infection of the frontal and nasal sinuses, from osteomyelitis of the skull, or from a compound fracture. Infection from the middle ear may spread up through the tegmen tympani in which case the surface of the bone is eroded, or by the veins, when no external lesion can be seen either on the bone or the cerebral surface. *Distant infection* most often comes from a septic focus in the lung, usually bronchiectasis; sometimes there is empyema. It is probable that infection spreads from the lung to the brain by the vertebral system of veins. This would explain the fact that there are no abscesses in other organs. The abscess is often single, the common site being the white matter of the frontal lobe (Fig. 652).

The abscess cavity is filled with pus in which there may be staphylococci, streptococci, or pneumococci. Bacillus pyocyaneus is often present, giving the pus a greenish color. The common site in middle-ear cases is the temporo-sphenoidal lobe, sometimes the cerebellum. The latter is much the more

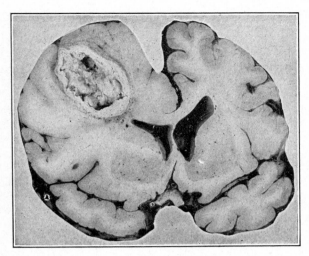

Fig. 652.—Single metastatic brain abscess in the frontal lobe secondary to an abscess of the lung. The right ventricle is dilated.

serious because of the frequency of meningitis, probably due to the depth of the cerebellar folia. When the infection comes from the frontal and nasal sinuses the frontal lobe is involved. A well-formed capsule is produced at the end of three weeks by fibroblasts in the adventitia of vessels. It is only after the formation of this capsule that an operation can be undertaken with hope of success. The best results are those obtained in abscess secondary to middle-ear infection, the worst in cases secondary to lung abscess. It is remarkable how silent a brain abscess may be for a considerable time, especially if it is in the temporo-sphenoidal lobe. The temperature may be normal, the pulse is slow (abnormally so), and there may be very little leukocytosis. The cerebrospinal fluid is usually normal, apart from increased pressure, but if the abscess approaches the surface polymorphonuclears may appear in the fluid, due to seepage of toxic material quiescent for many months, but eventually it will rupture into a ventricle or reach the surface and set up a fatal meningitis.

The threat of a brain abscess is two-fold: (1) spreading infection and (2) the increased intracranial pressure produced by a space-occupying lesion. The first of these can be controlled by antibiotics which have naturally reduced the incidence of the condition as well as that of the middle-ear infection which so often precedes it. The second can only be arrested by surgical intervention.

The earliest recognizable phase of cerebral infection is *acute, localized, nonsuppurative encephalitis* (Botterell). This is characterized by headache, some pyrexia, and focal disturbances, but not the drowsiness which heralds the development of a space-occupying lesion. If the condition is recognized it can be arrested by massive doses of those antibiotics and sulfonamides which pass readily into the cerebrospinal fluid.

Sinus Thrombophlebitis.—Infection reaches the venous sinuses of the dura mater by spread from some neighboring focus. The wall of the sinus becomes inflamed (phlebitis), and thrombosis follows as a matter of course. The *lateral sinus* is infected from the middle ear and mastoid, so that this is the vessel most often involved. The *superior longitudinal sinus* is infected from erysipelas and other septic conditions of the scalp. The *cavernous sinus* is infected from septic foci in the nose, face, orbit, and sphenoidal air sinus; carbuncle of the face is especially dangerous in this respect.

The *thrombosis tends to spread from one sinus to another, and from the lateral sinus down the jugular vein,* which can be felt as a hard and tender cord. The infection may spread outward, causing meningitis or cerebral abscess. The great danger, however, is the softening and liquefaction which occur in the infected thrombus. At any moment a piece of the softened clot may be dislodged, carried by the jugular vein to the right side of the heart, and thence to the lungs where it is arrested. The inevitable result is the formation of a pulmonary abscess, followed later by pyemia. For this reason ligation of the jugular vein must be done before any direct attack upon an infected lateral sinus can be attempted.

The *clinical course* of sinus thrombophlebitis is very different from that of cerebral abscess. In the former it is stormy and tempestuous compared with the calm and peace of the latter. High fever, rigors, and chills are common, owing to the continual discharge of septic material into the blood stream.

MENINGITIS

Infection may reach the meninges by the blood stream, from the brain, or from neighboring foci of infection in the middle-ear, nasopharynx, accessory nasal sinuses, etc. Meningitis may complicate fracture of the base of the skull, particularly the anterior cranial fossa with involvement of the nasal fossæ and ethmoidal sinuses. In such cases the fatal infection may come from infected sinuses through the fracture line many years after the accident. Almost any pathogenic organism may cause meningitis and even fungi have been known to do so, but there are only four common ones; these are the *meningococcus, streptococcus, pneumococcus,* and *tubercle bacillus.* The first three are pyogenic and cause purulent inflammation, so that the pathological changes are practically identical.

Meningococcal Meningitis.—This is the commonest form of meningitis. The disease is usually sporadic, but may become epidemic. For this reason it is known as epidemic cerebrospinal meningitis. The epidemiology is quite different from that of an ordinary infectious fever, for there is seldom more than one case in a family, and it is difficult to trace the contagion. The explanation is that the receptivity of the throat is high, while that of the meninges is low. There are always far more carriers than patients, and a carrier epidemic precedes and accompanies a case epidemic.

The *mode of infection* of the meninges is a matter of doubt. The disease is certainly spread from one person to another as a throat infection, as can be readily shown by taking swabs of the throats of a community during an epidemic. The difficulty is to decide by what route the meningococcus passes from the nasopharynx to the meninges. It may possibly spread through the lymphatics in the cribriform plate of the ethmoid and thus reach the subarachnoid space, but neither the organisms nor any sign of inflammation can be found in the ethmoid in fatal cases. It seems more likely that infection is by the bloodstream, for the meningococci can be found in the blood in about one-third of the early cases; sometimes, indeed, they are confined to the blood and never reach the meninges (meningococcal septicemia). It may be that the meninges are infected primarily from the blood, but it is difficult to explain the fact that in fulminant cases where the patient dies within twenty-four hours the blood and the fluid in the ventricles contain meningococci, yet the meninges are normal. It appears more likely that a metastatic focus is set up in the choroid plexus, from which the microörganisms are poured into the ventricles. First a choroiditis and then an ependymitis is produced, the cocci living on the ependymal lining of the ventricles, which is an epithelial structure like the lining of the nasopharynx. The flow of fluid carries pus and bacteria into the basal cisterns and down the spinal canal as well as to a varying extent up into the cerebral subarachnoid space. In infants, especially those brought up on the bottle, the brain is very soft, so that the sulci and cerebral subarachnoid space are easily closed by the increased pressure, and the pus collects entirely in the basal cisterns, giving the *posterior basic type of meningitis* seen only in infants.

Lesions.—The brain is covered with a purulent exudate, confined to the subarachnoid space and therefore most abundant in the sulci (Fig. 653). The meningeal vessels are greatly dilated. The exudate on the surface of the cerebrum is most marked in the frontal and parietal regions, but the bulk of

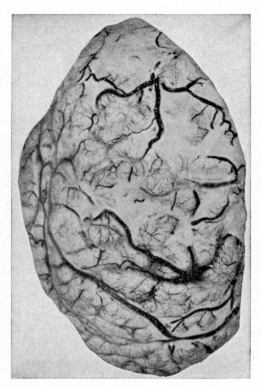

FIG. 653.—Acute meningococcal meningitis. The meningeal vessels are greatly dilated. Scattered over the surface are large opaque areas of purulent exudate.

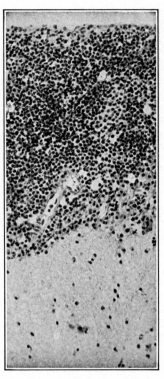

FIG. 654.—Acute meningitis. The subarachnoid space is packed with inflammatory cells. × 160

the exudate is to be found at the base, where it fills the interpeduncular space, passes forward along the optic nerves, backward into the great cisterns and upward along the middle and anterior cerebral arteries. In the spinal canal the exudate is largely confined to the posterior surface of the cord, an effect of gravity. The ventricles are moderately dilated and filled with turbid fluid, the choroid plexus is hyperemic, and the lining of the ventricles roughened.

Microscopically the subarachnoid space is filled with a purulent exudate consisting of polymorphonuclear leukocytes with a few lymphocytes and large mononuclear phagocytes (Fig. 654). Fibrin is seldom marked. The vessels are greatly distended and there may be small hemorrhages. Meningococci are present both inside and outside the leukocytes. The brain and cord are not affected, although the exudate may penetrate the perivascular sheaths for a little distance. The only place where there is any inflammation is under the ependyma and in the choroid plexus.

The rest of the body shows little change, for the meningococcus has difficulty in establishing itself in the tissues, although it flourishes on the surface of the upper respiratory tract and in the ventricles and subarachnoid space. The nasopharynx shows congestion, edema, and an infiltration with lymphocytes and plasma cells. In rare cases the meningococcus may cause endocarditis, pericarditis, arthritis, adrenal hemorrhage, etc.

Cerebrospinal Fluid.—Lumbar puncture shows the pressure to be raised owing to a marked increase in the amount of fluid formed. The fluid is tubid, but in the earliest stage it may be almost clear. The protein content is high, above 0.3 per cent and sometimes as high as 0.8 per cent. The sugar is diminished and may be absent, owing to the fermentative action of the meningococcus.

The film shows the cells to be polymorpho-nuclears, but as recovery sets in, their place is gradually taken by large mononuclear phagocytes (macrophages) and finally by lymphocytes. The meningococci are usually intracellular, but some may be extracellular. They are gram-negative diplococci, bean-shaped and indistinguishable in smears from the gonococcus. They are seldom numerous and sometimes none can be found. A puru-lent fluid in which no organisms can be found is almost certainly meningococcal. When culturing the fluid, at least a cubic centimeter should be used; it is useless to take a mere loopful. The result of culture rather than the gross appearance of the fluid is the true measure of the progress of the case.

Relation of Symptoms to Lesions.—In severe cases there may be a *hemorrhagic rash on the skin* and mucous membranes, a condi-tion known as spotted fever. Most of the cerebral symptoms, such as *headache* and *vomiting*, are due to increased intra-cranial pressure. *Stiffness* and *retraction of the neck*, the most characteristic part of the clinical picture, is caused by irritation at the posterior part of the base of the brain. It reaches its most extreme degree in the poste-rior basic meningitis of infants where the retraction may be so great that the head may actually touch the back, a condition of *opisthotonos*. *Strabismus* (squint) and *dip-lopia* (double vision) may be present due to involvement of the third, fourth, and sixth nerves at the base of the brain. The heightened intracranial pressure is due partly to an increased outpouring of fluid, partly to interference with the normal absorption from the cerebral subarachnoid space. This interference is caused by blockage of the eliminating apparatus (arachnoid villi and Pacchionian bodies) by the purulent exudate; the accumulation in the basal cisterns which tends to push the brain up against the roof of the skull probably plays a part. Lumbar puncture, and still better cisternal puncture, will help to relieve this state of affairs. If the fluid is not absorbed it will accumulate in the ventricles which become dilated, but a true internal hydrocephalus due to block-ing of the openings in the roof of the fourth ventricle is not common in adults. In infants it is a frequent and fatal complica-tion, the great compressibility of the very soft brain of the infant being the most im-portant factor.

It is obvious that the above account ap-plies to a case which has not been treated with chemotherapy. There are few acute bacterial infections in which the outlook has been more favorably affected by modern therapy instituted at an early stage than meningococcal meningitis.

Meningococcal Septicemia.—In every case of meningococcal meningitis there is prob-ably an element of septicemia, but the term meningococcal septicemia is usually reserved for those cases in which there is a blood infection without a corresponding infection of the meninges. It is an extrameningeal meningococcal infection. Meningitis may sometimes develop after the septicemia has been in progress for a number of weeks; this is called meningitis tarda. The course of meningococcal septicemia varies enormously. The fulminating cases may be incredibly rapid, and in these the infection may be so heavy that large numbers of meningococci can be seen in the blood smears. As Herrick remarks: "No other infection so quickly slays." In other cases the infections may go on for weeks and even months, blood cultures being repeatedly positive. In the more severe septicemic cases a hemorrhagic rash is likely to be present. Herrick describes the case of a soldier who walked into hospital at 4 p.m. and was dead at 8 p.m., the body covered with a purpuric rash. In other cases the infection may go on for weeks or even months, blood cultures being repeatedly posi-tive. In the more severe septicemic cases a hemorrhagic rash is likely to be present.

One of the most dreaded complications of acute meningococcemia is massive bilateral hemorrhagic necrosis of the adrenals, par-ticularly in infants and very young children. This results in fatal circulatory collapse due to destruction of the adrenal cortex, a con-dition known as the *Waterhouse-Friderichsen syndrome*. In older patients there may be multiple small areas of hemorrhagic necrosis due to thrombosis of the sinusoids, with the possibility of complete recovery (Thomison and Shapiro). The explanation of the mas-sive necrotizing lesions of the adrenal is not as simple as might be supposed, for they are not due to an overwhelming meningococcal infection with accompanying suppuration. It seems more likely that they are a manifestation of an immunological or hypersensitivity reaction to the meningococcus, a matter which has already been discussed on page 998.

Other Forms of Suppurative Meningitis.— *Pneumococcal meningitis* may be primary or secondary to infection in the middle-ear, nasal sinuses or lung. The disease is very acute. The morbid anatomy is the same as that of meningococcal meningitis. The purulent cerebrospinal fluid contains large numbers of pneumococci, so that the diagnosis can readily be made from a smear. The fibrinogen is much increased, and the fluid may even clot spontaneously. With modern chemotherapy the prognosis is much better in children than in adults, for in the adult there is a marked formation of a fibrinous exudate which causes obstructive hydrocephalus. *Streptococcal meningitis* is usually secondary to middle-ear or sinus infection, but occasionally it may be primary. The organism may be Streptococcus hæmolyticus, Streptococcus viridans or Streptococcus mucosus. The last-named usually comes from the ear and causes the formation of a characteristic sticky mucoid exudate. The morbid anatomy and the condition of the cerebrospinal fluid are the same as in the other two forms of acute meningitis. Streptococci are usually present in large numbers in the fluid. *Staphylococcal meningitis* is rare, and the organisms are present in very small numbers. *Influenza bacillus meningitis*, better called Pfeiffer's bacillus meningitis, is the fifth commonest form in America, although much less common in Britain. It is suppurative, commonest in children, and used to be very fatal. With broad spectrum antibiotics if the diagnosis is made early (a conveniently vague expression) it is said that the disease can be treated successfully in nearly every case. Typhoid and paratyphoid bacilli and Bacillus coli are occasional causes of meningitis. Still more rare are Bacillus pyocyaneus, Bacillus anthracis, Bacillus mallei, Friedländer's pneumobacillus, Micrococcus catarrhalis, actinomyces and a streptothrix.

Tuberculous Meningitis.—Tuberculous infection of the meninges may be primary (in

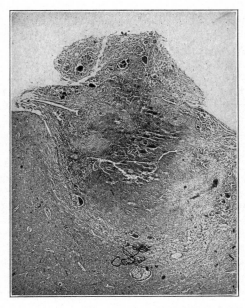

Fig. 655.—Small tuberculous lesion of the brain discharging into the subarachnoid space. Several giant cells can be seen.

the sense that it is the first active lesion to manifest itself), or it may be part of a general miliary tuberculosis. The infection reaches the brain by the blood stream, and it is usually believed that the meninges are primarily involved. It can be shown experimentally, however, that the meninges are very resistant to blood infection, even when large numbers of tubercle bacilli are injected into the carotid artery. On the other hand, they are readily infected when the injection is made directly into the subarachnoid space. Rich has shown that in many cases of tuberculous meningitis it is possible to demonstrate a tuberculous lesion in the brain, the choroid plexus, and even the meninges, and this lesion he regards as the primary source of the meningeal infection. The lesions are often multiple, but they may be no larger than a pea, so that the brain has to be cut into very thin slices if they are to be demonstrated. When one of these lesions is sufficiently superficial to discharge bacilli into the subarachnoid space or the ventricles, heavy infection of the meninges at once results (Fig. 655). The lesion may open into a blood vessel, causing general miliary tuberculosis (Fig. 656), or the Pac-

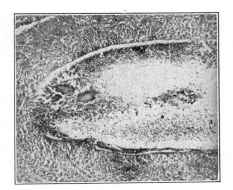

Fig. 656.—Tuberculous lesion in the brain rupturing into a blood vessel. Giant cells can be seen in the lumen of the vessel.

chionian bodies may be infected from the subarachnoid space and the bacilli pass in this way into the superior longitudinal sinus. Other workers do not agree with Rich, and believe that the meninges are infected from the blood stream. Beres and Meltzer examed 28 cases of tuberculous meningitis. In only 6 were there cortical tubercles which might have caused the meningitis, and in 11 there were tubercles in the choroid plexus.

Lesions.—The type of lesion varies with the massiveness of the infection. If the dose is small the principal lesion is the miliary tubercle, but if it is large there may be an abundant nonspecific exudative reaction with the formation of a creamy or greenish somewhat gelatinous exudate at the base of the brain extending from the chiasma in front to the cerebellum behind, filling up the spaces (Fig. 657) and glueing together the surfaces. The tubercles are covered up by this exudate, but they can usually be seen on the upper surface of the cerebellum, on the velum interpositum, and along the line of the vessels as they pass up to the cortex. Sometimes almost no exudate or tubercles can be detected unless a very careful examination be made of the base of the brain with a hand lens. In these cases it is difficult to understand why the patient should have died. A possible explanation is the frequent presence of microscopic lesions very close to the hypothalamus, a vital center. The convolutions are flattened and the sulci narrowed owing to the hydrocephalus which is nearly always present, and which is caused by the

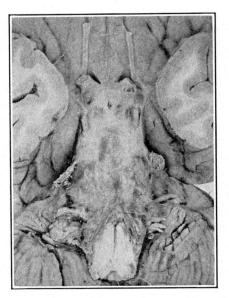

Fig. 657.—Tuberculous meningitis. The exudate covers the base of the brain.

thick exudate over the roof of the fourth ventricle. The ependymal lining of the dilated ventricles is roughened and granular ependymitis resembling that seen in cerebral syphilis is not uncommon (Fig. 658). When the brain is hardened and cut into very thin slices it is often possible to demonstrate small tuberculous lesions in the superficial part of the cortex or in the wall of the ventricle. Sometimes these lesions may be in the cord instead of the brain.

Microscopically the picture is a mixed one, partly tuberculous and partly inflammatory in nature. Definite, typical tubercles are usually conspicuous by their absence and the same is true of giant cells. Diffusely arranged epithelioid cells and areas of caseation necrosis are the characteristic features. Tubercle bacilli can be seen in appropriately stained sections. When the reaction is more acute the subarachnoid space is filled with lymphocytes, plasma cells and polymorphonuclears, but here again patches of necrosis indicate the nature of the process. The walls of the vessels are thickened and infiltrated with inflammatory cells. The *brain* is remarkably free from inflammatory lesions, but in places the infection may extend for a short distance into the cortex.

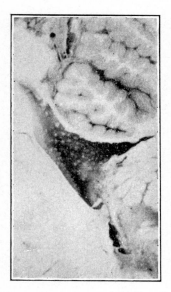

FIG. 658.—Tuberculous granular ependymitis.

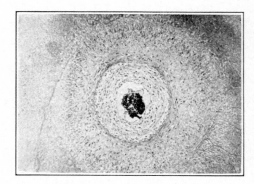

FIG. 659.—Endarteritis in treated tuberculous
meningitis. × 65.

The primary focus in the brain shows a typical picture of tuberculosis with giant cell formation. Tuberculous necrotic foci can often be found in the choroid plexus and velum interpositum.

Streptomycin treatment, by prolonging the survival period in those cases which do not recover, has greatly changed the picture at postmortem. Tuberculous granulation tissue replaces the cellular exudate, and this becomes converted into a dense layer of hyalinized connective tissue enclosing necrotic foci at the base of the brain. Hydrocephalus is a prominent feature due to obstruction in the aqueduct or the foramina of Luschka. In other cases the hydrocephalus is of the communicating type. Large meningeal tuberculomas composed of epithelioid tubercles with giant cells are a prominent feature, and similar large lesions are seen in the choroid plexus (Terplan).

Arterial changes, whilst occasionally seen before the days of chemotherapy, have become of much greater importance since the use of streptomycin has so greatly prolonged the life of these patients. The acute tuberculous arteritis commonly seen in the circle of Willis is transformed into a proliferative endarteritis with varying degrees of stenosis (Fig. 659). In some of the cases in my department in Toronto the structure of the vessels was so altered by tuberculous granulation tissue that they were only recognized by persistence of the internal elastic lamina. There is nothing to suggest that the intrathecal use of streptomycin is responsible for the endarteritis, which is due entirely to the prolongation of life. The great importance of the arterial lesions is that they cause multiple brain softenings, which in turn are responsible for a variety of focal cerebral symptoms. There may be massive necrosis of the corpus striatum.

From what has just been said it might be thought that modern therapy merely prolonged life long enough for arterial obstructive lesions to develop. Nothing could be farther from the truth. The early use of streptomycin and isoniazid in combination with para-aminosalicylic acid has transformed a disease with a mortality of 100 per cent into one in which a survival rate of less than 80 per cent suggests that the treatment was at fault. There is, however, a high incidence of detectable calcification, especially in the basal meninges, and it remains to be seen how this will affect the ultimate prognosis.

Cerebrospinal Fluid.—As the tuberculous process has an aptitude for producing both endarteritis and constrictive exudates around what has been called that most eloquent part of the central nervous system, the midbrain, early diagnosis has become of paramount importance, whereas formerly it was only of academic interest. The diagnosis is made by examination of the cerebrospinal fluid.

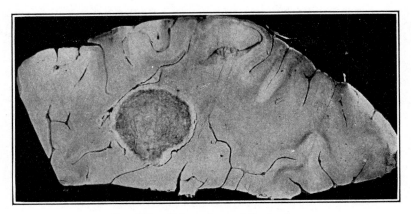

Fig. 660.—Tuberculoma of the brain.

The clinical picture in poliomyelitis, epidemic encephalitis, and a deep brain abscess may closely resemble that of tuberculous meningitis, and unfortunately the spinal fluid findings are rather similar, but there are slight though important differences. The pressure is raised, and the fluid is clear or opalescent, almost never turbid. When allowed to stand a fine *web of fibrin* forms. This is very characteristic of tuberculous meningitis and is never seen in encephalitis and brain abscess, but a web sometimes forms in poliomyelitis and syphilitic meningitis. The *protein* is increased to a greater degree in tuberculous meningitis than in the other three. The *sugar* is decreased and sometimes disappears; in poliomyelitis and brain abscess it is normal, and in encephalitis it may be above normal (0.07 to 0.09 per cent). Estimation of sugar is therefore of great use in distinguishing between these easily confused conditions. The *chlorides* are low (normal: 120 to 130 m.Eq/liter). This is the most valuable of all the chemical tests, for no other condition gives a really low reading. Just to prove that no test is perfect, in the very exceptional case the chloride level is normal. The *cells* average from 50 to 200 per c.mm. (normal: 5 or less, though in children it may be higher). The cell count is usually below 50 in encephalitis and brain abscess, but in poliomyelitis it may be similar to tuberculous meningitis. The predominant cell is the lymphocyte, but in acute reactions, especially in children, there

may be as many polymorphonuclears as lymphocytes. The demonstration of the *tubercle bacillus* is the conclusive proof of the nature of the condition. Both the web and the centrifuged deposit should be examined.

Relation of Symptoms to Lesions.—Paralysis of the cranial motor nerves, especially the oculomotor, may be caused by the exudate at the base of the brain, so that ptosis (drooping of the upper lid), squint, and diplopia are common. Stiffness and retraction of the neck are symptoms common to any meningeal irritation involving the base of the brain and the upper spinal meninges. Cortical irritation may lead to spasms and convulsions. The acute hydrocephalus which is of such constant occurrence is responsible for symptoms of compression terminating in coma.

TUBERCULOMA.—This is a rather rare slow-growing circumscribed tuberculous lesion, often multiple, usually occurring in children, and easily mistaken for a tumor of the brain. It may become as large as a walnut (Fig. 660). It generally forms a firm spherical mass, but softening may sometimes occur with the formation of a tuberculous abscess. *Microscopically* the center is caseous, with epithelioid and giant cells at the margin. The prognosis is bad, for operative interference is nearly always followed by tuberculous meningitis or general miliary tuberculosis.

TUBERCULOMA EN PLAQUE.—Tuberculoma en plaque is a very rare tuberculous lesion occurring only in adults. There is a tuberculous meningo-encephalitis of very chronic character, with the formation of a flat plaque on the surface of the fronto-parietal cortex. The symptoms are those of tumor, i.e., headache, vomiting and Jacksonian epilepsy, with the addition of fever.

Spinal Epidural Tuberculoma.—This is a granuloma between the spinal cord and the vertebral column. It is naturally associated with tuberculosis of the vertebræ, and equally naturally it is likely to produce compression of the spinal cord.

Sarcoidosis.—Sarcoidosis is not mentioned in this place because of its resemblance to tuberculosis, but rather because of its difference. It is a granulomatous disease of young persons involving most commonly the meninges, the region of the floor of the third ventricle and the pituitary. The gross appearance varies widely, from a slight diffuse thickening of the meninges to gray infiltrating masses easily mistaken for tumor. It differs from tuberculosis in that massive direct invasion of the brain from the subarachnoid space is common, the course is frequently benign and self-limited, and operative interference fails to activate the process (Aszkanazy).

VIRUS DISEASES

A large number of known viruses can attack the central nervous system, sometimes setting up an inapparent infection, frequently causing meningitis or nonparalytic poliomyelitis, less often encephalitis or encephalomyelitis. The stools are the best source of the poliomyelitis virus (3 types), the Coxsackie virus (25–30 types), and the Echo viruses (28 types). Throat swabs are also used. In mumps, herpes, and other nonenteroviral infections, the cerebrospinal fluid should be examined.

Viruses with a special affinity for the central nervous system are *neurotropic* and cause some of the most serious diseases which afflict that system. There are some viruses which primarily attack the nervous system, *e.g.*, poliomyelitis, rabies, distemper of dogs, Borna disease of horses. Others do not ordinarily involve the nervous system, but when injected into the brain of an animal they produce serious or fatal results; examples are herpes febrilis, salivary gland disease of guinea pigs, and vaccinia. There is still a third group of very common febrile diseases (measles, chicken pox, smallpox, vaccinia) in which injury of the nervous system occurs on rare occasions, usually during convalescence. Neurotropic viruses are peculiar in that they may reach the central nervous system *via* peripheral nerves (cranial and spinal), traveling actually in the axis cylinder of the nerve fiber. Moreover they diffuse throughout the entire nervous system (central, peripheral and visceral), as bacteria spread throughout the vascular system in septicemia. Thus, when the virus of rabies is inoculated into the brain it can be recovered from the peripheral nerves some days later, although if a nerve is cut across, the distal part remains free from infection. That the virus may travel by way of the axons is demonstrated by the fact that when the virus of poliomyelitis is inoculated into the sciatic nerve of one leg it can be recovered from the opposite motor cortex, thus following the decussation of the motor path. We now believe, however, that clinical poliomyelitis is due to a hematogenous infection of the central nervous system.

The *three cardinal lesions* of virus diseases of the central nervous system are *inclusion bodies, cellular necrosis*, and *inflammation*. Not all of these need be present and unfortunately none of them is specific for viruses. It is very difficult to say how long a virus may remain in the nervous system once it has gained entrance. There may be more than fancy in von Economo's conception of the "encaged virus," which once having got in cannot get out again. It may do no harm until some accessory factor takes a hand, as in the case of herpes febrilis. Many of the viruses produce inclusion bodies in the affected nerve cells, *e.g.*, rabies, poliomyelitis, and Borna disease of horses. These and other fundamental matters have already been considered in the general discussion on viruses in Chapter 13.

Reference has already been made to the way in which neurotropic viruses can travel along nerve fibers. This ability depends to some degree on the age of the individual. A neurotropic virus, which in young mice can travel from the nose to the olfactory region of the brain and thence to the thalamus and cortex causing fatal encephalitis, is held up in the olfactory region in older animals. This is probably due to the gradual development of a local immunity to the virus.

Two great classes of lesions produced by neurotropic viruses may be distinguished. (1) Non-suppurative encephalitis or myelitis in which the infecting agent enters and *destroys certain groups of nerve cells.* Poliomyelitis, rabies, herpes, louping ill in the sheep, Borna disease in the horse (equine encephalomyelitis) are characteristic examples; epidemic encephalitis may be included with reserve, and possibly herpes zoster. (2) Encephalomyelitis in which the essential lesion is a primary *demyelination of nerve fibers.* The evidence that this group is caused by a virus is not absolute, only suggestive. An acute disseminated encephalomyelitis of this type may be primary, or it may follow the specific infectious fevers or vaccination. The demyelination, shown by the Weigert-Pal method, is striking and widespread. The question naturally suggests itself as to whether such demyelinating diseases as disseminated sclerosis and Schilder's disease should be included in this group. These latter diseases, however, are slowly progressive, whereas encephalomyelitis, if not fatal, ends in recovery. Our knowledge regarding the essential mechanism of demyelination and the question whether it is due to one or several classes of agent is still too rudimentary to justify us in concluding that it is due to a virus infection in every instance. In addition to the destructive and demyelinizing lesions, both groups show perivascular collections of round cells. In Group I at least a proportion of these represent a true inflammatory reaction to the virus, all the more likely because polymorphonuclears are abundant in so typical an example as poliomyelitis. In Group II they are probably secondary to the myelin destruction, being proliferated microglial scavengers.

Encephalitis.—Inflammation of the brain may be bacterial or viral. Bacteria cause a *suppurative encephalitis* in the form of small abscesses scattered throughout the brain, which may be microscopic or visible to the naked eye. This occurs in pyemia due to various pyogenic bacteria, and in bacterial endocarditis, where the lesions are often microscopic. Such conditions are terminal, and therefore not of great clinical interest.

Virus encephalitis constitutes a group of diseases, some of which are epidemic. In some the lesions represent a non-suppurative inflammation characterized by perivascular collections of macrophages, lymphocytes and plasma cells with accompanying degeneration of nerve cells. In others, particularly the postinfectious types, demyelination is the outstanding feature. The principal examples of virus encephalitis are: (1) type A encephalitis (von Economo), (2) type B encephalitis (St. Louis), (3) equine encephalomyelitis, and (4) acute disseminated encephalomyelitis.

Type A (Lethargic) Encephalitis.—This is also known as epidemic encephalitis and encephalitis lethargica. Other forms of encephalitis may be epidemic associated with lethargy, and as this type was first described by von Economo in Vienna in 1917, it is often known by his name. It appeared like a bolt from the blue in 1917, spread all over the world in pandemic form, returned more than once to a locality, and then vanished. Fresh cases are very seldom seen now. On general grounds it must be assumed that the disease is due to a virus, but this has never been proved.

Lesions.—The gross appearance of the brain is not characteristic. Microscopically the chief lesion is the familiar perivascular collars of chronic inflammatory cells (Fig. 661). In contrast to poliomyelitis there are no polymorphonuclears, no inflammatory foci, no areas of necrosis. Congestion is marked, and small hemorrhages are frequent. The lesions are most numerous in the periaqueductal region of the midbrain, but they are also marked in the basal ganglia, pons and medulla. The cerebral and cerebellar cortex are not affected. Degeneration and disappearance of the pigmented cells of the substantia nigra in the midbrain is a striking feature in the chronic stage, and there is also cellular degeneration in the globus pallidus. These structures are stations on the extrapyramidal tract, the primitive motor pathway, and the lesions serve to explain the motor helplessness and rigidity.

The *cerebrospinal fluid* shows no characteristic changes except that the sugar content tends to be high, due to an accompanying hyperglycemia.

Symptoms.—To attempt to give an adequate account of the symptomatology of epidemic encephalitis would be ludicrous in a textbook of pathology, for almost every known neurological symptom may be pro-

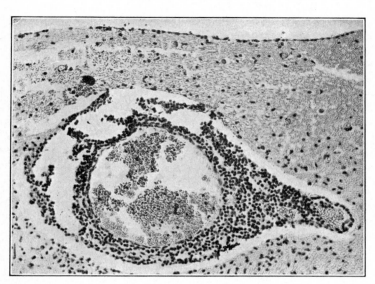

FIG. 661.—Epidemic encephalitis. Collar of cells around inflamed vessel in floor of fourth ventricle. The cells are in the true perivascular space. × 200.

duced. Moreover the epidemic gradually changed its clinical manifestations. Winnipeg was visited by two epidemics, both of which I studied, the first in the winter of 1919–1920, the second at the beginning of 1923. In the *first epidemic* the patient was dull, lethargic, somnolent, and showed oculomotor disturbances. He would lie like a log in bed with drooping lids or closed eyes, the lines of expression all ironed out, sunk in a stupor which no external stimuli could penetrate, the flash and speed of the mind gone, the dim rushlight of reason hardly flickering. In the *second epidemic* the picture had changed completely. Body and mind were now keyed to full activity. The muscles were in a state of constant movement, which was paralleled by a condition of mental excitement. Words came in a torrent, rationally at first, but drifting away into delirium. Occupation formed the main topic of conversation: the teacher was continually teaching, the merchant was casting up accounts, the builder planning new houses. The first picture was akinetic, the second hyperkinetic. It must be noted, however, that more than one-half the 1923 cases developed lethargy and somnolence sooner or later.

In addition to fever and somnolence, oculomotor palsies were extremely common, causing diplopia, strabismus, and ptosis. The hyperkinesia manifested itself by every variety of choreiform and athetoid movement, as well as clonic spasm of various kinds. Rigidity, a "muscle-bound" condition, was present in the acute stage, but was far more pronounced in chronic encephalitis, giving the well-known condition of *Parkinsonism* or *postencephalitic paralysis agitans*, with its mask-like face, stoop, flexed arms and wrists, and mincing steps. Some 20 per cent of the cases developed some degree of Parkinsonism. Other postencephalitic conditions which may be mentioned were narcolepsy and oculogyric crises (sudden attacks in which the eyes are fixed in a conjugate position). Among the most distressing of the sequelæ in children were profound emotional and moral disturbances, with disintegration of the mind and character.

Type B (St. Louis) Encephalitis.—During the late summer of 1933 an epidemic of encephalitis broke out in St. Louis and the surrounding district, which has been called encephalitis B. There was a recurrence in 1937. While resembling lethargic encephalitis, it appears to be more closely related to an epidemic reported from Japan in 1924.

Indeed, it is identical with the latter clinically and pathologically, although it reacts differently serologically. The disease differs from the lethargic forms in the following respects. Somnolence is uncommon, convulsions are frequent, there is a remarkable absence of the usual oculomotor palsies (ptosis, strabismus, diplopia), there are no sequelæ, the lesions are at higher levels (frequently in the cerebrum), there is no special localization in the midbrain. There were none of the tragic sequelæ of lethargic encephalitis. Monkeys and mice are successfully infected by intracerebral inoculation of brain tissue and also by the intranasal route. The St. Louis convalescent serum protects these animals against the St. Louis virus, but not against the virus from the Japanese cases. The disease is probably transmitted by mosquitoes.

Equine Encephalitis.—Horses suffer a fatal form of encephalomyelitis, a virus disease which appears in epidemic form. In 1938 there was a widespread epidemic of this disease in the United States and Canada. In a number of instances persons, particularly children, fell ill on farms where there were sick horses, and in fatal cases the same virus was found in the human patient and the horse. The human disease runs a very severe clinical course, with a fairly high cell count in the cerebrospinal fluid. In the late summer and during the autumn of 1941 over 1000 cases occurred in Manitoba and Saskatchewan due to the so-called Western strain of virus, and 1080 cases in North Dakota. At autopsy the picture is that of an acute disseminated encephalomyelitis with intense congestion, perivascular collections of polymorphonuclears, and in places an acute arteritis. In addition there is neuronal degeneration and areas of actual necrosis. The lesions are widely distributed throughout the cortex, basal ganglia, pons, medulla, and cervical cord. The cerebrospinal fluid cell count is rarely above 100 per c. mm., mainly lymphocytes, with a moderate increase in proteins. The polymorphonuclear exudate is reflected in the cerebrospinal fluid, which shows a high cell count in which from 60 to 90 per cent of the cells may be polymorphonuclears.

The disease is readily transmissible to mice by intracerebral injection of brain tissue. Human infection is probably due to mosquitoes, but this has not been proved. Specific antibodies are found in the blood of domestic birds and mammals during an epidemic. Chickens and pigeons seem to serve as a reservoir of the infection. The virus can be transmitted to these birds not only by mosquitoes but also by ticks. The latter vector can pass on the virus to their offspring for innumerable generations. The common crow is perhaps the main reservoir for the virus, which is transmitted both to horses and man by mosquito vectors. The evidence is conclusive that this is a virus disease; this is not true of the lethargic form of encephalitis.

There are two varieties of the disease, known as Eastern and Western. The *Eastern form*, prevalent in the Atlantic United States, Massachusetts in particular, is the more virulent. The cells both of the inflammatory exudate and the cerebrospinal fluid in the Eastern form are mainly polymorphonuclears, whereas in the *Western form* they are mainly lymphocytes. The mosquitoes responsible for the spread of the two types are of different species. Wild birds are supposed to be the reservoir hosts of the Eastern virus.

Mumps Meningoencephalitis.—Encephalitis caused by the virus of mumps is not infrequent. Indeed some workers believe that a mild degree of encephalitis occurs in the majority of cases of mumps. There may or may not be evidence of parotitis. The disease is rarely fatal. The lesions are rather meningeal than cerebral, as reflected by the very high lymphocytic count in the cerebrospinal fluid. The disease must not be confused with the encephalitis which may follow rather than accompany mumps, as is mentioned in connection with the encephalitis following fevers.

Acute Disseminated Encephalomyelitis.—The very occasional development of encephalitis as a result of one of the infective fevers has long been recognized. During recent years there has been a marked increase in the number of cases of acute and widespread involvement of the central nervous system either following some febrile disorder or occurring spontaneously. As these cases all have a similar if not common pathology, characterized by scattered patches of perivascular demyelinization associated with an inflammatory reaction, they may conveniently be considered under the heading of acute disseminated encephalomyelitis. Three main types may be distinguished: (1) post-vaccinal encephalitis, (2) encephalitis following infectious fevers, and (3) spontaneous encephalomyelitis.

Post-vaccinal Encephalitis.—This complication has come into prominence since 1922, particularly in England and Holland. It is the most dangerous form of disseminated encephalomyelitis, with a mortality of from 25 to 50 per cent. The incidence in England is 1 in 50,000 vaccinations, while in Holland it is 1 in 5000. The onset, usually about the eleventh day after vaccination, is acute and the course rapid, with fever, vomiting, headache, squint, and sometimes upper motor neurone paralysis. It is possible that the vaccine virus is not directly responsible for the encephalitis, but may activate a virus lying dormant in the body. This is not so far-fetched as it sounds, for it is known that 80 per cent of normal guinea pigs harbor a virus in the salivary glands, which when injected into the brain produces a fatal encephalitis. Perhaps a more reasonable explanation is that the reaction is an allergic one to the antecedent virus.

Secondary Encephalitis. — Encephalitis may occur not as a primary disease but as a complication of one of the viral fevers. Most often it is a sequel to *measles*. More rarely it follows other virus diseases such as mumps, chicken-pox, and whooping cough. Post-measles encephalomyelitis may be more of a myelitis than an encephalitis. The characteristic symptoms are paraplegia, first flaccid and later spastic, incomplete or dissociated anesthesia, and loss of sphincter control. Fortunately these symptoms are usually only temporary. Encephalitis may complicate *epidemic Asian influenza*. It arises about the fourth to the tenth day after the onset, when the patient seems to be recovering or to have recovered from the initial illness, being characterized by impairment of consciousness, few or no localizing signs, but an extremely abnormal encephalogram, with pronounced delta activity. The disease

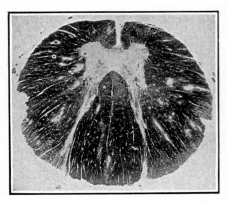

Fig. 662.—Post-vaccinal encephalomyelitis; myelin sheath stain. × 7.

may present as a psychotic outburst, or in some cases as an aseptic meningitis.

Primary Encephalomyelitis.—This disease seems to have become considerably more common in recent years. The prognosis is very much better than in encephalitis lethargica, for recovery is the rule and serious sequelæ are quite uncommon. In adults the clinical picture suggests a myelitis, while in children it is more a meningo-encephalitis. In the cerebral form there are symptoms of meningeal irritation, convulsions, or hemiplegia. Even with marked meningeal symptoms the cerebrospinal fluid is often normal, but the cell count may be increased. The spinal symptoms are pain and paresthesias in the legs, weakness and even temporary paralysis of the legs, with loss of the deep reflexes but a positive Babinski sign. Nystagmus is common, but diplopia, so characteristic of epidemic encephalitis, is very rare and the cranial nerves usually escape.

Lesions.—In all forms of acute disseminated encephalomyelitis the essential lesion is perivascular demyelinization (Fig. 662). The lesions are scattered in patchy form through the gray and white matter of the brain and cord. They are most marked in the pons, medulla, and the lumbar region of the cord, in contrast to the lesions of epidemic encephalitis which are most numerous in the midbrain. The demyelinization is best seen when the tissue is stained with iron hematoxylin or Weigert's myelin stain, the lesions standing out as pale patches on a black background. These lesions are very similar to those of disseminated sclerosis, but the removal of the myelin is extraordinarily rapid. Perivascular inflammatory cells are also present and these cells may form a broad zone outside the adventitia extending for some distance into the brain substance, quite unlike the compact collars of cells seen in epidemic encephalitis. The pale areas may contain many scavenger cells (compound granular corpuscles) derived from the microglia.

Aseptic Meningitis.—Just as acute pyogenic meningitis is not a specific entity but a clinical syndrome caused by various bacteria, so aseptic meningitis is a syndrome caused by a wide variety of viral agents. It is characterized by an acute onset, fever, headache, stiffness of the neck, and a high lymphocytic pleocytosis in the spinal fluid. In North America the principal viruses responsible are those of poliomyelitis, the Coxsackie virus (group B), herpes simplex, mumps, lymphocytic choriomeningitis, and the Echo or orphan group of viruses. The viruses involved seem to change from year to year. The meningitis of poliomyelitis will be considered in the discussion of that disease. Aseptic meningitis is more rarely encountered in infectious hepatitis, cat-scratch disease, measles, varicella and infectious mononucleosis. The condition may be simulated by leptospirosis, tuberculous meningitis and antibiotic-treated purulent meningitis. In Toronto about equal numbers of cases are due to poliomyelitis and Coxsackie group B virus, but perhaps in the majority of cases no virus can be identified (McLeod *et al.*). The technique of inoculating suckling mice with viruses or growing them on a monolayer tissue culture of monkey kidney or human thyroid cells with the production of specific cytopathogenic changes in the tissue cells has made rapid laboratory identification much more possible. Although the various forms are very similar, a few words may be devoted to lymphocytic choriomeningitis, Coxsackie group B infection, mumps and the Echo group.

Lymphocytic Choriomeningitis.—This descriptive term indicates that in man a remarkably high lymphocytosis (mean cell count of 700) in the cerebrospinal fluid is the chief laboratory finding, and that in the experimental animal the inflammatory lesions are in the leptomeninges and the choroid plexus with little evidence of a diffuse encephalitis. The commonly used prefix "benign" indicates that in the human subject the mortality is extremely low, although the rare case of fatal encephalitis has been reported. In the guinea pig, on the other hand, inoculation with cerebrospinal fluid from a human case results in a rapidly fatal illness. The infection occurs spontaneously in mice. While the disease is rare in Canada, there may be localized outbreaks among persons in close contact with infected mice, although the mode of transmission to man is not known. In the experimental animal lesions are present not only in the leptomeninges and choroid plexus, but also in the liver, kidney and adrenal, suggesting that the virus is mesodermotropic rather than neurotropic, thus explaining the usual absence of encephalitis. The fact that neutralizing antibodies have been demonstrated in 10 per cent of normal persons suggests that a subclinical or extraneural infection may not be uncommon.

Coxsackie Group B Meningitis.—In Ontario about 20 per cent of cases of aseptic meningitis are due to this virus (McLeod *et al.*). The Coxsackie virus consists of two groups, A and B. Group A causes herpangina in the animal, while Group B causes epidemic pleurodynia (Bornholm disease) in the animal and aseptic meningitis in man. The virus is pathogenic for the suckling mouse but not for the adult. In the suckling mouse group A produces a characteristic myositis, whilst group B gives rise to lesions of the central nervous system and the viscera. In Toronto about equal numbers of cases of aseptic meningitis were found to be due to the poliomyelitis virus and the Coxsackie group B virus.

ECHO Meningitis.—The so-called Echo group of viruses owes its fanciful name to the fact that members of it may cause enteritis, in tissue culture they produce *c*ytopathogenic changes, they are apparently confined to the *h*uman subject (fecal material of children), and for the most part they are not pathogenic, so that they have been described as orphans in search of a disease.

These four features add up to ECHO. They are also known as the *orphan group* of viruses. Two members of the group, type 6 and 7, are known to cause epidemics of aseptic meningitis in children. Moreover type 9 infection may be associated with a rubella-like rash. The condition is widespread in England and Europe. In the summer of 1956 an extensive outbreak occurred in Toronto, characterized by an abrupt onset, low fever, headache, neck rigidity, a rubelliform maculopapular rash, and muscle pain. The disease is of short duration, with complete recovery in the course of four to six days. The incidence is highest in children under the age of ten years. There is a very marked spinal fluid pleocytosis, sometimes as high as 2000 cells per c.mm. Early in the disease there may be a high neutrophil count. The Echo type 9 virus in the spinal fluid is pathogenic for suckling (not adult) mice, producing a myositis similar to that seen in Coxsackie group A infection in suckling mice.

Acute Anterior Poliomyelitis.—Poliomyelitis or infantile paralysis is an acute infectious disease of the central nervous system which may appear in endemic or in epidemic form. The *age incidence* may vary. In the past it has been a disease of young children, not of infants as the name suggests, adults usually being protected by an acquired immunity the result of a minimal or subclinical infection. In recent times the disease has become commoner among adults, perhaps by reason of children escaping the infection. In isolated populations such as the Eskimos poliomyelitis attacks all ages equally. In crowded primitive areas where hygiene and sanitation are undeveloped the disease is still one of infancy, even young children having already become immunized by the universally prevalent infection.

An epidemic usually begins about the end of June and disappears with the first onset of cold weather. In spite of this clear-cut seasonal incidence which suggests an insect carrier, there is no doubt that the disease is spread by personal contact. The carrier is not a patient, but a healthy person who harbors the virus in his nasopharynx or intestine. When a person develops the disease the virus in the throat at once loses its virulence, so that there is little danger of infection from the patient himself. More than one case seldom develops in a household. An epidemic of poliomyelitis is preceded by a carrier epidemic during which the virulence becomes raised. When this becomes sufficiently high, invasion of the nervous system occurs and a true epidemic begins, lasts a few months, and then rapidly disappears. During an epidemic the incidence of infection with *poliovirus* is much greater than the incidence of the disease.

The *host range* of the viral infection is remarkably restricted, for the usual strain will infect only the monkey and chimpanzee in addition to man. In the chimpanzee the infection produced by the oral route usually remains asymptomatic (subclinical), the animals becoming intestinal carriers.

Virology.—The general features of the virus which causes acute anterior poliomyelitis have already been considered on page 344 in Chapter 13 on virus infections. There we saw that there are three main antigenic types of virus, type I being the chief cause of epidemics, whereas type II is usually responsible for endemic and sporadic cases. The history of our knowledge of the virus is interesting. It was in 1908 that Landsteiner demonstrated conclusively that the disease was due to a virus, but during the next 40 years matters were practically at a standstill until 1949, when Enders, Weller and Robbins succeeded in growing the virus in large quantity on human embryonic tissue and on monkey adult organs. As the virus has a particular preference for the cells of primates, kidney epithelium of the monkey is used. Tell-tale *cytopathogenic changes* can be seen in the epithelial cells in the course of three or four days, while with fluorescent antibody technique (immune globulin labelled with fluorescein) the virus antigen can actually be visualized in the cytoplasm in the incredibly short space of five hours after massive inoculation (Buckley). It was the triumph of tissue culture which made possible the large scale commercial production of polio vaccine. It is now becoming clear that several members of the enterovirus family besides poliovirus can cause mild paralytic poliomyelitis (lower motor neurone paralysis), such, for example as Coxsackie A virus. It is probable that the proportion will increase as the impact of the polio-vaccination program begins to be felt.

In the past various ideas have been advanced as to: (1) the mode of spread of infection from one individual to another, and (2) the means by which the virus reached the central nervous system. These views need not be recapitulated, for there is now general agreement: (1) that man is the principal and perhaps the only reservoir of infection, (2) that intermediate vectors such as insects play no significant role, as was long believed, and (3) that the virus is conveyed in oropharyneal secretions or bowel excreta of healthy carriers rather than from patients suffering from the clinical disease. The infection is primarily one of the alimentary rather than the respiratory tract as we used to believe. The virus is excreted in the stools for several weeks, even though high antibody levels develop in the blood. If infection is from intestinal discharges, there is no more point in avoiding large crowds, or closing moving picture theaters, schools and churches, as has been done in the past, than there would be in the case of typhoid fever. Indeed the same precautions would seem to be desirable in the two diseases.

It used to be thought from experimental work on the monkey that the route by which the virus spreads from the original site of infection to the central nervous system was along the axis cylinders of nerves. While this can occur, serving to explain the spread up and down the cord, it has now been displaced by the concept of *viremia*. Invasion of the blood stream probably develops in every case, only to be quenched as a rule by circulating antibodies. It is only when these are not forthcoming in in sufficient quantity that the central nervous system becomes involved.

The *course of the disease* may be divided into three stages. In the *first or alimentary stage* the virus multiplies in the epithelial cells of the intestinal mucous membrane for about five days. The *second or viremic stage* may then develop, lasting for another five days. This is a period of uneasy truce, the virus trying to invade the central nervous system, but usually being prevented by circulating antibodies. Such cases are examples of silent infection, but any overexertion, fatigue or trauma may tip the balance against the defense. Peripheral injury can set up reactions which are visible under the microscope in the segment of the spinal cord from which the site of the peripheral lesion is innervated, changes which may render the nerve cells vulnerable to the action of a virus already present. For this reason it is not advisable during an active epidemic to subject children to such procedures as tonsillectomy or immunizing intramuscular inoculation. The *third or neural stage*, that of invasion of the gray matter (*polios*, gray) of the spinal cord and brain, may never develop if the immunological barrier in the blood is sufficiently strong. Antibody of low titer in the form of gamma globulin may prevent paralysis for a few weeks if given *before* exposure to the virus. Once invasion of the nervous system has occurred the progress of the virus cannot be influenced in any way. The immunity which follows the disease is life-long, immune bodies can be demonstrated in the blood during the remainder of the patient's life, and a second attack is therefore very rare.

Lesions.—The lesions are always widely distributed throughout the central nervous system, although the symptoms (monoplegia, etc.) may suggest a very limited involvement. The lumbar enlargement of the cord is the most frequent site of lesions, followed by the cervical enlargement. The most marked lesions are in the anterior horn, but the posterior horn is also involved. Although the disease is called a myelitis, the brain is invariably involved in cases that come to autopsy. The severe cerebral lesions are confined to the brain stem (medulla, pons, reticular formation and midbrain), they are slight or absent in the basal ganglia, and practically never found in the cerebral cortex with the exception of the precentral gyrus. Ependymitis in the floor of the fourth ventricle is not infrequent. In addition to the cord lesions there is involvement of the dentate nucleus of the cerebellum, the Gasserian ganglion, posterior root ganglia, and anterior and posterior nerve roots. It is evident that the virus has spread far and wide through the central nervous sys-

74

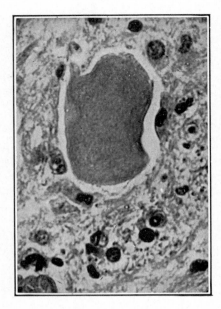

FIG. 663.—A large degenerated ganglion cell in poliomyelitis. The cell has lost its nucleus and its Nissl's granules. × 600.

tem. The lesions are both inflammatory and degenerative. The inflammatory lesions are the result, not the cause, of the degeneration. Sometimes, however, as in the brain stem, inflammation may be much more evident than any demonstrable neuronal degeneration.

The cord is swollen on account of edema, and bulges when cut across. The gray matter may be hyperemic. The meninges are congested and may show slight inflammatory change, but this is seldom marked, thus agreeing with the absence of marked cellular changes in the cerebrospinal fluid. The so-called meningeal symptoms characteristic of the preparalytic stage are apparently not due to meningeal inflammation, as can be shown convincingly in the experimental animal.

The *inflammatory lesions* are best studied in the gray matter of the anterior horn of the spinal cord (anterior poliomyelitis) and in that of the pons and medulla, but the white matter does not escape. There is great congestion and hemorrhages are frequent. The vessels are surrounded by collars of inflammatory cells similar to the perivascular collars in epidemic encephalitis. In addition to the perivascular lesions, diffuse and focal collections of inflammatory cells are present in the interstitial tissue. The focal collections may show necrosis. For the first few days the inflammatory cells are polymorphonuclears. These are then replaced by small round cells which have the appearance of lymphocytes, but when stained with silver they are seen to be microglia. Only the naked nuclei are stained in a hematoxylin and eosin preparation, but the silver brings out all the characteristic processes of the microglia cell. There is an enormous proliferation of microglia at an early stage of the disease; many of the cells lose their processes and become converted into neuronophages (see below). The astrocytes do not proliferate in the acute stage, but form the subsequent scar.

The *degenerative lesions* chiefly affect the *motor cells of the anterior horn* of the spinal cord, although the *cells of the posterior horn*, *Clarke's column*, and the *posterior root ganglia* may also suffer. Every degree of degeneration may be seen, from loss of Nissl's granules (chromatolysis) and eccentricity of the nucleus to complete disappearance of the cell (Fig. 663). Not a single ganglion cell may be seen in the section. The destruction is due to the invasion of the nerve cells by the virus. The process of cell death and disintegration may be incredibly rapid, as can be seen in the experimental animal. This agrees with the suddenness and completeness of the paralysis. The dead cells may be surrounded and invaded by phagocytes, a process known as neuronophagia. Most of the neuronophages are Hortega cells (microglia), but some polymorphonuclears may be seen. Degenerative changes are never marked in the brain, although the inflammatory lesions may be severe. Intranuclear inclusions are present in degenerating nerve cells in the early stage, but not when the cell has become necrotic (Hurst); the material must be fixed in sublimate formol and stained with Giemsa or eosin methylene blue.

The *nerves* show early demyelination and relatively minor changes in the axis cylinders. The lesions in the nerves are less severe and extensive than those in the muscles. It is possible that the virus may act directly on the nerves and even on the muscles (Denst and Neubuerger).

It would appear from the important work of Carey and his associates that one of the earliest changes is in the *motor end plates* when stained by the gold method, particularly in the respiratory muscles such as the diaphragm and intercostals. This change varies from a granular degeneration to complete dissolution. In the intercostal muscles of a girl, aged three, who died within thirty-six hours of the onset of symptoms, there was complete absence of motor end plates in 5978 denuded axons among 6109 that were counted. The motor axons degenerate, and it is important to note that the spread is centripetal, not centrifugal as when a motor nerve is severed. All this suggests that the virus may attack the nerve endings independently of the attack on the motor cells in the spinal cord.

The *end result*, seen when the cord is examined long after the acute illness, is atrophy of the anterior horn on one or both sides. The nerve cells are replaced by astrocytes, and there is well-marked gliosis and fibrillar formation. The motor fibers arising from the destroyed cells disappear, as can be seen in sections stained with Weigert's myelin sheath stain. The paralyzed muscles show atrophy, fatty infiltration, and replacement by connective tissue.

Lesions in other organs have been described, but it is difficult to know if they are related to the virus of poliomyelitis. *Myocardial lesions* are not uncommon (Saphir and Wile). These consist of perivascular infiltrations of polymorphonuclears and lymphocytes, together with loss of striations and nuclear degeneration in the muscle fibers. Both the cardiac lesions and the electrocardiographic changes which accompany them are strikingly similar to those found in potassium deficiency. It is possible that some of these lesions may be caused by one of the Coxsackie viruses, which may give a clinical picture resembling that of poliomyelitis.

Relation of Symptoms to Lesions.—Five main clinical varieties of response to infection by the virus are possible. (1) *Infection without symptoms* owing to the abundant formation of antibodies. This is the commonest occurrence, with infection being confined to the alimentary canal. Such persons are carriers. (2) *Abortive form*, in which there is no evidence of invasion of the nervous system, but merely symptoms of a general infection such as fever, malaise, headache, nausea, constipation or sore throat. This is the commonest form of the clinical disease. (3) *Non-paralytic form*, in which to the above signs and symptoms are added stiffness and pain in the back and neck caused by an aseptic meningitis. Recovery is rapid and complete. The diagnosis in this stage depends on a healthy clinical suspicion and lumbar puncture. It is evident that none of these varieties really deserve to be called poliomyelitis, because the gray matter of the cord is not inflamed. (4) *Paralytic poliomyelitis*, this being the classic form of the disease. When paralysis develops, usually on the second or third day, it attains its maximum at once, and as a rule shows no subsequent extension. This may be attributed to the rapid development of immunity. Only one arm or leg may be involved, or both legs (paraplegia). In addition to motor weakness, pain is a constant symptom. This is usually pain on passive movement, but there may be spontaneous pain in a limb. (5) *Bulbar poliomyelitis*, the most fatal form, is marked by such bulbar symptoms as facial paralysis, difficulty in swallowing, and failure of the respiratory and vasomotor centers. In this type there may be no spinal symptoms. In the fatal cases there is often a marked rise of blood pressure.

There is little or no opportunity for autopsy examination in the preparalytic stage, but observations on the experimental animal suggest that the so-called *meningeal irritation* (stiffness of the neck, irritability) is not due to inflammatory changes in the meninges, in spite of the fact that the cell count in the spinal fluid is highest at this stage. The initial *"systemic"* symptoms, such as fever, drowsiness, anxiety, heightened sensibility to pain, headache, and vomiting, may be explained by involvement of the thalamus and hypothalamus. The *pain* is probably due to lesions in the posterior root ganglia and in the posterior roots themselves. The *paralysis* is easily explained by the destruction of the motor cells in the anterior horn. Groups of motor cells may be picked out while neighboring groups are spared, and the lesions may be much more marked in the anterior horn on one side or may be confined to that side. This serves to explain the fact that the paralysis may be confined to one limb or even to one muscle or group of muscles. The virus appears to spread up and down the cord rather than across it, probably along the axis cylinders. Facial nerve palsy and paralysis of other cranial nerves are due to lesions in the brain stem. Difficulty in swallowing with regurgitation of fluids through the nose (paralysis of the palate), respiratory failure (to which death is usually due), and other signs of *bulbar paralysis* are caused by lesions in the medulla The *increased blood pressure* is due to bilateral nerve cell degeneration in the reticular formation of the medulla in an area corresponding with the upper half of the fourth ventricle (Löblick).

The *cerebrospinal fluid* in the paralytic form shows a moderate pleocytosis of not more than 200 to 300 lymphocytes per c. mm. The protein is normal or slightly elevated at first, rising later, as the cell count falls, to 300 mg. per 100 cc. In the non-paralytic form or the pre-paralytic stage the cell count is much higher, with polymorphonuclears predominating. When paralysis develops the cell count begins to drop and become lymphocytic. The spinal fluid of tuberculous meningitis can be distinguished from that of poliomyelitis by the presence of a fibrin web, the decrease of sugar and particularly of chlorides, and the much greater increase of protein, as well as the occasional finding of tubercle bacilli.

Prevention by Vaccine.—Effective immunization against the virus (all three types) for a time at least can be effected by means of two different forms of vaccine both made from tissue culture. (1) *Killed-virus vaccine* (formalinized), associated particularly with the name of Salk, given as three intramuscular injections, the first two one month apart and the third after three or six months. The vaccine produces a marked reduction in the oro-pharyngeal viral infection, but not on the discharge of natural virus in the feces. Antibody formation is stimulated after the second or third injections, but inoculations are not desirable in the midst of an epidemic for reasons already indicated. The immunity produced is limited in time. The killed-virus vaccine prevents paralytic poliomyelitis, but not poliomyelitis infection. (2) *Live* but *attenuated virus vaccine*, associated with the name of Sabin, is administered orally, can be given in the middle of an epidemic, and appears to give a lasting protection, although time alone will tell. The live virus vaccine, which is the younger brother of the killed virus vaccine, has the advantage that it spreads widely from the bowel of vaccinated to unvaccinated children, and thus establishes widespread protection. Several millions of children have received this vaccine, more particularly in the U.S.S.R., Czechoslovakia, and Mexico. We have already seen that gamma globulin can protect against paralysis for a few weeks.

Coxsackie Virus Infection.—The Coxsackie group of viruses, named for the village on the Hudson River in New York State where the virus was first isolated by Dalldorf in 1947 from a patient with paralytic poliomyelitis, belongs to the much larger group of *enteroviruses* which occur in the feces of infected persons. The other genera in the family are the 3 poliomyelitis viruses and the 20 ECHO viruses. There are 30 distinct types, but these fall into 2 groups, known as A and B. The main biological character of the virus is that it is pathogenic only for suckling mice and hamsters in whom immunity has not yet developed, not for older animals of these species nor for monkeys, thus differing sharply from the virus of poliomyelitis. For this reason it has been called the *suckling mouse virus*. This virus and other close antigenic relatives have been iso'ated from the stools and nasopharyngeal secretions of patients with signs of meningeal irritation and diagnosed as non-paralytic poliomyelitis and aseptic meningitis. The virus is widely distributed in the United States, and Rhodes and his associates have isolated both Coxsackie and poliomyelitis viruses from children and adult contacts in Toronto.

Group A viruses in suckling mice produce severe, widespread myositis, while in the human subject they may cause herpangina and three-day fever. *Herpangina* most often affects children, and is characterized by headache, fever, sore throat, and shallow herpetiform ulcers of the fauces, soft palate and pharynx. *Three-day fever* is the similar condition without ulcers, but with myalgia of the back and limbs.

Group B infection is responsible for aseptic meningitis and Bornholm disease. These conditions have already been referred to on page 1167. *Bornholm disease* is so-called by reason of an extensive epidemic on that island. It is also called *epidemic pleurodynia* myalgia. The first symptom is an alarmingly sudden attack of pain in the chest which can be excruciating, is exaggerated by movement, and may last a number of days. Abdominal pain may be confused with that of acute appendicitis, and sometimes there is pain in a shoulder or extremity. *Aseptic meningitis* is a frequent complication, or it may occur more frequently as a primary condition, the diagnosis being confirmed by the isolation of the virus from the cerebrospinal fluid. *Myocarditis* has been reported in the new-born infants of infected mothers. It will be recalled that myocarditis is a rather frequent complication of poliomyelitis.

Herpes.—Herpes is a disease caused by one of the filter-passing viruses. It is characterized by the formation of small vesicles. There are two distinct forms: (1) herpes zoster or shingles in which the vesicles follow the distribution of a sensory nerve, and (2) herpes simplex in which there is no such distribution. An attack of the former is followed by lasting immunity, but in the case of the latter there is no immunity. They are caused by entirely different viruses.

Herpes Zoster.—This is an inflammatory condition of the posterior root ganglia or the Gasserian ganglion, known to the public as *shingles*. It is the sensory analogue of poliomyelitis: the type of lesions in the nervous system and the condition of the cerebrospinal fluid is the same in the two diseases. Usually only one ganglion is involved, most often in the dorsal region. The eruption is always unilateral, running in a zone (zoster) as far as the middle line, and is preceded by neuralgic pains, which in old people may be very persistent and severe. The vesicles begin as papules, and

may leave some scarring. The *lesions* in the ganglia are similar to those in the anterior horn in poliomyelitis, *i.e.*, congestion, hemorrhage, perivascular collections of lymphocytes, and degeneration of ganglion cells with neuronophagia. There is Wallerian degeneration of the nerve fibers in the posterior roots, in the peripheral nerves, and in the posterior columns.

Intranuclear inclusions have been found not only in the dorsal root ganglia and sympathetic ganglia, but also in the esophageal mucosa, the myenteric plexus of the stomach, and in the cells in necrotic focal lesions in the pancreas, adrenal and ovary (Cheatham). It would appear that the distribution of the virus may be widespread and that it enters the body by the sympathetic nerves of the respiratory and gastrointestinal tracts, migrates to the dorsal root ganglia, and reaches the skin by centrifugal spread along the peripheral nerves. *The visceral and cutaneous lesions resemble those of varicella (chicken pox)*, and *it is probable that the viruses of the two diseases are identical*, the varicella lesions resulting from hematogenous spread in a non-immune person, while those of zoster result from neurogenous spread in a person with humoral immunity. Zoster or shingles seems to be due to the reactivation of a latent chicken pox virus. But there remains the problem: Where has the latent virus been hiding, and what allows the chicken pox virus to escape?

Herpes Simplex.—This is the common form of herpes which may complicate pneumonia and other fevers (herpes febrilis). It usually occurs on the lips (herpes labialis), but may be on the cornea or external genitals. It differs from herpes zoster in being recurrent, not following the line of nerves, and causing no change in the cerebrospinal fluid. When the virus of herpes simplex is inoculated into the cornea of a rabbit it sets up a fatal encephalitis. In rare instances it may cause a similar condition in man. In whichever part of the body the virus is inoculated, it passes along the axis cylinders until it reaches the central nervous system, where its presence can be detected by the appearance of the Lipschütz bodies which have already been described in Chapter 13. These bodies are found in the epithelial cells at the site of inoculation (skin, cornea), as well as in the nerve cells. The lesion in man is inflammation of a sensory nerve ganglion.

Rabies.—Rabies or hydrophobia is an excellent example of a disease caused by a *neurotropic virus*, which is transmitted to man by the bite of a rabid animal, usually a dog, sometimes a wolf. The vampire bat in South America in the vicinity of Trinidad can convey the infection both to cattle and man by its bite. The virus is excreted by the parotid and other salivary glands, so that the saliva of the animal is the source of infection. The general behavior of the virus has already been considered on page 345, but a few points may be recapitulated here. The *principal symptoms* are spasm of the muscles of deglutition and generalized convulsions. The patient is unable to swallow even water, the mere sight of which may precipitate violent spasms. This, of course, is the origin of the word *hydrophobia* (fear of water), an origin which is lost in the mists of antiquity. The disease, once developed, is believed to be uniformly fatal, although it can be prevented with astonishing success. The virus does not reach the central nervous system by the blood stream, as is the case with poliomyelitis, but along the axis cylinders of the afferent nerves from the point of inoculation. It is rather humbling to our pride to learn that Morgagni came to this conclusion in 1769 purely from clinical observation, a concept which was confirmed for snake venom in the experimental animal in 1781. The *incubation period* varies widely between two and sixteen weeks, with an average of about twelve weeks. It has long been believed that the length of the incubation period is governed by the distance of the bite from the central nervous system. The validity of this belief has now rather been called in question.

The *lesions* are entirely microscopic, consisting of cell degeneration, phagocytosis of the degenerating cells, and perivascular collections of lymphocytes and plasma cells. The worst lesions are those in the posterior horn of the spinal cord (compare with the lesions of poliomyelitis) and the posterior root ganglia. The pathognomonic feature is the presence of acidophilic *Negri bodies*

with a blue center in the cytoplasm of the ganglion cells of the hippocampus major, as well as the cells of the medulla and cerebellum. In a suspected case the dog is sacrificed and the hippocampus examined for Negri bodies.

It is quite amazing that the *method of prevention* used at the present day is that introduced by Pasteur who was naturally ignorant of the nature of the infection, and that the strain of virus used is Pasteur's "fixed virus," which has been maintained in rabbits since 1882. The success of the preventive treatment will depend on how soon the diagnosis is made before the symptoms appear. Unfortunately the vaccine consists of foreign (rabbit) brain material containing the virus, and occasionally this may sensitize the person and produce an allergic encephalomyelitis as the result of an antigen-antibody reaction, the antibodies being produced against nerve tissue products. This matter is discussed again on page 1182.

LOUPING ILL.—Although this is a virus disease of sheep, it may be considered here because of the interest of its lesions. As the Scotch name indicates, it is characterized by progressive incoördination and cerebellar ataxia. The disease can be reproduced both in the mouse and monkey. In the monkey there is a diffuse encephalomyelitis, but the principal lesion is a massive destruction and astonishing disappearance of the Purkinje cells of the cerebellum. The virus has the same strange selective action on these cells as the virus of poliomyelitis has on the motor cells of the anterior horn of the spinal cord. Laboratory workers in contact with the virus are said to have developed mild infections.

NON-VIRAL TYPES OF ENCEPHALITIS

Lead Encephalitis.—In the chronic lead poisoning of children (see Chapter 19), one of the most dreaded complications is lead encephalitis. This differs from other varieties of encephalitis in that it takes the form of an extreme cerebral edema caused by the presence of lead in the brain. A similar condition can be produced experimentally in animals by the continued administration of small quantities of lead. The brain is remarkably swollen, the cerebral convolutions are flattened, the ventricles are compressed, and the medulla is pressed down into the spinal canal. The cerebrospinal fluid pressure may be 700 mm. of water as compared with the normal pressure of 120 mm.

Drug Encephalitis.—It has long been known that a hemorrhagic encephalitis may follow the use of arsphenamine compounds and the sulfonamide group in hypersentivie individuals. It would now appear that a similar form of encephalopathy may develop in the course of long-continued treatment with streptomycin and para-aminosalicylic acid (Cavanagh). The lesions take the form of areas of anemic necrosis in the cortex and subjacent white matter, with an intense microglial reaction and large numbers of foam cells filled with lipid. The basic vascular lesions are proliferation of the capillary endothelium, hyaline thrombi plugging these vessels, and ring hemorrhages. Similar lesions are seen in the arsphenamine and sulfonamide cases. It is probable that the attack falls on the hypersensitive vascular endothelium.

Cerebral Toxoplasmosis.—Although this condition is caused by a protozoön parasite, Toxoplasma (page 360), it may be considered here. The infection occurs mainly in the newborn and young children (intra-uterine infection), but occasionally in adults. In the newborn the protozoa probably come from the mother who has a smouldering low-grade infection. At a later age it seems likely that the source of infection is an eye affected by toxoplasmosis. In children the clinical picture is that of encephalitis, but in adults, in spite of the presence of focal necrotic lesions in the brain, there are usually no cerebral symptoms. The lesions in the main are areas of granulomatous inflammation with the parasites within nerve cells (Fig. 664), foci of softening, and gritty patches and streaks. The most remarkable feature, both in children and adults, is the presence of calcification which may be extreme in degree and visible radiologically.

MYELITIS

Acute inflammation of the spinal cord is rather rare. It may be *traumatic*, due to injury of the spine, or *infective*, due to septic

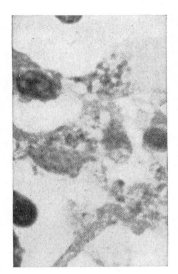

Fig. 664.—Cerebral toxoplasmosis: parasites within nerve cells.

embolism, to the infective fevers, or to syphilis. The *syphilitic* form is discussed in connection with syphilis of the nervous system. There is usually complete paralysis below the site of the lesion. This is usually in the lumbar region, so that the legs show a flaccid lower motor neurone paralysis with loss of deep reflexes and loss of sphincter control. There may be anesthesia below the lesion and hyperesthesia at the level of the lesion. If the lesion is in the cervical region both arms and legs will be paralyzed, but while the arms show a lower motor neurone paralysis, the legs develop an upper motor neurone type of paralysis, as the lower neurones remain intact.

Lesions.—The inflammation is usually confined to one or at the most a few segments of the cord; this is called *transverse myelitis*, because the entire thickness of the cord is involved. Occasionally the inflammation may be diffused throughout the cord; this is *disseminated myelitis*. The affected part is soft and flattened, the distinction between gray and white matter is lost, and liquefaction may occur. *Microscopically* there is great destruction of nerve cells and nerve fibers, of gray and white matter. Among the débris are large numbers of scavenger cells derived from the microglia. Perivascular collections of inflammatory cells are present in the surrounding tissue. The degeneration of the nerve fibers can be demonstrated in early cases by Marchi's method and in old cases by the Weigert myelin sheath stain.

SYPHILIS OF THE NERVOUS SYSTEM

Syphilis of the nervous system used to be a matter of the greatest importance and much space was devoted to it in these pages. Chemotherapy has changed the picture completely, and the account of the pathological changes has been correspondingly curtailed. The lesions may take four forms: gumma, meningoencephalitis, tabes dorsalis and general paresis.

Gumma.—A gumma is a firm gray mass usually arising from the meninges and extending into the brain, producing the clinical picture of a cerebral tumor. It is almost never seen now.

Syphilitic Meningoencephalitis.—This is a diffuse inflammation of the meninges extending into the brain. It is most marked at the base of the brain, and involves the cranial nerves, particularly the third, fourth and sixth, with accompanying ptosis, strabismus and diplopia. The perivascular sheaths are also filled with a similar exudate, and it is these which constitute the encephalitis. *Syphilitic myelitis* is a much more distinct entity than syphilitic encephalitis, and is indeed the commonest form of myelitis. It is of the transverse type, limited to a few segments. Thrombosis of the diseased vessels is probably a major etiological factor, as a result of which there is softening of the cord and marked destruction of nerve cells and fibers. *Syphilitic arteritis* is a marked feature of all the lesions. The adventitia is infiltrated with round cells and the intima is uniformly thickened. The result of this endarteritis obliterans is to produce great narrowing or actual closure of the lumen, which leads naturally to thrombosis. Aneurysm formation is not a result of cerebral syphilis, for the diffuse thickening does not weaken the vessel as do the patchy lesions of syphilitic aortitis. There may be a gummatous process around the vessel, a gummatous arteritis.

Cerebrospinal Fluid.—In acute syphilitic meningitis the reaction is severe and there is often a lymphocytosis of 500 or more. This high cell count is very suggestive of syphilitic meningitis. The protein content is high, the Wassermann reaction is positive, and the colloidal gold curve may be of the paretic or mid-zone types. A gumma causes much slighter changes; the Wassermann and colloidal gold reactions are weak or negative, and the lymphocytosis and protein increase are slight. If the lesions are chiefly vascular, the fluid may be practically normal.

Tabes Dorsalis.—Tabes dorsalis or locomotor ataxia is a syphilitic disease of the cord, a late manifestation usually coming on from ten to fifteen years after the primary infection, although the interval may occasionally be as short as two years. The indirect evidence that the disease is syphilitic is conclusive, but treponema pallidum has very seldom indeed been found in the cord, nerve roots or ganglia, and the lesions bear no resemblance to the ordinary changes produced by syphilis.

Lesions.—The true tabetic lesion is a degeneration and disappearance of the posterior columns of the cord and their replacement by neuroglial tissue. This lesion can be recognized with the naked eye. The pia over the dorsal columns is thickened and adherent. The surface of these columns is no longer convex, but flattened or concave, and on the cut surface they are gray and translucent so that they stand out clearly from the rest of the white matter. It is the wasting of the dorsal columns which gives the disease its name (*tabes*, wasting). The posterior nerve roots are atrophied and shrivelled in comparison with the plump anterior roots, but this distinction is not so easy to recognize.

The *microscopic change* is seen in sections stained with Weigert's myelin sheath stain or the simpler iron hematoxylin. The normal white matter is stained black, but the degenerated posterior columns remain unstained (Fig. 665). The lesions are usually most marked in the lumbar region, but in the so-called cervical tabes they are confined to the cervical region. The first change is a demyelinization, and droplets of myelin can be demonstrated by the Marchi method or Scharlach R. The axis cylinders

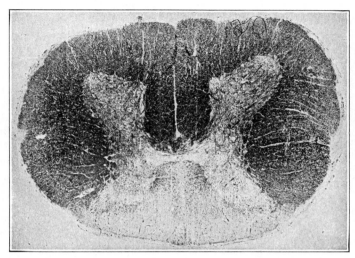

FIG. 665.—Tabes dorsalis: degeneration of posterior columns. (Weigert's myelin sheath stain.)

become disintegrated, and in time the whole of the medullary sheath disappears. There is proliferation of astrocytes and a replacement gliosis. Similar changes are seen in the posterior nerve roots and in the optic nerve.

Relation of Symptoms to Lesions.—Sensory disturbances include paresthesias, pain, and loss of muscle and vibration sense. The patient feels as if he were walking on something soft like cotton wool. "Lightning pains" of extreme severity shoot down the legs. The first effect of the lesion seems to be to set up violent impulses in the pain sensibility fibers and in the posterior nerve roots. There is also objective disturbance of pain sensibility in the shape of analgesia of the back and legs, so that the pain of lumbar puncture is not felt. The pain fibers end at once in the posterior horn of gray matter, and the second relay of fibers does not pass up in the posterior columns, from which it is evident that the interference must be in the posterior roots, not in the spinal cord. There is loss of muscle sense or sense of position, so that when the eyes are shut the position of the foot is unknown, and the patient sways when standing (Rombergism). The vibration sense is lost, so that he cannot feel the vibration of a tuning-fork placed on the shin. As both muscle sense and vibration sense impulses pass up in the posterior columns, it is natural that they should be lost.

Incoordination is due to interference with the muscle sense. As the patient is not sure of the position of his feet, he walks unsteadily and with a wide base (locomotor ataxia), lifting his feet high and throwing them down forcibly (stamping gait). *Loss of deep reflexes* in the legs is due to interference with the short fibers which anastomose directly around the cells of the anterior horn. The reflex arc is thus broken and the deep reflexes lost. The knee-jerk depends on the integrity of the third and fourth lumbar segments, and the Achilles jerk on the fifth lumbar and first sacral. In very low lesions the knee-jerk is preserved but the Achilles jerk is lost. The *light reflex* in the pupil is commonly lost, though contraction on accommodation is retained (Argyll-Robertson pupil). The nerve center for the pupillary reflex is the oculomotor nucleus in the midbrain, but the lesion is in the subependymal region of the aqueduct of Sylvius. In *optic atrophy* the optic nerve shows the same kind of lesion as the posterior nerve roots, but the way in which the lesion is produced is uncertain. The *visceral crises* are severe paroxysms of pain referred to various viscera (gastric, laryngeal, etc.). The cause is not known. The *trophic disturbances* are the most difficult to explain. The best known

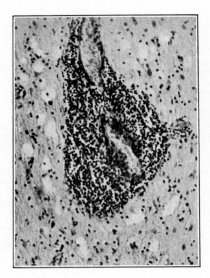

Fig. 666.—Perivascular cuffing in general paresis. × 85.

are *Charcot's joint* (a painless disorganization of one of the large joints), and the painless perforating ulcer of the foot. Possibly the analgesia which allows the parts to be severely traumatized may be more responsible than any loss of trophic nerve impulses.

Cerebrospinal Fluid.—There is lymphocytosis of from 10 to 50 per c.mm. In tabetic crises, possibly attended by meningeal irritation, there may be hundreds of cells with many polymorphonuclears. The protein is slightly increased. The colloidal gold curve is of the luetic type. The Wassermann reaction is positive in about 70 per cent of cases. In an old case of many years' duration the fluid may be practically normal.

General Paresis.—This disease, also known as general paralysis of the insane and dementia paralytica, is the most fearful of all the results of syphilitic infection. The lesions are the direct result of the action of the treponemata, for the latter can be demonstrated in the cerebral cortex. The symptoms appear from ten to fifteen years after the primary infection. Similarly the juvenile form due to congenital syphilis appears about the age of ten years. Fortunately antibiotic therapy has completely changed the outlook. What follows applies only to the untreated case.

Lesions.—The skull cap is thick, and there may be subdural hemorrhage with the formation of a thick membrane (pachymeningitis hæmorrhagica). The brain is small, with marked atrophy in the fronto-parietal region. The convolutions are wasted, the sulci widened, and there is a great compensatory excess of cerebrospinal fluid. The pia is thickened and adherent over the frontal lobe, so that when it is stripped off there is tearing or "decortication" of the surface. The lateral ventricles show a compensatory dilatation. The floor of the fourth ventricle is finely granular, giving it a frosted appearance, and the lateral ventricles may show the same condition to a lesser degree.

The *microscopic picture* is a mixture of syphilitic inflammation and tissue downfall. The meninges are densely infiltrated with lymphocytes and plasma cells. (1) The *inflammatory lesions*, which are most marked in the cerebral cortex and the floor of the fourth ventricle, consist of dense perivascular collections of lymphocytes and plasma cells, the latter being especially numerous and characteristic (Fig. 666). These lesions are found throughout the entire thickness of the cortex. There may also be a diffuse infiltration of inflammatory cells. These lesions are to be attributed to the irritation produced by the treponemata.

(2) The *degenerative lesions* are quite as marked, but they are more difficult to recognize unless one happens to be an expert neuropathologist. The general architecture of the cortex is completely lost, and the different layers can no longer be made out. There is great outfall of cells, especially in the frontal and parietal regions. Most of the pyramidal cells may have disappeared. Those which remain show every degree of degeneration.

(3) *Neuroglial proliferation* is marked, especially in the superficial layer of the cortex and in the walls and floor of the ventricles. The astrocytes multiply and form a dense feltwork of fibers (Fig. 667). These are responsible for the pial adhesions and the decortication. In the floor of the fourth ventricle the glial proliferation causes an irregular heaping up of the floor (Fig. 668). This is the cause of the granularity already described. The granulations are covered by

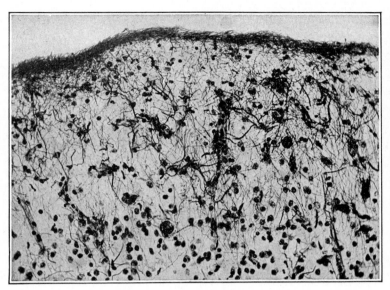

Fig. 667.—Cortical gliosis in general paresis. (Victoria blue.) × 150.
(Boyd, *Pathology for the Physician.*)

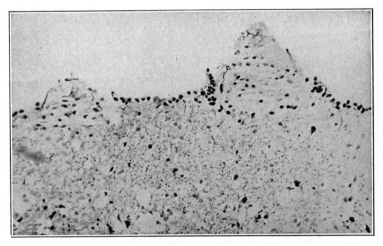

Fig. 668.—Granular floor of fourth ventricle in general paresis. The ependyma is desquamated from the mounds of neuroglia. × 175.

ependyma, but some of the summits may be bare. The microglia also proliferates (Fig. 669), giving rise to large numbers of "rod cells" (Fig. 670), which form an intermediary stage between the microglial cell and the compound granular corpuscle. In sections of the cerebral and cerebellar cortex and of the basal ganglia the Prussian blue reaction shows iron-containing pigment in the cyto-plasm of these cells and in perivascular spaces. The combination of the prolifera-tion of "rod cells" and the presence of iron pigment in their cytoplasm is pathognomonic of general paresis.

Relation of Symptoms to Lesions.—The name dementia paralytica describes the disease fairly well, because there is a general motor weakness, and if left to itself the con-

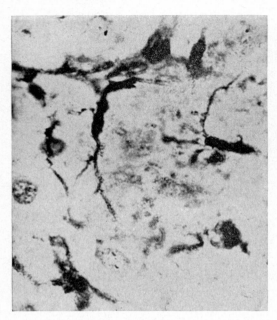

Fig. 669.—Hypertrophy and coarsening of microglial cells in cerebral cortex in general paresis. Silver impregnation. × 600. (Kindness of Dr. Mary Tom.)

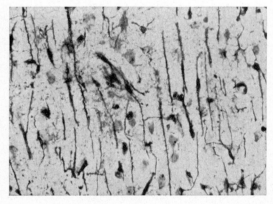

Fig. 670.—Rod cells formed from microglia in general paresis. Silver impregnation. × 200. (Kindness of Dr. Mary Tom.)

dition progresses remorselessly to complete dementia. The mental disorder first affects the faculties of judgment, reason, self-control and there is an accompanying loss of moral sense. As Oppenheim says, the work of deterioration begins first in the higher life of the mind and soul. As the dementia increases, the mental structure crumbles to the ground. Delusions of grandeur lead to a remarkable euphoria which contrasts strangely with the sad reality. The last stage is one of complete dementia. Tremors of the face, lips, and tongue are common. The speech is thick and characteristically slurring. The pupillary reflex is of the Argyll-Robertson type, with loss of reaction to light, but not to accommodation. Peculiar epileptiform or apoplectiform seizures ("paralytic seizures") may occur in which loss of consciousness may be followed by transient monoplegia or hemiplegia. Weakness of the muscles (paresis) is a constant feature of the disease, but never absolute paralysis.

Cerebrospinal Fluid.—The cells number from 30 to 100, and polymorphonuclears are often present, especially during convulsive seizures. The protein is increased. The Wassermann reaction is positive and intense in from 96 to 100 per cent of untreated cases. The colloidal gold reaction gives a paretic curve.

FUNGUS INFECTIONS

The brain and meninges are occasionally invaded by a variety of fungi. Unfortunately these infections are very resistant to any form of therapy at present available, so that the diseases which they cause are usually fatal.

Cryptococcosis.—This uncommon condition is caused by a yeast known as Cryptococcus neoformans or Torula histolytica (Fig. 669). It belongs to the group Blastomycetes. The resulting disease therefore also goes by the names of *torulosis* and European blastomycosis, in contrast to the North American and South American varieties of blastomycosis which rarely invade the central nervous system. The cerebral lesion is a meningo-encephalitis, and the infection is secondary to a lesion in the lung or elsewhere. The lesions may resemble those of tuberculosis, consisting of lymphocytes, epithelioid cells and giant cells, but the characteristic feature is the presence of large numbers of yeast-like cells, which are also present in the spinal fluid, from which they can be readily cultured. A curious feature is the presence of numerous cysts containing the organisms in the superficial layers of the cortex. These cysts are usually

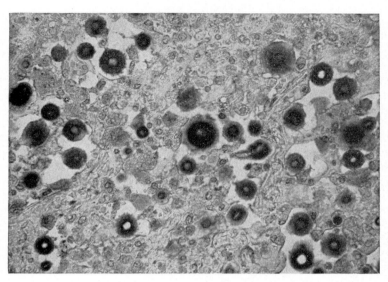

Fig. 671.—Cryptococcosis neoformans. The thick capsules of the organisms have been preserved by mounting in glycerin-jelly, omitting dehydration. Alcian blue stain. (Kindness of Dr. R. W. Mowry.)

microscopic in size, but they may be large enough to be seen with the naked eye. The clinical picture simulates that of tuberculous meningitis, but it is more chronic in character.

Mucormycosis.—This appears to be a new disease (Baker). The first report of the cerebral form appeared in 1943, the pulmonary form in 1948. Cases have now been observed in all parts of the United States, Canada and England, and the disease is probably world-wide. It is caused by certain fungi, especially Rhizopus, that are common contaminants of laboratory cultures and are not ordinarily pathogenic. The increasing frequency of the disease is probably due to the use of antibiotics, which reduce the number of bacterial infections but permit fungus invasion. Cortisone, ACTH, and antileukemic drugs also favor the development of the mycosis, as do diabetes and leukemia.

The fungus enters the nose and leads to sinusitis, orbital cellulitis and meningo-encephalitis. It grows rapidly, and is characterized by broad, branching, non-septate hyphæ known as rhizoids. A unique feature of the infection is a great affinity for arteries, the fungus penetrating the tough muscular walls and growing in the lumen, where it incites thrombosis with resulting infarction. There is thrombosis of the ophthalmic and internal carotid arteries, with cerebral softening. The organisms extend deeply into the brain, producing a mycotic encephalitis. The patients have been of all ages, from six months to sixty-five years. The duration of the fatal illness may be as short as one day, an astonishing fact considering that the infecting agent used to be regarded as nonpathogenic.

Other fungi may invade the central nervous system, usually from the lung. Of these infections only *coccidioidomycosis* and *histoplasmosis* need be mentioned. Both produce granulomatous lesions resembling those of tuberculosis. There is a chronic basilar meningitis, which may be associated with cerebral abscesses. Coccidioidomycosis is much more often encountered than histoplasmosis. The general characteristics of these fungi have already been considered in Chapter 12.

DEMYELINATING DISEASES

In our discussion so far we have found it convenient and not too difficult to classify the disorders of the central nervous system and collect them in groups for study. Such, for instance, are the cerebral ischemias due to vascular occlusion, viral and fungal infections, bacterial infections of the meninges, and, presently to be considered, benign and malignant neoplasms. Unfortunately there remains a large and heterogeneous collection of conditions of unknown etiology, which defy satisfactory classification and are referred to vaguely as degenerative diseases of the nervous system. From this large collection it seems justifiable to separate off at least two groups which we may refer to as the demyelinating and the metabolic diseases. This still leaves a large group which we must call degenerative, or in some cases nutritional.

On page 1124 we have already considered some of the general characteristics of the myelin sheath of nerve fibers both in the central nervous system and in the peripheral nerves, its peculiar ring-like structure as seen with the electron microscope, its chemical composition, and the staining methods by which it can be studied. When a peripheral nerve is cut, the myelin of the distal portion undergoes Wallerian degeneration. In pernicious anemia there may be subacute combined degneration of the spinal cord. A *true* demyelinating disease, as Adams and Kubik point out in their fine analysis of the subject, is characterized by (1) destruction of the myelin sheaths; (2) relative sparing of axis cylinders, as well as other elements such as nerve cells and neuroglia; (3) perivascular and subpial infiltrations of lymphocytes and plasma cells which are not secondary to the myelin degeneration. To these may be added the following (Adams): (4) conversion of the degenerating myelin into sudanophilic cholesterol esters and fats; (5) extreme hyperplasia of astrocytes; (6) multiple foci varying extremely in size; (7) absence of pathological changes in other organs. The combination of these qualities is remarkable and suggestive.

By far the most important member of the demyelinating group is *multiple sclerosis*, with which may be included *Schilder's encephalitis periaxialis diffusa*, a rare disease. To these must be added the acute conditions known as the *leukoencephalopathies*, namely acute disseminated encephalomyelitis and acute necrotizing hemorrhagic leukoencephalitis, these forbidding names being merely a description of the distribution and type of the lesions.

Pathogenesis.—Although the etiology of the human demyelinating diseases is unknown, we may allow ourselves some speculation about their nature and the mode of their production. The lesions which most closely resemble them are those of experimental encephalomyelitis in animals produced by the intracerebral injection of brain or spinal cord material in conjunction with Freund's adjuvant (a water-in-oil emulsion of killed mycobacteria). The attachment of central nervous system material to the foreign protein of the adjuvant seems to create a new antigen which is foreign to and therefore unrecognized by the body with a resulting delayed type of allergic reaction. The most striking feature of this seemingly *allergic encephalomyelitis* is demyelination. Typical allergic lesions can be produced many weeks after remission of an acute attack simply by means of electrolysis of the cerebral cortex, showing that the potentiality for relapse is constantly present (Bogdanove and Clark). This is of particular interest in view of the exacerbations and remissions which are such a baffling feature of human multiple sclerosis.

In human disease a similar combination of demyelination and inflammatory reaction is seen in the encephalomyelitis which on rare occasions follows vaccination against rabies and smallpox, and which sometimes complicates measles, chickenpox and smallpox after an interval of a few days. In addition to the fact that these are virus diseases it should be noted that the rabies vaccine contains central nervous system material, so that the reaction may with every justification be regarded as allergic in character. The resulting *lesions* are similar to those of the acute leukoencephalopathies, by virtue of their tiny or even microscopic size, their wide dissemination, their perivenous demyelination, and the infiltration of these areas and of the meninges with lymphocytes and plasma cells. It is true that these lesions do not resemble those of chronic multiple sclerosis or Schilder's disease, but we have a connecting link in the form of acute multiple sclerosis, which is marked by an acute onset, a succession of outbreaks, and lesions that are macroscopic in size like those of chronic multiple sclerosis, together with perivenous demyelination and lymphocytic infiltration as well as infiltration of the meninges. These lesions may be identical with those of post-rabies inoculation encephalomyelitis, which we may with confidence ascribe to an allergic reaction to the breakdown products of myelin similar in nature to the Arthus reaction.

It would appear then that at the present time an allergic process is the best working hypothesis for the baffling human demyelinating diseases as defined above, at least for the acute forms. Occasional intermediate or mixed cases are suggestive that the chronic forms should also be included. We still await isolation of the antigenic substances responsible, as well as the etiological factor or factors which trigger the mechanism.

Multiple Sclerosis.—This condition, also known as *disseminated* or *insular sclerosis,* is a chronic disease of the nervous system, characterized by curious remissions and relapses, and by the presence of multiple patches of sclerosis scattered diffusely throughout the gray and white matter of the brain and spinal cord. It is now one of the commoner diseases of the nervous system. The incidence varies greatly in different countries. It is commonest in Switzerland, quite common in England, France, and Germany, fairly common in Canada and the United States, rare in South America, and unknown in China and Japan.

Etiology.—The amount of time and money which has been expended in the effort to determine the factor or factors responsible for multiple sclerosis is beyond computing. Every possible type of agent has been accused, but the case against none of them has been proved. As we have just seen in our consideration of the group of demyelinating diseases in general, perhaps more may be said in favor of an auto-immune type of reaction affecting particularly the myelin sheaths than for any other concept. It is possible that persons with a general hypersensitivity may react only in the central nervous system, the reaction being between a tissue-bound antibody and a circulating antigen, and that the acute disease may confer on the central nervous system a form of tissue sensitivity which makes it vulnerable to further attacks (Bogdanove and Clark). Such a concept would serve to explain the very puzzling remissions and exacerbations which are so characteristic a feature of multiple sclerosis and which make a correct evaluation of therapeutic measures so difficult.

It has been suggested that degeneration of the *oligodendroglia cells* may be a primary factor in producing demyelination (Lumsden). The interfascicular oligodendrocytes, as opposed to the perineuronal ones, are the most numerous of the glial cells. There is a constant turn-over of myelin lipids in the brain, and this may prove to be the chief function of the oligodendrocytes, whose processes form a continuous membrane that may constitute a sheath outside the myelin sheath. It may well be that an antigen-antibody union on the surface of these membranes may result in selective damage to the cells and to the related myelin sheaths. This of course still leaves unanswered the question as to the nature of the agent responsible for the formation of antibody.

Precipitating factors, more particularly infective fevers or local trauma, sometimes seem to play a part in the onset of the disease or in a relapse after a remission. In occasional cases there is an undoubted familial incidence, suggesting an inherited predisposition which makes a person more susceptible to the unknown causal agent (McAlpine and Compston).

Lesions.—The lesions are scattered widely through the white matter of the brain and cord, and can be seen and felt in the fresh specimen as well-defined gray translucent patches. The lesions are very numerous in the brain, being especially well marked in the pons, medulla, and cerebellar peduncles. A dense periventricular sclerosis is common under the ependyma of the lateral ventricles and the third ventricle. There are patches in the optic nerve and optic chiasma. In the cord the lesions are most marked in the lateral columns (pyramidal tracts), but they are also present in the posterior columns.

The *microscopic picture* varies with the stage of the disease. If the autopsy is done during the *early stage,* which is seldom possible, the medullary sheaths are found to be

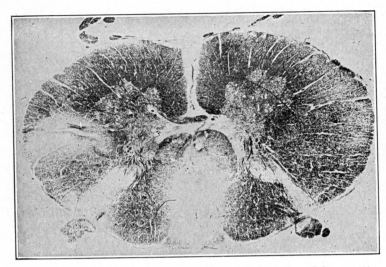

FIG. 672.—Multiple sclerosis. There are irregular asymmetrical patches of degeneration in the posterior and lateral columns. (Weigert's myelin stain.) × 8.

breaking up into droplets of myelin which can be stained with fat stains (osmic acid, Scharlach R), and the vessels are surrounded by collars of cells. Some of these cells are true inflammatory cells (lymphocytes and plasma cells), but others are compound granular corpuscles filled with droplets of myelin. The lesions are very similar to those of postvaccinal encephalitis, but in multiple sclerosis the production of the lesions is a much more gradual process. A characteristic feature is the development of a large amount of esterified cholesterol, probably due to an enzyme deficiency. This is also seen in Schilder's disease. In the *advanced stage*, the stage usually seen at autopsy, there are multiple neuroglial scars surrounding the blood vessels, chiefly in the white matter and to a lesser extent in the gray matter. In Weigert-Pal sections the scarred areas appear white on a black background (Fig. 672). In these patches of sclerosis the axis cylinders may be wonderfully intact, thus accounting for the remarkable remissions of symptoms which may take place. Some of the axis cylinders degenerate and others disappear entirely. The astrocytes proliferate enormously, and the nerve fibers are replaced by a dense glial network. There is a remarkable absence of secondary degeneration above and below the lesions, so that the patches of degeneration remain isolated. In this respect the disease differs entirely from tabes which is a system degeneration, *i.e.*, a condition affecting an entire system of fibers. Evidence of inflammation such as perivascular collars of cells is entirely lacking in the late stages of the disease.

Relation of Symptoms to Lesions.—The patient, usually between the age of fifteen and thirty-five years, suffers from a great variety of sensory and motor disturbances, many of which are curiously and characteristically fleeting. There are paresthesias of various kinds in the hands and feet, spastic paralysis of the upper motor neurone type with exaggerated deep reflexes and a positive Babinski sign, loss of the abdominal reflex, and transient disturbance of the organic reflexes. The well-known *Charcot triad* of nystagmus, intention tremor, and staccato speech are late manifestations of incoördination. The cranial nerves may be affected, causing sudden blindness, pallor of the temporal side of each optic disc, and oculomotor palsies. The patient is absurdly cheerful, considering the progressive and incurable nature of his ailment. Although progressive, the most surprising remissions often occur, during which most of the symptoms may disappear.

One of the most remarkable but easily overlooked features is the difference between the signs and symptoms of the disease. When you encounter a patient with bilateral loss of reflexes in both legs but loss of sensation on only one side, think of multiple sclerosis. This outstripping of symptoms by signs is rarely if ever seen in other neurological disorders.

The lesions are much more widespread than the severity of the symptoms would suggest. "Sclerosis creates multa, but not multum," as Oppenheim puts it. The comparative integrity of the axis cylinders explains the unexpected way in which such serious symptoms as paralysis or loss of vision may suddenly clear up. Lesions in the pyramidal tracts at different levels are responsible for the spastic paraplegia, exaggerated deep reflexes, and positive Babinski sign. The sensory changes are due to the lesions in the posterior columns. The absence of muscular atrophy and reaction of degeneration is to be expected from the fact that the anterior horns escape serious injury. The cerebellar incoördination, evidenced by nystagmus, intention tremor and scanning speech, is caused by lesions in the cerebellar peduncles which cut off the coördinating influences which play on the motor centers in the mid-brain and pons. The temporary loss of vision and the pallor of the temporal side of the discs are due to lesions of the optic chiasma or optic nerve. Diplopia, strabismus, and ptosis are caused by patches of sclerosis in the midbrain. These lesions, however, are different from the ordinary demyelinating lesions, for they include complete or incomplete degeneration of the axons of the nerve, a true optic neuritis. Perhaps some peculiar property of the myelin of the optic nerve is the determining feature.

The overaction of emotional expression is naturally difficult of explanation. According to Tilney and Riley the paleothalamus is related to the expression of the emotions. Now the paleothalamus is that part of the thalamus which borders the third ventricle and is covered by the ependyma. A dense sclerosis of this periventricular region is a very constant finding. It may be that a release of this center from control is responsible for the emotional overaction.

Occasional cases of *acute* or *subacute* multiple sclerosis are fatal in a few weeks or months. These are marked by an acute onset and course, but sometimes they are followed by a remission, and a relapsing chronic course. The acute onset may be characterized by headache, vomiting, and delirium due to involvement of the brain stem, the optic nerves, and the spinal cord. These are the cases which serve as connecting links with such a condition as acute disseminated encephalomyelitis, but which may eventually develop into chronic multiple sclerosis.

Cerebrospinal Fluid.—With one exception this shows little change. There is a mild lymphocytosis in the early cases and a slight increase of protein, but in the advanced sclerotic stage these changes are absent. The exception is the *colloidal gold reaction*, which in about one-half the cases *gives a paretic curve*, though the Wassermann reaction is always negative.

Schilder's Disease. Encephalitis Periaxialis Diffusa.—This rare condition, which affects children and young adults, closely resembles multiple sclerosis in its pathology, but it involves the cerebral hemispheres, not the brain stem and spinal cord. The disease is essentially a demyelinization of the white matter of both hemispheres, the gray matter escaping untouched. The affected areas are soft and gelatinous, gray and translucent. The process usually starts in the occipital lobes and spreads forward, but it may begin in any part of the cerebrum. The *microscopic features* are similar to those of early multiple sclerosis and post-vaccinal encephalitis, *i.e.*, demyelinization with destruction of the axis cylinders, perivascular collars of scavenger cells, and early gliosis. There is marked secondary degeneration of the affected paths. The cause of the condition is unknown.

The onset is acute and the course rapidly progressive but some cases may recover. The *symptoms* correspond with the lesions to a degree never seen in disseminated sclerosis. There is *early blindness* of cerebral type (occipital lobe), *deafness* (temporal lobe), *sensory disturbances* and loss of sense of position (parietal lobe), *spastic paralysis* (motor area), and *mental deterioration*

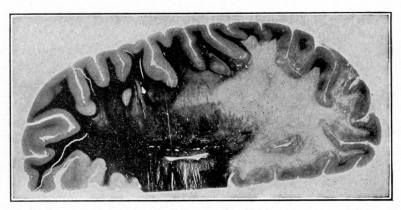

FIG. 673.—Section of a cerebral hemisphere in Schilder's disease. The normal white matter is stained black, while the degenerated area is completely unstained. Weigert's myelin stain. (Kindness of Dr. J. W. Kernohan in Sheldon, Doyle and Kernohan, courtesy of Arch. Neurol. and Psychiat.)

(frontal lobe). Convulsions are common. The combination in a child of progressive blindness, progressive spastic paralysis, and progressive mental failure is pathognomonic.

Morbid Anatomy.—The disease is essentially an affection of the white matter of the cerebral hemispheres. The gray matter of the cortex overlying the lesions is not involved. As a rule, the lesions are remarkably symmetrical in the two hemispheres. The affected areas are soft and gelatinous, gray and translucent in appearance, though becoming darker when kept in formalin, and are quite unlike the ordinary white matter from which they are sharply demarcated. The disease usually commences in the occipital lobes and spreads forward by contiguity, but it may begin in any part of the cerebrum (Fig. 673).

Acute Disseminated Encephalomyelitis.— This is an acute inflammation of the white matter of the brain or spinal cord or both, a leukoencephalomyelitis. It is related to infections, particularly those which are viral in nature. Thus it may develop after small-pox vaccination, inoculation against rabies, or during one of the viral exanthemata of childhood, chief of which is measles. Some cases with no clear history of a preceding infection and resembling acute multiple sclerosis should apparently be included in the group (Miller and Evans).

Etiology.—By far the commonest form of the disease is that which follows smallpox vaccination in children, but, as we have seen, it may follow or complicate other viral infections, more particularly measles. This does not mean that the lesions are necessarily caused directly by the virus. Owing to the resemblance of the lesions to what is observed in allergic encephalomyelitis produced in the experimental animal, it is believed that they may represent an auto-immune response of the white matter to some antigenic agent.

Lesions.—In fatal cases the three striking features of the lesions are their minute character, usually less than 1 mm. in diameter, their widespread distribution, and their acuteness. The lesions are small zones of demyelination around the smaller veins, more particularly in the subpial and subependymal regions, regions which are highly vascular. Another striking feature is perivascular collections of lymphocytes, plasma cells and histiocytes in the Virchow-Robin spaces. In those cases which recover completely it is to be presumed that the lesions are reversible.

Clinical Picture.—This is very variable. In the usual post-vaccinal cases, which develop symptoms within a week or ten days after vaccination, the onset is abrupt, with fever, headache, vomiting and evidence of meningeal irritation. This may be followed by the development of flaccid paralysis of the limbs, loss of sphincter control, together with nystagmus, occular palsies and changes in the pupil due to involvement of the brain stem. In the cerebrospinal fluid there is an increase of protein and lymphocytes. The post-vaccinal cases may have a mortality as high as 30 or even 50 per cent, death following deep coma. In the cases following measles the mortality is about 10 per cent, but less than half of those who survive make a complete recovery.

Acute Necrotizing Hemorrhagic Encephalomyelitis.—This formidable and forbidding title merely represents an attempt to condense all the pathological features of a condition into one brief phrase. The onset is fulminating and apoplectic with death ensuing within forty-eight hours, the extensive lesions in one or both hemispheres are necrotic or semifluid, with numerous small hemorrhages, and a violent perivascular inflammatory reaction both in the necrotic lesions and the meninges so that the spinal fluid contains many polymorphonuclears and the protein content is high. The cause and nature of the condition is unknown, but the acute hemorrhagic necrosis involving the vessels suggests some type of allergic reaction.

METABOLIC DISORDERS

It is easy to criticize the concept of metabolic diseases of the nervous system. It is hardly an exaggeration to say that every disturbance of metabolism is reflected to some extent in the brain, and it is certainly true that a metabolic disorder with cerebral manifestations severe enough to kill the patient may yet give rise to no gross or microscopic lesions which can be recognized, as we see in the case of diabetic coma, uremia, and other disorders of metabolism. Nevertheless it is convenient to consider a small group of cerebral disorders under the heading of metabolic disturbance, the outstanding examples being Wilson's disease, amaurotic familial idiocy together with other storage diseases, and porphyria.

Wilson's Disease. Hepato-Lenticular Degeneration.—This rare condition was first described by Kinnier Wilson in 1912 as progressive lenticular degneration. It is familial, affects young people, and is progressively fatal. There is a characteristic *clinical triad* of nervous system involvement,

liver involvement, and greenish pigmentation along the margin of the cornea. The *clinical manifestations* may be mainly neurological or mainly hepatic. The chief *neurological features* are muscular rigidity, tremor of the Parkinson type, difficulty with articulation, and marked emotionalism, features suggestive of a corpus striatum lesion. Usually the facies are expressionless and fixed owing to the rigidity, the mouth kept open so that saliva dribbles from it, but now and again a fatuous smile passes slowly across the face, or there are spasms of silent weeping. *Disturbance of hepatic function* is evidenced by prolonged fatigue, and by ascites and other signs of cirrhosis of the liver. Wilson recognized the association of two lesions apparently completely dissociated from one another, namely degeneration of the lenticular nucleus and cirrhosis of the liver. What he did not recognize, for it was not demonstrated until thirty-three years later, was that there was a factor common to both lesions, namely a greatly increased copper content in both the brain and the liver. The *green coloration of the cornea*, known as the *Kayser-Fleischer ring*, is also due to a deposition of copper. There is an increased aminoaciduria and an increased excretion of dicarboxylic amino acid peptides from renal tubular epithelium damaged by copper deposits.

The *lesions* in the brain and in the liver are associated with a *greatly increased copper content*. The change in the basal ganglia varies from a mere brownish (coppery) discoloration or a moth-eaten appearance to complete softening and cavity formation. The disease is confined to the corpus striatum, the change being most marked in the putamen, and to a lesser degree in the globus pallidus and caudate nucleus. The neighboring optic thalamus, which has much the same blood supply as the lenticular nucleus, escapes untouched. The nerve cells and fibers in the involved area disappear. Deposits of copper are apparent as a black precipitate on staining. The walls of the cavity contain a thick network of neuroglia. The cirrhosis of the liver is of the multilobular type, but in Wilson's original cases there was no clinical evidence of this lesion. There is marked irregularity in size and staining of the liver cell nuclei even in lobules containing no copper. The renal tubular epithelium may be damaged owing to deposits of copper.

We now know that the disease is *an inborn error of copper metabolism*. The decisive factor in the expression of the disorder is the genetic component, the abnormal gene having to be present in a double dose for the disease to become manifest clinically (Bearn). The familial incidence and the absence of the disease in parents points to a recessive mode of inheritance. The homozygous patients have an inborn disturbance of copper metabolism. The disease naturally has variants, so that occasionally the clinical picture may be one of hepatic cirrhosis rather than of lenticular degeneration, the crucial factor in the recognition of the variants being objective biochemical tests.

The *essence of the disorder* is an increased copper content of the body associated with an increased excretion of copper in the urine. When copper is administered to a normal person, the copper is first attached to the albumin fraction of the serum protein, but within twenty-four hours it is transferred from the albumin to the globulin fraction, becoming firmly bound in a protein complex known as ceruloplasmin because of its blue color. In Wilson's disease this transfer from albumin to globulin does not take place, the copper remaining loosely associated with the albumin fraction. Presumably it is this copper which is deposited in the brain, liver, kidney and cornea. There is therefore a low serum level of ceruloplasmin, and a test for this lowering of level is the most reliable and valuable diagnostic method in the early stages of the disease when treatment is most likely to be effective. Normally from 90 to 95 per cent of serum copper is bound to globulin in the form of ceruloplasmin and only 5 to 10 per cent to serum albumin. It would appear that the inborn error of metabolism in Wilson's disease is a defect in the synthesis of ceruloplasmin, resulting in the deposition of copper in the organs already mentioned, where it gives rise to the characteristic lesions and thus to the clinical symptoms which Wilson was the first to relate to the lesions. It must be admitted, however, that the levels of serum

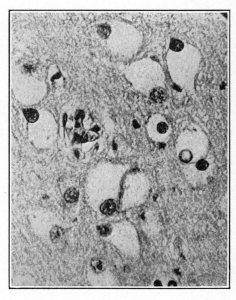

FIG. 674.—Amaurotic family idiocy. The cortical nerve cells are greatly distended with lipid, which displaces the nucleus to one side. × 375.

ceruloplasmin and copper vary considerably in different cases, and in the very occasional case they have been reported as normal.

Knowledge that the essence of the disease is the accumulation of copper in certain organs has made it possible to take tentative steps in the direction of therapy. Dimercaprol (BAL) forms a stable complex with copper and causes it to be excreted in the urine in large amounts, and penicillinase has been found to be even more effective.

Amaurotic Family Idiocy.—This fortunately very rare condition, also known as *Tay-Sachs disease*, is in essence a developmental failure in a specific enzyme system which leads to a progressive accumulation of lipid in the cells of the brain, cord and retina. It occurs in an infantile, a juvenile and a late form. The infantile form is practically confined to Jewish children, appears about the sixth month, and invariably ends fatally, usually in the course of 2 years.

The first-born are rarely affected, but when one child has had the disease the subsequent children seldom escape The symptoms are idiocy, muscular weakness, and rapidly developing blindness (amaurosis), so that the disease is well named. There is a characteristic cherry-red spot at the macula. The brain is small and hard. There is widespread degeneration of the cells and fibers of the cerebral cortex, the anterior and posterior horns of the cord, and the posterior root ganglia. The affected cells both in the brain and in the retina are filled with lipid (Fig. 674).

The *retinal lesions* responsible for the amaurosis are of the same character as those in the brain. The cherry-red spot is due to the fact that at the macula the retina is extremely thin, so that it is easily penetrated by the red reflex of the normal choroid, but immediately around this spot there is an abundance of nerve cells loaded with lipid which interferes with the choroid reflex.

The *nature of the disease* is a lipid storage (ganglioside) comparable to that of Gaucher's and Niemann-Pick's disease (sphingomyelin). All three conditions show the same age, racial and familial features. Of the three forms of Tay-Sachs disease the infantile has just been described. The *juvenile form* occurs in non-Jewish as well as Jewish children, appears between the ages of four and seven years, lasts much longer, and may not be associated with a cherry-red spot in the retina. The *late form* develops about the time of puberty or later, it is not confined to Jews, it causes no mental change, the retinal lesions are absent, it lasts for many years, and is usually only recognized at autopsy. It is evident that in these later cases the genetic defect and therefore the metabolic disorder is much less pronounced.

NUTRITIONAL DEFICIENCEIS

Many disturbances in nutrition must result in corresponding disturbance in cerebral function. The two most clear cut examples are subacute combined degeneration of the spinal cord due to deficiency of vitamin B_{12} and Wernicke's encephalopathy due to deficiency of thiamin. To these may be added pellagra due to niacin deficiency, although involvement of the skin and bowel is likely to overshadow that of the brain.

Subacute Combined Degeneration.—This nervous disease, characterized by paresthesias of the hands and feet and spastic paralysis of the legs, is closely related to pernicious anemia. Nearly every case sooner or later develops a macrocytic hyperchromic type of anemia, even though there may not be a full-fledged blood picture of pernicious anemia. The condition, which is not uncommon, affecting those of late middle age, is the result of a deficiency in vitamin B_{12}, itself based on the gastric defect responsible for the pernicious anemia. That the cord lesions are not due to the anemia is shown by the fact that the nervous symptoms may develop long before there is any sign of anemia. It is a progressive condition, but can be arrested by vitamin B_{12}. In rare cases combined degeneration of the spinal cord has been known to complicate other conditions, such as leukemia and gastric cancer.

Lesions.—These are most marked in the mid-dorsal region, with ascending secondary degeneration in the cervical cord and descending secondary degeneration in the lumbar cord. The lesions are symmetrical, and involve the posterior columns, crossed and direct pyramidal tracts, and the cerebellar tracts (Fig. 675). In the early stage and in remissions they are confined to the dorsal columns. They can be seen as translucent patches with the naked eye. It is not a system disease; the lesions are formed by the fusion of many small patches. There is first demyelinization with complete destruction of the medullary sheaths, followed later by disappearance of the axis cylinders. In the more recent lesions there is a complete absence of neuroglial proliferation, but in old lesions there may be some degree of secondary gliosis.

Relation of Symptoms to Lesions.—There is exact correspondence between the lesions and symptoms. The earliest symptom is numbness and tingling at the tips of the fingers and toes, a feeling of "pins and needles." Later there may be sensory loss, ataxia, and loss of the sense of position. The knee-jerks may be lost. All of these are posterior column symptoms. In other cases there are lateral column symptoms, *i.e.*, spastic paralysis, exaggerated deep reflexes, and a double Babinski sign. The end-stage is one of flaccid paralysis with complete sensory loss and paralysis of the sphincters; this corresponds with disappear-

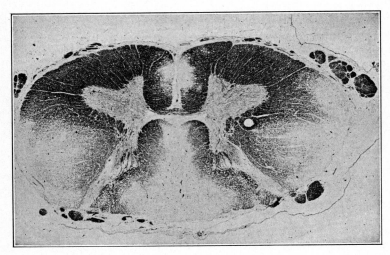

FIG. 675.—Subacute combined degeneration of the cord. Marked degeneration in the posterior columns, the crossed pyramidal and direct pyramidal tracts, and the right indirect cerebellar tract. (Weigert's myelin stain.) × 8.

ance of all the long tracts in the dorsal region. It sometimes happens that the neurological symptoms develop before there are any changes in the blood or bone marrow. In such cases it is useful to examine mouth washings, for the cells of the oral epithelium show marked nuclear polymorphism and the presence of giant nuclei, changes which are known to occur in these cells in pernicious anemia.

Wernicke's Encephalopathy.—This rare condition, known also as *acute superior hemorrhagic polioencephalitis*, is marked clinically by paralysis of the eye muscles, mental confusion, stupor or excitement, and usually death within a few days. The lesions are curiously restricted. The corpora mammillaria are constantly affected; in addition there may be lesions in the hypothalamus, thalamus, and periaqueductal gray matter. The gross lesions are congestion and hemorrhage. Death is not due to the lesions in the mammillary bodies, but to a profound disturbance of carbohydrate metabolism with accompanying hypoglycemia. The characteristic *microscopic lesion* is vacuolation and disintegration of the intercellular tissue with preservation of the nerve cells. It is as if these cells had remained intact in the center of an area of brain softening (Fig. 676). The smaller vessels are narrowed by

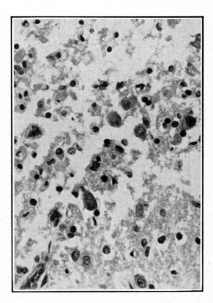

FIG. 676.—Mammillary body in Wernicke's encephalopathy.

reason of a marked increase in the cellularity of their endothelium. The condition presents a clear-cut pathological entity, but one which is easily overlooked at autopsy unless borne in mind. The hemorrhagic lesions in the walls of the third ventricle and aqueduct and the floor of the fourth ventricle are well brought out by Pickworth's benzidine stain, as is beautifully shown in Campbell and Biggart's paper. When Wernicke originally described the condition in 1881 he ascribed it to alcoholism, but it is now believed to be a deficiency disease, because similar lesions can be produced experimentally by vitamin B_1 deficiency. The alcohol supplies abundant calories but no vitamin B, as we have already seen to be the case in alcoholic cirrhosis of the liver. It is really cerebral beriberi, and can be cured rapidly and completely in the early stages by injections of thiamin.

PELLAGRA.—This example of avitaminosis is due to a deficiency in niacin or nicotinic acid. The clinical picture is marked by involvement of the skin, the bowel and the brain, with the development of the triad known as the three D's, namely dermatitis, diarrhea and dementia. The dementia is caused by neuronal degeneration involving the ganglion cells of the brain and the posterior and lateral columns of the spinal cord. The cord lesions may closely resemble those of subacute combined degeneration, so that it is possible that deficiency of some other member of the B complex in addition to niacin, such for instance as B_{12}, may also be involved.

IDIOPATHIC DEGENERATIONS

Having disposed of the demyelinating, the metabolic and the nutritional disorders of the central nervous system, we are left with a large, heterogeneous and highly unsatisfactory group of degenerative conditions to which the term idiopathic may appropriately be applied, because their etiology, their pathogenesis, and even their essential nature remains unknown. A reference to the table of contents at the beginning of this chapter will show that the majority are known by men's names, a striking tribute to our ignorance of these conditions.

Chronic Motor Neurone Degeneration.— Three different clinical entities, all of them rare, may be grouped under this heading, for in all of them the underlying basis is a primary degeneration of the motor neurones, upper or lower or both. They are all variants of one pathological process. In *progressive atrophy* the lesion is in the anterior horn, in *bulbar palsy* it is in the bulbar centers, and in *amyotrophic lateral sclerosis*

both the upper and lower motor neurones degenerate. There is no involvement of the sensory side. The cause of the condition is unknown and its nature uncertain. It occurs in persons over middle age, there is nothing inflammatory about it, and it seems to be a pure degeneration, a gradual neuronal decay, an abiotrophy. It is possible that a food deficiency, vitamin or otherwise, may be responsible. In all three forms there is progressive muscular weakness with atrophy and fibrillary tremors in the affected muscles. The basis of *Little's disease* (congenital palsy of children) is an agenesis of the upper motor neurone, so that it will be taken as an addendum to the present group.

It is now becoming apparent that the disease may have a genetic basis, although precipitating factors such as fatigue, infection or trauma may determine early localization of the manifestations of the condition. The most remarkable support for the genetic concept comes from a study of the incidence of amyotrophic lateral sclerosis in the Chamorros, natives of Guam and others of the Marianas Islands in the Pacific (Kurland). Amongst the 30,000 Chamorros the disease is 100 times as common as in the United States and other countries. About 1 per cent of the adults suffer from the condition, which is responsible for some 10 per cent of the deaths. There is a much higher incidence in young people, and multiple cases in the same family are of common occurrence. This familial feature has also been reported in other countries. It is suggested that an inherited disturbance of motor neurone metabolism may be the basis of the disease.

Another remarkable example of a degenerative disease of the nervous system with an apparently genetic basis is Kuru, a disease of the natives of New Guinea (p. 1193).

1. *Amyotrophic Lateral Sclerosis.*—This disease comes on in middle life, though by no means in the senile period. Rarely it may occur in youth. *Both the upper and lower motor neurones are involved.* There is atrophy of the anterior horns in the cord with great disappearance of the motor cells and wasting of the anterior nerve roots; the condition of the nerve roots should be compared with what is found in tabes. The

remaining anterior horn cells show every degree of degeneration. The pyramidal tracts are degenerated, and there is corresponding degeneration of the large Betz cells in the motor cortex. Late in the disease the motor nuclei in the pons and medulla degenerate. There is marked atrophy of the affected muscles. The change is spotty, not diffuse, many of the fibers being comparatively intact. These are innervated by the nerve cells which have escaped destruction. There is a replacement fibrosis.

The *chief symptoms* are weakness, wasting and fibrillary tremors of the muscles. The amyotrophy begins in the small muscles of the hands (thenar, hypothenar and interossei), and spreads to the forearm and shoulder. Spasticity of the legs, exaggerated deep reflexes and a positive Babinski sign due to an upper motor neurone lesion may appear even earlier. Symptoms of bulbar paralysis (see below) complete the picture at the end. The patient seldom survives more than three years, death being due to bulbar paralysis.

2. *Progressive Muscular Atrophy.*—This is amyotroph`c lateral sclerosis without clinical evidence of an upper motor neurone lesion, although at autopsy the lateral columns may show some degeneration. The disease is much rarer than the preceding form. The fibrillary tremors form the most striking feature of the clinical picture. As the bulbar centers are spared, the patient may drag out an existence for many years.

3. *Progressive Bulbar Palsy.*—The condition may be purely bulbar, or may be the end-stage of an amyotrophic lateral sclerosis. The motor nuclei of the pons and medulla are involved, *i.e.*, the seventh, ninth, tenth, eleventh and twelfth nerves. The clinical picture is best described by the alternative name, *glosso-labio-pharyngeal paralysis.* The first symptom is difficulty in articulation with loss of the labials. Owing to the weakness of the lips they are at first held in a peculiarly stiff manner; after a time the mouth remains permanently open. The tongue wastes and shows marked fibrillary tremors. There is paralysis of the palate and the pharynx, so that swallowing becomes impossible. The upper part of the face escapes.

Cerebral Palsy.—The condition of *congenital spastic diplegia* or *Little's disease* is due to an upper motor neurone degeneration, or rather to an *agenesia* or failure of development on the part of the motor cortical cells and the pyramidal tracts. The convolutions in the motor area are small and atrophic (*microgyria*). There is an association with premature birth, but this is not a causal factor. *There may be a history of rubella in the mother during the first trimester of pregnancy.* The symptoms usually appear, about a year after birth. The picture is purely motor. The child walks with a "cross-legged" or "scissors" gait, with great spasticity of the legs. The deep reflexes are exaggerated and there is a double Babinski sign. There may be slight involvement of the arms.

Spastic cerebral paralysis or *birth palsy* is quite a different condition from Little's disease, and is due to a meningeal hemorrhage at the time of birth. A monoplegia or hemiplegia is commoner than diplegia, and the paralysis is evident soon after birth. A gross lesion is always present.

Parkinson's Disease.—Some thirty years ago two forms of Parkinson's disease used to be encountered. The first was a sequel of the epidemic encephalitis lethargica which was so prevalent at that time. Sad reminders of that fact are still encountered, but fresh cases no longer develop. Once developed it remains stationary. The second form, known as *paralysis agitans*, is that originally described by Parkinson.

Parkinson's disease ("the shaking palsy") is a perfect example of disease of the extrapyramidal system, and will therefore be described in some detail. The *clinical picture* was drawn more than a hundred years ago by Parkinson with the hand of a master. The classical triad of symptoms are rigidity, tremor, and an attitude of flexion. (1) The *rigidity* results in a general absence of motor activity; there are none of the little movements depending on a healthy corpus striatum. It involves all the voluntary muscles, until at last the unhappy sufferer becomes as rigid as a block of marble. Articulation and swallowing become difficult, and finally there is complete anarthria and extreme dysphagia. The rigidity gives the face the familiar *Parkinsonian mask*. The mouth cannot be closed and the saliva drools down the chin. (2) The *tremor* affects the fingers and hands, giving a cigarette-rolling movement. It is present when the part is at rest, disappearing for a few minutes with movement. To use Parkinson's own words: "Commencing in one arm the wearisome agitation is borne until beyond sufferance, when by sudden changing of the posture it is for a time stopped in that limb." The writing and finer manipulations are affected for "the hand fails to answer with exactness the dictates of the will. The tremor is dependent on the integrity of the pyramidal tract for it disappears in a limb paralyzed as the result of a stroke, only to reappear as the power returns. (3) The whole attitude is one of *flexion*. The head is flexed on the chest, the body is bowed, the arms and wrist are flexed, the knees are bent. As the center of gravity is thrown forward he has to walk on the forepart of the feet, and comes to assume an overhanging position. "He is irresistibly impelled to take much quicker and shorter steps, and thereby to adopt unwillingly a running pace." An advanced example of the disease can be diagnosed at a glance.

Lesions.—The lesions take the form of degenerative changes in the corpus striatum, especially disappearance of the large motor cells of the globus pallidus. More than this it is not possible to say. The changes are not confined to the globus pallidus, so that it is not justifiable to regard the condition as a pure syndrome of the globus pallidus. The cause of the degeneration is not known; possibly it is in the nature of a senile atrophy. Edema, degeneration, and fibrosis have been described in the muscle spindles (neuromuscular bundles) of the small muscles of the thumb. The rigidity and tremor are evidently the result of the lesions in the corpus striatum. Intracytoplasmic inclusions are present in the pigmented cells of the substantia nigra in 86 per cent of the idiopathic cases and 44 per cent of the postencephalitic cases (Lipkin).

The possibility of a relation to trauma has been a matter of much dispute. Undoubtedly severe injury to the head may be followed after a latent interval by the appearance of tremors, due probably to destructive lesions in the basal ganglia caused by a wave of cerebrospinal fluid set up by the blow. These post-traumatic cases, however, do not present all the features of Parkinson's disease, and they may occur at a much earlier age.

Since 1952 first surgical and later chemotherapeutical methods have been directed against the globus pallidus in the treatment of Parkinson's disease (Cooper). What has been called chemopallidectomy, *i.e.*, the application of alcohol to the pallidus through a burr-hole in the skull, has given considerable relief in selected cases. Even more modern electronic methods have also been tried.

Postencephalitic Parkinsonism presents the same clinical picture as that which has just been described, but the course is usually not progressive. In spite of this similarity it is not a corpus striatum disease, for the degenerative lesions are in the substantia nigra and the red nucleus. The pigmented cells of the former may largely disappear. It is therefore a disease of the extrapyramidal system.

KURU.—Every now and then the investigator has the thrill of discovering a new disease, a thrill which may not be shared by the medical student who may think that he has to learn its details, which is certainly not the case. Although the reader will never see a case of Kuru, the clinical features are so arresting, the genetic basis so clear, the lesions so well defined, and the possible relationship to other obscure diseases of the central nervous system so suggestive that a brief account seems justified. Clinically the condition closely resembles Wilson's disease, but there is no involvement of the liver, nor any evidence of disturbed copper metabolism, so that it seems preferable to consider it with the idiopathic group of degenerations. It is akin to Parkinson's disease and other chronic progressive heredofamilial degenerative disorders of the nervous system, particularly the cerebellar and spinal ataxias and degenerations involving the corpus striatum.

Kuru, an acute progressive degeneration of the central nervous system confined to the Fore people in the Eastern Highlands of New Guinea, was first described in 1957 by Gajdusek and Zigas. The word kuru indicates trembling from fear and cold, so that the condition is known as "the shaking disease." It is the cause of over 50 per cent of the deaths in the community, and kills 1 per cent of the population every year, this figure at times reaching from 5 to 10 per cent. This astounding incidence may be explained on a heredofamilial basis, for in this isolated community marriage with close kinsmen is preferred. The chief victims are adult females, but almost one-quarter are children of both sexes. Adult males are frequently murdered on suspicion of being sorcerers responsible for the illness, a practice which serves to maintain a balance in the sex population.

The *clinical picture* is amazingly uniform. The first symptom is locomotor ataxia, which may be accompanied by pains in the leg. As the ataxia becomes more severe a distinctive tremor appears involving the trunk, extremities, and head. An early feature is a marked emotionalism with inappropriate and excessive laughter. The women and children are happy and euphoric. Dysarthria and a very blurred, slurred speech develops. Convergent strabismus is a late symptom. A curious feature is that the disease becomes static during pregnancy, followed by rapid deterioration after delivery. Towards the end the patient is completely incapacitated, with urinary and fecal incompetence and dysphagia leading to starvation. The condition is often fatal in from three to six months. The cerebrospinal fluid is normal, as are all other laboratory tests.

The *lesions* are entirely microscopic (Klatzo *et al.*). There is widespread neuronal degeneration, with loss of myelin especially in the spinocerebellar and corticospinal tracts. The characteristic and unusual cellular lesion is a striking degree of cytoplasmic vacuolation, giving a curious soap-bubble appearance (Fowler and Robertson). A similar appearance is seen in louping-ill of sheep, in which muscular incoordination is also very marked (page 1174). An intense astroglial and microglial proliferation accompanies the neuronal degeneration, these changes being particularly marked in the cerebellum and the extrapyramidal system. Degeneration is also present in the anterior horn cells, inferior olive, thalamus and pontine nuclei. Finally, plaques are encountered in the cerebellum in about half the cases studied, and sometimes in the basal ganglia and cerebral cortex. There are no lesions in any other tissues.

What all this means is at present a complete mystery. It seems quite possible, however, that "studies on Kuru, by virtue of the remarkable incidence of the disease may significantly contribute to the better understanding of many degenerative disorders within the central nervous system" (Klatzo *et al.*) At present we may presume that the disease is a manifestation of an inborn error in metabolism resulting from a genetic predisposition.

HUNTINGTON'S CHOREA.—This rare disease has an extremely marked hereditary tendency, 962 cases in the United States having been traced back to half a dozen individuals who migrated to that country in the seventeenth century, but it does not appear until middle life. The two chief *symptoms* are involuntary movements and tremors of choreiform character, and mental deterioration going on to dementia. Two *lesions* have been described: (1) atrophy of the cortical nerve cells and their associated fibers; (2) destruction and disappearance of the cells of the putamen and caudate nucleus (neostriatum) with comparative escape of the globus pallidus. The mental deterioration is evidently due to the extensive cortical changes, and the choreiform movements may be attributed to the loss of controlling influences from the neostriatum.

SYDENHAM'S CHOREA.—Although Sydenham's chorea is an inflammatory rather than a degenerative condition and bears no relation to the chorea of Huntington, it may for convenience be considered in this place.

St. Vitus' dance, as it used to be called, is one of the commonest of nervous disorders, yet its pathology is still obscure. It usually occurs in girls, and nearly always before the age of twenty years. Chorea is a manifestation of rheumatic fever, but it may not be preceded by a definite arthritis, for rheumatic manifestations in childhood are not necessarily arthritic. The *symptoms* take the form of sudden, irregular, involuntary movements. The disease runs its course in a few weeks and rarely ends in death. The *lesions* in the fatal cases are remarkably insignificant. There is marked hyperemia, a moderate perivascular lymphocytosis, and slight degeneration of nerve cells. These changes are most marked in the cerebral cortex and the basal ganglia, especially the neostriatum.

FRIEDREICH'S ATAXIA.—This rare familial disease belongs to the group of the abiotrophies, in which slow degeneration of several of the tracts of the nervous system occurs without any obvious reason. It is a disease of the young. The distribution of the lesions resembles that in subacute combined degeneration, for the disease is a combined degeneration affecting both posterior and lateral columns (Fig. 677). Friedreich's disease offers an unusually interesting example of the explanation of neurological symptoms by the pathological lesions. Owing to the lesions in the posterior columns there is loss of the deep reflexes and of deep muscle sense, the latter partially accounting for the ataxia, which affects the arms as well as the legs. But there is a large cerebellar element in the ataxia ("cerebellar reel"), due to involvement of the direct cerebellar tract. Lesions

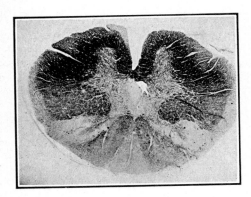

FIG. 677.—Friedreich's ataxia. × 7.

in the pyramidal tracts cause muscular weakness and a positive Babinski sign, even though the knee-jerks are lost. A characteristic deformity of the foot (high arch and hammer toe) and scoliosis are probably due to the pyramidal tract degeneration causing asymmetrical weakness of the muscles during the period of growth. Nystagmus and scanning speech are characteristic features, but their method of production is not obvious. Although posterior column sclerosis is present in both of the spinal ataxias (Friedreich's and locomotor), the former presents none of the lightning pains and other sensory disturbances which are so characteristic of tabes, a significant fact which suggests that the cause of these disturbances should be looked for outside the spinal cord.

Syringomyelia.—This is another rare disease of the earlier part of life depending on a perversion of development. It is therefore often associated with spina bifida and other congenital anomalies. The outstanding symptoms are *dissociated anesthesia* (loss of sensibility to pain and temperature with preservation of touch), *muscular atrophy in the arms, a spastic condition of the legs*, and certain so-called *trophic lesions*.

Lesions.—The essential lesion is a gliosis in the gray commissure and the base of the posterior horns in the lower cervical and upper dorsal region. This new-formed glial tissue becomes softened and liquefied so that a tubular cavity is formed (*syrinx*, a tube, the same word as syringe) (Fig. 678). The process may extend through the entire length of the cord, and even up into the brain stem. The cavity is separate from the central canals of the cord. The affected part is large, soft and flattened. The cavity is often lined by a layer of ependyma. It should be remembered that ependymal cells are merely specialized neuroglial cells, and that they may proliferate, giving rise to a gliosis, just as they may form an ependymal glioma. In the latter tumor the cells tend to surround tiny cavities, and it is possible that a similar tendency may explain the cavity formation in syringomyelia. All this is very theoretical, but there is nothing

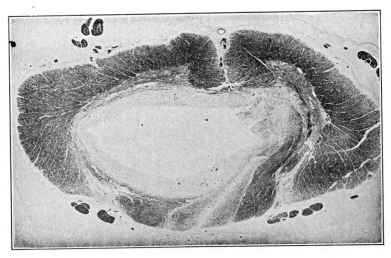

FIG. 678.—Syringomyelia. Marked cavity formation in the center of the cord, with surrounding zone of gliosis. (Weigert's myelin stain.) × 8.

better to put in its place. We may regard the process, then, as a benign neoplasia of glial tissue, in which ependymal cells possibly play a prominent part.

Relation of Symptoms to Lesions.—The *dissociated anesthesia* is observed in the arms, as the lesion is commonly in the cervical cord. The fibers for pain and temperature cross in the gray commissure, and are therefore caught in the destructive process. Most of the touch fibers pass up in the posterior columns of the same side and therefore escape. This explains the dissociation of the anesthesia. *Spasticity* of the legs with some loss of power is due to pressure on the pyramidal tracts in the cervical region. In the arms there is *muscular atrophy* of the lower motor neurone type, similar to that seen in progressive muscular atrophy. As the pathological process seldom involves the anterior horns, the reason for this atrophy is obscure. The *trophic lesions* are still more obscure. The name is unfortunate, for it is is probable that the root of the trouble is not the cutting off of hypothetical trophic influences from the cord, but the anesthesia which permits the tissues to be unduly traumatized. Thus burns on the hands are of common occurrence, as the patient is insensitive to heat. The best known example is the *Charcot joint*, usually the shoulder or elbow. Its chief characteristic is its extreme painlessness, although the joint is completely disorganized and may become dislocated. Such an insensitive joint must receive much trauma against which there is now no protective mechanism, and this may lead to the remarkable disintegration characteristic of the condition.

HYDROMYELIA.—This is a simple dilatation of the central canal of the cord. It may affect the whole or only part of the canals. It may be associated with hydrocephalus, and is related to that condition rather than to syringomyelia.

PICK'S CONVOLUTIONAL ATROPHY.—This is a very rare form of agenesia which manifests itself in the presenile period (fifty to sixty years). The brain is shrunken, and shows extreme symmetrical localized atrophy of parts of the cerebrum. The change is most marked in the frontal region, but in a case of the writer's the occipital convolutions were also extremely small. The atrophy is not arteriosclerotic or senile in character. The condition is progressive, and is accompanied by marked dementia. It is the phylogenetically younger parts of the brain which are most affected.

ALZHEIMER'S DISEASE.—In this presenile condition the distinctive microscopic features of the atrophic brain are senile plaques and neurofibrillary changes. The plaques consist of an acellular argyrophilic center surrounded by distorted neuroglial and nerve fibers. The neurofibrils become thickened, fragmented, and finally disintegrate. With the periodic acid-Schiff stain the senile plaques are seen to consist of amorphous as well as cellular and fibrillary elements (Margolis). The amorphous material is PAS-positive, whereas the other elements are PAS-negative. The plaques seem to be the result of the deposition of colloids in the ground substance of the cortex, the cellular components being probably reacting glial cells.

INTRACRANIAL TUMORS

Tumors within the cranial cavity may be divided into two great groups, intracerebral and extracerebral. The *intracerebral group* comprise the gliomas, metastatic carcinoma, and a few miscellaneous tumors such as hemangioma. The *extracerebral group*, far more favorable from the surgical standpoint, comprise the meningiomas, acoustic neuromas, and tumors of the pituitary and craniopharyngiomas which have already been considered in connection with the pituitary body.

The various intracranial tumors may also be divided into a clinically more benign group of slow growth and a much more malignant group, a distinction obviously of great clinical importance. To the *more benign group* belong meningioma, acoustic nerve tumor, pituitary adenoma, cerebellar astrocytoma, ependymoma, blood vessel tumors, and congenital tumors. The important members of the *malignant group* are glioblastoma and medulloblastoma, as well as cerebral astrocytoma to a much less marked degree.

GLIOMA

For practical purposes nearly all the tumors of the brain are neoplasms of the interstitial tissue, *i.e.*, gliomas. Of the three varieties of interstitial tissue, the microglia never gives rise to tumors, and the oliogdendroglia very seldom does, so that practically all the gliomas arise from the astrocytes. It must be noted that although some of the gliomas are among the most malignant of tumors, they never give rise to metastases. If large celloidin sections of the entire tumor and the surrounding brain tissue are made it will be found that in about one-third of the cases the glioma is relatively circumscribed, the microscopic limits corresponding fairly closely with the visible limits. About 60 per cent are diffuse, with microscopic limits extending widely beyond the grossly visible limits. This is true of all cerebral astrocytomas. There may be multicentric growth, but this is practically confined to the glioblastomas. About 30 per cent of gliomas are bilateral.

For many years the accepted classification of the gliomas was that proposed by Bailey and Cushing in 1926. This was based on the assumed resemblance of the various cells in the gliomas to embryonic cells recognizable in the differentiation of the developing nervous system. Such terms as astrocytoma arising from astrocytes, astroblastoma from astroblasts, and spongioblastoma (now called glioblastoma) from spongioblasts, were and still are in common use. It is well known, however, that an intermingling of different types of cells can be found in the different tumors, which destroys the idea of specificity. Kernohan's concept that the cells in the more rapidly growing gliomas represent different phases of dedifferentiation rather than undifferentiation appears much more satisfying. Astrocytoma, astroblastoma and glioblastoma multiforme would then represent different degrees of malignancy of the same type of neoplasm, astrocytoma Grade 1 corresponding with the classical astrocytoma, astrocytoma Grade 2 with astroblastoma, and astrocytoma Grade 3 and 4 with glioblastoma multiforme. The four adult types of cells in the central nervous system are astrocytes, ependymal cells, oligodendroglial cells and nerve cells. Each of these, in that order of frequency, may give rise to tumors of varying degrees of anaplasia and malignancy.

In support of the view that the common forms of glioma are variations of one basic type is the observation of Zimmerman and Maier that all the usual varieties can be induced in mice by the intracerebral implantation of pellets of a chemical carcinogen such as methylcholanthrene. A single tumor may consist of astrocytic, spongioblastic and oligodendrocytic parts. By homologous subcutaneous transplantation of such mixed tumors it has been possible to establish pure lines of the individual neoplasms. From a single tumor it has been possible to develop an ependymoma, an astrocytoma, and an oligodendroglioma.

A peculiar feature of the gliomas which we have already noted is that, no matter how malignant they may be, they do not metastasize outside the central nervous system. They make up for this, however, by showing a tendency to seeding throughout the subarachnoid space, both cerebral and spinal, a tendency which is much more marked in the case of the medulloblastoma. The reason why they do not metastasize appears to be that they do not invade the blood vessels, nor are there lymph spaces in the brain which communicate with the general lymphatic system. When the gliomas are implanted in the eye, the peritoneal cavity or the subcutaneous tissue of the experimental animal they grow readily.

Glioblastoma Multiforme.—This is the commonest and most malignant of the gliomas. It is a tumor of middle life, and is seldom found outside the cerebral hemispheres. It is not infrequently multiple—an unusual occurrence in a malignant tumor. If not treated, it rapidly kills the patient. The tumor is soft, gray, ill-defined, vascular, and often shows evidence of degeneration such as necrosis, hemorrhage, and cyst formation. Degeneration of the central part often gives the tumor a false appearance of encapsulation; in reality it is highly invasive, and the surgeon's great difficulty is to know where the tumor ends and normal brain begins (Fig. 679).

The *microscopic appearance* is characteristically varied. The tumor is highly cellular, and the cells are very pleomorphic, varying greatly in size and shape, recalling the varied cytological picture in osteogenic sarcoma of bone. This pleomorphism justifies the name "multiforme," which is applied to the common form of glioblastoma, in contrast to a rarer polar form of glioblastoma,

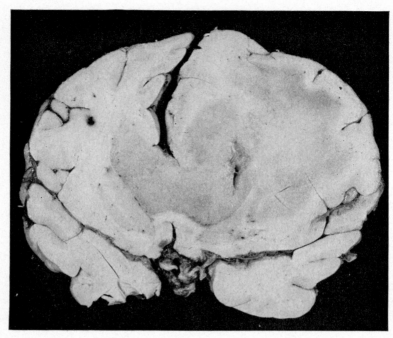

FIG. 679.—Glioblastoma multiforme, showing massive infiltration of right and left frontal lobes
(University of Alabama Medical School.)

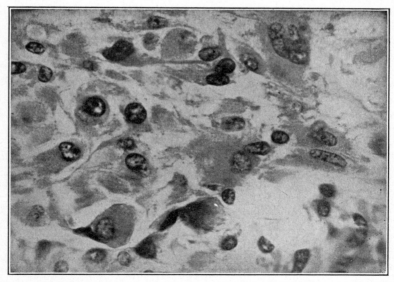

FIG. 680.—Glioblastoma multiforme.   The cells vary greatly in shape: some are round, some are elongated,
and some are pear-shaped.   × 700.

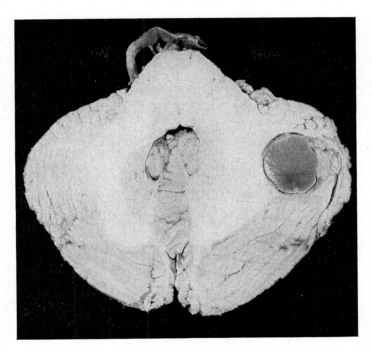

Fig. 681.—Cystic astrocytoma of cerebellum in a nine months old child. Histologically the lesion was well differentiated. (University of Alabama Medical School.)

in which the cells have a single process. Some of the cells are round or oval, some pear-shaped, some elongated (Fig. 680). They are bipolar spongioblasts when stained by Cajal's gold-sublimate method. There are also tumor giant cells with many nuclei. Mitoses are common. There are no glial fibers, for the spongioblast does not produce such fibers. The vascular endothelium often shows a remarkable proliferation so that the lumen of the vessels may be filled with masses of cells. This change may be observed in still normal tissue beyond the limits of the tumor. One can but guess at the significance of such a change. Around the tumor there is usually well-marked gliosis.

Astrocytoma.—The astrocytoma is a comparatively benign tumor. The average time of survival after operation is six years (Cushing), and many of the patients appear to be completely cured. The tumor blends so gently with the surrounding tissue that no line of demarcation can be drawn. It is usually much firmer than the glioblastoma owing to the fibrils of which it is composed.

The tumor may occur in any part of the brain. A common site is the cerebellum, especially in children. A distinction must be drawn between astrocytoma of the cerebrum in adults and astrocytoma of the cerebellum in children. The latter is the purest form of astrocytoma, often shows cyst formation, and is the most satisfactory glioma known to the surgeon. Most of the lesion may be represented by a cyst, with only a small nubbin of tumor left in the wall (Fig. 681). Small intraneoplastic cysts may be due to degeneration, but larger cysts, which are often outside the tumor, contain fluid which appears to be a transudate from the surface, and which rapidly accumulates after the cyst is aspirated. Astrocytoma of the cerebrum in adults may be much more cellular, and in places there may be an apparent transition towards glioblastoma.

The *microscopic picture* in a typical case forms a striking contrast to the glioblastoma (Fig. 682). The cells are few, and are uniform in size and shape. Sometimes, how-

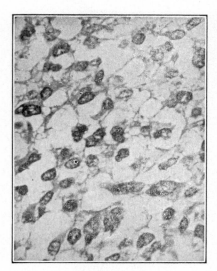

FIG. 682.—Astrocytoma. × 500.

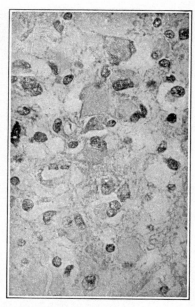

FIG. 683.—Degenerated astrocytes in astrocytoma. × 400.

ever, as the result of degenerative changes there is swelling and hyalinization of the cell body, and displacement of the nucleus to the side (Fig. 683). As already mentioned, in the cerebrum the tumor may be more cellular, and mitoses may occasionally be seen. The cells are separated by numerous glial fibrils, which are well stained with phosphotungstic acid hematoxylin, but are best shown by the gold method (Fig. 684). Neoplastic astrocytes, being often packed together, may be much more elongated than those of the normal brain. Moreover, they may be lacking in vascular footplates, ("sucker feet") which are always present in normal astrocytes. Blood vessels are not numerous. A feature characteristic of astrocytoma is the survival of occasional nerve cells in the midst of the tumor; this must be attributed to lack of destructive power on the part of the tumor. Calcification is not uncommon, and may be seen in the roentgen-ray picture. There is no gliosis around the tumor, and it may be very hard to tell the limits of the growth.

Medulloblastoma.—This highly malignant and rapidly-growing tumor usually occurs in children in the mid-line of the cerebellum (roof of fourth ventricle). It is, indeed, the commonest and the most malignant of the brain tumors of childhood, and it occurs exclusively in the cerebellum. It forms a

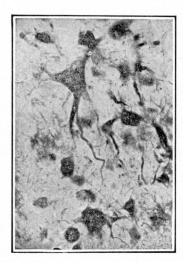

FIG. 684.—Astrocytoma; Cajal's gold-sublimate method. × 300.

soft reddish-gray mass which may fill the cavity of the fourth ventricle, producing marked hydrocephalus. It is the killing tumor of the child, just as glioblastoma is the killing tumor of the adult. In view of the fact that a tumor in the roof of the fourth ventricle of a child may be the extremely malignant medulloblastoma or the extremely

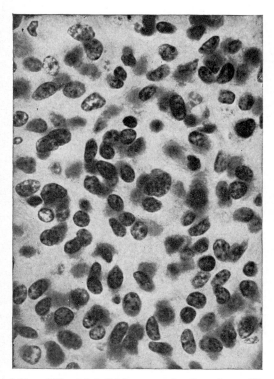

FIG. 685.—Medulloblastoma, showing the undifferentiated character of the tumor. × 700. (Boyd, *Pathology for the Physician.*)

innocent astrocytoma, biopsy confirmation of the tumor type is of great importance. The latter can be treated with complete success, whereas if the former is interfered with it is likely to be spread throughout the subarachnoid space. The medulloblastoma is the only glioma which penetrates the pia and invades the subarachnoid space diffusely. The *microscopic picture* is completely undifferentiated, like that of a round cell sarcoma (Fig. 685). The tumor is extremely cellular and there are no fibrils. The cells are round, but some may be carrot-shaped. The cells may be grouped around blood vessels, forming "pseudorosettes." These differ from the true rosettes of an ependymoma in having no lumen in the center.

Ependymoma.—This tumor is considerably more rare than the three preceding ones. It resembles the medulloblastoma in usually occurring in children and in the roof or floor of the fourth ventricle, but differs from it in being much less malignant and more highly differentiated. It may grow in the cerebrum close to the lateral or third ventricle. The tumor is fairly firm, and calcification, evident in the roentgen-ray picture, is quite common. *Microscopically* the tumor consists of ependymal cells or more primitive

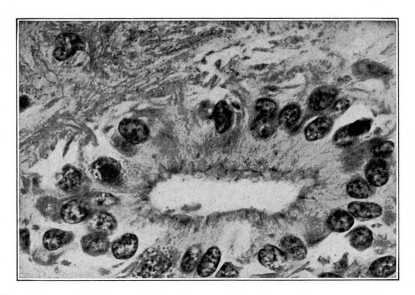

FIG. 686.—Ependymona of fourth ventricle in a boy, aged two years. The tumor cells are grouped around a lumen. Blepharoplasts can be seen in the cytoplasm close to the lumen. × 1000.

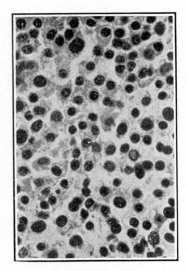

FIG. 687.—Oligodendroglioma.   × 500.

ependymal spongioblasts; the latter are tadpole-shaped, with an elongated tail. As the normal function of ependymal cells is to line a cavity, some of the tumor cells are grouped around small canals; these groups are known as rosettes, and when present in typical form are pathognomonic of ependymoma (Fig. 686). Between the nucleus and the lumen the cytoplasm may contain tiny rods known as blepharoplasts. These are characteristic of ependymal cells, being the remains of chromatin granules at the base of the cilia.

OLIGODENDROGLIOMA.—A very rare tumor of the oligodendroglia, confined to the cerebral hemispheres of adults. Although extremely cellular (Fig. 687), it is slow growing, and shows a marked tendency to perivascular calcification, which can be recognized in the roentgen-ray picture. In ordinary sections the cell bodies are represented by clear spaces like vegetable cells. To prove the nature of the tumor the cell processes must be stained with silver.

SHEATH TUMORS

It has already been pointed out that it is convenient and logical to divide intracranial tumors (with the exception of pituitary tumors which have already been considered in Chapter 35) into brain tumors proper and tumors of the sheaths of the brain. The latter comprise the meningioma and the acoustic nerve tumor.

Meningioma.—This is an innocent tumor (although rarely it may become malignant) and it constitutes one of the commonest forms of intracranial neoplasm. It may be related to trauma. I have seen a meningioma develop at the exact site of a traumatic scar four years after a blow on the head. There is about one meningioma to every four gliomas. The term meningioma is hardly satisfactory from a histogenetic standpoint, but it has the advantage of being noncommittal. The tumor arises from groups of mesothelial cells which cover the arachnoid villi and the Pacchionian bodies, and

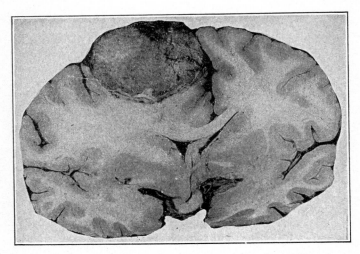

FIG. 688.—Meningioma. The tumor has formed a large depression for itself in the hemisphere, and has caused much distortion of the brain.

may be regarded as a meningeal fibro-blastoma. On account of their mode of origin the tumors are usually situated near the superior longitudinal sinus in the fronto-parietal region, but they may grow from the falx cerebri, or at the base of the skull in the anterior and middle cranial fossa.

The *gross appearance* is very characteristic, for the tumor presses on the brain from the outside and forms a deep bed for itself, from which in the autopsy room it can be readily shelled out (Fig. 688). In the operating room, however, things are far less simple, and the surgeon may readily lose his patient from hemorrhage from large vessels which pass between the highly vascular overlying bone and the tumor. The meningioma is usually much firmer than the glioma. It is adherent externally to the dura. It remains encapsulated, and does not penetrate the pia nor infiltrate the brain, so that it lends itself to surgical removal. *Microscopically* it consists of elongated fibroblastic cells often showing a whorled arrangement (Fig. 689). The whorls may undergo hyaline degeneration and form little masses like epithelial pearls. These may become calcified and resemble corpora amylacea, giving an appearance known as psammoma bodies or brain sand (*psammos*, sand), and on this account the tumor used to be known as a *psammoma*. In rapidly-growing tumors the cells may be rounder and much less differentiated. Occasionally fat may be present (*lipo-meningioma*). *Local changes in the skull* may be of great help in diagnosis. In about 25 per cent of cases there is bony thickening over the tumor which can be detected radiologically and sometimes clinically. This is due to penetration of the dura by the tumor and invasion of the skull, with ossification of the stroma of the invading tumor. In rare cases there may be erosion and perforation of the bone in place of thickening.

It is now realized that the ultimate prognosis is by no means as favorable as has been supposed. In many instances there is recurrence after an interval of years, due evidently to incomplete removal. Details of such cases will be found in Cushing's fine monograph on the meningiomas. The mere fact that extensive infiltration of bone is so frequent indicates that the tumor is not as

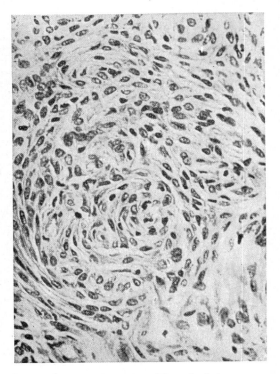

Fig. 689.—Meningioma. The whorled arrangement of the elongated cells is plainly shown. × 400.

benign as might be imagined from the microscopic picture.

Acoustic Nerve Tumor.—This is the second of the sheath tumors, and it resembles the meningioma in many respects. Occurring in the cerebello-pontine angle and growing from the sheath of the acoustic nerve, it forms a firm, round, well-encapsulated tumor, which presses on the brain stem and produces marked distortion and displacement of that structure (Fig. 690). A similar tumor sometimes grows on the roots of the spinal nerves. There is difference of opinion regarding the origin and nature of these tumors. It is usually regarded as a fibroblastoma arising from the perineurium of the nerve, but Masson believes that it is a tumor of the cells of the sheath of Schwann. It is identical in structure with the perineurial fibroblastomas (solitary neuromas) growing on peripheral nerves. The subject is discussed further in connection with tumors of nerves. *Microscopically* it consists of elongated nuclei

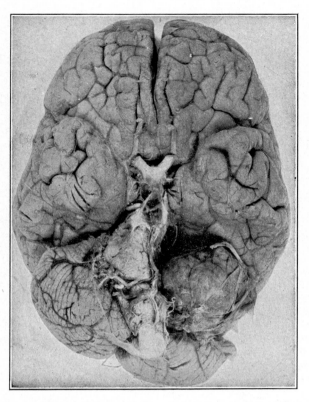

FIG. 690.—Acoustic nerve tumor. The tumor has produced marked distortion of the brain stem.

often arranged side by side so as to produce a characteristic banded or "palisade" appearance (Fig. 691). There may also be eddies or whorls of cells. The outline of the cells is vague, and the background is fibrous in character, probably collagen.

The *clinical effects* are *facial palsy* and *nerve deafness* (seventh and eighth nerves), and the usual signs of intracranial tumor. These effects are the result of involvement of the fifth, seventh and eight nerves, as shown by numbness along the jaw and side of tongue, some facial weakness, and deafness. In addition there are the usual signs of intracranial tumor. An important feature is a nearly invariable *increase of the protein in the cerebrospinal fluid*, although in one of our cases it was normal. It can at least be said that a normal fluid in a posterior fossa tumor nearly always means an intracerebellar lesion. The protein increase may be attributed to blockage of the circulation of cerebrospinal fluid to the spinal subarach-noid space or to compression of the venous channels draining the choroid plexus.

Although these tumors are so well encapsulated and lie completely outside the brain substance, operative treatment in the past has been attended by an appalling mortality. This is due to the proximity of the tumor to the brain stem. In the operation of simple enucleation of these tumors, the finger tears the tumor from the brain stem, injuring the delicate structure, an injury which is intensified by the packing necessary to check the profuse hemorrhage. In cases coming to autopsy, softening and small hemorrhages can be demonstrated in the pons and medulla. Even a simple suboccipital decompression is attended by a high mortality. Here the explanation is rather different. Owing to the position of the tumor, pressure on the aqueduct of Sylvius is of common occurrence, with a resulting hydrocephalus and pressure on the posterior cranial fossa. This pressure is

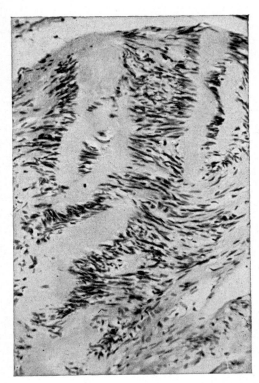

FIG. 691.—Neurinoma, showing characteristic palisading of nuclei. × 150. (Boyd, *Pathology for the Surgeon*, courtesy of W. B. Saunders Co.)

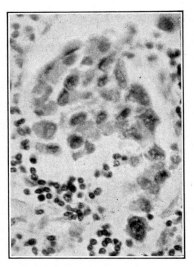

FIG. 692.—Pinealoma, showing the two types of cells. × 400.

minimized by the rough, inelastic tentorium cerebelli, but the moment that a subtentorial decompression is performed the full force of the hydrocephalus is exerted on the delicate brain stem. The method of intracapsular enucleation has greatly lessened the mortality from the operation.

MISCELLANEOUS INTRACRANIAL TUMORS

Pinealoma.—This is a very rare tumor which grows from the pineal body. It occurs for the most part in the second decade, and is marked by symptoms of involvement of the corpora quadrigemina (oculomotor palsies, deafness), and pubertas praecox, *i.e.*, precocious sexual development and adiposity. Whether these endocrine disturbances are of pineal origin or are due to destructive lesions in the region of the pineal and the wall of the third ventricle is open to debate.

Hydrocephalus is marked owing to the position of the tumor. The tumor may be regarded as an "adenoma" of the pineal, for it consists of the two types of cells normally present, very large pineal cells and small round neuroglial cells (Fig. 692). Now that the pineal gland is no longer regarded as the seat of the soul, it has become difficult to ascribe any function to it, although it does appear to produce a powerful lightening agent to which the name of *melatonin* has been given, as it acts on the melanocytes of the skin.

GANGLIONEUROMA.—This is perhaps the rarest of brain tumors. It is composed of adult nerve cells, and is more likely to be found outside the brain, *e.g.*, in the adrenal medulla (page 997).

Retinoblastoma.—This tumor is sometimes called *glioma of the eye*, but it contains no glial fibers, and as it seems to develop from the retinal anlage of the embryo it seems better to call it a retinoblastoma (Fig. 693). Owing to the presence of "rosettes" of columnar cells, it has been regarded as a *neuroepithelioma*. It is the second commonest tumor of the eye, malignant melanoma being the commonest. It is locally destructive, and in the later stages may metastasize to lymph nodes and in-

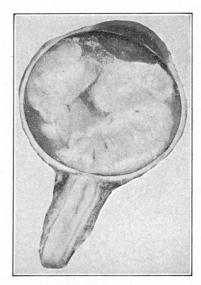

FIG. 693.—Retinoblastoma.

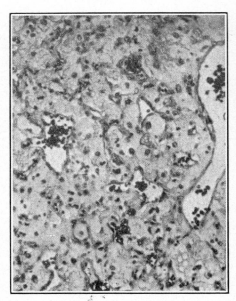

FIG. 694.—Lindau's disease. × 85.

ternal organs, thus proving that it is not a glioma. The tumor consists of small round cells consisting of little more than nuclei, with hardly any cytoplasm and no fibrils. The rosettes when present are characteristic circular structures composed of columnar cells which probably have a tendency to develop into rods and cones. They are often absent. The tumor presents three striking clinical characteristics: (1) over 90 per cent of the cases occur before the fourth year, so that it may be regarded as of congenital origin; (2) it is bilateral in 20 per cent of cases; (3) it displays a remarkable and tragic familial tendency, 10 children out of 16 in one family having died of this tumor.

Hemangioma.—Vascular tumors of the brain can be divided into (1) angiomatous malformations and (2) hemangioblastomas. Each group includes a general systemic disorder as well as the local cerebral lesion. The first condition is a *cavernous angiomatosis of the brain*; it is associated with a similar condition of the skin and with congenital glaucoma. The second is a *capillary angiomatosis of the cerebellum* and is associated with similar lesions of the retina and some of the viscera. The kidneys and the pancreas may be cystic. This angiomatosis of cerebellum and retina is known as *Lindau's disease*. In one case which I studied the

mother, a brother and a sister suffered from lesions both of the cerebellum and retina. In this case the pancreas was a mass of cysts, and many were present in the renal cortex. It is hereditary in character, occurring in one family in three generations. Sometimes the lesions are in the medulla or cord instead of the cerebellum; they never occur in the cerebrum. The tumor is composed of angiomatous spaces between which are xanthoma-like cells filled with lipid (Fig. 694).

Cholesteatoma.—This rare tumor is of developmental origin, arising from epithelial implantations which occur in the development of the embryo. The common site is under the pia, but it may be in the substance of the brain or in one of the ventricles. Depending on the time that the cellular anlage is cut off, the capsule may be either purely epidermal or dermal with hair follicles. In the later case the tumor will be a *dermoid cyst* with the usual buttery contents and wisps of hair. In the much commoner epidermal form the lesion is covered by stratified epidermal cells, which become desquamated and cornified. The *gross appearance* is highly characteristic, and has earned for the lesion the name of *pearly tumor* (Fig. 695). The tumor is globular, and the surface is smooth, silky, of a mother-of-pearl luster,

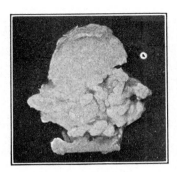

Fig. 695.—Pearly tumor (cholesteatoma.)

and may present pea-sized elevations. The surface can be picked off in flakes. *Microscopically* the tumor consists of layers of polygonal cells filled with granules, fatty material, and cholesterol crystals.

Metastatic Tumors.—When a diagnosis is made of tumor of the brain it must not be forgotten that the tumor may be secondary. By far the commonest site of the primary tumor is the lung, a possible route of transmission being the vertebral system of veins as well as the systemic circulation. Next in frequency comes the breast, followed in my experience by the large intestine and malignant melanoma of the skin. The tumors are usually multiple. When small they remain spherical and circumscribed, but when large and infiltrating they are irregular in shape. Necrosis and hemorrhage are common.

The *clinical picture* is often confused by the multiplicity and wide distribution of the tumors. Involvement of the meninges may give symptoms and signs of meningeal irritation. The course of the disease is apt to be more acute than in the case of a primary tumor. It is of importance to realize that the signs and symptoms may be entirely cerebral, with the primary neoplasm remaining completely silent. This is particularly likely to happen in the case of bronchogenic carcinoma.

Diffuse involvement of the meninges may be the result of invasion of the subarachnoid space by a glioma (usually a medulloblastoma) or a secondary tumor (often a melanoma); sometimes the melanoma seems to originate in the meninges. A mantle of tumor cells may cover the brain and even

the cord, and tumor cells may be found in the spinal fluid obtained by lumbar puncture. The methods of exfoliative cytology which have proved of such value in other regions of the body may enable a diagnosis of metastatic tumor to be made even in the absence of widespread meningeal involvement. The best results are obtained with wet stained films (McCormack *et al.*). The sugar values in the cerebrospinal fluid are likely to be low. The method is also of value in primary brain tumors.

Subacute Cerebellar Disease Associated with Cancer.—This strange and puzzling syndrome, if such it can be called, has nothing to do with cerebellar metastases. The tumor is usually an ovarian carcinoma, but it may be in the lung, breast or uterus. It is known that bronchogenic carcinoma is occasionally associated with peripheral neuropathy. The relationship of cerebellar symptoms with cancer of a distant organ was at first considered to be casual, but it is now regarded as causal although inexplicable. The first evidence of cerebellar involvement is unsteadiness in gait, then clumsiness of the hands and dysarthria of speech. Diplopia is an early symptom, which may be followed by nystagmus and shooting pains in the legs. In a few weeks or months the patient is bed-ridden. Death usually takes places within a year. The rapidity of onset and the progress of cerebellar symptoms may naturally suggest disseminated sclerosis or a cerebellar tumor. The cells and protein of the cerebrospinal fluid are increased and associated with a strong colloidal gold reaction suggestive of multiple sclerosis. The outstanding *microscopic lesion* is a widespread degeneration or loss of the Purkinje cells, which may be so great that few of these cells can be found. The *pathogenesis* is completely obscure, although it has been suggested that the cancer may produce some by-product which interferes with the metabolism of vitamins. It is possible that the tumor cells may compete for material released in the Krebs energy cycle, material that is necessary for the metabolism of cells in the central nervous system. The association of cancer of the pancreas with wandering venous thrombosis (Trousseau's syndrome) may be recalled. The scattered literature on the subject will be found in Greenfield's monograph, *The Spino-Cerebellar Degenerations*, pages 72 to 74.

Relation of Symptoms to Lesions.—Intracranial tumors, whether intracerebral or extracerebral, primary or secondary, may manifest themselves in two ways: (1) general effects, often known as *cardinal signs*, due to increased intracranial pressure, and (2) local effects, which are *focal signs due to disturbed specific brain function*. As we shall see, tumor cells may or may not be present in the spinal fluid.

General Effects.—The problem of increased intracranial pressure has already been discussed in an earlier part of this chapter. The tumor is a space-occupying lesion, but the *edema* which often accompanies it may increase the effect many times. *Secondary hydrocephalus* is perhaps the most important effect, for it is largely responsible for the increased intracranial pressure, and therefore for the classical (though late) symptoms of brain tumor, *i.e.*, headache, vomiting, and optic neuritis. Tumors in the posterior fossa are most likely to cause severe hydrocephalus, but a tumor in any position may produce some dilatation of the ventricles. A tumor in the posterior fossa may block the opening of the aqueduct of Sylvius or may press on the great vein of Galen as it curves around the splenium of the corpus callosum. The vein drains the choroid plexus, and pressure upon it leads to an increased production of cerebrospinal fluid and hydrocephalus. But a tumor in any part of the cranial cavity may cause hydrocephalus. This is probably due to pressure of the brain stem containing the narrow aqueduct of Sylvius against the hard edge of the tentorium cerebelli. *Distortion of the lateral ventricle* by the tumor is a common occurrence, and this can be detected by means of ventriculography, *i.e.*, filling the ventricles with air and taking a roentgen-ray picture. Displacement of a calcified pineal gland in the *x*-ray film is another indication of a space-occupying lesion. The *increased intracranial pressure* causes flattening of the convolutions and obliteration of the subarachnoid space. At operation the brain may not show the normal pulsation. The *optic neuritis* is due to the fluid in the

subarachnoid space being forced into the lymph spaces in the sheath of the optic nerve; this interferes with the venous return, and the result is edema and hemorrhage which give the ophthalmoscopic picture of choked disc and optic neuritis. When the intracranial pressure is high, clusters of arachnoid cells may penetrate the dura and appear on its cranial surface as nodular outgrowths. *Hemorrhage* into a glioma is common, and may cause a sudden exacerbation of symptoms or even death. The *skull* may show a characteristic mottling like beaten silver in the roentgen-ray picture from pressure of the convolutions, due to increased intracranial pressure. In meningioma there may be an even more characteristic local hyperostosis of the overlying bone.

Local Effects.—Local effects may show themselves as symptoms which suggest at an early date the presence and location of a brain tumor. Thus tumors of the frontal lobe are associated with deterioration of the personality, those of the temporal lobe with dreamy states and so-called uncinate fits characterized by unpleasant odors and a feeling of unreality, those of the occipital lobe with visual hallucinations such as scintillating lights. The onset of symptoms may be sudden, such as a stroke due to hemorrhage in the tumor (Fig. 696) or to occlusion of a vessel and thrombosis, but the commonest sudden symptom in the adult is convulsions. The recognition of these early manifestations of cerebral tumor is of great importance. If one waits for the development of such classical signs as vomiting and optic neuritis it is too late for successful neurosurgery. It may be noted that most of the tumors in childhood occur in and around the cerebellum, and that one-third of these are benign.

Spinal Fluid.—The cellular findings in the cerebrospinal fluid may or may not be of value. A pleocytosis, *i.e.* an increase in the cell count, always means something. We must decide, however, whether the increased count is due to tumor cells or merely to a lymphocytosis, the result of meningeal irritation. Moreover, in secondary carcinoma cancer cells may be present without a pleocytosis, and carcinomatous involvement of the meninges may cause a lymphocytic

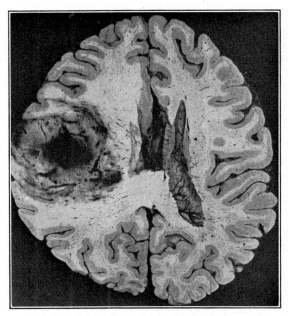

FIG. 696.—Glioblastoma showing hemorrhage in center.

pleocytosis without there being any cancer cells in the spinal fluid. Pleocytosis is most commonly found in glioma, but tumor cells are rarely seen in the fluid, whereas they are frequently found in secondary carcinoma (Fig. 697). A falling spinal fluid glucose level is highly suggestive of carcinomatous menigitis, and the search for tumor cells should be intensified.

SPINAL CORD TUMORS

Tumors of the spinal cord, although rare in comparison with tumors of the brain, are of more frequent occurrence than is commonly supposed; most of them are missed. The majority develop slowly, especially those of the extramedullary variety. The tumor may be (1) *extramedullary* or (2) *intramedullary;* the extramedullary tumors may be (a) *extradural* or (b) *intradural.*

Extramedullary Tumors.—These tumors are frequently benign in character, and there may be an interval of several years between the root symptoms and the appearance of any sign of pressure on the cord. Even when marked pressure has developed there may be little or no degeneration of the cord. *Neurofibromas* are the commonest, followed

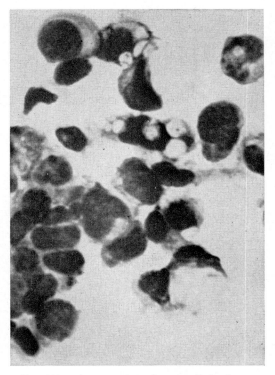

FIG. 697.—A group of carcinoma cells in the cerebrospinal fluid. × 1,150 (primary in bronchus). (McMenemey and Cumings, courtesy of Jour. Clin. Pathology.)

by meningiomas, and then by intramedullary tumors, of which the most frequent are ependymomas. *Extradural tumors* are uncommon. They are often sarcomatous in character, arising either from the outer surface of the dura or from the vertebrae. *Intradural tumors* form the main bulk of spinal cord tumors. The growth is usually benign in character, being either a *meningioma* or a *perineurial fibroma* of the nerve roots similar in character to the acoustic nerve tumor. The tumor is usually oval, seldom grows to a large size, and shows absence of the normal cord pulsation. The cord may be seriously compressed, but is seldom invaded by the tumor.

Dumb-bell tumors do not constitute a special class, but the term is a convenient descriptive one. The tumor is partly in the spinal canal, partly outside it, with the connecting link passing though an intervertebral foramen. It may arise intraspinally and grow out, or arise extraspinally and grow in. It usually originates from the meninges or nerve roots, but may grow from any tissue in this region. A lump may be detected in the cervical region. Compression symptoms develop, with the usual spinal fluid changes associated with compression.

Intramedullary Tumors.—These tumors are *gliomas*. Practically all the forms which have been described as occurring in the brain may be found in the cord. Perhaps the commonest is the *ependymoma*, which arises from the ependymal cells of the central canal. The tumor extends up and down the cord rather than horizontally, and the overlying dura may appear normal. Absence of pulsation indicates the lesion when the surgeon opens the spinal canal.

Relation of Symptoms to Lesions.—Although the cord is much compressed, generally from the side, it is remarkable how few pressure changes develop. It is for this reason that removal of these tumors is often attended with such satisfactory results, especially in the case of extramedullary tumors. In some cases, however, there may be myelitis, hemorrhage and degeneration.

There are three cycles in the life history of any spinal tumor. The *first* or *root cycle* is the longest, and the symptoms are unilateral in the early stage; there is first irritation and then compression of the nerve roots. The *second cycle* is characterized by the Brown-Séquard syndrome, with paralysis of motion and deep sensation on the side of the tumor, loss of pain and temperature sense on the opposite side. The syndrome is present in extramedullary but not intramedullary growths. The *third cycle* is one of paralysis of the organic reflexes (bladder and rectum), and the deep reflexes, together with vasomotor and trophic disturbance. The *cerebrospinal fluid* may show the "compression syndrome" if the canal is blocked. In the *cul-de-sac* below the obstruction the characters of the fluid are as follows: (1) massive spontaneous coagulation; (2) xanthochromia or yellow coloration of the fluid; (3) marked increase in the protein; (4) no corresponding increase in the cells. This is known as the *Froin syndrome*, of which only the last two features may be present. The presence of a block can also be shown by the *Queckenstedt sign* (absence of the normal rise in spinal pressure when both jugular veins are compressed). The exact site may sometimes be determined by the intraspinal injection of lipiodol followed by radiography. Lumbar puncture is, therefore, of great value in the diagnosis of suspected spinal cord tumors.

THE PERIPHERAL NERVES

Injury and Repair.—The effects of injury can be best studied in section of a peripheral nerve. Attention may be confined to one of the individual fibers of which the nerve is composed. When a nerve fiber is divided from its cell of origin the distal part undergoes the changes known as *Wallerian degeneration*, which have already been described in connection with the general pathology of the nervous system. It will be recalled that all three components of the fiber share in thse changes. The axis cylinder disintegrates and disappears, the medullary sheath breaks up into droplets of myelin, and the cells of the sheath of Schwann proliferate and exert a phagocytic action on the degenerated myelin. Similar changes occur in the proximal part up to the first node of Ranvier.

But combined with the degenerative

changes there is soon evidence of attempts at *repair*, just as inflammation of any tissue may pass imperceptibly into regeneration. The proliferated Schwann cells in both proximal and distal ends become arranged in the form of a tube along which new axis cylinders may grow out once more to the periphery. For long there was great difference of opinion as to whether the regeneration was *peripheral*, the new fibers being laid down by the Schwann cells (neurilemma) and joining up later with the proximal end, or *central*, the new fibers being formed as outgrowths from the divided proximal end. Modern opinion is entirely in favor of the central view, but it must be admitted that it is sometimes difficult to account for the speedy return of function which may follow division of a nerve on the hypothesis that the new fibers have grown from the site of the lesion to the motor or sensory end-organ concerned.

In the course of a few days the axis cylinder proceeds to grow out as a bulbous process in search of the missing distal end. This search will be unsuccessful if the distance between the two ends is more than an inch, or if the ends are separated by scar tissue. The surgeon may transplant a piece of nerve to close the gap when it is unduly large, but this piece merely acts as a bridge along which the new fibers may travel to the distal part. When the bulbous end of the axis cylinder reaches the distal portion it puts out fine fibrils which grow down the tubular sheath formed by the proliferated Schwann cells. These fibrils reëstablish the continuity of the pathway and become clothed again, with the assistance of the Schwann cells, by a medullary sheath. The rate of growth varies from one case to another, with an average of perhaps 1 to 3 mm. per day. If the distance is too great to be bridged or if the part supplied by the nerve has been amputated, the axis cylinder may coil up so as to form a nodule capped by fibrous tissue. Such a mass at the ends of a nerve, composed of nervous and fibrous tissue, is called an *amputation neuroma* (stump neuroma). Some degree of sensation may reappear fairly quickly, but complete restoration of function, even when the cut ends are brought into accurate apposition,

seldom occurs in less than three or four months.

The process which has just been described is only seen in the peripheral nerves. In the central nervous system the fibers do not possess a sheath of Schwann, so that while Wallerian degeneration takes place as before, real repair is impossible.

A different type of reaction is the *segmental degeneration of Gombault*, which occurs in incomplete lesions of varying cause. This is a periaxial demyelination involving one or more segments accompanied by a proliferation of phagocytic histocytes. The axis cylinders may appear to remain intact, but their conducting power may be impaired or lost, just as an electric current may be short-circuited without the wire being cut.

Neuritis.—The structure of the peripheral nerves is simple and the method of reaction in disease is limited. Perhaps for these very reasons the subject of neuritis is as confused and complex as any in the entire field of neuropathology. This confusion is well reflected in the various systems of classification and nomenclature which have been suggested and employed. Indeed the very term "neuritis" is a misnomer, for the lesions are degenerative rather than inflammatory in character, and are described better as neuropathy than neuritis.

At the present time there is no perfect nor even generally accepted classification of neuritis. At the risk of oversimplification we shall recognize two main groups of disturbance in the peripheral nerves: (1) primary or idiopathic acute polyneuropathy, in which involvement of the nerves is widespread and in which a disturbed immunological mechanism may be at fault; (2) secondary "neuritis," in which some causal factor can be recognized or suggested, and in which one or several nerves may be involved.

Acute Primary Polyneuropathy.—In 1859 Landry described a condition of "acute ascending paralysis," in which first the legs, then the arms, then the muscles of the trunk, and finally those of respiration were paralyzed. The condition, which came to be known as *Landry's paralysis*, was not necessarily ascending, for in some cases it would commence in the face and pass down-

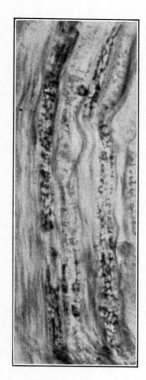

FIG. 698.—Demyelination in toxic neuritis. × 150.

ward. In 1916 Guillain and Barré described a condition of polyneuritis which developed in the wake of upper respiratory infections, grippe, skin abscesses, or infectious mononucleosis. What came to be known as the *Guillain-Barré syndrome* was marked by a slowly ascending flaccid motor paralysis associated with sensory disturbances such as paresthesias and severe root pains. Recovery was usual in a matter of months. In the occasional fatal cases lesions were said to be present in the brain, meninges and cord as well as in the nerves and nerve roots. The *cerebrospinal fluid* showed an *albumino-cytological dissociation*, the total protein content being considerably raised, while the lymphocytes were normal or only slightly increased in number.

It would now appear that the Guillain-Barré syndrome is the same condition as Landry's paralysis, and the former name has replaced the latter (Haymaker and Kernohan). It is a diffuse radiculoneuronitis which may commence in any peripheral nerve, spinal or cranial, motor or sensory, but generally begins in the limbs. Death is due to respiratory failure caused by involvement of the intercostal nerves. The cranial nerves are usually affected, as shown by dysphagia, dysarthria or aphonia. In the peripheral nerves the most marked lesions are found at the beginning of the spinal nerves, with progressive destruction of the myelin sheath which breaks up into droplets of myelin (Fig. 698), and later of the axis cylinders and the sheath of Schwann. If the patient lives sufficiently long the microscopic picture is one of final devastation.

The polyneuropathy has followed prophylactic inoculation against rabies, typhoid, tetanus, pertussis, etc. There is no real justification for the common name *infective neuritis*, although some features of the syndrome suggest a viral etiology, and an Echo virus has been isolated from the cerebrospinal fluid and feces. It would appear, rather, to be a manifestation of *hypersensitivity* to a variety of antigenic stimuli, rather than to direct infection with some one virus (Kisch). The cases may be divided into three groups: (1) those associated with or following viral or bacterial infections; (2) those following the parenteral administration of foreign proteins (immunization procedures, blood transfusion); (3) those in which there is no evident antecedent. The common denominator seems to be an *allergic reaction*. Strong support for this concept has been provided by the discovery that it is possible to produce an *experimental allergic neuritis* (EAN) (Waksman and Adams). When rabbit sciatic nerve or root ganglia are used the lesions are confined to the roots, the ganglia, and the peripheral nerves, with none of the changes in the central nervous system and meninges which characterize the experimental allergic encephalomyelitis (EAE) produced by sensitizing the animal by inoculations of brain or spinal cord together with a suitable adjuvant. Whether we can apply the experimental evidence to human polyneuritis is a matter which must be left to the future to decide. The all-important question still left unanswered is the nature of the antigen which acts on the sensitized myelin.

Carcinomatous neuropathy and *neuromyo-*

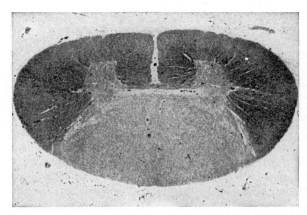

Fig. 699.—Carcinomatous neuropathy. Entire section of the lumbar spinal cord stained for myelin sheaths, showing extensive degeneration in the posterior column. (Case Records of the Massachusetts General Hospital in New Engl. J. Med.)

pathy may be included tentatively in this group, because of the possibility that nervous tissues or muscles may be sensitized to some product of the neoplasm (Brain and Henson). It is a primary sensory neuropathy with muscular changes associated with carcinoma. Cancer of the lung is most often at fault, but the condition is also found with other primary sites, such as the ovary, prostate, rectum, and breast. Neurologic changes tend to occur without relation to stages of the neoplastic growth. Symptoms may appear at least three years before tumor is even suspected. *Sensorimotor symptoms* can develop and totally vanish six months before direct evidence of cancer is apparent. There may be sensory peripheral neuropathy without motor symptoms. They are associated with degeneration and loss of neurones in the posterior root ganglia, breakdown of myelin sheaths in the posterior roots and peripheral nerves and loss of myelin in the posterior columns of the cord (Fig. 699). We have already seen that subacute cerebellar disease with widespread degeneration or loss of the Purkinje cells may be causally associated with cancer (page 1207). The condition is, of course, a baffling enigma. There is no relation between the onset, severity, or progression of the neuropathic symptoms and the size or rate of growth of the carcinoma.

"*Brachial neuritis*" is a rather common but little understood disorder which may be included in this group. It is a unilateral involvement of the brachial plexus which occurs at the height of a serum reaction or folowing some mild infection. Why it should involve the brachial plexus and only on one side is a complete mystery. Such a distribution is more characteristic of the second group of neural disturbances.

Secondary Neuritis.—It is natural that the peripheral nerves should be exposed to the action of a variety of injurious agents. Some of these will cause a true inflammation of the nerve, whilst others produce degenerative changes. It is convenient because of long usage to use the term neuritis to include these various conditions.

Trauma is one of the commonest causes of peripheral nerve injury. Traumatic neuritis may be the result of a wound, of sudden stretching, or of compression against an underlying bony surface or from pressure by a crutch. Exposure to cold may be included in this group. The effect is a localized neuritis.

Heavy metals may have an affinity for nerves and cause a polyneuritis. Of these lead and arsenic are amongst the most important. The motor fibers are especially vulnerable to lead. In arsenical poisoning both motor and sensory fibers, especially in their distal portion, are likely to be affected. The lesion is a patchy segmental degeneration of the Gombault type already mentioned.

Diphtheritic neuritis, which is more likely

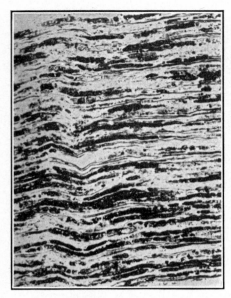

Fig. 700.—Demyelination in alcoholic neuritis.
× 75. (Boyd, *Pathology for the Physician.*)

to develop in children than in adults, is naturally attributed to the action of the diphtheria toxin on local peripheral nerves. Early in the disease this is no doubt true, and serves to explain the paralysis of the palate and of accommodation which are so characteristic. But after the disease is gone and forgotten a very different picture may develop, which is of great interest to us in view of the foregoing discussion. After a delay of three or four months the symptoms of a generalized sensory-motor polyneuritis may develop, often without evidence of a preceding local neuritis. This has all the earmarks of the allergic polyneuropathy already discussed, and the cerebrospinal fluid shows the albumin-cellular dissociation which is so characteristic of that immunological disturbance.

Deficiency neuritis is best illustrated in the case of *beri beri* due to thiamine deficiency. The sensory-motor nerves to the limbs are involved, and may show all degrees of change from mild segmental demyelination to advanced Wallerian degeneration. *Alcoholic neuritis* is also dependent on deficiency of B vitamins, not on the toxic action of the alcohol. Demyelination may be pronounced (Fig. 700).

Ischemic neuritis may be a polyneuritis due to vascular occlusion. Narrowing of the lumen of nutrient arteries to the peripheral nerves in polyarteritis nodosa is responsible for the neuritic pains so common in that disease. The nerves show corresponding degeneration of myelin. The most distinctive clinical feature is the asymmetrical distribution of the lesions, although occasionally it may be symmetrical, and sometimes only a single nerve is involved. Pressure neuritis (from crutch, *etc.*) may be due to ischemia as well as trauma.

Metabolic disorders may be associated with polyneuritis, possibly through interference with the metabolism of myelin. *Acute porphyria* is a mysterious and fortunately rare malady which presents clinical features suggestive of polyneuritis. It generally begins with symptoms suggestive of an ascending paralysis, such as pain and weakness in the extremities. Other features are colicky abdominal pains, mental symptoms, and epileptic seizures. The urine is a port-wine red, but may be colorless, only turning the characteristic color when exposed to sunlight. The condition is really an acute exacerbation of a chronic condition characterized by the passage of a porphyrin in the urine. The *nervous system lesions* are degeneration of the peripheral and sympathetic nerves, and of cells in the anterior horns and various parts of the brain. Degenerative lesions are also found in the liver, spleen, kidneys and muscles. The general subject of porphyria is discussed in detail on page 398.

Diabetic neuritis, like that of acute porphyria, may be regarded as belonging to the metabolic group. In about 4 per cent of poorly controlled diabetics sensory symptoms develop in the lower limbs, such as burning pains in the calves and paresthesias in the feet. Much more rarely there is a generalized polyneuropathy involving all the extremities, with both motor and sensory disturbance. Even single nerve trunks are sometimes affected. Finally it is possible that the *carcinomatous neuropathy* already discussed should be placed in the group of metabolic disorders.

Tumors.—The tumors of nerves form a remarkably confusing and complex subject regarding which a large amount might be said without adding very much to the reader's knowledge. The chief cleavage of opinion is as to which constituent of the nerve the neurinoma or ordinary nerve tumor arises from. This is commonly believed to be the connective tissue of the perineurium, and the tumor is, therefore, called *perineurial fibrcma* or *fibroblastoma*. On the other hand Masson and others maintain that it arises from the cells of the sheath of Schwann, and call it a *schwannoma*. Disregarding controversy and employing generally accepted terms the following main types may be recognized: (1) neurofibroma (perineurial fibroma, neurinoma, schwannoma), a conventional name indicating a nerve tumor resembling a fibroma without regard to its cell of origin; (2) neurofibromatosis (Von Recklinghausen's disease); and (3) neurogenic sarcoma.

No matter which view may be adopted, an examination of the different tumors will show the following common features: long, slender, wire-like fibers with elongated nuclei which have a tendency to be arranged in parallel or palisade fashion (Fig. 701); in addition to the palisading, which always suggests a nerve sheath origin, the nuclei may be grouped in eddies and streams. The more benign the tumor, the more pronounced are these features. The palisading is perhaps best seen in the acoustic nerve tumor and the similar tumors which occur in the spinal nerve roots, while the whorls are characteristic of meningioma. In the more malignant forms these characters naturally tend to be lost.

Neurofibroma.—This is a benign tumor which forms a round or fusiform firm white mass on the course of one of the larger nerves. It is attached to the sheath of the nerve, but the nerve fibers are not incorporated in the tumor, so that the term perineurial fibroma appears to be justified. *Microscopically* it is composed of long slender cells, the elongated nuclei of which are arranged in palisades or show whorls and eddies.

Neurofibromatosis: Von Recklinghausen's Disease.—In this peculiar and often familial condition there are large numbers of tumors, sometimes several hundreds of them, growing from the fine cutaneous nerves, so that the

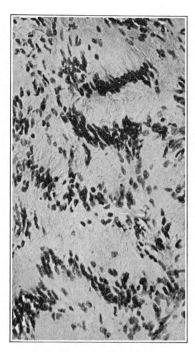

FIG. 701.—Neurofibroma (Schwannoma) showing palisading of nuclei. × 225.

condition is also known as multiple neurofibromata. They form soft nodules in the skin (*molluscum filrosum*), and may be distributed over the entire body. The skin is often pigmented in patches, or there may be groups of brown spots like freckles. Moreover some members of a family may develop nerve tumors, while others only have spots of pigment. Peculiar soft overgrowths of connective tissue may occur, causing great enlargement of a limb, a form of elephantiasis. Megacolon, giant appendix, and other similar overgrowths have been described in connection with similar lesions of the visceral nerves. It seems justifiable to regard the condition as more of a connective-tissue reaction that is part of a general process than as a simple tumor, neurofibromatosis rather than neurofibroma. Acoustic nerve tumor and meningioma may be associated with the condition, and there is always some intermingling of perineurial fibromatous tissue. *Microscopically* the same general picture is seen once again, but the structure is much more mixed. The

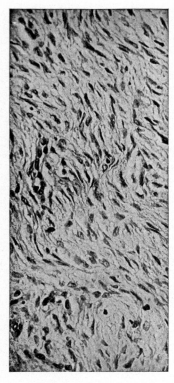

FIG. 702.—Neurogenic sarcoma showing the fasciculated arrangement. × 300.

characteristic tissue has a tangled or reticular structure, *which suggests a malformation rather than a neoplasm;* this tissue does not show palisading or whorls. It often undergoes a jelly-like hyaline degeneration. Superimposed on this reticular tissue is a varying amount of tissue of neurofibromatous type with palisades and whorls. When special stains are used nerve fibrils can be seen passing through the mass; this never occurs in a neurofibroma. It would appear that in von Recklinghausen's disease all the elements composing the nerve are involved in some degree, possibly due to failure of the insulating function of the sheath of Schwann.

Neurogenic Sarcoma.—Malignant tumors may arise from neurofibromas and from neurofibromatosis. The resulting tumor is called a *malignant schwannoma* by those who believe that the cell of origin is the Schwann cell. About half the cases arise in

persons with von Recklinghausen's disease. They occur at a younger age in the female, a fact which probably has a hormonal basis. The majority develop along a recognizable peripheral nerve. They form single, slowly-growing, infiltrating tumors, usually in the subcutaneous and intermuscular tissue of the arm and leg, the commonest location being the thigh. More rarely they occur in the viscera. *Microscopically* the tumor consists of elongated cells or fibers arranged in interlacing bundles and whorls showing a "curly" arrangement, in contrast to the parallel disposition of the fibers of a fibroma, an appearance always suggestive of a neurogenic origin (Fig. 702). There is not the palisading of a neurofibroma, the cells are more swollen, and there may be mitotic figures. The earliest evidence of malignancy is said to be the presence of large hyperchromatic nuclei.

DEFECTS OF DEVELOPMENT

The development of the central nervous system is indeed complex, and it is small wonder that many errors may occur during its course. It is convenient to attribute these errors to genetic mutation of unknown origin, but we are becoming aware of certain external factors which may play a part in the early stages of development. Amongst these may be mentioned German measles and perhaps other virus disease in the first trimester of pregnancy, irradiation from atomic bomb fallout or *x*-radiation, and cerebral hypoxia from various causes.

Brain.—*Anencephaly* is a condition in which the cranial vault is deficient and practically the entire brain is missing with the exception of some nervous tissue at the base of the posterior cranial fossa. The spinal cord may be absent except for some flattened plates of nerve tissue, yet the nerves are well developed, as is the body in general. The explanation of this is not evident. There is a remarkable atrophy of the adrenal cortex in the anencephalic monster; the nature of this atrophy is discussed in Chapter 36. The condition is incompatible with life. There may be a deficiency in the skull, usually in the line of a suture, with protrusion of the contents of the cranial cavity. A protrusion of the meninges is called a *meningocele*, which is a sac filled with cerebrospinal fluid and communicating with the subarachnoid space. An *encephalocele* is a protrusion of the brain, substance, a condition often associated with and dependent upon hydrocephalus. *Microcephaly* is a condition in which the brain usually the cerebral hemispheres, remains small. The convolutions may not develop, a condition of *microgyria*. *Porencephaly* is a lack of development of a superficial part of a hemisphere; the resulting space is filled with fluid, covered by membranes, and usually communicates with the lateral ventricle.

Tuberous Sclerosis.—This is a congenital condition in which tumor-like masses of neuroglia are scattered throughout the brain. The masses vary in size from that of a pea to that of a walnut. In the areas the cells are chiefly large astrocytes. The condition is often associated with congenital malformations and tumors in other organs, more particularly with rhabdomyoma in the heart, sebaceous adenomas in the skin, and embryoma in the kidney.

Arnold-Chiari Malformation.—This is a deformity of the hind-brain associated with congenital hydrocephalus in which there is a displacement of parts of the cerebellum and brain stem through the foramen magnum into the upper part of the vertebral canal. The displaced structures form a tongue-like process and the fourth ventricle is greatly elongated (Fig. 703). The modern view is that the displaced tissue plugs the foramen magnum, and that the *hydrocephalus* is due to the inability of the cerebrospinal fluid to pass around the brain stem and reach the cerebral subarachnoid space (Russell and Donald). There is perhaps more to be said for Chiari's original opinion, expressed in 1891, that the displacement of the brain stem is the result and not the cause of the hydrocephalus, which itself is due to embryonal atresia of the foramina in the roof of the fourth ventricle. The pulsating choroid plexus of the embryo acts like an unvalved pump, forcing the hind-brain into the vertebral canal (Gardner).

SPINAL CORD.—The spinal canal may remain entirely open especially in the lumbar region, a condition known as *rhachischisis* and often associ-

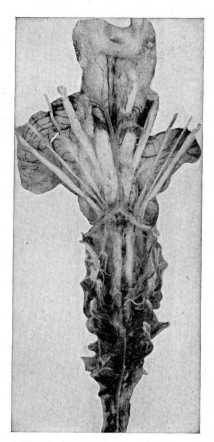

Fig. 703.—Arnold-Chiari malformation. (Boyd, *Pathology for the Surgeon*, courtesy of W. B. Saunders Co.)

ated with anencephaly. *Spina bifida* is a much more common and important condition, in which the neural arches remain open, but the canal is closed by the soft parts. The contents of the canal are protruded under the skin to form a soft mass which at once calls attention to the condition. Sometimes there is no protrusion and swelling to indicate the defect, so that the lesion is hidden, a condition known as *spina bifida occulta*. Its presence is indicated by a patch of hair on the wrinkled skin covering the defect; this hair may resemble a small tail. As the lower part of the canal is the last to close, spina bifida is commonest in the lumbo-sacral region. As a rule five or six vertebræ are involved, sometimes only one. The condition occurs about once in every 1000 births. The contents of the sac may be of three varieties: (1) meningomyelocele, (2) meningocele, (3) syringomyelocele. In the *meningomyelocele* (myelocele), which is the common form, the cord and the nerves of the cauda equina are spread out on the wall of the sac to which they are attached, producing a dimple of the skin known as the umbilicus. In the *meningocele*, which usually occurs in the sacral region, the sac is formed by a hernial protrusion of the arachnoid, the cord or cauda equina remaining within the vertebral canal. The *syringomyelocele* is a rare form in which there is great distention of the central canal and thinning of the cord tissue, so that the wall of the sac is the wall of the canal and is lined by ependymal cells. Spina bifida is often associated with congenital hydrocephalus. *Sacrococcygeal tumors* of developmental origin occur at the lower end of the spinal canal. Some of these are true teratomata, containing well-formed adult tissue. Dermoid tumors, lipomas and cysts may be present either inside or outside the canal. Other tumors appear to arise from remains of the neurenteric canal. The chief *symptoms* are paralysis of the bladder and rectum, weakness in the muscles of the legs leading to clubfoot, trophic ulcers, etc.; these are caused by pressure on the nerve centers. In spina bifida occulta the symptoms appear to be due to a fibrous cord stretching from the skin through the vertebral defect to be attached to the termination of the cord. As the vertebral column grows faster than the cord, it is evident that there will be an increasing degree of traction on the cord with the production of symptoms which may be very puzzling until the defect is discovered.

Sacrococcygeal Pilonidal Sinus.—This is a lesion which arises in the mid line in relation to the skin dimple at the tip of the coccyx, and has long been regarded as due to an error in development involving a remnant of the medullary canal. For this reason it is included in this place for convenience but without justification, as will soon become apparent. A sinus tract may extend from the dimple deep into the tissues, sometimes as far as the vertebral bodies. This tract can readily become infected owing to the anatomical site of the lesion, and very extensive dissections and excisions of large blocks of tissue have been performed with the object of removing a congenital channel lined by epidermis, only to be followed by recurrence.

This view has now been challenged, and an alternative concept has been suggested on good grounds that the condition may be of *acquired* rather than developmental origin (Patey and Scarff, Davage). Pilonidal means a nest of hair, and the hair which forms a striking feature of the lesion was supposed to arise from the epidermis lining the sinus. A similar lesion, an infective and granulomatous reaction to buried hair, (customers' hair) has been reported on barbers' hands. This interdigital pilonidal sinus may be considered an occupational disease of barbers. The hairs do not arise from the wall of the sinus, for they are short and without bulbs, as was noted by the early observers one hundred years ago, they lie free in granulation or scar tissue, and they may be surrounded by foreign body giant cells. It is believed that the *initial phase* of the process is the introduction of bacteria into the tissues with resulting infection and sinus formation, followed by the entrance of hairs into the sinus with the production of a foreign body granulomatous reaction and subsequent epithelization of the sinus from the surface. The hairs may be sucked in by negative pressure resulting from the alternating pressure and relaxation of the soft tissues of the internatal region against the coccyx during prolonged sitting. The condition has indeed been called "jeep disease" by army surgeons. The sinus is therefore an acquired lesion produced by infection rather than a pre-existing lesion which becomes infected. The civilized practice of using toilet paper may contribute to the retention of broken ends of hair mixed with fecal residue in the internatal cleft. It is of interest to note that pilonidal sinus is very uncommon in India, where personal cleansing after defecation is by means of water; toilet paper is never used by the native population, such use being looked down upon as very unhygienic.

The importance of this change in concept is that in the past extensive dissections to remove in entirety a mythical congenital sinus have resulted in extensive scarring and prolonged hospitalization for a condition which in its primary stages carries a trifling disability. When the cases are treated early by means of conservative measures such as hot fomentations and appropriate antibiotics, the average period of hospitalization is reduced to a few days (Klass). The age incidence of pilonidal sinus is of interest, for the condition is sharply limited to a distinct age group of between fifteen and thirty. This age incidence is at variance with that of congenital lesions, and the sharp drop in incidence at the age of thirty must indicate a naturally self-limiting condition. The lesion is much more common in the male, particularly in young soldiers.

REFERENCES

ADAMS, C. W. M.: J. Path. & Bact., 1959, 77, 648. (Staining of myelin.)

ADAMS, R. D. in *Allergic Encephalomyelitis*, edit. by Kies, M. W. and Aloord, E. C., Springfield, Ill., 1959. (Human demyelinating diseases.)

ADAMS, R. D. and KUBIK, C. S.: Am. J. Med., 1952, 12, 510. (Demyelinating diseases.)

ASZKANAZY, C. L.: J. Neuropath. & Exper. Neurol., 1952, 11, 392. (Sarcoidosis of central nervous system.)

BAKAY, L.: *The Blood-Brain Barrier*, Springfield, Ill., 1956.

BAKER, R. D.: J.A.M.A., 1957, *163*, 805. (Cerebral mucormycosis).

BEARN, A. C.: Am. J. Med., 1957, *17*, 747. (Wilson's disease.)

BERES, D. and MELTZER, T.: Am. J. Path., 1938, *14*, 59. (Tuberculous meningitis.)

BIRSE, SHEILA H. and TOM, MARY I.: Neurology, 1960, *10*, 101. (Cerebral infarction in ruptured intracranial aneurysms.)

BOGDANOVE, L. H. and CLARK, G.: J. Neuropath. & Exper. Neurol., 1957, *16*, 57, (Allergic encephalomyelitis.)

BOTTERELL, E. H. and DRAKE, C. G.: J. Neurosurg., 1952, *9*, 348. (Brain abscess.)

BRAIN, R. and HENSON, R. A.: Lancet, 1958, *2*, 971. (Carcinomatous neuromyopathies.)

BUCKLEY, S. M.: Am. J. Path., 1957, *33*, 691. (Cytopathology of poliomyelitis virus in tissue culture.)

CARMICHAEL, R.: J. Path. & Bact., 1950, *62*, 1. (Congenital aneurysms.)

CARRINGTON, K. W.: J. Mich. State Med. Soc., 1959, *58*, 373. (Hydrocephalus.)

CAVANAGH, J. B.: J. Clin. Path., 1953, *6*, 128. (Drug encephalitis.)

CHEATHAM, W. J.: Am. J. Path., 1953, *29*, 401. (Herpes zoster.)

COOPER, I. S.: *The Neurosurgical Alleviation of Parkinsonism*, Springfield, Ill., 1956.

CUMINGS, J. N.: J. Clin. Path., 1959, *12*, 489. (Chemistry of the cerebral lipids.)

DALLDORF, G., SICKLES, G. M., PLAGER, H. and GIFFORD, R.: J. Exper. Med., 1949, *89*, 567. (Coxsackie virus.)

DAVAGE, O. N.: Am. J. Path., 1954, *30*, 1191. (Pilonidal sinus.)

FIELDS, W. T. and HALPERT, B.: Am. J. Path., 1953, *29*, 677. (Brain stem hemorrhage in intracranial hypertension.)

FAZEKAS, J. F.: Am. J. Med., 1958, *25*, 89. (Pathological physiology of cerebral dysfunction.)

FISHER, M.: Can. Med. Ass. J., 1953, *69*, 257. (Strokes).

————.: Arch. Neurol. & Psychiat, 1951, *65*, 346; 1954, *72*, 187. (Cerebral softening.)

FOWLER, M. and ROBERTSON, E. G.: Aust. Ann. Med., 1959, *8*, 8. (Kuru.)

GAJDUSEK, D. C. and ZIGAS, V.: Am. J. Med., 1959, *26*, 442. (Kuru.)

GARDNER, W. J.: Cleveland Clinic Quart., 1959, *26*, 206. (Arnold-Chiari malformation.)

GERSCHENFELD, H. M., ZADUNAISKY, J. A. and DEROBERTIS, E. P. D.: Neurology, 1959, *9*, 412. (Function of astroglia in water-ion metabolism.)

GLASER, G. H.: Arch. Neurol. and Psychiat., 1952, *67*, 745. (Systemic lupus lesions in central nervous system.)

GLYNN, L. E.: J. Path. & Bact., 1940, *51*, 213. (Congenital aneurysms.)

GREEN, J. B., *et al.*: New Eng. J. Med., 1957, *256*, 220. (Cerebrospinal fluid transaminase in cerebral infarction.)

GREENFIELD, J. G., BLACKWOOD, W., McMENEMEY, W. H., MEYER, A. and NORMAN, R. M. *Neuropathology*, London, 1958.

HAYMAKER, W. and KERNOHAN, J. W.: Medicine, 1949, *28*, 59. (Landry-Guillain-Barré syndrome)

HERRICK, W. W.: Arch. Int. Med., 1919, *23*, 409. (Meningococcal meningitis.)

HURST, E. W.: J. Path. & Bact., 1929, *32*, 457; 1931, *34*, 331. (Experimental poliomyelitis.)

HUTCHINSON, E. C. and YATES, P. O.: Lancet, 1957, *1*, 2. (Caroticovertebral stenosis.)

HUTCHINSON, E. C. and STOCK, J. P. P.: Lancet, 1960, *2*, 445. (Carotid sinus syndrome.)

KERNOHAN, J. W. and SAYRE, G. P.: *Tumors of the Central Nervous System, Atlas of Tumor Pathology*, Armed Forces Institute of Pathology, Washington, D. C., 1952.

KERNOHAN, J. W., *et al.*: Proc. Staff Meet., Mayo Clinic, 1949, *24*, 71. (Classification of gliomas.)

KISCH, A. L.: New Eng. J. Med., 1958, *258*, 83. (Guillain-Barré syndrome.)

KLASS, A. A.: Can. Med. Ass. J., 1956, *75*, 737. (Pilonidal sinus.)

KLATZO, I., GAJDUSEK, D. C. and ZIGAS, V.: Lab. Invest., 1959, *8*, 799. (Pathology of Kuru.)

KOVACS, E.: J. Pediat., 1955, *46*, 691. (Nucleases in the cerebrospinal fluid.)

KURLAND, L. T.: Proc. Staff Meetings, Mayo Clinic, 1957, *32*, 449. (Epidemiology of amyotrophic lateral sclerosis.)

LIPKIN, L. E.: Am. J. Path., 1959, *35*, 1117. (Cytoplasmic inclusions in Parkinsonian states.)

LUMSDEN, C. E.: Brit. Med. J., 1951, *1*, 1035. (Pathology of multiple sclerosis.)

MAGOUN, H. W.: *The Waking Brain*, Springfield, Ill., 1958.

MARGOLIS, G.: Am. J. Path., 1953, *29*, 588. (Alzheimer's disease.)

McCORMACK, L. J.: Am. J. Clin. Path., 1953, *23*, 470. (Secondary tumors of brain.)

McMENEMEY, W. H. and CUMINGS, J. N.: J. Clin. Path., 1959, *12*, 400. (Cerebrospinal fluid in intracranial tumors.)

PATEY, D. H. and SCARFF, D. W.: Lancet, 1948, *2*, 13. (Pilonidal sinus.)

PENFIELD, W.: *Cytology and Cellular Pathology of the Nervous System*, New York, 1932.

POTTER, J. M.: Brain, 1959, *82*, 367. (Cerebral arterial spasm.)

QUASTEL, J. H. and SCHOLEFIELD, P. G.: Am. J. Med., 1958, *25*, 420. (Biochemical aspects of cerebral dysfunction.)

RICH, A. R. and McCORDOCK, H. A.: Bull. Johns Hopkins Hosp., 1929, *44*, 273; 1933, *52*, 5. (Tuberculous meningitis.)

RICHARDSON, J. C. and HYLAND, H. H.: Medicine, 1941, *20*, 1. (Spontaneous subarachnoid hemorrhage.)

ROSS, R. S. and McKUSICK, V. A.: Arch. Int. Med., 1953, *92*, 701. (Aortic arch syndrome.)

ROTHENBERG, S. F. and CORDAY, E.: J.A.M.A., 1957, *164*, 2005. (Transient cerebral strokes.)

RUSSELL, DOROTHY, S.: *Observations on the Pathology of Hydrocephalus*, London, 1949.

RUSSELL, DOROTHY, S. and DONALD, C.: Brain, 1935, *58*, 203. (Arnold-Chiari syndrome and hydrocephalus.)

RUSSELL, DOROTHY, S. and RUBINSTEIN, L. J.: *Pathology of Tumors of the Nervous System*, London, 1959.

SABIN, A. B.: J.A.M.A., 1959, *171*, 863. (Attenuated poliomyelitis vaccine.)

SAPHIR, O. and WILE, S. A.: Am. J. Med. Sci., 1942, *203*, 781. (Myocarditis in poliomyelitis.)

SPRIGGS, A. I.: J. Clin. Path., 1954, *7*, 122. (Malignant cells in cerebrospinal fluid.)

STEHBENS, W. E.: J. Path. & Bact., 1959, *78*, 179. (Medial defects of cerebral arteries.)

STEINER, J. W. and GELBLOOM, A. J.: Arthritis and Rheumatism, 1959, *2*, 537. (Rheumatoid lesions in central nervous system.)

TERPLAN, K. L.: Am. J. Path., 1953, *29*, 616. (Tuberculous meningitis and streptomycin therapy.)

THOMISON, J. B. and SHAPIRO, J. L.: Arch. Path. 1957, *63*, 527. (Adrenal lesions in acute meningococcemia.)

TOMLINSON, B. E.: J. Clin. Path., 1959, *12*, 391. (Cerebral infarction in subarachnoid hemorrhage.)

TORACK, R. M., TERRY, R. D. and ZIMMERMAN, H. M.: Am. J. Path., 1959, *35*, 1135. (Cerebral fluid accumulation.)

WAKSMAN, B. H. and ADAMS, R. D.: J. Exper. Med., 1955, *102*, 213; J. Neuropath and Exper. Neurol., 1956, *15*, 293. (Allergic polyneuropathy.)

WINDLE, W. F.: *Biology of Neuroglia*, Springfield, Ill., 1958.

ZIMMERMAN, H. M. and MAIER, N.: Am. J. Path., 1949, *25*, 801. (Gliomas.)

Chapter 43

The Bones

General Considerations
  STRUCTURE AND FUNCTION
  BONE FORMATION
    Osteosclerosis
    Pathological Calcification
    Pathological Ossification
  BONE RESORPTION
    Osteoporosis
    Osteomalacia
  REPAIR OF BONE
    Healing of a Fracture
    Fate of a Bone Graft
Inflammations
  ACUTE OSTEOMYELITIS
  CHRONIC OSTEOMYELITIS
    Brodie's abscess; typhoid
      osteomyelitis
  TUBERCULOSIS
    Pott's Disease
  SARCOIDOSIS
  SYPHILIS
Aseptic (Ischemic) Necrosis
  LEGG-PERTHES' DISEASE, ETC.
Osteodystrophies
  OSTEITIS FIBROSA
    Focal Form

FIBROUS DYSPLASIA
PAGET'S DISEASE
RICKETS
OSTEOMALACIA
SENILE OSTEOPOROSIS
RENAL OSTEODYSTROPHY
RADIATION OSTEODYSTROPHY
HYPERTROPHIC OSTEO-
  ARTHROPATHY
HYPEROSTOSIS FRONTALIS
  INTERNA
CONGENITAL OSTEODYSTROPHIES
  Osteogenesis Imperfecta
  Achondroplasia
  Hereditary Chondrodysplasia
  Marfan's Syndrome
  Osteopetrosis
Skeletal Reticuloses
  NON-LIPID HISTIOCYTOSES:
    HISTIOCYTOSIS-X
    Schüller-Christian Disease
    Letterer-Siwe Disease
    Eosinophilic Granuloma
  LIPID HISTIOCYTOSES
    Gaucher's Disease
    Niemann-Pick Disease

Bone Tumors
  OSTEOGENIC TUMORS
    Benign Osteoblastoma
    Osteosarcoma
    Parosteal Sarcoma
  CHONDROGENIC TUMORS
    Chondroma
      Benign chondroblastoma
      Chondromyxoid fibroma
    Chondrosarcoma
  COLLAGENIC TUMORS
    Giant Cell Tumor: Osteo-
    Fibrosarcoma
  MYELOGENIC TUMORS
    Ewing's Tumor
    Reticulum Cell Sarcoma
    Plasma Cell Myeloma
  TUMOR-LIKE PROCESSES
    Hamartomas
      Osteoma, osteochondroma,
      enchondroma, angioma,
      aneurysmal bone cyst
    Bone Reactions
      Osteoid osteoma, non-osteo-
      genic fibroma, ossifying
      fibroma, giant-cell epulis
  METASTATIC TUMORS

GENERAL CONSIDERATIONS

Structure and Function.—"Bone is a specialized type of connective tissue, characterized by the presence of cells with long branching processes (*osteocytes*) which occupy cavities (*lacunae*) and fine canals (*canaliculi*) in a hard dense matrix consisting of bundles of *collagenous fibers* in an amorphous ground substance (*cement*) impregnated with *calcium phosphate* complexes" (Pritchard). Bone is not a dead inert structure solely concerned with rigidity, but a living tissue actively concerned with metabolic processes, especially those involving calcium and phosphorus. It is hard by reason of the deposition of a complex mineral substance consisting mainly of calcium phosphate and carbonate in the soft organic matrix, which is the intercellular substance. Bone is the calcium and phosphorus reservoir of the body, a reservoir which contains 99 per cent of the total body calcium and 90 per cent of the phosphorus. There is a constant circulation between the skeletal reservoir and the body fluids and tissues, a circulation which can be traced by means of the radioactive isotopes, Ca^{45} and P^{32}.

Calcium, as we have just seen, is stored overwhelmingly in the bones, a mere 1 per cent being available for the soft tissues, where it is mainly intracellular, with only one-tenth of that amount in the blood and extracellular fluid. The very small amount which is not in the bones plays a vital role in body function. for it affects enzyme activity, cell membrane permeability, cardiac rhythm, and neuromuscular excitability. The calcium in the blood is maintained at a remarkably constant level of between 9 to 11 mg. per 100 cc., with an average of 10 mg. A fall in the level of serum calcium may produce tetany and death, while hypercalcemia results in functional disturbances and cardiac effects. The serum calcium and phosphorus maintain a delicate inverse equilibrium with one another; when one goes up the other

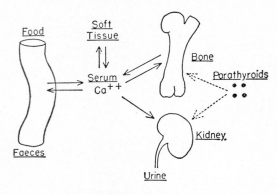

Calcium   Regulation

Fig. 704.—Factors involved in serum calcium regulation. (Copp, courtesy of Am. J. Med.)

goes down. This reciprocal relationship is
expressed by the formula Ca × P = 10 ×
3 = 30. A minor change in clacium results
in a major disturbance of health, but a
marked change in phosphorus causes only a
slight disturbance.

Calcium is readily absorbed from the upper
part of the small intestine, provided adequate amounts of calciferol (vitamin D_2) or
dehydrotachysterol (AT_{10}), a derivative of
irradiated ergosterol, are available. The
serum calcium level depends on a balance
between calcium added from intestinal absorption and bone absorption, and calcium
lost from the blood by excretion in urine and
feces and deposition in bone salts (Fig. 704).

Phosphorus must always be considered together with calcium in relation to bone,
where 90 per cent of the phosphorus of the
body is stored. Like calcium it is essential
for neuromuscular activity, and in addition
it is concerned with the maintainance of
H-ion concentration in body fluids, and with
the conservation and transfer of energy in
the intermediate metabolism of carbohydrates, proteins, lipids and various enzymes.
The absorption of phosphorus from the intestine is stimulated by an abundance of fat
in the diet, but only slightly by vitamin D.

The *metabolism of calcium and phosphorus*
in relation to bone must be considered as a
whole. When we speak of calcification we
mean of course the deposition of calcium
phosphate and not merely calcium. The
metabolism of calcium and phosphorus is

said to be influenced by 14 different factors.
Chief among these are parathyroid hormone
and vitamin D, but such hormones as estrogens, androgens, adrenal corticoids, thyroxin, and those of the anterior pituitary may
all play a part. The parathyroid glands
play a decisive role in the hemeostatic regulation of the calcium ion concentration of the
blood, but even in the absence of the parathyroids a fairly constant though low concentration of calcium ions is maintained.

The *absorption* and *excretion* of bone minerals in general are affected by phosphatase
activity, vitamin C and renal function. Upset of these metabolic regulators may result
in a number of diseases of bone which we
shall discuss presently. Chief among these
are osteitis fibrosa cystica, osteoporosis with
marked deficiency both in the *formation* of
matrix and the resorption of bone, osteomalacia and rickets with deficient *calcification* of the matrix, and Paget's disease. When
the complexity of the entire mechanism is
considered it becomes almost a matter of
surprise that anyone has normal bones.

Like all other tissues, bone consist of cells
and intercellular ground substance or matrix.
These have distinguishing characteristics
which are not seen elsewhere. The *cells* are
of three kinds:

(1) *Osteocytes*, the ordinary bone cells
lodged in the lacunae of the matrix. The
peculiar characteristics of the osteocyte is
that it is incapable of mitosis, its days are as
numbered as those of the red blood cell, it
has no hope of posterity, and it must therefore be removed together with the surrounding bone before any new bone can be formed.

(2) *Osteoblasts*, which are osteogenic cells
of a specific nature but not completely differentiated. They form a more or less continuous investment for the bone in the deep
layer of the periosteum, in the Haversian
canals, and in the endosteum. The osteoblasts have unlimited power of rapid reproduction, as if to compensate for the deficiencies of their children, the osteocytes, in
this respect. Osteoblasts, when multiplying
rapidly produce the enzyme, *alkaline phosphatase*, which splits organic phosphate compounds and liberates phosphate ions, thus
upsetting the local calcium-phosphate balance and causing the precipitation of calcium

salts in the ground substance. The phosphatase level of the serum may be raised either in excessive bone formation or in bone destruction, for in both of these increased osteoblastic activity comes into play.

(3) *Osteoclasts*, or bone phagocytes, are large cells lying in Howship's lacunae on the surface under the periosteum, spaces perhaps produced by these cells. The osteoclast is often multinucleated and it is from it that the foreign body giant cell is derived.

The *ground substance*, or matrix, is unique in containing the calcium-phosphate-carbonate complex which gives the skeleton its needed rigidity. This complex, as we have already seen, is precipitated in the ground substance by the action of alkaline phosphatase, which is controlled in turn by osteoblastic activity. The uncalcified organic matrix is called *osteoid*. It becomes bone with the precipitation of bone salts.

We may well ask how it is that bone cells, buried as they are in a dense calcified intercellular substance, are still able to maintan life and to continue the manufacture of phosphatase. Bone has solved this problem by the development of canaliculi, which connect the lacunae that house the osteocytes, communicate with the capillaries, and carry tissue fluid containing oxygen, food, calcium and phosphorus to the cells, thus providing the material without which phosphatase cannot function. Originally the canaliculi contain processes of the osteocytes, which may thus be said to "hold hands" together. "Cartilage cells, by contrast, can endure in frigid isolation, because their nutriment reaches them through the mucopolysaccharide matrix" (Collins and Curran).

In a state of health there is a normal equilibrium between nutrients reaching the bone and metabolites leaving it. The nutrients are chiefly proteins for the organic matrix, and calcium and phosphorus for the mineral complex. The health of the bone, therefore, will be effected not only by conditions in the bone itself, but also by the state of the blood, of the absorptive mechanism (the bowel) and the excretory mechanism (the kidneys). The vascularity of the part has much to do with the condition of the bone. Increased vascularity leads to decalcification and rarefaction, decreased vascu-

larity to increased density and osteosclerosis, while complete cutting off of the blood supply results in necrosis.

The *blood supply* to a bone comes from two sources: (1) the nutrient artery, by far the more important of the two, accounting for the richly vascularized medulla, and (2) penetrating periosteal vessels to the relatively avascular cortex, which is very vulnerable to pressure. It is evident that an acute inflammatory process accompanied by edema may cut off the blood supply from the nutrient artery with resulting ischemia which may lead to widespread necrosis, as is seen in acute osteomyelitis.

Bone Formation.—The complex problem of *ossification* will not be discussed here. It may be defined as "the process of connective tissue differentiation in which is laid down a strong and compact system of collagen fibers, blended with a non-fibrillar ground of mucopolysaccharides and enclosing living cells whose cytoplasmic processes ramify and interconnect with one another or with the periosteal or endosteal surfaces through minute calculi" (Collins and Curran). Calcium salts are readily deposited in this specialized material. Ossification may be endochondral or intramembranous in nature. *Endochondral ossification* is a replacement of cartilage by bone, and is the type of normal skeletal growth. *Intramembranous ossification* is the development of bone in a noncartilaginous connective tissue field, and is the method of osteogenesis in pathological ossification both in skeletal and extraskeletal sites.

Of greater interest to the pathologist is the distinction between woven and lamellar bone.

Woven bone is immature bone, contains an irregular lattice of coarse interlacing bundles of collagen fibers best shown with silver staining, and has a rich mucopolysaccharide content, so that it is PAS-positive, in this respect resembling cartilage. It is seen in pathologically-formed bone when the bone has been violently reactivated, as in fractures. *Lamellar bone* is mature bone as seen in the adult skeleton. The fibers are in fine bundles that run parallel with one another. Lamellar bone replaces the degenerated cartilage in endochondral ossification and woven bone in ossification in membrane. It is poor

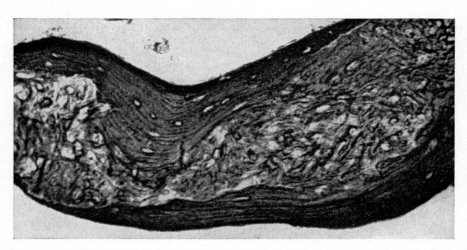

Fig. 705.—A newly formed bone trabecula stained with silver to show the contrasting reticulum patterns of the woven-bone centrum and the later parallel-fibered lamellar bone that has been laid upon it. × 200. (Collins, *Modern Trends in Pathology*, courtesy of Butterworth and Co. Ltd.)

in mucopolysaccharide, so that it is PAS-negative. Both woven and lamellar bone may be present in the same section of tissue (Fig. 705).

The much-debated question as to the part which the periosteum plays in bone formation will be discussed in connection with the repair of a fracture. Sometimes *metaplastic ossification* (to be distinguished from metastatic calcification) may occur, owing to a tissue other than osteoid becoming transformed into bone. In this way there may be bone formation in the walls of arteries, in the scars of abdominal wounds, and in the tonsil. It is hard to find a satisfactory explanation of this process.

Calcification is the term applied to the deposition of calcium in tissue which is not osteoid. The process is discussed again on the next page. *Metastatic calcification* occurs when calcium is removed from the bones as the result of some rarefying process and is deposited in other tissues. Hyperparathyroidism affords one of the best examples.

The *formation of bone* is regulated by a number of factors, of which the most important are hormones and vitamins. *Growth* of bone is controlled by *hormones* from the pituitary, thyroid, adrenal cortex, parathyroid, and male and female gonads. It is small wonder that this delicate hormonal balance is often upset, the result being usu-ally underproduction with rarefaction, but occasionally overproduction with osteosclerosis. An interesting example of the influence of a hormone on bone formation is the striking deposition of *medullary* bone in female birds during the pre-ovulatory stage of the egg-laying cycle. This is seen in the pigeon, chicken, duck, sparrow and parakeet. In the female parakeet there may sometimes be an *exophytic* hyperostosis widely distributed throughout the skeleton, due apparently to an excess of estrogen (Schlumberger). As regards vitamins, which have been called extrinsic hormones, it may be said that excess of vitamin A leads to osteoporosis and pathological fractures, that vitamin B complex stimulates and accelerates the formation of callus in fractures, and that vitamin C stimulates osteoblasts and its lack leads to scurvy and arrest of skeletal growth, while deficiency of vitamin D, due to lack of absorption of calcium from the intestine, results in rickets in the child and osteomalacia in the adult.

It seems probable that other still unknown factors, possibly dietary in character, may interfere with the formation of bone, especially in the earlier stages of postnatal development. In this connection the experimental work of Ponseti on the production of *lathyrism* in young rats is of particular interest. When a diet containing 50 per cent of the seeds of Lathyrus odoratus (sweet pea) was fed to rats during the first few weeks of life, degeneration of the mucopolysaccharides of the ground substance of the epiphyseal plates was produced, together with a loosening and detachment of tendinous and ligamentous insertions. The cartilaginous matrix loses its cohesion and becomes fibrillated. The animals develop many types of spinal deformity as well as lesions of the intervertebral discs. Further work of this kind may throw some much needed light on the pathogenesis of the group of the *aseptic necroses* in young people (page 1235), for similar lesions are seen in the lathyritic rats. The sweet pea diet is deficient in amino-acids, especially methionine. Lathyrism can be induced experimentally by various synthetic vitriles such as aminoacetonitrile (Selye). In acute experimental osteolathyrism produced in weanling rats by the administration of aminoacetonitrile there is a constant and marked decrease in the glycogen content of the cells of the lathyric epiphyseal cartilage (Karnovsky). It is of interest that weakness and spasticity of the legs is a feature of epidemic lathyrism in countries where famines force the population to consume a high proportion of legumes in their diet. A general review of the subject of lathyrism will be found in Selye's monograph

Osteosclerosis.—Local increased density of bone is of common recurrence, but it is due to local causes. Thus it is seen in chronic osteomyelitis and syphilis, in degenerative arthritis, where there is local mechanical stress, and above all in conditions of decreased vascularity. Considering how easily the balance of systemic regulating factors may be upset, it might be expected that generalized osteosclerosis would be of common occurrence. This is not so. Hypoparathyroidism and too liberal a supply of fluorine (fluorosis) are perhaps the only conditions associated with an overformation of bone involving the entire skeleton.

Pathological Calcification. — Pathological calcification may occur in normal tissue as the result of the blood being flooded with calcium (metastatic calcification), or it may represent the deposition of calcium in tissue which is injured, degenerating or dead (dystrophic calcification). *Metastatic calci-*

fication may be induced by repeated injections of parathyroid hormone, or it may occur in decalcifying diseases of bone such as the osteoporosis of forced immobility (poliomyelitis, etc.), osteomalacia, general carcinomatosis of bone, and multiple myeloma. The calcium is either removed from the bones or not laid down there, but deposited in other tissues, more particularly the kidneys. *Dystrophic calcification*, in which the calcium is laid down in dying or dead tissue without any reference to the blood calcium, is much more common. Both phosphate and carbonate are deposited in practically the same proportion as is found in bone. There is a tendency for any dying or dead tissue and accessible to the body fluids to become calcified. Necrosis and hyaline changes are the two chief antecedents of calcification.

In the course of our studies we have encountered many examples of pathological calcification. Some of the more important of these are the following: caseous tuberculous areas in which the infection has died out, arteriosclerosis, particularly Mönckeberg's sclerosis, healed endocarditis and pericarditis, phleboliths in veins, degenerating uterine fibroids, lithopedion (calcified fetus from a tubal pregnancy), renal convoluted tubules in mercuric chloride poisoning, and very many others.

Pathological Ossification.—Pathological ossification, also called *metaplastic ossification*, is the extra-skeletal formation of true bone. It is entirely unrelated to pathological calcification. There is a metaplasia of non-osseous into osseous tissue, but without the preliminary formation of osteoid. The new new bone develops as membrane bone, with an accumulation of mucopolysaccharides, alkaline phosphatase in the early stage, and the formation of woven bone which is gradually replaced by lamellar bone with parallel laminæ. The most striking examples are seen in the repair of fractures, in myositis ossificans, both traumatic and progressive, and in osteogenic bone tumors. Other examples of heterotopic ossification are old lesions of pulmonary tuberculosis, tuberculous lymph nodes, leiomyomas of the uterus, epithelial tumors of the bladder, calcareous arteries, and scars of the abdominal wall. The pathogenic factors responsible for this peculiar metaplasia are multiple and obscure, for a discussion of which the article by Collins and Curran should be consulted.

Resorption of Bone.—There is no tissue in the body which is capable of so much overgrowth or on the other hand so much resorption as bone. The cause of the resorption may be general (hyperparathyroidism) or local (pressure, etc.). It occurs in old age, from disuse, as the result of acute and chronic inflammation, and due to tumor and aneurysm. The removal of the excess callus of a fracture and of a sequestrum (dead bone) are excellent examples. Bone undergoing resorption is softer, more easily cut, and bleeds more readily because of its greater vascularity. It can be recognized in the roentgen-ray picture by the decreased density of the shadow.

There are two chief factors in the resorption of bone: (1) vascular resorption, and (2) the action of osteoclasts. (1) *Vascular resorption* is the powerful factor. In ordinary compact bone the blood vessels run longitudinally in a series of channels called the Haversian canals, around which the bony lamellae are grouped, and transversely from the periosteum in Volkmann's canals. Persistent vascular dilatation is followed by widening of the canals at the expense of the bone, and if inflammatory granulation tissue is formed within them, as in tuberculosis, the resorption becomes very marked, a condition of *rarefaction* or *osteoporosis*. Primary removal of the calcium salts, as in hyperparathyroidism, is also followed by widening of the canals and the formation of granulation tissue within them, but these changes have now become effects rather than causes of the resorption of bone. This primary removal of calcium is known as *halisteresis* (*hals*, salt; *steresis*, privation) or osteolysis. It would appear that in primary vascular resorption the mechanism by which the calcium is removed and the canals widened is a physico-chemical one. In inflammation there are probably local changes in the hydrogen-ion concentration that lead to solution of calcium and the production of narrow zones of decalcification around the vessels which allow the vascular canals to become dilated. Any

local excessive production of carbon dioxide tends to cause solution of calcium, for the solubility is affected directly by the carbon dioxide tension of the blood and tissue fluids. The reaction which takes place at the line of contact of dead and living bone is of this nature, although inflammation is also a factor here. For these reasons only well-vascularized living bone can be resorbed quickly. Dead bone is resorbed slowly by osteoclasts.

(2) *Osteoclasts* may be absent or they may dominate the process. The osteoclast or bone phagocyte is a large cell with strongly acidophilic and granular cytoplasm; it is often multinucleated, containing a few or a large number of nuclei (Fig. 706). It is from the osteoclasts that the foreign body giant cells of bone are derived. It may show a fringed or toothed border (brush border) along the edge in contact with bone. Howship's lacunæ on the surface under the periosteum are produced by the osteoclasts. The phagocytic action of osteoclasts is most readily studied in the removal of small fragments of bone which have become separated. Large foreign body giant cells are formed for this purpose. It is probable that decalcification must first occur before the osteoclast can exert its phagocytic action. This chemical change is brought about by the tissue juices, possibly by the osteoclasts themselves.

Osteoporosis.—Bone consists of an organic protein matrix laid down by osteoblasts, and an inorganic calcium complex (calcium-phosphate-carbonate) deposited in the matrix from the serum. Theoretically, therefore, osteoporosis might be due to: (1) excessive bone resorption, (2) insufficient deposition of the calcium complex, and (3) inadequate formation of the protein matrix.

In actual practice generalized bone deficiency of metabolic origin may take three forms. (1) *Generalized osteitis fibrosa*, where there is excessive bone resorption associated with compensatory new bone formation. The condition may be due to (*a*) hyperparathyroidism or (*b*) renal glomerular failure with phosphate retention. (2) *Osteomalacia*, where the calcium complex is not deposited in the protein matrix owing to calcium deficiency. There is abundant formation of pale-staining osteoid tissue with correspond-

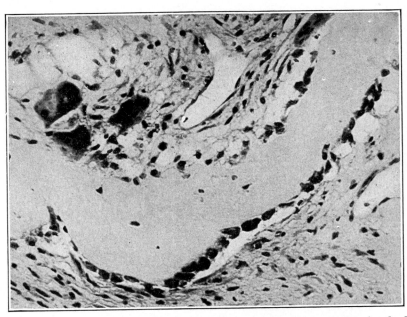

Fig. 706.—Three multinucleated osteoclasts above and to the left of a bone trabecula, the lower margin of which is lined by osteoblasts. × 300.

ing osteoblastic activity. The condition may be due to (a) deficient calcium absorption from the intestine, or (b) various renal tubular deficiencies resulting in excessive loss of calcium in the urine. (3) *Osteoporosis*, where there is poor formation of the protein matrix of bone, but normal calcium deposition and bone resorption. Osteoporosis may occur in a variety of clinical conditions, of which three deserve special mention. (a) *Atrophy of disuse*, seen in paralysis or immobilization of a limb, expecially in paraplegics. Osteoblasts lack the normal stimulus of stresses and strains, so that bone formation is diminished. The calcium is excreted in the urine and may give rise to the formation of stones in the kidney or bladder, thus explaining the frequent association of poliomyelitis and urinary calculi. (b) *Gonadal deficiency*. As osteogenesis is under the control of gonadal hormones, it is natural that osteoporosis should develop as a result of the loss of either estrogens or androgens. The former is much commoner owing to the occurrence of the female menopause. Indeed *"postmenopausal osteoporosis"* is the commonest metabolic bone disorder (Albright and Reifenstein). *Senile osteoporosis*, with its brittle bones and tendency to fractures, is for the most part gonadal in origin. It should be noted that osteoporosis also occurs in men with eunuchoidism and in young women with ovarian agenesis. (c) *Hypercorticoidism*. Osteoporosis is a feature of Cushing's syndrome, which is due to hypersecretion of adrenocortical hormone with glyconeogenic activity, a hormone which appears to inhibit the activity of osteoblasts. It has been suggested that a mechanism common to all causes may involve the action of glucocorticoids on bone-tissue (Urist). The benefit of gonadal hormones in the treatment of osteoporosis may be due to suppression of secretion of adrenal corticoid hormones, rather than a direct action on bone. Osteoporosis is known to develop in patients who have been on large amounts of corticoids for a prolonged period.

The *end results* of osteoporosis demand serious consideration, for the condition is an almost constant feature of the later years of life, being more pronounced in women, and it is likely to increase as the population

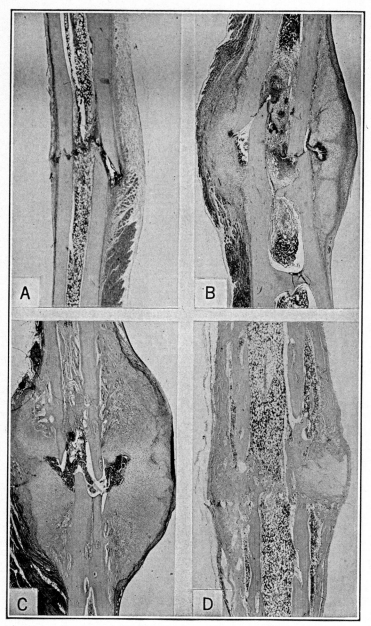

FIG. 707.—Healing of experimental fractures. × 14. *A*, Three days (subperiosteal osteoblasts); *B*, seven days (osteoid); *C*, fifteen days (abundant callus); *D*, six weeks (diminished callus being converted into bone). (Boyd, *Pathology for the Surgeon*, courtesy of W. B. Saunders Company.)

becomes older (Yendt). The trabeculæ are reduced in number and thickness although completely calcified, so that there is *too little bone*. The effect on the skeleton will naturally be quite different from that of osteomalacia, where there is insufficient calcification rather than deficient bone formation. In osteoporosis we may expect *compression fractures of the vertebræ, spinal deformities*, and *loss of height*. In osteomalacia, on the other hand, there is bending of the softened bones, with deformities of the leinless and pelvis which will be considered in a later section. *Back pain*, when it does occur in osteoporosis, is usually acute in onset and incapacitating, occurring either spontaneously or during mild vertebral strain. *Fracture of the neck of the femur* due to a minimal degree of trauma, the fracture causing a fall rather than a fall causing the fracture, is a frequent and tragic occurrence in elderly females.

The *radiological* feature of osteoporosis of the spine is demineralization, which is unfortunately nonspecific. Anterior wedging and compression of vertebral bodies is often present, and the spinous processes may be crowded together. The skull is usually not affected, perhaps because it is little affected by stress and strain.

Osteomalacia.—In this condition, which is considered more full in relation to the osteodystrophics, the osteoblasts manufacture sufficient matrix, but this does not all become calcified. The trabeculæ are therefore normal in size and number, but strips of uncalcified matrix, known as osteoid seams, can be seen along the margins. It is a defect in calcification, not a defect in growth. The serum calcium and inorganic phosphate are likely to be lower than normal, while the weakening of the bone stimulates osteoblastic activity with resulting elevated serum alkaline phosphatase levels. In osteoporosis, on the other hand, normal serum calcium, inorganic phosphate and alkaline phosphatase may be expected.

Repair of Bone.—The repair of bone is best studied in the healing of a fracture, either in human material or in experimental fractures in animals. Adult bone cells have lost the power of proliferation so that they play no part in the regeneration of bone.

Repair is carried out entirely by the osteoblasts which line the deep layer of the periosteum, the endosteum, and the Haversian canals. The deep cellular layer of the periosteum is a striking structure which must be seen to be appreciated. It is much more abundant in young bone, and can be seen to react exuberantly after a fracture. Osteoblasts are present both in the periosteum and the surface layer of bone, so that repair can occur either with or without the periosteum. The essential function of the periosteum is to supply the outer part of the bone with blood. Removal or separation of the periosteum is apt to be followed by death of this part of the bone.

Healing of a Fracture.—This takes place in three stages: First *granulation tissue* forms in the exudate between the broken ends of bone then *osteoid tissue* is formed, and finally *calcium salts* are deposited with the production of bone. (1) As a result of the fracture, blood and a varying amount of exudate are poured out between and around the ends of bone. This is invaded by cells and new capillaries, and a kind of granulation tissue is produced. The proliferating cells are osteoblasts, derived for the most part from the deep layer of the periosteum. The proliferation of osteoblasts is of an extraordinarily rapid and massive character; indeed, there is no other non-malignant process which is quite comparable with it (Fig. 707, *A*). (2) In the course of four or five days the osteoblasts form trabeculæ around central spaces which become Haversian canals. This is osteoid tissue, *i. e.*, tissue resembling bone in its structural arrangement but with no calcium salts in its homogeneous matrix (Fig. 707, *B*). The osteoid tissue, also known as *callus*, becomes increased in amount so as to act as a splint. By the end of the second week it is remarkably abundant (Fig. 707, *C*). (3) Finally calcium is laid down, and the ends are knit together by rigid, fully formed bone (Fig. 707, *D*). Low blood calcium produced by deficient diet does not slow the rate of healing or lead to non-union. In the immediate neighborhood of the fracture the bone cells die. Near the fracture the osteogenic cells proliferate in massive fashion, and may form cartilage instead of bone. This cartilage formation is most marked when there is movement or separation of the fragments. The new cartilage is invaded and replaced by bone. This is ossification in cartilage, as compared with the process just described which corresponds to ossification in membrane.

Changes in the hydrogen ion concentration influence the process. The pH is first acid, favoring decalcification. At the end of a week it changes to the alkaline side, with resulting deposition of calcium. A week later phosphatase is liberated by the osteoblasts; this causes deposition of calcium and phosphorus in the osteoid tissue.

The new material formed at the site of the fracture is known as *callus* on account of its hardness. In the later stages it may become calcified, but at first it is osteoid in character. Some of it is *external*, ensheathing the broken ends like solder; some is *intermediate*, forming a direct union between the fractured surfaces; some is *internal*, filling the marrow cavity. The internal and external callus is removed by osteoclasts, and the bone undergoes a process of molding which goes on for months, and results in a rearrangment of the lamellæ to meet the new stresses. If the gap between the fragments is not bridged by osteogenic cells in a certain time, fibroblasts will fill the gap with fibrous tissue, the matrix of which has no special affinity for calcium salts (non-union or fibrous union).

Fate of a Bone Graft.—When a piece of bone is transplanted by the surgeon to another position the greater part of it dies. Dead bone can be easily recognized under the microscope from the shrivelled appearance of the bone cells and the fact that large numbers of the lacunæ are empty. The part of bone bathed by the body fluids remains alive, *i.e.*, the surface, the lining of the medullary cavity, and the Haversian canals. The cells in these places are osteoblasts, so that osteoblastic activity is soon apparent. But much more striking, especially in the earlier stages, is bone removal. New vessels from the surrounding tissue grow along the Haversian canals, so that the bone becomes revascularized and is at the same time absorbed. Multinucleated osteoclasts also attack the graft, and many foreign body giant cells may be formed. The removal of the

graft is gradually brought about by the two great processes already studied, *i. e.*, vascular absorption and osteoclastic activity. In the course of six months if the graft has no function to perform it is merely represented by an atrophic mass of fibrous tissue. But a bone graft should be regarded as an implant rather than a transplant, because the implanted bone powerfully induces osteogenesis in the host tissues. It is this still mysterious property which renders the "transplantation" of bone of such great value to the orthopedic surgeon. The new bone formation is intramembranous ossification. If the transplant becomes a functioning structure, as when it is in continuity with another bone, osteoblastic activity is combined with absorption, and gradually it becomes the dominant process. The graft may finally become converted into living healthy bone. If the graft is taken from an animal of another species, none of the osteoblasts will survive.

INFLAMMATIONS

Acute Osteomyelitis.—The term osteomyelitis indicates inflammation of bone and bone marrow. But it is really an inflammation of the soft parts of bone, *i. e.*, the contents of the medullary cavity and the Haversian canals, together with the periosteum. It is a boil in a bone. The calcified portion takes no active part in the process, but it suffers secondarily from the loss of blood supply, and a greater or less portion may die.

Etiology.—The predisposing causes are age, sex and trauma. The great majority of acute infections of bone occur during the period of active growth, being commonest between the ages of two and ten years. The disease is 3 times as common in *boys* as in girls, probably because the former are more liable to trauma. A history of *trauma*, either a blow or a strain, is common, but may of course be purely coincidental. When a wrench is applied to a growing bone, the part mostlikely to give way is the metaphysis, in which an effusion of blood may occur, offering a suitable nidus to any bacteria carried to the part.

The *exciting* cause is one of the pyogenic organisms, usually Staphylococcus aureus, less frequently S. albus, and occasionally streptococcus, pneumococcus, and typhoid bacillus, the last named causing chronic rather than acute inflammation (page 274). Coccidioides immitis, a fungus found mostly in California, may cause *coccidioidal osteomyelitis*, the fungus entering the body through the skin and respiratory tract. Osteomyelitis may be: (1) hematogenous, or (2) non-hematogenous in origin. In the non-hematogenous form the infection may come (*a*) from without, or (*b*) extension. In *children* and adolescents (those with growing bones) osteomyelitis is due to a hematogenous infection. The staphylococcus often enters the blood stream through the skin, and it is common to find a healing boil if the whole body is carefully examined. In other cases the throat, teeth, and tonsils may be suspected.

In *adults* hematogenous infection is rare. When it does occur the disease is much less acute. Infection is most likely to be introduced from without, as in a compound fracture, gunshot wound, etc. In children also the infection may be local in origin, as in osteomyelitis of the mandible from an infected tooth, or inflammation of the mastoid process from middle-ear suppuration.

Lesions.—The description which follows applies to the hematogenous osteomyelitis of children untreated with antibiotics. The bones most often affected are the femur and tibia (much exposed to trauma and strain), followed by the humerus. The infection starts in the metaphysis—the part of the shaft which borders on the epiphyseal line in a growing bone.

The initial lesion is a focal suppuration abscess of the cancellous bone at the end of the shaft. Infection *spreads* rapidly in two directions: (1) along the medullary cavity, and (2) outward to the cortex. Pus is formed beneath the periosteum and lifts that membrane from the bone, at the same time making its way along the outside of the shaft. Many of the vessels are found to be thrombosed, and the septic thrombi form the chief menace of osteomyelitis, namely the formation of pyemic abscesses throughout the body. The denuded surface of dead bone has an opaque white appearance and does not bleed when scraped. The fatty tissue of the marrow is destroyed and is converted

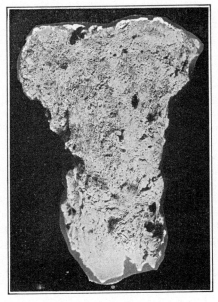

Fig. 708.—Osteomyelitis of upper end of tibia showing new bone formation and cloacæ.

into an oily pus. The *adjacent joint* is often filled with a sterile serous effusion. Sometimes the infection may pass to the epiphysis, perforate the articular cartilage, and invade the joint, setting up a suppurative arthritis.

The dead bone becomes separated from the living by the action of osteoclasts, forming a *sequestrum*, which can be lifted out freely when it is exposed at operation. But in the meantime the periosteum is not inactive. Although it is separated from the bone, some of the cells of the osteogenic layer usually survive, and when the acuteness of the infection is past these osteoblasts lay down new bone over the sequestrum in the form of a *new case* or *involucrum*. The involucrum is perforated here and there by *cloacæ* or sewers through which passes the pus produced by the irritation of the dead bone. (Fig. 708). Nature is unable to deal with this state of affairs, and the dead shaft remains locked up within the rigid involucrum without any chance of being absorbed.

Osteomyelitis of the spine usually commences in the neural arches of the vertebræ, although in the cervical region it is more likely to start in the vertebral bodies. When it begins in the neural arches the pus spreads backward, when it begins in the bodies it spreads forward, and may cause a retropharyngeal abscess. Death is likely to result from septic meningitis.

Relation of Symptoms to Lesions.—Acute hematogenous osteomyelitis is a disease of children, commonest in boys in the first or second decade. It is a disease of growing bones, rarely seen in the adult. It commences with the signs of an acute infection, *i.e.*, chills, high fever, rapid pulse, leukocytosis, and positive blood culture. There is severe pain and tenderness at the end of one of the long bones, due to the extreme tension within the unyielding bone caused by the violent inflammation, together with redness, swelling, and edema. Death may occur from septicemia or pyemia (endocarditis, abscesses in the kidneys, etc.), or, if treatment is inadequate, the disease may become chronic. As the initial lesions are confined to the soft parts of the bone, there are no characteristic roentgen-ray changes in the earlier stages of the disease.

The above account applies to the disease before the days of chemotherapy. With the advent of antibiotics osteomyelitis has become a medical rather than a surgical disease. The description which follows also applies to untreated cases.

Chronic Osteomyelitis.—If acute osteomyelitis is not adequately treated, the condition may become chronic and drag on until the patient dies of amyloid disease. But it may be more or less chronic from the beginning, with no definite history of an acute attack. Such a condition is known as a *Brodie's abscess*, a chronic circumscribed focus of suppuration at the upper end of the tibia, lower end of femur, upper end of humerus, and occasionally elsewhere. During periods of quiescence there is a small cavity surrounded by dense bone and containing a little serous fluid, but during periodic exacerbations the cavity is filled with pus from which staphylococci may be isolated. *Typhoid osteomyelitis* is a chronic infection which usually appears about two months after the acute illness, but there may be an interval of several years. The bacilli have been isolated twenty years after the original infection. The upper end of the tibia, the ribs and the sternum are the common sites.

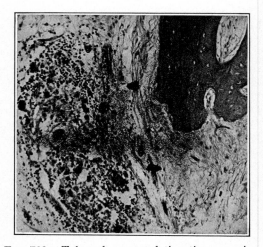

Fig. 709.—Tuberculous granulation tissue causing erosion of bone. Several giant cells can be seen.

Tuberculosis.—Tuberculosis of bone is a chronic osteomyelitis occurring in early life, displaying an excess of bone destruction over bone formation, yet with a tendency toward limitation of spread and spontaneous healing. The disease begins in spongy bone, and is commonest in the vertebræ, the small bones of the hands and feet, and the ends of the long bones including both metaphysis and epiphysis. As in the case of acute osteomyelitis, the region of the knee (lower end of femur and upper end of tibia) is a common site. There may be more than one focus; in the vertebral column this is the rule, not the exception. The infection is usually hematogenous, being carried to the spongy bone by the blood stream from a distant focus in lung. lymph nodes, etc., although occasionally no evident focus can be found. Trauma probably plays a part in inducing the bacilli to settle down, as can be shown experimentally, but the trauma must be mild. A severe injury such as a fracture calls forth such a rapid reparative reaction that the bacilli have no chance to establish themselves. Sometimes the infection spreads from a joint to the epiphysis by way of the perivascular lymphatics. Bone and joint tuberculosis are often associated; the primary lesion may be in either structure.

Lesions.—The lesions are of two main types: (1) There may be little or no caseation, but an abundant formation of soft tuberculous granulation tissue (Fig. 709). This exerts an erosive action, as a result of which the Haversian canals are enlarged and the outer and inner surfaces of the bone are eaten away. Osteoclasts assist in the work of destruction; but it is not a wholesale destruction. Branching trabeculæ of bone are left, the interspaces being filled with granulation tissue. This is a process of rarefaction or osteoporosis to which the name of *caries* is given. (2) There may be marked softening, destruction of bony trabeculæ, and caseation, which may be followed by the formation of tuberculous pus and a *cold abscess*. This type of lesion is characteristically seen in tuberculosis of the vertebræ. Although the lesions of tuberculosis are essentially destructive there may be a limited amount of osteosclerosis and formation of new bone. The periosteal osteogenic activity characteristic of osteomyelitis is never seen in tuberculosis, unless a septic element has been superadded.

The infection may *spread* down the medullary cavity so that most of the shaft is involved. It may spread through the epiphyseal cartilage, or if it starts in the epiphysis it may perforate the articular cartilage and invade the joint; the articular cartilage may be completely separated from the underlying bone. It may spread to the periosteum, where it forms a subperiosteal abscess. The soft parts then become involved, with the formation of a *cold abscess* which discharges through a sinus on to the skin.

Tuberculous dactylitis is a condition in which a metacarpal or one of the phalanges develops a fusiform swelling as a result of diffuse involvement of the medulla. The interior of the shaft is absorbed and new bone is laid down on the surface by the periosteum, so that the shaft appears to be expanded.

Tuberculosis of the Vertebræ.—This is also known as *Pott's disease of the spine.* The vertebræ are the commonest bones affected by tuberculosis. The disease occurs especially in young children, and usually begins in the center of the body of a vertebra which is supplied by a branch of the posterior spinal artery. Discrete lesions are often present in several adjoining vertebræ. The

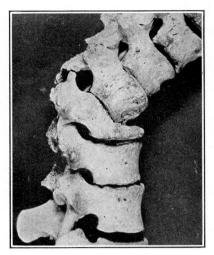

A

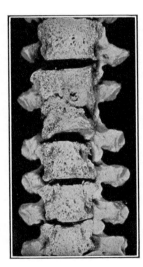

B

Fig. 710.—*A*, The central form of tuberculosis of the spine. The body of one vertebra is destroyed and collapsed, causing backward curvature of the spine.

B., Peripheral form of tuberculosis of the spine with surface involvement of many of the vertebral bodies.

center of the bone becomes caseous and the disease spreads to and destroys the intervertebral discs, but spares the transverse processes, spines, and articular processes. The destruction of the discs is of special importance, because in secondary carcinoma of the vertebræ, which often presents a radiological picture very similar to that of tuberculosis, the discs are hardly ever involved. The bodies collapse in front, while the spines remain intact behind, so that an acute curvature develops with its convexity pointing backward. (Fig. 710A). This form of curvature is known as *kyphosis*. In the rather rare *peripheral* form of adults the disease is confined to the anterior surface of the vertebræ, an area supplied by branches from the intercostal arteries; there is little or no deformity, but a large number of vertebræ may be involved. (Fig. 710B).

In children there is usually evidence of *pressure on the cord*. This is not due to the angling of the spine, but to the formation of tuberculous granulation tissue or to an accumulation of pus under the posterior common ligament which presses on the cord. It is remarkable how even severe pressure symptoms such as paraplegia may clear up when the weight is taken off the spine.

A *cold abscess* often develops and this may trek in almost any direction, although it is unable to travel directly backward owing to the posterior common ligament. It soon escapes at the sides of the vertebræ, and is then free to travel at will. In the *cervical* region it may form a retropharyngeal abscess or may appear at the side of the neck. In the *dorsal* region it may spread along a rib; when it comes to the surface it is very liable to be mistaken for primary disease of the rib unless the spine is carefully examined. In the *lumbar* region the pus enters the sheath of the psoas muscle, and passes down as a *psoas abscess* into the iliac fossa and under Poupart's ligament; it may then point at the saphenous opening or may pass down the thigh as far as the popliteal space. The pus may enter the sheath of the iliacus instead of the psoas; it will then point above Poupart's ligament. In any of these sites mistakes in diagnosis are frequent. When the abscess discharges on the surface a mixed infection develops, and the clinical picture changes very much for the worse with hectic temperature and rapid wasting. *Amyloid disease* may now develop, or the patient may die of general miliary tuberculosis.

The *course* of the disease varies. As the spine is seldom at rest there is a strong tendency to progression. If the patient is kept absolutely at rest on his back under the best hygienic conditions an astonishing recovery may follow with firm fibrous union between the vertebræ. These remarks apply to the patient who was treated before the advent of the chemotherapy of tuberculosis. The outlook now is naturally very much brighter.

Sarcoidosis.—The contentious matter of the nature and etiology of sarcoidosis, in particular in relation to tuberculosis, has already been discussed in Chapter 11. Suffice it to say here that the disease is a granuloma of uncertain etiology which, although prolonged in its course, has a strong natural tendency to healing. The skeletal lesions are not common, nor do they cause any serious disability. They are of interest in that they give a characteristic roentgenographic picture, which may be of value in the diagnosis of generalized sarcoidosis.

The disease may occur at all ages, but is commonest in the second and third decades. The most *frequent sites* are the phalanges of the hands and feet, the metacarpals and metatarsals, the wrist and ankle, and the long bones in that order. The earliest x-ray change is an increased coarseness of the trabecular pattern of the terminal phalanges, followed later by the development of multiple, small, punched-out areas of rarefaction. As sarcoid lesions do not become caseous, there is no cavitation, nor is there reactive sclerosis at the periphery, sequestrum formation, nor involvement of joints. The *microscopic picture* is that of sharply circumscribed collections of epitheloiid cells with multinucleated giant cells. In the late stages the lesions become fibrosed. The condition formerly described as osteitis tuberculosa multiplex or cystic tuberculosis of bone is simply sarcoidosis of bone.

Syphilis.—When I was a student, syphilis of bone was a disease of great importance, and had continually to be kept in mind in the differential diagnosis of bone lesions. Those days are gone forever, and modern chemotherapy has changed a common type of lesion into a rarity, so that we may dispose of the subject with welcome brevity.

Syphilitic disease of bone is an inflammation, an osteitis, just as tuberculosis is a special form of inflammation. It *differs from tuberculosis* in the following respects: (1) it affects the diaphysis of long bones rather than the articular ends, (2) the joint is seldom involved, and (3) osteosclerosis with new bone formation is much more prominent than osteoporosis or rarefaction. The bones most commonly affected are the tibia, sternum, cranium, and the bones of the face, especially the nose and palate. The disease may be of the acquired or congenital form. The lesions may appear in the earlier or the later stages. In the earlier stages there is likely to be a periostitis; in the late stages gummatous formation is not uncommon. The two usual manifestations of bone syphilis are the periosteal node and diffuse osteitis. The *periosteal node* is the characteristic lesion. It takes the form of a localized, firm, painful, tender swelling most frequently seen on the subcutaneous border of the tibia. The spirochetes appear to settle in the deeper vascular layer of the periosteum, and an abundant cellular granulation tissue is formed around the vessels not only in the periosteum but also in the mouths of the Haversian canals. The tension produced by this new tissue within the bony canals is responsible for the nocturnal boring pains alluded to by the Psalmist.

In *diffuse osteitis* the greater part of the shaft or the entire bone is involved from the periosteum to the medulla and from one articular cartilage to the other. New bone is laid down by the osteoblasts under the periosteum causing marked uniform thickening of the shaft, on the walls of the dilated Haversian canals causing greatly increased density of the bone, and in the medulla causing obliteration of that cavity. The entire bone is now dense and heavy.

Of the other osseous lesions mention may be made of gummatous destruction of the bones of the nose and hard palate, so that the bridge of the nose falls in at the root (*saddle-nose*), and there may be a large perforation of the palate. It may avoid embarrassment to remember that not every saddle-nose is caused by syphilis.

Congenital Syphilis.—The skeletal lesions of congenital syphilis might have demanded a chapter of their own in the past. Suffice it to say here that of the endless lesions which used to be seen, mention may be made of those in the epiphyses, the phalanges, the tibia, and the nose and palate. *Syphilitic epiphysitis* is a highly characteristic lesion seen at autopsy on the newborn. The normal thin, gray, epiphyseal line of the upper end of the tibia or the lower end of the femur becomes broad, irregular and yellowed in color. The normal cartilage is replaced by necrotic granulation tissue, so that the epiphysis is readily detached by slight trauma during life. The *x*-ray appearance is diagnostic. Antisyphilitic treatment quickly brings reunion and normal ossification. The "*saber-blade*" tibia is thickened, compressed laterally, and curved forward. The *phalanges* show a spindle-shaped swelling. The *nose* and *palate* may present the same lesions as in the acquired form.

ASEPTIC (ISCHEMIC) NECROSIS OF BONE

The condition now to be described has a large number of names which have greatly confused the subject. This confusion was inevitable, because information has accumulated piece-meal with regard to lesions in a variety of bones to which different names were applied in the belief that each was a separate entity. These lesions were described, largely on radiological appearances, by men whose names have been attached to the condition, with the somewhat absurd result that a list of the varieties rather resembles the index of a dictionary of medical biography. Some of these names or eponyms have become hallowed by such long usage that they are best retained.

The condition is a quiet necrosis of the epiphyses occurring in childhood and adolescence. As its nature is obscure the process goes by a variety of descriptive names. In former editions of this book it was called non-suppurative epiphysitis. Aseptic necrosis is now in common use, but ischemic necrosis is the more rational and informative. The lesions are of clinical importance not because of any marked disability which they produce, but because they are so *easily mistaken for bone tuberculosis*, especially in the hip and spine. The points the various forms have in common are as follows: (1) They always occur in the young, usually between

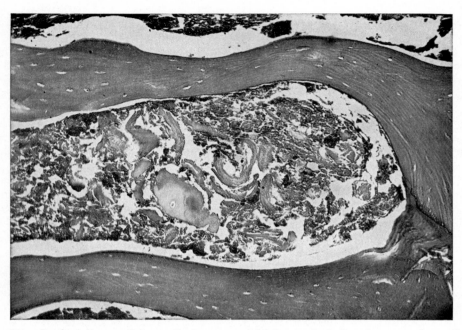

Fig. 711.—Perthes' disease. Between the two arms of this bone spicule there is a mass of necrotic débris with flakes of bone and soft tissue intermixed. (× 180.) (Aegerter and Kirkpatrick, *Orthopedic Diseases,* courtesy of W. B. Saunders Co.)

the ages of five and fifteen. (2) They affect epiphyses which have not yet fused and which are subject to special strain. (3) Symptoms are either slight or entirely absent. (4) The radiogram shows marked changes, such as flattening, fragmentation and increased density.

The *etiology* is uncertain. It seems probable that interference with the epiphyseal blood supply is an important factor, but no satisfying explanation has been forthcoming as to the cause of the ischemia. The epiphyseal portions of the bones are largely surrounded by cartilage, and even under normal conditions have a limited blood supply. A factor which may well prove to be of importance in the case of Perthes' disease, which is aseptic (ischemic) necrosis of the head of the femur, is the fact that between the age of three and eight years the blood supply of the proximal femoral epiphysis comes through the small group of lateral epiphyseal vessels without complementary supply from the round ligament or the metaphyseal vessels. Negro children on the other hand seem to preserve the vessels of the ligamentum teres, and for this reason, per-

haps, appear to be practically immune to Perthes' disease. The possibility of a low-grade infection has been suggested, but for this there is no definite evidence.

Lesions.—The femoral head and the tibial tubercle are the common sites in the long bones, while in the small bones the lesions are most frequent in the scaphoid, semilunar and metatarsals. In the early stage the evidence of necrosis is afforded by complete disappearance of the osteocytes, leaving the lacunæ as empty tombs, but with retention of the architecture of the bone. Soon a reactive hyperemia in the surrounding living bone and an invasion of osteoclasts commence resorption of the dead bone and its reconversion into new living bone by the activity of osteoblasts. This combination of resorption and apposition has been well termed "creeping substitution," as a result of which the original architecture is preserved to a remarkable degree. In this stage the bone is still soft, so that the head of the femur may become flattened as the result of weight-bearing. Finally the process of healing is completed.

Legg-Perthes' disease, often known as

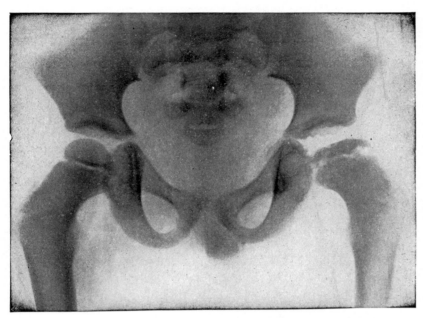

FIG. 712.—Perthes' disease: extreme flattening of the head of the femur. (Boyd, *Pathology for the Surgeon*, courtesy of W. B. Saunders Co.)

Perthes' disease, is the commonest form of aseptic necrosis. The lesion is confined to the head of the femur, usually in boys between the age of five and ten years. There is often a history of recent injury. The bony nucleus of the epiphysis is fragmented, so that it may resemble particles of mortar. (Fig. 711). As a result the head of the femur becomes flattened and splayed out. When healing occurs the fragments coalesce, and the bone regains some of its structure, but the flattening is permanent. The x-ray picture is absolutely characteristic, and it is by means of it that a final diagnosis is made (Fig. 712). The *earliest symptom* is a limp, accompanied by little or no discomfort. There is slight restriction of mobility. The condition *must be distinguished from early tuberculosis.*

Köhler's disease is aseptic necrosis of the *tarsal scaphoid*, and again there is a limp and slight pain on walking. The radiogram shows a scaphoid diminished in size, flattened, and of increased density. *Osgood-Schlatter's* disease involves the *tubercle of the tibia,* usually between the ages of twelve and sixteen years. It may follow direct trauma or sudden strain through the ligamentum patellæ. *Sever's disease* affects the posterior epiphysis of the *os calcis*, the lesion being probably due to strain on the bone acting through the tendo Achilles. *Kienböck's disease* is necrosis of the *carpal semilunar*, and is confined to adults. There is a history of trauma to the hand. *Kümmell's disease* or *post-traumatic spondylitis* occurs as the result of injury to the back due to a fall from a height on the feet or buttocks, or the impact of a heavy weight on the shoulders. After some months local symptoms develop, and the radiogram shows marked decalcification of a single vertebra with collapse of the vertebral body and the production of kyphosis.

OSTEODYSTROPHIES

The osteodystrophies, as their name implies, are disturbances in the growth of bone. The great majority are acquired, but a few are congenital. Some are due to lack of vitamins, others to overproduction of hormones, while in the case of perhaps the majority the cause is quite unknown. For the names of this amorphous group the table of contents at the beginning of this chapter may be consulted. These names naturally prove confusing to the reader, not to mention the author. There may be a difference of opinion as to the desirability of the use of eponyms in medicine, but it seems easier to remember almost any man's name than to try to recall the difference between chondrodysplasia, dyschondroplasia and chondro-osteodystrophy.

The outstanding fault in osteodystrophy may be: (1) disturbance in the growth of cartilage; (2) disturbance in the osteogenic-osteolytic balance; (3) disturbance in the deposition of hydroxyapatite in the cartilaginous matrix or in osteoid tissue (Follis). With regard to *disturbed growth of cartilage*, this may be in the direction of too little or too much. *Disturbance in the osteogenic-osteolytic balance* may be evidenced by: (1) *osteoporosis*, with decrease in the number and thickness of calcified trabeculæ, as shown by rarefaction in the *x*-ray film but without decalcification, due to decreased osteoblastic activity; (2) *osteosclerosis*, with increase in the number and width of the trabeculæ and width of the cortex, due to increased osteoblastic activity; or (3) *osteitis fibrosa*, due to increased osteolytic activity. A number of isolated *renal tubular defects*, some of which have a hereditary background, are associated with an inability to resorb metabolites such as water, phosphorus, glucose, amino acids and calcium from the glomerular filtrate, thus causing rickets in the child and osteomalacia in the adult. The varied disease syndromes are merely exaggerations of the normal pattern, again in terms of too little or too much (Follis).

The radiologist naturally occupies a commanding position in determining the location and the nature of lesions of bone. The *x*-ray *picture* is a reflexion of the gross anatomy and pathology of bone, although it suffers the handicap of being a two-dimensional shadow of a three-dimensional structure. It reveals, however, the two basic features of bone pathology, namely undue formation and undue absorption of bone substance. The basic pathology of bone resolves itself into these two elements: too little or too much. Unfortunately both may be combined at different times in the same case. For a demon-

stration of what an *x*-ray picture can show in bone disease the student should consult the superb collection of pictures in Snapper's *Medical Diseases of Bones*.

Osteitis Fibrosa.—This condition, also known as *osteitis fibrosa cystica*, may occur in a general or focal form. The two bear no relation to one another, although in both there may be the development of giant cell tumors. The focal form is confined to young people, whilst the general form may occur at any age. It is with the general form, sometimes called *von Recklinghausen's disease of bone*, that we are concerned at present. It is very much rarer than the focal variety.

It was in 1901 that von Recklinghausen gave the first accurate account of osteitis fibrosa, and in 1904 Askanazy reported a case associated with a parathyroid tumor, but a quarter of a century elapsed before the significance of this association was recognized. The bone lesions are a *manifestation of hyperparathyroidism*, due usually to an adenoma but occasionally to hyperplasia of the parathyroids. The *biochemical changes* are similar to those produced by the administration of parathyroid extract, and the osteoporosis and other bone changes can be reproduced experimentally in animals by continued administration of the extract. The calcium removed from the bones appears in the blood, and the *blood calcium* rises from 10 mg. per 100 cc. to 15 or 20 mg. The *phosphorus* is below normal (3 mg. per 100 cc.), because the renal threshold for phosphorus is lowered by excess parathyroid hormone. Normally the calcium and phosphate ions of the blood and calcium phosphate of the bones are in a state of equilibrium and are subject to the law of ionic dissociation, *i. e.*, concentration of the ions, if altered, must vary inversely with each other, so that excess of calcium ions causes fall of phosphate ions. If, however, renal insufficiency develops, as it is apt to do in the later stages of the disease, the phosphorus may be retained and the level in the blood may return to normal. The low serum phosphorus is particularly valuable for differentiating hyperparathyroidism from such decalcifying diseases as widespread metastatic carcinoma of bone in which the blood may be flooded with calcium. In osteitis fibrosa the serum alkaline phosphatase is considerably raised, although less so than in Paget's disease. There may be metastatic calcification of the arteries, and deposition of calcium in the renal pelvis with calculus formation. Large quantities of calcium are excreted in the urine, so that there is a negative calcium balance. *The results of removing the parathyroid tumor* may be among the most dramatic of postoperative phenomena; the blood calcium falls below normal so that there may be danger of tetany, the bone pains may be abolished immediately, the giant cell tumors may diminish in size in the course of a few weeks, the renal calculi may break into fragments which are passed into the bladder, there is a marked gain in weight, and cripples may throw away their crutches.

Lesions.—In advanced cases the highly porous bones may be much deformed and curved; they may be so soft that they can be cut with a knife, and the compact bone may be greatly thinned by the formation of cysts. (Fig. 713*A*.) These, however, are not necessarily present, so that osteitis fibrosa is a more correct name than osteitis fibrosa cystica. The cysts may contain watery fluid or gelatinous masses. Abundant callus is found at the site of a recent fracture. The *microscopic appearance* is supposed to be specific, but a similar histological picture may be met with in other diseases, as pointed out above. There is resorption of bone with marked osteoporosis. (Fig. 713*B*.) This goes hand in hand with vigorous new formation of young fibrous tissue which occupies the dilated Haversian canals and takes the place of the resorbed bone. The marrow is also fibrosed. Some of this connective tissue may become converted into osteoid tissue, and formation of new bone can be detected with rows of osteoblasts lining the spaces in the bone, but resorption always outstrips ossification and osteoclasts and giant cells form easily recognizable clumps. The formation of *multiple giant cell tumors* or *osteoclastomata* is a characteristic feature of the disease. These may be minute or they may form quite large tumors which can be detected clinically. The new connective tissue is poorly vascularized, so that degeneration, softening, and cyst formation may occur. The lesions are

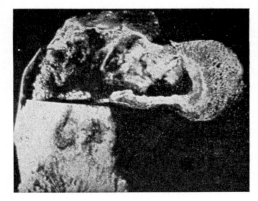

A

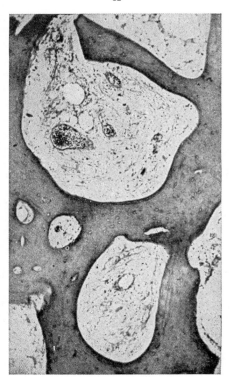

B

Fig. 713.—*A*, Osteitis fibrosa. The neck of the femur is converted into a large cystic cavity.

B, Osteitis fibrosa, showing the marked osteoporosis and resorption of bone. × 50.

at first in the form of circumscribed patches and are most marked at the ends of the growing bones, but in time they may fuse. The patient may die of osteogenic sarcoma, but this tendency is not nearly so marked as in Paget's disease.

Relation of Symptoms to Lesions.—The advanced clinical picture is easy to recognize, but the early stages may severely tax the diagnostic ability of the physician. The three principal symptoms are *bone pains, tumor-like swellings and deformity* of the bones, and *spontaneous fractures.* Of these, fracture is the most striking and often is the first sign of bone disease. The fracture heals more readily than might be expected from the rarefied condition of the bone, but this may be explained by the fact that bone formation is also active. Owing to the softening of the bones they may become markedly bowed, and in severe cases the most extreme deformities may develop. The bones most often affected are the humerus, femur, and tibia, in that order. The disease is progressive and fatal unless diagnosed and treated correctly. The roentgen-ray pictures show widespread local rarefaction and sometimes cyst formation. The bones have a translucent and honeycombed appearance, of the resorbed bone. The marrow is also the marrow is enlarged, and the periosteum normal. The chemical changes in the blood, which are all-important, have already been described.

Focal Form of Osteitis Fibrosa.—This is very much commoner than the generalized form. It bears no relation to that condition, for it is unconnected with hyperparathyroidism and the blood calcium and plasma phosphatase are normal. It occurs at the end of one or more of the long bones during their period of growth and is often first discovered through a spontaneous fracture. Cyst formation is common, as is the formation of a giant cell tumor. It is probably a perversion of the normal process of removal of calcified cartilage by vascular connective tissue preparatory to the formation of true bone. This matter will be discussed in connection with giant cell tumor of bone.

Fibrous Dysplasia of Bone.—Attention has been drawn by Lichtenstein and Jaffe to a condition which may readily be confused with osteitis fibrosa cystica. It appears to be a congenital anomaly in development resulting in tumor-like malformation of bone, and has been appropriately named fibrous dysplasia. One or several bones may be involved. Of 134 cases reviewed by Pritch-

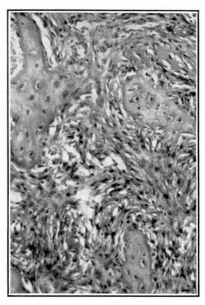

FIG. 714.—Fibrous dysplasia of bone. × 160.

ard only 28 were monostotic. Where the condition is multiple the lesions tend to be unilateral. The most common site is the upper end of the femur, which is often bowed outward. Fibrous dysplasia appears most commonly in early life, and the greatest activity is during the growth period. Many cases are asymptomatic, but pathological fracture may occur. Almost any bone may be involved. I have seen one case in which two adjoining ribs presented huge swellings mistaken for giant cell tumor, and another in which there was cyst formation in the skull. In the severe forms, usually occurring in childhood, there may be extraskeletal anomalies such as pigmentation of the skin, premature sex development in females, premature growth, and hyperthyroidism. These are known collectively as *Albright's syndrome.*

The affected part of the bone is expanded and the cortex is thinned, the interior being filled with rubbery, sometimes gritty, fibrous connective tissue. The *microscopic appearance* of the connective tissue varies; in some places it may be cellular, with spindly cells arranged loosely in whorls (Fig. 714), while elsewhere it may be densely collagenous. New trabeculæ of bone may be formed through metaplasia of the connective tissue,

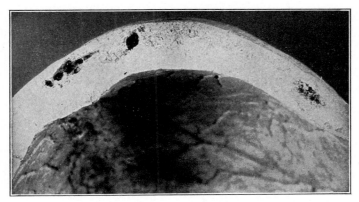

FIG. 715.—*A*, Paget's disease of the skull; great thickening of the bone and cyst formation. Water ran steadily through the thick skull cap.

thus accounting for the grittiness referred to above. In addition there may be small cysts, occasional hemorrhage, and giant cells. In the *x*-ray film there is a localized rarefaction which is readily mistaken for cyst formation.

Paget's Disease.—This condition, also known as *osteitis deformans* (although not nearly so deforming as von Recklinghausen's disease), was first described by Sir James Paget in 1876. It is usually regarded as a rarity, but Schmorl, examining the entire skeleton in his autopsies, collected 138 cases in the course of five years. There is first softening and later overgrowth of bone; during the period of softening characteristic deformities develop. A number of bones are usually affected, but the disease may remain confined to one bone for many years. The former or polyostotic variety is common, but the latter or monostotic form is relatively rare, often remaining subclinical. The monostotic form is commonest in the tibia, the polyostotic is most frequent in the sacrum and vertebræ. It is not certain if they are variations of the same disease.

Lesions.—The bones commonly affected are the skull, vertebræ, and bones of the leg. In Schmorl's material the spine (including the sacrum) was most frequently involved. At first the bones are soft and easily cut with a knife; it is at this stage that the deformities occur. Later the bone becomes hard and of increased thickness. There is a thick deposit of subperiosteal bone on the long bones and

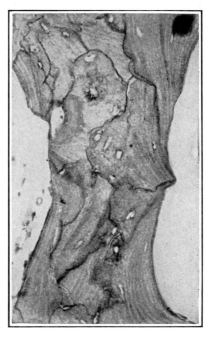

FIG. 715.—*B*, Paget's disease of bone showing mosaic appearance. × 200.

on the skull, and the surface is rough and irregular. In spite of the thickening the new bone is of a porous character, as can be demonstrated by pouring water into the thick skull cap through which it runs as through a sieve. The thick, hard, curved bones are very characteristic of Paget's disease. The thickening is most strikingly seen on the cut surface of the skull cap, and a pathological diagnosis can readily be made from it alone. (Fig. 715*A*.) *Microscopically* there is first a replacement of the original bone by connective tissue, and then a substitution of finely porous cancellous bone which gradually becomes harder. Absorption and apposition go on together, but the latter outstrips the former so that the bone becomes thick though still finely porous. One of the most characteristic features of the microscopic picture is the great number and *irregular arrangement of the lamellar systems*, which is seen in no other disease of bone. This gives what is known as a *mosaic* structure (Fig. 715*B*), due to variously shaped areas of new and old bone fitted together like pieces in a jig-saw puzzle. These pieces are not arranged around vascular canals to form Haversian systems; there is no formation of an "osteon." The cement lines are wide, prominent and irregularly scalloped. Cyst formation is very rare, and so is the formation of giant-cell tumors. The medullary cavity is filled with fibrous tissue. In about 10 per cent of cases sarcoma develops and kills the patient. This may be fibrosarcoma or osteogenic sarcoma. Fibrosarcoma, which is the commoner, arises from the new cellular connective tissue. The osteogenic sarcoma is not identical with the classic form, and may show great numbers of tumor giant cells. There are often multiple foci of sarcoma in different bones.

The *nature of the condition* is uncertain. By some it is believed to be a variation of osteitis fibrosa occurring at a later age, but the blood calcium and phosphorus are normal, the alkaline phosphatase is higher, and there is no parathyroid hyperplasia. Edholm, Howard and McMichael have demonstrated that in generalized Paget's disease *the bone blood flow is greatly increased*, sometimes up to twenty times the normal. This produces the same effect on the general circulation as do free arteriovenous communications, with resulting congestive heart failure. This effect is not seen in the localized form. It is of interest to note that Paget considered the bones to be hyperemic, and in one of his original cases the heart was dilated at autopsy. Other guesses have been

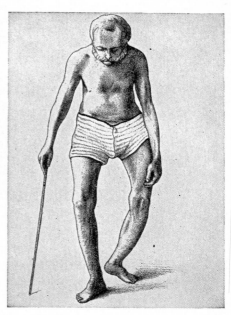

Fig. 716.—Paget's disease. A picture of one of Paget's original cases. (Sir James Paget, *Medico-chirurgical Transactions*, 1877.

made, but they are too baseless to be mentioned.

Relation of Symptoms to Lesions.—The disease usually begins over the age of forty. It may be familial. I know of two families in each of which three cases occurred. The legs are generally first affected, but the earliest change may be in the skull. The softened bones are bent, the femur outward, the tibia forward. They become hardened again in this position and look as if they had been bent by the hands of a giant. Persistent bone pains in the legs may appear before the deformity. The head enlarges, and the patient presents himself with a history that he has to buy hats of ever-increasing size. The head comes to present a very characteristic appearance, for it is a triangle with the base above, the face escaping almost completely. Occasionally the bones of the face are greatly thickened (*leontiasis ossea*). A kyphosis or posterior curvature of the softened spine is very common and reduces the height of the patient. The general appearance in the advanced stage of Paget's disease is highly characteristic. The short squat figure with bent shoulders, curved back, sunken chest, and great head hanging forward, as it waddles along with bowed legs, out-turned toes, and the aid of a stick, is a living justification for the name osteitis deformans (Fig. 716). The roentgen-ray picture is characteristic even before any deformity has appeared. The affected bones are thick and dense, although the medullary cavity is widened, and the vault of the skull presents a peculiar serrated (cock's comb) appearance which is pathognomonic. The disease is progressive, but, unlike osteitis fibrosa, does not usually shorten life. There is, however, a fairly strong tendency to the development of *osteogenic sarcoma*. When that tumor occurs over the age of fifty years it is almost always associated with Paget's disease. Arteriosclerosis is often very marked. *The serum alkaline phosphatase is very high, and may be over 100 units.*

Rickets.—Rickets is a form of osteodystrophy completely different from those already considered, because it is a manifestation of a vitamin deficiency. Avitaminosis D leads to changes in the bones which are different in different age periods, but which yet present fundamental similarities. In children the resulting disease is rickets, in *adults* it is *osteomalacia*. In both the bone trabeculæ are surrounded by broad zones of osteoid tissue, but in children there are additional changes at the junction of bone and cartilage in the growing ends of long bones.

Etiology.—Deficiency of four factors has to be considered: calcium phosphorus, vitamin D, and light. *Phosphorus deficiency* is more serious than *calcium deficiency*. *Vitamin D* facilitates the absorption of calcium and phosphate from the intestine. Light, or rather the short wave ultraviolet rays, activates the sterols in the skin and converts them into vitamin D.

These four deficiency factors must be considered collectively, for they often act together. Thus an amount of calcium in the diet sufficient to prevent rickets becomes insufficient when the phosphorus is also lowered, even though only to a moderate degree. The two seem to work hand in hand. The same is true of the action of light. When rats are fed on a rickets-producing diet they can be protected by being rayed for two minutes each day with the mercury-vapor-

quartz lamp. In actual practice rickets is a disease of the slums of large cities especially in countries which get little sunshine. Here all four factors are at work: the food is deficient in quality as well as quantity (calcium, phosphorus, and vitamin D) and there is a deficiency of ultraviolet light. The fault lies in the quality rather than the quantity of the food. A child may be starved and emaciated, yet show no sign of rickets, while a plump baby may be markedly rachitic. A diet almost exclusively of carbohydrates or proteins will produce rickets, but the addition of cod-liver oil will cure the disease. If the child gets a proper diet and sufficient sunlight, cod-liver oil is never necessary. Rickets is a disease of bottle-fed babies, except in the case of Negro children whose dark skin prevents the light from activating the ergosterol.

Lesions.—The essential rachitic lesion is an abundant formation of *osteoid tissue* which fails to become calcified. The bones are therefore soft and the epiphyses can be cut with a knife. The degree of involvement of the ends of the long bones is proportionate to the rapidity of growth of the epiphyseal cartilage. The most rapid growth occurs at the junction of the ribs and costal cartilages, the lower end of the femur, and the upper end of the humerus in that order. The widening of the epiphyseal line can be seen with the naked eye; it may be 10 or 15 mm. in diameter and is markedly irregular. It is widening not only in depth but also laterally, thus accounting for the nodular swellings of the ribs and at the ends of the long bones.

The *microscopic picture* is one of osteoid tissue formation without calcification. The cartilage cells are not arranged in rows as in normal growing bone, and the zone of proliferating cartilage may be ten times as deep as normal, sending out prolongations into the metaphysis which give the line the irregularity so characteristic of the gross appearance. (Fig. 717.) The zone of preparatory calcification is almost completely free of calcium. Beyond this there is a broad zone of osteoid tissue containing trabeculæ and resembling bone morphologically, but without the all-important lime salts. The osteoid tissue extends out to the perichondrium, where it causes the characteristic thickenings

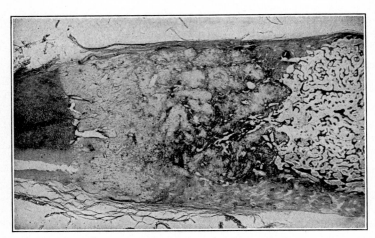

Fig. 717.—Rickets. There is extreme widening of the epiphyseal line and thickening of the bone in this region. There is complete absence of calcification of the osteoid tissue. × 7.

observed clinically. The bosses on the skull and the new periosteal and endosteal bone are also composed of this same material. When healing occurs there is active calcification of the osteoid tissue so that dense bone is formed. In course of time much of this new bone (rickety rosary, etc.) disappears.

Relation of Symptoms to Lesions.—Rickets is a disease of infancy and early childhood covering the period from six months to two years, but the bony changes then instituted may persist for the rest of the patient's life. It is a disorder of calcium and phosphorus metabolism, and examination of the blood shows that either there is a low serum calcium with a rather low inorganic phosphate or normal calcium with very low phosphate. Among the constitutional symptoms are anemia, enlargement of the spleen and lymphoid tissue, flabbiness of the muscles, sweating, and poor formation of the teeth. The bony changes are the combined result of defective calcification and excessive proliferation of epiphyseal cartilage. The bones are soft, so that the femur bends outward, the tibia forward, and the spine backward (kyphosis) or laterally (scoliosis). The constant pull of the tendo Achilles on the foot in the sitting position may produce a curved sabre-shaped tibia. In the softened pelvis the promontory of the sacrum is pushed forward and the acetabula inward, giving the same narrowed pelvic inlet as is seen in osteomalacia and

constituting an insuperable obstacle to normal delivery in later life. The sternum is pushed forward (*pigeon breast*), leaving a vertical groove on each side of the thorax. The epiphyseal proliferation gives rise to a series of nodules at the costo-chondral junctions (the *rickety rosary*), and to nodular swellings at the wrists, knees, and ankles. Bones developed in membrane also suffer, and there is heaping up of spongy bone (bossing) in the frontal and parietal regions so that the skull becomes square, giving to the brow a lofty and intellectual appearance which is seldom justified (Fig. 718). There may be thinning of the back of the skull where the head rests on the pillow, a condition known as *craniotabes*. This is due to absorption of the non-calcified osteoid tissue from pressure. In the *roentgen-ray picture* the normal thin epiphyseal line is broad and irregular; periodic examination of this line forms a convenient method of estimating the effects of treatment, and has been much used in experimental work.

The disease which has just been described is classical rickets, a nutritional deficiency disease, but it is largely a disease of the past due to environmental factors which have been corrected. The rickets encountered at the present day, at least in North America and England, is likely to be due to primary metabolic abnormalities dependent on renal defects, often hereditary in character. It is

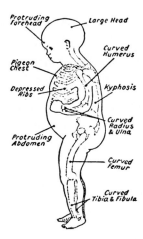

FIG. 718.—Clinical features of severe rickets. (Harris, *Vitamins in Theory and Practice*, courtesy of Cambridge University Press.)

rickets due to nature rather than to nurture (Dent). This condition is described under the heading of renal osteodystrophy, but first it will be convenient to discuss osteomalacia, which is rickets in the adult.

Osteomalacia.—Osteomalacia is a softening of bone after growth is completed. Like rickets, it is due to vitamin D deficiency, which prevents the absorption of calcum from the bowel. It is a very rare disease in North America, is fairly common in Europe particularly during wartime, and is extremely common in North China with its absence of sun, although in tropical South China the abundant sunshine prevents both osteomalacia and rickets. In osteomalacia and also in rickets calcium is not laid down in the bones because of lack of vitamin D, whereas in osteitis fibrosa, the condition with which osteomalacia may be confused clinically, the calcium is removed from the bones on account of too great parathyroid activity, the other great regulator of calcium metabolism. Osteomalacia often comes on during pregnancy owing to the great drain on the calcium of the woman's bones which occurs at that period. Starvation may be a factor, as was strikingly evident in Europe during both World Wars. The disease is one of middle life, and is almost confined to women who are pregnant or exhausted by much childbearing. The bones commonly affected are the lumbar vertebræ, pelvis, and the bones of the legs. Osteomalacia provides a good example of the difficulty of drawing correct conclusions regarding the osteodystrophies. The parathyroids may be enlarged, but it is almost certain that the hyperplasia is secondary and not primary, an attempt to offset the deficient calcification of the bones. The same *secondary parathyroid hyperplasia* is seen in rickets.

One group of incomplete fractures in the softened bone is known under the designation Milkman's disease, or better, *Milkman's syndrome*. The curious eponym does not refer to an occupational hazard to which the deliverer of milk is exposed, but to the writer who first described the condition. These incomplete fractures are usually bilateral, even symmetrical, and may involve such unusual sites as the scapula. The condition is also peculiar in that it does not respond to small doses of vitamin D, whereas osteomalacia does, unless caused by renal defects.

Senile Osteoporosis.—Reference has already been made to this condition in relation to the general subject of bone resorption. In the later period of life, particularly in women after the menopause, the bones tend to become rarefied. Bone absorption may be particularly marked in the vertebral column. The condition is due to a defect in the reparative mechanism of bone, the probable basis of which is the endocrine imbalance of later life, especially in the female. The notable feature of the blood chemistry is the lack of any abnormal findings. The absence of an elevation in the serum alkaline phosphatase serves to distinguish this condition from osteomalacia and from many metastatic tumors of bone.

Renal Osteodystrophy.—This rather indefinite term is preferable to that of *renal rickets*, hallowed by long usage. It signifies "an extraordinarily intricate series of reactions of the skeleton to the presence of renal insufficiency" (Stanbury). It seems justifiable to divide the cases into two main groups, glomerular rickets and tubular rickets, depending on which parts of the nephron are mainly involved. If the condition develops in childhood, as is usually the case, the result will be rickets, if in adults it will be osteomalacia. All forms of renal rickets and osteomalacia are vitamin D-resistant, that is to say they require enormous doses of vitamin D for their control. This feature is due to an inability to retain vitamin D owing to diminished reabsorption of phosphates and vitamin rather than an inability to use the vitamin.

Glomerular rickets, also known as *azotemic renal osteodystrophy*, is caused by destruction of both glomeruli and tubules, but with glomerular function, including phosphate excretion, suffering most. The condition may complicate chronic glomerulonephritis or chronic pyelonephritis. The skeletal changes are those of rickets in children and osteomalacia in the adult.

Tubular rickets is characterized by softening of the bones with accompanying deformities and interference with growth which may result in renal dwarfism. The condition seems to be a hereditary defect which prevents vitamin D from activating alkaline phosphatase in the tubular epithelium, so that there is deficient tubular reabsorption of phosphates with resulting interference in bone formation. Several varieties of renal tubular osteodystrophy are recognized at the present time (Snapper and Nathan). Suffice it to mention the *Fanconi syndrome*, in which there is impaired reabsorption of phosphate, probably in both proximal and distal tubules. The very short proximal convoluted tubule connected with the glomerulus by a narrow "swan neck" has already been described on page 611.

Radiation Osteodystrophy.—Radioactive elements have unfortunately a special affinity for the matrix and crystals of bone, where they remain for long periods of time. Replacement may occur on the surfaces or within the lattice structure of the crystals. Bone is continually being renewed by erosion and deposition, so that radioactive crystals may become isolated, giving a spotty distribution of discrete foci of intense concentration after exposure to radioactive isotopes. These may emit both beta rays and penetrating gamma rays, the half-lives of which vary from fractions of a second to many thousands of years. These constitute not only a direct hazard to bone, but also to the body in general if they should enter the circulation. In the bones there is danger of

damage to the bone marrow and the initiation of malignant tumors. In addition there is direct damage to the bone cells, both osteoblasts and osteocytes, with resulting interference with growth and repair.

The outstanding challenge of internal radiation is the enormously delayed latent period in the development both of radiation osteodysplasias and of malignancy following the retention of minutes amounts of radioactive elements, a period in the case of malignancy which may extend as long as thirty years.

The *source* of radioactive elements may be: (1) diagnostic radiation; (2) therapeutic radiation; (3) the abuse of fluoroscopic devices in shoe stores; (4) the use of radioactive material in industrial plants; (5) chain-reacting uranium piles; and (6) the explosion of atomic (fission) and hydrogen (fusion) bombs.

Atomic radiation is a special example of internal radiation, because much of the danger is from material which is ingested. In this respect radioactive strontium (Sr^{89}) is of primary importance, because it is deposited in bone, where it has a half-life of twenty-five years (Kulp *et al.*). Atomic and hydrogen bomb explosions release débris containing Sr^{90} into the stratosphere. After being fairly uniformly distributed in all latitudes this dust passes into the lower atmosphere, whence it is washed to earth by rain. Plants take up the radioactive strontium along with calcium, and cows eat the contaminated grass. Human beings ingest the strontium mainly in milk products and vegetables. Fish contaminated by explosions of fission and fusion bombs at sea are also a source of danger. Once the strontium is ingested by man it is deposited in the bones.

HYPERTROPHIC OSTEO-ARTHROPATHY.—This condition, also known as *Marie's disease*, is largely due to deficient oxygenation of the tissues, especially when associated with the absorption of toxins. It is met with, therefore, in such *pulmonary conditions* as bronchogenic carcinoma, bronchiectasis, chronic phthisis, empyema, and in congenital heart disease. A *primary, idiopathic familial form* may occur in which no focus of disease can be found elsewhere in the body. There is a subperiosteal formation of new bone with thickening of the bones of the hands and feet, and a lesser involvement of the long bones. The corresponding joints may show swelling and thickening of the synovial membrane. *Clubbing of distal phalanges* (fingers and toes) may be part of osteo-arthropathy or may occur apart from that condition, especially in subacute bacterial endocarditis. The clubbing is largely due to thickening of the soft tissues, probably from edema due to deficient oxygenation. The nails are thickened and characteristically curved, with or without an accompanying thickening of the phalanges.

HYPEROSTOSIS FRONTALIS INTERNAE.—This obscure condition, also known as metabolic craniopathy, is characterized by a peculiar bossy thickening of the inner table of the frontal bone associated with metabolic and psychotic disturbances. The cranial capacity is decreased, with resulting atrophy of the frontal lobes. The radiological appearance is readily recognized. The metabolic changes are those of pituitary dysfunction, particularly obesity, virilism and menstrual disorders, and may precede the bony changes. In 99 per cent of the cases the patients are women, usually after the menopause. There may be no metabolic or psychotic symptoms, and the bony lesions may be discovered by chance at autopsy. The etiology is unknown.

Congenital Osteodystrophies.—Some
osteodystrophies are obviously acquired, whilst others are congenital. Thus rickets and the osteitis fibrosa of hyperparathyroidism belong to the first group, osteogenesis imperfecta to the second. With many others, however, it is not possible to state with certainty whether the basis of the dystrophy was present at birth and genetic in origin. The congenital defect may apparently be in the osteoblasts, as in osteogenesis imperfecta, in the osteoclasts or chondroblasts, as in osteopetrosis, in a failure of endochondral ossification, as in achondroplasia, or of intramembraneous ossification, as in dysostosis cleidocranialis. Any step in the complex process may be defective or absent. If the fault lies in the germ plasm the osteodystrophy will be hereditary.

Osteogenesis Imperfecta.—This rare condition, also known as *fragilitas ossium*, is an affection of childhood in which the bones are imperfectly ossified. There is a marked hereditary and familial tendency. The child may be born dead with multiple fractures acquired in utero, it may be born alive and die afterwards from many fractures produced during delivery, or it may be born apparently healthy and only show evidence of brittleness during childhood and adolescence. There is a tendency for the condition gradually to disappear. A remarkable feature of the disease is that many of the patients have *blue sclerotics;* the color is due to partial visibility of the choroid through the sclerotic owing to some defect in that coat. Blue sclerotics may be associated with brittle bones in one member of the family, while the others have blue sclerotics but no special tendency to fractures. *Otosclerosis* may develop after the age of twenty years. The blood calcium and phosphorus are normal. The parathyroid glands may be enlarged. In one very severe case in a still born baby which I examined the enlargement was very noticeable. In addition to the fractures there may be bony swellings, especially in the temporal region so that the ears are turned out and down, and sometimes in the frontal or occipital regions. The ossification of the skull may be so incomplete that it is a mere membranous bag or a few bony plates; if ossification has proceeded further the skull may present a large number of Wormian bones. The teeth are poorly calcified and may be translucent. The bones are very light and fragile. *Microscopically* the trabeculæ are narrow and widely separated. Few osteoblasts can be seen, and it is possible that there may be a deficiency of phosphatase production.

ACHONDROPLASIA.—This is another rare defect in ossification, confined to bones ossified in cartilage, *i.e.*, long bones and base of skull; the rest of the skull and bones of the face develop normally. The child may die shortly after birth or may grow up as a *stunted dwarf* with short arms and legs, normal trunk, large head, depressed bridge of nose, and squat hands with fingers of equal length (*trident hand*) (Fig. 719). The shortness of the bones is due to failure of the epiphyseal cartilage to function. The epiphyses are enlarged and with the short diaphysis give the bone the appearance of a collar stud. The indrawing of the nose is due to relative shortening of the base of the skull from imperfect ossification. *Microscopically* the cells of the epiphyseal cartilage are large, are not arranged in rows, and show an undisciplined tendency to grow in all directions; there is no evidence of active ossification. The disease, which is often familial, is

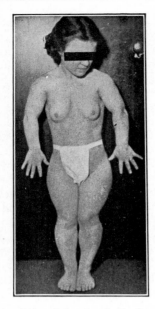

Fig. 719.—Achondroplastic dwarf.

probably due to some endocrine disorder. Dachshunds are achondroplastic dogs selectively bred.

HEREDITARY CHONDRODYSPLASIA.—This rare condition parades under a bewildering variety of names, some familiarity with which is desirable, because few writers seem to favor the same one. It is known as *multiple cartilaginous exostoses*, *multiple congenital osteochondromata*, and *diaphyseal aclasis*. Some of these names suggest a neoplastic condition, others an osteodystrophy. In essence it is a *disturbance of the growth of cartilage and bone*, in the course of which multiple tumors of bone and cartilage develop. In rare cases these may undergo malignant change.

The disease, which is about three times as common in males as in females, begins in early life. As the names imply, the hereditary factor is extremely marked, indicating that the defect lies in the germ plasm. Typical lesions have been traced through as many as 5 generations. In a review of over 1100 cases a hereditary element was evident in 64 per cent (Stocks and Barrington). In this series transmission was by the father in 73 per cent and by the mother in 27 per cent of the cases.

The multiple growths in the bones are merely incidental, not the essence of the disease. They are as a rule first noticed during the first decade of life. Almost any bone in the body may be involved, but those affected are, in their order of frequency, the femur, tibia, humerus, fibula, radius, ulna, phalanges, ribs, scapula, and pelvic bones. It will be noted that the flat bones as well as the long bones may be affected by the disease. The bones of the face and skull are rarely involved; they are laid down in membrane, not in cartilage. Only the bones ossified in cartilage are affected, flat bones as well as long bones. The two chief changes are deformities from retardation of growth and multiple exostoses. The growth retardation may affect any bone developed in cartilage and sometimes only one part of a bone, *e.g.*, acromion process of scapula. The radius or tibia may not grow properly while the ulna or fibula does, with resulting bowing of the bones. The radius becomes a bent bow; the ulna serves as its tight string. The exostoses appear on the shaft of the bones, often as the result of injury to the periosteum. At first they consist of cartilage, but later they may be completely ossified. There may be great numbers of these exostoses. Swellings may develop in the region of the epiphyseal lines, causing enlargement of the ends of the bones. The disease ceases when skeletal development is complete. Nothing is known as to the cause of the condition.

MARFAN'S SYNDROME.—In this remarkable condition, also known as *arachnodactyly* or *spider fingers*, there are anomalies of skeletal growth and of the mesenchymal tissue of the cardiovascular system. Marfan's original report in 1896 dealt with an extraordinary elongation of the distal parts of the extremities in a five-year-girl. Today the syndrome includes a tendency to great height, long and thin hands and feet, (Fig. 720), spinal curvatures, funnel or pigeon chest, dolicocephaly and bossing of the frontal bones, weakness of muscles, scanty subcutaneous fat, anomalies of the lens and other parts of the eye, defects of the cardiac septa, and medionecrosis of the aorta and pulmonary artery with a tendency to the formation of dissecting aneurysm which is often fatal (Tung and Liebow). It is evident that in this disease, as in osteogenesis imperfecta, the defect of mesenchymal development is by no means confined to the skeleton. The hereditary element may be very pronounced. Thus Bowers reports a family in which 31 cases of the disease occurred in the course of 6 generations. In the 17 members known to have been examined medically there was dislocation of the lens in 94 per cent, dolicocephaly in 94 per cent, arachnodactyly in 70 per cent, and clinical evidence of aortic disease in 15 per cent. The incidence of these stigmata did not change appreciably from one degeneration to the next in the fourth, fifth, and sixth generations. The syndrome was apparently transmitted by a single pleiotropic abnormal gene, the expression

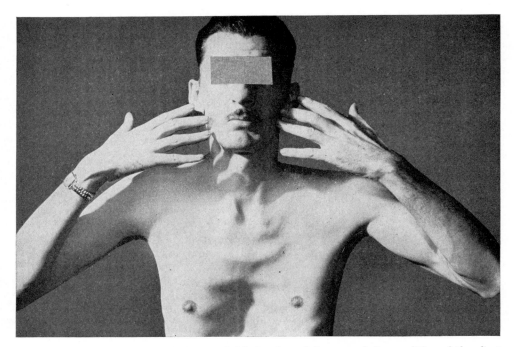

Fig. 720.—Marfan's syndrome. The long and thin hands and fingers and the condition of the chest are highly characteristic. (Kindness of Dr. Harold G. Pritzker.)

of that gene resulting in an abiotrophy of the cardiovascular system.

Osteopetrosis.—This extremely rare condition is also known as *Albers-Schönberg's* disease and *marble bones.* The disease shows a strong familial tendency. It is characterized by excessive calcification of osteoid tissue and absence of true ossification as shown by lack of bone lamellæ and of osteoblasts. The bones therefore lose their elasticity and fractures are common. The condition occurs in childhood or can be traced back to that period. In the roentgen-ray picture the normal structure of bone is replaced by a homogeneous, intensely dense, marble-like appearance. The principal features may be catalogued as follows: All the bones are very dense, particularly the ends of the long bones; narrowing of the cranial foramina causes optic atrophy and other cranial nerve disturbances; narrowing of the medullary cavity leads to osteosclerotic anemia; hydrocephalus, interference with dentition, and enlargement of the liver and spleen may be present. The cause of the condition is unknown.

SKELETAL RETICULOSES

Over the years a number of different groups of clinical conditions with associated pathological lesions have been described in which proliferation of the cells of the reticuloendothelial system with or without accumulation of lipid material is the dominant feature. In some of these the striking lesions were in the bones, while in others it was only realized later that the bones may be involved. For convenience of study they may be taken to constitute one large group, consisting, however, of two divisions which are unrelated. The first division is the *non-lipid reticuloses* consisting of eosinophilic granuloma, Schüller-Christian disease and Letterer-Siwe disease. The second division is the *lipid reticuloses*, namely Gaucher's disease and Niemann-Pick disease. These are regional manifestations of a disturbance of lipid metabolism associated with hyperlipemia; they are, indeed, lipid-storage diseases or lipidoses.

It is the first division, the *non-lipid reticuloses* which are in no sense primary disorders of lipid metabolism although characterized by deposits of lipids, with which we are more particularly concerned in connection with diseases of bone. The process is a *granulo-*

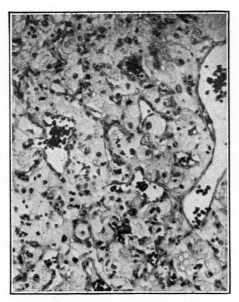

FIG. 721.—Schüller-Christian disease with giant cells. × 500.

matous rather than a neoplastic one and the cell principally involved is the histiocyte, so that Lichtenstein has suggested the generic title of *histiocytosis X* for the group of three non-lipid reticuloses. The eponyms by which two of the members of the group are known have served a useful purpose to denote clinical syndromes, but they do not necessarily indicate separate and distinct pathological entities. The clinical manifestations seem to depend largely on the effect of the age of the patient on the reactions. The younger the age, the more acute and malignant the process (Dennis and Rosahn). The histiocytosis, which is the basic lesion, may be localized to one bone or disseminated widely.

Schüller-Christian Disease.—This condition, known also as *Hand-Schüller-Christian disease* from the various observers who have reported cases, is a rare manifestation of histiocytosis. Christian emphasized the occurrence of a curious and at first inexplicable triad: (1) defects in the membranous bones, especially the skull; (2) exophthalmos; and (3) diabetes insipidus. These, however, need not be present. The condition is a syndrome rather than a disease, in which the basic lesion is an accumulation of histiocytes which

are loaded with lipids (Fig. 721.) Giant cells are common. Eosinophils are present early in the disease, so that the similarity to eosinophilic granuloma becomes obvious. The *bone defects* are due to *erosion produced by periosteal deposits of lipophages*, the *exophthalmos* to *deposits in the orbit*, and the *diabetes insipidus* to *deposits around the pituitary*. The pituitary lesion may also cause dwarfism. *Almost any organ* in addition to the bones may be affected. Lesions in the lungs may result in pulmonary fibrosis. The disease shows great variations in its course, the localization of the lesions, and the clinical manifestations. It generally affects young adults, and may be very chronic in character, lasting for years. The younger the age of onset, the worse is the prognosis. In early childhood it is rapidly fatal. The lipid is *cholesterol* contained in foam or xanthoma cells. The condition is not a true xanthomatosis, which is characterized by xanthomas of the skin and a clear cut disturbance of cholesterol metabolism.

Letterer-Siwe Disease.—This can probably be regarded as *Schüller-Christian disease in infants*. It is rare over the age of two years. The disease runs a rapid and fatal course marked by a skin eruption, hepatomegaly, splenomegaly, lymphadenopathy and progressive anemia. There is no secondary lipidization of the granulomatous lesions because of the acuteness of the process. Biopsy of the sternal marrow shows complete replacement by histiocytes. In rare instances the lesions may change in character to those of Schüller-Christian disease. It is evident that Letterer-Siwe disease can be regarded as the acute and infantile form of histiocytosis-X, while Schüller-Christian disease is the chronic form developing at a later age.

Eosinophilic Granuloma.—This is a painful inflammatory lesion of bone occurring at a young age and easily mistaken for osteomyelitis, tuberculosis and Ewing's tumor (Jaffe and Lichtenstein). The lesions may occur in any bone, but they are most frequent in the skull, ribs, vertebræ and long bones. The distribution is therefore similar to that of multiple myeloma and secondary carcinoma, and as the x-ray picture may also be similar, mistakes in diagnosis may readily occur. The age incidence, however, is quite different, for eosinophilic granuloma is a *disease of children and young adults*, most of the cases occurring before the age of twenty-one years.

The *lesion* is soft, expands the body, and consists of histiocytes, numerous eosinophilic polymorphonuclears, and sometimes giant cells arranged around cholesterol crystals which originate in areas of necrosis and hemorrhage. Some of the stromal cells take up the lipid and become foamy. As the lesions mature the eosinophils tend to decrease in numbers and finally disappear, while the lipophages become more numerous, but eventually these also are replaced by fibrous tissue which becomes ossified. The essential element in the lesion appears to be sheet-like collections of histiocytes, so that it must be regarded as a skeletal histiocytosis similar in nature to Schüller-Christian disease and Letterer-Siwe disease in spite of its benign course (Farber).

Lipid Histiocytoses.—In the group of the reticuloses of bone just described the presence of lipid (cholesterol) in the histiocytes must be regarded as coincidental. The group now to be considered represents a primary disturbance in the metabolism of certain complex lipids, kerasin and sphingomyelin in particular, with accumulation of these lipids in the reticuloendothelial cells throughout the body as well as in the bones. The two principal examples of the condition, Gaucher's disease and Niemann-Pick disease, have already been described in Chapter 40, so that only the skeletal lesions will be referred to here.

Gaucher's Disease.—Involvement of the skeleton is said to be constant in Gaucher's disease, and in one form of the disease the lesions are mainly osseous. The condition is often familial, and all the affected members of the family may suffer from the skeletal form of the disease. The femur, vertebræ and sternum are principally affected. Perhaps the commonest lesion is a bottle-shaped conical swelling of the lower part of the shaft of the femur with erosion of the cortex. Sternal puncture reveals the presence of the characteristic huge Gaucher cells distended with *lipid (kerasin)*, which stains only faintly or not at all with Sudan or Scharlach R.

Niemann-Pick Disease.—In this rare variety of lipid-storage disease, which is almost confined to Jewish infants, the histiocytes of every organ in the body may be loaded with lipid. There are no localized bone lesions, but the marrow is diffusely infiltrated with lipid-filled cells.

TUMORS OF BONE

In studying the difficult subject of bone tumors it is desirable to determine the constituents of the bone from which the various tumors arise. In many cases this is possible; in some it is difficult or impossible. Bone is a connective tissue which happens to be impregnated with lime salts. Anatomically it consists of periosteum, bone and bone marrow, while at each end of the growing bone there is epiphyseal cartilage. The periosteum consists of *fibrous tissue* and *osteoblasts*. The bone contains adult *bone cells* which are end-products incapable of proliferating and giving rise to a tumor, *osteoblasts*, and *osteoclasts*. The marrow consists of *marrow cells*, which need not be particularized further, and reticular or *reticuloendothelial cells*. In general terms, which will be subject to subsequent analysis, it may be said that the periosteal fibroblasts may give rise to fibrosarcoma, the osteoblasts to osteoma and osteogenic sarcoma, the osteoclasts to giant cell tumor, the cartilage cells to chondroma and chondrosarcoma, the marrow cells to multiple myeloma, and the reticular or reticuloendothelial cells to Ewing's tumor. It is convenient to consider the innocent and malignant tumors separately.

Endless classifications of primary bone tumors have been suggested by the three persons involved in the diagnosis, namely the clinician, the pathologist and the radiologist. Indeed there would seem to be almost as many classifications as there are writers on the subject. Some sort of classification is essential, because there is no field in which it is so important that the surgeon, the radiologist and the pathologist speak the same language. One's outlook on the subject depends largely on whether one is by nature a lumper or a splitter. In the Registry of Bone Sarcoma of the American College of the Surgeons there are 8 subvarieties of osteogenic sarcoma (osteosarcoma), which seems to be carrying splitting to an extreme. Lichtenstein remarks that he is reluctant to open his book on bone tumors with a classification "lest those not versed in the complexities of their pathological anatomy be frightened away or discouraged at the onset," and then he proceeds to do so.

The best type of classification, as originally suggested by Ewing, is that based on the tissue of origin, when that can be determined. A practical application of this principle is to recognize 4 main series of tumors, namely *osteogenic, chondrogenic, collagenic* and *myelogenic*, arising respectively from the osteoblast, the chondroblast, the collagenoblast (fibroblast), and the marrow reticulum (Aegerter and Kirkpatrick). The individual members of these groups will be found in the outline at the beginning of this chapter. As a rule the type cell can be identified by virtue of the intercellular ground substance it produces, be it osteoid, hyalin or collagen. In addition to the four main groups there are the *tumor-like processes*, which include *reactive lesions* that may be osteogenic or collagenic, and *hamartomas* that may be osteogenic, chondrogenic or collagenic. And finally there are the *secondary* or *metastatic* tumors, which are far commoner than primary tumors, and should always be suspected in a case of bone tumor in the latter half of life. Aegerter and Kirkpatrick point out that by excluding the tumor-like hamartomas, which are localized exaggerations of intramembranous bone formation and the reparative reactions to bone injury and other idiopathic lesions of unknown mechanism, the number of true primary bone tumors become relatively few and easy to remember.

Osteogenic Tumors.—The osteogenic series of bone lesions are characterized, as their name indicates, by the production of an intercellular substance which is recognizable as *osteoid*. Of the 6 members of the series only 3 are true neoplasms (benign osteoblastoma, osteosarcoma and parosteal sarcoma), 2 are hamartomas (osteoma and osteochondroma), and 1 is an idiopathic type of bone reaction (osteoid osteoma).

Benign Osteoblastoma.—It is unfortunate to have to begin our consideration of true bone tu-

mors with this example, because it seems to be very uncommon, and it is so readily confused with similar lesions parading under such names as ossifying fibroma and fibrous osteoma, lesions which are more related to the osteodystrophies than to neoplasms. It would indeed appear that a true bone-forming benign tumor is a rarity. The benign osteoblastoma is a comparative newcomer (Lichtenstein). Most patients are between ten and twenty-five years old. The common location is the vertebral column, followed by the short bones of the hand or foot. Pain in the back, or down the legs from pressure on nerves, is a frequent symptom. The *gross appearance* suggests a malignant tumor, especially osteogenic sarcoma, the consistence being gritty or sclerotic in places. *Microscopically* the basic tissue consists of a loosely fibrillar and highly vascular matrix rich in osteoblasts (Jaffe). In some areas the nests or sheets of osteoblasts are the conspicuous feature, while in other areas of the same lesion there is an abundance of intercellular osteoid material. The importance of the lesion lies in the fact that it may be confused with other conditions such as osteoid osteoma, osteosarcoma, and giant-cell tumor.

Osteosarcoma.—With the exception of multiple myeloma, osteosarcoma is the commonest and the most malignant of primary bone tumors. It is more generally called *osteogenic sarcoma*. Ewing, who introduced that term, used it to indicate that the tumor is "arising from bone" rather than "bone-forming," just as bronchogenic carcinoma signifies a carcinoma arising from a bronchus. Others use osteogenic to mean bone-forming, but the tumor cells may be less mature than the osteoblast and therefore unable to form osteoid. For this reason osteosarcoma seems a preferable term, comparable to chondrosarcoma and fibrosarcoma.

This is the *most common* and the *most malignant of bone tumors*. It is *a disease of the second and third decades* (10 to 30 years), and is very rarely seen after the age of 50 years. It may be noted that Ewing's tumor also occurs chiefly in childhood and adolescence, giant-cell tumors are commoner in the third decade and multiple myeloma generally occurs after the age of 40 years. The site of election of osteosarcoma is at the end of the long bones (metaphysis), giant cell tumor at the epiphysis, Ewing's tumor in the shaft of the long bones, and multiple

myeloma in the flat bones. Over 70 per cent of cases of osteosarcoma occur in the lower limb. The order of frequency is as follows: femur, tibia, humerus, pelvis, fibula. It hardly ever occurs in the forearm. A history of trauma is common but not so constant or convincing as in Ewing's tumor. Nothing is more difficult than to judge the relationship of trauma to tumor. There is no relation between fracture and any form of bone tumor. Martland has pointed out that osteogenic sarcoma may develop in those whose bones have become highly radioactive. In a group of girls who died from the ultimate effects of swallowing highly radioactive substances while painting the dials of luminous watches, 27 per cent of the deaths were due to osteogenic sarcoma. It was calculated that in the year 3491 A.D. the skeleton of one of these girls would still be giving off 185,000 alpha particles per second, each of these travelling at the rate of 180,000 miles per second.

The *gross appearance* depends on the stage. The first symptom is pain due to involvement of the sensitive periosteum, and this may precede the appearance of a tumor by weeks or months. When the tumor is well developed there is a fusiform mass at the end of the bone which fades away on to the shaft, giving a "leg of mutton" appearance. (Fig. 722.) At first the disease is confined to the bone, with involvement of the shaft, the medulla, and the periosteum, but in the later stages the periosteum is perforated with rapid dissemination of the growth in the soft parts. There is a coincident absorption and deposition of bone; the original shaft is absorbed, but tumor bone is laid down in the subperiosteal space by the osteogenic tumor cells. It is curious to note that the innocent giant cell tumor is destructive (osteolytic), while the very malignant osteogenic sarcoma forms new bone. This formation, however, is quite patchy, so that pathological fracture is likely to occur in the later stages. As the periosteum is lifted up from the bone by the tumor the vessels which enter the shaft from the periosteum are drawn out in parallel vertical lines, which form a scaffolding on which the new bone is laid down. Fine spicules are therefore found radiating outward from the central mass, and in the roentgen-ray picture these give a very character-

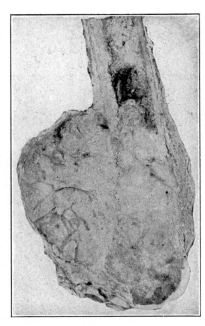

FIG. 722.—Osteogenic sarcoma of lower end of femur. The tumor has destroyed the shaft, and is both medullary and periosteal in distribution.

istic "sun-ray" effect. The consistence of the tumor varies with the amount of bone formed, which may be much or little. The tumor may be very soft and sarcomatous, or firm and fibrous, or hard and bony. The usual color is gray, but the tumor may be highly vascular and hemorrhagic, and may present cysts filled with blood. Necrosis and softening are common.

The *microscopic picture* is extraordinarily varied, so that different cases differ widely, and in a single case there may be the same pleomorphism as is seen in glioblastoma multiforme of the brain. The *tumor cells* are osteoblasts, and three types may be seen. (Fig. 723.) (1) The most constant and characteristic form is a small spindle cell with hyperchromatic nucleus and poorly-defined cytoplasm. If the tissue is poorly fixed and stained, the cytoplasm may not be detected, so that the cells appear round, but an osteogenic sarcoma is never a round cell tumor. (2) Other cells may be large and spindle-shaped or polyhedral. Mitoses are numerous in these cells. (3) Giant cells are often present. These may be tumor cells or

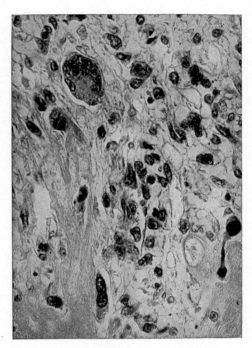

Fig. 723.—Osteosarcoma showing the characteristically pleomorphic picture and a typical tumor giant cell. × 300.

foreign body giant cells. The tumor giant cells may be mononuclear or may contain a small number of large nuclei. The cells have a more irregular, atypical, and neoplastic appearance than the foreign body giant cells. The latter are present when there is much bone destruction, and especially after an exploratory operation. The *intercellular substance* is as characteristic as the cells. It may be hyaline and fibrous, cartilaginous, myxomatous, osteoid, or osseous. Thus there may be formation of tumor bone. It is important for the pathologist to distinguish between tumor bone and true bone. Tumor bone is atypical and poorly formed, it blends with the stroma of the tumor, and it presents no bordering line of osteoblasts. When the stroma is largely fibrous, the sarcoma is of the sclerosing type. Calcium can be recognized by its dark blue color when stained with hematoxylin. If the blood vessels are very abundant, the tumor is said to be of the telangiectatic type. Invasion of the thin-walled vessels is common, and tumor cells may form the actual walls of the blood si-

nuses. The limb must therefore be handled with great gentleness. It is easy for metastases to be set up at the time of operation. Preliminary radiation of the tumor, by closing the vessels, diminishes this danger to a considerable degree.

The *x-ray picture* should always be taken into consideration in conjunction with the gross and microscopic appearance. The *chief features* are as follows: (1) Combined central and subperiosteal involvement. Benign tumors are either inside or outside the old cortex; malignant tumors are both. At the extreme margin of the tumor there is a little lip of reactive bone which represents the last line of defense of normal osteoblasts retreating in circular formation as the tumor advances under the periosteum (Codman triangle). (2) Presence of the old shaft. The shaft, although permeated by the tumor, is not displaced. In giant cell tumor the shaft is destroyed, and in Ewing's tumor it is greatly thickened. (3) Invasive character. The edge is irregular, never rounded and smooth as in giant cell tumors. (4) Osteolytic and osteoblastic. In the great majority of cases there is both bone destruction and bone formation. Bone formation usually takes the form of radiating spicules (sunray appearance), but this is by no means constant. (5) Involvement of the soft parts.

Spread takes place mainly by the blood stream, as is natural from the vascular arrangement just described. Metastases usually occur in the lungs, but if the tumor emboli pass the pulmonary capillaries they may lodge in other organs. It is important to note that secondary growths in other bones are very rare; *multiple bone tumors suggest Ewing's tumor in the young and multiple myeloma in the middle aged.* Metastatic carcinoma must not be forgotten. The lymph nodes are sometimes involved, but any enlargement is usually inflammatory. There is marked local invasion, and when the periosteum is perforated the tumor spreads rapidly through the soft parts and causes stretching of the skin.

The *prognosis* is extremely grave. Osteosarcoma is the most malignant tumor arising from bone. Early diagnosis is not easy, and after the true nature of the condition has been determined the usual survival period is

not more than eighteen months. The reason for this grim outlook is the early formation of pulmonary metastases. By the time the diagnosis has been made it is more than probable that tumor cells are growing in the lung. As we shall see, the behaviour of the tumor and the outlook for the patient is very different in the variety of bone sarcoma next to be considered.

PAROSTEAL SARCOMA.—Quite distinct from the central or classic type of osteosarcoma is the bone-forming tumor which develops in relation to the surface of bone and specifically in relation to the periosteum and the immediate parosteal connective tissue (Fig. 724). It was named parosteal sarcoma by Geschickter and Copeland in 1950, a term which prevents confusion with periosteal fibrosarcoma. It has also been called *juxtacortical osteogenic sarcoma* (Jaffe). This tumor is relatively uncommon, it has a much better prognosis than central osteosarcoma, and it is distinctive in other ways.

The tumor is *confined to the long bones*, and in at least half the cases it arises in the metaphysis of the lower end of the femur, growing into the soft tissue rather than into the bone. In consistence it varies from firm to hard. The *microscopic picture* is apt to be confusing, for it is common to find fields suggestive of fibrosarcoma, of chondrosarcoma and of osteosarcoma all in the same lesion. Sometimes the appearance is deceptively benign and the cells may appear innocent, just as the face of a dangerous criminal may appear innocent.

The *prognosis* is very different from that of central osteosarcoma. It is a slowly growing tumor, and it may be present for a number of years before a correct diagnosis is made. If the diagnosis is made reasonably early and the proper treatment carried out, a cure may be expected in the great majority of cases. Recurrence after local resection is frequent, the microscopic picture becomes more malignant, and pulmonary metastases are fairly common, although these may not become apparent for some years after removal of the recurring tumor.

Chondrogenic Tumors.—The chondrogenic series forms a confused and confusing group. It comprises two well defined entities, chondroma and chondrosarcoma, and two rare variants of chondroma, benign chondroblastoma and chondromyxoid fibroma. The condition known as endochromatosis, multiple enchondromata or hereditary multiple exostoses is a hamartoma, an error in devel-

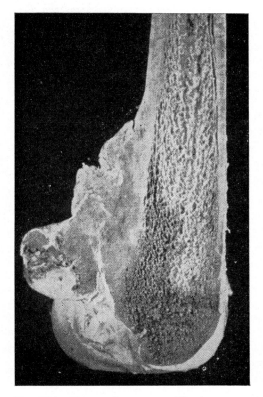

FIG. 724.—Parosteal sarcoma. The tumor mass blends with the cortex, which has become thickened, but the marrow cavity has not been invaded. (Jaffe, *Tumors and Tumorous Conditions of the Bones and Joints*, Lea & Febiger.)

opment rather than a neoplasm, and has already been considered in connection with the osteodystrophies.

CHONDROMA.—Cartilaginous tumors may arise from the epiphyseal cartilage or from the cartilage which precedes the developing bone, islands of which may remain unabsorbed. They occur during the growing period, and are *commonest in the short bones* of hands and feet where they may be multiple. Single chondromas of large size may grow from the scapula, pelvis, neck of femur, and other bones. These single tumors often undergo myxomatous and cystic degeneration, and are then liable to show malignant change into a *chondrosarcoma* especially when interfered with. *It may be easier to detect this change from the clinical behavior and the gross appearance at operation (invasion, etc.) than from the microscopic structure.* Invasion of the veins and metastases to the lungs confirms the malignant character of the change. A chondroma may grow on the surface or the interior of the bone. The latter form, known as an *enchondroma*, may cause expansion of the shaft, and when combined with cystic degeneration may give a roentgen-ray picture closely simulating that of giant cell tumor. The condition known as mutliple cartilaginous exostoses or chondrodysplasia is considered in connection with the bone dystrophies.

Microscopically, the chondroma consists of cartilage cells of varying age and size. Most of these are sufficiently mature to produce characteristic hyalin. In other areas the cells are less mature, smaller, distorted by fixation, and there is no hyalin formation. If the pathologist confines his attention to such an area or block of tissue he may make the serious mistake of calling the lesion a chondrosarcoma. *It is in such circumstances that consultation with the radiologist and clinician is so valuable and indeed imperative.*

Two other benign tumors of cartilage have been separated from the chondroma group. These are known as benign chondroblastoma and chondromyxoid fibroma. Both are distinctly rare. *Benign chondroblastoma* is a neoplasm of the *epiphyses of adolescents*. The only other bone tumor which characteristically involves the epiphysis is the giant cell tumor, and it does so only after the epiphysis has ossified. The tumor arises from young chondroblasts in the deep portion of the enchondral plate, manifests itself soon after puberty, invades the nucleus of the adolescent epiphysis, and may erode the articular cartilage, so that slowly increasing joint pain is the only symptom. *Microscopically*, the young chondroblasts are larger than normal cartilage cells. It produces little hyalin in many areas, so that the tumor is highly cellular, suggesting a malignant neoplasm. In other areas hyalin is very evident, together with myxoid and collagenous tissue. Some giant cells are usually present. *Chondromyxoid fibroma*, which would be better called *fibromyxoid chondroma*, is probably a variant of chondroblastoma, which arises from a group of immature chondroblasts left behind in the *metaphysis* after epiphyseal ossification is complete. This would explain the site, the more advanced age, and the fact that although pain is the outstanding feature, the joint is not usually involved. *Microscopically*, as the name indicates, the chondroblasts lie in a hyaline stroma which may be mainly myxomatous or mainly fibrous.

CHONDROSARCOMA.—Chondrosarcoma may arise de novo or as a malignant change in a benign chondroma. It is more than possible that in the latter instance the tumor has been malignant from the beginning. Chondrosarcoma is quite *different from osteosarcoma in respect to* (1) site, (2) age group, (3) microscopic appearance, and (4) prognosis. It is half as common as osteosarcoma. About 75 per cent of the cases involve the trunk or the upper ends of the humerus and femur. Generally speaking, the nearer a cartilaginous tumor is to the trunk, the more likely it is to be malignant. Cartilaginous tumors of the small bones are rarely malignant. Chondrosarcoma is unusual under the age of thirty-five, the incidence rising with the years, in striking contrast with the earlier age period of osteosarcoma. Moreover it is a slowly growing tumor.

Morbid Anatomy.—The tumor forms a firm rounded mass, grayish-white in color, which tends to be lobulated. The consistence varies much, depending on the histological structure. Some parts may be very firm and other parts equally soft. The *microscopic appearance* varies greatly in different parts of the section and in different parts of the tumor. Some areas are well differentiated and present the appearance of a benign chondroma. *There is perhaps no tumor in which the microscopic picture can be more misleading*, and in which it is so important for the surgeon to take cognizance of the gross appearance at operation (evidence of invasion, consistency) and the roentgenographic evidence. In other areas the cells may be highly anaplastic with great variation in size and absence of regular arrangement. Mitoses are never numerous, for the cells appear to divide by amitotic division. *Osteosarcoma contains neoplastic elements of all the tissues involved in normal bone formation, whereas in chondrosarcoma the elements are entirely cartilaginous.* Myxomatous degeneration may be very marked, a change highly suggestive of malignancy in a cartilaginous tumor, and one which is responsible for the soft consistency of some areas.

The situation may be summed up by saying that it may be impossible for the pathologist to arrive at a correct diagnosis from the microscopic appearance alone. *A benign chondroma may look malignant and a chondrosarcoma may appear benign.* The following *clinical features* are suggestive of malignancy (O'Neal and Ackerman): (1) Cartilaginous tumors of the pelvis, ribs, sternum and vertebræ; (2) large peripheral tumors, particularly if greater than 8 cm. in diameter; (3) enchondromas of the long bones, exclusive of those of the bones of the hands and feet—an enchondroma of a long bone which has perforated the cortex is practically certain to be malignant; (4) tumors which grow rapidly during adolescence, or which continue to grow after the age of twenty years at an accelerated rate, or which first develop during adult life. Multiple cartilaginous exostoses have a tendency to become malignant.

The *prognosis* forms an interesting contrast to that of osteosarcoma. Growth is slow compared with the rapid rate of osteosarcoma, and metastases are late. On the other hand the tumor is much more likely to recur at the site of operation than is the case with osteosarcoma.

Collagenic Tumors.—A variety of conditions parading under such names as ossifying fibroma and non-osteogenic fibroma have in the past been regarded as connective tissue tumors of bone, but are now known to be reactive lesions. The two true neoplasms composed of a fibroblastic stroma are giant cell tumor and fibrosarcoma.

GIANT CELL TUMOR.—In the general welter of confusion represented by the subject of bone tumors, the most enigmatic and controversial lesion is that known as giant cell tumor, sometimes referred to, especially by British writers, as *osteoclastoma.* There is difference of opinion on practically every aspect of the subject. It is, indeed, rather an amusing experience to read the opinions of the various experts on the views of other experts, often expressed with the ardor of religous fanaticism, especially with regard to two main aspects of the subject: (1) what constitutes a giant cell tumor? and (2) what is its origin?

(1) There can be little doubt that in the past many lesions with giant cells were wrongly regarded as giant cell tumors. Among these so-called "variants" of giant cell tumor which have been taken out of the general grab-bag of bone lesions with multinucleated giant cells may be mentioned the "brown tumors" of hyperparathyroidism, solitary bone cyst, aneurysmal bone cyst, non-osteogenic fibroma, chondroblastoma and chondromyxoid fibroma (Jaffe, Lichtenstein and Portis). The giant cell tumors of tendon sheaths and synovial membranes are quite unrelated to the bone tumors, being granulomatous rather than neoplastic in nature. The same is true of the myeloid epulis of the jaw. Here again *resemblance does not denote identity*, and the lesion should not be classed as an osteoclastoma. It is now recognized that the presence of giant cells alone cannot be taken as justification for a diagnosis of giant cell tumor, *i.e.*, true osteoclastoma, any more than the presence of lymphocytes indicates the nature of an inflammatory lesion. It is evident that giant cells are encountered in a variety of benign lesions of bone, and we have already seen that they are not uncommon in osteogenic sarcoma. This elimination of variants has cut down the number of true giant cell tumors very greatly, but has left a considerably more formidable neoplasm which is not nearly as benign as I was taught when I was an undergraduate.

(2) The *origin* of the tumor has been and still is a matter of endless debate. The lesion is composed of a fibroblastic stroma interspersed with multinucleated giant cells. Lichtenstein states that the giant cells are not derived from osteoclasts. The very name osteoclastoma indicates that others believe they are identical. Again, are these cells the cause or the consequence of the resorption of bone which is the chief characteristic of the tumor? If the stromal cells are regarded as immature osteoclasts, much of the difficulty can be removed.

Morbid Anatomy.—The tumor develops in young adults, usually before the age of thirty years, at or near the ossified epiphyseal line of a tubular bone in which enchondral growth has been completed. The lower end of the femur and the upper end of the tibia are the most common sites, accounting for as much

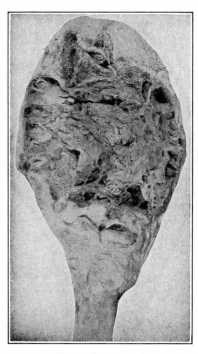

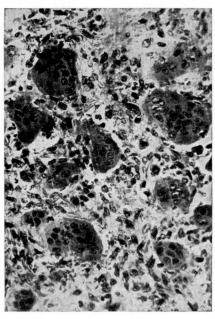

Fig. 725B.—Giant cell tumor of bone. The multinucleated giant cells are unusually numerous. × 225.

Fig. 725A.—Giant cell tumor of the upper end of the tibia. The material expanding the end of the bone is soft, red and resembles blood clot.

as 50 per cent of the cases, followed by the lower end of the radius. Sometimes the short tubular bones of the hand or foot may be involved, but the flat bones very seldom indeed. Growth extends in both directions, into the epiphysis and into the metaphysis. The epiphyseal location is of value in differentiating the lesion from bone cysts in the x-ray film.

The center of the bone is expanded, and the cortex often reduced to a mere shell, so that a spontaneous fracture may first attract the attention of the patient to the condition which may be painless although often accompanied by deep-seated pain. Fairly thick bone trabeculæ are left traversing the cystic lesion like beams supporting a crumbling building. This arrangement, best seen in the dried and macerated specimen from which the soft tissue has been removed or in the operating room when the soft parts are curetted away, is responsible for the soap-bubble appearance (see below). The *roentgen-ray picture* is highly characteristic, and from it a diagnosis can usually readily be made. It shows a rarefied, multicystic, or trabeculated appearance as if the mass was composed of large bubbles, thinning of the cortex, and sharp limitation of the lesion from the surrounding bone and soft parts.

The *gross appearance* in an advanced case, fortunately seldom seen at the present day, is that of a soft, dark red, hemorrhagic mass, sometimes with yellow areas. There may be great expansion of the end of the bone (Fig. 725A). The *microscopic picture* varies in different cases and in different parts of the same tumor. In all instances, however, *two types of cell* can be recognized: (1) spindle shaped or oval cells, which have, probably incorrectly, been termed stromal cells, but are really the basic mononuclear cells of the tumor; (2) multinucleated giant cells of osteoclast type, which are the largest of all giant cells (Fig. 725B). It has already been suggested that the giant cells may represent a development of the mononuclear spindle cells, perhaps representing an absorption phase of activity. In determining the neoplastic nature of the lesion attention must be paid not to the giant cells but to the mononuclear so-called stromal cells. These must show neoplastic characters to justify a diagnosis of giant cell tumor (Aegerter).

The tumor must not be regarded as a completely benign tumor, for it may show a varying degree of *leaning towards malignancy*. This can best be gauged by a study of the mononuclear cells. On this basis Jaffe, Lichtenstein and Portis have introduced the idea of grading of the tumors. In *Grade I* lesions, which constitute 50 per cent of the cases, giant cells are numerous in all fields, spindle cells predominate, and there are very few mitoses. These cases have a benign course. In *Grade II* the picture is intermediate in type. These cases tend to recur after removal. *Grade III* is a small group in which the mononuclear (stromal) cells are atypical, hyperchromatic, and show numerous mitoses, while the giant cells are small, few in number, and show the same anaplastic changes as the stromal cells. These tumors are frankly malignant, recur after removal, and may metastasize to a distance. Finally there are occasional examples in which the histological appearance is completely benign, yet metastasis to the lungs occurs, and these metastases also present a benign picture, yet result in the death of the patient.

FIBROSARCOMA.—This is the least common and least malignant of the connective tissue tumors of bone. It may originate in the periosteum or the medullary cavity, the two types being of equal frequency. The *periosteal type* grows mainly by expansion, producing a concave defect in the bone. Reactive bone may be formed, giving the Codman triangle. In the *medullary form* an oval defect is produced in the interior of the bone. The site of the tumor may be metaphysis or diaphysis, the former being somewhat the commoner. Any bone may be involved. The tumor is solid, firm, and whitish in color. The slowly growing forms develop a pseudocapsule. The *microscopic picture* is the same as that of a fibrosarcoma of the soft parts, with fusiform fibroblasts showing varying degrees of anaplasia in a collagenous matrix.

Myelogenic Tumors.—The three members of this group Ewing's tumor, reticulum cell sarcoma and plasma cell or multiple myeloma are all malignant tumors. It is believed that all three types are derived eventually from the marrow reticulum.

EWING'S TUMOR.—It was in 1920 that Ewing separated this tumor from the general group of bone sarcomas under the heading of endothelial myeloma. It forms about from 10 to 15 per cent of all malignant bone tumors (including giant cell tumors in the total). The *clinical history* is characteristic, but may be suggestive of osteomyelitis, a disease for which this condition is sometimes mistaken both by the clinician and the pathologist. The patient is usually between the ages of five and fifteen years, and the disease is quite rare above thirty years. There is often a history of trauma, followed shortly by pain, at first intermittent but later continuous, fever, and the appearance of a swelling. When the swelling is incised a soft necrotic cellular material is obtained which is easily mistaken for pus. The occasional occurrence of a moderate leukocytosis still further adds to the difficulties of diagnosis. The *roentgen-ray picture* shows diffuse involvement of the greater part of the shaft. There is a combination of bone formation and bone destruction; formation in the early stage, destruction later. The new bone on the surface may present a laminated appearance like the layers of an onion. One of the most striking characteristics of the tumor is its *response to radiation;* it may melt away just like a lymphosarcoma, only to return again later. This characteristic is of great diagnostic value.

There can be little doubt that some of the cases described in the literature as Ewing's tumor are really examples of metastatic growths. In most of these cases the diagnosis is based merely on a biopsy or roentgen-ray report, whereas no case can be finally accepted without a complete autopsy examination. This truth is strikingly demonstrated by a case reported by Willis in his monograph on the *Spread of Tumors*, in which a patient presented all the clinical, radiological and pathological (gross and microscopic) evidence of Ewing's tumor, and yet proved at autopsy to be a case of adrenal neuroblastoma with widespread metastases in the bones.

The *gross appearance* is that of a very soft disintegrating tumor resembling brain tissue.

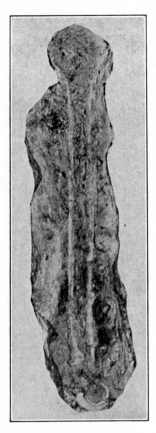

FIG. 726A.—Ewing's tumor of humerus. The growth is characteristically diffuse, involving the entire shaft. There were secondary growths in several other bones. (Boyd, *Pathology for the Surgeon*, courtesy of W. B. Saunders Co.)

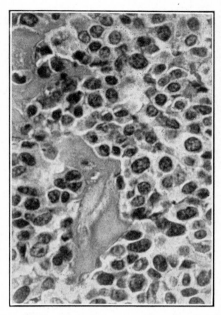

FIG. 726B.—Ewing's tumor. Tumor cells are replacing the bone, fragments of which can be seen at left of picture. × 600.

The bones most often involved are tibia, humerus, femur, fibula, clavicle, and os calcis in that order. The tumor starts in the medullary cavity, from which it invades and widens the bone canals, expands the cortex, and irritates the periosteum to lay down successive layers of new bone. This is normal bone laid down parallel to the surface, not tumor bone laid down at right angles to the surface as in osteogenic sarcoma. The tumor involves the metaphysis and the adjoining diaphysis or the diaphysis alone, in striking contrast to the location of giant cell tumor. The bulk of the tumor is subperiosteal, the medullary cavity becoming narrowed or even occluded by new reactive bone (Fig. 726A). Owing to the formation of new bone, pathological fracture is rare.

The *microscopic picture* is that of a round cell sarcoma. The cells are round or polyhedral, very uniform in appearance (*cellular monotony*), with a round nucleus and indistinctly defined cytoplasm which stains poorly. (Fig. 726B.) They are closely packed together, and are arranged in sheets or columns, but may be grouped around blood spaces so as to give an angio-endotheliomatous appearance. There is no intercellular substance, in striking contrast to osteosarcoma. The microscopic appearance gives little help in determing the *nature of the tumor*. Ewing originally called it an endothelial myeloma, in the belief from the occasional peritheliomatous arrangement that it arose from vascular endothelium. The feeling now is that it arises from the reticular cells of the marrow, and that Ewing's tumor and reticulum cell sarcoma are variants of the same tumor, but PAS-positive glycogen granules in the cytoplasm serve to distinguish the former from the latter.

Spread occurs within the shaft both longitudinally and transversely by means of the

bone canals, which in decalcified sections are seen to be filled with tumor cells. Distant spread occurs to the lungs, lymph nodes, other organs, and other bones. The bone metastases are of the greatest importance in differential diagnosis. They are hardly ever seen in osteosarcoma. In multiple myeloma there is usually multiple involvement of bones when the patient is first seen, but in Ewing's tumor the patient comes with a single tumor, the secondary growths not developing for several months. These growths are commonest in the skull, vertebræ, sternum, scapula, and ilium, *i.e.*, the flat bones containing red marrow. The *prognosis* is very bad, although the disease may sometimes be held in check for several years by means of radiation.

RETICULUM-CELL SARCOMA.—This is defined as a solitary malignant tumor of bone arising from reticular cells of the marrow. The distribution is on the whole similar to that of Ewing's tumor, with more frequent involvement of the metaphyses. The average age is considerably higher, and it is less than half as common. It is an osteolytic lesion with progressive destruction of bone. *Microscopically* the picture is similar to that of reticulum cell sarcoma of soft tissue. The cells show wider variations in size than those of Ewing's tumor, many of them being quite large. With silver stains a network of reticulin fibers can be demonstrated between the cells. It will be gathered that the histological distinction between solitary reticulum cell sarcoma and Ewing's tumor may be very difficult. As with other bone tumors, the radiological and clinical features of the case must be taken into account. The differentiation is of great practical importance, because reticulum cell sarcoma is *highly radiosensitive*, the growth is slow and the prognosis is much more favorable than is the case with Ewing's tumor.

PLASMA CELL MYELOMA.—This condition, which is a tumor of bone marrow rather than of bone and is commonly called *multiple myeloma*, is unique among neoplasms by reason of the remarkable aberrations in protein metabolism which accompany it. It is a neoplastic proliferation of the cells which normally produce gamma globulins, so it is natural that these globulins and others re-lated to them are present in excess quantity. Some of low molecular weight are excreted by the kidneys, where they may produce renal damage, with serious and sometimes fatal impairment of renal function. The *clinical picture* may therefore be conveniently considered under 3 headings: (1) the tumor mass with its effects on the bone and the bone marrow; (2) the excessive production of serum proteins; (3) damage to the kidneys.

The Tumor.—The gross and microscopic features of the neoplasm will be considered under the heading of lesions. It may be said here that plasma cell myeloma is a more common disease than was formerly thought, largely due to improved diagnostic techniques such as bone marrow aspiration, filter-paper electrophoresis, recognition of the significance of red cell rouleaux formation, etc. It is more frequent in the male and in the Negro. The *age incidence* is in striking contrast to that of Ewing's tumor, 80 per cent of the cases occurring over the age of forty years. It is primarily a disease of the flat bones, and the outstanding symptom is slowly developing *pain*, particularly in the back (vertebræ), the thoracic cage, and the pelvis. Although in rare cases there may be a solitary tumor, at least for a considerable period, in the usual case almost all the bones become involved. The cells appear to exert a lytic action on the bone, so that erosion is marked and *pathological fractures* are common. Huge amounts of calcium may be freed from the bones, with resulting hypercalcemia and metastatic calcification, particularly in the kidneys.

Widespread replacement of the marrow by rank weeds of tumor cells (myelomatosis) is responsible for *anemia* in the majority of cases, late if not early, and sometimes serious in degree. *Bleeding* from mucous membranes is common, particularly in the form of epistaxis. This may be due to thrombocytopenia caused by destruction of megakaryocytes, or to interference with normal fibrinogen formation by the abnormal proteins. Marrow aspiration will show tumor cells in the sternal marrow, even though there is no evidence of a tumor mass or of destruction of bone. This is a valuable method in doubtful cases, but it must not be carried too far, for the presence of plasma cells in the marrow is now known not to be confined to myeloma; and the biopsy findings may be responsible for a mistaken diagnosis.

Serum Proteins.—Plasma cell myeloma is associated with a profound change in protein synthesis, both quantitative and qualitative, the total serum proteins rising to 10 mg. or higher, with a gamma globulin wave many times the normal height. The most common biochemical finding is a distorted serum electrophoretic pattern, with marked inversion of the albumin-globulin ratio. Large amounts of abnormal serum globulins are produced by tumor cells whose metabolic activities are greatly altered. These are known as *myeloma globulins.* About 5 per cent of myeloma globulins are cryoglobulins. The ultracentrifuge is needed to distinguish some of the myeloma proteins from macroglobulins. In addition there is a copious excretion in the urine of a unique protein, the *Bence Jones* protein, which differs in many respects from the myeloma globulins. It was recognized in the urine over 100 years ago by Bence Jones from the fact that it appears as a cloud when the urine is heated to 55°C., disappears at 85° or on boiling, but reappears on cooling. The reason it is found in the urine and not in the serum is that its molecular size (37,000) is only half that of albumin, so that it can readily escape through the glomerular filter. This protein has been extracted from the tumor cells, and when injected intravenously into rabbits it appear in the urine. It is present in the urine in less than 50 per cent of the cases of myeloma. Being a product of marrow cells, it is not surprising that it is sometimes found in leukemia and secondary carcinoma of bone.

A remarkable feature is the extreme variability in the serum protein patterns of different patients. The patient with myeloma never has a normal serum pattern, and the particular pattern for each patient remains unaltered throughout the course of his disease. The primary function of plasma cells is the synthesis of gamma globulins, and it seems probable that individual plasma cells or nests of cells (clones of cells) produce their own specific protein. It is postulated that all the neoplastic plasma cells in a particular case stem from a single cell or group of cells, thus producing their own particular protein. The myeloma cell behaves in the same way as an antibody-forming cell under constant stimulation, suggesting a constant and therefore endogenous stimulus, possibly related to an auto-immune reaction. The *red cell rouleaux* formation in the blood and in marrow smears, which is a valuable diagnostic feature, is probably due to coating of the erythrocytes by the abnormal gamma globulins. One result is a shortened life span of the red cells. The *sedimentation rate* is increased in 90 per cent of cases, again presumably due to coating of the erythrocytes with abnormal serum globulins. A curious feature is the fact that although plasma cells are antibody factories, yet there is *deficient antibody production* in plasma-cell myeloma. There is therefore *increased susceptibility* to *bacterial infections*, especially the pneumonias, and this may antedate any clinical evidence of myelomatosis by months or even years.

Amyloidosis occurs in about 25 per cent of the cases. The amyloid is generally in unusual sites such as the intestine, voluntary muscle and bone, while the spleen, liver and kidney are often not involved. It is not colored with the usual stains for amyloid and is therefore referred to as atypical amyloid or paraamyloid. Amyloid deposits may occur in the tumors themselves, where they are often surrounded by giant cells (Dahlin and Dockerty). Amyloid is a glycoprotein, a compound of carbohydrate and protein, and there can be little doubt that the abnormal serum proteins are responsible for the "tissue proteinosis" of myeloma amyloidosis.

More detailed information regarding the complex biochemical disturbances produced by plasma-cell myeloma will be found in the reviews by Putnam and Osserman.

The Kidney.—The *myeloma kidney* is one in which renal lesions may or may not lead to renal failure. Renal function is impaired in about two-thirds of the cases, and this may be so severe as to lead to uremia and death. Large numbers of tubules may be filled and distended with casts of abnormal protein, often associated with giant cell formation (Fig. 727). The casts which are remarkably large and dense, are PAS-positive, thus differing from nearly all other

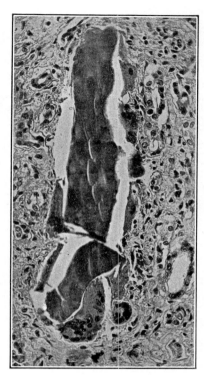

Fig. 727.—Bence-Jones protein in kidney. × 150.

casts. There is loss or lysis of the basement membrane containing the casts. Renal failure is not necessarily caused by tubular obstruction, for it may occur without the presence of Bence Jones casts. Metastatic calcification or *nephrocalcinosis*, which may be severe, cannot be expected to improve the functional capacity of the kidney. But no matter how great the damage to the kidney and how severe the degree of renal failure, arterial hypertension is never a complication.

Lesions.—Plasma cell myeloma is commonly referred to as *multiple myeloma*, for obvious reasons. In rare cases, however, it may occur as *solitary plasma cell myeloma*, the cells of which are well differentiated rather than neoplastic. After a lapse of years, however, the solitary myeloma may become multiple. Finally, there may be only a diffuse infiltration of tumor cells, a *myelomatosis*, without the formation of any discrete neoplasms. In such cases it is natural that tumor cells may appear in the blood, constituting a *plasma cell leukemia*. This

may also develop in the terminal stages of multiple myeloma. Indeed myeloma might be regarded as a plasma cell aleukemic leukemia with severe bone involvement.

The most striking feature is the multiplicity of the lesions, as indicated by the name. The flat bones containing red marrow are first involved, *i.e.*, sternum, ribs, vertebræ, skull, and pelvis; lesions may appear later in the long bones. Lesions distal to the elbow and knee are extremely rare. It is not possible to say with certainty if the lesions are primarily multiple or if one is primary and the others secondary. The condition is comparable with lymphatic leukemia, in which the bone marrow throughout the body is involved.

The *gross appearance* is that of soft gray tumors of the marrow, which are at first localized and produce marked destruction of the bone. (Fig. 728.) It is a pure rarefying lesion with no formation of new bone. It may be noted, however, that spontaneous fractures heal readily and with good callus formation. Later the entire marrow cavity is filled with gray or red tumor tissue.

Microscopically the tumor consists of plasma cells. These may be easily recognized as such by the abundant cytoplasm and the eccentric position of the nucleus (Fig. 728), but they do not show the characteristic staining with pyronin, the nucleus is likely to be larger, and there is seldom a perinuclear halo. As the normal plasma cell differentiates from its reticulum cell precursor, ribonucleic acid accumulates in the cytoplasm, being distributed in the form of Palade granules on the endoplasmic reticulum. It is this which is responsible for the cytoplasmic basophilia and the pyroninophilia of the classical plasma cell. As plasma cell myeloma is a malignant neoplasm, it is natural that some of this mechanism fails to function normally. There is great variation of cell types in different cases, from those in which the tumor cells closely resemble normal plasma cells to those in which the cells are larger, irregular in outline, contain two or more nuclei, with no suggestion of plasma cells, a picture which may readily be mistaken for that of Ewing's tumor. These bizarre cells used to be regarded as atypical erythroblasts and myeloblasts, which were

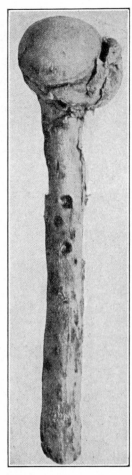

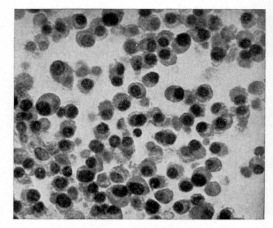

Fig. 729.—Plasma cell myeloma.   × 500.

Fig. 728.—Plasma cell myeloma. Numerous punched-out cavities in the shaft of the humerus. (Kindness of Dr. H. M. Vango from Boyd, *Pathology for the Surgeon*, courtesy of W. B. Saunders Co.)

supposed to constitute special forms of multiple myeloma. A much truer cytological picture is now given by marrow puncture and smear than by surgical biopsy, for by this means the distortion produced by fixation and dehydration is avoided.

The *roentgen-ray picture* is usually characteristic. The bone lesions are purely destructive and they are localized, so that radiologically they appear as round, punched-out, clear-cut areas in a number of bones. Occasionally there is merely diffuse decalcification without any localized lesions. Owing to the rarefaction the cortex may be destroyed, so that pathological fractures are

very common. The effect of radiation is similar to that in Ewing's tumor and lymphosarcoma. The lesions melt away marvellously, but soon reappear.

Spread is principally to the other bones. Metastases to the internal organs, especially the liver and spleen, are not common. The spleen may be enlarged even without metastases. Curiously enough, metastases are almost never found in the lungs.

The *prognosis* is very variable, with an average survival period after the condition is recognized of twenty to twenty-four months. Occasionally this period has been as long as ten years, and in such cases the cytological picture is well differentiated. Whether the course is short or long, the disease always proves fatal.

Mouse Myeloma.—A spontaneous transmissable plasma cell myeloma in mice has proved a boon to the laboratory investigator. The original tumor occurred in a single mouse, but it was transmissable to other mice of the same strain. The condition simulates human multiple myeloma as regards bone lesions and histological picture, as well as hyperglobulinemia with an abnormal serum protein electrophoretic pattern. In one strain there is even formation of Bence-Jones protein, with blockage of the renal tubules by casts of this material.

Tumor-Like Processes.—A true tumor, whether in bone or elsewhere, is a progressive, continuous proliferation of cells. A *hamartoma* (*hamartia*, error) is a spontaneous growth which produces an excessive number of cells that reach maturity and then cease to reproduce, so that growth is self-limited. In many cases the resulting lesion seems to represent a simple exaggeration of a normal physiological process. A number of bone lesions commonly regarded as tumors are hamartomatous rather than neoplastic in nature. Other lesions seem to represent *bone reactions* to stimuli of uncertain nature. Such are osteoid osteoma, and nonosteogenic fibroma.

HAMARTOMAS.—The general concept of a hamartoma is outlined above. Examples of such lesions are osteoma, osteochondroma, enchondroma, angioma, and aneurysmal bone cyst.

Osteoma is a localized exaggeration of intramembranous bone formation, so that no formation of cartilage is possible. It therefore occurs in bones formed by intramembranous ossification, particularly the inner or outer tables of the skull. Once formed it remains static, and gives rise to no symptoms. It is an *exostosis*, not a true tumor.

Osteochondroma is a perversion in growth direction, and is formed by enchondral growth, so that it does not occur in bones developed in cartilage. It is therefore the antithesis of osteoma. The lesion is identical with the lesions of hereditary multiple exostoses or hereditary chondrodysplasia, already described on page 1248, except that it it solitary and is not hereditary.

Enchondroma is a circumscribed mass of cartilage, which pushes the bone aside but does not invade it. A group of cartilage cells apparently become separated from the epiphysis in childhood or adolescence, so that the lesion develops in the metaphysis of cylindrical bones, including the ribs, the great majority occurring in the short bones of the hands and feet.

Angioma (hemangioma) of bone rarely causes symptoms, but if sufficiently careful search of the skeleton is made at autopsy, it proves to be not uncommon. The principal sites are the vertebral bodies and the skull, but occasionally it occurs in the metaphyses of the long bones. The angioma consists of masses of cavernous blood vessels lined with endothelium in a loose connective tissue stroma. It produces marked lysis of the

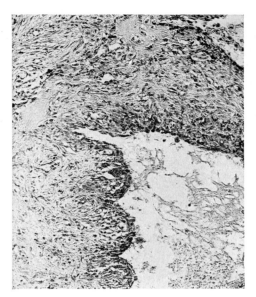

FIG. 730.—Aneurysmal bone cyst of scapula. × 50. (Kindness of Dr. N. B. G. McLetchie.)

surrounding bone. The lesion is highly vulnerable to irradiation therapy.

Aneurysmal bone cyst has an unfortunate name, for the lesion has nothing to do with aneurysms. It is a solitary cyst on the surface of bone filled with blood and lined by a highly vascular connective tissue containing many engorged and dilated vascular channels (Fig. 730). It may occur at any age, chiefly in the second and third decades, the common site being the vertebræ. Like angioma, it erodes the surrounding structure, and may result in fracture or hemorrhage with the formation of a hematoma. It is often mistaken for other conditions such as giant cell tumor or even sarcoma, so that there is real danger of overtreatment. There is great difference of opinion as to the nature of the condition, but it seems reasonable to suppose that it is the result of a rapidly growing angioma (Hadders and Oterdoon), although some of the experts reject this idea.

Reactive Lesions.—The conditions to be considered in this group deserve even less to be considered as true neoplasms than do the hamartomas.

Osteoid osteoma is a sharply circumscribed lesion consisting of a center of osteoid surrounded by new bone trabeculæ. It is at

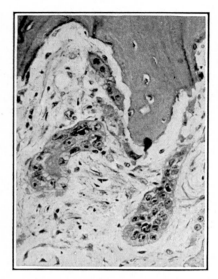

FIG. 731.—Secondary carcinoma of bone. × 250.

first cellular, later osteoid, and finally calcified atypical bone. It is a rather common condition, occurring in any bone and anywhere in the bone, but, as in the case of so many true tumors of bone, most frequently in the tibia and femur. The usual age incidence is ten to twenty-five years. *Pain* is the principal complaint, at first nagging and intermittent, later persistent, and finally intense. It is generally diagnosed as chronic osteomyelitis or bone abscess. The *x-ray picture* is characteristic, consisting of a central rarefied area surrounded by a dense zone of sclerosis. The nature and pathogenesis of the condition is unknown. In spite of its name it is certainly not a true neoplasm.

Non-osteogenic fibroma, also called *non-ossifying fibroma*, is in essence a focal area of deossification (as opposed to decalcification) in which the bone is replaced by fibrous tissue. It usually develops during adolescence near the ends of the shaft of the long bones of the lower limb. It is a slowly expanding lesion, seldom exceeding 5 cm. in diameter, and causing bone absorption with the risk of pathological fracture. The *gross appearance* is that of a yellow, gray or brown mass of soft consistence. *Microscopically* there are sheets or bundles of fusiform fibroblasts together with varying numbers of large macrophages filled with lipid or with hemosiderin as well as foreign body giant

cells. It is obvious that such a lesion may be mistaken for giant cell tumor, fibrous dysplasia, one of the lipid reticuloendothelioses, etc. The microscopic picture is consistent with that of a healed infarct, and local ischemia may be a factor in the pathogenesis of the condition. In about half the cases there are no symptoms, any pain is mild, and the lesion is usually discovered incidentally in roentgenograms made for other bone diseases.

Ossifying Fibroma is a vague lesion in which a fibrous matrix contains spicules or masses of osteoid and bone. As traumatic and ischemic injuries of bone may present a similar combination of fibroblastic proliferation and bone formation, and as the lesion may closely simulate fibrous dysplasia of bone, it will be obvious that ossifying fibroma must remain a somewhat nebulous entity, regarding which further information must be sought in the monographs of Jaffe, Lichtenstein and others devoted to bone tumors.

Giant Cell Epulis has been grouped in the past with giant cell tumor of bone, but it is a reparative granuloma, the result of a local reaction, not in any sense a true tumor. The meaning of the word epulis is "upon the gum," and the epulis grows in relation to the teeth, usually involving the mandible between the ages of 10 and 25. It consists of soft, spongy, reddish tissue made up of spindle cells and limited numbers of small multinucleated giant cells probably called forth by hemorrhage in the interior of the bone. The giant cells therefore do not form an integral part of the tumor in spite of the misleading name.

METASTATIC TUMORS.—Secondary tumors of bone are most likely to occur in carcinoma of the breast, prostate, kidney (hypernephroma), and lung, but many other malignant tumors may be the starting-point of secondary deposits. (Fig. 731.) Cancer of the thyroid gland deserves special mention. The bones commonly affected are the ribs, vertebræ, sternum, skull, and the upper end of the femur and humerus. In all of these bones the marrow is of the red variety and is well vascularized. In the shaft of a long bone the metastasis is often at the site of the nutrient artery. From all this it is evident that the usual mode of infection is by the blood stream, and not by lymphatic permeation as used to be thought. The deposit is formed in the medullary cavity. Roentgen-ray evidence goes to show that most of the tumors are purely osteolytic, the destruction not being associated with any bone formation. A round well-defined lesion is seen similar to that of multiple myeloma, although not quite so punched-out in character. Hypernephroma affords a perfect example of an osteolytic process. Breast cancers are for the most part osteolytic, but a few are osteoblastic. Cancers of the prostate, on the other hand, are almost entirely oseoblastic, so that the lesions appear sclerotic in the roentgen-ray picture. A large amount of new bone is formed, which may obliterate the shaft and even form projections on the surface. Even here there is probably an associated osteolytic process, for fractures may occur. In the osteolytic form fractures are common, and may be the first sign of bone disease. It is rather remarkable that in spite of the destruction of bone, the fracture may heal satisfactorily. The blood picture may suggest a correct diagnosis. There is a leuko-erythroblastic anemia, with normoblasts and myeloblasts in the smear.

It may be of some help to the student to have an indication of the more common locations of tumor and tumor-like lesions of bone, which are as follows. *Skull:* metastases. *Ribs, sternum and vertebræ:* metastases and multiple myeloma. *Long bones (epiphyses):* giant cell tumor, benign chondroblastoma. *Long bones (metaphyses):* osteochondroma, enchondroma, osteosarcoma, chondrosarcoma, non-osteogenic fibroma, fibrous dysplasia. *Long bones (diaphyses):* osteoid osteoma, Ewing's tumor. *Carpus and tarsus:* giant cell tumor, benign chondroblastoma. *Hands and feet:* enchondroma, osteochdonroma.

REFERENCES

AEGERTER, E. and KIRKPATRICK, J. A., JR.: *Orthopedic Diseases*, Philadelphia, 1958.
AEGERTER, E. E.: Am. J. Path., 1947, *23*, 283. (Giant cell tumor.)
BOWERS, D.: Ann. Int. Med., 1959, *51*, 1049. (Marfan's syndrome.)
COLLINS, D. H. and CURRAN, R. C.: in *Modern Trends in Pathology*, ed. D. H. Collins, London, 1959. (Pathological ossification.)
DAHLIN, D. C. and DOCKERTY, M. B.: Am. J. Path., 1950, *26*, 581. (Amyloidosis in plasma cell myeloma.)

DAMESHEK, W. and GUNZ, F.: *Leukemia*, New York, 1959. (Plasma cell myeloma.)
DENNIS, J. W. and ROSAHN, P. D.: Am. J. Path., 1951, *27*, 627. (Skeletal reticuloses.)
EDHOLM, O. G., HOWARD, S. and McMICHAEL, J.: Clin. Science, 1945, *5*, 249. (Pathogenesis of Paget's disease.)
EWING, J.: Surg., Gynec. & Obst., 1939, *68*, 971. (Classification of bone tumors.)
FARBER, S.: Am. J. Path., 1941, *17*, 625. (Eosinophilic granuloma.)
FOLLIS, R. H., JR.: Am. J. Med., 1957, *22*, 469. (Osteodystrophies.)
GESCHICKTER, C. F. and COPELAND, M. M.: Ann. Surg., 1951, *133*, 790. (Parosteal sarcoma.)
HADDERS, H. N. and OTERDOON, H. J.: J. Path. and Bact., 1956, *71*, 193. (Aneurysmal bone cyst.)
JAFFE, H. L.: *Tumors and Tumorous Conditions of the Bones and Joints*, Philadelphia, 1958.
JAFFE, H. L., LICHTENSTEIN, L. and PORTIS, R. B.: Arch. Path., 1940, *30*, 993. (Giant cell tumor.)
KARNOVSKY, M. J.: Lab. Invest., 1960, *9*, 639. (Glycogen in lathyrism.)
KULP, J. L., ECKELMANN, W. R. and SCHULERT, A. R.: Science, 1957, *125*, 219. (Strontium-90 in man.)
LICHTENSTEIN, L.: *Bone Tumors*, St. Louis, 2nd Ed., 1959.
————: Cancer, 1956, *9*, 1044. (Benign osteoblastoma.)
————:. Arch. Path., 1953, *56*, 84. (Histiocytosis X.)
O'NEIL, L. W. and ACKERMAN, L. V.: Cancer, 1952, *5*, 551. (Chondrosarcoma.)
OSSERMAN, E. F.: New Eng. J. Med., 1959, *261*, 952 and 1006. (Clinical aspects of plasma cell myeloma.)
PONSETI, I. V.: J. Bone and Joint Surg., 1954, *36-A*, 1031. (Lathyrism.)
PRITCHARD, J. J. in BOURNE, G. H: *The Biochemistry and Physiology* of Bone, New York, 1956.
PUTNAM, F. W.: New Eng. J. Med., 1959, *261*, 902. (Biochemical disturbances in plasma cell myeloma.)
SCHLUMBERGER, H. G.: Am. J. Path., 1959, *35*, 1. (Hyperostosis in the female parakeet.)
SELYE, H.: Rev. Canad. de Biologie, 1957, *16*, 1. (Lathyrism.)
SNAPPER, I.: *Bone Diseases in Medical Practice*, New York, 1957.
SNAPPER, I. and NATHAN, D. J.: Am. J. Med., 1957, *22*, 939. (Rickets and osteomalacia.)
STANBURY, S. W.: Brit. Med. Bull., 1957, *13*, 57. (Azotemic renal osteodystrophy.)
STOCKS, P. and BARRINGTON, A.: Eugenics Laboratory Memoir, 1925, *22*. (Hereditary chondrodysplasia.)
THOMSON, A. D. and TURNER-WARWICK, R. T.: J. Bone and Joint Surg., 1955, *37-B*, 266. (Skeletal sarcomata and giant cell tumor.)
TUNG, H. L. and LIEBOW, M. A.: Lab. Invest., 1952, *1*, 382. (Marfan's syndrome.)
URIST, M. R.: Clin. Research, 1958, *6*, 377. (Osteoporosis.)
YENDT, E. R.: Post-grad. Med., 1957, *22*, 38. (Osteoporosis.)

Chapter 44

The Joints

General Considerations
Acute Arthritis
  SUPPURATIVE
  NON-SUPPURATIVE
Tuberculous Arthritis
Chronic Arthritis
  RHEUMATOID ARTHRITIS
  ANKYLOSING SPONDYLITIS
    Aortitis and Carditis
  REITER'S SYNDROME
  OSTEOARTHRITIS

Gout
  PRIMARY
  SECONDARY
Miscellaneous Arthropathies
  CHARCOT'S DISEASE
  HEMOPHILIC JOINT
  LOOSE BODIES
Tumors of Joints and Tendon
  Sheaths
  MALIGNANT SYNOVIOMA

PIGMENTED VILLO-NODULAR
  SYNOVITIS
  Diffuse Villo-nodular Syno-
    vitis
  Localized Nodular Teno-
    synovitis
Cysts Connected with Joints
Lesions of the Intervertebral Discs
  HERNIATION OF NUCLEUS
    PULPOSUS
  PROTRUSION OF DISC

GENERAL CONSIDERATIONS

A JOINT is a structure of peculiar delicacy, and one which responds only too readily to injurious stimuli. When we consider the amount of stress and strain, not to mention abuse in sports, to which the joints are subjected in the course of a long life, it is little wonder that disease of the joints is amongst the commonest of clinical disorders. Man was not originally designed to stand upright, so it is but natural that the weight-bearing joints, namely those of the lower limbs and vertebral column, should be amongst the principal sufferers.

The structures which enter into the formation of a joint are the articular surfaces of bone covered by hyaline cartilage, the epiphyses, in some cases the epiphyseal cartilage and metaphysis, and the synovial membrane. The most striking feature of the microscopic appearance of articular cartilage is the preponderance of intercellular substance over cells, the chondrocytes lying quietly in lacunæ in the ground substance. The nourishment of the articular surface is a matter of great importance, for articular cartilage is singularly devoid of blood vessels. The lateral articular area is furnished with a delicate perichondrium continuous with the synovial membrane and containing numerous capillaries, but the central area possesses no perichondrium, the surface being formed of clear matrix containing no cells. The nourishment of the superficial layers of the

central articular area is dependent entirely on the synovial fluid.

This low threshhold of nourishment must be borne in mind when we interfere with the natural function of the joint. If force is required to place a joint in a given position, and if that position (forced position) is maintained during immobilization, the temporary stiffness that is natural may persist and be followed by clinical and x-ray evidence of joint degeneration. Salter and Field have shown that continuous compression of living hyaline cartilage in the rabbit and monkey is followed by changes varying from superficial necrosis to loss of the full thickness of cartilage. (Fig. 732). This *pressure necrosis of cartilage*, which may develop within 6 days in the experimental animal, is the result of interference with the diffusion of nutritive fluid through the intercellular substance of the cartilage. The lesion, which probably cannot be repaired, may interfere with the growth of the epiphyses or act as the starting point of osteoarthritis. It is difficult to detect the damage clinically, because the lesion is occult and painless. The possibility of the applicability of these findings in the experimental animal to the human subject is self-evident.

The protein content of the synovial fluid is less than half of that of the lymph, and this probably accounts for the feeble powers of resistance of this part of the articular cartilage, the readiness with which it degenerates, and the extreme slowness or ab-

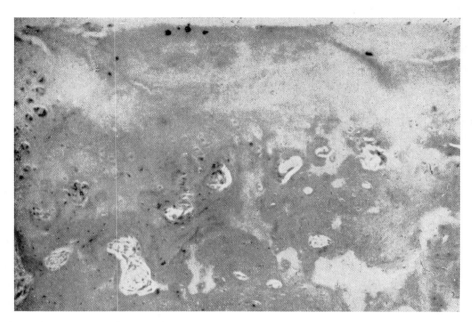

Fig. 732.—Pressure necrosis of cartilage showing loss of nuclear staining power in the chondrocytes of all layers, disappearance of superficial and transitional zones, and hypertrophy of subchondral bone. The edge of the lesion is seen at the left of the figure. (Salter and Field, courtesy of J. Bone and Joint Surg.)

sence of repair. Experimental destructive lesions of the lateral part are followed by rapid and abundant formation of cartilage, whereas in the central part there is little or none. The regenerative power of the lateral area is reflected in the "lipping" of cartilage which we shall encounter in chronic arthritis.

The synovial membrane is lined in the parts most remote from the articular edges by a single layer of endothelial-like cells, but nearer the articular edges this layer is very deficient, so that it offers no obstruction to absorption from the joint cavity. At the margin, and especially in the villi which occur chiefly in this region, the membrane contains great numbers of cells filled with globules of mucin which can readily escape into the joint cavity owing to the deficiency in the endothelial lining, an escape which is greatly facilitated by movements of the joint. So abundant are these mucinous cells in the synovial villi that they have been called "synovial glands." In chronic arthritis portions of the membrane may become detached and continue their secretion within the joint cavity.

Injection experiments show that colloidal solutions are absorbed by the lymphatics in the synovial membrane, and that this absorption is greatly facilitated by passive involvement of the joint or by allowing the animal to move about for a few hours. This is a point which may be worth considering in view of our tendency to immobolize a joint swollen with fluid for a period of time.

The word joint obviously means a place where two things are joined together, the things in question being bones. But the joining may belong to one or other of two very different categories, the first fibrocartilaginous, the second synovial.

Fibrocartilaginous Joints.—Here the skeletal elements are united by fibrocartilage, which is separated from the bone on either side by thin plates of hyaline cartilage. The classic example of such a joint is that which separates and unites two vertebræ, that is to say the intervertebral disc. These discs consist of two elements, the nucleus pulposus and the annulus fibrosus. The *nucleus pulposus* at birth is almost purely mucoid, containing some notochordal cells and some fine strands of fibrous tissue derived from the annulus fibrosus. With the passage of the years this tissue gradually replaces the notochordal tissue, until the entire disc becomes converted into fibrocartilage. The nucleus pulposus is a shock-absorbing mechanism, as well as playing an important part in fluid interchange. The difference in structure which characterizes the nucleus of the baby as compared with that of an old man serves to explain in part the difference in mobility of the spine in the two cases. The adult disc is avascular, depending on diffusion for its nutrition, probably through the plates of hyaline cartilage.

The annulus fibrosus binds the vertebral bodies together, and permits motion between them by reason of the spiral arrangement of its fibers. Pathological changes in the intervertebral discs consist of degenerative changes in the nucleus pulposus and the annulus fibrosus (Armstrong). It is doubtful if rupture of the annulus fibrosus with herniation of the nucleus pulposus occurs in a normal disc. Compression of the vertebræ with fracture of a hyaline plate results in forcing of nuclear material into the vertebral body before there is any suggestion of tearing of the annulus. We shall return to these matters in the discussion of lesions of the intervertebral discs with the attendent serious disability which may accompany these lesions (page 1298).

Synovial Joints.—A synovial joint consists of two cartilage-covered bones joined in a mutual embrace. As compared with the fibro-cartilaginous joint, the synovial joint is designed for free movement.

The articular cartilages are separated by a thin layer of synovial fluid, and when the joint is at rest the articular cartilages are in direct contact. If movement is fast enough, intra-articular pressure builds up, and the cartilages become separated by a thin film of lubricating fluid which now takes up the friction. The viscous nature of the synovial membrane is due to hyaluronic acid, a non-sulfated mucopolysaccharide. The effects of friction are maximal at the beginning and the end of movement (Gardner). *Use-destruction,* usually referred to as *wear and tear,* is inevitable during movement, the articular cartilage becoming slowly and in-

evitably worn away. This process is exaggerated by movements with heavy loads, by the decrease in the viscosity of the synovial fluid (too thin oil) which accompanies ageing, and by damage to the articular structures. We shall see that *osteoarthritis* may be an exaggerated form of use-destruction, in which the metabolism of the spinal fluid and of the articular cartilage play a part of prime importance.

ACUTE ARTHRITIS

Acute inflammation of a joint is caused either by bacterial infection or by trauma, such as a blow or sprain. *Trauma* gives rise to a mild though acute inflammation. The joint is swollen, the swelling being due partly to an increase of synovial fluid which may become cloudy or blood-stained, partly to inflammatory swelling of the synovial membrane which is congested and infiltrated with leukocytes. The *bacterial infections* may be suppurative or non-suppurative.

Suppurative Arthritis.—The common infecting organisms are staphylococci and streptococci. The infection may spread from the bone as in acute osteomyelitis, or may be introduced from without by a perforating wound of the joint. In pyogenic infections such as pneumonia and meningococcal meningitis there may be suppuration of one or more joints.

In suppurative arthritis the *synovial membrane* is hyperemic, swollen, soft, and infiltrated with pus cells. The cells lining the surface are cast off, and fibrin is deposited on the raw surface. The *synovial fluid* is milky or frankly purulent, crowded with polymorphonuclear leukocytes, and usually contains the infecting organisms. The *articular cartilage* becomes eroded and the underlying bone is exposed, causing great pain when the joint is moved. The *ligaments* are softened and give way, so that the joint becomes completely disorganized and is often dislocated. The *capsule* may then rupture, the pus making its way into the periarticular tissues. This is a picture of the most severe form of suppurative arthritis. In other cases the infection is milder and may be localized to the synovial membrane (*acute synovitis*), with little or no destruction of the joint. When there has been destruction of tissue there will be fibrous union (*ankylosis*), and if the articular surfaces are destroyed the union may be cartilaginous or bony.

Gonococcal arthritis used to be one of the common forms of suppurative arthritis, occurring in about 2 per cent of cases of gonorrhea a few weeks or even months after the original urethral infection, and usually confined to a few large joints, more particularly the knee. With the advent of chemotherapy gonorrhea has fallen from its high estate, and the arthritis which used to complicate its course has changed accordingly. The form likely to be seen today is a mild inflammatory swelling during the active phase of the genital infection. It probably represents a transient synovitis which leaves no permanent disability. We shall return to the subject of arthritis associated with urethritis in connection with Reiter's syndrome (page 1283).

Non-suppurative Arthritis.—Most examples of acute arthritis are non-suppurative, the inflammation is confined to the synovial membrane (acute synovitis), there is no destruction of tissue and therefore no permanent stiffness. *Traumatic synovitis* due to a strain is a good example of the condition. The synovial membrane is swollen, juicy, and congested, and infiltrated with inflammatory cells, while the synovial fluid is increased in amount, cloudy, and contains desquamated endothelium and small numbers of leukocytes. *Rheumatic arthritis* is the acute non-suppurative arthritis of *rheumatic fever*, which is discussed on page 265. Several joints are affected one after the other. There is an acute synovitis with excess of turbid fluid in the joint. Extreme tenderness is characteristic of the swollen and acutely inflamed joint. There is some involvement of the subsynovial and periarticular tissue and ligaments, and rheumatic nodules similar in structure to the Aschoff bodies in the heart may be present in the subcutaneous tissues. The inflammation usually undergoes complete resolution, but if there is severe involvement of the periarticular tissue, some permanent stiffness may result. The *etiology* of rheumatic fever remains an enigma. Although acute episodes develop 10 to 20 days after upper respiratory infections due to group A beta hemolytic streptococci, organisms cannot be recovered from involved tissues or body fluids other than the pharynx. The streptococci certainly seem to initiate the process but the exact mechanism of the process remains obscure. It may well be an antigen-antibody immune reaction involving connective tissue protein. Early treatment of upper respiratory streptococcal infection certainly prevents rheumatic fever attacks.

TUBERCULOUS ARTHRITIS

Tuberculosis of the joints is a disease of children, and is usually secondary to tuberculosis of the adjacent bone. When it occurs in an adult it is more likely to be primary in the synovial membrane, infection being carried by the blood stream from some distant focus. Bone tuberculosis has a strong tendency to spread to the corresponding joint, so that bone and joint tuberculosis are commonly combined. The bone lesion is in the metaphysis close to the epiphyseal cartilage, and from there the infection spreads outward along the vessels and reaches the synovial membrane. Or it may destroy the epiphyseal cartilage, invade the epiphysis, penetrate the articular cartilage, and in this way reach the joint. Trauma is said to be a predisposing factor, but as usual this is difficult to prove. The joints commonly affected are the hip and knee, followed by elbow, shoulder, and ankle.

Lesions.—All the joint structures and the adjacent bone are involved if the disease is not arrested, but in the adult the main lesion may be a tuberculous synovitis for a considerable time. The *synovial membrane* may resemble that of rheumatoid arthritis, but is even thicker and more voluminous, so that it may fill the entire cavity. It is gray in color and may show tubercles on the surface or only when the mass is incised. Gelatinous degeneration is common and caseation may occur in the late stages. Microscopically it usually presents a classical picture of tuberculous granulation tissue with epithelioid tubercles and numerous giant cells. The *fluid* is usually scanty but highly fibrinous, so that it contains flakes of fibrin which may develop into foreign bodies known as *melon-seed bodies* or *rice bodies*. Occasionally there

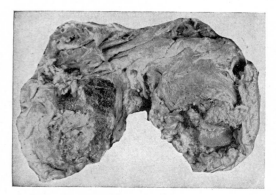

FIG. 733.—Tuberculosis of the knee joint. The articular cartilage of the femur is eaten away and the underlying bone is eroded.

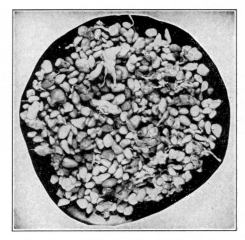

FIG. 734.—Melon-seed bodies in a joint.

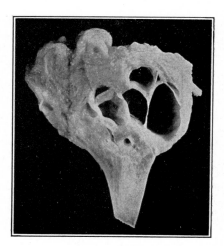

FIG. 735.—Cyst of external semilunar cartilage.

is abundant serous effusion (hydrops) with comparatively little synovial thickening; in these cases there may be large numbers of melon-seed bodies. The *articular cartilage* is attacked both from above and below, just as in rheumatoid arthritis. The synovial membrane, or rather the granulation tissue into which it is converted, creeps over the articular surface, becomes adherent to it, and sends vessels into it, so that the cartilage becomes eaten away and the underlying bone is exposed (Fig. 733). The cartilage is also attacked by granulation tissue from below, and instead of being eaten away it may become separated in flakes or even as a complete cast of the articular surface. The *bone* shows the rarefying osteitis which has already been studied in connection with tuberculosis of bone. The initial lesion is in the red marrow, and the absorption of bone is really secondary. The *periarticular soft parts* are involved later. The ligaments are softened and finally destroyed, so that the joint may be dislocated. The muscles and other periarticular tissues undergo gelatinous degeneration, a change which is largely responsible for the *white swelling* so characteristic of tuberculous arthritis. When the gelatinous tissue undergoes caseation and liquefaction a tuberculous abscess (cold abscess) is formed, the contents of which are not true pus but liquefied necrotic tissue. If this is open or perforates the skin, the whole picture is changed, and mixed infection runs riot through all the tissues in and around the joint. *Caries sicca* is a rare form

of the disease which usually affects the shoulder joint and pursues a slow course with no effusion, quiet absorption of the bone, and the formation of dense fibrous adhesions.

The termination is very variable. At almost any stage the disease may be arrested. This may result in mere stiffness, but when the articular surface is destroyed there will be fibrous or bony ankylosis. Amyloid disease may complicate prolonged secondary infection, or general miliary tuberculosis may terminate the picture.

Relations of Symptoms to Lesions.—Pain, an early and constant symptom, is due to erosion of the articular cartilage. It is worse when the patient drops off to sleep, because then the watchful muscles which hold the joint rigid are off their guard. The joint is swollen and has a characteristic fusiform contour. Much of the enlargement is caused by the swelling of the synovial membrane, but in the later stages the gelatinous swelling of the periarticular soft tissues plays a part. Limitation of movement, the earliest physical sign, is a natural sequel to any inflammatory lesion in a joint. Muscular spasm is an attempt to keep the part at rest. Early atrophy of the surrounding muscles is partly due to disuse.

CHRONIC ARTHRITIS

The term chronic arthritis has come to be used in a special sense. It does not mean, as the name suggests, a chronic inflammation of the joint, but a slow, progressive, crippling disease. It is not generally realized that this is the greatest single cause of prolonged disability in the world today. Thus in Sweden 9 per cent of all cases of permanent pensionable invalidity are due to arthritis, while in the state of Massachusetts the cases of disability number 140,000, compared with 25,000 from tuberculosis. In the United States it is estimated that some 4,500,000 persons suffer from chronic arthritis, and that 200,000 are totally disabled. The Metropolitan Life Insurance Company of New York estimates that the disease is responsible for an annual loss of 7,500,000 weeks of work and costs $200,000,000. The English figures are very similar. The groups are rheumatoid arthritis and osteoarthritis, which are sometimes included under the common heading of arthritis deformans, a name only too well justified. Rheumatoid arthritis has also been called chronic infective and proliferative arthritis, the last name indicating the proliferation of synovial membrane which is the dominant characteristic. Osteoarthritis is also called degenerative arthritis and hypertrophic arthritis because of the overgrowth of perichondral tissue resulting in "lipping" of cartilage and bone around the joint. It must be noted, however, that synovial membrane and cartilage are relatively simple structures which may respond to stimuli either by proliferation or degeneration, and that the same end result may be produced by a variety of agents, and the same agent may produce a variety of gross appearances. Foci of round cell infiltration in the synovial membrane do not necessarily spell infection, and the most intense inflammation may be present as the result of non-infective lesions. All of which indicates how difficult it is to reach conclusions regarding the etiology of chronic arthritis.

Rheumatoid Arthritis.—*Clinical Picture.*—Rheumatoid arthritis commonly occurs in women of between twenty and forty years, *i. e.*, during the period of reproductive activity. It is 3 times as common in women as in men. The onset is gradual and insidious, the commonest initial symptom being morning stiffness, but in children it may be quite acute, with multiple arthritis, fever, leukocytosis and enlargement of the spleen and lymph nodes, a condition known as *Still's disease*. A practically identical condition in adults, except that there is leukopenia in place of leukocytosis, is somewhat unjustifiable dignified by the name of *Felty's syndrome*. In rheumatoid arthritis the small joints of the hands and feet are the chief sufferers, but the larger joints may be involved later, the hip usually escaping. The course of the disease is marked by remissions and exacerbations, and at any time it may be arrested, but the injury to the joint is permanent, and the hands and feet are twisted, gnarled, and crippled for life. About 20 per cent recover completely, 60 per cent are left with minor disabilities, and 20 per cent remain severely disabled. The affected joints show a doughy spindle-shaped swelling, and the overlying skin may be tight and glossy. Ulnar deviation of the hand is a characteristic deformity. In from 15 to 20 per cent of the cases careful search will reveal the presence of *painless subcutaneous nodules* similar to those which are so characteristic of rheumatic fever. The usual site is the dorsal surface of the forearm a short distance below the olecranon. (Fig. 736.) They vary in size from seed-like bodies to nodules as large as an olive. They may persist for months and years and then disappear. The subcutaneous nodule is not found in osteoarthritis. There are often

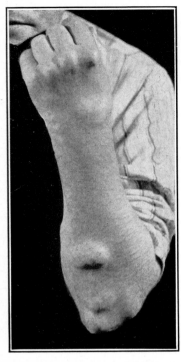

FIG. 736.—Subcutaneous nodules in rheumatoid arthritis. (Kindness of Dr. A. J Blanchard, Sunnybrook Hospital, Toronto.)

general signs suggestive of chronic infection such as malaise, occasional fever, anemia, palpitation, sweating, increased sedimentation rate and a general toxic appearance.

When we think of rheumatoid arthritis we are apt to conjure up the classic case of the text-books, the middle-aged woman whose joints become stiff and painful on movement, especially in the early morning or after resting for any length of time. Large as well as small joints are involved, at first a few and then many. Periods of relative quiescence are followed by remorseless progression, with a course gradually but surely downhill. After several years of struggle, she becomes restricted to a hobbling existence in the house, with final confinement to bed, resulting ankylosis, and many years of helplessness. The gloomy picture painted above is largely accounted for by the fact that most physicians do not see the patients who recover, because they do not return. If a complete follow-up of a large group of cases is instituted a very

different picture from the classsic one is revealed. At least 50 per cent of the patients when first seen have no real disability and still remain in that state after five years. Of those with mild or moderate disability some 50 per cent have improved after five years and have returned to their usual work or to modified employment. It is evident that in very many cases the body has an inherent ability to correct the disordered physiology and put out the fire, the ashes of which are represented by the lesions. Since skilled therapy seems to assist this natural healing tendency, it becomes important to make the diagnosis at as early a stage as possible.

The classical case is only too easy to diagnose. It is quite otherwise with the early case, for rheumatoid arthritis is a protean disease which may mimic several others. A really good laboratory test was needed to help the clinician. The red cell sedimentation rate is frequently increased, but it is within normal limits in up to 20 per cent of cases when they are first seen and in 5 per cent of children in an active stage of the disease. There may be outstanding changes in the plasma proteins, including a drop in albumin, a rise in globulin and fibrinogen, and an early but moderate increase in the C-reactive protein. Unfortunately none of these is specific.

A *specific agglutination test* has now been developed which is positive in a high percentage of cases of chronic arthritis, but negative in normal persons and in other forms of arthritis. The serum has the ability to agglutinate a variety of suspended particles. At first sheep erythrocytes sensitized by rabbit antiserum were used. Later sheep red cells were coated with tannic acid and sensitized with human gamma globulin. When the diluted serum of a chronic arthritic is added to such a preparation agglutination occurs. The test is positive both in the adult and the juvenile forms. It is said not to be affected by remissions, but this appears to be wrong in many instances, for even a strongly positive test can revert to a negative. The agglutination titer is highest in patients with disease of long duration. The explanation given for a positive test is the presence of a *rheumatoid factor* in the blood. It has also been suggested that an inhibitor of the agglutination-activating factor present in most normal sera is lacking in rheumatoid arthritis. The rheumatoid factor can now be isolated by precipitation in the cold combined with ultracentrifugation. It is a macroglobulin with a sedimentation constant of about 19 S, and appears to be an antibody or a circulating antigen-antibody complex. Its concentration in the blood and the synovial fluid is to a large extent a measure of the severity of the disease.

The *latex fixation test* is a further advance in technique, because it is not only as reliable as the various sheep cell agglutination tests, but it also has the advantage of being simple, very inexpensive, and quick (Plotz and Singer). It involves the use of a suspension of latex particles mixed with borate buffer and gamma globulin. Only a drop of serum is needed, a positive result being indicated by an aggregation of the latex particles visible to the naked eye. The latex particles in the system act simply as inert carriers of gamma globulin, and the same is true of the red cells in the erythrocyte-tannic acid system. Globulin-coated bentonite particles give equally good or even better results.

In one large series the latex fixation test was positive in 84 per cent of cases of clinically evident rheumatoid arthritis, whereas it was negative in over 96 per cent of cases of joint disease, including gout, other than rheumatoid arthritis. The serological agglutination reactions indicating the presence of the rheumatoid factor may also be present in the occasional case of disseminated lupus erythematosus, polyarteritis nodosa, and scleroderma, suggesting the possibility of some kind of relationship between rheumatoid arthritis and those members of the group of collagen diseases. This also brings up the question of a possible relationship between the rheumatoid factor and the L. E. factor. The rheumatoid factor, as we have just seen, is a macroglobulin associated with a protein complex of high molecular weight, but the L. E. factor is a much smaller globulin component. Both substances may occur in the same patient.

The *site of origin* of the rheumatoid factor has been conclusively demonstrated by the use of Coons' fluorescent-antibody method (Mellors *et al.*). As human gamma globulin

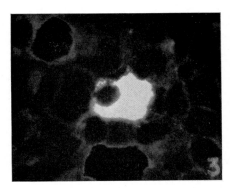

Fig. 737.—Synovial membrane. A mature plasma cell with an extremely eccentric unstained nucleus and cytoplasm containing rheumatoid factor. × 100. (Mellors, Humer, Corcos and Korngold, courtesy of J. Exper. Med.)

heated to 62°C. for ten minutes reacts specifically with the rheumatoid factor, it is possible to prepare a histochemical reagent for detecting the factor by conjugation of the product with fluorescein isothiocyanate. In fresh frozen tissue treated with this reagent the sites containing the rheumatoid factor show an apple green fluorescence when viewed with ultraviolet light. The rheumatoid factor is found exclusively in the tissues of patients with rheumatoid arthritis, and is confined to plasma cells in the synovial villi and the subcutnaeous nodules, as well as the plasma cells and reticulum cells of the germinal centers of some lymph nodes (Fig. 737). In the synovial membrane only a small number of plasma cells are stained, but in the affected follicles all of the reticulum cells show the reaction. The results do not prove that the factor is an antibody, but the distribution of the factor is just what would be expected if it were indeed an antibody.

The same fluorescent technique can be used to demonstrate the site of interaction between the rheumatoid factor and the tissue reactant. Fluorescein conjugates from rheumatoid blood serum give specific fluorescence with a component in the areas of fibrinoid necrosis in subcutaneous rheumatoid nodules removed from a patient with rheumatoid arthritis (Taylor and Shepperd). It is thought that the tissue reactant is probably a gamma globulin, and that this reacts with the rheumatoid factor, which seems to be an autoantibody to the tissue reactant.

Etiology.—An enormous amount has been written about the causation of rheumatoid arthritis, a sure indication that little is known about the subject. A satisfying answer to the question still eludes us. That does not prevent us from making some guesses. The pathological lesions produced in the experimental animal by immunological techniques resemble those of rheumatoid arthritis, as well as those of lupus erythematosus, rheumatic fever, polyarteritis nodosa, dermatomyositis, and scleroderma, conditions grouped under the heading of collagen diseases. Most of these patients have an elevated serum gamma globulin, which serves to support the view that the process is an immunological one. The main bone of contention is the possible relation of the arthritis and extraarticular lesions to bacterial infection. For many years it was believed that these lesions were the direct result of focal streptococcal infection in the tonsils, teeth and sinuses, so that countless tonsils and teeth were removed, with no obvious benefit in the vast majority of cases.

As Collins suggests, the arthritis may be due to a combination of *minimal metastatic bacterial infection with tissue hypersensitivity.* The sensitization may be the result of a series of minor infections or a chronic focus which periodically discharges a few bacteria into the blood. These are quickly removed from the blood, and at no time do they arrive at the joint in sufficient numbers to produce conventional metastatic lesions. All the time, however, the tissues are becoming sensitized, until finally one bacteremic episode culminates in a definite arthritis. Regarding the relationship of rheumatoid arthritis to rheumatic fever there is sharp difference of opinion. It is true that the lesions resemble each other, both being characteristic of the collagen group of diseases, but this is insufficient ground for suggesting a common etiology.

Rheumatic fever is like a violent but short-lived storm during which intensive treatment with cortisone can provide maximum protection until the storm blows over. The situation is entirely different with regard to rheumatoid arthritis. Here cortisone is not some new all-powerful, curative agent, as at first appeared to be the case, but merely something which suppresses the manifestations of the disease. To confuse the issue still further, aspirin appears to be as efficient as cortisone when the cases are followed for a sufficient period of time.

A sustained *allergic reaction* in the tissues has been suggested as the only satisfactory explanation of this chronic, often life-long, inflammatory process involving the connective tissues not only in the joints but all over the body (Dressner). Such a concept has a strong appeal. It focusses attention on the antibody-like rheumatoid factor and its associated gamma globulin. Unfortunately we are now confronted with the unpleasant fact that patients suffering from *agammaglobulinemia* suffer from arthritis far more frequently than should be the case. Each of these patients is unable to produce circulating antibody, gamma globulin and plasma cells. Moreover, the rheumatoid factor could not be demonstrated in any of these cases, although three developed subcutaneous nodules which were characteristic both clinically and histologically. This situation presents a conundrum which defies solution at the present time. It is perhaps important to mention that among the patients having both rheumatoid disease and agammaglobulinemia, extensive destruction of the joints has not been observed. Possibly this puzzling combination of agammaglobulinemia and clinical rheumatoid arthritis may be taken as pointing toward an infectious etiological agent, since agammaglobulinemia is known to be associated with an inordinate susceptibility to infection. One may be permitted to speculate what would have happened to our thinking about the cause of syphilis if the discovery of the Wassermann reaction had preceded the discovery of Treponema pallidum.

The possibility of *conditioning factors* must be taken into consideration. One such factor is undoubtedly the action of steroid hormones, as first suggested to Hench by the amelioration of symptoms which occurred during pregnancy or an attack of jaundice and which suggested the use of adrenal cortical steroids, more particularly cortisone (compound E) and hydrocortisone (compound F). A temporary deficiency of adrenal corticoids may allow the joints to become sensitized and damaged during the reversible phase of the disease. That there is no absolute adrenal deficiency due to loss of integrity of the adrenal cortex is shown by the fact that ACTH, the pituitary hormone which stimulates the cortex, produces the same beneficial results as cortisone itself.

A number of investigators, amongst whom Hench is especially worthy of mention, believe that the disease is not a manifestation of bacterial infection but rather a basic biochemical disturbance of unknown character. This disturbance may be accidentally corrected for a time by a number of apparently unrelated events, of which the chief are jaundice and pregnancy, in which there is probably some underlying biochemical change common to them all. Marked and sometimes startling amelioration of the arthritic symptoms occurs during the first trimester of pregnancy in about 90 per cent of cases. Even tubal pregnancy is effective. The relief ends a few weeks after delivery. Equally effective relief may be provided by hepatitis accompanied by jaundice in from 80 to 96 per cent of cases. The level of serum bilirubin needs to be above 6 mgm. per 100 cc. Hemolytic jaundice appears to be ineffective. When these figures are considered it becomes evident that the Achilles' heel of rheumatoid arthritis may well lie in "potential reversibility."

The *psychological aspects* of rheumatoid arthritis are getting increasing attention (Cormier and Wittkower). In some respects it appears to be a stress disease, associated particularly with environmental stress, especially poverty, grief and family worry. Its severity is said to be proportional to the degree of impairment in the capacity to express aggression. The patients are often overactive as children, but become inhibited later in life. Here again there is evidently room for disturbance in adrenal function. It is perhaps significant that rheumatoid arthritis is relatively uncommon amongst psychotics in mental hospitals.

Lesions.—The synovial membrane is primarily affected, so that the disease might be called synovioarthritis in contrast to osteoarthritis. If the joint is opened in the operat-

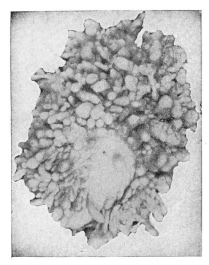

FIG. 738.—Synovial fringes in chronic arthritis.

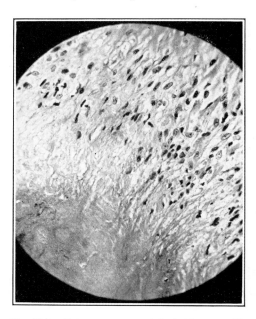

FIG 739.—Subcutaneous nodule in rheumatoid arthritis, showing necrosis and palisading.

ing room the *synovial membrane* is seen to be congested, edematous, redundant, and swollen so as to form pulpy masses or fringes and tags (Fig. 738). *Microscopically* it consists of vascular granulation tissue infiltrated with leukocytes and mononuclear cells of various kinds, with sometimes great numbers of plasma cells. (Fig. 739). There is often palisading of superficial synovial cells. The surface may be covered by a thin layer of necrotic material containing leukocytes. The *synovial fluid* is increased in amount and may be cloudy in character owing to the large number of the cells which it often contains. The mucin of the synovial fluid is similar to the mucin of the intercellular ground substance, consisting of hyaluronic acid bound to protein, and is probably produced by the numerous mast cells of the synovial membrane (Asboe-Hansen). The mast cells are known to be the source of heparin, which is closely related to hyaluronic acid. The cells which float in the fluid are degranulated mast cells. In rheumatoid arthritis the viscosity of the fluid is reduced owing to depolymerization of the hyaluronic acid.

The disease may be arrested at this stage, remaining a mere synovitis. Usually, however, the *articular cartilage* is involved. It is attacked both from above and below. The synovial membrane grows over it from the side, forming a thick vascular covering or *pannus* which becomes adherent to the cartilage and eats it away. The idea that pannus creeps over the surface of the articular cartilage and burrows under it may be quite wrong. It is possible that the destruction of the cartilage is due to dedifferentiation of the cartilage with accompanying disintegration in a similar fashion to the changes seen in the other collagen diseases (Collins). The cartilage is also attacked from below by granulation tissue which is formed in the superficial layers of the epiphysis as part of the inflammatory reaction. As a result of this combined attack the cartilage is destroyed. Adhesions are formed between the two layers of pannus covering the articular surfaces, and the joint cavity may be obliterated. Fibrous ankylosis of the joint develops and in time the ankylosis may become bony. The *periarticular tissue* shares in the inflammatory swelling and edema. The *muscles* of the part undergo marked atrophy; the extensors of the fingers are especially affected, so that the swollen fingers show a characteristic flexion. It has been shown by Steiner and his associates that this atrophy is the result of an inflammatory nodular polymyositis involving widely separated muscles. When first described these muscle lesions were thought to

be specific for rheumatoid arthritis, but Ogryzlo has found identical lesions in a wide variety of conditions, so that they must be regarded as non-specific. The *subcutaneous nodules* bear a striking resemblance to the similar nodules found in rheumatic fever, and provide the best picture of the microscopic lesion of rheumatoid arthritis. There is a large area of central necrosis surrounded by a zone of large mononuclear cells arranged in radial palisade fashion (Fig. 738). The arterioles in the surrounding tissue often show obliterating endarteritis and deposits of fibrin under the endothelium. The perineurium of the peripheral nerves may show multiple inflammatory lesions similar in type to the subcutaneous nodules.

Extraarticular Lesions.—Extraarticular lesions in addition to those just enumerated may be found at autopsy. These are particularly liable to occur in what has been described as *malignant rheumatoid arthritis*, cases of severe, prolonged illness with unsuccessful long-term cortisone therapy (Bevans *et al.*). Granulomatous and necrotic lesions in all stages of evolution and healing may be found in the pleura, pericardium, myocardium, diaphragm, kidneys and lungs. The principal lesion is a *fibrinoid necrosis of the small vessels*, a *vasculitis*. Coalescence of a number of these lesions may give a picture which may be mistaken for the lesions of rheumatic fever, but there is an absence of the Aschoff bodies and other hall-marks of that disease. There may be large non-bacterial vegetations on the valves. In one series of 25 cases 14 presented cardiac lesions (Baggenstoss and Rosenberg). With regard to a possible relationship of rheumatoid arthritis to rheumatic fever the interesting fact may be noted that pathological studies seem to indicate a frequent coexistence of the two diseases, whereas most clinical studies fail to do so. A critical evaluation of the pathological data appears to favor the view that there is only slightly greater than fortuitous coincidence of heart disease of the true rheumatic fever type in rheumatoid arthritis (Sokoloff).

There seems to be an increased incidence of vascular lesions of the polyarteritis nodosa type. This increase has been attributed by some writers to the prevalent use of long-

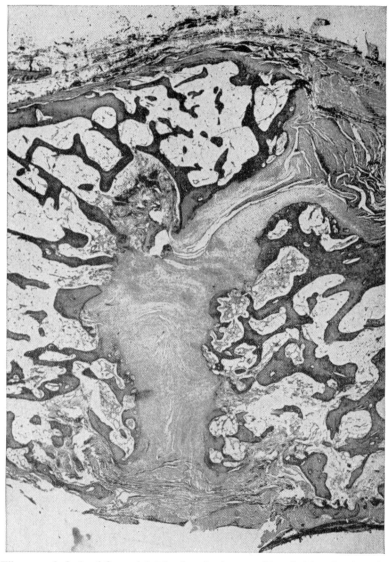

Fig. 740.—Fibrous ankylosis of finger joint in chronic rheumatoid arthritis. Section of proximal inter-phalangeal joint of fourth finger. There has been great destruction of cartilage and subchondral bone on both sides of the joint. The process is still active as may be seen by the vascular granulation tissue in the marrow with lymphocytic foci (best seen above center, in base of the phalanx, to the left), Cellular fibrous tissue joins the two bones and obliterates two-thirds of the joint space. H. and E. × 11. (Collins, *The Pathology of Articular and Spinal Diseases*, courtesy of Edward Arnold & Co.)

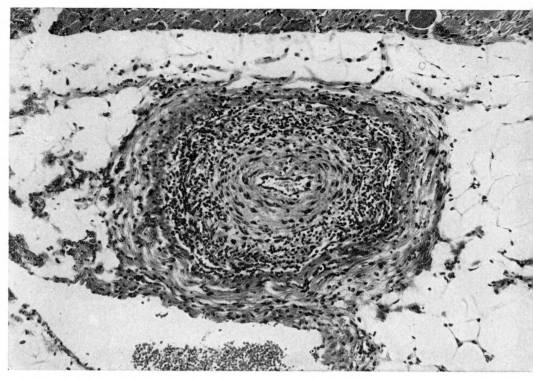

FIG. 741.—Rheumatoid arteritis. An artery supplying skelital muscle, showing proliferation of intima fibroblasts and infiltration with inflammatory cells. × 150. (Kindness of Drs. C. P. Handforth and J. F L. Woodbury, Halifax, Nova Scotia.)

term cortisone therapy. It seems to constitute a true *rheumatoid arteritis*, most often encountered in the myocardium, skeletal muscles, peripheral nerves, and alimentary tract (Fig. 741). Perhaps even more significant is an *acute venulitis*, which is more likely to be observed in biopsy material from acute cases (Kulka). Patients treated with steroids may show a fulminant vasculitis related to resurgence of disease activity during reduction in dosage of the drug. Changes in the *pituitary* have been described which may be significant. The mucoid cells (basophils and some chromophobes) are those which contain mucoprotein granules that stain with the PAS method. In rheumatoid arthritis these cells undergo a degeneration comparable to the change (Crooke-Russell cells) seen in Addison's disease (Pearse). *Lymphadenopathy* is frequent, enlarged nodes being found in about 30 per cent of cases. These are not necessarily related to the joints affected, and the lesions seem to represent systemic manifestation of rheumatoid disease. Follicular hyperplasia and sinus catarrh are the common changes, and the histological picture may simulate and be mistaken for giant-follicle lymphoma (Cruickshank), or even for Hodgkin's disease or reticulum cell sarcoma. *Amyloidosis* occurs as a systemic manifestation of the disease in nearly 10 per cent of cases. It may be due to a combination of hyperglobulinemia and liberation of chondroitin-sulfuric acid through destruction of cartilage.

The Relation of Symptoms to Lesions.—Swelling of the joint, a very constant feature is due partly to effusion into the joint, partly to changes in the periarticular tissues which have already been described. The joint has a peculiar doughy feel, and there is no development of osteophytes at the margin of the bones, a prominent cause of limitation of movement in osteoarthritis. The later disability and deformity is due partly to fibrous adhesions between the articular surfaces partly to the changes in the muscles, tendons and ligaments. Radiological examination may detect erosion of bones at the insertion of capsule into bone (Fig. 742). This and periosteal new bone formation along the shaft near the affected joint are the two most useful nonspecific indications of rheumatoid arthritis. Osteoporosis occurs earlier, but it is even less specific, being present in any condition producing disuse of a limb.

We have already seen that rheumatoid arthritis is a systemic disease, affecting many organs and tissues, although it is usually only the joint lesions which produce the disability. The patients often show signs suggestive of chronic infection. They are pale, pasty and unhealthy looking; they suffer from malaise, irregular attacks of pyrexia, palpitation and sweating; the sedimentation rate is increased and there is loss

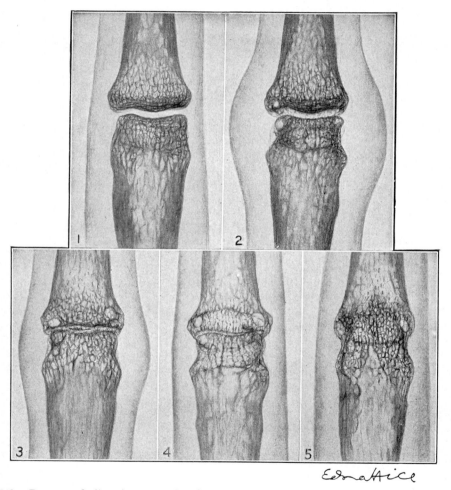

Fig. 742.—Roentgen findings in progressive rheumatoid arthritis. *1.* Normal proximal phalangeal joint of finger. There is no periarticular swelling. Note normal density of bone, and absence of cyst-like cavities. *2.* Early rheumatoid arthritis. Note the fusiform soft tissue (periarticular) swelling with some haziness of the joint space. *3.* Further progress of the disease with narrowing of the joint space indicating destruction of cartilage, demineralization of the bone and beginning formation of small bony cysts near the joint margin. *4.* As the disease advances, further demineralization occurs, with further narrowing and almost complete obliteration of the joint space, with diminution of the soft tissue swelling. *5,* Late stage: The joint space may entirely disappear (indicating complete destruction of the cartilage); there is bony ankylosis with some increase in the mineralization of the bone as compared with 4. The soft tissue swelling may disappear as in this instance. (Hollander, *Arthritis and Allied Conditions,* Lea & Febiger.)

of weight and strength. A characteristic macular rash, usually involving the limbs and trunk, is not uncommon, especially in Still's disease in children (Isdale and Bywaters). These features, while suggestive of infection, are of course no conclusive. They may merely indicate a disordered metabolism. The erythrocyte agglutination and the latex fixation reactions have already been discussed. A curious feature of the disease is a tendency to periodic remissions and exacerbations. It must be remembered that only some 10 per cent of the cases go on to serious crippling, and that there is a pronounced tendency to healing under rest and therapy such as gold, cortisone and hydrocortisone, aspirin, and phenylbutazene (butazolidin).

Ankylosing Spondylitis (Marie-Strümpell). —This chronic disabling disease of the spine, first described by Pierre Marie in 1898 and known as Marie-Strümpell spondylitis, presents one of the most challenging problems in the entire confusing arthritic group.

It is, however, very much commoner in males (15 to 1), usually beginning before the age of thirty. The etiology is uncertain, but certain features point to a chronic infection, *viz.*, low grade fever, tachycardia, high sedimentation rate, weight loss and wasting of muscles. Romanus suggests that the lesions are the result of infection starting in the prostate and seminal vesicles and extending by the vertebral system of veins and lymphatics first to the sacro-iliac joints and later to the spine, so that he calls the disease *pelvospondylitis ossificans*. About one-third of the cases of Reiter's syndrome (urethritis, peripheral arthritis and conjunctivitis) ultimately develop ankylosing spondylitis (page 1283). Those interested in the roentgenographic changes in the spine and pelvis during the earlier stages of ankylosing spondylitis will find a wealth of material in the monograph by Romanus and Ydén. The relationship of the condition to rheumatoid arthritis remains to be clarified, but the weight of evidence at present favors the concept that the two diseases are separate entities. The high male sex incidence, the negative serological reactions for the rheumatoid factor whether with sensitized sheep cell agglutination, latex fixation or bentonite

flocculation, and the absence of that rheumatoid hallmark, the connective tissue necrotizing nodule, are some of the more striking differences (Graham).

Lesions.—The essential lesions occur in the joints of the vertebral column. There is a *synovitis*, with increased vascularity, proliferative changes in the synovia, and infiltration of the tissues with lymphocytes and plasma cells. Later the *articular cartilage* is destroyed, fibrous adhesions are formed, and there is eventual bony fusion. Some of the earliest and most characteristic changes occur in the *sacro-iliac joints*, which may be demonstrated long before the onset of symptoms in the back. There is destruction and narrowing of the joint space, which appears in roentgen films as a fuzziness of the opposed surfaces of the bones. Later in the disease there is calcification followed by ossification of the various vertebral ligaments including the anterior spinal ligament and *finally the intervertebral discs* with bony ankylosis. Gradually the disease process may spread upward to the thoracic and finally the cervical spine. The condition now is well described by the term *"poker back."* The rigidity is extreme, the normal spinal curvatures are lost, and the cervical spine is curved into a bow which forces the miserable man's head down until his chin touches his chest. The state of the patient when these changes are complete can be better pictured than described.

Although the progress of the disease can be as relentless as described, the process may be arrested at any stage. *Involvement of the large peripheral joints* (hip, knee, shoulder, etc.) occurs in 15 to 25 per cent of cases, the lesions closely resembling those of rheumatoid arthritis and causing permanent disability. An acute inflammatory reaction is present in the peripheral joints in 50 to 60 per cent of cases, but in most of these the symptoms are transitory, and there are no permanent ill effects. Whether the disease is merely a special expression of rheumatoid arthritis or is a separate pathological entity remains a matter of dispute. While the condition resembles rheumatoid arthritis in many respects, the calcification of ligaments, predominance in males, lack of response to gold therapy and infrequency of streptococcal agglutinins in the blood are quite distinct from that disease.

Relation of Symptoms to Lesions.—Pain, an early and constant symptom, is due to erosion of the articular cartilage. It is worse when the patient drops off to sleep, because then the watchful muscles which hold the joint rigid are off their guard. The joint is swollen and has a characteristic fusiform contour. Much of the enlargement is caused by the swelling of the synovial membrane, but in the later stages the gelatinous swelling of the periarticular soft tissues plays a part. Limitation of movement, the earliest physical sign, is a natural sequel to any inflammatory lesion in a joint. Muscular spasm is an attempt to keep the part at rest. Early atrophy of the surrounding muscles is partly due to disuse, partly to the effect of the infection. It has been customary to employ radiotherapy in the hope of arresting the progress of the disease, but the leukemogenic power of ionizing radiation has begun to make itself felt in this connection. In one series there were 5 cases of rapidly progressive acute myeloid leukemia developing after this form of treatment (Graham). The interval between the initial treatment and the diagnosis of leukemia varied between eight months and eight years, with an average of five years. The risk increases with the size of dose and the number of courses of radiation therapy.

Spondylitis with Aortitis and Carditis.— One of the features which serves to distinguish ankylosing spondylitis from rheumatoid arthritis is the occasional association with lesions of the aortic valve, aorta and myocardium and corresponding symptoms. In such cases in addition to the spondylitis there is frequently involvement of the peripheral joints. Since the first two cases were reported by Bauer *et al.* in 1951, many others have been published, and it would appear that the condition is not the rarity it was at first believed to be. Thus in 519 cases of ankylosing spondylitis Graham and Smythe found 24 instances of aortic insufficiency developing some years after the onset of the spondylitis. The condition is distinct from rheumatic heart disease (no clear history of rheumatic fever, no Aschoff bodies, valves other than the aortic rarely involved), from

"rheumatoid heart disease" (no nodular granulomatous lesions in the pericardium, myocardium, endocardium or valves identical in structure with the subcutaneous rheumatoid nodule), and from syphilis (tests for Treponema infection negative).

The *lesions*, both gross and microscopic, closely resemble and are easily mistaken for those of syphilis. There is marked dilatation of the aortic valve ring producing aortic incompetence, the free margins of the aortic valve cusps are thickened and rolled, with partial fusion of the commissures in some cases (Fig. 742), and thickening and longitudinal wrinkling of the intima of the aorta. *Microscopically* the adventitia shows infiltration with lymphocytes and plasma cells as well as endarteritis obliterans of the arterioles, the media replacement of the elastica by scar tissue, and the intimal fibrous thickening. Why the lesions should mimic those of syphilis so perfectly we cannot at present say. The *clinical picture* is one of aortic regurgitation with diastolic murmur and wide pulse pressure, cardiac enlargement, conduction changes, substernal pain and congestive heart failure.

Reiter's Syndrome.—In 1916 Reiter described the triad of arthritis, urethritis and conjunctivitis which came to be known by his name. In historical justice it should be mentioned that Sir Benjamin Brodie reported 6 cases of the same triad in his book on *Diseases of the Joints* published in 1818. Indeed, if ever there was an eponym which was unjustified, it is that of Reiter's disease. Ford remarks that "Reiter's paper made a negligible if not misleading contribution to the subject." Reiter described a single case in a German officer who developed an abacterial purulent urethritis after an attack of abdominal pain and diarrhea, and in whom he claimed to have isolated a spirochete from the blood. The urethritis is abacterial, presumably venereal in origin. In other cases the arthritis and conjunctivitis follow diarrhea, dysenteric or otherwise, rather than urethritis. One of the many puzzling features of the disease is the fact that the postenteric cases are the rule in Scandinavia and France, whereas a venereal origin is common in England and North America (Ford). The patients often complain of only two of the

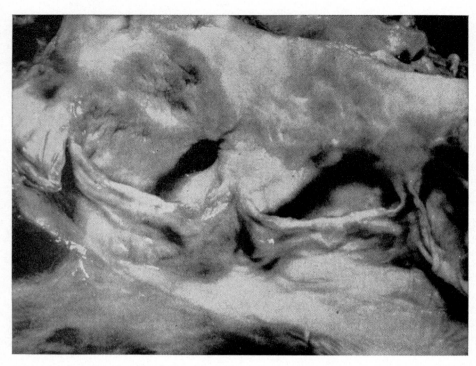

Fig. 743.—Aortic valve, showing thickening of the cusps, rolled free margins, thickening and separation of the commissures. The intima of the sinuses of Valsalva and ascending aorta is irregularly thickened and wrinkled. (Ansell, Bywaters, and Doniach, courtesy of Brit. Heart Jour.)

triad of symptoms. For the present it seems justifiable to regard the condition as a definite entity of unknown etiology, more closely related to ankylosing spondylitis than to rheumatoid arthritis. Indeed about one-third of the cases eventually develop some degree of spondylitis, whilst the majority clear up completely. The condition must not be confused with gonorrheal arthritis, which is a suppurative inflammation in which gonococci can be removed from aspirated synovial fluid or biopsied synovial tissue. Since the advent of antibiotics true, gonococcal arthritis has become a rarity.

Clinical Picture.—A migrating polyarthritis usually develops shortly after the appearance of a urethral discharge or an attack of diarrhea. The joints most frequently affected are in succession the knee, ankle, hip, and small joints of the hands and feet. These become swollen and painful. The characteristic ophthalmic lesion is a severe conjunctivitis, but iritis has been reported in over 10 per cent of cases. Involvement of the skin is common in the form of a discharging keratotic dermatitis (keratodermia), with flat pustules which may rupture and develop a thick horny crust. This is most marked on the soles of the feet, which may be intensely red from acute inflammation. Sacro-iliac arthritis is a late development in from 20 to 30 per cent of cases. The threat of ankylosing spondylitis has already been mentioned.

Osteoarthritis.—In its typical form this degenerative joint disease, better named *degenerative arthritis*, differs from rheumatoid arthritis in almost every respect. It is as common in men as in women, especially the form which affects the hip joint; it is a disease of the later period of life; there are no general symptoms; there is no evidence of a toxic factor; the large joints are commonly involved, often only one joint; there is no true ankylosis. The hip joint (*morbus coxæ senilis*) offers an excellent example of the monoarticular form occurring in elderly men. The small joints of the hands and feet may also be involved, and it is in them that the clinical manifestations can be more readily studied. The knuckles become greatly swollen and knobby. *Heberden's nodes*, which are much commoner in women, are often present; these are small bony outgrowths at the sides of the terminal phalangeal joints. In the early stage the node is a soft nodule containing a bead of mucoid material, and arises as the result of degeneration of the periarticular soft tissue with subsequent ossification. Movement may be much limited by osteophytic outgrowths, but there is no ankylosis.

Osteoarthritis is perhaps the oldest of all known diseases. It was present in our primitive ancestors, as can be seen in the illustration on page 6 of Brugsch's monograph on rheumatic diseases showing evidence of the disease in bones discovered in Nubian caves dating back to 8,000 or 10,000 B.C. Still more ancient are the osteoarthritic lesions found in the bones of prediluvial animals such as the dinosaurs. It is evident that the present-day prevalence of the disease cannot be blamed entirely on modern conditions of life.

Etiology.—The cause of the degeneration is unknown. It is a slow involutional process often associated with marked arteriosclerosis, so that local ischemia may play a part. It is always difficult to form a correct judgment of the relation of trauma to any pathological process, but the common idea that trauma is an etiological factor, especially in hip joint disease, appears reasonable. If a joint is continually exposed to trauma, as in professional athletes (*e. g.*, baseball catcher) or in the course of a trade, it may show the characteristic changes. Degenerative arthritis appears to be a process associated with the ageing of the tissues of the joints. It may be described as *"wear and tear" arthritis*. Similar changes are found in the knee joint in routine autopsies with increasing frequency with advancing age. The primary lesion appears to be a loss of chontroitin sulfate from the ground substance of the articular cartilage. The collagen fibrils are left unsupported, so that they are vulnerable to the mechanical effects of trauma and wear and tear. Erosion of cartilage in these knee joints is commonest over areas of contact subjected to the greatest movement, strain, weight bearing, and injury. As a result of gradual loss of elasticity in the articular cartilage the subchondral bone is no longer protected from the irregular localized effects of weight and pressure, and the changes characteristic of degenerative arthritis result. Age may therefore act in two ways: (1) by reducing the elasticity and (2) by representing trauma spread over a period of years. Similar lesions are present in horses and mules. Loss of cartilage is the primary lesion, followed by bone production which is secondary but has given the name of *hypertrophic arthritis* to the disease.

Once cartilage destruction sets in, the evolution of arthritis has begun. There is no longer harmony between form and function. The process of osteoarthritis or degenerative

	RHEUMATOID ARTHRITIS	OSTEOARTHRITIS
SEX:	Common in female.	Equally common in male.
AGE:	Generally under forty years.	Generally over forty years.
ONSET:	Gradual but sometimes acute.	Always gradual.
JOINT LESIONS:	An inflammatory condition of synovial membrane. Early lesions in metacarpo-phalangeal joints and wrists; symmetrical and migratory.	A degenerative condition of cartilage and bone. Early lesions in terminal interphalangeal joints, hips, and knees; often unilateral and fixed.
GENERAL SYMPTOMS:	Toxic symptoms, fever, loss of weight, anemia, low basal metabolic rate.	No constitutional disturbances.
LOCAL SIGNS:	Local signs of inflammation, marked deformity, extreme atrophy of muscles, swelling of soft parts, subcutaneous nodules, fibrous or bony ankylosis. Marked pain. Complete crippling in 10 per cent.	No local inflammation, deformity not marked, muscular atrophy only from disuse, soft parts not swollen, Heberden's nodes and no true ankylosis. Little or no pain. Complete crippling rare.

arthritis is thus a vicious circle of changing mechanical conditions and attempts at structural adaptations (Collins).

Lesions.—Osteoarthritis is a degeneration of articular cartilage and bone; in this it differs from rheumatoid arthritis which is primarily an inflammation of synovial membrane. The *cartilage*, both its cells and matrix, degenerate, and the smooth surface becomes roughened. The cartilage cells swell, burst, and disappear, and the matrix undergoes a perpendicular fibrillation which accounts for the velvety surface. The softened cartilage is gradually worn away until the underlying bone is exposed. In a hinge joint (elbow, knee) the process of attrition is irregular, so that parallel furrows and ridges are formed. The periphery of the cartilage has a much better blood supply than the central part and survives the general downfall. The *bone* degenerates together with the cartilage, but the exposed surface undergoes a curious process of condensation and hardening, as a result of which it becomes polished like ivory. This appearance is known as *eburnation* (*eburneus*, ivory), and no really satisfactory explanation of the process can be given at present. Deep to the condensed layer the bone is degenerated, rarefied, and becomes absorbed, so that the greater part of the head and neck of the femur may disappear. In addition to central atrophy there is peripheral proliferation. *Cartilaginous excrescences* are formed at the margin of the articular cartilage which resemble candle drippings and cause *lipping* of the edge of the joint. They increase the available articular surface and may be compensatory in character. They tend to become ossified and osteophytes are also formed farther out, so that the atrophied head of the bone is surrounded by a ring of excrescences which greatly limit movement. It is because of these changes, which form a striking feature in the roentgen-ray picture, that this variety is sometimes called by the misleading name of the hypertrophic form of chronic arthritis. In osteoarthritis of the spine osteophytes may *press on the nerve roots* as they emerge from the foramina, giving rise to referred pains. *Thinning of the intervertebral discs* is a feature of diagnostic importance in the *x*-ray film, as it does not occur in ankylosing spondylitis. The *synovial membrane* may become fibrous and fatty, and sometimes presents shaggy fringes which may be changed into cartilage and become detached to form the foreign bodies known as *joint mice*. The *ligaments* share in the general degeneration and dissolution, so that dislocation may occur finally.

GOUT

It is impossible to name a more fascinating disease at the present time than gout, or one with a more exciting history, distinguished patient clientele, or intriguing therapeutic story. One of the chief reasons why gout is such a household name is that so many of the great ones of the world in medicine, literature, religion, science and politics have suffered from an affliction which has provided plentiful material for cartoonists and humorists. It would almost seem as if, in the past at least, genius and gout went hand in hand, and that an excess of uric acid acted on the brain as well as on the joints.

The disease has been known since the earliest times, although under the name of *podagra*, a Greek derivation from *pous*, foot and *agra*, attack. The history of its therapy is also remarkable. *Colchicine*, one of the most effective and truly specific drugs in the entire pharmacopeia, was used for podagra 1500 years ago. By the 15th century it had lost its popularity owing to a confusion of meadow saffron or colchicum, from which colchicine is derived, with yellow saffron which has no medicinal value. It owes its reinstatement in modern times to a quack in the French Army under Napoleon. The remarkable thing about colchicine is that it is not a general analgesic, it does not relieve other types of pain or inflammation, it is of no value in any other form of arthritis, and it is not a uricosuric agent like probenecid (Benemid) which inhibits the reabsorption of uric acid, so that it has no effect on the excretion nor on the synthesis of that substance. The remarkable benefit which it produces in an acute attack is indeed an enigma.

Etiology.—In considering the cause of gout we have to remember that the disease may present itself in one or more of three very different aspects; namely the *acute attack*, the *intercritical period*, and *chronic gout*. The essence of gout is an overproduction of uric acid through a fault in intermediary purine metabolism. The defect is an inherited one, an inborn error of metabolism. Many members of the family who are free from symptoms may have hyperuricemia, just as the siblings of a case of sickle cell anemia may show the sickle cell trait. The strong *hereditary tendency* with its genetic basis, a tendency which was recognized by the Father of Medicine, is probably related to the very marked sex incidence, over 95 per cent of the patients being men. The genetic defect, which may indicate a minute variation in the DNA code, may well represent the lack of a specific enzyme. In man the end product of nitrogenous metabolism is urea, except for small quantities of uric acid formed in the breakdown of nucleoproteins. Birds, on the other hand, excrete nearly all their nitrogenous wastes as uric acid, and the same is true of reptiles. Renal failure in man is associated with uremia, but in birds with uricemia, which may be accompanied by gout. Gout is easily produced in birds merely by ligation of the ureters. The insolubility of uric acid in comparison with urea is of value to birds and reptiles by permitting development of the embryo in a hard shell. Uric acid is excreted through the kidneys as a dilute solution, from which water is absorbed, leaving the uric acid as a solid mass in the allantois. If soluble urea had been evolved, the embryo would have died in the egg from uremia. Birds and reptiles have retained this uricotelic mechanism into adult life. The metabolic defect in gout may be regarded as a partial reversion to the normal situation in birds and reptiles, namely, a significant *uricotelic* component in a predominantly *ureotelic* species (Talbott). The articular vice of uric acid is its low solubility in an acid medium.

The existence of a *miscible* or *metabolic pool* of uric acid is shown by the use of radioactive isotopes. The pool is the amount of uric acid in the tissues which can mix promptly with uric acid injected intravenously. The course of the latter can be followed by labelling it isotopically with N^{15} and measuring the amount excreted in the urine. From this the amount in the miscible pool can be calculated, an amount which may vary widely with little or no change in the blood uric acid level. The normal average content of the pool is around 1,000 mg. of uric acid, more or less, of which one-sixth is in plasma water and five-sixths in extravascular water. The *turnover rate* of labelled uric acid in the miscible pool varies from 0.6 to 0.9 pools per day with different workers.

In gouty persons the miscible pool is increased to 2 to 4 times the normal, even though the blood uric acid (normal between 2.4 and 6.4 mg. per 100 ml. of serum) is only slightly raised, while the turnover rate is considerably less than normal. These findings are quite independent of symptoms. Sometimes the increase is almost unbelievable. Stetten records one very severe case of twenty-five years' duration in which the pool on one occasion was 18,450 mg. and on another 31,000 mg. After several months of treatment with acetylsalicylic acid causing uricosuria the pool had dropped to 2,084 mg. with no change in the blood uric acid. Cincophen, an ancient remedy for gout, the salicylates, and to an even greater degree Benemid increase the excretion of uric acid in the urine, presumably by decreasing the amount absorbed by the renal tubules. This naturally not only decreases the miscible pool but increases the turnover rate. We have already seen that this effect is not shared by colchicine.

Increased knowledge of the chemical basis of gout and an appreciation of the fact that it is a genetically determined error of metabolism in which there is an excessive biosynthesis of uric acid and other purines is a pleasant piece of mental furniture for the student, which gives us a better understanding of the development of the lesions, but it does not help to explain the mechanism of the acute attack or of the curious periodicity of such attacks. For this we must invoke what have been called *precipitating factors* or *agents*. The classical and time-honored examples of these are purine-rich foods, which precipitate an acute attack. Beer and such red wines as port are much more dangerous than whisky; perhaps for this reason gout is a rare disease in Scotland. A friend of mine received the first indication that he was a victim of gout when the drinking of a glass of sherry before lunch was followed quickly by an attack of mental confusion associated with a high blood serum uric acid; at a later date there was severe unilateral renal hemorrhages. The acute attack of arthritis may come on without obvious cause. It may be preceded for a few days by marked uric acid retention. It would be nice to think that the acute attack represents a sudden precipitation of urates in the synovial membrane of the affected joint. Even if this were true we would be left wondering why the big toe should be picked out and why there should be so marked a systemic upset. Physical and psychic trauma are said to have a precipitating effect, even the wearing of too tight shoes.

Perhaps the pathogenesis of primary gout may be summed up by saying that the disease is the result of the interplay of many environmental factors, including diet, with a genetic factor, an inborn error of metabolism involving uric acid.

Clinical Picture.—Reference has already been made to the three phases of the disease in which the patient may be seen for the first time. They seem to have nothing in common.

The *acute attack* is the classic form described by writers of genius and drawn by cartoonists. Sydenham, himself a life-long sufferer from the malady, likened the pain to an angry dog gnawing his great toe. "The victim goes to bed and sleeps in good health. About two in the morning he is awakened by a severe pain in the great toe. The pain is like that of dislocation, and yet the parts feel as if cold water were poured over them. . . . Now it is a violent stretching and tearing of the ligaments, now it is a gnawing pain, and now a pressure and tightening. So exquisite and lively meanwhile is the feeling of the part affected that it cannot bear the weight of the bed clothes or the jar of a person walking in the room." The suddenness of onset is one of the mysteries of the disease. The joints chiefly affected are the metastarso-phalangeal joint of the great toe, (although in only 40 per cent of cases in the first attack), the fingers and the knee. The joint is acutely swollen, the overlying skin tense and shiny, and a sys-

temic reaction characterized by fever, chills, malaise, anorexia, headache, tachycardia, and a leukocytosis up to 20,000 may easily lead to a mistaken diagnosis of septic infection. The usual age of onset is around forty years, but the first attack may occur in childhood or old age. For the pathologist to be unable to explain so dramatic a clinical picture is more than humiliating.

The *intercritical period* represents the interval between acute crises. It may last for months or several years, the patient presenting no evidence of being a victim of gout unless articular deformities have developed. An athlete with gout in ancient times is said to have won an Olympic Marathon in the intercritical period. In spite of this period of calm, the uric acid situation remains unchanged.

The stage of *chronic gout* is one of deformites and subcutaneous tophi, which will be described in connection with the morbid anatomy. These lesions do not necessarily indicate that an active process is still in progress.

The facies of the gouty patient is often characteristic. The complexion is ruddy and the face plethoric owing to innumerable dilated venules, mainly in the malar area.

Lesions.—In writing of the morbid anatomy of gout one must naturally distinguish between the acute attack and the chronic lesions. As regards *acute gout* it is hardly an exaggeration to say that we know no more today about the underlying lesion than did Sydenham when he wrote his classic account of the torture of an attack of gout in 1683. No one has ever looked into the interior of the acutely inflamed joint, nor can the victim be expected to submit readily to a joint biopsy. There is reason to believe that urate crystals are deposited in the synovial membrane early in the disease (Fig. 744).

Chronic gout is due to the formation of masses of urate crystals in the joint structures and eventually in the kidney. These are caused by the excessive endogenous production of uric acid. Most American students regard the mechanism as metastatic in nature, the urate being deposited in the tissues because too much is presented by the blood, whereas European workers favor the idea of a dystrophy, urate being deposited

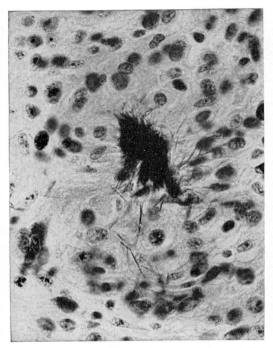

Fig. 744.—Deposits of urate crystals in synovial membrane with cellular reaction in acute gout. (Sokoloff, courtesy of Metabolism.)

in the tissues as the result of a primary pathological change (Sokoloff).

Crystals of biurate of sodium are laid down in the superficial layers of the articular cartilage as white chalky deposits rather like drops of paint, an appearance from which the name gout is derived (Latin *gutta*, a drop), the original clinical name being podagra, a Greek derivation from *pous*, foot and *agra* attack. The sheaves of needle-shaped crystals are usually surrounded by an area of necrosis. It is not certain whether the necrosis precedes or follows the deposition of the crystals. It has been suggested that crystals may enter the cartilage from the synovial fluid. The synovial membrane and capsular structures are also involved, and synovitis develops at an early stage, as is revealed by joint biopsy. Deposits are formed in the subchondral bone. The principal results are: (1) disintegration of cartilage with the development of an osteoarthritis; (2) massive obliteration of the joint by urates, and (3) chronic tophaceous synovitis.

Tophi are masses of crystals which accumulate in the soft tissues around the joints, particularly the toes and fingers. Similar deposits occur in the cartilage of the free margin and helix of the ear and occasionally in the eyelid. As tophi are painless, they are easily overlooked. The overlying skin may become ulcerated, and chalky material is discharged containing the characteristic crystals. A useful diagnostic procedure is to prick a suspected tophus with a needle, and look for the crystals under the microscope. Tophus formation is a feature of soft tissue deposits and is not seen in cartilage. Some idea of the deformities which may develop can be gathered from Figs. 745 and 746 and the illustrations of the paper by Lichtenstein and his associates. Periarticular tophi are composed of fibroblasts, polymorphonuclears, lymphocytes, and foreign body giant cells arranged around a central core of urate crystals with eventual fibrosis (Fig. 747). As the crystals are water-soluble, they must be fixed in a non-aqueous solution such as absolute alcohol. They are brilliantly anisotropic with polarized light. It would appear that recurring deposits of urate crystals in minute amounts over the years may precede the formation of tophi.

The *radiological findings* vary from normal structure to advanced deforming changes. The patient may have a number of acute attacks and be incapacitated, yet after a lapse of ten years the *x*-ray picture may show no irreparable damage. Punched out areas may form a striking feature owing to tophus deposits in the bone marrow. First the subchondral bone is involved, this is followed by erosion of the articular cartilage with narrowing of the joint space, and finally complete obliteration of the joint with sclerosis.

The *kidneys* are the only vital structures likely to be affected, with renal failure as the commonest cause of death. Deposits of urates in the pyramids with resulting interstitial inflammation result in severe degeneration of the lower part of the tubules which contain blood and pigment casts, a true lower nephron gout nephrosis. Deposits of urates in the kidneys are found in most longstanding cases of gout. The picture may simulate chronic glomerulonephritis or pyelonephritis. Gross hematuria, sometimes

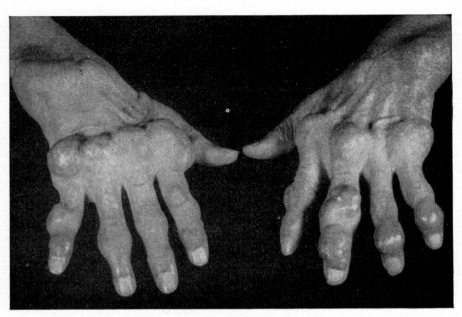

FIG. 745.—Marked formation of gouty tophi in the hands of a man who was supposed for years to have rheumatoid arthritis, and was treated as such. (Boyd, *Pathology for the Physician.*)

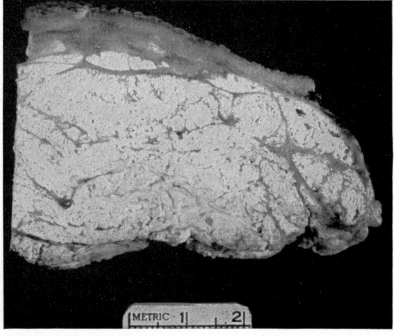

FIG. 746.—Masses of urate crystals forming subcutaneous tophus. (Boyd, *Pathology for the Physician.*)

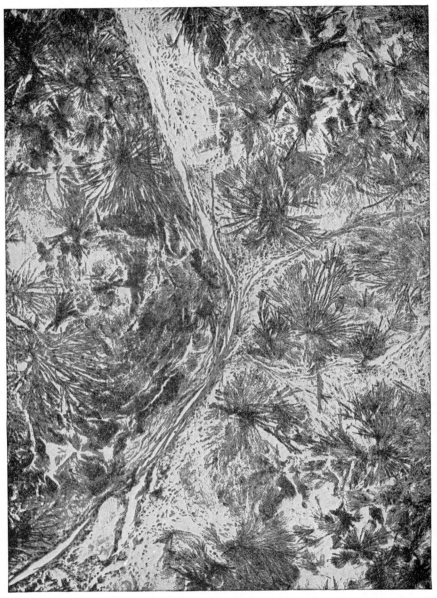

Fig. 747.—Urate crystals in gouty tophus of long standing. The crystalline masses are enveloped by fibrous tissue. Alcohol-fixed tissue. (Collins, *The Pathology of Articular and Spinal Diseases*, courtesy of Edward Arnold & Co.)

alarming in degree, may be the first thing to draw attention to the kidneys.

Secondary Gout.—It is possible to arrive at a common clinical end result as the result of more than one distinct metabolic aberration. The long chain of enzymatic reactions required for metabolic synthesis and degradation may be interrupted at different points. So it is with gout, in which either of two alternate pathways of purine synthesis may be augmented, although the resulting clinical manifestations, the recurrent acute arthritis and the chronic tophaceous deposits, are very much the same (Gutman *et al.*). *Primary gout* is a genetically determined error of metabolism in which excessive biosynthesis of uric acid and other purines occurs by *direct* metabolic pathways not involving increased formation and breakdown of nucleic acid. *Secondary gout*, on the other hand, is an acquired complication of certain hemopoietic disorders in which there is an accelerated turnover of nucleic acids in relation to the overproduction of one or another type of blood cell, with as a result an excessive biosynthesis of uric acid and other purines by *indirect* metabolic pathways. It is known that hyperuricemia and uricosuria may occur in the augmented turnover of nucleic acids in the leukemias, particularly chronic granulocytic and acute leukemia, in the myeloproliferative diseases, notably myeloid metaplasia and polycythemia vera, and occasionally in secondary polycythemia and still other hemopoietic disorders. That the predominant pathways of uric acid biosynthesis are different in primary and secondary gout is shown by the sharp contrast between the rapid peak of glycine-N^{15} incorporation into uric acid in the primary form compared with the slow peak in the secondary form.

Relation of Symptoms to Lesions.—In the normal person all the uric acid in the miscible pool appears to be in solution, but in the gouty patient most of it is in the solid phase in the form of tophi. There seems to be a continuous process of solution and precipitation taking place between the tophi and the body fluid analagous to the interchange of calcium and phosphate between bone and plasma, the latter interchange governed by the parathyroid hormone. In gout a fraction larger than normal of the dietary amino acids seems to be converted into uric acid, thus increasing the miscible pool, although not necessarily the serum uric acid. From what has already been said it is evident that the morphological basis of the acute arthritis is not understood. It is difficult to relate deposits of urates in the synovial membrane with the dramatic local picture and still less with the systemic reaction. Moreover, injections of uric acid in gouty subjects do not produce an acute attack, nor does colchicine, so effective in acute gout, lower the serum uric acid level. There must be some precipitating factor which so far eludes us. The pain may be caused in part by an acute effusion into the joint cavity as well as by edema of the surrounding soft tissues. In chronic gout, on the other hand, there may be the most extensive urate deposits with tophaceous reaction but with no pain or other symptoms of inflammation, yet at any time an acute attack may supervene.

The reader desirous of a more detailed account of the many fascinating aspects of the gout problem is referred to Talbott's monograph and to the May, 1957, number of Metabolism.

MISCELLANEOUS ARTHROPATHIES

CHARCOT'S DISEASE.—The peculiar condition known as Charcot's disease of joints may develop in the course of tabes dorsalis and occasionally it complicates syringomyelia, so that it has been called a *neuropathic arthropathy*. It may develop at a fairly early stage of tabes, and usually affects the large joints of the lower limb (hip, knee, and ankle) owing to the preponderatingly lumbar distribution of the tabetic lesions in the cord. In syringomyelia it is more common in the upper limb for a similar reason. As a rule only one joint is involved. The onset is insidious, but the patient may suddenly discover that the joint is much swollen. This swelling may develop quite rapidly. The further progress is a story of destruction and disintegration until the joint may be completely disorganized and flail-like, so that a hinge joint like the knee or elbow can be moved in every direction. Although grating and crunching can be felt in the joint there is a complete and remarkable *absence of pain*. Sometimes the process of destruction is very rapid, reaching its maximum in the course of a few weeks, after which the disease may become stationary. The head of the femur has been known to disappear in the course of six weeks. This quickness of action, so unlike ordinary osteoarthritis, is one of the most puzzling features of the disease. The *lesions* are essentially degenerative and destructive, especially in the acute cases where it would appear as if some powerful solvent had dissolved away first the articular surface and then the bone, leaving a ragged stump and disconnected fragments. The synovial membrane may develop villous and polypoid tags. When the acute stage is past numerous osteophytes may form a fringe around the joint and in the capsule. It seems probable that during the stage of attrition large numbers of osteoblasts are set free in the joint cavity and become implanted in the capsule and periarticular tissues where they form new bone. The *nature of the condition* is very obscure. The pathology does not remotely resemble that of syphilis. It is commonly supposed to be due to loss of hypothetical trophic influences on the joint on account of the cord lesion. It appears more probable that a loss of joint sensibility which may develop both in tabes and syringomyelia exposes it to trauma and attrition which in some obscure way bring about the rapid osteoarthritis characteristic of Charcot's disease.

HEMOPHILIC JOINT.—In hemophilia an osteoarthritis may develop as the result of repeated hemorrhages into one of the large joints. The patient is of course a male, and the first hemorrhage occurs in early childhood. The knees, the elbows and the ankles in that order are the joints most commonly affected, for a reason which it is easy to guess. The cartilage becomes eroded and fibrillated, the bone is exposed, periarticular osteophytes are formed, and the synovial membrane is thickened and fringed.

LOOSE BODIES.—Three forms of loose bodies in joints may be found in such conditions as tuberculosis, osteoarthritis and Charcot's disease, and loose bodies may occasionally occur in an apparently normal joint. These three varieties are fibrinous bodies, fibrous and fatty bodies, and cartilaginous bodies. (1) *Fibrinous loose bodies* occur chiefly in tuberculous joints, and also in synovial sheaths and bursæ affected by tuberculosis. They take the form of small, round or oval bodies like melon-seeds or rice-grains, and may be present in large numbers (Fig. 734, p. 1272). It is difficult to say if they are formed as the result of some fibrinous change on the surface of the synovial membrane or if they are deposited from fluid rich in fibrin. (2) *Fibrous and fatty loose bodies* are formed from villous tags of synovial membrane which become detached in tuberculous arthritis and osteoarthrosis, in both of which conditions the membrane is often marked by numerous fringes. Some of the bodies may still be attached by a slender pedicle. (3) *Cartilaginous loose bodies* may arise in three different ways. (*a*) A cartilaginous osteophyte may be detached in osteoarthrosis and particularly in Charcot's disease. (*b*) A loose body occurring in an otherwise normal joint has always been a puzzling phenomenon, but it appears probable that it is a fragment of articular cartilage which has become detached as the result of direct trauma or of muscular or ligamentous strain. (*c*) Synovial chondromata may develop in tags of synovial membrane and become detached.

TUMORS OF JOINTS AND TENDON SHEATHS

Tumors of joints are rare, in striking contrast to the extreme frequency of inflammatory lesions. Moreover, it is by no means easy to be certain as to what should be included in the group. The only lesion whose neoplastic character is agreed upon is the malignant synovioma, and, curiously enough, it seldom grows in the interior of a joint, but rather from its surroundings. It is when we come to the benign tumors, and particularly those of tendon sheaths, that the subject becomes almost hopelessly confused, for some of the endless names which have been used, such as giant cell tumor and benign synovioma, suggest a neoplasm, while others, such as villo-nodular synovitis, indicate a belief that the lesion is non-neoplastic. We shall use the latter term, defending the inclusion of the condition under the heading of tumors by emphasizing that the subject is still an enigma, for which no one has the certain answer. We shall begin with the only undoubted neoplasm, the malignant synovioma.

Malignant Synovioma (Synovial Sarcoma). —This is a not uncommon tumor. For long it was regarded as a rarity, but this was because it passed unrecognized, being diagnosed as adenocarcinoma, fibrosarcoma, reticulum cell sarcoma, endothelial sarcoma, etc. The reason for these errors is explained by the histological structure. The tumor develops in relation to the synovial membrane of joints, bursæ and tendon sheaths, but it is seldom found within these structures. About 75 per cent of the cases occur in the lower limb, mostly in the neighborhood of

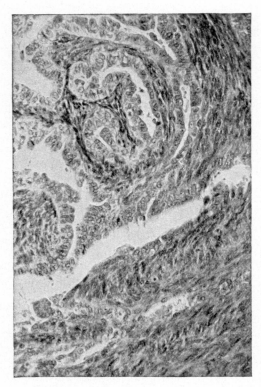

FIG. 748.—Malignant synovioma showing the sarcomatous and pseudoepithelial elements. × 175. (Boyd, *Pathology for the Surgeon,* courtesy of W. B. Saunders Co.)

the knee, including the popliteal fossa, and the lower part of Hunter's canal.

The tumor may have a deceptively circumscribed appearance, which lulls the suspicion of the surgeon, because the neighboring tissues are compressed into a pseudocapsule. Invasion of the joint is unusual. It is generally spongy and friable, but occasionally it is firm. The cut surface is gray, with yellow areas of necrosis and red or brown areas of recent or old hemorrhage.

The *microscopic appearance* varies greatly in different cases and even in different parts of the same tumor, a fact responsible for the various pathological diagnoses to which reference has already been made. The tumor presents two elements, which may be referred to as the sarcomatous and the pseudoepithelial. The *sarcomatous element* consists of fusiform or anaplastic cells, which correspond to the outer part of the synovial membrane. The *pseudoepithelial elements* consist of larger and more differentiated cells. They are grouped in cords or epithelium-like sheets, but the really characteristic arrangment is around slit-like spaces or short tubes so as to give a pseudoglandular appearance (Fig. 748). These cells secrete a mucinous material into the spaces. Giant cells containing blood pigment or lipid may be present. Preponderance of pseudoepithelial elements and giant cells indicates differentiation and a favorable prognosis (Wright). Unfortunately the vast majority of the tumors are poorly differentiated and lacking in giant cells, with a corresponding prognosis.

The tumor is of slow growth, and it may have been present for months or even a year or two before it is seen by the surgeon. At first swelling is the only symptom, and it is only later that pain brings the patient to the surgeon. *The clinical picture is entirely misleading, and the tumor is a highly treacherous one.* It has a strong tendency to recur after removal, and an equally strong tendency to metastasize to the lungs and occasionally to the regional lymph nodes. In a series of 104 collected cases, only 3 patients were alive and free from metastases at the end of five years after treatment (Haagensen and Stout).

Pigmented Villo-nodular Synovitis.—This descriptive term was introduced by Jaffe *et al.* in 1941 to signify a benign proliferative lesion of the synovial membrane of joint and tendon sheaths (tenosynovitis), which seems to start as a yellowish brown villous or nodular proliferation of the lining tissues. The pigmentation is due to varying amounts of hemosiderin and lipid owing to the hemorrhage which is apt to occur. *Microscopically* the new formation consists of polyhedral cells, histiocytes, giant cells, collagenous stroma, and deposits of hemosiderin. The polygonal cells and histiocytes sometimes contain large amounts of hemosiderin and lipid. It is convenient to consider separately the lesions of the joints which tend to be diffuse, and those of the tendon sheaths which are nodular.

Diffuse Villo-nodular Synovitis.—This is a rather rare condition involving the knee and only very occasionally other joints. Th greater part or the whole of the synovial membrane is brown in color, and presents on its surface villous projections (Fig. 749A) which may fuse into grape-like nodular masses (Fig. 749B). The lesion may also take the form of a *localized nodular synovitis*, sometimes as a single nodule. These also are pigmented, the color varying from pale yellow to chocolate brown. In the course of time the synovial proliferation may lead to the erosion of the articular surface, which may be responsible for some of the symptoms. *Microscopically*, two pathological processes seem to be recognizable, the one

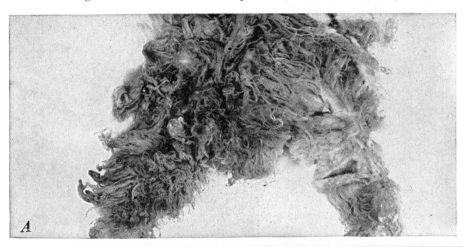

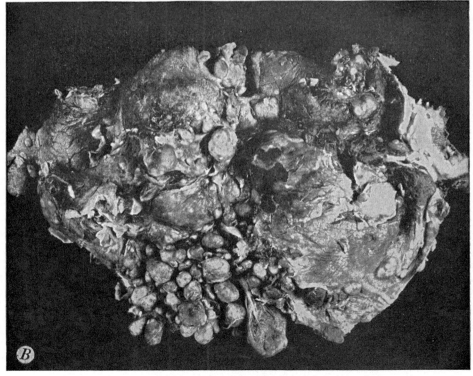

Fig. 749.—*A*. Pigmented villo-nodular synovitis of knee joint in the villous stage.
Fig. 749.—*B*. Nodular form of diffuse villo-nodular synovitis. (Jaffe, *Tumors and Tumorous Conditions of the Bones and Joints*, Lea & Febiger.)

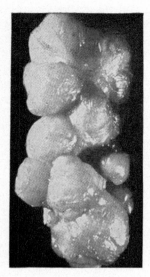

FIG. 750.—Localized nodular tenosynovitis. A
strikingly nodular lesion (enlarged 2½ times) removed
from finger. (Jaffe, *Tumors and Tumorous Conditions
of the Bones and Joints*, Lea & Febiger.)

tumor-like, the other inflammatory. The
various histological elements which have
already been enumerated are all present,
intracellular lipid and hemosiderin sometimes
dominating the picture. The *clinical picture*
is one of monoarticular arthritis characterized by painful exacerbations and remissions.
The painful attack is likely to be due to
hemorrhage, sometimes profuse, from the
villi into the joint cavity. This may or may
not be caused by trauma. The duration of
the condition varies from a few weeks to
many years. There are no constitutional
disturbances.

Localized Nodular Tenosynovitis.—This is
the condition commonly called *giant cell
tumor of tendon sheaths* and *benign giant cell
synovioma*, terms which serve as a justification for its inclusion in a discussion of tumors
of tendon sheaths. It appears to be basically
the same process as we have just studied in
diffuse synovitis, although presenting many
differences. It is much more common, it is
largely confined to the palmar surface of the
fingers and thumb, with occasional involvement of the toes, it presents as a firm nodule
which may be present for a long time before
its increase in size brings the patient to the
doctor, and it is more frequent in women.

The *lesion* takes the form of a golden or
reddish-brown nodular mass, superficially
very different from diffuse villo-nodular synovitis (Fig. 750). The variation in the gross
appearance of the two lesions may well be
related to their different physical environment (Sherry and Anderson). It is natural
for the villous pattern of growth to be maintained in the capacious synovial pockets of
the knee, whereas in the very limited space
of the tendon sheaths the new growth is
subjected to the shearing movements of the
tendons, which cause the villous processes to
fuse and force them into the sheath tissues.
Microscopically, the lesion consists of the
same elements as make up the villonodular
synovial proliferation in the large joints.
Focal collections of macrophages filled with
hemosiderin may dominate the picture (Fig.
750). An occasional abundance of giant
cells is responsible for the misleading term
giant cell tumor, for the condition has no
relation to giant cell tumor of bone. The
picture varies much in different cases and in
different parts of the same specimen, but the
basic fact emerges that the lesion as a whole
is the result of the fusion of individual
smaller nodules, and progresses by way of
an initial villous pigmented stage, through
an intermediate nodular and cellular stage
with slit-like clefts and spaces lined by
synovial endothelium, to a collagenous and
fibrous end stage (Jaffe).

The *pathogenesis* of the various forms of
villo-nodular synovitis and tenosynovitis is
naturally a subject on which diametrically
different opinions are expressed. Is the lesion a neoplasm or is it a reaction to an
irritant? If the former view is correct it
should be called a benign synovioma, if the
latter is true it is a synovitis. The multi-
formity of the cellular elements, the fact
that the spaces and clefts bordered by synovial lining cells are due to entrapment of
villous proliferations and are devoid of mucoid secretion which is so characteristic of
true synovial neoplasms, and the natural
course of the lesions towards fibrosis and
encapsulation, seems to favor the concept of
inflammation. The difficulty is to suggest
the etiological agent responsible.

In the case of villo-nodular synovitis of a
large joint, the presence of blood might be

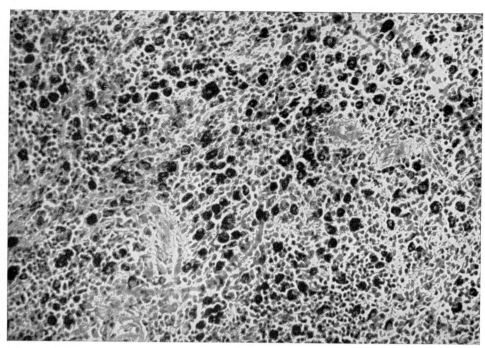

Fig. 751.—Nodular tenosynovitis showing pigment-filled macrophages in a tendon-sheath lesion. ($\times$ 160.) (Sherry and Anderson, courtesy of J. Bone & Joint Surg.)

an important factor. The synovitis of hemarthrosis, such as is seen in the hemophilic joint, presents a similar picture of inflammation. Repeated injections of autologous blood into the knee joints of dogs produce an appearance closely resembling that of villonodular synovitis (Young and Hudacek). The question is: Where does the blood come from? Trauma has been blamed in a number of cases. It has been suggested that a vascular neoplasm in the nature of an angioma may be responsible for repeated hemorrhages into the joint, perhaps precipitated by trauma. Even if these suggestions are accepted we are left with the problem of the nodular masses in the tendon sheaths which are so much more common than the lesions in the large joints.

CYSTS CONNECTED WITH JOINTS

The cyst may or may not communicate with a joint. A cyst in the neighborhood of a joint is likely to fall into one of three groups. (1) *Cysts due to distention of a bursal*

sac which may or may not normally open into the joint cavity. (2) Cysts formed by hernial protrusion of the synovial membrane through gaps in the capsular ligaments. Such a cyst is called a *Baker's cyst,* which almost always develops in connection with the knee, appears in the popliteal space, and may make its way down the leg after the manner of a cold abscess. (3) *Cysts of the semilunar cartilages* of the knee, usually the external, occasionally the internal (Fig. 735, page 1272). The cyst is multilocular, the contents are gelatinous, and a preceding history of trauma is common. Some of the cysts may have an endothelial-like lining. The lesion appears to be the result of a gelatinous degeneration of the fibrocartilage with cyst formation, so that the pathogenesis is similar to that of ganglion (page 1312). The cyst lining is probably formed by modified fibroblasts. Some writers believe that the cysts are developmental in character, arising from portions of the synovial membrane included in the semilunar cartilage.

82

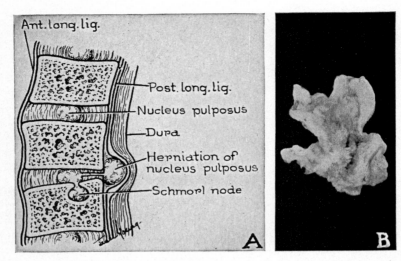

FIG. 752.—*A*, herniated nucleus pulposus and Schmorl node. *B*, herniated disc removed at operation.
(Peet and Echols, courtesy of Arch. Neurol. and Psychiat.)

LESIONS OF THE INTERVERTEBRAL DISCS

When we consider the important joints of the body we are apt to forget the intervertebral discs. And yet there is perhaps no part of the body where strain and movement are so constant, and where impairment of movement, especially when associated with pain, so cripples the full enjoyment of life.

Each disc consists of: (1) the nucleus pulposus, a highly elastic semi-fluid mass compressed like a spring between the vertebral surfaces; (2) the annulus fibrosus which surrounds and confines the turgid nucleus; (3) the cartilage plate which separates the nucleus from the vertebral body. Lesions may develop in any of the three constituents. Owing to man's upright position the discs are subjected to constant strain for which they were not originally intended, so that degeneration in later life is commoner than in any other organ, with corresponding loss of the normal cushioning function.

The nucleus pulposus is the essential part of the disc, and it is it which plays the chief role in pathological changes. In youth it presents a very marked elastic turgor, depending on the fluid content of the tissue, which seems to depend on the very high concentration of hyaluronic acid that serves to maintain the viscosity. With age this turgor gradually diminishes, and is completely lost in various degenerations. As the nucleus loses its fluidity and becomes desiccated and solid, the disc loses its firmness and becomes fragile and easily torn. Later the whole disc swells and is converted into a sodden mass like lumps of porridge. The spinal curvatures of advancing age are the consequence of degeneration of the discs.

The two chief pathological conditions related to the discs are (1) herniation of the nucleus pulposus into the bodies of the vertebræ, sometimes associated with spinal deformities, and (2) posterior prolapse into the spinal canal.

1. **Herniation of Nucleus Pulposus.**—The most frequent lesion, but one of minor clinical significance, is the Schmorl node (Fig. 752), which was present in 38 per cent of 3,000 vertebral columns removed by Schmorl at autopsy. It is the combined result of the internal pressure of the nucleus and weakening of the cartilage plate or the vertebral body by injury or disease. As the result of tearing of the cartilage plate (as in compression fracture) the turgid nucleus pulposus bulges into the body of the vertebra and may occupy the greater part of it. The vertebra may be weakened by osteoporotic change as in osteomalacia, again allowing prolapse and ballooning of the nucleus. In

adolescent kyphosis the primary lesion is in the discs, which are riddled with multiple remains of the notochord; fine tears appear in the cartilage, and, as the substance of the nucleus pushes its way out, these tears enlarge into wide fissures, so that there are multiple prolapses over the entire spine.

2. **Protrusion of Disc.**—The significant lesions are those to which the names of posterior *herniation, protrusion* and *prolapse* of the disc or its nucleus are attached. The lesions which give rise to symptoms are in the great majority of cases in the discs between the fifth lumbar vertebra and the sacrum or between the fourth and fifth lumbar vertebræ. Similar lesions in the cervical spine may cause neurological disturbances such as brachial neuritis and neurological syndromes in the neck and arm. Protrusions of the disc occur at the sites of maximum anterior spinal curvature, both in the lumbar and the cervical regions, that is to say, the region between the fourth lumbar and first sacral, and between the fifth and seventh cervical vertebræ. Various terms, such as nuclear herniation, annular protrusion, etc., are employed to indicate the various elements of the disc primarily involved, but these are apt to prove confusing. It is better to say that changes in the annulus, the nucleus or both are responsible for the disc lesions. The turgor of the nucleus pulposus is largely due to the elasticity of the annulus fibrosus which comprises it. Local loss of this elasticity may lead to local herniation of the nucleus. Degeneration of the nucleus as well as of the annulus begins after the second decade, with inspissation and gradual conversion of the gelatinous ground substance into formed elements. Such a change is normal at sixty years of age but pathological at thirty. This is comparable to the relation of the ageing process to osteoarthritis. The most severe extrusion will occur when the nucleus has lost none of its turgor, but the annulus has been damaged by trauma. The common lesion found at operation is a *backward displacement of the lateral part of the disc into the spinal canal* (Fig. 752), pressing on and stretching the nerves in the canal.

Etiology.—The etiological factors in disc protrusion have been analyzed by O'Connell in 500 cases operated on by him at Saint Bartholomew's Hospital, London. Injury was the apparent factor in 59 per cent, pregnancy and labor in 5.8 per cent, physical weakness after illness or operation in 1.2 per cent, and in 34 per cent no factor was discovered. The trauma may be sudden, as in a fall from a height, but usually it was the repetitious trauma of heavy labor, such as lifting or digging. The patients were for the most part between the ages of twenty-one and forty years, and 66 per cent were males. The sex incidence may be attributed to the frequency of occupational trauma in the male. The importance of pregnancy and labor is enhanced when it is realized that this factor was operative in 17 per cent of the female patients. O'Connell suggests that corpus luteum hormone, which is well known to cause relaxation of the pelvic joints during pregnancy, may also affect the lumbar intervertebral joints, thus favoring protrusion of a disc. To these more obvious causes it seems reasonable to add such intangible factors as congenital defects and degenerative lesions of the discs.

In a notable paper on the discs in low back pain Harris and Macnab point out that the spine acts as an integral whole. Just as the stability of a coupling unit depends on the integrity of all its components, so that damage to one affects all, so damage to one part of the vertebral column may lead to changes in other structures in the column. Macnab made a detailed gross and microscopic examination of the discs and posterior articulations in 123 lumbar spines removed at autopsy in my department in Toronto. Between the vertebræ there are two sets of joints, anterior and posterior. The anterior joints are the intervertebral discs, the posterior articulations are joints of the ordinary type, their capsule being in close relation to the nerve roots as they pass through the intervertebral foramina. Changes which affect one set of joints are likely to be reflected in the other set. Thus loss of substance of the nucleus by herniation into a vertebral body will upset the delicate balance, and damage first the annulus and then the posterior joints and ligaments. Tears in the posterior spinal ligaments which are supplied with sensory nerves may be an

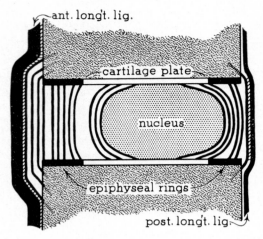

FIG. 753.—Diagram of fibers of annulus. Note the outermost annulus fibers are attached to the vertebral body just above the epiphyseal ring. These fibers are strong anteriorly and laterally, but are few in number posteriorly. This anatomical peculiarity probably accounts for the fact that lipping is seen anteriorly and laterally on the vertebral bodies, but very rarely posteriorly. (Kindness of Dr. Ian Nacnab.)

important factor in the production of the back pain. Instability of the disc resulting from loss of turgor of the nucleus will permit backward and forward movement of the vertebral bodies on flexion and extension. This applies a repeated strain on the anterior fibers of the annulus at their attachment to bone (Fig. 753). Ossification of the annulus occurs at this point. This bony excrescence gradually increases in size and gives rise to the radiological appearance of lipping of the vertebral bodies, sometimes erroneously referred to as osteoarthritis of the spine. The name *spondylosis* is applied to this complex of disc and posterior joint lesions (Brain). Subluxation of the posterior joints is common. Every stage of degenerative arthritis may be seen. The locking of a loose body in one of these joints will precipitate a sudden attack of lumbago. The concept of spondylosis, therefore, comprises more than that of a simple disc lesion.

Relation of Symptoms to Lesions.—The chief clinical features are *low back pain* and *sciatica.* "Though lumbago and sciatica carry little threat to life, they may interfere greatly with living" (O'Connell). The posterior longitudinal ligament and the annulus

fibrosus are supplied with sensory nerve fibers, and the low back pain is due to tearing of either of these structures or to stretching of the torn ligaments by the herniated nucleus pulposus. The lower limb symptoms are due to compression and stretching of nerves by the protruded disc. This may be brought about in one of three ways. (1) A large mass of disc tissue may fill the canal and compress all the nerve roots. (2) Usually only a relatively small mass of extruded tissue enters the spinal canal, presses on the nerve roots, anterior or posterior, and stretches instead of displacing the relatively taut nerve in its strong dural sheath. Tension rather than pressure is the important factor in producing the pain. (3) In rare instances sudden displacement of a large mass may injure the roots. One of the characteristic features of herniated disc pain is that it is aggravated by mechanical conditions. This is readily understood when the stretched and taut intraspinal nerves are kept in mind. Spasm of the muscles of the back is a marked feature, and in some cases there may be back disability from spasm of the erector spinæ without accompanying pain. It is possible to localize the lesion accurately by clinical findings in 75 per cent or more of all cases. Successful diagnosis without the use of a myelogram is possible through the elimination of other conditions giving a similar clinical picture by means of physical and x-ray examination. Excision of the protruded disc is required in only a small proportion of cases.

REFERENCES

ANSELL, B. M., BYWATERS, E. G. L. and DONIACH, I.: Brit. Heart J., 1958, *20*, 507. (Aortic lesions of ankylosing spondylitis.)

ARMSTRONG, J. R.: *Lumbar Disc Lesions*, 2nd ed., Edinburgh, 1958.

ASBOE-HANSEN, G.: Ann. Rheumatic Dis., 1950, *9*, 149. (Synovial fluid in rheumatoid arthritis.)

BAGGENSTOSS, A. H. and ROSENBERG, E. F.: Arch. Path., 1943, *35*, 503. (The heart in rheumatoid arthritis.)

BRAIN, R.: Lancet, 1954, *1*, 687. (Spondylosis.)

BRUGSCH, H. G.: *Rheumatic Diseases, Rheumatism and Arthritis*, Philadelphia, 1957.

COLLINS, D. H.: *The Pathology of Articular and Spinal Diseases*, Baltimore, 1949.

CORMIER, B. M. and WITTKOWER, E. D.: Can. Med. Ass. J., 1957, *77*, 533. (Psychological aspects of rheumatoid arthritis.)

CRUICKSHANK, B.: Scot. Med. J., 1958, *3*, 110. (Lymphadenopathy in rheumatoid arthritis.)

DRESSNER, E.: J. Chronic Diseases, 1957, *5*, 612. (Etiology of rheumatoid arthritis.)

FORD, D. K.: Bull. Rheum. Dis., 1958, *8*, 159, Ann. Rheum. Dis., 1953, *12*, 177. (Reiter's Syndrome.)

GARDNER, E.: Lab. Invest., 1959, *8*, 1160. (Joint physiology.)

GOOD, R. A., ROTSTEIN, J. and MAZZITELLO, W. F.: J. Lab. & Clin. Med., 1957, *49*, 343. (Rheumatoid arthritis and agammaglobulinemia.)

GRAHAM, D. C.: Can. Med. Ass. J., 1960, *82*, 671. (Ankylosing spondylitis.)

————: Arch. Int. Med., 1960, *105*, 51. (Leukemia following *X*-ray therapy for ankylosing spondylitis.)

GRAHAM, D. C. and SMYTHE, H. A.: Bull. Rheum. Diseases, 1958, *9*, 171. (The carditis and aortitis of ankylosing spondylitis.)

GUTMAN, A. B.: Am. J. Med., 1960, *29*, 545. (Gout: an inborn error of metabolism.)

GUTMAN, A. B., YÜ, T. V. and WEISSMANN, B.: Trans. Ass. Am. Phys., 1956, *69*, 229. (Secondary gout.)

HAAGENSEN, C. D. and STOUT, A. P.: Ann. Surg., 1944, *120*, 826. (Malignant synovioma.)

HANDFORTH, C. P. and WOODBURY, J. F. L.: Can. Med. Ass. J., 1959, *80*, 86. (Cardiovascular lesions in rheumatoid arthritis.)

HARRIS, R. I. and MACNAB, I.: J. Bone & Joint Surg., 1954, *36B*, 304. (Low back pain.)

JAFFE, H. L.: *Tumors and Tumorous Conditions of the Bones and Joints*, Philadelphia, 1958.

JAFFE, H. L., LICHTENSTEIN, L. and SUTRO, C. J.: Arch. Path., 1941, *31*, 731. (Pigmented villonodular synovitis.)

KULKA, J. P.: J. Chronic Dis., 1959, *10*, 388. (Vasculitis in rheumatoid arthritis.)

LICHTENSTEIN, L., SCOTT, H. W. and LEVIN, M. H.: Am. J. Path., 1956, *32*, 871. (Pathology of gout.)

MELLORS, R. C., et al.: J. Exper. Med., 1959, *110*, 875. (Cellular origin of the rheumatoid factor.)

O'CONNELL, J. E. A.: J. Bone & Joint Surg., 1951, *33-B*, 8. (Intervertebral disc lesions.)

OGRYZLO, M. A.: Arch. Path., 1948, *46*, 301. (The muscles in rheumatoid arthritis.)

PEARSE, A. E. G.: Lancet, 1950, *1*, 954. (Pituitary changes in rheumatoid arthritis.)

PLOTZ, C. M. and SINGER, J. M.: Am. J. Med., 1956, *21*, 888, 893. (Latex fixation test in rheumatoid arthritis.)

ROMANUS, R.: *Pelvo-Spondylitis Ossificans in the Male and Genito-Urinary Infection*, Stockholm, 1953.

ROMANUS, R. and YDÉN, S.: *Pelvo-spondylitis Ossificans: a Roentgenological and Clinical Guide to its Early Diagnosis*, Copenhagen, 1955.

SALTER, R. B. and FIELD, P.: J. Bone & Joint Surg., 1960, *42-A*, 31. (Continuous compression on living articular cartilage.)

SCHMORL, G.: Klin. Wchnschr., 1929, *8*, 1243. (The intervertebral discs.)

SHERRY, J. B. and ANDERSON, W.: J. Bone & Joint Surg., 1955, *37-A*, 1005. (Villonodular synovitis of tendon sheaths.)

SOKOLOFF, L.: Metabolism, 1957, *6*, 230. (The pathology of gout.)

————.: Am. Heart J., 1953, *45*, 635. (Heart disease in rheumatoid arthritis.)

STETTEN, DE W., JR.: Bull. New York Acad. Med., 1952, *28*, 664. (The metabolic defect in gout.)

TALBOTT, J. H.: *Gout*, New York, 1957.

TAYLOR, H. E. and SHEPHERD, W. E.: Lab. Invest., 1960, *9*, 603. (Reaction of autologous rheumatoid serum with subcutaneous rheumatoid nodules.)

WRIGHT, C. J. E.: J. Path. & Bact., 1952, *64*, 585. (Malignant synovioma.)

YOUNG, J. M. and HUDACEK, A. G.: Am. J. Path., 1954, *30*, 799. (Experimental pigmented villonodular synovitis.)

Chapter 45

The Muscles

General Considerations
Myositis
   Acute Polymyositis:
      Dermatomyositis
   Myositis Ossificans
     Traumatic
     Generalized
Lesions Due to Ischemia
   Anterior Tibial Syndrome

Volkmann's Contracture
Dupuytren's Contraction
Congenital Torticollis
Myoneural Junction Disorders
   Myasthenia Gravis
   The Myotonias
Muscular Dystrophies
Miscellaneous Myopathies
   Familial Periodic Paralysis

Paroxysmal Hemoglobinuria
Tumors
   Rhabdomyoma
   Granular Cell Myoblastoma
Tendons
   Tenosynovitis
   Ganglion
   Bursitis
   Tumors

GENERAL CONSIDERATIONS

The muscular system presents a paradox to the pathologist. The skeletal muscles, known to the layman as "the flesh," constitute from 40 to 45 per cent of the body weight, yet this is a field with which the pathologist is least familiar. The only modern book in English devoted to diseases of muscle in general is that by Adams, Denny-Brown and Pearson, to which the reader is referred for further information. The bulk of the muscles itself makes the choice of material for microscopic examination difficult, particularly in view of the fact that there are 434 voluntary muscles in the body. In this connection it may be added that this chapter is concerned only with the voluntary muscles, not with plain muscle, myocardium, etc.

Each muscle is composed of innumerable fibers, which are really hollow tubes filled with sarcoplasm in which fibrils are formed. The enclosing sheath of the tube, the sarcolemma, is nucleated, and the so-called fiber is in reality an elongated multinucleated cell which is a complex structural, metabolic and functional unit. The essential living element of the fiber is the sarcolemmal nucleus. When it is destroyed regeneration of the fiber within the sarcolemmal sheath does not take place, and the whole structure is treated as a foreign body. Repair begins with proliferation of the nuclei. With the electron microscope the mitochondria and the sarcoplasmic reticulum become prominent. These contain the enzymes which control muscle contractility, including those of the Krebs cycle. The most striking feature of the muscle fiber is its dependence upon innervation by the motor neurone. For this reason disorders of muscle may have their origin (1) in motor nerve cells (acute poliomyelitis, chronic progressive muscular atrophy), (2) in nerve fibers (polyneuritis), (3) at the myoneural junction (myasthenia gravis, myotonia congenita), and (4) in the muscles themselves (primary muscular atrophy). Such a relationship is unique in the entire field of pathology. Small wonder that the pathology of muscles is complex and confusing.

Function.—The essential function of the fiber is of course contraction and relaxation in response to a stimulus from the motor neurone. Muscle is a unique organ in that it is capable of converting stored chemical energy into mechanical energy to perform work in the cell. When we look at a muscle fiber under the microscope it looks calm and tranquil, but we now know that it is a seething mass of chemical activity in which electrolytes are continually passing into and out of the cell. The contractile protein of muscle appears to consist of at least two basic proteins, myocin and actin, bound in a complex called *actomycin* (AM), which is considered to be the structural protein of the myofibrils, containing the many enzymes necessary for muscle metabolism.

The charge which is fired by the neuronal spark is *adenosine triphosphate* (ATP), the energy-rich organic phosphate compound which in the resting muscle is strongly adsorbed to the actomycin complex, its three negative charges being probably neutralized by three potassium positive ions (Szent-Gyorgyi). When the volley of motor nerve impulses reaches the muscle fibers, the ATP-AM linkage is broken. ATP is liberated, and its breakdown provides energy for muscular contraction. During contraction the actomycin threads can shorten by 60 per cent. This must involve some sort of intermolecular rearrangement within a system composed of actin, myocin, and adenosine triphosphate, and adsorbed ions. When ATP is added to artificially prepared threads of actomycin in the proper ionic environment they shrink so quickly as to suggest contraction (Szent-Gyorgyi). In their relaxed state muscle fibers contain 2 per cent of protein and 98 per cent of water. Contracted fibers, on the other hand, contain 50 per cent of protein and 50 per cent of water, so that there is an enormous loss of water during contraction.

In the metabolism of muscle *potassium* undoubtedly plays an important part, although one at present little understood. Contraction of the fibers causes potassium to move out of muscle, while in hyperpotassemia there is a movement of the element into the muscle. *Both potassium loss and potassium intoxication may cause paralysis. Periodic paralysis* appears to be intimately linked with the potassium metabolism of the body, since low serum potassium levels are noted during an attack.

The enzyme *glutamic oxaloacetic transaminase* is present in greatest concentrations in cardiac and skeletal muscle. Destruction of this tissue will liberate the enzyme into the serum. It is well known that this occurs in myocardial infarction, and an estimation of the serum level is a reliable method of determining the presence of acute myocardial injury. It must be remembered that necrosis of some other tissues, the liver in particular, may be accompanied by an increase of the enzyme in the serum.

As skeletal muscle cells are particularly rich in transaminase, attention is being paid to the enzyme activity in the serum in various diseases affecting muscle either primarily or secondarily (Pearson). This matter will be discussed later in this chapter, but it may

be said here that *significant elevation of the serum transaminase* may occur in primary muscular dystrophy and in polymyositis, but not in muscular atrophy due to poliomyelitis or lower motor neurone degeneration. It is in the juvenile forms of dystrophy, particularly in the pseudohypertrophic form in children, that the serum estimation of transaminase is most useful. In slowly progressive cases in the adult the level may be quite normal.

A few words may be devoted to some *general reactions* of striated muscle to disease and injury. *Motor denervation* is accompanied by an early loss of potassium and glycogen. Some months later in the experimental animal the muscle fibers become replaced by fat. The fat appears to be formed from undifferentiated cells, there being no real transformation of muscle fibers into fat cells. *Atrophy of muscle* may be due to three main causes: (1) disuse; (2) chronic joint disease, where impressions from the diseased joint pass to the motor nerve cells and there induce changes which give rise to what is really a neuropathic atrophy; (3) disease of the motor nerve cells, as in poliomyelitis and progressive muscular atrophy. *Regeneration of muscle* is supposed to begin with proliferation of sarcolemmal nuclei and regeneration of healthy fibers. It has been shown, however, that at least after mild injury in the experimental animal the fibers lose their contractile myofibrils, but reform them quickly within the sarcolemmal tube without actual proliferation of muscle nuclei. After the injection of P^{32} the regenerating fibers quickly incorporate the isotope into the RNA, but not into the DNA of the newly formed fibers (Kitiyakara and Angevine). Myofibrils are laid down in the tube formed by the proliferating sarcolemma. In true muscular dystrophy the power of regeneration of the fibrils is lost, so that there is no nuclear proliferation. In most types of polymyositis, on the other hand, some degree of regeneration can take place, as is evidenced by the multinucleated cytoplasm.

MYOSITIS

Inflammation of muscle may occur in many different ways and be caused by many different etiological agents. Thus pyogenic infection may spread from a neighboring focus and cause a suppurative lesion. In septicemia there may be widespread involvement of muscles with abscess formation. In gas gangrene the muscles are destroyed by anærobic bacteria. The muscles may be involved in rheumatic fever, rheumatoid arthritis and other generalized conditions. They may be attacked by animal parasites and even viruses. In this place we shall consider none of these conditions, but shall confine our attention to the much more perplexing myositis problem defined by Steiner in 1903 as "an acute, subacute or chronic disease of unknown origin characterized by a gradual onset of vague and indefinite prodromata followed by edema, dermatitis and multiple muscle inflammation." In the intervening years little has been added to this description.

Acute Polymyositis: Dermatomyositis.— Two main forms of the condition so well outlined above by Steiner may be distinguished, the one *acute* or *subacute*, affecting mainly children, *involving the skin as well as many muscles*, and running a self-limited course, while the other is of a *chronic* character, *without skin manifestations*, and more common in adults than in children. The former is known as dermatomyositis or acute polymyositis, the latter as chronic polymyositis. Whether these two should be regarded as one and the same disease is naturally a very moot point.

Acute dermatomyositis is a severe non-suppurative inflammation of many muscles. The onset in the child is usually gradual, with lassitude and pains in the muscles suggesting trichiniasis, but fever if present is of low grade. The muscles of the shoulder girdle are usually the first involved, but soon the proximal muscles of all the limbs become extremely tender, swollen and weak. Weakness out of proportion to wasting is the hall mark of this disease of muscle. The pain may become so acute that the patient is unable to move in bed. A characteristic feature is an erythematous rash, varying from bright to dusky red and even blue, involving the face and neck, and spreading to the trunk and the extensor surfaces of the limbs. The rash may precede or accompany involvement of the muscles. A non-pitting edema of the skin is a frequent feature, and swelling of the face is common. A persistent sore throat may precede the onset of weakness by many weeks, a point of interest with regard to pathogenesis. Creatinuria is frequent and sometimes extreme in degree. Death may occur from involvement of the respiratory muscles with resulting pneumonia. After a period of many weeks recovery may set in. Occasionally the child is left a permanent invalid with atrophy of the limbs and rigidity of the muscles.

Chronic myositis is naturally more insidious in its onset. The chief early symptom is weakness, but tenderness and quite marked edema may develop. The condition has been called *generalized myositis fibrosa*. There is usually no skin involvement, but occasionally redness and a scaly erythema may develop. It is possible that this condition is quite unrelated to acute dermatomyositis, and that it should not be considered in this connection.

Lesions.—The lesions in the striated muscles, including the heart, are very striking. Grossly they are pale and atrophic, whilst microscopically they show all degrees of change from loss of cross-striation to complete disintegration. In sections which I have studied one gets the impression that the ground substance which holds together the fibers and the individual fibrils of those fibers has become dissolved and everything is falling to pieces. At an earlier stage the fibers are swollen and hyaline. The cells of the sarcolemma may be enlarged, rounded and multinucleated, and are possibly engaged in an attempt at repair. Myelin sheath degeneration of the peripheral nerves is frequent, perhaps due to interference with the ground substance between the fibers. Recovery of the muscle is indicated by the presence of small fibers with large vesicular sarcolemmal nuclei and evidence of regenerating myofibrils (Walton and Adams).

The lesions of dermatomyositis are not confined to muscle. The name itself indicates that the skin is also often involved. The disease appears to belong to the group of collagen degenerations, being characterized by the triad of vasculitis, fibrinoid necrosis of connective tissue, and degeneration of

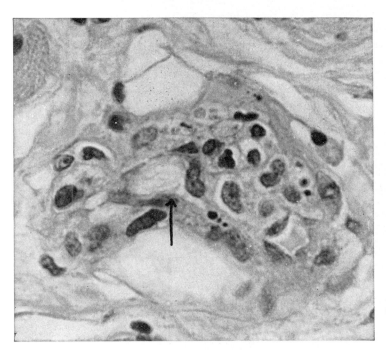

Fig. 754.—Acute dermatomyositis. Mesenchymal cells form a cuff around a small vessel whose lumen is indicated by an arrow. (Kindness of Dr. N. G. B. McLetchie.)

muscle (McLetchie and Coward). It may be noted that the creatinuria which characterizes acute dermatomyositis is much more intense than that which is encountered in other collagen diseases. Fibrinoid necrosis of connective tissue is a prominent feature not only in muscle, but also in the skin. Vasculitis, mainly proliferative in type, may be much in evidence in the various lesions, with cuffs of undifferentiated mesenchymal cells around the small arteries, the walls of which are often involved in fibrinoid necrosis (Fig. 753). Even in the acute form in children there is usually a rather remarkable paucity of inflammatory cellular response.

The exact nature and cause of dermatomyositis is not known, as is true also of the other collagen diseases. It is believed, however, that a vascular hypersensitivity to more than one variety of antigen, probably bacterial in nature, plays a major part in the pathogenesis of the condition.

Myositis Ossificans.—There are two kinds of so-called ossifying myositis, which bear no relation to one another. They are the traumatic and the progressive forms.

Traumatic Myositis Ossificans.—This is a not uncommon condition which may be the result of repeated injury to a muscle or a single severe injury, especially when accompanied by hemorrhage. A good example is the development of bone in the adductor muscles of the thigh in riders. It is possible that osteoblasts are detached as a result of the trauma and become implanted in the muscle where they form bone, but it is also possible that there may be a metaplasia of fibrous tissue into bone, especially when there has been hemorrhage and tissue destruction. The formation of bone which occasionally takes place in the edges of a laparotomy wound might be explained on this basis. The great practical importance of the condition is the danger that it may be mistaken for an osteogenic sarcoma of bone invading the muscle.

Progressive Myositis Ossificans.—This is a very rare progressive disease, which commences in childhood and slowly kills the patient. The first lesions take the form of doughy and sometimes painful swellings, particularly in the muscles of the back and neck. These swellings subside, leaving areas of fibrosis in which bone is gradually formed. The progress of the disease is marked by exacerbations and remissions. Large bony plates are formed, and the body may finally be enclosed in a sheath of bone which makes all movement impossible and leads to the death of the patient from respiratory paralysis. The disease appears to be some obscure disorder of the bone-forming power of the tissues possibly with some genetic basis, for not only does it develop in early childhood, but congenital bony defects such as microdactylia in the hand and absence of a phalanx in the great toe are often present.

LESIONS DUE TO ISCHEMIA

There are many features in common between the lesions in muscle provoked by trauma and those produced by ischemia due to vascular occlusion. Not only the muscle fibers but also connective tissue sheaths, blood vessels, nerves, and sensory organs all suffer to a degree proportionate to the intensity of the etiological factor. It is a pannecrosis of whole muscle. The two conditions which may be ascribed to ischemia are the anterior tibial syndrome and Volkmann's contracture.

Anterior Tibial Syndrome.—This condition, which was first described in 1943, is an excellent example of the statements quoted above. The patient is a young adult male who, without previous training, has been engaged in athletic exercises such as running, jumping or kicking a football, or in long marching. There is a rapid development of aching pain, firm swelling, and paralysis of the pretibial muscles. This may be accompanied by a low-grade fever and a moderate leukocytosis. The muscles involved are the tibialis anterior, the extensor digitorum longus and extensor hallucis longus, all contained in the tight anterior tibial compartment with its rigid walls, the interosseous membrane, fibula and tibia behind and the anterior tibial fascia in front. There may be evidence of involvement of the anterior tibial nerve (Charter), and the end result may be permanent paralysis.

When the anterior crural fascia is incised the acutely swollen muscles bulge into the wound. The affected muscles are at first soft, friable and reddish-gray in color, but after a few weeks they become white and fibrosed. The *microscopic picture* resembles that of acute injury to muscle. The fibers are swollen and degenerated and are separated by extravasated blood and a reactive exudate. Phagocytosis of dead fibers and extensive regenerative activity at the margins of the lesion go hand in hand, ending finally in replacement fibrosis. The picture is that of an acute infarct, similar in all respects to an infarct of the myocardium except that it is more extensive. It may be noted in passing that the lesion is an excellent demonstration of the fact that gangrene is *not* synonymous with death *en masse*, for here death of tissue (necrosis) could not be more massive, but there is no suggestion of gangrene for the simple reason that infection with putrefactive organisms is lacking.

The *pathogenesis* of the condition is uncertain. The most probable explanation is that strenuous exercise of an untrained muscle liberates excess quantities of metabolites, which lead to swelling of the muscle. It is known that prolonged activity of a muscle can lead to a 20 per cent increase in its bulk owing to accumulation of fluid in the tissue spaces (Hughes). The increased pressure causes venous stasis, which intensifies the swelling, and finally the pressure leads to occlusion of the arteries with resulting ischemic necrosis (but not gangrene). Incision of the anterior tibial fascia relieves the condition.

The common condition known to athletes and their coaches as *"shin splints"* is probably a minor manifestation of the anterior tibial syndrome. It occurs in runners and broad jumpers at the beginning of their training. The affected muscles are firm, swollen and painful when the ankle is moved, but the condition stops short of ischemic necrosis.

Volkmann's Contracture.—This condition, called originally by Volkmann ischemic contracture, usually occurs in young people and affects the muscles of the forearm. It is commonly associated with the pressure of splints or a tourniquet or with hemorrhage resulting from a fracture. Within a few hours of the receipt of injury burning pain develops in the hand or forearm. This is followed by contracture of the fingers which become fixed in the flexed position. If the muscle is exposed when the condition is fully developed it is hard, homogeneous, yellowish in color and is not recognizable as skeletal muscle. *Microscopically* the nuclei and cross-striations are lost, there may be an infiltration of inflammatory cells and phagocytes at the margin of the area, and the picture is one of infarct, similar to that of a cardiac infarct. Later the part becomes fibrosed.

Volkmann originally (1872) believed that the cause of the condition was direct pressure on the arteries. In 1914 the ischemic theory was given up, and the view substituted that venous obstruction was the causal factor (J. B. Murphy). A return has now been made to the idea that the condition is essentially ischemic in nature, due usually to arterial spasm resulting from injury to the wall of the vessel. An identical picture, both pathological and clinical, can be produced in the rabbit by ligating the arteries to a limb.

Dupuytren's Contraction.—Although this is not a lesion of muscle, nor are there grounds for supposing that the condition is the result of ischemia, it may be considered here for the sake of convenience.

Owing to thickening, hardening and shortening of the palmar fascia the fingers may become progressively flexed on the palm, so that normal use of the hand is impossible. The etiology is unknown. The microscopic picture is one of active prolifera-tion of fibroblasts which may be mistaken for fibrosarcoma, with dense collagen formation.

Congenital Torticollis.—This is a condition due not to ischemia, but rather to excessive congestion of muscle. The wry-neck usually develops about the age of four years. In these cases the history goes back to the so-called "sternomastoid tumor of infancy," which generally appears about ten days after birth. A spindle-shaped swelling develops in the sternocleidomastoid; this is peculiarly hard and feels like cartilage. The swelling persists for two or three months and is then gradually absorbed, disappearing entirely in four to six months after birth. If the muscle is now excised it is found to consist entirely of fibrous tissue with complete replacement of the muscle fibers. The neck lengthens rapidly in the fourth year, and as the fibrosed muscle is unable to grow, the head is pulled over to that side—a condition of congenital wryneck. The sterno-cleidomastoid tumor is produced as the result of acute venous obstruction due to pressure on the veins during labor, rendered permanent by thrombosis of the veins. When the artery to a muscle is tied experimentally or the artery and vein together, the result is simple atrophy. But when the vein above is tied, the arterial supply being left intact, the muscle becomes acutely swollen, hard and tender, and very cyanosed. The fibers disintegrate and the muscle is densely infiltrated with round cells. In the course of a few months such a muscle is

SPECIAL MUSCLE LESIONS SECONDARY TO VASCULAR DISORDERS

Condition	Differential Features
Anterior tibial syndrome (Ischemic etiology)	Painful swelling and paralysis of pre-tibial muscles. Lesions similar to a massive acute infarct.
Volkmann's Contracture (Ischemic etiology)	Usually damaged forearm muscles cause flexion of fingers. Microscopic changes similar to cardiac infarct.
Dupuytren's Contraction (non-muscular lesion)	Finger flexion secondary to fibrotic shortening of palmar fascia. Differentiate microscopically from a fibrosarcoma.
Congenital Torticollis (muscle congestion)	Shortening of sternocleidomastoid due to focal fibrotic scar following previous acute venous obstruction.

completely replaced by fibrous tissue. When the vein alone is obstructed the autolytic products from the breaking down muscle fibers are not carried away from the part and appear to stimulate proliferation of fibroblasts. The marked edema of the muscle also favors the formation of fibrous tissue.

Some of the important features of the foregoing lesions are summarized in the table on page 1307.

MYONEURAL JUNCTION DISORDERS

The delicate trophic relationship which exists between a striated muscle fiber and its motor nerve is a biological puzzle. In life the axis cylinder of a motor nerve is not merely a wire-like core, but a stream of liquid nutrients constantly flowing from that bio-chemical factory, the nerve cell, to reactive elements in the muscle cell, the nucleus of which is a concentration of special enzyme systems and metabolites. On stimulation of a nerve fiber *acetylcholine* is exploded in minute amounts at the myoneural junction, causing contraction. The enzyme, *cholin-esterase*, which is present both in muscle and the circulating blood, rapidly breaks down any excess of acetylcholine, thus limiting its effect to the desired point.

It is difficult to say with certainty which diseases of muscle are due to a breakdown of this delicate mechanism, but it would appear that myasthenia gravis may with confidence be placed in this category, and perhaps also the myotonias such as myotonia congenita and myotonia dystrophica.

Myasthenia Gravis.—This disease with the ominously descriptive name is characterized by great weakness, most marked in the muscles of the face, but shared to a lesser extent by the other muscles. Those innervated from the brain stem are affected first and most seriously, with drooping of the eyelids, blank and expressionless face, nasal voice, and difficulty in swallowing. The disease may begin with sudden weakness of a single muscle, or nearly every *voluntary* muscle in the body may be involved. *Plain muscle and myocardium are not affected.* After the muscle has been used a few times it rapidly loses its power of contraction, only

to regain it as rapidly with rest. This is the reverse of what is seen in the myotonias. In extreme cases the limbs are so weak and easily fatigued (myasthenia) that they can hardly be lifted, and death from respiratory paralysis comes as a welcome relief.

No lesions to explain this astonishing weakness can be found in the motor nerve cells, nerves, or muscles. This is the most puzzling of all the confusing features of this clinical enigma. It is true that changes in the muscles such as degeneration of individual fibers and collections of lymphocytes ("lymphorrhages") may be present, but these appear to be secondary in character. Biopsy of neuromuscular junctions shows multiplication and elongation of the end-plates even when the muscle is histologically normal. Multiplication occurs in other muscular diseases, but *elongation of end-plates* seems to be peculiar to myasthenia gravis (Bickerstaff and Woolf). This increases the synaptic area. When degenerative changes in the muscle have developed, there is excessive collateral sprouting of the terminal axous.

The *pathogenesis* of the disease is still an unknown quantity, in spite of the enormous amount of work which has been devoted to the problem. The functional abnormality is undoubtedly a failure of neuromuscular transmission, a breakdown, apparently, of the response of the motor endplates. There may be a deficient synthesis or liberation of acetylcholine at the motor end-plates, or an increased breakdown of acetylcholine due to over-activity of cholinesterase. In the myasthenic muscle there seems to be a continuing block due to some unknown substance liberated in the normal process, perhaps choline, with resultant blocking of the end-plates (Viets).

The *relation of myasthenia gravis to the thymus* is another problem, although there seems to be no doubt that some such relationship does exist. The thymus may contain and release a blocking substance, and after many years irreversible changes may develop at the myoneural junction. The existence of a humoral mechanism is suggested by the fact that in some cases the babies of myasthenic mothers are born with the disease, which clears up in a few days or weeks. It has been aptly said, however, that if the thymus is indeed a member of the endocrine orchestra, its notes are so muffled that no one has been able to distinguish them. The thymus is likely to show either a neoplasm (*thymoma*) or, more frequently, the presence of *lymphoid germinal centers* in the medulla, which are not there normally (Castleman and Norris). It is presently safe to say that either germinal centers or neoplasm are present almost uniformly in myasthenia gravis. It does not follow that removal of the thymus will necessarily benefit the patient, although this is a contentious subject, discussion of which would be out of place here.

The Myotonias.—The pathognomonic feature of myotonia is prolonged contraction of a muscle after cessation of the stimulus. The fibers are unable to relax. The condition is therefore the reverse of myasthenia gravis. When a movement is repeated a number of times the muscles warm up, and normal contraction and relaxation may then occur, myotonia returning again after rest. The myotonia may involve all the muscles, or it may appear to be confined to a few, although in such cases electromyography may show the condition to be more widespread. There are two rare clinical conditions characterized by a *failure of the muscle to relax*. These are (1) myotonia congenita, and (2) myotonia dystrophica. In the past these have been considered to be distinct and different entities, but there is now a tendency to regard the congenital and dystrophic forms as parts of a single disease process. They are placed under the heading of myoneural junction disorders, not because there is any evidence that such is their nature, but on account of the striking contrast which myotonia presents to myasthenia gravis. The real nature of the myotonias is completely obscure. The condition persists after spinal anesthesia and blocking of the motor nerve, so the mechanism involved seems to be intrinsic in the muscle.

Myotonia congenita or *Thomsen's disease* is a hereditary and familial but non-progressive condition in which the mytonia is often associated with hypertrophy of the muscles involved so that it might be called *myotonia hypertrophica* in contrast to myotonia dystrophica. It usually manifests itself in early childhood. The characteristic feature is a painful stiffening of the hypertrophied muscles after prolonged rest. The grasp of the hand may not be relaxed for from thirty to sixty seconds.

Myotonia dystrophica or *Steinert's disease* is also hereditary and familial, but it does not develop until the third or fourth decades, and dystrophy and wasting take the place of the hypertrophy of the congenital form. The myotonia may precede the atrophy by two or three years.

THE MUSCULAR DYSTROPHIES

This peculiar group of diseases of muscle appears to represent a genetic disorder of muscle metabolism. The dystrophies have several clinical divisions which we shall not go into here, but the basic pathology is the same. The disease generally begins in childhood, shows a very marked familial tendency so that several children in the family may be affected, attacks only the males, but is transmitted only by the females. The large muscles concerned with fixation (shoulder girdle, hip) are chiefly affected, the small muscles concerned with active and fine movement (hand, etc.) usually escape. This is the opposite to what occurs in progressive muscular atrophy, which of course is due to a lesion of the anterior horn cells of the spinal cord.

The largest group is known as *pseudo-hypertrophic muscular dystrophy* because of the remarkable enlargement of the muscles of the calf and later of the shoulder girdle. The bulging muscles, especially the gastrocnemei, give a misleading impression of strength, so that in my student days in Edinburgh the proud mother put her boy in kilts, only to learn later that all is not gold that glitters. The great symptom is muscular weakness. Owing to paralysis of the gluteal muscles the child cannot rise from the floor in the usual way, but has to "climb up his legs".

The *facio-scapulo-humeral group* differs from the pseudo-hypertrophic dystrophies as follows: (1) Both sexes are involved equally; (2) the age of onset may be in late adult life as well as in childhood; (3) there is primary involvement of the shoulder girdle, with

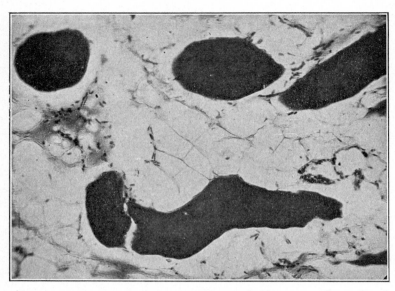

FIG. 755.—Pseudohypertrophic muscular dystrophy. The muscle fibers are swollen and are largely replaced by fat. × 140.

spread to the pelvic girdle many years later; (4) pseudohypertrophy of the muscles is very rare.

Lesions.—These involve the muscles and interstitial tissue. In the common pseudo-hypertrophic form the muscles are large and firm; the gastrocnemius, deltoid, supra-spinatus, and infraspinatus are most often affected. Other muscles are markedly atrophic. In the early stages the muscle fibers may be swollen, with loss of striations and increase of the sarcolemma nuclei, but later the fibers become atrophic. In this stage there may be a marked increase of the interstitial tissue, and great deposits of fat may occur between the muscle fibers. (Fig. 755). It is to these deposits of fat that most of the enlargement (pseudohyper-trophy) is due. The exact cause of these deposits is not known, but indirect evidence suggests that they may be due to pituitary disturbance.

Biochemical Lesion.—What we may call the biochemical lesion of the muscular dystrophies is loss of storage of creatine by the atrophic muscle, with excessive urinary loss of creatine, but reduction in the daily excretion of creatinine (Lilienthal and Zier-

ler). Over 95 per cent of the body's creatine, synthesized by the liver, is stored in the fibers of the skeletal muscles, where it is broken down with the formation of creati-nine. In health any creatine in the serum is excreted by the renal glomeruli but re-absorbed by the tubules, so that none appears in the urine. If the synthesis of creatine is maintained at a normal rate but the storage power in the muscles is lowered, the excess of creatine in the blood is too great to be absorbed by the tubules, so that creatinuria develops. As it is not converted into creatinine in the atrophic muscle there is a reduction in the daily excretion of creatinine in the urine. It is the urine which gives evidence of loss of muscle mass.

The *serum glutamic oxaloactic transaminase* has already been discussed. In muscular dystrophy an elevated serum level of this enzyme corresponds closely, although by no means perfectly, with the rate of progression of the disease. There is a high rate of correlation between the juvenile form of muscular dystrophy and an increase in serum transaminase. This is particularly marked when some of the muscles show pseudohypertrophy.

MISCELLANEOUS MYOPATHIES

A number of unrelated conditions do not readily fall into any of the groups already discussed, and may conveniently be considered here. Some, such as *athrogryposis*, a congenital condition characterized by generalized atrophy of muscles resulting in a fixed position of the limbs of the infant, are too rare for our purpose.

Familial Periodic Paralysis.—Nothing could be further from the slow progressive myopathies we have been considering than the condition which now demands our attention. It is well named, for not only is it often familial and therefore hereditary, as is true with so many disorders of muscle, but by far its most striking characteristic is the fact that the attacks of muscular weakness are periodic or occasional, and that in the intervals the muscles appear to be normal and the patient perfectly well. Frequently he may awake from sleep and find that he is unable to move. The intervals between attacks may be a matter of days, or weeks, or even years. In this and other respects the condition recalls the state of affairs in gout.

The essence of the condition is undoubtedly a *genetic anomaly of potassium metabolism*, although what determines the periodicity of the aberration remains a mystery. *Muscle biopsies* taken during an attack show the myofibrils to be pressed apart by an amorphous mass giving the fiber the appearance of a sieve. This represents an increase in intracellular fluid caused by a shift of potassium ions from the serum to within the cells. It is small wonder that such fibers have lost the power of contraction. The attacks are associated with a drop in the serum potassium level from a normal of 18 to 22 mg. per 100 cc. to as low as 5 mg.

Paroxysmal Myohemoglobinuria.—This rare condition is worthy of mention because of its resemblance to familial periodic paralysis. It is marked by a paroxysmal paralysis with dark urine related to exercise, a familial character, and a male (sex-linked) inheritance. Myohemoglobin is a ferrous-protein complex closely related to hemoglobin and present in the sarcoplasm of striated muscle. Its function appears to be that of a short-time oxygen reservoir which tides the muscle over from one contraction to the next by releasing oxygen to the oxydase systems in the fibers. As the molecular weight of myoglobin is only one-quarter that of hemoglobin, it is readily filtered into the urine. The attack comes on with some of the suddenness of periodic paralysis, and it may be accompanied by fever, nausea and vomiting. The precipitating factor is usually physical exertion. The urine is Burgandy red or almost black due to the presence of abundant myohemoglobin. The affected muscles are swollen, hard and tender, and the fibers are said to show acute necrosis. As a result the serum transaminase may rise to 15 times the normal level.

TUMORS

In the study of muscle tumors we encounter a curious paradox. Striated muscle, the most abundant tissue in the body, is very rarely the site of tumors, either primary or metastatic, whereas tumors of plain muscle are among the commonest of neoplasms. The confused subject may be considered in relation to two tumors, rhabdomyoma and granular cell myoblastoma.

Rhabdomyoma. — Rhabdomyoma (*rhabdos*, a rod or stripe) is the benign tumor of striated muscle. As a matter of fact there is some doubt if such a tumor of voluntary muscle really exists. Tumors containing beautifully developed cross-striated fibers (Fig. 143, page 244) are not found in voluntary muscle, but in developmental tumors arising early in life in the vagina, bladder and kidney (Wilms' tumor). They seem to originate from embryonic mesenchymal tissue with the potency for aberrant differentiation of muscle fibers.

Rhabdomyosarcoma is a rare highly malignant tumor of striated muscle. It is composed of cells of all shapes and sizes, but predominantly fusiform. Identification of the tumor is often extremely difficult, for cross-striations are either absent or very hard to distinguish on account of the highly anaplastic character of the growth.

Granular Cell Myoblastoma.—There is no tumor regarding which there is more difference of opinion than the one about to be considered. These differences refer to (1)

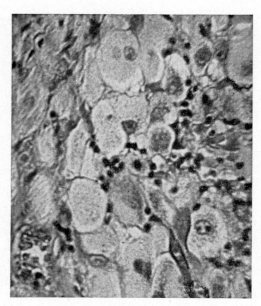

Fig. 756.—Granular cell myoblastoma of abdominal wall. The cytoplasm is coarsely granular and the cell boundaries indistinct. × 425. (Courtesy Dr. Leo Lowbeer from Boyd, *Pathology for the Surgeon*, courtesy of W. B. Saunders Co.)

the origin of the lesion, and (2) whether or not it is a true tumor. About one-third of the cases arise in the tongue. Of the remainder not more than 5 per cent occur in voluntary muscle. The tumor usually remains quite small, with an average size of 1 to 5 cm., being essentially benign. *Microscopically* it consists of polygonal cells with characteristic highly granular cytoplasm (Fig. 756). The granules have a high lipid content, so that the lesion used to be confused with a xanthoma. It is believed by some to originate from the cells of the sheath of Schwann, not from muscle fibers. Still others believe that the lesion is not a neoplasm, but represents a degeneration, which may be the result of trauma to which the tongue is so much exposed. From all of this it will be evident that hardly a worse name than myoblastoma could have been invented.

THE TENDONS

Tenosynovitis.—The tendons are nonvascular and therefore immune to inflamma-

tion, but the tendon sheaths at the wrist and ankle are often infected. All the usual forms of inflammation are met with in the tendon sheaths. *Traumatic tenosynovitis* occurs in piano players, typists, and others whose tendons are subjected to excessive use. Fibrin is laid down on the wall of the sheath and the surface of the tendon, so that cracking is felt when the tendon is used. If effusion occurs, an elongated swelling appears in the line of the tendon. *Suppurative tenosynovitis* may result from spread of infection from a septic process in the fingers. *Gonorrheal tenosynovitis* may be dry, serous, or suppurative. *Tuberculous tenosynovitis* resembles tuberculous arthritis. There may be an abundant formation of tuberculous granulation tissue causing a "white swelling" like that seen in tuberculosis of a joint. Or there may be abundant serous effusion (hydrops) with only limited production of granulation tissue, but abundant deposits of fibrin which are rubbed off by the play of the tendon, so that large numbers of melonseed bodies are formed.

Ganglion.—This is a cystic swelling which develops in connection with a tendon sheath. The common position is the back of the wrist, but it may occur on the dorsum of the foot and rarely on the outer aspect of the knee. It is attached to the tendon sheath or the joint capsule, but does not communicate with these cavities. It appears to commence as a proliferation of the connective tissue of the sheath; this undergoes mucoid degeneration with the formation of numerous small cysts which fuse to form one large cyst filled with soft mucoid material. Although we have spoken of a cyst, it is not a true cyst, for there is no endothelial lining. The condition known clinically as *compound palmar ganglion* is a tuberculous tenosynovitis.

Bursitis.—A bursa, which is a sac lined by synovial membrane and containing synovial fluid, may be the seat of inflammation or tuberculosis. *Traumatic bursitis* is usually caused by chronic and repeated irritation ("housemaid's knee", "student's elbow"), but occasionally it is due to a blow. The bursa is distended with serous fluid (hydrops), and in course of time the wall becomes thickened and covered with ridges and tags. The latter may be detached, forming melon-seed bodies. *Infective bursitis* is caused by a perforating wound or direct spread of infection from the adjacent joint. *Tuberculous bursitis* may take the form of hydrops with melon-seed bodies, or the bursa may be filled with granulation tissue, which eventually undergoes softening and liquefaction.

Tumors.—Tumors of tendon sheaths have already been considered in connection with tumors of joints (page 1293).

REFERENCES

ADAMS, R. D., DENNY-BROWN, D. and PEARSON, C. M.: *Diseases of Muscle,* New York, 1953.

BICKERSTAFF, E. R. and WOOLF, A. L.: Brain, 1960, *83,* 10. (Motor endplate in myasthenia gravis.)

CARTER, A. B., RICHARDS, R. L. and ZACHARY, R. B.: Lancet, 1949, *2,* 928. (Anterior tibial syndrome.)

CASTLEMAN, B. and NORRIS, E. H.: Medicine, 1949, *28,* 27. (The thymus in myasthenia gravis.)

HUGHES, J. R.: J. Bone and Joint Surg., 1948, *30-B,* 581. (Anterior tibial syndrome.)

KITIYAKARA, A. and ANGEVINE, D. M.: Am. J. Path., 1960, *37,* 613. (Regeneration of injured striated muscle.)

LILIENTHAL, J. L., JR. and ZIERLER, K. in THOMPSON, R. H. S. and KING, E. J.: *Biochemical Disorders in Human Disease,* London, 1957, p. 445.

MCLETCHIE, N. G. B. and COWARD, N. B.: Can. Med. Ass. J., 1957, *76,* 1018. (Dermatomyositis.)

PILLSBURY, D. M., SHELLEY, W. B. and KLIGMAN, A. M.: *Dermatology,* Philadelphia, 1956.

STEINER, W. R.: J. Exper. Med., 1903, *6,* 407. (Dermatomyositis.)

SZENT-GYORGI, A.: *Chemistry of Muscle Contraction,* New York, 1947.

VIETS, H. R.: Am. J. Med., 1955, *19,* 658. (Pathogenesis of myasthenia gravis.)

WALTON, J. N. and ADAMS, R. D.: *Polymyositis,* Edinburgh, 1958.

Chapter 46

The Skin

General Considerations
Normal Histology
Definition of Terms
Skin Biopsy
Hyperplasias
Seborrhoeic Keratosis
Senile Keratosis
Verruca Vulgaris
Molluscum Contagiosum
Callus and Corn
Acanthosis Nigricans
Ichthyosis
Disturbances of Pigmentation
Xeroderma Pigmentosum
Nonspecific Inflammations
Lesions of the Epidermis
Eczema
Psoriasis
Dermatitis Herpetiformis
Pemphigus
Lesions of the Dermis
Scleroderma
Circumscribed
Diffuse

Lupus Erythematosus
Localized (Discoid)
Disseminated
Urticaria Pigmentosa
Erythema Multiforme
Granuloma Annulare
Necrobiosis Lipoidica
Diabeticorum
Lichen Planus
Panniculitis
Erythema induratum
Specific Inflammations
Impetigo Contagiosa
Tumors of the Epidermis
Epidermoid Carcinoma
Basal Cell Carcinoma
Preinvasive Carcinoma
Bowen's Disease
Precancerous Lesions
Tumors of the Appendages
Sweat Gland Tumors
Spiradenoma or Hydradenoma
Papillary Syringocystadenoma
Papillary Hydradenoma

Sebaceous Gland Tumors
Sebaceous Adenoma
Tumors of Hair Follicles
Adenoid Cystic Epithelioma
Keratoacanthoma: *Molluscum*
Sebaceum
The Melanomas
Nevus
Blue Nevus
Malignant Melanoma
Melanoma in Childhood
Tumors of the Dermis
Sclerosing Hemangioma
Kaposi's Hemangiosarcoma
Glomangioma
Granuloma Pyogenicum
Myoepithelioma
Myocosis Fungoides
Cysts of the Skin
Milium
Colloid Milium
Skin Manifestations of Internal Diseases

This chapter is intended for the pathologist, more especially the resident in surgical pathology, not for the overburdened undergraduate student with his crowded timetable. The undergraduate might well read the section on such common skin diseases as seborrhoeic keratosis and psoriasis, and he must study those on tumors of the epidermis and in particular the melanomas, both benign and malignant.

GENERAL CONSIDERATIONS

The skin is a very remarkable structure. It is moist, supple, elastic and durable. The cells of the epidermis are continually multiplying, but the epidermis itself does not increase in thickness, because the surface cells are dying and dead though remaining united to one another like tiles on a roof, tiles which are continually blown away by the wind and continually replaced by new ones. The living cells are shielded by the very thin but tenacious film of dead cells against extremes of heat and cold, trauma, bacteria and viruses. This film is continually kept in good condition by the secretions poured out by the glands of the skin. Actually the skin is a sieve rather than a continuous layer, for it is perforated by hair follicles and by the openings of sweat and sebaceous glands. Despite its thinness (on the forehead the epidermis is only 0.006 mm. thick) the skin effectively protects the delicate internal structures and fluids and forms the almost perfectly fortified frontier of a closed world. Just as the cerebrospinal fluid is a mirror in which are reflected many disorders of the central nervous system, so the skin mirrors sickness and health, youth and age, due in large part to changes in the physical state of the mucopolysaccharides of its ground substance.

In structure seemingly simple, although in reality complex, the skin appears to surpass even the liver in the multiplicity of its functions. In addition to its protective function it controls the fluid content of the tissues, it is an efficient insulator and heat regulator, it both synthesizes cholesterol and converts it into vitamin D, and it is the most extensive and varied of the sense organs.

The skin is the largest organ of the body, constituting 16 per cent of body weight in the adult and covering 19,000 square centimeters; it is the most readily observed; it is the most accessible for biopsy, and yet until recently the study of its lesions have been largely left by the general pathologist to the specialist in skin pathology.

Normal Histology.—The skin consists of epidermis, dermis and epidermal appendages. Pathological lesions may develop in one or more of these elements. The *epidermis* consists of four layers: (1) a basal layer of single cells, with hyperchromatic nuclei which normally show a few mitoses indicating the activity of growth, the mitoses being more abundant when the biopsy is taken during the night, when growth is rapid; (2) a thick prickle cell layer, the rete malpighii; (3) a thin granular layer consisting of diamond-shaped cells filled with granules; and (4) a surface layer, the stratum corneum, consisting of dead keratinized cells which have lost their nuclei. In the palms and soles there is in addition a stratum lucidum composed of several layers of clear cells without nuclei. Interspersed among the basal cells are dendritic cells, the melanoblasts (melanocytes), whose function it is to form melanin. Some of these cells contain melanin pigment, others do not. The amount of pigment varies greatly with varying conditions. The function of melanin is to protect the body against the actinic rays of ultraviolet light.

The *dermis* or *corium* projects into the epidermis as dermal papillae which alternate with downward projections of epidermis, the rete pegs. The dermal papillae vary greatly under conditions of disease as to length, width, vascularity, fluid content and density of collagen. It is in the dermis that the true gel-like character of the ground substance was first recognized. This is the mucopolysaccharide, hyaluronic acid, on which so much of the physical character of the skin depends. The hyaluronic acid is acted on (depolymerized) by the enzyme hyaluronidase, which is, therefore, a spreading factor that governs the permeability of the skin. An increase of permeability will facilitate the spread of chemicals, bacteria and viruses. The permeability is under endocrine control, being decreased by estrogens and increased by cortisone.

The *epidermal appendages* are the sweat and sebaceous glands, the hair follicles and nails. The *sweat glands* open for the most part on the surface. The secretory coiled part lies in the dermis and is lined by cuboidal cells, external to which there is a layer of flattened contractile myoepithelial cells. The secretion is thin and watery. It may be of interest to note that sweat glands are only numerous in mules, donkeys and humans. The sweat glands in the axilla, groin, nipple and genital region are known as *apocrine glands*, because part of the cytoplasm is separated during secretion (*apo*, from and *krino*, I separate). They are much larger than the ordinary sweat glands (eccrine glands), and are lined by tall columnar cells, the cytoplasm of which is markedly acidophilic. Their ducts are usually connected with hair follicles. The *sebaceous glands* arise for the most part from the hair follicles to which they are attached. The cells become converted into fatty material which is liberated as secretion with total destruction of the cells (*holocrine gland*). Lesions which are greasy in character due to overactivity of the sebaceous glands are described as *seborrhoeic* in character. Or the secretion may be drier and mixed with exfoliated cells from the ducts and follicles, in which case it will form crusts. As sebaceous glands are filled with fatty material, fat-soluble chemicals and oils can penetrate the epidermal barrier via their ducts and reach the dermis. On the other hand the fatty secretion on the surface serves to protect the underlying living cells from bacteria and water-soluble poisons. The *arrector pili* smooth muscles are attached to the hair follicles. Contraction of these muscles causes the hair to be erected and expels the sebaceous secretion.

When the histopathologist studies a section of the skin he looks first at the epidermis as a whole to determine its thickness, and then in turn at the various layers of the epidermis for changes in quality and quantity, at the rete pegs, at the dermal papillae, the dermis and the epidermal appendages.

Definition of Terms.—Certain expressions are in common use in skin pathology and

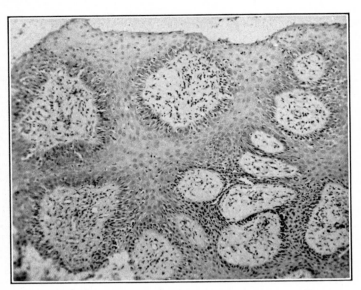

Fig. 757.—Artefact. Owing to tangential cutting the dermal papillæ appear to be embedded in the epidermis. × 110.

need to be defined. *Acanthosis* (*akantha*, a spine or thorn), is a hyperplastic thickening of the prickle cell layer, the rete malpighii. *Spongiosis* signifies intercellular edema in the rete malpighii, and is usually associated with acanthosis owing to increased nutrition of the rete cells. *Hyperkeratosis* is thickening of the stratum corneum. It is associated with increase in thickness of the stratum granulosum. *Parakeratosis* signifies imperfect keratinization with retention of nuclei in the horny layer, and is associated with loss of the granular layer. *Dyskeratosis* is a term applied to changes in the epidermis suggestive of developing malignancy, *e.g.* hyperchromatism, loss of cell polarity and increase in the number of mitoses, changes which may be summed up in two descriptive words, *atypicality* and *jumbling*, the latter referring to loss of the normal orderly cell arrangement.

Skin Biopsy.—No attempt will be made in this place to give an account of the innumerable conditions which have been described and named as skin diseases, of which there are over 300. Attention will be confined mainly to those lesions in which skin biopsy with microscopic examination may be of diagnostic value. The microscopic examination of minute pieces of skin is an art which requires much experience. The difference between lesions may be quantitative rather than qualitative, and such terms as cellular infiltration, edema, acanthosis and dyskeratosis are continually recurring. The taking of the biopsy specimen is important, for it may be very difficult for the pathologist to orientate the tiny lesion properly. The surgeon or dermatologist should place the tissue with the cut surface downward on a piece of blotting paper. The specimen is transfixed with a hypodermic wire stilette which remains as a marker up to the time of embedding. This prevents confusing artefacts due to tangential cutting such as are shown in Figure 757.

The lesions to be discussed will be considered under the headings of (1) hyperplasias, (2) pigment disturbances, (3) non-specific inflammations, (4) specific inflammations, (5) neoplasms, (6) cysts, and (7) cutaneous manifestations of systemic disorders. It will soon become apparent that this rigid compartmentation is artificial and cannot always be maintained.

HYPERPLASIAS

Seborrhoeic Keratosis.—This hyperplasia is also known as senile wart (*verruca senilis*)

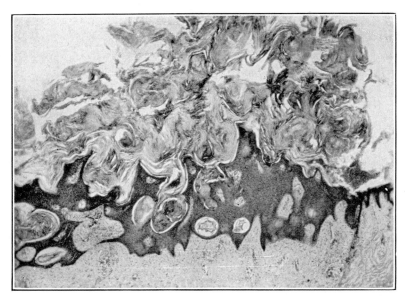

Fig. 758.—Seborrhoeic keratosis. Extreme hyperkeratosis on surface and keratotic plugs in depths of epidermis. × 45.

and basal cell papilloma. *The condition is one of the most important in dermatological pathology,* for it is common, it is frequently mistaken by the clinician for a pigmented mole or melanoma, and by the inexperienced pathologist for a basal cell carcinoma. The lesions, often in large numbers, occur on exposed parts of the body usually in persons over middle age. They are small, raised and wart-like, frequently pigmented to a marked degree, and the soft, greasy surface is responsible for the descriptive term seborrhoeic (*sebum,* tallow, *rhoia,* a flow). They have been likened to a piece of gum stuck on the surface.

The *microscopic appearance* is distinctive, but it is singularly difficult to present a word picture or convey a correct impression of this appearance. The lesion is entirely epidermal, which differentiates it from the common intradermal nevus. The sharply delimited patch of thickened epidermis gives an appearance of being "stuck on" when the slide is held up to the light. There is a marked degree of acanthosis, but the lower limit of the thickened rete malphighii is level, in sharp contrast to the downgrowths so characteristic of basal cell carcinoma. A subtle change has overtaken the various

layers of the rete, for the cells have now a curious uniformity, giving at first glance a suggestion of basal cells, but on closer scrutiny being clearly of the prickle cell variety. Even the basal layer has lost its usual characteristics. On the surface there may be a marked degree of hyperkeratosis (Fig. 758), but the hyperkeratotic material has often been desquamated, so that the descriptive title may appear to be unjustified. Perhaps the most arresting feature is the formation of sharply demarcated eosinophilic nests or plugs of laminated keratin at different levels of the rete, giving an impression of an inverted papilloma. This must on no account be mistaken for epidermoid carcinoma. There is keratosis in the depths as well as on the surface. Even under low magnification this feature often enables the correct diagnosis to be made without difficulty. The keratinization of the nests, in which prominent granules of keratin are produced, is preceded by the conversion of the somewhat hybrid-type cells into fully mature squamous prickle cells. (Fig. 759). The rete tends to be penetrated by dermal papillae, as a result of which there may be an interlacing of epithelial pegs and dermal papillae which has

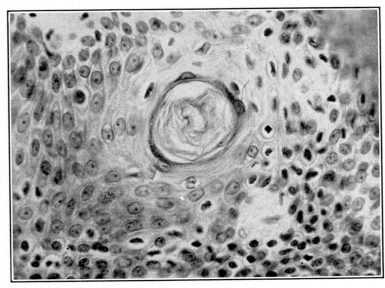

FIG. 759.—Seborrhoeic keratosis. Keratotic nest or plug next to basal layer. × 475.

been described as "bridging" of the pegs. Melanin pigment may be present in considerable amount in the epithelial cells, accounting for the dark color of the clinical lesion. It must be emphasized that the lesion shows no tendency to a malignant change. The terms senile wart and verruca senilis are unfortunate, because the lesions may occur in young persons, and the name is apt to be confused with senile keratosis. It is better, therefore, to avoid these terms.

Senile Keratosis.—In spite of the similarity of name, this is a very different condition from the preceding one. The lesions are small and firm, occurring principally on the face and the backs of the hands of elderly persons, but they may also develop in younger people much exposed to the sun *e.g.*, farmers and sailors. The condition is a *premalignant* one, with a strong tendency to develop into epidermoid carcinoma. *Microscopically* there is again hyperkeratosis, but the essential change is an irregular and atypical proliferation of the cells of the rete malphighii with hyperchromatic nuclei, loss of cellular polarity, and many mitoses (dyskeratosis). In many cases the picture may suggest a carcinoma in situ. The upper part of the dermis may show a dense infiltration with chronic inflammatory cells and many plasma cells, a state of affairs which should always suggest the possibility of a malignant change in the overlying epidermis.

Verruca Vulgaris.—The common wart is the result of invasion of the epithelial cells by a specific virus. It is a disease principally of adolescence and early adult life affecting particularly the fingers, palm and forearm. The warts occur in crops owing to autoinoculation. A particularly troublesome variety is the *plantar wart*, which causes painful pressure on the sensory nerve endings. This lesion occurs at pressure points on the sole, the commonest site being under the head of the second metatarsal. It must not be confused with a corn. The *microscopic changes* are papillary acanthosis with marked hyperkeratosis, an unusual degree of parakeratosis so that many nuclei can be seen in the stratum corneum, vacuolization of the cells of the rete and widening of the rete pegs (Fig. 760). The cells are swollen and mitoses are numerous. Intracellular bodies are usually present which may be interpreted either as keratotic degeneration or as true cytoplasmic inclusions.

Certain warts from the hands and feet differ clinically from other warts from the same sites in that they have a smooth margin, relatively less keratinization, and a surrounding erythematous halo. Suspensions of these warts yield virus-like particles under the electron microscope. They also possess esoinophilic intranuclear inclusion bodies and characteristic vacuolated cytoplasmic masses (Bunting *et al.*).

Molluscum Contagiosum.—This is a contagious condition caused by a virus and characterized by the development of small, white, waxy, almost transparent raised nodules on the skin especially of children. They may last for months or years and then disappear spontaneously. Softening occurs, and a cheesy material can be squeezed out through a small opening in the skin. The stimulation of the virus causes the prickle cells first to proliferate and then to degenerate. As a result of the proliferation the rete pegs project as bulbous swellings down into the corium (Fig. 761). These swellings, which may be so massive as to be referred to as lobules, compress the dermal papillae into thin septa. The elevated lesion bulges the surrounding epidermis outward so that it comes to assume the shape of a cup. Degeneration of the greatly enlarged prickle cells is accompanied by the appearance of the really characteristic feature, the *molluscum bodies*. These are rounded eosinophilic hyaline masses which develop in the de-

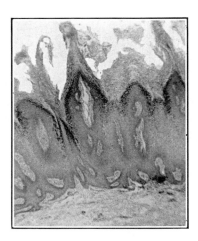

FIG. 760.—Verruca vulgaris. Papillary acanthosis and hyperkeratosis are marked.

generated cells displacing the nucleus to one side, and represent the elementary bodies of virus disease (Fig. 762). When an emulsion of the elementary bodies is injected into the skin of human volunteers, typical molluscum lesions develop in the course of two or three weeks. The egg-shaped glistening bodies, which can readily be squeezed out of the softened center of the lesion and are sometimes referred to as molluscum bodies, really represent the degenerated cells.

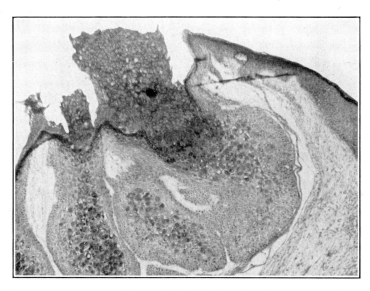

FIG. 761.—Molluscum contagiosum. The epithelial lobules, the elementary bodies, and cup-shaped expansion of the epidermis can be seen.

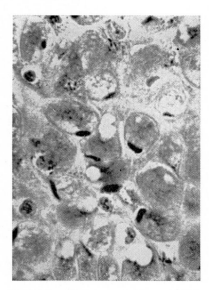

Fig. 762.—Molluscum bodies. × 500.

Callus and Corn.—In both of these lesions there is hyperkeratosis with marked thickening of the stratum corneum. In the corn or clavus keratinization is developed as a dense localized plug.

Acanthosis Nigricans.—The lesions are dark colored and warty in character, usually in the axilla, groin, elbows and knees. In adults there is a peculiar and unexplained association with abdominal cancer. The *microscopic appearance is* indicated by the descriptive name. The acanthosis takes a papillary form, accounting for the warty appearance, and hyperkeratosis is often more marked than acanthosis. The most characteristic feature is a dense melanin pigmentation of he basal layer of cells of the epidermis.

Ichthyosis.—The name, which means *fish skin*, is highly appropriate, for the surface is covered with large lamellae resembling fish scales. Most cases are congenital. *Microscopically* the disease is another example of hyperkeratosis in extreme form, with thining of the rete malphighii and absence of the granular layer, thus reversing the usual relationship of the granular and horny layers.

DISTURBANCES OF PIGMENTATION

The pigment of the skin is melanin produced by the melanoblasts intercalated between the basal layer, of cells of the epidermis. The amount of pigment varies in different races. At least in the lower animals and probably in man the melanin granules can move along branching processes of the melanoblasts, so that the pigment passes from the deeper to the superficial layers of the epidermis. The complex problem of melanosis has already been discussed on page 402, so that only brief mention will be made of it here. The pigment is produced by the action of an enzyme, tyrosinase, on a substrate, tyrosin. The melanin can be stained black by silver stains. The presence of the enzyme can be demonstrated in melanoblasts, either pigmented or non-pigmented, by the dopa reaction.

Melanin is the great protector of the skin against the actinic rays of the sun. It is increased in Addison's disease; it is deficient or absent in *albinism*, a congenital condition in which there is no pigment in the skin, hair, and eyes. *Leukoderma* is a patchy form of albinism, although the term is also used in a different sense. *Vitiligo* is an acquired form of leukoderma. Albinism may occur in the negro. When the negro albino lives in the tropics the situation becomes acutely serious, because such a person is unable to expose his unprotected skin to the fierce sun.

Xeroderma Pigmentosum.—This very serious hereditary disease of the skin is characterized by hypersensitivity of the epidermis to ultraviolet light. It usually develops in childhood, sometimes in the first year of life. In the later stages the skin is dry and atrophic with mottled pigmentation so that the lesions resemble those of chronic radiation dermatitis. In addition to the marked destructive changes in the skin there is a pronounced tendency to the development of basal cell and epidermoid carcinoma, so that the condition is *strongly precancerous*. The *microscopic picture* is complex. Hyperkeratosis is associated with marked atrophy of the rete malpighii, although in the later stages there may be patchy acanthosis. Melanin is increased in the basal layers of the epidermis, and numerous melanophores are seen in the superficial layers of the dermis. These layers also show marked destruction both of collagen and elastic fibers. All of these changes, including the tendency to develop carcinoma, may be attributed to an inherited sensitivity to ultraviolet light.

NONSPECIFIC INFLAMMATIONS: DERMATOSES

This is an indefinite and ill-defined group, and many of the conditions described here might well be considered under other headings. Indeed the term dermatoses merely means skin diseases. A convenient subdivision is into lesions mainly of the epidermis and lesions mainly of the dermis.

The *etiology* of very many of the nonspecific inflammations of the skin is obscure or unknown. In disease elsewhere the investigator has to try to answer the questions how, why and what. Unfortunately in the pathology of the skin he must often content himself with the third of these. The dermatologist must think in different terms from the internist, for he has to deal with the most sensitive organ in the body. *External irritants* must be considered, especially those concerned with occupation, more particularly cleansing agents. Or the irritant may be *blood-borne*, as in the case of drug dermatitis. *Undue sensitivity to light* may play a part, and photosensitivity may be induced by certain drugs or by circulating porphyrins. Multiplicity of facts must often be considered. Three factors which may act in conjunction or alone are the allergic, the psychogenic and the hormonal. The *allergy* may be to food, drugs, or animal and plant substances, the antigen-antibody reaction taking place in the skin. Beauty aids, more particularly nail lacquer, permanent wave solutions, hair dye, and lipstick in that order are frequent causes of allergic dermatitis. The *psychogenic factor* often plays a part in skin allergies, just as it does in asthma. It is persons predisposed to emotional conflicts and nervous tension who are likely to suffer from eczema and seborrheic dermatitis. Finally the *hormones*, particularly those of the sex glands and adrenals, exert a profound influence on the skin, hair follicles, and sebaceous glands. The waxing and waning of gonadal function are mirrored in the skin and its pilo-sebaceous sytem. Thus androgens stimulate surface epithelium and sebaceous glands, tending to produce hyper-keratosis and seborrhea, whereas estrogens have the contrary action, giving the soft skin of the female.

Lesions of the Epidermis

Eczema. Dermatitis.—These terms signify a nonspecific allergic response of the skin to a wide variety of agents which may act from the outside or through the vessels. The histological picture is correspondingly indefinite. In the acute varieties the lesions are essentially epidermal. Edema, both intercellular and intracellular, result in the formation of vesicles and bullae either in the rete malpighii or under the stratum corneum. These contain a few lymphocytes. In the subacute and particularly in the chronic varieties there is often marked acanthosis with elongation of the rete pegs, together with an inflammatory exudate in the corium consisting of a variety of cells, including eosinophils and histiocytes.

Psoriasis.—This is a chronic inflammatory disorder marked by the presence of reddish-brown papules and plaques covered with layers of silvery scales. When the scales are scraped away fine bleeding points become apparent which correspond to the apices of the underlying dermal papillae. The important *microscopic lesions* are in the epidermis. The horny layer is thickened at the expense of the granular layer, and parakeratosis is marked with air spaces between the layer of parakeratotic cells, an arrangement to which the silvery appearance of the scales is due. The rete malpighii overlying the dermal papillae is extremely thinned, and as these papillae are elongated and club-shaped with dilated capillaries, it is natural that bleeding should occur when the scales are removed (Fig. 763). The rete pegs are also elongated, thin above and thickened below. There is a varying degree of inflammatory exudate in the upper part of the corium, particularly in the papillae. Polymorphonuclear leukocytes migrate through the epidermis and form *micro-abscesses of Monroe* in the stratum corneum or just beneath it.

Dermatitis Herpetiformis.—As the name implies, the essential lesions in this disease are vesicular. The vesicles are situated in

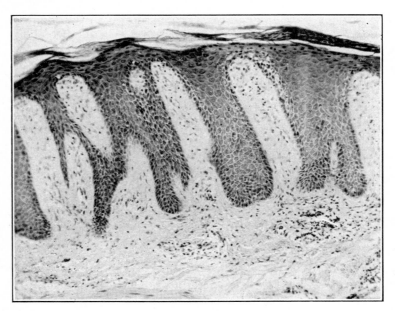

Fig. 763.—Psoriasis. The parakeratotic layer of epidermis is thick and scaly, the dermal papillæ are bulbous and edematous, interdigitating with deep rete pegs, the suprapapillary epidermal plate is thinned, and the corium and papillæ contain a scanty inflammatory exudate. × 125.

the deeper layers of the epidermis and may be subepidermal. There is little intercellular or intracellular edema. The really characteristic feature is the presence of large numbers of eosinophils, both in the vesicles and in the underlying dermis. The blood often shows a marked eosinophilia.

Pemphigus.—The characteristic feature of this serious and usually fatal disease is the formation of groups of large bullae, which may appear at intervals of weeks or months. The bullae develop deep in the epidermis or in the subepidermal tissue. They contain clear or cloudy fluid and soon rupture. The dermis may or may not show inflammatory changes. It will be seen that it may be difficult or impossible to distinguish between the lesions of pemphigus and dermatitis herpetiformis from microscopic examination. The reason for the fatal outcome is not clear, nor is the cause of the disease known. Possibly it is a virus infection akin to foot-and-mouth disease in animals.

Lesions of the Dermis

Scleroderma.—Scleroderma may occur in two very different forms, the one circum-scribed and benign, the other diffuse and frequently fatal. It is difficult to be certain if these are manifestations of the same disease, but there is not doubt that occasionally the circumscribed may pass into the diffuse form. In *circumscribed* scleroderma (*morphea*) firm white patches develop in the skin. These increase in size, but later become stationary and finally disappear, leaving an inconspicuous area of atrophic skin. The *diffuse* form is a very different story. From a local beginning, often on the face and neck, the condition spreads far and wide, until the greater part of the skin becomes hidebound. In the course of time symptoms due to visceral lesions are apt to develop.

The *microscopic lesions* of both forms, whether confined to a few patches in the skin or scattered through the viscera, are similar in essence. *It is a disease of collagen and its cement substance.* The early lesions are inflammatory in nature, with lymphocytic infiltration and swelling of the collagen fibers which are separated by edema. At a later stage all evidence of inflammation may be absent, the collagen fibers atrophy and become compressed into dense compact masses,

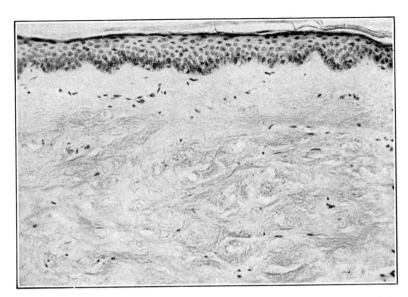

Fig. 764.—Scleroderma. Dense collagen, loss of appendages, atrophy of epidermis and flattening of rete pegs. × 150.

the elastic tissue is diminished, the skin appendages disappear except for a few atrophic sweat glands, and the blood vessels of the corium are thickened and their lumen narrowed (Fig. 764). The epidermis tends to be atrophied with flattening of the rete pegs.

Diffuse scleroderma may be regarded as a form, albeit an atypical form, of the group of diffuse collagen disease. Sclerosing lesions have been described in a great variety of organs, *e.g.*, heart, esophagus, bowel, kidneys, lungs, thyroid gland, and muscles. In all of these locations, in addition to overgrowth of connective tissue, there is degeneration and atrophy of muscle and occlusion of vessels. The disease is, therefore, not strictly a dermatosis, but a progressive systemic sclerosis (Beerman). Calcium deposits (calcinosis) may occur in the degenerated collagen. The cardiac symptoms may be so marked that the term *scleroderma heart disease* has been applied. When the lesions are limited to the hands there may be *acrocyanosis* (*akron*, extremity) resembling that of Raynaud's disease. *Esophagitis* with chronic ulceration is frequent. *Intestinal symptons* may be marked. There may be *renal failure with hypertension.*

Whilst the renal lesions are by no means constant there are usually numerous small infarcts in the cortex, with intimal proliferation in the interlobular arteries and hyalinization of the afferent arterioles and glomerular capillaries (Swarm and Germuth). If the clinical picture resembles malignant hypertension the vessels may show the necrotizing arteritis characteristic of that condition.

Lupus Erythematosus.—As in the case of scleroderma this disease may occur in a chronic localized benign form and in an acute disseminated often fatal form, characterized not only by widespread involvement of the skin but also by the presence of numerous visceral and vascular lesions. *Diffuse lupus erythematosus*, which is one of the diffuse collagen diseases, may develop from the localized form, or the visceral lesions may antedate the cutaneous ones. The characteristic L.E. cell is present in the blood of the discoid as well as the disseminated form, although much less constantly. Disseminated lupus has already been described on page 115.

The *localized* or *discoid* variety consists of small reddish macules usually situated on the nose and cheeks which become confluent

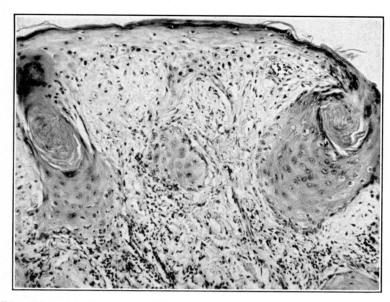

FIG. 765.—Discoid lupus erythematosus. The most striking change is the keratotic plugging of the hair follicles. Other features are colliquative degeneration of the basal layer of cells and atrophy of all layers of the epidermis, smudgy degeneration of collagen in the upper left quadrant, and a cellular infiltrate extending from the superficial to the deep layers of the dermis. × 75.

and resemble the open wings of a butterfly. It may involve any part of the skin. The lesion enlarges peripherally, with healing and scarring in the center, so as to assume a saucer-like or discoid form. The earliest *microscopic change* is dilatation of the vessels in the upper part of the corium, with extravasation of leukocytes and later lymphocytes and monocytes. Secondary changes in the epidermis and acanthosis alternating with atrophy of the epidermis, keratotic plugging of the hair follicles and sweat ducts, and liquefaction necrosis of the basal cell layer (Fig. 765). In a lesion on the face of a young women this picture is characteristic of discoid lupus. In the acute disseminated variety the changes are similar, but the dilatation of vessels and liquefaction of the basal cell layer are more marked and there is atrophy of the prickle cell layer. All of these changes are due to the basic lesions in the corium. Exposure to strong sunlight may precipitate a change from the discoid to the disseminated form.

Urticaria Pigmentosa.—This peculiar and distinctive disease commonly makes its appearance during the first year of life. At first the lesions may be typically urticarial in type (wheals associated with itching), but later they take the form of pigmented macules scattered over the entire skin. The pathognomonic features of the *microscopic picture* is the presence of great numbers of *mast cells* in the upper layers of the corium. The specific granules of these cells are not colored by hematoxylin and eosin, but stain intensely with an aniline dye such as toluidin blue. The cells tend to be perivascular in arrangement. Focal collections of mast cells are also found in the spleen, lymph nodes and thymus. The pigmentation is due to the presence of increased amounts of melanin in the deep layers of the epidermis. Subepidermal edema, the characteristic feature of simple urticaria and responsible for the itching, is likely to be present. *The whealing which occurs at the site of local stimulation is believed to be due to the release of histamine from the mast cells.* In rare instances generalized flushing of the skin has been reported, due, it has been suggested, to the release of serotonin from mast cells (Birt and Nickerson).

Urticaria.—Simple urticaria is character-

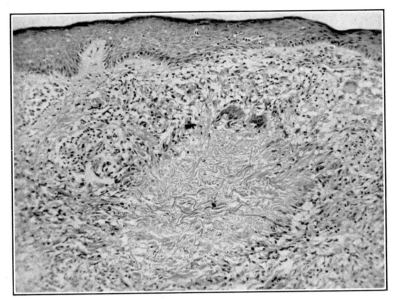

Fig. 766.—Granuloma annulare. Necrobiosis, histiocytes and giant cells in corium. × 110.

ized by the presence of transient wheals accompanied by itching. The *microscopic* basis of the wheal is edema of the superficial layers of the corium. The collagen fibers, which are swollen and pale, are widely separated by edema fluid, the dermal papillæ are widened and the rete pegs flattened.

Erythema Multiforme.—The name implies that erythema is a principal feature, and that the lesions are multiform in character, macules, papules, vesicles and bullæ. It is an acute self-limited disease, more common in young adults, and associated with symptoms suggesting general infection, *e.g.*, fever sore throat, and enlargement of the spleen and lymph nodes. The principal *microscopic change* is edema of the dermal papillae, with swelling of the collagen, dilatation of vessels, and marked perivascular infiltration of leukocytes. When vesicles are present there will be edema of the epidermis.

Granuloma Annulare.—This condition is very different from the other dermatoses which have been described so far. It takes the form of small firm nodules arranged usually in a ring-like or annular manner, for the most part on the hands and feet of young persons. The lesions may develop slowly or suddenly, and they may persist for months

or years. The *microscopic picture* closely resembles that of the subcutaneous nodules of rheumatic fever and rheumatoid arthritis, except that the lesions are confined to the corium. The center of the nodule presents a picture of necroboisis or coagulation necrosis rather than the fibrinoid necrosis of rheumatic lesions, and the ghostly outlines of collagen fibers can be traced uninterrupted through this region (Fig. 766). The central necrotic area is surrounded by palisaded rows of histiocytes and fibroblasts exactly as in the rheumatic nodule. An occasional multinucleated giant cell (not a typical Langhans' cell) may be seen, but, as in the case of the rheumatic nodule, there are no Aschoff cells. The picture must not be mistaken for tuberculosis. There is no true caseation and no true epithelioid cells. The etiology of granuloma annulare is at present unknown.

Necrobiosis Lipoidica Diabeticorum. — This diease is characterized by lipid deposits in an area of degenerated collagen in the dermis. In spite of the name, diabetes is present in only 80 per cent of the cases. The lesions, usually on the legs, take the form of circular or irregular plaques with a yellow center and violaceous periphery. The *micro-*

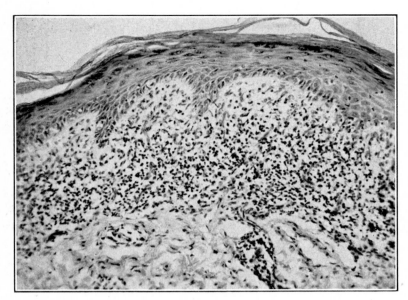

Fig. 767.—Lichen planus. Zone of lymphocytes in dermis, saw-tooth rete pegs, marked granular layer and hyperkeratosis. × 110.

scopic picture suggests that of an imperfectly developed granuloma annulare. The degeneration of collagen is not so complete (necrobiosis), the fibers being swollen, granular and partly fragmented, so that they may extend in various directions. At the periphery of this area there is a chronic inflammatory exudate with epithelioid cells and foreign-body giant cells. Two characteristic features are vascular changes and lipid deposits. The vessels show endarteritis, fibrosis, narrowing of the lumen and occasional thrombosis. These changes account for the degeneration of the collagen. Scarlet red staining of frozen sections reveals numerous granules of lipid between the cells. The changes in the vessels and the lipid deposits serve to differentiate the lesions from those of granuloma annulare.

Lichen Planus.—In this disease there are characteristic, small, multiple, angular, flat-topped (planus) or umbilicated nodules usually limited to the flexor aspects of the wrists and forearms and the legs immediately above the ankles. The *microscopic picture* is also characteristic. In the upper part of the cornium there is a sharply limited band-like infiltrate of lymphocytes and other chronic inflammatory cells which hugs the epidermis

and may be mistaken for lymphoblastoma (Fig. 767). In addition there is hyperkeratosis, a characteristic increase in the stratum granulosum, acanthosis with elongated pointed rete pegs which have been likened to a saw-tooth, and liquefaction degeneration of the basal cell layer.

Lichen Sclerosus et Atrophicus.—This lesion with the high sounding name consists of flat white papules like those of lichen planus, but with black horny plugs at the openings of the sweat glands and hair follicles, developing later into depressions. *Microscopically* there is marked keratotic plugging of the openings of the ducts and follicles with hyperkeratosis, but atrophy of the rest of the epidermis. The sclerosis is observed in the dermis and resembles that of scleroderma except for the absence of blood vessel changes and the fact that the texture is looser, more edematous, and less homogeneous.

Panniculitis.—As the name implies, this is not a condition affecting the skin proper, but rather the layer of subcutaneous fibrous and fatty tissue (*pannus*, cloth). A number of forms have been distinguished, but only two will be described. *Nodular, nonsuppurative, relapsing, febrile panniculitis*, known as *Weber-Christian disease*, is marked by development of crops of indurated, tender nodules in the subcutaneous fat. As healing occurs they leave a depression in the skin. *Microscopically* panniculitis may present three stages: the first is the acute inflammatory, the second the macrophagic, and the third the fibroblastic. The first stage, of short duration, is marked by an infiltration of acute inflammatory cells, mainly polymorphonuclear, but without suppuration. In the second stage, which provides the characteristic picture, the cells are mainly phagocytic histiocytes which are invading and engulfing the fat cells. They are, therefore, very swollen with foamy cytoplasm. A few foreign-body giant cells may be present. In the third stage fibroblasts replace the macrophages, collagen is laid down, and fibrous tissue formed. Neither the corium nor epidermis are involved. The etiology is unknown.

Erythema induratum (Bazin's disease) is a form of panniculitis in which indurated bluish-red nodules develop usually in the calves of the legs. As a rule they are associated with tuberculous lesions in other organs, but the relation to tuberculosis is rather indefinite. The *microscopic picture* is tuberculoid rather than characteristically tuberculous, and caseation is often absent. There is fat necrosis associated with a nonspecific chronic inflammatory reaction.

SPECIFIC INFLAMMATIONS

Inflammation of the skin may be caused be bacteria (tuberculosis, syphilis, etc.), fungi (blastomycosis, etc.), viruses (smallpox, etc), and animal parasites (scabies, etc.). These have already been described in the section on Principles of Pathology, but impetigo may be considered here.

Impetigo Contagiosa.—This contagious disease caused by pyogenic cocci, both staphylococci and streptococci, is a good example of inflammation confined to the epidermis. Exposed parts such as the face and hands are affected, often as the result of scratching. The bacteria penetrate the horny layer from without. First a vesicle and then a pustule develops between the stratum corneum and rete malpighii, polymorphonuclears wandering through the epidermis from the vessels of the corium. Intercellular edema may be marked in the rete, and the pus cells are readily seen. When the pustule ruptures it is covered with a crust of fibrin.

TUMORS OF THE EPIDERMIS

As the skin is of such complex structure it is natural that a wide variety of tumors should arise from it. Thus there may be tumors of epidermal and mesodermal origin, tumors of the skin appendages, pigment cells, nerves, vessels, muscles, and lymphoid tissue. Some of these tumors have already been described in the section on tumors in Chapter 9, because they are neoplasms which are not confined to the skin. Others which are primarily tumors of the skin will be considered here. There is bound to be some overlapping with regard to the hypertrophies and neoplasms. Thus some writers will include verruca senilis (seborrheic keratosis) with the former and others with the latter group.

Epidermoid Carcinoma.—This type of tumor may arise from squamous cell epithelium wherever it occurs. It may also originate from columnar epithelium, especially when that epithelium has undergone squamous metaplasia as in the bronchus. It has already been considered on page 230.

It may be noted here that *spontaneous healing* of multiple squamous cell carcinoma may occur in rare instances (Currie and Smith). In one such case the condition was present for twenty-one years. These tumor are widely distributed on the face, ears and limbs, and develop into malignant ulcers which heal spontaneously. There is often a familial history. At least some of the tumors appear to arise from hair follicles, and it has been suggested that the sebaceous glands may secrete a weak carcinogen derived from fatty-acid breakdown products of their secretion.

Basal Cell Carcinoma.—*Rodent Ulcer.*—This is a variety of squamous cell carcinoma which differs both clinically and pathologically from typical epidermoid cancer. It is relatively benign, of remarkably slow growth, and does not involve the regional lymph nodes. It presents the anomaly of a tumor which is relatively undifferentiated and is yet of low malignancy. Being undifferentiated it responds well to radiation, but not if it has infiltrated the underlying bone. *The distribution is highly characteristic.* The lesion occurs on the upper part of the face about the cheek, nose, and ear, above a line drawn between the tip of the ear and the angle of the mouth. It is, however, by no means confined to this region, and may occasionally occur on other parts of the skin. Not

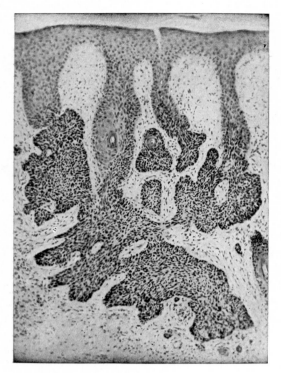

FIG. 768.—Basal cell carcinoma. The basal cell character of the growth is evident. × 90.

infrequently rodent ulcers are multiple, the skin of an area (usually the face) developing a tumor-forming tendency (Fig. 107, page 206). Exposure to bright sunlight appears to be a causal factor. In Australia where the light is very strong and the humidity very low the disease is extremely common. As many as 50 cases a day may be seen in the out-patient department at Sydney. The conditions in Australia are peculiar, for it is a country with a tropical sun in which there is is nothing but white labor. In other tropical countries those who are continually exposed to the brilliant glare have colored (protected) skins. It is interesting to note that the large Italian element in the labor population in Australia is relatively immune. The disease is much commoner at the north end of New Zealand than in the south. The tumor slowly erodes the deeper tissues, and in this way may cause great destruction of the nose, the contents of the orbit, etc. For this reason it is commonly called *rodent ulcer.*

The *microscopic appearance* is quite different from that of epidermoid carcinoma.

It consists of solid masses of darkly-stained cells which extend down into the dermis (Fig. 768), although often no connection with the epidermis may be seen in a given section. The columns extend down to a uniform level, and their ends have an expanded club-shaped appearance. This gives a geographic arrangement of capes, bays and promontories. There is none of the eosin-staining so characteristic of epidermoid carcinoma, no cell nests, no cornification. There are usually no mitotic figures, but they may occur in the more rapidly-growing forms. Melanin pigment may be so abundant as to be misleading. Occasional variations in this uniform picture may occur. Thus the structure may become lacy, cysts may form due to edema and liquefaction of the stroma, whilst in the rare *basosquamous type* there are nests of squamous cells like epithelial pearls.

The *origin* of the tumor has been a matter of dispute. The term basal cell carcinoma indicates the belief that the origin is from the basal cell layer of the epidermis. It seems probable that many of these tumors arise from the hair follicles or their anlage. Wallace and Halpert, indeed, have suggested the name *trichoma*. It is of interest to recall that while most of the malignant epithelial growths of the skin mimic the pattern of the epidermis, practically all the benign growths mimic the pattern of the skin appendages. This is true of the so-called basal cell carcinoma.

BOWEN'S DISEASE.—This is an intraepidermal carcinoma rarely developing into an invasive squamous cell carcinoma. It is an example of preinvasive carcinoma. There is acanthosis with elongation of the rete pegs, but the basal layer is intact. The characteristic feature is the atypical character of the epithelial cells, many of which show marked vacuolization with a cytoplasmic halo surrounding the nucleus, an appearance similar to that of Paget cells in Paget's disease of the breast. The scaly patches occur on the trunk and the extremities.

Preinvasive Carcinoma.—This condition, also called *intraepithelial carcinoma* and *carcinoma in situ,* may be observed in a number of locations, such as the stomach and bronchus, but to the pathologist concerned with the diagnosis of biopsy specimens the sites of paramount importance are the cervix and the skin. In order to justify this diagnosis

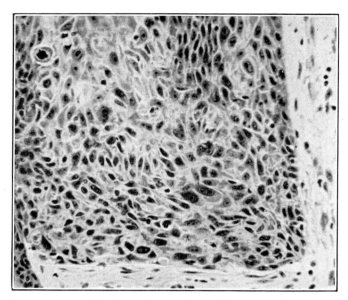

Fig. 769.—Preinvasive carcinoma. Dyskeratosis as evidenced by disorderly arrangement of cells (loss of polarity), variation in size and chromatic character of nuclei, and mitoses. × 250.

the various layers of the epidermis should show evidence of dyskeratosis, *i.e.* cellular unrest and malignant transformation such as acanthosis, hyperchromatism, loss of cell polarity (jumbling of cellular arrangement), and increased number of mitoses (Fig. 769). When only the basal layers are involved the condition should be regarded merely as basal cell hyperplasia. There is no invasion of the dermis, nor is there any guarantee that this will occur, but the picture must arouse apprehension. More particularly is this the case when marked lymphocytic infiltration of the underlying dermis suggests the action of some agent released from the proliferating cells of the epidermis.

Precancerous Lesions.—It is in the epidermis that the lesions known by the somewhat ambiguous name of precancerous can most readily be observed. Although all writers do not agree with this statement, a precancerous lesion should be distinguished from carcinoma in situ or intraepithelial carcinoma. The former is not yet cancer, whereas the latter lesion, in the opinion of the pathologist, is a definite cancer although not yet invasive. Bowen's disease is an example of carcinoma in situ. Senile keratosis, as well as leukoplakia, kraurosis vulvæ and radiation dermatitis which presents the same histological picture, xeroderma pigmentosa and junctional nevus are all examples of true precancerous lesions. They are in no sense malignant, but they have a tendency to develop into cancer and must alarm the clinician for that reason.

TUMORS OF THE APPENDAGES

Sweat Gland Tumors.—The nomenclature of tumors of the sweat glands is extremely complex and confusing because of the varied microscopic picture. Their names are legion, and each writer seems to delight in inventing new ones. For a detailed consideration of the subject the reader must consult works on skin pathology, although Gates, Warren and Warvi in their full review of the subject rather discourage this by remarking that "the literature is confusing and largely casuistic." Three common terms with their derivations may be mentioned. These are spiradenoma (*speira*, a coil), syringoma (*syrinx*, a tube), and hydradenoma (*idros*, sweat).

The tumors are adenomas which are usually solid but may be cystic. Rarely carcinoma may develop, but this is of low malignancy and only locally invasive.

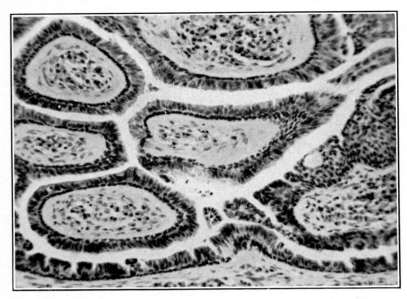

FIG. 770.—Sweat gland tumor. This is a papillary syringocystadenoma with papillary processes in a dilated duct. The double layer of cells lining the cyst can be distinguished. × 200.

Spiradenoma or *Hydradenoma*, the commonest of the tumors, also known as *cylindroma*, an ambiguous and confusing term, is a disease, often hereditary, characterized by multiple tumors of the skin. When these occur on the scalp they may cover the head like a wig or turban, so that the lesion is known as a *turban tumor*. The *microscopic picture* is one of sharply limited cell masses and stands in which are embedded alveolar spaces lined by cuboidal epithelium, each mass being surrounded by a hyaline membrane. The cells in the center have large pale nuclei and represent the secreting type; they are surrounded by a palisade of cells with small dark nuclei, which appear to be myoepithelial in nature. These tumors must not be mistaken for basal cell carcinoma, in which the pattern of growth is quite different.

Papillary Syringocystadenoma, as its name implies, arises from the duct of the gland. The duct is dilated, and the resulting cyst contains numerous villus-like projections covered by a double layer of cells, the outer layer being myoepithelial and the inner layer secreting cells (Fig. 770).

Papillary Hydradenoma is an adenoma of apocrine glands occurring almost exclusively on the labia majora and perineum of women. Into a cyst-like lumen project numerous papillary processes covered by a single layer of cylindrical, eosinophilic, secreting cells like those of an apocrine gland. The picture resembles that of cystic lobular hyperplasia of the breast.

Sebaceous Gland Tumors.—This group is as simple as the sweat gland group is complex, for the only one which deserves mention is *sebaceous adenoma*. The lesion is more a hyperplasia of the glands than a true tumor. It occurs as small yellow papules chiefly on the nose, checks and forehead. The microscopic picture is simple overgrowth of the sebaceous glands. Tuberous sclerosis of the cerebral cortex may be associated with multiple sebaceous adenomas. In rare cases locally infiltrating carcinoma has been described.

Tumors of Hair Follicles.—*Adenoid Cystic Epithelioma.* This lesion, also known as *trichoepithelioma* and *Brooke's tumor*, is believed to arise from the hair follicles. It forms multiple smooth tumors on the face and chest, occurs at a much earlier age than basal cell carcinoma for which it may be mistaken, and forms a heaped-up lesion on the surface. The lesion consists of solid

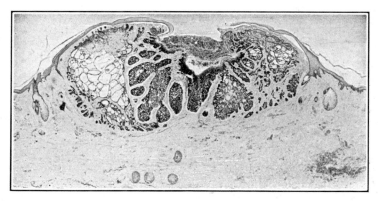

Fig. 771.—Adenoid cystic epithelioma showing cystic spaces. Note the resemblance to rodent ulcer. × 14.

masses of dark cells like those of a basal cell carcinoma and cystic spaces lined by squamous stratified epithelium and filled with keratin (Fig. 771). The tumor is quite benign and does not infiltrate the surrounding tissue.

Basal cell carcinoma is believed by some to arise from the cells of the hair follicle. This matter has already been discussed on page 1328.

Keratoacanthoma: Molluscum Sebaceum.— This common skin lesion is only a pseudotumor, not a true neoplasm. It is included here because in the past it has been regarded as an atypical form of squamous cell carcinoma as indicated by the term *self-healing carcinoma.* Some writers use the name keratoacanthoma, others call the lesion molluscum sebaceum; both are descriptive, as we shall see. The special importance of the condition is the ease with which it may be mistaken for squamous cell carcinoma, not only by the clinician, but also by the pathologist. It must not be confused with adenoid cystic epithelioma, which more resembles basal cell carcinoma.

The most striking clinical feature of the lesion, which commonly occurs as a solitary nodule on the cheek or nose in persons over forty years of age, is its rapid growth for from four to eight weeks, followed by slow involution (self-healing) in the course of from two to four months. Striking clinical and microscopic illustrations of this remarkable sequence of events will be found in the paper by Calnan and Haber. The nodule

rarely attains a diameter greater than 1 cm. It is dome-shaped, with a central horny plug or crust. There is no true ulceration, nor enlargement of the regional lymph nodes.

The lesion starts with hyperplasia of a group of hair follicles, which leads to hyperkeratosis and acanthosis. (It will be recalled that acanthosis is a hyperplastic thickening of the prickle cell layer). The hyperkeratotic areas fuse into one central mass, some of which may disintegrate to form a crater, while the acanthotic areas represent an irregular invasion of the dermis. From this account it will be realized how appropriate is the term keratoacanthoma, except that the suffix suggests a neoplasm. Microabscesses may develop later in the downgrowing mass. It is important to note that the downgrowth, which is in truth a molluscum or skin tubercle, never extends deeper than the hair follicles and sebaceous glands of the area, a useful point in diagnosis.

A suggestion as to the possible nature of the condition may be obtained from consideration of the skin cancer produced in rabbits by painting with carcinogens. Not all of such tumors behave as true carcinomas, for some regress spontaneously. The latter lesions may present an identical clinical microscopic picture to that of human keratoacanthoma, as can be seen in the illustrations in Ghadially's paper. In these cases there is an abnormal proliferation of hair follicles and sebaceous glands which is invasive but not malignant, a condition reminiscent of cholecystitis glandularis pro-

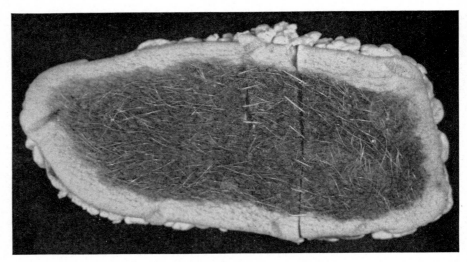

Fig. 772.—Intradermal nevus. Flat pigmented hairy lesion on posterior aspect of thigh of a fourteen-year-old boy, present since birth. (University of Alabama.)

liferans in the gallbladder (page 825). In the human subject it may be that a mild carcinogenic stimulus acting on a group of resting hair follicles triggers a growth which ceases when the normal cycle of hair growth, known to continue for about thirty days, returns to the resting phase.

THE MELANOMAS

Nevus.—A nevus is a mole. It is usually pigmented, but may not be; the color varies from gray to brown or jet black. A pigmented nevus must be distinguished from other pigmented lesions of the skin such as pigment spots, seborrheic keratosis, and dermatofibroma in which there is an increase of melanin on the surface and hemosiderin in the deeper parts. A microscopic distinction of importance is drawn between the intradermal nevus (the common mole) and the junctional nevus (see below). The former remains benign and the latter may become malignant. In the gross a distinction can also be drawn. The intradermal nevus is raised and hairy, while the junctional nevus is flat and may give the appearance of a drop of brown paint with a spreading margin, especially when it is becoming malignant. The nevus varies greatly in size, being usually quite small, but sometimes covering a large area of the body (Fig. 772).

Nevi are so common that nearly everyone has at least one tiny one, and the average person has over 20 pigmented moles. They are usually situated on the face, neck or back, but they may occur anywhere. Rarely a nevus occurs in the pigmented part of the eye. A nevus is a congenital condition, but it may not be apparent at birth, and many pigmented moles do not appear until adult life. It seems probable that the lesions are under the influence of and may be activated by steroid hormones. The great majority of nevi pursue an uneventful course. They may grow slowly for a time, remain quiescent for a long period, and gradually atrophy. The beginning of a *malignant change* may be indicated by the presence of a pink halo caused by the inflammatory reaction which accompanies such a change, increase of size and pigmentation, and itching. The dangerous sites are the palm, the sole, the digits (especially in the region of the nails), the genitals, the anus, and places exposed to continued trauma. The transformation is often slow and insidious, for melanoma enters by stealth like a thief in the night, but any sudden increase in the rate of growth should at once arouse a suspicion of malignancy.

Histogenesis.—The mode of origin of the nevus has been and still is a matter of endless debate. The older views, having been discarded, may be passed by. At the present time two theories hold the field, the epidermal (epithelial) and the neurogenic. For the arguments in support of the former the reader is referred to the article by Allen, for those in support of the latter to the papers by Masson. The controversy revolves around two points: (1) the nature of the melanoblasts, (2) the question as to whether additional structures are involved in the production of the nevus.

Even a cursory examination of a few surgical sections will suggest the possibility that the groups of nevus cells in the dermis represent downgrowths from the epidermis which have become cut off and isolated. The champions of the epidermal school hold that melanoblasts are merely epithelial cells which possess the power of forming pigment, that these proliferate in the basal layer of the epidermis and penetrate into the underlying dermis, where they may become cut off from their source of origin. The process may be arrested at any stage, but in each case the resulting lesion is a nevus.

The epidermal theory is so simple and satisfactory that, by comparison, the neurogenic theory appears complex and far-fetched, if not fantastic. But the body itself is complex, and many features of even normal development (e.g., the eye) appear to be fantastic. The basic fact to be faced is that some structures and arrangements only become apparent with perfect fixation, trichrome stains and silver impregnation of cytoplasm. Anyone who has seen a demonstration by Pierre Masson of Montreal illustrated by color photomicrographs of breath-taking perfection has a new world of structure revealed to him which is invisible with hematoxylin and eosin staining, and which cannot be reproduced with complete satisfaction in black and white illustrations.

In brief outline Masson's views are as follows. A fully developed nevus is a cutaneous malformation in which the two principal components are melanoblasts and the nerves of the dermis. The former come from above, the latter from below. Melanoblasts are cells resembling monocytes which occur in the basal layer of the epidermis. They are dopa-positive by reason of the melanogenase they contain, and may be pigmented or non-pigmented. (For discussion of the dopa reaction see page 402.) The pigment is rendered prominent by Fontana silver staining. Melanoblasts transfer their pigment to adjoining epidermal cells and to dermal macrophages that become melanophores or pigment carriers, which are dopa-negative but Fontana-positive. The melanoblasts gradually lose their melanin and enzyme

and are carried to the surface. They are replaced by young cells.

In the nevi of infants there is overproduction of melanoblasts and melanin. The melanoblasts may separate the malpighian cells from the basement membrane. There is marked excretion of melanin into the underlying dermis, where it is taken up by melanophores. Thus is formed the *junctional nevus*, (epidermal or marginal nevus), which is the characteristic nevus of childhood. Or there may be a dropping down of cells, an Abtropfung as it was called by Unna, in which groups of melanoblasts penetrate the basement membrane, at first hanging like drops from a roof, then becoming detached and falling down into the dermis, a new basement membrane forming above the cell clusters (Fig. 773). Some of the melanoblasts arise from such derivatives of the epidermis as the hair follicles and the sebaceous and sweat glands. As long as the migration of melanoblasts goes on the lesion is known as a *compound nevus*. When the Abtropfung has ceased and all connection with the epidermis has disappeared the lesion becomes an *intradermal nevus* (dermal nevus). This is the common nevus or mole of adult life. So far the process is identical with that described by the epidermal school.

There now occurs a multiplication of the cells of the sheath of Schwann in the cutaneous nerves. The schwannian cells break through the membrane which surround them and invade the connective tissue. They form a layer of cells separated from the melanoblasts by a zone of normal tissue. The melanoblasts seem to exert an attraction on the schwannian cells, for the former grow down and the latter grow up, till they meet in the dermis and merge together. The nevus tissue, which is derived from two distinct sources, now becomes a single structure, a neuronevus (Fig. 773).

The *natural history of the nevus* demands attention. From the age of three or earlier changes begin which transform the juvenile into the adult nevus. These changes are most marked shortly before puberty. At a very early stage there is a gradual depigmentation of the melanoblasts. At puberty and in the adult only those cells in the superficial region of the papillary dermis are pigmented and dopa-positive. The pigment has been taken up by the dopa-negative melanophores. The depigmented melanoblasts cannot be distinguished from the schwann cells. The cells of the lesion are now of two varieties. Near the epidermis they are round or polygonal, whilst deeper they are more elongated and arranged in anastomosing fascicles. These two types may be called the epithelioid and the fasciculated; one or other type may predominate.

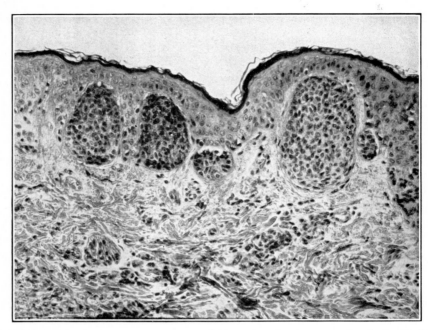

FIG. 773.—Intradermal neuronevus. The process of Abtropfung has been completed. In the dermis there
is a proliferation of cells of nervous origin. (Kindness of Professor Pierre Masson.)

Masson remarks that the nevus shows the cytological and histiogenetic properties that are specific for schwannian tissue. These are not apparent in thin sections stained with hematoxylin and eosin, they are more readily seen in trichrome stained material, and are most obvious in thick sections impregnated with silver nitrate for the demonstration of cytoplasm.

Other workers support the view of Masson regarding the dual origin of nevi from intraepidermal melanoblasts and proliferated schwannian cells (Berkheiser and Rappoport).

Malignant change when it does occur is *most likely to affect the junctional nevus after puberty.* It is exceptional in the intradermal form. It would appear that the neuroid element has an inhibitory effect on the tendency to malignancy.

Microscopic Appearance.—From the discussion on pathogenesis it is evident that the histological picture will depend on whether the nevus is intradermal, junctional or compound.

The *intradermal nevus* is the common form in the adult. It represents the completed stage of development, and is correspondingly quiescent. Nests and cords of closely packed "nevus cells" occupy the superficial layers of the dermis and sometimes the dermal papillæ (Fig. 774). The cells in superficial lesions are large, pale and polyhedral, but in the deeper lesions they are more fusiform and it is here that connections with nerve structures may be detected. The nests and sheets of cells are circumscribed, but at their lower limit they tend to trail off in an undecided manner which must not be mistaken for malignant invasion. The amount of melanin varies greatly. The pigment is contained in dopa-positive melanoblasts and in more peripheral fusiform dopa-negative melanophores. The overlying epidermis is not involved in the process, but may be either unduly papillary or flat.

The *junctional nevus* (epidermal nevus, marginal nevus) presents a highly distinctive appearance (Fig. 775). In the deeper layers of the rete, often in the rete pegs, there are sharply circumscribed collections of large loosely arranged cells (melanoblasts), some of which are sprinkled with melanin granules. The corium is not involved. The lesions may be limited to one spot or there may be alternating nevoid and normal portions of epidermis over an area of some size. The importance of the junctional nevus lies in the fact that it is this variety which is liable to develop into malignant melanoma after puberty. The presence of alternating or "skip" lesions may explain apparent recurrence of the melanoma after surgical removal (Allen and Spitz). This may not be a true recurrence but rather activation of outlying junctional nevi.

The *compound nevus* is a combination of the junctional and intradermal forms (Fig. 776). Nearly all intradermal nevi before puberty show this combination. In the adult it is very much less frequent, and it is these cases which hold the threat of possible malignancy.

Blue Nevus.—This is in an entirely different class from the other members of the group. It is the blackest of pigmented lesions and the most benign, in general less than 1 cm. in diameter, occurring in childhood and persisting unchanged throughout life. The usual sites are the face, the back of the hands and feet, and the soles. The *Mongolian spot* is a rather larger lesion at the lower end of the spine. The color fades about the third or fourth year of life. Both

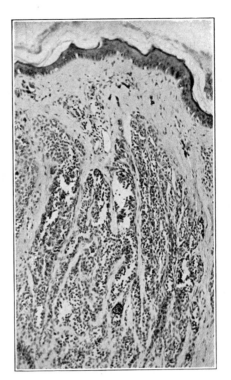

Fig. 774.—Intradermal nevus. The nevus cells are in the dermis and have no connection with the epidermis. × 100.

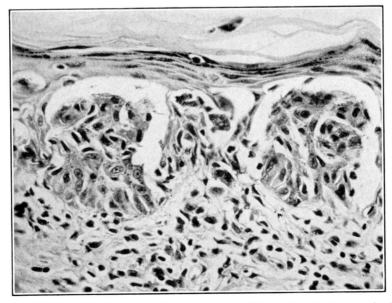

Fig. 775.—Junctional nevus. The melanoblasts, which were filled with melanin granules in the original section, are confined to the deeper layers of the epidermis. The smaller cells in the underlying dermis are inflammatory in nature. × 375.

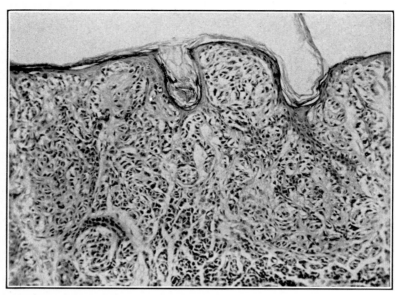

Fig. 776.—Compound nevus of combined juctional and intradermal type. The junctional changes in the epidermis are marked. There is direct continuity between the nevus cells in the epidermis and dermis. × 150.

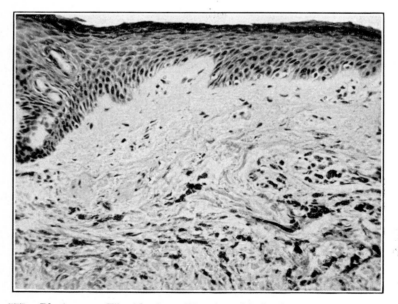

Fig. 777.—Blue nevus. Fibroblastic proliferation with deeply situated pigment cells. The epidermis is unaffected. × 175.

PLATE XX

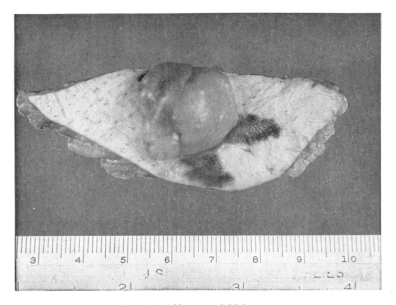

Junctional Nevus and Melanoma.

The nevus presents an appearance of two drops of dark oil in the skin. The large red mass is the melanoma, which microscopically was almost lacking in pigment, the surface being inflamed and ulcerated.

of these rare lesions consist of interlacing fasciculi of spindle cells amongst which are interspersed pigmented cells. Some of these are melanoblasts, dopa-positive and containing fine granules of melanin. They are situated in the deeper region of the skin, and are surrounded by heavily pigmented melanophores (Fig. 777). On account of the type of cells, their position and the presence of pigment, the lesion may be mistaken microscopically for a dermatofibroma containing hemosiderin granules. The differentiation can readily be made by means of the Prussian blue reaction for iron. *The blue nevus hardly ever becomes malignant,* nor are there any changes in the overlying epidermis.

Malignant Melanoma.—This highly malignant tumor is usually referred to merely as melanoma. It arises from melanoblasts in a nevus of the skin (Plate XIX) or in the pigmented coat of the eye. On the palms, soles and genitalia no preëxisting nevus may be evident clinically, but the possibility of a junctional nevus cannot be excluded. In rare instances a melanoma may originate in other locations such as the mucous membrane of the rectum, the nose or the meninges. It seems probable that malignant melanomas are under the influence of steroid hormones. *Nevi only become malignant after puberty,* and pregnancy has a bad influence on the course of the tumor. On the other hand the prognosis after surgical removal is a good deal worse in men than in women, especially in lesions of the head and neck (Allen and Spitz). The incidence is about the same in the two sexes. It may be noted that pigmented tumors are common in white and gray horses but quite rare in dark horses. It is said that if a white horse lives long enough it is almost certain to die of melanoma. It has also been said that a farmer could paint his fences with the pigment from the metastatic melanomata in a white horse, but I cannot vouch for this statement; it might depend on the length of the fences.

In the secondary growths the tumor cells continue to form pigment in enormous quantities. As much as 300 grams of melanin have been extracted from a liver filled with metastases. In rapidly growing tumors the pigment may escape into the blood (melanemia) and be excreted in the urine (melanuria). In rare cases there is a diffuse staining of the lining cells of the blood vessels and serous membranes.

Microscopic Structure.—The melanoma of the skin develops from the junctional type of nevus, although it would be unwise to say that this is invariably the case. Both the nuclei and cytoplasm of the nevus cells show suggestive changes. The proportion of nucleus to cytoplasm in increased, the nucleolus is enlarged, hyperchromatism is present, and mitoses may be observed. The cytoplasm is often vacuolated and sprinkled with fine melanin granules, and the cells become loosened and may be surrounded by a clear halo so as to have a resemblance to Paget cells. These changes extend throughout the epidermis as far as the stratum corneum, a highly suggestive appearance. (Fig. 778). Epidermal hyperplasia is nearly always present and must not be mistaken for squamous cell carcinoma.

Invasion of the dermis is indicated by the presence of circular or polyhedral cells with abundant spongy cytoplasm and fine pigment granules. The tumors cells may form small clusters in the subepidermal lymphatics, a grim indication of the early stage at which lymphatic dissemination of the tumor may occur. A subepidermal zone of inflammatory cells, mostly lymphocytes, is always suggestive of a malignant change. In the fully developed melanoma the large tumor cells in the dermis often show an alveolar arrangement, the groups being separated by a fine stroma (Fig. 779), but no tumor presents a more varied histological picture, and it may simulate a squamous or basal cell carcinoma, an adenocarcinoma, and, if the cells become fusiform, a fibrosarcoma. Pigmentation is usually marked, but this feature is very variable, and in one part of the tumor the cells may be loaded with melanin, while in another part they contain none. The melanoblasts may liberate their pigment, which is then taken up by phagocytic melanophores.

Spread.—A melanoma is important not because of any local disturbance it produces, for usually it remains small; it kills by producing widespread metastases. The tumor

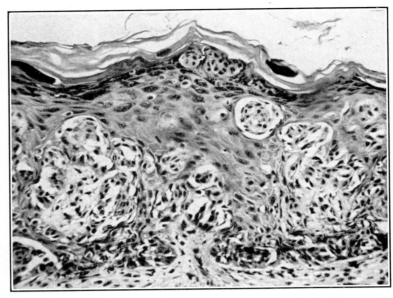

FIG. 778.—Junctional nevus showing malignant transformation. The junctional change involves all layers of the epidermis, the nevus cells are loosened, and some are surrounded by a clear halo. × 175.

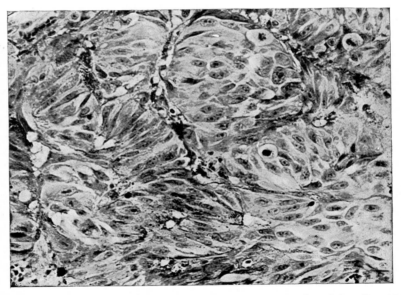

FIG. 779.—Malignant melanoma in skin showing characteristic acinar grouping of the cells. × 275. (Boyd, *Pathology for the Surgeon*, courtesy of W. B. Saunders Co.)

cells spread by the lymphatics to the regional lymph nodes and by the blood stream to distant parts, although in melanoma of the eye there is no lymph spread. The tumor spreads mainly and at first exclusively by the lymphatics; the regional lymph nodes soon become enlarged. Blood spread is a late event, and may be absent nearly until the end. When it does occur it is usually very wide, so that hardly an organ may escape. The skin is a common site of metastases. Secondary growths appear early in the skin; multiple growths of the skin even though non-pigmented should suggest a search for a primary melanoma. A history of loss of an eye from disease and an enlarged liver should suggest an ocular melanoma.

Melanoma in Childhood.—Melanoma in the child must be differentiated from adult melanoma (Spitz). The two are similar microscopically, with the exception of the fact that in about half the juvenile cases giant cells are present. But there is a world of difference in their clinical behavior. The juvenile melanomas, in spite of their apparent malignancy, remain localized in the majority of cases. With the arrival of puberty this difference disappears, and the tumors show the same tendency to metastasize as in the adult. It would appear that some inhibitory factor exists before puberty which prevents the spread of the tumor. It is natural to suggest that such an influence is hormonal in character.

Tumors of the Dermis

Many tissues and cells mingle in the dermis. There is fibrous tissue, blood and lymph vessels, nerves, plain muscle and lymphoid tissue. Fibromas and fibrosarcomas, hemangiomas and lymphangiomas, neuromas and neurofibromas, leiomyomas and lymphoblastomas are described elsewhere in this book. A few special types of tumor will be considered here.

Sclerosing Hemangioma.—This tumor is the result of the conversion of a capillary angioma into a solid cellular mass by proliferation of the stroma. Traces of the original vascular lumens can still be distinguished. It is a small, hard, non-encapsulated lesion of the corium, usually occurring on the extremities. It is composed of large, irregular, fusiform cells running in many directions and interlacing. It may be highly cellular, or may have abundant collagen and few cells, so that it has been called a *dermatofibroma*. An important feature is the ill-defined margin with infiltration of the surrounding tissue, and the cellular forms are easily mistaken for melanoma and neurofibroma. Phagocytic histiocytes often contain hemosiderin and lipids. The Prussian blue reaction for iron will readily distinguish the pigment from melanin. The capillaries of the angioma become obliterated, while segregated groups of endothelial cells remain. Accumulations of lipid and hemosiderin are probably extracted from the circulating blood (Gross and Wolbach), although to a lesser degree they may be derived from hemorrhages.

Kaposi's Multiple Hemorrhagic Hemangiosarcoma.—This is a very rare form of angiosarcoma of the skin, usually on the hands and feet. The disease is very much commoner in men than women, and usually in Italians and Jews. The lesions consist of many foci of capillary clusters in a stroma of malignant spindle-shaped cells. The course of the disease varies greatly. The vascular nodules may undergo involution and form atrophic pigmented scars, or lesions may develop in distant portions of the skin and in nearly every organ of the body the tumor is highly radiosensitive in the early stage.

Glomangioma. Glomus Tumor.—The word glomus means a conglomeration of minute arteries and veins. In the dermis of the extremities, particularly in the fingers and toes, there is an arteriovenous shunt by which the blood passes directly from the arteries into the veins without first passing through the capillaries. The channel along which the blood flows is lined by endothelium and surrounded by a mantle of large "epithelioid" or glomus cells; in addition there may be plain muscle fibers, while a rich plexus of non-medullated nerve fibers passes between the various cells. The epithelioid cells merge through a series of transitional forms with the typical spindle-shaped smooth muscle cells of the artery and vein. They appear to be derived from the pericytes of Zimmermann, specialized cells which are

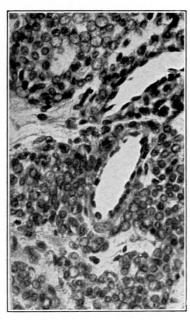

Fig. 780.—Glomus tumor; glomus cells surrounding vascular channel. × 225.

wrapped around the capillaries in all parts of the body and merge with the smooth muscle fibers. The entire mechanism constitutes a neuromyoarterial glomus, whose function appears to be to act as a kind of manometer controlling the circulation in the extremities and therefore the local temperature.

For the last one or two centuries the existence of "painful subcutaneous tubercles" in the extremities has been well recognized, but it was Masson who first in 1922 showed that these tumors arose from the glomus mechanism in the skin. Clinically these tumors are small, of slow growth, benign, confined to the extremities (common in the arm) and often situated under the finger nails, exquisitely tender, and characterized by paroxysms of burning pain during which the subungual lesions have a cyanotic appearance which is practically pathognomonic. Simple excision affords miraculous relief. A glomus tumor, however, may not be painful or even tender, depending probably on the amount of nerve fibers. *Microscopically* the tumor consists of a tangled mass of vessels surrounded by a fibrous capsule, and presenting the various elements (endothelial lining, glomus cells, plain muscle, and nonmedullated nerve fibers) already described in the normal glomus (Fig. 780).

Granuloma Pyogenicum.—This poorly named lesion is also known as *telangiectatic granuloma*, a much better term. It is a small, soft, red or bluish-red nodule, either pedunculated or sessile, which is highly vascular and bleeds readily. It often occurs at the site of an injury. *Microscopically* the nodule consists of numerous newly formed capillaries and vascular spaces in a loose edematous stroma. (Fig. 781). At first the picture is one of granulation tissue with superadded infection. Later the appearance becomes almost purely angiomatous with little evidence of infection, so that the lesion may be taken for a hemangioma and finally for a dermatofibroma.

Myoepithelioma.—*Myoepithelium* is the term applied to the elongated, flattened, contractile cells which are found external to the secreting cells of certain glands, more particularly the mammary, sweat, salivary, and lacrimal glands. Neoplasms consisting mainly or in part of myoepithelium have been recognized in the breast, and proliferation of myoepithelial elements is marked in certain mixed salivary gland tumors. Tumors of the skin, really tumors of sweat glands, may consist mainly of myoepithelial elements with an admixture of glandular cells (Hartz, Sheldon). A rare variant is the *clear cell myoepithelioma*, in which the cells are clear because they are filled with glycogen (Lever and Castleman). It must be noted that the term myoepithelioma does not indicate that the tumor is a malignant one, although at one time epithelioma was synonymous with squamous cell carcinoma.

Mycosis Fungoides.—Various forms of lymphoblastoma such as leukemia, lymphosarcoma and Hodgkin's disease may involve the skin secondarily. The variety known as mycosis fungiodes is a primary skin disease, although the internal organs may be affected later. It begins as a scaly eruption, with itching as a frequent symptom. After a period of months or years evidence of infiltration of the skin becomes apparent with the formation of elevated plaques. Finally

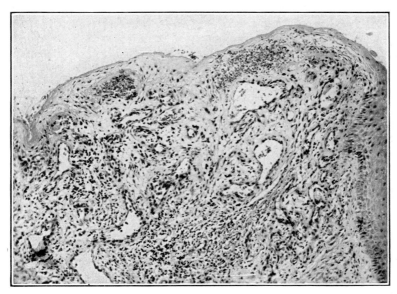

Fig. 781.—Granuloma pyogenicum. The projecting lesion consists of vascular spaces in edematous stroma. × 110.

the fungoid or tumor stage develops. The disease, like the other lymphoblastomas, is invariably fatal. The *microscopic picture* in the infiltrative and fungoid stages is marked by a pleomorphism which may closely resemble that of Hodgkin's disease. The masses of cells in the dermis contain reticulum cells, histiocytes, polymorphonuclears, eosinophils, and giant cells. The last named are more indefinite in character than the Reed-Sternberg cells of Hodgkin's disease, having an appearance of cells clumped together, so that they may be called "pseudo-giant cells."

Wood ticks and the *venom of insect bites* may cause lesions of the skin easily mistaken microscopically for mycosis fungoides and Hodgkin's disease. To add to the confusion the epidermis often shows pseudo-epitheliomatous hyperplasia which may simulate early epidermoid carcinoma.

Cysts of the Skin

Dermal cysts may be dermoid, epidermal and sebaceous, and milium.

Dermoid cysts are easily recognized microscopically, because the wall is composed of skin with its appendages, *e. g.*, sebaceous glands, hair follicles and hair. They may be called trichosebaceous cysts. *Epidermal cysts* form the common and important variety. Most of the cysts called by the clinician sebaceous cysts are classified by the pathologist as epidermal cysts. True *sebaceous cysts*, commonly known as *wens* and occurring on the scalp, are the result of obstruction of the ducts of sebaceous glands and are lined by sebaceous cells. Epidermal cysts may arise *de novo* from the dermal appendages, they may result from squamous metaplasia of sebaceous cysts, or they may be traumatic owing to fragments of epidermis being displaced into the dermis as the result of trauma or operation (implanation cysts), or from the presence of a foreign body such as a splinter or thorn.

The *epidermal cyst* is lined by squamous epithelium, and the contents are greasy keratin, squames which accumulate as they cannot be shed, fat and cholesterol. The cyst may rupture or leak into the tissues, where the contents excite a granulomatous reaction characterized by the presence of histiocytes, foreign body giant cells, cholesterol clefts, and the tell-tale squames (Fig. 782). At this stage the lining of the cyst may have disappeared, so that the true

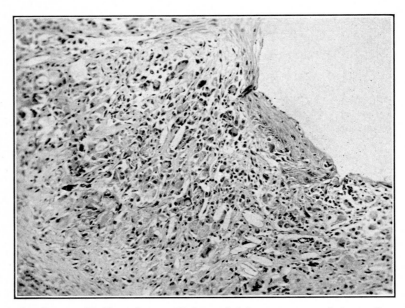

Fig. 782.—Ruptured epidermal cyst. Cholesterol clefts, squames, and giant cell reaction.

character of the lesion may not be recognized. There may be pronounced proliferation of the epithelium lining the dermal cysts with a simulation of carcinoma. Many of the cells may die but preserve their form and arrangement as is seen in an infarct of the kidney. This is known by the somewhat fanciful name of *mummifying epithelioma*. In other cases the cells become calcified, and the lesion is then a *calcifying epithelioma*. In rare cases there may be the development of a true carcinoma from the lining of a dermal cyst.

MILIUM.—This is a tiny white lesion of the *epidermis* no larger than a millet seed occurring in crops on the skin of the face, eyelid and genitalia. Each milium consists of a horny cyst developed in connection with the hair follicles, and may represent either a hyperkeratosis of the epithelium of the follicle or the retention products of sebaceous glands.

COLLOID MILIUM.—This condition is also known as colloid pseudomilium to distinguish it from the much more common true milium with which it has no relation, for it is a lesion of the *dermis*, not the epidermis. It takes the form of groups of lemon-yellow nodules the size of a millet seed or pin's head usually on the face and the backs of the hands of elderly persons. It represents a degeneration of the collagen and elastic tissue of the dermis. *Microscopically* the lesions

are sharply defined hyaline or colloid masses in the dermal papillæ suggesting deposits of amyloid, which stain intensely blue with thionine, although remaining unstained with ordinary connective tissue stains. It seems probable, although not certain, that the material is a mixture of collacin and elacin, collacin being a degeneration product of collagen, as elacin is a similar product of the elastin of which elastic fibers are composed.

SKIN MANIFESTATIONS OF INTERNAL DISEASES

The skin is a mirror of the health of the body. In this mirror may be reflected a wide variety of internal disorders. The skin has indeed been described as a mast from which signals of distress are flown. The subject is so vast that it would be absurd to attempt to do more than merely to allude to it here. Details can be found in Wiener's book.

Disorders of the *endocrine glands* may manifest themselves in the skin. Examples are the pigmentation of Addison's disease, the cutaneous and subcutaneous infiltration of myxedema, the hypertrichosis of adrenal cortical tumors, and the striæ of Cushing's disease. The pigmentation of *hemochromatosis* and *jaundice* becomes visible in the skin. *Pregnancy* is also associated with skin pigmentation and increased secretion of the sebaceous glands. In the *lymphoblastomas* such as lymphatic leukemia and Hodgkin's disease there may be infiltrations in the skin. *Metabolic disorders* such as diabetes and the lipidoses may be associated with xanthomatous skin lesions. The rash of the *acute exanthemata* is the most characteristic feature of these infections. The dermatological manifestations of the *chronic granulomata* such as syphilis and leprosy may be pathognomonic. Erythema induratum and crops of fleabitten petechiæ point to tuberculosis and subacute bacterial endocarditis respectively. Skin rashes, characteristic or otherwise, may be the result of *drug intoxication*. And so on, and so on. Actually, practically all systemic disorders may have cutaneous signs and symptoms.

All of which proves, if proof were needed, that the skin is indeed one of the most remarkable and important structures in the entire body.

REFERENCES

ALLEN, A. C.: Cancer, 1949, *2*, 28. (Histogenesis of nevi.)

ALLEN, A. C. and SPITZ, S.: Cancer, 1953, *6*, 1. (Nevi and melanoma.)

BEERMAN, H.: Am. J. Med. Sci., 1948, *216*, 458. (Diffuse scleroderma.)

BERKHEISER, F. W. and RAPPOPORT, A. E.: Am. J. Path., 1952, *28*, 477. (Histogenesis of nevi.)

BIRT, A. R. and NICKERSON, M.: Arch. Dermatol., 1959, *80*, 311. (Flushing of skin with urticaria pigmentosa.)

BUNTING, H., STRAUSS, M. J. and BOXFIELD, W. G.: Am. J. Path., 1952, *28*, 985. (Verruca vulgaris.)

CALNAN, C. D. and HABER, H.: J. Path. and Bact., 1955, *69*, 61. (Molluscum sebaceum; keratoacanthoma.)

CURRIE, A. R. and SMITH, J. F.: J. Path. and Bact., 1952, *64*, 827. (Spontaneous-healing squamouscell carcinoma.)

GATES, O., WARREN, S. and WARVI, W. N.: Am. J. Path., 1943, *19*, 591. (Tumors of sweat glands.)

GHADIALLY, F. N.: J. Path. and Bact., 1958, *75*, 441. (Keratoacanthoma in man compared with experimental lesions in the rabbit.)

GROSS, R. E. and WOLBACH, S. B.: Am. J. Path., 1943, *19*, 533. (Sclerosing hemangioma.)

HARTZ, P. H.: Am. J. Clin. Path., 1946, *16*, 385. (Myoepithelioma.)

LEVER, W. F. and CASTLEMAN, B.: Am. J. Path., 1952, *28*, 691. (Myoepithelioma.)

LEVER, W. F.: *Histopathology of the Skin*, Philadelphia, 2nd ed., 1954.

MASSON, P.: Cancer, 1951, *4*, 9. (Histogenesis of nevi.)

ORMSBY, O. S. and MONTGOMERY, H.: *Diseases of the Skin*, Philadelphia, 8th ed., 1948.

SHELDON, W. H.: Arch. Path., 1941, *31*, 326. (Myoepithelioma.)

SWARM, R. L. and GERMUTH, F. G., JR.: Am. J. Path., 1953, *29*, 577. (Diffuse scleroderma.)

WALLACE, S. A. and HALPERT, B.: Arch. Path., 1950, *50*, 199. (Basal-cell carcinoma.)

WIENER, K.: *Systemic Associations and Treatment of Skin Diseases*, St. Louis, 1947.

Chapter 47

Dental Pathology

General Considerations
Dental Caries
Periapical Tissue Infection
  Acute Apical Periodontitis
  Dental Granuloma
  Rarefying Osteitis
Periodontal Disease
  Gingivitis

Acute necrotizing gingivitis
Periodontitis
Periodontosis
**Extension of Odontogenic
  Infection**
  Osteitis
  Deep Neck Infections
  Maxillary Sinusitis

Focal Infection
Cysts of the Jaws
  Radicular Cyst
  Follicular Cyst
  Anterior Median Cyst
Odontogenic Tumors of the Jaws
  Odontomas
  Ameloblastoma:
    Adamantinoma

ALTHOUGH the care of the teeth belongs to the dental profession, the well-educated doctor should know at least something of the principal diseases of these structures, more particularly dental caries, periapical abscess and periodontitis, as well as of the more common cysts and odontogenic tumors of the jaws. A mere outline of these various conditions is all that is attempted in the following pages, for my own knowledge of dental disease takes me no farther. The pathology of the soft parts of the mouth has already been discussed in Chapter 25, where such conditions as inflammation, the granulomata, and neoplasms are considered.

GENERAL CONSIDERATIONS

The teeth are homologous to the dermal scales of certain fish, and to such appendages of the mammalian skin as the hair and nails. A hair is a horny structure composed of epithelial cells resting on a papilla of connective tissue containing blood vessels and nerves. A tooth is a calcified structure formed by epithelial cells resting on a papilla of connective tissue; the outer part of this dental papilla becomes calcified to form the dentin, the inner part remaining as the dental pulp supplied with vessels and nerves.

A tooth is composed of four structures: (1) enamel, (2) dentin, (3) pulp (the formative tissue of the dentin), and (4) cementum. The *enamel* is the hardest of animal tissues, but it is brittle and easily fractured. The *dentin* forms the main bulk of the tooth; it is strong and elastic, therefore not readily broken. Such a specialized tooth as the elephant's tusk consists of dentin without any covering of enamel, as it is designed for digging and fighting, functions for which toughness is needed and brittleness is undesirable. The dentin is traversed by great numbers of fine channels known as the dentinal tubules which pass from the pulp outward to the inner surface of the enamel and cementum. As the dentin is formed from the dental connective tissue papilla it is mesodermal in origin.

The *pulp* represents the remains of the formative organ of the dentin. The outer layer next the dentin contains specialized tall columnar connective cells, the *odontoblasts*, with long cytoplasmic fibrils which extend into the dentinal tubules; these are the only columnar connective tissue cells in the body. In addition to the odontoblasts, the pulp contains numerous ordinary connective tissue cells and abundant blood vessels, lymphatics, and nerves. The nerves end around the odontoblasts, but do not penetrate into the dentin, so that the odontoblasts form a connecting link between the sensitive dentin and the nerves. The nerves of the pulp respond in only one way when the dentin is stimulated by touch, heat or cold, and that is by pain. It is evident from what has been said that the constitution of the pulp enables that structure to develop a marked inflammatory reaction against bacterial infection, whereas no such reaction is possible in the avascular and acellular dentin and enamel.

The *cementum*, which closely resembles bone histologically, covers the dentin in the root portion of the tooth, and meets the enamel at the gingival line. It furnishes an attachment for the strong connective tissue fibers which fasten the root of the tooth to the bone of the alveolus.

The *peridontal membrane* or *pericementum*, which may be regarded as the periosteum of the tooth, is the fibrous connection between the bone and the cementum of the root. It is abundantly supplied with nerves which are responsible for the sensation felt when the tooth is touched. Atrophy of this membrane is followed by loosening of the tooth in its socket. Its normal functions may be summarized as nutrition, retention, cushioning, and tactile sense.

Three features in the anatomical arrangements are worthy of special mention in view of their possible relation to the development of disease. (1) The pulp is contained in a rigid space, which does not permit expansion. (2) Circulation is of the endarterial type, so that the tissue supplied is prone to infarction. (3) The blood vessels of the pulp are wide and anastomose freely, but they are of capillary structure, and it is difficult to distinguish between arterial and venous channels. Circulatory collapse is therefore readily brought about. These three features serve to account for the frequency with which death of the pulp occurs after the onset of an acute pulpitis. The absence of tactile sensory nerve endings in the dentin perhaps serves to explain why a patient is unable to locate an early toothache with accuracy.

DENTAL CARIES

Caries or dental decay is the most prevalent of all the diseases of the teeth. It has existed from prehistoric and early historic times. It is found in the teeth of Egyptian mummies. It is world-wide in its distribution, but certain races are remarkably exempt, *e.g.*, African natives and Eskimos. When these peoples adopt the diet of civilization, however, they develop caries. The teeth are the hardest structures in the body, yet, under modern living conditions, the most perishable. The etiology of caries is a singularly complex subject involving a large number of factors both local and constitutional, a consideration of which will be

85

postponed until the process itself has been described. Caries is primarily a disease of childhood, adolescents and young adults. The greatest susceptibility is at the period of the eruption of the teeth, the maximum incidence being in the interval of transition from the deciduous to the permanent teeth. The disease is commonest in the molars, then the upper incisors, then the bicuspids; the lower incisors and canines are rarely affected.

Lesions.—Dental caries is a unique process unlike any other in human pathology. It must not be confused with caries of bone, which is an inflammatory reaction to infection, for we have already seen that neither the enamel nor the dentin contains the vessels and connective tissue cells without which an inflammatory reaction is not possible. Caries may take either of two forms. The first, commonest between the ages of ten and sixteen, involves pits and fissures on the surface of the tooth, there is a very small point of entrance, and the progress is very rapid. The second, which occurs in late adolescence, involves the smooth surface of the tooth, the point of entrance is large, and the progress of the disease is correspondingly slow.

The tissues affected by caries are the enamel, the dentin, and the cementum, with secondary infection of the pulp. The enamel consists almost wholly of inorganic material (salts), whereas the dentin consists of 30 per cent organic matter (collagen and elastin). The pathogenesis of cavity formation in these two structures will differ accordingly. The mineral salts of the enamel are soluble in acids, and it is by acids that they are dissolved in caries. These acids are produced from the carbohydrates of the food by acid-forming bacteria, and the opportunity for the acids to act is afforded by the presence of fissures or defects on the occlusal surface (Fig. 783). In other cases the process commences on the lateral surface at the point of contact of two contiguous teeth, both of the teeth being commonly affected. The acid (lactic, malic, formic, acetic) dissolves the cement substance of the enamel at the bottom of the fissure, and a localized area of disintegration is produced which is wedge-shaped, with the

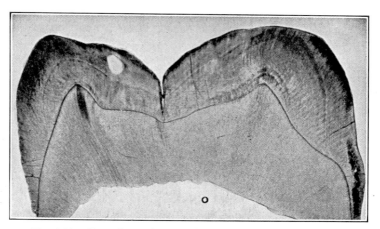

FIG. 783.—Deep fissure in enamel of occlusal surface. (Noyes.)

apex at the surface and the base toward the enamel-dentin junction. When the process reaches the dentin it proceeds more rapidly and more widely, spreading laterally along the line of junction owing to the branching of the dentinal tubules, and deeply into the dentin along the line of these tubules. The inorganic matter is here also dissolved, and again the area of disintegration is wedge-shaped, but this time with the base at the enamel-dentin junction and the apex toward the pulp. The bacteria spread readily along the dentinal tubules, so that the pulp is always potentially infected in every case in which the dentin is involved (Fig. 784). The organic matrix of the dentin is digested by proteolytic ferments of bacteria, which are either the original invaders or organisms of another group representing a secondary infection. As a result of the combined process a large area of dentin may be destroyed with the formation of a cavity of considerable size, although the original lesion in the enamel may still be quite small. Eventually the remainder of the enamel may cave in, resulting in a sudden marked enlargement of the cavity. The process is a steadily progressive one, as neither the enamel nor the dentin is capable of resistance or repair, although a formation of "secondary dentin" may be laid down between the dentin and the pulp, reducing the size of the pulp cavity; even this reaction is impossible in a devitalized tooth. The pain of caries is due to the inflam-

matory reaction which results from infection of the pulp.

Etiology.—The essence of dental caries is decalcification of the inorganic salts of which the tooth is for the most part composed. It is a local process or chain of processes determined by a number of local factors. These may be exciting or predisposing. There is general agreement that the *exciting cause* is bacterial infection with acid-producing organisms, which cause fermentation of refined carbohydrates retained as food débris in stagnant areas around the teeth with the elaboration of organic acids that attack the enamel. Rats reared in a germ-free environment develop no caries, despite being maintained on a "cariogenic" diet for a period of five months. When the mouth is touched with a swab containing enterococci, belonging to the same family as lactobacilli and capable of elaborating lactic acid, all the animals develop caries (Orland *et al.*). *Lactobacillus acidophilus* has been incriminated in particular, but it is highly probable that other acid-producing organisms may also be responsible in bringing about digestion of the organic matrix of the dentin.

Of *predisposing causes* it is quite evident that a *faulty diet* is all-important. Caries is essentially a disease of civilization, although primitive peoples are not free of it, nor were prehistoric peoples. It is the diet of civilization, particularly finely ground white flour, sugar and starchy foods, which is the culprit.

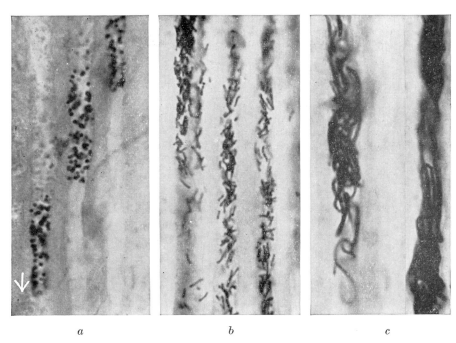

a b c

FIG. 784.—Microörganisms in different dentinal tubules of the same carious tooth (Gram stain). Magnification × 900.

  a.—Tubules containing groups of cocci.

  b.—Tubules containing a large number of short rods (bacilli).

  c.—Tubules containing tortuous filaments. (Courtesy of W. H. G. Logan in Boyle, *Kronfeld's Histopathology of the Teeth,* Lea & Febiger.)

Two striking examples of this truth come to mind. (1) The inhabitants of the Swiss village of Goms, high in the Alps, remained unchanged and completely isolated for two thousand years untouched by war or pestilence. They were farmers who lived on the produce of the soil and the meat of cattle. Wheat and fruit did not grow because of the high altitude. The native population was practically free of caries. Then came a road, a railway and stores with modern food stuffs, and at once dental decay became prevalent, with the incidence highest close to the railroad and lowest far up in the mountains. (2) In the little island of Tristan da Cunha, isolated in the south Atlantic, there is a community of white people with less caries than anywhere else in the world, and on this island no cereals can be grown owing to an infestation with rodents. It is of interest to note that there is not a single tooth brush on the island. In concentration camps dental decay ceases, possibly because of the absence of sugar in the diet.

Anatomical defects in the shape of occlusal fissures in the enamel give the bacteria the opportunity to work unmolested with no danger of the acids they produce being washed away by the saliva. These defects may have a genetic basis, for there is evidence of a *hereditary susceptibility* or resistance to the disease. *Local hygiene* plays a part. While it is not true that a clean tooth is necessarily a healthy one, it stands to reason that continued removal of food débris will tend to prevent the establishment of the conditions favorable to the development of caries. The saliva is a local factor which may be of great importance. In some mouths lactobacilli fail to flourish even when repeatedly introduced. This may depend on the pH of the saliva, or on other salivary factors so far undetermined. When caries begins on a smooth enamel surface it is due to the formation of a *dental plaque*, a colony of bacteria which becomes attached to the surface as the result of some property of the saliva. The acids formed under this plaque are prevented from diffusing, and act locally on the enamel. Thus *immunity to caries* may be due to faultless enamel, or to the fact that the environmental conditions are inimical to the growth of saprophytes in spite of the presence of deep fissures in the enamel. From the above brief review it is evident that we can agree with the statement that "the complete story of the causation of dental caries cannot yet be written" (Appleton).

Fluorine in drinking water has an inverse relationship to the incidence of caries in a community. Before this was discovered a direct relationship had been recognized between the concentration of fluorine in water and the occurrence of *mottled enamel*. If the teeth are only slightly affected, the enamel is dull, opaque, and chalky white, in more severe cases the enamel shows a yellow or light brown discoloration, while in the worst cases it is dark brown or almost black. The concentration of fluorine in the drinking water depends on the fluorine contained in the soil in the form of soluble fluorides of calcium, sodium and potassium. The condition develops during the period of enamel formation, and is present when the teeth erupt. The surface of the tooth is generally smooth and even, although histologically the enamel structure is defective, with incomplete calcification of the enamel rods and the deposition of brown pigment between the rods.

Mottling when pronounced is unsightly and even disfiguring, but, in spite of their defective structure, mottled teeth are strangely resistant to caries. High fluoride concentrations in the water supply which result in mottling are not necessary for the prevention of caries. The teeth of children who throughout life have used drinking water containing 1 part per million of fluoride show little or no mottling, yet the caries rate is as low as in children in a high fluoride area, and about one-third as much as in children brought up on fluoride-free water. The topical application of a solution of sodium fluoride to the teeth has given good results. Fluoride adsorbed or bound in the enamel or dentin lowers the solubility of these tissues to acids and thus prevents the onset of dental decay. It can also inhibit enzymatic processes of bacteria, the acid products of which serve to initiate the carious process.

"If we are to prevent caries we must seek to break the chain of processes which cause the lesion" (Darling). This, of course, is easier said than done. It is not a simple matter to eliminate all stagnation of food, to neutralize all lactic acid, or to inhibit all enzymes. The use of fluoride in drinking may be a faltering step in the right direction.

PERIAPICAL TISSUE INFECTION

We have already seen that when the integrity of the enamel is destroyed, infection readily passes along the dentinal tubules to reach the pulp. The result may vary from a mild pulpitis to severe suppuration, necrosis and gangrene of the pulp. The infection tends to extend through the apical foramen which admits the vessels and nerves, and may set up an acute periodontitis or a chronic apical periodontitis (dental granuloma).

Acute Apical Periodontitis.—This is likely to take the form of an abscess at the root of the tooth. The abscess may remain circumscribed as a *root abscess* (Fig. 785), or the suppuration may spread into the surrounding bone with the formation of an *alveolar abscess*. Such an abscess tends to discharge into the mouth either on the lingual or the labial side of the alveolar process. When the abscess is in the mandible, it may discharge on the skin surface. The regional submaxillary lymph nodes are swollen and tender.

Dental Granuloma.—A *dental granuloma* or *chronic apical periodontitis* is a condition characterized by the formation of a mass of chronic inflammatory tissue around the apex of a tooth (Fig. 786). It therefore contains polymorphonuclear leukocytes, lymphocytes, plasma cells, mononuclear phagocytes, and fibroblasts in varying proportion, and is surrounded by a connective tissue capsule which blends with the healthy periodontal membrane, thus uniting the "growth" to the tooth. More distinctive is the presence of masses of squamous epithelium, probably derived from the "paradental epithelial debris" of Malassez (Fig. 787). These are ce

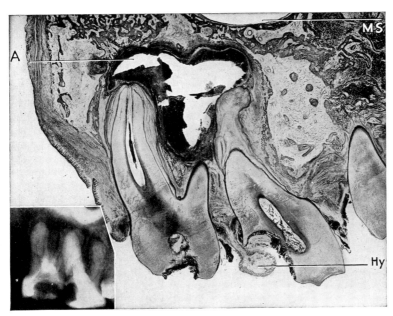

FIG. 785.—Exacerbation of chronic periapical inflammation and formation of an acute abscess. Mesio-distal section through the posterior portion of the maxilla. Second and third molar with decomposed infected pulps. The roentgenogram in the lower left corner shows the carious destruction of the crowns and the extensive periapical bone destruction. *A*, abscess cavity extending over the lingual roots of both molars; *MS*, floor of the maxillary sinus; *Hy*, hyperplastic gum tissue located in the cavity of the distal side of the second molar (gingival polyp). (Boyle, *Kronfeld's Histopathology of the Teeth*, Lea & Febiger.)

clusters found almost constantly in the periodontal membrane, and represent the remains of the enamel organ which extends as an epithelial sheath around the root (sheath of Hertwig) before the eruption of the tooth. The epithelial masses may proliferate as the result of the chronic irritation, and finally undergo cystic degeneration to form dental or radicular cysts (Fig. 788). The granuloma seldom if ever undergoes spontaneous resolution. The fibrous capsule and proliferated epithelium must be eradicated. In the majority of cases the affected tooth can be saved by adequate root canal therapy and resection of the apical lesion.

Rarefying Osteitis.—If the virulence of the infection and the acuteness of the reaction is less than in alveolar abscess but greater than in granuloma the result may be the condition known as rarefying osteitis. The inflammatory exudate at the apex of the tooth is not limited by a fibrous membrane, so that it infiltrates the adjoining bone. Thrombosis of the small nutrient vessels results in is-

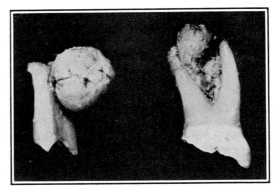

FIG. 786.—Two examples of dental granuloma. (Hill, *Oral Pathology.*)

chemic necrosis of bone and the formation of small sequestra with a foreign body giant cell reaction. If the exudate extends to the surface, it forms the subacute swelling known as a *gumboil*. In the upper jaw the osteitis process may destroy the floor of the antrum and set up a *maxillary sinusitis*.

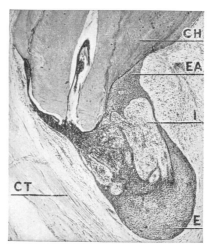

Fig. 787.—Dental granuloma, showing a solid mass of epithelium at the root end. *E*, epithelial proliferation; *I*, inflammatory cell infiltration between the epithelial strands. (Boyle, *Kronfeld's Histopathology of the Teeth*, Lea & Febiger.)

PERIODONTAL DISEASE

The periodontium comprises the investing and supporting tissues which surround the tooth, namely, the periodontal membrane, the gingiva and the alveolar bone. Disease affecting these structures may be inflammatory, degenerative, or a combination of inflammation and degeneration.

Gingivitis.—The gingiva is the mucous membrane covering the alveolar processes and surrounding the neck of each tooth. It resembles the skin both in its histology and in its pathological reactions. Gingivitis is therefore analagous to dermatitis. It may be caused by trauma (food impaction between the teeth, excessive or improper use of the toothbrush, calcareous deposits on the teeth in contact with the gingival tissue), bacterial infection, the excessive use of tobacco (pipe and cigarettes), and systemic disturbances such as general infections and the acute infective fevers. The great majority of cases occur in unclean mouths, and are associated with an accumulation of *calculus* in the gingival crevice. Indeed calculus is often the main source of irritation. Calcium salts are deposited from the saliva in such organic material as desquamated epithelial cells, food débris, mucin from the saliva, and masses of

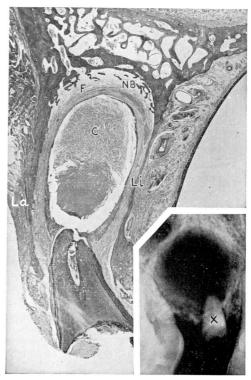

Fig. 788.—Radicular cyst formed at the apex of retained root fragment. The roentgenogram shows a large round area of bone destruction. Upper cuspid; aged fifty-six years. *C*, cyst cavity containing cholesterol; *F*, fibrous capsule; *NB*, trabeculæ of new bone; *La*, *Li*, thin labial and lingual bone plates. (Kronfeld, Australian Dental Congress.)

microörganisms. The first deposits are on the crowns of the teeth, and then in the gingival crevices. They are most marked on the lower anterior teeth opposite the openings of the submaxillary and sublingual glands and the upper posterior teeth opposite the opening of the parotid duct. The deposit can be removed by the use of the tooth brush within twelve hours, but not after that time.

The *lesions* resemble those of dermatitis. The connective tissue papillæ are elongated and close to the surface so that their distended capillaries readily rupture. If the surface epithelium is eroded by trauma or ulceration, bleeding from the gums may be expected. In the severe cases there is a marked infiltration of the tunica propria and the epithelium with polymorphonuclears together with edema. In the chronic cases, due to continued infection or mechanical trauma, the gingiva becomes markedly thickened and elevated owing to hyperplasia of the epithelium and connective tissue so that it bulges between and around the teeth. Hyperplastic gingivitis may be associated with hyperplasia of adenoid tissue and habitual mouth breathing. The continued administration of dilantin may lead to marked gingival hyperplasia for reasons at present unknown.

Acute Necrotizing Gingivitis.—This is often called *trench mouth*, because of its prevalence in the trench warfare of World War I. It is a necrotizing inflammation which detroys the gingiva between the teeth and results in the production of a gray pseudomembranous slough. It does not occur in a mouth lacking teeth. Pain, a fetid odor to the breath, and bleeding from the affected gum at the slightest touch, are among the distressing clinical features.

The *etiology* is obscure. Vincent's fusiform bacilli and various spirochetes are readily demonstrated, but it is not certain what part they play in the process, for the condition is not contagious, nor can it be transmitted from one person to another. Local depression of resistance from nutritional deficiency, debilitating disease, or some unknown factor seems to be a necessary antecedent.

The Achilles heel of the oral mucosa is the gingival sulcus, the shallow groove around the tooth bounded on one side by the tooth and on the other by the squamous epithelium of the gingiva. It is here that the soft tissues meet the tooth, and it is here, if the epithelium is damaged, that infection can reach the deeper periodontal tissue along the lymphatics of the periodontal membrane. Reference to the gingival sulcus brings us to the subject of periodontitis.

Periodontitis.—This very common condition used to be known as *pyorrhea alveolaris*, but that was a misnomer, for pyorrhea signifies a flow of pus, and most periodontal lesions have no visible purulent discharge. The condition is entirely unrelated to caries. Caries is a disease of the teeth, and is most likely to develop in the young. Periodontitis is a disease of the surroundings of the

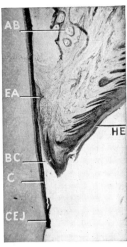

FIG. 789.—Normal gingival crevice. The depth of the crevice is practically zero. *CEJ,* cementoenamel junction; *C,* cementum; *BC,* bottom of gingival crevice located on the cementum; *EA,* epithelial attachment to the cementum; *HE,* hornification of the gingival epithelium; *AB,* alveolar bone. (Boyle, *Kronfeld's Histopathology of the Teeth,* Lea & Febiger.)

teeth, and develops after the age of thirty-five. In Tristan da Cunha, where caries is almost nonexistent, periodontal disease is quite prevalent.

Periodontitis is a chronic, progressive, inflammatory destruction of the periodontal tissue, and it is the greatest single cause of loss of teeth in the adult. The starting point is the formation of a *periodontal pocket,* which is at first an apparently innocent deepening of the normal gingival sulcus around the tooth. This seems to be the result of a persistent chronic gingivitis. Excessive lateral stress to a tooth due to malocclusion may also play a part (Figs. 789 and 790). Infection and inflammation extend along the lymphatics of the periodontal membrane. Proteolytic enzymes from the disintegrating leukocytes of the inflammatory exudate cause dissolution of the gingival fibers and the collagen fibers of the periodontal membrane. The formation of ulcers and minute abscesses leads to rapid detachment of the tissue along one side of the tooth. The resulting pocket, narrow at the opening on the surface but becoming wider toward the bottom, is filled with necrotic

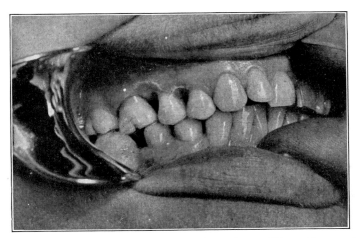

FIG. 790.—Deep periodontal pockets on mesial of first molar and second bicuspid upper, due to traumatic occlusion of lower second molar. (Gabel, *American Textbook of Operative Dentistry.*)

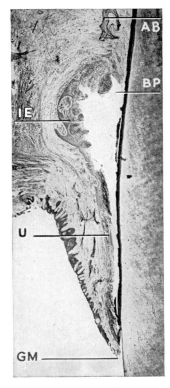

FIG. 791.—Periodontitis on the labial side of an upper cuspid. The arrow indicates the direction of the occlusal stress. On the labial surface there is a supracrestal pocket of about 7 mm. in depth; on the lingual surface the depth of the crevice is minimal. General view of the cuspid. Labio-lingual section. *GM*, gingival margin; *BP*, bottom of pocket on the labial side; *PM*, periodontal membrane; *AB*, alveolar bone. (Boyle, *Kronfeld's Histopathology of the Teeth*, Lea & Febiger.)

epithelium which provides an ideal culture medium for bacteria, so that a vicious circle is set up. Epithelium proliferates along the tooth surface, migrating toward the apex of the tooth (Fig. 791). The bone underlying the pocket is in a state of low grade chronic osteitis with osteclastic bone resorption, but no necrosis. With resorption of much of the alveolar process and destruction of the periodontium, loss of the tooth is inevitable unless adequate treatment is instituted, namely removal of the outer wall to the bottom of the pocket.

Periodontosis.—Periodontosis, as its name suggests, is a degenerative rather than an inflammatory process. It is as unusual as periodontitis is common. The supporting structures of the teeth are alveolar bone, cementum and periodontal membrane. Normally these can withstand not only the strain of mastication, but also unusual stresses and forces, the bone responding by increasing in density and the periodontal membrane becoming exceedingly strong. But this ability to respond varies from person to person, and it also varies with the state of health and nutrition. Failure to respond to functional stress leads to the condition known as *diffuse atrophy of alveolar bone*, with resorption of the bone supporting the apical two-thirds of the root of the tooth and conversion of the periodontium into loose connective tissue (Fig. 792). The inevitable result is loosening of the teeth with so-called *migration* and *lateral drifting*. The factors responsible are guessed at rather than known. The condition is most common in adolescence and early maturity, particularly in the female. This suggests a lack

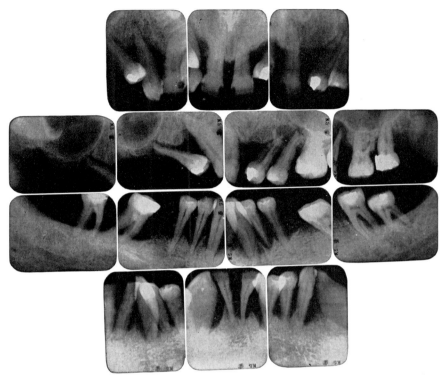

Fig. 792.—Radiograph showing extensive loss of supporting bone and drifting teeth which is the end result of long standing periodontal disease. An extreme loss of bone jeopardizes the wearing of dentures. (Kerr and Ash, *Oral Pathology*, Lea & Febiger.)

of androgenic steroid hormones. It is well known that ascorbic acid is necessary for the health of connective tissues, so that vitamin C deficiency has been suggested. Other nutritional as well as genetic factors have been suggested. In short we know little or nothing definite about the etiology and pathogenesis of periodontosis.

EXTENSION OF ODONTOGENIC INFECTION

Infection from a neglected periapical abscess may spread to surrounding structures and there cause serious damage. Three complications which deserve notice are osteitis, deep neck infections, and maxillary sinusitis.

Osteitis.—Inflammation of the jaws may be due to infection from a root canal, along the periodontal structures, or from the socket of an extracted tooth. This complication has largely disappeared owing to the use of antibiotics. A serious form of the

disease is that which follows radiation therapy of intra-oral cancer. In the jaws the sequestrum is rarely entirely surrounded by new bone (involucrum), which forms only beneath it and at the sides. As a result, when the sequestrum becomes separated it is extruded on the surface and healing occurs with remarkable rapidity.

Heavy therapeutic doses of radiation in the oral cavity present an especial dental problem. The destruction of the major salivary glands causes a severe xerostomia with consequent drop in pH of the remaining saliva. There follows a severe and rapid decalcification of remaining teeth which in turn leads to exposure of dental pulps and consequent infection. Instead of the usual local osteitis, a full blown *osteomyelitis* is likely to develop in the ischemic bone. This is one situation where the dentist may recommend extracting all remaining teeth prior to the radiation therapy.

Deep Neck Infections.—Any oral infection may spread into the face or down into the neck. It may take the form of localized abscess or a spreading cellulitis. An *abscess*, caused as a rule by staphylococci, is likely to arise from a periapical abscess, occasionally from an osteomyelitis. It will open either on the oral mucosa or on the skin. *Cellulitis*, called a phlegmon when severe, is a spreading inflammation of the connective tissue of the face and neck caused by fibrinolytic streptococci. The starting point is usually the lower jaw, but the infraorbital region may be involved from a maxillary tooth. It is through the loose connective tissue that the streptococci make their way most readily, and this is most abundant in the carotid sheath and in the lateral pharyngeal, submaxillary, sublingual and retropharyngeal spaces. These spaces are formed by the deep cervical fascia and its extensions. It is this fascia which governs the spread of infections in the neck. It ensheaths all the neck muscles and thus protects them. The fascial space superficial to the myohyoid muscle is large and extends across the neck to the other side, whereas the space deep to the muscle is much smaller and does not cross to the other side. *Ludwig's angina* is a rare form of severe phlegmon which involves the whole neck. Although usually a complication of one of the streptococcal fevers, it may occasionally arise from a mandibular molar tooth infection.

Maxillary Sinusitis.—Infection of the maxillary sinus or antrum usually comes from the nose, but in 10 per cent or more of cases it is said to be of dental origin. The roots of the first molar and second premolar and usually those of the second molar are immediately under the floor of the antrum, so that it is not remarkable that a periapical abscess of these teeth should occasionally discharge into the cavity and set up a sinusitis, either acute or chronic.

FOCAL INFECTION

The term focal infection as commonly used does not indicate merely a focus of infection but signifies the setting up of secondary infection at a distance from the original lesions. With such a focus there are the following theoretical possibilities: (1) The bacteria may pass into the lymphatics and cause lymphadenitis of the regional lymph nodes. (2) They may enter the blood stream, multiply there, and set up an acute or chronic septicemia. (3) They may not multiply in the blood, but may settle in some distant part and multiply there. This is what is usually known as focal infection. (4) They may remain localized, but their toxins may be absorbed and set up degenerative and fibrotic changes in distant organs.

There has been difference of opinion as to the common type of dental infection involved. Chronic periapical infection (root abscess, dental granuloma) used to be the most popular, but this has now been replaced by periodontal infection for the following reasons. (1) Periodontal lesions are commoner than dental granuloma. (2) There is a greater contact area with adjacent vascular and lymphatic channels. (3) Mechanical trauma is constantly present because of chewing. (4) The dental granuloma is a physically protected area where many organisms are destroyed and the numbers entering the blood stream are minor compared to those derived from mechanical pumping of teeth adjacent to a periodontal pocket.

The observations and conclusions of Fish and MacLean on the relation of oral streptococci to focal infection are remarkably interesting. They found that cultures from the roots of extracted teeth, irrespective of the condition of the tooth, always showed streptococci, although there was no microscopic evidence of inflammation in the periapical tissue. The conclusion they draw is that the germs gain entrance to the root during extraction. In chronic infection the streptococci are confined to a necrotic nidus surrounded by leukocytes or they may take refuge in the dental canals. Thus a position of stalemate is established: the leukocytes are killed if they go in and the streptococci are killed if they venture out. The organisms do not live in the living dental and paradental tissues, but they irritate them with their toxins. Fish and MacLean made the remarkable observation that streptococci appear in the blood within five minutes of extracting teeth in patients with periodontitis, and even chewing hard candies has the same effect of pumping germs from the infected gums into the blood. The blood soon becomes sterile, sometimes in ten minutes.

The crux of the problem of focal infection can be expressed in one question: Does transient bacteremia cause or aggravate systemic conditions? (Mitchell and Helman.) Almost every conceivable lesion has at one time or another been attributed to foci of infection in connection with the teeth. The following list of diseases is less open to criticism than the lengthy lists often drawn up by the enthusiastic advocates of focal infection; rheumatoid arthritis, myositis, endocarditis, nephritis, iritis and iridocyclitis. The problem is usually attacked from the angle of the patient suffering, say, from arthritis, and, as might be expected, roentgen-ray examinations will often reveal the presence of a quiet periapical granuloma. It is even more instructive to investigate the matter primarily from the dental standpoint. More than one large survey of university students with dental granulomas revealed by roentgen-ray films has been made, and such a survey has always showed that the persons with dental foci of infection have no more arthritis or heart disease than do the normal controls.

The concept of focal infection due to dental disease is not a new one for, as already mentioned in connection with the etiology of rheumatoid arthritis, the King of Assyria was advised by his physician 2500 years ago to have his teeth extracted because of the pains he suffered in his head and limbs. Since the day in 1910 when Sir William Hunter of London in an address to the medical students of McGill University first popularized the idea that dental infection might be responsible for inflammatory lesions in distant structures such as the heart, joints and muscles, the views of the medical and dental professions have fluctuated widely and wildly in relation to the subject. At one time removal of pulpless teeth for arthritis and rheumatism was as popular as removal of the appendix for discomfort in the right iliac fossa and of the ovaries for chronic pain in the female pelvis. The pendulum has now swung in the opposite direction. At the present time generalizations are dangerous as well as foolish. It is certainly the case that the relationship of dental infection with rheumatic and rheumatoid lesions has been greatly exaggerated, and that pulpless teeth with poorly filled root canals and chronic periapical infection may be completely harmless. It is equally true that just as a tuberculous bronchial lymph node may infect a distant kidney or bone, so may periapical infection result in inflammatory lesions of joints and other structures, especially in persons with a tendency, familial or otherwise, to systemic streptococcal infections with resulting lesions. The difficulty is to judge the frequency of this occurrence and to decide whether removal of infected teeth is likely to benefit the distant lesions. It would seem that each case must be decided on its own merits rather than on doubtful generalizations.

CYSTS OF THE JAWS

The true cysts of the jaws, which may be compared with cysts of the skin, arise from embryonal epithelial remnants. In the development of the tooth the crown is formed from the enamel organ. Downward extensions of the epithelium of the enamel constitute the sheath of Hertwig from which the apex of the tooth is derived. The tooth erupts towards the surface not continuously but in a series of fits and starts. With each of these bursts of growth little clusters of cells from the sheath of Hertwig are carried upwards with the connective tissue of the periodontal membrane. These clusters persist throughout the life of the tooth as the "epithelial débris" of Melassez, from which originate the lining of the dental cysts as well as the epithelial tumors of the jaws.

Of the epithelial cysts of the jaws, two, the radicular and the follicular, are odontogenic, being derived from epithelium that has been connected with the development of the tooth, whilst the third, the anterior median cyst, is derived from other epithelial remnants.

Radicular Cyst.—These cysts, also called *periodontal cysts*, are the most frequent of any that occur in the mouth. They are generally associated with chronic apical infection and develop in relation to a dental granuloma. The continued irritation of the infection appears to stimulate the remaining nests of cells of Hertwig's sheath (epithelial débris) to proliferate and fuse with the granuloma forming what has been termed an epitheliated granuloma. The center of the mass becomes necrosed, then liquefied, and finally converted into a cyst lined by squamous epithelium. The contents may be fluid or semi-solid containing cellular débris with cholesterol clefts and foreign body giant cells. If the infection remains active, the epithelium is destroyed, the lesion is surrounded by a fibrous wall, and the cyst remains small. If, however, the infection dies down, the epithelial wall persists, the cyst continues to grow expansively, and displaces the surrounding structures.

Follicular Cyst.—This lesion, also known as a *dentigerous cyst*, occurs in young persons and arises from the follicle of the developing tooth. It is always associated with an embedded tooth. The follicle consists of an inner epithelial lining and an outer connective tissue covering. If the follicle becomes detached from the crown, though adhering to the neck of the tooth, fluid collects between the crown and the follicle with the formation of a cyst and pressure atrophy of the alveolar bone. The cyst is similar in structure to the radicular variety, being lined by squamous epithelium with fluid or semi-solid contents, cholesterol clefts, and giant cells. As there is usually no inflammatory element, the cyst can continue to grow and may attain a very large size. If infection should occur, the epithelium is destroyed and the cyst remains small. A point of great clinical significance between radicular and dentigerous cysts is that the radicular cyst has no neoplastic potential, while the follicular cyst is the source of about one-third of ameloblastomas.

Anterior Median Cyst.—This lesion is not connected with a tooth and is therefore not an odontogenic cyst. It occurs in the midline of the maxilla, and may take one of two forms. The first is lined by squamous epithelium, the second by columnar ciliated epithelium. The squamous epithelium is derived from islands of cells which remain at the line of closure of the three parts of the developing palate, whilst the columnar ciliated epithelium is derived from the nasal part of the developing palatine duct. In both of these instances, therefore, the cysts arise from embryonal epithelial remnants.

This anterior median cyst is only one of half a dozen developmental cysts that differ only in anatomical position, and in which the lining epithelium may be either squamous or pseudostratified ciliated columnar.

ODONTOGENIC TUMORS OF THE JAWS

Tumors of the jaws may be odontogenic or non-odontogenic. Odontogenic tumors arise from the tooth or from embryonic structures from which the tooth originates. Non-odontogenic tumors are tumors of bone such as fibroma, fibrosarcoma, osteogenic sarcoma, giant cell tumor, etc. All of these have been described elsewhere.

Odontogenic tumors may be divided somewhat arbitrarily into odontomas and ameloblastomas or adamantinomas. The odontomas are tumors obviously connected with the teeth, whereas the ameloblastoma is a tumor of the jaw originating from epithelial remnants of the enamel organ, but with no obvious connection with a tooth. Many subdivisions and varieties of these tumors are recognized, but they concern the dental rather than the medical student.

Odontomas.—These lesions hardly deserve to be classified as true neoplasms, but rather as overgrowths of enamel, dentin, cementum, or a combination of these. They seem to originate in a disturbance of the dental follicle during the development of the tooth. If this disturbance occurs early, the enamel forming the crown is affected, if late, the dentin and cementum are involved. An enameloma, cementoma and dentinoma are recognized. The *enameloma* is the result of disturbance of the enamel organ during development. If this occurs before the enamel has begun to calcify, the tumor may be composed entirely of epithelial cells. The lesion is usually a mass of enamel attached to the tooth. The *cementoma* is much the commonest of the odontomas. It consists of a mass of cementum attached to the root of the tooth. It is an osteoma of dental origin. The *dentinoma* is an overgrowth of the root, and is the rarest of the odontomas.

Ameloblastoma: Adamantinoma.—This tumor has already been described on page 236, but reference must be made to it here. It is a rare tumor which, if untreated, may grow to an enormous size with extreme destruction of the jaw. It may be mainly solid or mainly cystic. The tumor is usually innocent, but there may be invasion and rarely metastases. The microscopic picture varies to a marked degree. When differentiation of the enamel organ is advanced there is an outer palisade layer of columnar cells, the ameloblasts, and a central core of "star cells" with large vacuoles and connecting cytoplasmic bridges (Fig. 132). In other cases the picture resembles that of a basal cell carcinoma. The *origin* of the tumor is considered to be from offshoots of cells from the enamel organ. Others consider that, at least in the basal cell type, the origin may be from the basal layer of the oral epithelium with which a continuity may be established.

REFERENCES

APPLETON, J. L. T.: *Bacterial Infection with Special Reference to Dental Practice*, Philadelphia, 4th ed., 1950.

DARLING, A. I.: Brit. Dent. J., 1959, *107*, 287. (Caries.)

FISH, E. W. and MACLEAN, I.: Brit. Dent. J., 1936, *61*, 336. (Focal infection.)

GABEL, A. B. edit: *Am. Textbook of Operative Dentistry*, 9th ed., Philadelphia, 1954.

HARDWICK, J. L.: Brit. Dent. J., 1960, *108*, 9. (Caries.)

HILL, T. J.: *Oral Pathology*, 4th ed., Philadelphia, 1949.

KERR, D. A. and ASH, M. M. Jr: *Oral Pathology*, Philadelphia, 1960.

KRONFELD, R.: *Histopathology of the Teeth*, 4th ed., edited by P. E. Boyle, Philadelphia, 1955.

MITCHELL, D. F. and HELMAN, E. Z.: J. Am. Dent. Ass., 1953, *46*, 32.

ORLAND, F. J., et al.: J. Am. Dent. Ass., 1955, *50*, 259. (Experimental caries in germ-free rats.)

Index

When more than one reference is given the principal reference is indicated by **heavy-faced type**, unless both are of equal importance.

A

ABDOMINAL wall, desmoid tumor of, 858
    lipoma of, 857
Abscess, 57
    alveolar, 1348
    cold, 1234
    healing of, 74
    of brain, 1153
    of liver, 814
    of lung, 653
    of tooth, 1348
    perinephritic, 589
    psoas, 428
    retropharyngeal, 705
    subphrenic, 854
Acanthosis, 1316
    nigricans, 1320
Acardiac fetus, 254
Acarus scabiei, 374
Achalasia of esophagus, 714
    of intestine, 777
Achlorhydria, 1046
Achondroplasia, 1247
Achylia gastrica, 1046
Acid-base balance, 552
Acid-fast bacilli, chromogenic, 661
Acid mucopolysaccharides, 80
Acids, corrosive, 427
Acoustic nerve tumor, 1203
Acromegaly, 978
Acrocyanosis, 1323
Actinomycosis, 317
    abdominal, 318
    cervicofacial, 317
    of intestine, 757
    of liver, 814
    of lung, 662
    thoracic, 318
Acute anterior poliomyelitis, 1168
Acute arthritis, 1270
Acute bacterial endocarditis, 463
Acute leukemia, 1082
Acute massive collapse of lung, 674
Acute necrotizing gingivitis, 1351
Adamantinoma, **236**, 1357
Adams-Stokes syndrome, 473
Addison's disease, 988
    idiopathic, 112
    pigmentation, in, 990
    relation of symptoms to lesions, 990
Adenocarcinoma, 232
Adenoid cystic epithelioma, 1331
Adenolymphoma of parotid, 711
Adenoma, 228
    of adrenal cortex, 995
    of bronchus, 691
    of kidney, 612
    of pancreas, 848

Adenoma, of parathyroid, 1029
    of pituitary, 973
    of thyroid, 1021
Adenomyosis of uterus, 906
Adenosine triphosphate, 1302
Adenoviruses, 336, 343
Adhesions, fibrinous, 74
    fibrous, 74
Adrenal, adenoma of, 995
    aldosterone, 982
    amyloidosis, 999
    carcinoma of, 995
    cortisone, 983
    ganglioneuroma of, 998
    glucocorticoids of, 982
    insufficiency, acute, 987
        chronic, 988
    massive hemorrhage of, 998
    mineralocorticoids, 982
    myelolipoma of, 999
    necrosis of, 998
    neuroblastoma of, 996
    nitrogen hormones of, 984
    noradrenalin, 984
    pheochromocytoma of, 997
    relation to pituitary, 984
    secondary tumors of, 998
    virilism, 993
Adrenocorticotrophic hormone, 979
Adreno-genital syndrome, 879, 903
Afibrinogenemia, 1078
Africa, cancer in, 195
Agammaglobulinemia, 101, **1043**
    and rheumatic arthritis, 1276
Agglutination test in rheumatoid arthritis, 1274
Agnogenic myeloid metaplasia, 1069, **1100**
Agranulocytosis, 1086
Air embolism, 146
Alarm reaction, 986
Alastrim, 338
Albers-Schönberg's disease, 1249
Albinism, 1320
Albright's syndrome, 1240
Alcohol, ethyl, 429
    methyl, 429
Alcoholic hyaline bodies, 796, 799
Alcoholism in hepatic cirrhosis, 796
Aldosteronoma, 994
Aldosterone, 982
Aldosteronism, 982
    primary, 993
    secondary, 994
Aleukemic leukemia, 1078
Alkaline phosphatase, 552
    in Paget's disease, 1243
Alkalis, caustic, 427
Alkylating agents as carcinogens, 185

Alleles, 432
Allergic encephalomyelitis, 1182
Allergy, 97, 102, 105
Alloxan diabetes, 833, **839**
Alpha cell tumor, 849
Alveolar abscess, 1348
Alveolar-capillary block, 633
Alveolar cell carcinoma, 690
    membranes of, 633
Alzheimer's disease, 1196
Amaurotic family idiocy, 1188
Amebic abscess of liver, 814
Amebic dysentery, 753
Ameloblastoma, 1357
Amniotic fluid embolism, 147
Ampulla of Vater, 828
Amylase, serum, 832, 836
Amyloid, 88
    degeneration of liver, 818
    nephrosis, 573
    staining reactions, 88
Amyloidosis, 88
    in plasma cell myeloma, 1262
    in rheumatoid arthritis, 1280
    localized, 93
    of adrenal, 999
    of myocardium, 490
    of spleen, 1101
    pathogenesis of, 93
    primary, 92
    secondary, 90
Amyotrophic lateral sclerosis, 1191
Anaerobic spore bearers, 311
Anamnestic reaction, 275
Anaphylaxis, 103
Anemia, aplastic, 1068
    chlorosis, 1054
    classification of, 1044
    congenital spherocytic, 1056
    Cooley's, 1062
    dibothriocephalus latus, 1051
    erythroblastic, 1062
    gastrectomy, 1052
    hemolytic, 1054
    immune antibody, 1063
    in glomerulonephritis, 566
    in Hodgkin's disease, 1117
    iron deficiency, 1052
    leuko-erythroblastic, 1069
    macrocytic, 1045
    malignancy, 1070
    microcytic hypochromic, 1052
    myelophthisic, 1069
    of chronic infection, 1070
    of chronic renal disease, 1070
    of lead poisoning, 1070
    of malignancy, 1070
    of pregnancy, 1052, 1070
    osteosclerotic, 1069
    pernicious, 1045
    pyridoxine deficiency, 1054

Anemia, secondary, 1069
  sickle cell, 1059
  sprue, 1051
Anencephalic fetus, 981
Anencephaly, 253, **1216**
Anenploidy, 875
Aneurysm, aortic, 532
  arteriovenous, 536
  atheromatous, 533
  dissecting, 534
  intracranial, 1147
  of sinus of Valsalva, 535
  syphilitic, 533
Aneurysmal bone cyst, 1265
Aneurysms, 532
Angina pectoris, 471
Angioma, 245, **540**
  capillary, 245
  cavernous, 245
  of bone, 1265
Angiomatosis, capillary of cere-
  bellum, 1206
  cavernous of cerebrum, 1206
Animal parasites, 355
Anisocytosis, 1047
Anitschkow myocyte, 454
Ankylosing spondylitis, 1282
  aortic lesion in, 457
Ankylostoma duodenale, 362
Anoxia, 164
  anemic, 164
  anoxic, 164
Anoxic nephrosis, 578
  pathogenesis of, 582
Anterior median cyst of jaw, 1356
Anterior spinal artery occlusion,
  1146
Anterior tibial syndrome, 1306
Anthracosis, 649
Anthrax, 311
Antibodies, 85, 99
  blocking, 1040
  fluorescent-labelled, 99
Anticoagulants, 127
Antidiuretic hormone, 551
Antigen-antibody complexes, 103
Antigens, 98
Anti-hemophilic factor, 1077
Anus, imperforate, 253
Aorta, aneurysm of, 532
  coarctation of, 478
  medionecrosis of, 516
  rheumatic disease of, 456
Aortic arch syndrome, **524**, 1138
  insufficiency, 486
  stenosis, 486
Aortitis, rheumatic, 456
  rheumatoid, 531
  syphilitic, 528
  undetermined etiology, 531
Aplastic anemia, 1068
Apocrine glands, 1315
Apoplexy, 1142
Appendicitis, acute, 758
  chronic, 761
  obliterans, 762
Appendix, carcinoid of, 772
  foreign bodies, 763
  in measles, 762
  mucocele of, 762
  oxyuris vermicularis, 763
Arachnodactyly, 1248
Argyll-Robertson pupil, 1177

Argyria, 405
Armanni-Ebstein lesion, **22**, 842
Arnold-Chiari malformation, 1133,
  1217
Arrhenoblastoma, 935
Arsenic poisoning, 428
Arterial hypertension, 517
Arterial spiders, 789
Arteries, blood supply, 501
  distributing, 501
  elastic, 501
Arteriolar necrosis, 522
Arteriolar nephrosclerosis, 593
  benign, 594
  malignant, 597
Arterioles, 501
Arteriosclerosis, 502, 516
Arteriolosclerosis, aging, 517
  benign, 520
  hypertension, 517
  malignant, 522
  pulmonary, 671
Arteriosclerotic heart disease, 471
Arteriovenous aneurysm, 536
  of lung, 672
Arteriovenous fistula, 536
Arteritis, acute, 527
  giant cell, 524
  rheumatic, 531
  syphilitic, 531
  temporal, 524
Arthritis, acute, 1270
  chronic, 1273
  degenerative, 1284
  gonococcal, 1271
  non-suppurative, 1271
  rheumatic, 1271
  rheumatoid, 1273
  suppurative, 1270
  tuberculous, 1271
Arthropods, 374
  transmission of infection by, 375
Arthus reaction, 104
Asbestosis, 651
Ascaris lumbricoides, 364
Ascending reticular system, 1124
Aschoff body, 266
Ascites, dropsical, 857
  exudative, 857
  in liver disease, 789
Ascorbic acid, 383
Ascorbic acid deficiency, 81
  in repair, 70
Aseptic meningitis, 1167
Aseptic necrosis of bone, 1235
Askanazy cells, 1017
Aspergillosis, 327
  of lung, 664
Aspergillus fumigatus, 327
Asterixis, 788
Asteroid inclusions, 47
Asteroid lesions in sarcoidosis, 292
Asthma, bronchial, 106, **627**
  relation of symptoms to lesions,
  628
Astrocytes, 1127
Astrocytoma, 1199
Astroglia, 1127
Atelectasis, 673
  compression, 674
  congenital, 673
  obstructive, 674
Atherosclerosis, 502

Atherosclerosis, age in, 513
  blood lipids in, 506
  ceroid in, 505
  cold in, 507
  electron microscopy in, 508
  ground substance in, 510
  heredity in, 514
  hormones in, 514
  hypertension in, 513
  intimal hemorrhage in, 504, 513
  lesions of, 502
  lipids in, 503
  mast cells in, 514
  mural thrombosis in, 511
  pathogenesis of, 505
  production of, 136
  relation to diet in, 508
  stress in, 513
  vessel wall in, 510
  vitamin deficiency, 515
Athrogryposis, 1311
Atmospheric pressure, 410
Atom, components of, 412
Atomic bomb radiation, 423
  effect on bone, 1246
Atomic energy, 413
Atomic fall-out, 1246
Atopy, 105
ATP, 31, 1302
Atrial septal defects, 475
Atrio-ventricular node, 446
Atrophy, 250
Auto-antigens, 109
Auto-immunity, 109
  and blood diseases, 1089
  disease, 109
Autolysis, 25, 27
Autosomal dominant inheritance,
  436
  recessive inheritance, 436
Autosome anomalies, 880
Axillary vein thrombosis, 134
Ayerza's disease, 672
Azo compounds, carcinogenic, 185

B

Bacillary dysentery, 277, **753**
Bacillus anthracis, 311
Bacillus pyocyaneus, 270
Backward failure, 496
Bacteremia, 84
Bacteria, classification, 261
  host defense against, 260
Bacterial endocarditis, 457
  subacute, 458
Bacteriophage, 334
Bacterium coli, 270
Bacteroides infection, 270
Baker's cyst, 1297
Balantidium coli, 356
Banti's disease, 1095
Barlow's disease, 386
Baron von Munchausen syndrome,
  483
Bartonella anemia, 103
Bartonella bacilliformis, 314
Basal cell carcinoma, 232, 1327
Basophil leukocyte, 1038
Basophilic stippling, 1035
Bauxite fibrosis, 651
Bazin's disease, 1327
B.C.G., 291

stridium botulinum, 314
etani, 313
velchii, 312
udy swelling, 17
bbing of fingers, 673, 1247
agulation of blood, 126
agulation time, 1075
arctation of aorta, 478
-carcinogens, 195
ge, 196
hronic irritation, 197
liet, 196
eredity, 196
rauma, 197
ccidioides immitis, 323
ccidioidomycosis, 322
of lung, 663
hnheim on inflammation. 36
lchicine, 1286
in gout, 1286
ld abscess, 1234
ld, common, 342, 622
liform bacteria, 269
litis, chronic ulcerative, 749
llagen disease, lesions of brain,
147
llagen diseases, 86
    biochemical changes in, 115
    cortisone, 115
llagen fibers in healing, 70
llagenic tumors of bone, 1257
llapse of lung, acute massive,
574
lloid milium, 1342
loboma, 441
mmon cold, 342, 622
mplement fixation test, 299
mpound nevus, 1335
mpound palmer ganglion, 1312
ncussion, 1151
ndyloma acuminatum, 938
ngenital cystic kidney, 616
ngenital cystic lung, 692
ngenital defects, 432
ngenital heart disease, 473
    relation of symptoms to
        lesions, 480
ngenital spherocytic anemia,
    1056
    relation of symptoms to
        lesions, 1057
ngenital syphilis of bone, 1235
ngenital torticollis, 1307
ngestion, venous, 161
ngestive splenomegaly, 1095
ngo red test, 95
nn's syndrome, 993
nstitution in disease, 442
ntrecoup, 1151
oley's anemia, 1062
ombs test, 1041, **1055**, 1065
pper absorption in Wilson's dis-
    ease, 806
or bovinum, 486
orn, 1320
oronary arteries, 446
oronary artery occlusion, 463
    cholecystitis and, 467
    mast cells in, 466
    pathogenesis of, 463
    relation of symptoms to
        lesions in, 470
orpora amylacea, 25, 1129

Corrigan pulse, 486
Corrosive acids, 427
Cortisone, 983
Councilman bodies, 346
Courvoisier's law, 827
Coxsackie group B meningitis,
    1167
Coxsackie, infection, 1172
    viruses, 337
Craniopagus, 253
Craniopharyngioma, 974
Cranioschisis, 253
Craniotabes, 1244
C-reactive protein, 265, 452
Creatine loss in muscular
    dystrophy, 1310
Cretinism, 1013
Crohn's disease, 751
    relation of symptoms to
        lesions, 753
Crooke's hyaline change, 992
Crow's feet hemorrhages, 1135
Crush syndrome, 581
Cryoglobulinemia, 1042
Cryptococcus neoformans, 321
    of brain, 1180
    of lung, 664
Cryptococcosis, 321
Curling's ulcer, 171, **723**, 730
Cushing's syndrome, 973, 979, **991**
Cyclops, 253
Cylindroma, 1330
Cyst, anterior median, 1356
    Baker's, 1297
    dentigerous, 1356
    dermal, 1341
    epidermal, 1341
    follicular, 1356
    mesenteric, 857
    of semilunar cartilage, 1297
    periodontal, 1355
    radicular, 1355
    sebaceous, 1341
Cystic disease, of kidney, 616
    of lung, 692
Cystic hygroma, 246, 707, 1106
    hyperplasia of breast, 943
    lymphangioma, 707
Cysticerus cellulosae, 369
Cystitis, 863
    cystica, 863
    interstitial, 863
Cystosarcoma phyllodes, 949
Cysts connected with joints, 1297
Cysts of jaws, 1355
    of skin, 1341
Cytogenetics, 874
Cytology, exfoliative, 215
Cytomegalic inclusion disease,
    348, 644
Cytoplasmic inclusions, 15

D

DYCTYLITIS, tuberculous, 1233
Death, sudden, 472
Deficiency diseases, 377
    hepatitis, 794
Degeneration, fatty, 18
    hyaline, 24
    hydropic, 17
    lipoidal, 20
    mucoid, 23

Degenerative arthritis, 1284
Dehydration, 156
Demyelinating diseases, 1181
Dental caries, 1345
    granuloma, 1348
    osteitis, 1353
    plaque, 1348
    pulp, 1344
Dentigerous cyst, 1356
Dentin, 1344
Dentinoma, 1356
Dermal cyst, 1341
Dermatitis herpetiformis, 1321
Dermatofibroma, 1339
Dermatomyositis, acute, 1304
Dermatopathic lymphadenitis,
    1107
Dermatoses, nonspecific, 1321
Dermis, tumors of, 1339
Dermoid cyst of ovary, 931
    of skin, 1341
Dermoids, inclusion, 248
Desmoid tumor, 236, **858**
Desoxyribonucleic acid, 11
DeQuervain thyroiditis, 1016
Diabetes, bronzed, 395
Diabetes insipidus, 976, 1098
Diabetes mellitus, adrenal in, 840
    arterial lesions in, 843
    glycogen infiltration of islets
        in, 841
    hemochromatosis and, 844
    heredity in, 838
    Kimmelstiel-Wilson lesion in,
        842
    Kussmaul breathing in, 845
    nature of, 837
    obesity in, 839
    pancreatic lesions in, 840
    papillitis necroticans in, 842
    pituitary in, 840
    relation of symptoms to
        lesions, 844
    renal lesions in, 842
    retinal lesions in, 843
Diabetic glomerulosclerosis, 573
    retinopathy, 843
Diapedesis of leukocytes, 37
Diaphysial aclasis, 1248
Diazo reaction, 275
Dibothriocephalus latus anemia,
    1051
Dicumarol, 127
Diet in relation to repair, 67
Diffuse collagen diseases, 86
Diphtheria, **279**, 703
Diphyllobothrium latum, 370
Dissecting aneurysm, 534
Disseminated lupus erythematosus,
    155, 525
    sclerosis, 121, **1183**
Distomum pulmonis, 373
Diuretics, 612
Diverticulum, Meckel's, 764
    of bladder, 870
    of bowel, 763
    of esophagus, 715
Diverticulitis, 764
Diverticulosis, 763
DNA, 12
    in neoplasia, 174
Dopa reaction, 402
Dorothy Reed cells, 1115

Dracunculus medinensis, 367
Drosophila, mutations by radiation, 422
Drug encephalitis, 1175
Drug-induced hemolytic anemia, 1058
Dubin-Johnson disease, 811
Dubin-Spring disease, 811
Ductus arteriosus, patent, 478
Duodenal diverticula, 741
ulcer, 732
Duodenum, carcinoma of, 740
Duplication of alimentary tract, 779
Dupuytren's contraction, 1307
Duran-Reynals' phenomenon, 262
Dusting powder granuloma, 62
Dust-reticulation, 649
Dysentery, amebic, 753
bacillary, 276, 753
relation of lesions to symptoms, 277
Dysgerminoma, 936
Dyskeratosis, 1316
Dysphagia, 720
Dystrophia adiposa-genitalis, 976
Dystrophy, muscular, 1309

E

East African endomyocardial fibrosis, 480
Eburnation, 1286
Ecchymoses, 164
Echerichia coli, 270
Echinococcus alveolaris, 372
Echinococcus cyst, 372
ECHO meningitis, 1167
ECHO viruses, 337
Eclampsia, 576, **917**
arteriolar vasoconstriction, 918
Ectopea cardis, 253
Eczema, 1321
Edema, cachectic, **160**
cardiac, 159
causes, of, 158
famine, 160
hereditary, 160
inflammatory, 159
lymphatic, 159
of lung, 668
pulmonary, 160
renal, 160
tissue changes, in, 157
Eisenmenger complex, 477
Elastic hyperplasia of arterioles, 520
Electricity, 409
burns, 409
Electrocardiogram, 449
Electrolytes, 152
Electron microscopy of cancer cells, 177
Electrons, 412
Elementary bodies, 333
Elephantiasis, 367, 1105
Ellis classification of nephritis, 556
Embolism, 138
air, 146
amniotic fluid, 147
fat, 144
mesenteric, 778
paradoxical, 143

Embolism, pulmonary, 141
tumor, 209
Embryoma of kidney, 615
Emphysema, atrophic, 680
centrilobular, 677
compensatory, 680
interstitial, 680
obstructive, 675
panlobular, 676
spontantous mediastinal, 681
Empyema, 694
Enamel, 1344
Enameloblastoma, 236
Enameloma, 1356
Encephalitis, acute, localized, non-suppurative, 1154
drug, 1175
equine, 1165
lead, 1174
lethargic, 1163
periaxialis diffusa, 1185
post-vaccinal, 1166
secondary, 1166
type A, 1163
type B, 1164
Encephalomalacia, 1139
Encephalomyelitis, acute disseminated, 1165, **1186**
acute necrotizing hemorrhagic, 1187
allergic, 1182
primary, 1166
Enchondroma, 1256
Endarteritis, acute, 528
Endocardial fibroelastosis, 479
Endocarditis, acute bacterial, 463
bacterial, 457
marantic, 482
syphilitic, 529
terminal, 482
thrombotic non-bacterial, 482
Endocervicitis, 903
Endometrial cysts, 926
hyperplasia, 899
sarcoma, 913
stromatosis, 902
Endometrioma of umbilicus, 858
Endometriosis, 900
chocolate-colored cysts, 901
Endometritis, 902
puerperal, 902
Endomyocardial fibrosis, East African, 480
Endoplasmic reticulum, 14
Entamoeba histolytica, 355
Enteric cysts, 779
Enteritis, catarrhal, 746
pseudomembranous, 747
regional, 751
staphylococcal, 747
terminal, 751
uremic, 751
Enterobius vermicularis, 364
Enterocolitis, pseudomembranous, 746
Enterogenous cysts, 765
Enteropathy, exudative, 751
Enteroviruses, 337
Eosinophil leukocyte in inflammation, 41
Eosinophilia, 1038
Eosinophilic granuloma, 1250
Ependymoma, 1201

Epidermal cysts of skin, 1341
Epidemic hemorrhagic fever, 3
Epidermoid carcinoma, of skin, 1327
spontaneous healing, 1327
Epididymis, spermatic granulor 881
Epididymitis, gonorrheal, 881
non-gonorrheal, 881
Epignatus, 247, 254
Epilepsy, 1152
temporal lobe lesions, 1153
Epiphysitis, syphilitic, 1235
Epithelial crescent, 560
Epithelial invasion, benign, 20
Epithelioid cells, 61
Epulis, 1257
Equine encephalomyelitis, 116
Ergastroplasm in neoplasia, 18
Erysipelas, 264
Erythema induratum, 1327
multiforme, 1325
Erythremia, 1071
Erythroblastosis fetalis, 918, 10
Erythrocyte, 1034
abnormal forms of, 1035
development of, 1034
enzymes of, 1034
life span of, 1035
Erythrocytosis, 1071
Erythromelalgia, 537
Erythroprotein, 1034
Esophageal varices, 716
Esophagitis, 713
Esophagus, achalasia of, 704
carcinoma of, 717
cicatriceal stricture of, 714
congenital anomalies of, 719
diverticula of, 715
heterotopic gastric mucosa in 719
leiomyoma of, 719
peptic ulcer of, 713
scleroderma of, 713
spontaneous rupture of, 719
structure and fucëtion of, 71
varices of, 716
Ewing's tumor, 1259
Exfoliative cytology, 215
cancer of cervix, 911
fluorescent microscopy in,
in gastric carcinoma, 739
Exophthalmic goiter, 1008
Exophthalmos, 1012
Extradural abscess, 1153
Extradural hemorrhage, 1148
Exudate, 157

F

Facio-scapulo-humeral muscu
dystrophy, 1309
Fallopian tube, structure of, 92
carcinoma of, 924
cysts of, 924
Fallot, tetralogy of, 476
Familial periodic paralysis, 131
Fanconi syndrome, 1246, 611
Farcy, 281
Farmer's lung, 652
Fat cyst of liver, 795
Fat embolism, 144
of lung, 671

necrosis, 28
of breast, 961
, staining of, 20
ty cysts, 20
ty degeneration, 18
of liver, 818
ty infiltration, 19
ism, 439, 1059
·y's syndrome, 1273
1ale genital tract, anomalies of,
39
mentation, 14
lgen reaction, 11
or hepaticus, 789
er, 154
1uses of, 155
inical picture, 156
unction of, 156
rin cap, 576
rin formation in inflammation,
2
rinoid, 86, 113, 266
ecrosis, 86
in rheumatoid arthritis, 1278
rinolysis, 135
·oadenoma of breast, 948
·ocystic disease, 845
·oids, of cervix, 905
· uterus, 903
roma, 236
f ovary, 932
romyxoid chondroma, 1256
·osarcoma, 240, 1259
·eriosteal, 1259
·ous dysplasia of bone, 1240
ller's myocarditis, 488
·ria bancrofti, 366
·edinensis, 367
inguinis hominis, 366
riasis, 366
1 tapeworm, 370
ula, 58
cal, 58
·-bitten kidney, 460
1s, 375
s, 375
id balance, disturbance of, 156
id, intercellular, 150
1tracellular, 150
1travascular, 150
kes, 373
orescence and glomerulo-
ephritis, 557
orescence technique in rheu-
1atoid arthritis, 1274
orine in relation to dental
1ries, 1348
my liver, 31
al embolic glomerulonephritis,
56
al infection due to dental
isease, 1354
ic acid, 390, 1046
in macrocytic anemia, 391
icular cyst of jaw, 1356
icular hyperkeratosis, 379
icular lymphoma, 1112
d poisoning, 276
infection type, 276
toxin type, 276
amen ovale, patent, 475
ward failure, 496
cture, healing, 1229

Fragilitas ossium, 1247
Frambesia, 304
Freezing, death from, 408
Frei-Hoffman test, 347
Freund's adjuvant, 109
Friedländer's bacillus, 279
pneumonia, 640
Friedreich's ataxia, 1194
Fröhlich's syndrome, 975
Froin syndrome, 1210
Frostbite, 408
high altitude, 408
Fungi, principal pathogenic, 329
Fungus infections, 316

G

GALLBLADDER, carcinoma of, 828
cholesterolosis of, 822
empyema of, 821
hydrops of, 821
strawberry, 823
structure and function of, 819
Gallstones, 825
mixed, 826
pure cholesterol, 826
pure pigment, 826
Gamma bodies, 347
Gamma globulins, 100
Ganglioneuroma, 247, 998, 1205
Gangrene, 28
dry, 29
gas, 30, 312
moist, 29
of lung, 653
Gas gangrene, 30, 312
Gastric polyposis, diffuse, 740
ulcer, 728
Gastritis, 724
acute, 725
atrophic, 726
chronic, 726
giant hypertrophic, 726
Gaucher's disease, 1097, 1251
Gee's disease, 766
General adaptation syndrome, 986
General paresis, 1178
relation of symptoms to lesions,
1179
Generalized myositis fibrosa, 1304
Genes, 432
Genetic radiation hazards, 422
Genital tract, tuberculosis of, 882
Geographic cancer, pathology of
urinary calculus, 866
Geography of cancer, 194
German measles, 341
relation to congenital defects,
341
Ghon lesion, 288
Giant cells, 45
Giant follicle lymphoma, 112
Giant-cell arteritis, 524
Giant-cell epulis, 1266
Giant-cell pneumonia, 644
Giant-cell tumor, 1257
of tendon sheaths, 1296
Gigantism, 977
Gilbert's disease, 810
Gingival sulcus, 1351
Gingivitis, 1350
acute necrotizing, 1351
Girdle of Venus, 529

Gitterzellen, 1129, 1140
Glanders, 280
Glandular fever, 1088
Glioblastoma multiforme, 1197
Glioma, 1196
Gobulin-fluorescein staining, 177
Globulins, abnormal, 1042
in collagen diseases, 115
Glomangioma, 542, **1339**
Glomerular obsolescence, 595
Glomerular rickets, 1246
Glomerulitis, focal, 566
Glomerulonephritis, acute, 558
basement membrane, 561
chronic, 561
diffuse, 555
etiology of, 556
lesions of, 558
membranous, 568
relation of symptoms to lesions,
562
subacute, 560
urinary changes in, 566
Glomerulosclerosis, diabetic, 573
intercapillary, 573
Glomoid hyperplasia of pulmonary
vessels, 672
Glomus jugularis, tumor of, 707
Glomus tumor, 1339
Glossitis, 704
syphilitic, 704
Glottis, edema of, 624
Glucagon, 833
Glutamic oxaloacetic transaminase,
450, 786, 1303, 1310
Glutathione stability test for drug
sensitivity, 1059
Glycogen, cardiac, 451
infiltration, 21
myocardial, 450
Glycogen nephrosis, 22
of kidney, 22
of liver, 22
Glycogen storage disease, 818
of heart, 23
Goiter, diffuse colloid, 1005
exophthalmic, 1008
geographic pathology, 1004
lymphadenoid, 1016
nodular, 1006
relation of symptoms to lesions,
1001
Golgi apparatus, 10
Gombault, segmental degeneration
of, 1211
Gonococcal infections, 268
arthritis, 269
Gonorrheal epididymitis, 881
salpingitis, 921
urethritis, 871
Gout, 1286, 1287
acute, 1288
chronic, 1288
clinical picture, 1288
renal lesions in, 1289
etiology, 1286
kidney in, 1289
lesions, 1288
primary, 1292
relation of symptoms to lesions,
1292
secondary, 1292
tophi, 1289

Gout, uric acid, 1287
Grading of tumors, 204
Gram's stain, 256
Granular cell myoblastoma, 1311
Granulation tissue, 58, 72
Granuloma annulare, 1325
   dental, 1348
   pyogenicum, 1341
Granulomas, 61, 63
   bacterial, 61
   beryllium, 62
   dusting powder, 62
   foreign body, 62
   infective, 61
   lint, 62
   mycotic, 61
Granulosa cell tumor, 933
Graphite fibrosis of lung, 651
Graves' disease, 1008
Grawitz tumor, 613
Ground itch, 363
Ground substance, 79
Guarnieri bodies, 333, 338
Guillian-Barré syndrome, 1088,
   1212
Guinea worm, 368
Gumboil, 1349
Gumma, 303
Gynecomastia, 943
   in liver disease, 789

H

HABITUS, 443
Hair follicle tumors, 1330
Half-life, radioactive, 415
Halisteresis, 1226
Hamartoma of bone, 1265
   of lung, 691
Hamman-Rich syndrome, 646
Hand-Schüller-Christian disease,
   1250
Hanot's hypertrophic cirrhosis, 801
Hashimoto's disease, 112, 1016
Healing, hormonal control of, 72
   of abscess, 74
   of collagen fibers, 70
   of granulation tissue, 72
   of wound, 68
   primary union, 69
   secondary union, 72
Heart block, 473
   blood supply of, 446
   conducting system of, 446
   congenital rhabdomyoma of, 492
   function of, 448
   glycogen storage disease of, 23
   myxoma of, 492
   rheumatic disease of, 451
   secondary tumors of, 492
   structure of, 445
   tumors of, 491
Heart disease, congenital, 473
   hypertensive, 473
Heart failure, 495
Heart failure cells, 163, 667
Heat loss, 154
   production, 154
   stroke, 407
Heberden's nodes, 1285
Heinz bodies, 1058

Hemangioendothelioma, 541
   benign, 541
   malignant, 541
Hemangioma, 245, **540**
   capillary, 540
   cavernous, 540
   of bone, 1265
   of brain, 1206
   sclerosing, **540**, 1339
Hemangiopericytoma, 541
Hemangiosarcoma, multiple
   hemorrhagic, 1339
Hematemesis, 720
Hematocele, 894
Hematoidin, 165, **394**
Hematoma, 164
Hematoporphyrin, 393
Hematosalpinx, 923
Hematoxylin bodies, 118
Hematuria, 619, **870**
Hemobilirubin, 809
Hemochromatosis, **395**, 805, 844,
   850
   exogenous, 806
Hemoglobin, 393
Hemoglobin C disease, 1063
   E disease, 1063
Hemoglobins, abnormal, 1036
Hemoglobinuria, 1063
   March, 1063
   paroxysmal cold, 1064
   paroxysmal nocturnal, 1063
Hemolytic anemia, 1055
   acquired, 1063
   drug-induced, 1058
   Coombs test in, 1055
   hereditary, 1056
Hemolytic disease of newborn,
   1064
Hemophilia, 1076
Hemophilic joint, 1293
Hemophilus ducreyi, 306
   influenzæ, 306
   pertussis, 306
Hemopericardium, 495
Hemorrhage, 164
   arrest of, 165
   cerebral, 1142
   secondary, 165
Hemorrhagic diseases of newborn,
   1077
Hemorrhoids, 779
Hemosiderin, 165
Hemosiderosis, **394**, 506
   idiopathic pulmonary, 668
   transfusional, 395
Hemothorax, 696
Henoch's purpura, 1075
Heberden's nodes, 1285
Hepar lobatum, 815
Heparin, 127
Hepatic coma, 788
Hepatic lobule, 782
Hepatic vein, thrombosis, 814
Hepatitis, chronic, 121
   deficiency, 794
   infectious, 791
   infective, 346
   lupoid, 793
   relation of symptoms to lesions,
      792
   serum, 346, 791

Hepatitis, subacute necrosis
   nodular hyperplasia, 791
   toxic, 793
   viral, 346, 791
Hepato-cellular failure, 787
Hepato-lenticular degeneration
   806, **1187**
Hepato-renal syndrome, 581
Hepatoma, 816
Hereditary blood diseases, 438
   chondrodysplasia, 1248
   defects, 439
   hemoglobinopathies, 1059
   mental diseases, 441
   metabolic disorders, 439
   neuromuscular disorders, 440
   skeletal defects, 440
Heredity in cancer, 441
   in disease, 431
Hermaphroditism, 895
Hernia, 774
Herniation of nucleus pulposu
   1298
Herpes simplex, 339, **1173**
   zoster, 339, **1173**
   relation to varicella, 1173
Hertwig, sheath of, 1355
Heterologous transplantation
   cancer, 198
Heterotopia, 253
Hexokinase hypothesis, 833
Hiatus hernia, 715
Hibernoma, 238
Hilus cell tumor of ovary, 935
Hirschsprung's disease, 777
Histiocytes, 44
Histiocytoses, skeletal, lipid,
Histiocytosis X, 1250
Histoplasma capsulatum, 325
Histoplasmin skin reaction, 3
Histoplasmosis, 323
   of lung, 664
   primary, 325
   progressive, 325
Hodgkin's disease, 1114
   anemia in, 1117
   granuloma, 1116
   paragranuloma, 1116
   prognosis of, 1117
   relation of symptoms to
      lesions, 1116
   sarcoma, 1116
Homeostasis, 149
Hookworm, 362
Hormonal-dependent tumors
Hormones, adrenocorticotrop
   970, 979
   antidiuretic, 971
   as carcinogens, 191
      in relation to ground su
         stance, 81
   general discussion, 964
   gonadotrophic, 971
   growth, 970
   in relation to repair, 67
   oxytocin, 971
   thyrotrophic, 970, 979
Horner's syndrome, 1141
Horse-shoe kidney, 619
Houssay phenomenon, 840
Hunner stricture of ureter, 8
   ulcer, 863
Huntington's chorea, 1194

tchinson's teeth, 304
aline degeneration, 24
  of arterioles, 520
aline membrane disease, 669
aluronidase, 52, **80**
latid cyst, 371
latid disease of liver, 815
latidiform mole, 247, **914**
lradenoma, 1330
lrocele, 893
lrocephalus, 1133
  ommunicating, 1133
  ternal, 1133
lrocyanic acid, 429
lrogen bomb radiation, 424
lromyelia, 1196
lronephrosis, 861
lropericardium, 495
lrophobia, 345, 1174
egri bodies in, 345
eventive inoculation, 345
lropic degeneration, 17
lrops, congenital, 1066
lrosalpinx, 921
lrothorax, 696
groma, cystic, 1106
ercalcemia of infants, 610
ercholesterolemia, 1098
ercholesterolemic spleno-
  egaly, 1098
erchromic macrocytic anemia,
  046
eremia, arterial, 161
ergammaglobulinemia, 101
erglycemia, 837
erkeratosis, 1316
ernephroma, 613
elation of symptoms to lesions,
  615
erostosis frontalis internæ, 1247
erparathyroidism, 1027, 1238
erpituitarism, 977
romegaly, 978
gantism, 977
erplasia, 251
ersensitivity, 102
naphylactic, 103
acterial type, 105
ellular, 105
inical features of, 106
elayed, 105
a syphilis, 105
sions of, 106
o foods, 105
o plants, 105
berculin type, 105
ersplenism, **1058**, 1087, 1094
ertension, arterial, 517
arctation of aorta, 519
ndocrine, 518
ssential, 519
eredity, 520
olyarteritis nodosa, 519
ulmonary, 671
elation of kidney to, 601
nal, 518
tinal lesions in, 599
ascular, 519
ertensive encephalopathy,
  1142
eart disease, 473
ertrophic osteoarthropathy,
246

Hypertrophy, 251
  adaptive, 251
  compensatory, 251
  physiological, 251
Hypervitaminosis A, 380
Hypervitaminosis D, 382
Hypoadrenalism, 987
Hypogammaglobulinemia, 1043
Hypoparathyroidism, 1029
Hypopituitarism, 974
Hypopotassemia, 153
Hypoprothrombinemia, 383
Hypospadias, 895
Hypothermia, 408

I

ICHTHYOSIS, 1320
Icterus gravis, 1064
  neonatorum, 812
Idiopathic cardiac hypertrophy,
  473
Idiopathic thrombocytopenic
  purpura, 111
Ileitis, regional, 753
Immunity, 97
  acquired, 98
  passive, 98
  species, 98
  tissue, 101
  to viral infections, 333
  tumor, 197
Impetigo contagiosa, 1327
Inborn errors of metabolism, 435,
  439
Incisural sclerosis, 1153
Inclusion congenital, 248
  dermoids, 248, 253
  disease, 348, 644
  implantation, 248
Inclusions, cytoplasmic, 15
Infarction, 139
  of heart, 140
  of kidney, 140
  of spleen, 140
  pulmonary, 141
Infarct of bowel, 778
  of brain, 1138
  of heart, 467
  ot kidney, 603
  of liver, 813
  of lung, 671
  of prostate, 888
  of spleen, 1101
Infarcts of placenta, 918
Infection, 81
  changing picture of, 257
  localization of, **52**, 81
  recovery from, 84
  spread of, 84, 259
Infectious mononucleosis, 1088
Infective granuloma, 61
Infective hepatitis, 346
Inflammation, allergic, 59
  blood plasma in, 38
  catarrhal, 59
  causes of, 35
  chemotaxis in, 39
  chronic, 60
  definition of, 35
  degenerations in, 55
  diapedesis of leukocytes in, 37
  eosinophils in, 41

Inflammation, fibrinous, 59
  general discussion of, 54
  giant cells in, 45
  influence of cortisone in, 59
  localization of infection, 52
  lymph of exudate, 50
  lymphocytes, in, 42
  macrophages, in, 44
  mast cells in, 41
  membranous, 59
  neutrophils in, 40
  phagocytosis in, 47
  plasma cells in, 43
  relation of symptoms to lesions,
    54
  serotonin in, 40
  serous, 59
  serous membranes, 55
  tissue changes in, 55
  vascular phenomena in, 36
Inflammatory exudate, cells of, 40
  lymph of, 50
Influenza, etiology of, 342
  hemagglutination test for, 343
  relation of symptoms to lesions,
    643
  swine, 343
Influenzal pneumonia, 641
Inheritance ot disease, 435
  dominant, 436
  recessive, 436
  sex-linked, 437
Insensible water, 151
Insulin, 832
Intercapillary glomerulosclerosis,
  574, 842
Intercellular substance reactions,
  79
Interferon, 335
Intermediate tumors, 226
Internal environment, 149
  pathology of, 152
Interstitial fluid, 150
Interstitial nephritis, acute,
  diffuse, 584
Intervertebral disc, herniation of,
  1299
  lesions of, 1298
  prolapse of, 1299
  protrussion of, 1299
Intestinal diverticula, 763
  lipodystrophy, 767
  obstruction, 775
    acute, 776
    chronic, 777
    organic, 775
    paralytic, 775
  pneumatosis, 779
Intestine, achalasia, 777
  actinomycosis, 757
  benign tumors of, 769
  carcinoid tumor of, 772
  carcinoma of, 770
  developmental defects of, 779
  infarction of, 778
  malignant tumors of, 770
  multiple polyposis, 769
  obstruction of, 775
  pneumatosis of, 779
  polyposis of, 769
  structure and function of, 744
  tuberculosis of, 753

Intracellular fluid, 150
    inclusions, 333
Intracranial aneurysms, 1147
    atherosclerotic, 1148
    congenital, 1147
    mycotic, 1148
    hemorrhage of newborn, 1149
    pressure, increased, 1135
    suppuration, 1153
    tumors, 1196
        relation of symptoms to
            lesions, 1208
Intradermal nevus, 1334
Intraepithelial carcinoma, 1328
Intralobar sequestration, 693
Intravascular fluid, 151
Intussusception, 774
Involucrum, 1231
Iodine metabolism, 1001
    radioactive, 1003
    trap, 1001
Ionization, 414
Ionizing radiation, 412
    in carcinogenesis, 186
Iron, absorption of, 394
    deficiency anemia, 1052
    duodenal mucosal block, 396
    storage disease, 396
Irradiation pneumonitis, 645
Ischemia, 164
Ischemic obsolescence, 596
Ischiopagus, 254
Islet cell tumors, 848
Isotopes, as tracers, 414
    in therapy, 415
    radioactive, 414

J

JAUNDICE, 397
    acholuric, 809
    familial hemolytic, 810
    hemolytic, 810
    hepatocellular, 810
    obstructive, 809
    symptoms of, 811
Jaws, cysts of, 1355
    odontogenic tumors of, 1356
    osteitis of, 1353
Jejunal ulcer, 735
Joints, cysts of, 1297
    fibrocartilaginous, 1269
    structure and function of, 1268
    synovial, 1270
    tumors of, 1293
Junctional nevus, 1334
Juxtaglomerular apparatus, 548,
    553

K

KAHN precipitation test, 299
Kala-azar, 1100
Kangri cancer, 186
Kaposi's sarcoma, 542, 1339
Karyorrhexis, 26
Kayser-Fleischer ring, 1187
Keloid, 73
Keratinizing metaplasia, 379
Keratoacanthoma, 1331
Keratomalacia, 379

Keratosis, seborrheic, 1316
    senile, 1318
Kernicterus, 1066
Kidney, adenoma of, 612
    bilateral cortical necrosis of, 603
    carcinoma of, 613
    congenital anomalies of, 618
    congenital cystic, 616
    embryoma of, 615
    function of, 550
    infarct of, 603
    needle biopsy of, 555
    phosphate-losing, 609
    phosphate-retaining, 609
    potassium-losing, 608
    relation to hypertension, 601
    salt-losing, 608
    solitary cyst of, 617
    structure of, 546
    tuberculosis of, 591
    water-losing, 608
Kienbock's disease, 1237
Kimmelstiel-Wilson lesion, **574**,
    842
Klinefelter's syndrome, 434, 877
Koch phenomenon, 287
Köhler's disease, 1237
Kraurosis vulvæ, 939
Krukenberg tumor, 931
Kümmell's disease, 1237
Kuru, 1193
Kussmaul breathing, 845
Kveim test, 294
Kwashiorkor, 377, **795**
Kyphosis, 1234

L

LANDRY's paralysis, 1211
Langhans cells, 61, 916
Laryngitis, 624
    diphtheric, 624
    syphilitic, 624
    tuberculous, 624
Larynx, carcinoma of, 625
    papilloma of, 625
Lateral drifting of teeth, 1352
Latex fixation test, 1275
Lathyrism, 1224
Laurence-Moon-Biedl syndrome,
    976
Lead encephalitis, 1174
Lead poisoning, 406, **428**
    anemia, 1070
L.E. cell, 119
Left ventricular failure, 497
Legg-Perthes' disease, 1236
Leiomyoma, 243
    of uterus, 903
Leiomyosarcoma, 243
Leishmaniasis, 359
Lenticular degeneration, progres-
    sive, 806, **1187**
Leontiasis ossea, 1242
Lepra cells, 295
Lepromin test, 298
Leprosy, 295
    lepromatous form, 295
    tuberculoid form, 296
Leptocytes, 1062
Leptospira canicola, 813
Leptospirosis ictero-hemorrhagiæ,
    305

Letterer-Siwe disease, 1098, 125
Leukemia, acute, 1082
    etiology of, 1085
    in mice, 189
    lymphatic, 1080
    monocytic, 1083
    myelogenous, 1079
    plasma cell, 1083
    relation of symptoms to lesio
        1083
    transmissable mouse, 1085
    vertical transmission of, 1085
Leukocytes, 1037
    biochemistry, 1038
    emigration of, 37
    function of, 1038
Leukoderma, 1320
Leuko-erythroblastic anemia, 10
Leukoplakia of bladder, 863
    of vulva, 939
Leukosis, fowl, 1085
Leydig cells, 873
Libman-Sacks endocarditis, 117
Lichen planus, 1326
Lichen sclerosus et atrophicus,
    1326
Light, 408
    hypersensitiveness, 409
    ultraviolet, 409
Lightening, 410
Lindau's disease, 1206
Linitis plastica, 737
Lint granuloma, 62
Lip, angioma of, 703
    carcinoma of, 702
    syphilis of, 703
Lipase, serum, 832
Lipid histiocytoses, 1251
Lipiodal degeneration, 20
Lipochromes, 405
Lipodystrophy, progressive, 21
Lipoid nephrosis, 568
    pneumonia, 644
Lipoid-storage diseases, 1097
Lipomelanotic reticular hyper-
    plasia, 1107
Liposarcoma, 242
Lipotropic factors, 18
Lithopedion, 924
Little's disease, 1192
Little strokes, 1137
Liver, abscess of, 754, 814
    actinomycosis of, 814
    acute yellow atrophy of, 791
    alkaline phosphatase, 787
    amebic abscess of, 814
    ammonia intoxication, 789
    amyloid degeneration of, 818
    arterial spiders of, 789
    atrophy of, 819
    benign tumors of, 818
    cavernous hemangioma of, 81
    cholangioma of, 817
    chronic venous congestion of,
        813
    circulation of, 784
    cirrhosis of, 796
    developmental defects of, 819
    endocrine imbalance, 789
    fat cysts of, 795
    fatty degeneration of, 818
    flap, 788
    flukes, 373

r, foamy, 819
nction of, 784
nction tests of, 785
ycogen storage in, 818
utamic oxaloacetic trans-
 aminase, 786
emangioma of, 818
epatoma of, 816
ydatid cysts of, 815
farction of, 813
icrovilli of, 783
ecrosis of, 790, 793
eedle biopsy of, 787
utmeg, 813
olycystic disease of, 819
ostmortem changes in, 819
ost-necrotic cirrhosis of, 792
rimary carcinoma of, 816
iedel's lobe of, 819
rcoidosis of, 814
rcoma of, 818
histosomiasis of, 816
condary carcinoma of, 817
lerosis of, 806
ace of Disse, 783
ructure of, 782
philis, acquired, of, 815
congenital, of, 815
berculosis of, 815
ar pneumonia, 635
complications of, 637
relation of symptoms to
 lesions, 638
lized nodular tenosynovitis,
 96
-jaw, 313
omotor ataxia, 1176
ler's syndrome, 645
e bodies in joints, 1293
 cartilaginous, 1293
 fatty, 1293
 fibrinous, 1293
in-Levi syndrome, 975
ing ill, 1174
er motor neurone lesions, 1126
er urinary tract, congenital
 omalies, 872
vig's angina, 264, 705
, abscess of, 653
tinomycosis of, 662
ute massive collapse of, 674
veolar cell carcinoma of, 690
terio-venous aneurysm of, 672
pergillosis of, 664
astomycosis of, 662
own induration of, 667
ccidioidomycosis, of, 663
ngenital anomalies of, 692
yptococcosis of, 664
ema of, 668
abolism of, 671
 embolism of, 671
ke, 373
action of, 633
ngrene of, 653
moid hyperplasia of vessels
 of, 672
toplasmosis of, 664
aline membrane disease of,
 669
postatic congestion of, 668
opathic hemosiderosis of, 668
arction of, 671

Lung, mucormycosis of, 665
 nocardiosis of, 663
 phycomycetes infection of, 665
 sarcoidosis of, 666
 secondary tumors of, 692
 streptothricosis of, 663
 structure of, 632
 syphilis of, 662
 tuberculosis of, 654
Lupoid hepatitis, 793
Lupus erythematosus, 115, 525,
 1323
 discoid, 115
 disseminated, 115
 lesions in central nervous
 system, 1147
 localized, 1323
 systemic, 115, 525
Lutembacher's disease, 475
Luschka's crypts, 825
Lycopodium granuloma, 855
Lymphadenitis, acute, 1106
 chronic, 1106
 dermatopathic, 1107
 mesenteric, 1106
Lymph node, biopsy of, 1104
 fungus infections of, 1109
 lymphogranuloma venereum
 of, 1109
 sarcoidosis of, 1109
 secondary tumors of, 1118
 structure of, 1103
 syphilis of, 1109
 tuberculosis of, 1107
 tumors of, 1109
Lymphadenoid goiter, 111, 1016
Lymphadenopathy, 1119
Lymphangioma, 246, 1106
Lymphangitis, 1105
Lymphatic leukemia, 1080
 obstruction, 159, 367
Lymphatic system, function of,
 1104
 structure of, 1103
Lymphedema, 1105
Lymphocytic choriomeningitis,
 1167
Lymphocyte in inflammation, 42
Lympho-epithelioma, 232
Lymphogranuloma inguinale, 347
 venereum, 347, 1109
Lymphoma, benign, 1118
 macrofollicular, 1112
Lymphopathia venereum, 1109
Lymphosarcoma, 1110
 of stomach, 740
Lysozyme, 749

M

MacCallum patch, 453
Machinery murmur, 476
Macrocheilia, 246, 1106
Macrofollicular lymphoma, 1112
Macroglobulinemia, 1043, 1090
Macroglossia, 246, 1106
 in amyloidosis, 93
Macrophages in inflammation, 44
Macula densa, 549
Malabsorption syndrome, 765
Malakoplakia, 870
Malaria, 356
 blackwater fever, 358

Malaria, lesions, 358
Maldevelopments, 252
Malformations, 252
Malignancy, characteristics of, 201
Malignant arteriolosclerosis, 522
 granuloma, 623
 melanoma, 1337
 nephrosclerosis, retinal lesions,
 599
 pustule, 311
 synovioma, 1293
 thymoma, 1120
Mallory hyaline bodies, 796, 799
Mallory-Weiss syndrome, 720
Malta fever, 307
Marble bones, 1249
March hemoglobinuria, 1063
Marchiafava-Micheli syndrome,
 1063
Marfan's syndrome, 635, 1248
Marie's disease, 1246
Marie-Strümpell spondylitis, 1282
Mast cell, 1038
 function of, 44
Mast cells in allergic reactions,
 107
 in coronary thrombosis, 466
 in urticaria pigmentosa, 1324
Mastitis, acute, 961
 chronic, 943
 plasma cell, 962
Maxillary sinusitis, 1354
Measles, 339
 appendix in, 762
 German, 341
 giant-cell formation, 340
Meckel's diverticulum, 764, 858
Meconium ileus, 777, 846
Mediastinal cysts, 698
 teratoma, 698
 tumors, 698
Medionecrosis of aorta, 516
Mediterranean anemia, 1062
Medulloblastoma, 1200
Megakaryocytes in purpura, 1073
Megaloblast, 1048
Megaloureter, 861
Meigs' syndrome, 696, 932
Melanin, 402
 inhibitors, 403
Melanoblasts, 402
Melanocyte-stimulating hormone,
 403
Melanoma, 1332
 in childhood, 1339
 malignant, 1337
Melanosis, 403
 coli, 404, 779
Melasma, 403
Melon-seed bodies, 1271
Membranes of cell, 12
Mendel, Gregor, 431
Mendelson's syndrome, 653
Meningeal hemorrhage, 1148
 extradural, 1148
 subarachnoid, 1149
 subdural, 1149
Meninges, diffuse malignancy of,
 1207
Meningioma, 1202
Meningitis, aseptic, 1167
 Coxsackie group B, 1167
 ECHO, 1167

Meningitis, influenza bacillus, 1158
  meningococcal, 1155
  pneumococcal, 1158
  streptococcal, 1158
  tuberculous, 1158
Meningocele, 1217
Meningococcal infections, 267
Meningococcal meningitis, 1155
  relation of symptoms to
    lesions, 1157
Meningococcal septicemia, 1157
Meningococcemia, 268
Meningomyelocele, 1217
Menstruation, 896
  endometrial changes, 897
Mental disease, hereditary, 441
Mesangium, 547
Mesenteric cysts, 857
Mesenteric vascular occlusion, 778
Metabolism, inborn errors of, 439
Metachromasia, 80
Metaplasia, 249
  connective-tissue, 250
  endothelial, 250
  epithelial, 250
Metastases, cancer to cancer, 213
  distribution of, 212
Metchnikoff, 34, 48
Methemoglobinemia, 1036
Mexican hat cell, 1059
Micro-abscesses of Monroe, 1321
Microcephaly, 1217
Microcytic hypochromic anemia,
  1052
Microsomes, 10
Microglia, 1129
Microgyria, 1217
Middle lobe syndrome, 631
Middle meningeal hemorrhage,
  1148
Migrating thrombophlebitis in
  carcinoma of pancreas, 848
Migration of teeth, 1352
Mikulicz cell, 623
Mikulicz's disease, 712
  syndrome, 712
Milium, 1342
  colloid, 1342
Milk alkali syndrome, 610
Milkman's disease, 1245
  syndrome, 1245
Milroy's disease, 160
Mitochondria, 13
  in cancer, 180
Mitosis, 176
Mitral insufficiency, 485
  stenosis, 483
Modified inheritance, 436
Mole, 1332
Molecular disease, 10, 1037
  hereditary, 433
Molluscum bodies, 1319
  contagiosum, 342, 1319
  fibrosum, 1215
  sebaceum, 1331
Mönckeberg's sclerosis, 515
Mongolian idiocy, 434
  spot, 1335
Mongolism, 880
Moniliasis, 326
Monocyte, 1038
Monocytic leukemia, 1083
Mononucleosis, infectious, 1088

Monro, micro-abscesses of, 703
Monsters, 253
Morbus coxae senilis, 1284
Morphea, 1322
Mosaic structure, 1242
Mottled enamel, 1348
Mouse leukemia, 1085
Mouse myeloma, 1264
Mouth, carcinoma of, 703
M S H, 990
Mucin, connective tissue, 24
  epithelial, 24
Mucinous cystadenoma of ovary,
  926
Muco-epidermoid carcinoma, 234
  tumors, 710
Mucoid carcinoma, 234
Mucoid degeneration, 23
Mucormycosis, 327
  of brain, 1181
  of lung, 665
Mucoviscidosis, 845
  of liver, 846
  of lungs, 846
  of meconium ileus, 846
  of pancreas, 845
  of sweat glands, 846
Multiple cartilaginous exostoses,
  1248
Multiple myeloma, 1261
  amyloidosis in, 1262
  Bence Jones protein in, 1262
  kidney in, 1262
  mouse, 1264
  serum proteins in, 1262
Multiple sclerosis, 121, **1183**
  relation of symptoms to
    lesions, 1184
Mummifying epithelioma, 1342
Mumps, 347
  meningoencephalitis, 1165
Muscular dystrophies, 1309
  facio-scapulo-humeral group,
    1309
  pseudohypertrophic muscular,
    1309
Muscle lesions secondary to vascular disorders, 1307
Muscle, adenosine triphosphate,
  1302
  atrophy of, 1303
  glutamic oxaloacetic trans-
    aminase, 1303
  potassium, 1303
  regeneration of, 1303
  structure and function of, 1302
  tumors of, 1311
  worm, 365
Mutation, 435
Myasthenia gravis, 1308
  acetylcholine in, 1308
  cholinesterase, 1308
  relation to thymus, 1308
Mycetoma, 320
Mycobacterium lepræ, 295
Mycobacterium tuberculosis, 281
Mycosis fungoides, 1340
Myelin sheath, 1124
Myelitis, 1175
  disseminated, 1175
  transverse, 1175
Myelofibrosis, 1086
Myelogenic tumors, 1259

Myelogenous leukemia, 1079
Myeloid metaplasia of spleen,
  agnogenic, 1069, 1099
Myelolipoma of adrenal, 999
Myeloma globulins, 1262
Myeloma kidney, 617, 1262
  multiple, 1261
  plasma cell, 1261
Myeloproliferative disease, 1085
Myiasis, 375
Myoblastoma, 245
  granular cell, 1311
Myocardial degenerations, 489
Myocardial infarct, 467
  glutamic oxaloacetic trans-
    aminase, 469
  loss of glycogen in, 470
  mural thrombus in, 468
  succinic dehydrogenase in, 4
  without coronary occlusion,
    469
Myocarditis, 488
  deficiency, 490
  diphtheritic, 489
  Fiedler's, 488
  granulomatous, 489
  idiopathic, 122
  isolated, 488
  syphilitic, 489
  toxic, 489
  tuberculous, 489
  viral, 489
Myocardium, amyloidosis of, 49
  potassium deficiency, 491
  vitamin deficiency, 490
Myoepithelioma, 1340
Myo-epithelium, 941, 1340
Myohemoglobinuria, paroxysma
  1311
Myoneural junction disorders,
  1308
Myositis, 1303
  acute, 1304
  chronic, 1304
Myositis ossificans, progressive,
  1305
  traumatic, 1305
Myotonia congenita, 1309
  dystrophica, 1309
Myxedema, 1013
  laboratory features, 1014
  pituitary, 1014
  primary, 1014
Myxoma, 237
Myxosarcoma, 237, 242

N

NABOTHIAN follicles, 903
Nagana, 359
Necator americanus, 362
Neck, cysts of, 706
  deep infections of, 1354
  lymphoblastoma of, 707
  secondary carcinoma of, 708
  tumors of, 707
Necrobiosis lipoidica diabeticoru
  1325
Necrosis, 25
  coagulation, 26
  fat, 28
  liquefaction, 27

edle biopsy of kidney, 555
  of liver, 787
egri bodies, 345, 1174
eisseria infections, 267
eoplasia, 173
  DNA in, 174
  nature of, 174
eonatal thrombocytopenic pur-
    pura, 1074
ephritis, acute diffuse inter-
    stitial, 584
  radiation, 567
ephrocalcinosis, 610, 866
ephrosis, acute tubular, 577
  amyloid, 573
  anoxic, 578
  chronic glomerular, 567
    relation of symptoms to
      lesions, 570
  glomerular capillary basement
    membrane, 569
  glycogen, 22
  hemoglobinuric, 578
  lipoid, 568
  lower nephron, 578
  of pregnancy, 576
  sucrose, 23
  toxic, 583
  traumatic tubular, 578
ephropathy, vacuolar, 584
ephrosclerosis, benign, 594
  malignant, 597
  relation of symptoms to lesions,
    600
  senile, 599
ephrotic syndrome, 568
euritis, 1211
  acute porphyria, 1214
  brachial, 1213
  deficiency, 1214
  diabetic, 1214
  diphtheritic, 1213
  ischemic, 1214
  secondary, 1213
  traumatic, 1213
erve cell, 1123
  fiber, 1124
  erves, tumors of, 1214
euroblastoma, of adrenal, 996
eurofibroma, 237, 1215
eurofibromatosis, 1215
eurogenic sarcoma, 241, 1216
euroglia, 1126
euroma, plexiform, 237
euromyopathy, carcinomatous,
    181, 1212, 1213
euronal degeneration, 1125
euronophagia, 1125
europathic arthropathy, 1292
europathy, carcinomatous, 1212
eurosarcoma, 241
eutropenia, primary splenic, 1087
eurotropic viruses, 344, 1162
evus, 1332
  blue, 1335
  compound, 1335
  histogenesis of, 1332
  intradermal, 1334
  junctional, 1334
  natural history of, 1333
iacin, 389
  pathology, 389
  physiology, 389

Nicotinic acid, 389
Niemann-Pick disease, 1098, 1251
Night-blindness, 379
Nipple, bleeding from, 961
Nissl's degeneration, 1125
Nocardiosis, 319
  of lung, 663
Non-disjunction, 875
Non-osteogenic fibroma of bone,
    1266
Noradrenalin, 984
Noradrenalism, 995
Nose, malignant granuloma of, 623
  syphilis of, 623
  tuberculosis of, 623
Nuclear energy, 412
Nucleic acids, 11
Nucleus, 13
  pulposus, 1269
    herniation of, 1298
Nutmeg liver, 163
Nyctalopia, 379

O

Ochronosis, 405
Odontogenic cysts of jaw, 1355
  tumors of jaw, 1356
Odontoma, 236, 1356
Oligodendroglia, 1129
Oligodendroglioma, 1202
Onion skin arterioles, 118
Onkocytoma, 711
Ophthalmia neonatorium, 269
Orchitis, 881
  mumps, 882
  traumatic, 881
Orthostatic albuminuria, 619
Organelles, 10
Organisers, chemical, 247
Organization of thrombus, 74
Ornithosis, 343
Oroya fever, 314
Orthostatic albuminuria, 619
Osgood-Schlatter's disease, 1237
Osler nodes, 460, 461
Osmotic pressure, 151, 153
Ossification, metastatic, 1225
  pathological, 1225
Ossifying fibroma, 1266
Osteitis deformans, 1241
Osteitis, dental, 1353
  fibrosa, 1238
    focal, 1240
    general, 1238
  rarefying, 1349
Osteoarthritis, 1284
Osteoarthropathy, hypertrophic,
    1246
Osteoblastoma, benign, 1252
Osteoclastoma, 1239, 1257
Osteochondroma, 1265
Osteoclasts, 1226
Osteodystrophies, 1237
  congenital, 1247
Osteodystrophy, radiation, 1246
  renal, 1245
Osteogenesis imperfecta, 1247
Osteogenic sarcoma, 1252
  x-ray appearance, 1254
Osteogenic tumors, 1252
Osteoid, 1223, 1229
  osteoma, 1265

Osteoma, 238, 1265
Osteomalacia, 381, 1226, 1229,
    1245
Osteomyelitis, acute, 1230
  chronic, 1232
  coccidioidal, 231
  of spine, 1231
  typhoid, 1232
Osteopetrosis, 1249
Osteoporosis, 1226
  senile, 1245
Osteosclerosis, 1247
Ovary, abscess of, 933
  adrenal-like tumors of, 936
  arrhenoblastoma, 935
  Berger tumor of, 936
  Brenner tumor of, 937
  carcinoma of, 930
  dermoid cyst of, 931
  dysgerminoma of, 937
  fibroma of, 932
  follicular cysts of, 925
  granulosa cell tumor of, 933
  hilus cell tumor, 935
  hormones of, 925
  Leydig cells of, 924
  lutein cysts of, 926
  mucinous cystadenoma of, 926
  Reinke crystalloids of, 924
  sarcoma of, 933
  secondary carcinoma of, 931
  serous cystadenoma of, 927
  structure of, 924
Oxytocin, 971
Oxyuris granuloma, 364
  vermicularis, 364

P

Pacemaker of heart, 446
Paget's disease of bone, 1241
  relation of symptoms to
    lesions, 1242
Paget's disease of breast, 956
  extramammary, 957
Painful subcutaneous nodules,
    1340
Painless subcutaneous nodule,
    1273
Palade granules, 14
Palmer erythema, 789
Pancoast syndrome, 691
Pancreas, alpha cell tumor, 849
  amylase, 832
  annular, 851
  beta cell tumor, 848
  carcinoma of, 847
  congenital anomalies of, 850
  endocrine function of, 832
  exocrine fucётion of, 832
  glucagon, 833
  hemochromatosis of, 850
  insulin, 832
  islet cell tumors of, 848
  islets of Langerhans, 831
  lipase of, 832
  obstruction of duct, 850
  structure of, 831
  trypsin of, 832
  Zollinger-Ellison syndrome,
    848
Pancreatic duct, obstruction of,
    850

Pancreatitis, acute hemorrhagic, 833
  alcoholism, 835
  chronic relapsing, 836
  fat necrosis, 835
  relation of symptoms to lesions, 835
Panniculitis, 1326
Papain, 81
Papillary hydradenoma, 1330
  syringocystadenoma, 1330
Papillitis necroticans, **589**, 842
Papilloma, mucous, 228
  squamous, 227
Paradental epithelial debris, 1348
Paradoxical embolism, 143
Parakeratosis, 1316
Paralysis agitans, 1192
Parametritis, 902
Parasitic fetus, 254
Parasitism, 354
Parathyroid, adenoma of, 1029
  carcinoma of, 1030
  primary hyperplasia of, 1029
  secondary hyperplasia of, 1029
Paratyphoid infection, 276
Parkinson's disease, 1192
  postencephalitic, **1164**, 1193
Parkinsonism in Wilson's disease, 1187
Parosteal sarcoma, 1255
Parotid gland, adenolymphoma of, 711
  carcinoma of, 710
  tumors of, 708
Paroxysmal cold hemoglobinuria, 110, 1064
  myohemoglobinuria, 1311
  nocturnal hemoglobinuria, 1063
Parovarian cyst, 937
Parthenogenesis, 247
PAS reaction, 15, 21
Pasteurella infections, 308
  pestis, 310
  tularensis, 308
Patent ductus arteriosus, 478
Pathogenicity, 256
Paul-Bunnell test, 1089
Pearly tumor, 1207
Pediculi, 375
Pel-Ebstein fever, 1117
Pellagra, 389, 1191
Pelvic cellulitis, 902
Pelvo-spondylitis ossificans, 1282
Pemphigus, 1322
Penetrance, 436
Penis, carcinoma of, 893
Peptic ulcer, 728
  blood groups, 728
  complications of, 734
  etiology of, 729
  malignant change in, 733
  of esophagus, 713
  relation of symptoms to lesions, 734
Periapical dental infection, 1348
Periarteritis, acute, 527
  nodosa, 523
Pericardial coelomic cyst, 699
Pericarditis, 492
  acute idiopathic, 493
  cholesterol, 495
  chronic constrictive, 494

Pericarditis, relation of symptoms to lesions, 495
  rheumatic, 456
  tuberculous, 494
  uremic, 495
  viral, 494
Pericementum, 1345
Pericytes of Zimmermann, 540
Perinephritic abscess, 589
Perineurial fibroma, 1215
Periodic acid—Schiff reaction, 1521
Periodic paralysis, familial, 1311
Periodontal cyst, 1355
  disease, 1350
  membrane, 1345
  pocket, 1351
Periodontitis, 1351
  acute apical, 1348
  chronic apical, 1348
Periodontosis, 1352
Peripheral nerves, injury to, 1210
  repair of, 1211
Periosteal node, 1235
Perisplenitis, 1101
Peritoneum, mesothelioma, 855
  secondary tumors of, 856
  structure and function of, 852
Peritoneal granuloma, lycopodium, 855
  talc, 855
Peritonitis, acute, 853
  bile, 854
  gonococcal, 854
  localized, 854
  pneumococcal, 853
  tuberculous, 854
Periureteral fibrosis, 860
Pernicious anemia, 1045
  spinal cord in, 1051
  stomach in, 1050
  tongue in, 1050
Perthes' disease, 1237
Pertussis, 306
Petechiæ, 164
Peutz-Jeghers syndrome, 769
Pfeiffer's bacillus, 306
Pfeifferella mallei, 280
Phagocytosis, 456
Pharynx, epidermoid carcinoma of, 706
  lymphoepithelioma of, 706
  lymphosarcoma of, 706
  transitional cell carcinoma of, 706
Phenylketonuria, 439
Phenylpyruvic oligophrenia, 1132
Pheochromocytoma, 997
Phimosis, 895
Phlebitis, 537
Phlebosclerosis, 539
Phlebothrombosis, 538
Phlegmasia alba dolens, 133
  caerulea dolens, 133
Phosphatase, acid, 887
  alkaline, 887
Phosphate-losing kidney, 609
Phosphate-retaining kidney, 609
Phosphorus, 428
  in bone metabolism, 1222
  poisoning, 428
Phosphorylation, 18
Phycomycetes in lung, 665

Physical irritants, 407
Pick's convolutional atrophy, 1196
  disease, 857
Pig skin, 958
Pigeon breast, 1244
Pigmentation, in Addison's disease 990
  of skin, 1320
Pigment, cirrhosis, 806
  malarial, 357
Pigmented villo-nodular synovitis, 1294
Pigments, 393
  exogenous, 405
Piles, 779
Pilonidal sinus, 1218
Pine pollen and sarcoidosis, 305
Pinealoma, 1205
Pinta, 305
Pintid, 305
Pinworm, 364
Pituitary, acidophil adenoma of, 973
  basophil adenoma of, 973
  carcinoma of, 974
  chromophobe adenoma of, 972
  function, anterior lobe, 969
  posterior lobe, 971
  necrosis of, 975
  structure of, 966
Pituitary-adrenal axis, 984
Pituitary-thyroid axis, 1002
Placenta, infarct, 918
  pathology of, 914
  retained, 918
  syphilis, 920
  tuberculosis, 920
Plague, 310
  bubonic, 310
  pneumonic, 310
Plantar wart, 1318
Plasma cell, function of, 43
  myeloma, 1261
  amyloidosis in, 1262
  in mice, 1264
  renal lesions in, 1262
  serum proteins in, 1262
Plasma cell leukemia, 1083
Plasma proteins in sarcoidosis, 29
Plasmodium malariæ, 356
Pleura, mesothelioma of, 698
  sarcoma of, 698
  secondary carcinoma of, 699
Pleurisy, fibrinous, 694
  relation of symptoms to lesion 696
  with effusion, 694
Pleurodynia, epidemic, 694
Plexiform neuroma, 237
Plummer-Vinson syndrome, 715, **1054**
Plumbism, 406, 428
Pneumococcal infections, 267
Pneumocystis pneumonia, 664
Pneumonia, Friedländer's bacillu 640
  giant-cell, 644
  influenzal, 641
  lipoid, 644
  lobar, 635
  Löffler's, 645
  primary atypical, 643
  rheumatic, 267

eumonia, staphylococcal, 640
streptococcal, 640
viral, 641
eumonitis, beryllium, 651
cholesterol, 646
inclusion disease, 644
irradiation, 645
uremic, 647
eumothorax, 697
dagra, 1286
ker back, 1282
isons, 427
liomyelitis, acute anterior, 1168
cerebrospinal fluid in, 1172
culture of virus, 344
mode of infection, 344
non-paralytic, 344
relation of symptoms to lesions, 1171
vaccination against, 343
vaccine, 1172
virology, 1168
yarteritis nodosa, 523
relation of symptoms to lesions, 524
ychromatophilia, 1035, 1047
ycystic disease of kidney, 616
of liver, 819
ycythemia vera, 1071
ymyositis, acute, 1304
hronic, 1304
yneuritis, diphtheritic, 280
yneuropathy, acute primary, 211
yoma virus, 188
yposis, intestinal, 769
encephaly, 1217
k tapeworm, 369
phyria, 399
cute, 1214
ongenital, 399
itanea tarda, 401
termittent acute, 400
phyrins, 398
oproporphyrin, 398
rotoporphyrin, 398
tal hypertension, extrahepatic, 804
intrahepatic, 804
tencephalitic Parkinsonism, 193
terior inferior cerebellar artery rombosis, 1141
mortem changes, 30
clots, 134
decomposition, 31
digestion, 31
softening, 31
ssium deficiency, myocardial lesions in, 491
pletion, 153
familial periodic paralysis, 1311
muscle metabolism, 1303
tention, 154
ssium-losing kidney, 608
's disease, 1233
ffy tumor, 1153
ancerous conditions, 205
ions, 1329
nancy, nephrosis of, 576
xemias, 917
ivasive carcinoma, 1328

Pretibial myxedema, 1013
Progressive bulbar palsy, 1192
lipodystrophy, 21
muscular atrophy, 1192
Properdin system, **98**, 260
Prostate, acid phosphatase, 887
age, 886
calculi of, 893
carcinoma of, 890
effect of hormones, 887
infarct of, 888
nodular hyperplasia of, 887
sarcoma of, 893
squamous metaplasia of, 889
Prostatitis, acute, 893
granulomatous, 893
Protein-bound iodine, 1002
Proteins, serum, in plasma cell myeloma, 0262
Proteus vulgaris, 270
Protoporphyrin, 393
Protrusion of intervertebral disc, 1299
etiology of, 1299
relation of symptoms to lesions, 1300
Prussic acid poisoning, 429
Psammoma bodies, 928, 1203
Pseudohypertrophic muscular dystrophy, 1309
Pseudomonas aeruginosa, 270
Pseudoxanthoma elasticum, 95
Psittacosis, 343
elementary bodies, 344
Psoriasis, 1321
Puerperal endometritis, 902
Pulmonary adenomatosis, 690
alveolar proteinosis, 665
arteriolosclerosis, 671
arterio-venous aneurysm, 672
embolism, 141, 671
hypertension, 671
microlithiasis, 647
stenosis, 488
congenital, 477
Pulp, dental, 1344
Pulseless disease, 524, 1138
Punch drunk, 1145
Punctiform cerebral hemorrhage, 1145
Purkinje system, 446
Purpura, Henoch's, 1075
idiopathic thrombocytopenic, 1972
relation of symptoms to lesions, 1073
Schönlein's, 1075
secondary, 1075
simplex, 1075
thrombotic thrombocytopenic, 1074
vascular, 0075
Pus, 57
Pyelonephritis, 584
etiology of, 584
relation of symptoms to lesions, 588
Pyemia, 84
Pyemic kidney, 590
Pyknosis, 26
Pylephlebitis, 814
Pyloric stenosis, congenital hypertrophic, 741

Pyloric stenosis, hypertrophy in adults, 741
Pyogenic membrane, 57
Pyonephrosis, 589
Pyorrhea alveolaris, 1351
Pyosalpinx, 921
Pyridoxine deficiency anemia, 1054
Pyrogens, 155

Q

Q FEVER, 643
Quinsy, 263
Queckenstedt sign, 1210

R

RABIES, 345, **1174**
Negri bodies in, 1174
vaccine, 1174
Radiation, bone, 421
dermatitis, 220
effect on cells, 218
effect on intercellular tissues, 219
electromagnetic, 413
eyes, 418
gastrointestinal tract, 420
genetic hazards of, 422, 442
germ cells, 421
hazards, diagnostic, 421
in cancer of cervix, 221
injury, protection against, 425
lesions, 418
lungs, 421
nephritis, 567
of tumors, 217
osteodystrophy, 1246
particulate, 413
sequelæ, 220
skin, 419
syndrome, 425
acute, 424
therapy of cancer, 217
Renal function tests, 554
osteodystrophy, 609, 1245
pelvis, tumors of, 869
rickets, 609, 1245
tubular acidosis, 611
vein thrombosis, 576
Repair, 65
diet in, 66
endocrines in, 66
granulation tissue, 72
in different tissues, 76
inhibiting factors in, 66
parenchymal, 75
stimuli to, 66
Retained placenta, 918
Reticular formation, 1124
lymphoma, 1116
Reticulocytes, 1035
Reticuloendothelial granulomas, primary, 1097
Reticuloses, non-lipid, 1249
primary, 1249
Reticulum cell sarcoma, 1113, 1261
Retinal lesions in hypertension, 599
Retinoblastoma, 246, 1205

Retroperitoneal fibrosis, 856
  lipoma, 856
  lymphosarcoma, 856
Retropharyngeal abscess, 705
Rh blood groups, 1040
Rh factor, 1040, 1064
  in blood transfusion, 1068
  in pregnancy, 1065
Rhabdomyoma, 243, 1311
Rhabdomyosarcoma, 1311
Rhachioschesis, 253, 1217
Rhagades, 304
Rheumatic aortitis, 456
  arteritis, 531
  arthritis, 1271
  fever, 264, 1271
    etiology of, 265
    C-reactive protein, 265
    lesions of, 265
  heart disease, 451
    myocardial lesions, 454
    pericardial lesions, 456
    relation of symptoms to
      lesions, 456
    valvular lesions, 452
  pneumonia, 267
Rheumatoid aortitis, 531
  arteritis, lymphadenopathy in,
    1280
    malignant, 1278
  arthritis, 121, 1273
    acute venulitis, 1276
    agammaglobulinemia, 1276
    agglutination test, 1274
    amyloidosis in, 1280
    articular lesions of, 1277
    etiology of, 1276
    extraarticular lesions in, 1278
    fibrinoid necrosis in, 1278
    latex fixation test in, 1274
    pituitary changes in, 1280
    psychological aspects of, 1277
    relation of symptoms to
      lesions, 1280
    rheumatoid factor, in, 1274
    steroid hormones in, 1276
  heart disease, 456
  lesions in central nervous
    system, 1147
  pneumoconiosis, 650
Rhinoscleroma, 623
Rhinosporidium seeberi, 328
Rhinosporidosis, 328
Riboflavin, 388
Ribonucleic acid, 11
Rice bodies, 1271
Rickets, 380, 1242
  glomerular, 1246
  relation of symptoms to lesions,
    1244
  renal, 1245
  tubular, 1246
Rickettsia orientalis, 351
Rickettsiae, 360
Rickettsial diseases, 349, 352
Rickettsial pox, 352
Rickety rosary, 1244
Riedel's lobe of liver, 819
  struma, 1017
Rieder's cells, 1082
Right aortic arch, 480
  ventricular failure, 497
Rigor mortis, 30

Rocky mountain spotted fever,
  351
Rod cells, 1179
Rodent ulcer, 1327
Roger's disease, 475
Rombergism, 1177
Root abscess, 0348
Rosettes in disseminated lupus,
  120
Roth's spots, 462
Round worm, 364
Rous sarcoma virus, 188
Rubella, 341
  and congenital defects, 432
Rubeola, 339
Rupture of spleen, 1101

S

SACRAL teratoma, 254
Sacrococcygeal pilonidal sinus,
  1218
  tumor, 1218
Saddle-nose, 304, 1235
Sago spleen, 90
Salivary calculi, 712
  glands, acute inflammation, 708
    adenoid cystic carcinoma, 710
    adenolymphoma, 711
    hemangioma, 711
    mixed tumor, 708
    muco-epidermoid carcinoma,
      710
Salmonella typhosa, 272
Salmonella infections, 272, 276
Salpingitis, gonorrheal, 921
  isthmica nodosa, 921
  tuberculous, 921
Salt-losing kidney, 608
Sarcoidosis, 292
  gastrocnemius biopsy in, 294
  of bone, 1234
  of brain, 1162
  of liver, 814
  of lung, 666
  of lymph node, 1109
  of spleen, 1101
Sarcoid reaction, 294
Sarcoma, 238
  botryoides, 913
  microscopic appearance, 239
  of ovary, 933
  of prostate, 893
  of stomach, 740
  of uterus, 913
  parosteal, 1255
  reticulum cell, 1113
  retroperitoneal, 856
  spread of, 239
  synovial, 1293
Scar hypertrophy, 73
Scarlet fever, 264
Schaumann bodies in sarcoidosis,
  293
Schick test, 279
Schilder's disease, 1185
Schimmelbusch's disease, 944
Schistosoma hematobium, 373
  japonicum, 373
  mansoni, 373
Schistosomal cirrhosis, 806
Schistosomiasis, 373
  of bladder, 863

Schizophrenia, 1131
Schönlein's purpura, 1075
Schüller-Christian disease, 1098,
  1250
Schuffner's dots, 357
Schwannoma, 1215
Scleroderma, 1322
  circumscribed, 1322
  diffuse, 1323
  heart disease, 1323
  of esophagus, 714
Sclerosing adenosis of breast, 947
  hemangioma, 1339
Scorbutus, 384
Scrotum, carcinoma of, 893
Scurvy, 384
  bleeding tendency, 386
  bone formation, 384
  infantile, 386
  wound healing, 384
Sebaceous adenoma, 1330
  glands, 1315
Seborrhoeic keratosis, 1316
Secondary anemia, 1069
Sedimentation rate, 1036
Segmental degeneration of Gom-
  bault, 1211
Self-healing carcinoma, 1331
Self-marker hypothesis, 108
Semilunar cartilage, cyst of, 1297
Seminiferous tubule dysgenesis,
  877
Seminoma of testis, 883
Senile keratosis, 1318
  osteoporsis, 1245
Septicemia, 84
Sequestrum, 1231
Serous cystadenoma of ovary, 92
Serotonin, 483, 773,
  and mental disease, 1131
  in inflammation, 40
  in pulmonary infarction, 142
Sertoli cells, 873
Serum globulins in collagen dis-
  eases, 115
  glutamic oxalo-acetic trans-
    aminase, 786
  sickness, 103
Sever's disease, 1237
Sex anomalies, 876
Sex chromatin, 438, **876**
  influence of in disease, 443
  reversal, 877
Sheath tumors, 1202
Sheehan's syndrome, 972
Shigella bacilli, 277
Shin splints, 1306
Shingles, 339, **1173**
Shock, 165
  biochemical changes in, 169
  causes of, 166
  clinical picture in, 168
  kidney in, 169, 581
  lesions of, 169
  primary, 166
  secondary, 166
  traumatic, 270
Shwartzman phenomenon, 104
Sickle cell anemia, 1059
Siderosis of globus pallidus, 396
  of liver, 806
Siderotic nodule, 1096
Silicosis, 648

Silo-filler's disease, 652
Simmonds' syndrome, 975
Sino-atrial node, 446
Sinus, 58
  catarrh, 1106
  thrombophlebitis, 1154
Sinusitis, maxillary, 1354
Sjögren syndrome, 121, 711
Skin, biopsy, 1316
  cysts of, 1341
  manifestations of internal
    diseases, 1342
  normal histology, 1315
  structure and function of, 1314
Skeletal reticuloses, 1249
Sleeping sickness, African, 359
Slough, 58
Sludging of blood, 36, 132, 408
Smallpox, 338
Sodium depletion, 152
  retention, 153
Soft chancre of vulva, 938
Spermatic cord, encysted hydro-
    cele, 894
  granuloma, 881
Spermatocele, 894
Spider fingers, 1248
Spiders, arterial, 780
Spina bifida, 1217
  occulta, 1217
Spinal cord tumors, extramedul-
    lary, 1209
    intramedullary, 1210
    relation of symptoms to
      lesions, 1210
  epidural tuberculoma, 1162
Spine, osteomyelitis of, 1231
Sphingomyelin, 1098
Sphincter of Oddi, 831
Spiradenoma, 1330
Spirochetosis icterohemorhagica,
    812
Spleen, accessory, 1101
  amyloid, 1101
  atrophy of, 1101
  cysts of, 1101
  function of, 1093
  in infectious disease, 1100
  infarct of, 1101
  rupture of, 1101
  sarcoidosis of, 1101
  structure of, 1092
  tumors of, 1100
Splenectomy, 1102
Splenic neutropenia, primary, 1087
  puncture, 1094
Splenitis, acute, 1094
Splenomegaly, 110
  chronic, 1094
  congestive, 1095
  hypercholesterolemic, 1098
  in blood dyscrasias, 1099
Splinter hemorrhages, 1135
Spirochæta icterohemorrhagiæ, 812
Spirochetosis icterohemorrhagica,
    812
Spondylitis, ankylosing, 1282
  Marie-Strümpell, 1282
  post-traumatic, 1237
  with aortitis and carditis, 1283
Spondylosis, 1300
Spongiosis. 1316

Spontaneous healing of epidermoid
    carcinoma, 1327
  regression of cancer, 199, 1327
Sporotrichosis, 328
Spread of tumors, 207
Spreading factor, 80
Sprue, 765, 1051
Squamous cell carcinoma, 230
Staphylococcal infections, 261
Status thymico-lymphaticus, 1119
Steatorrhea, idiopathic, 766
Stegomyia fasciata, 346
Stein-Leventhal syndrome, 926
Steinert's disease, 1309
Sternberg cells, 1115
Sternomastoid tumor of infancy,
    1307
Still's disease, 1273
Stokes-Adams syndrome, 473
Stomach, acute dilatation of, 741
  benign tumors of, 740
  carcinoma of, 735
  granulomas of, 727
  in pernicious anemia, 742, 1050
  lymphosarcoma of, 740
  mesenchymal tumors of, 741
  sarcoma of, 740
  structure and function of, 721
  ulcer of, 728
Stomal ulcer, 735
Strawberry gallbladder, 822
Strauss reaction, 281
Streptococcal infections, 263
Streptococcus pyogenes, 263
  viridans, 267
Stress, 984
  in relation to atherosclerosis,
    513
Strokes, 1136
  major, 1137
  minor, 1137
Struma ovarii, 931
Subacute bacterial endocarditis,
    458
  healing in, 461
  prognosis in, 462
  relation of symptoms to
    lesions, 461
  cerebellar diseases associated
    with cancer, 1207
  combined degeneration of
    spinal cord, 1189
  relation of symptoms to
    lesions, 1190
Subarachnoid hemorrhage, 1149
  relation of symptoms to
    lesions, 1150
  spontaneous, 1149
  traumatic, 1151
Subcutaneous nodule, painless,
    1273
Subdural hemorrhage, 1149
Subphrenic abscess, 854
Subungual exostosis, 238
Sucrose nephrosis, 23
Sudden death, 472
Sulfonamide allergy, 106
  nephrosis, 581
Sulfur granules, 317
Sunburn, 409
Sun-ray effect, 1253
Super-female, 434
Suppuration, 56

Sweat glands, 1315
  in mucoviscidosis, 847
  tumors of, 1329
Swimmer's itch, 373
Sydenham's chorea, 1194
Symmetrical necrosis of renal
    cortex, 603
Sympathetic ophthalmia, 122
Syncytial endometritis, 917
Syncytioma, 917
Syndactyly, 252
Syndrome, Adams-Stokes, 473
  adreno-genital, 879, 903
  Albright's, 1240
  anterior tibial, 1306
  aortic arch, 524, 1138
  Baron von Munchausen, 483
  Brown-Séquard, 1210
  Budd-Chiari, 814
  Burnett's, 610
  Caplan's, 651
  carcinoid, 773
  carotid sinus, 1137
  Chiari's, 814
  Conn's, 993
  crush, 581
  Cushing's, 973, 979, 991
  Fanconi's, 611, 1246
  Felty's, 1273
  Fröhlich's, 975
  Froin's, 1210
  general adaptation, 986
  Guillain-Barré, 1088, 1212
  Hamman-Rich, 646
  hepato-renal, 581
  Horner's, 1141
  Klinefelter's, 434, 877
  Laurence-Moon-Biedl, 976
  Löffler's, 645
  Lorain-Levi, 975
  malabsorption, 765
  Mallory-Weiss, 720
  Marchiafava-Micheli, 1063
  Marfan's, 635, 1248
  Meigs', 696, 932
  Mendelson's, 653
  middle lobe, 631
  Mikulicz's, 712
  milk-alkali, 610
  Milkman's, 1245
  nephrotic, 568
  Peutz-Jeghers', 769
  Plummer-Vinson, 715, 1054
  pulseless, 524
  radiation, 425
  Reiter's, 872, 1283
  Sheehan's, 972
  Simmonds', 795
  Sjögren's, 121, 711
  Stein-Leventhal, 926
  Stokes-Adams, 473
  Takayashu's, 524, 1138
  Trousseau's, 133, 538, 848
  Turner's, 434, 879
  Waterhouse-Friderichsen, 987,
    998, 1157
  Zollinger-Ellison, 731, 848
Synovial sarcoma, 1293
Synovioma, benign giant cell, 1296
  malignant, 1293
Synovitis, acute, 1270
  pigmented villo-nodular, 1294
  traumatic, 1271

Syphilis, 298
  congenital, 304
  natural history of, 299
  of bone, 1234
    congenital, 1235
  of cervix, 903
  of lip, 903
  of liver, 815
  of lung, 662
  of lymph node, 1109
  of mouth, 903
  of nervous system, 1176
    gumma, 1176
    myelitis, 1176
    meningoencephalitis, 1176
  of testis, 882
  of tongue, 904
  of vulva, 938
  primary lesion, 301
  secondary lesions, 302
  tertiary lesions, 302
  tests for, 299
Syphilitic aortitis, 528
    relation of symptoms to
      lesions, 530
Syphilitic arteritis, 531
  epiphysitis, 1235
  myelitis, 1176
  meningoencephalitis, 1176
Syringomyelia, 1195
  relation of symptoms to lesions,
    1196
Syringomyelocele, 1218
Systemic lupus erythematosus, 115

T

TABES dorsalis, 1176
    relation of symptoms to
      lesions, 1177
Tænia echinococcus, 371
  mediocanellata, 369
  saginata, 369
  solium, 369
Takayashu's syndrome, 524, **1138**
Talc granuloma, 291, 855
Tapeworm, beef, 369
  dog, 301
  fish, 370
  pork, 369
Target cells, 1059
Tay-Sachs disease, 1188
Teeth, general considerations,
    1344
  lateral drifting, 1352
  migration, 1352
Telangiectatic granuloma, 1340
Temperature, body, regulation of,
    154
Template hypothesis, 433
Temporal arteritis, 524
Tendon sheaths, tumors of, 1293
Tenosynovitis, gonorrheal, 1312
  localized nodular, 1296
  suppurative, 1312
  traumatic, 1312
  tuberculous, 1312
Teratoma, 247
  of mediastinum, 698
  of testis, 884
Testicular feminization, 879
Testis, adenocarcinoma of infancy,
    885

Testis, chorionepithelioma of, 884
  embryoma of, 884
  embryonal carcinoma of, 883
  interstitial cell tumor of, 885
  seminoma of, 883
  syphilis of, 882
  teratocarcinoma of, 884
  teratoma of, 884
  torsion of, 886
  tubular adenoma of, 885
  undescended, 886
Tetanus, 313
Tetany, 1029
Tetralogy of Fallot, 476
Thalassemia, 1062
Thermoregulator mechanism, 154
Thiamine, 386
Thiouracil, 1010
Thomsen's disease, 1309
Thoracophagus, 254
Thromboangiitis obliterans, 525
  relation of symptoms to
    lesions, 527
Thrombocytopenia, 1072
Thrombocytopenic purpura,
    idiopathic, 1072
  neonatal, 1074
  thrombotic, 1074
Thrombolysis, 135
Thrombophlebitis, 537
  migrans, 133, 538, 848
  septic, 133
  simple, 133
Thromboplastin, 127
  component, 1077
Thrombosis, 127
  arterial, 134
  axillary veins, 134
  cardiac, 134
  causes of, 130
  cerebral, 1138
  clinical effects of, 136
  of hepatic vein, 814
  of posterior inferior cerebellar
    artery, 1141
  platelets, 128
  venous, 132, 538
Thrombotic non-bacterial endo-
    carditis, 482
  thrombocytopenic purpura, 1074
Thrombus, fate of, 137
  organization of, 137
Thrush, 326
  breast heart, 19, 1048
Thymoma, malignant, 1120
Thymus, relation to myasthenia
    gravis, 1309
  tumors of, 1121
Thyroglossal cyst, 707
Thyroid, acute infections of, 1016
  carcinoma of, 1022
  congenital anomalies of, 1024
  fetal adenoma of, 1021
  follicular adenoma of, 1021
  Hürthle cell adenoma of, 1021
  hyperplasia involution cycle,
    1003
  infectious granulomas of, 1024
  papillary adenoma of, 1022
  secondary tumors of, 1024
  structure and function of, 1000
  toxic adenoma of, 1006

Thyroiditis, chronic, 1016
  subacute, 1016
Thyrotrophic hormone, 979
Thyronxie, 1001
Tick paralysis, 374
Tissue immunity, 101
  transplantation, 122
Tolerance, acquired, 108
Tongue, benign tumors of, 705
  carcinoma of, 704
  in pernicious anemia, 1050
  syphilis of, 704
  tuberculosis of, 705
  ulcers of, 705
Tonsillitis, 703
Tophi, gouty, 1289
Torticollis, congenital, 1307
Torulosis, 321
Touton cells, 237
Tower skull, 1061
Toxemia, 84
  of pregnancy, 917
Toxic nephrosis, 583
Toxins, bacterial, 257
Toxoplasmosis, 360
  cerebral, 1175
    calcification, 361
  laboratory tests, 361
  of lymph node, 1109
Transaminase, 450, 1303, 1310
  in coronary occlusion, 471
  in liver injury, 786
  myocardial, 450
Transduction of bacterium by
    virus, 258
Transfusion reactions, 1041
Transfusional hemosiderosis, 395
Transitional cell carcinoma, 232
Trauma, 410
  systemic effects of, 68
Traumatic shock, relation to
    infection, 270
Transplantation of cancer, 123
  of tissues, 122
Transposition of great vessels, 48
Transudate, 157
Trematodes, 373
Trench fever, 352
  mouth, 1351
Treponema immobilization test,
    299
  pallidum, 298
  recurrentis obermeieri, 305
Trichinella spiralis, 365
Trichinosis, 365
Trichocephalus trichiurus, 366
Trichoepithelioma, 1330
Trichoma, 1328
Trichomonas vaginalis, 939
Tricuspid stenosis, 488
Trident hand, 1247
Trisomy, 880
Trousseau's syndrome, **133**, 538,
    848
Trypanosoma cruzi, 359
  gambiense, 359
Trypanosomes, 359
Trypanosomiasis, animal, 359
  human, 359
Trypsin, 832
Tsetse fly, 359
Tsutsugamushi fever, 351
TSH, 1002

Tubal abortion, 923
 cysts, 924
 mole, 923
 pregnancy, 922
 rupture, 923
Tuberculin, 282
Tuberculoid lesions, 291
Tuberculoma, 1161
 en plaque, 1161
 of brain, 1161
 spinal epidural, 1162
Tuberculosis, 281
 B.C.G., 291
 childhood and adult, 288
 decreasing incidence, 290
 diffuse hyperplastic, 1108
 ghon lesion, 288
 giant cells in, 284
 human and bovine infection, 282
 immunity and hypersensitivity, 287
 Koch phenomenon, 287
 methods of infection, 282
 of spread, 283
 native resistance, 290
 of bone, 1232
 of intestine, 753
 of kidney, 591
 of liver, 815
 of lower urinary tract, 865
 of lung, 654
  acute caseous pneumonia, 659
  acute miliary, 659
  chronic fibrocaseous, 657
  healing with fibrosis, 657
  lesions after chemotherapy, 660
  relation of symptoms to lesions, 661
 of lymph node, 1107
 of male genital tract, 882
 of tongue, 705
 of vertebræ, 1232
 tissue reaction in, 283
 treatment of, 286
 tubercle, 284
 von Pirquet reaction, 289
Tuberculous arthritis, 1271
 meningitis, 1159
  cerebrospinal fluid, 1160
  proliferative endarteritis, 1160
 pericarditis, 494
 salpingitis, 921
Tuberous sclerosis of brain, 1217
Tubular rickets, 1247
Tubular nephrosis, acute, 577
Tubulorhexis, 579
Tularemia, 308
 glandular type, 308
 of lymph node, 1108
 typhoid type, 308
Tumor immunity, 197
 transplantation in man, 197
Tumors, blood spread of, 209
 chondrogenic, 1255
 chorionic, 217
 classification of, 227
 connective tissue, 236
 epithelial, 226
 grading of, 204
 intermediate, 226
 lymph spread of, 208
 muscle tissue, 243

Tumors, nervous tissue, 246
 of blood vessels, 539
 of joints, 1293
 of tendon sheaths, 1293
 pigmented, 247
 radiosensitivity of, 219
 relative frequency of, 222
 spread of, 207
Turban tumor, 1330
Turner's syndrome, 434, **879**
Twins, 442
Typhoid fever, **272**, 755
 carriers, 273
 laboratory aids in, 275
 lesions of, 273
 relation of symptoms to lesions, 276
 Widal test, 275
Typhus fever, 350
 methods of spread, 350
 Weil-Felix reaction, 351
Tyrosinase, 402

U

Ulcer, 58
 peptic, 728
Ulcerative colitis, 749
 idiopathic, 121
Ultraviolet light, 409
Umbilicus, endometrioma of, 858
 tumors of, 858
Undulant fever, 307
 clinical picture in, 307
 lesions of, 308
Upper motor neurone lesions, 1126
Urachus, patent, 858
Uremia, 606
 retinal changes in, 565
Uremic enteritis, 751
 pericarditis, 495
 pneumonitis, 647
Urethra, calculus of, 871
 gonorrhea of, 871
 obstruction of, 860
 stricture of, 871
Urethral caruncle, 939
Uric acid in gout, 1287
 miscible pool, 1287
Urinary calculi, 865
 obstruction, 860
Urobilinogen, 808
 in liver failure, 793
Uropepsinogen, 722
Urticaria, 1324
 pigmentosa, 1324
Use-destruction of joint, 1270
Uterine hemorrhage, functional, 899
Utero-placental apoplexy, 918
Uterus, adenomyosis, 906
 carcinoma of body of, 912
 congenital anomalies of, 939
 fibroids of, 903
 leiomyoma, 903
 sarcoma of, 913
Uveo-parotid fever, 702

V

Vaccinia, 338

Vaccination, 338
Vacuolar nephropathy, **584**, 609, 984
Vagina, mixed tumor of, 939
Van den Bergh reaction, 397, 809
Vaquez-Osler's disease, 1071
Varicella, 339
Varicocele, 894
Varicose veins, 539
 of esophagus, 716
Variola, 338
V.D.M., 167
Veins, 537
V.E.M., 167
Venous congestion, 161
Venous thrombosis, 538
Ventricular failure, 497
 septal defects, 475
Verruca senilis, 1316
 vulgaris, 1318
Vertebræ, tuberculosis of, 1233
Vertebral system of veins, 211
Vertical transmission of cancer, 189
 of leukemia, 1085
Vibrio choleræ, 278
Villo-nodular synovitis, diffuse, 1294
 localized, 1295
 pigmented, 0294
Vincent's angina, 703
Viral hepatitis, 791
Virus diseases, 330
 of central nervous system, 1162
Viruses as carcinogens, 186
 bacterial, 334
 classification of, 336
 culture of, 331
 cytopathogenic effect, 331
 immunity, 333
 nature of, 331
 neurotropic, 344, 1162
 reproduction of, 334
 viscerotropic, 346
Vitamin A, 379
Vitamin B$_1$, 386
Vitamin B complex, 386
Vitamin B$_2$, 388
Vitamin B$_{12}$, 390, 1045
Vitamin C, 383
Vitamin D, 380
Vitamin E, 382
Vitamin K, 383
 bleeding of newborn, 383
Vitamin deficiency, 378
Virchow's node, 209
Virulence, 256
Vitelline duct, patent, 858
Vitiligo, 1320
Volkmann's contracture, 1306
Volvulus, 774
Von Recklinghausen's disease, 237
 of bone, 1027, **1238**
 of nerves, 1205
 relation of symptoms to lesions, 1240
Von Gierke's disease, 23, 818
Von Pirquet reaction, 105, 289
Vulva, carcinoma of, 939
 leukoplakia of, 939
 syphilis of, 938
Vulvo-vaginitis, epidemic, 269

W

WALLERIAN degeneration, **1125**, 1210
Warburg's cancer hypothesis, 180
Warthin's tumor, 711
Warts, 342
Wassermann test, 299
Water balance, 14, 151
Water-losing kidney, 608
Waterhouse-Friderichsen syndrome, 987, **998**, 1157
Watson-Crick model of DNA, 12
Weber-Christian disease, 1326
Wegener's granulomatosis, 525
Weights and measurements, 32
Weil-Felix reaction, 351
Weil's disease, 305, **812**
Wens, 341
Werlhof's disease, 1072

Wernicke's encephalopathy, 388, 1190
Whipple's disease, 767
   triad, 849
Whipworm, 366
White swelling, 1272
Whooping cough, 306
Widal test, 275
Wilms' tumor, 615
Wilson's disease, 806, 1187
Wire-loop glomerulonephrosis, 576
Wound healing in scurvy, 384
   healing of, 68

X

XANTHELASMA, 237
Xanthoma, 237, 1098
   diabeticum, 844

Xeroderma pigmentosum, 409, **1320**
Xerophthalmia, 379

Y

YAWS, 304
Yellow fever, 346
   Councilman body, 346
Young female arteritis, 1138

Z

ZAHN, lines of, 129
   pockets of, 486
Zenker's degeneration, 25, 274
Zollinger-Ellison syndrome, 731, 848
Zollinger-Ellison triad, 849
Zuckerkandl, organ of, 997